Exam Preparatory Manual for Undergraduates

PATHOLOGY

FIFTH EDITION

Ramadas Nayak MBBS MD

Former Head
Department of Pathology
Kasturba Medical College, Mangaluru
Manipal Academy of Higher Education
Karnataka, India

Former Professor and Head
Department of Pathology
Yenepoya Medical College
Mangaluru, Karnataka, India
askdr.nayak@gmail.com

Rakshatha Nayak MBBS MD DNB

Assistant Professor
Department of Pathology
Kasturba Medical College
Mangaluru, affiliated to Manipal Academy of Higher Education
Karnataka, India

Foreword

K Ramnarayan

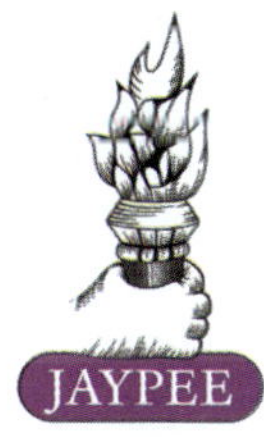

JAYPEE BROTHERS MEDICAL PUBLISHERS
The Health Sciences Publisher
New Delhi | London

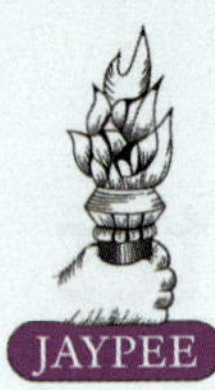

Jaypee Brothers Medical Publishers (P) Ltd.

Headquarters
Jaypee Brothers Medical Publishers (P) Ltd.
EMCA House
23/23-B, Ansari Road, Daryaganj
New Delhi - 110 002, India
Landline: +91-11-23272143, +91-11-23272703
+91-11-23282021, +91-11-23245672
Email: jaypee@jaypeebrothers.com

Corporate Office
Jaypee Brothers Medical Publishers (P) Ltd.
4838/24, Ansari Road, Daryaganj
New Delhi 110 002, India
Phone: +91-11-43574357
Fax: +91-11-43574314
Email: jaypee@jaypeebrothers.com

Overseas Office
J.P. Medical Ltd.
83 Victoria Street, London
SW1H 0HW (UK)
Phone: +44 20 3170 8910
Fax: +44 (0)20 3008 6180
Email: info@jpmedpub.com

Website: www.jaypeebrothers.com
Website: www.jaypeedigital.com

Inquiries for bulk sales may be solicited at: jaypee@jaypeebrothers.com

Exam Preparatory Manual for Undergraduates—Pathology

First Edition: 2015
Second Edition: 2017
Third Edition: 2019
Fourth Edition: 2020
Reprint: 2021
Fifth Edition: **2025**

ISBN 978-93-5696-974-2

Printed at Sanat Printers

Dedicated to

Late Sri Lakshman Nayak
and
Late Smt Meera Nayak
(Parents of Dr Ramadas Nayak)
Students who inspired us,
Patients who provided the knowledge,
Our teachers, friends, well-wishers, and family members,
who encouraged and supported us.

Foreword

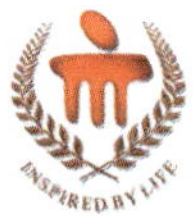

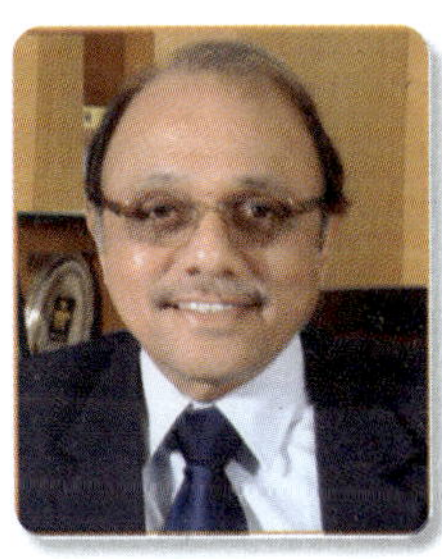

"Any intelligent fool can make things bigger and more complex," said Albert Einstein. To make things understandable and appealing is the persisting and daunting task of a passionate teacher. It is in this context that Dr Ramadas Nayak's book assumes a considerable significance. In this book, he has provided conceptual clarity that it is both astounding and amazing.

The veritable qualities of a review book include simplicity, structure, sequence, and standardization. To this, must be added another 's', i.e., sympathy—sympathy for the reader who is grappling with the essentials. Dr Nayak's endeavor to have all these qualities in the book is a testimony of his expertise and experience as an effective and exemplary teacher.

I am delighted to write this Foreword to *Exam Preparatory Manual for Undergraduates—Pathology*, which, I am certain, will be an invaluable resource for students and teachers in pathology.

K Ramnarayan
MBBS MD (Path) PG Dip. Higher Education
Vice-Chancellor
Manipal Academy of Higher Education
Manipal, Karnataka, India

Preface to the Fifth Edition

We are proud to present the fifth edition of *Exam Preparatory Manual for Undergraduates—Pathology*, which has gained popularity since its first edition. This edition includes additional features to help students understand the subject and score well in examinations. It is organized to incorporate modifications suggested by the new "Competency-based Medical Education" (CBME).

As the saying goes, "Change is inevitable," and this book has undergone changes to meet students' needs. Pathology is a rapidly expanding, ever-changing, and interesting field in medicine. This book aims to present vast knowledge of pathology in a clear manner for undergraduate and postgraduate medical students and those in paramedical courses. It provides a sound understanding of disease mechanisms, which is foundational for basic science. The book includes colored illustrations, tables, text boxes, and flowcharts to simplify complex information. The understanding of molecular pathology has greatly increased, and this is highlighted in relevant chapters. This edition is completely revised, updated, better illustrated, and a comprehensive manual for excelling in pathology examinations. Each chapter has been updated to include all core and noncore competencies as per CBME guidelines. Some figures and illustrations have been replaced with higher-quality images. We have used clear and simple language to ensure accessibility for students from diverse educational backgrounds. Some illustrations, text, and boxes are available online. Scenario-based multiple-choice questions are included at the end of each chapter.

Organization

This book consists of 27 chapters divided into three sections: General Pathology, Hematology, Transfusion and Clinical Pathology, and Systemic Pathology.

Section 1—General Pathology: Covers basic pathologic mechanisms, including cell injury and adaptation, inflammation and healing, infections and infestations, hemodynamic disorders, immunopathology, neoplasia, genetic and pediatric diseases, environmental and nutritional diseases, and basic diagnostic cytology.

Section 2—Hematology, Transfusion and Clinical Pathology: Includes hematology introduction, disorders of red and white blood cells, hemostasis disorders, blood banking and transfusion, and clinical pathology. For detailed knowledge of hematology and clinical pathology, students can refer to **Essentials in Hematology and Clinical Pathology** by Dr Ramadas Nayak and Dr Sharada Rai.

Section 3—Systemic Pathology: Addresses diseases of various organ systems, including cardiovascular, respiratory, gastrointestinal, hepatobiliary, pancreatic, urinary, male and female genitals, breast, endocrine, musculoskeletal, skin, and central nervous system disorders.

Usage Guidance

- **CC (core curriculum) and NC (noncore curriculum):** Highlighted in a box with lines.
- **Bold words:** Emphasize key terms to remember.
- **Questions:** Commonly expected pathology questions are provided, with frequently asked questions in red and less frequent ones in blue.
- **Illustrations and figures:** Essential for answering theory questions that require diagrams.
- **Definitions:** Provided in yellow boxes for frequent viva and theory questions.
- **Pathogenesis:** Presented with flowcharts and text for better understanding.
- **Classification:** Only essential classifications for examinations are included.
- **Morphology:** Gross and microscopic findings are highlighted in boxes.
- **Clinical cases:** Incorporates common scenario-based (clinical-oriented) questions.
- **Interpretation of laboratory results:** Includes skills for interpreting urinary findings, renal and liver function tests, and cerebrospinal fluid analysis.

This book serves as a rapid review source for undergraduate and postgraduate students, featuring numerous illustrations, photographs, tables, text boxes, and flowcharts for easy understanding.

We recommend using this book to understand basic knowledge and refresh it during examinations. Most importantly, we thank our students, whose needs drive the continuous improvement of this manual.

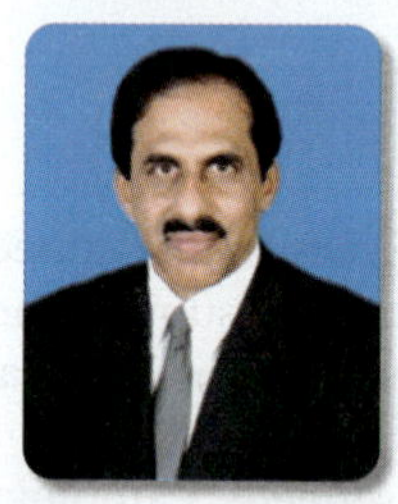

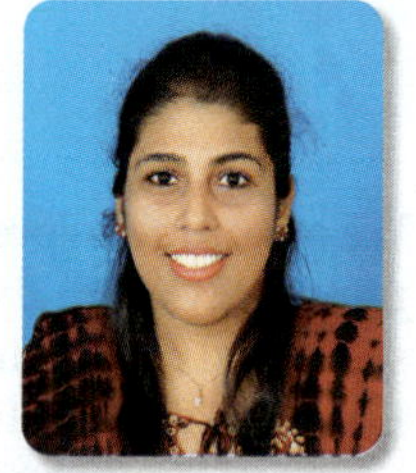

Ramadas Nayak

Rakshatha Nayak

Preface to the First Edition

Pathology is a rapidly-expanding and ever-changing field and lays the foundation for understanding diseases. This book is an endeavor to present the vast knowledge of pathology in a lucid manner for the second year medical and dental students, and those undergoing training in paramedical courses. My aim is to provide a sound knowledge of pathology and hence give insight into etiology, pathogenesis, pathology and the disease course. Every attempt has been made to present information in a simplified text augmented with the use of colored illustrations.

Organization

This book consists of 23 chapters and is organized into two sections namely general pathology and systemic pathology.
Section 1—General pathology: It provides an overview of the basic pathologic mechanisms underlying diseases including cellular adaptations, inflammation, tissue repair, chronic inflammation, hemodynamic disorders, immunological disorders, neoplasia, and genetics.
Section 2—Systemic pathology: It deals with chapters devoted to diseases and disorders of various organ systems including vascular, cardiac, respiratory, gastrointestinal, liver and biliary tract, pancreas, kidney, male and female genital tract, bones, endocrines, skin, and central nervous system. For hematology section, readers are requested to refer to *Rapid Review of Hematology* authored by Dr Ramadas Nayak and Dr Sharada Rai and *Essentials in Hematology and Clinical Pathology* by Dr Ramadas Nayak, Dr Sharada Rai and Dr Astha Gupta.

After many years (more than 34 years) of teaching undergraduates, I found that undergraduate students find it difficult to understand, remember and answer the questions during examinations, in a satisfying way. There are many pathology textbooks, but undergraduates face difficulty to refresh their knowledge during examinations. This encouraged me to write a book to fill the niche, to provide basic information to an undergraduate in a nutshell. The text provides all the basic information the student will ever need to know. Keywords are shown in bold words so that the student can rapidly go through the book on the previous day or just before the examination. Most students are fundamentally "visually oriented." As the saying "a picture is worth a thousand words", it encouraged me to provide many illustrations.

How to use this book

I recommend that this book to be used by all students for understanding the basic knowledge and refresh their knowledge during examinations. The readers are requested to give more emphasis on word in bold letters that represents the keywords to be remembered. One of the aims of the students after getting undergraduate degree is to fetch a good ranking in the postgraduate entrance examination. Most graduates cannot answer multiple choice questions (MCQs) in entrance examination by just reading the usual textbooks in pathology. In this book, text boxes have been designed at the sides of main text that provide information useful in answering these MCQs. These boxes also provide commonly expected pathology questions during undergraduate examination. This book can serve as a source of review of general and systemic pathology for even postgraduates in pathology.

About 350 illustrations, 82 gross photographs, 162 photomicrographs, 152 tables, 3 X-rays, and a clinical photograph have been incorporated for easy understanding of the subject. Appendices provide various important bodies and its associated conditions, important cells in various lesions and pathognomonic structures in diseases.

Ramadas Nayak

Acknowledgments

- Our sincere thanks to all our family members, especially Smt Rekha Nayak, Ms Rashmitha Nayak, Mr Ramnath Kini, Master Rishab Kini, Mr U Ramnath Nayak (Chartered Accountant), and Ms Aradhya Nayak, for patiently accepting our long preoccupation with this work.
- We are indebted to Dr Ramdas M Pai (Chancellor), Dr HS Ballal (Pro-Chancellor), Lt Gen (Dr) MD Venkatesh (Vice-Chancellor), and Dr Dilip G Naik (Pro Vice-Chancellor) of Manipal Academy of Higher Education, Manipal, Karnataka (India), for their support. We are grateful to our beloved Dr Unni Krishnan, Dean, Kasturba Medical College, Mangaluru, Karnataka (India), for his constant support and encouragement.
- We are thankful to all our friends who contributed fantastic images for this book. Our sincere thanks go to Dr Sharada Rai, Professor of Pathology, Kasturba Medical College (Mangaluru), Manipal Academy of Higher Education, Manipal.
- We would like to express our gratitude to all our friends, colleagues, and undergraduate and postgraduate students in the Department of Pathology at Yenepoya Medical College and Kasturba Medical College, Mangaluru, who helped us in different stages of preparing the manuscript. Thank you to all those who provided support, discussed ideas, read drafts, offered comments, and assisted in editing, proofreading, and graphic designing.
- A special thanks to Shri Jitendar P Vij (Group Chairman), Mr Ankit Vij (Managing Director), Mr MS Mani (Group President), of M/s Jaypee Brothers Medical Publishers (P) Ltd, New Delhi, India, for publishing the book in the same format as wanted, well in time. We are grateful to Shri Jitendar P Vij, for unmasking our talent as authors.
- We would like to offer a huge appreciation to the wonderful work done by Dr Madhu Choudhary (Director–Educational Publishing), Ms Pooja Bhandari [Director–Production (Books and Journals)], Mr Ajay Kumar Sharma [Deputy General Manager (Books and Journals)], Ms Sunita Katla (Executive Assistant to Group Chairman and Publishing Manager), Ms Samina Khan (Executive Assistant to Director–Educational Publishing), Dr Aditya Tayal (Editorial Manager–Content Strategy), Mr Rajesh Sharma (Production Coordinator), Ms Seema Dogra (Cover Visualizer), Ms Neha Verma (Graphic Designer–Cover), Mr Laxmidhar Padhiary (Quality Controller), Mr Jagvir Singh Tomar (Typesetter), and Mr Rajesh Gurkundi (Graphic Designer) of M/s Jaypee Brothers Medical Publishers (P) Ltd, New Delhi, India.
- We thank Mr Venugopal V (Director–Digital Sales), and Mr Gajanan Prabhu (Bengaluru) of M/s Jaypee Brothers Medical Publishers (P) Ltd, for taking this book to every corner of Karnataka.
- Last but definitely not least, a thank you to our undergraduate and postgraduate students. Without you, we would not write. You make all our books possible.

  There are many more people we could thank, but space, and modesty compel us to stop here.

Images Contribution

We express our heartfelt gratitude to all of our friends who generously provided the necessary images for this publication:

- Dr Sharada Rai (Professor), Dr Shikha Jayasheelan (Assistant Professor), Dr Vatsala KB (Assistant Professor), Department of Pathology, Dr Jagadish Rao PP (Professor and Head, Department of Forensic Medicine and Toxicology, Honorary State Medicolegal Consultant), Dr Suresh Kumar Shetty (Professor of Forensic Medicine and Toxicology, Honorary State Medicolegal Consultant, and Associate Dean), Dr Sonali Ullal (Associate Professor of Radiology), Dr Sriram Bhat M (Professor of Surgery), and Dr Archith Boloor (Additional Professor of Medicine), Kasturba Medical College (Mangaluru), Manipal Academy of Higher Education, Manipal, Karnataka, India.
- Dr Anuradha CK Rao (Professor), Dr Sushma Belurkar (Additional Professor), and Dr Kanthilatha Pai (Associate Dean and Professor), Department of Pathology, Kasturba Medical College, Manipal Academy of Higher Education, Manipal, Karnataka, India.
- Dr Surendra Nayak Kapadi, Department of Histopathology, Ministry of Health, Maternity Hospital, Sabah Area, Kuwait.
- Dr Reba Philipose T (Professor and Head), Dr Sandhya I (Professor of Pathology), Dr Muktha R Pai (Former Professor and Head), Dr Arvind P (Associate Professor), Dr Priyanka Shetty (Assistant Professor), Dr Lovely George (Associate Professor), and Dr Ashwin Polnaya (Professor of Radiology), AJ Institute of Medical Sciences and Research, Mangaluru, Karnataka, India.
- Dr Krishnaraj Upadhyaya (Professor), Dr Supriya P (Associate Professor), Dr Renuka Patil (Associate Professor), Dr Divya Ail (Associate Professor), Dr Swaroop Raj (Professor), Dr Vidya Rekha Kamath (Assistant Professor), Dr Indra Puthran (Professor), Dr Shariff MH (Professor), Dr Gloria Venissa Quadros (Assistant Professor), Dr Anjali Vijay (Assistant Professor), Dr Ariya S (Assistant Professor), Dr Vasudeva Prabhu, Dr Shabeera Shamsuddin, Dr Akib Avaru, Dr Hiba Jaleel, Dr Mary Netheya and Dr Prema Saldanha (Professor and Head), Department of Pathology, Dr Malathi M (Professor and Head), Dr Siddharth Biswas (Professor), Dr Madan K (Assistant Professor), Dr Christina Avril Goveas, Dr Loretta Ann Pereira (Assistant Professor), Department of Oncopathology, and Dr Sahana KS (Professor and Head), Department of Pediatrics, Yenepoya Medical College, Mangaluru, Karnataka, India.
- Dr Mahesh Karigoudar, Dr Karigoudar Diagnostic Laboratory and Blood Bank, Vijayapur, Karnataka, India.
- Dr Rashmi MV (Professor and Head) and Dr Niranjana Murthy B (Medical Superintendent and Professor), Department of Pathology, Siddaganga Medical College and Research Institute, Tumakuru, Karnataka, India.
- Dr Leena Dennis Joseph (Professor), Dr Sandhya Sundaram (Professor and Head), and Dr Archana B (Assistant Professor), Department of Pathology, Sri Ramachandra Institute of Higher Education and Research, Chennai, Tamil Nadu, India.
- Dr Arundhathi S, Additional Professor, Department of Pathology, All India Institute of Medical Sciences, Mangalagiri, Andhra Pradesh, India.
- Dr Shashikala P (Professor and Head), Department of Pathology, SS Institute of Medical Sciences and Research Centre, Davanagere, Karnataka, India.
- Dr Sheela Devi CS, Professor and Head, Department of Pathology, JSS Medical College, JSS Academy of Higher Education and Research, Mysuru, Karnataka, India.
- Dr S Sankar (Principal and Professor of Pathology), Government Medical College, Kottayam, Kerala, India.
- Dr Ramesh Chavan (Professor) and Dr Ashwini Ratnakar (Assistant Professor), Department of Pathology, Jawaharlal Nehru Medical College, KLE (Deemed to be University), Belagavi, Karnataka, India.
- Dr Jayaprakash Shetty (Vice-Dean, Professor and Head, Department of Pathology) and Dr Kisan Prasad HL (Professor of Pathology), KS Hegde Medical Academy, Mangaluru, affiliated with Nitte University, Mangaluru, Karnataka, India.
- Dr Seethalakshmi NV (Professor), Dr Bindu MR (Professor), Dr Indu R Nair (Additional Professor), and Dr Meera Subramanian (Senior Lecturer), Department of Pathology, Amrita Institute of Medical Sciences, Kochi, Kerala, India.
- Dr Feroz M (Professor and Head), Dr Asiq Sideeque N (Professor), Dr Jayalakshmi PS (Professor), and Dr Nisha TG (Associate Professor), Department of Pathology, MES Medical College, Perinthalmanna, Kerala, India.
- Dr Supriya Gireesan (Professor and Head), Department of Pathology, Calicut Medical College, Kozhikode, Kerala, India.
- Dr Nandeesh BN and Dr Anita Mahadevan (Professor and Head), Department of Neuropathology, National Institute of Mental Health and Neurosciences (NIMHANS), Bengaluru, Karnataka, India.

- Dr Rajeevan K (Professor) and Dr Deeshma T (Associate Professor), Department of Pathology, Malabar Medical College, Kozhikode, Kerala, India.
- Dr Jayaram N Iyengar (Managing Director) and Dr Ananth Vikas, Anand Diagnostic Laboratory (A Neuberg Associate), Neuberg Anand Reference Laboratory, Bengaluru, Karnataka, India.
- Dr Shruthi M Krishna (Consultant Ocular Pathologist and In-Charge), Center for Ocular Pathology and Education (COPE), Narayana Nethralaya, Bengaluru, Karnataka, India.
- Dr Ajit Nambiar (Director and Head), Pathology and Laboratory Medicine, Karkinos Health Care, Ernakulam, Kerala, India.
- Late Dr Prasanna Shetty B (Professor and Head) and Dr Sulatha Kamath (Professor), Department of Pathology, MS Ramaiah Medical College, Bengaluru, Karnataka, India.
- Dr Sathyavathi R Alva (Professor and Head), Dr Navya BN (Professor), Dr Gopinath Rajesh (Associate Professor), Dr Anjali Rao K (Assistant Professor) and Dr Bharathi M (Professor), Department of Pathology, KVG Medical College and Hospital, Sullia, Karnataka, India.
- Dr Jayaprakash CS (Professor) and Dr Umashankar T (Professor and Head), Department of Pathology, Father Muller Medical College, Mangaluru, Karnataka, India.
- Dr Alok Sharma (Director) Renal Pathology and Electron Microscopy, National Reference Laboratory, Dr Lal PathLabs Ltd, New Delhi, India.
- Dr Narayana Murthy C (Professor and Head), Department of Pathology, Basaveshwara Medical College and Hospital, Chitradurga, Karnataka, India.
- Dr Vijay Shankar S (Professor of Pathology), Adichunchanagiri Institute of Medical Sciences, Adichunchanagiri University, Nagamangala, Karnataka, India.
- Dr Jayashree K (Professor and Head) and Dr Rekha A Nair (Professor), Department of Pathology, Regional Cancer Institute, Thiruvananthapuram, Kerala, India.
- Dr Parvathi Devi GK (Professor and PG Co-ordinator) and Dr Kodandaswamy (Professor), Department of Pathology, Sri Siddhartha Medical College, affiliated with Siddhartha (Deemed to be University), Tumakuru, Karnataka, India.
- Dr Veena Shenoy (Associate Professor, and Residency Program Director), Department of Pathology, The University of Mississippi Medical Center, Mississippi, USA.
- Dr Dayananda S Biligi (Professor), Department of Pathology, Bangalore Medical College and Research Institute, Bengaluru, Karnataka, India.
- Dr Parth Goswami, Assistant Professor of Pathology, All India Institute of Medical Sciences, Rajkot, Gujarat, India.
- Dr Santosh KV, Consultant Pathologist, Metropolis Healthcare Limited, Bengaluru, India.
- Dr Vinit Anand (Professor and Head), Dr Vaibhav Nayak (Professor), Dr Indudhara PB (Professor), Dr Ganga H (Associate Professor), and Dr Harshitha KS (Senior Resident), Subbaiah Institute of Medical Sciences, Shivamogga, Karnataka, India.
- Dr Annie Jojo (Head and Senior Consultant), Department of Pathology, Lisie Hospital, Ernakulam, Kerala, India.
- Dr Francisco Couto (Director and Professor of Pathology), Dr RGW Pinto (Professor and Head), Dr Premila de Sousa Rocha (Associate Professor), Dr Suresh RS Mandrekar, Dr Shruti U Shetye (Tutor), Dr Merline Augustine (Tutor), and Dr Priyanka Raghuvir Mashelkar (Formerly Tutor), Department of Pathology, Goa Medical College, Goa, India.
- Dr Nischita Budihal (Professor and Head), Department of Pathology, Sri Siddhartha Institute of Medical Sciences and Research, Tumakuru, Karnataka, India.
- Dr Tanuj Kanchan (Professor), Department of Forensic Medicine and Toxicology, All India Institute of Medical Sciences, Jodhpur, Rajasthan, India.
- Dr Vandana Kamath (Associate Professor of Pathology), Christian Medical College, Vellore, Tamil Nadu, India.

Contents

SECTION I: General Pathology

1. Introduction to Pathology 3
   - Definitions and Terms 3
   - Role of a Pathologist in Diagnosis and Management of Disease 5
   - History and Evolution of Pathology 9

2. Cell Injury and Adaptation 14
   - Types of Cellular Responses to Injury 14
   - Cell Injury 14
   - Types of Cell Injury 16
   - Necrosis 16
   - Apoptosis 22
   - Other Pathways of Cell Death 27
   - Mechanisms of Cell Injury and Cell Death 28
   - Cellular Adaptations to Stress 38
   - Intracellular Accumulations 43
   - Extracellular Deposits: Pathologic Calcification 50
   - Hyaline Change 52
   - Mucoid Degeneration 53
   - Cellular Aging 53

3. Inflammation and Healing 60
   - Inflammation 60
   - Acute Inflammation 63
   - Mediators of Inflammation 73
   - Morphological Types/Patterns of Acute Inflammation 80
   - Outcomes of Acute Inflammation 82
   - Chronic Inflammation 83
   - Systemic Effects of Inflammation 88
   - Tissue Repair 91
   - Cell Proliferation and Cell Cycle 91
   - Stem Cells 93
   - Factors that Influence Wound Healing 97
   - Examples of Tissue Repair and Fibrosis 98

4. Infections and Infestations 106
   - Mycobacterial Infections 106
   - Spirochete Infections 111
   - Bacterial Diseases 114
   - Viral Diseases 115
   - Rickettsial Infections 117
   - Chlamydial Infections 117
   - Fungal Infections and Opportunistic Infections 118
   - Mycetoma 120
   - Parasitic Diseases 121
   - Malaria 122
   - Other Infections 127

5. Hemodynamic Disorders, Thromboembolism, and Shock 129
   - Edema 129
   - Disorders of Perfusion 134
   - Shock 138
   - Hemostasis and Thrombosis 145
   - Thrombosis 149
   - Embolism 155
   - Infarction 161

6. Immunopathology, AIDS, and Amyloidosis 165
   - Immunity 165
   - Hypersensitivity Reactions 169
   - Major Histocompatibility Complex Molecules 181
   - Immunology of Transplantation 183
   - Autoimmune Diseases 188
   - Systemic Lupus Erythematosus 189
   - Other Autoimmune Disorders 194
   - Immunodeficiency Syndromes 196
   - Acquired Immunodeficiency Syndrome 197
   - Amyloidosis 205

7. Neoplasia 215
   - Nomenclature of Neoplasms 216
   - Characteristics of Benign and Malignant Neoplasms 220
   - Epidemiology of Cancer 229
   - Genetic Lesions in Cancer 232
   - Molecular Basis of Cancer 234
   - Etiology of Cancer: Carcinogenic Agents 254
   - Clinical Aspects of Neoplasia 261
   - Laboratory Diagnosis of Cancer 264
   - Examples of Benign Tumors 269

8. Genetic and Pediatric Diseases 272
   - Basics of Genetics 272
   - Genetic Disorders 278

- ❖ Cytogenetic Abnormalities and Mutations in Childhood *281*
- ❖ Tumors and Tumor-Like Lesions of Infancy and Childhood *283*
- ❖ Storage Diseases *285*

9. Environmental and Nutritional Diseases 288

- ❖ Environmental Pollution *288*
- ❖ Effects of Tobacco *291*
- ❖ Effects of Alcohol *292*
- ❖ Malnutrition *293*
- ❖ Obesity *296*
- ❖ Common Vitamin Deficiencies *299*

10. Basic Diagnostic Cytology 306

- ❖ Diagnostic Role of Cytology *306*
- ❖ Methods for Obtaining Specimens *307*
- ❖ Techniques in Exfoliative Cytology *311*
- ❖ Fine Needle Aspiration Cytology *313*
- ❖ Fnac Appearance of Some Common Lesions *314*
- ❖ Other Cytology Techniques *315*

SECTION II: Hematology, Transfusion and Clinical Pathology

11. Introduction to Hematology and Disorders of Red Blood Cell 319

- ❖ Normal Hematopoiesis *320*
- ❖ Anticoagulants *321*

Red Blood Cell Disorders 324

- ❖ Anemia *324*

Anemias of Impaired Red Cell Production 329

- ❖ Iron Deficiency Anemia *329*
- ❖ Megaloblastic Anemia *334*
- ❖ Aplastic Anemia *341*

Increased Red Cell Destruction (Hemolytic Anemias) 342

- ❖ Hereditary Spherocytosis *344*
- ❖ Glucose-6-Phosphate Dehydrogenase (G6PD) Deficiency *346*
- ❖ Hereditary Defects in Hemoglobin *347*
- ❖ Thalassemia *347*
- ❖ β-Thalassemia Major *348*
- ❖ β-Thalassemia Minor/Trait *351*
- ❖ α-Thalassemia *352*
- ❖ Sickle Cell Anemia *352*
- ❖ Sickle Cell Trait *357*
- ❖ Immunohemolytic Anemias *357*

Anemias of Blood Loss 361

- ❖ Approach to the Diagnosis of Hemolytic Anemia *361*

12. Disorders of White Blood Cell, Lymph Node, and Spleen 365

Non-neoplastic Disorders of White Cells 365

- ❖ Quantitative Disorders of Leukocytes *365*
- ❖ Qualitative Disorders of Leukocytes *370*
- ❖ Infectious Mononucleosis (Glandular Fever) *370*

Neoplastic Proliferations of White Cells 371

- ❖ Acute Leukemia *371*
- ❖ Acute Lymphoblastic Leukemia/Lymphoma *373*
- ❖ Acute Myeloid Leukemia *375*
- ❖ Myeloproliferative Neoplasms *378*
- ❖ Chronic Myeloid Leukemia *378*
- ❖ Polycythemia or Erythrocytosis *381*

Lymph Node and Spleen 382

- ❖ Lymph Node *382*
- ❖ Non-Hodgkin Lymphomas *384*
- ❖ Hodgkin Lymphomas *391*
- ❖ Splenomegaly *397*
- ❖ Plasma Cell Neoplasms *398*

13. Bleeding Disorders: Hemorrhagic Diathesis 406

- ❖ Normal Hemostasis *406*
- ❖ Bleeding Disorders *406*
- ❖ Bleeding Disorders Caused by Vessel Wall Abnormalities *407*
- ❖ Bleeding Disorders due to Reduced Number of Platelets: Thrombocytopenia *407*
- ❖ Coagulation Disorders *409*
- ❖ Disseminated Intravascular Coagulation *414*

14. Blood Banking and Transfusion.................................. 422

- ❖ Blood Group System *422*
- ❖ Transfusion Medicine *425*

15. Clinical Pathology 438

- ❖ Hemoglobin Estimation *438*
- ❖ Peripheral Blood Smear *440*
- ❖ Hematocrit (Packed Cell Volume) *443*
- ❖ Erythrocyte Sedimentation Rate *445*
- ❖ LE Cell Test *447*
- ❖ Bone Marrow Examination *447*
- ❖ Osmotic Fragility Test *449*
- ❖ Urine Analysis *450*
- ❖ Body Fluids *462*
- ❖ Peritoneal Fluid *464*
- ❖ Cerebrospinal Fluid Examination *465*
- ❖ Semen Analysis *467*
- ❖ Thyroid Function Tests *468*
- ❖ Renal Function Tests *471*
- ❖ Liver Function Tests *472*
- ❖ Sputum Examination *476*

SECTION III: Systemic Pathology

16. Cardiovascular Disorders 479

Vascular Disorders 479

- Arteriosclerosis *479*
- Atherosclerosis *479*
- Aneurysms and Dissection *487*
- Hypertensive Vascular Disease *492*
- Vasculitis *495*
- Vascular Tumors *498*

Heart Disorders 499

- Heart Failure *499*
- Rheumatic Fever and Rheumatic Heart Disease *503*
- Ischemic Heart Disease *508*
- Myocardial Infarction *512*
- Infective Endocarditis *523*
- Noninfected Vegetations *528*
- Cardiomyopathy *528*
- Pericarditis and Pericardial Effusion *532*
- Congenital Heart Disease *536*
- Cardiac Myxoma *539*

17. Respiratory Disorders 541

- Pneumonia *541*
- Lung Abscess *547*
- Obstructive Lung Diseases *548*
- Tuberculosis *559*
- Sarcoidosis *568*
- Pneumoconioses *569*
- Lung Tumors *574*
- Metastatic Tumors *584*
- Miscellaneous *585*
- Pleural Tumor *586*

18. Oral Cavity and Gastrointestinal Tract 589

- Oral Cavity *589*
- Salivary Gland Neoplasms *591*
- Odontogenic Tumors *594*

Gastrointestinal Tract 595

- Esophagus *595*
- Stomach *597*
- Intestine *612*
- Polyps of Colon *630*
- Genetic Tumor Syndromes *633*
- Colorectal Adenocarcinoma *635*
- Acute Appendicitis *642*

19. Hepatobiliary and Pancreatic Disorders 646

Liver 646

- Bilirubin Metabolism *646*
- Jaundice *647*
- Hepatic (Liver) Failure *651*
- Viral Hepatitis *653*
- Alcohol-Related Liver Disease *664*
- Nonalcoholic Fatty Liver Disease *672*
- Cirrhosis *673*
- Portal Hypertension *675*
- Inherited Metabolic Liver Diseases *678*
- Autoimmune Cholangiopathies *680*
- Liver Abscesses *682*
- Malignant Neoplasms of Liver *682*
- Metastatic Tumors *687*

Gallbladder 688

- Cholelithiasis (Gallstones) *688*
- Cholecystitis *693*
- Carcinoma of the Gallbladder *696*

Pancreas 696

- Pancreatitis *696*
- Pancreatic Carcinoma *704*
- Interpretation of Liver Function and Viral Hepatitis Serology Panel *706*

20. Kidney and Urinary Tract Disorders 710

- Histology of the Kidney *710*
- Glomerular Diseases *712*
- Nephritic Syndrome *716*
- Nephrotic Syndrome *721*
- Glomerular Lesions Associated with Systemic Diseases *734*
- Diseases Affecting Tubules and Interstitium *737*
- Acute Kidney Injury *742*
- Acute Tubular Injury *744*
- Chronic Kidney Disease *746*
- Vascular Diseases of the Kidney *748*
- Horseshoe Kidneys *751*
- Cystic Diseases of the Kidney *751*
- Urolithiasis (Renal Calculi, Stones) *754*
- Urinary Tract Obstruction (Obstructive Uropathy) *757*
- Malignant Tumors of the Kidney *759*
- Nephroblastoma (Wilms Tumor) *763*
- Urothelial Tumors *764*
- Common Urinary Abnormalities in a Clinical Specimen *770*

21. Male Genital Tract Disorders 774

Testis 774

- Cryptorchidism *774*
- Testicular Tumors *775*

Penis 784

- Tumors of the Penis *784*

Prostate 788

- Prostatitis *788*

- ❖ Benign Prostatic Hyperplasia *789*
- ❖ Male Infertility *797*

22. Female Genital Tract Disorders.................................. 799

Cervix 799
- ❖ Normal Structure *799*
- ❖ Inflammations of the Cervix *799*
- ❖ Premalignant and Malignant Neoplasms of the Cervix *800*

Uterus 807
- ❖ Menstrual Cycle *807*
- ❖ Endometriosis *808*
- ❖ Endometrial Hyperplasia *810*
- ❖ Endometrial Carcinoma *812*
- ❖ Uterine Leiomyomas *815*
- ❖ Uterine Leiomyosarcoma *817*

Ovaries 817
- ❖ Ovarian Tumors *817*
- ❖ Epithelial Tumors *818*
- ❖ Germ Cell Tumors *826*
- ❖ Sex Cord-Stromal Tumors *831*
- ❖ Metastatic (Secondary) Tumors *833*

Gestational Disorders 833
- ❖ Gestational Trophoblastic Disease *833*

23. Breast Disorders.. 842
- ❖ Female Breast *842*
- ❖ Benign Epithelial Lesions *842*
- ❖ Carcinoma of the Breast *844*
- ❖ Types of Breast Carcinoma *849*
- ❖ Invasive (Infiltrating) Carcinoma *850*
- ❖ Paget Disease of the Nipple *855*
- ❖ Fibroepithelial Tumors of Breast *858*
- ❖ Male Breast *861*

24. Endocrine Disorders.. 863

Thyroid Gland 863
- ❖ Autoimmune Thyroid Disease *863*
- ❖ Thyrotoxicosis *866*
- ❖ Hypothyroidism *869*
- ❖ Diffuse and Multinodular Goiters *870*
- ❖ Thyroid Neoplasms *874*
- ❖ Follicular Cell-Derived Neoplasms *874*

Diabetes Mellitus 882
- ❖ Laboratory Diagnosis of Diabetes *893*

Parathyroid Glands 896
- ❖ Hyperparathyroidism *896*
- ❖ Hypoparathyroidism *898*

Adrenal Glands 898
- ❖ Adrenal Cortex *898*
- ❖ Adrenal Neoplasms *903*
- ❖ Adrenal Medulla *904*
- ❖ Multiple Endocrine Neoplasia Syndromes *907*

25. Bones, Joints, and Soft Tissue Tumors......................... 910
- ❖ Infections—Osteomyelitis *910*
- ❖ Paget Disease of Bone (Osteitis Deformans) *914*
- ❖ Bone Tumors *915*
- ❖ Rheumatoid Arthritis *926*
- ❖ Osteoarthritis *928*
- ❖ Gout and Gouty Arthritis *931*
- ❖ Healing of a Fracture *933*
- ❖ Soft Tissue Tumors *936*
- ❖ Tumors of Adipose Tissue *936*
- ❖ Fibroblastic/Myofibroblastic Tumors *939*
- ❖ Skeletal Muscle Tumors *941*
- ❖ Smooth Muscle Tumors *942*
- ❖ Peripheral Nerve Sheath Tumors *943*
- ❖ Tumors of Uncertain Origin *945*

26. Skin Disorders... 949
- ❖ Carcinoma Precursors *949*
- ❖ Squamous Cell Carcinoma *950*
- ❖ Basal Cell Carcinoma *951*
- ❖ Melanocytic Neoplasms *953*

27. Disorders of the Central Nervous System and Eye........ 960
- ❖ Meningitis *960*
- ❖ Interpretation of Cerebrospinal Fluid Findings *964*
- ❖ Tumors of Central Nervous System *966*
- ❖ Gliomas *967*
- ❖ Embryonal Tumors *973*
- ❖ Meningiomas *975*
- ❖ Metastatic Tumors *977*
- ❖ Eye *977*

Bibliography *981*

Index *983*

Competency Table

Number	COMPETENCY The student should be able to	Core Y/N	Chapter number	Page number
PA1.1	Describe the role of a pathologist in diagnosis and management of disease	Y	1	5
PA1.2	Enumerate common definitions and terms used in pathology	Y	1	3
PA1.3	Describe the history and evolution of pathology	N	1	9
PA2.1	Demonstrate knowledge of the causes, mechanisms, types and effects of cell injury and their clinical significance	Y	2	14
PA2.2	Describe the etiology of cell injury. Distinguish between reversible-irreversible injury—mechanisms; morphology of cell injury	Y	2	15, 16, 28
PA2.3	Intracellular accumulation of fats, proteins, carbohydrates, pigments	Y	2	43
PA2.4	Describe and discuss cell death—types, mechanisms, necrosis, apoptosis (basic as contrasted with necrosis), autolysis	Y	2	16, 22, 28
PA2.5	Describe and discuss pathologic calcifications, gangrene	Y	2	50
PA2.6	Describe and discuss cellular adaptations—atrophy, hypertrophy, hyperplasia, metaplasia, dysplasia	Y	2	38
PA2.7	Describe and discuss the mechanisms of cellular aging and apoptosis	N	2	53
PA2.8	Identify and describe various forms of cell injuries, their manifestations and consequences in gross and microscopic specimens	Y	2, 3	58, 105
PA3.1	Describe the pathogenesis and pathology of amyloidosis	Y	6	205
PA3.2	Identify and describe amyloidosis in a pathology specimen	N	6	209
PA4.1	Define and describe the general features of acute and chronic inflammation including stimuli, vascular and cellular events	Y	3	60
PA4.2	Enumerate and describe the mediators of acute inflammation	Y	3	73, 86
PA4.3	Define and describe chronic inflammation including causes, types, nonspecific and granulomatous; and enumerate examples of each	Y	3	83
PA5.1	Define and describe the process of repair and regeneration including wound healing and its types	Y	3	91
PA6.1	Define and describe edema, its types, pathogenesis and clinical correlations	Y	5	129
PA6.2	Define and describe hyperemia, congestion, hemorrhage	Y	5	134, 137
PA6.3	Define and describe shock, its pathogenesis and its stages	Y	5	138
PA6.4	Define and describe normal hemostasis and the etiopathogenesis and consequences of thrombosis	Y	5	149
PA6.5	Define and describe embolism and its causes and common types	Y	5	155
PA6.6	Define and describe ischemia/infarction its types, etiology, morphologic changes and clinical effects	Y	5	161
PA6.7	Identify and describe the gross and microscopic features of infarction in a pathologic specimen	Y	5	163
PA7.1	Define and classify neoplasia. Describe the characteristics of neoplasia including gross, microscopy, biologic, behavior and spread. Differentiate between benign from malignant neoplasms	Y	7	215, 216, 220

Number	COMPETENCY The student should be able to	Core Y/N	Chapter number	Page number
PA7.2	Describe the molecular basis of cancer	Y	7	234
PA7.3	Enumerate carcinogens and describe the process of carcinogenesis	Y	7	254
PA7.4	Describe the effects of tumor on the host including paraneoplastic syndrome	Y	7	261
PA7.5	Describe immunology and the immune response to cancer	N	7	251
PA8.1	Describe the diagnostic role of cytology and its application in clinical care	Y	10	306
PA8.2	Describe the basis of exfoliative cytology including the technique and stains used	Y	10	307
PA8.3	Observe a diagnostic cytology and its staining and interpret the specimen	Y	10	314
PA9.1	Describe the principles and mechanisms involved in immunity	Y	6	165
PA9.2	Describe the mechanism of hypersensitivity reactions	Y	6	169, 169
PA9.3	Describe the HLA system and the immune principles involved in transplant and mechanism of transplant rejection	Y	6	181, 183
PA9.4	Define autoimmunity. Enumerate autoimmune disorders	Y	6	188
PA9.5	Define and describe the pathogenesis of systemic lupus erythematosus	Y	6	189
PA9.6	Define and describe the pathogenesis and pathology of HIV and AIDS	Y	6	197
PA9.7	Define and describe the pathogenesis of other common autoimmune diseases	N	6	194
PA10.1	Define and describe the pathogenesis and pathology of malaria	Y	4	122
PA10.2	Define and describe the pathogenesis and pathology of cysticercosis	Y	4	124
PA10.3	Define and describe the pathogenesis and pathology of leprosy	Y	4	106
PA10.4	Define and describe the pathogenesis and pathology of common bacterial, viral, protozoal and helminthic diseases	N	4	114
PA11.1	Describe the pathogenesis and features of common cytogenetic abnormalities and mutations in childhood	N	8	281
PA11.2	Describe the pathogenesis and pathology of tumor and tumor-like conditions in infancy and childhood	N	8	283
PA11.3	Describe the pathogenesis of common storage disorders in infancy and childhood	N	8	285
PA12.1	Enumerate and describe the pathogenesis of disorders caused by air pollution, tobacco and alcohol	Y	9	288, 291, 292
PA12.2	Describe the pathogenesis of disorders caused by protein calorie malnutrition and starvation	Y	9	293
PA12.3	Describe the pathogenesis of obesity and its consequences	Y	9	296
PA13.1	Describe hematopoiesis and extramedullary hematopoiesis	Y	11	320
PA13.2	Describe the role of anticoagulants in hematology	Y	11	321
PA13.3	Define and classify anemia	Y	11	324
PA13.4	Enumerate and describe the investigation of anemia	Y	11	325
PA13.5	Perform, identify and describe the peripheral blood picture in anemia	Y	15	440
PA14.1	Describe iron metabolism	Y	11	329
PA14.2	Describe the etiology, investigations and differential diagnosis of microcytic hypochromic anemia	Y	11	331, 332, 333
PA14.3	Identify and describe the peripheral smear in microcytic anemia	Y	11	332

Number	COMPETENCY The student should be able to	Core Y/N	Chapter number	Page number
PA15.1	Describe the metabolism of vitamin B_{12} and the etiology and pathogenesis of B_{12} deficiency	Y	11	334
PA15.2	Describe laboratory investigations of macrocytic anemia	Y	11	337
PA15.3	Identify and describe the peripheral blood picture of macrocytic anemia	Y	11	337
PA15.4	Enumerate the differences and describe the etiology and distinguishing features of megaloblastic and non-megaloblastic macrocytic anemia	N	11	339
PA16.1	Define and classify hemolytic anemia	Y	11	342
PA16.2	Describe the pathogenesis and clinical features and hematologic indices of hemolytic anemia	Y	11	344
PA16.3	Describe the pathogenesis, features, hematologic indices and peripheral blood picture of sickle cell anemia and thalassemia	Y	11	347, 352
PA16.4	Describe the etiology pathogenesis, hematologic indices and peripheral blood picture of acquired hemolytic anemia	Y	11	357
PA16.5	Describe the peripheral blood picture in different hemolytic anemias	Y	11	344
PA16.6	Prepare a peripheral blood smear and identify hemolytic anemia from it	Y	11	344
PA 17.1	Enumerate the etiology, pathogenesis and findings in aplastic anemia	N	11	341
PA17.2	Enumerate the indications and describe the findings in bone marrow aspiration and biopsy	N	15	447
PA18.1	Enumerate and describe the causes of leukocytosis leucopenia lymphocytosis and leukemoid reactions	Y	12	365, 384
PA`18.2	Describe the etiology, genetics, pathogenesis classification, features, hematologic features of acute and chronic leukemia	Y	12	371, 378, 384
PA19.1	Enumerate the causes and describe the differentiating features of lymphadenopathy	Y	12	382
PA19.2	Describe the pathogenesis and pathology of tuberculous lymphadenitis	Y	12	383
PA19.3	Identify and describe the features of tuberculous lymphadenitis in a gross and microscopic specimen	Y	12	383
PA19.4	Describe and discuss the pathogenesis, pathology and the differentiating features of Hodgkin's and non-Hodgkin's lymphoma	Y	12	384, 391, 397
PA19.5	Identify and describe the features of Hodgkin's lymphoma in a gross and microscopic specimen	Y	12	392
PA19.6	Enumerate and differentiate the causes of splenomegaly	Y	12	397
PA19.7	Identify and describe the gross specimen of an enlarged spleen	Y	12	397
PA20.1	Describe the features of plasma cell myeloma	Y	12	398
PA21.1	Describe normal hemostasis	Y	13	406
PA21.2	Classify and describe the etiology, pathogenesis and pathology of vascular and platelet disorders including ITP and hemophilias	Y	13	407, 408, 411
PA21.3	Differentiate platelet from clotting disorders based on the clinical and hematologic features	Y	13	413
PA21.4	Define and describe disseminated intravascular coagulation, its laboratory findings and diagnosis of disseminated intravascular coagulation	Y	13	414
PA21.5	Define and describe disseminated intravascular coagulation, its laboratory findings and diagnosis of vitamin K deficiency	Y	13	414

Number	COMPETENCY The student should be able to	Core Y/N	Chapter number	Page number
PA22.1	Classify and describe blood group systems (ABO and RH)	Y	14	422
PA22.2	Enumerate the indications, describe the principles, enumerate and demonstrate the steps of compatibility testing	Y	14	426
PA22.4	Enumerate blood components and describe their clinical uses	Y	14	428
PA22.5	Enumerate and describe infections transmitted by blood transfusion	Y	14	430
PA22.6	Describe transfusion reactions and enumerate the steps in the investigation of a transfusion reaction	Y	14	431, 434
PA22.7	Enumerate the indications and describe the principles and procedure of autologous transfusion	Y	14	435
PA23.1	Describe abnormal urinary findings in disease states and identify and describe common urinary abnormalities in a clinical specimen	Y	15, 20	450, 770
PA23.2	Describe abnormal findings in body fluids in various disease states	Y	15	462, 464, 465
PA23.3	Describe and interpret the abnormalities in a panel containing semen analysis, thyroid function tests, renal function tests or liver function tests	Y	15	467, 468, 471, 472
PA24.1	Describe the etiology, pathogenesis, pathology and clinical features of oral cancers	N	18	590
PA24.2	Describe the etiology, pathogenesis, pathology, microbiology, clinical and microscopic features of peptic ulcer disease	Y	18	600
PA24.3	Describe and identify the microscopic features of peptic ulcer	Y	18	603
PA24.4	Describe and etiology and pathogenesis and pathologic features of carcinoma of the stomach	Y	18	605
PA24.5	Describe and etiology and pathogenesis and pathologic features of tuberculosis of the intestine	N	18	615
PA24.6	Describe and etiology and pathogenesis and pathologic and distinguishing features of inflammatory bowel disease	Y	18	621
PA24.7	Describe the etiology, pathogenesis, pathology and distinguishing features of carcinoma of the colon	Y	18	635
PA25.1	Describe bilirubin metabolism, enumerate the etiology and pathogenesis of jaundice, distinguish between direct and indirect hyperbilirubinemia	Y	19	646
PA25.2	Describe the pathophysiology and pathologic changes seen in hepatic failure and their clinical manifestations, complications and consequences	Y	19	651
PA25.3	Describe the etiology and pathogenesis of viral and toxic hepatitis—distinguish the causes of hepatitis based on the clinical and laboratory features. Describe the pathology, complications and consequences of hepatitis	Y	19	653
PA25.4	Describe the pathophysiology, pathology and progression of alcoholic liver disease including cirrhosis	Y	19	664
PA25.5	Describe the etiology, pathogenesis and complications of portal hypertension	Y	19	675
PA25.6	Interpret liver function and viral hepatitis serology panel. Distinguish obstructive from nonobstructive jaundice based on clinical features and liver function tests	Y	19	649, 706
PA26.1	Define and describe the etiology, types, pathogenesis, stages, morphology and complications of pneumonia	Y	17	541
PA26.2	Describe the etiology, gross and microscopic appearance and complications of lung abscess	Y	17	547

Number	COMPETENCY The student should be able to	Core Y/N	Chapter number	Page number
PA26.3	Define and describe the etiology, types, pathogenesis, stages, morphology and complications and evaluation of obstructive airway disease (OAD) and bronchiectasis	Y	17	548, 556
PA26.4	Define and describe the etiology, types, pathogenesis, stages, morphology microscopic appearance and complications of tuberculosis	Y	17	559
PA26.5	Define and describe the etiology, types, exposure, environmental influence, pathogenesis, stages, morphology, microscopic appearance and complications of occupational lung disease	Y	17	569
PA26.6	Define and describe the etiology, types, exposure, genetics environmental influence, pathogenesis, stages, morphology, microscopic appearance, metastases and complications of tumors of the lung and pleura	Y	17	574
PA26.7	Define and describe the etiology, types, exposure, genetics environmental influence, pathogenesis, morphology, microscopic appearance and complications of mesothelioma	N	17	586
PA27.1	Distinguish arteriosclerosis from atherosclerosis. Describe the pathogenesis and pathology of various causes and types of arteriosclerosis	Y	16	479
PA27.2	Describe the etiology, dynamics, pathology types and complications of aneurysms including aortic aneurysms	Y	16	487
PA27.3	Describe the etiology, types, stages pathophysiology, pathology and complications of heart failure	Y	16	499
PA27.4	Describe the etiology, pathophysiology, pathology, gross and microscopic features, criteria and complications of rheumatic fever	Y	16	503
PA27.5	Describe the epidemiology, risk factors, etiology, pathophysiology, pathology, presentations, gross and microscopic features, diagnostic tests and complications of ischemic heart disease	Y	16	508, 512
PA27.6	Describe the etiology, pathophysiology, pathology, gross and microscopic features, diagnosis and complications of infective endocarditis	Y	16	523
PA27.7	Describe the etiology, pathophysiology, pathology, gross and microscopic features, diagnosis and complications of pericarditis and pericardial effusion	Y	16	532
PA27.8	Interpret abnormalities in cardiac function testing in acute coronary syndromes	Y	16	522
PA27.9	Classify and describe the etiology, types, pathophysiology, pathology, gross and microscopic features, diagnosis and complications of cardiomyopathies	N	16	528
PA27.10	Describe the etiology, pathophysiology, pathology, features and complications of syphilis on the cardiovascular system	N	4, 16	113, 532
PA28.1	Describe the normal histology of the kidney	Y	20	710
PA28.2	Define, classify and distinguish the clinical syndromes and describe the etiology, pathogenesis, pathology, morphology, clinical and laboratory and urinary findings, complications of renal failure	Y	20	742
PA28.4	Define and describe the etiology, precipitating factors, pathogenesis, pathology, laboratory urinary findings progression and complications of chronic renal failure	Y	20	746
PA28.5	Define and classify glomerular diseases. Enumerate and describe the etiology, pathogenesis, mechanisms of glomerular injury, pathology, distinguishing features and clinical manifestations of glomerulonephritis	Y	20	712

Number	COMPETENCY The student should be able to	Core Y/N	Chapter number	Page number
PA28.6	Define and describe the etiology, pathogenesis, pathology, laboratory, urinary findings, progression and complications of IgA nephropathy	Y	20	732
PA28.7	Enumerate and describe the findings in glomerular manifestations of systemic disease	Y	20	734
PA28.8	Enumerate and classify diseases affecting the tubular interstitium	Y	20	737
PA28.9	Define and describe the etiology, pathogenesis, pathology, laboratory, urinary findings, progression and complications of acute tubular necrosis	Y	20	744
PA28.10	Describe the etiology, pathogenesis, pathology, laboratory findings, distinguishing features progression and complications of acute and chronic pyelonephritis and reflux nephropathy	Y	20	737, 740
PA28.11	Define classify and describe the etiology, pathogenesis pathology, laboratory, urinary findings, distinguishing features progression and complications of vascular disease of the kidney	Y	20	748
PA28.12	Define classify and describe the genetics, inheritance, etiology, pathogenesis, pathology, laboratory, urinary findings, distinguishing features, progression and complications of cystic disease of the kidney	Y	20	751
PA28.13	Define classify and describe the etiology, pathogenesis, pathology, laboratory, urinary findings, distinguishing features progression and complications of renal stone disease and obstructive uropathy	Y	20	754, 757
PA28.14	Classify and describe the etiology, genetics, pathogenesis, pathology, presenting features, progression and spread of renal tumors	Y	20	759
PA28.15	Describe the etiology, genetics, pathogenesis, pathology, presenting features and progression of thrombotic angiopathies	N	20	750
PA28.16	Describe the etiology, genetics, pathogenesis, pathology, presenting features and progression of urothelial tumors	N	20	764
PA29.1	Classify testicular tumors and describe the pathogenesis, pathology, presenting and distinguishing features, diagnostic tests, progression and spread of testicular tumors	Y	21	775
PA29.2	Describe the pathogenesis, pathology, presenting and distinguishing features, diagnostic tests, progression and spread of carcinoma of the penis	Y	21	786
PA29.3	Describe the pathogenesis, pathology, hormonal dependency presenting and distinguishing features, urologic findings and diagnostic tests of benign prostatic hyperplasia	Y	21	789
PA29.4	Describe the pathogenesis, pathology, hormonal dependency presenting and distinguishing features, diagnostic tests, progression and spread of carcinoma of the prostate	Y	21	792
PA29.5	Describe the etiology, pathogenesis, pathology and progression of prostatitis	N	21	788
PA30.1	Describe the epidemiology, pathogenesis, etiology, pathology, screening, diagnosis and progression of carcinoma of the cervix	Y	22	800, 805
PA30.2	Describe the pathogenesis, etiology, pathology, diagnosis and progression and spread of carcinoma of the endometrium	Y	22	812
PA30.3	Describe the pathogenesis, etiology, pathology, diagnosis and progression and spread of carcinoma of the leiomyomas and leiomyosarcomas	Y	22	815

Number	COMPETENCY The student should be able to	Core Y/N	Chapter number	Page number
PA30.4	Classify and describe the etiology, pathogenesis, pathology, morphology, clinical course, spread and complications of ovarian tumors	Y	22	817
PA30.5	Describe the etiology, pathogenesis, pathology, morphology, clinical course, spread and complications of gestational trophoblastic neoplasms	Y	22	833
PA30.6	Describe the etiology and morphologic features of cervicitis	N	22	799
PA30.7	Describe the etiology, hormonal dependence, features and morphology of endometriosis	N	22	808
PA30.8	Describe the etiology and morphologic features of adenomyosis	N	22	810
PA30.9	Describe the etiology, hormonal dependence and morphology of endometrial hyperplasia	N	22	810
PA31.1	Classify and describe the types, etiology, pathogenesis, pathology and hormonal dependency of benign breast disease	Y	23	842
PA31.2	Classify and describe the epidemiology, pathogenesis, classification, morphology, prognostic factors, hormonal dependency, staging and spread of carcinoma of the breast	Y	23	844
PA31.3	Describe and identify the morphologic and microscopic features of carcinoma of the breast	N	23	850
PA31.4	Enumerate and describe the etiology, hormonal dependency and pathogenesis of gynecomastia	N	23	861
PA32.1	Enumerate, classify and describe the etiology, pathogenesis, pathology and iodine dependency of thyroid swellings	Y	24	870
PA32.2	Describe the etiology, cause, iodine dependency, pathogenesis, manifestations, laboratory and imaging features and course of thyrotoxicosis	Y	24	866
PA32.3	Describe the etiology, pathogenesis, manifestations, laboratory and imaging features and course of thyrotoxicosis/hypothyroidism	Y	24	869
PA32.4	Classify and describe the epidemiology, etiology, pathogenesis, pathology, clinical laboratory features, complications and progression of diabetes mellitus	Y	24	882
PA32.5	Describe the etiology, genetics, pathogenesis, manifestations, laboratory and morphologic features of hyperparathyroidism	N	24	896
PA32.6	Describe the etiology, pathogenesis, manifestations, laboratory, morphologic features, complications and metastases of pancreatic cancer	N	19	704
PA32.7	Describe the etiology, pathogenesis, manifestations, laboratory, morphologic features, complications of adrenal insufficiency	N	24	901
PA32.8	Describe the etiology, pathogenesis, manifestations, laboratory, morphologic features, complications of Cushing's syndrome	N	24	899
PA32.9	Describe the etiology, pathogenesis, manifestations, laboratory and morphologic features of adrenal neoplasms	N	24	903, 904
PA33.1	Classify and describe the etiology, pathogenesis, manifestations, radiologic and morphologic features and complications of osteomyelitis	Y	25	910
PA33.2	Classify and describe the etiology, pathogenesis, manifestations, radiologic and morphologic features and complications and metastases of bone tumors	Y	25	915

Number	COMPETENCY The student should be able to	Core Y/N	Chapter number	Page number
PA33.3	Classify and describe the etiology, pathogenesis, manifestations, radiologic and morphologic features and complications and metastases of soft tissue tumors	Y	25	936
PA33.4	Classify and describe the etiology, pathogenesis, manifestations, radiologic and morphologic features and complications of Paget's disease of the bone	N	25	914
PA33.5	Classify and describe the etiology, immunology, pathogenesis, manifestations, radiologic and laboratory features, diagnostic criteria and complications of rheumatoid arthritis	N	25	926
PA34.1	Describe the risk factors pathogenesis, pathology and natural history of squamous cell carcinoma of the skin	Y	26	950
PA34.2	Describe the risk factors pathogenesis, pathology and natural history of basal cell carcinoma of the skin	Y	26	951
PA34.3	Describe the distinguishing features between a nevus and melanoma. Describe the etiology, pathogenesis, risk factors morphology clinical features and metastases of melanoma	N	26	954
PA34.4	Identify, distinguish and describe common tumors of the skin	N	26	949
PA35.1	Describe the etiology, types and pathogenesis, differentiating factors, CSF findings in meningitis	Y	27	960
PA35.2	Classify and describe the etiology, genetics, pathogenesis, pathology, presentation sequelae and complications of CNS tumors	Y	27	966
PA35.3	Identify the etiology of meningitis based on given CSF parameters	Y	27	964
PA36.1	Describe the etiology, genetics, pathogenesis, pathology, presentation, sequelae and complications of retinoblastoma	N	27	977

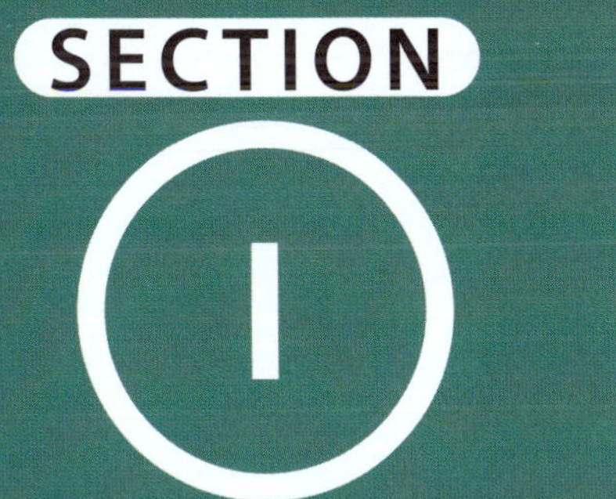

General Pathology

Section Outline

1. Introduction to Pathology
2. Cell Injury and Adaptation
3. Inflammation and Healing
4. Infections and Infestations
5. Hemodynamic Disorders, Thromboembolism, and Shock
6. Immunopathology, AIDS, and Amyloidosis
7. Neoplasia
8. Genetic and Pediatric Diseases
9. Environmental and Nutritional Diseases
10. Basic Diagnostic Cytology

Introduction to Pathology

Chapter Outline

- Definitions and Terms
- Role of a Pathologist in Diagnosis and Management of Disease
- History and Evolution of Pathology

DEFINITIONS AND TERMS

PA 1.2 (CC): Enumerate common definitions and terms used in pathology.

Definition: Pathology is the **scientific study (logos) of disease (pathos)**. It mainly focuses on studying of the structural, biochemical, and functional changes in cells, tissues, and organs in disease.

Learning Pathology

The study of pathology can be divided into general pathology and systemic pathology.

- **General pathology:** It deals with the study of mechanisms, and basic reactions of cells and tissues to abnormal stimuli and inherited defects. These reactions are usually not tissue specific. For example, acute inflammation in response to bacterial infections produces a very similar response in most tissues.
- **Systemic pathology:** This deals with the changes in specific diseases/responses of specialized organs and tissues.

Scientific Study of Disease

The disease process is studied under the following aspects. The standard definitions and terms used in pathology are also mentioned below:

Etiology

The etiology is the origin of the disease. It includes the underlying **causes** and modifying factors responsible for the initiation and progression of the disease process. It describes why a condition arises or what sets the disease process in motion. Etiology refers to why a disease arises. The causative factors of a disease can be divided into two major categories: Genetic (e.g., inherited or acquired mutations, and disease-associated gene variants, or polymorphisms) and acquired (e.g., infectious, chemical, hypoxia, nutritional, physical).

- **Causative agents:** Some diseases are closely linked with etiologic factors, and these etiological factors are said to be the causative agents for the disease. For example, microbial pathogens are considered the causative agents of infectious illness: *Mycobacterium tuberculosis* causes pulmonary tuberculosis, human immunodeficiency virus causes HIV disease, *Entamoeba histolytica* causes amebic dysentery. These diseases cannot develop without pathogens in the body; however, this does not mean that all individual exposed to infection will have the same consequences because many host factors affect the clinical course.
- **Etiological factors:** Even when there is a strong link between disease and etiologic agent, only proportions of the individuals exposed to the etiological factor may develop the disease. For example, if an individual consume large quantities of alcohol he/she may develop liver cirrhosis. In this case, alcohol consumption is considered to be the cause, yet only proportions of individuals who drink alcohol heavily will develop cirrhosis. The concept of one etiologic agent as the cause of one disease is not applicable to the majority of diseases. The exact causes of most disorders remain incompletely understood.
- **Multifactorial:** Most common diseases are multifactorial due to combination of causes (several different etiologic factors that contribute to their development), i.e., inherited genetic susceptibility and various environmental triggers (e.g., coronary heart disease, hypertension, diabetes, and cancer). For example, coronary heart disease is a result of the interaction of genetic predisposition, elevated blood pressure, exposure to cigarette smoke, diet, and many other lifestyle factors acting together. None of these individual factors can be said to cause the disease.

- **Idiopathic:** When the **cause of the disease is unknown**, a condition is said to be **idiopathic.**
- **Iatrogenic:** If the **cause of the disease is** the result of an **unintended or unwanted medical intervention**, the resulting condition is said to be **iatrogenic.**
- **Risk factor:** When the link between a causative/etiologic factor and development of a disease is less than certain but the probability is increased when the factor is present, it is called a risk factor. The identification of risk factors is important for the prevention of the disease.

Pathogenesis

Pathogenesis refers to the steps in the development or evolution of a disease from the initial stimulus to the ultimate expression of the manifestations of the disease. Pathogenesis deals with **mechanisms of development, progression of disease** and the sequence of physiologic events that follow the exposure of cells or tissues (i.e., from the beginning of any disease process) to an injurious agent (initial contact with an etiologic agent/causative factor). It is a dynamic interplay of changes in cell, tissue, organ, and systemic function. It produces cellular, biochemical and molecular abnormalities and ultimate expression of a disease. The study of pathogenesis is a main focus of pathology. With the present advances in technology, it is possible to identify the changes occurring at cellular and molecular level that give rise to the specific functional and structural abnormalities of any particular disease. Thus, it describes how a disease process develops or evolves. This knowledge is helpful for designing new therapeutic approaches. In summary, pathogenesis is a description of how etiologic factors alter physiologic function and lead to the development of clinical manifestations in a particular disorder or disease. Thus, pathogenesis describes how a disease develops.

Pathophysiology: In pathology, the study and diagnosis of disease is performed through examination of organs, tissues, cells, and bodily fluids. Physiology is the study of the mechanical, physical, and biochemical functions of living organisms. Together, as pathophysiology, the term refers to the study of abnormalities in physiologic functioning (i.e., physiological changes) of an individual or an organ due to a disease.

- **Latent period:** Few causative agents produce signs and symptoms of the disease immediately after exposure. Usually, etiological agents take **some time to manifest the disease** (e.g., carcinogenesis) and this time period is called as the latent period. It varies depending on the disease.
- **Incubation period:** In disorders caused by infectious (due to bacteria, viruses, etc.) agents, the **period between exposure and the development of disease** is called the incubation period. It usually ranges from days to weeks. Most of the infectious agents have characteristic incubation period.
- It is essential to know the etiology and pathogenesis of the disease to understand the disease as well as to develop rational treatment. There are diseases that morphologically appear similar (e.g., a malignant tumor of an organ), but they have different molecular differences (e.g., mutations and epigenetic changes). This helps in precision (or personalized) medicine in which therapies are designed for each individual's disease rather than disease as such.

MORPHOLOGIC CHANGES

All diseases start with structural changes (pathologic changes) in cells. **Rudolf Virchow** (known as the **father of modern pathology**) proposed that injury to the cell is the basis of all disease. Morphologic changes refer to the **gross and microscopic structural changes** in cells or tissues affected by disease. **Lesion** is the term used for the characteristic changes in tissues and cells produced by disease in an individual. The term **"pathology"** (pathological feature) is **sometimes used synonym with morphology.** Now morphology is routinely supplemented by analysis of protein expression and genetic alterations.

Gross

Many diseases have characteristic gross pathology and a fairly confident diagnosis can be given before light microscopy. For example, serous cystadenoma of ovary usually consists of one cystic cavity containing serous fluid (*refer* **Fig. 22.26A**); cirrhosis of liver is characterized by total replacement of liver by regenerating nodules (*refer* **Figs. 19.19A and B**).

Microscopy

Light microscopy: Abnormalities in tissue architecture and morphological changes in cells can be studied by light microscopy.

- **Histopathology:** Sections are routinely cut from tissues and processed by paraffin-embedding. The sections are cut from the tissue by a special instrument called microtome and examined under light microscope. In certain situations (e.g., histochemistry, rapid diagnosis), sections are cut from tissue that has been hardened rapidly by freezing (frozen section). The sections are stained routinely by hematoxylin and eosin.
  - **Pathognomonic abnormalities:** If the **structural changes are characteristic of a single disease or diagnostic of an etiologic process,** it is called as **pathognomonic.** Pathognomonic features are those features which are restricted to a single disease, or disease category. The diagnosis should not be made without them. For example, **Aschoff bodies** are pathognomonic of **rheumatic heart disease** and **Reed-Sternberg cells** are pathognomonic of **Hodgkin lymphoma** (*refer* **online Tables 15.21 to 15.23**).
- **Cytology:** The cells from cysts, body cavities, or scraped from body surfaces or aspirated by fine needle from solid lesions can also be studied under light microscope. This study of cells is known as cytology and is used widely especially in diagnosis and screening of cancer.
- **Histochemistry (special stains):** Histochemistry (*refer* **Table 2.11**) is the study of the chemistry of tissues, where tissue/cells are treated with specific reagent so that the features of individual cells/structure can be visualized, e.g., **Prussian blue reaction for hemosiderin** (*refer* **Fig. 2.31**).

- **Immunohistochemistry and immunofluorescence:** Both utilize antibodies (immunoglobulins with antigen specificity) to visualize substances in tissue sections or cell preparations. Former uses **monoclonal antibodies** linked chemically to enzymes (*refer* **Figs. 23.17A to C**) and latter uses **fluorescent dyes.**

Electron microscopy: Electron microscopy (EM) is useful to study the changes at ultrastructural level, and for the demonstration of viruses in tissue samples in certain diseases. The most common diagnostic use of EM is for the interpretation of biopsy specimen from kidney (*refer* **Fig. 20.17A**).

Functional Derangements and Clinical Manifestations

Functional Derangements

The effects of genetic, biochemical and structural changes in cells and tissues are **functional abnormalities**. For example, excessive secretion of a cell product (e.g., nasal mucus in the common cold); insufficient secretion of a cell product (e.g., insulin lack in diabetes mellitus).

Clinical Manifestations

The functional derangements produce clinical manifestations of disease, namely symptoms and signs.

Symptoms: The subjective feelings of an abnormality in the body are called as symptoms. It is any change in the body or its functions as perceived by the patient. The symptoms are subjective experience of disease and can only be described to an observer by the affected patient.

Signs: Manifestations of disease that are observed by physician/observer are termed signs of disease and is an objective evidence of a disease. For example, the feeling of nausea is a symptom, whereas vomiting is objectively observed and is a sign. Signs are apparent to observers, whereas symptoms may be obvious only to the patient.

Laboratory tests and investigations: Some signs and symptoms (e.g., fever, headache) are nonspecific and do not indicate a specific cause. In such situation further clinical examination and, often, laboratory tests (biochemical analysis, hematological, microbiological, cytological examination, etc.) and investigations (e.g., X-ray, diagnostic imaging) may be required to know the possible causes of the signs and symptoms.

Diagnosis: It is the art or act of identifying (determine the cause) a disease (pathological condition) from its signs and symptoms. Many diseases/disorders are characterized by a particular constellation of signs and symptoms, the knowledge of which is essential for accurate detection and diagnosis.

Syndromes: Diseases characterized by **multiple abnormalities** (symptom complex) are called syndromes. A syndrome is a group (collection) of medical signs, symptoms, laboratory findings, and physiological disturbances occurring together that are often associated with a particular disease or disorder. For example, carpal tunnel syndrome; irritable bowel syndrome; Klinefelter syndrome, Down syndrome.

Prognosis

The prognosis forecasts (predicts) the known or likely **course (outcome) of the disease** and, therefore, the fate of the patient.

Complications

It is a **negative pathologic process** or event occurring **during the disease** which is not an essential part of the disease. It usually aggravates the illness. For example, perforation and hemorrhage are complications which may develop in typhoid ulcer of intestine.

Sequelae

It is a pathologic condition **following as a consequence of a disease**. For example, intestinal obstruction following healed tuberculosis of intestine, mitral stenosis following healed rheumatic heart disease.

Remission and Relapse/Exacerbation

Some diseases may pass through several cycles/alteration of remission and relapse/exacerbation. For example, inflammatory bowel disease (Crohn disease and ulcerative colitis), and some autoimmune diseases. An exacerbation is characterized by a relatively sudden increase in the severity of a disease or any of its signs and symptoms. A remission is characterized by a decline in severity of the signs and symptoms of a disease. If a remission is permanent, the patient is said to be cured.

Various steps involved in study of disease are presented in **Figure 1.1.**

ROLE OF A PATHOLOGIST IN DIAGNOSIS AND MANAGEMENT OF DISEASE

PA 1.1 (CC): Describe the role of a pathologist in diagnosis and management of disease.

Pathology is a branch of medicine involved in understanding the cause of disease, the processes involved in testing the disease and the reporting of diagnostic tests.

Q. Describe the role of a pathologist in diagnosis and management of disease.

Subdivisions of Pathology

The study of pathology can be divided into different branches (disciplines) and subspecialties (**Table 1.1**).

Anatomic Pathology/Histopathology

In anatomic pathology, microscopic examination is an essential tool for the study. It includes histopathology, cytopathology and autopsy. Histopathology is the classic

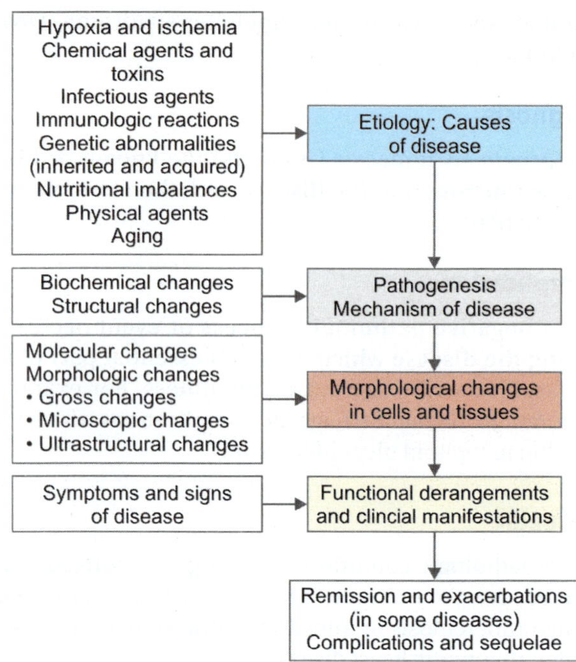

Fig. 1.1: Steps involved in study of disease.

and most useful method of study. The term histopathology is used synonymously with anatomic pathology or morbid anatomy. Modern anatomic pathology is divided into subspecialities, such as renal pathology, dermatopathology, gastrointestinal pathology, cardiac pathology, pulmonary pathology, neuropathology, gynecologic pathology, breast pathology, oral pathology, etc.

Surgical Pathology

It deals primarily with the study of structure changes in tissues/organs removed from the living patients by biopsy or surgical resection. Surgical pathology includes both gross or naked eye examination referred to as gross or macroscopic changes, as well as examination of processed tissue under a compound light microscope. Intraoperative examination is done by use of frozen tissue sections and is employed for rapid diagnosis.

Microscopic examination: It requires tissues be cut with a microtome into thin sections that can be stained with routine stains, such as hematoxyline and eosin (H & E). Two types of sectioning methods are most commonly used: *frozen sections* and *paraffin-embedded* or *permanent sections*.

- **Frozen sections:** Frozen sections are cut by using cryostat (microtome in a refrigerated chamber) or freezing microtome from tissue that has been hardened rapidly by freezing (hence termed frozen section). They can be prepared rapidly (within minutes) during the course of surgery while the patient is still under anesthesia (for details *refer* page 265).
- **Permanent sections:** In most instances, pathologists rely on the study of better-preserved tissue by conventional permanent tissue sections with paraffin embedding technique stained with hematoxylin and eosin. These are prepared from tissues that have been fixed, dehydrated and embedded in paraffin wax as a supporting medium prior to sectioning. Though it needs more time for preparation (about 24 hours), permanent sections have several advantages over frozen tissue sections. These include thinner (typically 5 μm) and better-quality sections without any freezing artefacts. They permit greater certainty of interpretation. Some tissues (e.g., those containing fat or bone) cut poorly as frozen sections but may be

TABLE 1.1 Major pathology disciplines and roles.

Discipline/subspecialty	*Role*
Anatomic pathology	
• Histopathology	Study of disease in human tissue samples (e.g., in cancer management through the staging and grading of tumors)
• Cytopathology	Study of disease in individual cells
• Forensic pathology	Determination of cause and manner of death for legal purposes
• Autopsy	Determination of cause and manner of death
Hematology	Study of the blood and bone marrow
Clinical pathology also called laboratory medicine	It is largely concerned with analysis of blood and other fluids and involves, for instance, clinical biochemistry, microbiology, and hematology
• **Chemical pathology** (clinical biochemistry)	Study of the biochemical tests to diagnose and treat patients. Also to understand the biochemical basis/mechanisms of the body related to disease. Body fluids, such as blood or urine are used for screening, diagnosis, prognosis and management through chemical and biochemical tests
• Medical microbiology	Study of infection
Molecular and genetics pathology	Study of the molecular and genetic basis of diseases and heritable conditions. Variety of tests of molecules within organs, tissues or bodily fluids are performed
Immunopathology	Study of the immunologic basis of disease
Transfusion medicine	Study of the collection, preparation, storage, and clinical use of blood products

satisfactorily studied in permanent sections. H & E may be further supported by numerous special stains (histochemistry) for specific tissue components (e.g., mucus, glycogen, collagen, bacteria, and fungi) in certain situations.

- **Ancillary staining and analytical methods:** Histochemistry (special stains), immunohistochemistry, and electron microscopy are ancillary technique in surgical pathology that may be helpful or necessary supplements for diagnosis.
  - **Special stains** may aid in the diagnosis of one or another type of tumor (i.e., differential diagnosis) and classification. Examples include special stains for mucins, amyloid, lipids and glycogen.

Surgical pathology helps to diagnose a disease and determine a treatment plan and has a definitive role in tumor diagnosis. With very few exceptions, definitive therapy for cancer should not be undertaken in the absence of a tissue diagnosis.

Role of Pathologists

Diagnosis

Diagnostic role is a **key aspect of pathology laboratories.** Pathologist examines the changes in the tissue samples/ biopsies of the body (removed at surgery or autopsy), in the cells obtained from needle-aspirated specimens, in blood and other body fluids/secretions (including urine, cerebrospinal fluid, sputum, pleural/ascitic/pericardial fluid and synovial fluid). Some of these changes in test show the causes (e.g., lepromatous leprosy with positive lepra bacilli in the tissue sections, malarial parasites in the peripheral blood smear, *Candida albicans* in vaginal smear).

Tumor Grading, Staging, and Prognosis of Disease

Pathologists helps in clinical care by assessing disease severity and prognosis. For example, determining the tumor staging [e.g., the well-known **TNM system** (*refer* pages 263-4)] and grading of a cancer to estimate tumor prognosis by histopathology; this information determines the precise type and severity (stage) of the cancer. Staging attempts to measure the extent of spread of a malignant tumor within a patient on the basis of tumor size, lymph node involvement, and the presence of other metastases. **Tumor grading is a tumor's degree of differentiation** and growth rate, often graded as I to III where III represents the least differentiated, fastest dividing tumors and presumed to have the worst prognosis.

Management of the Disease

Some of the test are fundamental in deciding and managing treatment plans for patients. Examples include, use of antiestrogenic agents in estrogen receptor-positive breast cancers. A newer approach has been to target the HER2/*neu* antigen (*refer* **Fig. 23.17C**) which is overexpressed in certain breast and ovarian cancers. The HER2/*neu* antigen is targeted by a therapeutic agent, trastuzumab (Herceptin, Genentech) consisting of a humanized monoclonal antibody that binds to the HER2/*neu*. A complete and accurate pathology report is crucial for precise diagnosis and to decide the best treatment plan for patient. In the present era, importance is given to **identify markers that help to predict the response to new and different therapeutic modalities**.

Monitor the Response to Treatment

Pathology reports may be helpful in monitoring the clinical response to treatment. For example, analyzing blood levels of markers of renal function (renal function tests) in patients with renal failure, minimal residual disease in lymphomas after treatment.

To Comment of Excision Margin in Surgical Specimens

An important concern in surgical pathology is the **adequacy of tumor excision**. Depending on the tissue or type of excision or resected specimen, this decision can be made on either frozen or permanent sections. It is necessary to know the **distances between the edges of the tumor and the excision (resection) margins**. If the tumor forms a discrete mass and the margins of the specimen are well/ clearly recognizable/defined, then determination of excision margins is usually straightforward. Examples of tumors whose excision is likely to have clearly recognizable margins include tumors arising in the gastrointestinal tract, lung, and skin. Excision margins should be identified and painted with ink before any dissection, thus permitting accurate measurement of these distances microscopically. All lymph nodes associated with a cancer specimen need to be dissected out, described along with their location, and processed for histology.

Other roles: Pathology plays a number of other key roles. One is **quality assurance** within the healthcare system. Pathologists routinely supervise the laboratory to ensure pathology results are appropriate and of the highest standard.

Cytopathology

Cytopathology consists of study of exfoliated cells [i.e., cells shed off from the lesions (exfoliative cytology)] scraped, or brushed cells or fine-needle aspiration cytology (FNAC) of superficial and deep-seated lesions for diagnosis. These can be a rapid, efficient, and low-risk technique for establishing an accurate diagnosis. Role of a cytopathologist in diagnosis and management of disease are discussed in Chapter 10.

Forensic Pathology and Autopsy

This includes the study of organs and tissues removed at postmortem (autopsy) for medicolegal work and for determining the underlying sequence and cause of death. Forensic pathology is integral to legal system. By this, the course of events that occurred in the patient during life and the probable cause of death can be ascertained. Postmortem anatomical diagnosis helps the clinician to enhance their knowledge about the disease and their judgment. Forensic autopsy is done for medicolegal purposes. In postmortem examination 'the dead teach the living' and has an important role in patient care, around the world.

Hematology

Hematology deals with the study of diseases of blood. It includes laboratory hematology and clinical hematology. The hematological diseases include disorders of the red and white blood cells, platelets and the coagulation system. It may be non-neoplastic, certain inflammatory diseases, benign or malignant disorders. Red blood cell (RBC) disorders include disorders of hemoglobin (anemia, such as iron deficiency, sickle cell disease) and white blood cell (WBC) disorders include quantitative disorders of white blood cells and malignant disorders, such as leukemia, lymphoma or myeloma. The disorders of platelets (e.g., thrombocytopenia) and disorders of blood coagulation (e.g., hemophilia) are also part of hematology. Hematologists receive blood samples for checking any abnormalities. They examine the blood film for any abnormality (e.g., anemia, leukemia) and also perform a bone marrow aspiration and biopsy. Common hematologic test is a complete blood count (CBC), which includes white blood cell count, red blood cell count, platelet count, hematocrit/red blood cell volume (HCT), hemoglobin concentration (HB), differential white blood count and red blood cell indices. Other examples of hematologic tests include prothrombin time (PT), and partial thromboplastin time (PTT).

Clinical Pathology (Laboratory Medicine)

Clinical pathology includes analysis of various fluids including blood and body fluids, such as urine, semen, cerebrospinal fluid (CSF) and other body fluids. Such analysis may be qualitative, semiquantitative or quantitative. Wide range of laboratory test results assist clinicians in their diagnosis and treatment of disease. These results help hospital departments including intensive care, operating theaters, special care baby units and oncology.

Clinical Biochemistry

This includes quantitative determination of various biochemical constituents in serum and plasma, and in other body fluids. There is some overlapping between clinical pathology and clinical biochemistry.

Microbiology

This includes the study of disease-causing microbes. Depending upon the type of microorganism studied, it is further developed into bacteriology, parasitology, mycology, virology, etc.

Immunology

In this, abnormalities in the immune system of the body comprising of immunology and immunopathology are studied.

Medical Genetics

It deals with the relationship between heredity and disease. It is useful in blood grouping, inborn errors of metabolism, chromosomal aberrations in congenital malformations and neoplasms, etc.

Molecular Pathology

Most of the diseases can be diagnosed by the morphological changes in tissues. But, with the present advances in diagnostic pathology, we realize that cellular disturbances develop due to alterations in molecules (genes, proteins, and others) that influence the survival and behavior of cells. Thus, in the present modern pathology, it is necessary to understand the cellular and molecular abnormalities that give rise to diseases. The detection and diagnosis of abnormalities at the molecular level (i.e., DNA of the cell) is performed by molecular pathology. Molecular pathology has revealed the biochemical basis of many diseases, mainly congenital disorders and cancer. These techniques can detect changes in a single nucleotide of DNA and include in situ hybridization, polymerase chain reaction (PCR), etc. In situ hybridization can detect the presence of specific genes or their messenger RNA in tissue sections or cell preparations. Minute quantities of nucleic acids can be amplified by the use of the polymerase chain reaction. DNA microarrays can be used to determine patterns of gene expression (mRNA). These methods are used for research purposes as well as a part of diagnostic pathology reports. Molecular pathology, for example, using nucleic acid probes with or without amplification by the polymerase chain reaction is used to detect expression of specific tumor genes or gene mutations.

Transfusion Medicine

This branch ensures adequate stocks of safe blood when needed for blood transfusions. The blood bank/center confirms that the donated blood is the right match for the patient's blood group. This branch deals with blood and transplant service providing vital support for blood transfusion, organ and stem cell transplantation.

HISTORY AND EVOLUTION OF PATHOLOGY

PA 1.3 (NC): Describe the history and evolution of pathology.

Medicine is as old as humankind. In the beginning of mankind, there was a desire and need to know about the causes, mechanisms and nature of diseases. This knowledge was gained over the centuries from supernatural beliefs to the present knowledge of modern pathology. Pathology has evolved over the years as a distinct discipline or branch apart from others, such as anatomy, medicine, surgery, etc. For an undergraduate beginner in pathology, it is necessary to know brief review of history of pathology and personalities with their outstanding contribution.

Prehistoric Times to Medieval Period

During prehistoric time; religion, magic and medical treatment were quite linked to each other. It was believed that the disease was the outcome of 'curse from God' or it had supernatural origin from 'evil eye of spirits.' The disease was treated by priests through prayers and sacrifices, and magicians by magic power. Some ancient superstitions still exist in some parts of the world.

Religious and magical belief: The link between medicine and religion was firmly believed throughout the world. This has resulted in belief in different societies that there are gods and goddesses of healing. For example, *Dhanvantri* was considered as the deity of medicine in India, and orthodox Indians' belief in *Mata Sheetala Devi* as the pox goddess. Same way Greeks had *Aesculapius* and Apollo as the principal gods of healing.

Philosophical and rational approach: This approach was by the methods of observations and this followed the earlier religious and magical beliefs. This philosophical concept to all-natural phenomena was introduced by Greek philosophers namely *Socrates, Plato* and *Aristotle*.

Hippocrates: The real practice of medicine began with the great Greek clinical genius *Hippocrates* (460–370 BC). He is regarded as 'the father of medicine' and he dissociated medicine from religion and magic. He revolutionized the practice of medicine and established the basic foundations of the role of the physician. He studied patient's symptoms and described methods of diagnosis. He recorded his observations on cases and his writings called Hippocratic Corpus remained for nearly two thousand years as the mainstay of learning of medicine. However, Hippocates too propagated the prevailing concept on mechanism of disease based on disequilibrium of our basic humors (water, air, fire, and earth). Later this concept was abandoned. Hippocrates set standards for patient care and the physician's attitudes and philosophies that persist today. Many aspects of the Hippocratic approach to medicine are still with us today. Hippocrates rational and ethical attitudes in practice and teaching of medicine are being respected by the medical profession and *'Hippocratic oath'* is taken by all medical students at the time of entry into practice of medicine.

After Hippocrates, Greek medicine reached Rome (now Italy). After 146 BC, Rome controlled Greek world and dominated in ancient Europe. Many terms in medicine have their origin from Latin language which was the official language of countries included in ancient Roman empire (Spanish, Portuguese, Italian, French and Greek languages have their origin from Latin). Hippocratic teaching was propagated in Rome by Roman physicians. Prominent among them are *Cornelius Celsus* (53 BC to AD 7) and *Claudius Galen* (AD 130–200).

- Celsus first described four cardinal signs of inflammation namely rubor (redness), tumor (swelling), calor (heat), and dolor (pain).
- Galen postulated humoral theory, later called Galenic theory. According to this theory, the illness was considered as due to imbalance between *four humors* (or body fluids)—blood, lymph, black bile (believed at that time to be from the spleen), and biliary secretion from the liver.

In India, in the centuries before and after Hippocrates, the hypothesis of disequilibrium of four elements of the body (Dhatus) similar to Hippocratic doctrine was mentioned in ancient Indian medicine books during AD 200. Susruta (Sushruta Samhita) and Chakara (Charaka Samhita) produced encyclopedic founding works of Ayurvedic medicine. Charaka listed 700 plant-derived medicines/ remedies and surgical sciences was documented by Sushruta.

Backwardness during Medieval period: During Middle Ages (or medieval period that lasted from the 5th to the 15th century), there was marked backwardness in medicine. During this period, there were widespread and devastating epidemics. This resulted in reversal of the process of rational thinking back to supernatural concepts and divine punishment for 'sins.' The dominant belief was that life was due to influence of vital substance under the control of soul *(theory of vitalism)*. During this period, the dissection of human body was strictly forbidden because it was considered to hurt the 'soul.'

Human Anatomy and Era of Gross Pathology

Renaissance period: The backwardness during Medieval period was followed by the Renaissance period (i.e., revival of learning). This began from Italy in late 15th century and spread to whole of Europe. During this period, there was quest (an attempt to achieve something) for advances in art and science. There was freedom of thought and emphasis on philosophical and rational attitudes again.

Human Anatomy

- The development of human anatomy took place at the beginning of this period with the art works and **drawings of human muscles and embryos** by famous Italian painter **Leonardo da Vinci** (1452–1519).
- **Vesalius (1514–1564) dissected human body** of freshly executed criminals. His pupils, Gabriel Fallopius (1523–1562) described human oviducts (Fallopian tubes) and Fabricius discovered lymphoid tissue around the intestine of birds (bursa of Fabricius).
- The special human anatomic dissection in the form of **postmortem** came into practice in various parts of ancient Europe.

Microscope

- **Antony van Leeuwenhoek** (1632–1723), a cloth merchant by profession in Holland, during his spare time **invented** the first ever **microscope** by grinding the lenses. He also introduced histological staining using saffron to examine muscle fibers.
- **Marcello Malpighi** (1624–1694) observed the **presence of capillaries** by using microscope. He described the malpighian layer of the skin, and lymphoid tissue in the spleen (malpighian corpuscles). **Malpighi is known as 'the father of histology.'**

Morbid Anatomy

Morbid anatomy (pathologic anatomy) is a branch of medical science concerned with the study of the structure of diseased organs and tissues.

- **Giovanni B Morgagni** (1682–1771): The beginning of study of morbid anatomy was by Italian anatomist, pathologist, *Giovanni B Morgagni* (1682–1771). He was an excellent teacher in anatomy, a prolific writer and a practicing clinician. Morgagni dismissed the ancient humoral theory of disease and published his life-time experiences based on 700 postmortems and their corresponding clinical findings. Thus, he laid the foundations of clinicopathologic methodology in the study of disease. He introduced the concept of clinicopathologic correlation (CPC), establishing a coherent sequence of cause, lesions, symptoms, and outcome of disease.
- **Sir Percival Pott** (1714–1788) was a famous surgeon in England. He **described tuberculosis of the spine** (Pott's disease). He was also **first to identify occupational cancer** (cancer of scrotal skin) in the chimney sweeps in 1775 and discovered chimney soot as the first chemical carcinogenic agent.
- During the latter part of 18th Century, **John Hunter** (1728–1793) who was a student of Sir Percival Pott became the greatest surgeon-anatomist of all times. His elder brother **William Hunter** (1718–1788) was a reputed anatomist-obstetrician. These brothers **developed the first museum of comparative anatomy and pathology** in the world by collecting surgical specimens and arranged them into separate organ systems. This museum knows as the Hunterian Museum, now housed in Royal College of Surgeons of London.
- **Edward Jenner** (1749–1823) who demonstrated **inoculation in smallpox.**
- **Matthew Baillie** (1760–1823) is a prominent English pathologist published first-ever systematic textbook of morbid anatomy in 1793.
- **Era of gross pathology**:
  - **Richard Bright** (1789–1858) described non-suppurative nephritis which was later termed as glomerulonephritis or **Bright's disease.**
  - **Thomas Addison** (1793–1860) gave an account of chronic adrenocortical insufficiency and was termed as **Addison's disease.**
  - **Thomas Hodgkin** (1798–1866) observed the complex of chronic enlargement of lymph nodes, often with enlargement of the liver and spleen, which was later called **Hodgkin's disease** (presently known as Hodgkin lymphoma).
  - **Xavier Bichat** (1771–1802) in France described that organs were composed of tissue and divided the study of morbid anatomy into General Pathology and Systemic Pathology.
  - **RTH Laennec** (1781–1826), a French physician had numerous discoveries. These include **description of several lung diseases** (tubercles, caseous lesions, miliary lesions, pleural effusion, and bronchiectasis), **chronic sclerotic liver disease** (later called Laennec's cirrhosis) and **invented stethoscope.**
  - **Carl F von Rokitansky** (1804–1878) is a self-taught German pathologist who **performed nearly 30,000 autopsies** himself. He described acute yellow atrophy of the liver, wrote monograph on diseases of arteries and congenital heart defects. Unlike most other surgeons during that time, Rokitansky did not do clinical practice of surgery but instead introduced the concept that pathologists should confine themselves to making diagnosis which became the accepted role of pathologist later.

Era of Technology Development and Cellular Pathology

Correlation of clinical features with autopsy findings: Up to middle of the 19th century, the major method of study of disease was by correlating clinical manifestations of disease with gross pathological findings at autopsy.

Advances in Pathology

In the 19th century, sophistication in surgical techniques led to advancement in pathology. The anatomist-surgeons of earlier centuries got replaced largely with surgeon-pathologists. **In later half of the 19th century, pathology became a diagnostic discipline** with the evolution of cellular pathology. This was closely linked to technology advancements in machinery for cutting thin tissue sections, improvement in microscope, and development of dyes for staining.

Identification of Microorganisms

- French chemist **Louis Pasteur** (1822–1895) **discovered the disease-causing microorganisms** and this replaced the prevailing theory of spontaneous generation of disease and firmly established **germ theory of disease.**
- In 1873, **GHA Hansen** (1841–1912) in Germany identified **Hansen's (lepra) bacillus** as the first microbe that caused leprosy (Hansen's disease).

Immunity and Phagocytosis

- The **basis of immunization** was initiated by **Edward Jenner** while studying infectious diseases.
- **Metchnikoff** (1845–1916), a Russian zoologist, **discovered phenomenon of phagocytosis** by human defense cells against invading microbes.

Staining

Developments in chemical industry lead to switching over from earlier dyes of plant and animal origin to **synthetic dyes**. In 1856, **Perkin** prepared first synthetic dye namely aniline violet. This led to emergence of a viable dye, industry for histological and bacteriological purposes. Various pioneers who contributed the use for dye are as follows:

- **Paul Ehrlich** (1854–1915), German physician, conferred Nobel prize in 1908 for his work in immunology. He described **Ehrlich's test for urobilinogen** using **Ehrlich's aldehyde reagent** and staining techniques of cells and bacteria. These developments led to the foundations of clinical pathology.
- **Christian Gram** (1853–1938), Danish physician, used **crystal violet for staining bacteria**.
- **DL Romanowsky** (1861–1921), Russian physician, developed **stain for peripheral blood film** using eosin and methylene blue derivatives.
- **Robert Koch** (1843–1910), German bacteriologist **described Koch's postulate and Koch's phenomena**. He also developed techniques of fixation and staining for identification of bacteria. He **discovered tubercle bacilli** in 1882 and cholera vibrio organism in 1883.
- **May-Grünwald** in 1902 **and Giemsa** in 1914 developed **stains for blood and bone marrow**. They applied them for classification of cells in blood and bone marrow.
- **Sir William Leishman** (1865–1926) in 1914 described **Leishman's stain for blood smear/films** and observed Leishman-Donovan bodies (LD bodies) in leishmaniasis.
- **Robert Feulgen** (1884–1955) described **Feulgen reaction for DNA staining**. This laid the foundations of cytochemistry and histochemistry.

Technical Advances

Advances in techniques and machinery led to development and upgrading of microtomes for obtaining thin sections of organs/tissues and staining by dyes for enhancing detailed study of sections. The presence of cells in thin sections of non-living object cork was first demonstrated by Robert Hooke in 1667. In the 19th century, FT Schwann (1810–1882) was, the first neurohistologist, and Claude Bernarde (1813–1878), was pioneer in pathophysiology.

Histopathology

Till the end of the 19th century, the study of morbid anatomy was confined largely to autopsy-based study and thus remained as a retrospective science.

Rudolf Virchow (1821–1905) in Germany **first did the microscopic examination of diseased tissue at cellular level.** This became as the histopathology method of investigation. Virchow hypothesized cellular theory and is aptly known as **"father of cellular pathology"**. According to him:

- All cells come from other cells.
- Disease is an alteration of normal structure and function of these cells.

This led to sound foundation of diagnostic pathology based on microscopy and was followed and promoted by numerous brilliant successive workers. This gave birth to biopsy pathology. Other discoveries by Rudolf Virchow are:

- **Virchow's triad:** Virchow described etiology of thrombosis [(Virchow's triad namely (i) slowing of blood-stream, (ii) changes in the vessel wall and (iii) changes in the blood itself)].
- **Virchow's lymph node:** Metastatic spread of tumor of carcinoma stomach to supraclavicular lymph node.
- **Components and diseases of blood** (fibrinogen, leukocytosis, leukemia).

Frozen section: **Julius Cohnheim** (1839–1884), student of Rudolf Virchow, **described the concept of frozen section** examination while the patient was still on the operation table.

The concept of surgeon and physician as pathologist started in the 19th century and it continued as late as the middle of the 20th century in most clinical departments. During this period, biopsy pathology work was assigned to some faculty member in the clinical department. The notable pathologists of the first half of 20th century had background of clinical training and these include **James Ewing** (1866–1943), **AP Stout** (1885–1967) and **Lauren Ackerman** (1905–1993) in United States of America; **Pierre Masson** (1880–1958) in France, and **RA Willis** in Australia.

Landmarks in Modern Pathology

- **Karl Landsteiner** (1863–1943) **described major human blood groups** in 1900 and is considered **"father of blood transfusion"**. He was awarded Nobel prize in 1930.
- **Ruska and Lorries** in 1933 **developed electron microscope**. This helped to identify the ultrastructure of cell and its organelles.
- **George N Papanicolaou** (1883–1962), a Greek-born, American pathologist is known as '**father of Exfoliative cytology**'. In 1930s, he developed **exfoliative cytology for early detection of cervical cancer**.
- **William Boyd** (1885–1979), psychiatrist-turned pathologist was by an **eminent teacher-author in pathology during 20th century**. His textbooks, namely 'Pathology for Surgeons' (first edition, 1925) and 'Textbook of Pathology' (first edition, 1932), dominated and inspired the few generations of students of pathology all over the world due to **his flowery language and lucid style**.
- **MM Wintrobe** (1901–1986) **discovered hematocrit technique**.

Modern Pathology

In the latter half of 20th century and during 21st century, advances made it possible to **study diseases at genetic and molecular level**. The evidence based and objective diagnosis may enable the physician to institute targeted therapy. The major benefit due to these advances in molecular biology are in the field of diagnosis and treatment of genetic disorders, immunology and in cancer. Some of the discoveries are as follows:

- **Albert Coons** in 1940s discovered *immunofluorescence techniques*.
- **Watson and Crick** in 1953 described **the** *double helix* **structure of DNA** of the cell.
- **Tijo and Levan in 1956, identified chromosomes and their correct number in humans** (46 = 23 pairs).
- **Nowell and Hagerford in 1960,** identified **Philadelphia chromosome** t(9;22) in chronic myeloid leukemia. This was the first chromosomal abnormality detected in any cancer.
- **In situ hybridization** (ISH) was introduced in 1969. In this, a labeled probe is used to detect and localize specific RNA or DNA sequences **'in situ'** (e.g., in the original place). Its **later modification uses fluorescence microscopy** (FISH) to detect specific localization of the defect on chromosomes.
- **Recombinant DNA technique** was developed in 1972 using restriction enzymes to cut and paste part/bits of DNA.
- **Kary Mullis** in 1983, introduced **polymerase chain reaction** (PCR). In this multiple copy of DNA fragments can be done and this has revolutionized the diagnostic molecular genetics. PCR analysis is more rapid than ISH, can be automated by thermal cyclers and requires less amount of DNA for the test.
- **Barbara McClintock** invented **flexibility and dynamism of DNA** by for which she was awarded Nobel prize in 1983.
- **Ian Wilmut** and his colleagues at Roslin Institute in Edinburgh in 1997, performed **mammalian cloning**. By using this technique, they performed the somatic cell nuclear transfer to create the clone of a sheep named Dolly. However, reproductive cloning for human beings is very risky and absolutely unethical.
- **Stem cell research:** It started in 2000s by harvesting the primitive stem cells isolated from embryos and maintaining their growth in the laboratory. There are two types of stem cells in humans, namely (i) embryonic stem cells and (ii) adult stem cells. Stem cells have many applications in the treatment of many human diseases, such as Alzheimer's disease, diabetes, cancer, strokes, etc. In future, stem cell therapy may be able to replace whole organ transplant and stem cells 'harvested' from the embryo may be used as a replacement of damaged tissue/organ. Hematopoietic stem cells are being used for many diseases of the hematopoietic system.
- **Human Genome Project (HGP):** It consisted of a consortium of countries and was completed in April 2003. By HGP, it is possible to read nature's complete genetic blueprint used in making of each human being (i.e., gene mapping). Clinical trials by gene therapy for the treatment of some single gene defects have resulted in some success, especially in hematological and immunological diseases. Future developments in genetic engineering may be able to design new and highly effective individualized treatment options for genetic diseases and also may suggest preventive action against diseases.
- **Uses of Human Genome Project:** It is listed in **Box 1.1**.

BOX 1.1: Uses of human genome project.

The understanding of the genome provides clues for:

- **Etiology** of cancers, Alzheimer's disease, etc.
- Defining the **pathogenesis** of a disease and to study the disease processes at **molecular level.**
- **Susceptibility** of an individual to a variety of illnesses, e.g., carcinoma breast, disorders of hemostasis, liver diseases, cystic fibrosis, etc.
- Precise new ways to **prevent** a number of diseases that affect human beings.
- To **diagnose and treat** disease. Target genes for treatment and management of diseases.
- **Human development and anthropology:** Analysis of similarities between DNA sequences from different organisms helps to **study evolution.**
- **Researcher:** By visiting the human genome database on the World Wide Web, researcher can examine what other scientists have written about the gene.

Telepathology and Virtual Microscopy

Q. Write a short note on telepathology and virtual microscopy.

Telepathology is defined as the **practice of diagnostic pathology at a distance**. In this, a remote pathologist (receiving side) utilizes tissue specimens, histological, cytological electronic (digital) images which are transferred over a telecommunication network from a different location (sending side).

Components: The various components of telepathology network include:

- A conventional light microscope
- Devise to capture the image, i.e., a camera mounted on a microscope
- Telecommunication link between the sending and receiving sites
- A work station at the receiving site with a high-quality video monitor

Advantages/benefits: Telepathology makes it **faster and easier to share medical images**. Pathologists in different locations can view images simultaneously and discuss diagnoses through teleconferencing. Pathologist can consult pathologists who are specialized in area of concern, such as liver pathology or lung pathology. It allows pathologists, surgeons and radiologists to communicate with each other over diagnostic dilemmas and overcoming the barrier of distance.

Main Categories of Telepathology

The types of telepathology include:

Static image-based systems

In this static telepathology, images are captured from a digital camera connected to a microscope. An image area is selected and transmitted. A limited number of images (1 to 40) are captured and stored in the hard drive of the computer or compact disc-read only memory (CD-ROM) for transmission. It is economical, simple and requires only a standard telephone and internet connection. Disadvantage is that selection of field for images should be done by expert and if done by a non-expert may miss the important areas.

Virtual slide systems

Pathology specimen slides are scanned and high-resolution digital images created for transmission.

Real-time systems

This is also termed robotic interactive telepathology and dynamic pathology. In this, the recipient pathologist remotely guides a robotically controlled motorized microscope by means of a joystick (a device that can be moved forwards, backwards and sideways to control a machine or computer) and view 'real-time' images on a high-resolution monitor. The section can be viewed entirely and this eliminates the inadequate or inappropriate selection of fields. These instruments allow the remote user to move the microscopic field in any direction, to change magnifications, and even to change the focus (particularly useful for cytological preparations). The resolution of the images is practically the same as that obtained with the actual slide under the microscope. This technique is suitable for routine histological preparations, immunostains, cytology preparations, and electron micrographs.

Lesions: Term used for describing the more or less circumscribed pathological changes in tissues and cells produced by disease.

Remission: It is the process of conversion from active disease to quiescence. Some of the chronic diseases are interspersed by periods of quiescence when the patient is relatively in good health.

Relapse: It is the process in which the signs and symptoms of disease reappear.

Normal cell is capable of handling physiological demands and maintains a steady state called homeostasis.

The fixative most commonly used in histopathology for surgical specimens is: 10% formalin.

Stain commonly used for Histopathological examination of slides: Hematoxylin and Eosin (H&E).

The most common fixatives:

- For light microscopy is 10% neutral buffered formalin (4% formaldehyde in phosphate-buffered saline).
- For electron microscopy, glutaraldehyde (2.5% solution in phosphate buffered saline).

Cell Injury and Adaptation

CHAPTER OUTLINE

- Types of Cellular Responses to Injury
- Cell Injury
- Types of Cell Injury
- Necrosis
- Apoptosis
- Other Pathways of Cell Death
- Mechanisms of Cell Injury and Cell Death
- Cellular Adaptations to Stress
- Intracellular Accumulations
- Extracellular Deposits: Pathologic Calcification
- Hyaline Change
- Mucoid Degeneration
- Cellular Aging

TYPES OF CELLULAR RESPONSES TO INJURY

Depending on the nature of the stimulus/injury, the cellular responses can be mainly divided into four types (**Box 2.1** and *refer* **online Fig. 2.1**).

BOX 2.1: Types of cellular responses to injury.

1. Cellular adaptations: Hypertrophy, hyperplasia, atrophy and metaplasia
2. Cell injury
   - Reversible cell injury
   - Irreversible cell injury
3. Intracellular accumulations
4. Pathologic calcification

Different stages of cellular responses to stress and injurious stimuli are shown in **Flowchart 2.1**.

CELL INJURY

PA 2.1 (CC): Demonstrate knowledge of the causes, mechanisms, types and effects of cell injury and their clinical significance.

Definition: Cell injury is the functional and morphologic effect of stresses due to a variety of etiological agents on the cell. It produces changes in its internal and external environment.

Cellular injury occurs when a stress exceeds the cell's capability to adapt. Injured cells may either recover **(reversible injury)** or die **(irreversible injury)**.

Flowchart 2.1: Different stages of cellular responses to stress/injury.

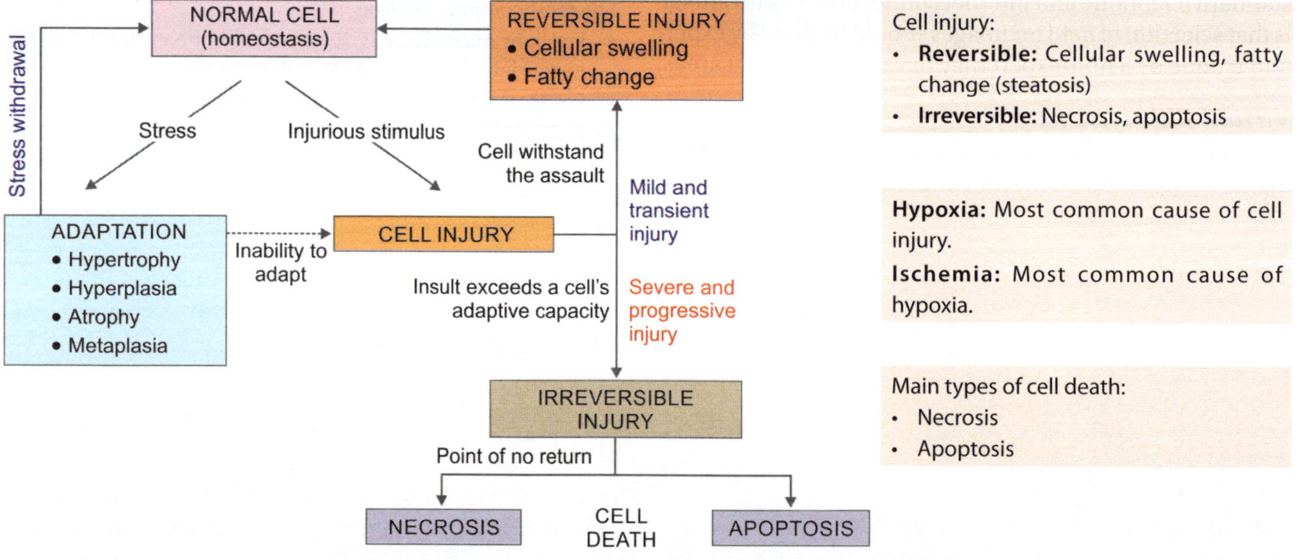

Cell injury:
- **Reversible:** Cellular swelling, fatty change (steatosis)
- **Irreversible:** Necrosis, apoptosis

Hypoxia: Most common cause of cell injury.

Ischemia: Most common cause of hypoxia.

Main types of cell death:
- Necrosis
- Apoptosis

Causes (Etiology) of Cell Injury

PA 2.2a (CC): Describe the etiology of cell injury.

Q. Write a short note on the causes of cell injury.

The causes of cell injury range from gross physical trauma (e.g., road traffic accident), to a single gene defect (e.g., enzyme deficiency resulting in specific metabolic disease). Following are the main categories of causes of cell injury.

A. **Hypoxia and ischemia:** Hypoxia refers to **inadequate oxygenation of tissue** and ischemia means reduced blood supply. Both are the **most common cause of cell injury**. Both reduce the oxygen supply to the tissues, and ischemia, in addition, produces deficiency of essential nutrients and accumulation of toxic metabolites in the tissue affected. Causes of hypoxia are:
   - **Decreased blood flow** is called **ischemia** and results from an arterial obstruction. This obstruction may be due to thrombosis, embolism, atherosclerosis or external compression of vessel. In ischemia, the cells cannot generate ATP by aerobic metabolism, but ATP is inefficiently produced anaerobically. Ischemia causes chemical and pH imbalances, accompanied by increased formation of free radical species.
   - **Inadequate oxygenation of the blood** (hypoxemia): It may be due to lung disease, decreased perfusion of tissues (e.g., cardiac failure, hypotension shock), decreased oxygen-carrying capacity of the blood (e.g., anemia), severe blood loss, carbon monoxide poisoning.

   Mechanism of injury: Hypoxia causes cell injury by **reducing aerobic oxidative respiration** and **decreasing the synthesis of adenosine triphosphate** (ATP).

   Outcome: Depending on the severity of the hypoxia, cells may adapt, undergo reversible injury, or die (irresistible injury).

B. **Physical agents:** These include the following:
   - Mechanical trauma (e.g., blunt/penetrating/crush injuries, road accidents, gunshot wounds).
   - Thermal injury: Extremes of temperature (burns and deep cold).
   - Radiation (ionizing radiation and nonionizing radiation).
   - Electric shock.
   - Pressure changes: Sudden changes in atmospheric pressure.

C. **Chemical agents, toxins and drugs:**
   - Heavy metals and chemical poisons (e.g., arsenic, mercuric salts or cyanide).
   - Simple chemicals (e.g., hypertonic concentrations of glucose or salt).
   - Strong acids and alkalies.
   - Oxygen at high concentrations is toxic.
   - Environmental and air pollutants (e.g., insecticides, pesticides and herbicides).
   - Industrial and occupational hazards (carbon monoxide and asbestos).
   - **Social/lifestyle choices:** Addiction to narcotic drugs and alcohol and cigarette smoking.
   - Therapeutic drugs.

D. **Infectious agents:** Infections caused by viruses, bacteria, fungi, rickettsiae, protozoa, metazoa, and other parasites. The mechanism by which these infectious agents cause injury varies.

E. **Immunologic reactions:** Generally, immunity protects the host against various injurious agents but it may cause lethal cell injury.
   - **Autoimmunity:** Immune reactions to endogenous self-antigens are responsible for autoimmune diseases.
   - **Hypersensitivity reactions and other immune reactions (anaphylactic reactions):** Heightened immune reactions to many external agents (e.g., microbes and environmental agents).

F. **Genetic derangements:** Genetic defects may cause cell injury because of:
   - Deficiency of functional proteins (e.g., enzyme defects in inborn errors of metabolism).
   - Accumulation of damaged DNA or misfolded proteins.

G. **Nutritional imbalances:** It may due to deficiency or excess of nutrients.
   - **Nutritional deficiencies:**
     - Protein-calorie deficiencies (e.g., starvation, marasmus, kwashiorkor).
     - Deficiencies of specific vitamins, minerals (e.g. anemia), or of trace elements.
   - **Nutritional excesses:**
     - Excess of cholesterol predisposes to atherosclerosis.
     - Obesity is associated with increased incidence of several important diseases, such as diabetes and cancer.
     - Hypervitaminosis.

H. **Aging:** Cellular aging or senescence in aging decreases the ability of cells to respond to stress and, eventually it results in the death of cells and the individual.

I. **Idiopathic:** Cause is not known. For example, most common type of hypertension (90%) is idiopathic (or essential) hypertension where we do not know the cause.

J. **Iatrogenic causes:** Iatrogenic means owing to a physician. Examples include untoward effects of administered therapy (drugs, radiation).

The Progression of Cell Injury and Death (refer online Fig. 2.2)

All the stresses and noxious influences produce their effects on the cell first at the molecular or biochemical level.

These early changes are minute and can only identified with highly sensitive methods of examination. The histochemical, ultrastructural, or biochemical techniques detect these changes within minutes to hours after injury. A time lag exists between the stress and the morphologic changes of cell injury or death. The changes observed by light microscopy or the naked eye may take considerably longer (hours to days) time to appear.

TYPES OF CELL INJURY

PA 2.2b (CC): Distinguish between reversible-irreversible injury and morphology of cell injury.

Two types: Cell injury may be broadly divided into two types: **(1) reversible and (2) irreversible (cell death).** Reversible injury may progress to an irreversible stage and result in cell death.

Reversible Cell Injury

Reversible injury is the stage of cell injury during which the deranged function and morphology of the injured cells can return to normal if the causative stimulus is removed. If the stimulus is acute and brief (or short-lived) or mild, the cell injury produces changes in the cells which are reversible up to a certain point.

Light microscope features of reversible cell injury: Two patterns of reversible cell injury namely **cellular swelling and fatty change**.

Cellular Swelling

It was originally applied to the gross appearance of the organ involved but is now applied to the microscopic appearance. It is closely related to **hydropic change, cloudy swelling, and vacuolar degeneration**. Cellular swelling represents disturbances in protein and water metabolism. Being a manifestation of a disturbance in protein metabolism, it is also called **albuminous degeneration**.

Causes: It may be caused by many forms of **mild injury** but is usually due to bacterial toxins, chemical poisons, and malnutrition. It is due to changes in ion concentrations and fluid homeostasis. There is an increased flow of water into the cells which results in increased water content of injured cells.

MORPHOLOGY

- **Organs involved:** Kidney, liver, heart and muscle.
- **Gross:** The organ affected is slightly enlarged due to swelling of its cells. The organ appears pale because of the compression of blood vessels by the swollen cells. The cut surface has a cloudy appearance and is opaque.
- **Microscopy:** The best example is the cellular swelling of highly specialized cells of the convoluted tubule of the kidney. The cell is swollen and projects unevenly into the lumen of the tubule. As the process advances the cytoplasm breaks down and its granular material gets discharged into the lumen of the tubule. These granules are proteinaceous in nature.

Subcellular changes in reversibly injured cells (*refer* online Fig. 2.3): In reversibly injured cells, several subcellular changes occur.

- **Endoplasmic reticulum (ER):** Cellular (hydropic) swelling leads to the **distension of ER cisternae** due to the accumulation of fluid. Additionally, **membrane-bound polysomes can disaggregate,** and they may detach from the surface of the rough ER.
- **Mitochondria:** In cases of ischemic injury, where there is a poor supply of oxygen by the blood, mitochondria exhibit **swelling**.
- **Plasma membrane:** Reversibly injured cells may display focal extrusions of the cytoplasm, resulting in the formation of **blebs on the plasma membrane**.
- **Nucleus:** Reversible injury to the nucleus is characterized by segregation of fibrillar and granular nucleolar constituents.

Steatosis (Fatty Change)

It is explained on pages 44-6.

Irreversible Cell Injury/Cell Death

If the cell is exposed to continuous injurious stimulus or if the injury is severe, the cells undergo cell death. **The mechanism of cell death depends on the nature and severity of the injury.** Two main types of cell death: **Necrosis and apoptosis.**

- **Necrosis:** Always a pathologic process.
- **Apoptosis:** May be physiological or pathological.

NECROSIS

PA 2.4a (CC): Describe and discuss cell death—types, mechanisms, necrosis, apoptosis (basic as contrasted with necrosis), autolysis (*refer* page 28).

Cell death develops as a manifestation of irreversible cell injury. **Two main types of cell death are necrosis and apoptosis. They differ in their mechanisms, morphology, and roles in physiology and disease** (*see* **Table 2.4**). Severe injury (e.g., loss of oxygen and nutrient supply, toxins, various infections, trauma) cause severe damage to mitochondria with depletion of ATP and rupture of lysosomal and plasma membranes. It produces a rapid and uncontrollable form of death and is called "accidental" cell death. The morphological manifestation of inevitable end result of severe damage is **necrosis**. The necrosis occurs accidentally because the injury is so severe to be repaired and many cellular constituents fail or fall apart. It is not regulated by specific signals or biochemical mechanisms (in contrast to apoptosis). When cell death occurs by necrosis, it elicits a local inflammatory response that clears the "scene of the accident." Apoptosis is "regulated" cell death. It is mediated by specific molecular pathways that are activated under specific circumstances. These pathways kill the cells with surgical precision. It is without inflammation or the associated collateral damage.

Q. Define necrosis. Describe the various types of necrosis, causes and pathology of each with suitable examples. Add a note on gangrene.

Necrosis is a pathologic process characterized by localized area of death in a living tissue as a **consequence of severe injury.** It is caused by the progressive degradative action of enzymes following harmful injury.

Definition: Necrosis is rapid, uncontrolled, **"accidental" and unregulated form of cell death.** The morphologic manifestation of accidental cell death is termed necrosis. It results from damage to cell membranes and loss of ion homeostasis.

The necrotic cells cannot maintain integrity of membrane and their contents including **cellular enzymes** leak out and **ultimately digest the cell.** This bring out acute **inflammatory reaction** and subsequent repair process in the surrounding tissue (local host reaction), which itself may produce further cell injury. The enzymes which digest the cell are derived from lysosomes of either dying cells themselves or from leukocytes recruited as part of the inflammatory reaction.

Main causes of necrosis: These include ischemia (loss of oxygen supply)/reperfusion injury, exposure to microbial toxins, burns, chemical and physical injury.

MORPHOLOGY (FIG. 2.4)

Injured cell in necrosis show changes in the cytoplasm and nuclei and the general changes are as follows:

Cytoplasmic Changes

Cytoplasm of the necrotic cells have **increased eosinophilia** and have **glassy, homogeneous** appearance. The routinely used hematoxylin and eosin (H&E) stain contains blue dye hematoxylin and red dye eosin. Increased eosinophilia (i.e., red appearance) is due to increased binding of eosin to denatured cytoplasmic proteins and loss of basophilic ribonucleic acid (RNA) in the cytoplasm. Homogeneous appearance is due to the loss of glycogen particles. When enzymes have digested cytoplasmic organelles, the cytoplasm becomes vacuolated (due to digested the cell's organelles by enzymes) and gives a "moth-eaten" appearance **(Fig. 2.4).**

Nuclear Changes

These may take up one of three patterns and are the result of breakdown of DNA and chromatin.

- **Pyknosis:** Shrinkage of nucleus which appears **shrunken and deeply basophilic** (similar to ink drop). It is also observed in apoptosis.
- **Karyorrhexis:** The pyknotic nucleus can subsequently undergo **fragmentation into many smaller fragments.** This change is called karyorrhexis.
- **Karyolysis:** Progressive **fading (dissolution) of basophilic staining of the nuclei** because of digestion of DNA by deoxyribonuclease (DNase) activity and leads to a ghost nuclei.

As the time passes (1 or 2 days), the nucleus in the necrotic (dead) cell totally disappears.

- **Electron microscopic findings (Fig. 2.4):** These include discontinuities in plasma and organelle membranes, marked dilation with the **appearance of large amorphous densities in the mitochondria,** disruption of lysosomes, and presence of **intracytoplasmic myelin figures.** Myelin figures are rolled-up or scroll-like arrangement of a lipid bilayer within a cell and this superficially resemble the myelin sheath of nerves.
- **Fates of necrotic cells:** After necrosis, these necrotic cells may either persist for some time or may be **digested by enzymes and disappear.** Dead cells may be replaced by myelin figures, which may be either phagocytosed by other cells or may undergo further degradation into fatty acids. These fatty acids can bind calcium salts and the **necrotic cells may become calcified (dystrophic calcification).**

Morphological Patterns/Types of Tissue Necrosis (Box 2.2)

Stimuli that cause necrosis produce diverse and recognizable histologic and cytologic patterns. Most of the types of necrosis have distinctive gross appearances except fibrinoid necrosis which is identified only by microscopic examination.

Coagulative Necrosis

Q. Write a short note on coagulative necrosis.

It is the common type, in which the **outline of dead tissues (underlying tissue architecture) is preserved (at least for few days). Infarct** is a localized area of coagulative necrosis. Coagulative necrosis is characteristic of infarcts (areas of necrosis caused by ischemia) in **all solid organs except the brain.**

Causes: Ischemia caused by obstruction in a vessel.

Mechanism: Ischemia denatures and coagulates structural proteins and enzymes. This blocks the proteolysis of the dead cells. Coagulation causes the protein albumin to change from a gelatinous, transparent state to a firm, opaque state, similar to that of a cooked egg white.

MORPHOLOGY

Gross

Organs affected: Coagulative necrosis is characteristic of **infarcts** (areas of necrosis caused by ischemia) **in all solid organs except the brain.** More frequent in organs supplied by end arteries with limited collateral circulation such as **heart** (*refer* **Fig. 16.26**), **kidney (Fig. 2.5A), spleen** (*refer* **Fig. 5.26A) and limb (dry gangrene)** (*refer* **Fig. 2.11A).**

Appearance: The appearance of necrotic tissue is described as coagulative necrosis because **it resembles the coagulation of proteins that occurs upon heating.** The necrotic tissues appear firm and slightly swollen. Involved region appear **dry, pale, yellow and firm.** Probably, the injury denatures both structural proteins and enzymes. This can prevent the proteolysis of the dead cells. **It is wedge-shaped in organs like kidney (Fig. 2.5A) and spleen** (**Fig. 5.26A**). The area of coagulative necrosis is called an infarct.

Microscopy (Figs. 2.5B and C, and refer Fig. 16.27F)

Indistinct outline of dead tissue. In coagulative necrosis, the normal cells are converted into their **'tomb stones',** i.e., outlines of

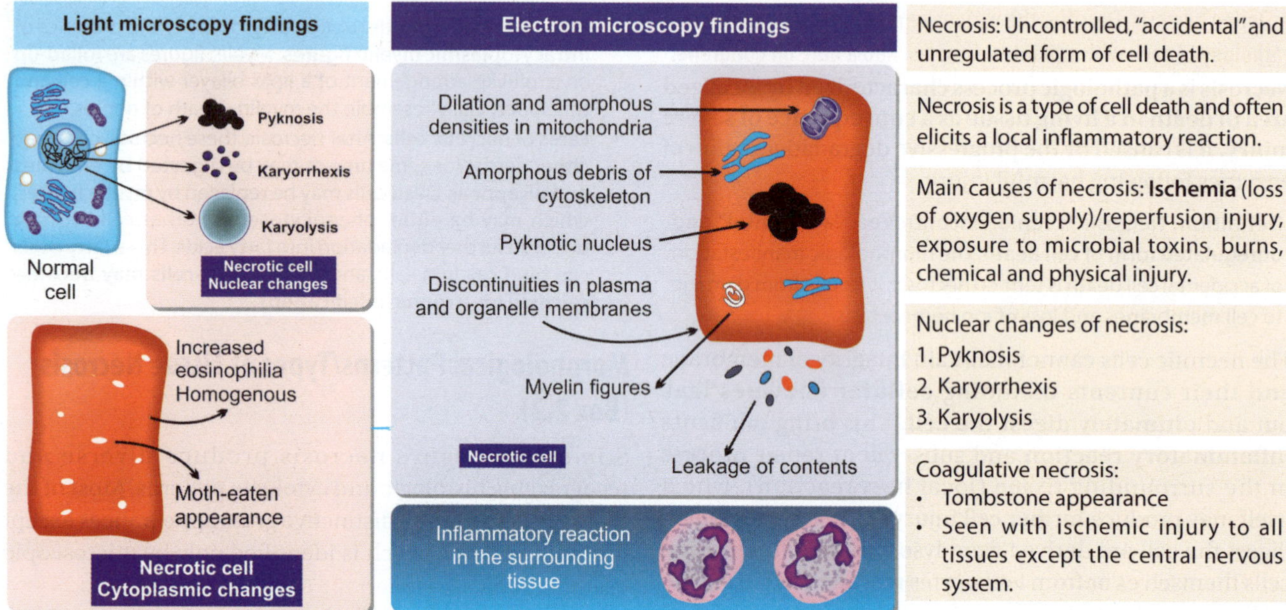

Fig. 2.4: Diagrammatic appearance of morphological changes in necrosis.

BOX 2.2: Morphologic patterns of necrosis (example).

1. Coagulative necrosis (e.g., myocardial infarct)
2. Liquefactive necrosis (colliquative necrosis) (e.g., abscess)
3. Caseous necrosis (e.g., tuberculosis)
4. Fat necrosis (e.g., acute pancreatitis)
5. Fibrinoid necrosis (e.g., immune mediated vasculitis)
6. Gangrene (gangrenous necrosis) (e.g., atherosclerosis, diabetes)
7. Gummatous necrosis (e.g., syphilis)

the cells are maintained and the cell type can still be recognized but their cytoplasmic and nuclear details are lost. The cells are swollen and have more eosinophilic cytoplasm than the normal. **Nucleus may be either absent or show karyolysis. Leukocytes surround the site of necrosis** and the lysosomal enzymes of the leukocytes digest the necrotic cells. The resulting cellular debris are then removed by phagocytosis by infiltrating neutrophils and macrophages.

Liquefactive Necrosis (Colliquative Necrosis)

Q. Write a short note on liquefactive/colliquative necrosis.

In this type of necrosis **dead tissue** rapidly **undergoes softening** and transforms into a **liquid viscous mass**.

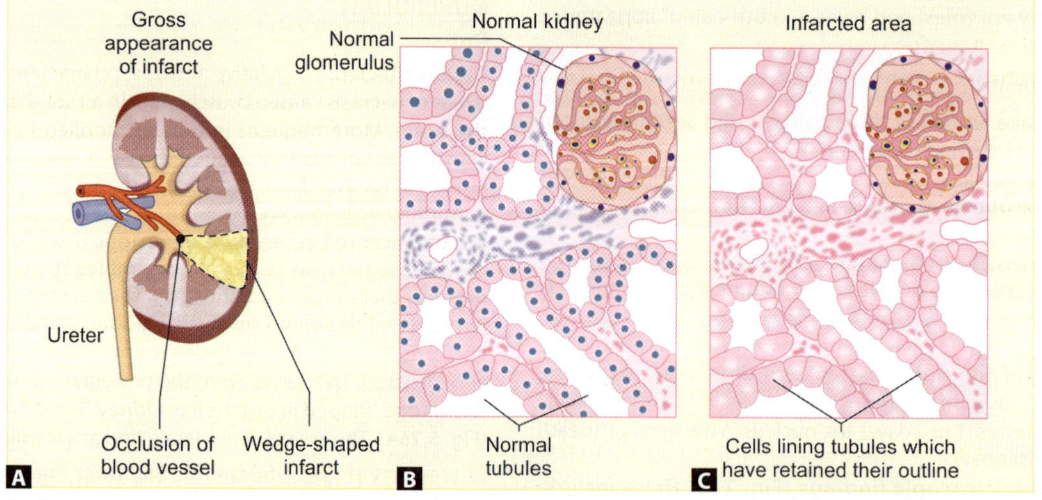

Figs. 2.5A to C: Diagrammatic appearance of gross and microscopy of infract kidney: (A) Gross appearance of infarct of kidney (within dotted lines); (B) Microscopy of normal kidney; (C) Microscopic appearance of infarcted area of kidney. Infarcted area shows necrotic cells with preserved cellular outlines with loss of nuclei. The glomerulus is not affected.

Causes:

- **Ischemic injury to central nervous system (CNS)**, i.e., neurons and glial cells in the brain.
- **Suppurative infections:** Infections by bacteria, e.g., *staphylococci, streptococci*, and *Escherichia coli*) or occasionally fungus which stimulate the quick accumulation of inflammatory cells, and the enzymes liberated from these leukocytes digest ("liquefy") the tissue.

Mechanism: Pyogenic bacteria attract neutrophils into the area. Liquefaction of the dead tissue is due to digestive action of the hydrolytic enzymes (hydrolases) or the abundant lysosomal enzymes released from dead cells (autolysis) and leukocytes (heterolysis).

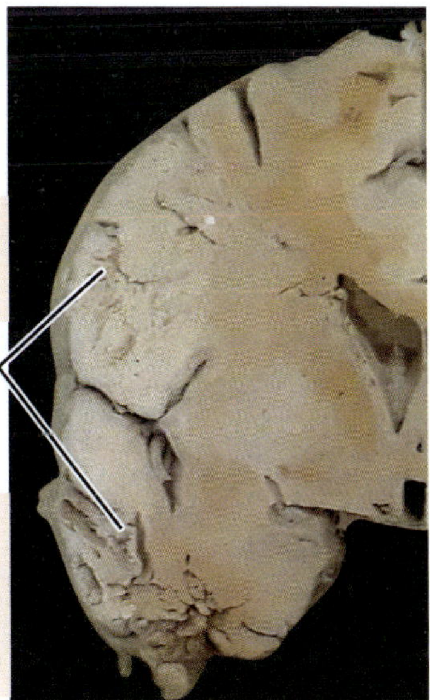

Fig. 2.6: Liquefactive necrosis. An infarct in the brain shows soft necrotic area with dissolution of the tissue forming a cavity.

MORPHOLOGY

Gross

The necrotic cells are completely digested and is converted into a viscous liquid that is eventually removed by phagocytes. The involved area appear **soft with liquefied center containing necrotic debris.** Later when it is cut into, the area of liquefaction necrosis exudes pus and leaves a hole or cystic space in the tissue.

Organs affected are:

- **Ischemic injury to brain:** Necrotic area is soft and center shows liquefaction **(Fig. 2.6)**. The reason for liquefactive necrosis in brain may be the **presence of rich digestive hydrolytic (abundant lysosomal) enzymes** (or different hydrolases specific to cells of the CNS) **and lipids, and also the presence of little connective tissue** in the brain.
- **Abscess anywhere:** The **bacterial infection** causes acute inflammatory reaction and the resulting necrosis of tissue produces the liquid viscous material which is frequently **thick, creamy yellow** and is called **pus** or **purulent exudate. The localized collection of pus is termed abscess.**
- It is also seen in wet gangrene (*refer* **Fig. 2.11B**) and pancreatic necrosis.

Microscopy

Pus consists of liquefied necrotic cell debris, dead leukocytes and macrophages (scavenger cells) filled with phagocytosed material. It is surrounded by proliferating fibroblasts and capillaries (granulation tissue).

Caseous Necrosis

Q. Write a short note on caseous necrosis.

It is a distinctive type of necrosis which shows **combined features of both coagulative and liquefactive necrosis.**

Cause: Characteristic of **tuberculosis** and is due to the type IV hypersensitivity reaction. It may also occur in certain types of fungal infections (e.g., histoplasmosis). It is **due to the presence of high lipid content in the cell wall in these organisms** (e.g., lipopolysaccharides such as mycolic acid in tuberculosis).

Mechanism: The dead cells disintegrate, but the debris is not digested completely by hydrolases and persist indefinitely as amorphous, coarsely granular, eosinophilic debris. Unlike, the necrotic cells neither lose their cellular outlines like in coagulative necrosis nor do not disappear by lysis like in liquefactive necrosis.

MORPHOLOGY

Gross

Organs affected: Tuberculosis may involve any organ, most common in **lung** and **lymph node.**

Appearance: The causative organisms are attacked by numerous lipid-containing macrophages. Necrosis of these macrophages produces a solid, amorphous, cheesy mass. Necrotic area appears **yellow-white, soft, friable, granular** and resembles **dry, clumpy cheese**, hence the name caseous (**cheese-like**) necrosis (**Fig. 2.7 and** *refer* **Fig. 17.20A).** This appearance is partly due to the effects of lipopolysaccharides present in the capsule of the tubercle bacilli, *Mycobacterium tuberculosis*.

Microscopy

- Focal lesion of tuberculosis is a **granuloma (Fig. 2.8, and** *refer* **Figs. 3.17 and 17.19)** which may be **caseating (soft granuloma) or noncaseating (hard granuloma).** The necrosis is found in the center of foci of tuberculous granuloma.
- **Caseous necrosis** is a collection of fragmented or lysed cells and appears as **eosinophilic, amorphous (meaning shapeless/poorly defined/structureless), coarsely granular material.** In contrast to coagulative necrosis, there is **complete obliteration of the tissue architecture** and it is not possible to identify the cellular outlines. The central caseous necrosis is surrounded by epithelioid cells (modified macrophages having slipper-shaped vesicular nuclei), Langhans type giant cells (nuclei arranged in a horse-shoe pattern), foreign body type giant cells, peripheral mantle of lymphocytes and fibroblasts forming granuloma.
- Caseous necrotic material **may undergo dystrophic calcification.**

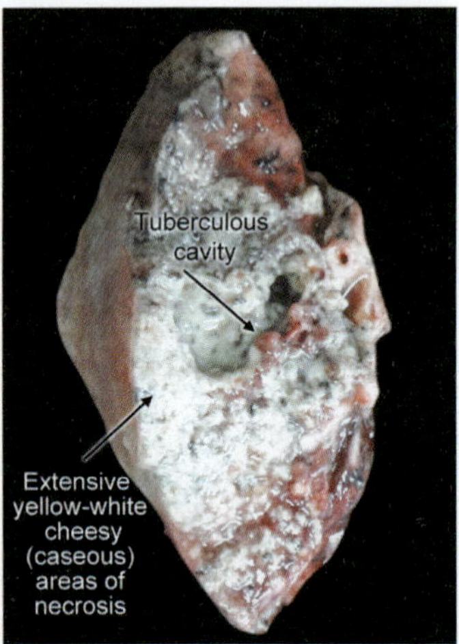

Caseous necrosis occurs in tuberculosis (most common), fungal infections (histoplasmosis, coccidiodomycosis).

Caseous = cheese-like

Fig. 2.7: Gross appearance of caseous necrosis. Lung shows cavity with caseous necrosis.

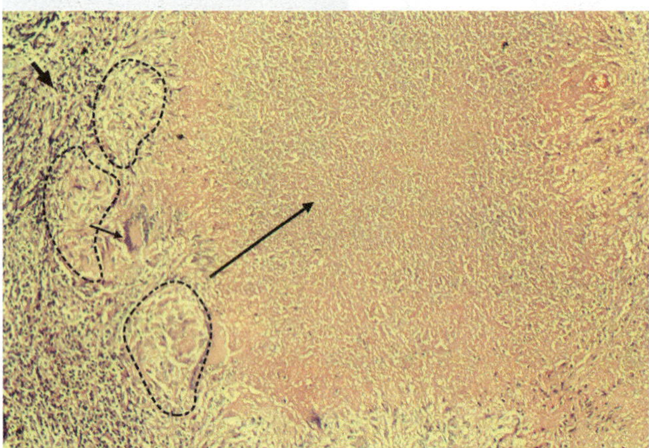

Fig. 2.8: Microscopic appearance of a caseous necrosis. It is tuberculous granuloma showing an area of central necrosis (long arrow) surrounded by multiple Langhans-type giant cells (small arrow), epithelioid cells within dotted lines, and lymphocytes (thick arrow).

Fat Necrosis

Q. Write a short note on fat necrosis.

It refers to **focal areas of fat destruction**, which affects adipose tissue. It occurs mainly at anatomic locations rich in fat.

Types: Fat necrosis may be enzymatic or traumatic.

1. **Enzymatic fat necrosis:** Occurs in adipose tissue around acutely inflamed pancreas (in **acute pancreatitis**) or abdominal trauma.
   - **Mechanism:** In pancreatitis, the enzymes (one of them is lipase) leak from acinar cells into the substance of the pancreas and the peritoneal cavity and causes tissue damage. Phospholipases and proteases attack plasma membranes of adipocytes and release intracellular triglycerides. Lipase destroys fat cells, splits the triglyceride esters within fat cells and liberates free fatty acids which combine with calcium (also magnesium, and sodium ions) and form calcium soaps (fat saponification).

MORPHOLOGY

Gross

Appears as opaque, **chalky-white areas (Fig. 2.9A)** embedded in otherwise normal adipose tissue. This helps both the surgeon and the pathologist to grossly identify the lesions.

Microscopy

The necrotic **fat cells appear pale with shadowy outlines surrounded** by basophilic calcium deposits and an inflammatory reaction **(Fig. 2.9B)**.

2. **Traumatic fat necrosis:** Occurs in **tissues with high fat content** (like in **heavy, pendulous breast and thigh**) following severe trauma. It may also occur following **radiation**, **surgery or removal of breast implants**. In traumatic fat necrosis, triglycerides and lipases are released from the injured adipocytes. In the breast,

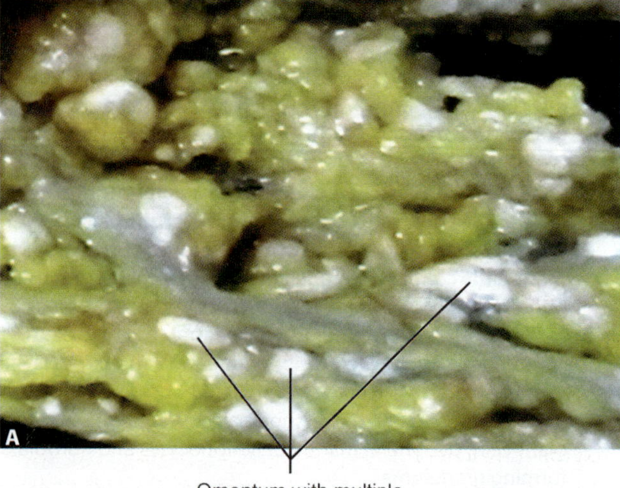

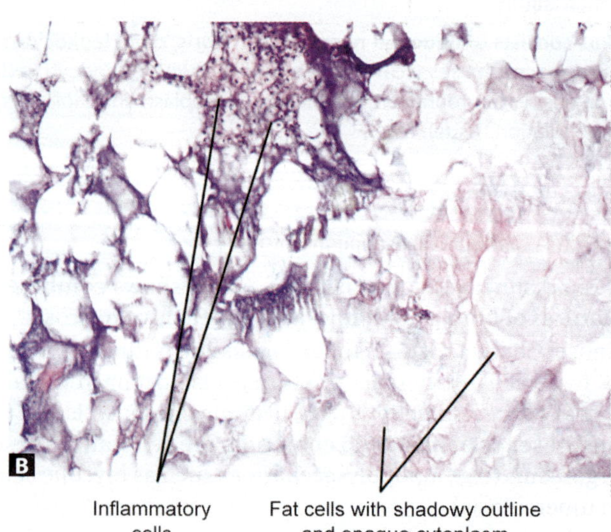

Figs. 2.9A and B: (A) Omentum shows multiple chalky-white areas of fat necrosis caused by acute pancreatitis; (B) Fat necrosis shows necrotic fat cells in the right lower part and inflammatory reaction between normal (left upper area) and area of fat necrosis.

traumatic fat necrosis is common and may mimic a tumor, particularly if calcification has occurred.

Fibrinoid Necrosis

It is a **special form of necrosis detected on light microscopic examination**. Characterized by **deposition of pink-staining (fibrin-like) proteinaceous material** in the tissue matrix with a **staining pattern similar to fibrin**. It obscures the underlying cellular detail.

Causes: Usually seen in **immune-mediated** (deposition of antigen-antibody complexes in the wall of vessels) **vascular injury/vasculitis** (e.g., polyarteritis nodosa), **malignant hypertension, Aschoff bodies** in rheumatic heart disease, placenta in **preeclampsia**, or **hyperacute transplant rejection** (transplant organs undergoing rejection).

Microscopy

The fibrinoid necrosis appear as brightly eosinophilic, hyaline-like deposit in the vessel wall **(Fig. 2.10)**. It is better appreciated under phosphotungistic acid hematoxylin (PTAH) stain.

Gangrene (Gangrenous Necrosis)

Q. Define gangrene. Mention its types and differences between them.

Definition: It is **massive necrosis with superadded putrefaction** (superimposed decomposition by bacteria).

It is similar to postmortem decomposition except that only a portion of the body is dead. It is **not a distinctive type of cell death**, but is commonly used in clinical practice.

Types: Two types, namely **dry and wet gangrene**. A variant of wet gangrene known as **gas gangrene** is **caused by clostridia** (gram-positive anaerobic bacteria).

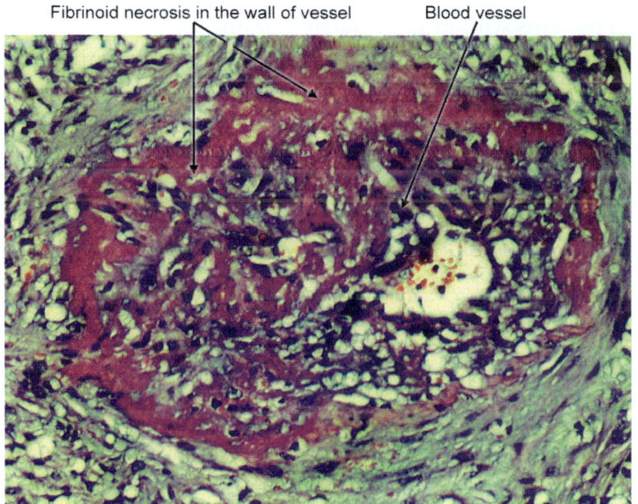

Fig. 2.10: Fibrinoid necrosis in the wall of blood vessel [Phosphotungistic acid hematoxylin (PTAH) stain].

Dry Gangrene

Q. Write a short note on dry gangrene.

Causes: Arterial occlusion (e.g., atherosclerosis), thromboangiitis obliterans (Buerger's disease), Raynaud's disease, trauma, and ergot poisoning.

Sites: It usually involves a **limb**, generally the distal part of lower limb (leg, foot, and toe).

MORPHOLOGY

Gross

Affected part is **dry, shrunken** (shriveled) and **dark brown or black** resembling the **foot of a mummy**. The black color is due to the liberation of hemoglobin from hemolyzed red blood cells. The hemoglobin is acted upon by hydrogen disulfide produced by bacteria and forms **black iron sulfide**. The gangrene spreads slowly to the point where the blood supply is adequate to keep the tissue viable. A **line of demarcation** is seen between gangrenous and adjacent normal area **(Fig. 2.11A)**.

Microscopy

The necrosis **(coagulative type)** shows smudging of soft tissue and overlying skin. The **line of demarcation consists of granulation tissue with inflammatory cells.**

Wet Gangrene

Q. Write a short note on wet gangrene.

Causes: Due to the venous blockage (e.g., strangulated hernia, intussusception or volvulus). Diabetic patients may develop both dry (due to atherosclerosis of tibial and popliteal arteries) and wet gangrene. It usually follows a minor injury to toe or foot. Diabetic gangrene is due to high glucose content in the necrosed tissue which favors the growth of bacteria.

Sites: Occurs in **moist tissues or internal organs** (e.g., bowel, lung, mouth, etc.).

MORPHOLOGY

Gross

The affected part is **soft, swollen, cold, putrid and black/dark (Fig. 2.11B). No clear line of demarcation.** It produces a foul odor due to the presence of pus.

Microscopy

It shows liquefactive type of necrosis and occurs when neutrophils invade the site.

Q. Write a short answer on gas gangrene.

Gas gangrene: Special type of wet gangrene caused by infection with a gas forming anaerobic *Clostridium perfringens*. These organisms enter into the tissues through open contaminated wounds (e.g., muscles, complication of operative procedures on colon). It produces hydrolytic enzymes and a necrotizing toxin. Toxins produced by them cause local necrosis. Grossly, the affected area is swollen, edematous, painful and crepitant due to accumulation of gas bubbles of carbon dioxide within the tissues.

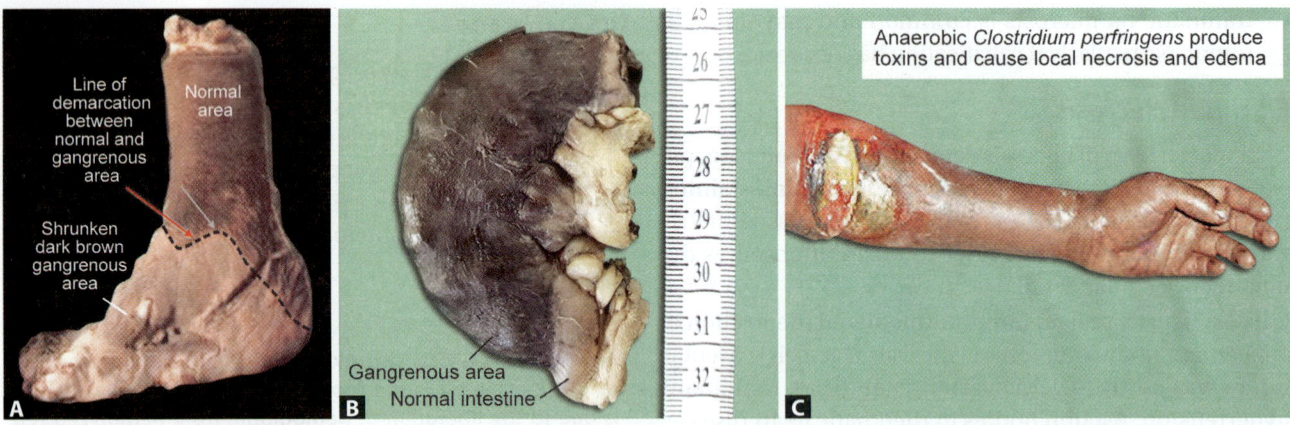

Figs. 2.11A to C: (A) Dry gangrene of left leg shows dry shrunken discolored gangrenous foot separated from adjacent normal area by a line of demarcation (dotted line); (B) Wet gangrene of small intestine; (C) Gas gangrene in upper limb.

TABLE 2.1 Differences between dry and wet gangrene.

Characteristics	*Dry*	*Wet*
General features		
Common site	Limbs	Bowels
Examples	Gangrene of lower limb due to atherosclerosis	Volvulus, intussusception
Etiological factors		
Cause of ischemia	Arterial obstruction	Commonly venous obstruction
Rate of obstruction	Slow	Abrupt
Gross features		
Appearance of involved part	Shriveled, dry (mummification) and black	Swollen, soft and moist/wet
Line of demarcation	Clear cut between gangrenous and healthy part	Not clear cut
Spread	Slow	Rapid
Prognosis	Fair	Poor due to severe septicemia

Gas bubbles are formed by fermentation of sugars by bacterial toxins **(Fig. 2.11C)** and edema and are also absorbed causing severe systemic manifestations. The hydrolytic enzymes and toxins destroy connective tissue and cellular membranes and cause bubbles of gas to form in muscle cells. It can be fatal if enzymes lyse the membranes of red blood cells, destroying their oxygen-carrying capacity.

Differences Between Dry and Wet Gangrene (Table 2.1)

Q. List the differences between dry and wet gangrene.

Gummatous Necrosis Enzymatic

The necrotic tissue is firm and rubbery and is usually found in syphilis (*refer* page 114).

Laboratory Detection of Necrosis

Whenever there is necrosis, there is **leakage of intracellular proteins through the damaged cell membrane** which ultimately **reaches the circulation**. Thus, it is possible to detect tissue-specific necrosis using blood or serum samples. Examples include (i) cardiac muscle contains a unique isoform of the contractile protein troponin, (ii) hepatic bile duct epithelium contains the enzyme alkaline phosphatase, and (iii) hepatocytes contain transaminases. Necrosis of these tissues elevate the serum levels of these proteins and are **useful markers of tissue damage.** Cardiac-specific troponins can be detected in the blood 2 hours after myocardial cell necrosis, before any microscopic changes of myocardial infarction. It is very sensitive and highly specific. Hence, serial measurement of serum cardiac troponins plays main role in the diagnosis and management of patients with myocardial infarction.

Ultrastructural differences between reversible and irreversible injury is presented in **Table 2.2**.

APOPTOSIS

PA 2.4b (CC): Describe and discuss cell death—mechanisms of apoptosis (basic as contrasted with necrosis).

Q. Write long essay on definition, causes and the mechanism of apoptosis.

Q. Write a short note on apoptosis.

Definition: Apoptosis is a **pathway of (programmed) cell death induced by a tightly regulated suicide program.** It is characterized by **activation of intrinsic enzymes of the cell that degrade its own nuclear DNA and proteins** (both nuclear and cytoplasmic).

Fragments of the apoptotic cells (apoptotic bodies) break and fall off from the cells and hence named apoptosis

Q. Describe the ultrastructural changes in reversible cell injury. List the differences between reversible and irreversible injury.

TABLE 2.2 Ultrastructural differences between reversible and irreversible injury.

Structure involved	*Reversible injury*	*Irreversible injury*
Plasma membrane changes	Blebbing, blunting, loss of microvilli	Discontinuities in plasma and organelle membrane
Mitochondrial changes	Swelling and appearance of small amorphous densities	Marked dilation with appearance of large amorphous densities (precipitated calcium), aggregates of fluffy material (denatures protein)
Endoplasmic reticulum	Dilation with detachment of polysomes	Swelling and fragmentation
Myelin figure (large intracellular whorled phospholipid masses)	May be present	Usually present
Nuclear changes	Disaggregation of granular and fibrillar elements	Pyknosis, karyolysis and karyorrhexis

[meaning "falling off" (mainly involved enzymes are caspases)]. In contrast to necrosis, the apototic cells and its fragments are cleared before there is leakage of cellular contents. Hence, apoptosis does not bring out an inflammatory reaction in the surrounding tissue.

Causes of Apoptosis

Apoptotic cell death is **not necessarily an indication of injury**. It may be occur in several physiological conditions as well as a pathologic process.

Physiological Situations

Removal of excess cells during embryogenesis (organogenesis) and developmental processes (e.g., disappearance of web tissues between fingers and toes).

Elimination of hormone-dependent cells after withdrawal of hormonal stimuli: Involution of hormone dependent tissues occurs by apoptosis due to decreased hormone levels (e.g., endometrial cell breakdown during the menstrual cycle, regression of lactating breast after withdrawal of breast-feeding and ovarian follicular atresia in menopause).

Cell turnover in proliferating cell populations: For example, immature lymphocytes in the bone marrow and thymus, B lymphocytes in germinal centers that fail to express useful antigen receptors (fail to produce high-affinity antibodies), and epithelial cells in intestinal crypts, to maintain a constant cell number (*homeostasis*).

Elimination of potentially harmful cells: In immunology, the clones of **self-reactive (autoreactive) lymphocytes** that recognize normal self-antigens are deleted by apoptosis.

Death of host cells that have served their useful purpose: For example, decline of leukocyte numbers at the end of immune and inflammatory response due to loss of survival signals as stimulus for activation of leukocytes, and lymphocytes at the end of an *immune response*.

In all of the physiologic conditions, cells undergo apoptosis because they are deprived of necessary survival signals (e.g., growth factors and interactions with the extracellular matrix), or they receive pro-apoptotic signals from other cells or the surrounding environment.

Pathological Conditions

Apoptosis **eliminates cells that are genetically altered or damaged beyond repair.** It is responsible for cell loss in many pathologic states. It is mainly due to activation of pro apoptotic proteins.

Elimination of mutant cells with damaged DNA: It is necessary that cells that have accumulated genetic defects during their lifespans must be eliminated. DNA may be damaged (either directly or through production of free radicals) by many injurious agents like ultraviolet (UV) light, ionizing radiation, cytotoxic anticancer drugs and hypoxia.

- ***p53* triggered apoptosis:** Mainly tumor-suppressor gene *p53* recognizes cells with damaged DNA and assesses whether it can be repaired. If the damage is too severe to be repaired, *p53* triggers apoptosis.
- **Destroying cells with dangerous mutations or with DNA damage beyond repair** by apoptosis **prevents the development of cancer.**
- In certain cancers, where *p53* is mutated or absent, the apoptosis is not induced in cells with damaged DNA.

Elimination of cells with excessively accumulated misfolded proteins: Mutations in the genes encoding proteins or extrinsic factors (damage due to free radicals) may result in accumulation of unfolded or misfolded proteins.

- Excessive intracellular accumulation of these abnormally folded proteins in the ER is known as **ER stress**, which results in apoptotic cell death.
- Apoptosis caused by the accumulation of misfolded proteins is found in several degenerative diseases of the central nervous system **(Alzheimer, Huntington, and Parkinson diseases)** and other organs.

Killing of viral infected cells: In viral infections, the infected cells are lost mainly due to apoptosis induced either by the virus (as in adenovirus and HIV infections) or by host human response by cytotoxic T lymphocytes (as in viral hepatitis).

Elimination of neoplastic cells/rejection of transplant: The T-cell-mediated mechanism is responsible for apoptosis in tumors and cellular rejection of transplants.

Elimination of parenchymal cells in pathologic atrophy: Obstruction of duct in the parenchymal organs like pancreas, parotid gland and kidney can lead to apoptosis of the parenchymal cells.

MORPHOLOGY

Electron Microscope

Q. Write a short note on morphology of apoptosis.

The ultrastructural features of apoptosis (**Fig. 2.12**) are:

Cell shrinkage: Cell size is reduced and the becomes dense eosinophilic.

Chromatin condensation and fragmentation: It is the **most characteristic feature** of apoptosia. Chromatin aggregates peripherally under the nuclear membrane. The nucleus may break up to produce two or more nuclear fragments.

Formation of cytoplasmic blebs and apoptotic bodies: Cell first shows extensive surface blebbing followed by fragmentation into membrane-bound apoptotic bodies. The **apoptotic bodies are composed of cytoplasm and tightly packed organelles, with or without nuclear fragments.**

Phagocytosis of apoptotic cells/bodies: The apoptotic bodies are rapidly ingested by phagocytes **(usually by macrophages)** and degraded by the lysosomal enzymes of phagocytes.

Light Microscopy

Apoptosis involves *single cells or small clusters of cells* in the background of viable cells. The apoptotic cells appear as round or oval mass having intensely **eosinophilic** cytoplasm. The **nuclei appear as fragments of dense nuclear chromatin.** Throughout the process, the cell contents are contained within an envelope formed by the original cell membrane. Because the cell contents do not spill into the extracellular tissue, apoptosis **does not elicit an inflammatory reaction** in the host.

Mechanisms of Apoptosis

Q. Write a short note on mechanism of apoptosis.

Apoptosis is regulated by biochemical pathway. The survival or apoptosis of many cells depends upon balance between **two opposite sets of signals** namely: **(1) death signal** (proapoptotic) and **(2) prosurvival** (antiapoptotic) **signals**. Unlike necrosis, apoptosis engages the cell's own signaling cascades and results in its own death (suicide). Apoptosis results from **activation of enzymes** called as **caspases** (i.e., they are *c*ysteine proteases that cleave proteins after *asp*artic residues). The caspases are a family of cysteine proteases that occur as inactive proenzymes. They must undergo enzymatic cleavage to become active. Therefore, the **presence of active caspases in the cells is a marker for apoptosis.**

Phases of Apoptosis

The process of apoptosis can be divided into (A) initiation phase and (B) execution phase.

A. Initiation Phase

Apoptosis is initiated by signals derived from two distinct pathways activated by distinct stimuli, namely: **(1) intrinsic or mitochondrial pathway (activated in cells under stress) and (2) extrinsic or death receptor pathway (which responds to signals from other cells).**

Intrinsic (mitochondrial) pathway of apoptosis (Fig. 2.13)

Increased mitochondrial permeability: Survival or apoptosis of cells is determined by the permeability of mitochondria. This pathway of apoptosis is due to increased permeability of the mitochondrial outer membrane. It is the **major mechanism and occurs** in a variety of **physiological and pathological apoptosis.** It is **activated by intracellular signals.** Increased permeability of the mitochondrial outer membrane releases death-inducing (pro-apoptotic) molecules from the mitochondrial intermembrane space into the cytoplasm.

Cytochrome c: Mitochondria are organelles that contain proteins such as cytochrome c that act as, a double-edged sword. Cytochrome c is essential for producing the energy (e.g., ATP) that is required for the viability of the cell, but when released into the cytoplasm (an indication that the cell is not healthy) **initiates apoptosis.** The release of pro-apoptotic proteins such as cytochrome c depends on the integrity of the outer membrane of the mitochondria. This integrity is tightly regulated by the BCL2 family of proteins.

BCL2 family (Table 2.3): Mitochondrial permeability is controlled by the *BCL2* family. The BCL-2 family is the cell's life/death switch. This *BCL2* family is named after *BCL2* (the name BCL stands for on B-cell lymphoma), a gene that is usually overexpressed due to chromosomal translocations

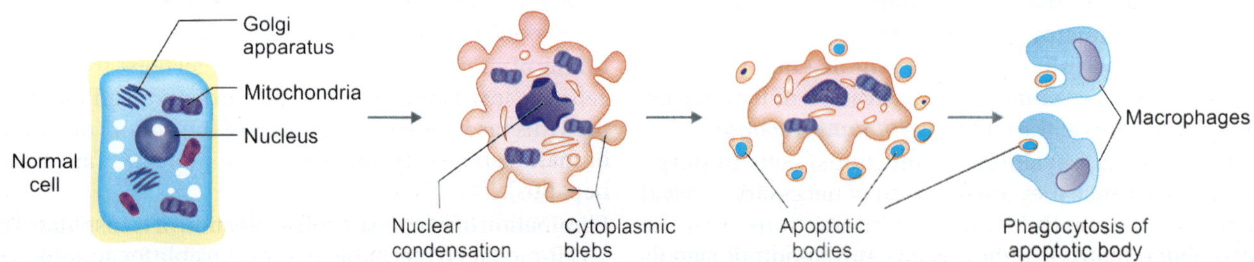

Fig. 2.12: Electron microscopic changes in apoptosis.

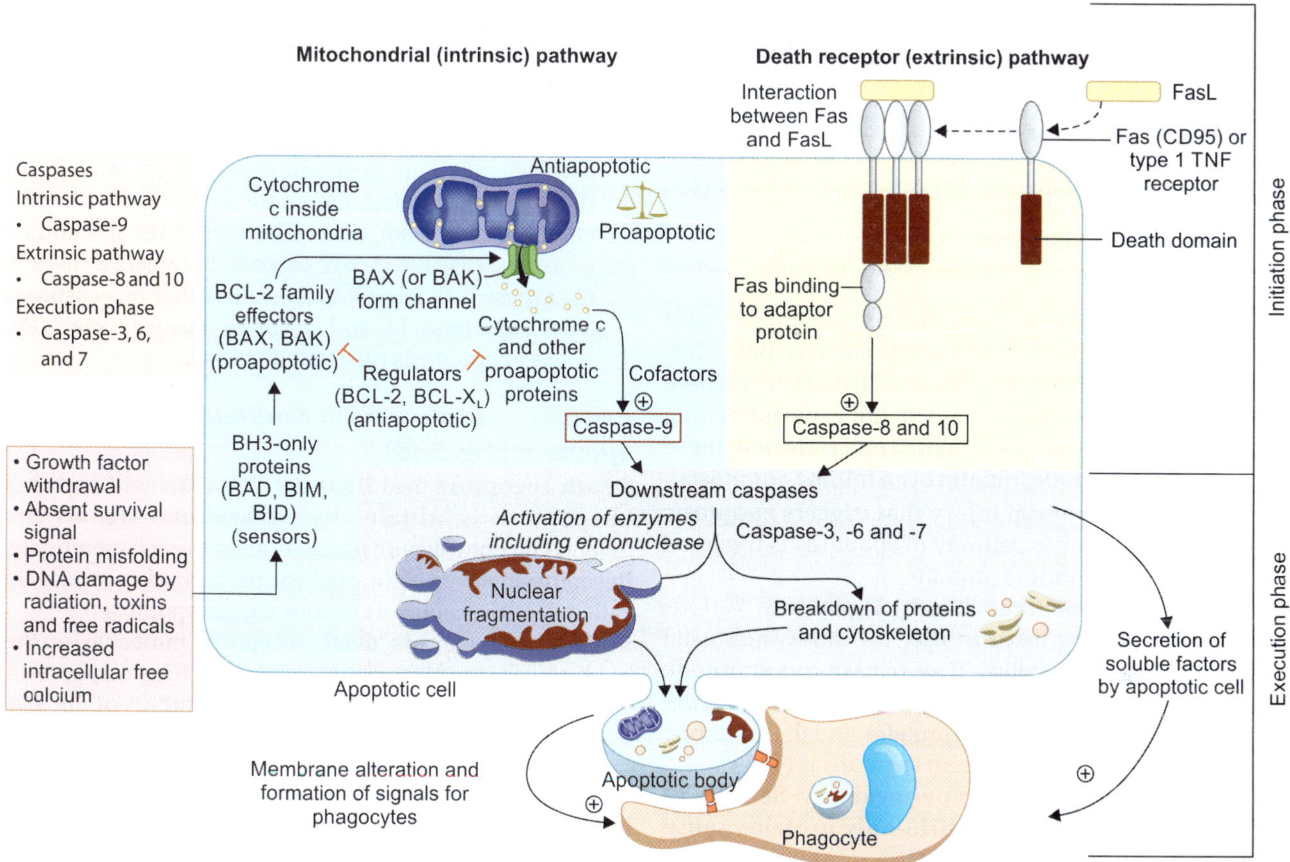

Fig. 2.13: Mechanisms of apoptosis. It consists of initiation and execution phases that activate caspases. The initiation phase may be activated by mitochondrial (intrinsic) or death receptor (extrinsic) pathways In the mitochondrial pathway, BH3-only proteins (e.g., BAD, BIM, BID) sense a lack of survival signals or DNA or protein damage. It activates effector molecules that increase mitochondrial permeability. The mitochondria become leaky. This causes leakage of substances such as cytochrome c from mitochondria into the cytosol and activates caspases. In the death receptor (extrinsic) pathway, signals from plasma membrane receptors lead to the assembly of adaptor proteins into a "death-inducing signaling complex" and activate caspases. Both the intrinsic and extrinsic pathways of the initiation phase activate the execution phase leading to apoptosis.

TABLE 2.3 BCL2 family proteins.

Antiapoptotic	*Pro-apoptotic*	*Regulated apoptosis initiators (BH3-only proteins)*
BCL2	BAX	BAD, BIM, BID, BIK, Puma, Noxa
BCL-XL	BAK	
MCL1		

and other aberrations in certain B-cell lymphomas. *BCL2* family genes are located on chromosome 18. The *BCL2* family has more than 20 members. They share one or more of four characteristic Bcl-2 homology (BH) domains (BH1–BH4) which are important determinants of their pro- versus antiapoptotic properties. This *BCL2* family may be divided into three subfamilies, depending on the number of BH domains namely (1) pro-apoptotic, (2) antiapoptotic function, and (3) regulated apoptosis initiators (sensors/BH3-only proteins) (**Table 2.3**).

1. **Antiapoptotic (i.e., prosurvival) *BCL family*:** The main members of this group are **BCL2, BCL-XL, and MCL1.** These proteins are present in the outer mitochondrial membrane, in the cytosol, and membrane of ER. They keep the mitochondrial outer membrane impermeable. Thereby, they **prevent leakage of cytochrome c and other death-inducing proteins into the cytosol.** Growth factors and other survival signals stimulate the production of antiapoptotic proteins. Thus they protect cells from apoptosis.
2. **Pro-apoptotic (i.e., antisurvival) *BCL family*: BAX and BAK** are the two members of this group within the outer mitochondrial membrane. On activation, BAX and/or BAK increase the mitochondrial permeability and allow cytochrome c leakage from the intermembranous space into the cytosol. Bak is mainly a mitochondrial protein. Bax is largely cytoplasmic.
3. **Regulated apoptosis initiators:** This group, includes BAD, BIM, BID, BIK, Puma, and Noxa. They are **sometimes called BH3-only proteins (sensors).** These proteins are sensor proteins of cellular stress and consequent damage. They maintain a peaceful

BOX 2.3: Causes of mitochondrial injury that triggers apoptosis (proapoptotic signals).

- **Absence/withdrawal of growth factor or survival signals.**
- **DNA damage:** For example, by radiation, cytotoxic anticancer drugs, hypoxia either directly or through free radicals.
- **Endoplasmic reticulum (ER) stress:** Due to accumulation of excessive amount of misfolded proteins.
- **Increased intracellular free calcium.**

balance (equilibrium) between antiapoptotic Bcl-2 (Bcl-xL, Mcl-1, etc.) and proapoptotic Bax/Bak. They prevent the initiation mitochondrial pathway of caspase activation in the cell. The mitochondrial default setting is prosurvival. When **upregulated and activated, these regulated apoptotic initiators can initiate apoptosis.**

Causes of mitochondrial injury that triggers apoptosis (Box 2.3): The intrinsic pathway of apoptosis is triggered through the bcl-2 family of proteins.

Steps in the intrinsic (mitochondrial) pathway: Various mitochondrial injury listed in **Box 2.3** causes increased mitochondrial permeability. They **release pro-apoptotic molecules (death inducers) into the cytoplasm**. Thus, the balance shifts to pro-apoptotic proteins and the apoptotic cascade is activated. The different steps are as follows:

- **Increased mitochondrial permeability: Sensors of the *BCL2* family** namely **BH3-only proteins** sense the lack of survival signals or DNA or protein damage **(Box 2.3).** They activate effector molecules that increase the permeability of mitochondria.
- **Blocking the function of antiapoptotic proteins:** Sensors of the ***BCL2* family** namely **BH3-only proteins also bind to and block the function of** protective **antiapoptotic proteins** namely ***BCL2*** and ***BCL-XL***. The synthesis of BCL2 and BCL-XL may be decreased because of an absence of survival signals.
- **Activation of pro-apoptotic BCL family:** The above-mentioned causes **(Box 2.3)** of mitochondrial injury activate several sensors of the *BCL2* **family** called BH3-proteins. They in turn **activate two critical pro-apoptotic *BCL2* family** effector proteins, namely ***BAX*** and ***BAK***.
- **Leakage of mitochondrial proteins into the cytosol:** ***BAX*** and ***BAK*** create channels in the mitochondria that **allow the release of several mitochondrial proteins from the inner mitochondrial membrane to leak out into the cytosol** (cytoplasm). One of these proteins is **cytochrome c.**
- **Activation of caspase-9: In the cytoplasm, cytochrome c** (Cyt c) **interacts with certain cofactors** (e.g., cytosolic apoptosis-activating factor-1 /Apaf-1) and procaspase-9 to form the *apoptosome.* The **apoptosome activates caspase-9.** The caspase-9 is the **critical initiator caspase of the mitochondrial pathway.** Its activation sets in an auto-amplification process. The cytoplasm of normal cells contains proteins that block the activation of caspases and function as physiologic **inhibitors of apoptosis (called IAPs)**. The normal function of the IAPs is to prevent the inappropriate activation of caspases, including executioners like caspase-3. IAPs keep cells alive and their inhibition permits initiation of the caspase cascade. Other mitochondrial proteins may enter the cytoplasm, **neutralize** these IAPs and initiate a caspase cascade. Active caspase-9 triggers a cascade of caspase activation and activates other pro-caspases (such as caspase-3,6, and 7). They mediate the execution phase of apoptosis (discussed below).

Extrinsic (death receptor-initiated) pathway of apoptosis (Fig. 2.13)

Death receptors and ligands: The extrinsic pathway of apoptosis is **initiated by extracellular signals** and involves receptor-ligand interactions at the cell membrane. Receptors involved in the extrinsic pathway of apoptosis are called death-receptors (i.e., they trigger apoptosis).

- **Many cells express "death-receptors" molecules on the surface of the plasma membrane that trigger apoptosis.** Most of these death receptors are **members of the TNF (tumor necrosis factor) receptor family.** These receptors contain a cytoplasmic domain called the **death domain,** named so because it brings out interaction with other proteins involved in cell death. The cytoplasmic tails of these death domains consist of docking (anchoring or binding) sites for the corresponding death domains of other proteins. In the extrinsic (death receptor) pathway, **apoptosis is initiated when** the **death receptors** present get **activated.**
- **Type I TNF receptor and Fas**: The **well-known** cell membrane **death receptors** are the (1) type I TNF receptor **(TNFR1)** and (2) Fas **(CD95)**. The **ligand for receptor TNFR1 is TNFα.** Fas death receptor is expressed mainly on activated T lymphocytes [cytotoxic T lymphocytes (CTLs)] and the **binding ligand for Fas is called Fas ligand (FasL/CD95L).** TNF-α is a soluble cytokine.

Steps in the extrinsic pathway: Various steps are as follows:

- **Binding of ligand with receptor**: Extrinsic pathway becomes activated when TNFR and Fas/CD95 bind to their corresponding ligands namely TNF-α and CD95L/FasL at the cell surface. FasL binding to its receptor is described in detail here.
- **Activation of caspases**: After binding to the ligand-activated receptors, the docking proteins stimulate downstream signaling molecules, especially procaspases-8 and -10. These inactive procaspases are converted to their active forms, **caspases-8 and -10**. In turn, these caspases activate downstream caspases in the execution pathway of apoptosis.
- The cytoplasmic death domains of Fas receptor bind to an **adapter protein.** This adapter protein also contains

BOX 2.4: Functions of the extrinsic pathway.

The extrinsic pathway of apoptosis is **involved in eliminating:**
- **Self-reactive lymphocytes** thereby avoiding autoimmunity. FasL is expressed on T-cells that recognize self-antigens and function to eliminate self-reactive lymphocytes.
- **Killing of target cells:** This is by some cytotoxic T lymphocytes (CTLs) that express FasL
  - **Virus-infected cells** through cytotoxic T lymphocytes.
  - **Tumor cells** through cytotoxic T lymphocytes (CTLs).

a death domain and is called the Fas-associated death domain (FADD). FADD in turn binds to pro-caspase-8 (an inactive form of caspase-8) via a death domain and generates active caspase-8.

The functions of the extrinsic pathway are listed in **Box 2.4.**

B. Execution Phase (Terminal Phase) of Apoptosis (Fig. 2.13)

- The above-mentioned two initiating pathways produce initiator caspases namely: (1) the **mitochondrial pathway activates initiator caspase-9**, and (2) the **death receptor pathway activates the initiator caspase-8 and 10**.
- The initiator caspases activate another series of caspases called **"effector," or "executioner," caspases (such as caspase-3, -6 and -7)** that mediates the final phase of apoptosis.
- **Caspase-3:** It is the most commonly activated effector caspase. It stimulates enzymes that cause fragmentation of the nucleus [e.g., caspase-activated DNase (CAD), which degrades chromosomal DNA] and also degrades components of the nuclear matrix. Caspase-3 also destabilizes the cytoskeleton as the involved cells begin to fragment into apoptotic bodies.

Removal of Apoptotic Cells

Phagocytosis

Apoptotic cells and bodies are engulfed and removed by phagocytic cells (mainly macrophages). The phagocytosis is so efficient that these dead cells and apoptotic bodies disappear within minutes. Even when the apoptosis is extensive their rapid removal prevents release of their cellular contents which may elicit inflammation.

Factors favoring phagocytosis: The apoptotic cells and apoptotic bodies undergo several changes in their membranes and produce signals that favor phagocytosis of these cells/bodies.

- **Expression of phosphatidylserine:** In healthy cells, **phosphatidylserine** is present on the inner leaflet of the plasma membrane. In cells undergoing apoptosis **phosphatidylserine** turns out and is expressed on the outer layer of the membrane causing easy recognition by receptors present on the macrophage.
- **Secretion of soluble factors: Apoptotic cells secrete soluble factors** (e.g., **thrombospondin**) that recruit phagocytes.
- **Natural antibodies and proteins of the complement system** may coat apoptotic bodies which aids in phagocytosis.

Diagnosis/Detection of Apoptosis

1. DNA fragmentation assay is carried out **by electrophoresis of genomic DNA**. Apoptosis produces **"step ladder pattern"** in contrast to smeared pattern seen in necrosis.
2. **T**erminal deoxynucleotidyl transferase biotin d-**U**TP **N**ick **E**nd **L**abeling (TUNEL) technique for in vivo detection of apoptosis.
3. Chromatin condensation seen by hematoxylin and eosin, Feulgen and acridine orange staining.
4. Estimation of:
   - Cytosolic cytochrome c
   - Activated caspase
   - Annexin V: Apoptotic cells express phosphatidylserine on the outer layer of plasma membrane because of which these cells are recognized by the dye Annexin.
   - Propidium iodide assay by flow cytometry/ fluorescent microscopy.

Disorders Associated with Dysregulated Apoptosis

Disorders with reduced apoptosis: It may allow the survival of abnormal cells.

- **Cancer:** Normally, cells with damaged (mutated) DNA are cleared in the body by undergoing apoptosis. Apoptosis may be reduced in some cancers. Best established role of BCL2 in protecting tumor cells from undergoing apoptosis is observed in follicular lymphoma.
- **Autoimmune disease.**

Disorders with increased apoptosis: This will cause an excessive loss of cells.

- **Neurodegenerative diseases (Alzheimer, Huntigton, Parkinson disease)**.
- **Ischemic injury:** In myocardial infarction and stroke.
- **Death of virus-infected cells:** Many viral infections, important being acquired immune deficiency syndrome (AIDS).

Q. List the differences between apoptosis and necrosis.

Differences between apoptosis and necrosis are summarized in **Table 2.4**.

OTHER PATHWAYS OF CELL DEATH

Necroptosis: It is a type of cell death that shows features of both necrosis and apoptosis. It is caspase-independent. It resembles morphologically necrosis and mechanistically apoptosis.

TABLE 2.4 Differences between apoptosis and necrosis.

Features	Apoptosis	Necrosis
Cause	Often physiological, means of eliminating unwanted cells; may also be pathological	Invariably pathological
Biochemical events	Energy-dependent fragmentation of DNA by endogenous endonucleases	Impairment or cessation of ion homeostasis
Lysosomes	Intact	Leak lytic enzymes
Morphology		
Extent	Single or small cluster of cells	Involves group of cells
Cell size	Cell reduced (shrinkage) and fragmentation to form apoptotic bodies with dense chromatin	Cell enlarged (swelling) and undergo lysis
Integrity of cell membrane	Maintained	Disrupted/lost
Nucleus	Fragmentation into nucleosome-size fragments	Pyknosis, karyorrhexis, karyolysis
Cellular contents	Intact; may be released in apoptotic bodies	Enzymatic digestion; may leak out of cell
Adjacent inflammatory response	None	Usual
Fate of dead cells	Ingested (phagocytosed) by neighboring cells	Ingested (phagocytosed) by neutrophil polymorphs and macrophages
DNA electrophoresis	DNA laddering is seen	Shows smearing effect
TUNEL staining	Positive	Negative

Pyroptosis: It is a type of programmed cell death accompanied by the release of fever (*pyro* refers to fever) producing cytokine IL-1 and bears some biochemical similarities with apoptosis.

Ferroptosis: It is a form of cell death that is triggered when excessive intracellular levels of iron or reactive oxygen species. It causes unchecked membrane lipid peroxidation.

Autolysis

PA 2.4c (CC): Describe, autolysis.

Autolysis (means self-lysis) is destruction of the cell by its own hydrolytic enzymes released from lysosomes. Autolysis is generally reserved for postmortem change. It develops rapidly in some tissues rich in hydrolytic enzymes such as pancreas and gastric mucosa. It occurs little slowly in tissues such a the heart, liver and kidney; and slow in fibrous tissue. Microscopically, the cellular details are lost and they appears as cells with homogeneous and eosinophilic cytoplasm.

Differences between necrosis and autolysis are listed in **Table 2.5**.

TABLE 2.5 Differences between necrosis and autolysis.

Features	Necrosis	Autolysis
Definition	Morphologic changes following cell death in living tissue	Self-digestion or disintegration of cells by enzymes liberated from own lysosomes
Occurrence	In living tissue	After death of cells
Inflammatory reaction	Present	Absent
Calcification	May occur	Absent

MECHANISMS OF CELL INJURY AND CELL DEATH

PA 2.2c (CC): Mechanisms of cell injury.

Q. Describe the biochemical and molecular mechanism of cell injury.

Q. Write a short essay on the mechanism (biochemical basis) of cell injury.

General Principles of Cell Injury

- **Cellular response to injury:** It depends on (1) the type of injury, (2) the duration of injury, and (3) the severity of the injury.
- **Consequences of injury:** It depends on (1) the type of cell involved, (2) the adaptability of the cell, (3) the status of the cell, and (4) the genetic makeup of the cell.
- **Targets and biochemical mechanism of cell injury:** Injurious stimuli that cause cell injury lead to complex cellular, biochemical, and molecular changes. Certain mechanism is common for most forms of cell injury and cell death. **Cell injury causes abnormalities in one or more vital cellular components (Fig. 2.14).** The main cellular components that are the targets of cell injury are

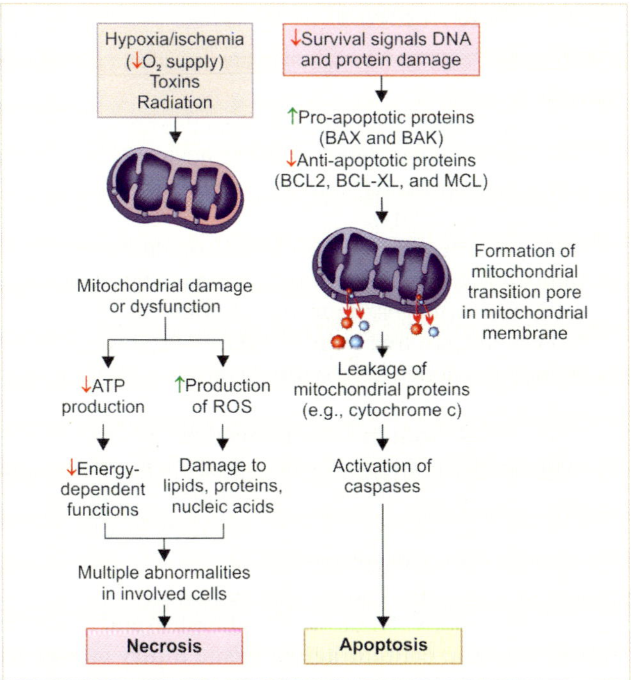

Fig. 2.14: Role and effects of mitochondria damage in cell injury and death. Mitochondria can be involved by various injurious stimuli. They can lead to necrosis or apoptosis.

(ATP: Adenosine triphosphate; ROS: reactive oxygen species).

mitochondria (mitochondrial damage/dysfunction), **cell membranes** (damage to cellular membranes), **the machinery involved in the synthesis of protein and secretion, and DNA** (damage to DNA and misfolding of proteins). The consequences of injury show distinct involvement of cellular components but are usually overlapping.

Mitochondrial Dysfunction and Damage

Production of ATP by mitochondria: Normally, ATP is produced in two ways. The **major pathway** of its production, particularly in nondividing cells (e.g., brain and liver), is by **oxidative phosphorylation of adenosine diphosphate and requires oxygen.** The **second minor method of production is the glycolytic pathway**, which can generate small amounts of ATP **in the absence of oxygen**. It uses glucose derived either from body fluids or from the hydrolysis of glycogen. Mitochondria produce ATP which is a life-sustaining energy and are also targets of many injurious stimuli. **Mitochondria are the main cellular component involved in all pathways that lead to cell injury and death.**

Causes of mitochondrial damage: Mitochondria are susceptible to almost all types of injurious stimuli. These include the reduced supply of oxygen and nutrients (because of **ischemia and hypoxia**), **toxins** (e.g., cyanide), and **radiation (Fig. 2.14).** Mitochondria can be damaged by an increase in cytosolic Ca^{2+}, ROS, and reduced oxygen supply. In some inherited diseases, mutations can occur in mitochondrial genes and may be associated with mitochondrial damage.

Major Consequences of Mitochondrial Damage

Three major consequences of mitochondrial damage are as follows:

1. **Reduced production and depletion of ATP: Failure of oxidative phosphorylation, leads to reduced production of ATP and depletion of ATP. ATP is** an energy source **needed for almost all enzymatic, biosynthetic, and degradative activities in cells.** Mitochondrial damage is associated with failure of oxidative phosphorylation and progressive depletion of ATP. Loss of ATP influences many cellular systems.
   - **Reduced activity of the plasma membrane ATP-dependent sodium pump (Na^+, K^+-ATPase):** This causes accumulation of sodium inside cells and with loss of potassium from the cell. The net solute gain results in the **intracellular accumulation of water.** This causes **cell swelling** and **dilation of ER.**
   - **Compensatory increase in anaerobic glycolysis:** If the supply of oxygen to cells is reduced (e.g., in ischemia), oxidative phosphorylation ceases. This leads to a decrease in cellular ATP and an associated increase in adenosine monophosphate (AMP). ATP depletion is associated with the alteration of cellular energy metabolism. There are increased rates of glycogenolysis and glycolysis to maintain energy supplies by producing ATP through the metabolism of glucose derived from glycogen. The glycogen stores get rapidly depleted. Glycolysis under anaerobic conditions results in the **accumulation of lactic acid with decreased intracellular pH**, and **reduced activity of many cellular enzymes.**
   - **Structural disruption of the protein synthetic apparatus:** Prolonged and severe depletion of ATP leads to structural disruption of protein synthetic apparatus. This causes the **detachment of ribosomes from the rough ER, dissociation of polysomes, and reduction in the synthesis of proteins.** There may also be **increased misfolding of protein.**
   - **Irreversible damage:** Ultimately, depletion of ATP causes irreversible damage to the membranes of the mitochondria and lysosomes. This produces **necrosis of the cell.** Necrosis is the main form of cell death due to hypoxia, but it may also cause apoptosis through the mitochondrial (intrinsic) pathway.
2. **Reactive oxygen species:** Abnormal oxidative phosphorylation also leads to the formation of reactive oxygen species (ROS). ROS produces many harmful effects (refer to the page 30 below).
3. **Leakage of mitochondrial proteins:** Mitochondrial damage often leads to the formation of high-conductance channels in the membrane of the mitochondria. These are called the mitochondrial permeability transition pores.

The mitochondria contain proteins such as **cytochrome c.** These are released into the cytoplasm through the channel (pores) formed. The leakage of mitochondrial protein is regulated by other proteins. The loss of survival signals and other pro-apoptotic BAX and BAK activate apoptosis by the intrinsic pathway. When mitochondria are healthy, they sustain life. But when damaged can activate numerous protective and pathologic reactions.

Oxidative Stress: Accumulation of Oxygen-derived Free Radicals

Q. Write a short note on free radical injury and its role in cell injury.

Free Radicals

Free radicals are **unstable chemical compounds** with a **single unpaired electron in an outer orbit (Fig. 2.15).**

Properties of free radicals: These are as follows:

- **Highly reactive:** Free radicals (unpaired electrons) are highly reactive and "attack" and modify adjacent molecules. These molecules can be inorganic or organic chemicals which are key components of cell membranes and nuclei. Examples include proteins, lipids, carbohydrates, and nucleic acids.
- **Unstable and rapidly destroyed:** Normally, free radicals produced in the cells are unstable and are rapidly destroyed.
- **Autocatalytic reactions:** When free radicals react with any molecules, they convert those molecules into free radicals. Thus, they initiate a chain of damage forming autocatalytic reactions.

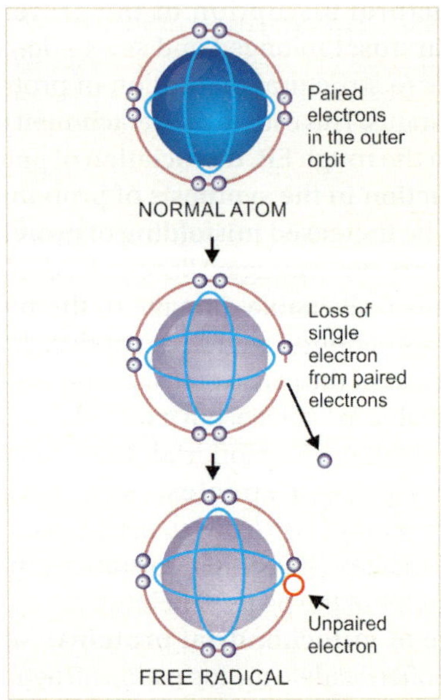

Fig. 2.15: Formation of free radical.

Types of Free Radicals

Q. Write a short note on free radical injury (including types of free radicals).

- **Oxygen-derived free radicals:** Reactive oxygen species (ROS) are oxygen-derived free radicals. ROS includes superoxide anion ($O_2^{\bullet}$), hydrogen peroxide (H_2O_2), and hydroxyl ions ($^{\bullet}OH$).
- **Reactive nitrogen species (nitric oxide derived free radicals):** Nitric oxide (NO) is generated by endothelial cells, macrophages, neurons, and other types of cells. NO can act as a free radical and can also be converted to highly reactive peroxynitrite anion ($ONOO^-$), NO_2, and NO_3^-.
- **Free radicals from enzymatic metabolism of exogenous drugs and chemicals:** Free radicals that are not ROS but have similar effects can be produced by enzymatic metabolism of exogenous chemicals or drugs. For example, CCl_4 can generate CCl_3.

Causes of free radical-mediated cell injury: It is seen in many types of injury. These include **chemical and radiation injury, hypoxia, cellular aging, tissue injury caused by inflammatory cells, microbial killing by phagocytes, and ischemia-reperfusion injury** (caused by to restoration of blood flow in ischemic tissue). Free radical injury is an important mechanism of cellular injury, especially by reactive oxygen species (ROS).

Oxygen-derived Free Radicals

Reactive oxygen species (ROS) are a type of oxygen-derived free radical. The **cell injury caused by ROS is called oxidative stress. Cell injury due to free radicals, particularly ROS is an important mechanism of cell damage.** It occurs in **many pathologic conditions.**

Normal production and degradation of ROS: Normally, ROS are **produced in cells during mitochondrial respiration and energy generation**. They are **degraded and removed by intracellular ROS scavengers.** These degradative defense systems **maintain a steady state in which free radicals may be present at low concentrations but do not cause cellular damage.**

Generation of Free Radicals

Accumulation (excess) of free radicals: It may be either **due to an increased rate of production or ineffective degradation** (decreased scavenging or removal)**.** The excess of free radicals causing cell injury is called oxidative stress. Oxidative stress is involved in various pathologic conditions. These include cell injury, cancer, aging, and some degenerative diseases (e.g., Alzheimer disease). Free radicals may be produced within cells in several ways **(Fig. 2.16)**:

1. **Reduction-oxidation (redox) reactions in all cells:** Reduction-oxidation (redox) reactions occur in the mitochondria during the normal metabolic processes

involved in the production of energy. During this process, ROS are produced in **small amounts in the mitochondria of all cells.** During the redox reaction, molecular oxygen is reduced in the mitochondria by the sequential addition of four electrons to H_2 to produce two water molecules. However, this reaction is imperfect and oxygen is only partially reduced. During this process, small amounts of partially reduced, highly reactive, short-lived toxic intermediates are produced. These have different numbers of electrons transferred from oxygen. These intermediates include:

a. **Superoxide anion** ($O_2^{\bullet}$ with one electron): During redox reaction, **superoxide anion** ($O_2^{\bullet}$) is produced when oxygen (O_2) is only partially reduced. These ROS are mainly involved in destroying phagocytosed material, like microbial pathogens, dead cells, etc.
b. **Hydrogen peroxide (H_2O_2 with two electrons).** It is formed spontaneously from superoxide anion and by the enzyme superoxide dismutase (SOD). Hydrogen peroxide (H_2O_2) is more stable than superoxide anion ($O_2^{\bullet}$) and is not particularly injurious. It is largely metabolized to H_2O by catalase. However, when there is excess peroxide, it may be converted to the very destructive and highly reactive hydroxyl radical ($^{\bullet}OH$).
c. **Hydroxyl radical ($^{\bullet}OH$ with three electrons):** These are formed by (1) radiolysis of water (caused, e.g., by ionizing radiation), and (2) H_2O_2 reaction with transition metals (have valence electrons in two shells instead of only one). Transition metals such as iron and copper are excellent catalysts that can easily donate or accept free electrons during intracellular reactions and catalyze the formation of free radicals. Transition metals ferrous iron (Fe^{2+}) or cuprous copper (Cu^{1+}) are involved in the Fenton reaction. Hydrogen peroxide (H_2O_2) in the presence of metals (e.g., Fe^{2+}) is converted by the Fenton reaction ($H_2O_2 + Fe^{2+} \rightarrow Fe^{3+} + {}^{\bullet}OH + OH^-$) to a **highly reactive free radical called hydroxyl radical ($^{\bullet}OH$).** Ionizing radiation and high doses of ultraviolet light can increase the production of ROS by hydrolyzing water into hydroxyl ($^{\bullet}OH$) and hydrogen ($H^{\bullet}$) free radicals.

2. **During inflammation in phagocytic leukocytes (*refer* Figs. 3.8 and 3.9):** ROS is produced in the activated leukocytes (mainly neutrophils) for the destruction of the ingested microbes and other substances produced during inflammation. During phagocytosis, **ROS is produced in the phagosomes and phagolysosomes** of the leukocytes (mainly neutrophils and macrophages) by a process similar to mitochondrial respiration. This process is called a **respiratory burst (oxidative burst).**
   a. **Superoxide ($O_2^{\bullet}$) and H_2O_2:** During the process of respiratory burst, the enzyme phagocytic oxidase [NADPH (nicotinamide adenine dinucleotide phosphate) oxidase, respiratory burst oxidase], present in the membranes of phagolysosomes, catalyzes the production of superoxide. This superoxide is converted to H_2O_2. Defects in superoxide production by leukocytic causes chronic granulomatous disease.
   b. **Hypochlorite (OCl^- or ClO^-):** Myeloperoxidase is abundant in leukocytes, especially neutrophils. **H_2O_2** is converted to the highly reactive compound (potent radical) hypochlorite by the enzyme myeloperoxidase. The hypochlorite is the **major component of household bleach**. This ROS released from phagocytic neutrophils is lethal for microorganisms and if released extracellularly, can also injure surrounding normal tissues.

Removal/Neutralization of Free Radicals (Fig. 2.16)

Q. Write a short note on antioxidants (mechanisms of removal/neutralization of free radicals).

Cells have different mechanisms to remove free radicals and thereby minimize their injurious effects. These mechanisms to remove free radicals include spontaneous breakdown and enzymatic and nonenzymatic mechanisms. The enzymatic and nonenzymatic systems that inactivate free radicals are sometimes called free radical scavengers.

Spontaneous breakdown: Free radicals are naturally unstable and usually undergo spontaneous breakdown. For example, $O_2^{\bullet}$ is unstable and degrades (dismutates) spontaneously to O_2 and H_2O_2 in the presence of water.

Enzymatic mechanisms: Many enzymes act as free radical-scavenging systems (detoxifying enzymes). They break down free radicals H_2O_2 and $O_2^{\bullet}$. These enzymes are located near the sites of production of the free radicals. These enzymes include the following:

- **Superoxide dismutases (SODs)** are enzymes found in many types of cells. The manganese-SOD is found in mitochondria and copper-zinc-SOD in the cytoplasm. These enzymes **convert superoxide ($O_2^{\bullet}$) into hydrogen peroxide** (H_2O_2)($2O_2^{\bullet} + 2H \rightarrow H_2O_2 + O_2$). **$H_2O_2$ is further degraded by catalase** (refer to below).
- **Glutathione peroxidases** are a family of enzymes and their main function is to protect cells from oxidative damage. The glutathione peroxidase 1 is the most abundant member of this family and is found in the cytoplasm of all cells. Reduced glutathione (GSH) is one of the most important scavengers of reactive oxygen species (ROS). Under normal conditions, reduced GSH constitutes up to 98% of cellular GSH. **GSH in conjugation with the glutathione peroxidase 1 catalyzes the breakdown of H_2O_2 to H_2O.** It is also involved in the breakdown of acetaminophen free radicals. The intracellular ratio of reduced glutathione (GSH) with oxidized glutathione (GSSG) (i.e., GSH: GSSG) indicates the oxidative state of the cell. It is an

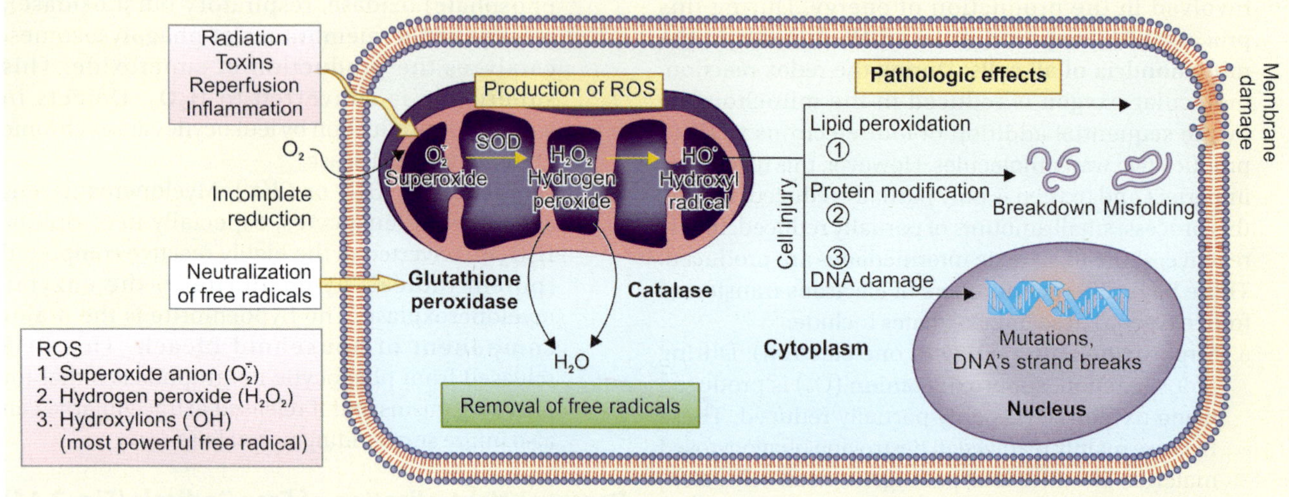

Fig. 2.16: The production removal, and role of reactive oxygen species (ROS) in cell injury. The generation of ROS is increased by various injurious stimuli. These free radicals are removed by spontaneous degradation and by different enzymatic systems. Increased production or inadequate removal leads to the accumulation of free radicals in cells. The free radicals may damage lipids (by peroxidation), proteins, and DNA.

(SOD: superoxide dismutase).

important marker of oxidative stress and indicates the cell's ability to detoxify ROS.

- **Catalase** is an enzyme present in peroxisomes. It catalyzes the **conversion of hydrogen peroxide (H_2O_2) free radicals into oxygen (O_2) and water (H_2O)**. It is **highly efficient** and can degrade millions of molecules of H_2O_2 per second.

Nonenzymatic mechanism: Serum, tissue fluids and cells have **antioxidant nonenzymatic mechanisms.** They protect against potentially harmful oxygen-derived free radicals **(Box 2.5).** Antioxidants can either block the formation of free radicals or inactivate (e.g., scavenge) free radicals once they have formed. The antioxidants may be exogenous or endogenous.

- **Exogenous antioxidants:** Examples include **vitamins E, A, and C** (ascorbic acid); β-carotene, **and sulfhydryl-containing compounds** (e.g., cysteine and glutathione).
- **Endogenous antioxidants:** Free metal iron and copper are reactive metals. They can catalyze the formation of ROS. Under normal conditions, the reactivity of these metals is minimized by binding these metal ions to storage and transport proteins (e.g., transferrin, ferritin, albumin, lactoferrin, and ceruloplasmin). This **prevents these metals from participating in reactions that produce ROS.**

BOX 2.5: Various types of antioxidants.

Enzymatic antioxidants
- Superoxide dismutase (SOD)
- Glutathione peroxidase
- Catalase

Nonenzymatic antioxidants
- **Exogenous:** Vitamin E, vitamin A, ascorbic acid, β-carotene, and sulfhydryl-containing compounds (e.g., cysteine and glutathione)
- **Endogenous:** Storage and transport proteins in the serum, such as transferrin, ferritin, albumin, lactoferrin, and ceruloplasmin

Pathologic Effects of Free Radicals (Fig. 2.16)

Reactive oxygen species (ROS) and other free radicals can cause cell injury in many diseases **by damaging multiple components of cells**. Free radicals can activate both **necrosis** and **apoptosis**. The main reactions that cause injury by free radicals are:

Peroxidation of membrane lipids: The double bonds in membrane lipids are susceptible to attack by free radicals. In the presence of O_2, the lipid-radical interactions due to oxygen-derived free radicals cause peroxidation of lipids within plasma and organellar membranes. These peroxides are themselves unstable and reactive and produce an autocatalytic chain reaction. **ROS damages plasma membranes and membranes of mitochondria and lysosomes.**

Crosslinking and other changes in proteins: Free radicals promote protein cross-linking (e.g., disulfide bonds). This results in increased degradation or loss of functional activity of proteins. Free radical reactions may also cause direct fragmentation of polypeptides. Damaged proteins may fail to fold properly. This triggers the unfolded protein response and increases the proteasomal degradation of unfolded or misfolded proteins. These are harmful to the cell.

DNA damage: Free radical radicals can produce several types of DNA damage. These include mutations and single- and double-strand DNA breaks. Such oxidative DNA damage may be seen in **apoptotic cell death, cell aging, and malignant transformation of cells.**

The major free radicals and their pathologic effects are summarized (*refer* **online Table 2.6).**

Membrane Damage (Fig. 2.17)

Initially, injury causes loss of selective membrane permeability. Ultimately, it leads to obvious damage to the membrane. Membrane damage consistently occurs in most forms of cell injury (except apoptosis).

Types of the membrane affected: Damage to cellular membranes may disturb the integrity and functions of all cellular membranes. The membrane damage may affect the **plasma membrane, mitochondrial membrane, or lysosomal membrane.**

Causes and biochemical mechanisms of membrane damage: These include the following:

- **Lipid peroxidation by ROS:** Oxygen free radicals (reactive oxygen species) damage the cell membranes by lipid peroxidation.
- **Decreased phospholipid synthesis:** The synthesis of phospholipids in cells may be reduced due to defective mitochondrial function or due to hypoxia and deprivation of nutrients. This decreases the production of ATP and affects energy-dependent biosynthetic pathways. Decreased phospholipid synthesis may also occur in all cellular membranes, including those of mitochondria.
- **Increased phospholipid breakdown:** Severe cell injury is associated with increased degradation of membrane phospholipids. This is probably due to the activation of calcium-dependent phospholipases by increased intracellular and mitochondrial Ca^{2+}. The breakdown of phospholipids leads to the accumulation of **lipid breakdown products**. These products include unesterified free fatty acids, acyl carnitine, and lysophospholipids. They have a detergent effect on membranes. These products may either be inserted into the lipid bilayer of the membrane or exchanged with membrane phospholipids. They can alter the permeability and electrophysiologic properties of the membrane.
- **Cytoskeletal abnormalities:** Cytoskeletal filaments connect the plasma membrane to the cell interior. This attachment may be damaged by the proteases activated by cytosolic Ca^{2+}. When the detachment is extreme, it causes swelling of cells, particularly in myocardial cells. This damage leads to detachment of the cell membrane from the cytoskeleton. These cells are susceptible to stretching and rupture. In ischemic cells, defects of the membrane may cause depletion of ATP and calcium-mediated activation of phospholipases. The bacterial

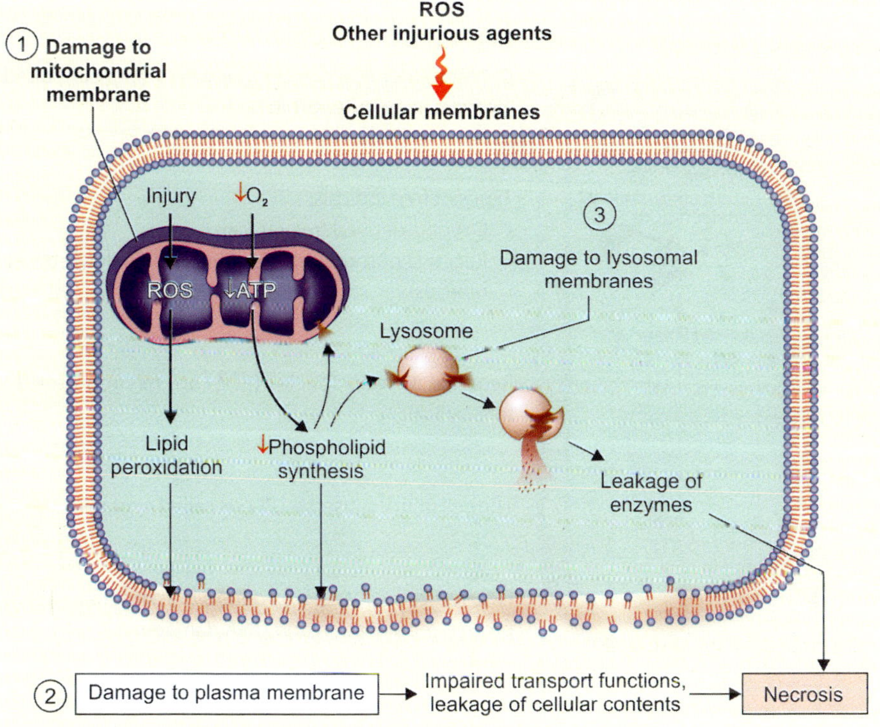

Mechanism of cell injury and cell death:
1. Mitochondrial dysfunction and damage
2. Oxidative stress
3. Membrane damage
4. Disturbances in calcium homeostasis
5. Endoplasmic reticulum stress
6. DNA damage

Consequences of mitochondrial dysfunction and damage.
- Reduced production and depletion of ATP.
- Formation of reactive oxygen species (ROS)
- Leakage of mitochondrial proteins (e.g., cytochrome c) that cause apoptosis

Fig. 2.17: Mechanism and effects of membrane damage.

toxins, viral proteins, lytic complement components, and physical and chemical agents can also directly damage the plasma membrane. Different biochemical mechanisms may damage the membrane **(Fig. 2.17)**:

Effects of membrane damage: Damage to different cellular membranes has varying effects on cells.

- **Damage of mitochondrial membrane:** This opens the mitochondrial permeability transition pore. This leads to **decreased production of ATP and release of proteins that initiate death by apoptosis.**
- **Damage of plasma membrane:** It leads to **loss of osmotic balance** and **entry of fluids and ions, and loss of cellular contents**. There may also be **leakage of metabolites** (e.g., glycolytic intermediates) that are important for the reconstitution of ATP. This may further deplete sources of energy.
- **Injury to lysosomal membranes**: It leads to **leakage of lysosomal enzymes into the cytoplasm** and activation of acid hydrolases in the acidic intracellular pH of the injured cell. These lysosomal hydrolases include RNases (degrade RNA), DNases (degrade DNA), proteases (degrade proteins), phosphatases (degrade phosphoproteins), and glucosidases (degrade glycogen). This **leads to necrosis of cells.**

Disturbance in Calcium Homeostasis

Normally, calcium ions act as second messengers in many signaling pathways. However, if **excessive amounts of calcium are released into the cytoplasm of the cells, it may cause cell injury. Normally, the concentration of free Ca^{2+}** in the **cytosol** (cytoplasm) is **much lower** (~0.1 µmol) **than extracellular** Ca^{2+} (1.3 mmol). Most of the intracellular Ca^{2+} is present within the mitochondria and the ER (endoplasmic reticulum).

Causes of increased cytosolic calcium: It occurs in **ischemia** and with **certain toxins**.

Mechanism of increased cytosolic calcium: Initially, the increase in cytosolic Ca^{2+} is due to the release from intracellular stores. Later, it is due to increased entry of calcium across the dysfunctional plasma membrane **(Fig. 2.18)**.

Mechanism of damage by calcium (Fig. 2.18): Excessive intracellular Ca^{2+} may cause cell injury by several mechanisms.

- **Opening of the mitochondrial permeability transition pore:** The accumulation of Ca^{2+} in mitochondria opens the mitochondrial permeability transition pore. This causes failure of ATP production.
- **Activating various enzymes (Fig. 2.18):** Increased cytosolic Ca^{2+} activates several enzymes with potentially

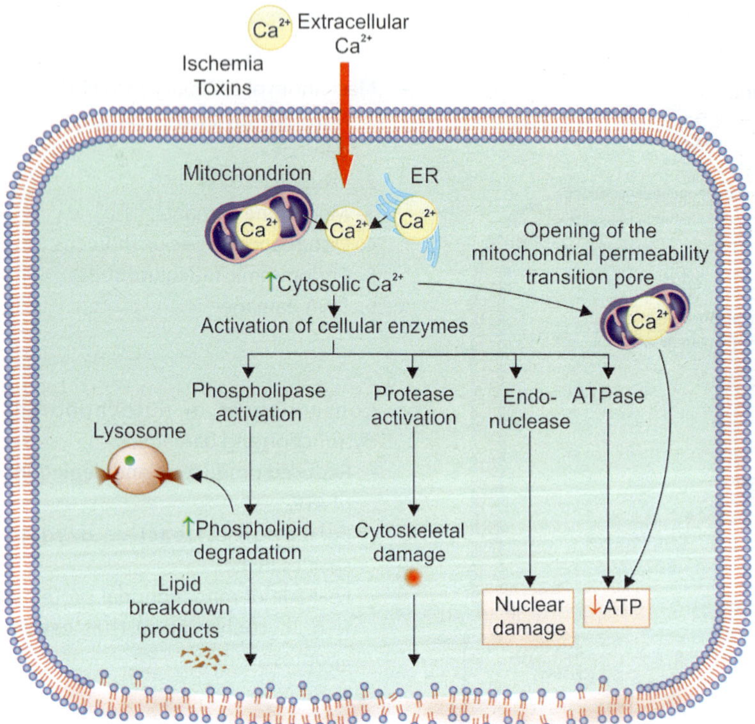

Fig. 2.18: Mechanism of cell damage due to increased cytosolic calcium. (ER: endoplasmic reticulum).

Free radicals
Unstable chemical compounds with a single unpaired electron in an outer orbit.

Types of free radicals:
- Oxygen-derived free radicals
- Reactive nitrogen species (nitric oxide derived free radicals)

Reactive oxygen species (ROS) are oxygen-derived free radicals.

The cell injury caused by ROS is called oxidative stress.

Free radicals cause peroxidation of membrane lipids, protein modification and DNA damage.

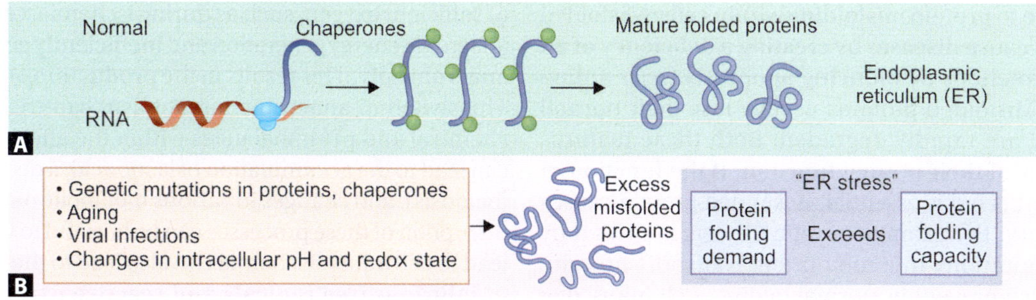

Figs. 2.19A and B: (A) Steps involved in the normal folding of newly synthesized protein in the endoplasmic reticulum; (B) Causes and mechanism involved in ER (endoplasmic reticulum) stress.

harmful effects on cells. These enzymes include ***phospholipases*** (causes membrane damage), ***proteases*** (causes breakdown of both membrane and cytoskeletal proteins), ***endonucleases*** (causes fragmentation of DNA and chromatin), and ***ATPases*** (accelerate ATP depletion).

Endoplasmic Reticulum Stress: The Unfolded Protein Response

Folding of protein (Figs. 2.19A and B): Every cell synthesizes proteins, folds them into proper three-dimensional configurations and delivers them to their desired places. **Protein must be correctly folded** and this folding **occurs in the endoplasmic reticulum**. The proper folding of newly synthesized proteins is **controlled by the chaperones in the ER**. But this process is imperfect, and some misfolded polypeptides are produced. These **misfolded proteins are transported into the cytoplasm and undergo proteolysis in proteasomes by ubiquitination**.

Endoplasmic reticulum (ER) stress: It occurs when the capacity of the ER to fold proteins becomes saturated. This causes an accumulation of misfolded proteins in the ER. The misfolded proteins accumulated in the ER induce the protective, adaptive cellular response with several alterations that are collectively called the **unfolded protein response (Fig. 2.20). This adaptive response activates signaling pathways that increase the production of chaperones**, increase proteasomal degradation of abnormal proteins, and slow translation of proteins. Thus, this response reduces the levels of misfolded proteins in the cell. However, if the quantity of **misfolded protein exceeds the capacity of adaptive response, additional signals are produced that activate proapoptotic sensors. This triggers apoptosis mainly by the mitochondrial (intrinsic) pathway.** This process is called *ER stress.*

Causes of intracellular accumulation of misfolded proteins: It may be due to **increased production of misfolded proteins or reduced cell's ability to** repair or **eliminate them.** The causes include genetic **mutations** in proteins and chaperons (with the production of abnormal

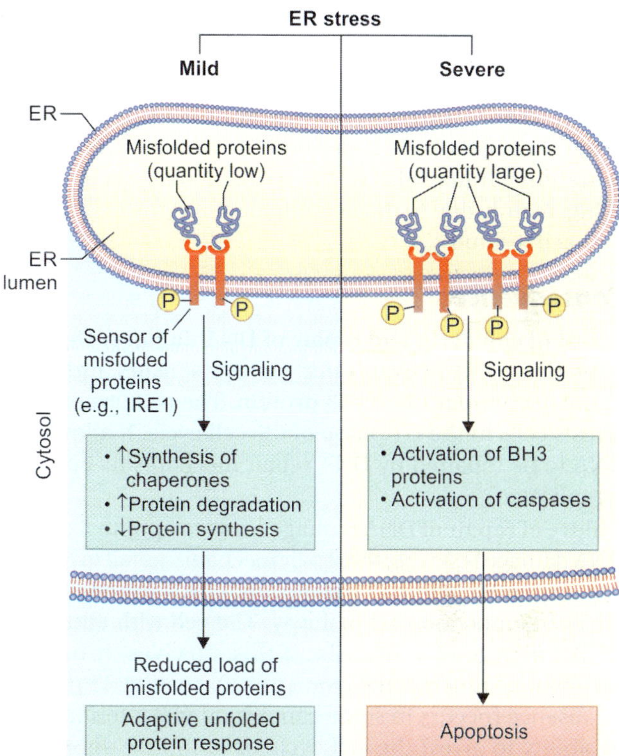

Fig. 2.20: The unfolded protein response and ER stress. The sensors such as the kinase IRE1 in the ER membrane detect misfolded proteins in the ER. This activates an adaptive unfolded protein response. This response can protect the cell from the harmful effects of the misfolded proteins. When the quantity of misfolded proteins is too large to be corrected, death by apoptosis occurs through the mitochondrial pathway.

(IRE1: inositol requiring enzyme-1)

proteins); **aging** (associated with decreased capacity to correct misfolding); **infections** (especially **viral infections** associated with the synthesis of large amounts of microbial proteins that exceed the capacity of proper protein folding); and **changes in intracellular pH and redox state**. The burden of misfolded proteins may be increased due to deprivation of glucose and oxygen, as in ischemia and hypoxia.

Diseases due to protein misfolding within cells: Misfolded protein may **cause diseases by creating a deficiency of an essential protein or by inducing apoptosis** (*refer* **online Table 2.7**). Misfolded proteins usually lose their normal activity and are rapidly degraded. Both these features lead to a loss of their normal function. If the function of the protein affected is essential, misfolded protein causes cellular injury. For example, cystic fibrosis is caused by inherited mutations in a membrane transport protein, some of which prevent its normal folding. Cell injury due to protein misfolding causes cellular abnormality in several neurodegenerative diseases.

Damage to DNA

Causes of DNA damage: It may be due to exposure of cells to **radiation, chemotherapeutic (anticancer) drugs, intracellularly generated ROS and acquisition of mutations**. It may also occur spontaneously as a part of aging, mainly due to the deamination of cytosine residues to uracil residues.

Consequences

Arrest of cell cycle and repair of DNA damage: Damage to nuclear DNA activates intracellular **sensors and leads to the accumulation of p53 protein.** The p53 protein first arrests cells in the G1 phase of the cell cycle. It allows the DNA to be repaired by DNA repair mechanisms before it is replicated.

Failure of repair of DNA damage leads to apoptosis: If the DNA damage is severe, the repair mechanisms fail to correct it successfully, and p53 triggers apoptosis usually by the intrinsic mitochondrial pathway. The cell with abnormal DNA undergoes apoptosis. If this survives, it has the potential to undergo malignant transformation. Mutations or absence (occurs in some cancers) of p53 interfere with its ability to arrest the cell cycle or to induce apoptosis. These cells with DNA damage may undergo various types of genomic alterations (e.g., chromosomal deletions) that may lead to neoplastic transformation.

Examples of Cell Injury and Necrosis

Hypoxia and Ischemia

Ischemia refers to a condition due to interrupted or diminished (insufficient) blood flow to a particular tissue or organ. This leads to a decreased supply of oxygen and nutrients to affected cells. **Ischemia is the most common cause of cell injury. In ischemia, the reduced blood flow is most often due to a mechanical arterial obstruction.** When tissue experiences ischemia, it can lead to tissue hypoxia (a reduced oxygen supply) or anoxia (a complete lack of oxygen). This lack of oxygen affects the ability of cells within the tissue to produce energy mainly ATP. Oxygen is required for oxidative phosphorylation and the generation of adenosine triphosphate (ATP). In the absence of sufficient oxygen, such as during ischemia, cells resort to anaerobic energy generation and **inefficiently generate ATP anaerobically.** This results in the **production of lactic acid.** The switch to anaerobic metabolism can trigger several chemical and pH imbalances within the affected tissue. It can lead to the accumulation of lactic acid, a decrease in pH (acidosis), and changes in various metabolic pathways. The disruption of these processes can be harmful to the cells and lead to cell injury. Ischemia can also lead to the **generation of injurious free radicals and reactive oxygen species.** These molecules can cause oxidative stress, damaging cellular structures and molecules, including proteins, lipids, and DNA.

Hypoxia vs. ischemia: In hypoxia, oxygen supply is reduced, but blood flow is maintained. This allows cells to continue producing energy through anaerobic glycolysis as a compensatory mechanism. In contrast, ischemia compromises the delivery of glycolytic substrates, leading to more severe cell injury because not only does aerobic metabolism cease (terminate), but anaerobic energy generation also fails. Hence, **ischemia causes more rapid and severe cell and tissue injury than hypoxia.**

Short periods of ischemia may not cause irreversible damage, and cells can recover if circulation is restored promptly. However, if ischemia persists for an extended period, it can lead to irreversible cell injury and cell death. The mechanisms of cell damage in prolonged ischemia can involve the activation of cell death pathways, such as apoptosis or necrosis.

Hypoxia-inducible factor (HIF): Cells subjected to the stress of hypoxia do not immediately die. They activate compensatory mechanisms driven by transcription factors from the hypoxia-inducible factor (HIF) family. HIF induces the synthesis of various proteins that help cells survive in low-oxygen conditions. Some of these proteins, such as vascular endothelial growth factor (VEGF), stimulate the growth of new blood vessels (angiogenesis) to improve oxygen supply, while others promote uptake of glucose and glycolysis as an alternative energy source. Anaerobic glycolysis can generate ATP in the absence of oxygen using glucose derived either from the circulation or from the hydrolysis of intracellular glycogen. Tissues with a greater glycolytic capacity due to the presence of glycogen (e.g., the liver and striated muscle) can survive the loss of oxygen and decreased oxidative phosphorylation better than tissues with limited glycogen stores (e.g., the brain).

Depletion of ATP: Prolonged or severe hypoxia and ischemia result in the depletion of ATP, which has several detrimental effects on cells. These effects include the failure of the sodium pump in the plasma membrane, a decrease in intracellular pH, changes in enzyme activities, increased generation of injurious free radical species (reactive oxygen species/ROS), and defects in protein synthesis.

Cells may recover from damage produced by short periods of ischemia if circulation is restored. However, long periods of ischemia lead to irreversible cell injury and death. In clinical practice, timely intervention to restore blood flow to ischemic tissues is crucial to minimize damage and prevent irreversible cell injury. **Ischemia is a common factor in conditions like myocardial infarction (heart attack) and stroke,** where prompt medical treatment is vital to reduce tissue damage and improve patient outcomes.

Mechanism of Ischemic Cell Injury (Fig. 2.21)

Ischemic cell injury following hypoxia or ischemia occurs when there is a decrease in blood supply and, consequently, oxygen delivery to tissues. This can lead to a cascade of events that ultimately result in cell damage and, in severe cases, cell death. Here's an overview of the mechanisms involved in ischemic cell injury.

Reduced ATP production: Intracellular oxygen levels drop, leading to a decline in oxidative phosphorylation and **reduced ATP production**. This ATP deficiency causes **initial reversible cell and organelle swelling and eventually cell death through necrosis**.

Hypoxia-inducible factor-1 (HIF-1): Cells have developed protective responses to cope with hypoxic stress. One of the key protective mechanisms is the induction of a transcription factor called hypoxia-inducible factor-1 (HIF-1). HIF-1 helps promote survival pathways, stimulate the formation of new blood vessels (angiogenesis), and enhance glycolysis, which is a less oxygen-dependent way of generating ATP.

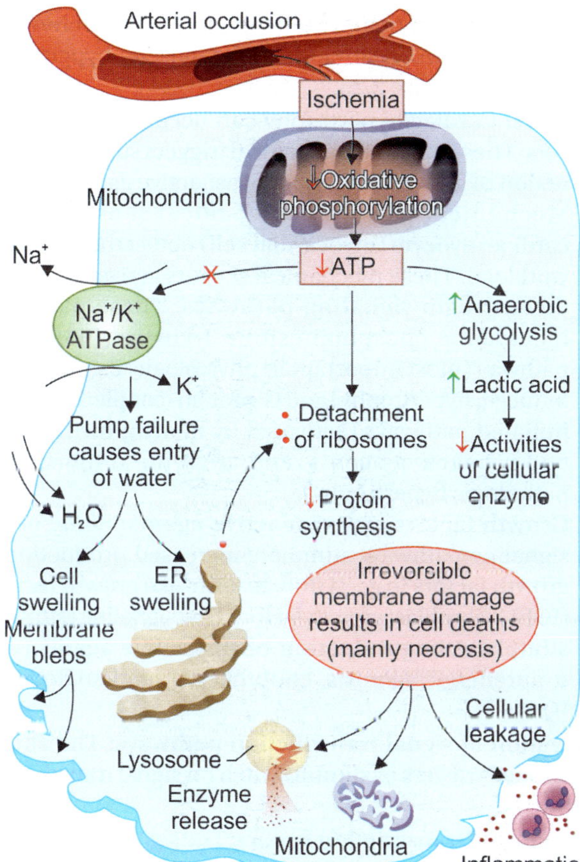

Fig. 2.21: Consequences of hypoxia and ischemia. It shows the functional and morphologic changes induced by hypoxia and ischemia.

Hypothermia: One of the most useful strategies in managing ischemic brain and spinal cord injuries is the induction of hypothermia. Lowering the core body temperature to around 92°F (33.5°C) can have several beneficial effects: reduces metabolic demands, decreases cell swelling, suppresses free radicals, and inhibits inflammatory response.

Ischemia-reperfusion Injury

Q. Write a short note on ischemia-reperfusion injury.

Ischemia-reperfusion injury is a **phenomenon that occurs when blood flow is restored to previously ischemic (lack of blood supply) but viable tissues.** It paradoxically results in increased cell injury and necrosis, rather than the expected recovery of reversibly injured cells. This paradoxical response can have significant clinical implications, particularly in cases of myocardial (heart) and cerebral (brain) ischemia.

Mechanism of reperfusion injury: Several mechanisms contribute to the exacerbation of cell injury during the reperfusion phase following ischemia:

- **Increased reactive oxygen species (ROS) production:** When blood flow is restored (reoxygenation) to ischemic tissues, there can be an excessive generation of ROS, such as superoxide radicals and hydrogen peroxide. This oxidative stress can further damage cells and tissues. **ROS produced by infiltrating leukocytes** may also contribute to the damage of vulnerable injured cells.
- **Calcium influx**: The influx of calcium ions into cells during reperfusion can cause injury. High levels of intracellular calcium can activate various enzymes and pathways that promote cell damage and cell death (*refer* **Fig. 2.18**).
- **Inflammation**: Ischemic injury triggers an inflammatory response, and this inflammation intensifies with reperfusion. Increased blood flow and oxygen supply can lead to the recruitment and activation of leukocytes in the affected tissues. These activated leukocytes release inflammatory mediators, such as cytokines and chemokines, which can contribute to additional tissue injury.
- **Activation of complement system**: The complement system is part of the immune system and plays a role in inflammation. During reperfusion, the complement system may also become activated, leading to the release of complement proteins that can contribute to tissue damage.

CELLULAR ADAPTATIONS TO STRESS

PA 2.6 (CC): Describe and discuss cellular adaptations: atrophy, hypertrophy, hyperplasia, metaplasia, and dysplasia (*refer* page 224).

Adaptation is a process of adjusting physiology, morphology, and behavior in response to new or altered circumstances. These circumstances may be internal and external in origin, in the physical and social environment. Cells adapt to their environment to escape and protect themselves from injury. An adapted cell is neither normal nor injured and its condition lies between these two states. Adaptive responses have limits and when stresses affects the essential cell function, it leads to cell injury.

Q. Write a short note on cellular adaptations.

When the cells are exposed to pathological stimuli (that may harm its normal structure and function), the cells can achieve a **new, steady altered state. This state allows them to survive** and continue to function in an abnormal environment. These **reversible changes** in the size, number, phenotype, metabolic activity or functions of cells in response to new or altered internal or external conditions or circumstances constitute **cellular adaptations.** The cellular response to persistent, sublethal stress reflects the cell's efforts to adapt. Cellular stress may be physiological or pathological. It may be either due to an increased functional demand or a reversible cellular injury. Physiologic adaptations develop in response to normal stimulation by hormones or endogenous chemical mediators (e.g., enlargement of the breast and uterus during pregnancy), or to the demands of mechanical stress (e.g., muscles). Pathologic adaptations occur to escape injury, but at the expense of normal function (e.g., squamous metaplasia of bronchial epithelium in smokers). Physiologic and pathologic adaptations can take several distinct forms. Types of adaptations are mentioned in **Box 2.1** and **Figure 2.1.**

Hypertrophy

Q. Write a short note on (definition, types/examples and mechanism) hypertrophy.

Definition: Increase in the size of the tissue or organ due to increase in the size of the parenchymal cells.

Causes (Box 2.6)

It is caused by increased functional demand/workload or by hormonal stimulation. **If the cause/stress is not relieved hypertrophy can progress to functionally significant cell injury.**

BOX 2.6: Causes of hypertrophy.

Physiological
- **Hypertrophy of skeletal muscle** (increased demand), e.g., the bulging muscles of body builders manual laborers, and athletes.
- **Hypertrophy of smooth muscle** (stimulation by hormones): e.g., growth of the uterus during pregnancy from estrogenic stimulation.

Pathological
- **Hypertrophy of cardiac muscle** (increased workload), e.g., left ventricular hypertrophy **(Figs. 2.22A to C)** due to hypertension or damaged valves (aortic stenosis/incompetence, mitral incompetence). In such cases, initially, hypertrophy improves function, but later this adaptation often fails and leads to heart failure.
- **Hypertrophy of smooth muscle:** Examples include
  - Hypertrophy of urinary bladder muscle in response to urethral obstruction [e.g., prostate hyperplasia **(Figs. 2.24A and B** and *refer* **Fig. 21.14)**]
  - Hypertrophy of the muscular layer of the stomach due to pyloric stenosis.

Mechanisms of Hypertrophy

Hypertrophy is due to increased synthesis of cellular proteins. Signals that elicit hypertrophic responses vary depending on the type of cell and circumstances. Understanding of mechanism of hypertrophy is based on studies of the heart. Steps involved in biochemical mechanisms of myocardial (cardiac muscle) hypertrophy are shown in **Figure 2.23**.

Triggers: Cardiac hypertrophy can occur in response to triggers. These include mechanical triggers such as stretch, the action of growth factors, and vasoactive agents.

- **Mechanical triggers:** Mechanical sensors in the cardiac myocyte (myocardial cell) detect the increased workload. These mechanical sensors activate complex downstream signaling pathways. These pathways include the phosphoinositide 3-kinase (PI3K)/AKT pathway (most important in physiologic, e.g., exercise-induced, hypertrophy) and G-protein-coupled receptor–initiated pathways (activated by many growth factors and vasoactive agents, and are more important in pathologic hypertrophy).
- **Growth factors and vasoactive agents:** Some of the signaling pathways stimulate increased production of growth factors [e.g., TGF-β, insulin-like growth factor 1 (IGF1), fibroblast growth factor]. Few signaling pathways stimulate the production of vasoactive agents (e.g., α-adrenergic agonists, endothelin-1, and angiotensin II).

Activation of signal transduction pathways: The above-mentioned triggers or stimuli switch on signal transduction pathways.

Activation of transcription factors: The signal transduction pathways activate transcription factors. These transcription factors include GATA4, nuclear factor of activated T cells (NFAT), and myocyte enhancer factor 2 (MEF2). These transcription factors induce the expression of genes that encode several cellular proteins.

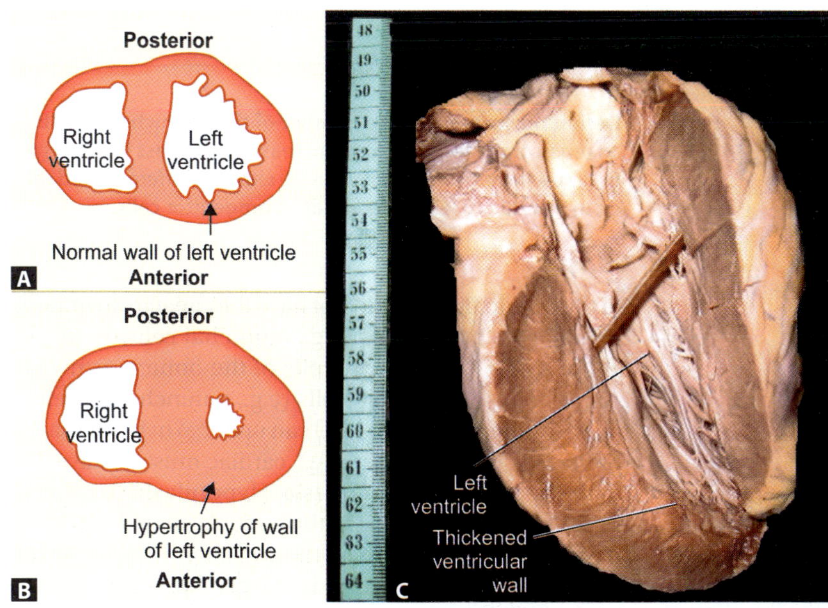

Figs. 2.22A to C: (A) Transverse section of normal heart; (B) Transverse section of heart with thickening of wall of the left ventricle due to hypertrophy; (C) Longitudinal section of heart with left ventricular hypertrophy.

Adaptations
Cellular stress may be physiological or pathological either due to an increased functional demand.

Cellular adaptations
- Hypertrophy
- Hyperplasia
- Atrophy
- Metaplasia

Hypertrophy
Increase in the size of the tissue or organ due to increase in the size of the parenchymal cells.

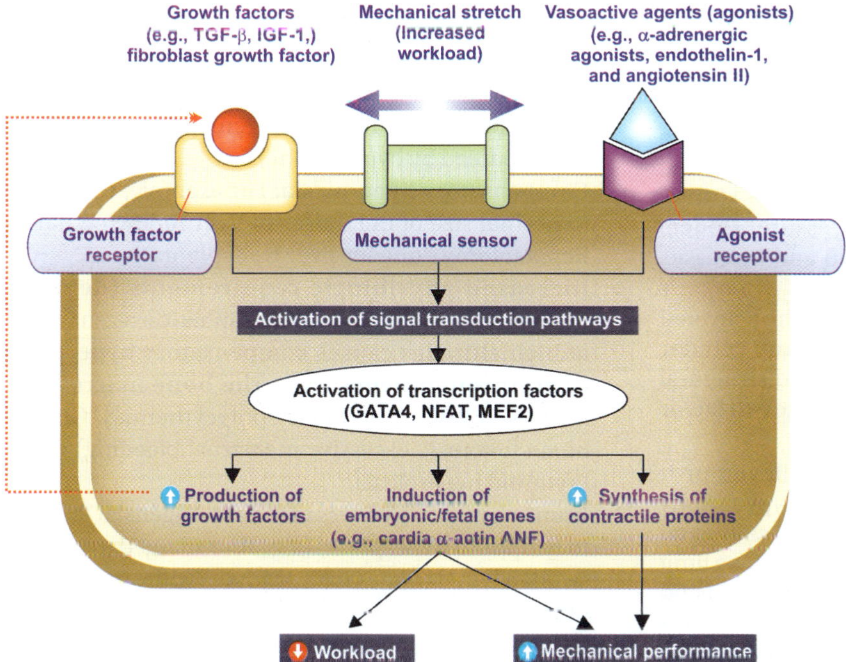

Fig. 2.23: Mechanisms of myocardial hypertrophy.
(ANF: atrial natriuretic factor; IGF-1: insulin-like growth factor; TGF-β: transforming growth factor-β)

In some organs both hypertrophy and hyperplasia may coexist (e.g., uterus during pregnancy).

Hypertrophied organ has no new cells, but has cells with increased size.

Physiological causes of hypertrophy
- Bulging muscles of body builders manual laborers, and athletes.
- Growth of the uterus during pregnancy from estrogenic.

Pathological causes of hypertrophy
Left ventricular hypertrophy due to hypertension or damaged valves (aortic stenosis/incompetence, mitral incompetence).
- Hypertrophy of urinary bladder muscle in response to urethral obstruction (e.g., prostate hyperplasia)
- Pyloric stenosis.

Consequences: These are as follows:
- **Increased synthesis of contractile proteins:** One result of the expression of genes is the synthesis of more proteins and myofilaments per cell. This increases the force generated with each contraction and makes the myocardial cell to meet increased work demand.
- **Induction of embryonic/fetal genes:** Some genes are normally expressed only during the early development of embryo and fetus. They are re-expressed in hypertrophied cells. Cardiac hypertrophy is also associated with a switch in gene expression from genes that encode adult-type contractile proteins to genes that encode fetal or neonatal forms. These fetal/neonatal are functionally distinct isoforms of the same adult proteins. For example, during hypertrophy, the α isoform of myosin myosin-heavy chain is replaced by the fetal β isoform of the myosin heavy chain. This β

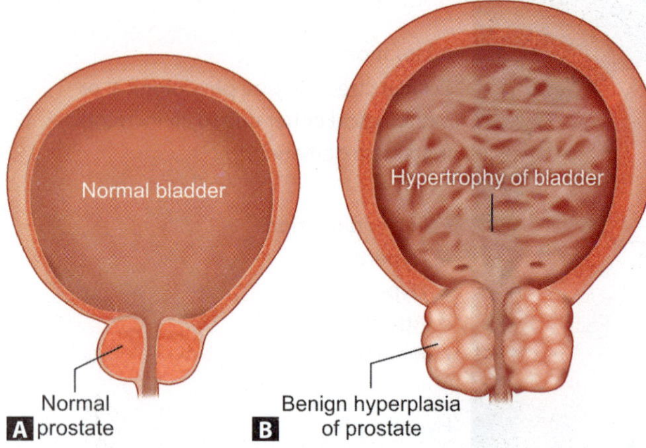

Figs. 2.24A and B: Cut section of prostate along with urinary bladder: (A) Normal prostate; (B) Enlarged prostate due to nodular hyperplasia. The urinary outflow obstruction results in hypertrophy of bladder muscle.

isoform produces a slower, more energetically efficient contraction.

Other proteins that are products of genes that participate in the cellular response to stress can also be altered in hypertrophic myocardial cells. For example, cardiac hypertrophy is associated with increased expression (re-expression) of the atrial natriuretic factor gene. Atrial natriuretic factor (ANF) is expressed in the embryonic heart, but not expressed after birth. ANF is a peptide hormone that causes salt secretion by the kidney and decreases blood volume and pressure. Hence, ANF reduces hemodynamic workload and increases mechanical performance.

- **Increased production of growth factors:** The activated genes also stimulate the synthesis of many cellular proteins. These include growth factors and structural proteins. **These growth factors stimulate growth factor receptors in cardiac myocytes.**

Regressive changes: If the stress is not relieved or it exceeds the adaptive capacity of the tissue hypertrophy can progress to cell injury. Whatever may be the cause and mechanism of cardiac hypertrophy, it finally reaches a limit beyond which enlargement of cardiac muscle mass is no longer able to cope with the increased burden. When this happens in the heart due to sustained hypertension, many regressive changes appear in the myocardial fibers. The most important change is the degradation, fragmentation and loss of myofibrillar contractile elements. In severe cases, myocytes undergo death. The result of these degenerative changes is dilation of the ventricle ultimately producing cardiac failure.

MORPHOLOGY

Gross

Involved **organ is enlarged.**

Microscopy

Increase in **size of the cells** as well as the **nuclei.**

Hyperplasia

Q. Write a short note on hyperplasia.

Definition: Increase in the number of the parenchymal cells in an organ or tissue, resulting in **increased size/mass of the organ or tissue.** Increase in number may be **either of differentiated cells or, in few due to less differentiated progenitor cells.**

Causes

All the cells in the body do not have the capacity to undergo hyperplasia. Labile cells (e.g., epithelial cells of the skin and mucous membranes, cells of the bone marrow and lymph nodes) and stable cells (e.g., parenchymal cells of the liver, adrenal, and thyroid) can undergo hyperplasia. But permanent cells (e.g., neurons, cardiac muscle) have little or no capability for hyperplasia. **Hyperplasia persists till the stimulus is present.** On the contrary, in neoplasia, the cells undergo proliferation with loss of growth-regulatory mechanism due to a change in the genetic composition of the affected cell.

Physiological hyperplasia: It occurs either due to hormonal stimulation or as compensatory process.

- **Hyperplasia due to hormones:** For example, hyperplasia of glandular epithelium of the **female breast at puberty, pregnancy and lactation**, hyperplasia of the uterus during pregnancy from estrogenic stimulation (also accompanied by hypertrophy).
- **Compensatory hyperplasia:** For example, restoration to normal size of the **donor in liver following partial hepatectomy done for liver transplantation.**
- **Increased physiologic requirements (demand-induced hyperplasia):** Low atmospheric oxygen tension at high altitudes causes compensatory **hyperplasia of erythroid precursors in the bone marrow** and increased RBCs (secondary polycythemia). Chronic blood loss (e.g., excessive menstrual bleeding) causes erythroid hyperplasia.
- **Immune responsiveness to many antigens:** It may lead to **lymphoid hyperplasia** (e.g., the enlarged tonsils and swollen lymph nodes in individuals with streptococcal pharyngitis).

Pathological hyperplasia: It occurs either due to **excess** endocrine stimulation or chronic injury/irritation.

- **Excessive hormonal stimulation** [e.g., **endometrial hyperplasia** (due to estrogen, *refer* **Figs. 22.15 and 22.16**)] and **benign prostatic hyperplasia** [due to androgens (**Figs. 2.24A and B** and *refer* **Figs. 21.12 and 21.13**)]. Enlargement of the male breast **(gynecomastia)** may occur in men with excess estrogens [e.g., following estrogen therapy for prostate cancer or in cirrhosis (liver is not capable of metabolizing endogenous estrogens and leads to their accumulation)].
- **Altered calcium metabolism in chronic renal failure:** It may lead to **parathyroid hyperplasia** to maintain blood levels of calcium.

- **Chronic injury/irritation:** Long-standing inflammation or chronic injury may lead to hyperplasia of affected areas especially in **skin or oral mucosa**.
- **Viral infections:** Certain viral infections, such as papillomaviruses cause skin warts and several mucosal lesions. These are accompanied by **hyperplasia of involved epithelium.**

Hyperplasia disappears if the signals that initiate it subsides. Pathological hyperplasia can progress to cancer, e.g., **endometrial hyperplasia can develop into endometrial cancer**.

Mechanism

- Hyperplasia is characterized by cell proliferation mostly of mature cell mediated **through stimulation by growth factor or hormones**.
- In some cases, the new cells may be derived from tissue **stem cells/less differentiated progenitor cells.**

MORPHOLOGY

Gross

Size of the affected organ is **increased**.

Microscopy

Increased number of cells with increased number of mitotic figures.

Atrophy

Q. Write a short note on atrophy.

Definition: Atrophy is the **reduced size of an organ or tissue** resulting from a decrease in the parenchymal cell size and number.

Causes

The atrophy of an organ differs from cellular atrophy. Reduced size of an organ may be due to reversible cell shrinkage or by irreversible loss of cells.

Physiological atrophy: Common in certain tissues during normal fetal development and in adult life.

- **During fetal development** (e.g., atrophy of embryonic structures such as **thyroglossal duct**).
- **During adult life:** It may be due to loss of endocrine stimulation or from senile arteriolosclerosis [e.g., involution of thymus, atrophy of **brain, gonads and heart** due to aging (senile atrophy)] and uterus after menopause.

Pathological atrophy: Local or generalized.

1. **Local**
   - **Disuse atrophy (decreased workload)** [e.g., atrophy of limb muscles immobilized in a plaster cast (as treatment for fracture) or after prolonged bed rest].
   - **Denervation (loss of innervation) atrophy** (e.g., loss of stimulatory signals leads to atrophy of muscle due to damage to the nerves (as in **poliomyelitis, motor neuron disease**).
   - **Ischemic (diminished blood supply)** *neuropathic atrophy* (e.g., brain atrophy produced by ischemia due to atherosclerosis of the carotid artery).
   - **Pressure atrophy:** Prolonged pressure in inappropriate locations may cause atrophy (e.g., atrophy of **renal parenchyma in hydronephrosis** due to increased pressure).
   - **Loss of endocrine stimulation** (e.g., **endometrium and breast** due to loss of hormonal signals **after menopause**).
   - **Absence of growth-stimulating (trophic) signals to maintain size and function:** For example, the adrenal cortex, thyroid, and gonads are maintained by trophic hormones from the **pituitary gland injury** (e.g., Sheehan syndrome) and undergo atrophy in their absence.
2. **Generalized: Starvation (inadequate nutrition) atrophy** [e.g., **severe acute malnutrition (SAM)**], leads to wasting (decreased mass) of skeletal muscle and adipose tissue.

Mechanisms

Atrophic cells have diminished function. Atrophy results from an imbalance in cellular protein pathway: (1) reduced synthesis and (2) increased degradation.

MORPHOLOGY

Gross

The **organ is small and often shrunken**.

Microscopy

The **cells are smaller in size** due to reduction in cell organelles. Such as mitochondria, myofilaments and endoplasmic reticulum. It is often accompanied by an increase in the number of autophagic vacuoles containing cell debris.

Q. List the differences between atrophy, hypertrophy and hyperplasia.

Differences between atrophy, hypertrophy and hyperplasia are listed in **Table 2.8.**

The term **hypoplasia** is used for the developmentally small size of an organ or tissue. **Aplasia** is the extreme failure of an organ or tissue development and shows only rudimentary tissue.

Metaplasia

Q. Write a short note on metaplasia (including types) with examples. What is its significance?

Definition: Metaplasia is a **reversible change** in which **one adult cell (differentiated) type (epithelial or mesenchymal) is replaced by another adult cell (differentiated)** type.

Some types of epithelial cells are more resistant than others to some insults. Thus, metaplasia is usually an adaptive response to persistent injury.

- Metaplasia is usually **fully reversible adaptive response** to **chronic persistent injury**. If the noxious stimulus is

TABLE 2.8 Differences between atrophy, hypertrophy and hyperplasia.

	Atrophy	*Hypertrophy*	*Hyperplasia*
Definition	Reduced size of an organ or tissue resulting from a decrease in cell size and number	Increase in the size of the tissue or organ due to increase in the size of cells	Increase in the size/mass of the organ or tissue due to increase in the number of cells
Size of the involved organ	Reduced	Increased/enlarged	Increased
Cells			
Number	Reduced	No change	Increased
Size	Reduced	Increased	No change
Organelles	Reduced	Increased	No change
Rate of cell division	–	–	Increased
Synthesis of DNA, RNA and protein	–	Increased	Increased

removed (e.g., cessation of smoking), the metaplastic epithelium may return to normal.

- Metaplasia is mainly **seen in association with tissue damage, repair and regeneration.**
- The **replacing cell type** is usually **more suited to a change in environment**. It usually occurs as an adaptation to persistent injury and the replacement cell type is better able to tolerate the injurious stimulation than the original cell type.

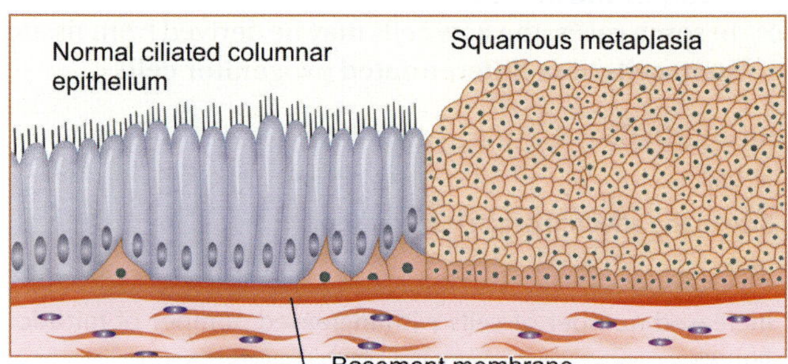

Fig. 2.25: Squamous metaplasia in which columnar epithelium (left) is replaced by squamous epithelium (right).

Types and Causes of Metaplasia

Metaplasia is divided into two types: (1) Epithelial and (2) Mesenchymal.

Epithelial Metaplasia

Epithelial metaplasia is of two types: squamous (more common) and columnar metaplasia.

Squamous metaplasia: Usually, squamous epithelium replaces chronically irritated, or stressed, glandular epithelium. In squamous metaplasia, the original epithelium is replaced by squamous epithelium. Metaplasia usually involves the replacement of glandular epithelium with squamous epithelium.

- **Respiratory tract** [e.g., chronic irritation due to tobacco smoke and vitamin A (retinoic acid) deficiency, the normal ciliated columnar epithelial cells of the trachea and bronchi undergo squamous metaplasia **(Fig. 2.25)**]. Though the squamous epithelial lining is more durable, important mechanisms of protection against infection of the columnar epithelium namely mucus secretion and the ciliary action are lost. Thus, in most situations, it is an undesirable change. If the stimulus that predispose to metaplasia persists, it can initiate malignant transformation in metaplastic epithelium.
- **Cervix:** Squamous metaplasia in cervix is associated with chronic infection in the endocervix.
- **Ducts with stones:** In different locations such as bile duct, pancreas, salivary glands, prostate which are normally lined by simple columnar epithelium undergo squamous metaplasia.
- **Renal pelvis and urinary bladder:** They are normally lined by urothelium. In chronic infection and stones, it may undergo squamous metaplasia. If the stimulus that predispose to metaplasia persists, it can initiate malignant transformation in metaplastic epithelium.

Columnar metaplasia: Original epithelium is replaced by columnar epithelium.

- **Squamous to columnar: In Barrett esophagus, the squamous epithelium of the esophagus replaced by columnar cells** (*refer* **Fig. 18.8**) due to chronic reflux of highly acidic gastric contents into the lower esophagus.
- **Intestinal metaplasia:** The gastric glands are replaced by cells resembling those of the small intestine.

Under persistent stress, metaplasia can progress to dysplasia and cancer (e.g., Barrett esophagus may progress to adenocarcinoma of the esophagus).

Connective Tissue Metaplasia

Osseous metaplasia: Formation of new bone at sites of tissue injury is known as osseous metaplasia. Bone formation in muscle, known as **myositis ossificans**, occasionally occurs after intramuscular hemorrhage. Other examples include cartilage of larynx and bronchi in elderly

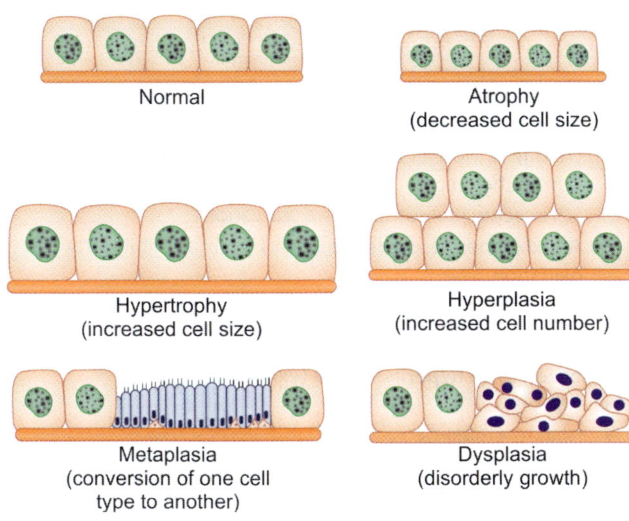

Fig. 2.26: Various types of cellular adaptations.

individual, scar of chronic inflammation of long duration, fibrous stroma of tumor (e.g., leiomyoma).

Mechanism

Develops due to the reprogramming of precursor cells (i.e., stem cells or undifferentiated mesenchymal cells) that are present in normal tissues. Metaplasia is usually fully reversible. If the noxious stimulus is removed.

Dysplasia is discussed on page 224.

Various types of cellular adaptations are diagrammatically shown in **Figure 2.26**.

INTRACELLULAR ACCUMULATIONS

PA 2.3 (CC): Intracellular accumulation of fats, proteins, carbohydrates, and pigments.

Metabolic derangements in cells may manifest as intracellular accumulation of abnormal amounts of various substances. The abnormal amounts of substances may accumulate either within the cytoplasm (within organelles especially lysosomes) or in the nucleus of the cell. These substances may be normal or abnormal, endogenous (synthesized by the affected cells) or exogenous (produced elsewhere), harmful (causing varying degrees of injury), or harmless (innocuous). Accumulation of the substance can cause reversible cell injury whereas more severe accumulation can lead to irreversible cell injury.

Mechanism of intracellular accumulation (Fig. 2.27): Four main pathways can lead to abnormal intracellular accumulations.

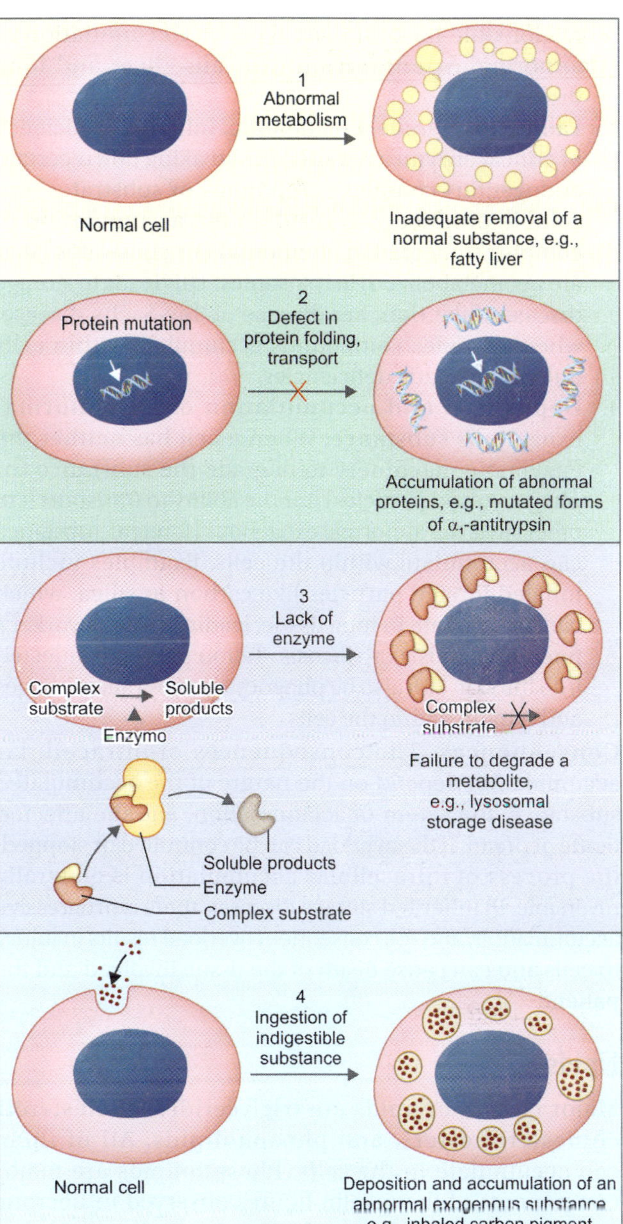

Fig. 2.27: Mechanisms of intracellular accumulation: (1) Due to abnormal metabolism (e.g., fatty change in the liver). (2) Mutations with alterations in protein folding and transport (e.g., mutated forms of α_1-antitrypsin), (3) A deficiency of critical enzymes (e.g., lysosomal storage diseases), (4) An inability to degrade phagocytosed particles (e.g., accumulation of carbon pigment, silica).

1. **Inadequate removal of a normal substance:** This may be secondary to defects in mechanisms of packaging and transport. For example, in the liver, abnormal metabolism of lipids can cause excessive accumulation of intracellular fat, known as fatty change or steatosis. It can occur due to abnormal lipid metabolism. It is often seen in conditions like alcoholic liver disease and nonalcoholic fatty liver disease (NAFLD) [currently termed metabolic-associated fatty liver disease (MAFLD)].
2. **Accumulation of an abnormal endogenous substance:** Genetic or acquired defects in the folding, packaging, transport, or secretion of an endogenous substance can lead to its accumulation. An example is the mutated forms of α_1-antitrypsin, a protein that inhibits enzymes

responsible for tissue breakdown. Accumulation of abnormal α_1-antitrypsin can cause liver and lung diseases.

3. **Failure to degrade a metabolite:** Inherited deficiency of critical enzymes required for breaking down certain endogenous complex compounds or substrates into soluble products can result in the accumulation of complex undegraded compounds or substrates (that are not metabolized) in lysosomes. This leads to storage diseases, like Gaucher disease or Tay-Sachs disease, where complex compounds accumulate within cells due to enzymatic deficiencies.
4. **Deposition and accumulation of an abnormal exogenous substance:** When a cell has neither the enzymatic machinery to degrade the substance (or phagocytosed particles) nor the ability to transport it to other sites, the abnormal exogenous (foreign) substance can accumulate within the cells. Examples include inhaled foreign particles like carbon or silica, which can accumulate in lung tissue, leading to coal worker's pneumoconiosis or silicosis. Tattoo pigments injected into the skin can also be phagocytosed by macrophages and remain within the cells.

Consequences: The consequences of intracellular accumulation depend on the nature of the accumulated substance, the extent of accumulation, and the affected tissue or organ. If the overload can be controlled or stopped, the process of intracellular accumulation is generally reversible. In inherited storage diseases, there is progressive accumulation, and the consequent overload results in injury to cells and can cause death of the tissue involved and the patient.

Lipids

Major classes of lipids are triglycerides, cholesterol/cholesterol esters, and phospholipids. All of them can accumulate in the cells. Phospholipids are major components of the myelin figures observed in necrotic cells. In addition to lipids, abnormal complexes of lipids and carbohydrates accumulate in the lysosomal storage diseases (*refer* pages 285-7).

Steatosis (Fatty Change)

Q. Write a short note on causes (etiology), pathogenesis, and morphology of fatty change/steatosis liver. Add a note on special stains for fat.

Definition: Steatosis is defined as the abnormal accumulation of triglycerides within the cytosol of the parenchymal cells. It is a manifestation of reversible cell injury.

Organs involved: Steatosis occurs in organs involved in fat metabolism namely the **liver**. It may also occur in the nonfatty organs such as the **heart, skeletal muscle, kidney** (lipoid nephrosis or minimal change disease), and other organs.

BOX 2.7: Causes of hepatic steatosis.

Disorders with hepatocyte damage
- **Alcoholic abuse:** Alcohol is the most common cause of fatty change in the liver and most of the fat deposited in the liver is from the diet.
- Sever acute malnutrition and starvation
- **Anoxia (anemia, cardiac failure):** Hypoxia inhibits fatty acid oxidation.
- Toxins (carbon tetrachloride, chloroform, etc.)
- Reye syndrome.

Disorders with hyperlipidemia (excess fat)
- Obesity
- Diabetes mellitus
- Congenital hyperlipidemia.

Fatty Liver

The liver is the most common site for steatosis because it plays a key role in fat metabolism. Depending upon the cause and amount of fat accumulation, steatosis may be mild and reversible, or severe producing irreversible cell injury and cell death.

Causes: The causes of steatosis of the liver are listed in **Box 2.7.**

Normal Fat Metabolism (Fig. 2.28)

Sources of free fatty acid: Normal hepatocytes contain some **amount of fat.** It is derived from the following sources:
- **From adipose tissue:** Free fatty acids released from adipose tissue.
- **From diet:** The dietary fat (chylomicrons and free fatty acids) absorbed from the GI tract enter the liver as free fatty acids.
- **From acetate in liver cells:** A **small quantity of fatty acids** is also synthesized **from acetate in the liver cells.**

Metabolism of free fatty acids in the liver: Free fatty acids are metabolized as follows:
- **Formation of triglycerides: Most free fatty acid is esterified to triglycerides** by the action of α-glycerophosphate.
- **Conversion into cholesterol, phospholipids, and ketone bodies: A small part of free fatty acid in the liver is converted into cholesterol, phospholipids, and ketone bodies**. The cholesterol, phospholipids, and ketones are used in the body.

Formation of lipoproteins: Most of the newly synthesized triglycerides are converted **into** lipoproteins, which require 'lipid acceptor protein'. Lipoproteins are secreted from the liver cells into circulation as plasma lipoproteins (**mainly chylomicrons and very low-density lipoprotein or VLDL**).

Pathogenesis of Fatty Liver

Various mechanisms are involved in the excess accumulation of triglyceride in the liver and one or more mechanisms may be responsible for steatosis of the liver.

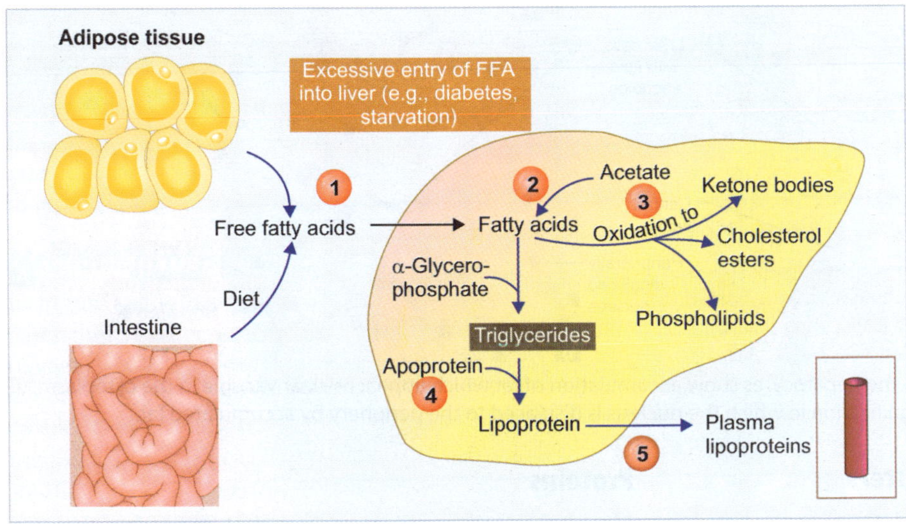

Fig. 2.28: Metabolism of lipids in the liver and various mechanisms that can produce accumulation of triglycerides in fatty liver.

Alcohol is the most common cause of steatosis of liver.

Special stains for fat
1. Sudan IV
2. Oil red O
3. Osmic acid
4. Sudan black

Organs involved in steatosis
- Liver
- Heart
- Skeletal muscle
- Kidney in lipoid nephrosis

1. **Excessive entry of free fatty acids (FFA) into the liver (1 in Fig. 2.28):** From peripheral stores FFA enters into the liver during **starvation and diabetes**.
2. **Defective metabolism of lipids:** This may be due to:
   - **Increased synthesis of fatty acids from acetate by liver (2 in Fig. 2.28).**
   - **Decreased oxidation of fatty acids into ketone bodies (3 in Fig. 2.28)** resulting in increased esterification of fatty acids into triglycerides.
   - **Decreased synthesis of apoproteins** (e.g., in CCl_4 **and protein malnutrition)** causes decreased formation of lipoproteins from triglycerides **(4 in Fig. 2.28)**.
3. **Defective excretion of lipoproteins:** A fatty liver may also develop due to a defect in the excretion of lipoproteins from the liver into the blood **(5 in Fig. 2.28).**

Mechanism of steatosis in alcoholic abuse: These are as follows:- Ethanol (1) increases lipolysis and thus delivers free fatty acids to the liver; (2) increases the synthesis of fatty acids, (3) decreases mitochondrial oxidation of fatty acids to ketone bodies, (4) raises triglyceride production, and (5) impairs the release of lipoproteins. All these metabolic consequences produce a fatty liver in alcohol abuse.

MORPHOLOGY

Q. Write a short note on gross and microscopy of fatty liver.

Fatty Liver

Gross (Fig. 2.29): Liver is enlarged with rounded margins. It is yellow, soft, and greasy to the touch.

Microscopy: Characteristically, **hepatocytes show numerous lipid vacuoles in the cytoplasm.** This is because, in the H & E stained section prepared by the paraffin-embedding technique, fat is dissolved in organic solvents (e.g., xylene/xylol) and appears as vacuoles.

- **Microvesicular steatosis:** Initially, fat is seen as small vacuoles in the cytoplasm around the nucleus (*refer* **Fig. 19.17A**).
- **Macrovesicular steatosis:** Later, as the process progresses, the vacuoles become larger. These vacuoles coalesce, creating clear spaces that displace the nucleus to the periphery of the cell (**Figs. 2.30A and B** and *refer* **Fig. 19.17B**). This gives a signet ring appearance and this should not be mistaken for signet ring cells seen in signet ring carcinoma (*refer* **Fig. 18.19**). the vacuoles pushing the nucleus to the periphery of the cell.
- **Special stains for fat:** Fat can be demonstrated in fresh unfixed tissue by frozen sections stained by fat stains. **Sudan IV or Oil Red-O** stains give an **orange-red color** to the fat. **Osmic acid** (is a fixative as well as a stain) and **Sudan black B** give a **black color.**

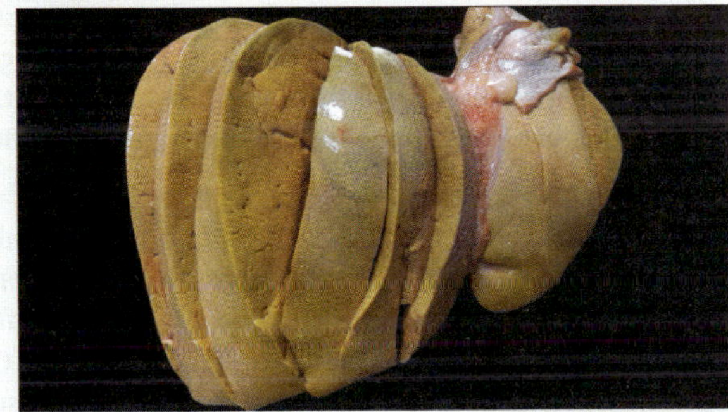

Fig. 2.29: Fatty liver showing liver with yellow color and sharp border.

Heart

Q. Write a short note on the heart in fatty change.

Lipid in the cardiac muscle can have **two patterns**:

1. **Alternate involvement:** Prolonged moderate hypoxia (e.g., severe anemia), creates grossly apparent bands of involved **yellow myocardium alternating with bands of darker, red-brown, uninvolved myocardium (tigered effect, tabby cat appearance).**
2. **Uniform involvement:** More severe hypoxia or some types of myocarditis (e.g., diphtheria infection) show more **uniform involvement of myocardial fibers.**

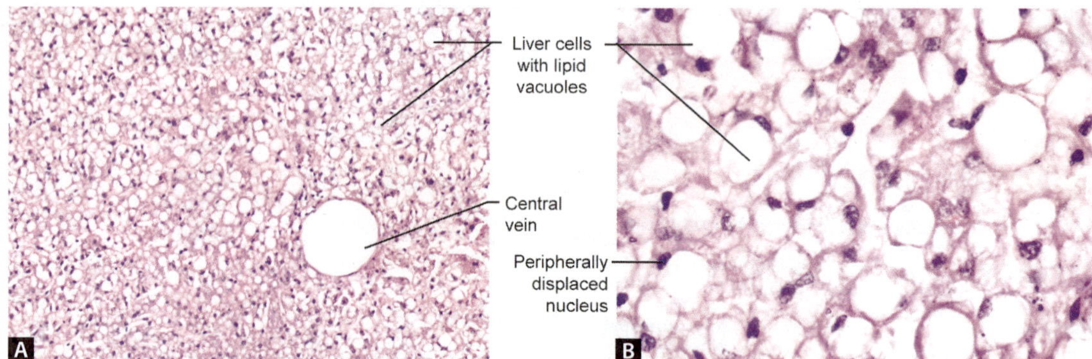

Figs. 2.30A and B: (A) Fatty liver in which the hepatocytes show accumulation of fat which appear as clear vacuole in the cytoplasm; (B) Hepatocytes at higher magnification in which the nucleus is displaced to the periphery by accumulated fat.

Cholesterol and Cholesterol Esters

Cholesterol is a double-edged sword. On the one hand, it is a critical component of all plasma membranes, where it plays a crucial role in maintaining membrane fluidity and integrity and is a precursor in steroidogenesis. On the other hand, its storage in excess is associated with atherosclerosis. Cellular cholesterol metabolism in cells is tightly regulated to ensure that there is a balanced synthesis and catabolism of cholesterol without significant intracellular accumulation. However, in pathological conditions, phagocytic cells may intracellularly accumulate lipids (triglycerides, cholesterol, and cholesteryl esters). It may be either due to increased intake or decreased catabolism of lipids. These pathological conditions are briefly discussed below.

Atherosclerosis: It is a disease of the **aorta and large arteries** characterized by the presence of **atherosclerotic plaques composed of smooth muscle cells and macrophages within the intima filled with lipid vacuoles. Most of the lipid is cholesterol and cholesterol esters** (*refer* **page 480**).

Q. Write a short note on xanthoma.

Xanthoma: It is a condition characterized by the **intracellular accumulation of cholesterol within macrophages** and leads to the **formation of tumor-like masses.** These xanthomas are often found in the subepithelial connective tissue of the skin and tendons producing tumorous masses. They **result from both acquired and hereditary hyperlipidemic states.** Microscopically, it consists of clusters of foamy cells in the subepithelial connective tissue of the skin and tendons.

Cholesterolosis: It is characterized by the **focal accumulation of cholesterol-laden macrophages in the lamina propria of the gallbladder.** The exact mechanism leading to cholesterolosis is not well understood is not known.

Niemann–Pick disease, type C: It is a genetic lysosomal storage disorder caused by mutations affecting an enzyme involved in cholesterol trafficking within the body. It is characterized by abnormal **accumulation of cholesterol in** various **organs.**

Proteins

Morphologically visible protein pathologic accumulation of protein can occur within the cells. It is less common than lipid accumulations.

Light microscopy: The intracellular accumulations of proteins appear as **rounded, eosinophilic droplets, vacuoles, or aggregates in the cytoplasm.**

Electron microscopy: The protein can appear as amorphous, fibrillar, or crystalline structures.

Causes of Intracellular Accumulation of Proteins

Excesses of morphologically visible accumulation of proteins within the cells (intracellular) may occur either because of **increased uptake or increased synthesis.** Examples are as follows:

Increased Uptake of Proteins

Reabsorption protein in proximal renal tubules: It occurs in **renal diseases associated with loss of protein in the urine** (proteinuria). In the kidney, normally, trace (small) amounts of protein (albumin) filtered through the glomerulus are reabsorbed in the proximal convoluted tubule by a process called pinocytosis. However, when there is heavy protein leakage (e.g., nephrotic syndrome) through the glomerulus, there is increased (excessive) reabsorption of the protein into vesicles. These vesicles containing this protein appear microscopically as pink hyaline droplets within the cytoplasm of the tubular epithelial cells. The process is reversible and with the control of proteinuria, the protein droplets are metabolized and disappear from the cell.

Excessive Synthesis or Accumulation of Proteins

- **Russell bodies:** Plasma cells synthesize immunoglobulins (a type of proteins). Whenever the plasma cells newly synthesize excessive amounts of **immunoglobulins** they can accumulate within the rough endoplasmic reticulum (RER) present in the cytoplasm of some plasma cells. The RER becomes distended with immunoglobulins and produces large, round, homogeneous eosinophilic (pink hyaline) inclusions called Russell bodies **(Fig. 2.33B)**.

- **Defective intracellular transport and secretion of critical proteins:** α_1-antitrypsin deficiency is a heritable disorder in which, mutations in the gene coding for α_1-antitrypsin yield an insoluble protein. The protein produced is significantly slow in the folding process and is not easily exported/secreted from the cells. This results in the accumulation of partially folded intermediates which aggregate in the ER of the cytoplasm of the liver cells and appear as eosinophilic globular deposits of a mutant protein. This results in the deficiency of the circulating enzyme and there is excessive digestion of elastic tissues which produces emphysema (*refer* page 548 of Chapter 17). In many of these diseases, the damage is not only due to the loss of protein function but also due to ER stress caused by the misfolded proteins.
- **Accumulation of cytoskeletal proteins**: The internal framework of a cell is composed of protein filaments known as cytoskeletal proteins. They provide structural support to the cells and drive the movement of the cell. There are several types of cytoskeletal proteins and are usually divided into three categories namely microfilaments [thin actin filaments (6–8 nm), thick myosin filaments (15 nm)], intermediate (10 nm) filaments and microtubules (20–25 nm in diameter), depending on the diameter and the composition of filaments. The intermediate filaments provide a flexible intracellular scaffold that organizes the cytoplasm and resists forces applied to the cell. The intermediate filaments are subdivided into five classes: (i) keratin filaments (characteristic of epithelial cells), (ii) neurofilaments (neurons), (iii) desmin filaments (muscle cells), (iv) vimentin filaments (connective tissue cells), and (v) glial filaments (astrocytes). Accumulations of keratin filaments and neurofilaments are observed in certain types of cell injury.
  - **Mallory's body or alcoholic hyaline** (*refer* **Fig. 2.33A and page 669): ** It is an eosinophilic cytoplasmic inclusion seen in liver cells and is characteristic of **alcoholic liver disease**. It appears as amorphous pink masses. They represent the intracellular accumulation of intermediate filaments of keratin (cytokeratin).
  - **Neurofibrillary tangle (tau protein):** It is found in cortical neurons of the brain of patients with **Alzheimer disease** and consists of neurofilaments and other proteins.
- **Aggregation of abnormal proteins:** Abnormal or misfolded proteins may aggregate and get deposited in tissues and interfere with their normal functions.

Intracellular or extracellular: The protein deposits may be intracellular, extracellular, or both. These aggregates of proteins may either directly or indirectly cause the pathologic changes.

- **Intracellular accumulation of misfolded proteins:** It may be due to either increased production of the misfolded proteins or reduced ability to eliminate them.
  - **Prion diseases**: These are neurodegenerative disorders (spongiform encephalopathies) caused by the accumulation of abnormally folded prion proteins. Abnormal prion proteins may be due to either inherited mutations or exposure to the aberrant form of the protein.
  - **Lewy bodies (α-synuclein):** They are observed in neurons of the substantia nigra of patients with Parkinson disease.
- **Extracellular accumulation of proteins:** Apart from abnormal intracellular accumulation, abnormal protein deposits can occur primarily in extracellular spaces in some disorders, such as certain forms of amyloidosis (*refer* pages 209-11).

Glycogen

Glycogen is a long-chain polymer of glucose. It is formed and mainly stored in the cytoplasm of the liver and to a lesser extent in muscles. Glycogen is a readily available energy source and when needed is depolymerized to glucose in a stepwise manner by a series of enzymes. These enzymes may be inactivated by mutation.

Causes

Excessive intracellular deposits/accumulation of glycogen can occur due to an abnormality in either glucose or glycogen metabolism.

Glycogen storage disease: Glycogen is degraded in steps by a series of enzymes. Deficient of any enzymes involved in any of these steps may be observed as an inborn (genetic) error of metabolism called a glycogen storage disease or glycogenosis.

Diabetes mellitus: Storage of glycogen in cells is normally regulated by blood glucose levels, and hyperglycemic states are associated with increased glycogen stores. Thus, in uncontrolled diabetes mellitus (a disorder of glucose metabolism) there is impaired cellular uptake of glucose, which results in high serum and urine glucose levels. It is accompanied by excessive accumulation of glycogen in hepatocytes, epithelial cells of the renal proximal tubules (renal tubules reabsorb the excess filtered glucose and store it intracellularly as glycogen), β-cells of the islets of Langerhans, and cardiac muscle cells.

MORPHOLOGY

Microscopy: In routine H & E stained sections, glycogen appears as **clear vacuoles within the cytoplasm** of the affected cells. Glycogen gets dissolved in aqueous fixatives and appears as vacuoles in the cytoplasm. Hence, **for its identification, tissues should be fixed in absolute alcohol.**

Special stains for glycogen: These include **Best's carmine or the periodic acid-Schiff (PAS)** which gives a **rose-to-violet color to the glycogen.** Diastase digestion of a parallel section before staining serves as a further control by hydrolyzing the glycogen.

Pigments

Q. Write a short note on various (exogenous and endogenous) pigments.

Definition: Pigments are **colored substances.** They are either **normal** constituents of cells (e.g., melanin), **or are abnormal** (e.g., carbon) and accumulate in cells.

Types of pigments (Table 2.9): Pigments may be exogenous (coming from outside the body), or endogenous (produced within the body itself).

Endogenous Pigments

Endogenous pigments are either normal constituents of cells or accumulate under special circumstances.

Melanin

Melanin is an endogenous, brown-black, nonhemoglobin-derived pigment. It is produced by the melanocytes and dendritic cells by the oxidation of tyrosine to dihydroxyphenylalanine by the enzyme tyrosinase. It is stored as cytoplasmic granules in the phagocytic cells namely melanophores. Normally, it is present in the **hair, skin, mucosa at some places, choroid of the eye, meninges, and adrenal medulla.** Various disorders of melanin pigmentation produce generalized and localized hyperpigmentation and hypopigmentation **(Table 2.10).**

Hemoglobin-derived Pigments

These are the **most important endogenous pigments.** These pigments are **hemosiderin, acid hematin (hemozoin), bilirubin, and porphyrins.**

Hemosiderin

Q. Write a short note on hemosiderin and hemosiderosis.

TABLE 2.9 Different types of pigments.

Endogenous pigments	*Exogenous pigments*
Melanin	• Carbon (anthracotic)
Hemoglobin derived pigments • Hemosiderin • Hematin (hemozoin) • Bilirubin • Porphyrins	• Tattooing • Arsenic • β-carotene
Lipofuscin (Wear and tear pigment)	
Melanin-like pigment: Seen in • Alkaptonuria • Dubin-Johnson syndrome	

TABLE 2.10 Causes of hyper- and hypopigmentation.

Generalized hyperpigmentation	*Generalized hypopigmentation*
1. **Addison's disease** 2. **Chloasma:** Hyperpigmentation on the skin of face, nipples, and genitalia during pregnancy 3. **Chronic arsenical poisoning** (raindrop pigmentation of the skin)	**Albinism:** Generalized hypopigmentation due to genetic deficiency of tyrosinase enzyme
Focal hyperpigmentation	***Localized hypopigmentation***
1. **Cäfe-au-lait spots** in neurofibromatosis and Albright's syndrome 2. **Peutz–Jeghers syndrome:** Focal perioral pigmentation 3. **Melanosis coli:** Pigmentation of the mucosa of the colon 4. **Tumors of melanocytes:** Benign (nevi) and malignant (melanoma) tumors 5. **Lentigo:** Premalignant condition	1. **Leukoderma:** Autoimmune disorder with localized loss of pigmentation of the skin 2. **Vitiligo:** Local hypopigmentation of the skin 3. **Acquired focal hypopigmentation:** Leprosy, healing of wounds, DLE, radiation dermatitis, pityriasis alba, pityriasis versicolor, idiopathic guttate hypomelanosis, etc.

Definition: Hemosiderin is a **hemoglobin-derived, golden yellow-to-brown, granular, or crystalline pigment** and is one of the major storage forms of iron. It is a degradation product of ferritin.

Causes: Local or systemic excess of iron causes hemosiderin to accumulate within cells.

- **Local excesses:**
  - **Bruise**
  - **Brown induration of the lung** in chronic venous congestion of the lung (*refer* **Fig. 5.7**).
- **Systemic excesses: Systemic overload of iron** is known as **hemosiderosis.** The main causes:
  - **Increased absorption of dietary iron.**
  - **Excessive destruction of red cells** (e.g., hemolytic anemias).
  - **Repeated blood transfusions.**

MORPHOLOGY

Site of Accumulation

Localized: Found in the **macrophages** of the involved area.

Systemic: Initially found in the **liver, bone marrow, spleen, and lymph nodes.** Later deposited in macrophages of other organs (e.g., skin, pancreas, kidney).

Microscopy: Appears as a **coarse, golden, granular pigment within the cytoplasm (within lysosome).**

Special stain for hemosiderin: Prussian blue (Perl's stain) histochemical reaction in which hemosiderin converts colorless potassium ferrocyanide to **blue-black** ferric ferrocyanide **(Fig. 2.31).**

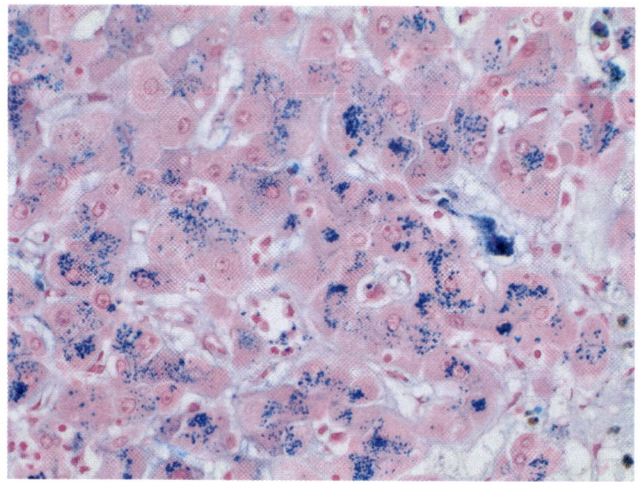

Fig. 2.31: Perl's stain. Liver with hemosiderin (blue) deposits.

Hemochromatosis: Severe accumulation of iron is associated with damage to the liver, heart, and pancreas. The triad of **cirrhosis of the liver, diabetes mellitus** (due to pancreatic damage), **and brown pigmentation of the skin** constitute **bronze diabetes.**

Hematin (hemazoin)

Hematin (hemazoin) is a brown-black pigment and is also known as a **malarial pigment.** It contains heme iron in ferric form in an acidic medium. It **does not stain positive by Prussian blue (Perl's) reaction,** probably because it forms a complex with a protein and is unable to react in the stain. Hematin pigment is seen commonly in **chronic malaria and mismatched blood transfusions.** It can be deposited in macrophages and in the hepatocytes.

Formalin pigment is formed in blood-rich tissues that are preserved in an acidic formalin solution.

Bilirubin is the normal major pigment found in bile. It is a **noniron-containing pigment derived from hemoglobin.**

Porphyrins are normal pigments **present in hemoglobin, myoglobin, and cytochrome.**

Lipofuscin

Q. Write a short note on lipofuscin and brown atrophy of the heart.

Lipofuscin (lipochrome) is an **insoluble, golden-brown, endogenous, intracellular pigment.** It is also called **lipochrome or "wear and tear pigment."**

Appearance: Microscopically, it appears as a **yellow brown** (brownish-yellow), **finely granular cytoplasmic pigment,** often present in the **perinuclear region.** When present in large amounts, it gives a brown appearance to the atrophic tissue, particularly the heart, which is called *brown atrophy.*

Tissues involved: It accumulates in various tissues undergoing slow, regressive changes. It is particularly prominent in the **heart (often called brown atrophy of the heart), liver, and brain** as a function of age or atrophy. It is seen in aging patients (old age), severe malnutrition, and cancer cachexia.

Composition: It is composed of a **mixture of lipids, phospholipids, and proteins. It is accumulated by accretion (a gradual increase) of peroxidized unsaturated lipids and oxidized cross-linked proteins.** The term lipofuscin is derived from the Latin word (*fuscus*, brown), and refers to brown lipid.

Significance: It **indicates a product of past free radical injury** and is derived through lipid peroxidation. Lipofuscin does not injure cells or their functions.

Alkaptonuria

Q. Write a short answer on ochronosis.

Homogentisic acid is a pathological black pigment formed in a rare metabolic autosomal recessive disorder termed alkaptonuria. It is characterized by a deficiency of an oxidase enzyme needed for the breakdown of homogentisic acid. This leads to the accumulation of homogentisic acid **pigment in the skin, connective tissue, cartilage, capsules of joints, ligaments, and tendons.** The pigment is melanin-like and the pigmentation is known as **ochronosis.** The homogentisic acid is excreted in the urine (homogentisic aciduria). The **urine** of patients of alkaptonuria, **if allowed to stand for some hours in the air, turns black** due to oxidation of homogentisic acid.

Exogenous Pigments

Carbon (coal dust): It is the most common exogenous pigment that is present as an air pollutant in urban regions. After inhalation, it is phagocytosed by macrophages present in the alveoli. These macrophages transport the pigment to regional tracheobronchial lymph nodes through lymphatic channels. Accumulation of the carbon pigment blackens the draining lymph nodes and lung parenchyma *(anthracosis).* In coal miners, the aggregates of carbon dust may elicit a fibroblastic reaction or produce emphysema. The lung disease is termed a *coal worker's pneumoconiosis.*

Tattooing: It is a form of localized, exogenous pigmentation of the skin. The pigments inoculated into the skin are phagocytosed by dermal macrophages. These macrophages remain at the site of inoculation for the rest of the lives of these individuals. The pigments usually do not elicit any inflammatory response.

Pigmentation of the liver may be caused by: (1) lipofuscin, (2) malaria pigment, (3) Wilson disease, (4) bile pigment, and (5) pseudomelanin.

Commonly used histochemistry (special stains) in histopathology are listed in **Table 2.11**.

Q. Write a short note on commonly used histochemistry (special stains) in histopathology.

TABLE 2.11 Commonly used special stains in histopathology.

Stain	*Substance*	*Interpretation*
Amyloid		
Congo-red under a polarizing microscope	Amyloid	Apple green birefringence
Carbohydrates		
Periodic acid-Schiff (PAS)	Glycogen, mucin, mucoprotein, glycoprotein, fungi, basement membranes of glomeruli and tubules	Magenta color
Mucicarmine/Best's carmine	Epithelial mucin, encapsulated fungi (cryptococcus)	Red color
Alcian blue	Acid mucin	Blue
Lipids		
Sudan III	Lipid	Orange
Oil Red O		Red
Osmium tetroxide		Brown black
Connective tissue		
Van Gieson	Extracellular collagen	Red
Masson's trichrome	Collagen, smooth muscle	Collagen-blue, smooth muscle-red
Phosphotungstic acid hematoxylin (PTAH)	Cross striation of skeletal muscles, glial filaments, fibrin	Dark blue
Verhoeff's elastic	Elastic fibers	Black
Microorganisms		
Gram's stain	Bacteria	Gram +ve = blue Gram –ve = red
Ziehl-Neelsen's (acid-fast) stain	Tubercle bacilli and other acid-fast organisms	Red
Fite-Faraco	Lepra bacilli	Red
Silver methenamine	Fungi	Black
Pigments and minerals		
Prussian blue stain (Perl's stain)	Hemosiderin	Blue
Masson Fontana	Melanin	Black
Von Kossa	Calcium	Black
Alzarine Red S	Calcium	Orange red
Rubeanic acid	Copper	Greenish-black

EXTRACELLULAR DEPOSITS: PATHOLOGIC CALCIFICATION

PA 2.5 (CC): Describe and discuss pathologic calcifications, gangrene (*refer* pages 21-2).

Q. Write a short note on pathologic calcification.

Calcification is the **deposition of calcium salt** and is a normal physiologic process during bone maturation and enamel formation. Pathologic calcification is the abnormal deposition of calcium salt and occurs in a wide variety of disease states.

Definition: Pathologic calcification is an **abnormal deposition of calcium salts in tissues other than osteoid or enamel.** It is also associated with the deposition of small amounts of iron, magnesium, and other minerals.

Types of pathologic calcification: It occurs in two ways namely **(1) dystrophic and (2) metastatic.**

Dystrophic Calcification

Q. Write a short note on dystrophic calcification.

In this type, **deposition of calcium salts** occurs locally **in injured or dead tissues, such as areas of necrosis of any type**.

Causes

In this type, **calcium metabolism is normal**. After cell injury, calcium from the blood leaves into the interstitial fluids and deposits extracellularly in injured tissues:

- **Necrotic tissue of any type:** Calcification occurs in **caseous, coagulative, liquefactive, enzymatic fat necrosis.** It also occurs in **dead eggs** of *Schistosoma*, cysticercosis, and hydatid cysts.
- **Advanced atherosclerosis:** Central necrotic core of advanced *atheromatous plaques* in the aorta and coronaries.
- **Heart valves:** Calcification can occur **in aging or damaged heart valves.**

Q. Write a short answer on Monckeberg's medial calcific sclerosis.

- **Monckeberg's medial calcific sclerosis:** Calcification in the **media of the muscular arteries (Fig. 2.32A)** in **old people**.
- **Psammoma bodies: Single necrotic cells on which several layers of mineral get deposited progressively to create a lamellated shape** called **psammoma bodies (Fig. 2.32B).**
- **Goiter of thyroid**
- **Gamna-Gandy bodies (*refer* to Fig. 5.11C):** They occur in **chronic venous congestion (CVC) of the spleen.** They appear as calcified deposits admixed with hemosiderin on fibrous tissue.

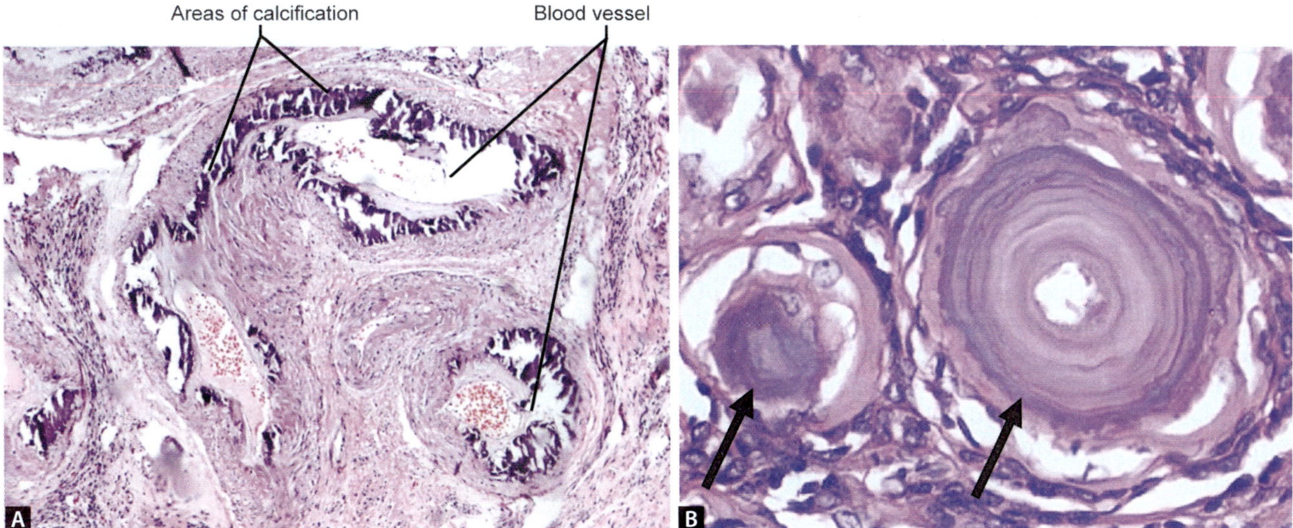

Figs. 2.32A and B: (A) Monckeberg's medial calcific sclerosis in which the tunica media of arteries in the myometrium of the uterus show calcification. The lumen of these vessels is not narrowed; (B) Meningioma with psammoma bodies (arrows).

- **Others**: **Dense old scars, and cysts (e.g., epidermal and pilar cysts of skin).**
- **Calcinosis cutis**: Shows irregular nodular **deposits of calcium salts in the skin and subcutaneous tissue**.

Dystrophic calcification develops slowly. This phenomenon can serve as a definite marker for areas of cell death (the site of dead cells) and is often used in diagnostic radiography for various medical conditions. For example, **mammography is based mainly on the detection of small calcifications in breast cancers; congenital toxoplasmosis,** an infection involving the central nervous system, is suggested when calcification is seen in an infant's brain.

Mechanism (*refer* online Flowchart 2.2): The exact pathogenic mechanisms responsible for dystrophic calcification are unknown.

MORPHOLOGY

Gross: The calcium salts appear as **fine, white granules or clumps.** They are often felt as gritty deposits.

Microscopy (Figs. 2.32A and B): Under the H&E stain, calcium salts appear as **basophilic, amorphous granular**, sometimes clumped material. They may be intracellular, extracellular, or seen in both locations. **Over time**, the calcified focus may form **heterotopic bone.**

Q. Write a short note on psammoma bodies.

Psammoma bodies: These are dystrophic calcifications, in which a **single necrotic cell** may constitute seed crystals that may become **surrounded by several layers of mineral (calcium) deposits.** The progressive accumulation of outer layers may create lamellated configurations. These are termed **psammoma bodies** because they resemble grains of sand. **Some papillary cancers (e.g., papillary carcinoma of the thyroid, serous papillary carcinoma of the ovary, papillary carcinoma of the kidney), and meningioma** are likely to develop psammoma bodies.

Asbestos bodies: In asbestosis, calcium and iron salts can be deposited surrounding long slender spicules of asbestos in the lung. This produces beaded **dumbbell-shaped structures** termed as asbestos bodies (*Refer* **to Figs. 17.26 and 17.27**).

Special stains for calcium: The calcium deposits appear black in the **silver impregnation method of von-Kossa**, and appear red in *alizarin red S*.

Significance of dystrophic calcification: It may be a sign of previous cell injury. However, it often causes organ dysfunction (e.g., in calcific valvular disease, atherosclerosis).

Metastatic Calcification

Q. Write a short note on metastatic calcification.

It is the **deposition of calcium salts in** apparently **normal tissues.** It is **associated with hypercalcemia secondary to deranged calcium metabolism.**

Causes of Hypercalcemia

Q. Write a short answer on the causes of metastatic calcification.

- **Increased secretion of parathyroid hormone (PTH):** It occurs in hyperparathyroidism due to parathyroid tumors and ectopic secretion of PTH-related protein by malignant tumors. PTH causes bone resorption and hypercalcemia.
- **Destruction (resorption) of bone tissue:** It may occur secondary to primary tumors of bone marrow (e.g., multiple myeloma, leukemia), diffuse metastasis to bone (e.g., carcinoma of breast), increased bone turnover (e.g., Paget disease), or immobilization.
- **Vitamin D-related disorders,** e.g., vitamin D intoxication and sarcoidosis (macrophages activate a vitamin D precursor).

- **Renal failure:** Causes retention of phosphate, leading to secondary hyperparathyroidism.
- **Less common causes:** These include aluminum intoxication (occurs in patients on chronic renal dialysis) and milk-alkali syndrome (due to excessive ingestion of calcium and absorbable antacids such as milk or calcium carbonate).

Mechanism: Metastatic calcification may occur throughout the body and is **found at the sites where there is excretion of acid by tissues.** This leads to the local production of an internal alkaline compartment (created by the excretion of acid by tissues). This results in the local production of hydroxyl ions. The hydroxyl **ions** can lead to the precipitation of calcium hydroxide and hydroxyapatite, forming a mixed salt. These salts are then deposited in the affected tissues. A. Mitochondria are the earliest involved organelle.

Sites affected: It mainly affects the **interstitial tissues of the (1) gastric mucosa, (2) kidneys (basement membrane of the renal tubules), (3) lungs, (alveolar septa of the lung) and (4) blood vessels** (on the internal elastic lamina of **systemic arteries, and pulmonary veins**).

MORPHOLOGY

The morphology of calcium deposits in metastatic calcification is similar to that seen in dystrophic calcification. They may occur as **noncrystalline amorphous deposits or**, at other times, as **hydroxyapatite crystals.** The specific appearance can vary depending on the affected tissue and the local conditions.

Significance: In most cases, the deposition of mineral salts in metastatic calcification does not produce clinical dysfunction or symptoms.

- **Massive lung involvement:** Occasionally massive deposition of calcium salts in the lungs can lead to significant radiographic (X-ray) changes. This can affect lung function and lead to respiratory compromise,
- **Kidney involvement (nephrocalcinosis):** Massive mineral deposits in the kidney, a condition referred to as nephrocalcinosis, may lead to renal damage.

The differences between dystrophic and metastatic calcification are presented in **Table 2.12**.

TABLE 2.12 Differences between dystrophic and metastatic calcification.

Features	*Dystrophic calcification*	*Metastatic calcification*
Tissue affected	Dead and degenerated tissue	Living tissue
Calcium metabolism	Normal	Deranged
Serum calcium level	Normal	Raised
Site of calcification	Necrosis (e.g., caseous necrosis), dead parasites, atherosclerotic plaque, etc.	Lung, mucosa of the stomach, kidneys, and blood vessels

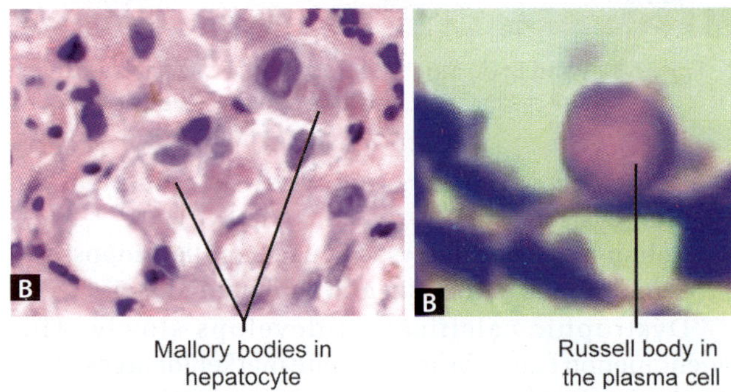

Figs. 2.33A and B: (A) Mallory bodies; (B) Russell bodies.

HYALINE CHANGE

Q. Write a short note on hyaline change (including definition and types).

Hyaline refers to an alteration **within cells or in the extracellular space**, which **appears as a homogeneous, glassy, pink** in routine histological sections stained with hematoxylin and eosin (H&E).

Causes (Table 2.13)

It consists of **different and unrelated lesions**. They have **nothing in common**. The term is etiologically not useful, but is widely used as a a descriptive microscopic term.

Intracellular Hyaline (Table 2.13)

Q. Write a short note on Russel body.

- **Mallory body (alcoholic hyaline) (Fig. 2.33A)** in the liver is alcoholic hyaline **composed of cytoskeletal filaments.**
- **Russell bodies** are **excessive accumulation of immunoglobulins in the rough endoplasmic reticulum of plasma cells (Fig. 2.33B).**
- **Hyaline droplets** in the proximal tubular epithelial cells of the kidney due to **excessive reabsorption of plasma proteins in proteinuria.**
- **Zenker's degeneration:** Hyaline change of rectus abdominis muscle (becomes glassy and hyaline) in **typhoid fever**.

Extracellular Hyaline (Table 2.13)

- Collagenous fibrous tissue in **old scars.**
- Hyaline change in **uterine leiomyoma (Fig. 2.34).**
- **Hyaline in renal arterioles** resulting from extravasated plasma protein and deposition of basement membrane material. It occurs in long-standing **hypertension and diabetes mellitus.**

TABLE 2.13 Examples of hyaline change.

Intracellular hyaline	*Extracellular hyaline*
1. Mallory bodies 2. Russell bodies (e.g., multiple myeloma) 3. Crooke's hyaline (present in basophil cells of the pituitary gland in Cushing syndrome) 4. Zenker's hyaline change	1. Collagenous fibrous tissue in scar 2. Hyaline change in uterine leiomyoma 3. Hyaline membrane in respiratory distress syndrome 4. Hyaline arteriosclerosis in diabetes and hypertension 5. Hyalinization of glomeruli in chronic glomerulonephritis 6. Corpora amylacea in the prostate, brain, and spinal cord in the elderly, old infarct of lung

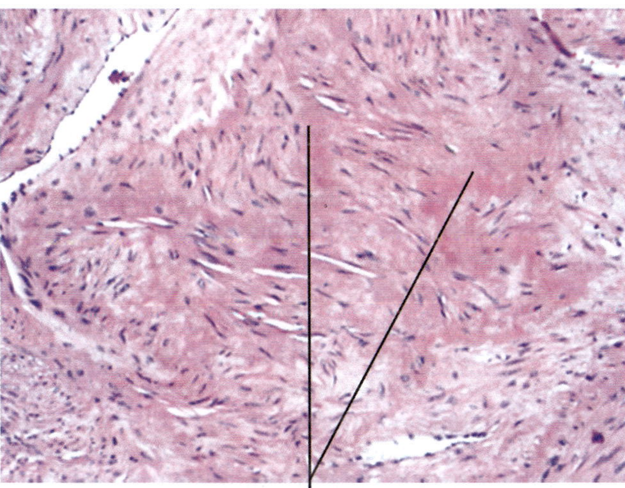

Fig. 2.34: Hyaline change in leiomyoma of the uterus.

- **Hyaline membrane in the lung** consists of plasma protein deposits along in alveoli in in respiratory distress syndrome.
- In **chronic glomerulonephritis**, the **glomeruli** show hyalinization.

Q. List the conditions in which Mallory bodies are seen.

Mallory hyaline/body was observed in the:
1. Alcoholic hepatitis
2. Indian childhood cirrhosis (ICC)
3. Primary biliary cholangitis
4. Wilson disease
5. Hepatocellular carcinoma
6. Focal nodular hyperplasia of liver

MUCOID DEGENERATION

- **Mucus is the viscid watery secretion** produced by mucous glands. It consists of a loose combination of proteins and mucopolysaccharides. Its main constituent is a glycoprotein called mucin.
- Mucus is produced by mitochondria and then they move to the Golgi apparatus, where they are converted into mucin. When this process is exaggerated with **excessive secretion of mucus** it is termed mucoid degeneration.
- Mucin is normally produced by both epithelial cells of mucous membranes and mucous glands and also by certain connective tissue cells, especially in the fetus (e.g., umbilical cord). Mucoid degeneration may involve both epithelial and connective tissue mucin. Usually, connective tissue mucin is termed as myxoid, i.e., mucus-like.
- Both epithelial and connective tissue **mucin are stained by alcian blue**. Epithelial mucin stains positively with periodic acid-Schiff (PAS) and connective tissue mucin is PAS negative and stains with colloidal iron.

Epithelial mucin: Examples of excessive epithelial mucin secretion are:
- **Catarrhal inflammation of the mucous membrane,** e.g., inflammation of the mucosa of the respiratory tract and gastrointestinal (GI) tract.
- **Obstruction,** e.g., mucocele of the gallbladder, appendix, and oral cavity.
- **Cystic fibrosis of the pancreas.**
- **Mucus secreting tumors,** e.g., GI tract and ovary.

Connective tissue mucin: Examples:
- **Mucoid or myxoid degeneration:** Examples of tumors include myxoma, neurofibroma, fibroadenoma, and sarcomas.
- **Dissecting aneurysm of aorta.**
- **Myxedema:** Myxomatous changes in the dermis.
- **Myxoid change in ganglion.**

CELLULAR AGING

PA 2.7 (NC): Describe and discuss the mechanisms of cellular aging and apoptosis (*refer* pages 22-27).

Cellular aging is **an inevitable process that begins from conception and continues till death**. It is the gradual, insidious, and progressive decline in the various physiological functions and structural changes of cells in almost all systems. Aging involves molecules, and different cell types (particularly postmitotic cells like neurons and cardiomyocytes, compared to rapidly dividing cells like those in the gut or skin), tissues, and organs. It includes a decline in muscular strength, cardiac function, nerve conduction, pulmonary capacity, glomerular filtration, and vascular elasticity. Cellular aging begins to unfold after the achievement of sexual maturity.

Significance of aging: Aging is **one of the strong independent risk factors for many chronic diseases.** These include **cancer, Alzheimer disease, ischemic heart disease, atherosclerosis, diabetes, and osteoarthritis.** Cellular aging may lead to the death of the cell or decreased capacity of cells to respond to injury and increase difficulties in maintaining physiological homeostasis.

Causes

Cellular aging is multifactorial and life span is subject to strong genetic and environmental influences.

Genetic abnormalities: They cause a progressive decline in cellular function and viability.

Environmental factors: Cellular aging is also caused by the accumulation of cellular and molecular damage because of exposure to exogenous influences. These include diet, social conditions, and the development of age-related diseases (e.g., atherosclerosis, diabetes, and osteoarthritis). They cause progressive accumulation of sublethal injury over the years at the cellular and molecular level. Reduced food intake without malnutrition [dietary restriction (DR)] promotes longevity in many species.

Mechanism of Cellular Aging

Mechanisms of cellular aging are **complex and multifactorial.** Many factors contribute to the manifestations of aging.

Cellular aging arises from the accumulation of damage (e.g., from free radicals), limited cell division (replicative senescence), impaired DNA repair, and disrupted protein balance.

Environmental and Metabolic Damage

Reactive Oxygen Species

One of the toxic products that cause damage to the cells that contribute to age-associated disease is free radicals mainly **reactive oxygen species (ROS)**. ROS may be either produced in excess, or there is a reduction of antioxidant defense mechanisms (*refer* pages 30-1). ROS is mostly generated endogenously in mitochondria. Important ROS include **superoxide, peroxide, and nitric oxide**. However, current data indicates that ROS is not a major factor involved in aging.

Excessive production of ROS may be due to environmental influences (toxins and ionizing radiation) and mitochondrial dysfunction. ROS can interact with and damage all cellular macromolecules. ROS can produce diverse lesions associated with aging. The oxidative damage may be an important cause of senescence in aging. These can damage nucleic acids (DNA damage causing breaks and genome instability), modify and inactivate proteins, and damage lipids. Damaged cellular organelles also accumulate as the cells age.

Reduction of antioxidants: To counter the effects **of ROS**, cells possess a network of antioxidant defenses that detoxify ROS and repair ROS-related damage (*refer* pages 30-34). These pathways include superoxide dismutases (SOD), catalase, glutathione peroxidase, thioredoxins, thioredoxin reductase, and many others. Oxidative stress occurs when ROS exceeds cellular defenses. **Reduction of antioxidant defense mechanisms** may occur with age.

Decline of mitochondrial function with aging: With age, mitochondria lose their efficiency. Mitochondria produce less ATP and more ROS. Decline of mitochondrial function contributes to major age-associated conditions. These include sarcopenia (loss of muscle mass and strength), insulin resistance and type 2 diabetes, cardiac dysfunction, neurodegeneration, etc.

DNA Damage

DNA damage: It can occur from **external** (physical, chemical, biological) and **internal factors** like ROS. It can affect the integrity of both nuclear and mitochondrial DNA. These **DNAs frequently undergo mutations**, which include base substitutions, copy number variations, and deletions or insertions. Many mutations occur spontaneously**.** DNA damage can be accelerated by both endogenous stresses (e.g., ROS) and exogenous insults (e.g., exposure to UV radiation, and chemotherapeutic agents).

DNA repair: DNA repair enzymes usually repair most of the DNA damage, but some persist. These persistent mutations accumulate as cells age. DNA repair plays a crucial role in the aging process. Next-generation DNA sequencing studies revealed 14 new mutations per year in hematopoietic stem cells, likely contributing to age-related issues, including cancer.

Defective DNA repair: Many protective repair responses counterbalance the metabolic damage in cells. One of them is endogenous DNA repair enzymes, which identify the DNA damage and repair most of it. However, some persist and accumulate as cells age, especially if repair mechanisms become inefficient over time. Common hematologic malignancies occur more frequently in older individuals. Many inherited syndromes are characterized by premature aging. These are caused by mutations in genes that encode DNA repair proteins. DNA repair mechanisms are defective in diseases such as **Werner syndrome and ataxia-telangiectasia**. Werner syndrome patients exhibit premature aging due to a defective DNA helicase, involved in DNA replication, repair, and unwinding. This enzyme's defect leads to rapid chromosomal damage accumulation, resembling cellular aging. Genetic instability in somatic cells is seen in other disorders with accelerated aging manifestations, like **Bloom syndrome** and ataxia-telangiectasia, where mutated genes encode proteins responsible for repairing double-strand DNA breaks.

Effects of DNA damage on aging: Accumulation of mutations in nuclear and mitochondrial DNA will ultimately **compromise the functional activities and survival of cells.** The effects of DNA damage include: (1) telomere dysfunction, (2) epigenetic alterations and changes in gene expression, (3) synthesis of defective proteins affecting protein homeostasis, (4) mitochondrial dysfunction leading to cell death, (5) cellular senescence (proliferative arrest) and stem cell loss and (6) impact on aging-related signaling pathways.

Cellular Senescence

Replicative senescence: Most normal cells, except for stem cells, have a **limited capacity for replication**. This limitation is often referred to as the "Hayflick limit." **Hayflick limit** is the number of times a normal human cell population will divide until cell division stops. **After a** certain **fixed number of divisions** (usually around 60–70 cell divisions), all these **cells enter a state known as replicative senescence.** Replicative senescence is the reduced capacity of cells to divide secondary to the progressive shortening of telomeres. **These cells** can no longer divide and become arrested in a nondividing **become arrested in terminally nondividing state.**

Aging and cellular replication: Aging is associated with the progressive replicative senescence of cells and is characterized by a decrease in the number of cell divisions that can occur over time. Cells from children typically have a greater capacity for replication compared to cells from older individuals. **Werner syndrome is a rare genetic disorder that mimics premature aging.** Individuals with Werner syndrome experience various age-related symptoms at an early age. Cells from patients with Werner syndrome often exhibit substantially lower replicative potential, which means they reach replicative senescence earlier than cells from healthy individuals.

Mechanisms of Cellular Senescence (Figs. 2.35A and B)

Two key mechanisms underlie cellular senescence:

Telomere attrition

Telomeres: These are **protective, short, repetitive sequences of DNA** (TTAGGG) present **at the end regions** of linear **chromosomes.** Telomeres **ensure the complete copying of chromosomal ends during the S-phase of the cell cycle** and protect them from fusion and degradation. They ensure the complete replication of chromosomes.

Shortening of telomere: *Telomere attrition* is the shortening and reduced effectiveness of telomere. **With each cell division in somatic cells, a small section of the telomere is not duplicated**. This causes telomeres to become progressively shortened **(Fig. 2.35)**. One mechanism of replicative senescence is the gradual (progressive) shortening of telomeres. **As telomeres become shorter, the unprotected chromosome ends are recognized as damaged DNA.** Once the ends of telomeres are completely eroded the ends of chromosomes are no longer protected. These ends are sensed in cells as broken DNA. This triggers a signal for **cell cycle arrest**. Telomere attrition can also lead to end-to-end chromosomal fusions and other types of genomic instability.

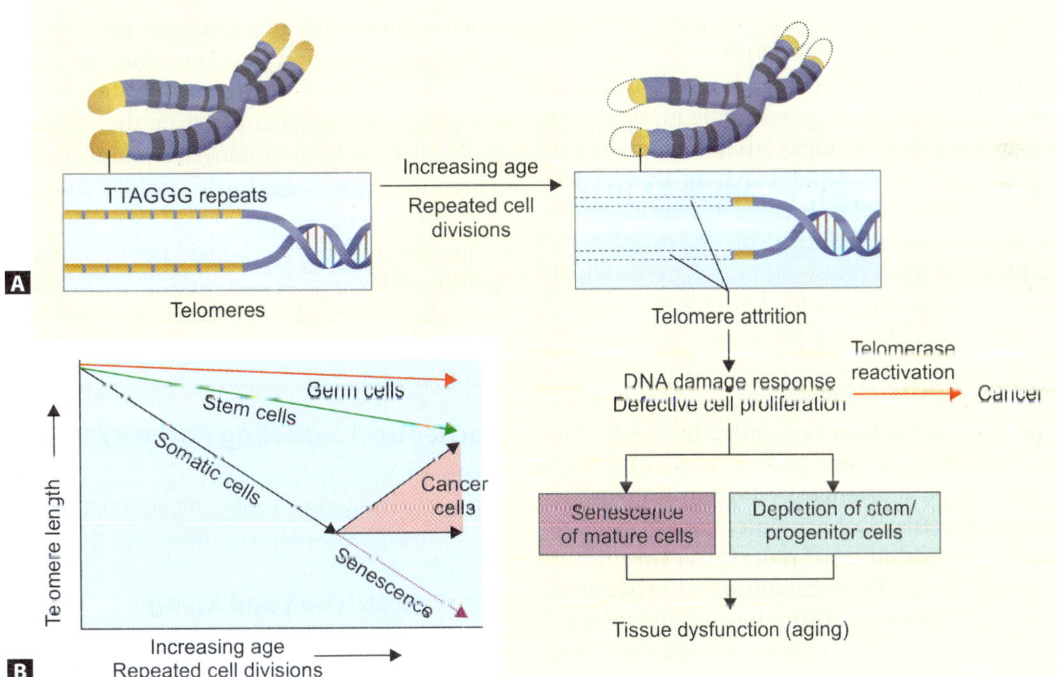

Figs. 2.35A and B: The role of telomeres and telomerase in replicative senescence of cells. Telomeres are the protective caps at the ends of linear chromosomes. They consist of repetitive DNA sequences (TTAGGG in humans) and associated proteins. (A) Telomere attrition. With each cell division, a portion of the telomere is lost. Repeated cell division is associated with aging. Each round of cell division leads to progressive shortening of telomeres at the end of chromosomes. When telomeres become critically short, they can no longer effectively protect the genetic material. They trigger senescence and loss of stem cell pools; (B) Telomere attrition is characteristic of somatic cells. Telomerase is an enzyme that can counteract telomere attrition. Germ cells and stem cells maintain their telomere length by expressing telomerase and are capable of unlimited replication. Cancer cells frequently activate telomerase and are thereby able to maintain telomeres.

Telomerase: Telomere length can be maintained by an enzyme called telomerase, which adds nucleotides to the ends of chromosomes. Telomerase is a specialized RNA-protein complex that uses its own RNA as a template for adding nucleotides to the ends of chromosomes.

- **Telomerase active in germ cells:** Telomerase is typically active in germ cells. The germ cells with high telomerase activity have extended replicative capacity **(Figs. 2.35A and B)**.
- **Telomerase is present at lower levels in somatic stem cells:** Shortening of telomeres also may decrease the regenerative capacity of stem cells.
- **Telomerase is absent in most somatic cells:** Therefore, as most somatic cells age, their telomeres become shorter and they exit the cell cycle. This results in an inability to generate new cells to replace damaged ones.
- **Telomerase reactivation in cancer cells:** In immortalized cancer cells, telomerase is usually reactivated and telomere length is stabilized. This permits the cells to proliferate indefinitely. It may be an essential step in the formation of cancer.
- **Inherited deficiencies in telomerase activities:** This may be observed in certain diseases, such as aplastic anemia (caused by to failure of hematopoietic stem cells), pulmonary and liver fibrosis, infertility, and premature graying of hair. These disorders are considered as "telomeropathies."

Activation of tumor suppressor genes

Activation of tumor suppressor genes, such as those encoded by the CDKN2A locus, plays a role in regulating replicative senescence. This locus encodes two tumor suppressor proteins, one of which is p16 or INK4a. The expression of p16 is correlated with a person's age in various human and mouse tissues. p16 controls the progression from the G1 phase to the S phase of the cell cycle, which helps protect cells from uncontrolled growth signals and promotes the cellular senescence pathway.

Altered Protein Homeostasis

All cellular proteins are collectively called the proteome. The proteome must be maintained properly to ensure normal cellular function and longevity. Protein homeostasis involves two mechanisms: (1) the **maintenance of proteins in their correctly folded conformations** (mediated by chaperones) and (2) the **degradation of misfolded, damaged, or unneeded proteins** by the autophagy-lysosome system and ubiquitin-proteasome system. These two degardaing systems are constantly subject to diverse challenges. Cellular proteins are constantly subject to diverse challenges. With aging, cells are not able to maintain normal protein homeostasis, because of impairment of both normal folding and degradation of misfolded proteins. Defective protein homeostasis results from impaired chaperone and proteasome functions. This leads to the loss of normal proteins and the accumulation of misfolded proteins.

Impairment of Normal Folding of Protein

With aging, there is increased turnover and decreased synthesis of proteins. This can result in an imbalance in protein homeostasis. Aging is associated with the impaired function of proteasomes. Proteasomes are responsible for the degradation of misfolded or damaged proteins. Aging is associated with the impairment of proteasome function, which can lead to the accumulation of misfolded proteins. Chaperones play a crucial role in promoting the correct folding of proteins. As we age, there can be a decline in the activity of chaperones, which further contributes to protein misfolding.

Defective Degradation of Misfolded Proteins

The proteasomal degradation of proteins is by degradation of misfolded proteins by proteasomes. Protein misfolding and aggregation can arise from various factors, including translational errors, oxidative damage, mutations, and genetic polymorphisms. These misfolded proteins can cause cellular injury. With aging there is also defective activity of chaperones.

Autophagy: It is one proteostatic mechanism that is closely linked to aging. The autophagy is a regulated process by which cells degrade damaged proteins in lysosomes. Autophagic function declines with age. Rapamycin has multiple effects and these include the promotion of autophagy. Rapamycin is a drug that inhibits the mTOR (molecular target of rapamycin) pathway. Administration of rapamycin increases the life span of middle-aged mice.

Consequences of abnormal protein homeostasis: Maintenance of proteostasis contributes to longevity. Abnormalities in protein homeostasis can have many effects on cell survival, replication, and functions. It can also lead to the accumulation of misfolded proteins, thereby triggering apoptosis.

Biochemical Signaling Pathways

Biochemical signaling pathways may also be involved in regulating the aging process. These include environmental stress such as calorie restriction and sirtuins.

Caloric Restriction and Aging

Caloric restriction refers to reducing calorie intake without malnutrition. Biochemical alterations associated with calorie restriction **may counteract aging, slow down aging, and prolong lifespan.** The caloric restriction may activate DNA repair. Caloric restriction is associated with decreased production of reactive oxygen species (ROS) by mitochondria and reduces ROS-associated damage in cells. Caloric restriction also leads to a reduction of overall adiposity, particularly visceral adiposity. Biochemical changes associated with calorie restriction affect signaling pathways that regulate cellular metabolism and reduce aging. These include:

- **Inhibitors of insulin-like growth factor (IGF):** IGF is produced in many cell types in response to growth hormone secretion by the pituitary gland. It involves a downstream network of kinases and transcription factors. IGF, as its name implies, mimics intracellular signaling by insulin and thereby informs cells of the availability of glucose, promoting an anabolic state as well as cell growth and replication. Insulin/IGF-I–like signaling (IIS) negatively regulates longevity. The actions of reduced IGF-1 signaling include: (i) lowering the rate of cell growth and metabolism, (ii) reduction in errors in DNA replication, (iii) better DNA repair and (iv) enhancing protein homeostasis.
- **Decreased mTOR (molecular target of rapamycin) activity:** mTOR is a nutrient-sensitive, protein kinase with conserved roles in limiting longevity. Through complex signaling pathways, mTOR phosphorylates many cellular targets and is a central controller of cell growth and aging. Genetic or pharmacologic inhibition of mTOR activity that decreases mTOR activity has been found to slow the aging process and increase life span (longevity). Rapamycin also suppresses neoplasia.

Partial inhibition of the above two pathways may switch cells from focusing on growth and proliferation to concentrating on repairing damage. These may prolong the lifespans. Caloric restriction modulates the activities of specific sirtuin proteins. It also decreases inflammation and upregulates DNA repair mechanisms.

Sirtuins

Sirtuins are a family of NAD-dependent protein deacetylases. There are at least seven types of sirtuins and are distributed in different cellular compartments. They play a role in adapting cellular functions to environmental stresses like food deprivation and DNA damage. **Sirtuins promote the expression of several genes whose protein products increase longevity.** These include proteins that inhibit metabolic activity, reduce apoptosis, stimulate the folding of proteins, and counteract the harmful effects of oxygen free radicals. Sirtuins also increase insulin sensitivity and glucose metabolism, making them potential targets for treating diabetes.

Functions of sirtuins: An increase in sirtuins, particularly sirtuin-6 has two functions: the sirtuins (1) contribute to metabolic adaptations of caloric restriction and (2) promote genomic integrity by activating DNA repair enzymes through deacylation. Probably a constituent of red wine may activate sirtuins and thus increase life span!

Hormesis: It is a biological phenomenon where exposure to low doses of a potentially harmful agent results in a beneficial effect on health, stress tolerance, growth, or longevity. The longevity associated with calorie restriction represents an example of hormesis.

Persistent Low-level Inflammation

As age advances there is accumulation of damaged cells, lipids, and DNA. These may activate the inflammasome (*refer* page 62) pathway, leading to persistent low-level inflammation. Persistent inflammation may be responsible for chronic diseases, such as atherosclerosis and type 2 diabetes. Cytokines produced during inflammatory reactions may themselves produce alterations in cells that promote aging. Chronic metabolic disorders may speed up the aging process. Stresses may accelerate aging probably by increased production of glucocorticoids.

Mechanisms of cellular aging are summarized in **Figure 2.36.**

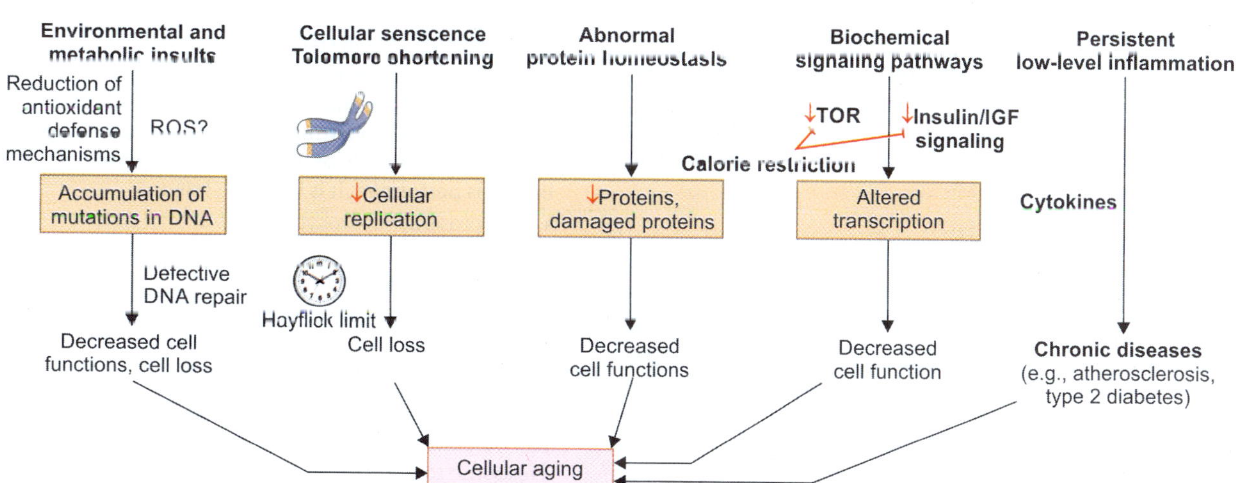

Fig. 2.36: Mechanisms of cellular aging. Multiple mechanisms are involved in cellular aging. Some environmental modifications, such as calorie restriction, counteract aging by activating various biochemical signaling pathways.

(ROS: reactive oxygen species; IGF: insulin-like growth factor; TOR: the target of rapamycin).

PA 2.8 (CC): Identify and describe various forms of cell injuries, their manifestations, and consequences in gross and microscopic specimens.

SCENARIO-BASED MCQs

1. A 56-year-old man comes for a routine checkup. On examination, he has a blood pressure of 160/100 mm Hg. If his hypertension remains untreated for years, the following cellular adaptations will most likely develop in his myocardium of the left ventricle:
   A. Hypertrophy B. Hyperplasia
   C. Metaplasia D. Atrophy
2. The uterus of a 25-year-old woman pregnant measures 30 × 14 × 12 cm. The enlargement of the uterus is brought out due to:
   A. Endometrial hyperplasia
   B. Myometrial smooth muscle hypertrophy
   C. Myometrial smooth muscle hypertrophy and hyperplasia
   D. Endothelial hyperplasia of uterine blood vessels
3. A 35-year-old man sustains a fracture of the right femur in a road accident. His right leg is placed in a plaster cast and has been immobilized for 6 weeks. On removing the plaster cast, the diameter of the right calf has decreased in size. The reduced size of calf muscle is most likely the result of the following alteration:
   A. Atrophy B. Myositis ossificans
   C. Hyaline change D. Hypoplasia
4. A 63-year-old man with a history of gastroesophageal reflux disease dies in the hospital following a massive stroke. At autopsy, representative sections are obtained from the gastroesophageal junction. Microscopic examination of these tissues shows an intestine-like epithelium composed of goblet cells and surface cells similar to those of incompletely intestinalized gastric mucosa. There is no evidence of nuclear atypia. Of the following, the changes in the esophagus describe the lesion as a process termed as:
   A. Columnar metaplasia B. Simple hyperplasia
   C. Complex hyperplasia D. Squamous metaplasia
5. A 40-year-old man, a chronic alcoholic is admitted to the hospital for severe abdominal pain over the past 12 hours. On examination, he is hypotensive and in shock. Laboratory studies show raised serum amylase. On explorative laparotomy grossly the mesentery showed multiple small foci of fat necrosis with calcification. The most likely event for this is:
   A. Acute cholecystitis
   B. Acute pancreatitis
   C. Acute hepatitis B hepatitis
   D. Infarction of small intestine
6. A 70-year-old man suddenly lost consciousness. On awakening 1 hour later, he could not speak or move her right arm. A head CT scan done two months later showed a large cystic area in the left parietal lobe. The pathologic processes that have most likely occurred in his brain are:
   A. Coagulative necrosis B. Fat necrosis
   C. Caseous necrosis D. Liquefactive necrosis
7. A 54-year-old male developed sudden retrosternal chest pain. His troponin levels were raised. He developed sudden cardiac arrest and died. On postmortem examination, the type of necrosis that can be observed on microscopic examination of the heart is:
   A. Caseous B. Fibrinoid
   C. Liquefactive D. Coagulative
8. A 48-year-old man complains of severe substernal chest pain for 2 hours. An ECG showed changes suggestive of an acute myocardial infarction. He was administered thrombolytic therapy with tissue plasminogen activator (t-PA) and this was followed by raised serum creatine kinase (CK) level. The event that most likely occurred in the myocardium after t-PA therapy is:
   A. Myofiber atrophy
   B. Reperfusion injury
   C. Increased synthesis of CK
   D. Regeneration of cardiac myocytes
9. On day 28 of her menstrual cycle, a 25-year-old woman experiences the onset of menstrual bleeding arche. The process that is most likely responsible for the initiation of shedding of her endometrial cells during bleeding is:
   A. Necrosis B. Apoptosis
   C. Caseous necrosis D. Liquefactive necrosis
10. A 57-year-old man has a lung carcinoma with metastases. He was treated with chemotherapy. One month later, microscopic examination of a metastatic lesion shows many foci in which individual tumor cells appear shrunken and deeply eosinophilic. The nuclei of these cells showed condensed aggregates of chromatin under the nuclear membrane. The pathologic process involving these shrunken tumor cells is most likely triggered by release of the substances from mitochondria into the cytosol is:
    A. BCL2 B. Catalase
    C. Phospholipase D. Cytochrome c
11. On physical examination of a 48-year-old chronic alcoholic man showed an enlarged liver. Enlargement of the liver was confirmed by an abdominal CT scan. A biopsy of the liver showed numerous cytoplasmic vacuoles. The special stain that is useful for demonstration of the nature of vacuole is:
    A. Sudan IV
    B. Congo red
    C. Periodic acid-Schiff stain
    D. Prussian blue reaction (Perl's stain)
12. A 12-year-old male child was suffering from β-thalassemia. He was regularly visiting the pediatrician. On physical examination, the skin of the child has a bronze color. A liver biopsy is performed. It is likely to show:
    A. Apoptosis of hepatocytes
    B. Councilman bodies
    C. Mallory bodies hepatocytes
    D. Hemosiderin in hepatocytes

Answers and Explanation

1. **The answer is A: Hypertrophy.** If hypertension is not treated for years, the left ventricle undergoes hypertrophy. Hypertrophy is a response to trophic signals or increased functional demand. Other options is a cellular adaptation that does not occur in the heart of a patient with long-standing hypertension. Hyperplasia and metaplasia never occur in heart muscles.

2. **The answer is C: Myometrial smooth muscle hypertrophy and hyperplasia.** The increase in uterine size during pregnancy is due to hypertrophy (an increase in the size) and hyperplasia (increase in number) of myometrial smooth muscle cells. The endometrium also increases in size, mainly through hyperplasia, but it is only a thin lining to the muscular wall and does not produce as much change in size. The endothelial hyperplasia of uterine blood vessels is a minor but essential component in this increase in size, but not the largest component.
3. **The answer is A: Atrophy.** Reduced workload due to plaster cast causes cells to shrink, a process called *atrophy*. The cells are smaller. Myositis ossificans is a connective tissue metaplasia that can occur in the muscle following fracture. But, it does not reduce the size of calf muscles. Hyaline change is a nonspecific, pink, glassy eosinophilic appearance of cells. Hypoplasia is a developmental anomaly characterized by the incomplete development or underdevelopment of tissue.
4. **The answer is A: Columnar metaplasia.** Metaplasia is the conversion of one differentiated cell to another differentiated tissue. In this case, the esophageal squamous epithelium is replaced by columnar epithelium due to chronic gastroesophageal reflux. The lesion shows an intestine-like epithelium composed of goblet cells and cells similar to those of incompletely intestinalized gastric mucosa. It is termed Barrett esophagus. Squamous metaplasia (choice D) occurs in the bronchial epithelium of smokers. Choices B, and C are changes that are most often described in the uterine endometrium.
5. **The answer is B: Acute pancreatitis.** Severe abdominal pain with elevated serum amylase favor acute pancreatitis. Lipase, released from pancreatic acinar cells during an attack of acute pancreatitis, leads to fat necrosis. Other options do not produce fat necrosis. Acute cholecystitis does not produce fat necrosis. Viral hepatitis does not cause necrosis in organs other than the liver. Intestinal infarction is a form of coagulative necrosis.
6. **The answer is D: Liquefactive necrosis.** The central nervous system tissues have high lipid content. In this case, stroke results in liquefaction necrosis as a consequence of ischemic injury. Coagulative necrosis usually occurs due to ischemia in most solid organs. Fat necrosis is seen in the pancreas and breast.
7. **The answer is B: Coagulative necrosis.** Sudden retrosternal chest pain with raised troponin levels is indicative of myocardial infarction. The morphologic appearance of the necrotic myocardial cells has traditionally been termed coagulative necrosis because of its similarity to the coagulation of proteins that occurs upon heating. Other options are different types of necrosis that are not seen in myocardial infarction.
8. **The answer is B: Reperfusion injury.** After myocardial infarction, the restoration of blood flow can prevent further cellular damage only if the existing cell damage is not great. However, the reperfusion of damaged cells generates oxygen-derived free radicals and produces a reperfusion injury. The raised levels of CK are indicative of myocardial cell necrosis. Myocardial fibers cannot regenerate to a significant degree, and atrophic fibers do not release significant CK. The CK is an intracellular enzyme that does not markedly leak from intact myocardial cells. t-PA induces thrombolysis to restore blood flow in occluded coronary arteries.
9. **The answer is B: Apoptosis.** The onset of menstruation is apoptosis brought out through hormonal stimuli. It involves the intrinsic (mitochondrial) apoptotic pathway. As hormone levels drop, the endometrium breaks down, sheds, and then regenerates. Necrosis is always pathological and menstruation is a physiologic process. Caseous necrosis is characteristic of granulomatous inflammation, most commonly seen with mycobacterial infection. Liquefactive necrosis occurs with acute bacterial infection or in the brain after ischemia.
10. **The answer is D: Cytochrome C.** The microscopic feature is typical of apoptosis produced by chemotherapeutic agents. The release of cytochrome *c* from the mitochondria is a main step in many forms of apoptosis and leads to the activation of caspases. BCL2 is an antiapoptotic protein that prevents the release of cytochrome *c* and thereby prevents caspase activation. Catalase is a scavenger of hydrogen peroxide. Phospholipases are activated during necrosis and damage the cell membrane.
11. **The answer is A: Sudan IV.** Numerous cytoplasmic vacuoles in a chronic alcoholic are due to steatosis (fatty change) of the liver. Fat can be demonstrated in cryostat (frozen) sections using special stains such as Sudan IV, oil red O, and osmic acid. Congo red is used for the demonstration of amyloid. Periodic acid-Schiff stain is for glycogen and Prussian blue reaction (Perl's stain) is for hemosiderin.
12. **The answer is D: Hemosiderin in hepatocytes.** β-thalassemia is a hereditary cause of hemolytic anemia. These patients are likely to develop hemosiderosis due to excessive deposition of hemosiderin. Hemosiderin is the storage form of iron. This pigment gets deposited in various organs such as the liver. The bronze color of the skin is also due to the deposition of hemosiderin in the skin. Apoptosis is not a feature of β-thalassemia. Councilman bodies are seen in viral hepatitis and Mallory bodies are mainly seen in alcoholic hepatitis.

Metaplasia
- Epithelial: Squamous and columnar metaplasia.
- Connective tissue metaplasia: Myositis ossificans.

Metaplasia: Most common is squamous metaplasia in the lungs of smokers.

Dystrophic calcification
- Normal serum calcium levels.
- Occurs in dead tissues (areas of necrosis).

Metastatic calcification
- Increased serum calcium levels
- Occurs in living tissues.
- Sites: Lungs (commonest site), stomach, pulmonary vein, systemic artery, and kidneys.

Lipofuscin
- Also known as "lipochrome," 'wear and tear' pigment, pigment of aging
- Indicator of free radical injury.
- Deposited mostly in heart and liver.

Inflammation and Healing

Chapter Outline

- Inflammation
- Acute Inflammation
- Mediators of Inflammation
- Morphological Types/Patterns of Acute Inflammation
- Outcomes of Acute Inflammation
- Chronic Inflammation
- Systemic Effects of Inflammation
- Tissue Repair
- Cell Proliferation and Cell Cycle
- Stem Cells
- Factors that Influence Wound Healing
- Examples of Tissue Repair and Fibrosis

INFLAMMATION

PA 4.1 (CC): Define and describe the general features of acute and chronic inflammation including stimuli, vascular and cellular events.

Q. Define inflammation. Mention the types and causes of acute inflammation. Explain the sequential vascular changes in acute inflammation.

Definition: Inflammation is a **complex local response of the living vascularized tissues to infections and tissue damage (injury).**

General Features of Inflammation

Purpose: Inflammation is **fundamentally a protective response** that is essential for survival, except for certain situations (e.g., hypersensitivity reactions). **It brings out cells** (phagocytic leukocytes) **and molecules that are necessary for host defense** (antibodies, and complement proteins) **from the circulation to the site of injury (where they are required).** These cells and molecules help **to eliminate the causative injurious agents** (e.g., microbes, toxins) **as well as the cells and tissues that died (necrotic tissue) from the original injury.** It also initiates the repair of damaged tissues.

Terminology: The suffix *-itis* is added after an organ that is involved in inflammation. For example, appendicitis (inflammation of the appendix), conjunctivitis (conjunctiva), and meningitis (meninges). Inflammation is distinct from infection. Infection is an invasion into the body by pathogenic microbes and their subsequent injury to the host, whereas inflammation is a response by the body to a variety of etiologic agents (infectious or non-infectious).

Q. Mention the types of inflammation. List the differences between acute and chronic inflammation.

Types of inflammation: Inflammation may be divided into **acute or chronic**. Sometimes, the term subacute inflammation is used to describe the inflammation between acute and chronic. Differences between acute and chronic inflammation are listed in **Table 3.1**.

TABLE 3.1 Differences between acute and chronic inflammation.

	Acute inflammation	*Chronic inflammation*
Onset	Rapid in onset (usually in minutes or hours)	May follow acute inflammation or be slow in onset (days)
Duration	Short duration. Lasts for hours or a few days	Longer duration; may be months
Predominant cells	Neutrophils (also called polymorphonuclear leukocytes)	Monocytes/macrophages, lymphocytes, and sometimes plasma cells
Main characteristics	Exudation of fluid and plasma proteins (edema) and the accumulation of leukocytes, predominantly neutrophils (also called polymorphonuclear leukocytes)	Inflammatory cells associated with the proliferation of blood vessels, continuing tissue destruction and fibroblast proliferation
Fibrosis	Usually mild and self-limited and can progress to a chronic phase	May be severe and progressive with fibrosis (the deposition of connective tissue)
Signs: Local and systemic	Prominent	Variable, usually modest

Cardinal Signs of Inflammation

Q. Mention the cardinal signs of inflammation and its mechanism.

The four **external manifestations of inflammation are** called **cardinal signs of inflammation** as first described by Roman encyclopedist **Celsus (Aulus Cornelius Celsus)** in the first century AD. A fifth clinical sign, **loss of function** (functio laesa), was later added by **Rudolf Virchow** (the father of modern pathology), in the 19th century. These cardinal signs are listed in **Table 3.2.**

Causes of (Stimuli for) Inflammation

Q. Mention the various causes of acute inflammation.

There are various causes of inflammation (**Box 3.1**), but the body responds to all of them in a similar manner.

Main Pathways in Acute Inflammation

Inflammatory response mainly consists of three elements.

1. **Vascular response (changes in blood vessels):** Locally increased blood flow and increased vascular permeability.
2. **Cellular response**: Recruitment and activation of a specific population of innate immune cells—polymorphonuclear leukocytes (PMNs, polys, neutrophils, etc.) to the site of inflammation.
3. **Effector cascades**: Activating pathways which release inflammatory mediators. For example, arachidonic acid pathways, and complement and coagulation pathways.

Inflammation is largely confined to the site of infection or damage but can develop some systemic manifestations (e.g., fever in bacterial or viral infections) (*refer* **online Fig. 3.1**).

Is inflammation always beneficial?

Beneficial: Normally, the inflammatory reaction is protective and beneficial.

Harmful: In some circumstances, the inflammatory reaction may cause disease and tissue damage.

TABLE 3.2 Cardinal signs of inflammation (Celsus).

Cardinal sign [Latin mnemonic (sign)]	*Mechanism*
1. Rubor (redness)	Increased blood flow and stasis
2. Calor (heat)	Increased blood flow with heat dissipation
3. Tumor (edema/swelling)	Increased vascular permeability causes the escape of protein-rich fluid from blood vessels into surrounding tissue
4. Dolor (pain)	Chemical mediators: Prostaglandins and kinins
5. Loss of function (functio laesa)*	Soluble mediators and leukocyte-mediated tissue damage

The first four (1 to 4) are described by Celsus. *Fifth (5) by Rudolf Virchow

BOX 3.1: Exogenous and endogenous causes of inflammation.

EXOGENOUS CAUSES

Infections (bacterial, viral, fungal, and parasitic) and **microbial toxins.**

Trauma (blunt, penetrating, or crush injuries)

Physical agents:

- Thermal injury (e.g., burns, frostbite or hyperthermia)
- Irradiation/radiation
- Electric shock
- Sudden changes in atmospheric pressure

Chemical injury:

- Strong acids and alkalies
- Insecticides, and herbicides
- Environmental toxins
- Pharmaceutical agents
- Oxygen, water, glucose, salt
- Drugs of abuse

Foreign bodies (e.g., sutures, talc, and tissue implants)

Nutritional derangements

ENDOGENOUS CAUSES

Tissue necrosis:

- **Ischemia:** Reduced blood flow and cause infarction in the heart (myocardial infarction), brain, and other tissues
- Anoxia

Immune reactions:

- Hypersensitivity reactions
- Autoimmune diseases
- Transplant organ rejection

Genetic derangements

- **Temporary local tissue damage:** For example, inflammatory reactions due to infections usually cause local tissue damage and are accompanied by pain and functional impairment. Usually, the harmful effects are self-limited with little damage and disappear after the inflammation subsides.
- **Excessive/prolonged inflammation:** In diseases where the inflammatory reaction is misdirected (e.g., against self-tissues in **autoimmune diseases**), or **life-threatening hypersensitivity reactions** to insect bites, drugs, and toxins, or is more prolonged (e.g., in **infections by microbes that resist eradication** such as tuberculosis, leprosy or chronic diseases such as rheumatoid arthritis, atherosclerosis), inflammation **can produce chronic diseases.**
- **Defective inflammation:** Too little inflammation, which is usually characterized by increased susceptibility to infections. It is usually seen leukopenia/neutropenia (reduced number of leukocytes) due to replacement of the bone marrow by cancers and suppression of the marrow by chemotherapies for cancer and graft rejection.

Recognition of Microbes and Damaged Cells

Recognition of microbes, necrotic cells, and foreign substances: The first step in inflammatory responses is the recognition of microbes, necrotic cells, and foreign substances. This recognition is by receptors on the cell surface (cellular receptors) and circulating proteins.

Cellular Receptors for Microbes

Recognition by sentinel cells in tissues: All tissues contain resident cells. The most important of these resident or sentinel cells are **tissue-resident macrophages, dendritic cells (cells in epithelia and all tissues that are involved in capturing microbes), and many other cells.** Their primary function is to **detect the presence of foreign invaders** (e.g., infectious **pathogens such as microbes)** or dead (necrotic) cells. These cells ingest and destroy the causes of that harm, and elicit the inflammatory reaction. The inflammatory reaction in turn recruits cells and proteins from the blood to complete the elimination process.

Pattern-Recognition Receptors (PRRs)

The presence of microbes and necrotic tissue is recognized by sentinel cells through receptors present in these cells.

Sites of receptors: The sentinel, host cells express receptors for microbial products. These receptors are present in multiple cell compartments: **on the surface** (recognize microbes in the extracellular space); in **endosomes** (in which ingested microbes are present); and **in the cytosol** (certain microbes may survive in cytoplasm). There are many cellular receptors that detect pathogens or the damage induced by them.

Pathogen-associated molecular patterns (PAMPs): The receptors in the host sentinel cells recognize molecular structures called **pathogen-associated molecular patterns** (PAMPs) that are part of many microorganisms but not of the host body's own cells. PAMPs structures include **mannose-rich oligosaccharides, peptidoglycans, and lipopolysaccharides of the bacterial cell wall, as well as unmethylated CpG DNA** commonly found in many pathogens. Hence, such cellular receptors for microbes are known as "pattern recognition receptors (PRRs)."

Types of receptors

The well-known of these PRRs are transmembrane proteins that belong to the family of *Toll-like receptors (TLRs).*

Q. Write a short note on Toll-like receptors (TLRs) and their importance.

Toll-like receptors (Fig. 3.2): They are named after the founding member, Toll, a gene that was discovered in Drosophila. TLRs are **in the plasma membranes and endosomes**. They are capable of **detecting PAMPs derived from extracellular and ingested microbes** like bacterial lipopolysaccharide (LPS, or endotoxin) or bacteria taken into phagosome by phagocytosis. There are 10 expressed TLR genes in humans. Each TLR recognizes a distinct set of molecular patterns. TLRs are single-pass transmembrane proteins. Their extracellular region is composed of leucine-rich repeat (LRR) such as CD14.

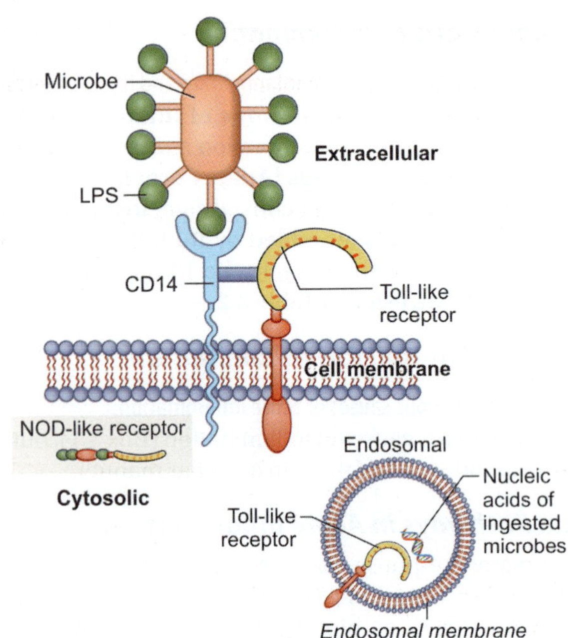

Fig. 3.2: Toll-like receptor.

[LPS: lipopolysaccharide; CD14: a member of the family of leucine-rich repeat (LRR) proteins].

- **Recognition of PAMPs:** Microbes have few highly conserved common molecular structures shared by entire classes of pathogens. These structures are called pathogen-associated molecular patterns (PAMPs) and are essential for the infectivity of these pathogens. TLRs recognize these PAMPs.
- **Cytokine production:** Once the microbes are recognized by these receptors, they stimulate the production of cytokines. These cytokines induce inflammation.

Sensors of Cell Damage

All cells contain cytosolic receptors such as *NOD-like receptors (NLRs).* They recognize various molecules that are liberated or altered as a consequence of cell damage. These cytosolic receptors are called **damage-associated molecular patterns (DAMPs).**

Molecules recognized by DAMPs: Examples of the molecules include uric acid (a product of DNA breakdown), ATP (released from damaged mitochondria), decreased intracellular K^+ concentrations (due to loss caused by injury to plasma membrane injury), DNA (when it is liberated into the cytoplasm and not sequestered in nuclei, as it should be normally), etc.

Activation of inflammasome and inflammation: A different sensor system consists of cytosolic *NOD-like* receptors (NLRs). On activation of NLRs, they recruit and activate a multiprotein complex called the *inflammasome.* NLRs recognize a wide range of stimuli, such as products of dead cells (e.g., uric acid, microbial products). It **stimulates the production of the cytokine interleukin-1** (IL-1). In turn, IL-1 recruits leukocytes and thus induces inflammation. The recruited leukocytes, phagocytes, and destroy dead cells. Gain-of-function mutations in the cytosolic receptors produce rare diseases known as *autoinflammatory syndromes* which are characterized by spontaneous inflammation. IL-1 antagonists are effective in the treatment of these disorders.

Inflammasome and associated disorders: Inflammasome is also responsible for inflammatory reactions to urate crystals (cause of gout), cholesterol crystals (in atherosclerosis), lipids (in metabolic syndrome and obesity-associated diabetes), and amyloid deposits in the brain (in Alzheimer disease). IL-1 plays a role in atherosclerosis and obesity-associated type 2 diabetes mellitus.

Circulating Proteins

If microbes escape the recognition by sentinel cells in tissues and they enter the circulation. In the circulation, microbes are recognized by several *plasma proteins*, such as **antibodies and members of the complement system**. These proteins can destroy circulating microbes and are recruited to tissue sites of infection. There they stimulate inflammatory reactions.

ACUTE INFLAMMATION

Q. Explain the sequential vascular changes/reactions of blood vessels/hemodynamic changes in acute inflammation.

Sequence of events in acute inflammation: Acute inflammation consists of two major components: (1) reaction of blood vessels (vascular changes/events); and (2) emigration of the leukocytes from the microcirculation [leukocytic (cellular) events]. Most of these **changes occur in postcapillary venules at the site of infection or tissue injury**. The walls of these vessels react to stimuli and allow the passage of fluid and proteins. Vasodilation slows the blood flow and sets the stage for the subsequent reactions. The increased vascular permeability allows the plasma proteins to enter the tissue site of injury. By transmigration, the leukocytes migrate from inside the vessels to the site of infection or necrosis. These leukocytes destroy the injurious agents and clean the damage. All these reactions are caused by cytokines and other molecules. These molecules are collectively called *inflammatory mediators*.

Reactions of Blood Vessels (Vascular Changes/Events)

Q. Define inflammation. Describe the vascular changes (reactions of blood vessels) in acute inflammation.

The vascular reactions of acute inflammation **(Figs. 3.3 and 3.4)** consist of (1) **changes in the flow of blood** (i.e., **changes in the vascular flow and caliber**) and (2) the **increased permeability of vessels**.

Purpose: Both the above reactions **maximize the movement of plasma proteins and deliver the circulating leukocytes out of the circulation and into the site of infection or tissue injury**. The main function of the inflammatory response is to eliminate injurious stimuli and remove injured tissue components, thus allowing the damaged tissue to undergo repair.

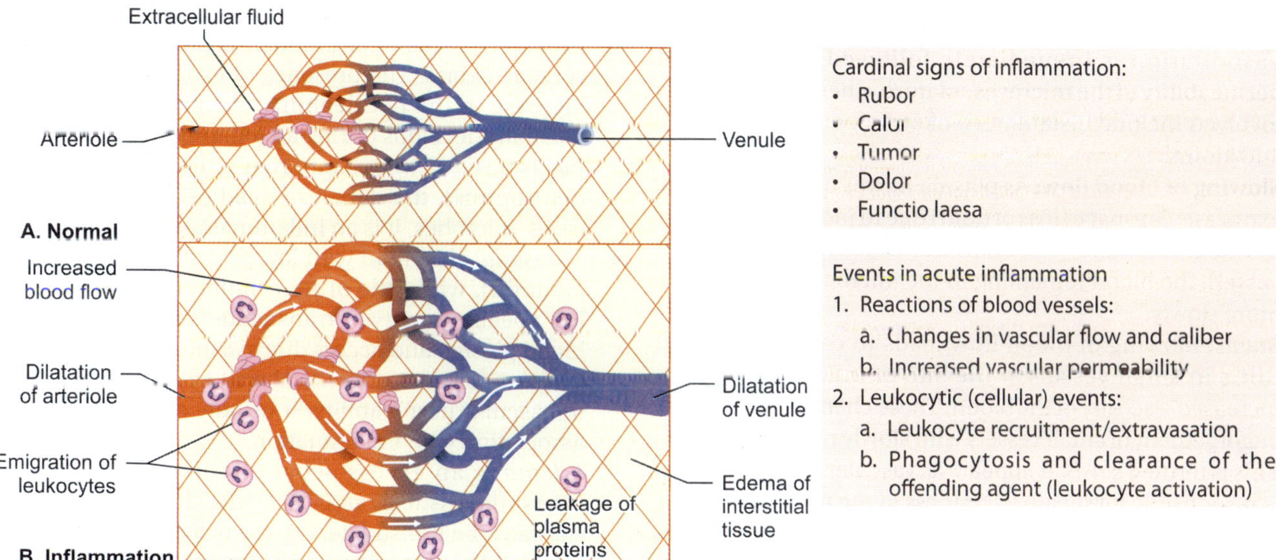

Fig. 3.3: Local features of acute inflammation, compared to normal are vasodilatation, increased blood flow, leakage of plasma fluid and proteins, and emigration of leukocytes.

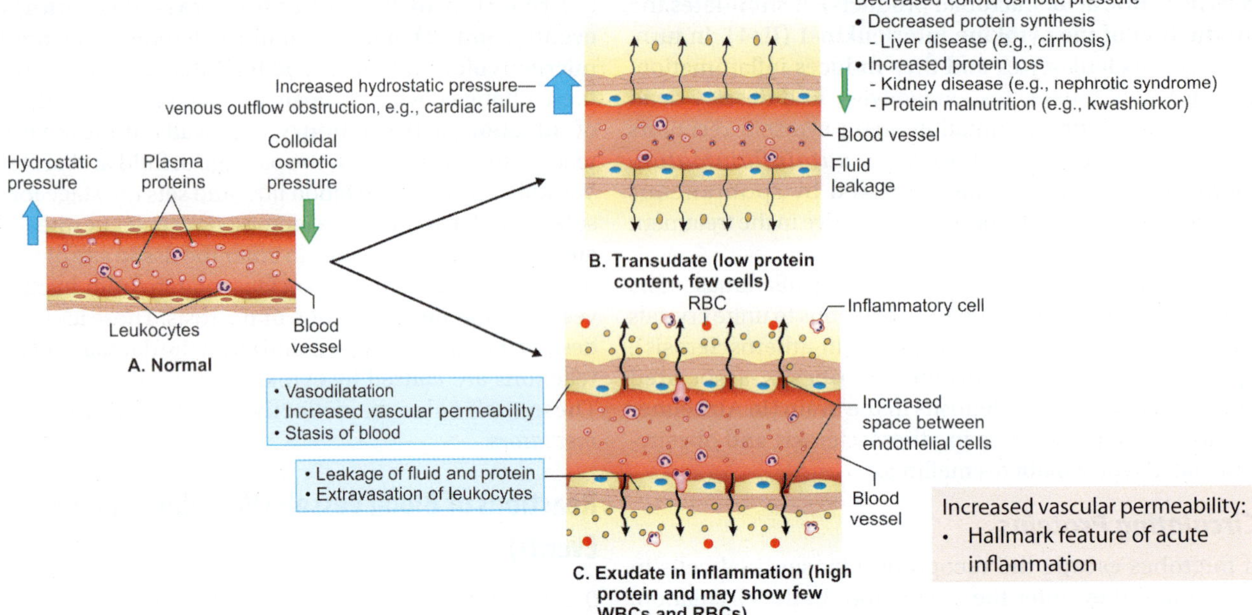

Figs. 3.4A to C: (A) Normal fluid exchange between blood and extracellular fluid; (B) Formation of transudate; (C) Formation of exudate in inflammation.

Changes in Vascular Flow and Caliber

Vasodilation: Vasodilation is one of the earliest features of acute inflammation; sometimes, it follows a transient constriction of arterioles. It results in **increased blood flow and increased blood volume** in the microvascular bed of the area. It is responsible for the externally seen **redness *(erythema)*** and **local heat** that are cardinal signs accompanying most acute inflammatory reactions. The most important chemical mediator causing vasodilation is **histamine.** Other mediators include **prostaglandins, kinins, and nitric oxide (NO)**.

Increased permeability of the microvasculature: Vasodilation is immediately followed by **increased permeability of the microvasculature.** Chemical mediators involved include histamine, leukotrienes, neuropeptides, and kinins.

Slowing of blood flow: As plasma moves outward into the extravascular space (loss of fluid) due to increased vascular permeability, and vasodilation (increased diameter of vessel), the blood remaining in the microcirculation flows more slowly.

Stasis: Slowing of blood flow leads to concentration of RBCs in small vessels at the site of inflammation and increased viscosity of the blood. These changes result in the engorgement of small vessels with slowly moving red cells. This is termed *stasis.* It appears as vascular congestion and is responsible for localized redness of the involved tissue.

Leukocyte events: As stasis develops, blood leukocytes (mainly neutrophils), accumulate along the endothelium of vessels. Simultaneously, endothelial cells are activated by mediators produced at sites of infection and tissue damage and these endothelial cells express increased levels of adhesion molecules. This leads to firm adhesion of leukocytes to the endothelium and is followed by the migration through the vascular wall into the interstitial tissue. It is described later on pages 66-8.

Increased Vascular Permeability (Vascular Leakage)

Q. Write a short essay on the mechanism of increased vascular permeability (vascular leakage) in inflammation.

Terminologies

- *Exudate* has a high concentration of protein and contains cellular debris. The presence of exudate indicates an increase in the permeability of small blood vessels. It usually develops during an inflammatory reaction.
- *Pus* is a *purulent* exudate rich in leukocytes (mostly neutrophils), the debris of dead cells, and, in many cases, microbes. It is an inflammatory exudate.
- *Transudate* is a fluid with low protein content (mostly albumin), with little or no cellular material, and has low specific gravity. A transudate is an ultrafiltrate of blood plasma and occurs due to osmotic or hydrostatic imbalance across the vessel wall without an increase in vascular permeability. It usually does not occur in association with inflammation.
- *Edema* is an excess accumulation of fluid in the interstitial tissue or serous cavities. It can be either an exudate or a transudate. **Escape of a protein-rich fluid** (exudate) **causes edema** and is one of the cardinal signs of inflammation. Differences between transudate and exudate are listed in **Table 3.3**.

TABLE 3.3 Difference between transudate and exudate.

Characteristics	*Transudate*	*Exudate*
Cause	Noninflammatory process	Inflammatory process
Mechanism	Ultrafiltrate of plasma, due to increased hydrostatic pressure with normal vascular permeability	Increased vascular permeability
Appearance	Clear, serous	Cloudy/purulent/hemorrhagic/chylous
Color	Straw yellow	Yellow to red
Specific gravity	<1.018	>1.018
Protein	Low, <2 g/dL, mainly albumin	High, >2 g/dL
Fibrin content and clot formation	Fibrin content is low and does not coagulate	Fibrin content is high and coagulates/clots spontaneously
Cell count	Low	High
Type of cells	Few lymphocytes and mesothelial cells	Neutrophils in acute and lymphocytes in chronic inflammation
Bacteria	Absent	Usually present
Lactate dehydrogenase (LDH)	Low	High
Examples	Seen in congestive cardiac failure	Pus
Character of edema	Pitting type	No pitting

Chemical mediators causing increased vascular permeability: Histamine, serotonin, C3a, and C5a (liberate vasoactive amines from mast cells, other cells), **bradykinin, leukotrienes C4, D4, E4,** platelet-activating factor (PAF at low concentration), neuropeptides (substance P).

Mechanism of Increased Vascular Permeability

Q. Describe the mechanism of increased vascular permeability.

Several mechanisms can cause increased vascular permeability:

1. **Contraction of endothelial cells:** It **creates an opening between the endothelial cells** and is the **most common mechanism of vascular leakage**. It occurs immediately after injury (15–30 minutes) and is usually short-lived and hence called an **immediate transient response**.
   - **Chemical mediators involved:** Histamine, bradykinin, leukotrienes, and the neuropeptide substance P.
2. **Direct endothelial injury:**
   - Direct injury or damage to the endothelium can be caused by severe injuries. This may be due to direct damage to endothelium as in burns, actions of microbes, and microbial toxins. One of the features of acute inflammation is leukocyte (mainly neutrophils) adhesion to endothelium. These neutrophils which adhere to the endothelium during inflammation may also indirectly cause injury to the endothelial cells and thus amplify the damage.
   - Direct endothelial injury produces necrosis and detachment of endothelial cells.
   - In most cases the increased vascular permeability begins immediately after injury and is sustained for several hours till the damaged vessels are either thrombosed or repaired. Hence, this type of response is called an **immediate sustained response.**
3. **Alterations in transcytosis:** The process of transport of fluids and proteins through the intracellular channels (called vesiculo-vacuolar organelle) in the endothelial cell is called transcytosis. These channels may be opened in response to certain factors that promote vascular leakage [e.g., vascular endothelial growth factor (VEGF)]. However, its contribution to vascular permeability in acute inflammation is not clear.

Q. Mention the differences between transudate and exudate.

Refer **Table 3.3.**

Leukocytic/Cellular Events

Q. Describe the leukocyte/cellular events in acute inflammation.

The leukocytic event **delivers leukocytes** capable of phagocytosis (neutrophils and macrophages) **to the site of injury**. Neutrophils are produced in the bone marrow. They are rapidly recruited to sites of inflammation and are short-lived. Macrophages (discussed on page 84) are slow to respond but are long-lived. Leukocyte events can be divided into **leukocyte recruitment and leukocyte activation.** The most important leukocytes are the phagocytic neutrophils and macrophages. They ingest and destroy bacteria and other microbes.

Leukocyte Recruitment/Extravasation

Normally, leukocytes move rapidly in the flowing blood. During inflammation, they slow down and escape to the site of injury (causative agent) in the extravascular space (outside the vessels).

Definition: Leukocyte recruitment to sites of inflammation (extravasation) is **the process of migration of leukocytes from the lumen of the vessel to the site of injury in the extravascular tissues.**

Type of leukocytes: Leukocytic (cellular) event in acute inflammation **delivers leukocytes** capable of phagocytosis **to the site of injury.** The main function of these leukocytes is the elimination of the causative agents and is an essential feature of inflammation. The most important phagocytic cells involved are leukocytes namely **neutrophils and macrophages**.

- **Neutrophils** are produced in the bone marrow. They are rapidly recruited to sites of inflammation and are **short-lived**.
- **Macrophages** (discussed under chronic inflammation on page 84) are slow to respond and recruit but are **long-lived**.

Steps in leukocyte recruitment/extravasation: Migration of leukocytes from the lumen of the blood vessel to the site of tissue injury is a multi-step process. It involves chemical mediators and is **controlled by adhesion molecules and cytokines.** This process can be divided into different phases **(Fig. 3.5)**.

1. **Leukocyte adhesion to endothelium** in which there is adhesion of leukocytes to endothelium at the site of inflammation.
2. **Leukocyte migration through the vessel wall:** The leukocytes escape between endothelium cells of the vessel wall into the extravascular tissue.
3. **Chemotaxis of leukocytes:** Leukocyte migrates in the extravascular tissue **toward the offending agent** due to chemotactic stimulus.

Different chemical molecules or mediators are involved in each of these steps.

Leukocyte Adhesion to Endothelium

Normal blood flow: Normally, blood flows from capillaries into postcapillary venules in an uninterrupted manner with the movement of circulating blood cells in parallel layers (called laminar flow). The circulating cells are moved by sweeping movement of laminar flow and prevent the blood cells from attaching to the vascular endothelium. RBCs being the smaller cells tend to move faster than the larger white blood cells. So, RBCs occupy the central axial column, and leukocytes are pushed out toward the wall of the vessel. The rapid movement of leukocytes in the flowing blood prevents them from attaching to the vascular endothelium. In inflammation, they should be stopped and then brought outside the vessels to the offending agent or the site of tissue damage. The sequence of leukocyte events in inflammation, occurring in the vascular lumen is discussed below.

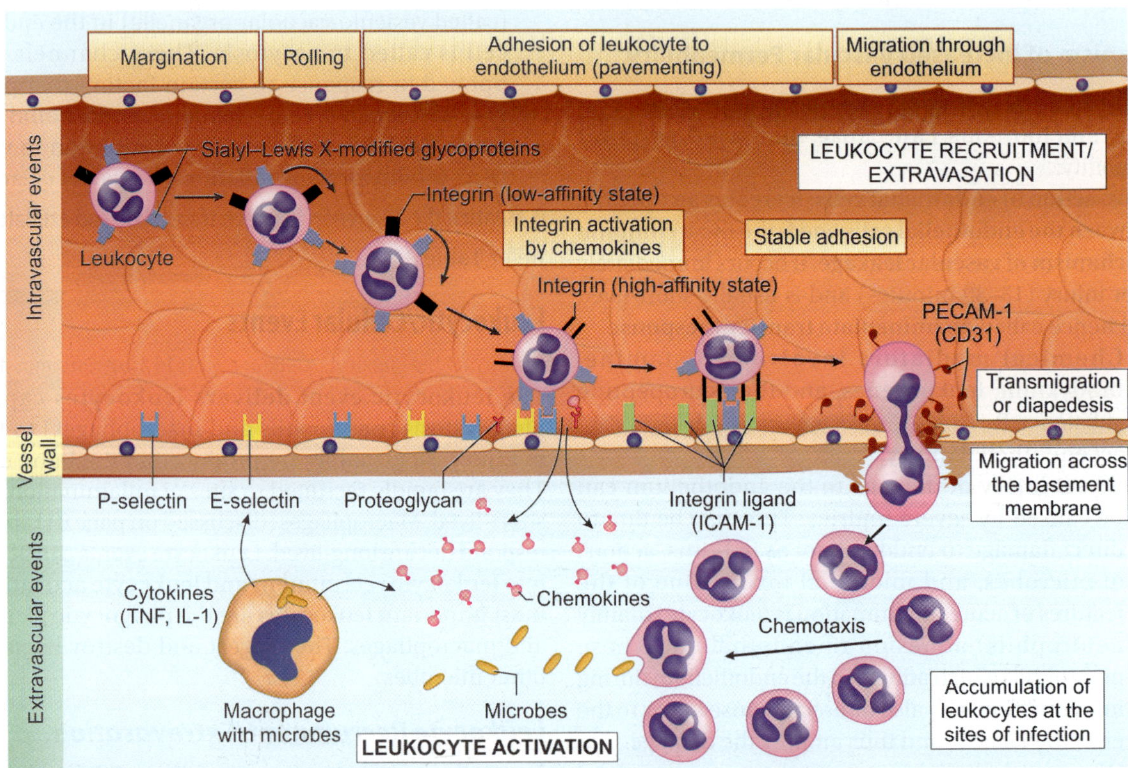

Fig. 3.5: Various steps of leukocyte migration through blood vessels. The leukocytes first roll, and then firmly adhere to endothelium, followed by transmigration across the endothelium. Leukocytes pierce the basement membrane and migrate toward chemoattractants from the source of injury. Selectins are involved in rolling; integrins in adhesion; and CD31 (PECAM-1) in transmigration.

Margination: During the early phase of inflammation, there is a slowing of blood flow (stasis) due to vasodilatation of the postcapillary venules, and loss of fluid due to increased vascular permeability at the margins of the vessels. The **leukocytes** (mainly neutrophils) being larger than red cells, **assume a peripheral position (column)** and **accumulate along the endothelial surface of vessels**. This process of leukocyte redistribution is termed margination.

Rolling and weak binding to endothelial cells: Marginated leukocytes can detect and react to changes in the vascular endothelium. Initially, the endothelial cells get activated by cytokines and other locally produced chemical mediators. These endothelial cells express adhesion molecules. **Initially, the leukocytes attach loosely/weakly to the endothelium** that is expressing adhesive molecules. Then the leukocytes detach and bind again to the endothelial surface and move along the endothelial surface with a mild jumping movement. This process of abrupt propelling (instead of smooth gradual) movement of leukocytes along the endothelial surface is termed rolling. The temporary binding of leukocytes to endothelial cells is also called **tethering**.

Q. Describe the role of selectins and integrins in acute inflammation.

- **Molecules involved in initial weak interaction between leukocytes and endothelial cells:** The attachment of leukocytes to endothelial cells is mediated by complementary adhesion molecules on leukocytes and endothelial cells. The expression of adhesion molecules is due to cytokines. The **involved molecules belong to the selectin** (lectin-like molecules, hence the name) **family of adhesive molecules and their complementary ligands (Table 3.4)**. The two major families of molecules involved in leukocyte adhesion are the selectins and integrins. **Selectins mediate the initial weak interactions between leukocytes and endothelium and integrins mediate firm adhesion** (described below).
  - **Selectins:** Selectins are receptors present on leukocytes and endothelium. They have an extracellular domain that binds sugars (hence the lectin part of the name). The three members of this family are E-selectin expressed on endothelial cells; **P-selectin present on platelets and endothelium; and L-selectin found on the surface of most leukocytes.** Their corresponding ligands are presented in **Table 3.4.**
- **Chemical mediators involved:** These include **cytokines such as (1) tumor necrosis factor (TNF), (2) interleukin-1 (IL-1),** and **(3) chemokines (chemoattractant cytokines)**. Cytokines are secreted by cells in tissues, in response to microbes and other injurious stimulus. The endothelial selectins (E-selectins) are activated after stimulation by cytokines and other mediators.

Firm adhesion of leukocyte to endothelium: After selectin-mediated rolling and weak binding, endothelium gets activated and leukocytes bind more firmly (adhesion) and finally come to rest at some point (**leukocyte arrest**). These leukocytes resemble pebbles over the endothelium (pavementing) and the bloodstream runs without disturbing them.

- **Molecules involved in firm adhesion of leukocytes to endothelium: Integrins** (family of leukocyte surface proteins) **and corresponding ligands (Table 3.5) are responsible for firm adhesion of leukocytes to endothelium I.**
- **Chemical mediators involved:** Endothelial cells are activated by **cytokines namely: TNF and IL-1**. They increase the expression of ligands for integrins on leukocytes **(Table 3.5)**. Drugs that block TNF leukocyte recruitment are used for the treatment of chronic inflammatory diseases. Chemokines are chemoattractant cytokines that cause leukocyte activation and **conversion of low-affinity** integrins **on leukocytes to high-affinity state** resulting in firm adhesion of the leukocytes to the endothelium.

Leukocyte Migration through Endothelium

Q. Write a short note on leukocyte transmigration.

Across the vessel wall and the endothelium: After the firm adhesion and arrest of leukocytes on the endothelial

TABLE 3.4 Selectins and complimentary selectin ligands involved in rolling.

Type of selectin (protein/ synonyms)	*Distribution of selectin*	*Ligand and their*	*Expression of ligand*
L-selectin (CD62L)	Neutrophils, monocytes, T cells (naïve and central memory) and B cells (naïve)	Sialyl-Lewis X/PNAd on GlyCAM-1, CD34, MAdCAM-1	On endothelium [high endothelial venule (HEV)]
E-selectin (CD62E)	Endothelium activated by cytokines (TNF, IL-1)	Sialyl-Lewis X (e.g., CLA) on glycoproteins	On neutrophils, monocytes, T-lymphocytes
P-selectin (CD62P)	Endothelium activated by cytokines (TNF, IL-1), histamine, or thrombin; platelets	Sialyl-Lewis X on PSGL-1 and other glycoproteins	

(GlyCAM-1: glycan-bearing cell adhesion molecule-1; MAdCAM-1: mucosal adhesion cell adhesion molecule-1; TNF: tumor necrosis factor; IL-1: interleukin-1; CLA: cutaneous lymphocyte antigen-1; PSGL-1: P-selectin glycoprotein ligand-1)

TABLE 3.5 Integrins along with complimentary ligands involved in endothelial-leukocyte adhesion.

Integrins(proteins/synonyms)	*Distribution of integrin*	*Complimentary ligands*	*Expression of ligand*
LFA-1 (CD11a:CD18/$\alpha_L\beta_2$)	Neutrophils, monocytes, T-cells (naïve, effector, memory)	ICAM-1 (CD54), ICAM-2 (CD102)	Expressed on endothelium and upregulated on activated endothelium
MAC-1 (CD11b:CD18/$\alpha_M\beta_2$)	Monocytes, macrophages, dendritic cells (DCs)		
VLA-4 (CD49d:CD29/$\alpha_4\beta_1$)	Monocytes, T-lymphocytes (naïve, effector, memory)	VCAM-1 (CD106)	

(ICAM: intercellular adhesion molecule; LFA-1: lymphocyte-associated function antigen; MAC-1: macrophage antigen1; VCAM: vascular cell adhesion molecule; VLA-4: very late antigen-4)

surface, the next step is the migration of leukocytes through the vessel wall.

1. **Transmigration or diapedesis:** Leukocytes eventually migrate through the vessel wall by squeezing through the intercellular junctions between the endothelial cells (i.e., by crawling between endothelial cells). This extravasation of leukocytes is termed **transmigration or diapedesis**. It occurs mainly in postcapillary venules because here the endothelial cells are capable of maximal retraction.
   - **Molecules involved:** These include a **member of the immunoglobulin (Ig) superfamily called CD31 or PECAM-1 (platelet endothelial cell adhesion molecule-1)** expressed on leukocytes and endothelial cells.
2. **Migration across the basement membrane:** Leukocytes penetrate (traverse) the basement membrane of the vessel by secreting collagenases (e.g., matrix metalloproteinases/MMPs). Usually, there is no injury to the vessel wall during leukocyte transmigration.

Chemotaxis of Leukocytes

Q. Define and write a short note on chemotaxis.

After exiting the circulation, leukocytes move in the extravascular tissues toward the site of injury by a process called chemotaxis. Leukocytes move toward the inflammatory stimulus in the direction of the chemical gradient of locally produced chemoattractants **(Fig. 3.6)**.

Definition: Chemotaxis is defined as the **directed process of migration of leukocytes along a chemical gradient.**

Movement of leukocytes in extravascular tissue: The leukocyte moves by extending filopodia (thin membrane protrusions that act as antennae for a cell to probe the surrounding environment) that pull the cell in the direction of extension. It is similar to an automobile with front-wheel drive pulled by the front wheels. Thus, the leukocytes migrate toward the inflammatory stimulus in the direction of the locally produced chemoattractants.

Chemoattractants: These are produced in response to infections and tissue damage and during immunologic reactions. These may be:

- **Exogenous: Soluble bacterial products** (e.g., peptides with N-formylmethionine termini).
- **Endogenous:**
  - Cytokines, mainly chemokine family (e.g., **IL-8**)
  - Complement components: **C5a, C3a**
  - Arachidonic acid metabolites of lipoxygenase pathway: **Leukotriene B_4 (LTB_4)**.

Accumulation of leukocytes at the sites of infection and injury: This is achieved by binding leukocytes to the extracellular matrix proteins through **integrins and CD44.**

Nature of leukocyte infiltrates*:* It varies with the age of the inflammatory response and the nature (type) of stimulus. **In most types of acute inflammation, neutrophils are predominant during the first 6–24 hours.** These are replaced by **monocytes in 24–48 hours**. Exceptions for this usual pattern of cellular infiltration are as follows:

- *Pseudomonas* bacteria: The cellular infiltrate consists of neutrophils for several (2–4) days.
- Viral infections: Lymphocytes may be the first cells to arrive.

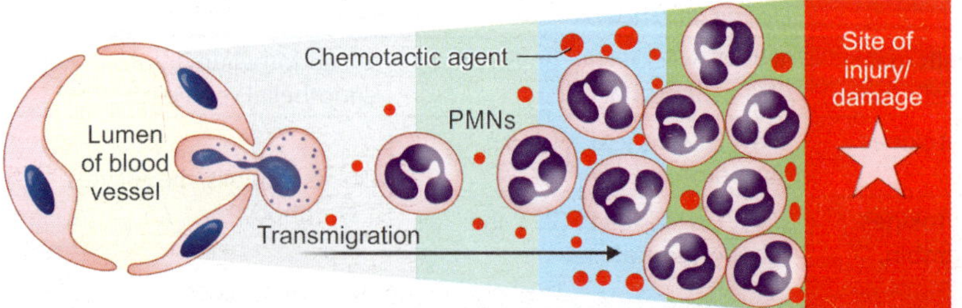

Acute inflammation: The main leukocyte involved is neutrophils (polymorphonuclear leukocytes—PMNs)

Chemotactic factors:
- Exogenous: Bacterial products
- Endogenous: C3a, C5a, LTB4, and IL-8

Fig. 3.6: Diagrammatic representation of chemotaxis in which the leukocytes migrate along a chemical gradient towards the site of injury or damage. (PMNs: polymorphonuclear leukocytes)

- Hypersensitivity reactions are dominated by activated lymphocytes, macrophages, and plasma cells.
- Allergic reactions and infections with certain parasites: Eosinophils may be the main cell type.

Clinical importance of leukocyte adhesion molecules: Three main types of leukocyte adhesion deficiency (LAD) have been identified. All are transmitted as an autosomal recessive disease and characterized by the inability of neutrophils to exit the circulation to sites of infection, leading to leukocytosis and increased susceptibility to infection.

Phagocytosis and Clearance of the Offending Agent (Figs. 3.7A to C)

Q. Write a short note on phagocytosis and its sequence of events.

Leukocyte activation: Recognition of microbes or dead cells by the receptors of recruited leukocytes (neutrophils and monocytes) at the site of infection or cell death initiates several responses in leukocytes together known as leukocyte activation. The most important functional responses of leukocyte activation are **phagocytosis and intracellular killing**.

Phagocytosis

The term phagocytosis was first used by Elie Metchnikoff. Many leukocytes **recognize, internalize, and digest** foreign material, microorganisms, or cellular debris by a **process termed phagocytosis**. The most important phagocytes in the body are *neutrophils* and *macrophages*.

Definition: Phagocytosis is defined as the ingestion of particulate material by phagocytic cells.

Steps in phagocytosis: It consists of three steps **(Figs. 3.7A to C):**

1. Recognition and attachment of the particle/injurious agent to be ingested by the leukocyte.
2. Engulfment with formation of a phagocytic vacuole.
3. Killing or degradation of the ingested material or microbe (intracellular destruction of microbes and debris).

Recognition and attachment

Receptors on the surface of phagocytic cells recognize components of microbes and necrotic cells. Leukocytes express several receptors that recognize external stimuli. These include (1) receptors for microbial products (e.g., Toll-like receptors-TLRs), (2) G protein-coupled receptors (recognize N-formyl methionine residues), (3) receptors for cytokines (for IFN-γ), (4) mannose receptors (binds to terminal mannose and fucose residues of glycoproteins and glycolipids present on microbial cell walls), (5) scavenger receptors (bind and ingest low-density lipoprotein (LDL) particles and a variety of microbes), and (6) receptors for opsonins (described below).

Q. Write a short note on opsonins and their role in inflammation.

Receptors for opsonins (phagocytic receptor): The efficiency of phagocytosis is increased if the microbes are coated *(opsonized)* with molecules called *opsonins*. The phagocytes also have specific receptors for opsonins.

Opsonins: These include IgG **antibodies, the C3b** breakdown **product of complement, and certain plasma lectins** (notably mannose-binding lectin) called collectins **(Table 3.6)**.

Bruton disease: Defect in the maturation of the B-cells leading to the absence of immunoglobulin production. Hence, there is **defective opsonization** in Bruton disease.

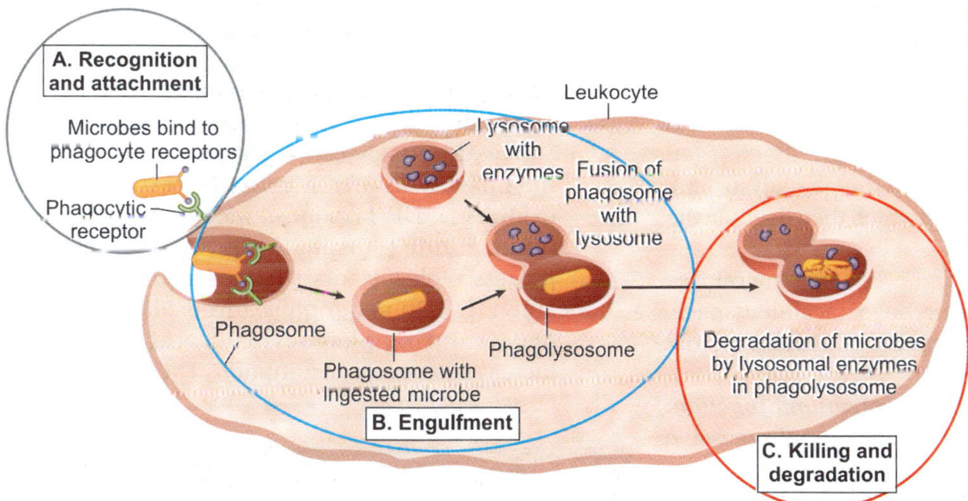

Chemotaxis is the directed process of migration of leukocytes along a chemical gradient.
Acute inflammation: Neutrophils predominate in the early stage and are replaced by monocytes after 24 hours.

Opsonization
Requires special chemical called opsonins.
These include complement proteins C3b, lectins and antibodies.

Figs. 3.7A to C: Different steps in phagocytosis: (A) Recognition and attachment which involves binding to receptors on the leukocyte membrane to injurious agent (e.g., bacteria); (B) Engulfment, formation of phagosome and fusion of lysosomes with phagocytic vacuoles to form phagolysosome; (C) Killing/degradation of ingested particles within the phagolysosomes by lysosomal enzymes and by reactive oxygen and nitrogen species.

TABLE 3.6 Different opsonins and their corresponding receptors on leukocytes.

Opsonin	*Receptor on leukocyte*
IgG antibodies	Fc receptor (FcγRI)
Complement components C3b	Type 1 and 3 complement receptors (CR1 and CR3)
Collectins	C1q
Others • Acute phase proteins (e.g., CRP) • Mannose-binding lectins	

Engulfment

The next step in phagocytosis is engulfment. In this step, pseudopods from the leukocytes extend around the object (injurious agent) and form a phagocytic vacuole. Phagocytosis is dependent on the polymerization of actin filaments present in the phagocytic cell. The polymerized actin filaments push the plasma membrane of the phagocyte forward.

Phagosome: After a microbe/particle is attached to receptors on phagocytes, **extensions of the plasma membrane of leukocytes form pseudopods surrounding the** foreign material/ **particle to be ingested** (e.g., bacterium, foreign material, injurious agent). The plasma membrane of leukocyte remodels to increase surface area and surround the foreign material. These pseudopods of plasma membrane form a phagocytic cup. The resulting phagocytic cup engulfs the foreign agent and forms a membrane-bound vesicle or vacuole called a phagosome. The plasma membrane then "zippers" around the opsonized particle and pinches off to form a vesicle or vacuole in the cytosol (cytoplasm) called a phagosome. The phagosome contains the ingested particle/microbe.

Phagolysosome: Then the membrane of the **phagosome** containing the foreign material **fuses with** the membrane of the cytoplasmic **lysosome to form a phagolysosome. Lysosomal granules are discharged** into this phagolysosome. Acid pH in the phagolysosome activates these hydrolytic enzymes, which then degrade the phagocytosed material.

During engulfment, the phagocyte also may release some contents of its granule into the extracellular space. They may damage innocent bystander (watcher) normal cells.

Clinical significance of defects in phagolysosome function: **Chédiak-Higashi syndrome** is an autosomal recessive condition characterized by:

- **Increased susceptibility to infections:** Due to **defective fusion of phagosomes with lysosomes in phagocytes.**
- Leukocyte abnormalities include neutropenia (decreased numbers of neutrophils), defective degranulation and delayed microbial killing, and peripheral blood smear consisting of **leukocytes with giant granules** (due to aberrant phagolysosome fusion).
- The gene associated with this syndrome encodes a **large cytosolic protein** called **LYST** (Lysosomal Trafficking Regulator), which **regulates lysosomal trafficking.**
- Bleeding disorders due to **defects in platelets.**

Killing and degradation

Q. Write a short note on free radicals and acute inflammation.

Intracellular destruction of microbes and debris: Killing and degradation of ingested microbial agents/particles occurs within neutrophils and macrophages. The most important microbicidal agents are: (1) **reactive oxygen species** (ROS), (2) **reactive nitrogen species derived from nitric oxide (NO)**, (3) **lysosomal enzymes,** and (4) **granule enzymes and other proteins**. These potentially harmful substances are normally sequestered in lysosomes and separated from the cell's cytoplasm to avoid damage to the phagocyte while it is performing its normal function.

1. **Reactive oxygen species (ROS)** (*refer* **pages 31-2):** Reactive oxygen species (ROS) are chemically reactive oxygen-derived free radicals. Normally, they are rapidly inactivated. However, increased production can cause cell injury. Phagocytosis stimulates an oxidative burst, with a sudden increase in oxygen consumption, glycogen catabolism (glycogenolysis), increased glucose oxidation, and production of reactive oxygen species (ROS). ROS are also called *reactive oxygen intermediates.* Types of ROS are presented in **Table 3.7**.
   Cell of origin: ROS are produced inside the leukocytes (neutrophils and macrophages).
   - **Mechanism of production of ROS (Figs. 3.8 and 3.9):** The free radicals are mainly produced in the phagolysosomes of neutrophils.
   - **Superoxide anion ($O_2^{\bar{\cdot}}$):** In neutrophil cell membranes of the phagocytic vacuole, phagocytosis rapidly activates a multicomponent electron transport enzyme called NADPH oxidase (also called **phagocyte oxidase**). NADPH oxidase is only active after its cytosolic subunit translocates to the phagolysosome membrane. NADPH oxidase oxidizes NADPH (reduced nicotinamide-adenine dinucleotide phosphate) to NADP. During the process, molecular oxygen is reduced to superoxide anion ($O_2^{\bar{\cdot}}$). In neutrophils, this oxidative reaction occurs during phagocytosis. NADPH oxidase increases oxygen consumption. The production of

TABLE 3.7 Types of reactive oxygen species.

Type of reactive oxygen species	*Nature of reactivity*
Superoxide anion ($O_2^{\bar{\cdot}}$, one electron)	**Weak**
Hydrogen peroxide (H_2O_2, two electrons)	**Weak**
Hydroxyl ions (•OH, three electrons)	**Highly reactive**

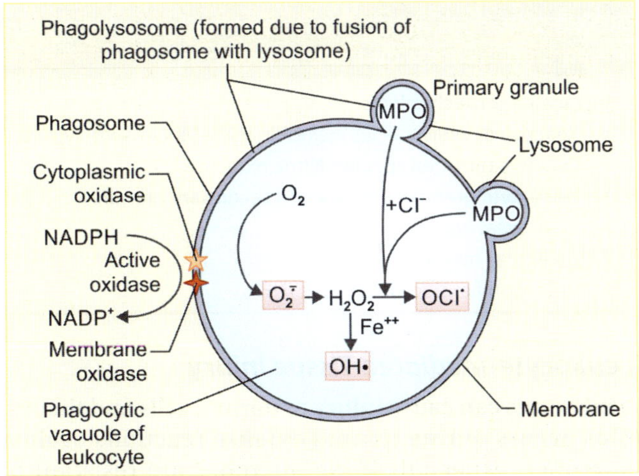

Fig. 3.8: Production of reactive oxygen species in leukocytes inside the phagocytic vacuole of leukocytes. In activated leukocytes, cytoplasmic components of the phagocyte oxidase enzyme assemble in the membrane of the phagosome. They form the active enzyme, which converts oxygen into superoxide ($O_2^{\bar{\cdot}}$) and H_2O_2. Myeloperoxidase (*MPO*), present in the granules of neutrophils, converts H_2O_2 to hypochlorite (OCl^-) and hydroxyl radical ($OH^{\cdot}$)

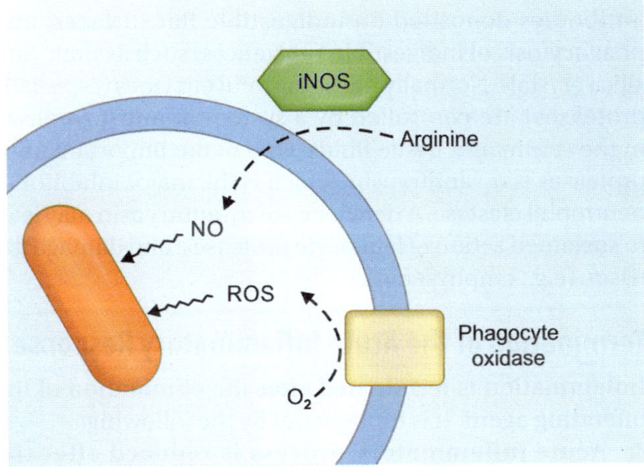

Fig. 3.9: Production of reactive nitrogen species. Nitric oxide (NO) can also kill ingested microbes.

(iNOS: inducible nitric oxide synthase; ROS: reactive oxygen species).

ROS associated with oxygen consumption is called the ***respiratory burst***.

- **Hydrogen peroxide (H_2O_2)**: $O_2^{\bar{\cdot}}$ is converted into hydrogen peroxide (H_2O_2) at the cell surface and in phagolysosomes, either spontaneously or through superoxide dismutase (SOD). The dismutation is a process of simultaneous oxidation and reduction.

$$O_2^{\bar{\cdot}} + 2H \rightarrow H_2O_2$$

  - **Hypochlorite radical (ClO^-):** The **amount of H_2O_2 produced is usually insufficient to kill most of the microbes** by itself (although superoxide and hydroxyl radicals may be sufficient to do so). However, the azurophilic granules of neutrophils containing the enzyme **myeloperoxidase** (MPO) can convert H_2O_2 into a powerful ROS (H_2O_2-MPO-halide system). H_2O_2 is stable and is a source for generating additional reactive oxidants. MPO in the presence of a halide anion such as Cl^-, converts H_2O_2 to **hypochlorite radical (ClO^-).** Hypochlorite is a **potent oxidant and antimicrobial agent** (NaOCl is the active component in chlorine bleach). Hypochlorite (ClO^-) destroys microbes either by **halogenation** (a chemical reaction that involves the addition of halogens, e.g., chlorine) or by proteins and **lipid peroxidation** (oxidative degradation of lipids). The **H_2O_2-MPO-halide system is the most powerful bactericidal system of neutrophils.**
  - After the oxidative burst, H_2O_2 is broken down to water and O_2 by catalase. Lysosomal acid hydrolases then digest the dead microorganisms.
- **Hydroxyl radical ($^{\bullet}OH$):** H_2O_2 is also converted to hydroxyl radical ($^{\bullet}OH$) which is also a **powerful destructive free radical** (bactericidal agent). This occurs slowly at physiologic pH. But if ferrous iron (Fe^{2+}) is present, the Fenton reaction rapidly converts H_2O_2 to $^{\bullet}OH$. Further reduction of $^{\bullet}OH$ produces water (H_2O).

Mode of action of ROS: Oxygen-derived free radicals bind to and modify cellular lipids, proteins, and nucleic acids. Thus, they destroy cells such as microbes.

Tissue damage: Oxygen-derived radicals may be released extracellularly from leukocytes and may produce tissue damage during inflammation. Serum, tissue fluids, and host cells have *antioxidant mechanisms* that can protect against tissue damage caused by these potentially harmful oxygen-derived radicals (*refer* pages 31-2).

2. **Reactive nitrogen species:** These are derived from nitric oxide (NO).

Q. Write a short note on nitric oxide in inflammation.

Nitrogen-derived molecules (Fig. 3.9): $NO^{\bullet}$ (Nitric Oxide) is a soluble gas. Phagocytes and endothelial cells produce $NO^{\bullet}$ and its derivatives. **$NO^{\bullet}$ is produced from L-arginine** by the action of nitric oxide synthase (NOS). This can also kill microbes (especially in macrophages) similar to ROS. The inducible (iNOS) type (one of the three types) is involved in microbial killing. iNOS is expressed when macrophages are activated by cytokines (e.g., IFN-γ) or microbial products. The iNOS produces NO within macrophages.

Mode of action: In macrophages, NO reacts with superoxide ($O_2^{\bar{\cdot}}$) produced by phagocyte oxidase to produce **highly reactive free radical peroxynitrite ($ONOO^-$).** Similar to ROS, they attack and damage the lipids, proteins, and nucleic acids of microbes.

3. **Leukocyte granule contents:** Leukocytes can also kill microorganisms by nonoxidative mechanisms

(without an oxidative burst). The contents of leukocyte granules can kill or destroy bacteria, other infectious agents, and ingested material. Phagocytic vesicles containing engulfed material (or microbial) may fuse with **granules of leukocytes and also with lysosomes.** **Neutrophils** have **two main types of granules**: specific and azurophilic. The contents of both types of granules are released when neutrophils are activated. These granules contain enzymes that degrade microbes and dead tissues and may also produce tissue damage.

i. **Smaller *specific*** (or secondary) granules: These granules contain lysozyme, collagenase, gelatinase, lactoferrin, plasminogen activator, histaminase, and alkaline phosphatase.
ii. **Larger *azurophil*** (or primary) granules: These granules contain myeloperoxidase, bactericidal factors (such as defensins), acid hydrolases, and a variety of neutral proteases (elastase, cathepsin G, nonspecific collagenases, proteinase 3).

Lysosomal enzymes: Phagocytic vesicles containing engulfed material in the neutrophil may fuse with the granules within the lysosomes. These ingested materials are destroyed in the phagolysomes by the actions of these enzymes.

Macrophages contain lysosomes filled with acid hydrolases (degrade the dead microorganisms), collagenase, elastase (kill bacteria), and phospholipase. All these enzymes can destroy ingested materials and cell debris.

4. **Neutrophil extracellular traps (NETs):** Activated neutrophils not only release the granule contents but also liberate **chromatin components, including histones**. They **form extracellular fibrillar networks called *neutrophil extracellular traps (NETs)*.**

Composition: NETs consist of a viscous meshwork of nuclear chromatin (includes histones and associated DNA) that binds and concentrates granule proteins such as antimicrobial peptides and granule enzymes. During the formation of NET, the nuclei of the neutrophils are lost, leading to the death of the neutrophils. NETs can be detected in the blood during sepsis. This is due to the widespread activation of neutrophils during sepsis.

Function: The microbes can be destroyed in these extracellular sites. NETs **concentrate antimicrobial substances at sites of infection and prevent the spread of the microbes** by trapping them in the fibrils. It is a non-phagocytic **mechanism of killing microbes**.

Significance: The nuclear chromatin in the NETs may be a source of nuclear antigens in systemic autoimmune diseases (e.g., lupus). In these patients, there is an immunological reaction against their own DNA and nucleoproteins.

Various mechanisms involved in the killing or degradation process during phagocytosis are presented in **Box 3.2**.

Leukocyte events in inflammation are summarized (*refer* **online Flowchart 3.1**).

BOX 3.2: Various mechanisms involved in the killing or degradation process during phagocytosis.

Intracellular mechanisms
- Reactive oxygen species including H_2O_2-MPO-halide system
- Reactive nitrogen species: Nitric oxide
- Leukocyte granule: Primary and secondary granules
- Lysosomal enzymes

Extracellular mechanisms
- Neutrophil extracellular traps (NETs)

Leukocyte-mediated Tissue Injury

Leukocytes can cause injury to normal cells and tissues. This occurs during normal defense reactions against microbes, especially if the microbes are resistant to destruction (e.g., mycobacteria). Leukocytes can produce tissue damage in autoimmune diseases or allergic diseases. **Mechanism of leukocyte-mediated tissue injury:** Leukocytes release the granule contents and lysosomes into the tissues. This usually happens when the activated leukocytes try to eliminate microbes and other injurious agents. The process is prominent when phagocytes come across materials that cannot be easily ingested. For example, antibodies deposited on indigestible flat surfaces, and phagocytosis of indigestible substances, such as urate and silica crystals. Normally, these harmful enzymes (especially proteases) are controlled by a system of **anti-proteases** in the serum and tissue fluids. One of the important anti-proteases is α_1-antitrypsin, which is the major inhibitor of neutrophil elastase. A deficiency of α_1-antitrypsin may lead to sustained action of leukocyte proteases, and damage the tissue (e.g., emphysema).

Termination of the Acute Inflammatory Response

Inflammation is terminated after the elimination of the offending agent. It is brought out by the following:

- **Acute inflammatory process is reduced after the causative agents are removed.** This is because of the following properties of the **chemical mediators of inflammation. The chemical mediators:**
  - Are produced only as long as the stimulus persists
  - Have a short half-life span
  - Are degraded after their release
- **Neutrophils also have a short life span** and die by apoptosis within hours to a day or two after leaving the bloodstream.
- There is a variety of **termination mechanisms** that stop the inflammatory process. These include:
  - A switch in the type of metabolite produced from arachidonic acid namely proinflammatory leukotrienes to anti-inflammatory lipoxins (*refer* page 74-5).
  - The liberation of anti-inflammatory cytokines [e.g., transforming growth factor-β (TGF-β) and IL-10] from macrophages and other cells.

MEDIATORS OF INFLAMMATION

PA 4.2 (CC): Enumerate and describe the mediators of acute inflammation.

Q. List chemical mediators of inflammation. Discuss the role of chemical mediators in inflammation.

Definition: Substances that initiate and regulate inflammatory reactions are called **mediators of inflammation**. Numerous mediators that are produced at the site of the reaction are responsible for inflammatory reactions.

General Properties of Chemical Mediators

Source of Mediators

Mediators of inflammation are produced either by cells at the inflammatory site or from plasma proteins. The main mediators of inflammation are listed in **Table 3.8**.

Cell-derived mediators: These are either **rapidly released from intracellular granules** (e.g., histamine in mast cell granules) **or are synthesized de novo** (e.g., prostaglandins and leukotrienes, cytokines) in response to a stimulus. They are produced mainly by **tissue macrophages, dendritic cells, and mast cells.** But platelets, neutrophils, endothelial cells, and most epithelia also secrete some inflammatory mediators.

Plasma-derived mediators: These are derived from circulating **inactive precursors** (e.g., complement proteins, kinins). They enter the site of inflammation and get activated, usually by a series of proteolytic cleavages.

General Features

Stimuli that bring out the production of mediators: Active mediators are produced only in response to various stimuli. These stimuli include **microbial products and substances released from necrotic cells.** Thus, inflammation is triggered only when and where it is required.

Short-lived: Most of the mediators have a short-lifespan. They quickly decay or are inactivated by enzymes, or scavenged or inhibited. These control mechanisms prevent excessive reactions.

Actions: They have tightly regulated and interrelated actions. One mediator can stimulate the release of other mediators. The secondary mediators may have similar, different, or even opposite actions.

Target: Most mediators act by **binding to specific receptors** on target cells. Target cell type varies depending on the type of mediator. They can act on one or a few or many diverse targets or may have different effects on different types of cells.

Cell-derived Mediators

Q. Write a short note on cell-derived mediators of inflammation.

TABLE 3.8 Main mediators of inflammation.

Mediators	*Actions*
CELL-DERIVED	
Vasoactive amines	
Histamine	• Vasodilation • Increased vascular permeability • Endothelial activation
Arachidonic acid (AA) metabolites	
Prostaglandins	• Vasodilation • Pain • Fever
Leukotrienes	• Increased vascular permeability • Chemotaxis • Leukocyte adhesion and activation
Cytokines	
TNF, IL-1, IL-6	• **Local:** Endothelial activation (expression of adhesion molecules) • **Systemic:** Fever, metabolic abnormalities, hypotension (shock)
Chemokines	Chemotaxis, leukocyte activation
Platelet-activating factor	Vasodilation, increased vascular permeability, leukocyte adhesion, chemotaxis, degranulation, oxidative burst
PLASMA PROTEIN-DERIVED	
Complement	• Leukocyte chemotaxis and activation • Direct target killing (membrane attack complex) • Vasodilation (mast cell stimulation)
Kinins	Increased vascular permeability, smooth muscle contraction, vasodilation, pain

(IL-1: interleukin-1; TNF: tumor necrosis factor; MAC: membrane attack complex).

Vasoactive Amines: Histamine and Serotonin

Vasoactive mediators **produce changes in blood vessel tone resulting in changes in blood flow**. Histamine and serotonin are the first mediators to be released during inflammation, which are stored as preformed molecules in cells.

Histamine

It is the **major vasoactive amine** a preformed vasoactive mediator. It is rapidly released from cells and is the **first mediator to be produced during inflammation.** It is responsible for the immediate transient response.

Source: Histamine is stored as a preformed molecule in the granules of **mast cells** (the richest source), **blood basophils, and platelets.** The mast cell is normally present in the connective tissue adjacent to blood vessels.

Stimuli: Mast cell degranulation and release of histamine occur may be triggered by various stimuli.

- **Binding of IgE antibodies to mast cells**: It occurs in immediate hypersensitivity (allergic) (type 1) reactions.
- **Products of complement**: These are called *anaphylatoxins* and include C3a and C5a.
- **Physical injury:** For example, trauma, cold, heat.
- **Other chemical mediators:** Neuropeptides (e.g., substance P) and cytokines (IL-1, IL-8).

Actions: (1) **Dilation of arterioles** and (2) **increase of the permeability of venules.** Its action on blood vessels is mediated through binding to histamine receptors called H1 receptors present in microvascular endothelial cells.

Serotonin (5-Hydroxytryptamine)

It is a preformed vasoactive mediator.

- **Source: Platelets,** some neuroendocrine cells (e.g., in the gastrointestinal tract).
- **Stimulus:** Platelet aggregation and antigen-antibody complexes.
- **Actions:** It is a **vasoconstrictor**. However, its role in inflammation is not clear.

Arachidonic Acid Metabolites (Prostaglandins, Leukotrienes, and Lipoxins)

Q. Write a short note on the role of arachidonic acid metabolites in inflammation.

Arachidonic Acid (AA)

Arachidonic acid-derived metabolites (Fig. 3.10) are the lipid mediators and consist of *prostaglandins* and *leukotrienes.*

Source: AA is a 20-carbon polyunsaturated fatty acid **present in plasma membrane phospholipids**. AA-derived mediators, also known as *eicosanoids* (from the Greek, *eicosa*, meaning 20, because they are derived from 20-carbon fatty acids). **AA is derived from cell membrane phospholipids mainly through the action of enzyme phospholipase A_2.** Eicosanoids bind to receptors on many cell types and **can mediate almost every step of inflammation.**

Stimuli: The enzyme phospholipase A_2 that acts on the cell membrane to produce AA is activated by

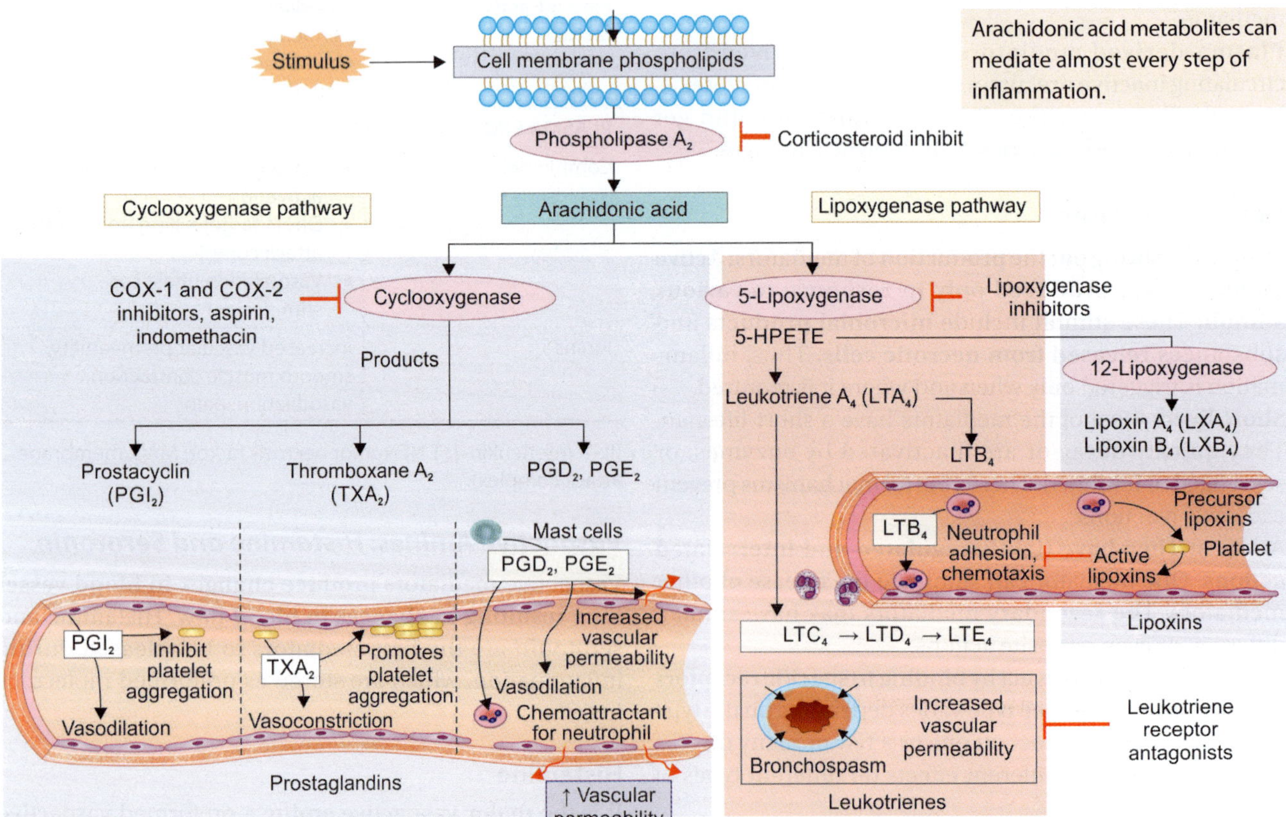

Fig. 3.10: Arachidonic acid metabolites involved in inflammation. The cyclooxygenase pathway generates prostaglandins (PGIs) and thromboxane (TXA_2). The lipoxygenase pathway forms lipoxins (LXs) and leukotrienes (LTEs).

(COX: cyclooxygenase; HETE: hydroxyeicosatetraenoic acid; HPETE: hydroperoxy eicosatetraenoic acid)

various inflammatory stimuli. These include **cytokines, complement products (e.g., C5a), and physical injury.**

Production of AA Metabolites

Arachidonic acids are generated by two major classes of enzymes, **cyclooxygenases** (which generate prostaglandins) and **lipoxygenases** (which produce leukotrienes and lipoxins).

Q. Write a short note on the role of prostaglandin in acute inflammation. Add a note on thromboxane A_2.

Prostaglandins: Products of cyclooxygenase pathway

The most important products of the cyclooxygenase pathway that are involved in inflammation are **prostaglandins.**
Terminology: Prostaglandins are named depending on the structure coded by a letter, as in PGD, PGE, and others, and a subscript numeral (e.g., 1, 2), which indicates the number of double bonds in the compound.
Source: Prostaglandins (PGs) are produced by **mast cells, macrophages, endothelial cells, and many other cell types.**
Synthesis: Prostaglandins and thromboxanes are produced from AA by the actions of two **cyclooxygenases, COX-1 and COX-2 (cyclooxygenases 1 and 2)** which differ in where these enzymes are expressed. COX-1 is produced in response to inflammatory stimuli and is expressed in most tissues. By contrast, COX-2 is induced by inflammatory stimuli and they produce prostaglandins in inflammatory reactions. However, COX-2 is low or absent in most healthy tissues.
Important prostaglandins in inflammation: These include **PGE_2, PGD_2, PGF_{2a}, PGI_2 (prostacyclin), and TXA_2 (thromboxane A_2).** Each is derived by the action of a specific enzyme on an intermediate in the pathway.
Effects: Prostaglandins are involved in the **vascular and systemic reactions of inflammation.**

- **Local effects:**
  - **PGD_2 and PGE_2: Vasodilation and increased permeability. PGD_2 is also a chemoattractant for neutrophils.**
  - **Thromboxane A_2 (TxA_2):** Platelets contain the enzyme thromboxane synthase. It produces TxA_2. TxA_2 is a **powerful platelet-aggregating agent and vasoconstrictor.**
  - **Prostacyclin (PGI_2):** Vascular endothelium does not have thromboxane synthase, but contains prostacyclin synthase. This enzyme forms prostacyclin (PGI_2) and its stable end product PGF_{1a}. Prostacyclin is **a vasodilator and a potent inhibitor of platelet aggregation.**
- **Systemic effects:** Prostaglandins are responsible for **pain and fever** in inflammation.

Leukotrienes: Products of lipoxygenase pathway

Source: Leukotrienes are produced by **leukocytes and mast cells by the action of lipoxygenase.**
Synthesis and their actions: Leukotrienes **are involved in vascular and smooth muscle reactions and leukocyte recruitment.** The production of leukotrienes involves multiple steps.

- First leukotriene A_4 (LTA_4) is synthesized.
- LTA_4 gives rise to LTB_4 or LTC_4.
  - **LTB_4:** It is produced by **neutrophils and some macrophages.** It is a **powerful chemotactic agent and activator of neutrophils.**
  - **LTC_4 and its metabolites, LTD_4 and LTE_4:** They are produced **mainly in mast cells.** They cause **severe vasoconstriction, bronchospasm** (important in asthma), and **increased permeability of venules.**

Lipoxin

They are also produced from AA by the lipoxygenase pathway.
Actions: Unlike prostaglandins and leukotrienes, the lipoxins suppress inflammation.

- Lipoxins **inhibit neutrophil chemotaxis and adhesion to endothelium.**
- They **inhibit the recruitment of leukocytes.**

Clinical Significance of AA Metabolites

- **Cyclooxygenase inhibitors:** Aspirin and other nonsteroidal anti-inflammatory drugs (NSAIDs), such as ibuprofen inhibit both COX-1 and COX-2. Thus, they inhibit prostaglandin synthesis.
- COX-1 is mostly constitutive (housekeeping) whereas COX-2 is inducible. However, in endothelium and CNS COX-2 is constitutively present.
- **Lipoxygenase inhibitors:** 5-lipoxygenase is not affected by NSAIDs. A drug that inhibits leukotriene production is useful in the treatment of asthma.
- **Corticosteroids:** They are broad-spectrum anti-inflammatory agents.
- **Leukotriene receptor antagonists:** These drugs block leukotriene receptors and prevent the actions of the leukotrienes. These are used in the treatment of allergic asthma and allergic rhinitis.

The main actions of arachidonic acid metabolites (eicosanoids) involved in inflammation are presented in **Table 3.9.**

TABLE 3.9 Main actions of arachidonic acid metabolites in inflammation.

Actions	*Eicosanoids (arachidonic acid metabolites)*
Vascular changes	
• Vasodilation	Prostaglandins PGI_2 (prostacyclin), PGE_1, PGE_2, PGD_2
• Vasoconstriction	Thromboxane A_2, leukotrienes C_4, D_4, E_4
• Increased vascular permeability	Leukotrienes C_4, D_4, E_4
Chemotaxis, leukocyte adhesion	Leukotriene B_4
Pain and fever	Prostaglandins

Cytokines and Chemokines

Q. Write a short note on cytokines.

Cytokines are proteins that function as **mediators in immune responses** and **inflammation (acute and chronic)**. They regulate inflammatory responses from initial changes in vascular permeability to resolution and restoration of tissue.

Source: Cytokines are produced by many types of activated cells. These include **activated lymphocytes and macrophages, endothelial, epithelial, and connective tissue cells**. They are produced at sites of tissue injury. Important cytokines involved in inflammation **(Table 3.10)** are discussed below.

Mode of action: Cytokines **act through specific receptors on target cells**. Cytokines may act in one of several modes: autocrine (act on the cells that produce them); paracrine (on neighboring cells); and endocrine (act through the bloodstream on distant cells).

Tumor Necrosis Factor and Interleukin-1

Tumor necrosis factor (TNF) and interleukin-1 (IL-1) are the **two major cytokines involved in inflammation.**

Source: TNF and IL-1 are produced mainly by **activated macrophages and dendritic cells.**

- **TNF**: It is also produced by T lymphocytes and mast cells.
- **IL-1**: It is also produced by some epithelial cells.

Stimuli: The stimuli for the secretion of TNF and IL-1 include **microbial products, necrotic cells**, and a variety of other inflammatory stimuli.

Actions in inflammation (Fig. 3.11): TNF and IL-1 contribute to the local and systemic reactions of inflammation.

- **Local effects of TNF and IL-1**
  - **Endothelial activation and leukocyte recruitment** Both TNF and IL-1 act on endothelium. **Increase in the expression of endothelial adhesion molecules mostly E- and P-selectins** and **ligands for leukocyte integrins.** These changes are required for the recruitment of leukocytes to sites of inflammation.
    - **Stimulate the production of other mediators.** These include other cytokines and chemokines, and eicosanoids.
    - **Increase the procoagulant activity of the endothelium.**
  - **Activation of leukocytes and other cells.**
    - **TNF increases the responses of neutrophils to other stimuli** such as bacterial endotoxin and stimulates the microbicidal activity of macrophages.
    - **IL-1:** It **activates fibroblasts to synthesize collagen** and **stimulates proliferation of synovial and other mesenchymal cells.** It also stimulates **Th17 responses**, which induce acute inflammation.
- **Systemic effects:**
  - **Systemic acute-phase reactions**: IL-1 and TNF (and IL-6) produce systemic acute-phase responses including fever in association with infection or injury. They also cause leukocytosis.
  - **Systemic inflammatory response syndrome** (SIRS): IL-1 and TNF can produce SIRS resulting from disseminated bacterial infection (sepsis) and other non-infectious serious conditions such as severe burns, trauma, and pancreatitis (discussed on page 90). TNF at high concentrations dilates blood vessels

TABLE 3.10 Cytokines involved in inflammation.

Cytokine	*Main sources*	*Main actions in inflammation*
In Acute Inflammation		
TNF*	Macrophages, mast cells, T lymphocytes	Expression of endothelial adhesion molecules and secretion of other cytokines; systemic effects (anorexia, fever, shock)
IL-1*	Macrophages, endothelial cells, and some epithelial cells	Similar to TNF; inflammatory cell activation; fever
IL-6*	Macrophages, other cells	Systemic effects (acute-phase response); stimulates hepatic synthesis of plasma proteins, including fibrinogen, and also acts on the hypothalamus to induce fever
Chemokines	Macrophages, endothelial cells, T lymphocytes, mast cells, other cell types	Recruitment of leukocytes to sites of inflammation (chemotaxis); leukocyte activation
In Chronic Inflammation		
IL-12	Dendritic cells, macrophages	Increased production of IFN-γ
IFN-γ	T lymphocytes, NK cells	Activation of macrophages (increased ability to kill microbes and tumor cells)
IL-17	T lymphocytes	Recruitment of neutrophils and monocytes

*Endogenous pyrogens.

(IFN-γ: interferon-γ; IL: interleukin; NK cells, natural killer cells; TNF: tumor necrosis factor).

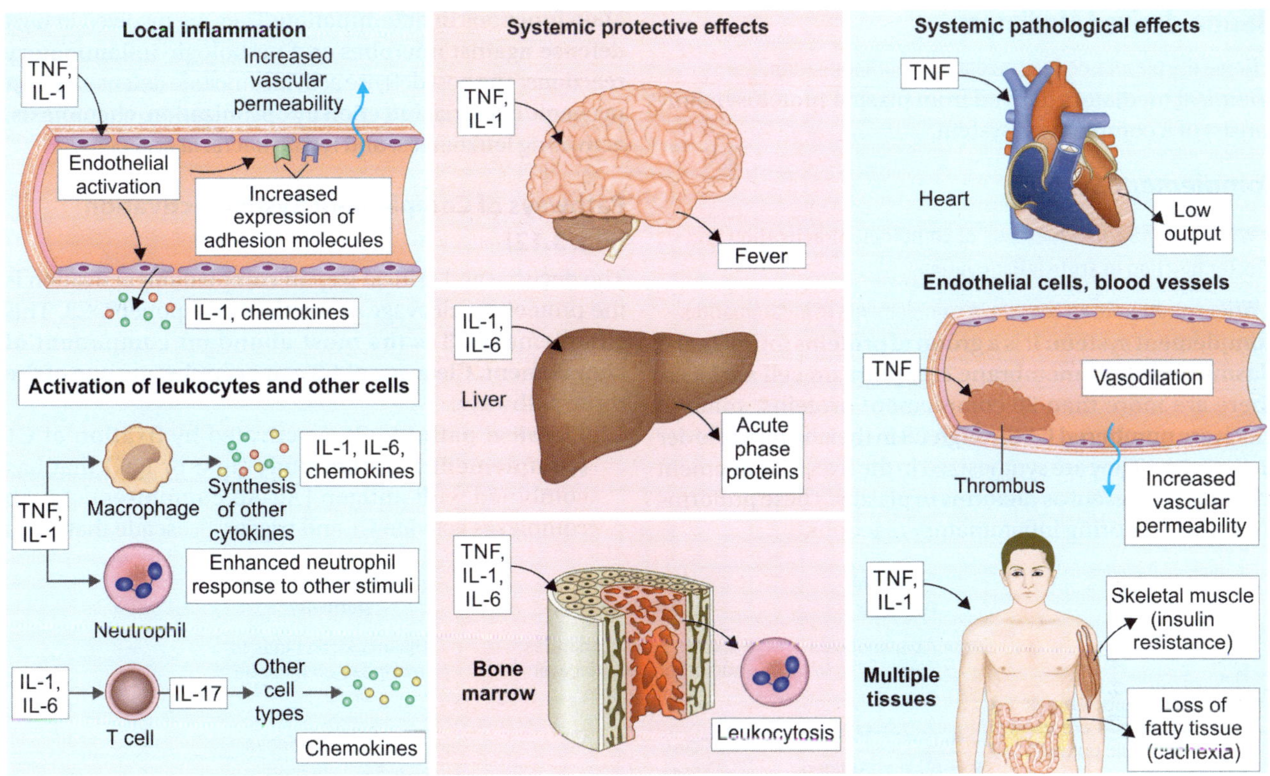

Fig. 3.11: Main local and systemic roles of cytokines in acute inflammation.

and reduces myocardial contractility. Both these reduce blood pressure in SIRS.

- **Suppresses appetite and cachexia**: TNF can regulate energy balance by promoting mobilizing lipids and protein and suppressing appetite. Hence, continuous production of TNF may lead to *cachexia*. Cachexia is a pathologic state characterized by loss of weight, atrophy of muscle, and loss of appetite (anorexia) and is observed in some chronic infections (e.g., tuberculosis) and cancers.

Clinical importance: TNF antagonists are effective in the treatment of chronic inflammatory diseases. Examples include rheumatoid arthritis, psoriasis, and some cases of inflammatory bowel disease. However, patients on TNF antagonists are more susceptible to mycobacterial infection, and this is due to the decreased ability of macrophages to kill intracellular microbes.

Chemokines

Chemotactic cytokines or chemokines are **small proteins (8 to 10 kD).** They mainly **act as chemoattractants for specific types of leukocytes** at the site of inflammation.

Classification: Chemokines are secretory proteins with four conserved cysteines (C) linked by disulfide bonds. Chemokines are classified into four major groups namely—(1) C-X-C chemokines, (2) C-C chemokines, (3) XC chemokines, and (4) CX3C chemokines.

Localization: Chemokines **bind to proteoglycans** and are thus **present at high concentrations on the surface of endothelial cells and in the extracellular matrix.**

Main functions: The two main functions of chemokines are as follows:

- **In inflammation**. The microbes and other stimuli induce the production of **inflammatory chemokines**. These **chemokines bind to leukocyte receptors**. They stimulate the following:
  - **Integrin-dependent attachment of leukocytes to the endothelium.**
  - **Chemotaxis.** They cause the migration of leukocytes in tissues to sites of infection or tissue damage.
- **Maintenance of tissue architecture**. Some chemokines are produced constitutively by stromal cells in tissues and are known as *homeostatic chemokines*. These chemokines **promote the localization of various cell types to specific anatomic regions.** For example, certain chemokines promote the localization of T and B lymphocytes to certain areas of the spleen and lymph nodes.

Other Cytokines in Acute Inflammation

- IL-6 produced by macrophages and other cells is involved in local and systemic reactions.
- IL-17 produced by T lymphocytes promotes neutrophil recruitment.

Plasma-derived Mediators

Q. Name the plasma-derived mediators of inflammation.

Chemical mediators derived from plasma proteins mainly consist of a complement system.

Complement System

Q. What are the three methods of complement activation and its effector function in acute inflammation?

Q. Write a short note on the role of complements in inflammation.

Complement system: It is **a group of proteins found in the plasma and their membrane receptors on cell surfaces.** There are more than 20 complement proteins, some of which are **numbered C1 through C9** in their historical order of discovery. They are synthesized in the liver. Complement proteins are present as preforms in plasms. These proforms are activated during inflammatory reactions.

Main functions in inflammation: They are involved in **host defense against microbes and pathologic inflammatory reactions.** The host defense activities include **defense against pyogenic bacterial infection by opsonization, chemotaxis, activating leukocytes, and lysing bacteria and cells.**

Pathways of Complement System Activation (Fig. 3.12)

The decisive and critical step in complement activation is the proteolytic cleavage of the third component, C3. This complement **C3 is the most abundant component of complement. Cleavage of C3 can occur by any one of the three pathways:**

1. **Classical pathway:** It is activated by **fixation of C1 (complement 1) to antibody** (IgM or IgG) that has combined with antigen (Ag-Ab complexes). Ag-Ab complexes activate C1 and trigger a cascade that leads

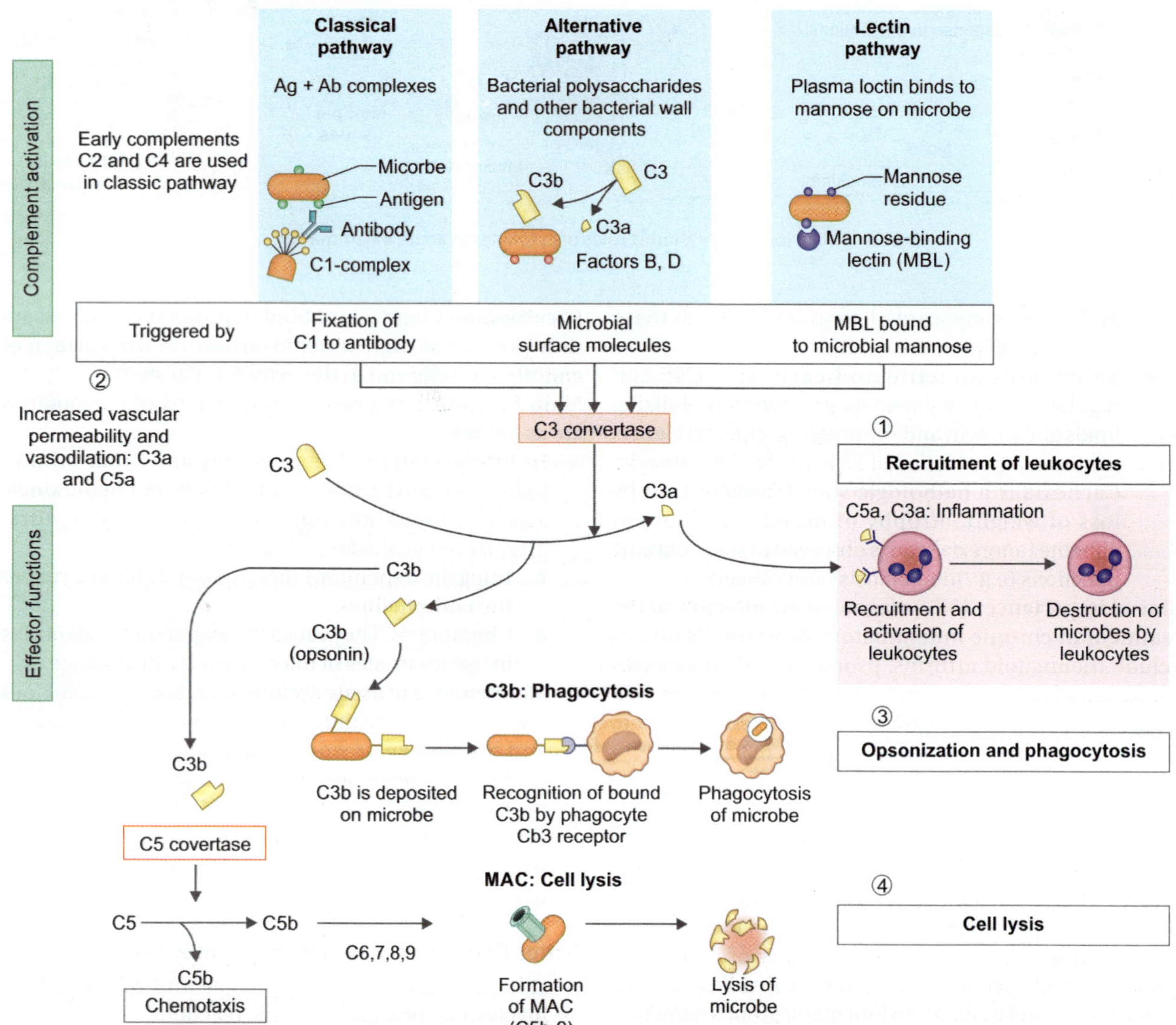

Fig. 3.12: The different pathways of activation and functions of the complement system. A critical step in the complement system by different pathways is the activation of C3. C3a and C5a also increase vascular permeability and vasodilation by relase of histamine from mast cells. (MAC: membrane attack complex).

to the formation of the membrane attack complex (MAC). Other activators include products of bacteria and viruses, protease

2. **Alternative pathway:** It is activated by **microbial surface molecules** [e.g., endotoxin from bacterial surfaces, or lipopolysaccharide (LPS)], **complex polysaccharides, cobra venom**, viruses, tumor cells, and other foreign substances, **in the absence of antibodies.**
3. **Lectin pathway:** In this pathway, plasma mannose-binding lectin binds to carbohydrates (mannose) on microbes and activates C1. In this pathway also, there is no role of antibody.

Steps in Complement Pathway

Formation of *C3 convertase:* All three pathways of complement activation lead to the formation of an enzyme called the *C3 convertase.*

Splitting of C3 by C3 convertase: C3 convertase splits C3 into two functionally distinct fragments namely C3a and C3b. C3a is released as an anaphylatoxin. C3b reacts with cell proteins to localize, or "fix," on the cell surface where complement is being activated. **C3b** and its degradation products on the surface of pathogens enhance phagocytosis. This process of coating a pathogen with a molecule that enhances phagocytosis is termed opsonization; the molecule that does this is called an **opsonin.**

Formation of *C5 convertase:* Then additional C3b binds to the previously produced fragments of complement to form *C5 convertase* (complex of C4b, C2a, and C3b). This C5 convertase cleaves C5 into C5a and C5b. It releases C5a (also an anaphylatoxin) and leaves C5b attached to the cell surface.

Formation of the membrane attack complex (MAC): C5b acts as the nidus for subsequent sequential binding of C6, C7, C8, and C9 (late components of complement) and forms the membrane attack complex (MAC). MAC is composed of multiple C9 molecules.

Assembly of MAC on target cells or microbes: The MAC directly inserts into plasma membranes. It results in the formation of a cylindrical transmembrane channel through the plasma membrane. This leads to lysis of cells or microbes.

Main Functions of Complements in Inflammation

1. **Recruitment of leukocytes: C5a**, and, to a lesser extent **C3a,** and C4a complement components (cleavage products of complements) stimulate recruitment of neutrophils and other leukocytes at the site of injury.
2. **Increased vascular permeability and vasodilation: C3a and C5a** stimulate the **release of histamine from mast cells.** This in turn increases vascular permeability and causes vasodilation. C3a, C4a, and C5a are called anaphylatoxins because their actions are similar to mast cell mediators involved in anaphylaxis.
3. **Promote opsonization and phagocytosis:** C3b and its cleavage product iC3b (inactive C3b) act as opsonins. When C3b is fixed to a microbial wall, it promotes phagocytosis by neutrophils and macrophages. The phagocytosis is achieved through surface receptors for these complement fragments on these phagocytes.
4. **Cell lysis:** The deposition of the membrane attack complex—MAC (C5b-C9) on cells, especially thin-walled microbes such as *Neisseria* bacteria creates pores. These holes in the cell membrane permit intracellular water and ions to leak out. This leads to the death (lysis) of the cells, Thus, patients with inherited deficiencies of the terminal components of complement or those treated with complement inhibitors are at high risk of disseminated infections with *Neisseria* species (meningococci and gonococci).

Regulation of complement system: The **complement activation is controlled by cell-associated and circulating regulatory proteins.** The regulatory proteins prevent the production of active complement fragments or remove the activated fragments that deposit on cells, thereby protecting the host from indiscriminate injury. These regulatory mechanisms include spontaneous decay, and proteolytic inactivation, by binding active components (e.g., C1 esterase inhibitor binds C1 to form inactive complex) and by cell membrane-associated molecules [e.g., decay accelerating factor (DAF), CD59].

Other Mediators of Inflammation

Platelet-activating Factor (PAF)

Q. Write a short note on the platelet-activating factor.

Platelet-activating factor (PAF) is another phospholipid-derived mediator.

Source: PAF is synthesized by various cell types namely: **platelets, basophils, mast cells, neutrophils, macrophages, and endothelial cells.**

Action: And has multiple inflammatory effects. However, its role in acute inflammatory reactions is not clear.

- **Vascular reactions:** PAF causes **vasoconstriction and bronchoconstriction. At low concentrations,** it produces **vasodilation and increased vascular permeability** at sites of tissue injury.
- **Cellular reactions: Increased leukocyte adhesion** to endothelium, **chemotaxis,** leukocyte degranulation, and oxidative burst.
- **Platelet aggregation:** PAF causes platelet aggregation.

Products of Coagulation

The link between coagulation pathway and inflammation: Almost all types of tissue injury that lead to clotting also induce inflammation, and inflammation causes changes in endothelial cells that increase the chances of abnormal clotting (i.e., thrombosis). It was observed that cleavage products of fibrin (fibrinopeptides) can stimulate inflammation. Many forms of tissue injury are associated with both clotting and inflammation. Inhibition of coagulation factors was found to reduce the inflammatory reaction to certain microbes. This indicates that there is a close association (link) between coagulation and inflammation. However, it is difficult to establish a cause-and-effect relationship and the significant role of products of coagulation in stimulating inflammation.

Protease-activated receptors (PARs): The link between coagulation and inflammation was supported by the discovery of *protease-activated receptors (PARs,* also known as the thrombin receptor). These PARs are **expressed on platelets and leukocytes**, which **are activated by thrombin**. The thrombin is the protease that cleaves fibrinogen to produce fibrin clot and causes powerful aggregation of platelets during the process of clot formation. However, the major role of the PARs is in platelet activation during clotting.

Kinins

Kinins are vasoactive peptides. They are formed from plasma proteins, called **kininogens** by the action of specific **proteases called kallikreins.** The enzyme kallikrein cleaves a plasma glycoprotein precursor, high-molecular-weight kininogen, to generate ***bradykinin.***

Actions of bradykinin: Their effects are like those of histamine (*refer* 73-4).

- **Increases vascular permeability, contraction of smooth muscle, and dilation of blood vessels.**
- **Pain:** It produces pain when injected into the skin.

Inactivation: The action of bradykinin is quick and short-lived. They are quickly inactivated by an enzyme called **kininase.**

Neuropeptides

Neuropeptides are small peptides (e.g., substance P, neurokinin A) produced in the central and peripheral nervous system.

Source: They are secreted by sensory nerves and various leukocytes.

Actions: These may be involved in the initiation and regulation of inflammatory responses. Substance P transmits pain signals and increases vascular permeability.

The most important mediators involved in acute inflammation are summarized in **Table 3.11** (*refer* **online Fig. 3.13**).

Q. Write a short note on the role of different mediators in different reactions of inflammation (For answers refer Table 3.11).

TABLE 3.11 Important mediators involved in acute inflammation.

The action of the mediator	*Name of the mediator*	*Source of the mediator*
Vasodilation	Histamine	Mast cells, basophils, platelets
	Prostaglandins	Mast cells, all leukocytes
Increased vascular permeability	Histamine and serotonin	Platelets
	C3a and C5a (liberate vasoactive amines from mast cells, and other cells)	Plasma (produced in the liver)
	Leukotrienes C_4, D_4, E_4	Mast cells, all leukocytes
Chemotaxis, leukocyte recruitment and activation	Cytokines (TNF, IL-1, IL-6)	Macrophages, lymphocytes, endothelial cells, mast cells
	Chemokines	Leukocytes, activated macrophages
	C3a, C5a	Plasma (produced in the liver)
	Leukotriene B_4	Mast cells, leukocytes
	Bacterial products (e.g., *N*-formyl methyl peptides)	Bacteria
Fever	IL1, TNF	Macrophages, endothelial cells, mast cells
	Prostaglandins	Mast cells, leukocytes
Pain	Prostaglandins	
	Bradykinin	Plasma protein
	Neuropeptides (substance P)	Leukocytes, nerve fibers
Tissue damage	Lysosomal enzymes	Leukocytes
	Reactive oxygen species	

(IL-1: interleukin-1; IL-6: interleukin-6; TNF: tumor necrosis factor).

Morphologic characteristics of acute inflammatory reactions: The general morphologic features of most acute inflammatory are **dilation of small blood vessels and accumulation of leukocytes and fluid in the extravascular tissue.** However, morphologic patterns vary. It depends on the etiologic agent, the severity of the reaction, and the particular tissue and site affected. Gross and microscopic appearances can often provide clues about the cause.

MORPHOLOGICAL TYPES/PATTERNS OF ACUTE INFLAMMATION

Q. Write a short note on morphological types/patterns of acute inflammatory reaction with suitable examples.

Serous Inflammation

Feature: It is characterized by **the accumulation of a thin serous (serum-like), protein-rich exudate (fluid).**

Sites affected: Serous fluid accumulates in **body cavities** such as the peritoneum, pleura, or pericardium or spaces created by tissue injury. **The accumulation of fluid in a mesothelium-lined cavity is called an *effusion*.** Pleural effusion occurs as a complication of lobar pneumonia. Inflammation of synovium (synovitis) produces an accumulation of fluid in joint cavities.

Appearance: The serous fluid is **sterile and usually does not contain large numbers of leukocytes.** The leukocytes are present in large numbers in purulent inflammation. **Serous exudate or effusion is yellow, straw-like in color.**

Mechanism of fluid accumulation: The fluid in the **body cavities** may be derived from the plasma (due to increased vascular permeability) or may be secreted by mesothelial cells (due to local irritation). **Skin blistering formed in burns or viral infection** is due to the accumulation of serous fluid within or immediately beneath the damaged epidermis.

Fibrinous Inflammation

Feature: Fibrinous inflammation is characterized by the **deposition of fibrin**. It develops as a result of the local activation of coagulation.

Sites affected: A fibrinous exudate is mostly observed with **inflammation in the lining of body cavities**, such as the **meninges, pericardium, and pleura**. When a fibrinous exudate develops on a serosal surface, such as the pleura or pericardium, it is known as fibrinous pleuritis or fibrinous pericarditis respectively. For example, fibrinous pericarditis (*refer* **Fig. 16.20**) is seen in rheumatic fever and is classically known as "**bread and butter**" pericarditis.

Mechanism of fibrinous inflammation: A marked **increase in vascular permeability** leads to the **escape of large molecules like fibrinogen from the lumen of the vessel** into the extravascular space. The fibrinogen accumulates within exudates, and if a procoagulant stimulus is present, it forms fibrin. The exudate is rich in fibrin and is called **fibrinous exudate**. Microscopically, fibrin appears as an eosinophilic or pink meshwork of threads or pink amorphous coagulum.

Consequences: These are as follows:

- **Resolution:** Fibrinous exudates may be resolved by the breakdown of fibrin (fibrinolysis) and cleared by macrophages.
- **Organization:** If fibrinous exudates are not resolved, **ingrowth of fibroblasts and blood vessels** may occur into the exudate. This process is called organization. This leads to scarring. This may be harmful. For example, an extensive organization within the pericardial cavity may obliterate the pericardial space and produce restrictive cardiomyopathy.

Suppurative or Purulent Inflammation: Abscess

Q. Write a short note on the abscess.

Feature: Purulent inflammation is characterized by the **production of pus** or purulent exudate. Microscopically, this exudate **consists of neutrophils, the liquefied debris of necrotic cells, and edema fluid.**

Etiology: The most common cause of purulent (*suppurative*) inflammation is **infection with bacteria that produce liquefactive necrosis** (e.g., staphylococci). These bacteria that produce localized suppuration are called **pyogenic** (pus-producing) bacteria. For example, acute suppurative appendicitis.

Abscesses: It is the **localized collections of purulent inflammatory exudates in a tissue**, an organ, or a confined space. They are produced by the deposition of pyogenic bacteria into a tissue. Abscesses have a central necrotic focus (consisting of necrotic leukocytes and necrotic parenchymal cells) surrounded by a zone of preserved neutrophils (e.g., boil caused by *Staphylococcus aureus*). Outside this zone, there may be vascular congestion and parenchymal and fibroblastic proliferation. In time the abscess may become walled off and replaced by connective tissue. If pus accumulates in hollow organs or pleural cavities, it is known as empyema.

Ulcer

Q. Write a short note on the ulcer.

Definition: An ulcer is defined as a local defect, or excavation, of the surface of an organ or tissue. An ulcer is **produced by the sloughing (shedding) of inflamed necrotic tissue.**

Injury to epithelial structures due to neutrophils and the mediators released by them (plus ROS and NO), can denude the epithelium leading to ulceration. This exposes the underlying connective tissue.

Common sites: Ulceration develops only when there is necrosis of tissue and resultant inflammation exists on or near a surface.

1. Mucosa of the mouth, stomach [(e.g., peptic ulcer of the stomach or duodenum (*refer* **Fig. 18.13**)], intestines (*refer* **Fig. 18.24**), or genitourinary tract.
2. Skin and subcutaneous tissue of the lower extremities (e.g., varicose ulcers).

Microscopy: Both acute and chronic inflammation may coexist in ulcers.

- **Acute stage:** During the acute stage, it shows severe infiltration of polymorphonuclear leukocytes and vascular dilation in the margins of the defect.
- **Chronic stage:** With time, the margins and base of the ulcer show scarring and infiltration by chronic inflammatory cells (lymphocytes, plasma cells, and macrophages).

Other Morphologic Patterns

Hemorrhagic inflammation: When inflammation is associated with severe vascular injury or deficiency of coagulation factors, it causes hemorrhagic inflammation, e.g., acute pancreatitis (*refer* **Fig. 19.44**) due to proteolytic destruction of vascular walls.

Catarrhal inflammation: Acute inflammation of a mucous membrane is accompanied by excessive secretion of mucus and the appearance is described as catarrhal, e.g., common cold.

Membranous inflammation: In this type, the epithelium is covered by a membrane consisting of fibrin, desquamated epithelial cells, and inflammatory cells, e.g., pharyngitis or laryngitis due to *Corynebacterium diphtheriae*.

Pseudomembranous inflammation: It is characterized by superficial mucosal ulceration covered by sloughed mucosa, fibrin, mucus, and inflammatory cells. For example, pseudomembranous colitis is due to *Clostridium difficile* colonization of the bowel, usually following broad-spectrum antibiotic treatment.

Necrotizing (gangrenous) inflammation: The combination of necrosis and bacterial putrefaction is gangrene (*refer* pages 21-2 and **Fig. 2.11**), e.g., gangrenous appendicitis.

Terminologies

Bacteremia: It is defined as a condition characterized by the presence of a small number of bacteria in the blood. They cannot be detected by direct microscopic examination of blood and are detected by blood culture (e.g., typhoid infection caused by *Salmonella typhi*).

Septicemia: It is defined as the presence of rapidly multiplying, highly pathogenic bacteria in the blood (e.g., pyogenic cocci/bacilli). It is usually associated with systemic effects such as toxemia and neutrophilic leukocytosis.

Pyemia: It is the dissemination of small septic emboli in the blood that produce their effects at the site of their lodgment. Thus, it can lead to pyemic abscesses or septic infarcts.

Cellulitis: It is the term used for diffuse inflammation of the soft tissues due to organisms, produced from spreading effects of substances like hyaluronidase released by some bacteria.

OUTCOMES OF ACUTE INFLAMMATION

Q. Write a short note on outcomes of acute inflammation.

Many variables may modify the outcome of inflammation. These include the nature and intensity of the injury, the site and tissue affected, and the response of the host. Typically, all **acute inflammatory reactions have one of the following outcomes (Flowchart 3.2):**

1. **Complete resolution.** Optimally, all effective inflammatory responses will: (i) limit the area of injury, (ii) clear (eliminate) the causative injurious agent and damaged tissue; and (ii) return the affected tissue to normal (i.e., restore normal tissue architecture and physiologic function). This process of **complete return of tissue architecture to normal following acute inflammation** is called *resolution* (e.g., resolution in lobar penumonia). It is the usual outcome that occurs:
   - When the injury is limited or short-lived
   - With no or minimal tissue damage/destruction
   - When the damaged (injured) parenchymal tissue is capable of regeneration.

   In the process of resolution, the cellular debris and microbes are removed by macrophages and the edema fluid is resorbed mainly through lymphatics.
2. **Abscess: A localized collection of pus is called an abscess.** If the area of acute inflammation is walled off

Flowchart 3.2: Outcomes of acute inflammation: (1) resolution, (2) suppuration, (3) healing by connective tissue replacement [healing by fibrosis and scarring (organization)], or (4) progression to chronic inflammation.

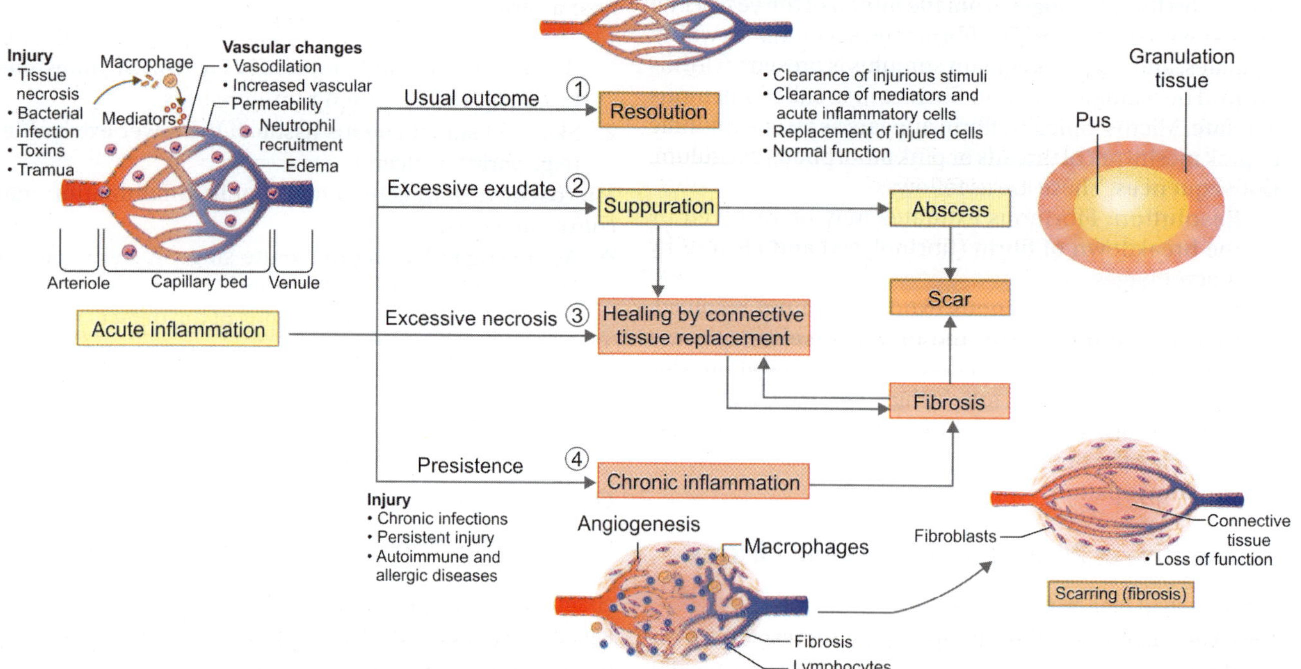

by inflammatory cells and fibrosis, neutrophil products destroy the tissue and form an abscess.

3. **Healing by connective tissue replacement (scarring, or fibrosis).** The process of **replacement of dead tissue by living tissue,** which matures to form scar tissue is known as **organization. Scarring or fibrosis occurs:**
   - In the presence of significant tissue destruction.
   - With inflammation in tissues incapable of regeneration.
   - When there is plenty of fibrin exudation in tissue or serous cavities (pleura, peritoneum) that cannot be removed or cleared.

   This process involves the growth of connective tissue into the area of tissue damage or exudate. The inflammatory region is converted into a mass of fibrous tissue (scar).
4. **Progression to chronic inflammation:** Chronic inflammation may follow acute inflammation, or it may be chronic from the beginning itself. Acute inflammation may progress to chronic when the acute inflammatory response cannot be resolved. This may be due to:
   - Persistence of the injurious agent or
   - Abnormality in the process of healing.

   Examples: (1) Bacterial infection of the lung may begin as acute inflammation (pneumonia). But when it fails to resolve, it can cause extensive tissue destruction and form a cavity with chronic inflammation known as **lung abscess.** (2) Acute osteomyelitis, if not treated properly may progress to **chronic osteomyelitis.** (3) Chronic inflammation with a persisting stimulus results in **peptic ulcer** of the duodenum or stomach, which may persist for months or years.

CHRONIC INFLAMMATION

PA 4.3 (CC): Define and describe chronic inflammation including causes, types, nonspecific, and granulomatous; and enumerate examples of each.

Definition: Chronic inflammation is defined as **inflammation of prolonged duration** (weeks or months) in which there are **varying combinations of (i) inflammation** (continued recruitment of chronic inflammatory cells), **(ii) tissue damage** (due to prolonged inflammation), **and (iii) attempt at healing** (to restore tissue integrity) **occur at the same time.**

Mode of development: Chronic inflammation may:
1. **Follow an acute inflammation,** which does not resolve (e.g., chronic osteomyelitis) or
2. **Begin as an insidious, low-grade, chronic, sometimes progressive** response without any prior (former) acute inflammatory reaction.

Causes of Chronic Inflammation

Q. What are the causes of chronic inflammation?

Chronic inflammation may occur in one of the following settings:

1. **Persistent infections by microorganisms:** Persistent infection by microbes that are difficult to eliminate (get rid of) elicit and produce chronic inflammation, e.g., mycobacteria, and certain viruses, fungi, and parasites. **Some agents may cause** a **distinct pattern of chronic inflammation** known as a **granulomatous reaction.** In some infections, acute inflammation may be incompletely resolved and progress into chronic inflammation. For example, bacterial infection of the lung can progress to a chronic lung abscess.
2. **Hypersensitivity and autoimmune diseases:** Chronic inflammation may be caused by **excessive and inappropriate activation of the immune system.**
   - **Autoimmune diseases:** In these diseases, immune reactions develop against the individual's own tissues (autoantigens/self-antigens). It causes a self-sustaining immune reaction and produces chronic tissue damage and inflammation. Examples include **rheumatoid arthritis** and multiple sclerosis.
   - **Allergic diseases:** In these diseases, chronic inflammation develops because of excessive immune responses against common environmental substances (e.g., **bronchial asthma**).
   - **Unregulated immune response** (e.g., inflammatory bowel disease).
3. **Prolonged exposure to potentially toxic injurious agents:** These toxic agents may be exogenous or endogenous.
   - **Exogenous:** For example, **silica** is a nondegradable, inanimate, exogenous material. If persons are exposed to inhalation of silica particles for a long time, it causes an inflammatory lung disease called **silicosis.**
   - **Endogenous: Atherosclerosis** is a disease of arterial intima, and probably represents a chronic inflammatory process partly due to endogenous toxic plasma **lipid components** (cholesterol and other lipids).

Morphologic Features

Q. Mention the morphological/histological features of chronic inflammation.

Acute inflammation manifests with vascular changes, edema, and predominantly neutrophilic infiltration. In contrast, chronic inflammation is characterized by the following features:
- **Mononuclear cells infiltrate:** These include **macrophages, lymphocytes, and plasma cells.**
- **Tissue destruction:** This may be caused due to the persistence of causative agents or by the inflammatory cells.
- **Healing by fibrosis:** Chronic inflammation shows attempts at healing. It is characterized by the replacement of damaged tissue by connective tissue. It is associated

with *angiogenesis* (proliferation of small blood vessels) and *fibrosis*. It leads to the formation of a *scar*.

Cells and Mediators of Chronic Inflammation

Q. Write a short note on the cells of chronic inflammation.

Chronic inflammation is characterized by the combination of: **(i) leukocyte infiltration, (ii) tissue damage, and (iii) fibrosis.** These microscopic features result from the local activation of several cell types and the production of mediators.

Role of Macrophages

Q. Mention the role of macrophages in chronic inflammation.

Macrophage is the predominant cell in chronic inflammatory reactions. They belong to the mononuclear phagocyte system.

Mononuclear Phagocyte System

The mononuclear phagocyte system consists of a class of cells that occur in various parts of the body. These cells have in common the property of phagocytosis. These cells are professional phagocytes whose primary function is to ingest and destroy particulate matter, microbes, and dead cells. The cells that make up the *mononuclear phagocyte system* are as follows:

Macrophages: Normally, macrophages are **diffusely distributed in most connective tissues.** These macrophages are the **dominant cells in most chronic inflammatory reactions.** These macrophages: (i) destroy foreign invaders and tissues, (ii) secrete cytokines and growth factors, and (iii) activate other cells, mainly T lymphocytes. They have many other roles in host defense, inflammation, and repair. Tissue macrophages have **abundant cytoplasm containing phagocytic vacuoles.** These phagocytic vacuoles may contain ingested material, as well as lysosomes and other organelles.

- **Circulating monocytes:** *Circulating cells* belonging to macrophage origin are known as *monocytes*. Blood monocytes measure 10–15 μm in diameter. They have **bean-shaped nuclei and finely granular cytoplasm.**

Tissue-resident macrophages: Apart from connective tissue, these macrophages are found in specific locations in organs. These locations include the liver (Kupffer cells), spleen, and lymph nodes (sinus histiocytes), central nervous system (microglial cells), and lungs (alveolar macrophages).

Origin of Macrophages (Figs. 3.14A and B)

Hematopoietic stem cells: Macrophages in tissues are derived **from hematopoietic stem cells in the bone marrow.**

Progenitors in the embryonic yolk sac and fetal liver: During early development, macrophages are derived **from progenitors in the embryonic yolk sac and fetal liver.** Tissue-resident macrophages (e.g., microglia and Kupffer cells) arise from the yolk sac or fetal liver early in embryogenesis. These tissue-resident macrophages stay for long periods and are replenished mainly by the proliferation of resident cells.

Macrophage Events in Inflammation

Monocytes: In inflammatory reactions, progenitors in the bone marrow give rise to monocytes.

Differentiation of monocytes into macrophages: Monocytes from bone marrow enter the blood, and migrate into various extravascular tissues. These monocytes differentiate **and transform into** a larger phagocytic cell known as tissue **macrophages.** The molecules involved in the entry of blood monocytes into tissues are similar to those

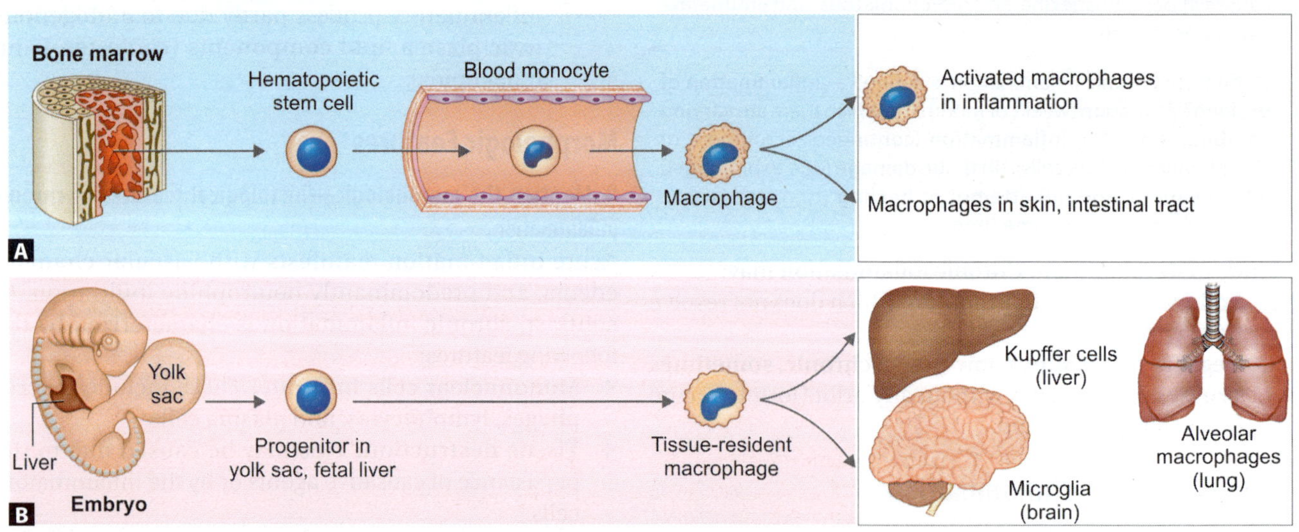

Figs. 3.14A and B: Maturation of mononuclear phagocytes: (A) During inflammatory reactions, most of the tissue macrophages are derived from hematopoietic stem cells; (B) Early in development, some tissue-resident macrophages are derived from embryonic precursors in the embryonic yolk sac and fetal liver.

involved in neutrophil emigration (e.g., adhesion molecules and chemokines).

Macrophages have a **longer life span** in tissues than other leukocytes. Therefore, macrophages are often the **dominant cells in inflammatory reactions within 48 hours of onset.**

Macrophage Activation (Fig. 3.15)

Tissue macrophages are activated by **two major pathways: (1) classical and (2) alternative.**

1. Classical macrophage activation

Classically activated are also called M1 macrophages.

Mediators of classical macrophage activation: This activation may be brought out by microbial products (e.g., endotoxin), T cell-derived signals (mainly cytokines such as IFN-γ), and foreign substances (e.g., crystals and particulate matter).

Products of activated macrophages: Classically activated macrophages produce nitric oxide (NO), and reactive oxygen species (ROS). They also upregulate lysosomal enzymes. All these increase their ability to kill/eliminate ingested organisms, and they secrete cytokines that stimulate inflammation.

Function: Phagocytosis.

2. Alternative macrophage activation

These alternatively activated cells are also called M2 macrophages.

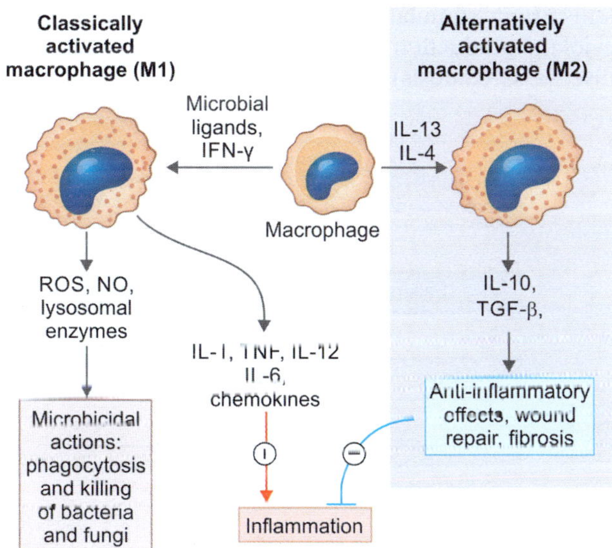

Fig. 3.15: Pathways of macrophage activation. Different stimuli activate tissue macrophages to develop into functionally two distinct populations of macrophages M1 and M2. Classically activated (M1) macrophages are activated by microbial products and cytokines, particularly IFN-γ. These macrophages phagocytose and destroy microbes and debris from dead tissues and can produce inflammatory reactions. Alternatively, activated (M2) macrophages are activated by other cytokines and these are important in tissue repair and the resolution of inflammation.

Mediators of activation: Alternative macrophage activation is brought out mainly by **cytokines** IL-4 and IL-13 produced by T-lymphocytes and other cells. They secrete growth factors that promote angiogenesis, activate fibroblasts, and stimulate collagen synthesis. They also inhibit inflammation

Function: These are not actively microbicidal. Their main function is **tissue repair**. They secrete growth factors and promote angiogenesis, activate fibroblasts, and stimulate collagen synthesis. They also inhibit inflammation.

Functions of Macrophages in Inflammation

These are as follows:

- **Phagocytosis:** The activated macrophage **ingests microbes and debris.** Their **products remove injurious agents** such as microbes and debris from dead tissues.
- **Initiation and propagation of inflammatory reactions:** Macrophages secrete mediators of inflammation, such as cytokines (TNF, IL-1, chemokines, and others) and eicosanoids (arachidonic acid metabolites). Through these products, macrophages initiate and propagate inflammatory reactions, and play a central role in inflammation.
- **Initiation of the tissue repair and scar formation and fibrosis.**
- **Feedback loop for defense against many microbes by cell-mediated immune response.** Macrophages display antigens to T lymphocytes and respond to signals from T cells. Thus, they set up a feedback loop for defense against many microbes by cell-mediated immune responses.

Role of Lymphocytes

Microbes and other environmental antigens activate T and B lymphocytes. These lymphocytes intensify and propagate chronic inflammation. The lymphocytes may be the predominant cells in autoimmune and other hypersensitivity diseases. Activated B lymphocytes and antibody-secreting plasma cells are usually seen in chronic inflammation.

Q. Write a short note on the T helper cell.

CD4+ T lymphocytes: These are important T lymphocytes. CD4+ T lymphocytes secrete cytokines that promote inflammation and influence the nature of the inflammatory reaction. There are three subsets of CD4+ T cells. These subtypes secrete different types of cytokines and produce different types of inflammation.

- **Th1 cells:** They produce the cytokine IFN-γ. This cytokine activates macrophages by the classical pathway.
- **Th2 cells:** They secrete IL-4, IL-5, and IL-13. These cytokines recruit and activate eosinophils and activate macrophages through alternate pathways. Involved in defense against helminthic infestation and allergic reactions.

- **Th17 cells:** They secrete IL-17 and other cytokines. These cytokines stimulate the secretion of chemokines responsible for recruiting mainly neutrophils into the reaction.

Other Cells in Chronic Inflammation

- **Plasma cells:** They are derived from activated B lymphocytes and produce antibodies either against foreign or self-antigens. Activated B lymphocytes and antibody-producing plasma cells are seen at the site of chronic inflammation (e.g., syphilis). In some chronic inflammatory reactions, the lymphocytes, antigen-presenting cells, and plasma cells form lymphoid follicles similar to those found in lymph nodes. Examples include in the synovium of patients with rheumatoid arthritis, in the thyroid in Hashimoto thyroiditis, and the gastric mucosa in *Helicobacter pylori* infection.
- **Eosinophils:** They are seen in immune reactions mediated by IgE and in parasitic infections. A **chemokine**, that **attracts eosinophil recruitment is eotaxin**. The granules of eosinophils contain a **major basic protein** that is toxic to parasites and also destroys the epithelial cells.
- **Mast cells:** They are distributed in connective tissues and participate in both acute and chronic inflammatory reactions. They are seen in allergic reactions to foods, insect venom, or drugs.
- **Neutrophils:** These are **characteristic of acute inflammation**. However, many forms of chronic inflammation that last for months, continue to show many neutrophils. These may be because of either the persistence of microbes or cytokines and other mediators produced by activated macrophages and T lymphocytes. For example, in **chronic bacterial infection of bone (osteomyelitis)**, a neutrophilic exudate can persist for many months. Sometimes, neutrophils are seen along with chronic inflammation and this pattern of inflammation is called **acute or chronic**.

PA 4.2 (CC): Identify and describe acute and chronic inflammation in gross and microscopic specimens.

Types of Chronic Inflammation

It can be divided into: (1) chronic nonspecific inflammation and (2) granulomatous inflammation.

Chronic Nonspecific Inflammation

It is chronic inflammation in which the injurious agent produces a nonspecific chronic inflammatory reaction. It consists of chronic inflammatory cells such as **macrophages, lymphocytes**, and sometimes plasma cells. There is no granuloma formation. Examples include **chronic osteomyelitis, chronic pyelonephritis, and chronic cholecystitis.**

Granulomatous Inflammation

Q. Define and classify granuloma. Write a short note on granulomatous lymphadenitis.

Definition: A **granuloma** is defined as a form of **chronic inflammation characterized by microscopic collections of activated macrophages** (that are transformed into epithelium-like/epithelioid cells), **often with T lymphocytes**. Sometimes, it is associated with central necrosis.

The term *granuloma* is derived from the macroscopic (gross) granular appearance of these inflammatory nodules. **Mechanism of granuloma formation (Fig. 3.16):** Granulomatous inflammation is a protective response that isolates a persistent offending agent, preventing it from disseminating and restricting inflammation. It usually occurs as an attempt to suppress causative agents that are difficult to eradicate and that induce strong T cell–mediated immune responses. For example, persistent microbes such as mycobacteria or some fungi. Granulomatous inflammation also develops against indigestible foreign bodies present in the tissue, in the absence of T cell–mediated immune responses. These foreign bodies are not immunogenic but are too large to be phagocytosed by macrophages (e.g., talc, silk sutures, asbestos, and other fibers). This results in persistent activation of the phagocytic cells. Granuloma also occurs with persistent infection, and chronic stimulation of macrophages due to persistent cytokine production in autoimmune diseases (e.g., Crohn disease, sarcoidosis).

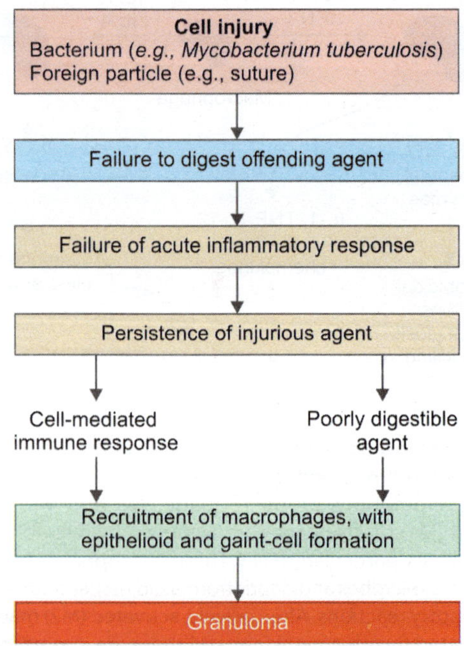

Fig. 3.16: Mechanism of granuloma.

MORPHOLOGY

Q. Write a short note on epithelioid cells and granuloma.

Granuloma (Figs. 3.17A to C)

Granuloma consists of the following types of cells when viewed under the usual hematoxylin and eosin preparations:

Epithelioid cells: These are the main cells of granulomatous inflammation. Epithelioid cells are the **activated (modified) macrophages that** vaguely **resemble squamous epithelial cells.** These epithelioid macrophages form nodular collections or aggregates at the site of an indigestible phagocytic stimulus.

- **Cytoplasm:** The epithelioid cells have **abundant, pale, pink, granular cytoplasm** with **indistinct cell borders,** often appearing to merge into one another.
- **Nucleus:** The **nucleus is oval or elongated** and may show the folding of the nuclear membrane. The nucleus is **less dense than that of a lymphocyte.**

Giant cells: Frequently, but not invariably, granulomas contain **multinucleated giant cells.** These are formed by the fusion of "frustrated" macrophages (epithelioid cells) in which their cytoplasm fuses to become syncytial multinucleated giant cells. They have abundant cytoplasm and have many small nuclei. Nuclei may be as many as 20 or more. They are found in the periphery or sometimes in the center of granulomas. There are several types of giant cells seen in granuloma.

- **Langhans giant cell:** When the **multiple nuclei of giant cells are arrayed around the cell's periphery in a horseshoe pattern,** the cell is called a Langhans giant cell. These giant cells may attain diameters of 40–50 µm.
- **Foreign body–type giant cell:** In this giant cell, the **multiple nuclei tend to be distributed haphazardly throughout the cytoplasm.** It occurs when there is a foreign agent (e.g., silica) or other indigestible material.

Lymphocytes: The aggregates of epithelioid macrophages are usually surrounded by a rim of lymphocytes (CD4+ T lymphocytes). The lymphocytes form a concentric ring or "collar" around the central core of macrophages, giant cells, and sometimes, necrotic debris. These lymphocytes are recruited to the site of inflammation by cytokines produced by activated macrophages and giant cells.

Necrosis: Sometimes granulomas are associated with central necrosis. For example, granulomas are associated with certain infectious organisms (classically *Mycobacterium tuberculosis*). In tuberculosis, a combination of hypoxia and free injury leads to a central zone of necrosis. Grossly, caseous necrosis appears as granular, and cheesy (*refer* to **Fig. 2.7**) and is therefore called **caseous necrosis.** Microscopically, caseous necrosis appears as amorphous, structureless, eosinophilic, granular debris (*refer* to **Fig. 2.8**). However, the granulomas in Crohn disease, sarcoidosis, and foreign body reactions do not have necrotic centers and are called *noncaseating (hard) granulomas*.

The outer rim of fibroblasts: Older granulomas in addition may show a rim of fibroblasts and connective tissue as the outermost layer. Granulomas may heal by producing extensive fibrosis.

Types of Granulomas

Depending on the pathogenesis granulomas are divided into two types:

1. **Foreign body granulomas:** It develops **against relatively inert foreign bodies** that do not stimulate any specific inflammatory or immune response (absence of T-cell-mediated immune responses). Examples of foreign bodies include **suture materials, talc** (associated with intravenous drug abuse), or other fibers that are large enough to be phagocytosed by a macrophage. Epithelioid cells and giant cells are closely found on the surface of these foreign bodies. The foreign material can usually be found in the center of the granuloma, particularly if seen with polarized light (appears refractile).
2. **Immune granulomas:** These are caused by various agents/microbes that can generate a persistent T-cell-mediated immune response. Immune granulomas usually develop when the causative agent is difficult to eliminate, such as a persistent microbe (e.g., *Mycobacterium tuberculosis*) or a self-antigen. In these granulomas, macrophages activate Th1 cells to produce cytokines, such as IFN-γ, which activates the macrophages. Granuloma in tuberculosis is referred to as a tubercle and usually shows central caseous necrosis (due to a combination of hypoxia and free radical-mediated injury) and is rare in other granulomatous diseases. Sometimes, it may be necessary to perform

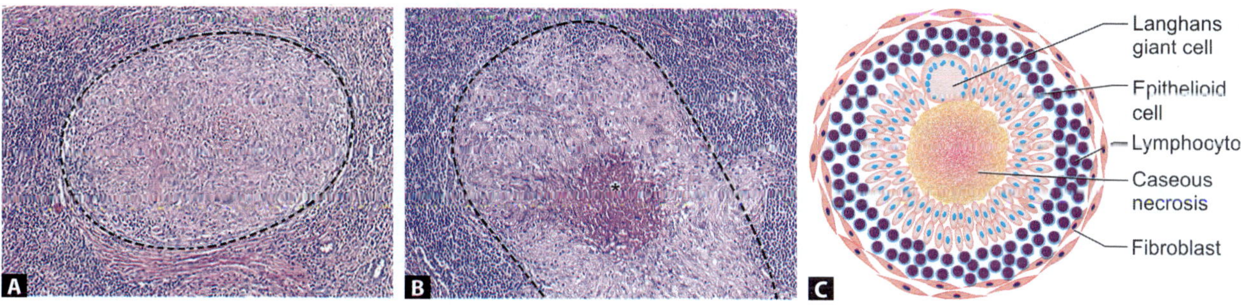

Figs. 3.17A to C: Microscopic appearance of a granuloma: (A) Tuberculous granuloma (dotted line) showing aggregate of epithelioid cells; (B) Tuberculous granuloma (dotted line) showing a central area of caseous necrosis (*) surrounded by epithelioid cells, and lymphocytes; (C) Diagrammatic representation of granuloma in tuberculosis showing central necrosis, surrounded by epithelioid cells, Langhans-type giant cells, lymphocytes, and an outer layer of fibroblasts.

TABLE 3.12 Examples of granulomatous inflammation.

Disease	*Cause*	*Tissue reaction*
Tuberculosis (*refer* **Fig. 3.17**)	*Mycobacterium tuberculosis*	Caseating granuloma (tubercle): central necrosis with amorphous granular debris surrounded by epithelioid cells, rimmed by lymphocytes, histiocytes, and fibroblasts. Occasional Langhans giant cells, presence of acid-fast bacilli
Leprosy (*refer* **Figs. 4.2A and B**)	*Mycobacterium leprae*	Acid-fast bacilli in macrophages; noncaseating granulomas
Syphilis	*Treponema pallidum*	Gumma: microscopic to grossly visible lesion. Consists of histiocytes; plasma cell infiltrate; and central necrotic cells without loss of cellular outline (coagulative necrosis)
Cat-scratch disease	Gram-negative *Bacillus*	Rounded or stellate granuloma containing central granular debris and neutrophils; giant cells rare
Sarcoidosis (*refer* **Fig. 17.22**)	Unknown etiology	Noncaseating granulomas with plenty of activated macrophages
Crohn disease (inflammatory bowel disease) (*refer to* **Fig. 18.35**)	Immune reaction against intestinal bacteria, self-antigens	Dense chronic inflammatory infiltrate with occasional noncaseating granulomas in the wall of the intestine
Foreign body granulomas	Talc, suture	Non-caseating granulomas with foreign body giant cell

additional tests/investigations to identify the etiologic agent in granuloma.

- Special stains, e.g., acid-fast stains for tubercle bacilli.
- Culture methods, e.g., in tuberculosis and fungal diseases.
- Molecular techniques, e.g., the polymerase chain reaction in tuberculosis.
- Serologic studies, e.g., in syphilis.

One of the causes of granulomatous lymphadenitis is tuberculosis. **Tuberculosis is the model of a granulomatous disease caused by infection. Always, tuberculosis should always be excluded as the cause when granulomas are identified.**

Examples of granulomatous inflammation are listed in **Table 3.12.**

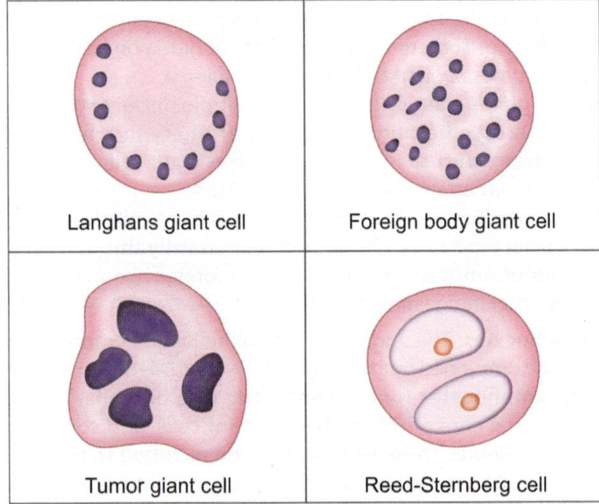

Fig. 3.18: Common types of giant cells (diagrammatic).

Giant Cell

Q. Write a short note on various types of giant cells and the conditions associated with them.

Definition: A cell with more than one nucleus is called a giant cell or multinucleated cell.

Types of giant cells (Fig. 3.18): Various types of giant cells and their associated conditions are mentioned in **Box 3.3.**

SYSTEMIC EFFECTS OF INFLAMMATION

Q. Write a short note on the systemic effects of inflammation.

Acute inflammation produces the cardinal signs of inflammation that are localized to the site of inflammation. However, many acute inflammations are **associated with cytokine-induced systemic reactions.** These include fever, leucocytosis, acute phase reactant proteins, lymphangitis-lymphadenitis, malaise, anorexia (reduced appetite, and shock.

Mediators: The systemic manifestations of inflammation develop as reactions to cytokines produced by leukocytes. These cytokines are produced in response to infections [stimulated by bacterial products such as lipopolysaccharides (LPS)] and other inflammatory stimuli. The most important **mediators of the systemic response** are **cytokines TNF, IL-1, and IL-6.** Other cytokines such as type I interferons are also involved in the reaction. Usually, the systemic reactions are more severe in acute than in chronic inflammation. This is because of increased levels of cytokine production in acute inflammation.

The systemic effects of inflammation consist of various clinical and pathologic changes and are briefly discussed below.

BOX 3.3: Types of giant cells.

PHYSIOLOGICAL
- Osteoclast
- Syncytiotrophoblast
- Megakaryocyte

PATHOLOGICAL

Fused macrophages
- **Foreign body giant cells:** These have multiple uniform nuclei scattered throughout the cytoplasm. They may be seen in reaction insoluble material
  - **Exogenous:** e.g., suture material, talc, etc.
  - **Endogenous material:** e.g., keratin (dermoid cyst of ovary, epidermal cyst), cholesterol, urate crystals (in gout)
- **Disorders of lipid metabolism:** Touton giant cells have vacuolated cytoplasm due to lipid, e.g. in xanthoma
- **Infective or inflammatory conditions:** Reaction to certain organisms [e.g., tuberculosis (Langhans giant cells in which nuclei are arranged in a horseshoe pattern), fungal infections, syphilis]
- **Fusion of cardiac histiocytes:** Aschoff giant cells in immune-mediated rheumatic heart disease.

Giant cells resulting from fusion of cells: Viral infection
- Epithelial giant cells, e.g., herpes virus infection (molding of nuclei to one another)
- Connective tissue, e.g., Warthin–Finkeldey giant cells in measles

Tumor giant cells: They have hyperchromatic nuclei of varying size and shape
- **Giant cell tumors:** Bone (Osteoclast like giant cell in giant cell tumor)
- **Reed-Sternberg cells:** Hodgkin lymphoma
- Giant cell variants of many malignant tumors, e.g., carcinoma of the lung
- Syncytiotrophoblasts like giant cell

Damaged muscle fibers: Regenerating sarcolemmal cells in damaged skeletal muscles

Fever

Fever is the elevation of body temperature, usually by 1–4°C. It is one of the **most common** and **classical manifestations of the systemic response**. This occurs especially when inflammation is due to an infection (e.g., bacteria, viruses). **Molecules that cause fever are called pyrogens**.

Mechanism: In infections, bacterial products (e.g., LPS) stimulate leukocytes to release the **cytokines IL-1 and TNF**. These cytokines stimulate the production of prostaglandins, particularly PGE_2, in the vascular and perivascular cells of the hypothalamus. PGE_2 acts on the hypothalamic thermoregulatory center (i.e., neurons in the preoptic nucleus of the hypothalamus) causing fever. NSAIDs, including aspirin, inhibit prostaglandin synthesis and thereby reduce fever.

Changes in the Leukocytes

Leukocytosis (*refer* Box 12.1): A total leukocyte count of more than 11,000/µL is termed leukocytosis. It is **common in inflammatory reactions,** especially those caused by **bacterial infections**. Leukocyte count may be **increased up to 15,000 or 20,000 cells/µL.** Sometimes, it may be extremely high reaching 40,000 to 100,000 cells/µL associated with more immature neutrophils in the blood (shift to the left). This extreme elevation may be like the white cell counts found in leukemia and are called **leukemoid reactions** (*refer* page 366-7). It is important to distinguish it from leukemia, which is a malignant disease.

- **Mechanism:** It is due to the increased release of leukocytes from the bone marrow caused by cytokines namely TNF and IL-1. Prolonged infection also causes leukocytosis by stimulating the release of hematopoietic growth factors called colony-stimulating factors (CSFs). The CSFs are released from macrophages, stromal cells, endothelial cells, and T lymphocytes in the marrow.

Neutrophilia: In most bacterial infections, there is an **increase in the blood neutrophil count** known as neutrophilia (*refer* to **Box 12.3**).

Lymphocytosis (*refer* to Box 12.8): An **absolute increase in lymphocyte count** is known as lymphocytosis. It is seen in **viral infections** (e.g., infectious mononucleosis, mumps, and German measles).

Eosinophilia (*refer* to Table 12.3): An **absolute increase in eosinophil count** is seen in **bronchial asthma, allergy, and parasitic infestations.**

Leukopenia (*refer* Box 12.2): It is an absolute decrease in the number of circulating white cells. It is associated with a few infections like **typhoid fever and some viruses, rickettsia, and certain protozoa.**

The Acute-Phase Response

Q. Write a short note on acute phase proteins/reactants.

The acute-phase response is the **production of plasma proteins, called acute-phase proteins**. These proteins are produced in the liver. The **levels of these proteins in the blood may be markedly raised (increase up to several hundred-fold)** as part of the response to inflammatory stimuli.

Types of acute-phase proteins. Three of the well-known acute phase proteins are: (a) **C-reactive protein (CRP), (b) fibrinogen, and (c) serum amyloid A (SAA) protein.** The synthesis of these proteins by hepatocytes is increased by cytokines, especially IL-6 (for CRP and fibrinogen) and IL-1 or TNF (for SAA). Acute-phase proteins such as CRP and SAA bind to the cell wall of the microbes and may act as opsonins and fix complement. During acute inflammation, acute-phase proteins have beneficial effects.

C-reactive Protein (CRP)

Q. Write a short note on C-reactive protein.

CRP is an **acute-phase reactant** synthesized mainly by the **liver.** Its synthesis is stimulated by several inflammatory mediators (mainly by cytokines, e.g., IL-6) acting on liver cells. CRP **augments the innate immune response** by binding to microbial (bacteria) cell walls or **may act as opsonins** and activate the classical complement cascade. They also bind chromatin and help in clearing necrotic cell nuclei. Its significance is as follows:

- **Raised serum levels of CRP** are a **marker for increased risk of myocardial infarction in patients with coronary artery disease**. Probably inflammation involving atherosclerotic plaques in the coronary arteries may predispose to thrombosis and subsequent myocardial infarction.
- **Plasma CRP** is a **strong, independent marker of risk for myocardial infarction, stroke, peripheral arterial disease, and sudden cardiac death**, even in healthy individuals.
- CRP is also a **useful marker for assessing the effects of risk reduction measures**, such as cessation of smoking, weight loss, exercise, and statins; each one of these reduces CRP levels.

Fibrinogen

Raised ESR: Fibrinogen binds to red cells and neutralizes the negative surface charge of red cells. This causes red cells to form stacks (rouleaux) and is responsible for the raised erythrocyte sedimentation rate (ESR). Thus, the measurement of the *erythrocyte sedimentation rate* is a simple test for detecting inflammation.

Serum Amyloid A (SAA) Protein

Serum amyloid-associated (SAA) protein is synthesized in the liver and circulates in the blood bound to high-density lipoproteins. It is an acute phase response. The production of SAA protein is **increased and prolonged** in **chronic inflammatory states** (e.g., chronic osteomyelitis, lung abscess, bronchiectasis, tuberculosis, leprosy). It **can cause secondary amyloidosis** (amyloidosis associated with chronic inflammation).

Other Acute Phase Proteins

- **Increased production of hepcidin:** *Hepcidin* is an iron-regulating protein that reduces the availability of iron to erythroid progenitors in the bone marrow. Inflammation is also associated with increased production of *hepcidin*. Thus, it reduces the availability of iron and is **responsible for the anemia occurring in association with chronic inflammation.**
- **Thrombopoietin:** It is the major growth factor for megakaryocytes (platelet precursors) in the bone marrow. It is also upregulated in systemic inflammation. It leads to an elevated platelet count (thrombocytosis)

Other Manifestations of the Systemic Response

Increased pulse and blood pressure; decreased sweating (due to redirection of blood flow from cutaneous to deep vascular beds, to minimize heat loss through the skin).
Rigors (shivering), chills, anorexia, somnolence (feeling drowsy), and malaise (lack of well-being). These are probably due to cytokines acting on brain cells.
Septic shock: In disseminated, severe bacterial/microbial infections (sepsis), the presence of large numbers of bacteria and their products in the blood stimulates the production of excessive amounts of several cytokines **(cytokine storm)**, notably TNF, IL-1, and IL-6. High blood levels of cytokines can lead to disseminated intravascular coagulation, hypotension, and metabolic disturbances (such as insulin resistance and hyperglycemia). This clinical trial is called *septic shock.*

Systemic Inflammatory Response Syndrome (SIRS)

Q. Write a short note on systemic inflammatory response syndrome (SIRS).

A **syndrome like septic shock** may occur **as a complication of non-infectious disorders** (non-microbial conditions), such as severe burns, trauma, pancreatitis, and other serious conditions. Both the infectious and non-infectious causes of shock can produce a similar set of clinical findings of systemic inflammation such as fever, tachycardia, tachypnea, leukocytosis, or leukopenia. In both settings, massive ***inflammatory reaction*** stimulates the **production of large quantities of several cytokines**, mainly **TNF and IL-1** (others IL-6 and platelet-activating factor [PAF]) into the systemic circulation. Marked blood levels of cytokines produce widespread clinical and pathologic abnormalities. Collectively these reactions are called *systemic inflammatory response syndrome (SIRS)*. Thus, **SIRS** can develop due to septic shock (by microbes) as well as a variety of other non-infectious insults.
SIRS is an exaggerated and generalized manifestation of a local immune or inflammatory reaction: SIRS is a hypermetabolic state characterized by two or more signs of systemic inflammation. These include **fever, tachycardia, tachypnea, leukocytosis, or leukopenia, in the setting of a known cause of inflammation.** SIRS is **often fatal.** Septic shock is triggered by microbial infections and is associated with severe systemic inflammatory response syndrome (SIRS). In septic shock clinical SIRS is so severe that it is associated with organ dysfunction, disseminated intravascular coagulation, hypotensive shock, and metabolic abnormalities such as insulin resistance and hyperglycemia. If severe and persistent, it may lead to organ failure and death.

TISSUE REPAIR

PA 5.1 (CC): Define and describe the process of repair and regeneration including wound healing and its types.

Q. Define the terms healing, regeneration, and repair.

Injury to cells and tissues **results in loss of cells and tissues.** It sets in inflammation (restricts tissue damage) and **initiates the replacement of lost tissue by living tissue** through the process of repair. This replacement is done by a transient increase in cellularity due to the proliferation of cells by either regeneration and/or scar formation.

Definition: Repair, sometimes called healing, is a **process of the restoration of tissue architecture and function after an injury.**

Types (*refer* online Figs. 3.19A and B): Repair (healing) of damaged tissues can occur by two types of reactions: **(1) regeneration and (2) scar formation.**

- **Regeneration:** It is defined as a process in which **lost tissue is replaced by tissue of a similar type.** It results in the complete restoration of lost or damaged tissue components and the affected tissue returns to a normal state. Thus both matrix composition and tissue architecture are fully restored. Regeneration occurs by the proliferation of residual cells that survive the injury and retain the capacity to generate the mature cells of that tissue. The cells that are responsible for regeneration may be mature differentiated cells or more commonly tissue stem cells.
- **Scar formation:** It is defined as a process in which **lost/damaged tissue is replaced by fibrous tissue or scar.** It occurs when the injured tissues are incapable of complete restitution, or when the supporting structures of the tissue are damaged. In scarring, repair occurs by the **deposition of connective (fibrous) tissue or excessive collagen.** The fibrous scar provides enough structural stability and the injured tissue is usually able to function. When **scarring occurs following chronic inflammation** (e.g., in the lungs, liver, kidney, and other parenchymal organs), it **is called fibrosis.**

Types of cells that proliferate during healing: Many types of cells proliferate during healing. These include the **remaining cells of the injured tissue** (to restore normal structure), **vascular endothelial cells** (to generate new vessels for supplying the nutrients required for the healing process), and **fibroblasts** (needed for the formation of fibrous tissue to fill defects that cannot be healed regeneration).

Factors Deciding the Pattern of Healing

The proportion of regeneration and repair process in healing depends on:

Intrinsic proliferative capacity of the tissue: According to the proliferative capacity of the cells, the tissues of the body can be divided into three groups:

1. **Labile (continuously dividing) tissues:** The cells of labile tissues **proliferate throughout life**, replacing the lost cells from stem cells. These tissues can regenerate after injury as long as the pool of stem cells is preserved Examples:
   - **Hematopoietic cells** of the bone marrow and **cells of lymph nodes and spleen.**
   - **Basal layers of surface epithelia** of the **skin, oral cavity, vagina, and cervix.**
   - **Columnar epithelium** of the **gastrointestinal tract and uterus.**
2. **Stable (quiescent) tissues:** Cells of stable tissue normally do not proliferate, but can **proliferate in response to injury or loss of tissue**. Examples:
   - **Parenchymal cells of solid organs:** For example, **liver, kidneys, pancreas, adrenal and thyroid.**
   - **Mesenchymal cells:** Fibroblasts, vascular endothelial cells, smooth muscle cells, chondrocytes, and osteocytes.
3. **Permanent (non-dividing) tissues:** Cells of these tissues **cannot proliferate after birth**. Injury to these tissues is irreversible because the cells cannot regenerate. In these tissues, repair is done by scar formation. Example:
   - **Neurons: Damaged neurons** are **replaced by** the proliferation of the **glial cells**
   - **Skeletal muscle** cells
   - **Cardiac muscle** cells.

   However, limited stem cell replication and differentiation can occur in some areas of the adult brain, and heart muscle cells can proliferate after myocardial necrosis.

The extent of tissue injury: The injury may be mild or severe.

- **Mild and short duration:** The damaged tissue is healed by regeneration without significant scarring.
- **Severe and chronic:** Healing occurs by fibrous tissue forming a scar.
  - Severe tissue injury damages both parenchymal cells and the extracellular matrix (ECM) framework
  - Chronic inflammation

CELL PROLIFERATION AND CELL CYCLE

Definition: Cell proliferation maintains a steady-state tissue homeostasis, and replaces dead or damaged cells.

Cell cycle: It is the **sequence of events that results in cell proliferation**. The proliferation of cells is characterized by DNA replication and mitosis. The cell cycle is a regulated process, which involves activators and inhibitors, as well as checkpoints.

Phases of the cell cycle (Fig. 3.20): It consists of (i) G_1 (gap 1, presynthetic), (ii) S (DNA synthesis), (iii) G_2 (gap 2, premitotic), and (iv) M (mitotic) phases.

Checkpoints: They check whether there is any damage to DNA and chromosomes in the replicating cells.

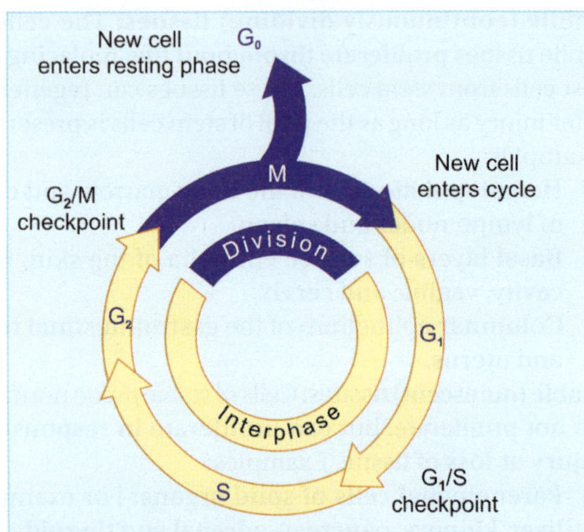

Fig. 3.20: Cell cycle showing different phases (G_0, G_1, G_2, S, and M). Cells from labile tissues (e.g., epidermis) may remain in cycle continuously; stable cells (e.g., liver cells) are quiescent but can enter the cell cycle; permanent cells (e.g., neurons) have lost the capacity to proliferate and cell cycle arrests in the G_1 phase or exit the cycle and are in G_0 phase.

These checkpoints make sure that only normal cells complete replication. There are two checkpoints:

1. **G_1/S checkpoint monitors the integrity of DNA before replication.**
2. **G_2/M checkpoint checks DNA after replication** and monitors whether the cell can safely enter mitosis.

Growth Factors

Q. Write a short note on growth factors.

Definition: Growth factors **stimulate the activity of proteins** that are **needed for cell survival, growth, and division.**

Cell proliferation occurs due to signals produced by growth factors and from the extracellular matrix. There are many different growth factors, some of them act on multiple cell types, and others are cell-selective. Various growth factors involved in wound healing and regeneration are listed in (*refer* **online Table 3.13**).

Mechanism of action: Growth factors induce cell proliferation by **binding to specific receptors**, and deliver positive growth signals to the target cells. These signals stimulate the **expression of genes** whose products have several functions which include: activation of the cell cycle, relief blocks that prevent cell cycle progression, prevention of apoptosis, and increases the synthesis of cellular components (nucleic acids, proteins, lipids, carbohydrates) needed for a mother cell to produce two daughter cells.

Signaling Mechanisms of Growth Factor Receptors

Q. Write a short note on different types of signaling.

The **receptor-mediated signal transduction** process is activated by the binding of ligands (e.g., growth factors and cytokines) to specific receptors. Receptor activation leads to the expression of specific genes.

Modes of signaling (Figs. 3.21A to C): Depending on the source of the ligand and the location of its corresponding receptors (i.e., in the same, adjacent, or distant cells), the modes of signaling can be divided into three types:

1. **Autocrine signaling:** In this, signaling molecules **act on the cells that secrete them.** For example, liver regeneration, the proliferation of antigen-stimulated lymphocytes, and tumors.
2. **Paracrine signaling:** In this type, a **signaling molecule is produced by one cell type, that acts on adjacent target cells** (usually of a different type) which expresses the appropriate receptor. For example, in repair, the factor

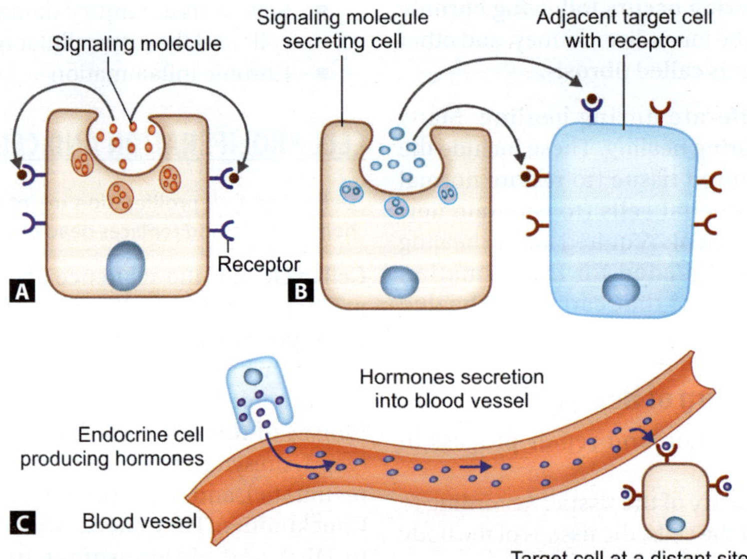

Figs. 3.21A to C: Modes of signaling: (A) Autocrine; (B) Paracrine; (C) Endocrine signaling.

produced by macrophage (one cell type) has a growth effect on fibroblast (adjacent target cells of different types).

3. **Endocrine signaling:** In this, hormones are produced by cells of endocrine organs, are usually carried by the blood, and act on **target cells that are at a distance 3 from the site of their synthesis**.

STEM CELLS

Q. Write a short note on stem cells. What are its subtypes?

Definition: Stem cells are characterized by two main properties (i) their **ability to self-renewal and (ii) capacity to generate differentiated cell lineages**.

Properties: Stem cells are maintained by self-renewal. It consists of two types of cell division:

1. **Asymmetric division:** All stem cells have the ability to undergo asymmetric cell division. In this type of mitosis (cell replication), the stem cell divides into two cells:
   i. **One daughter cell** enters a differentiation pathway and gives rise to a **mature cell type**.
   ii. The **other cell remains a stem cell** (undifferentiated) and retains the self-renewal capacity.
2. **Symmetric division:** In this type of cell division, both daughter cells retain **self-renewal capacity**. This type of division occurs under the following conditions:
   i. Early in embryogenesis- when stem cell populations are expanding.
   ii. Under stress conditions, such as in bone marrow repopulation after ablative chemotherapy.

Varieties of stem cells: There are two main varieties:

1. **Embryonic stem (ES) cells:** These are the most undifferentiated cells. They are present in the **inner cell mass of the blastocyst** (during the development of the embryo). They have almost limitless cell renewal capacity and can **give rise to every cell in the body**. Thus, they are *totipotent* and capable of giving rise to all mature cell lineages. ES cells can be induced under appropriate culture conditions to form specialized cells of **all three germ cell layers** (ectoderm, mesoderm, and endoderm).
2. **Tissue stem cells:** They are also called adult stem cells. In the tissues, these cells are found among the differentiated cells. They are protected within specialized tissue microenvironments called *stem cell niches*. These niches are found in many organs and are as follows:
   - **Bone marrow:** It contains two types of stem cells namely:
     - **Hematopoietic stem cells** (HSCs): They are **present in perivascular niches.** They can generate all the blood cell lineages and are used for the treatment of hematologic diseases. They can be collected directly from the bone marrow, peripheral blood after administration of certain colony-stimulating factors, and umbilical cord blood.
     - **Mesenchymal stem cells (MSCs):** They can generate chondrocytes, osteoblasts, adipocytes, myoblasts, and endothelial cell precursors depending on the tissue to which they migrate.
   - **Intestinal epithelium: The epithelial stem cells located in the crypts** immediately above Paneth cells in the small intestine or at the base of the crypt in the colon.
   - **Other sites:** These include the bulge region of **hair follicles, the limbus of the cornea, and the subventricular zone in the brain.**

Tissue stem cells have a **limited capacity to generate different cell types than ES cells.** They usually differentiate and produce only those cells normally found within a particular tissue (i.e., the tissue in which they reside). Injury to the tissue triggers signals that stimulate their proliferation and differentiation into mature cells. Thus, these stem cells repopulate the injured tissue. Tissue stem cells regenerate the injured tissues, especially when the differentiated cells that survive the injury have limited or no intrinsic proliferative capacity.

Healing by Regeneration

Regeneration is the **replacement of injured tissues by similar tissue. It returns an injured or lost tissue to its original state following inflammation.**

Cells that proliferate during regeneration: In the process of regeneration of injured cells and tissues proliferation of cells occurs. The **proliferation involves: (i) residual cells along with (ii) the development of mature cells from stem cells.** This proliferation is brought out by growth factors.

Type of cells capable of regeneration: Tissue regeneration can occur in parenchymal organs composed of cells that are capable of proliferation. Regeneration in **tissues or organs containing labile cells** (e.g., hematopoietic cells in the bone marrow, surface epithelia) or **stable cells** (e.g., liver, kidney, endothelial cells, fibroblasts). The new cells are derived from tissue stem cells and rapidly proliferating immature progenitors. However, in permanent tissues (e.g., neurons and cardiac muscle cells), the cells cannot regenerate and healing is only by forming scars.

Integrity of architecture: In regeneration, normal tissue architecture can be restored only if the residual tissue is structurally intact. For example, after partial surgical resection of the liver scars the remaining liver should have normal architecture.

- **Loss of framework: Regeneration is incomplete**, if the entire tissue, including the supporting framework, is damaged by infection or inflammation. This is accompanied by scarring. For example, the liver abscess is accompanied by extensive destruction of the liver and collapse of the reticulin framework. It leads to the formation of scars even though the remaining liver cells can regenerate.

Variation of regeneration: Regeneration varies in different types of tissues and with the severity of injury.

- **In epithelia of the intestinal tract and skin:** Regeneration is provided by the underlying **intact basement membrane.** The injured **cells are rapidly replaced by the proliferation of residual cells and differentiation of tissue stem cells.**
- **In parenchymal organs:** Tissue **regeneration usually is a limited process in parenchymal organs** which **consists of mature cells capable of proliferation,** except the liver. The **liver has an extraordinary capacity to regenerate.** Some regenerative capacity is seen in the pancreas, adrenal, thyroid, and lung. For example, the surgical removal of a kidney produces a compensatory response in the remaining kidney. This response consists of both hypertrophy and hyperplasia of proximal duct cells.

Liver Regeneration

The liver has a tremendous capacity to regenerate. This regenerative growth of the liver is observed after partial hepatectomy, which may be done for resection of the tumor in the liver or living-donor hepatic transplantation.

Mechanism of Regeneration of the Liver

Regeneration of the liver occurs by two mechanisms: (1) **proliferation of remaining hepatocytes** and (2) **regeneration from stem cells**. Which of these two mechanisms plays a dominant role depends on the nature of the hepatic injury.

The proliferation of residual hepatocytes following partial hepatectomy. The proliferation of the residual hepatocytes can regenerate up to 90% of the liver.

- **Cytokines and growth factors stimuli proliferation:** Hepatocyte proliferation in the liver is due to the combined actions of **cytokines and polypeptide growth factors**. Initially, cytokines (e.g., IL-6) produced by Kupffer cells act on hepatocytes and make the parenchymal cells competent to receive and respond to growth factor signals. During the next phase of regeneration, growth factors (e.g., HGF and TGF-α), produced by many cell types, act on the primed hepatocytes to stimulate their proliferation.

Liver regeneration from stem cells. Following chronic liver injury or inflammation, the proliferative capacity of hepatocytes is impaired. Hence, regeneration occurs from stem cells. In the liver, these stem cells are present in specialized niches called *canals of Hering* (the site where bile canaliculi connect with larger bile ducts).

Repair by Scarring (Connective Tissue Deposition)

If repair cannot be achieved by regeneration alone, the replacement of the injured cells occurs with connective tissue. This leads to the formation of a scar.

Conditions in which scarring occurs: Scarring may occur (i) with **severe tissue injury**, (ii) **chronic injury with damage to parenchymal cells and epithelia** as well as to the connective tissue framework, and (iii) **injury to nondividing cells.**

Scar: The term *scar* is typically **used in connection to wound healing in the skin.** But it may also be used to describe the **replacement of parenchymal cells in any tissue by collagen.** For example, scarring in the heart after myocardial infarction.

Steps in Scar Formation

Q. Write a short note on the steps of wound healing.

Scar formation can be best understood by studying the healing of skin wounds (refer to pages below). Various steps are briefly discussed below.

Hemostatic plug: Within minutes after a traumatic injury, a hemostatic plug is formed at the site of the injury. This comprises of platelets and stops bleeding. It also provides a framework (scaffold) for infiltrating inflammatory cells and the formation of a stable clot.

Inflammation: Whenever there is tissue injury, an inflammatory reaction begins. Next 6–48 hours, phagocytes namely **neutrophils followed by monocytes** (become macrophages in tissue) are recruited to the site of injury. These phagocytes try to get rid of the injurious agents and clear the debris (injured tissue). **Macrophages are the main cells involved in the process of repair.** Different macrophage populations (M1 and M2) (*refer* to page 84-5) clear causative microbes and necrotic (dead) tissue. The macrophages that are mostly involved in repair are the alternatively activated (M2) type. **Macrophages also promote inflammation and produce growth factors that stimulate the proliferation of many cell types in the repair.** Once the injurious agents and necrotic tissues are cleared, the inflammation resolves.

Macrophages play a central role in repair by clearing offending agents and dead tissue, providing growth factors for the proliferation of various cells, and secreting cytokines that stimulate fibroblast proliferation and connective tissue synthesis and deposition

Cell proliferation: In the next stage (takes up to 10 days), several cell types such as epithelial cells, endothelial and other vascular cells, and fibroblasts, proliferate and migrate to close the wound (that is cleaned by macrophage). Each cell type has different functions.

- **Epithelial cells:** The surrounding epithelial cells **migrate over the wound** to cover it. It occurs as a response to locally produced growth factors.
- **Endothelial and other vascular cells:** They proliferate and **form new blood vessels** and this process is termed **angiogenesis** (*refer* to below).
- **Fibroblasts:** These cells proliferate and migrate into the site of injury. They synthesize collagen fibers that **form scars.**

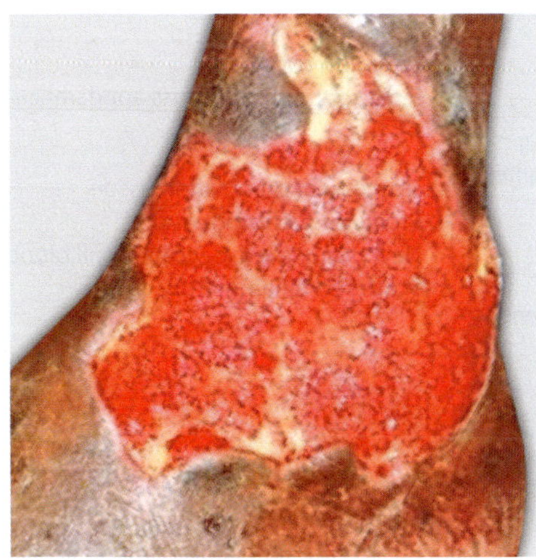

Fig. 3.22: Pink, soft, granular appearance of granulation tissue on the surface of healing wounds.

Q. Write a short note on granulation tissue.

Formation of granulation tissue: During the **first 24–72 hours** of the repair process, the proliferation of fibroblasts and vascular endothelial cells begins. A specialized type of tissue unique and **hallmark (characteristic) of healing wounds** is formed and is called granulation tissue (**Fig. 3.22**).

MORPHOLOGY

The *granulation tissue* consists of a combination of: **(i) proliferating fibroblasts, (ii) new blood vessels, and (iii) ECM.** The term derives from its **pink, soft, granular gross appearance** of granulation tissue observed below the scab of a healing skin wound. Microscopically **(Figs. 3.23A and B),** granulation tissue consists of:

- **Proliferating fibroblasts.**
- **New thin-walled, delicate small blood vessels** (angiogenesis). These are thin-walled, delicate, leaky capillaries, that allow the passage of plasma proteins and fluid into the extravascular space. This leakage of plasma proteins and fluid is responsible for edema often seen in granulation tissue.
- **Loose extracellular matrix (ECM).** The capillaries of granulation tissue are surrounded by a loose extracellular matrix.
- **Scattered inflammatory cells** mainly macrophages.

The **amount** of granulation tissue formed depends on: (i) the **size of the tissue deficit** created by the wound and (ii) the **intensity of inflammation.**

Remodeling: The **connective tissue** that has been **deposited by fibroblast is reorganized** and altered to **produce a stable fibrous** *scar*. This process of remodeling begins 2–3 weeks after injury and may continue for months or years.

Angiogenesis

Q. Write a short note on angiogenesis in repair.

Definition: Angiogenesis is the **process of formation of new blood vessels from existing vessels.**

Growth of capillaries: Granulation tissue consists of more capillaries per unit volume than any other tissue. During repair, restoring the capillary bed is required for the supply of oxygen and nutrients. New capillaries form by angiogenesis. Angiogenesis occurs by the sprouting of endothelial cells from pre-existing capillary venules and creates the granular appearance for which the tissue is named granulation tissue.

Significance of angiogenesis: Angiogenesis is important (i) at sites of injury for healing, (ii) in the development of collateral circulations at sites of ischemia, and (iii) for the growth (increase in the size) of tumors.

Regulation of angiogenesis during repair: Angiogenesis in wound repair is a tightly regulated process. Many angiogenic and antiangiogenic factors are involved in regulating vessel growth. The *vascular endothelial growth factor (VEGF)* is the most important proangiogenic mediator produced in wounds. VEGF stimulates wound angiogenesis.

Steps in Angiogenesis (Figs. 3.24A to D)

Angiogenesis involves the formation of new vessels from existing ones. Various steps in angiogenesis are as follows:

1. **Vasodilatation:** It occurs in nearby intact vessels at the site of injury. Vasodilatation occurs **in response to nitric oxide. It shows increased permeability of the pre-existing vessel caused due** to vascular endothelial growth factor (VEGF) at the site of injury. VEGF stimulates both the migration and proliferation of endothelial cells. VEGF is produced by macrophages in response to hypoxia,
2. **Separation of pericytes from the abluminal surface of blood vessels.** There is digestion of the basement membrane of the vessel by matrix metalloproteases.

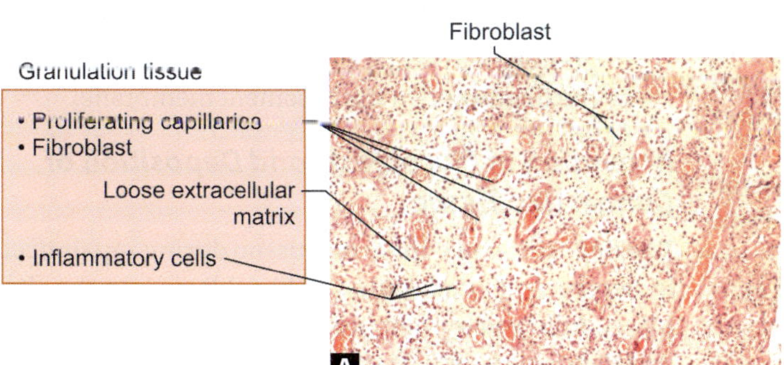

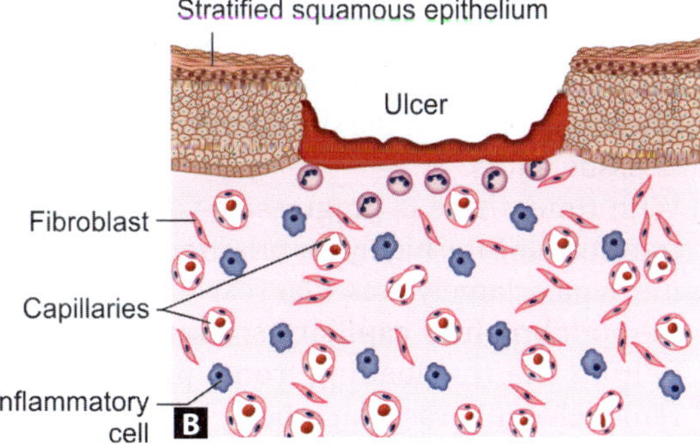

Figs. 3.23A and B: (A) H&E; (B) Diagrammatic. Microscopy of granulation tissue consisting of numerous blood vessels, fibroblasts, and edema.

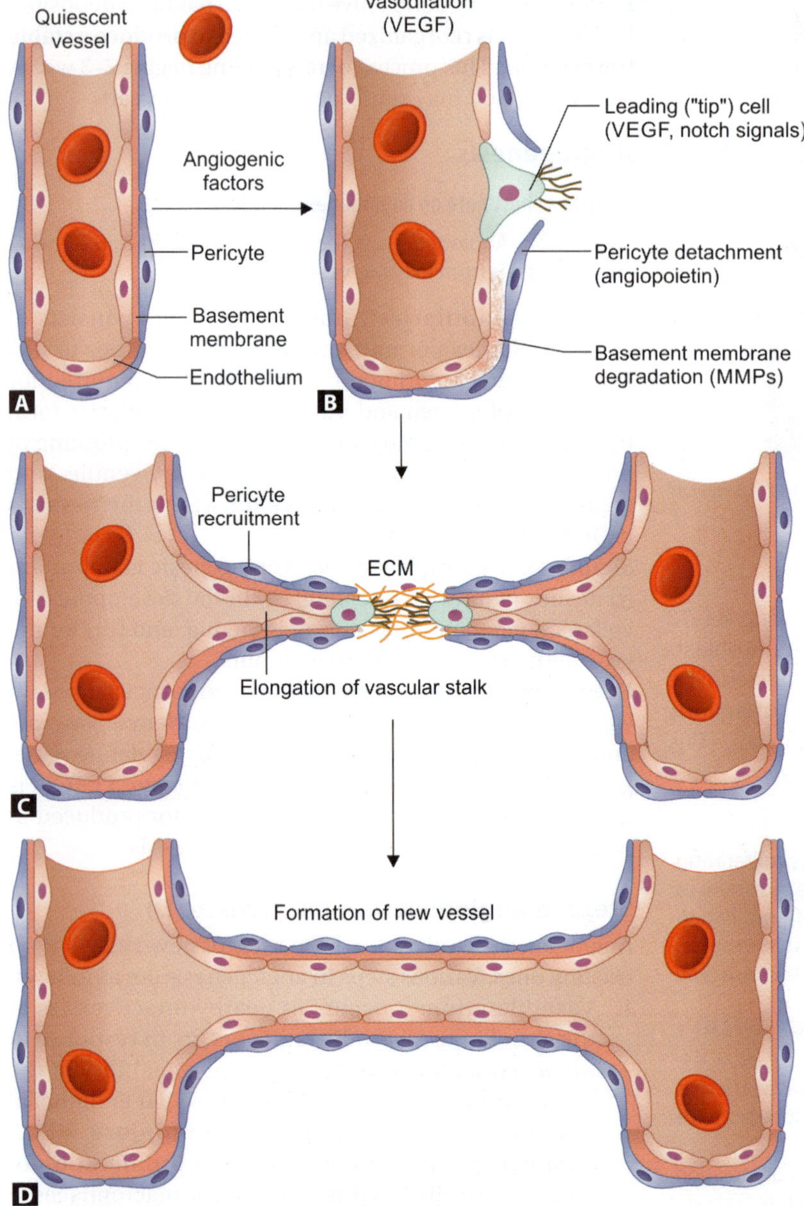

Granulation tissue
- Pink, soft, granular gross appearance

Microscopy of granulation tissue
- Proliferating fibroblasts.
- New thin-walled, delicate small blood vessels
- Scattered inflammatory cells

Figs. 3.24A to D: Steps in angiogenesis in tissue repair: (A) Normal blood vessel; (B) Vasodilatation: First, pericytes separate from the outer surface of the vessel. Then endothelial cells put out cell extensions, called pseudopodia, that move/grow and proliferate from the existing vessel to form capillary sprouts towards the site of injury/wound (angiogenic stimuli). Cytoplasmic flow enlarges the pseudopodia of endothelial cells, and eventually, the cells divide. Vacuoles are formed in the new daughter cells and they fuse to create a new lumen; (C) Endothelial cells proliferate, loosely following each other, and are presumably guided by pericytes. Maturation of vessel (stabilization) involves the recruitment of pericytes and smooth muscle cells to form the periendothelial layer; (D) The entire process continues till the blood-vessel sprouts encounter another capillary sprout, with which it will connect. Thus, it builds new circulatory systems. At its peak, granulation tissue is the most richly vascularized tissue in the body. Once repair is complete, most of the newly formed capillaries undergo apoptosis. It leaves a pale, avascular scar rich in collagen.

(ECM: extracellular matrix; MMPs: matrix metalloproteinases; VEGF: vascular endothelial growth factor).

This permits the formation of a vessel sprout at the site of basement membrane digestion.

3. **Migration and proliferation of endothelial cells** toward the site of injury caused due to fibroblast growth factors (FGFs), mainly FGF-2.
4. **Proliferation of endothelial cells** just behind the "tip" (leading front) of migrating cells. Endothelial cells at the leading front of the sprout migrate toward the area of tissue injury.
5. With time, there is progressive vascular regression, transforming the highly vascularized granulation tissue into a pale, largely avascular scar.
6. **Remodeling into capillary sprouts/tubes:** The cells behind the tip (leading front) proliferate and are remodeled into vascular tubes.
7. **Recruitment of periendothelial cells.** In parallel, pericytes (in small capillaries) or smooth muscle cells (in larger vessels) are recruited and remodeled. Finally, it leads to the **formation of mature vessels.**
8. **Suppression of endothelial proliferation and migration.** Formation of the mature vessel is followed by the deposition of the basement membrane.

Activation of Fibroblasts and Deposition of Connective Tissue

The deposition of connective tissue during repair occurs in two steps: (1) migration of fibroblasts into the site of injury, followed by their proliferation, and (2) production and deposition of ECM proteins.

As the healing progresses, the number of proliferating fibroblasts and new vessels decreases. However, the fibroblasts progressively synthesize and deposit an increased amount of ECM. Later the granulation tissue scaffolding is converted into a pale, avascular scar. The predominant mode of repair results in scar formation.

MORPHOLOGY
Scar or Fibrosis in Tissues

The scar is composed of inactive, spindle-shaped fibroblasts, dense bundles of collagen, fragments of elastic tissue, and other ECM components.

Special stains: To identify different protein constituents of scars and fibrotic tissues, special stains are useful.

- **Trichrome stain:** It contains three stains (hence its name), that stain red cells orange, muscle red, and collagen blue. Thus, it **detects collagen fibers in the scar tissue.**
- **Elastin stain:** It identifies delicate fibers of elastin, which is the major component of flexible elastic tissue.
- **Reticulin stain:** Reticulin is one of the extracellular matrix proteins of the connective tissue stroma of normal organs and is also present in early scars. It is composed of type III collagen.

By the end of the first month, the scar consists of acellular connective tissue without inflammatory infiltrate.

Remodeling of Connective Tissue

The outcome of the repair depends on the balance between synthesis and degradation of ECM proteins. After the formation of the scar, there is continuous remodeling. The remodeling (i) increases the strength and (ii) diminishes the size of the scar.

Increase of wound strength: It is **due to the cross-linking of collagen and the increased size of collagen fibers.** Also, the type III collagen deposited early in repair shifts to the more resilient type I collagen. In well-sutured skin wounds, the wound strength may attain 70–80% of normal skin by 3 months.

Diminishing the size of the scar: As the time passes, the scar shrinks. It is due to the action of **matrix metalloproteinases (MMPs).** Matrix metalloproteinases (MMPs) are a family of proteinases. They are named so because they are dependent on metal ions (e.g., zinc) for their activity. MMPs are produced by various types of cells such as fibroblasts, macrophages, neutrophils, synovial cells, and some epithelial cells. The synthesis and secretion of MMPs are regulated by growth factors, cytokines, and other agents. During scar formation, MMPs are activated to remodel the deposited ECM. This is followed by the inactivation of MMPs by the tissue inhibitors of metalloproteinases (TIMPs). Remodeling indicates that the equilibrium/balance between ECM synthesis (collagen deposition) and degradation has been restored.

Role of Macrophages in Repair

Q. Write a short note on the role of macrophages in inflammation/repair.

Macrophages are important cells involved in repair. Their functions in repair include:

- Clear the offending agents and dead tissue.
- Provide growth factors for the proliferation of various cells.
- Secret cytokines that stimulate fibroblast proliferation and connective tissue synthesis and deposition.

FACTORS THAT INFLUENCE WOUND HEALING

Q. List the factors that influence wound healing.

Factors that interfere with tissue repair may be extrinsic (e.g., infection) or intrinsic to the injured tissue, and systemic or local.

Q. Discuss the factors promoting and delaying the process.

Local Factors

Q. List the factors that delay healing.

Local Factors that Delay Wound Healing/Repair

1. **Infection:** It is the **single most important cause** of delay in healing. Infection causes persistent local tissue injury and prolongs inflammation.
2. **Mechanical factors: Movement (mobility) of the wounded area** may compress the blood vessels, separate the edges of the wound (dehisce), and can result in delayed healing. Increased local pressure or torsion may also delay healing.
3. **Foreign bodies:** Unnecessary sutures or foreign bodies (fragments of steel, glass), or even bone can delay healing.
4. **Size and type of wound: Large** excisional wounds or **wounds caused by blunt trauma.**
5. **Location of injury/wound:** A **wound over the skin covering bone** with little intervening tissue between skin and bone prevents wound contraction (e.g., skin over the anterior tibia or the cranium). The edges of skin lesions (e.g., burns) in such locations cannot be apposed. **Inflammation affecting tissue spaces** (e.g., pleural, peritoneal, synovial cavities) develops extensive exudates and may undergo resolution. But a larger amount of exudate may undergo organization (ingrowth of granulation tissue into the exudate, and forms a fibrous scar).
6. **The type of tissue:** Injury to **tissues composed of permanent cells** results in scarring.
7. **Poor perfusion:** Due either to **arteriosclerosis and diabetes or to obstructed venous drainage** (e.g., in varicose veins) impairs wound healing.

- **Varicose veins** of the legs **decrease venous drainage** and **can cause nonhealing ulceration.**
- **Bed sores (decubitus ulcers)** result due to prolonged, localized, pressure, which **diminishes both arterial and venous blood flow.**
- Wounds in **areas with poor blood supply**, such as the foot.

7. Ionizing radiation decreases the repair process.
8. Complications may delay wound healing.

Local Factors that Favor Wound Healing

Q. List the factors that promote healing.

1. **Size and type of wound: Small surgical incisions** or other injuries heal quickly with less scar formation.
2. **Good blood supply:** Wounds in areas with good blood supply, such as the **face**, heal **faster than** those with **poor blood supply**, such as the foot.
3. **Type of tissue injured:** Complete restoration can occur when there is a mild injury to **tissues composed of labile** (e.g., skin) **and stable** (e.g., hepatocytes) cells rather than permanent cells (e.g., myocardial infarct).
4. **Wounds in which edges are closely apposed.**

Systemic Factors that Impair Tissue Repair

1. **Nutritional status:** Nutritional **deficiencies** delay wound healing/repair. These include:
   - **Protein deficiency** (e.g., malnutrition).
   - **Vitamin C deficiency:** It inhibits collagen synthesis and delays healing.
   - **Trace elements:** Copper and zinc deficiency.
2. **Age:** Wound healing is rapid in young compared to in aged individuals. Healing capacity declines with age.
3. **Metabolic status: Diabetes mellitus** is a metabolic disease associated with delayed healing/tissue repair for many reasons, one of them being microangiopathy associated with diabetes. It is an important systemic cause of delayed wound healing.
4. **Circulatory status: Inadequate blood supply** (due to arteriosclerosis) or venous abnormalities (e.g., varicose veins) that retard venous drainage, and delay healing.
5. **Hormones: Exogenous glucocorticoids (corticosteroids) have anti-inflammatory effects.** Steroids inhibit the production of TGF-β (a cytokine that promotes collagen deposition). Steroids inhibit collagen and protein synthesis and **impair wound healing**. Thus, during the postsurgical period, the administration of glucocorticoids may prevent adequate healing of wounds. However, glucocorticoids are sometimes used (along with antibiotics) for treating corneal infections to reduce the likelihood of collagen deposition and vision loss.
6. **Hematological abnormalities:** Quantitative or qualitative defects in **neutrophils, bleeding disorders** (coagulation defects, thrombocytopenia) and **anemia** may slow the healing process.

Factors that affect wound healing are listed in **Table 3.14.**

TABLE 3.14 Factors that affect wound healing.

Factors that delay wound healing	
Local factors	***Systemic factor***
1. Infection 2. Mechanical factors 3. Foreign bodies 4. Large excisional wounds or wounds caused by blunt trauma 5. Wounds located in sites where edges cannot be approximated (e.g., wound over skin covering bone such as tibia) 6. Poor perfusion (blood supply) 7. Ionizing radiation decreases 8. Complications of wound healing	1. Poor general health (nutritional deficiencies): Protein deficiency (e.g., malnutrition), vitamin C deficiency, and deficiency of trace elements 2. Old age 3. Metabolic status, e.g., diabetes mellitus 4. Circulatory status, e.g., inadequate blood supply 5. Drugs, e.g., glucocorticoids 6. Hematological abnormalities. Quantitative or qualitative defects in neutrophils and bleeding disorders
Factors that favor wound healing	
Local factors	***Systemic factors***
1. Small surgical incisional or other injuries 2. Wounds in areas with good blood supply (e.g., face) 3. Mild injury to tissues composed of labile (e.g., skin) and stable (e.g., hepatocytes) cells 4. Clean wounds in which edges are closely apposed (sutured wound)	1. Good general health 2. Good nutrition including vitamin C 3. Younger age 4. Good circulatory status

EXAMPLES OF TISSUE REPAIR AND FIBROSIS

Two clinically important types of repair are discussed below namely (i) the healing of skin wounds (cutaneous wound healing), and (ii) fibrosis in injured parenchymal organs. Repair follows three connected processes in a sequence: (a) inflammation, (b) proliferation of epithelial and other cells, and (c) maturation of the connective tissue scar.

Healing of Skin Wounds

Wounds in the skin and extremities are easily accessible. Hence, their healing is studied extensively. Healing within hollow viscera and body cavities is less accessible for study, but usually parallels the repair sequence in the skin.

Classification: Healing of skin wounds can be classified into *healing by first intention (primary union),* and *healing by second intention (secondary union).* However, key events in both types of wound healing are identical.

1. **Healing by first intention (primary union):** It refers to epithelial regeneration with minimal scarring (e.g., well-apposed surgical incisions).
2. **Healing by second intention (secondary union):** It refers to larger wounds that heal by a combination of regeneration and scarring.

Healing by First Intention

Q. Describe the healing of a clean surgical wound (healing by first intention).

Definition: Healing of a **clean, uninfected surgical incision** in the skin joined with surgical sutures is known as healing by **primary union or by first intention**. It refers to epithelial regeneration with minimal scarring.

Primary healing occurs when injury involves only the epithelial layer, and the edges of a wound closely approximated surgically. Surgical incision causes **death of a minimum number of** epithelial and connective tissue **cells**. The **disruption of epithelial basement membrane** continuity is also **minimal**. Re-epithelialization occurs by regeneration and is excellent because epidermal cells need to migrate only a minimal distance. There is a **relatively thin scar**. This is the simplest type of cutaneous wound healing.

Stages in the Healing by First Intention (Figs. 3.25A to D)

The sequence of events in primary union is as follows:

Within the First 24 Hours

- **Formation of a blood clot:** Wounding causes the rapid activation of coagulation pathways and forms a **blood clot in the space between sutured margins.** Blood clot contains not only trapped red cells but also fibrin, fibronectin, and complement components. Clot serves to stop bleeding and acts as a support for migrating and proliferating cells. These cells are attracted by growth factors, cytokines, and chemokines released into the injured area. **Dehydration at the external surface of the clot** leads to the formation of a **scab** over the wound.
- **Neutrophil infiltration:** Within 24 hours of the wound, **neutrophils** appear at the margins of the incision. The migrating neutrophils use the support produced by the

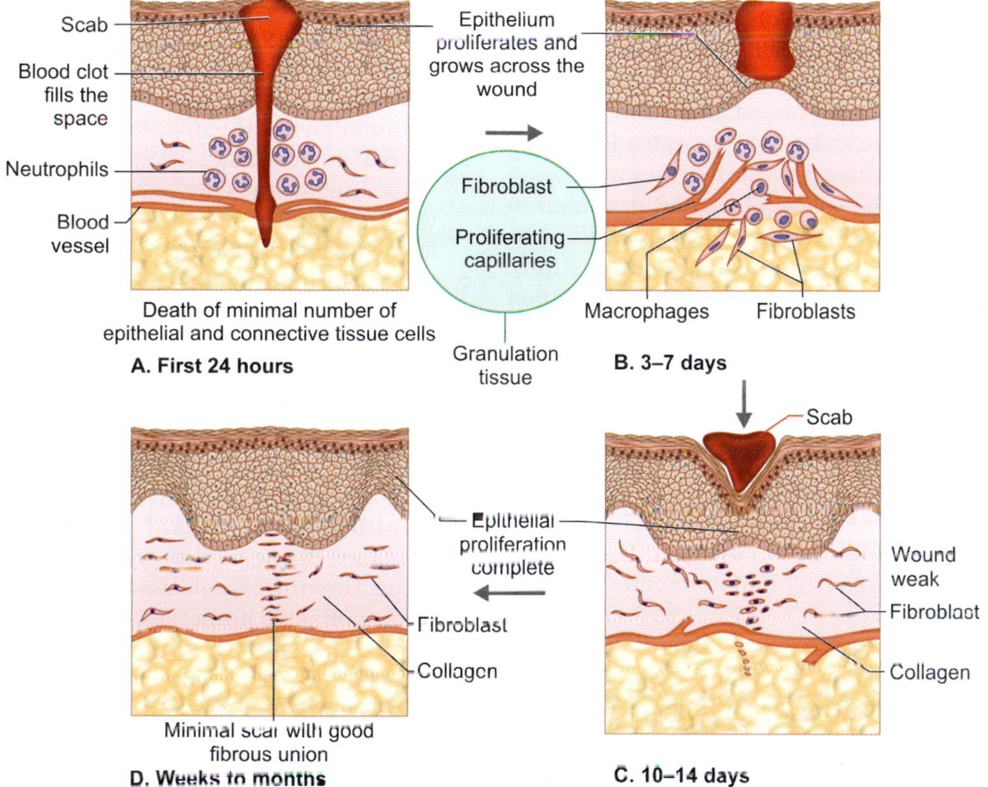

Figs. 3.25A to D: Healing by primary intention: (A) A wound with closely approximated edges and minimal tissue loss. The blood clots and fills the gap between the edges of the wound. Within 24 hours of the wound, neutrophils appear at the margins of the incision; (B) Neutrophils are largely replaced by macrophages. Epithelium at the edges proliferates fuses in the midline below the surface and epithelial continuity is re-established in the form of a thin continuous surface layer. Granulation tissue is formed and progressively invades incision space; (C) The epithelial proliferation is complete and the wound is weak. The leukocytic infiltrate, edema, and increased vascularity (angiogenesis) disappear; (D) Fibrosis with a small scar composed of acellular connective tissue without inflammatory cells. The scar is covered by intact, essentially epidermis. Collagen deposition along the line of stress and wound gradually achieves the tensile strength of normal skin.

fibrin clot. They **release proteolytic enzymes which clean out debris.**

- **Epithelial changes:** At the cut edges of the wound, the **basal cells of the epidermis** begin to show increased **mitotic activity. Epithelial cells from both the edges of the wound proliferate** and migrate across the wound along the dermis. This produces a thin but **continuous epithelial layer that closes the wound within 24–48 hours.**

By Day 3

- **Macrophages: Neutrophils are largely replaced by macrophages. Macrophages play a central cellular role in the repair process.** The macrophages clear extracellular debris, fibrin, and other foreign material. They promote angiogenesis and deposition of ECM.
- **Granulation tissue:** It begins to progressively invade incision space.
- The **epithelial cells fuse in the midline below the surface scab** and epithelial continuity is re-established in the form of a thin continuous surface layer.

By Day 5

- **Neovascularization and leakage of fluid from blood vessels: Granulation tissue fills** the **incision space/ wound and fills the wound area.** The neovascularization reaches its peak during this period. These new vessels of granulation tissue are leaky. They allow the leakage of plasma proteins and fluid from the intravascular region into the extravascular space. Thus, new **granulation tissue** is generally **edematous.**
- **Fibroblast proliferation and collagen deposition:** Fibroblasts progressively migrate into the granulation tissue. These fibroblasts proliferate and progressively lay down collagen and ECM.
- **Surface epidermis** achieves its **normal thickness** and differentiation. It matures with surface keratinization. The acute **inflammatory response** begins to **subside.**

During the Second Week

- **Increased accumulation of collagen:** During the second week, collagen accumulation and fibroblast proliferation continues.
- During the second week, the wound shows a substantial decrease or **disappearance of leukocytic infiltrate, edema, and increased vascularity (angiogenesis).**

By the End of the First Months

- **Scar:** The **scar is composed of acellular connective tissue without inflammatory cells.**
- **Normal surface epithelium:** The scar is covered by intact, essentially epidermis.
- **Tensile strength of the wound:** Collagen deposition along the line of stress and **wound gradually achieves a maximal of 80% of the tensile strength** of normal skin.

Healing by Secondary Union or by Second Intention

Q. Describe the mode of healing of the wound by the second intention.

Definition: Healing by **secondary union or by second intention** refers to the healing of a larger wound that is healed by a **combination of regeneration and scarring.** This wound has the following characteristics:

- Open with a **large tissue defect** on the skin surface.
- Having **extensive loss of cells and tissue.**
- The wound cannot approximated by surgical sutures.

Features of Healing by Secondary Intention (Figs. 3.26A to D)

It differs from primary healing in several aspects:

- **More exudate and necrotic tissue:** Larger wounds causing large tissue deficits show **more exudate and necrotic tissue.** The fibrin **clot or scab** formed at the surface of the wound is **large.** Full epithelialization of the wound surface is slow because of the larger gap.
- **More severe inflammatory reaction** because of larger tissue defect, more amount of necrotic tissue, exudate, and fibrin that must be removed.
- **More prone to secondary infection,** and inflammation-mediated injury.
- **Formation of larger amounts of granulation tissue.** The **larger defect requires more** amount of (abundant) **granulation tissue** to fill a large gap.
- **Increased scar tissue:** More volume of granulation tissue usually leads to extensive deposition of collagen with substantial scar formation. Ultimately, the scar formed is pale and avascular.
- **Loss of dermal appendages:** The skin appendages that have been destroyed in the region of the wound are permanently lost.
- **Wound contraction:** Open wounds contract and deform as they heal. It generally occurs in large surface wounds. It helps to close the wound by reducing the gap between the edges of the wound and the wound surface area. It is an important feature in healing by secondary union.
- **Myofibroblasts:** Wound contraction involves the formation of a network of *myofibroblasts* of granulation tissue. These myofibroblasts are modified fibroblasts that have contractile properties. They **have ultrastructural features of smooth muscle cells.** They contract in the wound tissue and are responsible for wound contraction.

Wound Strength

A major portion of the connective tissue in repair is fibrillar collagens (mostly type I collagen) which are responsible for the development of strength in healing wounds. The time for a skin wound to achieve its maximal strength is as follows:

- **At the end of the first week:** When sutures are removed from an incisional surgical wound, **wound strength** is about **10%** that of normal unwounded skin.

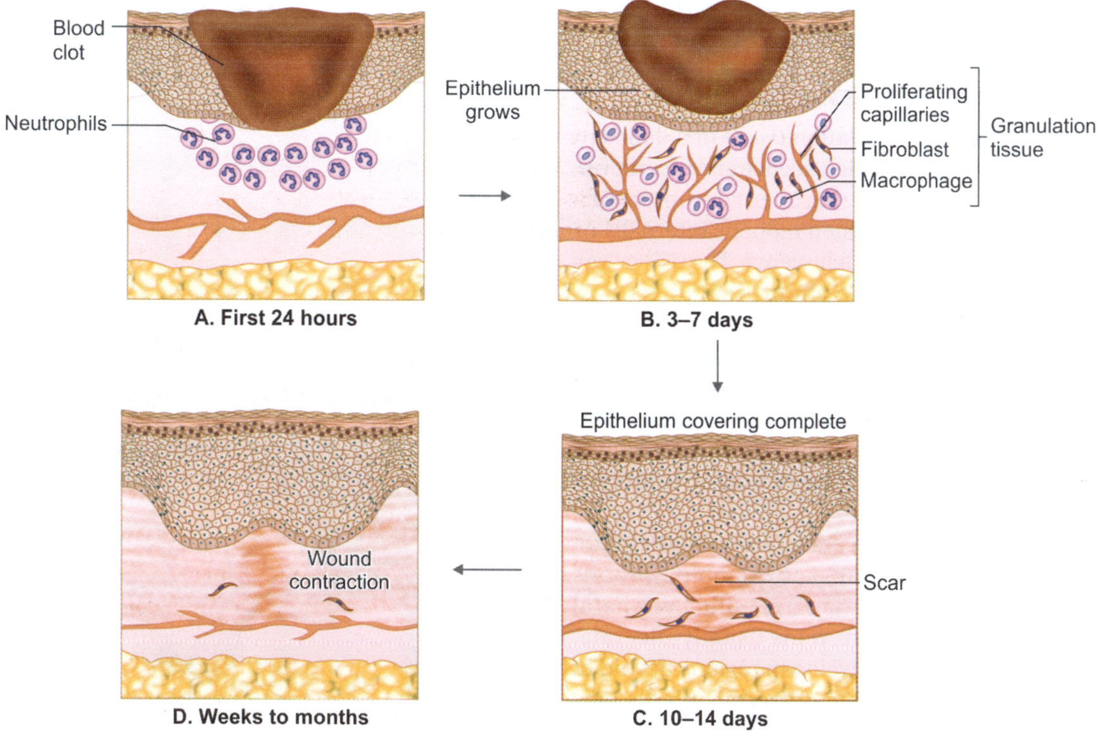

Figs. 3.26A to D: Healing by secondary intention: (A) There is a significant loss of tissue and the edges are far apart. Acute inflammation develops both at the edges and base; (B) The cell proliferation starts from the edges and a large amount of granulation tissue is formed; (C) The wound is covered on the entire surface by the epithelium. The collagen fibers are deposited; (D) Granulation tissue is replaced by a large scar. There is significant wound contraction.

- **Four weeks:** Wound strength quickly increases over the next 4 weeks, and then slows down.
- **Three months:** Wound strength **reaches 70–80% of the tensile strength** of unwounded skin.

Differences between healing by primary and secondary intention are discussed in **Table 3.15**.

Q. Compare/tabulate the differences between wound healing by primary and secondary intention with suitable diagrams.

TABLE 3.15 Differences between healing by primary and secondary intention.

Feature	Primary intention	Secondary intention
Nature of wound	Clean surgical wound	Unclean
Margins	Surgical clean margin	Irregular
Sutures	Used for apposition of margins	Cannot be used
Infection	Absent	May be infected
Amount of granulation tissue	Scanty at the incised gap and along the suture track	Abundant and fill the gap
Outcome	Neat linear scar	Irregular contracted scar
Complications	Rare	Infection and suppuration

Fibrosis in Parenchymal Organs

Scar versus fibrosis: Normal wound healing is associated with the deposition of collagen. **The scar is an altered organization of connective tissue matrix** (i.e., collagen fibers) **compared to normal, surrounding tissue. Fibrosis is an abnormal process characterized by the excessive deposition of collagen and other ECM components in internal organs in chronic diseases.** Fibrosis is the pathologic outcome of persistent injury and causes loss of function. Sometimes, the terms scar and fibrosis are used interchangeably. The basic mechanisms of fibrosis are similar to that of scar formation in the skin during tissue repair.

Fibrotic disorders: It is usually observed in persistent injurious stimuli, such as chronic infections and immunologic reactions. Fibrosis may produce severe organ dysfunction and even organ failure. **TGF β is an important fibrogenic agent.** Examples of fibrotic disorders include **cirrhosis of the liver**, systemic sclerosis (scleroderma), fibrosing diseases of the lung (e.g., idiopathic pulmonary fibrosis, **pneumoconioses**), **end-stage kidney disease,** and constrictive pericarditis.

Abnormalities in Tissue Repair

Q. Mention the complications of wound healing.

Complications in wound healing can be due to abnormalities in any of the basic processes involved in healing.

These include deficient scar formation, excessive formation of the repair components, and formation of contractures.

Inadequate Granulation Tissue Formation

Inadequate formation of granulation tissue or a deficient scar formation can cause **wound dehiscence** and **ulceration.**

1. **Dehiscence** (the wound splitting open) or rupture of a wound. When a surgical incision reopens internally or externally it is termed wound dehiscence. The risk factors for dehiscence are obesity, malnutrition, infections, and vascular insufficiency. Wound dehiscence is the most common life-threatening complication after abdominal surgery. It is due to increased abdominal pressure/mechanical stress on the abdominal wound from vomiting, coughing, or **ileus.** They can produce mechanical stress on the abdominal wound, leading to its rupture.
2. **Ulceration:** Wounds can ulcerate **due to inadequate angiogenesis** during healing. For example, wounds in the leg of patients with atherosclerotic peripheral vascular disease or varicose veins usually ulcerate. Non-healing wounds also develop in regions devoid of sensation. These **neuropathic or trophic ulcers** may be seen in diabetic peripheral neuropathy and nerve damage from leprosy.
3. **Incisional hernia** resulting from weak scars of the abdominal wall due to a defect caused by prior surgery. They are due to **insufficient deposition of the extracellular matrix or inadequate cross-linking in the collagen matrix.**

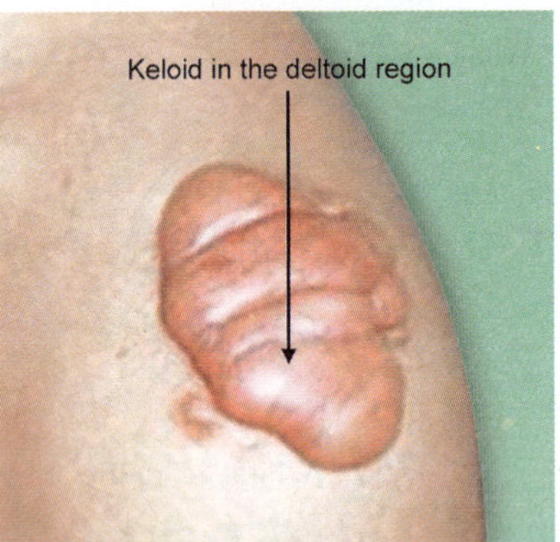

Fig. 3.27: Keloid in the upper arm.

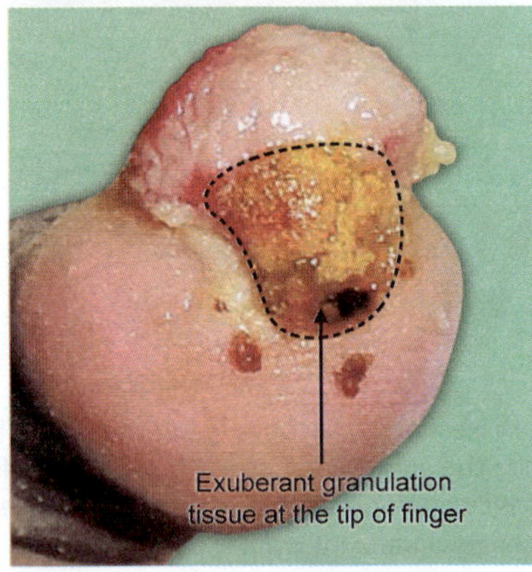

Fig. 3.28: Exuberant granulation (within dotted line) at the tip of the finger below the nail bed.

Excessive Scarring

Excessive formation of the components of the repair process can result in:

1. **Hypertrophic scar:** The **accumulation of excessive amounts of extracellular matrix,** mostly collagen may give rise to a raised scar at the site of the wound known as a hypertrophic scar. They usually develop after thermal or traumatic injury, which involves the deep layers of the dermis. These may grow rapidly. They contain abundant myofibroblasts but usually regress over several months.
2. **Keloid:** If the **scar tissue grows/progresses beyond the boundaries of the original wound and does not regress,** it is called a keloid **(Fig. 3.27).** Thus, a keloid is an exuberant scar that recurs with a still larger keloid after surgical excision.
3. **Exuberant granulation (Fig. 3.28):** This consists of the **localized formation of excessive amounts of granulation tissue.** Such exuberant granulation tissue projects above the level of the surrounding skin and prevents re-epithelialization. This mass formed is often named **proud flesh.** Excessive granulation must be removed by cautery or surgical excision to allow restoration of the continuity of the epithelium. Old terminology pyogenic granuloma or granuloma pyogenicum should be discouraged).
4. **Desmoids or aggressive fibromatoses:** Rarely, incisional scars or traumatic injuries may be followed by excessive proliferation of fibroblasts and other connective tissue elements. They are termed desmoids, or aggressive fibromatoses. These neoplasms lie in the interface between benign and malignant (though low-grade) tumors. These may recur after excision.

Excessive Contraction

A decrease in the size of a wound due to myofibroblasts is known as **contraction**. Contraction in the size of a wound is an important feature of the normal healing process. An **exaggeration of** this **contraction** is termed *contracture.* It produces deformities of the wound and the surrounding tissues. Contractures usually develop on the palms, the soles, and the anterior aspect of the thorax. The consequences of contractures are:

- **Compromise movements** [e.g., contractures that follow severe burns can compromise the movement of the involved region **(Fig. 3.29)** and joint movements].
- **Obstruction** [e.g., in GI tract contracture (stricture) can cause intestinal obstruction].

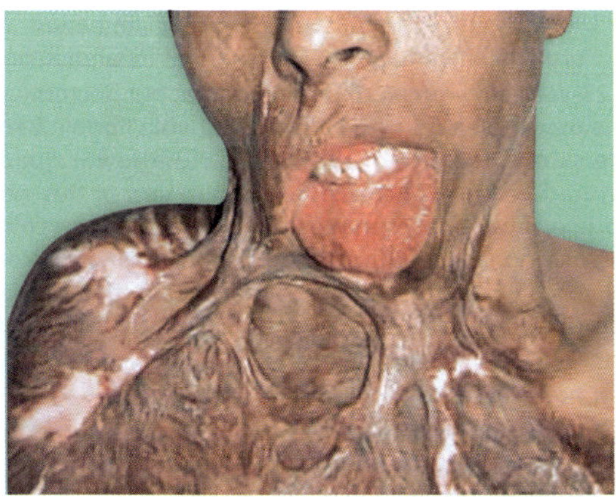

Fig. 3.29: Wound contracture—severe contracture of a wound on the neck and the right side of the neck.

Others

- **Infection** of wounds by microbes.
- **Epidermal cysts** can develop due to the persistence of epithelial cells at the site of wound healing.
- **Pigmentation** may develop due to either colored particles left in the wound or due to hemosiderin pigment.
- **Neoplasia** (e.g., squamous cell carcinoma may develop in Marjolin's ulcer, which is the scar that follows burns in the skin).

Defects in Healing: Chronic Wounds

Defects in healing and chronic wounds are observed in many clinical situations. These are due to local and systemic factors. Wounds can ulcerate if blood supply is inadequate or if vascularization is insufficient during healing. Common examples are as follows:

Venous leg ulcers: They occur usually **seen in elderly individuals** as a result of chronic venous hypertension, caused by severe varicose veins or congestive heart failure. These conditions are associated with a poor supply of oxygen leading to failure to heal.

Arterial ulcers: They occur in people with **atherosclerosis** of peripheral arteries or peripheral arterial disease, especially in diabetic patients. The ischemia interferes with repair and causes necrosis of the skin and underlying tissues.

Diabetic ulcers: They develop in the **lower extremities**, especially the feet. Diabetes is accompanied by small vessel disease (microangiopathy) that produces ischemia, and neuropathy and is prone to secondary infections. If the ulceration is left unchecked, it proceeds to infection of the underlying bone (osteomyelitis) and progressive loss of the extremity. Microscopically, these lesions show epidermal ulceration and extensive granulation tissue in the underlying dermis.

Pressure sores: These are characterized by areas of ulceration and necrosis of skin and underlying tissues due to prolonged compression of tissues against a bone. The sores are caused by mechanical pressure and local ischemia.

Neuropathic or trophic ulcers: Non-healing wounds also develop in regions devoid of sensation because of trauma or pressure. Constant pressure as little as 2–3 hours on the skin over a bony process can produce a local infarct. These ulcers can be both broad and deep, with the infection involving the underlying connective tissue. Neuropathic or trophic ulcers may be seen in diabetic peripheral neuropathy and nerve damage from leprosy.

Complications of wound healing are shown in **Flowchart 3.3.**

SCENARIO-BASED MCQs

1. **An 18-year-old girl sustains a cut in her left hand while cutting vegetables. The wound becomes infected by bacteria. The inflammatory response developed to bacterial infection. Of the following cells in the extravascular tissue, the bacteria are removed by:**
   A. Mast cell B. Macrophage
   C. T lymphocyte D. B lymphocyte
2. **A 60-year-old diabetic woman complained of a high fever with chills and a productive cough having yellowish sputum for the past 2 days. On auscultation of the chest, crackles are**

Flowchart 3.3: Complication of wound healing.

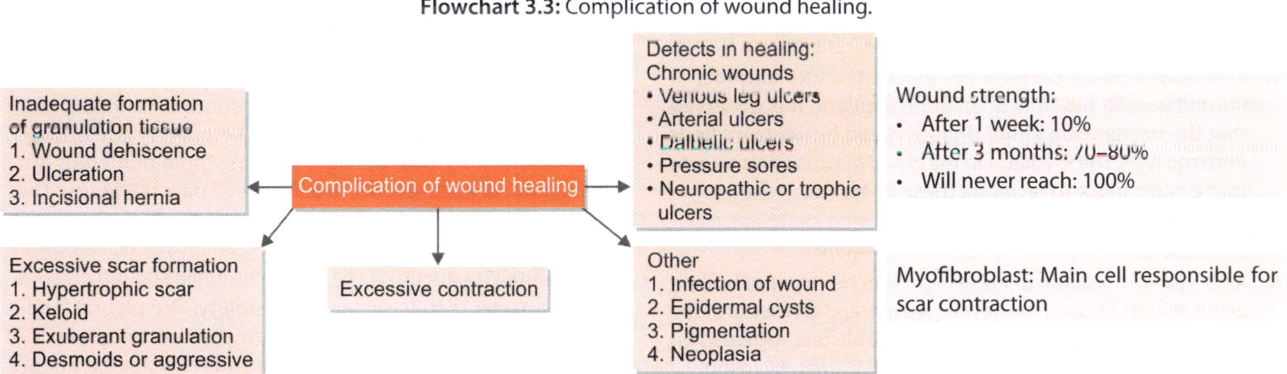

audible in the base of the left lung bases. A chest radiograph shows patchy pulmonary infiltrates in the left lower lobe. If her sputum is microscopically examined, the inflammatory cell type that is most likely to be seen is:

A. Neutrophils B. Macrophages
C. T lymphocytes D. Langhans giant cells

3. **A 65-year-old man with severe emphysema developed worsening right ventricular failure for the past 5 years. For the past 3 days, he has developed a fever and increasing dyspnea. A chest radiograph shows an accumulation of fluid in the pleural spaces. The fluid is obtained by thoracentesis. It has a specific gravity of 1.030 and microscopically shows numerous degenerating neutrophils. The most likely mechanism that caused fluid accumulation in pleural space is due to changes in:**
   A. Lymphatic pressure
   B. Vascular permeability
   C. Colloid osmotic pressure
   D. Leukocytic adhesion to the endothelial cells
4. **Mother of a 5-year-old child gives a history of recurrent infections with pyogenic bacteria in the child. These infections were found on culture including *Staphylococcus aureus* and *Streptococcus pneumoniae*. The infections are associated with neutrophilic leukocytosis. The child developed necrosis in the soft tissue. Microscopic examination of a biopsy from this area showed microbial organisms, but only very few neutrophils. An analysis of neutrophil function shows a defect in rolling. This child's increased susceptibility to infection is most likely due to a defect involving the molecule namely:**
   A. Selectins B. Integrins
   C. Leukotriene B4 D. Complement C3b
5. **A woman who is allergic to pollens in the flowers visits a neighbor's garden full of various types of flowers. During the visit, she inhales pollen from flowers. Within minutes, she develops congestion of the nose with abundant secretion from the nose. The mediator that is most likely to produce these symptoms is:**
   A. Bradykinin B. Histamine
   C. Complement C5a D. Interleukin-1 (IL-1)
6. **A 38-year-old woman takes acetylsalicylic acid (aspirin) for arthritis. Although her pain in the joint is reduced with this drug, the inflammatory process continues. The aspirin therapy relives her pain mainly through a reduction in the synthesis of the mediators namely:**
   A. Histamine B. Prostaglandins
   C. Leukotriene E4 D. Complement C1q
7. **In an experiment, bacteria are inoculated into aliquots of normal human blood with an anticoagulant. It is observed that the bacteria are either phagocytized by neutrophils or undergo lysis. The mediator in the blood plasma components that is most likely to facilitate these effects is:**
   A. Plasmin B. Fibrin
   C. Kallikrein D. Complement
8. **A 65-year-old woman unknowingly touches a pot of boiling water. Within 2 hours, she developed marked erythema of the skin of the fingers of her hand, and small blisters appeared on the finger pads. This morphological inflammatory response suggests:**
   A. Ulceration B. Serous inflammation
   C. Purulent inflammation D. Fibrinous inflammation
9. **A 25-year-old woman underwent an appendectomy. After one month, she detected a small palpable nodule beneath the skin at the site of the healed right lower quadrant sutured incision. Microscopic examination of this excised nodule shows macrophages, small lymphocytes, collagen deposition, and multinucleated giant cells. On polarized microscopy, a refractile material is seen in the nodule. The complications of the surgery that account for these findings are:**
   A. Chronic inflammation
   B. Granuloma formation
   C. Healing by second Intention
   D. Exuberant granulation tissue
10. **A 49-year-old man underwent laparoscopic hernia repair. Despite the small size of the incision, he has poor wound healing. On further inquiry, he reveals that his usual diet has poor nutritional value and is deficient in vitamin C. Synthesis of the following extracellular matrix components is most likely affected by this deficiency:**
    A. Elastin B. Laminin
    C. Integrin D. Collagen
11. **An 18-year-old man lacerated his left upper arm and required sutures. The sutures were removed 1 week later. Wound healing continued, but the site became disfigured over the next 2 months. The term used for the disfigured lesion at the wound site is known as:**
    A. A Resolution B. Dehiscence
    C. Organization D. Keloid formation
12. **A 60-year-old man suffers a massive heart attack and expires 24 hours later due to ventricular arrhythmia. Microscopic examination of the myocardium of the left ventricle would show an abundance of the following inflammatory cells:**
    A. Neutrophils B. Lymphocytes
    C. Macrophages D. Plasma cells

Answers and Explanation

1. **The answer is B: Macrophage.** Macrophages are phagocytic cells in tissues. They are derived from circulating blood monocytes. The other cells in the options listed are not phagocytic cells. B lymphocytes can differentiate into plasma cells and secrete antibodies that can neutralize infectious agents. Mast cells can release various inflammatory mediators. T lymphocytes are mainly seen in chronic inflammatory processes.
2. **The answer is A: Neutrophils.** The signs and symptoms are suggestive of acute bacterial pneumonia. It produces an acute inflammation with predominated neutrophils that fill alveoli. This gives rise to yellowish, purulent sputum. Langhans giant cells are seen with granulomatous inflammatory diseases such as tuberculosis. Macrophages become more numerous after initiation of acute events, usually after 2 days (48 hours). They clean up tissue and bacterial debris through phagocytosis. Mast cells participate in allergic and anaphylactic responses. Lymphocytes are observed in chronic inflammation
3. **The answer is B: Vascular permeability.** The pleural fluid is an exudate containing a significant amount of protein and degenerating neutrophils. This occurs due to increased vascular permeability (mainly in venules). When exudation occurs,

the protein content of the extravascular space increases, and extravascular colloid osmotic pressure increases. This causes the accumulation of extracellular fluid and is not the primary event. Leukocytic adhesion can not produce exudation. The lymphatics drain the proteinaceous fluid and reduce the amount of extravascular and extracellular fluid.

4. **The answer is A: Selectins.** Leukocyte rolling is the initial step of the leukocyte event in acute inflammation. Rolling depends on the interaction between selectins (P-selectin and E-selectin on endothelial cells, and L-selectin on neutrophils) and their corresponding sialylated ligands (e.g., sialylated Lewis X). Integrins are involved in the firm adhesion of leukocytes to the endothelial cells. Complement C3b acts as an opsonin that facilitates phagocytosis. Leukotriene B4 is a chemotactic agent.
5. **The answer is B: Histamine.** Histamine is found in mast cells present in the connective tissues next to blood vessels beneath mucosal surfaces in airways. The binding of an antigen (allergen) to IgE antibodies that are previously attached to the mast cells by the Fc receptor triggers mast cell degranulation. This releases histamine and causes increased vascular permeability and mucous secretions. Bradykinin is produced by the activation of the kinin system causes vascular permeability, smooth muscle contraction, and pain. Complement C5a is a powerful chemotactic factor for neutrophils. Interleukin-1 (IL-1) is produced by activated macrophages and mediates many systemic effects. These include fever, cachexia, and hypotension.
6. **The answer is B: Prostaglandins.** Prostaglandins are produced through the activation of the cyclooxygenase pathway of arachidonic acid metabolism. Aspirin and other nonsteroidal anti-inflammatory drugs block the synthesis of prostaglandins, which can produce pain. Complement C1q is produced in the early stage of complement activations. Histamine is mainly a vasodilator. Leukotrienes are produced by the lipoxygenase pathway and is not blocked by aspirin.
7. **The answer is D: Complement.** Activation of complement may occur through components of microbial cell walls such as polysaccharides (alternative pathway) or mannose (lectin pathway), or antibodies attached to surface antigens (classic pathway). An activated complement system produces various complement components. These include complement C5a (neutrophil chemoattractant); complement C3b (opsonin); and complement C5-9 (the membrane attack complex/MAC). The remaining options are more closely associated with the activation of the coagulation system. Fibrin is produced by the coagulation system, but not in an anticoagulation. Kallikrein generates bradykinin. Plasmin is generated from plasminogen and helps to lyse clots.
8. **The answer is B: Serous inflammation.** It is the mildest morphologic form of acute inflammation. A blister is a classical example of serous inflammation. It develops due to the exudation of fluid into the subcorneal or subepidermal space. Because the injury is mild, the accumulated fluid is relatively protein-poor. A protein-rich exudate results in fibrinous inflammation. Loss of the epithelium leads to ulceration. Acute inflammatory cells, mainly neutrophils, emigrate into a body cavity or space and form a purulent (suppurative) exudate. It is classically associated with liquefaction necrosis.
9. **The answer is B: Granuloma formation.** The polarizable material in the nodule is the suture, and a multinucleated giant cell (foreign body giant cells) is characteristic of a granulomatous reaction to foreign material. If a large, gaping wound is not closed by sutures, it can close the wound by the second intention. Chronic inflammation alone does not produce a localized nodule with giant cells. Exuberant granulation tissue does not appear as a nodule.
10. **The answer is 10 D: Collagen.** Vitamin C deficiency leads to scurvy. Vitamin C helps to cross-link fibrillar collagens to provide tensile strength. Though elastin is a fibrillar protein, it tends to regenerate poorly in scar tissue, even with adequate nutrition. Thus, a scar does not stretch like the skin around it. The other choices are not vitamin C-dependent.
11. **The answer is D: Keloid formation.** The healing process may be complicated by the exuberant production of collagen, giving rise to a keloid. It appears as a prominent raised, nodular scar. Dehiscence occurs when a wound pulls apart and is common with abdominal wounds. Organization occurs as granulation tissue is replaced by fibrous tissue. If normal tissue architecture is restored, it is termed resolution.
12. **The answer is A: Neutrophils.** These are the predominant cells seen during the first 24 hours. In this case, myocardial infarction elicits an acute inflammatory infiltrate of neutrophils. Macrophages are seen after 24 to hours in acute inflammation. All other cells mentioned in the option are seen in chronic inflammation.

SCENARIO-BASED ESSAY

Q. A 12-year-old boy presented with a sudden onset of abdominal pain, fever and vomiting. On abdominal palpation, tenderness is present at a point that lies one-third of the distance laterally on a line drawn from the umbilicus to the right anterior superior iliac spine (McBurney's point). He underwent surgery and recovered completely.

a. **What is the probable diagnosis? (Ans: Acute appendicitis).**
b. **Define inflammation (*refer* page 60). Enumerate cellular events of inflammation (*refer* pages 65-72).**
c. **Fate (outcomes) of acute inflammation (*refer* pages 82-3).**

PA 2.8 (CC): Identify and describe various forms of cell injuries, their manifestations, and consequences in gross and microscopic specimens.

Acute inflammation:
- Slectins: Rolling of neutrophils.
- Integrins: Firm adhesion of neutrophils to endothelium

Transmigration (diapedesis): Requires PECAM molecule or CD31.

H_2O_2-MPO-halide system is the most efficient bactericidal (killing bacteria) system of neutrophils.
O_2-dependent MPO system is most potent microbicidal system.

No granuloma in acute inflammation.

No necrotizing granuloma in leprosy.

Myofibroblast: Main cell responsible for scar contraction.

CHAPTER 4

Infections and Infestations

CHAPTER OUTLINE

- Mycobacterial Infections
- Spirochete Infections
- Bacterial Diseases
- Viral Diseases
- Rickettsial Infections
- Chlamydial Infections
- Fungal Infections and Opportunistic Infections
- Mycetoma
- Parasitic Diseases
- Malaria
- Other Infections

MYCOBACTERIAL INFECTIONS

Mycobacteria are bacteria that appear as slender, aerobic rods. They grow in straight or branching chains. Mycobacteria have a characteristic waxy cell wall composed of unusual glycolipids and lipids including mycolic acid. This wall is responsible for its acid-fast nature on staining. Acid-fast means that they will retain stains, even on treatment with a mixture of acid and alcohol. They are weakly gram-positive. Two important mycobacteria that cause granulomatous disease are *Mycobacterium tuberculosis (tuberculosis)* and *Mycobacterium leprae (leprosy).* Tuberculosis is discussed on pages 559-67 of Chapter 17. Nontuberculous mycobacteria (NTM) are mycobacteria other than *M. tuberculosis* and *M. leprae.* Of the 150 NTM species, the most frequent human pathogens are *Mycobacterium avium* complex (MAC).

Leprosy

PA 10.3 (CC): Define and describe the pathogenesis and pathology of leprosy.

Leprosy or **Hansen disease** (named after the discovery of the causative organism by Hansen), is a **chronic, granulomatous, slowly progressive, destructive infection** caused by ***Mycobacterium leprae***. Leprosy is one of the oldest human diseases and lepers were isolated from the community in the olden days.

Sites of involvement: *Mycobacterium leprae* mainly affects the **peripheral nerves, skin, and mucous membranes** (nasal) and results in disabling deformities.

***Mycobacterium leprae*:** The characteristic features of this mycobacteria are:

- **Slender, weakly acid-fast intracellular bacillus:** It closely resembles *Mycobacterium tuberculosis* but is less acid-fast.
- **Proliferates at low temperature of the human skin:** These bacilli prefer temperatures lower than those in internal organs. **Cannot be cultured** on artificial media or in cell culture. Lepra bacilli grow at sites where the temperature is below that of the internal organs. Examples: **Footpads of mice**, ear lobes of hamsters, rats, and other rodents. **Experimentally transmitted to nine branded armadillos** (they have low body temperature ranging from 32–34°C).
- **Antigen in lepra bacilli:** The bacterial cell wall contains mainly 2 antigens namely *M. leprae*-specific phenolic glycolipid (PGL-1) and lipoarabinomannan (LAM).

Mode of transmission: Leprosy has **comparatively low communicability**.

1. **Inoculation/inhalation:** Likely to be transmitted from person to person through **aerosols from** asymptomatic lesions in the **upper respiratory tract**. Inhaled *M. leprae*, is taken up by alveolar macrophages and disseminates through the blood, but replicates only in relatively cool tissues of the skin and extremities.
2. **Intimate contact:** It may be transmitted by intimate contact for many years with untreated leprosy patients. They shed many bacilli from damaged skin, nasal secretions, mucous membranes of the mouth, and hair follicles.

Source of infection: *M. leprae* is present in **nasal/respiratory secretions or ulcerated lesions of patients** suffering from leprosy.

Incubation period: Generally, 5–7 years.

Classification

Q. Classify leprosy.

A. Ridley and Jopling (1966) Classification (Table 4.1)

It **depends on the clinicopathological spectrum of the disease**, which is **determined by the immune resistance of the host (Flowchart 4.1)**. Leprosy is classified into five groups with two extreme or polar forms, namely—**tuberculoid and lepromatous types.**

Variants of leprosy: These include indeterminate and histoid leprosy.

Q. Write a short note on indeterminate leprosy.

- **Indeterminate leprosy:** It is an initial nonspecific stage of any type of leprosy. Pure neural leprosy with neurologic involvement is the main feature. The skin lesions of leprosy are not seen. Indeterminate leprosy and tuberculoid lesions are paucibacillary and their diagnosis is made together with clinical evidence (for microscopy *refer* page 110).
- **Histoid leprosy:** It is a **variant of lepromatous leprosy** in which the **skin lesions grossly resemble nodules of dermatofibroma** (a soft tissue tumor involving skin) and microscopically shows numerous lepra bacilli.

TABLE 4.1 Ridley and Jopling (1966) classification and associated immune response.

Group	*Immune response*
Tuberculoid leprosy (TT)	Polar form that has maximal immune response
Borderline tuberculoid (BT)	Immune response falls between BB and TT
Borderline leprosy (BB)	Immune response exactly falls between two polar forms of leprosy
Borderline lepromatous (BL)	Immune response that falls between BB and LL
Lepromatous leprosy (LL)	Polar form with the least immune response

B. WHO Classification

- **Paucibacillary:** All cases of tuberculoid leprosy and some cases of borderline type are paucibacillary. They do not show lepra bacilli on microscopic examination.
- **Multibacillary:** All cases of lepromatous leprosy and some cases of borderline type are multibacillary.

Pathogenesis

Ingestion of mycobacteria by macrophages and proliferation: After the inoculation, *M. leprae* is taken up by macrophages and disseminates in the blood. However, the mycobacteria **replicate mainly in relatively cool tissues** of the skin and extremities. Its proliferation occurs at 32–34°C, the temperature of the human skin.

Virulence depends on the properties of the mycobacterial cell wall: *Mycobacterium leprae* does not secrete any toxins. Its virulence depends on the properties of its cell wall (like that of *M. tuberculosis*) and immunization with BCG may provide some protection against *M. leprae* infection.

Cell-mediated immunity: An infected individual develops delayed-type hypersensitivity reactions (cell-mediated/type IV hypersensitivity reaction) to dermal

Flowchart 4.1: Ridley–Jopling classification of leprosy.

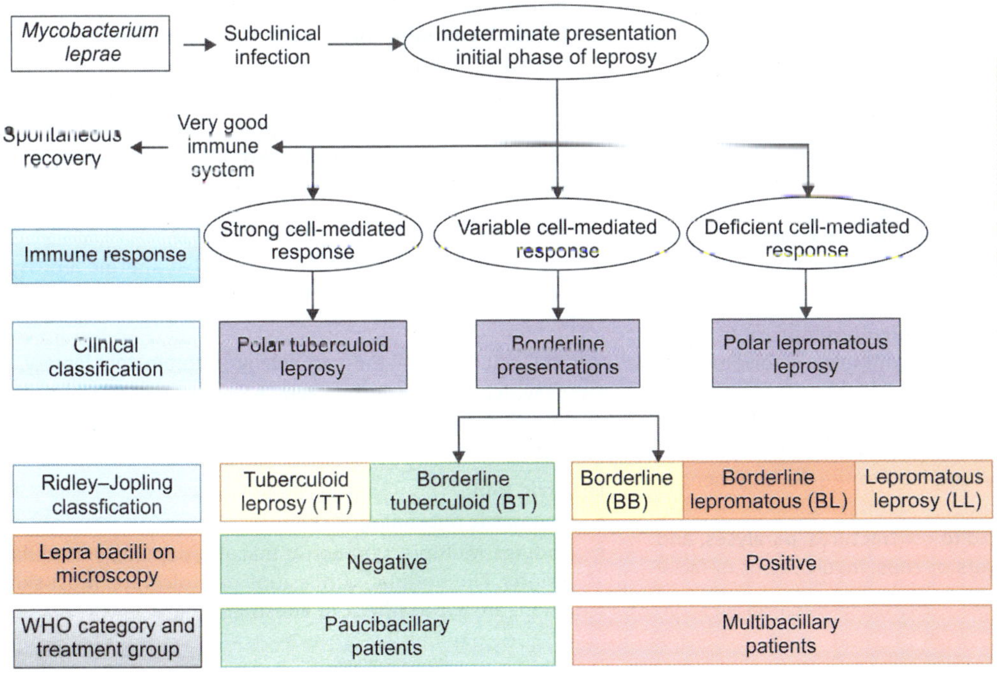

Mycobacterium leprae → Subclinical infection → Indeterminate presentation initial phase of leprosy

Very good immune system → Spontaneous recovery

Immune response	Strong cell-mediated response		Variable cell-mediated response		Deficient cell-mediated response
Clinical classification	Polar tuberculoid leprosy		Borderline presentations		Polar lepromatous leprosy
Ridley–Jopling classfication	Tuberculoid leprosy (TT)	Borderline tuberculoid (BT)	Borderline (BB)	Borderline lepromatous (BL)	Lepromatous leprosy (LL)
Lepra bacilli on microscopy	Negative		Positive		
WHO category and treatment group	Paucibacillary patients		Multibacillary patients		

Classification of leprosy:
1. Ridley and Jopling classification.
2. WHO classification: Paucibacillary and multibacillary.

Lepromatous leprosy (LL): Polar form with the least immune response.
Tuberculoid leprosy (TT): Polar form with maximal immune response.

Fite-Faraco stain: Modified Ziehl-Neelsen stain used for demonstration of lepra bacilli in tissue.

injections of **lepromin.** Lepromin is a bacterial extract obtained from lepra bacillus.

Different T-cell responses: *M. leprae* causes two different patterns of disease namely tuberculoid and lepromatous. They have different types of helper T-lymphocyte response to *M. leprae.* The **T-helper (Th1) lymphocyte response** to *M. leprae,* determines whether an individual develops a tuberculoid or lepromatous type of leprosy.

- **Tuberculoid leprosy:** These patients **have a Th1 response**. This is associated with the secretion of IL-2 and IFN-γ as well as a Th17 response. The IFN-γ is essential for an effective host macrophage response.
- **Lepromatous leprosy:** These patients have **a weak Th1 response** and, some have a **relative increase in the Th2 response.** This causes poor cell-mediated immunity and proliferation of lepra bacilli. Sometimes, antibodies may be produced against *M. leprae* antigens, but they are usually not protective. These antibodies may combine with free antigens leading to the formation of immune complexes. These can lead to the development of erythema nodosum, vasculitis, and glomerulonephritis.

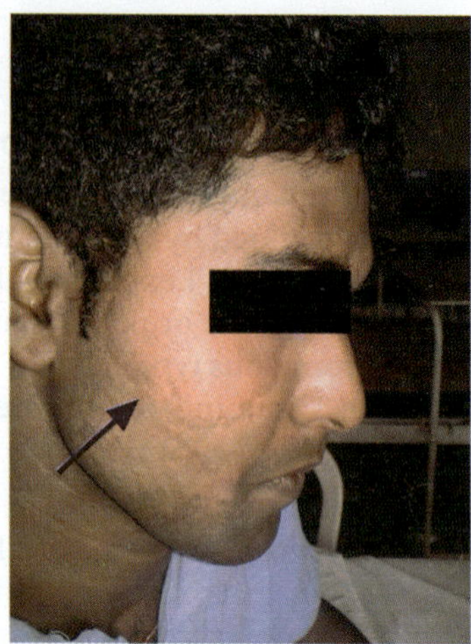

Fig. 4.1: Localized, well-demarcated, red or hypopigmented skin patches on the face (arrow).

MORPHOLOGY

Two extremes or polar forms of the diseases are the tuberculoid and lepromatous types. **M. leprae multiplies at temperatures** below the core human body temperature. Hence, the **lesions tend to occur in cooler parts of the body** (e.g., hands and face). Lesions show marked variations. It may vary from small, insignificant, and self-healing macules of tuberculoid leprosy to the diffuse, and disfiguring lesions of lepromatous leprosy. This marked variation in disease presentation is due to differences in immune reactivity.

Q. Write a short note on the morphology of tuberculoid leprosy.

1. Tuberculoid Leprosy

It is the **less severe form** of leprosy. The lesions of tuberculoid leprosy cause **minimal disfigurement** and are **not infectious.** It is **very slow in its course** and most patients die with leprosy.

Lesion in skin

- **Number of lesions: Single or very few lesions.**
- **Common sites:** Usually on the **face, extremities, or trunk**
- **Type: Localized, well-demarcated, flat, red or hypopigmented, dry, scaly, elevated, skin patches (Fig. 4.1)** having raised outer edges and depressed pale centers (central healing). As they progress they develop irregular shapes with induration.

Nerve involvement

- **The dominating feature of tuberculoid leprosy is nerve involvement.** They often show **asymmetric** involvement of large peripheral nerves.
- **Loss of sensation:** Nerve involvement causes **loss of sensation in the skin** and atrophy of skin and muscle. These affected parts are liable to trauma and lead to the development of **chronic skin ulcers.**
- **Consequences:** It may lead to **contractures, paralyses, and autoamputation of fingers or toes.** Involvement of facial nerve can lead to paralysis of the eyelids, with keratitis and corneal ulcerations.

Microscopy (Figs. 4.2A and B)

- **Granuloma:** These are well-formed, circumscribed, and **non-caseating** (no caseation). The term "tuberculoid leprosy" is used because the granulomas resemble those found in tuberculosis, It is seen in all involved sites and the dermis of skin. Granulomas are composed of **epithelioid cells** (modified macrophages), **Langhans giant cells, and lymphocytes.** though they **lack necrosis.**
- **Absence of Grenz zone:** Granulomas in the dermis extend to the basal layer of the epidermis (without a clear/Grenz zone).
- **Fite-Faraco** (modified Z-N stain for demonstration of lepra bacillus) stain generally **does not show lepra bacillus,** hence the name "**paucibacillary**" leprosy.
- **Perineural (surrounding nerve fibers) inflammation:** Nerve fibers are usually swollen and infiltrated with **lymphocytes (Fig. 4.2B).**
- **Strong T-cell immunity:** It is responsible for granuloma formation, without lepra bacilli.
- **Peripheral nerves:** They are surrounded by **granulomatous inflammatory reactions.** The destruction of small dermal nerve twigs may occur and is **responsible for the sensory deficit** associated with tuberculoid leprosy.

2. Lepromatous Leprosy

It is the **more severe form** and is also called **anergic leprosy,** because of the unresponsiveness (anergy) of the host immune system.

Q. Write a short note on the morphology of lepromatous leprosy.

Sites involved: These include **skin, peripheral nerves, anterior eye chamber, upper airways** (down to the larynx), **testes, hands, and feet.**

Lesion in skin

- **Symmetric thickening of skin.**
- **Nodules. Multiple, symmetric, macular, papular, or nodular lesions:** The nodular skin lesions may ulcerate. Most skin lesions are **hypoesthetic or anesthetic.**

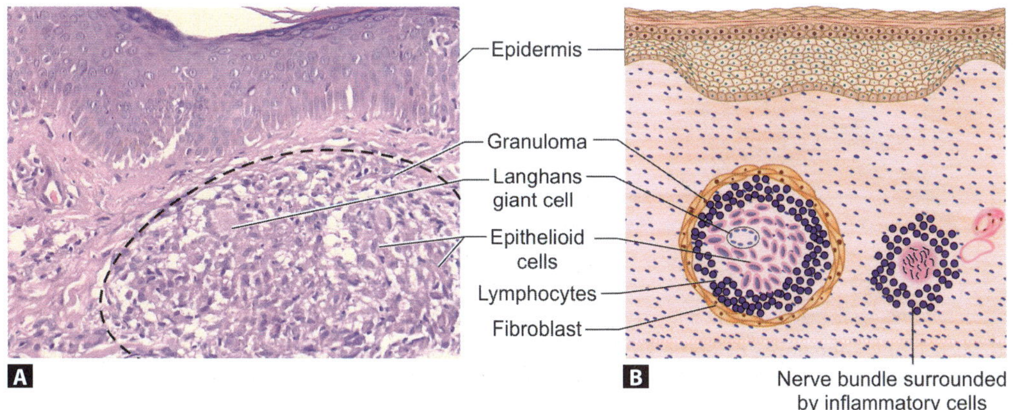

Figs. 4.2A and B: Microscopy of tuberculoid leprosy with circumscribed noncaseating granulomas (dotted line): (A) Photomicrograph; (B) Diagrammatic.

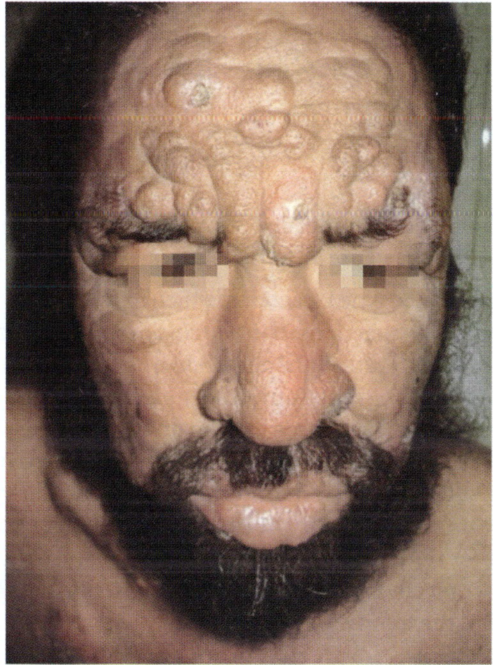

Fig. 4.3. Leonine facies of lepromatous leprosy.

- **Sites of lesions:** More severe involvement of the **cooler areas of skin** (e.g., earlobes, wrists, elbows, knees, and feet), than warmer areas (e.g., axilla and groin). Other sites include eyes, testes, nerves, lymph nodes, and spleen.
- **Leonine facies:** With progression, the **nodular lesions in the face and earlobes may coalesce** to produce a lion-like appearance known as **leonine facies (Fig. 4.3).** This may be accompanied by loss of eyebrows and eyelashes.

Peripheral nerves

- Particularly the **ulnar and peroneal nerves** are **symmetrically invaded** with mycobacteria.
- **Loss of sensation and trophic changes** in the hands and feet may follow the damage to the nerves.

Other sites

Testes: Usually, severely involved, leading to the destruction of the seminiferous tubules leading to **sterility**.

The anterior chamber of the eye: It may lead to **blindness.**

Upper airways: Chronic nasal discharge and voice change.

Microscopy of skin lesion (Figs. 4.4 and 4.5)

It shows **nodular or diffuse infiltrates of foamy macrophages containing numerous lepra bacilli.**

- **Flattened epidermis:** Epidermis is thinned and flattened (loss of rete ridges) over the nodules.
- **Grenz** (clear) **zone:** Beneath the epidermis, there is a **narrow, uninvolved "clear zone" of the dermis** (normal collagen) **called the Grenz zone (Figs. 4.4A and B).** It separates the epidermis from nodular accumulations of macrophages.

Q. Write a short note on the lepra cell.

- **Lepra cells (Fig. 4.5A):** The nodular lesions contain large aggregates of **lipid-laden foamy macrophages**. These are called lepra cells, or **Virchow cells**. These are filled with aggregates of acid-fast lepra bacilli (*M. leprae*). The aggregates or masses of acid-fast material inside the macrophage are called **"globi."**
- **Fite-Faraco (acid-fast) stain (Fig. 4.5B):** It shows **numerous lepra bacilli** ("red snappers") **within the foamy macrophages.** They may be arranged in a parallel fashion like **cigarettes in a pack**. Due to the presence of numerous mycobacteria, lepromatous leprosy is also referred to as **"multibacillary"**
- **Damage to peripheral nerves:** Widespread symmetrical invasion of the mycobacteria into Schwann cells and endoneural and perineural macrophages damages the peripheral nervous system. It **particularly involves the ulnar and peroneal nerves** where they approach the skin surface. Loss of sensation and trophic changes in the hands and feet develop following nerve involvement.
- *M. leprae* in sputum and blood. This may be observed **in advanced cases** of lepromatous leprosy,

3. Borderline Leprosy

Some individuals may have with intermediate form of disease, called **borderline leprosy.**

Borderline tuberculoid (BT) shows epithelioid cells and numerous lymphocytes with a narrow clear subepidermal zone. Lepra bacilli are few and found in nerves.

Borderline lepromatous (BL) shows predominantly histiocytes, few epithelioid cells, and lymphocytes. Numerous lepra bacilli are found.

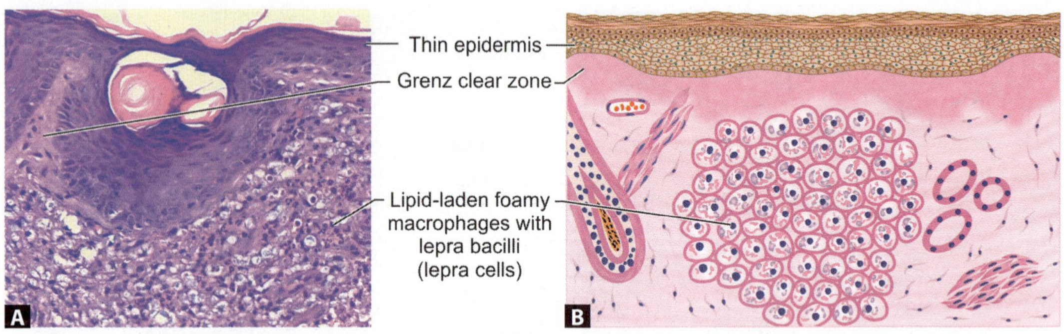

Figs. 4.4A and B: Microscopic appearance of lepromatous leprosy: (A) Photomicrograph; (B) Diagrammatic. The epidermis is thinned and the dermis shows dense collections of lepra cells. The epidermis is separated from the collections of lepra cells by an uninvolved Grenz zone.

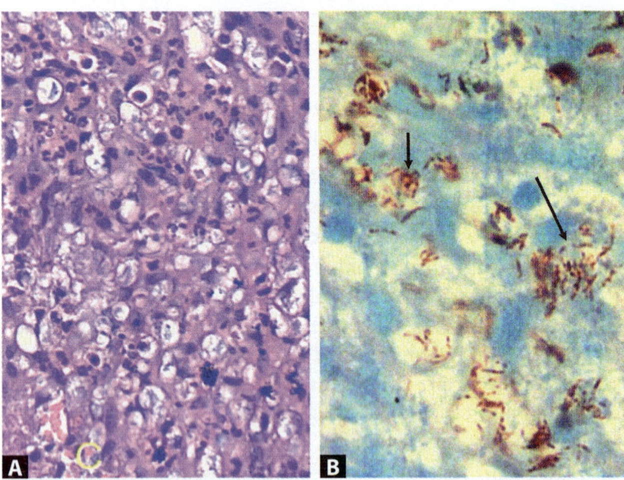

Figs. 4.5A and B: Lepromatous leprosy: (A) High power view showing foamy macrophages; (B) Acid-fast lepra bacilli within macrophages (Fite–Faraco stain) (arrows).

Mid-borderline (BB) or dimorphic form shows sheets of epithelioid cells without any giant cells. Few lymphocytes are found in the perineurium. Lepra bacilli are seen mostly in nerves.

4. Indeterminate Leprosy

Microscopically, features are nonspecific and few findings help in suspecting leprosy. These include (1) local infiltration of lymphocytes or mononuclear cells surrounding the skin adnexa (e.g., hair follicles and sweat glands) or around blood vessels, (2) involvement of nerve (if seen strongly favors the diagnosis), and (3) finding of lepra bacilli (which confirms the diagnosis).

Lepromin Test

It is **not a diagnostic test** for leprosy. It is **used for classifying leprosy** based on the immune response.

Procedure: An antigen extract of *M. leprae* called lepromin is intradermally injected.

Q. Write a short note on the lepromin test/Mitsuda reaction.

Reaction: (1) An **early positive reaction** appearing as an indurated area in 24–48 hours is called the **Fernandez reaction,** and (2) a **delayed granulomatous reaction** appearing after 3–4 weeks is known as the **Mitsuda reaction.**

Interpretation: (1) **Lepromatous leprosy shows** a **negative lepromin test** due to suppression of cell-mediated immunity. (2) **Tuberculoid leprosy** shows a **positive lepromin test** because of delayed hypersensitivity reaction.

Reactions in Leprosy

The immunity in leprosy may change spontaneously or following treatment.

Type I reaction: Borderline leprosy is the most unstable form of leprosy where immune status may shift up or down.

These are called type I reactions, which may be of **two types:**

1. **Upgrading reactions:** If immunity improves, the disease may shift towards tuberculoid leprosy.
2. **Downgrading reaction:** If the immunity decreases, the disease moves towards lepromatous leprosy.

Type II reaction or erythema nodosum leprosum: It **occurs mostly in lepromatous leprosy**, particularly when on treatment. Clinically, it presents with (1) tender red plaque or nodules and (2) fever, malaise, and arthralgia. Microscopically, it shows **necrotizing vasculitis and lepra bacilli in the foamy macrophages.**

Differences between lepromatous and tuberculoid leprosy are presented in **Table 4.2.**

Diagnosis of Leprosy

1. **Clinical examination:**
   - **Sensory testing**
   - Examination of peripheral nerve
2. **Demonstration of acid-fast bacilli: Skin smears prepared by slit** (split skin smears by splitting the skin) **and scrape method** (scrapings from cut edges of the dermis). *Mycobacterium leprae* can be demonstrated in split skin smears by splitting the skin, and in nasal smears by the following techniques:
   - **Acid-fast (Ziehl–Neelsen) staining.** The staining procedure is similar to that procedure employed for *M. tuberculosis* but can be decolorized by lower concentration (5%) of sulphuric acid (less acid-fast).

TABLE 4.2 Differences between lepromatous and tuberculoid leprosy.

Characteristics	*Lepromatous leprosy*	*Tuberculoid leprosy*
Clinical features		
Skin lesions	Symmetrical, multiple, ill-defined, macular, nodular	Asymmetrical, hypopigmented, well-defined macular
Disfigurement	Leonine facies, loss of eyebrows, pendulous earlobes, claw hands, saddle nose	Minimal disfigurement
Nerve involvement	Seen but with less severe sensory loss than tuberculoid	Common with sensory disturbances
Microscopy of skin lesions		
Type of lesion	Nodular or diffuse collections of lepra cells within the dermis	Noncaseating granulomas are composed of epithelioid cells and Langhans giant cells
Grenz/clear zone between inflammatory cells and epidermis	Present	Absent
Lepra bacilli	Plenty within the lepra cells as globular masses (globi)	Rare if any
Bacillary index	4 or 5	0
Other features		
Immunity	Suppressed-low resistance	Good immunity-high resistance
Lepromin test	Negative	Positive
Infectivity	High	Low
Complications	Erythema nodosum leprosum (ENL) may cause vasculitis, glomerulonephritis, and nerve damage	Nerve damage can lead to sensory disturbance, paralysis

3. **Skin biopsy:** Fite–Faraco staining procedure is a modified ZN procedure and is better for tissue sections **(Fig. 4.5B)**. Gomori methenamine silver (GMS) staining can also be used.
4. **Nerve biopsy**
5. **Molecular method: Polymerase chain reaction (PCR).**
6. *IgM antibodies to PGL-1 antigen.* Detected in 95% of cases of lepromatous leprosy but only in 60% of cases of tuberculoid leprosy.

SPIROCHETE INFECTIONS

Spirochetes are long, slender, corkscrew-shaped bacteria covered by a specialized cell envelope (membrane) called an outer sheath. This envelope may mask its antigens from the host's immune response. It also permits them to move by flexion and rotation.

Identification: Spirochetes have the basic cell wall structure of gram-negative bacteria. But, they stain poorly with the Gram stain. They cannot be detected by routine light microscopy. Specialized techniques, such as **darkfield microscopy or silver impregnation,** are required for their detection.

Diseases caused by spirochetes: They generally cause chronic and relapsing disease. Three spirochetes that cause disease are *Treponema*, *Borrelia*, and *Leptospira*.

Syphilis

Syphilis (lues) is a **chronic, sexually transmitted infection (STI)** caused **by spirochete *Treponema pallidum*.** It manifests with multiple clinical and pathologic presentations.

Etiology: Syphilis is caused by a spirochete Treponema pallidum (Fig. 4.6A). *Treponema pallidum* has the following characteristics.

- *T. pallidum* is a **thin, delicate, corkscrew-shaped spirochete**, that measures about 10 µm long with tapering ends and has about 10 regular spirals. It is very fragile and is killed by soap, antiseptics, drying, and cold.
- **Actively motile,** showing rotation around the long axis, backward and forward motion.
- **Cannot be grown in artificial media.**
- **Staining:** It does not stain with ordinary bacterial stains and *Treponema pallidum* is too slender to be seen in Gram stain. It can be visualized by **silver stains, dark-field examination, and immunofluorescence techniques.**

Source of infection: An **open lesion of primary or secondary syphilis.** Lesions in the mucous membranes or skin of the genital organs, rectum, mouth, fingers, or nipples.

Mode of transmission: These are through the following routes:

- **Sexual contact:** It is the **usual mode of spread.**

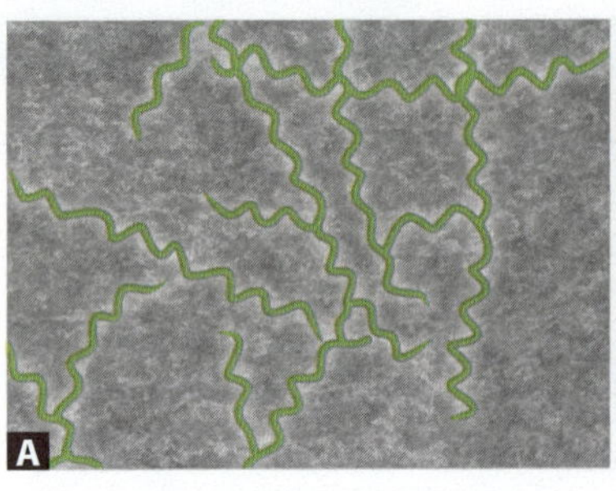

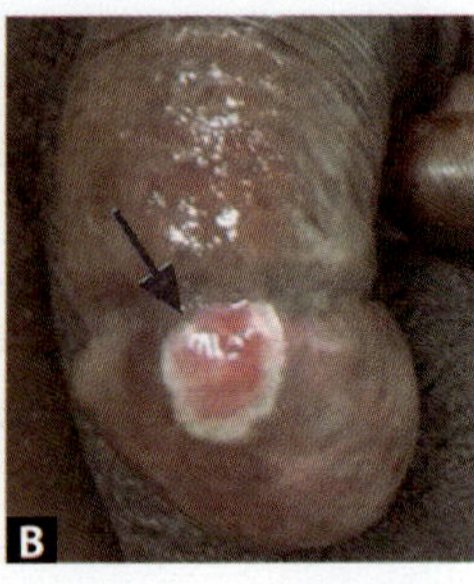

Figs. 4.6A and B: (A) Diagrammatic appearance of *Treponema pallidum* under Dark-field examination; (B) Primary chancre on glans penis (arrow).

- **Transplacental transmission**: It can also be transmitted by the mother suffering from active disease to the fetus (during pregnancy) or during delivery. It results in congenital syphilis.
- **Blood transfusion.**
- **Direct contact with the open lesion** is a rare mode of transmission.

Pathogenesis

Basic microscopic lesion: Irrespective of stage, the basic microscopic lesion of syphilis consists of:

- **Proliferative endarteritis:** It is a characteristic obstructive vascular lesion in which mononuclear infiltrates surround small vessels (arteries and arterioles) and is termed **periarteritis**. Much of the pathologic changes of syphilis can be due to the ischemia produced by these vascular lesions. The pathogenesis of endarteritis is unknown.
- **Mononuclear inflammatory infiltrate:** It consists predominantly of **plasma cells** (plasma cell-rich infiltrate) accompanied by **lymphocytes**.

Stages of Syphilis (Fig. 4.7)

Q. Write a short note on the stages of syphilis.

Treponema pallidum passes from the site of inoculation to regional lymph nodes, enters the systemic circulation, and disseminates throughout the body. Syphilis can be **(1) congenital or (2) acquired**. The course of acquired syphilis is divided into three stages: (i) primary syphilis, (ii) secondary syphilis, and (iii) tertiary syphilis. These **stages have distinct clinical and pathologic manifestations.**

Acquired Syphilis

Primary syphilis

Q. Write a short note on primary chancre.

Treponemes may spread throughout the body by blood and lymphatics even before the appearance of the primary chancre.

Primary chancre: It is the **classical lesion of primary syphilis**. Primary chancre develops about **3 weeks after contact** with an infected individual. It is **usually, painless** and often unnoticed.

MORPHOLOGY

Gross

Sites: Primary chancre occurs at sites of entry of *T. pallidum*. The primary chancre is located at the site of treponemal invasion.

- **Men:** It is on the **penis (Fig. 4.6B) or scrotum of 70% of men.**
- **Women:** It is on the **cervix, vulva,** and **vaginal wall of 50% of women.**

It may also be seen in the anus or mouth.

Hard chancre: It is a **single, firm, nontender (painless), slightly raised, red papule** (chancre) up to several centimeters in diameter. It erodes to create a **clean-based shallow ulcer.** Because of the induration surrounding the ulcer (creates a buttonlike mass), it is designated as a **hard chancre (Fig. 4.6B).**

Microscopy

Mononuclear infiltration: Primary chancre consists of a clean-based shallow ulcer with mononuclear infiltrate. This consists of **plasma cells,** with scattered macrophages and lymphocytes. These mononuclear cells are also seen surrounding the blood vessels (periarteritis).

Blood vessels with proliferative endarteritis (luetic vasculitis): It is characterized by endothelial cell proliferation which progresses to intimal fibrosis.

Demonstration of treponema: Plenty of treponemes can be demonstrated in the chancre by: (1) silver stains (e.g., Warthin-Starry stain) or (2) immunofluorescence techniques or (3) Dark-field examination.

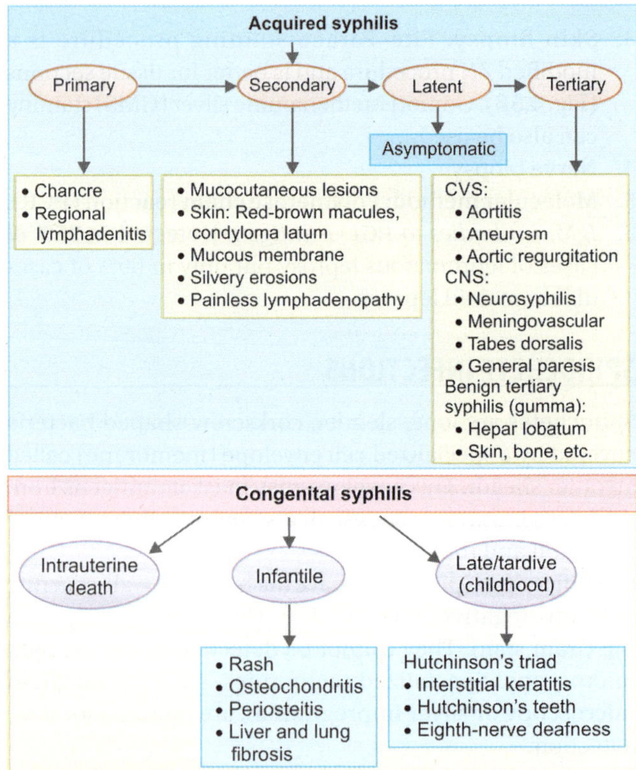

Fig. 4.7: Various manifestations of syphilis.
(CVS: cardiovascular system; CNS: central nervous system)

Regional lymphadenitis: It is due to nonspecific acute or chronic inflammation, plasma cell-rich infiltrates, or granulomas.

Fate: Primary chancre **heals in 3–6 weeks with/without therapy**.

Secondary Syphilis

Q. Write a short note on secondary syphilis.

This stage develops **2–10 weeks after the primary chancre** in approximately 75% of untreated patients. Its manifestations are due to systemic spread and proliferation of the spirochetes within the skin and mucocutaneous tissues.

MORPHOLOGY

Mucocutaneous Lesions

These are painless, superficial lesions that contain spirochetes and are infectious.

Skin lesions: These consist of the following:

- **Skin rashes:** They consist of **discrete red-brown macules** less than 5 mm in diameter, **but they may be maculopapular, follicular, scaly, pustular, or annular.** They are **more frequent on the palms of the hands** (*refer* **online Fig. 4.8A**), or **soles** of the feet.
- **Condylomata lata** (*refer* **online Fig. 4.8B**): These are **broad-based, elevated plaques** with numerous spirochetes. They are seen in moist areas of the skin, such as the **anogenital region (perineum, vulva, and scrotum), inner thighs, and axillae.**

Mucosal lesions: Usually occurs in the mucous membranes of the **oral cavity, pharynx, or genital region** (e.g., **vagina).** They appear as **silvery-gray superficial erosions.** These lesions contain numerous *T. pallidum* and are **highly infectious.**

Microscopy of lesions of secondary syphilis is similar to primary chancre, i.e., infiltration by plasma cells and endarteritis obliterans.

Painless Lymphadenopathy

Lymphadenopathy especially involves **epitrochlear nodes** and shows plenty of spirochetes.

Symptoms: Secondary syphilis may manifest with mild fever, malaise, and weight loss which may last for several weeks. Secondary syphilis lasts several weeks. The lesions subside even without treatment, and the patient enters the latent stage of the disease.

Asymptomatic neurosyphilis: It occurs in 8–40% of patients. Asymptomatic neurosyphilis with meningitis, visual changes, or hearing changes occurs in 1–2% of patients.

Tertiary Syphilis

Q. Write a short note on tertiary syphilis and its manifestations.

Asymptomatic latent phase: After the lesions of secondary syphilis have subsided patients enter an asymptomatic latent phase of the disease. The latent period may last for 5 years or more (even decades), but spirochetes continue to multiply. This stage is rare if the patient gets adequate treatment, but can occur in about one-third of untreated patients. Focal ischemic necrosis due to obliterative endarteritis is responsible for many of the processes associated with tertiary syphilis.

Manifestations: Three main manifestations of tertiary syphilis are: **(i) cardiovascular syphilis, (ii) neurosyphilis, and (iii) so-called benign tertiary syphilis.** These may develop alone or in combination.

Cardiovascular syphilis

PA 27.10 (NC): Describe the etiology, pathophysiology, pathology features, and complications of syphilis in the cardiovascular system.

Cardiovascular syphilis accounts for more than 80% of cases of tertiary syphilis. Probably immune response may be involved in its pathogenesis. It most **frequently involves the aorta** and is known as syphilitic aortitis.

MORPHOLOGY

Syphilitic aortitis: Accounts for more than 80% of cases of tertiary disease, and affects the **proximal aorta.**

Saccular aneurysm (*refer* pages 490-1) and aortic valve insufficiency: Occlusion of the vasa vasorum due to endarteritis leads to **necrosis and scarring of the aortic media** causing loss of elasticity, strength, and resilience. Gradual weakening and slow progressive **dilation of the aortic root and arch** causes **aortic valve insufficiency** and **aneurysms of the proximal aorta.** Syphilitic aneurysms are saccular and seen in the ascending aorta, which is an unusual site for the more common atherosclerotic aneurysms. On gross examination, the aortic intima appears rough and pitted (**tree-bark appearance**).

Myocardial ischemia: Narrowing of the coronary artery ostia (at the origin of the aorta) caused by subintimal scarring may lead to myocardial ischemia/infarction.

Neurosyphilis

It may be asymptomatic or symptomatic.

- **Asymptomatic neurosyphilis:** It accounts for about one-third of neurosyphilis cases. It is detected by **CSF examination**, which shows **pleocytosis (increased numbers of inflammatory cells), elevated protein levels,** or **decreased glucose.** Antibodies can also be detected in the CSF, which is the most specific test for neurosyphilis.
- **Symptomatic disease:** Takes one of several forms
  - **Chronic meningovascular disease:** Chronic meningitis involves the base of the brain, cerebral convexities, and spinal leptomeninges.
  - **Tabes dorsalis:** It is characterized by **demyelination of the posterior column, dorsal root, and dorsal root ganglia.**
  - **General paresis of insane:** Shows generalized brain parenchymal disease with **dementia**; hence called general paresis of insane.

Benign tertiary syphilis

It is characterized by the formation of nodular lesions called **gummas** in any organ or tissue. Gummas reflect the development of delayed hypersensitivity to the spirochete. Gummas are very rare and may be found in patients with acquired immune deficiency syndrome (AIDS).

MORPHOLOGY

Gumma

May be **single or multiple, white-gray, and rubbery.** They **vary in size** from microscopic lesions to large tumor-like masses.

Site: They occur in most organs but mainly involve:

- **Skin, subcutaneous tissue,** and the **mucous membranes of the upper airway and mouth.** They may produce nodular lesions or, rarely, destructive, ulcerative lesions.
- **Bone and joints:** It causes local pain, tenderness, swelling, and sometimes pathologic fractures.
- In the **liver,** scarring due to gummas may cause a distinctive hepatic lesion known as **hepar lobatum.**

Microscopy: The center of the gumma shows **coagulative necrosis,** surrounded by **plump, palisading macrophages, fibroblasts, and plenty of plasma cells.** Treponemes are scant in gummas.

Congenital Syphilis

Q. Write a short note on congenital syphilis.

Transplacental transmission: *T. pallidum* can cross the placenta and spread from the infected **mother to the fetus** (during pregnancy). Transmission occurs when the **mother is suffering from primary or secondary syphilis** (when the spirochetes are abundant). It can also be transmitted by a mother suffering from primary syphilis to a child during delivery. Because routine serologic testing for syphilis in done in all pregnancies, congenital syphilis is rare.

Manifestations: It can be divided into:

1. **Intrauterine death and perinatal death:** Congenital syphilis may result in intrauterine and perinatal death.
2. **Early (infantile) syphilis:** It manifests in the **first 2 years of life** and is often manifested by **nasal discharge** and congestion (**snuffles**). Other features are:
   - A **desquamating or bullous eruption/rash** can lead to epidermal sloughing of the skin, mainly in the hands, feet, around the mouth, and anus.
   - **Skeletal abnormalities.** These include:
     - **Syphilitic osteochondritis:** Inflammation of bone and cartilage is more distinctive in the nose. Destruction of the vomer causes the collapse of the nasal bridge. This produces characteristic **saddle nose deformity.**
     - **Syphilitic periostitis:** It involves the tibia and causes excessive new bone formation on the anterior surfaces and leads to **anterior bowing** or **saber shin.**
   - **Liver: Diffuse fibrosis** in the liver can develop and is called **hepar lobatum.**
   - **Lungs: Diffuse interstitial fibrosis** in the lungs can occur and the **lungs appear pale and airless (pneumonia alba).**
3. **Late (tardive) syphilis:** It **manifests 2 years after birth, and about 50% of untreated children with neonatal syphilis will develop late manifestations.** Its distinctive manifestations is **Hutchinson's triad.** It consists of (i) **interstitial keratitis.** (2) **Hutchinson's teeth** (they are like small screwdrivers or peg-shaped incisors, with notches in the enamel) and **eighth nerve deafness.**

Laboratory Diagnosis

Immunofluorescence of exudate from the chancre is important for the diagnosis of primary syphilis. Microscopy and polymerase chain reaction (PCR) are also useful.

Serological Tests

- **Nontreponemal antibody tests:** These tests measure antibodies to cardiolipin, a phospholipid present in both host tissues and *T. pallidum*. These antibodies are detected by the rapid plasma reagin and venereal disease research laboratory (VDRL) tests. False-positive VDRL test is found in certain acute infections, collagen vascular diseases (e.g., systemic lupus erythematosus), drug addiction, pregnancy, hypergammaglobulinemia of any cause, and lepromatous leprosy.
- **Antitreponemal antibody tests:** These measure antibodies, which react with *T. pallidum*. These include: (i) fluorescent treponemal antibody absorption test (FTA), and (ii) microhemagglutination assay for *T. pallidum* antibodies.

Jarisch–Herxheimer reaction: Treatment of syphilitic patients having a high bacterial load, by antibiotics can cause a massive release of endotoxins, and cytokine that may manifest with high fever, rigors, hypotension, and leukopenia. This **syndrome** is called the Jarisch–Herxheimer reaction, which **can develop not only in syphilis but also in other spirochetal diseases,** such as Lyme disease.

BACTERIAL DISEASES

PA 10.4 (NC): Define and describe the pathogenesis and pathology of common bacterial, viral, protozoal, and helminthic diseases.

Pyogenic Bacteria

They produce suppurative/purulent inflammation: Pyogenic inflammation is a type of inflammation characterized by increased vascular permeability and leukocytic infiltration, mainly of neutrophils. The neutrophils accumulate at the site of infection due to the release of chemoattractants from the "pyogenic" (pus-forming) bacteria. These bacteria are mostly extracellular gram-positive cocci and gram-negative rods.

MORPHOLOGY

Gross: The size of the lesion depends on the location of the lesion and the organism involved. The size of purulent lesions may range from tiny microabscesses to diffuse involvement of the involved organ or tissue.

Microscopy: It consists of pus, which is formed by masses of dying and dead neutrophils and liquefactive necrosis of the involved tissue.

Consequences: Depends on the site and causative organism. Examples include: Pneumococcal infection of the lung usually spares alveolar walls and causes lobar pneumonia that resolves completely; Staphylococci and *Klebsiella* infection of the lung destroys alveolar walls and form abscesses that heal with scar formation; bacterial pharyngitis resolves without sequelae, and untreated acute bacterial infection of a joint destroys the joint.

Bacteremia: It is an invasion of the bloodstream by bacteria and occurs when bacteria enter the blood. It occurs commonly as an integral part of some infections.

Pyemia: Septicemia is the presence of infective agents in the bloodstream. Pyemia is **septicemia due to pyogenic organisms**. Pyemia occurs when pathogenic organisms enter the bloodstream and form small aggregates (microemboli). They result in either pyemic abscesses or septic infarct in various organs.

Diphtheria

Diphtheria is caused by *Corynebacterium diphtheria*. *Corynebacterium diphtheria* is a slender gram-positive rod with clubbed ends.

Mode of spread: From person to person in respiratory droplets (respiratory diphtheria) or skin exudate (cutaneous diphtheria).

Incubation period: Commonly 3–4 days.

Types: Common types include:

1. **Respiratory diphtheria:** It causes pharyngeal infection. Inhaled *C. diphtheria* is carried in respiratory droplets that proliferate at the site of attachment on the mucosa. It produces exotoxin which causes necrosis of the epithelium and formation of a dense fibrinosuppurative exudate. The coagulation of this exudate on the ulcerated necrotic surface creates a tough, dirty gray to black, superficial membrane known as **pseudomembrane** (because it is not formed by viable tissue). When the membrane sloughs off, there is bleeding which may lead to asphyxia. With control of the infection, the pseudomembrane is either coughed-up or dissolved by enzymatic digestion. The toxin also damages the heart, nerves, and other organs.
2. **Cutaneous diphtheria:** It causes chronic ulcers with a dirty gray membrane without any systemic damage.

Immunization with diphtheria toxoid (formalin-fixed toxin): It stimulates the production of toxin-neutralizing antibodies which protect persons from the lethal effects of the toxin.

Gram-negative Bacterial Infections

Whooping Cough or Pertussis

Pertussis or whooping cough is a highly communicable acute bacterial disease of childhood, caused by the gram-negative coccobacillus ***Bordetella pertussis***. The wide use of the DPT (**D**iphtheria, **P**ertussis, and **T**etanus) vaccine has reduced the prevalence of whooping cough.

Incubation period: About 1–2 weeks.

Pathogenesis: *Bordetella pertussis* has a strong affinity for the bronchial epithelium and invades macrophages. *B. pertussis* proliferates and stimulates the bronchial epithelium to produce abundant tenacious mucus causing laryngotracheobronchitis. In severe cases, it causes bronchial mucosal erosion, hyperemia, and copious mucopurulent exudate. The toxin produced by the organism inhibits neutrophils and macrophages and paralyzes cilia. Within 7–10 days after exposure, the catarrhal stage of whooping cough begins and is the most infectious stage. Peripheral blood shows marked lymphocytosis (up to 90%) and enlargement of lymphoid follicles in the bronchial mucosa and peribronchial region.

Clinical features: It is characterized by **paroxysms of violent coughing** followed by a characteristic **loud inspiratory "whoop."** Other features include low-grade fever, rhinorrhea, conjunctivitis, and excess tear production. The condition is self-limiting but may cause death due to asphyxia in infants.

Bacillary dysentery (*refer* pages 616-7).

VIRAL DISEASES

Poliovirus Infection

Poliovirus causes an acute systemic viral infection. It can produce a wide range of clinical manifestations ranging from mild, self-limited infections to paralysis of limb muscles and respiratory muscles. Poliovirus is a spherical, unencapsulated **RNA virus** belonging to the enterovirus genus.

Mode of infection: Poliovirus infects only humans and is transmitted by the **fecal-oral route**.

Incubation period: About 10 days.

The vaccines [Salk formalin-fixed (killed) vaccine and the Sabin oral, attenuated (live) vaccine] have eradicated polio in India.

Pathogenesis: The polio virus is ingested and replicates in the mucosa of the pharynx, tonsils, and gut (Peyer patches in the ileum). From the mucosa, it spreads through lymphatics to lymph nodes and eventually the blood. Most poliovirus infections are asymptomatic. In nonimmunized patients, poliovirus infection causes a subclinical or mild gastroenteritis. In about 1% of infected patients, poliovirus secondarily invades the CNS and replicates in motor neurons of the spinal cord (spinal poliomyelitis) or brain stem (bulbar poliomyelitis).

MORPHOLOGY

Acute cases show mononuclear cell perivascular cuffs in the **anterior horn motor neurons of the spinal cord.**

Clinical Features

- **Spinal cord involvement:** When polio affects the motor neurons of the spinal cord, it destroys motor neurons and leads to paralysis.
- **CNS infection:** It causes meningeal irritation and shows features of aseptic meningitis.

Herpes Virus Infections

Herpes viruses are large encapsulated viruses with double-stranded DNA genomes. Herpes viruses cause acute infection followed by latent infection. During latent infection, the viruses persist in a noninfectious form with periodic reactivation and shedding of infectious viruses. Reactivation of the virus causes dissemination of the infection and tissue injury. There are eight types of human herpes viruses, belonging to three subgroups: the α-group (e.g., HSV-1, HSV-2); β-group (e.g., CMV, human herpesvirus-6), and the γ-group (EBV and KSHV/HHV-8).

Herpes Simplex Viruses

There are two types of herpes simplex viruses (HSV) namely—**HSV-1 and HSV-2.** They **differ serologically but are closely related genetically and cause a similar set of primary and recurrent infections.**

1. **Mucocutaneous lesions:**
   - HSV-1 and HSV-2 cause self-limited cold sores and gingivostomatitis.
   - **Blisters or cold sores:** Both viruses replicate at the site of entry of the virus (namely—the skin and the mucous membranes usually the oropharynx or genitals). They cause vesicular lesions of the epidermis. Fever **blisters or cold sores** are observed in the facial skin around mucosal orifices (lips and nose).
   - **Gingivostomatitis:** It is usually observed in children and is caused by HSV-1. The viruses spread to sensory neurons and are transported along axons to the neuronal cell bodies, where they establish latent infection.
   - **Genital herpes** is more often caused by HSV-2 than by HSV-1.
   - In immunocompetent individuals, primary HSV infection resolves, although the virus remains latent in nerve cells. During the latency period, the viral DNA remains within the nucleus of the neuron. Reactivation of HSV-1 and HSV-2 may occur with or without symptoms, and this reactivation causes the spread of the virus from the neurons to the skin or mucous membranes.
2. **Ophthalmic lesions:** Two forms of **corneal lesions may be produced: (1) herpes epithelial keratitis and (2) herpes stromal keratitis** (which can lead to corneal blindness).
3. **Nervous system:** HSV-1 can also produce encephalitis.

MORPHOLOGY

HSV-infected cells contain large, pink to purple **intranuclear inclusions** (Cowdry type A). HSV also produces inclusion-bearing multinucleated syncytia.

Rabies

Rabies is a viral disease causing **severe encephalitis** and transmitted to humans by the **bite of a rabid animal (usually a dog)**. Rabies virus is sensitive to and killed by ethanol, iodine preparations, and soap detergents.

MORPHOLOGY

Gross: External examination of the brain shows edema and vascular congestion.

Microscopy: It shows widespread neuronal degeneration and an inflammatory reaction which is most severe in the brainstem.

Negri bodies: These are the **pathognomonic** microscopic features. They are cytoplasmic, round to oval, eosinophilic inclusions that can be found in pyramidal neurons of the hippocampus and Purkinje cells of the cerebellum. Rabies virus can be identified within the Negri bodies by ultrastructural and immunohistochemical methods.

Clinical features: Rabies virus enters the CNS by ascending along the peripheral nerves from the wound site (bite of a rabid animal).

The incubation period usually ranges from **1 to 3 months** and it depends on the distance between the wound and the brain.

Symptoms

- **Nonspecific symptoms:** Rabies presents with nonspecific symptoms such as malaise, headache, and fever. **Local paresthesia around the wound** along with the above symptoms is diagnostic.
- **CNS excitability:** As the infection progresses, the patient develops severe CNS excitability. The slightest touch is painful and causes violent motor responses or even convulsions. Signs of meningeal irritation and flaccid paralysis may develop as the disease progresses.

- **Hydrophobia:** Contracture of the pharyngeal muscles on swallowing produces foaming at the mouth. This causes aversion/fear to swallow even water (hydrophobia).
- Produces coma and death from respiratory failure.

Measles (Rubeola)

Q. Write a short note on measles.

Measles is an **acute viral infection** caused by the measles (rubeola) virus. It **affects multiple organs** and causes a wide range of diseases ranging from mild, self-limited infections to severe systemic manifestations. It can produce severe disease in patients with defects in cellular immunity (e.g., with HIV or hematologic malignancy). Measles can be prevented by vaccines. Epidemics of measles occur among unvaccinated individuals. Diagnosis is by clinical features, by serology, or by detection of viral antigens in nasal exudates or urinary sediments.

Mode of transmission: Measles virus is transmitted by respiratory droplets.

Incubation period: 9–11 days.

Pathogenesis: The measles virus is a single-stranded RNA virus of the paramyxovirus family. Measles can replicate in many cell types such as epithelial cells and leukocytes. Initially, the virus multiplies within the respiratory tract and then spreads to local lymphoid tissues. Replication of the virus in lymphoid tissue is followed by viremia and systemic dissemination to many tissues. The tissues involved are conjunctiva, skin, respiratory tract, urinary tract, small blood vessels, lymphatic system, and CNS. Most children develop T-cell–mediated immunity to the virus which controls the viral infection and produces the measles rash. Hence, the measles rash is less common in patients with deficiencies in cell-mediated immunity. In malnourished, it may cause croup, pneumonia, diarrhea and protein-losing enteropathy, keratitis (producing scarring and blindness), encephalitis, and hemorrhagic rashes ("black measles"). Measles can cause transient immunosuppression, resulting in secondary bacterial and viral infections. Antibody-mediated immunity to measles virus protects against reinfection.

MORPHOLOGY

Measles rash: It is blotchy, reddish-brown and observed on the face, trunk, and proximal extremities. It is produced by dilated skin vessels, edema, and a mononuclear perivascular infiltrate.

Koplik spots: These are pathognomonic of measles and consist of ulcerated mucosal lesions in the oral cavity near the opening of the Stensen (parotid) ducts. They appear as small, irregular, bluish-white dots measuring 1 mm in diameter surrounded by erythema.

Lymphoid organs—Warthin–Finkeldey giant cells: Lymphoid organs show marked follicular hyperplasia, enlarged germinal centers, and randomly distributed multinucleate giant cells, called **Warthin–Finkeldey giant cells** (pathognomonic of measles). These giant cells have eosinophilic nuclear and cytoplasmic inclusion bodies. These are also found in the lungs and sputum.

RICKETTSIAL INFECTIONS

Rickettsiales are vector-borne obligate intracellular bacteria. These organisms have the structure of gram-negative, rod-shaped bacteria. However, they stain poorly with Gram stain.

Diseases produced: They cause epidemic and scrub typhus, spotted fevers (*Rickettsia rickettsia*), ehrlichiosis, and anaplasmosis.

- **Epidemic typhus:** Caused by *Rickettsia prowazekii.*
  - **Mode of transmission.** Transmitted from person to person by body lice.
  - **Clinical features:** Includes macular rash that progresses to a petechial, maculopapular rash on the entire body except the face, palms, and soles.
- **Scrub typhus:** Caused by *Orientia tsutsugamushi.*
  - **Mode of transmission.** By chiggers.
  - **Clinical features:** Include fever, headache, myalgia and cough, and associated lymphadenopathy from the chigger bite.
- **Rocky Mountain spotted fever:** Caused by *Rickettsia rickettsia.*
  - **Mode of transmission:** By dog ticks.
  - **Clinical features:** Begins as a nonspecific severe illness with fever, myalgias, and gastrointestinal distress. As the disease progresses widespread macular then petechial rash involving the palms and soles develop.

Pathogenesis: The manifestations of rickettsial infections are mainly due to infection of endothelial cells (especially those in the lungs and brain) which results in endothelial dysfunction and injury. Widespread endothelial dysfunction/injury can cause shock, peripheral and pulmonary edema, and disseminated intravascular coagulation, renal failure, and CNS manifestations (e.g., coma).

MORPHOLOGY

Characterized by small vessel lesions and focal areas of hemorrhage and inflammation in many organs and tissues.

Diagnosis: Rickettsial diseases are usually diagnosed clinically. Diagnosis is confirmed by serology or immunostaining of the organisms.

CHLAMYDIAL INFECTIONS

Chlamydia Trachomatis

It is a small gram negative bacterium and exists in two forms during its unique life cycle.

- **Elementary body:** It is an infectious, metabolically inactive form and has a spore-like structure. Host cells take up the elementary body by endocytosis and form endosomes. The bacteria prevent the fusion of the endosome and lysosome.
- **Reticulate body:** Inside the endosome of the host cell, the elementary body differentiates into a metabolically

active form, called the reticulate body. The reticulate body replicates and forms new infectious elementary bodies.

Diseases produced: *C. trachomatis* infection causes—(1) urogenital infections, (2) inclusion conjunctivitis (3) lymphogranuloma venereum, (4) ocular infection of children, trachoma.

Genital infection by *C. trachomatis* is the most common sexually transmitted bacterial infection in women.

MORPHOLOGY

C. trachomatis **urethritis** appears identical to gonorrhea. It produces mucopurulent discharge containing mainly neutrophils. **Lymphogranuloma venereum** contains a mixed granulomatous and neutrophilic inflammatory response. Chlamydial inclusions are seen in the cytoplasm of epithelial cells or inflammatory cells. Regional lymphadenopathy is common and shows granulomatous inflammatory reaction associated with irregularly shaped foci of necrosis containing neutrophils (**stellate abscesses**). With time, extensive fibrosis may cause local lymphatic obstruction, lymphedema, and strictures.

FUNGAL INFECTIONS AND OPPORTUNISTIC INFECTIONS

Fungi grow as multicellular filaments (mold) or individual cells alone or in chains (yeast). They have cell walls which gives them a shape.

- **Yeasts** are round to oval and reproduce by budding. Some yeasts (e.g., *Candida albicans*) produce buds that fail to detach and become elongated, producing a chain of elongated yeast cells called **pseudohyphae**.
- **Molds** are thread-like filaments (hyphae) that grow and divide at their tips. They can produce round cells known as **conidia**, which can easily become airborne, disseminating the fungus.
- Many fungi are dimorphic, i.e., they exist as yeast or molds, depending on environmental conditions (yeast form at human body temperature, and a mold form at room temperature).

Types of Fungal Infections

Fungal infections are also known as *mycoses.* Human fungal infections are divided into four major types:

1. **Superficial and cutaneous mycoses:** Common and limited to the skin, hair, and nails.
2. **Subcutaneous mycoses:** Involve the skin, subcutaneous tissues, and lymphatics.
3. **Endemic mycoses:** Caused by dimorphic fungi and can produce serious systemic illness in healthy individuals.
4. **Opportunistic mycoses:** They can cause life-threatening systemic diseases in immunosuppressed individuals.

Diagnosis

1. Histological examination.
2. **Culture:** Definitive identification of some requires culture.

Yeast

Q. Write a short note on candidiasis.

Candidiasis

Live as commensals: *Candida* species reside normally in the skin, mouth, gastrointestinal tract, and vagina. They usually live as commensals and seldom produce disease in healthy individuals.

Infection: Most *Candida* infections occur when the normal commensal flora breaches the skin or mucosal barriers. There are different strains of *Candida* of which *C. albican* is the most frequent cause of human fungal infections. These infections may be either limited to the skin or mucous membranes or may disseminate widely.

Pathogenesis: A single strain of *Candida* can live as commensal or may become pathogenic. *Candida* can shift between different phenotypes and phenotypic switching is the mechanism by which *Candida* adapts to changes in the host environment (e.g., produced by antibiotic therapy, the immune response, or altered host physiology).

- *Candida* produce many **adhesins** (e.g., integrin-like protein) which help them to adhere to host cells and are an important determinant of virulence.
- *Candida* produce many **enzymes** that contribute to invasiveness (e.g., aspartyl proteinases).

MORPHOLOGY

C. albicans may appear as yeast, pseudohyphae, and, less commonly, true hyphae, defined by the presence of septae. The pseudohyphae form consists of a chain of budding yeast cells joined end to end at constrictions. They represent an important diagnostic clue.

Superficial Candidiasis

Diabetic and burn patients are susceptible to superficial candidiasis.

Oral candidiasis: Most commonly candidiasis takes the form of a superficial infection on mucosal surfaces of the **oral cavity (thrush)**. The florid proliferation of the fungi creates gray-white, dirty-looking pseudomembranes. This form of candidiasis is found in newborns, debilitated people, children receiving oral steroids for asthma, following a course of broad-spectrum antibiotics (destroying competing normal bacterial flora), and HIV-positive patients.

Candida esophagitis is seen in AIDS patients and those with hematolymphoid malignancies.

Candida vaginitis is common and is seen in women who are diabetic, pregnant, or on oral contraceptive pills or on antibacterial agents (which alter the vaginal flora).

Cutaneous candidiasis: It may present as an infection of the nail (onychomycosis), nail folds (paronychia), hair follicles (folliculitis), moist, intertriginous skin, such as armpits or webs of the fingers and toes (intertrigo), and penile skin (balanitis). **In healthy** individuals, *Candida* can cause **vaginitis** and diaper rash (cutaneous candidal infection in the perineum of infants, the region in contact with wet diapers).

Invasive/Disseminated Candidiasis

It is caused by the dissemination of *Candida* into the bloodstream thereby spreading into various tissues or organs. It can develop especially in patients with indwelling intravenous lines or catheters or undergoing peritoneal dialysis. Severe disseminated candidiasis develops mostly in patients with neutropenia (e.g., due to acute leukemia, after chemotherapy, or hematopoietic stem cell transplantation). It may lead to shock and disseminated intravascular coagulation.

Cryptococcosis

Two species of *Cryptococcus* namely—*C. neoformans* and *C. gattii* can cause disease in humans. Both of them grow as encapsulated yeasts.

Species of *Cryptococcus*

1. ***Cryptococcus neoformans***

Source: *Cryptococcus neoformans* is present in the soil and bird (particularly pigeon) droppings. The mode of infection in humans is through inhalation.

Susceptibility: Though *C. neoformans* can cause meningoencephalitis in healthy individuals, more frequently it causes opportunistic infection in a patient with AIDS, leukemia, lymphoma, systemic lupus erythematosus, or sarcoidosis, and in immunosuppressed transplant recipients. Many of these patients receive high-dose corticosteroids, which is a major risk factor for *C. neoformans* infection.

2. ***Cryptococcus gattii***

Source: *C. gattii* is found in soil, and is acquired by inhalation. It causes disease in immunologically normal individuals and usually presents as large lesions producing mass effects or may mimic the radiologic appearance of a neoplasm.

Pathogenesis: Virulence factors of *Cryptococcus* that help it in evasion of host defenses are:

- **Polysaccharide capsule** of cryptococci prevents its phagocytosis by alveolar macrophages, and also leukocyte migration, and recruitment of inflammatory cells.
- **Melanin production:** Laccase in the yeast catalyzes melanin formation which (1) has antioxidant properties, (2) reduces phagocytosis, (3) counteracts the effects of antifungal agents, (4) binds iron, (5) and provides cell wall integrity.
- **Enzymes:** Such as serine proteinase may help in tissue invasion; mannitol dehydrogenase (produces mannitol) causes osmotic edema and inhibits the killing of the yeast by neutrophils and reactive oxygen species.

MORPHOLOGY

Cryptococcus has yeast form and has no pseudohyphal or hyphal forms. The cryptococcal yeast measures 5–10 µm and has a highly characteristic thick gelatinous capsule containing a polysaccharide.

Special stains: In tissues, the polysaccharide stains intensely red with periodic acid-Schiff and mucicarmine and is detected with antibody-coated beads in an agglutination assay. India ink preparations produce a negative image, and the thick capsule has a clear halo within a dark background.

Sites Involved

- **The lung is the primary site** of infection and it is **usually mild and asymptomatic**
- **Central nervous system (CNS): The major lesions produced by *Cryptococcus* are in the CNS, mainly involving the meninges, cortical gray matter, and basal nuclei.**

Host response to cryptococci is varied and depends on the immunity of the host.

- In immunosuppressed patients, there may not be any inflammatory reaction and gelatinous masses of fungi can grow in the meninges or expand the perivascular Virchow–Robin spaces within the gray matter, producing the soap-bubble lesions.
- In severely immunosuppressed patients, *C. neoformans* may widely disseminate to the skin, liver, spleen, adrenals, and bones.
- In nonimmunosuppressed individuals or those with the protracted disease, the fungi produce a chronic granulomatous reaction.

Molds

Aspergillosis

***Aspergillus* is a ubiquitous mold:** *Aspergillus fumigatus* is the most common pathogenic species of the fungus.

- It causes allergies (allergic bronchopulmonary aspergillosis) in healthy individuals.
- It produces serious sinusitis, pneumonia, and invasive disease in immunocompromised individuals.

Predisposing factors: These include conditions causing neutropenia and the use of corticosteroids.

Mode of transmission: *Aspergillus* species are transmitted as airborne conidia.

Pathogenesis: The lung is the major portal of entry. The small-sized (about 2–3 µm) spores of *A. fumigatus* reach the alveoli. Alveolar macrophages recognize conidia through TLR2 and the lectin dectin-1 receptors. Both receptors activate phagocytes to ingest and kill the conidia. In immunosuppressed states, conidia can produce hyphae and these hyphae invade tissues. Invasive aspergillosis is highly associated with neutropenia and impaired neutrophil defenses.

Virulence factors: *Aspergillus* produces many virulence factors. These include adhesins, antioxidants (e.g., melanin pigment, mannitol, catalases, and superoxide dismutases), **enzymes** (phospholipases, proteases), **and toxins.**

Lesions: The aflatoxin produced by *Aspergillus* species growing on the surface of improperly stored peanuts is a carcinogen and may cause **liver cancer**. Sensitization to *Aspergillus* spores can cause **allergic alveolitis. Allergic bronchopulmonary aspergillosis**, associated with hypersensitivity due to superficial colonization of the bronchial mucosa, may develop in patients with asthma.

MORPHOLOGY

Colonizing Aspergillosis (Aspergilloma)

It refers to the growth of the fungus within the cavities of the lung with minimal or no invasion of the tissues (the nose also is usually colonized). Lung cavities are usually the result of prior tuberculosis, bronchiectasis, old infarcts, or abscesses. Proliferating masses of hyphae form brownish "fungus balls" seen lying free within these lung cavities. Patients with aspergillomas usually present with recurrent hemoptysis.

Invasive Aspergillosis

It is an opportunistic infection that develops in immunosuppressed patients. The primary lesions are usually in the lung and appear as necrotizing pneumonia. They are sharply delineated, rounded, gray foci having hemorrhagic borders; they are called target lesions.

Aspergillus tends to invade blood vessels and may spread to involve the heart valves and brain.

Aspergillus **forms fruiting bodies (usually in lung cavities) and septate filaments, 5–10** μm **thick, branching at acute angles (40°).**

Mucormycosis (Zygomycosis)

Mucoromycotina is widely found in nature and does not harm immunocompetent individuals. But they can infect immunosuppressed individuals causing mucormycosis.

Mucormycosis (formerly zygomycosis) is an opportunistic fungal infection caused by bread mold fungi. These mold fungi include *Mucor, Rhizopus, Lichtheimia* (formerly *Absidia),* and *Cunninghamella.*

Predisposing factors: These include conditions causing neutropenia, use of corticosteroids, diabetes mellitus, iron overload, and breakdown of the skin barrier (e.g., in burns, surgical wounds, or trauma).

Pathogenesis

Mode of transmission: Mucormycotina is transmitted by airborne asexual spores. However, infection can occur through skin or ingestion.

Lesions: Inhaled spores usually produce infection in the nasal sinuses and the lungs.

MORPHOLOGY

Mucormycetes form nonseptate hyphae of variable width (ranging from 6 to 50 μm). They exhibit frequent right-angle branching, distinct from *Aspergillus* hyphae.

Sites involved: The three main sites of invasion are: (i) the nasal sinuses, (ii) the lungs, and (iii) the gastrointestinal tract, depending on the mode of transmission (i.e., inhalation or ingestion). In diabetic patients, the fungus may spread from the nasal sinuses to the orbit and brain, giving rise to **rhinocerebral mucormycosis.**

Lung involvement with mucoromycotina may be secondary to rhinocerebral disease, or it may be primary in patients with severe immunodeficiency.

Dimorphic Fungi

The important dimorphic fungi include *Blastomyces, Histoplasma*, and coccidioidomyces.

They grow as yeast in human tissue but as a hyaline mold when cultured in a laboratory at room temperature.

MYCETOMA

Q. Write a short note on Madura foot/mycetoma foot and its gross features.

Definition: Mycetoma is defined as a **chronic suppurative infection involving a limb, shoulder, or other tissues** and is **characterized by draining/discharging sinuses.** The discharging grains (material) consist of colonies of fungi or bacteria.

Types: Mycetomas can be divided into two main types depending on the causative agent namely—(i) **Eumycetoma** (fungal disease and comprises about 40% of cases) and (ii) **Actinomycetoma** (higher bacteria and comprises about 60% of cases).

Eumycetoma

- **Etiology:** It is a **chronic granulomatous fungal disease** caused by true fungi, *Madurella mycetomatis* or *Madurella grisea.*
- **Mode of infection:** The organisms are **inoculated directly from soil** into bare feet during agricultural work, from carrying of contaminated sacks on the shoulders, and into the hands from infected vegetation.

MORPHOLOGY

It involves the **skin and subcutaneous tissue.** After several months of infection, the affected site, most commonly the foot, manifests as an open area or break in the skin. The **affected part is swollen** and when the foot is affected, it is termed mycetoma pedis (mycetoma of the foot) or 'Madura foot' **(Fig. 4.9).** This was initially named **Madura foot**, after its discovery in the region called Madura in India. The infection extends deeply into the subcutaneous tissues, along the fascia, and eventually invades the bones. They **drain serosanguinous fluid containing granules through sinus tracts.** The size, color, and degree of hardness of granules depend on the etiologic species and are characteristic of mycetoma. The surrounding tissue shows a granulomatous reaction. The fungi stain positively with Gomori's methenamine silver (GMS) stain.

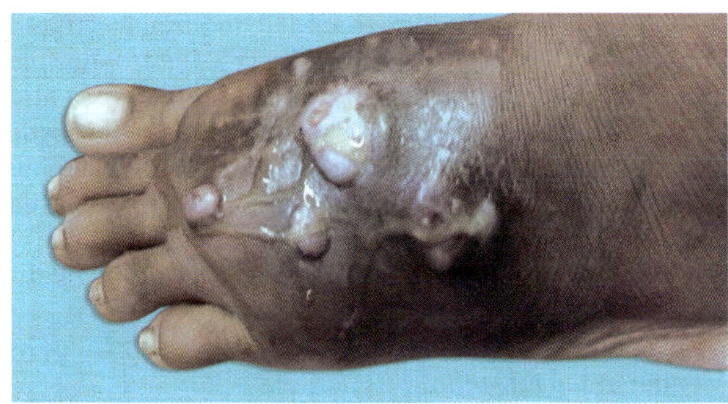

Fig. 4.9: Mycetoma (Madura foot) showing numerous sinuses discharging serosanguinous fluid.

Actinomycosis

Q. Write a short note on actinomycosis.

Actinomycosis is a chronic suppurative disease **caused by the anaerobic bacteria**, *Actinomycetes israelii*. It is **not a fungus.** The organisms are commensals in the oral cavity, gastrointestinal (GI) tract and vagina.

Mode of infection: Infection is always **endogenous in origin and not due to personal contact.** Break in mucocutaneous continuity, and diminished immunity due to some underlying disease favor the organism to invade, proliferate, and disseminate.

MORPHOLOGY

Depending on the anatomic location of lesions, actinomycosis is divided into four types:

1. **Cervicofacial actinomycosis:**
   - It is the most common form (60%) and has the best prognosis.
   - Infections gained through tonsils, carries teeth, periodontal diseases, or trauma following extraction of the tooth.
   - In the beginning, a firm swelling develops in the lower jaw (i.e., lumpy jaw). Later, the mass breaks down and forms abscesses and sinuses. Typically, the **sinus discharges yellow sulfur granules.** The infection may spread into the adjacent soft tissues and may destroy the bone.
2. **Thoracic actinomycosis:**
   - The infection of the lung is a result of aspiration of the organism from the oral cavity or extension of infection from abdominal or hepatic lesions.
   - Initially, lung lesions resemble pneumonia but as the disease progresses it spreads to the whole lung, pleura, ribs, and vertebrae.
3. **Abdominal actinomycosis:**
   - The common sites are the appendix, cecum, and liver.
   - The infection occurs as a result of swallowing the organism from the oral cavity or as an extension from the thoracic cavity.
4. **Pelvic actinomycosis:** It develops as a complication of intrauterine contraceptive devices (IUCDs).

Microscopy (Figs. 4.10A and B)

The following features are seen irrespective of the location of actinomycosis:

- **Granulomatous reaction with central suppuration:** There is a formation of abscesses in the center of lesions and the periphery of the lesions shows chronic inflammatory cells, giant cells, and fibroblasts.
- The **central abscess** contains a bacterial colony (sulfur granule) characterized by radiating filaments (called ray fungus) surrounded by hyaline, eosinophilic, club-like ends that represent immunoglobulins.
  - **Special stains for bacteria:** The organisms are gram-positive filaments and nonacid-fast (except Nocardia). They stain negatively with Gomori's methenamine silver (GMS) stain.

PARASITIC DISEASES

Protozoa

Protozoa are unicellular eukaryotic organisms. The protozoa are transmitted by insects or by the fecal-oral route.

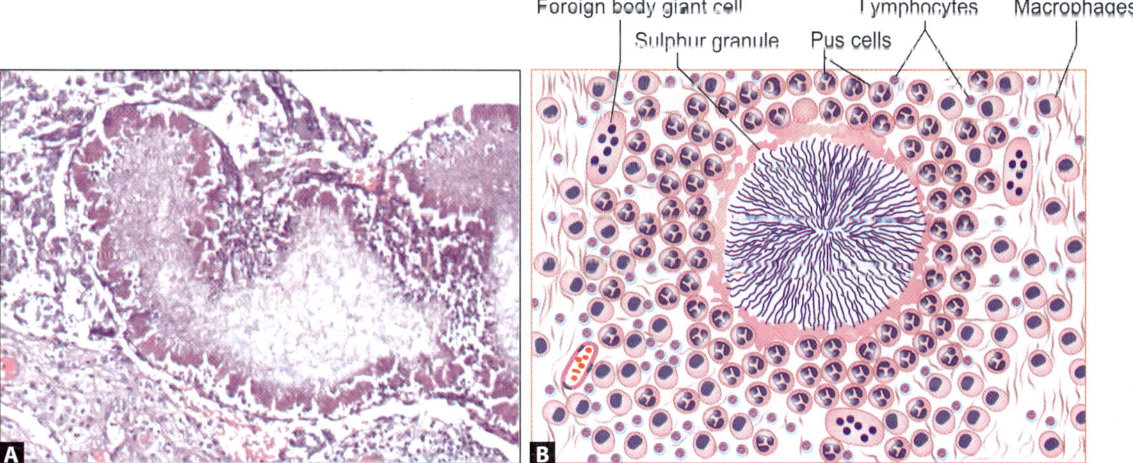

Figs. 4.10A and B: Microscopy of actinomycosis showing central bacterial colony surrounded inflammatory cells. (A) Hematoxylin and eosin; (B) Diagrammatic.

MALARIA

PA 10.1 (CC): Define and describe the pathogenesis and pathology of malaria.

- Malaria, caused by the intracellular parasite *Plasmodium*.
- *Plasmodium falciparum* (causes severe cerebral malaria) and the four other malaria parasites that infect humans (*P. vivax, P. ovale, P. knowlesi,* and *P. malariae*) are all transmitted by female anopheles mosquitoes.
- **Incubation period:** It varies with the type of species:
  - *P. vivax*—14 days (ranges 8–17 days)
  - *P. falciparum*—12 days (ranges 9–14 days)
  - *P. malariae*—28 days (ranges 18–40 days)
  - *P. ovale*—17 days (ranges 16–18 days).

Life Cycle and Pathogenesis (Fig. 4.11)

The life cycles of the *Plasmodium* species are similar.

- ***P. vivax, P. ovale, P. knowlesi, and P. malariae:*** They produce **low levels of parasitemia** and mild anemia.
- ***P. falciparum* infection:** It **produces high levels of parasitemia** and may lead to **severe anemia, cerebral symptoms, renal failure, pulmonary edema, and death.**

The life cycle of *Plasmodium* species is simple because it involves only humans and mosquitoes. However, the development of the parasite is complex, because it passes through several morphologically distinct forms. Malarial parasites pass their life cycle in two different hosts namely—(1) human (intermediate host) and (2) female anopheles mosquito (definitive host). A notable feature of the life cycle is the alternation of sexual and asexual phases in the two hosts. The asexual phase, called schizogony, occurs in the human. In the mosquito, first a sexual phase (gamogony) occurs; followed by another asexual reproductive phase (sporogony).

Human Cycle

It starts with the introduction of the infectious stage of *Plasmodium*, the *sporozoite* by the bite of the infected female anopheles mosquito. The mouthparts of male anopheles mosquitoes cannot penetrate human skin; hence, they feed solely on plant juices. The sporozoite is slender, elongated, and measures about 10–55 mm in length and about 1 mm in diameter. The *sporozoite* is found in the salivary glands of mosquitoes. During a mosquito bite, the mosquito takes a blood meal and sporozoites are released into the human's blood (1 in **Fig. 4.11**). The different stages of the human cycle are:

Exoerythrocytic Stage (Pre-erythrocytic Schizogony)

This stage occurs in the liver. Within minutes of entry of sporozoites (infectious stage) into the human blood, they attach to and invade liver cells (2 in **Fig. 4.11**). Within liver cells, malaria parasites multiply, and the spindle-shaped sporozoites become rounded and transform into trophozoites (feeding stage of the parasite). This trophozoite undergoes several nuclear divisions **(schizogony)** and transforms into pre-erythrocytic schizont. **Pre-erythrocytic schizont** contains several merozoites (3 in **Fig. 4.11**). About 30,000 *merozoites* (asexual, haploid forms) are released when each infected liver cell ruptures (4 in **Fig. 4.11**).

- During *P. falciparum* infection, rupture of liver cells usually occurs within 8-12 weeks.
- In contrast, *P. vivax* and *P. ovale* release weeks to months after initial infection.

The infection of the liver and development of merozoites is referred to as the exoerythrocytic stage. This stage is asymptomatic. Only a few liver cells/hepatocytes are infected by *Plasmodium*. Hence, liver damage does not occur in malaria. Some sporozoites of *P. vivax* and *P. ovale* do not develop further and may remain in the liver as hypnozoites. However, they can cause a relapse of malaria after many years.

Erythrocytic Stage (Fig. 4.11)

Once released from the liver, *Plasmodium* merozoites bind to the surface of red cells (5 in **Fig. 4.11**) and invade red blood cells (RBC) by penetration of the membrane. Within the red cells (erythrocytic stage) the parasites grow and hydrolyze hemoglobin through its enzymes.

Asexual forms (6 in **Fig. 4.11**): In the red blood cells, the parasite passes through the stages of asexual forms namely—trophozoite, schizont, and merozoite. These asexual forms of parasites can be demonstrated in the thick blood smears.

- *Trophozoite* is the first stage of the parasite in the red cell and is characterized by the presence of a single chromatin mass. First immature trophozoites (ring forms) are formed followed by mature trophozoites.
  - **Ring form:** Early trophozoite form is called ring form **(Fig. 4.11)**. It appears as a signet ring containing a central vacuole and peripheral thin rim of cytoplasm and a nucleus. Ring forms are the first asexual form that can be demonstrated in the peripheral blood. Ring form occupies one-third of RBC except in *P. falciparum*, where it occupies one-sixth of RBC. *Plasmodium* feeds on hemoglobin. The undigested products of hemoglobin metabolism such as hematin, excess protein, and iron porphyrin combine to form **malarial pigment (hemozoin pigment)**. The appearance of malarial pigment varies. Mostly it is brown-black and numerous (except in *P. vivax* it is yellowish-brown and in *P. falciparum*, it is few in number).
  - **Late trophozoite:** Ring form enlarges and appears more irregular due to amoeboid movement and transforms into late trophozoite or amoeboid form.
- *Schizont:* It is the next stage. Late trophozoites become compact, vacuoles disappear, pigments scatter

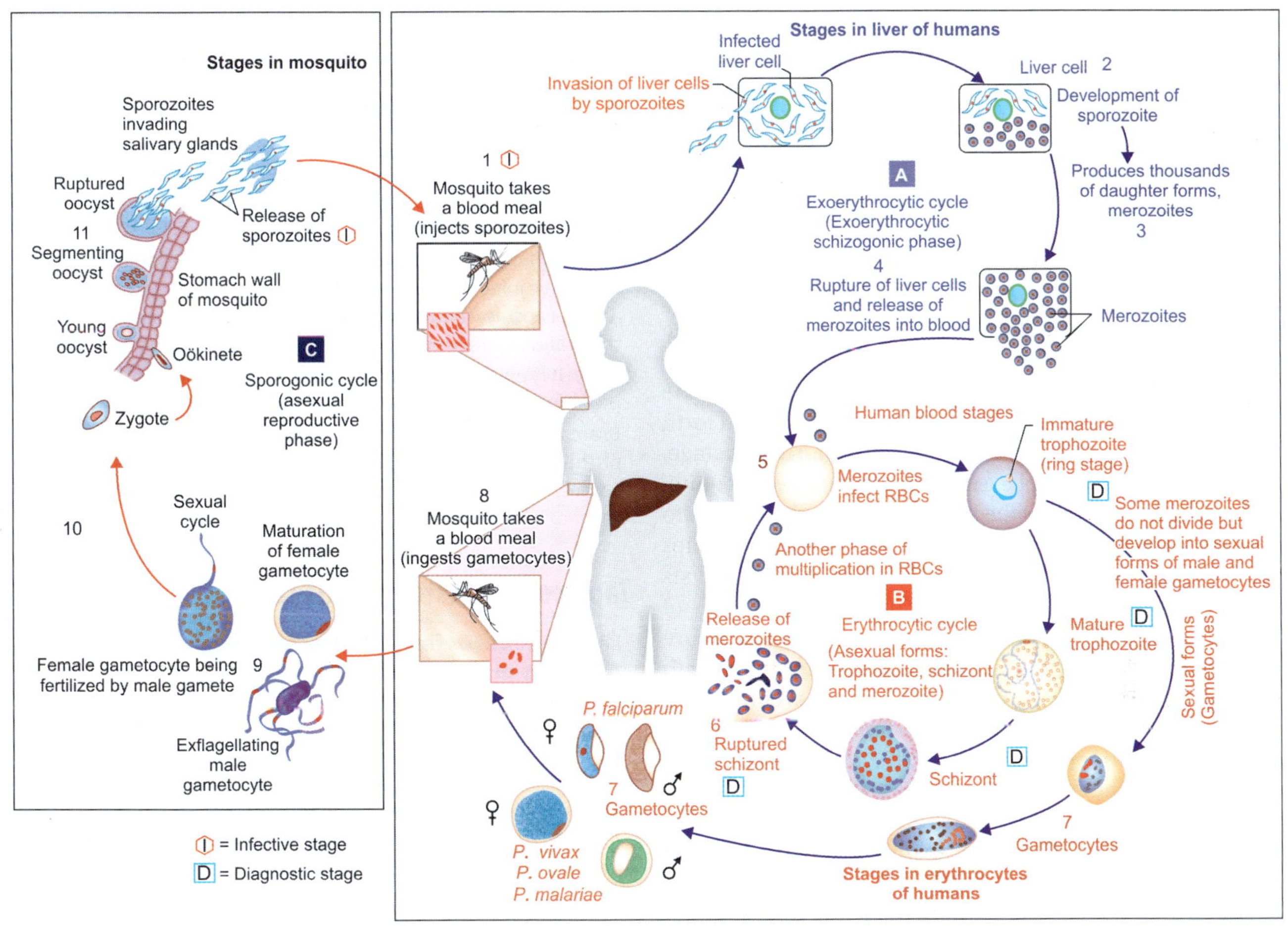

Fig. 4.11: Life cycle of malarial parasites (*refer* text for description).

throughout the cytoplasm, and the nucleus becomes larger and lies at the periphery. This form is called **schizont**. It shows multiple chromatin masses, each of which develops into a merozoite.

- *Merozoites*: Schizont undergoes multiple nuclear divisions (schizogony or merogony) and produces 6–30 daughter merozoites arranged in the form of a rosette. Lysis of the red cell containing merozoites occurs and the new merozoites infect additional red cells. The characteristic clinical features of malaria such as paroxysmal fever, chills, and rigors develop during the release of these merozoites into the blood. The periodicity of such paroxysms (every 48–72 hours) varies with the species of the malarial parasite. Ruptured RBCs release the daughter merozoites, malarial pigments, and toxins into the circulation. This is responsible for a malarial paroxysm of fever at the end of each erythrocytic cycle.

Sexual forms (7 in **Fig. 4.11**): Most malaria parasites within the red cells develop into merozoites. However, some parasites after entering into RBCs, under specific conditions instead of developing into trophozoites transform into sexual forms called gametocytes. The gametocytic development occurs in the blood vessels of organs such as the spleen and bone marrow and only the mature gametocytes appear in the peripheral blood. The gametocytes are round (except in *P. falciparum* in which they are crescent or banana-shaped). They are of two types namely (i) male gametocyte (or microgametocyte) and (ii) female gametocyte (or macrogametocyte). Microgametocytes are smaller in size and lesser in number, their cytoplasm stains pale blue, and the nucleus is larger, stains red and diffuse. In contrast, macrogametocytes are larger, and numerous, their cytoplasm stains deep blue, nucleus is small, red, and compact. Gametocytes neither cause any clinical illness nor they divide. Patients harboring gametocytes are considered carriers or reservoirs of infection. They play an important role in the transmission of the disease. These gametocytes infect the mosquito when a mosquito bites the infected human and takes its blood meal.

Malaria is more severe when caused by *Plasmodium falciparum* than the other *Plasmodium* species.

Mosquito Cycle (8 to 12 in Fig. 4.11)

A female anopheles mosquito during its blood meal from (8 in **Fig. 4.11**) an infected patient ingests both sexual and asexual forms of the parasite, but it is only the mature sexual forms (gametocytes) that are capable of development (hence considered as an infective form of the parasite to a mosquito). The asexual forms get digested. The nucleus of the male gametocytes divides into eight flagellated actively motile bodies called **microgametes**. Microgametes protrude out as thread-like filaments, lash out for some time and then, break free. This process is called **ex-flagellation** (9 in **Fig. 4.11**). Female gametocytes do not divide and do not undergo exflagellation but it matures to form one **macrogamete or female** gamete. The female gametocyte gets fertilized by the male microgamete and forms a nonmotile round **zygote** (10 in **Fig. 4.11**). The zygote transforms into a vermicular motile elongated form with an apical complex (the **ookinete** stage). Till this stage, the development takes place in the midgut of the mosquito. The ookinete penetrates the stomach wall of the mosquito and lies just beneath the basement membrane. It becomes rounded and forms an **oocyst** (11 in **Fig. 4.11**). Oocysts undergo sporogony (meiosis) and produce thousands of spindle-shaped **sporozoites**. The mature oocyst rupture and release the sporozoites. These **sporozoites migrate to the salivary gland** (12 in **Fig. 4.11**). Mosquito is considered as infective when the sporozoites are present in the salivary gland. Once infected, the mosquito remains infective throughout its life.

Mixed infection: Different species of *Plasmodium* can infect the same mosquito. This can transmit mixed infections to human beings.

MORPHOLOGY

Q. Write a short note on the morphology of *Plasmodium falciparum* in a peripheral blood smear.

Peripheral blood smear: Diagnosis of malaria infection can be made by examination of a Giemsa/Leishman-stained peripheral blood smear (**Fig. 4.12**). It **shows the asexual stages of the parasite within infected red cells.**

Spleen: *Plasmodium falciparum* infection produces **splenomegaly.** In chronic infections, the spleen becomes fibrotic and brittle, with a thick capsule. The parenchyma appears gray or black because of the granular, brown-black, faintly birefringent hemozoin pigment.

Liver: It is enlarged and pigmented. Kupffer cells contain malarial pigment, parasites, and cellular debris.

Brain: In **cerebral malaria** caused by *P. falciparum*, blood vessels of the brain show plugging of parasitized red cells. Around the vessels, there are ring hemorrhages and small focal inflammatory reactions called **malarial** or **Dürck granulomata.**

Tapeworms (Cestode Parasites)

PA 10.2 (CC): Define and describe the pathogenesis and pathology of cysticercosis.

Cysticercosis

Cysticercosis is an infection caused by larvae that develop after ingestion of eggs of a tapeworm namely—***Taenia solium*** (pork tapeworm/armed tapeworm). **Cysticercus is the resting stage of the larva in the intermediate host.**

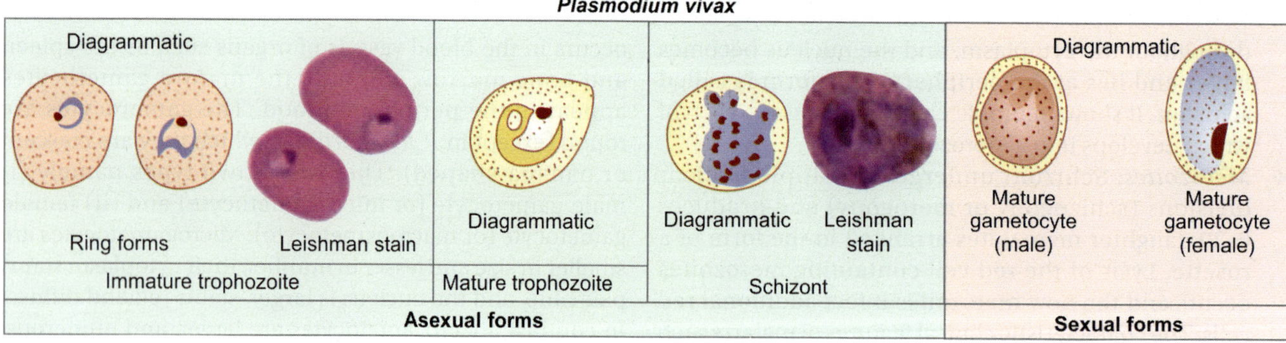

Fig. 4.12: Appearance of malarial parasite *(Plasmodium vivax and falciparum)* in human.

Taenia solium has a complex life cycle and requires two mammalian hosts: (1) a definitive host (in which the worm reaches sexual maturity—humans) and (2) an intermediate host (in which the worm does not reach sexual maturity—humans and pigs).

Mode of infection: *T. solium* can be transmitted to humans in two ways with distinct outcomes.

1. Ingestion of larval cysts called cysticerci (present in uncooked pork) or
2. Ingestion of eggs present in contaminated food/water.

Pathogenesis (Fig. 4.13)

- **Ingestion of cysticerci (larval cysts):** When larval cysts are ingested in undercooked pork by human beings, they attach to the intestinal wall and develop into mature adult tapeworms. They can grow to many meters in length. The life cycle of the parasite is completed with this mode of infection and cysticercosis does not develop. Adult tapeworms shed eggs in the feces of human beings.
- **Ingestion of eggs:** When intermediate hosts (pigs or humans) ingest eggs in food or water contaminated with human feces, the eggs develop into larvae, penetrate the gut wall, and enter the blood circulation. They spread to various sites like muscle, and brain and form **cystic larvae termed cysticercus cellulosae**.

MORPHOLOGY

Organs affected: Cysticerci may be found in any organ, but the more common locations include the **brain, skeletal muscles, skin, and heart.**

Number: The cysticercus can be single or multiple.

Appearance: Cysticercus consists of round to oval white to the opalescent cyst, 0.5–1 cm (often grape-sized) in diameter containing little, clear cyst fluid. It contains an invaginated scolex (which has four suckers) and a circle of birefringent hooks on its wall. They remain viable for a long time. Once the embryo dies, it induces a granulomatous reaction with eosinophils and may later show scarring and calcification, which may be visible by radiography.

Clinical features: Adult tapeworms in the intestine can produce abdominal pain, diarrhea, and loss of appetite.

Neurocysticercosis: The most serious manifestations of cysticercosis are due to the involvement of the brain (neurocysticercosis). Cerebral symptoms depend on the location of the cysts. It can produce epilepsy (convulsions), hydrocephalus, increased intracranial pressure, blurred vision, and other neurologic disturbances.

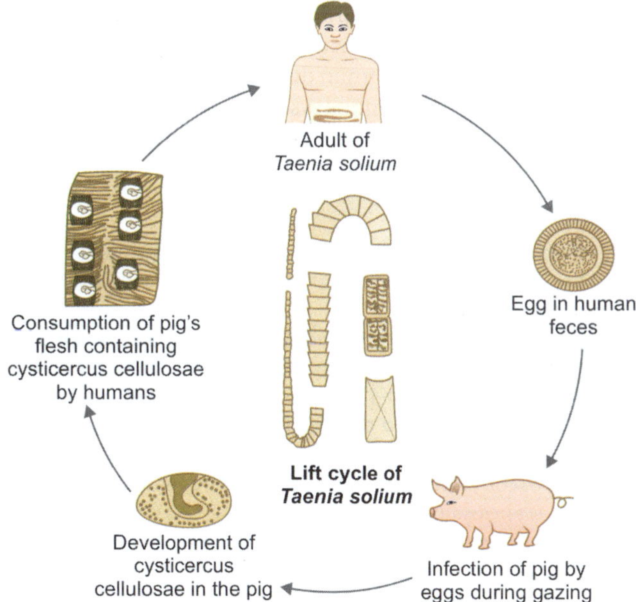

Fig. 4.13: Life cycle of *Taenia solium*.

Echinococcosis/Hydatid Disease

Hydatid disease is a parasitic infestation by cestode (tapeworms) ***Echinococcus granulosus***.

Life cycle: *Echinococcus granulosus* requires two mammalian hosts to complete its life cycle.

- **Definitive host** (in which the worm reaches sexual maturity)**:** Dog, jackal, and fox.
- **Intermediate host** (in which the worm does not reach sexual maturity)**:** Sheep, pig, goat, cattle, man (dead-end host).

Pathogenesis (Fig 4.14): Adult *Echinococcus granulosus* worm is found in the small intestines of dogs and other canines. The dog is infected by eating the viscera of sheep containing hydatid cysts. The adult worm in the small intestines of dogs discharges eggs in feces which are ingested by man, sheep, pigs, and other mammals. Man

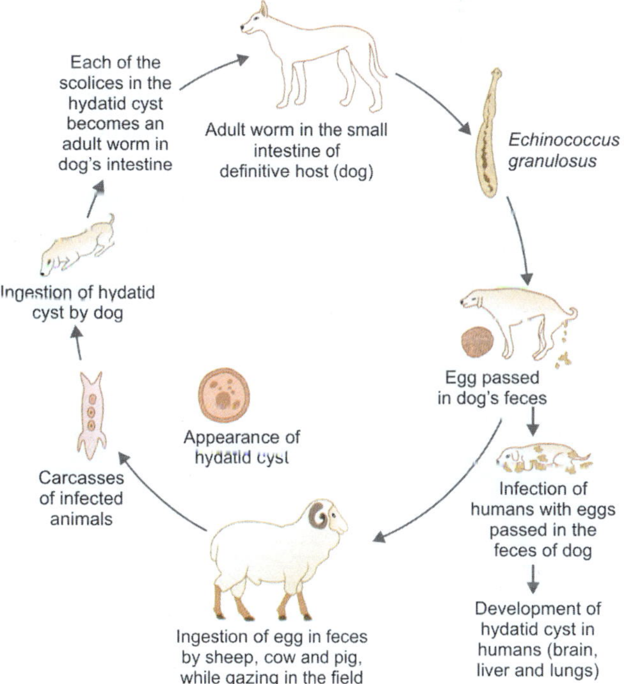

Fig. 4.14: Life cycle of *Echinococcus granulosus*.

acquires infection by: (i) handling dogs, and (ii) eating food/vegetables contaminated with eggs shed by dogs or foxes. The eggs hatch in the human duodenum and are carried to the liver by the portal venous system and other sites through systemic circulation. Those that are trapped in the hepatic sinusoids develop into hydatid cysts.

MORPHOLOGY

- **Sites:** About 65% of human *E. granulosus* cysts are found in the liver and 5–15% in the lung, 10–20% in bones and brain, or other organs.
- **Hydatid cysts (Fig. 4.15)** begin at microscopic levels and grow slowly. They may eventually attain a size over 10 cm in diameter in about 5 years. *E. granulosus* usually produces a unilocular hydatid cyst while *E. multilocularis* produces multilocular hydatid disease in the liver.
- **Microscopy:** The cyst wall consists of three distinguishable zones enclosing an opalescent fluid:
  1. **Pericyst (outer, capsular layer):** It shows an inflammatory reaction and consists of fibroblasts, giant cells, and mononuclear and eosinophils.
  2. **Ectocyst (intermediate opaque, non-nucleated layer):** It is distinctive and has innumerable delicate laminations.
  3. **Endocyst** (inner, nucleated, germinative layer with daughter cysts and scolices projecting into the lumen)**:** Daughter cysts can develop within the large mother cyst. They appear first as minute projections of the germinative layer that develop central vesicles and thus form tiny brood capsules. Degenerating scolices of the worm produce a fine, grain-like (sand-like) sediment within the hydatid fluid (hydatid sand).

Clinical Features

- **Liver:** Produces pressure effects due to cyst.
- **Cerebral:** Epilepsy
- **Renal:** Hematuria
- **Rupture of cyst:** The liberation of antigenic proteins in the hydatid fluid into the circulation produces eosinophilia and may even cause anaphylactic reactions.

Laboratory diagnosis: Casoni test.

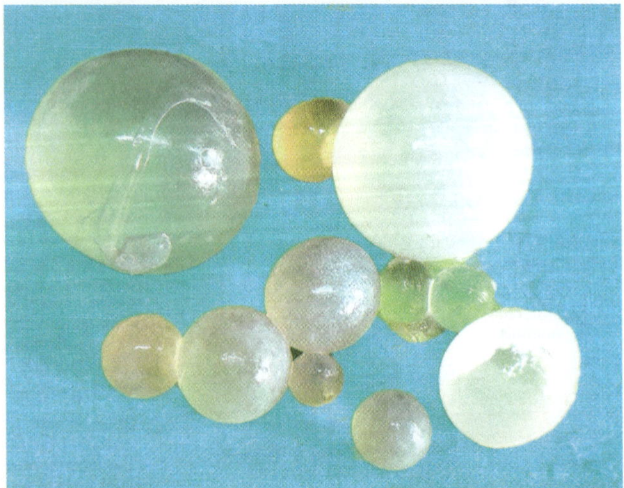

Fig. 4.15: Multiple unilocular hydatid cysts of varying sizes.

Filariasis

Filariasis is transmitted by mosquitoes and is caused by closely related nematodes, *Wuchereria bancrofti,* and *Brugia* species (*B. malayi*).

Diseases: Filariasis causes a spectrum of diseases.

1. Asymptomatic
2. Recurrent lymphadenitis
3. Chronic lymphadenitis with elephantiasis
4. Tropical pulmonary eosinophilia.

Pathogenesis

Pathogenesis: The definitive host is man and the intermediate host is mosquito. During the mosquito bite to humans, the infective larvae are released by mosquitoes into the tissues. They develop within lymphatic channels into adult males and females which mate and release microfilariae into the bloodstream. During the mosquito bite of the infected persons, the mosquitoes can take up the microfilariae. These microfilariae undergo further development in the mosquito and they become infective and transmit the disease to humans.

MORPHOLOGY

- In chronic filariasis, the adult parasites lodge in the lymphatics and stimulate fibrosis and the formation of granulomas around the adult parasites. Thus, chronic filariasis leads to **persistent lymphedema** of the extremities (*refer* **Fig. 5.4A**), scrotum, penis, or vulva.
- In severe and long-standing swollen legs may develop tough subcutaneous fibrosis and epithelial hyperkeratosis, termed **elephantiasis (Fig. 4.16A).** Adult filarial worms (live, dead, or calcified) are observed in the draining lymphatics or nodes. Microfilaria **(Figs. 4.16B and Fig. 5.4B)** is the embryo of *Wuchereria bancrofti* and can be seen in blood and body fluids.
- Filariasis can also cause hydrocele.

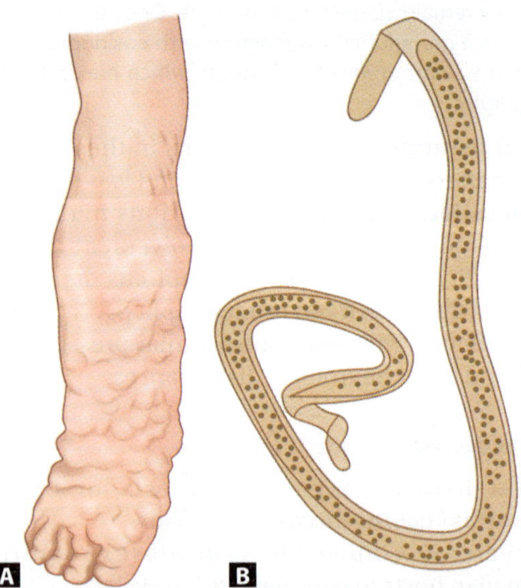

Figs. 4.16A and B: (A) Elephantiasis of leg; (B) Diagrammatic appearance of microfilaria (embryo of *Wuchereria bancrofti*).

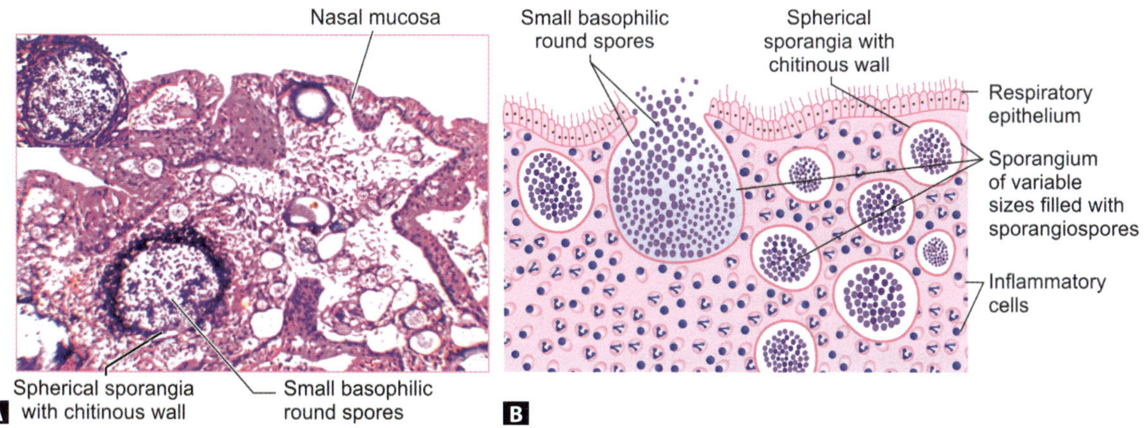

Figs. 4.17A and B: Rhinosporidiosis of nasopharynx showing spherical sporangia: (A) Hematoxylin and eosin (H & E); (B) Diagrammatic.

OTHER INFECTIONS

Rhinosporidiosis

Q. Write a short note on rhinosporidiosis.

Rhinosporidiosis is an inflammatory disease caused by *Rhinosporidium seeberi*. **Usually, it occurs in the nasopharynx as a polyp** but may also be observed in the larynx and conjunctiva. It is also observed in the oropharynx, rectum, and external genitalia.

It is endemic in India and Sri Lanka and sporadic in other parts of the world.

Microscopy (Figs. 4.17A and B)

- Structure of nasal mucosa.
- Many **spherical cysts called sporangia** measuring up to 200 nm in diameter and having **thick walls** (chitinous walls) are seen. Each of these cysts (i.e., sporangium) **contains numerous small basophilic round spores** of the size of erythrocytes. On rupture of a sporangium, the spores may be discharged into the submucosa or onto the surface of the mucosa.
- **Chronic inflammatory** (plasma cells, lymphocytes, histiocytes, neutrophils) **infiltrate** in the intervening and subepithelial layer.

Molluscum Contagiosum

Q. Write a short note on molluscum contagiosum.

Molluscum contagiosum is a common, **self-limited, highly contagious viral disease of the skin** caused by a double-stranded DNA poxvirus.

Mode of infection: Usually spread by **direct contact.** Common among children and young adults.

MORPHOLOGY

Lesions

The infection leads to **multiple lesions on the skin and mucous membranes,** with a predilection for the face, trunk, and anogenital areas. Individual lesions are **small, firm, smooth,** often pruritic, **pink to skin-colored, dome-shaped papules,** generally ranging in diameter from 2 mm to 4 mm. Fully developed lesions have a characteristic **central umbilication** and in a fully-developed lesion, a small amount of **cheesy (curd/paste-like) keratinous material can be expressed on pressing from the central umbilication.** This material if smeared onto a glass slide and stained with Giemsa may show diagnostic molluscum bodies.

Microscopy (Fig. 4.18)

The microscopic picture is characteristic.

- **Infected epithelial cells:** A typical lesion consists of a **sharply circumscribed** (delimited) **lobulated, cup-shaped mass** of proliferating infected epithelial cells of the epidermis growing down into the dermis.
- **Molluscum body:** As the infected epithelial cells differentiate within the mass, their **cytoplasm is gradually filled by viral inclusion.** These inclusions enlarge the epithelial cells and displace the nucleus. The viral inclusions are diagnostically specific structures (which appear ellipsoid) and are termed as **molluscum bodies**. The viral inclusions are found in cells of the stratum granulosum and the stratum corneum. Under hematoxylin and eosin stain, these inclusions appear **faintly granular eosinophilic in the blue-purple stratum granulosum** and **pale blue in the red stratum corneum.** These molluscum bodies contain numerous viral particles. Most lesions spontaneously regress.

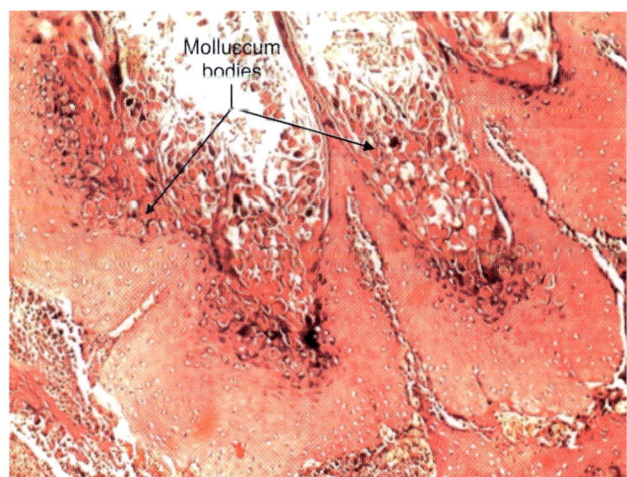

Fig. 4.18: Molluscum contagiosum. Epithelial cells of the epidermis show ellipsoid cytoplasmic inclusions.

SCENARIO-BASED MCQs

1. **A 29-year-old man presents to the dermatology outpatient department with maculopapular and nodular skin lesions. These lesions are mainly seen on his face, elbows, wrists, and knees. These lesions are has reduced to absent sensation. Microscopy of these lesions showed nodular aggregates of foamy cells (lipid-filled macrophages). Fite Feraco stain revealed numerous bacilli arranged in cigar bundles. The most likely diagnosis is:**

   A. Anthrax B. Hansen disease
   C. Neurofibroma D. Neurilemmoma

2. **A 22-year-old man attends the skin outpatient with a nontender ulcer on his penis for the past week. On enquiry, he revealed that he has multiple sexual partners and does not use barrier precautions. Physical examination showed a 0.7 cm lesion with a firm, erythematous, indurated base, and sharply demarcated borders. The lesion is scraped, and microscopic darkfield examination shows positive for motile spirochetes. Which of the following condition is responsible for the lesion?**

   A. Primary syphilis B. Gonococcal infection
   C. HIV infection D. Tuberculous ulcer

3. **A 65-year-old male has developed aortic root dilation and aortic insufficiency. He has a long history of unprotected sexual intercourse with multiple partners. The most likely disease that has produced the lesions in aorta is:**

   A. Primary syphilis B. Secondary syphilis
   C. Tertiary syphilis D. Congenital syphilis

Answers and Explanation

1. **Answer is B: Hansen disease (leprosy)-lepromatous form.** It is caused by *Mycobacterium leprae,* which infects peripheral nerves and skin. Diagnosis is made by biopsy of a skin lesion. Large aggregates of lipid-filled macrophages contain acid-fast bacilli demonstrated by the Fite Feraco stain. Cutaneous anthrax is caused by *Bacillus anthracis. It* produces a necrotic skin lesion with eschar at the site of inoculation. The other two options are tumors of peripheral nerves and they do not show foamy macrophages with acid-fast bacilli.
2. **Answer is A: Primary syphilis.** Infection with *Treponema pallidum* produces characteristic painless syphilitic chancres in the primary stage of syphilis. It is nontender with an indurated base and is known as hard chancre. Gonorrhea produces acute inflammation with abscess formation and mainly involves urethral region. HIV infection is also sexually transmitted disease but do not produce chancre. Tuberculous ulcer usually do not involve glans.
3. **Answer is C: Tertiary syphilis.** If infection with *Treponema pallidum is not* treated, it can progress to tertiary syphilis many years later. The most common manifestations of tertiary syphilis are aortitis (typically in the thoracic portion), neurosyphilis, and gummatous necrosis of several sites (e.g., skin, bone, and joint). Other stages of syphilis does not involve aorta. Congenital syphilis does not manifest with CVS abnormalities at the age of 65 years.

Leprosy (Hansen's disease): A chronic infectious disease caused by Mycobacterium leprae.

Leprosy affects the cooler parts of the body (e.g., the skin, mouth, respiratory tract, eyes, peripheral nerves, nodes and testis).

Classification of leprosy
- Ridley and Jopling (1966) Classification:
  - Olar tuberculoid (high resistance)
  - Olar lepromatous (low resistance)
  - Orderline towards either type.
- WHO classification:
  - Aucibacillary
  - Ultibacillary

Leprosy: Not a necrotizing granuloma.

Leprosy microscopy:
- Epromatous leprosy: Foam cells (multibacillary) and Grenz zone.
- Uberculoid leprosy: Epithelioid cell granulomas (paucibacillary).

Syphilis: (Sexually-transmitted) disease caused by spirochetes, Treponema pallidum.

Syphilis: Acquired (primary, secondary, and tertiary) or congenital.

Primary syphilis: Lesion is a chancre that appears on genitals or at extra-genital sites.

Secondary syphilis: Mucocutaneous lesions and painless lymphadenopathy.

Tertiary syphilis:
- Gummas (in the liver or testis).
- Diffuse lesions (cardiovascular and neurosyphilis).

Congenital syphilis: Saddle nose deformity, saber shin, Hutchinson's triad [peg-spaced incisor (Hutchinson's teeth), interstitial keratitis, and VIII nerve deafness]

Necrotizing granuloma Tuberculosis, syphilis, histoplasmosis, Cat's scratch disease.

Durck granuloma: cerebral malaria.

Hemodynamic Disorders, Thromboembolism, and Shock

Chapter Outline

- Edema
- Disorders of Perfusion
- Shock
- Hemostasis and Thrombosis
- Thrombosis
- Embolism
- Infarction

EDEMA

PA 6.1 (CC): Define and describe edema, Its types, pathogenesis, and clinical correlations.

Q. Define edema.

Definition: An **abnormal accumulation of fluid in the interstitial space within tissues is called edema.**

Q. Tabulate the differences between transudate and exudate.

Types of edema fluid: The edema fluid may be either transudate or exudate. The differences between transudate and exudate are presented in **Table 3.3**. Special forms of edema are listed in **Table 5.1**.

1. **Transudate:** It is a **protein-poor fluid** caused by **increased hydrostatic pressure or reduced plasma protein**. Transudate is observed in heart failure, renal failure, hepatic failure, and certain forms of malnutrition.
2. **Exudate:** It is a **protein-rich fluid** produced **due to increased vascular permeability** and is seen in **inflammation**.

Pathophysiologic Categories of Edema (Table 5.2)

Q. Classify and list the different pathophysiological categories (causes) of edema.

Edema may be localized or generalized in distribution.

Local/localized edema: It is **limited to an organ or part** (e.g., arm, leg, epiglottis, larynx).

- **Obstruction of vein or lymphatic:** For e.g., edema of limb (usually the leg) develops due to venous or lymphatic obstruction caused by **thrombophlebitis, chronic lymphangitis, resection of regional lymph nodes, filariasis,** etc.
- **Inflammation:** It is the **most common cause** of local edema. Burns cause prominent local edema by increasing local vascular permeability.

TABLE 5.1 Special forms of edema.

Terminology	*Body cavity involved*
Hydrothorax	Pleural cavity
Hydropericardium	Pericardial cavity
Hydroperitoneum (ascites)	Peritoneal cavity

- **Immune reaction:** For example, urticaria (hives), or edema of the epiglottis or larynx (angioneurotic edema).

Q. Discuss the causes and pathogenesis of generalized edema.

Generalized edema: It is **systemic in distribution** and affects visceral organs and the skin of the trunk and lower extremities.

- **Causes:** The main causes of generalized edema are due to disorders of fluid and electrolyte metabolism namely **(i) heart failure, (ii) nephrotic syndrome** (renal diseases with massive loss of serum proteins into the urine), and **(iii) cirrhosis of the liver**.
- **Anasarca:** It is a **severe form of generalized edema**. It is characterized by conspicuous fluid accumulation in subcutaneous tissues, visceral organs, and body cavities.

Normal fluid balance: The smallest vessels of the vascular system and the lymphatic vessels are termed *microcirculation.* Normally, the fluid flows out from the arteriolar end of the microcirculation into the interstitium. This is balanced by flowing in the fluid at the venular end. As fluid moves through the interstitial space, most of it returns to the capillary bed. Normally, a small amount of fluid (approximately 10% of the fluid) is left in the interstitium and is drained (absorbed) by the adjacent lymphatic vessels, and it reaches the general bloodstream via the thoracic duct. The **movement of water and salts between the intravascular and interstitial spaces is controlled by four distinct forces or pressures**. These include **(1) vascular**

TABLE 5.2 Pathophysiologic categories of edema.

Increased hydrostatic pressure

Impaired venous return

- Congestive heart failure
- Constrictive pericarditis
- Cirrhosis of liver (ascites)
- Venous obstruction or compression
  - Venous thrombosis
  - Compression of veins by external pressure (e.g., external mass)
- Prolonged postural (lower extremity) inactivity (e.g., prolonged standing)

Arteriolar dilation

- Heat
- Neurohumoral dysregulation
- Inflammation

Decreased plasma osmotic pressure (hypoproteinemia)

- Nephrotic syndrome (protein-losing glomerulopathies)
- Advanced disease of the liver (e.g., cirrhosis)
- Malnutrition
- Protein-losing gastroenteropathy

Lymphatic obstruction

- Inflammatory
- Neoplastic
- Post-irradiation
- Postsurgical

Sodium retention (hypervolemia)

- Excessive salt intake with renal insufficiency
- Decreased renal excretion of sodium
- Renal hypoperfusion
- increased renin-angiotensin-aldosterone secretion

Inflammation (increased capillary permeability)

- Acute and chronic inflammation
- Burns
- Angiogenesis
- Adult respiratory distress syndrome

hydrostatic pressure, (2) interstitial fluid colloid osmotic pressure, (3) plasma colloid osmotic pressure, and (4) interstitial fluid pressure. This delicate balance of forces is summarized by **Starling's hypothesis (Fig. 5.1)**. According to this, the net filtration is equal to the combined forces that favor filtration minus the combined forces that oppose filtration. Clinically, **vascular hydrostatic pressure** (the force that drives the fluid out of circulation) and **plasma colloid osmotic pressure** (the force that drives the fluid into circulation) are the **most important.**

Mechanism/Pathogenesis of Edema (Fig. 5.2)

Any mechanism, that interferes with the normal fluid balance (*refer* above), may produce edema. **Increased hydrostatic pressure or decreased colloid osmotic pressure** produces increased interstitial fluid. If the

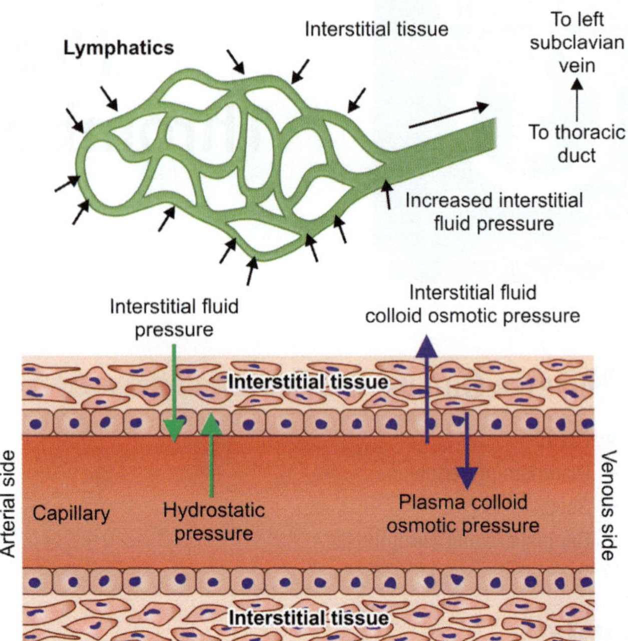

Fig. 5.1: Factors influencing the movement of fluid across capillary walls. Normally there is a balance between hydrostatic and osmotic pressure so that there is only little net movement of fluid into the interstitium. Mechanisms that can produce edema include increased hydrostatic pressure or diminished plasma osmotic pressure. Normally lymphatics in the interstitial tissue return much of the excess fluid into the circulation by way of the thoracic duct. If the fluid accumulated exceeds the capacity of lymphatic drainage also produces local edema.

movement of fluid into tissues (or body cavities) **exceeds lymphatic drainage**, the fluid accumulates in the interstitial tissue. Edema may also develop **when the permeability of capillaries is increased** and they "leak" fluid (e.g., inflammation). These pathophysiologic mechanisms may operate singly or in combination.

Increased Hydrostatic Pressure

Hydrostatic pressure at the capillary end of microcirculation drives the fluid out of the capillary into the interstitial tissue space. Any conditions, that increase the hydrostatic pressure, can produce edema. **Increases in hydrostatic pressure are usually caused by disorders that impair venous return.** The increased hydrostatic pressure **may be regional or generalized.**

Regional increase in hydrostatic pressure: The **local impairment in venous return** increases local hydrostatic pressure. Examples:

- **Deep venous thrombosis** in a lower extremity may produce regional **edema restricted to the distal portion of the affected leg.**
- **Postural edema** may be seen in the **feet and ankles** of individuals who stand in an erect position for a long duration.

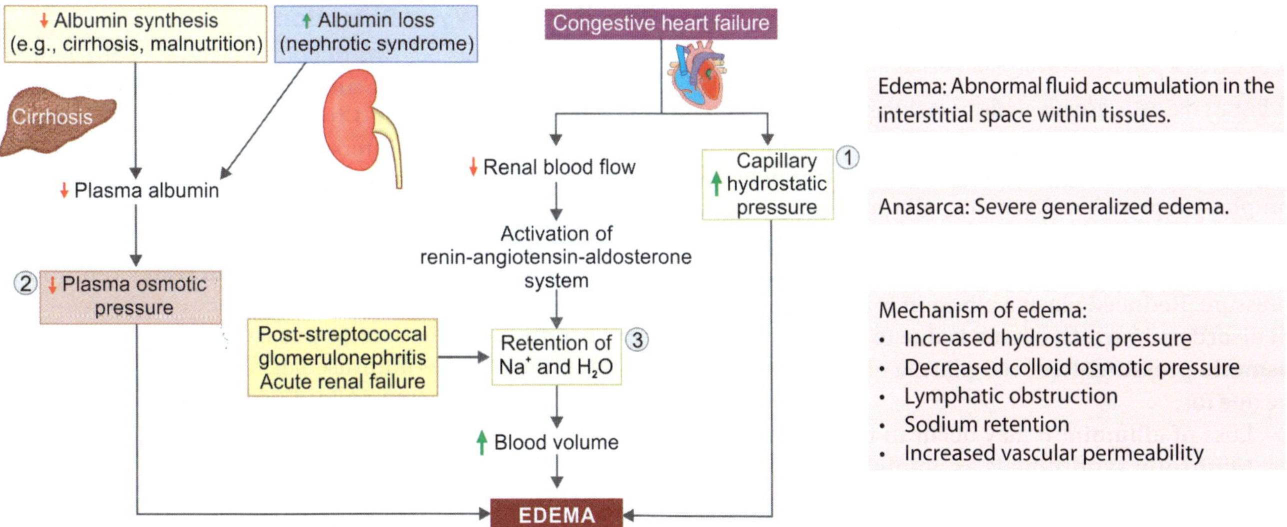

Fig. 5.2: Pathogenesis of systemic edema from congestive heart failure, renal failure, or reduced plasma osmotic pressure. Three mechanisms include (1) increased hydrostatic pressure, (2) reduced plasma osmotic pressure, and (3) retention of sodium (Na^+) and water (H_2O). Lymphatic obstruction is involved in localized edema.

Q. Mention the pathogenesis/mechanism of cardiac edema.

Generalized increase in hydrostatic pressure: It produces **generalized edema**. Most common cause is **congestive heart failure (CHF)**. Congestive heart failure is associated with a **systemic increase in venous pressure** and, thereby causes generalized edema. Most commonly congestive heart failure is associated with **ischemic heart disease**. However, almost any chronic cardiac disorder may lead to congestive heart failure. Congestive heart failure may be a **failure of the left ventricle, right ventricle, or both. Right-sided heart failure** results in the pooling of blood on the venous side of the circulation and increases the hydrostatic pressure in the venous circulation. This increases the movement of fluid into the interstitial tissue spaces. It shows characteristic **peripheral pitting edema. Left-sided heart failure** results in increased hydrostatic pressure in the pulmonary circulation and leads to **pulmonary edema**.

Mechanism of cardiac edema (Flowchart 5.1): The main cause of cardiac edema is congestive heart failure. Several factors increase the venous hydrostatic pressure in congestive heart failure. Reduced cardiac output in congestive heart failure leads to the following adaptive changes:

- Impaired return of venous blood to the heart leads to pooling of blood in the venous circulation and increases capillary hydrostatic pressure.
- Hypoperfusion of the kidneys. It decreases glomerular filtration and triggers the renin-angiotensin-aldosterone axis. This leads to the retention of sodium and water *(secondary hyperaldosteronism)*. This adaptation in patients with normally functioning hearts, increases cardiac filling and cardiac output, resulting in improved renal perfusion. However, patients with failing hearts usually cannot increase cardiac output in response to increases in cardiac filling. This leads to a vicious cycle of fluid retention, increased venous hydrostatic pressures, and worsening of edema. This cycle continues unless cardiac output is restored or renal water retention is reduced (e.g., by salt restriction or treatment with diuretics or aldosterone antagonists). Secondary hyperaldosteronism is also observed in generalized edema of noncardiac origin. These patients may also benefit from treatment with salt restriction, diuretics, and aldosterone antagonists.

Flowchart 5.1: Mechanism of generalized edema in congestive heart failure.

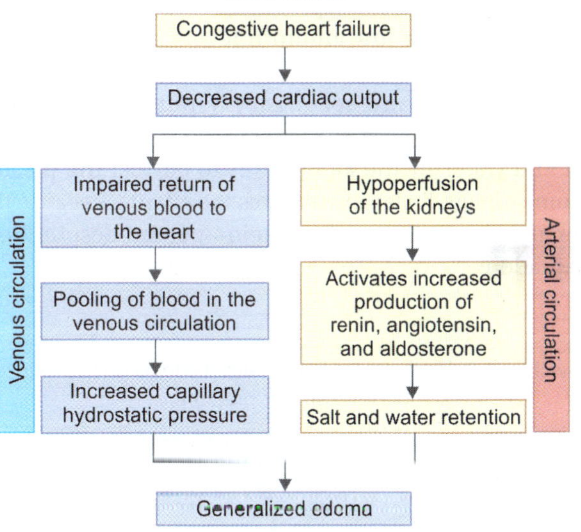

Pathologic consequences of chronic congestive heart failure are presented in (*refer* **online Fig. 5.3**).

Decreased Plasma Osmotic Pressure

Q. Discuss the pathogenesis of renal edema.

Q. Discuss the pathogenesis of edema in cirrhosis.

Plasma osmotic pressure normally tends to draw the fluid into the vessels. The **plasma osmotic pressure is dependent on plasma proteins.** Normally, **albumin** (major plasma protein) accounts for almost 50% of the total plasma protein and is the main contributor to colloid osmotic pressure. **Reduced plasma albumin is a common feature of disorders in which edema is due to decreased colloid osmotic pressure.** Reduced plasma albumin levels may be due to:

- **Loss of albumin:** It may occur in the **urine or stool. Nephrotic syndrome** is an important cause of **loss of albumin in the urine** (albuminuria). Nephrotic syndrome is associated with damage to glomeruli that allows albumin (and other plasma proteins) into the urine. **Malabsorption and protein-losing enteropathy** are characterized by **loss of protein in the stool**.
- **Reduced albumin synthesis:** It occurs in **severe liver diseases** (e.g., cirrhosis) and **protein malnutrition** (due to decreased intake of proteins).

Consequences of low albumin levels (Flowchart 5.2): It leads to edema, reduced intravascular volume, renal hypoperfusion, and secondary hyperaldosteronism. However, in these disorders, increased retention of salt and water by the kidney fails to correct the plasma volume deficit. It also exacerbates the edema, because the primary defect—low serum protein—persists despite these adaptations.

Flowchart 5.2: Mechanism of generalized edema due to reduced plasma osmotic pressure.

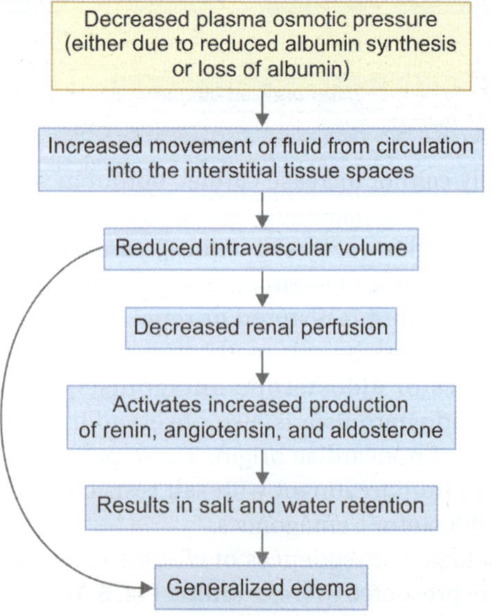

Sodium and Water Retention

Water represents 50–70% of body weight. It is distributed between intracellular and extracellular fluid (ECF) spaces (further divided into interstitial and vascular compartments). The interstitium contains about 75% of ECF. **Increased retention of sodium salt is invariably associated with retention of water.** Sodium and water retention may be a primary cause of edema.

Mechanism of edema in sodium and water retention. These include the following:

- **Increased hydrostatic pressure** due to increased plasma volume (intravascular volume).
- **Decreased plasma colloid osmotic pressure** due to decreased plasma protein concentration.

Causes: May be primary or secondary

- **Primary:** It is associated with a wide variety of disorders of the kidney such as **post-streptococcal glomerulonephritis and acute renal failure.**
- **Secondary:** It develops in disorders that decrease renal perfusion, the most important cause being **congestive heart failure.**

Lymphatic Obstruction

Q. Write a short note on localized edema.

Normally, lymphatics resorb fluid from interstitial spaces. Lymphatic obstruction causes impaired drainage of lymph from interstitial spaces and produces localized edema, called **lymphedema**.

Causes of lymphatic obstruction: Various causes of impaired lymphatic drainage are as follows:

- **Parasitic infestations:** In **filariasis** (caused by *Wuchereria bancrofti*), the parasite (**Fig. 5.4B**—microfilaria) may cause extensive obstruction of lymphatics and fibrosis of lymph nodes. If the block is in the inguinal region, it can produce edema of the external genitalia and lower limbs (upper arm if the axillary region is involved) which

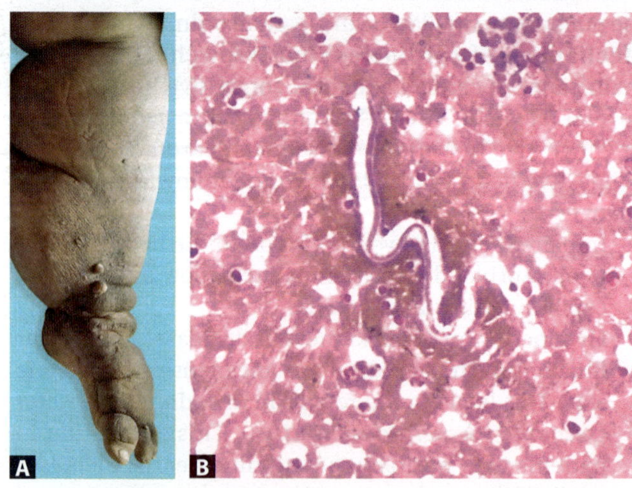

Figs. 5.4A and B: Elephantiasis due to obstruction of lymphatics (A) by *Wuchereria bancrofti* (microfilaria—B).

may be massive and resemble the leg of an elephant and is known as **elephantiasis (Fig. 5.4A and *refer* Fig. 4.16)**.

- **Invasive malignant tumors:** For example, **lymphedema of the breast** (edema of the overlying breast skin) develops due to infiltration and **blockage of superficial (subcutaneous) lymphatics by malignant cells.** It gives rise to a characteristic finely pitted appearance to the involved region of skin of the affected breast and is called ***peau d'orange*** (orange peel/orange skin) appearance.
- **Chronic inflammation of lymphatics** associated with fibrosis. For example, lymphedema occurs in the scrotal and vulvar regions due to **lymphogranuloma venereum**.
- **Damage by surgery/radiation:** Patients with breast cancer may develop severe edema of the upper arm as a complication of **surgical removal and/or irradiation of the breast** and **associated axillary lymph nodes.**
- **Pressure over lymphatic drainage from outside** (e.g., tumors obstructing thoracic ducts).
- **Hereditary disorder: Milroy's disease** is a hereditary disorder characterized by **abnormal development of lymphatics**. The edema may be seen in one or both lower limbs.

  Through lymph, proteins in the interstitial space are returned to circulation. So, **edema fluid** produced due to lymphatic obstruction has a **high protein** concentration. The increased protein content may **stimulate fibrosis** in the dermis of the skin and is **responsible for the induration found in lymphedema**.

MORPHOLOGY

Edema can be **easily detected on gross examination.** It may involve any organ or tissue but is **most common in subcutaneous tissues, the lungs,** and the **brain**. Microscopically, edema appears as a clear space, which separates the extracellular matrix.

Generalized Edema

Subcutaneous edema: Generalized edema is seen mainly in the subcutaneous tissues. It may be diffuse or more easily noticed in regions with high hydrostatic pressures. In most cases, the distribution of **edema is dependent on gravity** and is termed **dependent edema**. Thus, it is prominent in the legs when standing, and in the sacrum when recumbent (lying flat). **If pressure is applied** by a finger over substantially edematous subcutaneous tissue, it **displaces the interstitial fluid and leaves a finger-shaped depression.** This sign is called **pitting edema (Fig. 5.5).**

Edema of renal origin (e.g., nephrotic syndrome): It can **affect all parts of the body.** Initially, it is observed **in tissues with loose connective tissue matrix**, such as the **eyelids** (*refer* **Fig. 20.13**) and **scrotal region**. Edema in the eyelids is called **periorbital edema** and is a characteristic of severe renal disease.

Q. Write briefly on pulmonary edema.

Pulmonary Edema

Gross: The **weight of the lungs is increased** 2–3 times of normal weight. **The cut section** shows **frothy**, sometimes **blood-tinged**

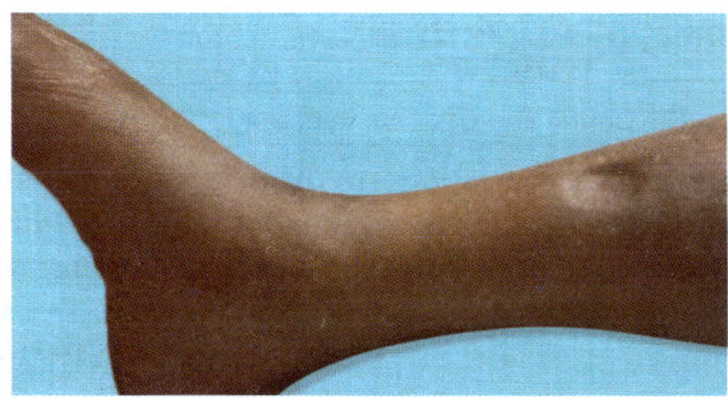

Fig. 5.5: Pitting edema in which when pressure by finger is applied, it displaces interstitial fluid and leaves a depression at that site.

fluid (due to a mixture of air, edema, and extravasated red cells) **oozing from the lung.**

Microscopy: The edema fluid is seen in the alveolar septa around capillaries and reduces the diffusion of oxygen. Edema fluid present in the alveolar spaces favors bacterial infection.

Brain Edema

It may be localized (e.g., in abscess or tumor) or generalized, depending on the nature and extent of the pathologic process or injury. In **generalized edema, the sulci are narrowed and the gyri appear swollen** and become flattened against the skull. The ventricular cavities are compressed and the brain expands and may herniate.

Clinical Consequences

They range from minimal effects to rapidly fatal effects.

Generalized subcutaneous tissue edema: It indicates the presence of an underlying **cardiac or renal disease**. Severe subcutaneous edema **may delay cutaneous wound healing or the clearance of skin infection.**

Pulmonary edema: It is a common clinical condition and is most commonly **caused by left ventricular failure**. Other causes include renal failure, acute respiratory distress syndrome, and pulmonary inflammation or infection.

Q. Write briefly on brain edema.

Cerebral/brain parenchymal edema: It is life threatening. In severe brain edema, the **brain substance may herniate** (extrude) **through the foramen magnum, or occlude the blood supply to the brainstem.** Both conditions may damage the medullary centers and lead to death.

Myxedema: It is a form of **non-pitting** edema involving the skin of the face and visceral organs **observed in hypothyroidism** (*refer* **page 869**). The edema is due to excessive deposition of glycosaminoglycans and hyaluronic acid, in the skin, subcutaneous tissue, and visceral organs.

Papilledema: Swelling of the optic nerve head is called papilledema. The concentric increase in pressure encircling the optic nerve produces stasis of venous outflow which leads to swelling of the optic nerve head. The causes are: (i) compression of the nerve (e.g., primary neoplasm of the optic nerve), and (2) raised cerebrospinal fluid pressure surrounding the nerve.

DISORDERS OF PERFUSION

PA 6.2a (CC): Define and describe hyperemia.

Hyperemia and congestion are disorders of perfusion characterized by locally increased blood volume within a tissue. But the underlying mechanisms are different.

Hyperemia

Q. Write a short note on hyperemia.

Definition: Hyperemia is an **active process** in which **arteriolar dilation** leads to increased **blood flow to a tissue/organ.**

Causes: It may be physiological or pathological.

- **Physiological:** Response to **increased functional demand.** For example, heart and skeletal muscle **during exercise.**
- **Pathological:** Seen in **inflammation** and is responsible for the two cardinal signs of inflammation namely **heat** (calor) and **redness** (rubor/**erythema**).

PA 6.2b (CC): Define and describe congestion.

Congestion

Q. Write a short note on chronic passive congestion.

Definition: Congestion is a **passive process** resulting from **impaired (reduced) venous outflow of blood** from a tissue/organ.

Types and causes: Congestion may occur systemically or locally.

- **Systemic:** Generalized increases in venous pressure, typically occur in **congestive heart failure** (e.g., coronary artery disease and hypertension). The congestion **mainly involves the liver, spleen, and kidneys.**
- **Local:** Examples include, congestion of leg veins due to **deep venous thrombosis (DVT)** results in **edema of the lower extremity**, and local congestion at various sites due to **compression of veins**, e.g., tight bandage, plasters, tumors, pregnancy, hernia, etc.

Onset: It may be acute or chronic congestion.

Acute Congestion

It develops during shock or sudden right-sided heart failure. It may occur in the **lungs and liver.**

MORPHOLOGY

Acute pulmonary congestion: It shows alveolar capillaries engorged with blood, edema of the alveolar septa, and intra-alveolar hemorrhage.

Acute hepatic congestion: It shows distention of the central vein and sinusoids with blood and centrally located hepatocytes may undergo necrosis. Periportal hepatocytes may develop fatty change because they experience less severe hypoxia due to their proximity to hepatic arterioles.

Chronic Venous Congestion (CVC)

It usually produces edema in the organ/tissue in which the venous outflow is reduced. **Congested tissues have a dusky reddish-blue color (cyanosis)** due to stasis of red blood cells (RBCs) and the accumulation of deoxygenated hemoglobin.

Chronic Venous Congestion of the Lung

Q. Write a short note on CVC lung (brown induration of lung).

Causes: These include:

- **Mitral stenosis** (e.g., rheumatic mitral stenosis).
- **Left-sided heart failure:** Chronic left-ventricular failure develops secondary to **coronary artery disease or hypertension.**

The mechanism of chronic venous congestion (CVC) of the lung is presented in **Flowchart 5.3.**

Q. Write a short note on heart failure cells and the special stain used for its demonstration.

Consequences: In chronic left-sided failure, the left heart cannot pump out the blood flowing from the lungs. This creates back pressure and chronic passive pulmonary congestion. This increases the pressure in alveolar capillaries and these capillaries become engorged with blood leading to chronic venous congestion (CVC) of the lung. This **increased pressure in capillaries** has four major consequences:

1. **Microhemorrhages:** The **wall of alveolar capillaries may rupture and produce minute hemorrhages into the alveolar space.** The hemoglobin from the RBCs released into the alveoli space breaks down and **liberates iron-containing hemosiderin pigment** (brown color). Hemosiderin is phagocytosed by alveolar macrophages. These **hemosiderin-laden macrophages** are known as **heart failure cells. Perl's stain** (a special stain for hemosiderin) imparts a blue-black color to hemosiderin in the cytoplasm.
2. **Pulmonary edema:** It is due to the forced movement of fluid from congested vessels into the alveolar airspaces.

Flowchart 5.3: Mechanism of chronic venous congestion of the lung.

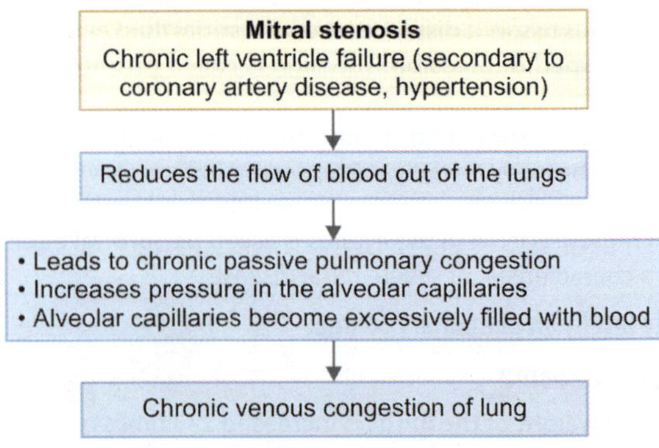

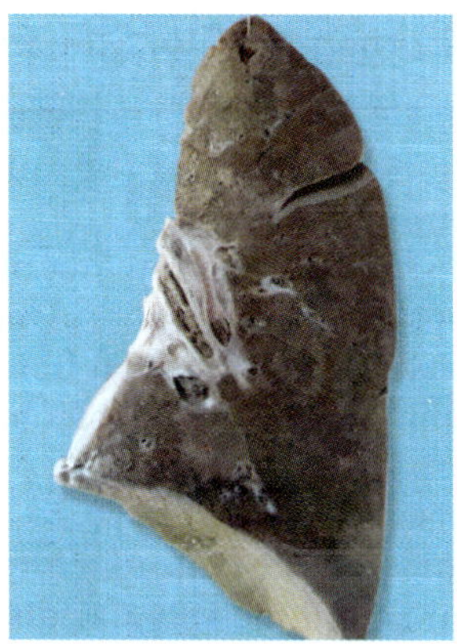

Fig. 5.6: Chronic venous congestion of lung showing brown induration of lung.

3. **Fibrosis:** It develops due to **increased fibrous tissue in the interstitium of the lung**. The combination of fibrosis and hemosiderin (iron) causes the **lungs to become firm and brown (brown induration)**.
4. **Pulmonary hypertension:** It is due to back pressure transmission of pressure from the alveolar capillaries to the pulmonary arterial system. This may lead to right-sided heart failure, and later to generalized systemic venous congestion.

MORPHOLOGY

Gross

The lung is **heavy. Cut section** (c/s) **rusty brown color** (due to hemosiderin pigment), **firm in consistency** (due to fibrosis), and is known as **brown induration of lung (Fig. 5.6).**

Microscopy (Figs. 5.7A and B)

- **Distension** and **congestion of capillaries** in the alveolar septa of the lung.
- **Thickened alveolar septa** due to an increase in the fibrous connective tissue and is responsible for the firm consistency of the lung.
- **Heart failure cells** are seen in the alveoli.

Chronic Venous Congestion of the Liver

Q. Write a short note on causes and gross and microscopic features of chronic venous congestion of the liver (CVC liver/nutmeg liver).

Causes: The hepatic veins empty into the inferior vena cava just inferior to the heart, so the liver is vulnerable to acute or chronic passive congestion. **Right-sided heart failure** is the most common cause. **Rare causes include constrictive pericarditis, tricuspid stenosis, and obstruction of the inferior vena cava and hepatic vein**. The mechanism of chronic venous congestion of the liver is presented in **Flowchart 5.4**.

MORPHOLOGY

Gross

The liver increases in size and weight and the **capsule appears tense. The cut section** shows **alternate** (combination of) **dark and light areas (Fig. 5.8)** and resembles a cross-section of nutmeg (**nutmeg liver**).

- **Congested centrilobular regions** (with hemorrhage and necrosis) appear **dark red-brown.** Congestion is most prominent around terminal hepatic venule (central veins) within hepatic lobules.
- **Periportal unaffected** (better oxygenated) **region** of the lobules appear **pale** and **may show fatty change.**

Microscopy (Figs. 5.9A and B)

Centrilobular region:

- **Congestion and hemorrhage** in the central veins (terminal hepatic venule) and adjacent sinusoids. The **severe central hypoxia may produce centrilobular hepatocyte necrosis.**
- **Thickening of central veins and fibrosis** in prolonged venous congestion.
- **Cardiac sclerosis/cardiac cirrhosis:** Prolonged (sustained) chronic hepatic venous congestion may lead to thickening of central veins and centrilobular fibrosis. Only in the most extreme cases of venous congestion (e.g., due to constrictive pericarditis or tricuspid stenosis), the fibrosis may be sufficiently generalized and severe resulting in cardiac sclerosis/cirrhosis.

Periportal region: It shows **fatty change** in hepatocytes.

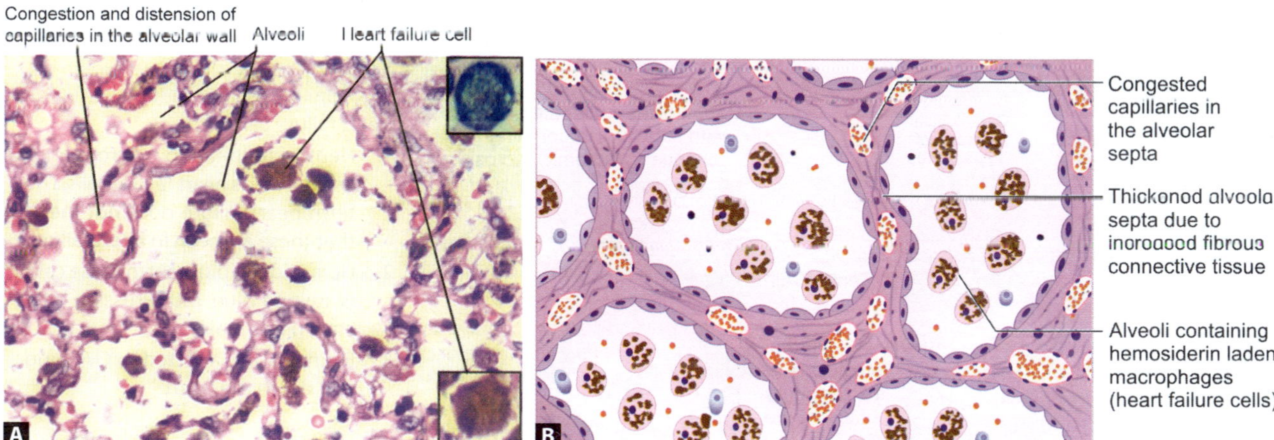

Figs. 5.7A and B: Chronic venous congestion lung: (A) Hematoxylin and eosin; (B) Diagrammatic section from lung shows thickened alveolar walls and hemosiderin-laden macrophages (heart failure cells) in the alveolar lumen Inset of A, lower right-hemosiderin-laden macrophage and upper left—Perl's stain imparting blue-black color to hemosiderin in the cytoplasm.

Flowchart 5.4: Mechanism of chronic venous congestion of the liver.

Right-sided heart failure (most common cause). Rare causes include constrictive pericarditis, tricuspid stenosis, etc.

↓

Increased pressure on right side of heart

↓

Systemic venous congestion

↓

Liver: Dilatation of central veins of liver. Transmission of increased venous pressure to the sinusoids

↓

Dilatation of sinusoids→ischemic necrosis of hepatocytes in the centrilobular region

↓

Chronic venous congestion of liver (nutmeg liver)

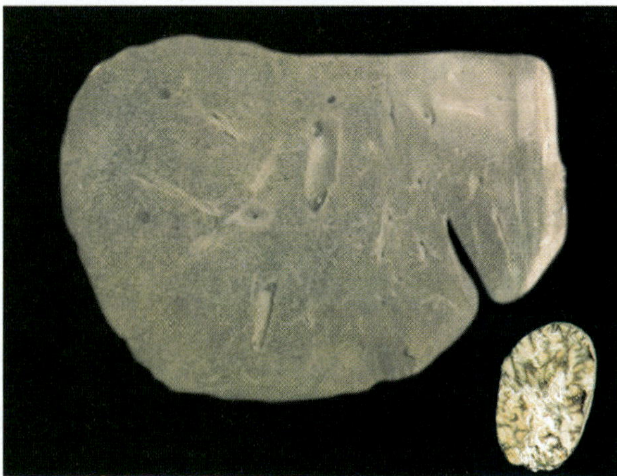

Fig. 5.8: Chronic venous congestion of the liver. The liver shows alternate dark and light areas and resembles the cut surface of a nutmeg (inset).

Congestive Splenomegaly (CVC Spleen)

Q. Write a short note on CVC spleen/congestive splenomegaly.

Congestion and enlargement of the spleen is called congestive splenomegaly.

Causes: Chronic obstruction to the outflow of venous blood from the spleen leads to higher pressure in the splenic vein.

- **Intrahepatic obstruction to blood flow: Cirrhosis of the liver** is the main cause (e.g., alcoholic cirrhosis, pigment cirrhosis).
- **Extrahepatic disorders:**
  - **Systemic or central venous congestion** (e.g., **tricuspid, or pulmonic valvular disease, chronic cor pulmonale, right heart failure, or following left-sided heart failure**). **Splenomegaly is only moderate** and rarely exceeds 500 g in weight.
  - **Obstruction of the extrahepatic portal vein or splenic vein.** It may be due to spontaneous **portal vein thrombosis**, which is usually caused by intrahepatic obstructive disease, or inflammation of the portal vein (pylephlebitis). Thrombosis of the splenic vein can also develop by infiltrating tumors arising in neighboring viscera, such as carcinomas of the stomach or pancreas.

MORPHOLOGY

Gross

Q. Write a short note on Gamna-Gandy bodies.

- Spleen is **enlarged, firm, and tense (Fig. 5.10)**. In long-standing chronic splenic congestion, spleen is **markedly enlarged** (1,000–5,000 g). **The capsule is thickened. The cut section oozes dark blood.**
- Enlarged spleen **may show excessive functional activity** termed **hypersplenism** leads to **hematologic abnormalities (e.g., thrombocytopenia pancytopenia).**

Microscopy (Figs. 5.11A to C)

- **Red pulp:** It shows **dilatation and congestion** in the early stages. Hemorrhage and fibrosis develop in later stages. **Capillarization of sinusoids** may occur, in which sinusoids get converted into capillaries.

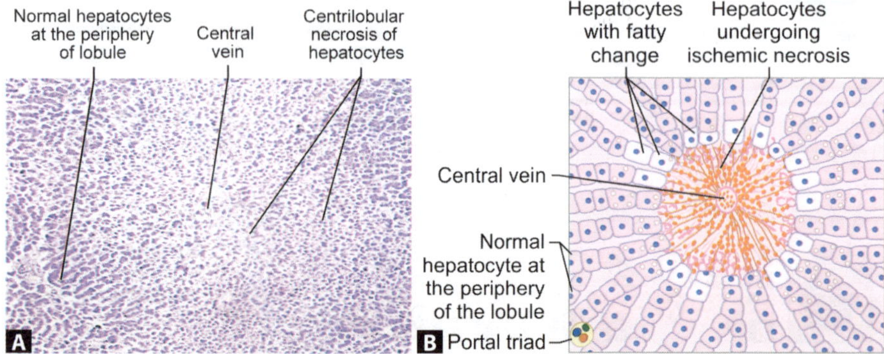

Heart failure cells:

1. Hemosiderin-laden macrophages are known as heart failure cells. The term heart failure does not mean that these are seen in heart failure.
2. Hemosiderin pigment in these cells is stained blue with Prussian blue stain (Perl's stain).
3. Found in lung affected by CVC lung and not in the heart.

Figs. 5.9A and B: Microscopy of chronic venous congestion of the liver: (A) Photomicrograph (H&E); (B) Diagrammatic. It shows centrilobular necrosis with degenerating hepatocytes surrounded by apparently normal hepatic parenchyma in the periportal region.

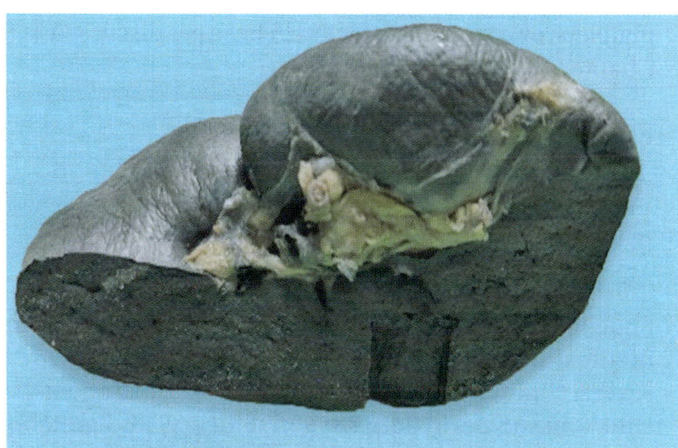

Fig. 5.10: Chronic venous congestion of the spleen shows an enlarged, firm, and tense spleen.

- **Thickened fibrous capsule and trabeculae.**
- **Gamna-Gandy bodies.** May show **Gamna-Gandy bodies (Fig. 5.11C),** which consist of **iron-containing, fibrotic, and calcified foci of old hemorrhage.**
- **Hypersplenism: Slowing of blood flow** from the cords to the sinusoids prolongs the exposure of the blood cells to macrophages in the spleen and leads to **excessive destruction of blood cells (hypersplenism).**

Hemorrhage

PA 6.2c (CC): Define and describe hemorrhage.

Definition: Hemorrhage (bleeding) is defined as the escape or extravasation of blood from vessels.

Etiology: The various causes of hemorrhage are:

1. **Trauma to the vessel wall:** The most common and obvious cause is trauma that **damages the blood vessels,** e.g., penetrating wounds in the heart or great vessels, during labor, etc.
2. **Vascular diseases:**
   - **Rupture of aneurysm:** Severe atherosclerosis may weaken the wall of the aorta (mainly abdominal aorta) and produce permanent abnormal dilatation of vessels called an aneurysm. These aneurysms may rupture and bleed into the retroperitoneal space. Aneurysm may be congenital due to a weak cerebral artery (berry aneurysm) and may rupture and cause subarachnoid hemorrhage.
   - **Inflammatory lesions of the vessel wall:** Infections (e.g., blood vessels traversing a tuberculous cavity in pulmonary tuberculosis of the lung) bleeding from chronic peptic ulcer, typhoid ulcers, polyarteritis nodosa, septicemia.
3. **Neoplastic invasion of vessels:** Invasive neoplasms may erode blood vessels and result in hemorrhage (e.g., hemorrhage following vascular invasion in carcinoma of the tongue).
4. **Hemorrhagic (bleeding) diatheses:** The risk of hemorrhage in these clinical disorders/conditions is increased and usually occurs spontaneously or follows an insignificant injury. There is **defective clot formation.** They have diverse causes, including inherited or acquired defects in vessel walls, platelets, or coagulation factors. Examples include purpura, scurvy, and acute leukemias. Scurvy is associated with capillary fragility and bleeding, due to the defective supporting connective tissue structures.
5. **Raised pressure within the vessels:** It may occur in systemic hypertension causing bleeding (e.g., cerebral and retinal hemorrhage), or high pressure in the veins (e.g., varicose veins legs or esophagus or pulmonary capillaries in chronic venous congestion of lung).

Manifestations: The bleeding may occur **externally** (exterior of the body), **or internally.** Internally blood may accumulate within a tissue (e.g., hematoma) into the serous cavities/body spaces **(Table 5.3)** or a hollow viscus. Hemorrhage may be manifested by different appearances and may have various clinical consequences. Terminology used in bleeding disorders is discussed on page 406.

Clinical significance: The blood loss may be acute (large and sudden), or chronic (small repeated blood loss may occur over some time).

Effects: The effect of hemorrhage ranges from trivial (e.g., bruise) to fatal (e.g., a massive retroperitoneal hematoma resulting from rupture of a dissecting aortic aneurysm).

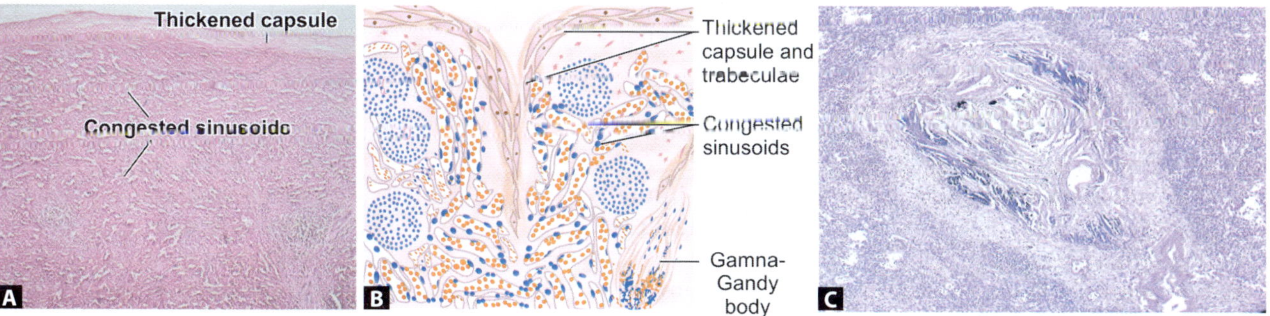

Figs. 5.11A to C: Chronic venous congestion of spleen: (A) H&E; (B) Diagrammatic. Shows thickened capsule, and dilated sinusoids; (C) Gamna-Gandy body.

TABLE 5.3 Terminologies and definition of hemorrhage.

Hemorrhage into various body cavities
• **Hemothorax:** Hemorrhage into the pleural cavity • **Hemopericardium:** Hemorrhage into the pericardial space • **Hemoperitoneum:** Bleeding into the peritoneal cavity • **Hemarthrosis:** Bleeding into a joint space
Hemorrhage in other sites
• **Petechiae:** Pinpoint hemorrhages (1–2 mm in diameter), usually in the skin or conjunctiva. • **Purpura:** Diffuse superficial hemorrhages in the skin They are slightly larger (>3 mm) than petechiae, but <1 cm in diameter. • **Ecchymosis:** A large superficial hemorrhage in the skin. It is larger (1–2 cm) and results from blood escaping through the endothelium into intact subcutaneous tissue. It is **purple at first**, then **turns green, then yellow** before resolving. This sequence of color changes is due to the progressive oxidation of bilirubin released from the hemoglobin of degraded RBCs. A good example of an ecchymosis is a "black eye." • **Hematoma:** Hemorrhage into soft tissue.

The effects of hemorrhage depend upon: (i) the amount (volume) of blood loss, (ii) the speed/rate of blood loss, and (iii) the site of hemorrhage.

- **Amount and the speed of hemorrhage**
  - Acute hemorrhage:
    - A sudden/rapid loss of up to 20% of the blood volume or slow loss of even larger amounts usually has little clinical effects in healthy adults because of compensatory mechanisms.
    - A sudden/acute loss of 33% of blood volume may lead to hypovolemic shock resulting in death.
    - Loss of up to 50% of blood volume gradually over 24 hours may not be fatal.
  - Chronic or recurrent loss of blood:
    - External bleeding: Bleeding into an internal cavity, as in gastrointestinal hemorrhage from a peptic ulcer (arterial hemorrhage) or esophageal varices (venous hemorrhage) or menstrual bleeding frequently leads to iron deficiency anemia due to loss of iron in hemoglobin.
    - Internal bleeding: Iron is efficiently recycled from phagocytosed red cells when the bleeding is internal (e.g., a hematoma). Hence, it does not produce iron deficiency anemia.
  - Jaundice: Extensive hemorrhages can occasionally produce jaundice due to the massive breakdown of red cells and hemoglobin.
- **Site of hemorrhage:** Bleeding may be trivial in the subcutaneous tissues. However, it can cause death if located in the brain.

Hemorrhagic diatheses: The risk of hemorrhage (often after an insignificant injury) is increased in various disorders. These are called *hemorrhagic diatheses*. These disorders may be due to inherited or acquired defects in vessel walls, platelets, or coagulation factors. These are discussed in the Chapter 13.

SHOCK

PA 6.3 (CC): Define and describe the shock, its pathogenesis, and its stages.

Q. Define and classify shock (enumerate the types of shock).

Shock is the most common, important, and very serious medical condition. It is the final common pathway for several clinical events, that are capable of causing death. **In shock, tissue perfusion, oxygen delivery, and metabolic waste removal do not meet tissue demands.** Characteristic features of shock are presented in **Flowchart 5.5.**

Cellular injury: Initially, the cellular injury in shock is reversible. However, prolonged shock in the end leads to irreversible tissue injury and is often fatal.

Definition: Shock is a pathological state in which diminished cardiac output or reduced effective circulating blood volume causes inadequate tissue perfusion (microcirculation) **of vital organs and leads to cellular hypoxia.**

Classification

Q. Classify shock.

Develops as a complication of several events: These events include severe hemorrhage, extensive trauma or burns, large myocardial infarction, massive pulmonary embolism, and severe microbial sepsis. According to etiology (cause), shock can be classified into three major general categories (**Table 5.4**).

Etiology

Q. Describe the etiology and pathogenesis of shock.

Flowchart 5.5: Characteristic features of shock.

Extreme and widespread failure of the circulatory system (either due to decreased cardiac output or reduced effective circulating blood volume)
↓
Systemic hypotension
↓
Life-threatening inadequate/impaired tissue perfusion (hypoperfusion)
↓
Tissue hypoxia
↓
Reversible cellular injury
↓
Irreversible tissue injury and organ failure
↓
Death

TABLE 5.4 Major types of shock.

Types of shock	*Principal mechanisms*	*Clinical example*
Hypovolemic shock	Inadequate blood or plasma or fluid volume	• Massive hemorrhage • Water loss (e.g., vomiting, diarrhea, severe gastroenteritis, massive burns, trauma)
Cardiogenic shock	Failure of the myocardial pump due to intrinsic myocardial damage, extrinsic compression, or obstruction to outflow	Myocardial infarction, ventricular rupture, arrhythmia, cardiac tamponade, pulmonary embolism
Shock associated with systemic inflammation	• Severe microbial infections • Bacterial sepsis • Fungal sepsis • Superantigens (e.g., toxic shock syndrome) • Trauma, burns, pancreatitis	Peripheral vasodilation and pooling of blood; endothelial activation/injury; leukocyte-induced damage; disseminated intravascular coagulation; activation of cytokine cascades
Others		
Neurogenic shock	Result of loss of vascular tone and peripheral pooling of blood	Anesthetic accident or a spinal cord injury
Anaphylactic shock	Acute widespread systemic vasodilation and increased vascular permeability results in tissue hypoperfusion and hypoxia	IgE-mediated hypersensitivity reaction

Q. List the main types of shock with suitable examples.

Hypovolemic Shock

Q. Write a short note on hypovolemic shock.

Hypovolemic shock results from **low cardiac output** due to:

- **Loss of blood** (e.g., **massive hemorrhage**).
- **Loss of plasma** (e.g., **severe burns**).
- **Loss of fluid: Vomiting, diarrhea, severe gastroenteritis,** e.g., cholera.

The pathogenesis of hypovolemic shock is presented in **Flowchart 5.6.**

Cardiogenic Shock

Q. Write a short note on cardiogenic shock.

Cardiogenic shock results from **low cardiac output** due to:

- **Intrinsic myocardial damage** (e.g., **massive myocardial infarction**, ventricular arrhythmias).
- **Extrinsic pressure or compression of the heart** (e.g., **cardiac tamponade**).
- **Obstruction to the outflow of blood from ventricles** (e.g., pulmonary embolism).

The pathogenesis of cardiogenic shock is presented in **Flowchart 5.6.** The left-sided heart failure also reduces the entry of blood from a pulmonary vein into the left atrium. This leads to the movement of fluid from pulmonary

Flowchart 5.6: Pathogenesis of hypovolemic and cardiogenic shock.

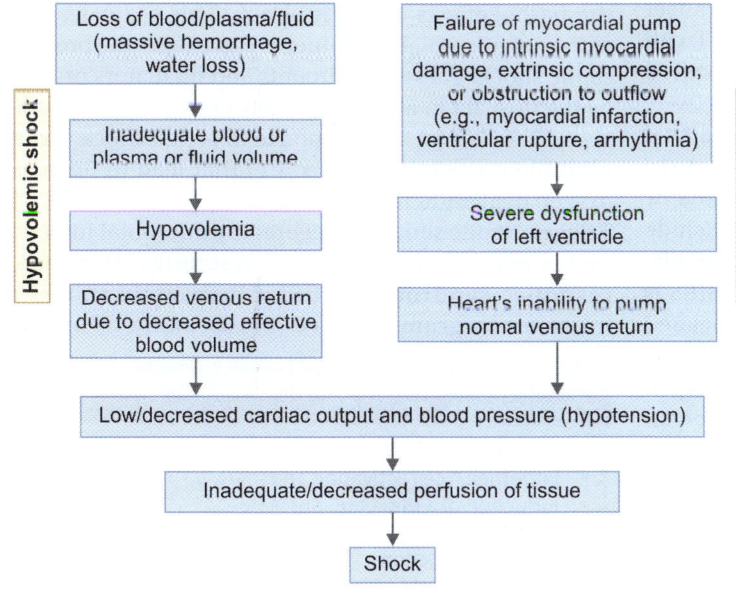

Causes of hypovolemic shock:
- Massive hemorrhage
- Severe burns
- Severe vomiting, diarrhea, severe gastroenteritis

Causes of cardiogenic shock:
- Massive myocardial infarction
- Ventricular arrythmias
- Cardiac tamponade
- Pulmonary embolism

Common sources of infection associated with septic shock: Pneumonia, peritonitis, pyelonephritis, abscess (especially intra-abdominal), primary bacteremia, etc.

vasculature into the pulmonary interstitial space and the alveoli resulting in **pulmonary edema.**

Sepsis, Septic Shock, and the Systemic Inflammatory Response Syndrome

These three conditions are interrelated and somewhat overlapping. The definition of these according to The Third International Consensus Definitions for Sepsis and Septic Shock (2016) is presented below.

Systemic Inflammatory Response Syndrome (SIRS)

Q. Write a short essay on systemic inflammatory response syndrome (SIRS).

Sepsis (disseminated, severe bacterial/microbial infections) **shows large numbers of bacteria and their products in the blood and produces septic shock.** A **syndrome similar to septic shock may occur as a complication of non-infectious disorders** (non-microbial/sepsis-like conditions), associated with systemic inflammation such as severe burns, trauma, pancreatitis, and other serious conditions.

The massive outpouring of inflammatory mediators from innate and adaptive immune cells: In both the septic (infectious) and non-infectious (SIRS) causing shock, there is a massive ***inflammatory reaction***. It stimulates the production of large quantities of inflammatory mediators from innate and adaptive immune cells. It produces **several cytokines, mainly TNF and IL-1** [others IL-6 and platelet-activating factor (PAF)] into the systemic circulation.

Effects of cytokines: Marked blood levels of cytokines produce widespread clinical and pathologic abnormalities. They produce **arterial vasodilation, vascular leakage, and venous blood pooling**. Collectively these reactions are called *systemic inflammatory response syndrome (SIRS)*. Thus, **SIRS** can develop due to septic shock (by microbes) as well as a variety of other non-infectious insults. In cancer patients treated with chimeric antigen receptor T-cell (CAR-T) therapy, a similar iatrogenic syndrome called *cytokine release syndrome* can develop.

Clinical features: SIRS is an exaggerated and generalized manifestation of a local immune or inflammatory reaction. SIRS is a hypermetabolic state characterized by two or more signs of systemic inflammation. These include **fever, tachycardia, tachypnea, leukocytosis, or leukopenia,** in the setting of a known cause of inflammation. SIRS is **often fatal.** The cardiovascular abnormalities associated with SIRS lead to tissue hypoperfusion, cellular hypoxia, and metabolic derangements. These can result in organ dysfunction and, if severe and persistent can cause organ failure and death.

Septic shock: It is **triggered by microbial infections** and is **associated with severe systemic inflammatory response syndrome** (SIRS). In septic shock, clinical SIRS is so severe that it is **associated with organ dysfunction, disseminated**

Flowchart 5.7: Common pathogenic mechanism of septic shock.

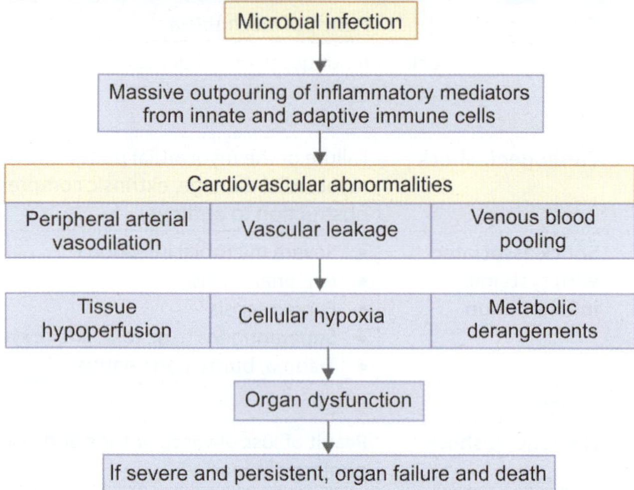

intravascular coagulation, hypotensive shock, and metabolic abnormalities such as insulin resistance and hyperglycemia. If severe and persistent, it may lead to organ failure and death **(Flowchart 5.7).**

Pathogenesis of Septic Shock

Q. Describe the pathogenesis of septic shock.

The incidence of shock is increasing. It is due to improvements in life support for critically ill patients, increased numbers of immunocompromised hosts (as a result of chemotherapy, immunosuppression, advanced age, or human immunodeficiency virus infection), and the increasing number of patients infected with multidrug-resistant organisms in the hospitals. The mortality rate in septic shock is about 50%.

Major Pathogenic Pathways in Septic Shock

Initiation of shock: Diverse microorganisms can initiate the pathogenesis of septic shock. This indicates that a variety of microbial constituents can trigger the process of septic shock. These constituents and mediators produced by the host act in an incompletely known way to produce septic shock. The host response to septic shock involves multiple mechanisms **(Box 5.1)** that lead to decreased oxygen delivery at the tissue level.

Trigger: Septic shock is **triggered by microbial infections and is associated with severe systemic inflammatory response syndrome (SIRS).** Most septic shocks are triggered by **gram-positive** (most common) **or gram-**

BOX 5.1: Major factors contributing to the pathogenesis of septic shock.

- Inflammatory and counter-inflammatory responses
- Endothelial cell activation and injury
- Induction of a procoagulant state
- Metabolic abnormalities
- Organ dysfunction

negative bacteria or fungi. Apart from microbes, SIRS may be triggered by other conditions such as burns, trauma, and/or pancreatitis.

The hallmark of septic shock: Similar to SIRS, in septic shock, there is a **massive outpouring of inflammatory mediators** from innate and adaptive immune cells that produce arterial **vasodilation, vascular leakage, and venous blood pooling.** These cardiovascular abnormalities result in tis**sue hypoperfusion, cellular hypoxia, and metabolic derangements** that lead to organ dysfunction and, if **severe and persistent, organ failure** and death. The **tissue hypoperfusion is** due to a **decrease in peripheral vascular resistance** as a result of **systemic arteriolar vasodilation, vascular leakage,** and **venous pooling of blood in the periphery**. Cardiac output may be normal or even increased in the early stages.

The common pathogenic mechanism of septic shock is presented in **Flowchart 5.7.**

Inflammatory and Counter-inflammatory Responses (Fig. 5.12)

Triggering of proinflammatory responses (reactions)

The proinflammatory responses are directed to eliminate the causative pathogen but are responsible for the organ/ tissue damage in septic shock.

- **Activation of receptors on cells of the innate immune system by microbial cell wall constituents:** In sepsis, several constituents of the microbial cell wall (e.g., bacterial peptides) engage receptors on the cells of the innate immune system. Examples include Toll-like receptors (TLRs) which recognize microbe-derived substances containing "pathogen-associated molecular patterns" (PAMPs), G-protein-coupled receptors that detect bacterial peptides, and C-type lectin receptors (e.g., dectins) that recognize fungal cell wall components.
- **Release of proinflammatory mediators:** The activation of the above-mentioned receptors on cells of the immune system triggers the **production of proinflammatory mediators.** These include:
  - **Cytokines** such as **TNF (tumor necrosis factor), IL-1, IFN (interferon), IL-12,** and **IL-18.** The concept of **"Cytokine storm"** postulated that, in response to an infectious stimulus, there was massive and rapid production of cytokines.
  - **Cytokine-like** mediators such as **high mobility group box 1 protein (HMGB1).**
  - **Elevated levels of markers of acute inflammation.** The inflammatory mediators cause raised levels of markers of acute inflammation such as **C-reactive protein and procalcitonin.** These are useful markers indicative of septic shock.
  - **Production of reactive oxygen species and lipid mediators** [e.g., prostaglandins, platelet-activating factor (PAF)].
- **Consequences of the released proinflammatory effector molecules.** These effector molecules produce the following effects:
  - **Upregulation of adhesion molecule on endothelial cells and further production of cytokine and chemokine**. The effector molecules **activate endothelial cells** (and other cell types) to **upregulate the expression of adhesion molecules**. This in turn **stimulates the production of cytokine and chemokine.**
  - **Activation of complement cascade by microbial components**. This results in the **production of anaphylatoxins (C3a, C5a), chemotactic fragments (C5a), and opsonins (C3b)**. All these products of the activated complement system contribute to the proinflammatory state.
  - **Activation of coagulation by microbial components. It is by** direct activation of factor XII and indirectly through altered endothelial function. This results in widespread activation of thrombin and may further increase inflammation by triggering protease activated receptors on inflammatory cells.

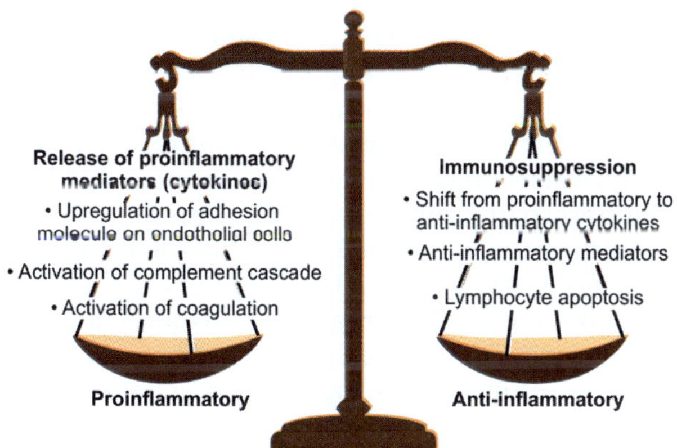

Fig. 5.12: Inflammatory and counter-inflammatory responses in septic shock.

Activation of counterregulatory immunosuppressive mechanisms

After the initial hyperinflammatory state produced by sepsis, inhibitory pathways will become activated. The inhibitory response **activates counter-regulatory immunosuppressive mechanisms**. This may involve both innate and adaptive immune cells. Thus, in a patient with sepsis, there may be an **oscillation between hyperinflammatory and immunosuppressed states** during their clinical course.

Mechanisms for the immune suppression in septic shock: These include an (i) shift from pro-inflammatory (Th1) to anti-inflammatory (Th2) cytokines, (ii) production of anti-inflammatory mediators (e.g., soluble TNF receptor, IL-1 receptor antagonist, and IL-10), (iii) widespread apoptosis

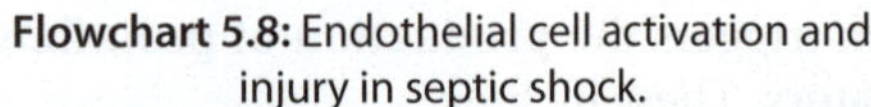

Flowchart 5.8: Endothelial cell activation and injury in septic shock.

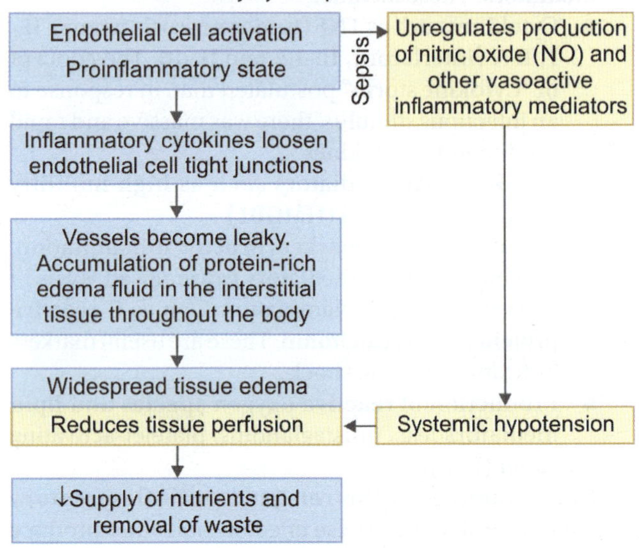

of lymphocytes, and (iv) the immunosuppressive effects of apoptotic cells.

Endothelial Cell Activation and Injury (Flowchart 5.8)

Widespread vascular leakage and tissue edema: In sepsis, the proinflammatory state and endothelial cell activation **upregulate the expression of adhesion molecules.**

- **Edema throughout the body: Loosening of endothelial cell tight junctions by inflammatory cytokines** makes the **vessels leaky throughout the body**. It results in **widespread accumulation of protein-rich fluid in the interstitial tissue**. This leads to tissue edema throughout the body.
- **Edema impairs tissue perfusion:** Edema affects both the supply of nutrients and the removal of waste. This **impairment of tissue perfusion** may be exacerbated by attempts to support the patient with intravenous fluids.

Systemic hypotension: Endothelial activation also **upregulates the production of nitric oxide (NO) and other vasoactive inflammatory mediators** (e.g., C3a, C5a, and PAF). These may cause **relaxation of vascular smooth muscle and produce systemic hypotension**

Induction of a Procoagulant State (Flowchart 5.9)

Sepsis causes the expression of many factors that favor coagulation or a procoagulant state.

Factors activating the coagulation system in sepsis

- **Activation of factor XII** by microbial components such as **endotoxin.**
- **Actions of proinflammatory cytokines (e.g., IL-6) that favor coagulation.**
  - Cytokines **increase the production of tissue factor** by monocytes and possibly endothelial cells.

Flowchart 5.9: Factors activating coagulation system in septic shock.

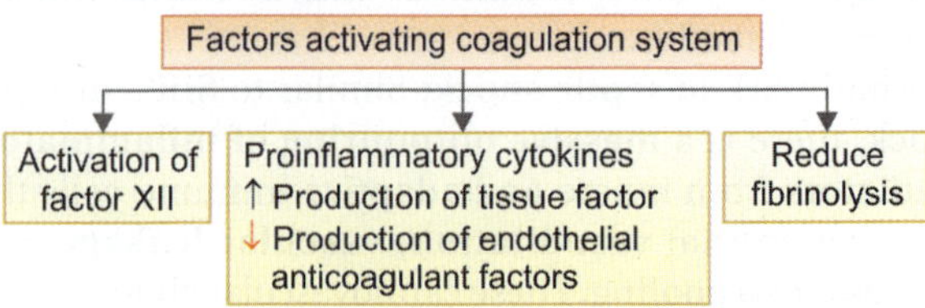

  - **Reduce the production of endothelial anticoagulant factors**, such as tissue factor pathway inhibitors, thrombomodulin, and endothelial protein C receptor.
  - **Reduce fibrinolysis** by **increasing the expression of plasminogen activator inhibitor-1.**

Consequences of activation of coagulation system

- **Diminished clearance of activated coagulation factors:** Vascular **leakage and tissue edema** reduce the flow of blood flow in the small vessels. This causes stasis of blood and reduces the clearing of activated coagulation factors.
- **Systemic activation of thrombin and the deposition of fibrin-rich thrombi in small vessels:** The above factors that favor procoagulant state activate thrombin and the deposition of fibrin-rich thrombi in small vessels, often throughout the body. This further reduces the tissue perfusion. The procoagulant state leads to **dangerous complications namely disseminated intravascular coagulation (DIC)** in about 50% of septic patients. In DIC, there is marked consumption of coagulation factors and platelets that lead to deficiencies of these factors. These patients with DIC develop **bleeding and hemorrhage.**

Metabolic Abnormalities

Patients with severe sepsis develop (i) insulin resistance and hyperglycemia, (ii) Decreased glucocorticoid production, and (iii) lactic acidosis.

1. **Insulin resistance and hyperglycemia:** In sepsis, these are **due to the action of proinflammatory cytokines** such as TNF and IL-1, **stress-induced hormones** (e.g., glucagon, growth hormone, and glucocorticoids), and **catecholamines.** These **molecules favor gluconeogenesis.** The proinflammatory cytokines suppress the release of insulin, promote insulin resistance in the liver and other tissues, and impair the surface expression of GLUT-4 (a glucose transporter). **Hyperglycemia decreases neutrophil function,** suppresses its bactericidal activity, and causes increased expression of adhesion molecules on endothelial cells.
2. **Decreased glucocorticoid production:** Initially, there is acute increased glucocorticoid production, and this is later followed by decreased production and functional deficiency of glucocorticoids. This may be

due to the reduced synthetic capacity of intact adrenal glands or adrenal necrosis *(Waterhouse-Friderichsen syndrome)* resulting from disseminated intravascular dissemination.

3. **Lactic acidosis:** Cellular hypoxia and diminished oxidative phosphorylation in sepsis may produce increased production of lactate and lactic acidosis.

Organ Dysfunction

Decrease the supply of oxygen and nutrients to the tissues: These are due to systemic hypotension, interstitial edema, and thrombi in the small vessels.

Mitochondrial damage: Oxidative stress causes damage to the mitochondria and impairs oxygen use.

Decreased contractibility of the myocardium and cardiac output: It is **due to increased levels of cytokines and secondary mediators.**

Adult respiratory distress syndrome: This may develop due to the increased vascular permeability and endothelial injury.

Multiorgan failure: Finally, the above factors lead to the failure of multiple organs, mainly the **kidneys, liver, lungs,** and **heart** resulting in death.

Prognosis: The severity and outcome of septic shock depend on several factors. These include: (i) the extent and virulence of the infection, (ii) the immune status of the host, (iii) the presence of other comorbidities, and (iv) the pattern and level of production of various mediators.

A group of proteins secreted by bacteria called **superantigens** also produce a syndrome similar to septic shock (e.g., *toxic shock syndrome*). Superantigens are polyclonal T-lymphocyte activators. They cause the release of high levels of cytokines. These will produce a variety of clinical features, ranging from a diffuse rash to vasodilation, hypotension, shock, and death.

The summary of various mechanisms involved in the pathogenesis of septic shock is presented in **Figure 5.13.**

Stages of Shock

Q. Describe three different/various stages of shock.

Shock is a progressive disorder, and if the underlying condition is not treated, it leads to death. Death is usually due to the failure of multiple organs. Stages of shock can be divided into three general phases.

1. **Nonprogressive (compensated/reversible) phase:** During the initial phase, homeostatic compensatory mechanisms **redistribute the blood supply** in such a way that the effective **blood supply to the vital organs is maintained**. This is achieved by neurohumoral

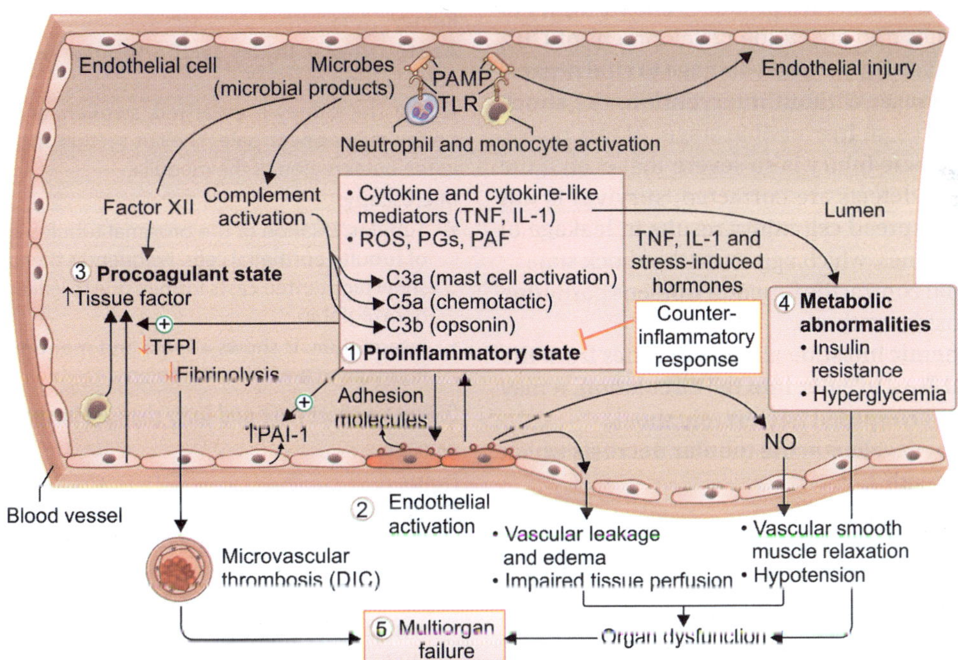

Fig. 5.13: Major pathogenic pathways involved in septic shock. Microbial products activate endothelial cells and cellular and humoral elements of the innate immune system. They initiate a cascade of events that lead to a proinflammatory and procoagulant state. There is activation of the complement system, neutrophils and macrophages, and factor XII. These are accompanied by metabolic changes that if not checked may lead to end-stage multiorgan failure. Major factors contributing to the pathogenesis of septic shock are: (1) Inflammatory and counter-inflammatory responses, (2) Endothelial cell activation and injury, (3) Induction of a procoagulant state, (4) Metabolic abnormalities, and (5) Organ dysfunction.

(DIC: disseminated intravascular coagulation; IL-1: interleukin-1; NO: nitric oxide; PAF: platelet-activating factor; PAI-1: plasminogen activator inhibitor-1; PAMP: pathogen-associated molecular pattern; PGs: prostaglandins; ROS: reactive oxygen species; TFPI: tissue factor pathway inhibitor; TLR: Toll-like receptor; TNF: tumor necrosis factor.)

mechanisms, which try to maintain cardiac output and blood pressure.

Compensatory changes: The neurohumoral mechanism maintains cardiac output and blood pressure. These neurohumoral compensatory changes are as follows:

- **Widespread vasoconstriction** except in vital organs. **Coronary and cerebral vessels** usually **maintain relatively normal blood flow and oxygen delivery**. Thus, blood is shifted from the skin to the vital organs (e.g., heart and brain). Cutaneous vasoconstriction produces the "shocky" skin coolness and pallor of the skin. Initially, septic shock can cause cutaneous vasodilation, and the patient may present with warm, flushed skin.
- **Fluid conservation by the kidney.**
- **Tachycardia.**

2. **Progressive phase: If the underlying causes are not corrected**, shock **passes to the progressive phase**. With worsening circulatory and metabolic derangement. It is characterized by **widespread tissue hypoperfusion** and **hypoxia.** The intracellular aerobic respiration is replaced by **anaerobic glycolysis, increased** production of **lactic acid,** metabolic **lactic acidosis, and** decreased tissue **pH.** This produces dilatation of arterioles, peripheral **pooling of blood into the microcirculation, and decreases** the **cardiac output. This in turn** produces **anoxic injury** to endothelial cells and favors the development of **DIC,** widespread tissue hypoxia, and **damage to vital organs.**
3. **Irreversible phase: Without intervention, the shock eventually** enters an **irreversible stage.** At this phase, **cellular and tissue injury is so severe** that even if the hemodynamic defects are corrected, **survival is not possible.** Widespread cell injury results in leakage of lysosomal enzymes, which aggravate the shock state.
   - **Myocardial contractile function worsens** partly due to nitric oxide synthesis.
   - If the **ischemic intestine allows microbes from the intestinal flora to enter into the circulation,** it may lead to **superimposed bacteremic shock.**
   - The patient develops **acute tubular necrosis** which results in death.

MORPHOLOGY (TABLE 5.5)

Q. Describe the morphological changes in various organs in shock.

Changes in Cardiogenic or Hypovolemic Shock

These are mainly due to hypoxic injury. Morphological changes are particularly evident in adrenals, kidneys, lungs, brain, heart, and gastrointestinal tract. **Fibrin thrombi** may develop in any tissue but is most commonly visualized in kidney glomeruli.

Adrenal

- **Lipid depletion in the cortical cell:** It is due to the conversion of the relatively inactive vacuolated cells to metabolically active cells. The active cells utilize stored lipids for the synthesis of steroids.

TABLE 5.5 Summary of main morphological features of shock.

Organ	*Changes*
Adrenal	Lipid depletion in the cortical cells
Kidney	Acute tubular necrosis (ATN)/acute renal failure
Lungs	Relatively resistant to hypoxic injury. However, septic shock shows diffuse alveolar damage (shock lung) with a hyaline membrane
Heart	Coagulative necrosis and contraction band necrosis
Liver	Congestion and necrosis of the centrilobular region of the liver
Brain	Encephalopathy (ischemic or septic) and cortical necrosis
Gastrointestinal tract	• Diffuse gastrointestinal hemorrhage • Erosions of the gastric mucosa and superficial ischemic necrosis in the intestine

- **Focal hemorrhage:** It occurs in the inner cortex of the adrenal in **severe** shock.
- **Massive hemorrhagic necrosis** of the entire adrenal gland is found in the Waterhouse–Friderichsen **syndrome**, which is **associated with severe meningococcal septicemia.**

Q. Write a short note on renal changes in shock.

Kidney

Acute tubular injury (acute tubular necrosis) is a major complication of shock.

Gross: The kidney is **enlarged, swollen**, and **congested.** The **cortex may appear pale.** The cut section shows blood pooling in the outer region of the medulla.

Microscopy:

- **Tubules:** Dilation of the proximal tubules and **focal necrosis of tubular epithelial cells.** Frequently, the tubular lumen may show **pigmented casts** formed due to leakage of hemoglobin or myoglobin.
- **Interstitium:** It shows **edema** and **mononuclear cells** in the interstitium and within tubules.

Q. Write a short note and lung changes in shock/diffuse alveolar damage.

Lungs

- Lungs are relatively resistant to hypoxic injury and are usually not affected in pure hypovolemic shock.
- However, when shock is due to bacterial sepsis or trauma, it shows **diffuse alveolar damage** which can lead to acute respiratory distress syndrome (ARDS), also known as shock lung.

Gross: The lung is **firm and congested. The cut surface** shows **oozing out** of **frothy fluid.**

Microscopy:

- **Edema:** It first develops around peribronchial **interstitial** connective tissue and later in the **alveoli.**
- **Necrosis:** Endothelial and alveolar epithelial cells undergo necrosis which leads to the formation of **intravascular microthrombi.**

- **Hyaline membrane:** It is usually seen lining the alveolar surface. It may also line alveolar ducts and terminal bronchioles.

Heart

Gross: It shows **petechial hemorrhages** in the epicardium and endocardium.

Microscopy: **Necrosis** of the myocardium is seen which may range from minute focus to large areas of necrosis. Prominent **contraction bands** are seen by light microscopy.

Liver

Gross: Liver is enlarged. The cut section shows a **mottled** (blotched) appearance due to the marked pooling of blood in the centrilobular region.

Microscopy: The centrilobular region of the liver shows **congestion and necrosis.**

Brain

Encephalopathy (ischemic or septic) and cortical necrosis.

Gastrointestinal Tract

Shock produces **diffuse gastrointestinal hemorrhage. Erosions of the gastric mucosa** and superficial **ischemic necrosis** in the intestine lead to gastrointestinal bleeding.

Changes in Septic Shock

- Septic shock can lead to **DIC** which is characterized by the **widespread** formation of fibrin rich **microthrombi**, particularly in the brain, heart, lungs, kidney, adrenal glands, and gastrointestinal tract.
- The utilization of platelets and coagulation factors in DIC produces **bleeding manifestations.** It may show **petechial hemorrhages** on the serosal surface and the skin.

Clinical Consequences

The clinical features of shock depend on the cause.

- **Hypovolemic and cardiogenic shock:** Usually present with features of hypotension and hypoperfusion. The features include **altered sensorium, cyanosis, oliguria, weak rapid pulse, tachypnea**, and **cool, clammy extremities.**
- **Septic shock:** The **skin initially may be warm and flushed** because of peripheral vasodilation.

The initial underlying cause that precipitated the shock may be life-threatening (e.g., myocardial infarction, severe hemorrhage, or sepsis). Later, the organ dysfunction involving **cardiac, cerebral, and pulmonary** function worsens the situation. The **electrolyte disturbances and metabolic acidosis** may further exacerbate the situation.

Patients who survive the initial complications may develop **renal insufficiency** characterized by a progressive decrease in urine output and severe fluid and electrolyte imbalances.

Prognosis

The prognosis depends on the cause and duration of the shock. Patients with hypovolemic shock may survive with appropriate management. Septic shock, or cardiogenic shock associated with massive myocardial infarction, usually has a high mortality rate.

HEMOSTASIS AND THROMBOSIS

PA 6.4a (CC): Define and describe normal hemostasis.

Hemostasis: It is a well-regulated physiological process by which blood is maintained in a liquid state inside the vessels, yet arrests bleeding at the site of vascular injury by forming a hemostatic clot.

Thrombosis: It is the pathologic counterpart of hemostasis. It is characterized by the formation of a clot (a thrombus) within vessels that have been damaged by a disease process.

Normal Hemostasis

Hemostasis is a **precisely well-regulated process that occurs at the site of traumatic vascular injury**. It leads to the formation of a blood clot, which serves to prevent or limit the extent of bleeding. **Hemostasis involves (i) platelets, (ii) clotting** (coagulation) **factors, and (iii) endothelium** of blood vessels.

Steps in Hemostasis

Hemostasis is initiated to arrest hemorrhage in response to vascular damage (injury) by forming a blood clot. It includes several sequences of events at a site of vascular injury (**Figs. 5.14A to D**).

Normally, blood vessels are lined by a smooth, non-thrombogenic endothelium. **Injury to the endothelium** causes transient vasoconstriction and **exposes highly thrombogenic subendothelial extracellular matrix** (ECM), **initiating platelet events.** These events form a hemostatic plug and prevent or limit any further hemorrhage at the site of vascular injury. The general sequence of events of hemostasis at a site of vascular injury is as follows:

Arteriolar Vasoconstriction

It occurs immediately after vascular injury and markedly reduces the flow of blood to the injured site. This vasoconstriction is transient and bleeding may resume if there is no activation of platelets and coagulation factors.

Mechanism: It is mediated by **reflex neurogenic mechanisms** and enhanced by the local secretion of factors such as **endothelin** (a powerful endothelium-derived vasoconstrictor).

Primary Hemostatic Plug

Platelets play an important role in hemostasis: Primary hemostasis is the term used for **platelet plug formation at the site of injury** (primary platelet plug). It occurs immediately within seconds of injury. It initially seals vascular defects and is **responsible for the arrest of bleeding from microvasculature.** A platelet plug provides a surface that binds and concentrates activated coagulation factors.

Mechanism: Damage or disruption of the endothelium lining the blood vessels after a traumatic vascular injury,

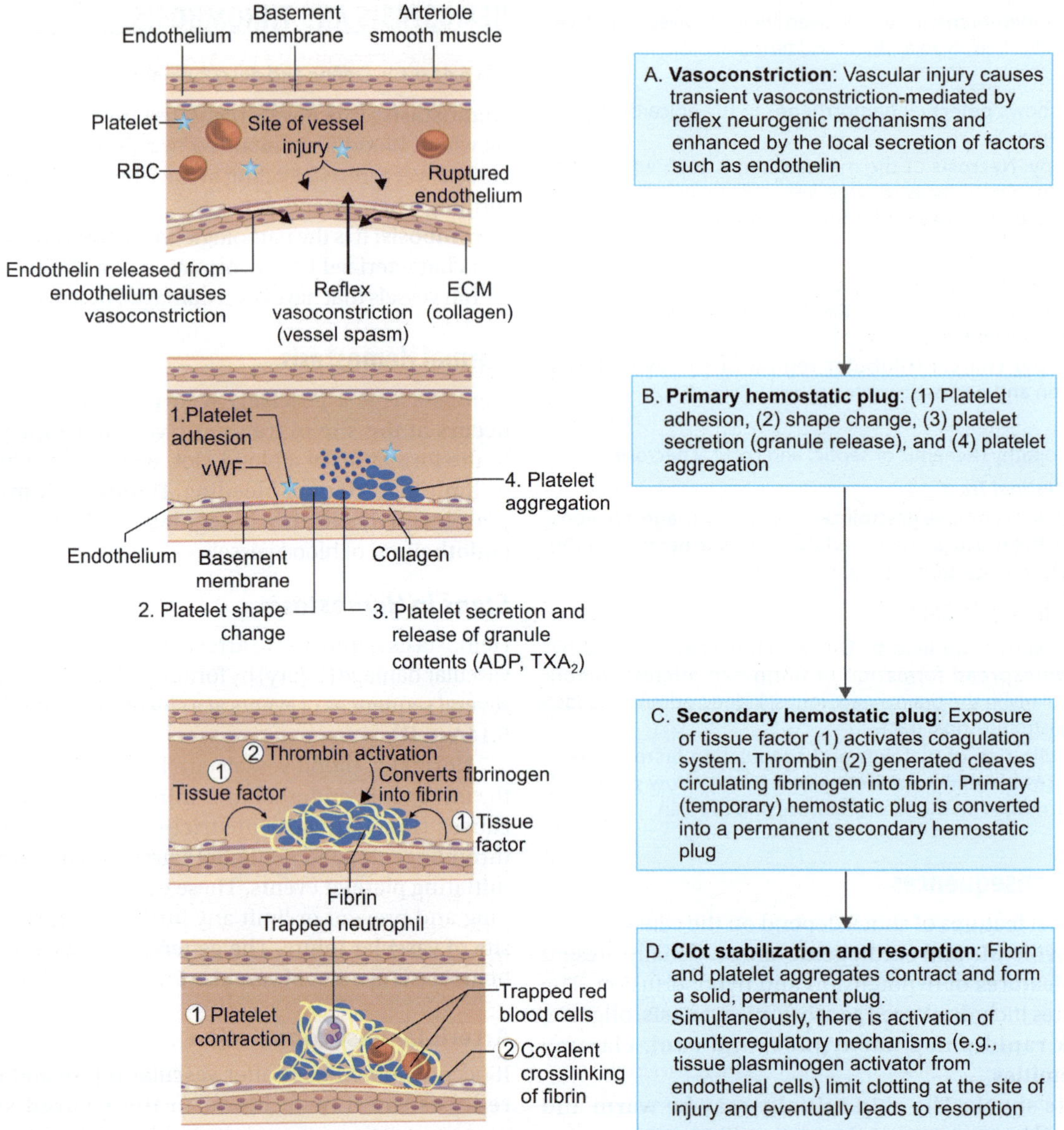

Figs. 5.14A to D: Different steps in hemostasis.

exposes subendothelial connective tissue, such as collagen. The collagen binds to the von Willebrand factor (vWF). vWF promotes platelet adherence and activation. These lead to the formation of a platelet plug. Primary hemostasis involves three steps: **Platelet adhesion and shape change, platelet secretion (granule release), and platelet aggregation.**

Platelet adhesion and shape change

- **Platelet adhesion at the site of vascular injury:** The initial step is the **adhesion of platelets** to subendothelial structures at the site of injury. The link between the surface of the platelet with exposed subendothelial collagen is brought out by the **von Willebrand factor.** vWF is synthesized by both endothelial cells and megakaryocytes (α-granules of platelets).
- **Platelet shape change:** Following the adhesion of platelets to the subendothelial region, there is a dramatic change in the shape of platelets. Platelets change their shape from round to spherical smooth discs to spiky "sea urchins" (animals that are typically small, spiny, and round) with protrusions, thereby markedly increasing the surface area. This change in the shape of the platelet is accompanied by **increased affinity for fibrinogen and** the **formation of coagulation factor complexes**.

Platelet secretion (release reaction), activation, and recruitment

Soon the platelets **release granule contents.** The processes of shape change along with the release of granule content are together known as **platelet activation.** Platelet activation is brought out by several factors, including the coagulation factor **thrombin and ADP**.

Platelet aggregation

Platelet aggregation (clumping together) follows platelet activation. The secreted products of platelets recruit additional platelets and cause platelet aggregation (i.e., bridging/adhesion of adjacent platelets). This process is mediated by fibrinogen which acts as an intercellular bridge between adjacent platelets. Activated platelets also produce the prostaglandin called thromboxane A_2 (TxA_2) which induces strong aggregation of platelets. These clumps of platelets formed quickly (within 3–7 minutes) stop bleeding from the site of injury and are known as **primary hemostatic plugs.** The process of primary hemostatic plug formation is termed **primary hemostasis.**

Secondary Hemostatic Plug

It is characterized by the deposition of fibrin at the site of vascular injury. This process takes an average of 3–10 minutes.

Exposure of tissue factor at the site of injury: Tissue factor binds and activates factor VII. This in turn activates a cascade of reactions that **generates thrombin**. Thrombin is a potent activator of platelets and causes additional platelet aggregation (of primary hemostatic plug) at the site of injury. The initial platelet aggregation is reversible. However, concurrent activation of thrombin stabilizes the platelet plug by causing further activation and aggregation which in turn promotes irreversible contraction of platelets. **Thrombin cleaves circulating fibrinogen into insoluble fibrin, thereby forming a fibrin meshwork at the site of vascular injury.** The platelets contract, and form an irreversibly fused mass. The fibrin formed from fibrinogen cements the platelets and produces a definitive secondary hemostatic plug. The red cells and leukocytes also get trapped in the fibrin meshwork and are found in hemostatic plugs. The process of conversion of the initial temporary primary hemostatic (platelet) plug into a permanent secondary hemostatic plug is known as **secondary hemostasis.**

The solid permanent plug so formed **prevents any further hemorrhage.** The hemostatic plugs/clots thus formed are confined to the site of injury by the fibrinolytic system. Subsequently, vascular repair is accomplished by thrombolysis and recanalization of the occluded site.

Clot Stabilization and Resorption

Polymerized [large number of units (monomers) bonded together] fibrin and platelet aggregates contract and form a solid, **permanent plug.** This prevents further hemorrhage. Simultaneously, there is activation of counter-regulatory mechanisms [e.g., tissue plasminogen activator (t-PA) released from endothelial cells] which limit clotting at the site of injury and eventually lead to resorption and tissue repair.

Failure of the hemostatic system to restore the integrity of an injured vessel causes bleeding. The inability to maintain the fluidity of blood results in thrombosis.

Functions of Normal Endothelium

Endothelial cells play an important role in both homeostasis and thrombus formation. They have both antithrombotic and prothrombotic (procoagulant) properties. The balance between these two opposing endothelial properties determines the thrombus formation. Ultrastructurally, endothelial cells contain Weibel Palade bodies.

Antithrombotic Properties (Fig. 5.15A)

Q. Write a short note on the antithrombotic properties of endothelium.

Normally, the endothelial cells have antiplatelet, anticoagulant, and fibrinolytic properties which prevent thrombosis (and also coagulation) **(Figs. 5.15A and B)**. These factors act together to prevent thrombosis and to limit clotting to sites of vascular damage. The antithrombotic properties of the endothelium can be divided into types of activities that are directed at (i) platelets, (ii) coagulation factors, and (iii) fibrinolysis.

Platelet Inhibitory Effects

Platelet inhibitory effects prevent platelet adhesion and aggregation by the following mechanisms:

Intact endothelium prevents THE adhesion of platelets (and plasma coagulation factors) to the highly thrombogenic subendothelial extracellular matrix (ECM).

Production of inhibitors of platelet aggregation by endothelial cells. Normal endothelium releases many factors that inhibit platelet activation and aggregation. The most important factors include **prostacyclin** (PGI_2), **nitric oxide (NO),** and **adenosine diphosphatase** (which degrades adenosine diphosphate—ADP).

Endothelial cells bind thrombin and inhibit thrombin's ability to activate platelets.

Anticoagulant Effects

Normal endothelium acts as a barrier. It protects the interaction of coagulation factors in the circulation with the tissue factor in vessel walls. Thereby it prevents coagulation. The endothelium expresses multiple factors that inhibit coagulation. These are as follows:

- **Thrombomodulin and endothelial protein C receptor: Thrombomodulin** present on the endothelial cells binds to thrombin **and endothelial protein C receptors on endothelial cells bind to protein C.** They form a complex on the endothelial surface. When thrombin is bound in this complex, it loses its ability to activate coagulation factors and platelets. Instead thrombin cleaves and activates protein C (a vitamin K–K-dependent protease) that requires a cofactor, protein S. Activated protein C/protein S complex is a powerful inhibitor of coagulation cofactors Va and VIIIa.

- **Heparin-like molecules:** They are found on the surface of the endothelium. They bind and activate **antithrombin III**. This in turn inhibits thrombin and factors IXa, Xa, XIa, and XIIa. Heparin and related drugs exert their anticoagulant effect by stimulating antithrombin III activity.
- **Tissue factor pathway inhibitor (TFPI):** Like protein C, TFPI requires protein S as a cofactor. TFPI binds and inhibits tissue factor/factor VIIa and prevents coagulation.

Fibrinolytic Effects

Normal endothelial cells synthesize tissue-type plasminogen activator (*t-PA*). It is a key component involved in fibrinolysis which degrades a thrombi whenever it is formed.

Prothrombotic Properties (Fig. 5.15B)

Q. Write a short note on the prothrombotic properties of the endothelium.

Endothelial cells may be damaged or activated in several ways. These include trauma, inflammation, infectious agents, hemodynamic forces, plasma mediators, and cytokines. The damaged or activated endothelial cells promote a prothrombotic state by its platelet, procoagulant, and antifibrinolytic effects.

Platelet-activating Effect

Endothelial damage exposes the subendothelial thrombogenic ECM and allows the adhesion of platelets from circulation to ECM. *von Willebrand factor (vWF)* produced by normal endothelial cells is an essential cofactor that helps platelet binding to matrix elements.

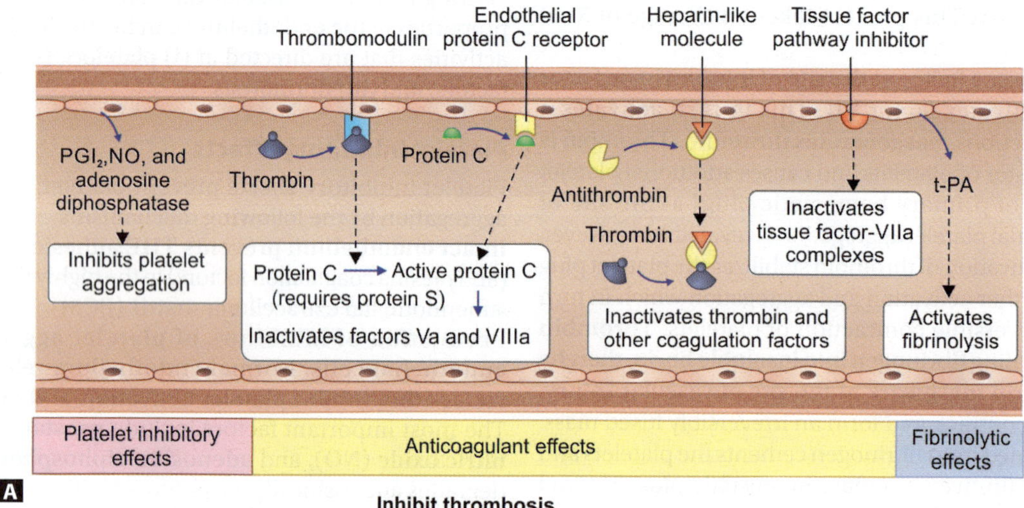

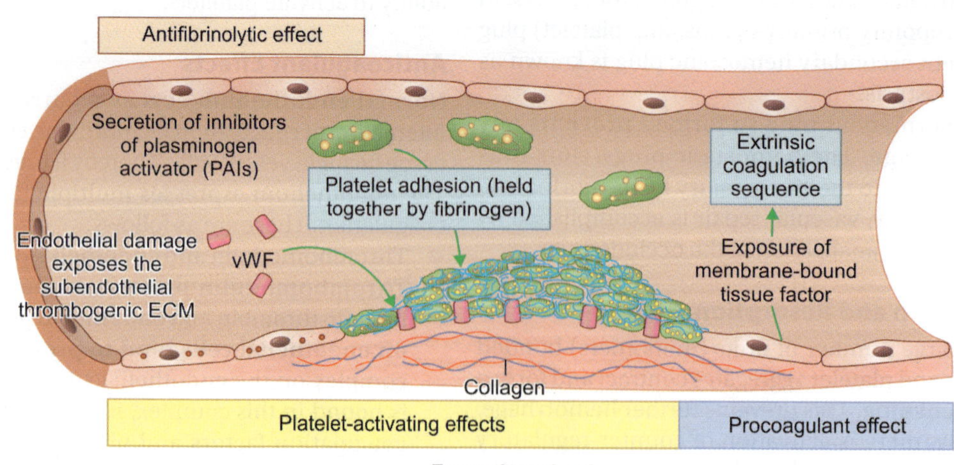

Figs. 5.15A and B: Endothelial factors that inhibit thrombosis (A), and that favor thrombosis (B).
(ECM: extracellular matrix; NO: nitric oxide; PGI2: prostacyclin; t-PA: tissue plasminogen activator; vWF: von Willebrand factor)

Procoagulant Effect

Endothelial cells synthesize tissue factors in response to cytokines [e.g., tumor necrosis factor (TNF) or interleukin-1 (IL-1)] or bacterial endotoxin. Tissue factor activates the extrinsic coagulation cascade. Activated endothelial cells increase the catalytic function of activated coagulation factors IXa and Xa.

Antifibrinolytic Effect

Endothelial cells secrete inhibitors of plasminogen activators (PAIs). They reduce fibrinolysis and tend to favor thrombosis.

Antithrombotic and prothrombotic properties of the endothelium are listed in **Table 5.6.**

TABLE 5.6 Antithrombotic and prothrombotic properties of endothelium.

*Antithrombotic properties (refer **Fig. 5.15A**)*	*Prothrombotic properties (refer **Fig. 5.15B**)*
Platelet inhibitory effects • Intact endothelium prevents adhesion of platelets • Acts as a barrier between platelets and subendothelial thrombogenic ECM • Produce inhibitors of platelet aggregation (e.g., PGI_2, NO, and adenosine diphosphatase)	**Platelet-activating effects** • Endothelial damage exposes the subendothelial thrombogenic ECM (extra-cellular matrix) • *von Willebrand factor (vWF)* produced by normal endothelial cells helps platelet binding to ECM
Anticoagulant effects • Heparin-like molecules • Thrombomodulin • Tissue factor pathway inhibitor (TFPI)	**Procoagulant effects** • Synthesis of tissue factor that activates the extrinsic coagulation cascade • Activated endothelial cells increase the catalytic function of factors IXa and Xa
The fibrinolytic effect through tissue-type plasminogen activator (tPA). It converts plasminogen to plasmin that cleaves fibrin	**Antifibrinolytic effects** through secretion of inhibitors of plasminogen activators (PAIs) which reduce fibrinolysis

THROMBOSIS

PA 6.4b (CC): Define and describe the etiopathogenesis and consequences of thrombosis.

Q. Define thrombus and describe the etiopathogenetic of thrombus.

Definition: Thrombosis (plural thromboses) is defined as the **process of formation of a solid mass in the circulating blood from the constituents of flowing blood.**

The **solid mass formed is called a thrombus (plural, thrombi).** It consists of an aggregate of coagulated blood containing platelets, fibrin, and trapped cellular elements of blood within a vascular lumen.

Etiology

Q. What is Virchow's triad? List its components.

Virchow's triad (Box 5.2 and Fig. 5.16). Three primary abnormalities can lead to the formation of a thrombus and constitute Virchow's triad.

Endothelial Injury (Changes in the Vessel Wall)

Normally, high blood flow rates in the heart and arterial circulation prevent the adhesion of platelets to the endocardium/endothelium and wash out any activated coagulation factors. **Endothelial injury** is important for the formation of a thrombus in the **heart or the arterial circulation**. The endothelial cell injury **promotes the adhesion of platelets at the site of injury and almost surely forms a thrombus in the heart or artery.** Endothelial injury may be either physical damage or endothelial activation (dysfunction).

Causes

Thrombus can occur in the heart, arterial and venous circulation. The triggers for arterial and venous thromboses tend to be different, but they share common risk factors. **Thrombi in the heart:** They develop **within the chambers of the heart on the endocardium.** The mural thrombosis (i.e., a thrombus adhering to the underlying cardiac wall). In the

BOX 5.2: Constituents of Virchow's triad.

1. **Endothelial injury** (changes in the vessel wall).
2. **Alteration in normal blood flow** (changes in the blood flow).
3. **Hypercoagulability of the blood** (changes in the blood itself).

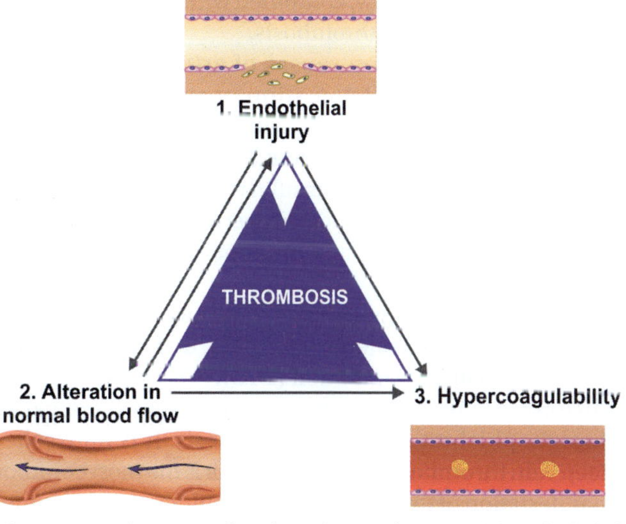

Fig. 5.16: Virchow's triad in thrombosis. These are (1) endothelial injury (the most important factor), (2) alteration in blood flow (stasis or turbulence), and (3) hypercoagulability.

heart, endocardial injury, especially when associated with changes in blood flow may cause a thrombus. Conditions in which mural thrombosis occurs include:

- **Myocardial infarction:** Mural thrombi occur **over areas of infarcted myocardium** with damage to the adjacent endocardium. They adhere to the left ventricular wall. The predisposition to thrombus formation is due to the **injured endocardium** and the altered blood flow in the segment of the myocardium affected by infarct. Thrombi may also develop following **catheter trauma**.
- **Atrial fibrillation:** Irregular atrial activity in atrial fibrillation **halts the atrial blood flow** and facilitates the formation of a mural thrombus, usually in the **left atrial appendage**.
- **Cardiomyopathy:** It may be associated with mural thrombi in the left ventricle.
- **Endocarditis: Small thrombi on the cardiac valves are called vegetations.** These thrombi develop on valves, usually mitral or aortic, that are damaged by bacterial infection (**bacterial endocarditis**) or inflammation (e.g., **Libman–Sacks endocarditis** in systemic lupus erythematosus). **Nonbacterial thrombotic endocarditis** are small, sterile thrombi (vegetations) on noninfected valve leaflets. They occur in chronic wasting states, such as advanced cancer, possibly reflecting a hypercoagulable state. Vegetations may also develop on **damaged valves** (e.g., due to rheumatic heart disease, or congenital heart disease).

Thrombosis in the arterial system: Conditions in which thrombosis occurs include:

- **Atherosclerosis: Ulcerated** atherosclerotic **plaque** is the **most common cause of arterial thrombus.** It most often affects atherosclerosis involving the **coronary, cerebral, mesenteric, and renal arteries, and arteries of the legs.** Thrombi are common in **aortic aneurysms,** in which the turbulent blood flow, combined with intrinsic vascular disease, promotes thrombosis.
- **Other less common causes of arterial thrombosis:** These include inflammation of arteries (arteritis), trauma, and blood disorders. Risk factors for thrombosis include metabolic syndrome, which typically includes obesity, hyperglycemia, insulin resistance, dyslipidemia and hypertension; advanced age; tobacco use; previous thrombosis; cancer; and immobilization after surgery or leg casting.
- **Capillaries:** Thrombi in capillaries may occur with **acute inflammatory lesions**, vasculitis, and **disseminated intravascular coagulation (DIC).**

Thrombosis in the venous system: It was once called thrombophlebitis or phlebothrombosis. It is now called **deep vein thrombosis** (DVT) because it is the most common manifestation of this disorder. It is a multifactorial disorder.

Mechanism of thrombi due to endothelial injury: Endothelial damage with loss of endothelium **exposes thrombogenic subendothelial ECM. Platelets adhere** to the site of endothelial injury and **release prothrombotic tissue factors.** There is a local depletion of antithrombotic factors like PGI_2. Severe endothelial injury may cause thrombus formation by exposing vWF and tissue factors.

Endothelial Activation or Dysfunction

A thrombus can develop without any physical disruption of the endothelium. Endothelial cells can respond to various stimuli (e.g., inflammation and other noxious stimuli) and also favor the formation of thrombus. The endothelium can adjust its steady-state (constitutive) functions and express newly acquired (inducible) properties. This is by **shifting the pattern of gene expression in endothelium to one that is both proinflammatory and prothrombotic.** This process (change) is referred to as endothelial activation or dysfunction.

Causes: Inducers of endothelial activation include **physical injury, infectious agents, turbulent** (abnormal) **blood flow, cytokines,** and other inflammatory mediators, metabolic abnormalities (such as hypercholesterolemia or homocysteinemia), and toxins absorbed from cigarette smoke.

Mechanism: Endothelial dysfunction can **disturb the balance between prothrombotic** and **antithrombotic activities of endothelium by:**

- **Procoagulant changes:** Activated endothelial cells downregulate the expression of coagulation inhibitors (e.g., thrombomodulin, endothelial protein C receptor), and tissue factor protein inhibitors. It also increases the expression of tissue factor
- **Antifibrinolytic effects:** Activated endothelial cells secrete plasminogen activator inhibitors (PAIs). They prevent fibrinolysis and downregulate the activity of t-PA and urokinase. These changes favor the development of thrombi.

Alterations in Normal Blood Flow

Normally, blood flows through a blood vessel in layers and the velocity of the layers varies. This normal blood flow is termed **as laminar (Fig. 5.17).** Blood in the center moves faster than blood in the outer layers. This is because, the

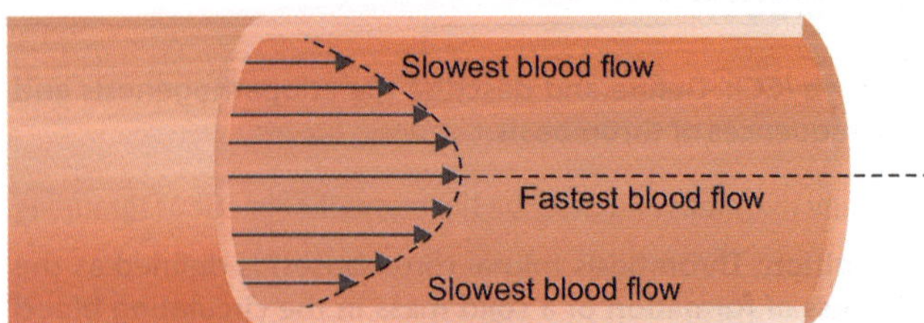

Fig. 5.17: Laminar blood flow in normal vessel. In laminar flow, all the elements of the blood move in streamlines that are parallel to the axis of the blood vessel. The layer of blood in contact with the vessel wall is slow-moving or motionless whereas the maximal velocity is observed in the blood that moves along the axis of the blood vessel.

blood in the center layer is in contact with blood only, whereas the outermost layer is also in contact with the intima of the blood vessel wall, which produces friction against the cellular components (platelets and other cellular elements) of the blood. Many blood cells stick or adhere to the intima from this outer layer because of minimal flow.

Causes

The causes of abnormal blood flow are turbulence and stasis.

Turbulence (disturbed movement of blood). The streamlined laminar flow may be disrupted by normal anatomy and by pathologic processes creating turbulent flow. Turbulent flow is an interruption in the forward current of blood flow by crosswise flow **(Figs. 5.18A and B)**. Turbulence results if **blood flows around an obstruction in the vessel or over a roughened intimal surface** (e.g., atheromatous plaque). **Turbulence contributes to thrombosis in arterial circulation and the heart.**

Stasis: It is a **major cause of venous thrombosis.**

A clinical disorder associated with turbulence and stasis

- **Heart:** (i) **Acute myocardial infarction** results in **focally noncontractile myocardium;** (ii) **arrhythmias/ atrial fibrillation** [e.g., rheumatic mitral stenosis in conjugation with disordered atrial rhythm (atrial fibrillation), it predisposes to mural thrombi in atria]; (iii) **dilated cardiomyopathy.**
- **Arteries: Ulcerated atherosclerotic plaques expose subendothelial ECM** and also cause **tubulance. Aneurysms** cause local stasis.
- **Veins:** Thrombi develop in the saphenous veins with **varicosities** or in deep veins.

Other causes: Hyperviscosity syndromes (e.g., with **polycythemia vera) and RBC disorders** (e.g., **sickle cell anemia)** can cause vascular occlusions and stasis.

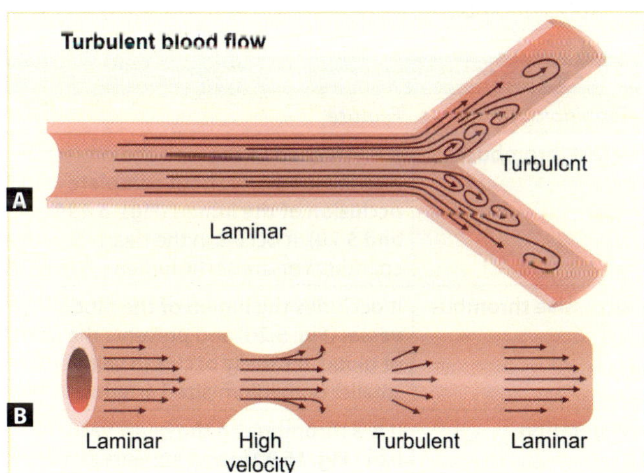

Figs. 5.18A and B: Turbulent flow: (A) At the bifurcation of a blood vessel; (B) Around the obstruction in the vessel.

Mechanism

Stasis and turbulence produce thrombus by the following mechanism:

- **Promote endothelial cell activation** and **increase the procoagulant activity,** partly by flow-induced changes in endothelial gene expression. Turbulent flow **forms countercurrents and local pockets of stasis.**
- **Brings platelets** and leukocytes **into contact with the endothelium.**
- Stasis **slows cleansing and dilution** of **activated clotting factors** and reduces the inflow of clotting factor inhibitors.

Hypercoagulability

Q. Write a short note on the causes of the coagulable state (primary conditions associated with increased risk of thrombosis).

Definition: Hypercoagulability (also known as thrombophilia) is a **systemic disorder associated with an abnormally high tendency to develop a clot/thrombus.**

Causes: Hypercoagulability **is usually caused by alterations in coagulation factors.** It is an **important risk factor for venous thrombosis** and is a less frequent contributor to arterial or intracardiac thrombosis. Disorders that lead to hypercoagulability can be divided into primary (genetic) and secondary (acquired) **(Table 5.7).**

Primary (Inherited) Hypercoagulability

If a young patient (<50 years of age) presents with thrombosis, inherited causes of hypercoagulability should be considered even when acquired risk factors are present. Inherited hypercoagulability is most commonly caused due to mutations in the factor V and prothrombin genes:

- **Factor V mutation:** It is also called the **Leiden** (Dutch city where it was first described) **mutation**. This mutation causes an amino acid substitution in factor V and mutated factor V is resistant to proteolysis by protein C. Thus, there is loss of an important antithrombotic counterregulatory mechanism. Factor V Leiden mutations are associated with an increased risk for **venous thrombosis.**
- **Prothrombin mutation:** A single-nucleotide substitution in the prothrombin gene leads to increased expression of the prothrombin gene. It is associated with an increased risk for **venous thrombosis.**
- **Rare causes:** Less common causes of primary hypercoagulable states include inherited deficiencies of anticoagulants such as antithrombin, protein C, or protein S.

Secondary (Acquired) Hypercoagulability

Secondary causes can be categorized as (i) high-risk, and (ii) elevated risk for thrombosis **(Table 7.2)**.

Factors contributing to acquired hypercoagulability

- **Trauma or cardiac failure: Stasis or vascular injury** is the most important factor.

TABLE 5.7 Major causes of hypercoagulable state.

A. Primary (genetic)
Common: Increased prothrombotic factors
• Factor V mutation: Factor V Leiden (substitution of Arg to Gln in amino acid residue 506; results in resistance to activated protein C)
• Prothrombin mutation (G20210A noncoding sequence variant; results in increased level of prothrombin)
• High levels of factors VIII, IX, XI, or fibrinogen (genetics not known)
Rare: Deficiency of antithrombotic (anticoagulant) factors
• Antithrombin III deficiency
• Protein C deficiency
• Protein S deficiency
Very rare
• Fibrinolysis defects
• Homozygous homocystinuria (deficiency of cystathione β-synthetase
B. Secondary (acquired)
High-risk for thrombosis
• Prolonged bed rest or immobilization
• Myocardial infarction, atrial fibrillation
• Tissue injury (e.g., surgery, fracture, burn)
• Disseminated intravascular coagulation
• Cancer
• Prosthetic cardiac valves
• Heparin-induced thrombocytopenia
• Antiphospholipid antibody syndrome
Elevated risk for thrombosis
• Nephrotic syndrome
• Hyperestrogenic states (pregnancy and postpartum)
• Oral contraceptive use
• Cardiomyopathy
• Smoking
• Sickle cell anemia

- **Oral contraceptive use and pregnancy:** It is associated with **increased hepatic synthesis of coagulation factors and reduced synthesis of antithrombin.**
- **Disseminated cancers:** They may release procoagulant tumor products (e.g., mucin from adenocarcinoma) and predispose to thrombosis.
- **Advancing age:** Increased platelet aggregation and reduced release of PGI_2 from endothelium predisposes to hypercoagulability.
- **Smoking and obesity:** They promote hypercoagulability by unknown mechanisms.

Two clinically significant conditions related to acquired hypercoagulable states are:

1. **Heparin-induced thrombocytopenia (HIT) syndrome:** It develops in up to 5% of patients treated with unfractionated heparin (for therapeutic anticoagulation). Autoantibodies formed in this condition bind complexes of heparin and platelet factor-4 (PF4). It leads to platelet activation, aggregation, and removal from circulation. It leads to a prothrombotic state.
2. **Antiphospholipid antibody syndrome:** This was **previously called the lupus anticoagulant syndrome.** It manifests as recurrent thromboses, repeated miscarriages, cardiac valve vegetations, and thrombocytopenia. In antiphospholipid antibody syndrome, the antibodies bind phospholipids, but the pathologic effects of the antibodies are mediated through binding to epitopes on proteins that interact with phospholipids. The antibodies frequently produce a false-positive serologic test for syphilis because the antigen in the standard assay for syphilis is embedded in the phospholipid cardiolipin.

Terminologies (Table 5.8)

Q. Write a short note on mural thrombi.

Types of thrombi: Thrombi may be **arterial or venous type**. Differences between arterial and venous thrombus are shown in **Table 5.9**.

MORPHOLOGY

Sites: Thrombi can occur anywhere in the cardiovascular system.

- **Arterial and cardiac thrombi:** They arise **at sites of endothelial injury or turbulence.**
  - **Cardiac thrombi** usually occur at sites of turbulence or endocardial injury. More common in the atrial appendages. Can also develop on the **endocardial surface over the site of acute myocardial infarction** (*refer* **Fig. 16.26**).
  - **Valves:** Thrombi on heart valves are called **vegetations** (*refer* **Fig. 16.32A**). They are more common on **mitral or aortic valves.**
  - **Arteries:** The aorta or larger arteries usually develop mural thrombi. Thrombi developing in the medium or smaller arteries are frequently occlusive. They develop (in decreasing order of frequency) in the **coronary, cerebral, and femoral arteries.** Arterial thrombi tend to be **white.**
- **Venous thrombi.** They usually occur at **sites of stasis.** Venous thrombosis (phlebothrombosis) is usually occlusive and forms a long cast of the lumen. They contain more trapped RBCs (and relatively few platelets). They are therefore known as **red or stasis thrombi.**

TABLE 5.8 Terminologies used in thrombi and their features.

Terminology	*Feature*
Mural thrombus	It is **attached to the wall** and projects into the lumen, **without complete occlusion of the lumen (Figs. 5.19B and 5.20).** It occurs in the heart chambers or the aortic lumen.
Occlusive thrombus	It **occludes the lumen of the blood vessel (Fig. 5.20)** and prevents the flow of blood. It usually occurs in veins or smaller or medium-sized arteries.
Vegetation	It is a **thrombus on the heart valve** (*refer* **Fig. 16.32A**) and appears as a polypoid mass projecting into the lumen (e.g., infective endocarditis).

TABLE 5.9 Differences between arterial and venous thrombus.

Characteristics	*Arterial thrombus*	*Venous thrombus*
Main cause	Injury to endothelium	Stasis
Rate of blood flow	Rapid	Slow
Usual type of thrombus	Mural	Occlusive
Common sites	Aorta, coronary, cerebral, and femoral arteries	Superficial varicose veins and deep veins of the leg
Gross		
Color	Gray-white	Red-blue
Lines of Zahn	More prominent	Less prominent
Composition	The friable meshwork of platelets, fibrin, RBCs, and degenerating leukocytes	More trapped RBCs and relatively few platelets
Propagation	Retrograde manner from point of attachment of thrombus (i.e., towards the heart)	In an antegrade manner from the point of attachment towards the direction of blood flow (i.e., towards the heart)
Effects	Ischemia causing infarction of area supplied by the artery containing thrombus	Thromboembolism, edema, and ulceration

Attachment: Thrombi are **attached focally to the intimal surface** of the vessel.

Size and shape: It depends on the site of origin and its cause.

Q. Write briefly on lines of Zahn.

Lines of Zahn

Both **gross and microscopy** of thrombus show **alternating light and dark retracted areas.** The light (pale or white) area consists of pale platelets held together by fibrin. The dark area is rich in red cells. These alternating laminations of light and dark are known as **lines of Zahn (Figs. 5.19A and B).** These lines are only found in thrombi that develop in flowing blood. Hence, they can distinguish antemortem thrombosis from the bland nonlaminated postmortem clots (formed in the postmortem state). Thrombi in the "low-flow" venous system superficially resemble postmortem clots, but usually show ill-defined laminations.

Layers in Thrombus

- **The first** layer of the thrombus on the endothelium/endocardium is a **platelet layer**.
- **On top of the platelet layer, fibrin** is precipitated to **form upstanding laminae** which anastomose to form an intricate structure that **resembles coral** (coralline thrombus). In **between the upstanding laminae** and anastomosing fibrin meshwork, the **red blood cells get trapped. Retraction of fibrin produces a ribbed appearance** on the surface of the thrombus.

Arterial thrombi: They are often occlusive, usually rich in platelets, and most commonly develop on a ruptured atherosclerotic plaque.

Venous thrombi (phlebothrombosis): These thrombi form in the sluggish venous circulation. Therefore, they contain more enmeshed red cells and are termed **red, or stasis, thrombi.** They are invariably occlusive and **form a long cast within the lumen of the vessel.** They often propagate toward the heart and are prone to give **rise to emboli.** They develop most commonly in the veins of the lower extremities (90% of venous thromboses).

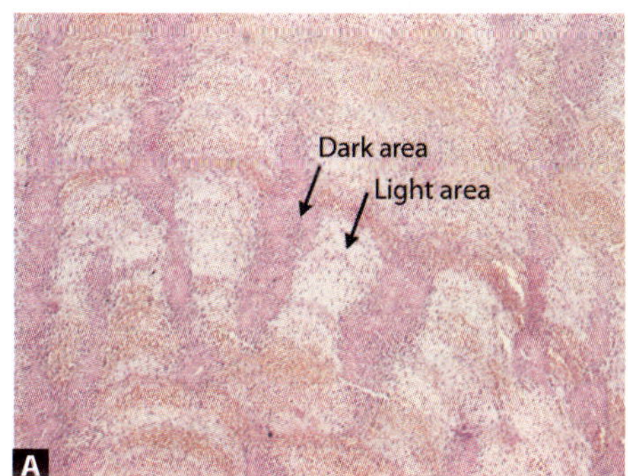

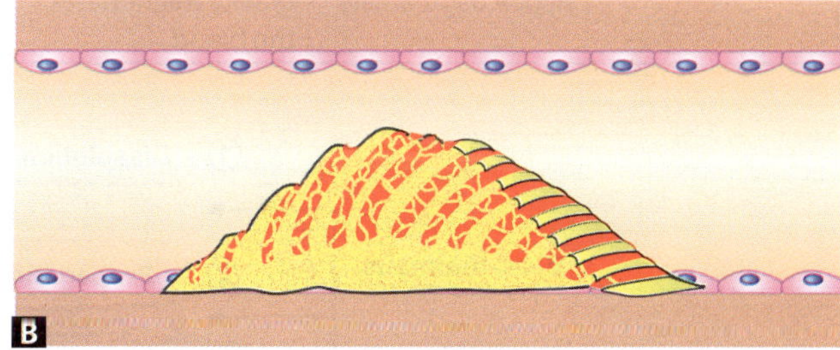

Figs. 5.19A and B: Appearance of thrombus: (A) Microscopic; (B) Diagrammatic showing alternating dark and light areas (lines of Zahn).

Postmortem Clots

Q. Describe the appearance of a postmortem clot.

Thrombus versus clot: A thrombus should be distinguished from a simple blood clot. The **clot is formed due to the activation of coagulation and can form in vitro or postmortem. Hematoma results from hemorrhage and then forms a clot outside the vascular system.** Determination of whether a clot is formed during life (antemortem thrombi) or after death (postmortem clot) is important in a medical autopsy and forensic pathology. Differences between antemortem venous thrombi and postmortem clots are listed in **Table 5.10**. After death, the red blood cells settle and produce two layers.

1. **Lower layer:** It contains **many RBCs**, which have settled by gravity and form a dark red lower portion. This has a **reddish and gelatinous** appearance which resembles **currant jelly**.
2. **Upper layer:** It is **poor in cells and is yellow-white**. It is firm representing coagulated plasma without red blood cells. It is called **chicken fat** because of its color and consistency.

TABLE 5.10 Differences between antemortem venous thrombi and postmortem clots.

Characteristics	*Antemortem venous thrombi*	*Postmortem clots*
Attachment to the underlying vessel wall	Focally attached to the underlying vessel wall	Usually not attached to the underlying vessel wall
Consistency	Dry, granular, firm, and friable	Gelatinous, soft, and rubbery
Shape	May or may not fit the vascular contours	Have the shape of the vessel in which it is found
Appearance	Alternate dark and white areas. They contain gray strands of deposited fibrin	Currant jelly and chicken fat appearance. Because of red cell settling, they have a dark red dependent portion and a yellow "chicken fat" upper portion
Lines of Zahn	Present	Absent
Mechanism	Changes in blood flow (stasis) and hypercoagulability	Occurs in stagnant blood in which gravity fractionates the blood

Fates of Thrombus (Fig. 5.20)

Q. Write a short note on the fate of the thrombus.

1. **Dissolution (lysis) of thrombi without any consequences: Newly formed thrombi may disappear** due to activation of fibrinolysis. This may lead to rapid shrinkage and complete dissolution of thrombi. **Old thrombi** are **more resistant to lysis**. This resistance to lysis has clinical importance, as the administration of fibrinolytic agents (e.g., t-PA in acute coronary thrombosis) is usually not effective unless given within a few hours of thrombus formation.
   If a patient survives an initial thrombotic event, during the following days to weeks the thrombus may undergo some combination of the following processes:
2. **Propagation of thrombi:** It is the **process in which thrombi grow and increase in size**. The thrombus which was initially **mural, may become an occlusive** thrombus. Irrespective of the site, thrombi tend to propagate toward the heart. Thus, **arterial thrombi grow retrograde** (towards the heart) from the point of attachment and **venous thrombi extend in the direction of blood flow** (towards the heart)**.** The propagating portion of a thrombus is usually poorly attached to the vessel wall. Therefore, thrombi are likely **to undergo fragmentation and** migrate through the blood as an **embolus**.

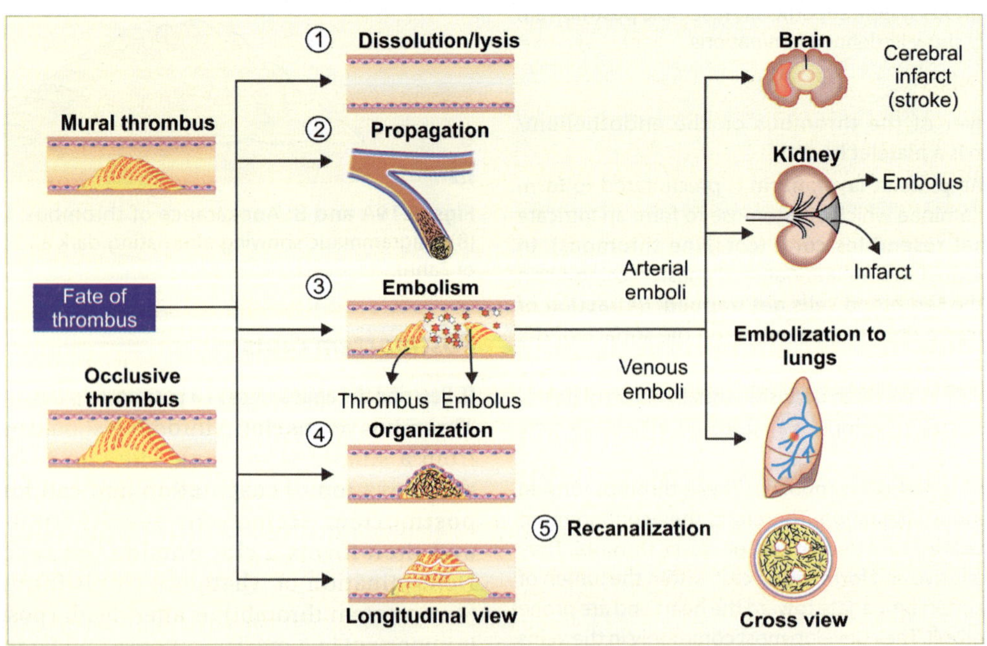

Fig. 5.20: Fate of thrombus.

3. **Embolization:** A portion or all of the thrombus may get detached from its site of origin and form emboli. These emboli can travel to other sites through the circulation and lodge in a blood vessel away from the site of thrombus formation. The **consequences depend on the site of lodgment.** Large venous thrombi may get detached and travel to the pulmonary circulation to the lungs as pulmonary emboli.
4. **Organization:** If thrombi are not dissolved (either spontaneously or by therapy), these older thrombi become organized **by the ingrowth of endothelial cells, smooth muscle cells, and fibroblasts.** Small, organized thrombi may be incorporated into the vessel wall.
5. **Canalization/recanalization:** In time, new capillary channels lined by endothelial cells may form an organized thrombus. These capillary channels may form thoroughfare channels and can re-establish the continuity of the original lumen to a limited extent.
6. **Mycotic aneurysm (*refer* pages 488 and 490):** Rarely, the central region of the thrombi may undergo enzymatic digestion due to lysosomal enzymes released from trapped leukocytes and platelets. If bacteremia develops, these thrombi may become infected and produce an inflammatory mass. This region of the vessel becomes weak and can produce mycotic aneurysm.

Refer **online Venous Thrombosis (Phlebothrombosis) along with Figures 5.21 and 5.22.**

Thrombophlebitis

Inflammation of the wall of the vein (thrombophlebitis) causes damage to the endothelium and **may lead to thrombus formation.** The thrombus formed is firmly attached to the wall of the vein and does not embolize. Sterile inflammation may be produced by direct trauma, chemicals, or ionizing radiation. Bacterial inflammation of veins may be produced in the veins near the infected areas.

Thrombophlebitis migrans (migratory thrombophlebitis or Trousseau syndrome). It is **characterized by recurrent thrombotic episodes** involving the superficial and deep veins, especially of the extremities. May develop as a **complication of deep-seated cancers** such as cancer of the **pancreas (tail and body), lung, stomach, and female genital tract.** First described by Trousseau who had pancreatic cancer, when he noticed it on himself and suggested that it was a **sign of visceral cancer.** It is known as Trousseau's syndrome.

Consequences of Thrombi

Thrombi are clinically important because they **obstruct arteries and veins** and also may **give rise to emboli.** Its consequences depend on the site of the thrombosis and embolization.

Obstruction of involved vessel: Thrombi can obstruct involved arteries and veins.

- **Arterial thrombi:** They may cause **infarctions** in the region supplied by the vessel involved in the thrombus. Occlusion at certain locations (e.g., a coronary artery, and cerebral vessels) can be life-threatening.
- **Venous thrombi:** Small venous thrombi may cause no symptoms. Larger thrombi can cause **congestion and edema in the region distal to obstruction** by thrombus. It predisposes the development of infections and varicose ulcers on the overlying skin. Forced dorsiflexion of the foot produces tenderness in the calf associated with DVT and is known as the **Homan sign.**

Embolization: Arterial, cardiac, and venous thrombi can undergo fragmentation and detach to form emboli. It is the **major complication** and these are thromboemboli. The consequences of an embolism depend on (1) the site of lodgment of emboli, (2) the tissue affected, and (3) the source of thromboemboli.

- **Arterial and cardiac thromboemboli:** The most common sites of lodgment of emboli are the brain, kidneys, and spleen because of their rich blood supply. The various effects are mentioned on page 157-8, (*refer* **Fig. 5.24**).
- **Venous emboli:** They may lodge in the lungs causing various consequences of **pulmonary embolism** (*refer* pages 156-7, and **Fig. 5.23**).

Disseminated intravascular coagulation (DIC): It is widespread thrombosis within the microcirculation. It may be sudden or insidious in onset. DIC occurs in various disorders ranging from obstetric complications to advanced malignancy. DIC is discussed in detail on pages 414-6 in Chapter 13.

EMBOLISM

PA 6.5 (CC): Define and describe embolism and its causes and common types.

Q. Define embolism. Mention the different types of embolism/embolus with examples.

Definition: An embolus is a **detached intravascular solid, liquid, or gaseous mass** that is **transported in the blood to a site distant from its point of origin.** It often causes tissue dysfunction or infarction at the site of lodgement.

Types of Emboli

Q. Mention different types of emboli.

The majority of emboli are derived from the dislodgement of thrombi—hence the term **thromboembolism** (i.e., a thrombi, or part of a thrombi, that is formed at one location and then travels to a distant site). Other less common types of emboli are fat, air or nitrogen, atherosclerotic debris (cholesterol emboli), tumor, or amniotic fluid.

Classification (Table 5.11): Emboli may be classified in different ways.

1. **Depending on the physical nature of the emboli, they may be classified as:**
   - **Solid: Thromboemboli, atheromatous material, tumor emboli,** tissue fragments, bacterial clumps or parasites, foreign bodies.

TABLE 5.11 Classification of emboli.

Physical nature: Solid, liquid, gaseous
Presence or absence of infection: Bland, infected
Source: Cardiac, vascular (arterial, venous, lymphatic)
Flow of emboli: Paradoxical, retrograde (moving backward), antegrade (moving forward)
System involved: Pulmonary, systemic emboli

- **Liquid: Fat, bone marrow, and amniotic fluid.**
- **Gaseous: Air** or nitrogen.

2. **Depending on whether the emboli is infected or not, it may be classified as (i) bland** (sterile) or **septic** (infected).
3. **Depending on the source and site of origin (Fig. 5.23):** The emboli may be **endogenous** (formed within the body) or **exogenous** (introduced from outside). Various sites of origin of emboli are as follows:
   - **Cardiac emboli:** They usually arise from the left side of the heart. Examples are emboli from (1) atrial appendage, (2) **left ventricle** in **myocardial infarction**, and (3) **vegetations on the valves in infective endocarditis.**
   - **Vascular emboli:** They may originate from an artery, vein, or lymphatic.
     - **Arterial** emboli (e.g., atheromatous plaque, aneurysms).
     - **Venous** emboli (e.g., deep vein thrombus, tumor emboli).
     - **Lymphatic** emboli (e.g., tumor emboli).
4. **Depending on the flow of emboli,** they may be of the following types:

   Q. Write a short note on paradoxical embolism.

   - **Paradoxical emboli:** They are rare and the **emboli originate** in the **venous circulation** and **bypass the lungs** by traveling **through a right-to-left shunt** such as an atrial septal defect (incompletely closed/patent foramen ovale) or interventricular defect. Then, they **enter the left side of the heart** and **block the blood flow to the systemic arteries** (*refer* pages 537-8).

   Q. Write a short note on retrograde embolism.

   - **Retrograde emboli: Emboli,** which **travel against the flow of blood** are known as retrograde emboli. For example, **prostatic carcinoma metastasis to the spine**. It occurs through **retrograde spread via intraspinal veins** which carry the emboli from large thoracic ducts and abdominal veins due to increased pressure in the body cavities (e.g., during coughing or straining).

Pulmonary Embolism

Q. Write a short note on pulmonary embolism.

Definition: Pulmonary embolism (PE) is defined as an **embolism in which emboli occlude the pulmonary arterial tree.**

Site of origin of emboli (Fig. 5.23): Deep leg vein thromboses (DVTs) are the source in more than 95% of cases of pulmonary emboli. Deep leg veins include popliteal, femoral, or iliac veins. Other sites include pelvic veins and vena cava. Most fatal ones arise from iliofemoral veins.

Risk of pulmonary embolism: The major risk factor is **after surgery**. The risk increases with advancing age, obesity, prolonged operative procedures, postoperative infection, cancer, and pre-existing venous disease.

The mechanism of pulmonary thromboembolism is presented in **Flowchart 5.10**.

Fate of pulmonary embolism: It depends on the size of the embolus.

1. **Resolution or organization: Small** pulmonary **emboli** may travel into the smaller branches of pulmonary arteries and may **resolve completely**. Most (60–80%) of them are clinically **silent**. Over time they become **organized** and are incorporated into the wall of the pulmonary vessel.
2. **Massive pulmonary embolism:** When emboli **obstruct 60% or more of the pulmonary circulation**, it is known as massive pulmonary embolism. It is one of the most dramatic fatal complications of DVT.

   Q. Write a short note on saddle embolism.

   - **Saddle embolus:** It is a **large pulmonary embolus that lodges at the bifurcation of the main pulmonary artery**. It produces acute massive obstruction of the blood flow to both lungs. This may lead to **acute right ventricular failure or shock.** Right ventricular failure reduces the left ventricular cardiac output

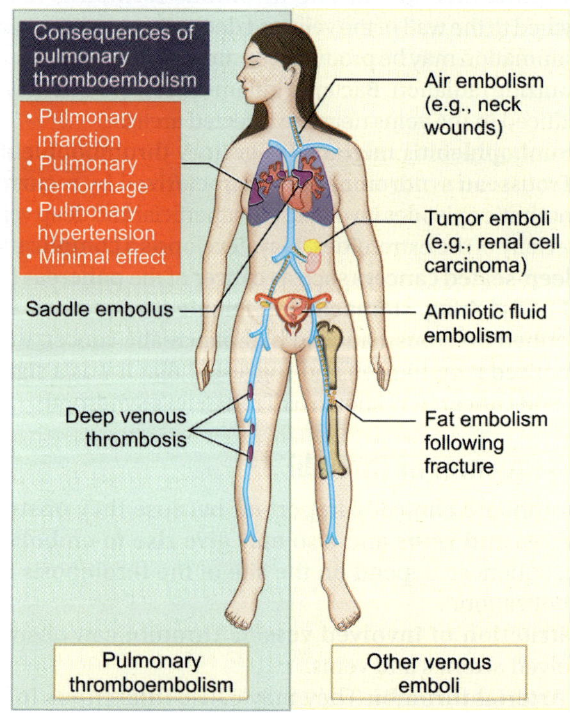

Fig. 5.23: Sources and effects of venous emboli.

Flowchart 5.10: Mechanism of pulmonary thromboembolism.

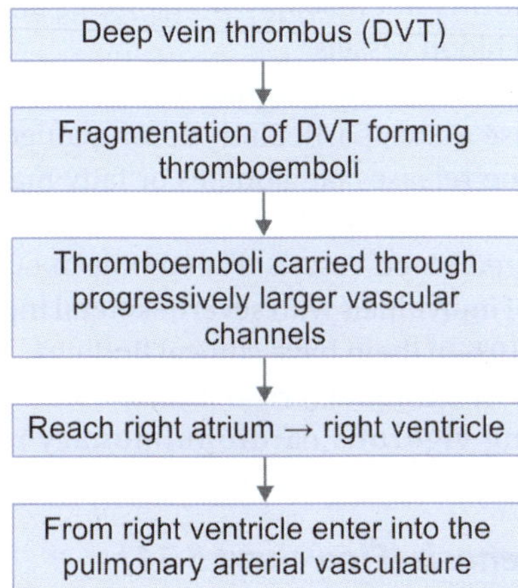

and produces sudden severe hypotension (or shock). It may result in **sudden death**.

3. **Multiple recurrent pulmonary emboli:** These **may fuse to form** a **single large mass.** Usually, the patient who has had one PE is likely to have recurrent emboli.
4. **Paradoxical embolism** (*refer* page 156). Rarely, a venous embolus pass through an atrial or ventricular defect and enters the systemic circulation.

Consequences (Fig. 5.23)

1. **Pulmonary infarction:** Most (about 75%) small pulmonary emboli do not produce infarcts. However, an embolus can **produce infarction in patients with congestive heart failure or chronic lung disease**.
   - **Gross (Fig. 5.26B):**
     - **Type:** Usually **hemorrhagic type, because of blood supply to the infarcted (necrotic) area by the bronchial artery**.
     - **Shape: Pyramidal** in shape with the base of the pyramid on the pleural surface. When the blood in the infarcted area is resorbed, the center of the infarct becomes pale.
     - **Fate:** Granulation tissue grows from the edges of the infarct resulting in the organization of the infarct and forming a **fibrous scar**.
   - **Clinical features:** Cough, stabbing pleuritic pain, shortness of breath, and occasional hemoptysis. Pleural effusion is a common complication and pleural fluid is often blood stained.
2. **Pulmonary hemorrhage: Obstruction of medium-sized pulmonary arteries** by emboli and subsequent rupture of these vessels can **result in pulmonary hemorrhage.**
3. **Pulmonary hypertension: Multiple recurrent pulmonary emboli may cause mechanical blockage of the arterial bed.** This may **result in pulmonary hypertension** and **right ventricular failure**.
4. **Minimal effect:** Obstruction of **small end-arteriolar branches** of the pulmonary artery by emboli usually **neither produces hemorrhage nor infarction.**

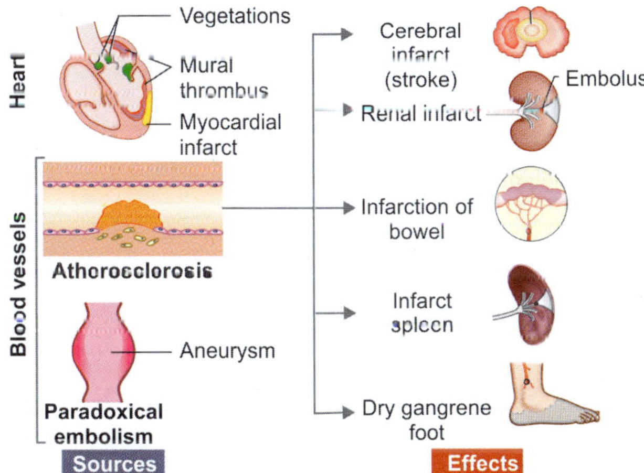

Fig. 5.24: Common sources and effects of systemic arterial emboli. It usually arises from the left side of the heart or major arteries. The usual consequence is either infarction or gangrene at the site of lodgment.

Systemic Thromboembolism

Definition: It is defined as an embolism in which **emboli occlude systemic arterial circulation.**

Systemic arterial embolism **usually produces infarcts** in the region supplied by the involved vessel.

Sources of Systemic Emboli (Fig. 5.24)

Heart: It is the most common source of systemic thromboemboli.

- **Intracardiac mural thrombi:** It is the most common source and is associated with thrombi over the **myocardial infarct** of the left ventricular wall. In **mitral stenosis, dilatation of the left atrium and atrial fibrillation predisposes to thrombus** and embolization. **Paradoxical emboli** are a rare source.
- **Vegetations (thrombi on heart valves):** For example, the source of vegetation in **bacterial endocarditis** (valvular vegetation from aortic or mitral valves) or prosthetic valves

Blood vessels: The source in the aorta or arteries is thrombi on **ulcerated atherosclerotic plaques** or from aortic **aneurysms.** In 10–15% of cases, the origin of systemic emboli is not known.

Site of lodgment: The arterial emboli can **travel almost anywhere and lodge in a wide variety of sites.** This is in contrast to venous emboli, which lodge mainly in one vascular bed namely the lung. The arterial emboli tend to **pass through the progressively narrow arterial lumen** and **lodge at points where the vessel lumen narrows abruptly** (e.g., at bifurcations or in the area of an atherosclerotic plaque).

Consequences: The consequences of systemic emboli depend on the (i) diameter of the occluded vessel, (ii) the presence or absence of a collateral blood supply, and (iii) the tissue's vulnerability to anoxia. **Thromboembolic** at the site of arrest may **grow (propagate) locally at the site of the arrest** and produce severe obstruction leading to **infarction of the affected tissues (Fig. 5.24)** or it may undergo **fragmentation and lysis. Major sites affected by arterial thromboemboli (Fig. 5.24)** are as follows:

1. **Lower extremity (75%):** Embolism to an artery of the leg may produce **gangrene**.
2. **Brain (10%):** Arterial emboli in the brain may produce **ischemic necrosis** in the brain (strokes).
3. **Intestine:** Emboli in the mesenteric vessels may produce **infarction of the bowel**.
4. **Kidney and spleen:** They are less commonly affected. Renal artery embolism may cause small peripheral **infarcts** in the kidney.
5. **Blood vessels:** Emboli originating from bacterial vegetation may cause inflammation of arteries and produce **mycotic aneurysms**.
6. Upper extremities are less commonly affected.

Paradoxical embolism: Rarely emboli arising in the systemic venous circulation bypass the lungs by traveling through an incompletely closed foramen ovale, atrial or ventricular septal defect. These emboli may enter the left-sided circulation and block flow through systemic arteries. Normally, left atrial pressure exceeds that in the right. Hence, most **paradoxical embolism** occurs when there is a right-to-left shunt.

Fat Embolism

Q. Describe fat embolism.

Fat and marrow embolus **consist of microscopic globules of fat with or without bone marrow (fatty marrow)** elements in the vasculature. The release of these elements into the circulation produces fat embolism.

Causes: The fatty marrow released from the following sources forms microscopic fat globules and enters into damaged blood vessels

- **Severe trauma to adipose tissue:** Severe trauma to adipose tissue, particularly accompanied by **fractures of bone** releases fat globules or fatty marrow (with or without associated hematopoietic marrow cells) into ruptured blood vessels. Fat embolism occurs in about 90% of individuals with **severe skeletal injuries**, but less than 10% of them have clinical findings.
- **Soft tissue trauma (crush injuries) and burns.**
- **During vigorous cardiopulmonary resuscitation** (probably they are of little clinical significance).

Pathogenesis (Flowchart 5.11)

Fat enters ruptured capillaries at the site of fracture/trauma. Hemorrhage into the marrow and subcutaneous fat may raise interstitial pressure above capillary pressure. This increased tissue pressure also forces fat into the circulation. Fat embolism syndrome involves both mechanical obstruction and biochemical injury.

Mechanical obstruction: Fat microemboli occlude the pulmonary and cerebral microvasculature, both directly and by triggering platelet aggregation.

Biochemical injury: The chemical composition of the fat present in the lung in fat embolism is different from that in adipose tissue. The mechanical obstruction alone cannot explain this difference. So, pathogenesis probably involves mechanical obstruction associated with biochemical injury. Free fatty acids are released from the fat globules causing local injury to endothelium. This along with platelet activation and granulocyte recruitment releases free radicals, protease, and eicosanoid. They enhance vascular damage.

Flowchart 5.11: Pathogenesis of fat embolism by mechanical obstruction and biochemical injury.

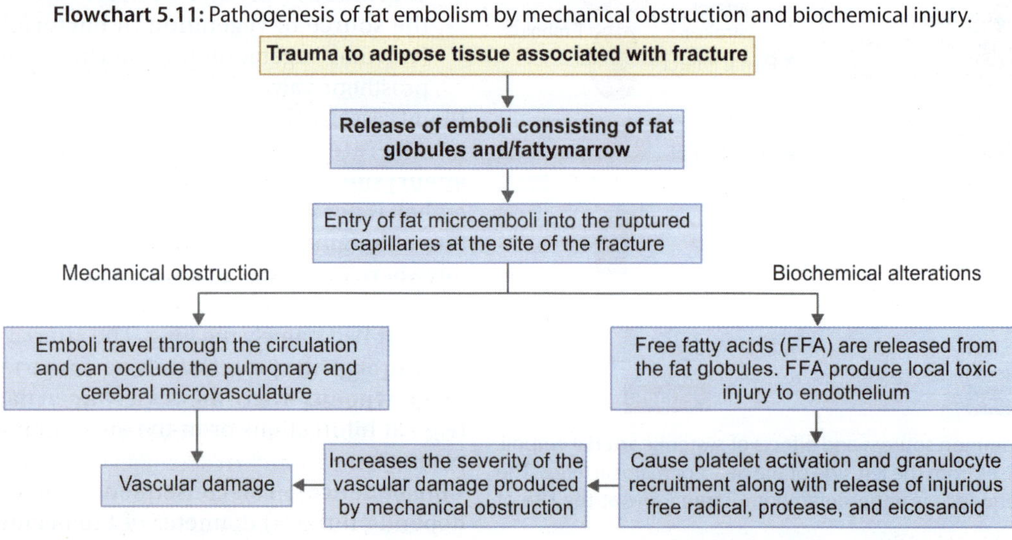

Consequences of Fat Embolism

It depends on the size and quantity of fat globules and whether the emboli are arrested in the pulmonary or systemic circulation.

Sites of arrest of fat emboli: Emboli in the venous side lodge **in the lungs. If emboli pass into the systemic circulation,** they may be arrested in the **brain, kidneys,** and other organs. The paradoxical fat emboli may reach systemic circulation (e.g., through patent foramen ovale) and get deposited in the brain, kidney, etc.

Manifestations: In **most of the cases** it is **asymptomatic. Sometimes**, it may clinically manifest as potentially **fatal fat embolism syndrome**. Fat embolism syndrome is the term applied when **the patient develops symptoms due to severe fat embolism.** The most severe form of fat embolism syndrome may be fatal and it develops in only a minority of patients (death in 10% of cases).

- **Time of development:** Signs and symptoms develop **1–3 days after the traumatic injury**.
- **Respiratory symptoms:** It causes pulmonary insufficiency and presents with sudden onset of **tachypnea, dyspnea, and tachycardia** which may lead to **respiratory failure**.
- **Neurologic symptoms:** These include **irritability, restlessness, delirium, and coma**.
- **Hematological findings:**
  - **Thrombocytopenia:** Rapid onset of thrombocytopenia produces **diffuse petechial rash** (found in 20–50% of cases) and may be a useful **diagnostic** feature. Thrombocytopenia is due adhesion of platelets to fat globules and subsequent aggregation or splenic sequestration.
  - **Anemia:** It is due to aggregation of red cells and/or due to hemolysis.
- **Chest radiography:** It shows diffuse opacity of the lungs and may progress to **opacification of lungs** (whiteout)—characteristic of **acute respiratory distress syndrome**.
- **Autopsy findings: Numerous fat globules** can be found impacted **in the microvasculature of the lungs (in pulmonary emboli) and brain** and sometimes other organs (in systemic emboli).
  - **Lung:** The lungs typically show the changes of **acute respiratory distress syndrome**.
  - **Brain:** The lesions include **cerebral edema, small hemorrhages**, and occasionally microinfarcts.
- **Demonstration of fat embolism:** Fat is dissolved during routine tissue preparations by the solvents (xylene/xylol) used in paraffin embedding. The microscopic demonstration of fat microglobules requires **frozen sections and special stains for fat** (e.g., Sudan III and IV, Oil Red O, and osmic acid).

Air Embolism

Q. Write a short note on air/gas embolism/Caissons disease/decompression sickness.

Air embolism **occurs when air enters into venous or arterial circulation**. These gas bubbles can coalesce and obstruct vascular flow and cause distal ischemic injury.

Causes

Venous air embolism: Air embolism into venous circulation may be caused due to:

- **Trauma/injury:** Air may enter the venous circulation through **neck wounds and chest wall injuries**.
- **Surgery/invasive procedures:** These include procedures such as **thoracocentesis, punctures of the great veins during obstetric or laparoscopic procedures**, or hemodialysis.
- **Criminal abortion.**

Arterial air embolism: Air embolism may occur in the **coronary artery during bypass surgery or** cerebral arterial circulation by neurosurgery in an upright "sitting position."

Amount of air required to have a clinical effect of air embolism: It is usually **more than 100 cc**. Amounts circulating air less than this have little consequences.

Mechanism: In the circulation, air/gas bubbles tend to coalesce to form frothy masses. They physically obstruct vascular blood flow in the right side of the heart, pulmonary circulation, and brain. This may lead to death.

Microscopy: Air bubbles are seen as empty spaces in capillaries and small vessels of the lung/brain.

Decompression Sickness

Decompression sickness is a unique form of gas embolism. It occurs when dissolved gasses (usually nitrogen) exit the solution and form bubbles inside the body on depressurization. Decompression sickness may be acute or chronic.

Acute Decompression Sickness

Risk factors: Acute decompression sickness develops when individuals are **exposed to sudden changes in atmospheric pressure**. This may be either from high atmospheric pressure to normal level or from normal pressure to low atmospheric pressure.

- **Exposure to high atmospheric pressure:** During descent, the atmospheric pressure is high. Risk factors include individuals exposed to increased atmospheric pressure, such as **scuba and deep-sea divers and underwater construction workers** (e.g., tunnels, drilling platform construction). It may also occur during **sport diving** (drowning is the first).
- **Exposure to low atmospheric pressure:** During ascent, the atmospheric pressure is low. For example, **unpressurized aircraft during rapid ascent.**

Mechanism of acute decompression sickness (Flowchart 5.12): During descent (e.g., during a deep-sea dive), the air is breathed at high pressure, and **large amounts of inert gas (particularly nitrogen) become dissolved in the blood, tissues, and body fluids.** When the individual (diver) ascends, this gas is released from the solution and exhaled.

Flowchart 5.12: Mechanism of acute decompression sickness.

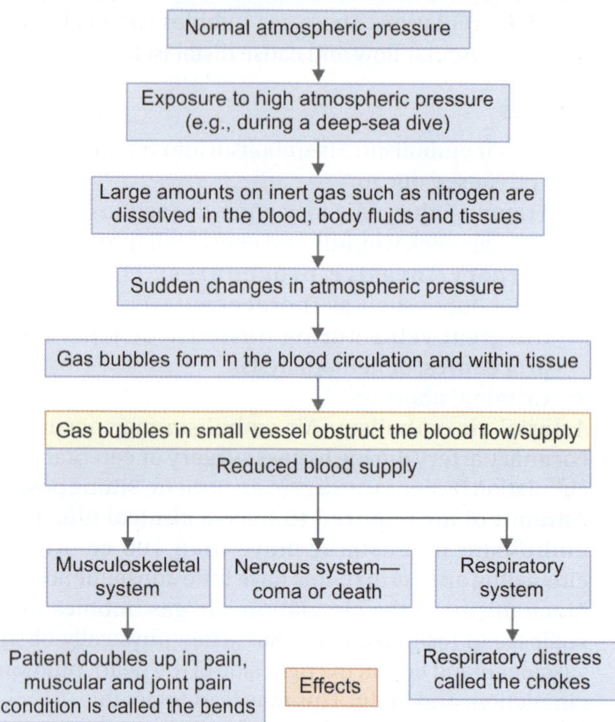

But, **if the individual then moves to a lower-pressure environment (i.e., ascends) too rapidly (i.e.,** decompresses suddenly), the **nitrogen expands in the tissues and bubbles out of solution** in the blood to form gas emboli. These gas bubbles in the circulation and within tissues, **obstruct blood flow and cause tissue ischemia.**

- **The bends:** Rapid formation of **gas bubbles within skeletal muscles and supporting tissues in and about joints** leads to a **painful condition** called the bends. It is characterized by temporary muscular and joint pain, due to obstruction of small vessels in these tissues. The patient doubles up in bed due to acute pain in joints, ligaments, and tendons.
- **The chokes (respiratory distress): Gas bubbles in the pulmonary vessels** cause **edema, hemorrhages, and focal atelectasis or emphysema**. This leads to respiratory distress.
- **CNS:** Bubbles in the central nervous system can cause loss of memory, ataxia, and visual disturbances. Severe involvement of cerebral blood may lead to the sudden onset of coma or even death.

Chronic Decompression Sickness (Caisson Disease)

Caisson disease (named for the pressurized underwater pressurized vessels/diving bells used during bridge construction) is a more **chronic form of decompression sickness.** Workers in these pressurized vessels may **develop both acute and chronic forms of decompression sickness.**

Characteristic features: Caisson disease is characterized by recurrent or persistent gas emboli. These gas emboli produce obstruction to blood flow. It causes foci of ischemic necrosis throughout the body, especially the skeletal system. In the bones, it produces multifocal (multiple foci of) **ischemic (avascular) necrosis.** The more commonly involved bone includes the **head of the femur, tibia, and humerus.** This complication was originally detected in construction workers in diving bells (caissons).

Treatment: The individuals affected by acute decompression sickness are treated by placing them in a high-pressure chamber. This forces the bubbled-out gas to go back into solution. Subsequent slow decompression allows gradual gas resorption and exhalation, thereby preventing the re-formation of obstructive bubbles.

Amniotic Fluid Embolism

Q. Write a short note on amniotic fluid embolism.

Amniotic fluid embolism **develops when amniotic fluid (along with fetal cells and debris) enters the maternal circulation.** The amniotic fluid entry occurs through a tear in the placental membranes and/or open (ruptured) uterine vein **(Fig. 5.25).**

Time of occurrence: It is a rare maternal threatening (80% fatal) unpredictable and unpreventable complication. It occurs **at the end of labor and the immediate postpartum period.**

Consequences: From the venous circulation, amniotic fluid emboli enter the right side of the heart and finally rest in the pulmonary circulation. Amniotic fluid has a high thromboplastin activity and initiates a potentially **fatal disseminated intravascular coagulation (DIC).**

MORPHOLOGY

Amniotic fluid contents within pulmonary vasculature: Amniotic fluid emboli are composed of squamous cells shed from fetal skin, lanugo hair, fat from vernix caseosa, and mucin derived from the fetal respiratory or gastrointestinal tract.

Other findings: These include **marked pulmonary edema, diffuse alveolar damage**, and features of DIC.

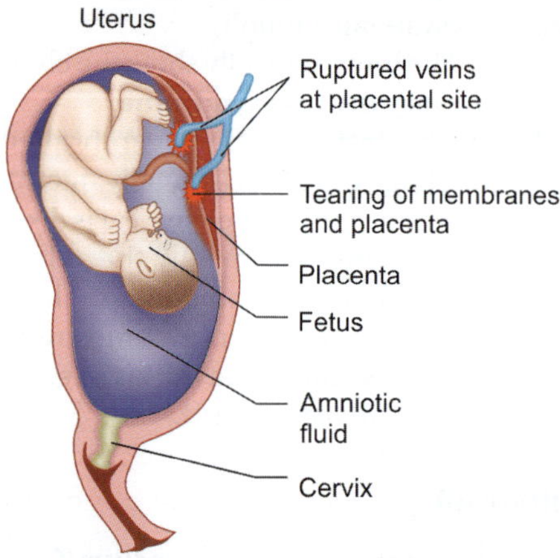

Fig. 5.25: Amniotic fluid embolism.

Clinical Features

- **Abrupt onset:** It develops during the immediate postpartum period. It is characterized by sudden onset of **severe dyspnea, cyanosis, and neurologic impairment ranging from headache to seizures.** This may be followed by the development of **shock, coma, and death.**
- **DIC:** If the patient survives the initial acute crisis, the patient develops bleeding due to disseminated intravascular coagulation (DIC) **secondary to the release of thrombogenic substances from amniotic fluid.**
- **Acute respiratory distress syndrome (ARDS): If the patient overcomes DIC, she is still at high risk of developing ARDS.**

Miscellaneous Pulmonary Emboli

- **Foreign bodies:** Various foreign substances may act as emboli.
  - **Talc emboli:** It may occur in intravenous drug abusers who use talc as a carrier for illicit drugs.
  - **Cotton emboli:** It may occur due to cleansing of the skin by cotton before venipuncture.
- **Schistosomiasis:** The ova of Schistosoma may gain entry into the circulation from the bladder or gut and lodge in the lungs.
- **Tumor emboli:** It may occur during hematogenous dissemination of cancer.
- **Atheromatous emboli** (cholesterol emboli): Fragments of atheromatous plaque may embolize.
- **Platelet emboli:** During the early stages of atherosclerosis, there is platelet deposition in the intimal surface of blood vessels. They may form platelet emboli.
- **Infective emboli:** In infective endocarditis, the vegetation seen on the diseased heart valves may become infected. These infected vegetations may break off and form infective emboli. Their effects are due to both emboli and infective agents that may weaken the wall of the vessel. It may lead to the formation of a **'mycotic' aneurysm** (*refer* page 490). **Mycotic is a misnomer because the infective agent is usually bacterial, not fungal.**

INFARCTION

PA 6.6 (CC): Define and describe ischemia/infarction, its types, etiology, morphologic changes, and clinical effects.

Q. Define infarct.

Definition: An infarct is a **localized area of ischemic necrosis caused by occlusion of the blood supply** of the affected tissue. It **develops distal to occlusion of an end artery. Infarction is the process of producing an infarct.**

Mostly infarct is a coagulative type of necrosis due to sudden occlusion of arterial blood supply. If the patient survives, the infarct heals with a scar. Common and important infarcts are shown in **Table 5.12.**

TABLE 5.12 Common and important infarcts.

Organ/tissue affected	*Infarction*
Heart	Myocardial infarction*
Brain	Cerebral infarction*
Lung	Pulmonary infarction
Bowel/intestine	Intestinal infarct
Ischemic necrosis of distal extremities	Gangrene

*most common

Causes of Infarction

Q. What are the causes of red and pale infarct? /Types of infarcts with examples.

Arterial causes: The most important causes are:

- **Occlusions of lumen:** It is the most common cause of infarction. It may be due to (1) arterial **thrombus** or (2) arterial **embolus (Fig. 5.24).**
- **Causes in the arterial wall:** Examples include local vasospasm, expansion of **atheromatous plaque secondary to hemorrhage into the plaque** (e.g., myocardial infarct following atherosclerosis of coronary artery), or thromboangiitis obliterans.
- **External compression of the vessel:** Examples include compression by a tumor, a dissecting aortic aneurysm, or edema within a confined space (e.g., in anterior tibial compartment syndrome).
- **Uncommon causes.**

Venous causes: These are rare causes of infarction.

- **Occlusions of the lumen of the vein** may be due to **(1) thrombus or (2) embolus.** Although venous thrombosis can cause infarction, it usually produces only congestion. Typically, it leads to the opening of the bypass channels and they provide sufficient outflow to restore the arterial inflow. Thus, infarcts due to venous thrombosis generally occur only in organs with a single efferent vein (e.g., testis or ovary).
- **Extrinsic vessel compression:** These include uncommon causes such as compression by a tumor, twisting of vessels (e.g., in testicular torsion or bowel volvulus), traumatic vascular rupture, and entrapment of vessel in a hernia sac **(strangulated hernia).**

Factors that Determine the Development of an Infarct

Q. Mention the factors that influence the development of an infarct.

The outcome of vascular occlusion may range from no or minimal effect to the death of a tissue (**organ dysfunction**) or sometimes the death of an individual. The **major factors** that determine the outcome of an infarct are:

1. **Nature of the vascular supply:** The anatomy of the vascular supply is one of the factors.
   - **Dual/parallel blood supply:** The most important factor that determines whether occlusion of an

individual vessel causes damage is the presence or absence of an alternative blood supply. Organs or tissues with double or parallel blood supply are **less likely to develop infarction**, e.g., lung, liver, hand, and forearm.

- **Lung:** It has a dual supply by the pulmonary and bronchial arteries. Thus, obstruction of the pulmonary arterioles does not produce lung infarction unless the bronchial circulation is also obstructed.
- **Liver:** It receives blood from the hepatic artery and the portal vein.
- **Hand and forearm:** It has parallel radial and ulnar arterial supply.

- **End-arterial blood supply:** The kidney and spleen have blood supply, which are end-arteries with little or no collaterals. Arterial obstruction in these organs usually causes tissue death and **infarction**.

2. **Rate of occlusion: Slow occlusion** is **less likely to produce infarction than rapid occlusion**. This is because it provides time to develop alternate (collateral) blood supply. For example, in the heart, small interarteriolar anastomoses, interconnect the three major coronary arteries. They normally carry minimal blood flow. When one coronary artery is slowly occluded (e.g., by an atherosclerotic plaque), flow in this collateral circulation may increase sufficiently to prevent infarction—even if the original coronary artery develops complete occlusion of the lumen.
3. **Vulnerability of tissue to hypoxia:** Different cell types vary in their susceptibility to injury by hypoxia. This is mainly due to differences in their basal metabolic needs.
   - **Neurons are highly sensitive to hypoxia**. They undergo necrosis **even if the blood supply is occluded for only 3–4 minutes.**
   - In the heart, **myocardial cells** are also quite sensitive to hypoxia, but **less sensitive than neurons**. Myocardial cells **die after only 20–30 minutes of ischemia**.
   - **Fibroblasts:** They may remain viable even after many hours of ischemia.
4. **Oxygen content of blood:** In a normal individual, partial obstruction of a small vessel may not produce any effect, but in a patient with anemia or cyanosis same may produce infarction.

Classification of Infarcts

Q. Write a short note on different types of infracts, their causes, and common sites of occurrence.

Infarcts are classified depending on their color (reflects the amount of hemorrhage), the presence or absence of microbial infection, and according to their age (**Table 5.13**).

TABLE 5.13 Classification of the infarct.

According to color	*Presence or absence of infection*	*According to the age of infarct*
White/pale (anemic)	Septic, when it is infected	Recent or fresh
Red (hemorrhagic)	Bland, when it is free of infection	Old or healed

Q. Mention the organs involved in the red and pale infarct.

White/pale infarcts: They occur

1. **With arterial occlusions**
2. **In solid organs with end-arterial circulation without a dual blood supply (e.g., heart, spleen, and kidney)**
3. **Tissue with increased density** which prevents the diffusion of RBCs from adjoining capillary beds into the necrotic area.

Red/hemorrhagic infarcts: They occur

1. With **venous occlusions** (e.g., torsion of testis or ovary). Red infarcts may also occur due to arterial and also contain coagulative necrosis. However, these infarcts also show bleeding into the affected area from adjacent vessels.
2. In **loose textured tissues** (e.g., lung) that allow red cells to diffuse through and collect in the necrotic zone.
3. In **tissues with dual (double) blood supply** (e.g., lung, liver) that allows blood flow from an unobstructed parallel blood supply into a necrotic zone. Also occurs in organs with extensive collateral circulation (**e.g.,** small intestine and brain).
4. **In tissues previously congested due to decreased venous drainage.**
5. **When blood flow is re-established after the occurrence of infarct:** It occurs when the blood flow is re-established to a site of previous arterial occlusion and necrosis. For example, in the heart, a red infracts may occur after an infarcted area is re-perfused following therapeutically induced lysis of an occluding thrombus or coronary angioplasty of an obstructed coronary artery.

Septic infarct: It develops when the necrotic tissue of an infarct contains pyogenic bacteria or becomes, infected. Emboli that arise from bacterial endocarditis (infected cardiac valve vegetations) are themselves infected, and the resulting infarcts are usually septic. A septic infarct may form a frank abscess.

MORPHOLOGY

Q. Write a short note on organs involved in pale and red infracts.

White/Pale Infarcts

Organs involved include the **heart, kidneys, spleen,** and dry gangrene of the extremities [foot or leg due to arterial occlusion (often occurs in diabetes) is a large pale infarct].

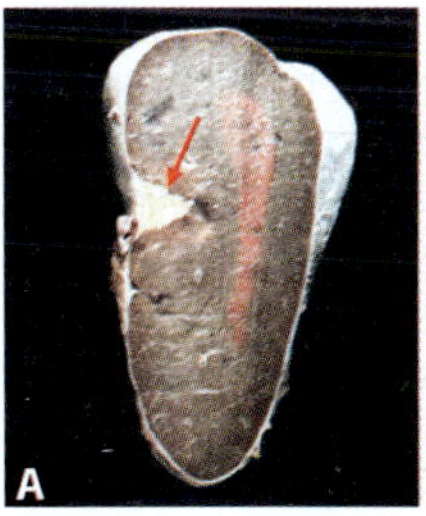

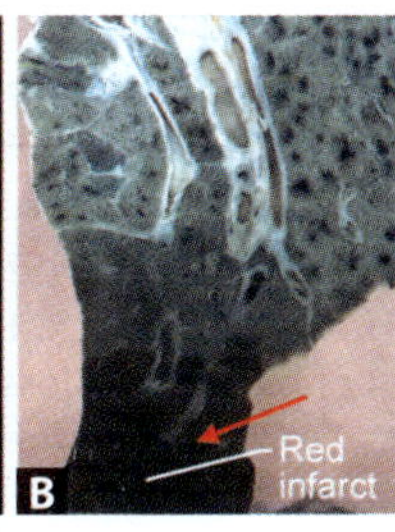

Infarct: Localized area of ischemic necrosis caused by occlusion of either the arterial blood supply or the venous drainage.

Figs. 5.26A and B: (A) Infarct spleen showing wedge-shaped pale/white infarct (arrow); (B) Lung showing sharply circumscribed, dark red to purple hemorrhagic infarct (arrow).

Gross:

- **Appearance:** White infarcts are usually **wedge-shaped (Fig. 5.26A). The occluded blood vessel** is **at the apex** and the **periphery/surface** of the organ **forms the wide base.** If the base is a serosal surface, it often shows an overlying fibrinous exudate.
- **Margins of infarct:** They may be irregular, because of blood flow from adjacent vessels. The **margins of acute infarcts are indistinct and slightly hemorrhagic.** As time passes, the edges become better defined by a narrow rim of hyperemia caused by inflammation.
- **As time passes**, infarcts in organs without dual circulation become progressively **paler, light yellow in color,** and more **sharply defined.**

Red/Hemorrhagic Infarcts

Gross (Fig. 5.26B): Appears as a **sharply circumscribed area of necrosis, firm** in consistency and **dark red to purple** in color.

Microscopy of Infarct

In most tissues, **both pale and red infarcts** characteristically show **ischemic coagulative necrosis.** In the brain, an infarct usually undergoes liquefactive necrosis and may become a fluid-filled cyst (referred to as a cystic infarct).

- **Coagulative necrosis:** Microscopic changes of **frank necrosis** appear after about **4–12 hours.**
- **Acute inflammation cells** infiltrate the necrotic area from the viable margins all-round the infarcts within a few hours. It becomes **prominent within 1–2 days.**
- Inflammation is followed by a **repair process,** which begins **at the preserved margins. The necrotic cells** in infarcts and extravasated red cells are **phagocytosed by macrophages.**
- In tissues composed of stable or labile cells, **parenchymal regeneration** can occur at the periphery where stromal architecture is preserved.
- **Granulation tissue** may **replace the infarcted area** which **matures to** form **scar tissue.**
- If the infarct is large (e.g., in the heart or kidney), the necrotic center may persist for months.

Septic infarctions: They may occur in two situations:

1. **Infection:** Infarct may get infected when it is **seeded by pyogenic bacteria**, e.g., infection of the pulmonary infarct.
2. **Septic emboli:** They contain organisms and can produce septic infarct, e.g., vegetations of bacterial endocarditis may cause septic infarct of spleen.

The organisms present in a **septic infarct** convert infarct into a frank **abscess.**

PA 6.7 (CC): Identify and describe various forms of cell injuries, their manifestations, and consequences in gross and microscopic specimens.

SCENARIO-BASED MCQs

1. **A 7-year-old boy has had increasing weakness and puffiness in his face. On physical examination, he has periorbital edema and pitting edema at the ankles. His blood pressure was normal and he is afebrile. Laboratory studies show marked albuminuria (more than 3.5 g/day). The mechanism of edema in this patient is mainly due to:**
   A. Decreased osmotic pressure
   B. Increased hydrostatic pressure
   C. Impaired lymphatic drainage
   D. Increased vascular permeability
2. **A 56-year-old with cancer in the right breast underwent a mastectomy with axillary lymph node dissection. Postoperatively, she developed marked swelling of the left arm that has persisted for 5 months. On physical examination, her right arm was not painful with movement or touch. In the right arm, there is neither tenderness nor redness, but it is enlarged with a doughy consistency. The most likely mechanism for these findings in the right arm is due to:**
   A. Cellulitis
   B. Lymphedema
   C. Phlebothrombosis
   D. Decreased plasma oncotic pressure
3. **A 68-year-old man with ischemic heart disease complains of increasing shortness of breath. He is a chronic smoker and a known diabetic. On physical examination, the patient has swollen legs, an enlarged liver, and fluid in the pleural cavities. The hemodynamic disorders responsible for enlarged livre are:**
   A. Deep venous thrombosis
   B. Arterial thromboembolism
   C. Chronic passive congestion
   D. Thrombosis of the hepatic vein
4. **A 42-year-old man had a history of long-standing rheumatic heart disease. He was diagnosed as having mitral stenosis. He dies in a car accident. At autopsy, mitral stenosis was noted. Microscopically, the lung showed "heart failure cells." These cells represent:**
   A. Cells found in right-sided heart failure
   B. Stasis of blood in the coronary arteries
   C. Macrophages laden with hemosiderin pigment
   D. Neutrophils with ingested RBCs
5. **A 40-year-old woman with third-degree burns over 70% of his body due to a sudden fire accident in the kitchen while cooking. He was admitted to the hospital in an unconscious state. She expires 24 hours later. The most likely cause of death is:**
   A. Hypovolemic shock
   B. Congestive heart failure
   C. Pulmonary saddle embolism
   D. Disseminated intravascular coagulation

6. **A 73-year-old woman is brought to the hospital in an unconscious state. Her blood pressure is 70/30 mm Hg. She is febrile (38°C/100.5°F) and tachypneic. Laboratory findings showed a total WBC count of 22,000/µL, 90% neutrophils on differential leukocyte count. Urinalysis showed numerous gram-negative organisms. The signs and symptoms in this patient are likely due to:**
   A. Septic shock
   B. Neurogenic shock
   C. Cardiogenic shock
   D. Hypovolemic shock
7. **An 81-year-old man had a fall and is hospitalized. He has a fracture in his right femoral trochanter. Two weeks later, his right leg is swollen, especially below the knee. He develops pain on movement of the leg. On palpation, there is swelling and tenderness. This patient is likely to develop complications namely:**
   A. Fat embolism syndrome
   B. Pulmonary thromboembolism
   C. Gangrenous necrosis of the foot
   D. Disseminated intravascular coagulation
8. **A 64-year-old man is recovering from surgery done to correct an abdominal aneurysm. Suddenly, he develops acute chest pain and dies. An autopsy showed a thromboembolus at the bifurcation of the left and right pulmonary arteries. The most likely cause of this patient's pulmonary thromboembolus is:**
   A. Bacterial endocarditis
   B. Deep venous thrombosis
   C. Paradoxical embolization
   D. Complicated atherosclerotic plaque

Answers and Explanation

1. **The answer is A: Decreased osmotic pressure.** This child has nephrotic syndrome with loss of albumin in the urine and hypoalbuminemia. It decreases plasma osmotic pressure, leading to the movement of intravascular water into the extravascular compartment and produce edema. Increased hydrostatic pressure is responsible for generalized edema due to heart failure. Options C and D are the causes of localized edema.
2. **The answer is B: Lymphedema.** The surgery for breast carcinoma disrupted lymphatic return. This has resulted in functional lymphatic obstruction and lymphedema of the arm. The lymphatic channels play an important in draining fluid and protein that have leaked into the extravascular tissues from the intravascular compartment. Cellulitis is caused by an infection of the skin and subcutaneous tissue. It shows redness, warmth, and tenderness indicative of inflammation. Phlebothrombosis produces swelling with pain and tenderness, but it is uncommon in the upper extremities. Decreased plasma oncotic pressure from hypoalbuminemia, leads to more generalized edema.
3. **The answer is C: Chronic passive congestion.** A generalized increase in venous pressure usually develops in chronic heart failure. This results in an increase in the volume of blood in many organs (e.g., liver, spleen, and kidneys). The liver is particularly susceptible to chronic passive congestion because the hepatic veins empty into the vena cava immediately inferior to the heart. Deep venous thrombosis and arterial thromboembolism do not produce hepatomegaly. Thrombosis of the hepatic vein (Budd-Chiari syndrome) may cause liver enlargement, but it is not a complication of congestive heart failure.
4. **The answer is option C: Macrophages laden with hemosiderin pigment.** The heart failure cells are macrophages laden with hemosiderin pigment seen in chronic venous congestion of the lung. Hemosiderin can be demonstrated by Perl's stain (Prussian blue reaction). Heart failure cells are neither seen in the lung in right-sided heart failure nor with stasis of blood in coronary arteries. These cells are not neutrophils.
5. **The answer is A: Hypovolemic shock.** Hypovolemic shock may be caused by loss of blood, fluid loss from severe burns, or diarrhea. In this case of burns, direct damage to the microcirculation increases vascular permeability. Patients with third-degree burns lose large amounts of plasma. The other choices are unlikely causes of death in a patient with severe burns.
6. **The answer is A: Septic shock.** Septic shock results from a systemic inflammatory response syndrome (SIRS). The most common cause of septic shock is septicemia with gram-negative organisms. It leads to dysfunction of multiple organs and hypotension. Clinical features include two or more signs of systemic inflammation (e.g., fever, tachycardia, tachypnea, leukocytosis, or leukopenia) in a patient with a known cause of inflammation. Neurogenic shock (choice B) can develop after an acute injury to the brain or spinal cord. Cardiogenic shock (choice C) occurs in advanced heart failure. Hypovolemic shock (choice D) develops following loss of blood or fluids.
7. **The answer is B: Pulmonary thromboembolism.** He has deep venous thrombosis. This occurred as a consequence of venous stasis from immobilization. The large, deep thrombi in leg veins can embolize the lungs (pulmonary thromboembolism), leading to death. Fat embolism can develop with fractures, but pulmonary manifestations usually occur 1–3 days after the multiple fractures. Gangrene usually develops from arterial, not venous, occlusion in the leg. Disseminated intravascular coagulation is not a common complication in patients with venous thrombosis of the extremities.
8. **The answer is B: Deep venous thrombosis.** One of the most common complications that occur post-surgical is the sudden death of a patient who appeared to be on the way to recovery. The cause of this is usually due to a massive pulmonary embolism. A large pulmonary embolus may lodge at the bifurcation of the main pulmonary artery (saddle embolus). This obstructs blood flow to both lungs. With acute obstruction blocking more than half of the pulmonary arterial tree, the patient develops severe hypotension and may die within minutes. The other choices are the causes of arterial embolism.

SCENARIO-BASED ESSAY

Q. A 64-year-old male presents with pedal edema and exertional dyspnea. On examination, the pedal edema is pitting in nature and there are destined jugular veins. Laboratory investigation showed hemoglobin of 3.5 g/dL. He is neither diabetic nor hypertensive. A clinical diagnosis of congestive heart failure is made.

a. **List the types of edema (*refer* pages 129-30).**
b. **Describe the pathophysiology of edema in the above clinical condition (*refer* page 131).**
c. **Describe the morphological consequences of this condition (*refer* pages 135-6).**

Lines of Zahn: Antemortem thrombi.

Chicken fat appearance: Postmortem clots

Immunopathology, AIDS, and Amyloidosis

Chapter Outline

- Immunity
- Hypersensitivity Reactions
- Major Histocompatibility Complex Molecules
- Immunology of Transplantation
- Autoimmune Diseases
- Systemic Lupus Erythematosus
- Other Autoimmune Disorders
- Immunodeficiency Syndromes
- Acquired Immunodeficiency Syndrome
- Amyloidosis

The normal immune system is essential for protection against infection. The immune system is like a double-edged sword. Though it is protective in most situations, sometimes a hyperactive immune system may cause fatal diseases.

IMMUNITY

PA 9.1 (CC): Describe the principles and mechanisms involved in immunity.

Definition: Immunity is **the host's resistance (defense mechanism) against invasion by any foreign antigen, including microorganisms**. The foreign antigens (agents) include toxins, chemicals, drugs, multicellular parasites, and transplanted foreign tissues.

Immune system: It consists of a collection of cells and molecules that defend the body against the numerous pathogens that individuals come across.

The Normal Immune Response

Types of immune response: There are two arms in the immune system namely innate and adaptive immunity (*refer* **online Fig. 6.1**).

Innate Immunity

General features of innate (also called natural, or native) immunity are presented in **Box 6.1**.

BOX 6.1: General features of innate immunity.

- Ready-made, first (initial) line of defense present by birth.
- Provides immediate (rapid) initial protection against an invading pathogen.
- Does not depend on the prior contact with foreign antigens or microbes.
- Lacks specificity, but is highly effective.
- No memory, and no self/non-self-recognition.
- Triggers the adaptive immune response.

Major Components of Innate Immunity

The major components are epithelial barriers that act as mechanical barriers and several plasma proteins.

Physical/anatomical barriers

Cells: These are as follows:

- **The epithelial barriers:** These include the epithelium lining of the skin, and gastrointestinal and respiratory tracts that block the entry of microbes.
- **Phagocytic cells:** It consists of mainly **neutrophils, and monocytes (macrophages in tissue)** in the blood. Phagocytic cells use several receptors to sense microbes and are called "microbial sensors" (pattern recognition receptors) (*refer* page 62).
    - **Pathogen-associated molecular patterns (PAMPs):** Microbes have few highly conserved common molecular structures shared by entire classes of pathogens. These structures are called **pathogen-associated molecular patterns** and are essential for the infectivity of these pathogens.
    - **Pattern recognition receptors (PRRs) (*refer* Fig. 3.2):** Phagocytic cells involved in innate immunity recognize PAMP using a group of cellular receptors (microbial sensors) called pattern recognition receptors. Damage-associated molecular patterns (DAMPs) are the substances released from injured

and necrotic cells. Pattern recognition receptors recognize these DAMPS molecules. Examples of PRRs:

- ♦ **Toll-like receptors (TLRs):** These are trans-membrane receptors. About 10 types of human TLRs have been identified. Each receptor recognizes a unique set of microbial patterns. For example, TLR2 recognizes various ligands (e.g., lipoteichoic acid) expressed by gram-positive bacteria, and TLR4 recognizes lipopolysaccharides (LPS) of gram-negative bacteria.
- ♦ **Others:** These include **receptors for mannose residues; NOD (nucleotide-oligomerization domain protein)-like receptors located in the cytoplasm and serve as intracellular sensors for microbial products; and opsonins.**

- ❖ **Dendritic cells:** These cells **function as antigen-presenting cells** to T-cells. They produce type I interferons (IFN) (e.g., IFN-α), which inhibit viral infection and replication (*refer* page 168).
- ❖ **Natural killer (NK) cells:** They defend against many viral infections and other intracellular pathogens (*refer* pages 168-9).

Soluble molecules in the blood and tissues

These include several proteins such as the **complement system,** and proteins that coat microbes and aid in phagocytosis (e.g., mannose-binding lectin and C-reactive protein).

Reactions of Innate Immune Immunity

- ❖ **Inflammation** and destruction of invading microbe
- ❖ **Antiviral defense** is mediated by **dendritic cells and NK cells.**

It also generates signals stimulating the subsequent, more powerful adaptive immune response.

Adaptive Immunity

Adaptive immunity is normally quiescent. If the innate immune system fails to protect against invading microbes effectively, the adaptive immune system responds (or *adapts*) or is activated. It generates powerful mechanisms for neutralizing and eliminating pathogens. The terms *immune system* and *immune response* are usually used for adaptive immunity. The adaptive immune response typically becomes fully active in 3–7 days. General features of adaptive (also called acquired, or specific) immunity are presented in **Box 6.2**.

BOX 6.2: General features of adaptive immunity.

- Second line of defense acquired during life
- Capable of recognizing both microbial and nonmicrobial substances
- Takes more time to develop and is more powerful than innate immunity
- Long-lasting protection
- Prior exposure to antigen is present
- Three characteristic features are (1) specificity, (2) diversity, and (3) memory.

Types of Adaptive Immunity

Adaptive immunity is of two types: humoral immunity, and cell-mediated (or cellular) immunity.

Q. Write a short note on humoral immunity.

1. **Humoral immunity:** It is mediated by soluble protein products called **antibodies**. These antibodies are produced by B lymphocytes (also called **B cells**). Antibodies can react with the specific antigen responsible for its production.
   - ■ **Function:** They protect against extracellular pathogens in the blood, mucosal organs, and tissues.

Q. Write a short note on cellular immunity.

2. **Cellular immunity (cell-mediated immunity):** It is mediated by **T lymphocytes** (also called T cells), **macrophages**, and their soluble products called **cytokines.**
   - ■ **Functions:** It produces a localized reaction to organisms, usually intracellular pathogens. It produces a defense against viruses, fungi, and intracellular bacteria by directly killing infected cells with cytotoxic T lymphocytes or activating phagocytes to kill the ingested microbes.

   Cell-mediated cytotoxicity is important in the lysis of virus-infected cells and in rejecting allograft and tumor cells. Other cytotoxic cells involved in cell-mediated immune response are null cells (NK). These NK cells can attack the target cells and kill them—an important immunoregulatory role, orchestrating and regulating the responses of other components of the immune system.

Different types of adaptive immunity and their differences are shown in **Table 6.1**. Both B and T lymphocytes express highly specific receptors for a wide variety of substances, called **antigens.**

Cells of the Immune System

The immune system cells consist of **lymphocytes**, specialized **antigen-presenting cells (APCs)**, and other cells such as **phagocytes and eosinophils.** The major cell types involved in adaptive immune responses are discussed below.

TABLE 6.1 Differences between two types of adaptive immunity.

Type	*Mediator*	*Protection against*
Humoral immunity	B lymphocytes which secrete antibodies	Extracellular microbes and their toxins
Cell-mediated (or cellular) immunity	T (thymus-derived) lymphocytes	Intracellular microbes

Naïve Lymphocytes

These mature lymphocytes have not encountered the antigen (immunologically inexperienced). After the lymphocytes are activated by recognizing antigens, they **differentiate into effector cells** (perform the function of eliminating microbes) and **memory cells** (live in a state of heightened awareness and are better able to combat the microbe in case it infects again).

T Lymphocytes

T (thymus-derived) lymphocytes develop from thymus precursors and become effector cells.

Distribution: Mature T-cells are found in (1) **peripheral blood** where they constitute **60–70% of lymphocytes** and (2) **T-cell zones of peripheral lymphoid organs** namely the paracortical region of lymph node and periarteriolar sheaths of the spleen.

Recognition of antigen: T-cells cannot recognize free or circulating antigens. They recognize a specific cell-bound antigen using an **antigen-specific T-cell receptor (TCR).**

T-cell markers: Leukocyte cell surface molecules are named systematically by assigning them a **'cluster of differentiation' (CD) antigen number** that helps identify them. **Primary T-cell associated CD molecules: CD1, CD3, CD4, CD5 and CD8. CD3** is involved in signal transduction, also known as **pan T-cell marker**. It is involved in T-cell activation.

Major classes of T lymphocytes: Naïve T-cells can differentiate into two subtypes, **CD4 and CD8.** Both subtypes serve as "coreceptors" in T-cell activation. They are called coreceptors because they work with the antigen receptor in response to antigen.

Q. Write a short note on the T helper cell.

- **CD4+ T-cell:** This subset of T-cells expresses CD4 molecules on their surface and are called **helper T-cells.** They are named so because they secrete soluble molecules (cytokines) that **stimulate (help) B cells to produce antibodies** and **help macrophages to destroy phagocytosed microbes.** They are **subcategorized as Th1, Th2, and Th17 CD4+ T-cells.** They **constitute about 60% of mature T-cells.** CD4+ helper cells play a main role in immunity and severe immune defects occur from their destruction as in human immunodeficiency virus (HIV) infection.
- **CD8+ T-cell:** This subset of T-cells expresses CD8 molecules and are called **cytotoxic/killer T-cells.** CD8+ T-cells function as cytotoxic T lymphocytes (CTLs) to **destroy host cells harboring microbes and tumor cells.** They **constitute about 30% of T-cells.**

When the antigen-presenting cells (APCs) present antigen to T-cells, CD4 molecules on T-cells recognize and bind only to class II MHC molecules and CD8 binds only to class I MHC molecules.

B Lymphocytes

B (bone marrow-derived) lymphocytes develop from precursors in the bone marrow. It **produces antibodies, that are the mediators of humoral immunity.**

Distribution: Mature B-cells **constitute 10–20% of the circulating peripheral lymphocyte population.** They are also present in bone marrow and **peripheral** (secondary) **lymphoid tissues** such as lymph nodes (cortex), spleen (white pulp), and mucosa-associated lymphoid tissues (pharyngeal tonsils and Peyer's patches of GIT).

Recognition of antigen: B lymphocytes (cells) recognize antigens using membrane-bound **B-cell receptor (BCR). It** has unique antigen specificity. They recognize antigens without requiring the MHC.

Functions of B-cells: The primary function of B-cells is to **produce antibodies.** After stimulation by antigen and other signals, B-cells differentiate into **plasma cells.** These cells secrete antibodies which are the mediators of humoral immunity. There are five classes of antibodies: **IgG, IgM, IgA, IgE, and Ig D.** The salient features of various antibodies are presented in **Table 6.2.**

Markers: B-cell markers include: CD10 (CALLA), CD19, CD20, CD21 (also called EBV receptor), CD23, CD79a.

The main classes of lymphocytes and their functions in adaptive immunity are presented in (*refer* **online Fig. 6.2**):

Natural Killer Cells

Q. Write a short note on natural killer cells.

Natural killer (NK) cells are innate immune cells. They are non-phagocytic **large** (a little larger than small lymphocytes) **granular** (numerous cytoplasmic **azurophilic granules) lymphocytes.** They constitute **about 5–15% of human peripheral lymphoid cells.** They arise from the same common lymphoid progenitor that gives rise to T and B lymphocytes.

Markers: They **do not bear the markers for T- or B-cells.** Two cell surface molecules, **CD16 and CD56,** are commonly used to identify them.

Functions: Natural killer (NK) cells provide **defense against many viral infections** and other **intracellular pathogens** and **have antitumor activity,** causing lysis of cells with which they react. Killing of the cells is performed without prior exposure to or activation by the microbes or tumors. Because of this ability, NK cells act as an early line of defense against viral infections and few tumors. They recognize abnormal cells in two ways:

1. **Antibody dependent cellular cytotoxicity (ADCC). NK cells** bear (CD16) immunoglobulin receptors (F,R) and **bind antibody-coated targets leading to the lysis of target cells.** This phenomenon is called antibody-dependent cell-mediated cytotoxicity (type IV).
2. **Killing of target cells through receptors (Figs. 6.3A and B):** NK cells have a variety of **surface receptors for MHC** (major histocompatibility complex) **class I.** These are of two types **inhibitory or activating receptors.**

TABLE 6.2 Salient features of antibodies (immunoglobulins).

Features	*IgM (millionaire's antibody)*	*IgG (subtypes: IgG1, IgG2, IgG3, IgG4)*	*IgA*	*IgE (reagin/ homocytotropic antibody)*	*IgD*
Approximately % of total Ig	5%	80% (maximum)	15%	Trace	Trace
Molecular weight	900,000 (maximum)	150,000	150,000–300,000	190,000	180,000
Type of heavy chain	μ	γ	α	ε	δ
Structure	Pentamer (maximum size)	Monomer	Dimer (in glandular secretions), monomer (in serum)	Monomer	Monomer
Complement activation	Yes (classical pathway)	Yes (classical pathway)	Activates alternate complement pathway	No	No
Transport across placenta	No	Yes	No	No	No
Half-life (days)	5	21	6	2	3
Main function	Primary immune response	• Secondary immune response • Functions as B-cell receptor	• Mucosal immunity • Highly effective at neutralizing toxins	Allergic diseases, defense against parasite infection, and anaphylactic reaction	Unknown

The function of NK cells is regulated by a balance between signals from these activating and inhibitory receptors (**Figs. 6.3A and B**).

- **Inhibitory receptors:** MHC class I molecules are normally expressed on healthy/normal host cells. NK cell inhibitory receptors recognize this self-class I MHC molecules on normal healthy host cells (MHC class I positive). They prevent NK cells from killing normal host cells by inhibiting the death pathway.
- **Activating receptors:** They recognize molecules that are expressed at high levels on stressed or infected cells. Infections (e.g., viral infections) and stress are associated with reduced expression of class I MHC molecules and increased expression of molecules that engage activating receptors. These activating receptors kill the target cell. Thus, NK cells kill cells infected by some microbes or cells that are damaged beyond repair. NK cells also secrete cytokines such as interferon-γ (IFN-γ) and provide early defense against intracellular microbial infections.

Antigen-presenting Cells

Many types of cells capture antigens and display them to lymphocytes. Of these, dendritic cells are the most important antigen-presenting cell (APC) involved in displaying protein antigens to naïve T-cells.

Dendritic Cells

As the name suggests these cells have numerous fine cytoplasmic processes that resemble dendrites. These are important antigen-presenting cells in the body and can be functionally of the following types:

Interdigitating dendritic cells (IDC): They are the **most important APCs** for initiating primary T-cell responses against protein antigens. **The common location is below the epithelial lining. Immature dendritic cells within the epidermis are known as Langerhans cells.**

Follicular dendritic cell: It is present in the germinal centers of lymphoid follicles in the spleen and lymph nodes (hence named as follicular dendritic cell).

Other Antigen-presenting Cells

Macrophages: They are **a part of the mononuclear phagocyte system.** Macrophages **process the antigens** present in the phagocytosed microbes and protein antigens. After processing, the **antigen is presented to T-cells** and thus, they function as APCs in T-cell activation. They are also effector cells in immunity. These include the following:

- **Cell-mediated immunity:** Macrophages are the main effector cells in certain types of cell-mediated immunity, the reaction that serves to eliminate intracellular microbes. In this type of response, T-cells activate macrophages and increase their capability to kill ingested microbes.
- **Humoral immunity:** Macrophages also participate in the effector phase of humoral immunity. Macrophages get activated by IFN-γ.
- **Phagocytosis:** Macrophages efficiently phagocytose and destroy microbes that are opsonized (coated) by IgG or C3b through their respective receptors.

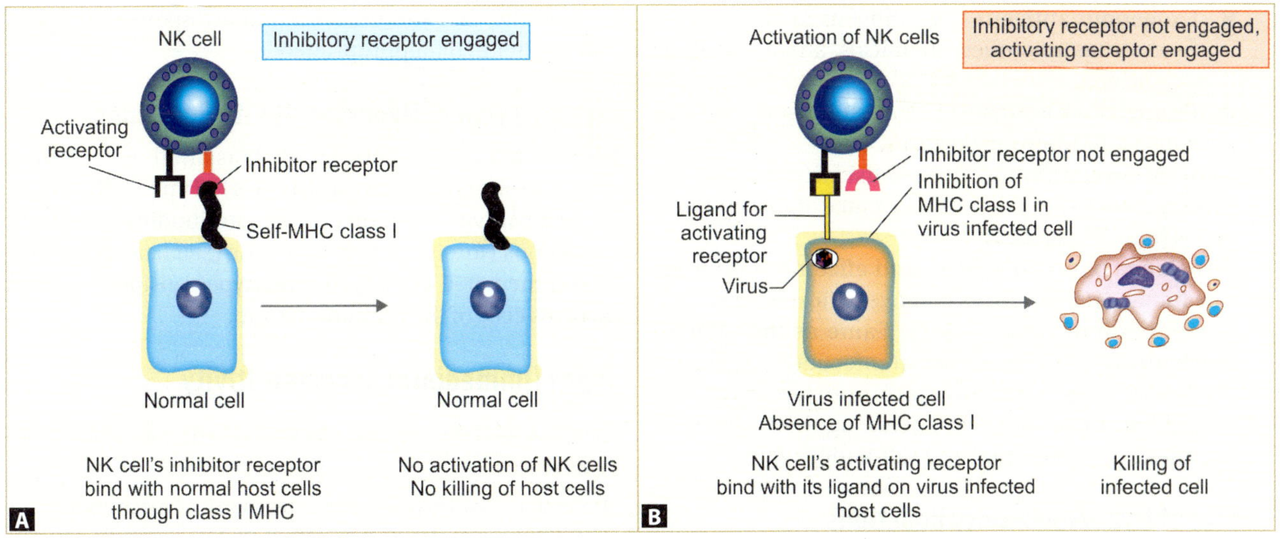

Figs. 6.3A and B: Activating and inhibitory receptors of natural killer (NK) cells: (A) Healthy host cells express self-class I major histocompatibility complex (MHC) molecules. These molecules are recognized by inhibitory receptors of NK cells. This prevents NK cells from killing healthy cells; (B) Infected and stressed cells have reduced expression of class I MHC molecules. Thus, the inhibitory receptors of NK cells are not engaged. There is expression of ligands for activating receptors. This results in the activation of NK cells and killing of infected cells/stressed cells.

Cytokines

Immune responses involve multiple interactions among many cells. These cells include lymphocytes, dendritic cells, macrophages, other inflammatory cells (e.g., neutrophils), and endothelial cells. Some of these interactions are cell-to-cell contact. However, many interactions and effector functions of leukocytes are mediated by **short-acting soluble small proteins** called **cytokines**. These cytokines represent the **messenger molecules of the immune system** and are involved in cell signaling. **Interleukins (ILs)** (play a role in communication between leukocytes) are a group of cytokines that regulate the immune and inflammatory responses.

Classification: Most of the cytokines have many effects and can be classified depending on their functions.

Cytokines of innate immunity: These cytokines are produced rapidly in response to microbes and other stimuli.

- **Sources:** Mainly secreted by macrophages, dendritic cells, and NK cells.
- **Actions:** Induce inflammation and inhibit replication of the virus (antiviral defense).
- **Cytokines.** TNF, IL-1, IL-12, type I IFNs, IFN-γ and chemokines.

Cytokines of adaptive immune responses: These are as follows:

- **Source:** These cytokines are produced mainly by CD4+ T lymphocytes in response to antigen and other signals.
- **Actions:** They promote lymphocyte proliferation and differentiation and activate effector cells.
- **Cytokines:** IL-2, IL-4, IL-5, IL-17, and IFN-γ.

Colony-stimulating factors: These cytokines stimulate hematopoiesis and are assayed by their ability to stimulate the formation of blood cell colonies from bone marrow progenitors. They increase leukocyte numbers during immune and inflammatory responses.

HYPERSENSITIVITY REACTIONS

PA 9.2 (CC): Describe the mechanism of hypersensitivity reactions.

Q. Classify and briefly describe hypersensitivity reactions.

Immune response is generally a protective process but sometimes it may be injurious. Immune reactions that lead to tissue injury are categorized under *hypersensitivity,* and the resulting diseases are termed *hypersensitivity diseases.* Hypersensitivity means that the **body responds to a particular antigen in an exaggerated fashion**, where it does not happen in normal circumstances. Thus, hypersensitivity is considered an immune response that is inappropriately triggered, excessive, or produces undesirable effects on the body.

Definition: Hypersensitivity reaction is a **pathological, excessive, and injurious immune response to antigen, leading to tissue injury, disease,** or sometimes death **in a sensitized individual**. The resulting diseases are named hypersensitivity diseases.

General Features of Hypersensitivity Disorders

The basic mechanism that triggers hypersensitivity is a specific antigen–antibody reaction or a specific antigen–lymphocyte interaction.

- **Priming or sensitization:** It occurs in **individuals who had previous contact with the antigen** (allergen).
- **Nature of antigens:** It may be **exogenous or endogenous** origin.

   - **Exogenous antigens** (e.g., antigens in dust, pollen, food, drugs, microbes, chemicals, and a few blood products).
   - **Endogenous antigens:** Self or autologous antigens **cause autoimmune diseases.**
- **Genetic susceptibility:** Hypersensitivity diseases are usually associated with the inheritance of susceptibility genes (e.g., HLA genes).
- **Imbalance between control and effector of immune mechanisms:** It produces damage to host tissues.
- **Mechanism of tissue injury:** Same as the effector mechanisms of defense against infectious pathogens. However, these reactions are poorly controlled, excessive, or misdirected (e.g., against normally harmless environmental and self-antigens).

Causes of Hypersensitivity Reactions

Hypersensitivity immune responses may be directed against different types of antigens. These include the following:

Autoimmunity: This is caused due to reactions against self-antigens. Normally, the immune system does not elicit an immune reaction against one's own antigens. This phenomenon is termed *self-tolerance* (i.e., the body "tolerates" its own antigens). Occasionally, there is a failure of self-tolerance. This results in reactions against one's own cells and tissues. This is called *autoimmunity.* The diseases caused due to autoimmunity are called *autoimmune diseases.*

Reactions against microbes: There are many types of reactions against microbial antigens that may cause disease.

1. **Excessive immune reaction or unusually persistent: T-cell responses against persistent microbes.** In some infections, the microbial antigen is unusually persistent (e.g., *Mycobacterium tuberculosis*). T-cell responses against such persistent microbes may give rise to severe inflammation, and cause tissue injury sometimes with the formation of granulomas. It is seen in tuberculosis and some other infections.
2. **Formation of immune complexes:** The microbial antigens elicit antibodies. These antibodies may bind to the antigens and produce immune complexes. These immune complexes may deposit in tissues and trigger inflammation (e.g., post-infectious glomerulonephritis).
3. **Cross-reactivity:** Rarely, do antibodies or T cells react with a microbe cross-react with a host tissue. This cross-reactivity is involved in the development of rheumatic heart disease. The SARS-CoV-2 coronavirus can induce a systemic inflammatory reaction that is an important cause of morbidity in COVID-19.

Reactions against environmental antigens: Individuals may be allergic to common environmental substances (e.g., pollens, animal dander, and dust mites), and therapeutic drugs. These are usually noninfectious, harmless antigens to all persons who are exposed to them. However, some individuals react against these antigens. Such individuals are prone to produce an unusual immune response.

In all these conditions, the immune response is triggered and maintained inappropriately.

Classification of Hypersensitivity Reactions

Hypersensitivity reactions are classified according to immune mechanisms **(Table 6.3)**. Type I, II, and III hypersensitivity reactions involve antibodies specific for exogenous (foreign) or endogenous (self) antigens. Type IV, cell-mediated or delayed-type, hypersensitivity reaction involves cells of the immune system.

Type I (Immediate) Hypersensitivity

Q. Write a short note on type I hypersensitivity reactions and their pathogenesis.

Definition: Type I hypersensitivity reaction is a type of **immediate immunological tissue reaction**. It generally **occurs rapidly (within 5–10 minutes) after the interaction of antigen** (allergen) **with IgE antibodies bound to the surface of mast cells in a sensitized person.**

Characteristics

- **Immediate reaction:** Type I hypersensitivity is also known as ***immediate hypersensitivity*** reaction because it occurs within minutes (5–10 minutes).
- **Antigen called allergen:** The environmental antigens that initiate or elicit type I reactions are known as **allergens** because it triggers allergy. **Environmental factors are important in the development of allergic diseases.** The resulting diseases are usually known as **allergic or atopic disorders.** Many allergens (e.g., house dust mites, pollens, animal danders, or molds) in the environment are **harmless for most individuals**. Allergens elicit significant IgE reactions only in **genetically predisposed individuals**, who are said to be **atopic.** An increased tendency to develop immediate hypersensitivity reactions is called *atopy.*
- **Mediated by IgE antibodies:** It **develops after the interaction of environmental antigens (allergens) with IgE antibodies** bound to **mast cells.** The injury in type I hypersensitivity reaction is mainly caused by Th2 cells, IgE antibodies, and mast cells (its mediators). The mediators released from mast cells act on blood vessels and smooth muscle. The cytokines from mast cells recruit and activate inflammatory cells.
- **Genetic susceptibility:** Immediate hypersensitivity reactions occur in **genetically susceptible individuals previously sensitized** to the antigen. There is a strong genetic or hereditary linkage regarding the IgE response to antigens (allergens). This genetic component involves both the ability to respond to an allergen and the general ability to produce an IgE antibody response. Most have higher levels of serum IgE and more IL-4-4-producing **Th2 cells than the general population.**

TABLE 6.3 Classification of hypersensitivity reaction according to the effector immune mechanism.

Type of hypersensitivity reaction	*Immune mechanisms*	*Examples of associated disorders*
Antibody-mediated		
Immediate (type I) hypersensitivity	• Production of IgE antibody and involvement of Th2 cells • Immediate release of vasoactive amines and other mediators from mast cells • Later recruitment of inflammatory cells	Local: Hay fever, bronchial asthma (atopic form), allergies, urticaria (hives) Systemic: Anaphylaxis
Antibody-mediated (type II) hypersensitivity	• Production of cytotoxic antibodies IgG, and IgM. They bind to an antigen on the target cell surface or fixed tissue. It leads to phagocytosis. • Lysis of target cell by activated complement or Fc receptors mediated inflammation.	Autoimmune hemolytic anemia; Goodpasture syndrome
Immune complex–mediated (type III) hypersensitivity	Antibodies (IgG, IgM, IgA) formed against exogenous or endogenous antigens. Form immune complexes usually in the circulation, deposition of antigen-antibody complexes in vascular beds leads to activation of complement system. Complement products recruit leukocytes and induce inflammation. Fc receptors of leukocytes release enzymes and other toxic molecules	Autoimmune diseases such as systemic lupus erythematosus (SLE), rheumatoid arthritis; some forms of glomerulonephritis; serum sickness; Arthus reaction
Cell-mediated		
Cell-mediated immune (type IV) hypersensitivity	• $CD4^+$ cytokine-mediated inflammation: Activated T lymphocytes release cytokines, inflammation, and macrophage activation CD4+ T lymphocytes of the Th1 and Th17 subsets produce cytokines and induce inflammation. • T cell-mediated cytotoxicity: CD8+ T cells kill virally infected cells, mismatched transplant cells, or tumor cells	Contact dermatitis; granulomatous diseases (tuberculosis, leprosy) Type 1 diabetes, Hashimoto thyroiditis

- **Severity:** Clinical manifestations depend on the site of antigen exposure and the extent of sensitization. It may be **mild** (e.g., seasonal rhinitis, hay fever), **or severe** debilitating (e.g., asthma), **or** even **fatal** (e.g., anaphylaxis).
- **Generalized or localized:** The reactions may be localized (e.g., asthma) or genialized (anaphylaxis) reactions.

Sequence of Events (Fig. 6.4)

Most type I hypersensitivity reactions follow a classical sequence of cellular responses. The following sequence of events occurs only in a genetically susceptible individual exposed to common environmental antigens:

During Initial Exposure to Antigen (Sensitization)

- **Exposure to sensitizing antigen (allergen):** Individuals are exposed to environmental allergens. They may be introduced by: **(1) inhalation, (2) ingestion, or (3) injection**. The antigen is taken up by dendritic cells (antigen-presenting cells) and presented to Naïve T cells.
- **Activation of Th2 cells:** In genetically susceptible individuals, antigens (allergens) strongly activate **Th2 cells.** These Th2 cells are a subset of CD4+ (helper) T-cells that **secrete several cytokines (e.g., IL-4, IL-5, and IL-13)** which are responsible for the reactions of type I hypersensitivity.
- **Production of IgE antibodies by B cells: IL-4 and IL-13** secreted by Th2 cells **stimulate antigen-specific B-cells (plasma cells) to secrete** cytotropic **IgE antibodies.** IL-5 activates eosinophils and recruits to the site of reaction. IL-13 also stimulates epithelial cells to secrete mucus.
- **Sensitization of mast cells by IgE antibody:** Mast cells are mainly concentrated near blood vessels and nerves and in subepithelial tissues (common sites of type I hypersensitivity). Mast cells have high-affinity receptors for the Fc portion of the epsilon (ε) heavy chain of IgE called FcεR1. **IgE antibodies** produced by plasma cells **attach to** the FcεR1 on the **mast cells.** These **IgE antibody-bearing mast cells are sensitized to react if antigens bind to these antibodies**. Basophils circulating in blood resemble mast cells and express FcεR1. These basophils may also contribute to immediate hypersensitivity reactions.

During Subsequent Exposure to Antigen (Activation Phase)

- **Binding of allergen to IgE molecules on mast cells during re-exposure:** When a sensitized individual (the

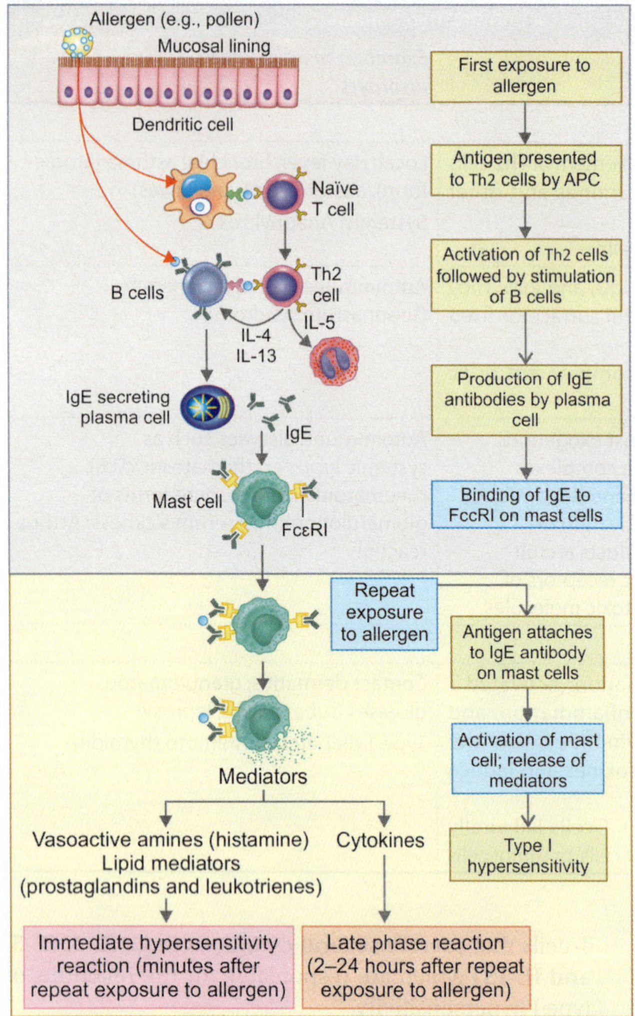

Fig. 6.4: Sequence of events in type I hypersensitivity. It is initiated by exposure to an allergen, which stimulates Th2 responses and IgE production, in genetically susceptible individuals. IgE binds to mast cells. On re-exposure to the allergen, the antigen binds to IgE on the mast cells and activates it to secrete the mediators. These mediators produce the manifestations of type I hypersensitivity. (APC: antigen-presenting cell).

mast cell has attached IgE antibodies) is subsequently re-exposed to the specific allergen, the allergen binds to antigen-specific IgE molecules on mast cells. It usually occurs at or near the site of entry of allergen entry.

- **Activation of mast cells and release of mediators:** The **antigen (allergen) binds** to more than one **IgE antibody molecule on mast cells and is termed cross-linking.** This generates signals leading to the secretion of various mediators from the mast cells **(mast cell degranulation).**

Mediators of Type I Hypersensitivity Reactions

It consists of three groups namely vasoactive amines, lipid mediators, and cytokines.

Vasoactive amines: These are preformed molecules and are released from mast cell granules. The most important is **histamine,** which is released within seconds or minutes of mast cell activation. Histamine causes **vasodilation, increased vascular permeability, smooth muscle contraction, and increased secretion of mucus.** Other mediators include proteases and other contents of mast cell granules.

Lipid mediators: These are **newly synthesized by activated mast cells** in the same pathways as do other leukocytes (arachidonic acid pathway, *refer* pages 74-5 and **Fig. 3.10**). These include prostaglandins and leukotrienes.

- **Prostaglandin D2 (PGD_2):** It is the most abundant mediator produced by the cyclooxygenase pathway in mast cells. It **causes severe bronchospasm and increased secretion of mucus.**
- **Leukotrienes:** These are produced by lipoxygenase pathways in mast cells. **LTC_4 and LTD_4** are the most powerful vasoactive and spasmogenic agents. They are more active than histamine in **increasing vascular permeability and producing contraction of bronchial smooth muscle. LTB_4 is a powerful chemotactic mediator** for neutrophils, eosinophils, and monocytes.

Cytokines: Activated mast cells secrete many cytokines that are **involved during the late-phase reaction.** These include **TNF and chemokines**, which **recruit and activate leukocytes.**

Two Phases of IgE Triggered Reactions

Type I hypersensitivity reaction has two well-defined phases namely (1) immediate response and (2) late-phase reaction.

Immediate Response

Time of development and duration: It usually develops **within 5–30 minutes after exposure** to an allergen and subsides within 60 minutes.

Mediators: Mast cell granule contents (vasoactive amines such as histamine) and **lipid mediators** mediate it (prostaglandins and leukotrienes **(Fig. 6.4)**.

Characteristics: These include **vasodilation, increased vascular permeability (leakage), and spasms of nonvascular smooth muscles.**

Late-phase Reaction

Time of development and duration: It usually **begins 2 to 8 hours** after the exposure to antigen. It may **last for several days.**

Mediators: It is mainly mediated by **cytokines.**

Characteristics: It is characterized by **inflammation and tissue injury.**

- **Dominant inflammatory cells:** These include **neutrophils, eosinophils, and lymphocytes,** especially Th2 cells. **These cells infiltrate involved tissues.** Inflammation is a major component of many allergic diseases, notably asthma and atopic dermatitis.

Hence, therapy is by anti-inflammatory drugs such as corticosteroids.

- **Tissue injury:** For example, damage to the mucosal epithelial cells.

Clinical Manifestations

Clinical manifestations of type I hypersensitivity reaction **vary in severity and intensity**. The route of exposure to antigen usually determines the nature of the reaction. It **may occur as a local reaction or as a systemic disorder.** Examples of type I hypersensitivity reactions are listed in **Table 6.4**.

Local reactions: They generally **occur at the particular site of exposure** and depend on the mode of exposure. For example, it develops in the skin following contact, the gastrointestinal tract following ingestion, or the lungs following inhalation of an allergen. Common examples include certain forms of bronchial asthma (bronchoconstriction), allergic rhinitis (hay fever), food allergies, hives (urticaria), and atopic dermatitis (eczema).

However, ingestion or inhalation of allergens can also produce systemic reactions if the allergen is absorbed into the circulation (e.g., peanut allergy). Sometimes, infants develop atopic dermatitis, followed, by allergic rhinitis and asthma later in life. These three disorders (atopic dermatitis, allergic rhinitis, and asthma) are form the *atopic triad.* Their sequential development is called the *atopic march.*

Systemic disorders: The protein antigens (e.g., in bee venom) or drugs (e.g., penicillin) that enter the circulation may produce a life-threatening allergic reaction called systemic *anaphylaxis***.** In a sensitized individual, the patient develops itching, urticaria (hives), and skin erythema within minutes of exposure to the allergen. This is followed rapidly by severe respiratory difficulty due to pulmonary bronchoconstriction and hypersecretion of mucus. Laryngeal edema may further enhance airway obstruction. It may also affect the musculature of the entire gastrointestinal tract, causing vomiting, abdominal cramps, and diarrhea. Without immediate intervention, systemic vasodilation will lead to a fall in blood pressure (anaphylactic shock).

TABLE 6.4 Examples of disorders caused by type I hypersensitivity reactions.

Localized type I hypersensitivity	*Systemic type I hypersensitivity*
• Bronchial asthma (atopic/extrinsic) • Allergic rhinitis, sinusitis (hay fever) • Allergic conjunctivitis • Urticaria • Atopic dermatitis/eczema • Angioedema • Allergic gastroenteritis (food allergy)	Anaphylaxis due to: • Drugs such as antibiotics (most commonly penicillin) • Bee stings • Insect bite • Foreign proteins (e.g., antisera) • Foods (peanuts, fish, and shellfish) • Food additives

The patient may progress to circulatory collapse and death within minutes.

Diagnosis of type I hypersensitivity: It is by typical clinical history and examination, skin-prick testing, and by measuring specific IgE in the serum.

Antibody-mediated (Type II) Hypersensitivity

Q. Write a short note on type II hypersensitivity reactions.

Definition: Type II hypersensitivity disorders are **caused by antibodies (IgG/IgM)**, which react with **target antigens on the surface of specific cells or other tissue components.**

Characteristics

Antibodies: The antibodies that mediate type II reactions are **IgG (usually) and IgM (rarely).**

Antigen: It may be endogenous or exogenous:

- **Endogenous antigens:** These antigens may be normal molecules **intrinsic to the cell membrane or extracellular matrix** (e.g., autoimmune diseases).
- **Exogenous antigens:** The exogenous antigens (e.g., drug metabolite) may get **adsorbed on a cell surface or extracellular matrix.** They may cause altered surface antigens.

Mechanism of Injury

In type II hypersensitivity, antibodies cause disease by any of the **three mechanisms** (1) **targeting cells for phagocytosis**, (2) **activating the complement system and inflammation**, or (3) **interfering with normal cellular functions**. The antibodies responsible for type II reactions are IgG and IgM antibodies capable of activating complement. IgG can also bind to phagocyte Fc receptors.

1. Opsonization and Phagocytosis (Fig. 6.5A)

- **Opsonization of target cells:** Opsonization is an immune process in which the foreign pathogens for elimination by phagocytes are coated by molecules called opsonins. The opsonin facilitates phagocytosis of the target (cell/microbe). The opsonins include immunoglobulin G (IgG and complement component C3b. In this mechanism, circulating cells, such as **red cells or platelets, become coated (opsonized) with autoantibodies, with or without complement proteins.**
- **Phagocytosis of target cells through receptors:** The opsonized target cells undergo **phagocytosis by neutrophils and macrophages.** These **phagocytes have receptors for the Fc fraction of IgG antibodies and breakdown products of the C3 complement protein.** These receptors on phagocytic cells **bind and ingest opsonized particles.**
- **Destruction of target cells in the spleen:** Opsonized blood cells (red cells, platelets) undergo destruction by macrophages in the spleen. Hence, splenectomy is of clinical benefit in some antibody-mediated diseases.

Clinical situations associated with antibody-mediated cell destruction

- **Transfusion reactions:** If blood from an incompatible donor is transfused to a recipient **(major blood group incompatibilities)**, cells from an incompatible donor react with preformed antibodies in the host (recipient), leading to its destruction of RBCs (intravascular hemolysis).
- **Hemolytic anemia of the fetus and newborn (erythroblastosis fetalis):** In this, there is an **incompatibility between fetal and mother red blood cells.** IgG anti-red blood cell antibodies from the mother cross the placenta and destroy fetal RBCs.
- **Autoimmune hemolytic anemia, neutropenia, and thrombocytopenia:** In these conditions, individuals produce antibodies against their own blood cells.
- **Drug-induced hemolytic anemia:** In this, a drug attaches to plasma membrane proteins of red cells, and antibodies are produced against the drug-protein complex. This in turn destroys red blood cells.

2. Activating the Complement System and Inflammation (Fig. 6.5B)

The inflammation may be produced by two mechanisms namely **(i) complement-mediated or (ii) Fc receptor-mediated inflammation.**

- **Complement-mediated inflammation:** In this type II hypersensitivity, **antibodies bound to tissue antigens activate the complement system** by the classical pathway. Products of activated complement have many actions, and one of them is the **recruitment of leukocytes** namely neutrophils and macrophages. Activated inflammatory cells (leukocytes) **cause injury by releasing lysosomal enzymes and generating toxic reactive oxygen species** (free radicals). They cause injury to target cells.
- **Fc receptor-mediated inflammation:** Leukocytes have Fc receptors (FcR) on the cell surface. It can bind the Fc portion of the antibody (immunoglobulin/Ig). Thus, **leukocytes attach the Fc portion of antibodies through its Fc receptors.** This leads **accumulation of leukocytes and inflammation.**

Clinical situations: This antibody-mediated inflammation produces tissue injury in some forms of **glomerulonephritis** (e.g., Goodpasture syndrome due to complement- and Fc receptor–mediated inflammation), **vasculitis caused by ANCA** (neutrophil degranulation and inflammation), pemphigus vulgaris (antibody-mediated activation of proteases), and **vascular rejection in organ grafts**.

3. Antibody-mediated Cellular Dysfunction

In this mechanism of type II hypertensives, the antibodies are directed against an essential protein. These antibodies impair or dysregulate the important functions of the target cell without directly causing cell injury or inflammation.

Clinical situations

- **Antibodies blocking the binding of vitamin B_{12} to intrinsic factors:** Intrinsic factor is required for absorption of vitamin B_{12} in the stomach. In **pernicious anemia, antibodies are directed against** an intrinsic factor that **prevents the absorption of vitamin B_{12}**. This leads to a deficiency of this vitamin and abnormal hematopoiesis. In pernicious anemia, antibody-mediated damage to gastric epithelial cells may also contribute.
- **Antibody-mediated stimulation of cell function (Fig. 6.5C):** Antibodies can also stimulate excessive cellular responses. For example, in **Graves disease, antibodies are present against the thyroid-stimulating hormone receptor** on thyroid epithelial cells. These antibodies stimulate thyroid epithelial cells to secrete thyroid hormones. This leads to hyperthyroidism.
- **Antibody- and complement-mediated damage:** Previously, it was thought that in **myasthenia gravis,** antibodies directed against acetylcholine receptors in the motor end plates of skeletal muscles block neuromuscular transmission. This results in muscle weakness, but without injury. However, recent findings have shown benefits with complement inhibition therapies. This suggests that **both antibody- and complement-mediated damage to motor end plates** may be involved in its pathogenesis. Examples of type II hypersensitivity diseases are presented in **Table 6.5.**

Immune Complex-mediated (Type III) Hypersensitivity

Q. Write a short note on type III hypersensitivity reactions.

Antigen–antibody complexes are termed immune complexes: Type III hypersensitivity reaction is an immune complex-mediated reaction.

Definition: Type III hypersensitivity reactions are **characterized by the formation of immune complexes in the circulation.** These complexes may **get deposited in blood vessels, leading to complement activation and subsequent self-sustaining acute inflammation.** The inflammatory cells recruited (neutrophils and monocytes) **release lysosomal enzymes,** generate **toxic free radicals, and cause tissue damage.**

General Characteristics

Antibodies: Type III hypersensitivity involves **complement-fixing antibodies namely IgG, IgM,** and occasionally IgA.

Antigen. It may be exogenous or endogenous.

- **Exogenous:** Various **foreign proteins** such as foreign serum protein injected (e.g., diphtheria antitoxin, horse anti-thymocyte globulin) or produced by an infectious microbe.
- **Endogenous: Antibody against self-components** (autoimmunity), e.g., nucleoproteins.

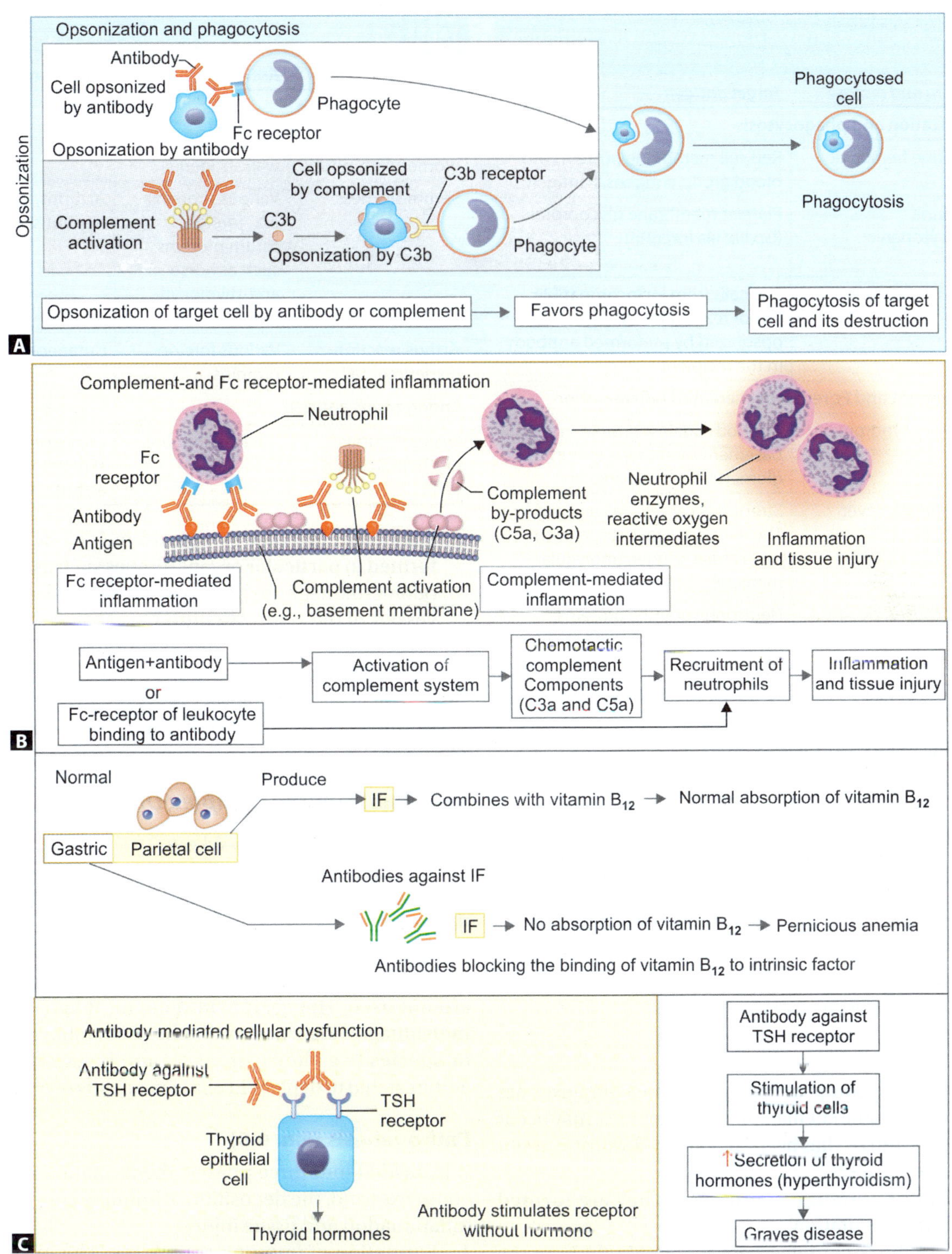

Figs. 6.5A to C: Various mechanisms of type II hypersensitivity reaction: (A) Opsonization and phagocytosis: The cells are opsonized by antibodies and complement components. They undergo phagocytosis followed by lysis of cells inside the phagocytes (e.g., macrophages in the spleen); (B) Complement and Fc receptor-mediated inflammation. Inflammation is induced by antibody binding to Fc receptors of leukocytes and by complement breakdown products; (C) Antibody-mediated stimulation of cell function. Pernicious anemia is due to antibodies blocking the binding of intrinsic factor (IF) with vitamin B_{12}. Autoantibodies bind against the thyroid-stimulating hormone (TSH) receptor and activate thyroid cells to produce excessive hormones and cause hyperthyroidism in Graves' disease.

TABLE 6.5 Examples of type II hypersensitivity (antibody-mediated) diseases.

Mechanism and disease	*Target antigen*
1. Opsonization and phagocytosis	
Autoimmune hemolytic anemia	Red cell membrane proteins (Rh blood group antigens, I antigen)
Autoimmune thrombocytopenic purpura	Platelet membrane glycoprotein (Gp IIb: IIIa integrin)
Transfusion reactions	The cells from an incompatible donor react with and are opsonized by preformed antibody in the recipient
2. Complement and Fc receptor-mediated inflammation	
Goodpasture syndrome	Antibody against protein in basement membrane kidney glomeruli and lung alveoli
Acute rheumatic fever	Streptococcal cell wall antigen. The antibody cross-reacts with myocardial antigen (molecular mimicry)
Vasculitis caused by ANCA	Neutrophil granule proteins, probably released from activated neutrophils
Pemphigus vulgaris	Antibody-mediated activation of proteases
3. Antibody-mediated cellular dysfunction	
Pernicious anemia	Antibody against the intrinsic factor of gastric parietal cells
Graves disease (hyperthyroidism)	Antibody against thyroid-stimulating hormone (TSH) receptor (agonistic antibodies)
Myasthenia gravis	Both antibody- and complement-mediated damage to motor end plates

(ANCA: antineutrophil cytoplasmic antibodies).

Sites of immune complex formation. The complexes are usually formed in the circulation, but sometimes, may occur at sites where antigen has been "planted" previously (in situ immune complexes).

- **Circulating immune complexes:** They are **formed within the circulation.**
- **In situ immune complex:** Less commonly, the immune complexes are formed at **extravascular sites** where antigens might have been previously planted.

Sites of immune complex deposition: The circulating antigen-antibody complexes once formed, are deposited in various tissues. The deposition may be systemic or local.

- **Systemic deposition:** Circulating immune complexes tend to be systemic. These complexes can deposit in blood vessels anywhere in the body (**in many organs**).

TABLE 6.6 Examples of immune complex-mediated diseases.

Disease	*Antigen*	*Manifestations*
Exogenous antigen		
Poststreptococcal glomerulonephritis	Streptococcal cell wall antigen(s)	Glomerulonephritis
Serum sickness	Various proteins, e.g., foreign serum proteins such as horse anti-thymocyte globulin	Arthritis, vasculitis, nephritis
Arthus reaction (experimental)	Various foreign proteins	Cutaneous vasculitis
Endogenous antigen		
Systemic lupus erythematosus (SLE)	Nuclear antigens	Glomerulonephritis, skin lesions, arthritis, others

- **Localized:** Immune complexes may be **deposited or formed in particular organs/tissues such as the kidney** (glomerulonephritis), **joints** (arthritis), and **small blood vessels of the skin (vasculitis)**.

Most pathogenic immune complexes are those that are produced in amounts and sizes that are not efficiently cleared by phagocytes in the spleen and liver.

Examples of immune complex disorders are listed in **Table 6.6**.

Systemic Immune Complex Disease

Q. Write a short note on serum sickness.

Serum sickness is a classic example of a systemic immune complex disease. It was once a frequent sequela that occurred after the administration of large amounts of foreign serum (e.g., serum from immunized horses used for protection against diphtheria). Nowadays, foreign serums are not used. Hence, it is infrequent. It **can develop in individuals who receive antibodies from other individuals or species** (e.g., horse or rabbit antithymocyte globulin administered to deplete T cells in recipients of organ grafts).

Pathogenesis (Fig. 6.6)

It is divided into three phases: the formation of immune complexes and, the deposition of immune complexes. and inflammation and tissue injury.

1. **Formation of immune complexes: The introduction of protein antigen initiates an immune response.** It results in the **formation of antibodies.** Antibodies usually form a week (7–12 days) after the injection of the foreign protein (exposure to the antigen) and these antibodies are secreted into the blood. The antibodies in the circulation react with the antigen that is still present and **form antigen-antibody (immune) complexes.** Most immune complexes are removed effectively before

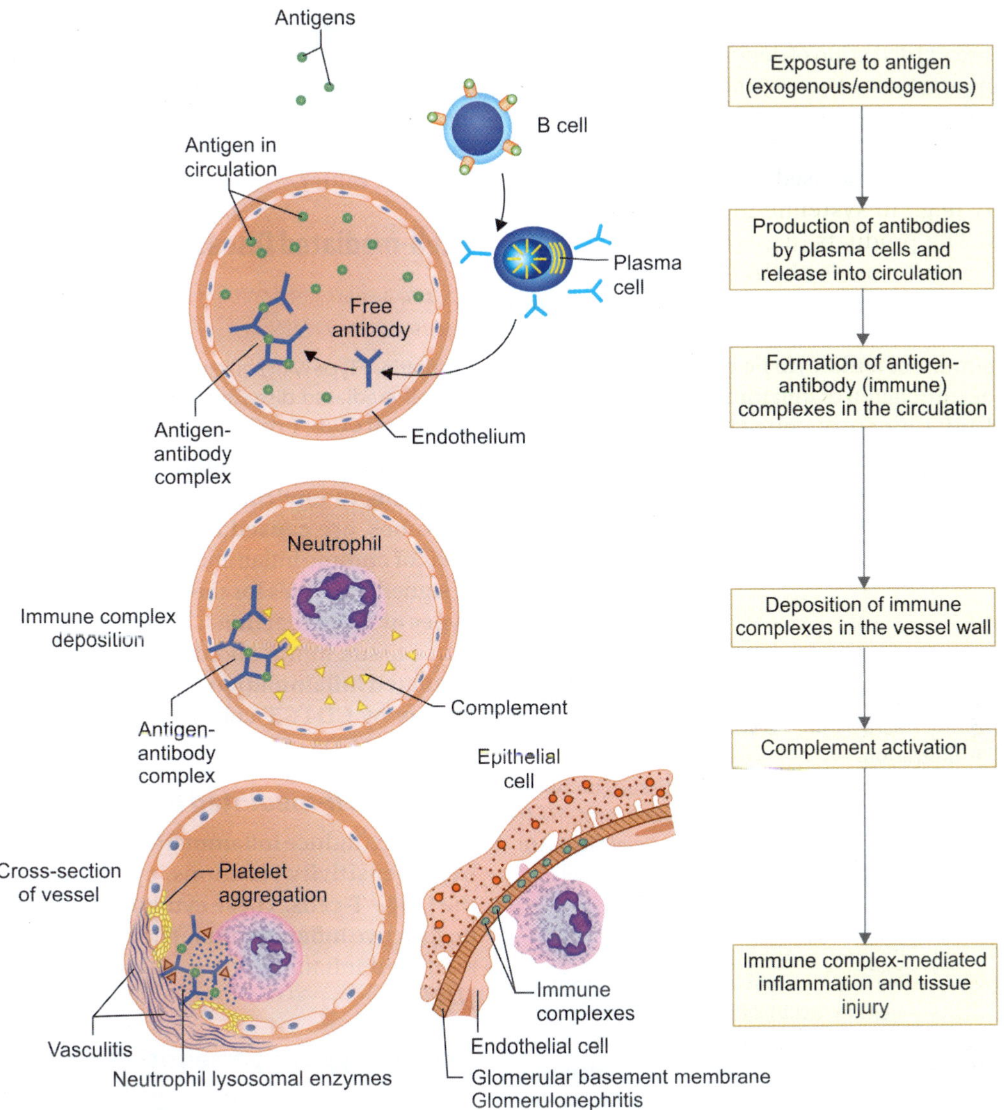

Fig. 6.6: Pathogenesis of systemic immune complex-mediated disease (type III hypersensitivity). Immune complexes are deposited in tissue to activate the complement system and recruit tissue-damaging inflammatory cells. The pathogenic ability of immune complexes to mediate tissue injury depends on size, solubility, net charge, and ability to fix complement.

they can cause tissue injury. In type III hypersensitivity, the immune complexes are not removed. Type III hypersensitivity results from the **failure** of the immune and phagocytic systems **to effectively remove antigen–antibody immune complexes** and is not tissue specific. It is not an immediate reaction. It occurs over several hours or longer (i.e., glomerulonephritis) and is usually an ongoing process.

2. **Deposition of immune complexes:** During the next phase, the **immune complexes are deposited in vessels.** The sites of immune complexes deposits are the areas where they become concentrated. They concentrate in organs where blood is filtered at high pressure to form other fluids (e.g., like urine and synovial fluid). Hence, the immune complex usually affects **glomeruli and joints.** The endothelium in these regions is usually fenestrated, thereby promoting the passage of immune complexes between endothelial cells. Usually, the **most pathogenic immune complexes are those of medium size, formed under conditions of slight antigen excess.** These deposits cause an inflammatory process leading to tissue injury.
3. **Inflammation and tissue injury:** Once deposited in tissues, **immune complexes initiate acute inflammatory reactions.** This develops approximately 10 days after antigen administration. Inflammatory reaction may be brought out by two mechanisms:
   - **Complement activation:** The antibodies involved are IgG or IgM. Both these antibodies activate complement by the classical pathway. Features

supporting evidence of complement-mediated injury are: (1) detection of deposition of complement proteins at the site of injury, and (2) consumption of complement during the active phase of the disease as evidenced by decreased serum levels of C3. The C3 level can be used as a marker for disease activity [e.g., in systemic lupus erythematosus (SLE)]. The products (e.g., chemotactic C5a) of complement causes chemotactic **recruitment of acute inflammatory cells** (neutrophils and monocytes) to the site.

- **Engagement of leukocyte Fc receptors:** This leads to the accumulation of inflammatory cells at the site.

Activated inflammatory cells (leukocytes) **release lysosomal enzymes, arachidonic acid products, and reactive oxygen species** which produce **tissue damage.**

Clinical features: Fever, urticaria, joint pains (arthralgias), lymph node enlargement and proteinuria appear during this phase.

MORPHOLOGY

General Features

- **Acute necrotizing vasculitis:** It is the **main feature** and is characterized by **necrosis of the vessel wall and intense neutrophilic infiltration.**
- **Fibrinoid necrosis:** It consists of necrotic tissue, immune complexes deposits, complement, and plasma protein. It produces a **smudgy eosinophilic appearance** (*refer* **Fig. 2.10**) at the site of the deposit and obscures the cellular detail.

Kidney

Features of immune complex deposits in the kidney.

- **Immunofluorescence microscopy:** It appears as **granular lumpy deposits** (*refer* **Fig. 20.8**) of immunoglobulin and complement.
- **Electron microscopy:** It appears as **electron-dense deposits** along the glomerular basement membrane (*refer* **Fig. 20.9**).

- **Acute serum sickness:** It is induced by administration of a single large dose of antigen. It presents with fever, rash, and arthritis. The lesions resolve as the immune complexes are cleared by phagocytes.
- **Chronic serum sickness:** It develops with repeated or prolonged exposure to an antigen. This occurs in many diseases, such as systemic lupus erythematosus (SLE), membranous glomerulonephritis, polyarteritis nodosa, and several other vasculitides. SLE is associated with persistent antibody responses to autoantigens.

Local Immune Complex Disease (Arthus Reaction)

Q. Write a short note on Arthus reaction.

Arthus reaction is a **local area of tissue necrosis usually in the skin.** It **results from acute immune complex vasculitis.** Arthus reaction can be experimentally produced by injection of an antigen into the skin of a previously immunized animal (with circulating antibodies against the antigen). As the antigen diffuses into the vascular wall, it **locally binds to the antibody and forms large immune complexes at the site of injection.** Within a few hours, edema, and hemorrhage, occasionally followed by ulceration develop at the site of the injection site. **Immune complexes deposited in the vessel walls cause fibrinoid necrosis and thrombosis leading to ischemic injury.**

T-cell-mediated Diseases (Type IV Hypersensitivity)

Q. Write a short note on type IV hypersensitivity reactions/delayed hypersensitivity reactions.

Definition: Type IV hypersensitivity is **mediated by T lymphocytes** (T-cell-mediated diseases). **Two types of T-cells are involved CD4+ and CD8+ T-cells.**

Importance: Many **autoimmune disorders, and pathologic reactions to environmental chemicals and persistent microbes, are caused by T-cells.** T-cell reactions are the basis of chronic inflammatory diseases. Many of the newly designed therapies for these diseases target T cells.

Types of T-cell reactions: Two types of T-cell reactions can cause tissue injury and disease. These are (1) **Cytokine-mediated inflammation** in which **cytokines are produced mainly by CD4+ T-cells** and (2) **Direct cell cytotoxicity caused** by **CD8+ T-cells.**

CD4+ T-cell-mediated Inflammation

Cytokines induce inflammation. In CD4+ T-cell-mediated hypersensitivity reactions, cytokines are produced by the CD4+ T-cells. These cytokines can cause chronic and destructive inflammation. The **classical example** of T-cell-mediated inflammation is ***delayed-type hypersensitivity (DTH).***

Delayed-Type Hypersensitivity

Delayed-type hypersensitivity (DTH) develops in response to antigenic exposure in a previously sensitized individual. In the DTH reaction, an antigen is injected into the skin. It leads to a detectable skin reaction within 24–48 hours. Since the **reaction is delayed** (by 24–48 hours) **after exposure to antigen,** it is termed delayed-type hypersensitivity (DTH). This contrasts with immediate hypersensitivity which occurs immediately.

Mechanism of CD4+ T-cell-mediated inflammation (Fig. 6.7)

- **Presentation of tissue antigen to naïve CD4+ T-cells.** On first exposure to a protein antigen, the antigen is taken up by dendritic cells. The **dendritic cell (antigen-presenting cell/APC) presents the antigens to naïve T-cells.**
- **Differentiation of CD4+ T-cells into effector Th cells (Th1 or Th17):** After the antigen is presented to naïve T cells, CD4+ T-cells are activated. CD4+ T-cells differentiate into effector cells namely Th1 and Th17. Classical T-cell-mediated hypersensitivity is a reaction

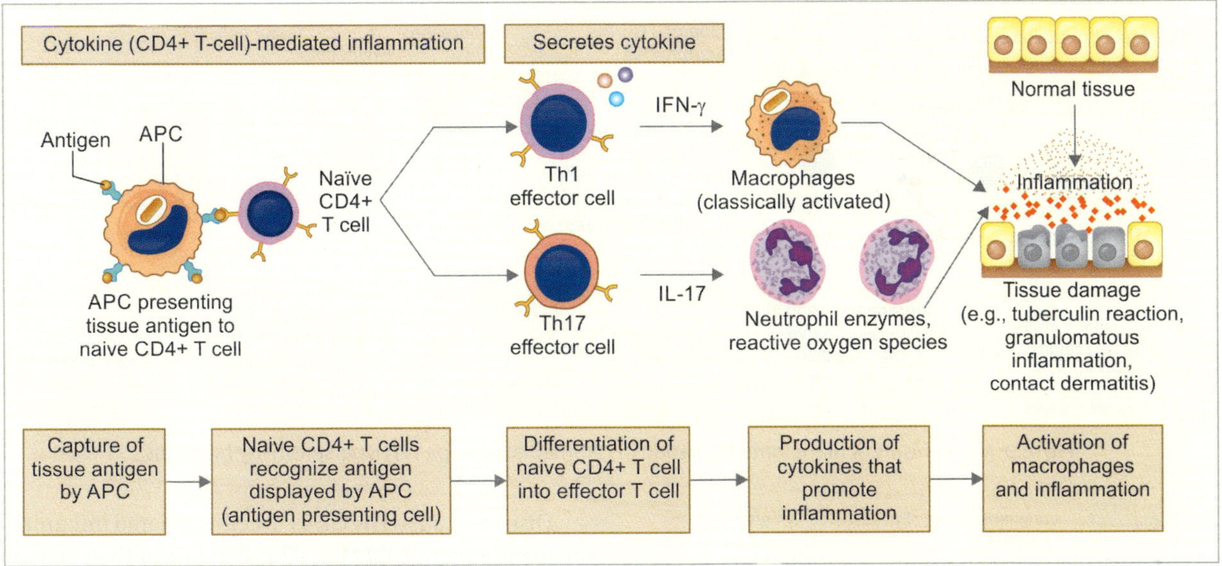

Fig. 6.7: Mechanisms of CD4+ T-cell mediated (type IV) hypersensitivity reactions. In delayed-type hypersensitivity reactions, antigens are presented to naïve T-cells by antigen-presenting cells (APC). Depending on the cytokines produced by APC, naïve T-cells may differentiate into CD4+ Th1 or Th17. Th1 cells secrete cytokines that activate macrophage leading to tissue injury. Th17 cells produce cytokines that produce inflammation by recruiting neutrophils. Both mechanisms produce tissue damage.

of Th1 effector cells. But Th17 cells also may be involved, especially when neutrophils are prominent in the inflammatory infiltrate.

- **Activated Th1 cells:** On repeat exposure to an antigen, **Th1 cells secrete cytokines, mainly IFN-γ.** These cytokines are responsible for many of the manifestations of delayed-type hypersensitivity. **IFN-γ–activates macrophages**. These macrophages are classically activated (M1) macrophages. They produce substances that destroy microbes and damage tissues and mediators that promote **inflammation.**
- **Activated Th17 cells:** They secrete cytokines (e.g., IL-17) that **promote inflammation** by recruiting more **neutrophils and monocytes** to the site of reaction.

Clinical Examples of CD4+ T-cell-mediated Inflammatory Reactions

Three examples of CD4+ T-cell-mediated inflammatory reactions are (i) tuberculin reaction, (ii) granulomatous inflammation, and (iii) contact dermatitis.

1. **Tuberculin reaction (Montoux test)** (*refer* **online Fig. 6.8): It is a classic example of delayed-type** hypersensitivity (DTH).
   - **Injection of purified protein derivative** (PPD): PPD, also called tuberculin, contains protein antigens of the *Mycobacterium tuberculosis* bacillus. In this test, **PPD is injected intracutaneously.**
   - **Positive reaction: In a previously sensitized individual, the injection site becomes red and indurated** in 8–12 hours. It reaches a peak (usually 1–2 cm in diameter) in 24–72 hours, and thereafter slowly subsides.
   - **Microscopy:** It shows the accumulation of mononuclear cells, mainly CD4+ T-cells and macrophages, around venules, producing perivascular "cuffing."
2. **Granulomatous inflammation: Prolonged DTH reaction against persistent microbes** (e.g., tubercle bacilli) **or other nondegradable** (foreign bodies) **injurious agents** may produce a special type of microscopic reaction known as **granulomatous inflammation. Mechanisms of granuloma formation in cell-mediated (type IV) hypersensitivity reactions are shown in Figure 6.9. Granuloma** is a **microscopic aggregate of epithelioid cells (Fig. 6.10), surrounded by a rim of lymphocytes.** Older granulomas are enclosed by a rim of fibroblasts and connective tissue.
3. **Contact dermatitis:** It is a common example of tissue injury due to DTH reactions. Contact with various environmental antigens (e.g., poison ivy, metals such as nickel and chromium, chemicals like hair dyes, cosmetics, and soaps) may evoke inflammation with blisters in the skin at the site of contact known as contact dermatitis. Probably, the environmental chemical binds to and structurally modifies self-proteins. These modified proteins are recognized by T-cells and elicit the reaction. The same mechanism causes many *drug reactions.* The drug (often a reactive chemical) alters self-proteins, including MHC molecules. These neoantigens are recognized as foreign by T-cells, leading to the production of cytokine and inflammation.

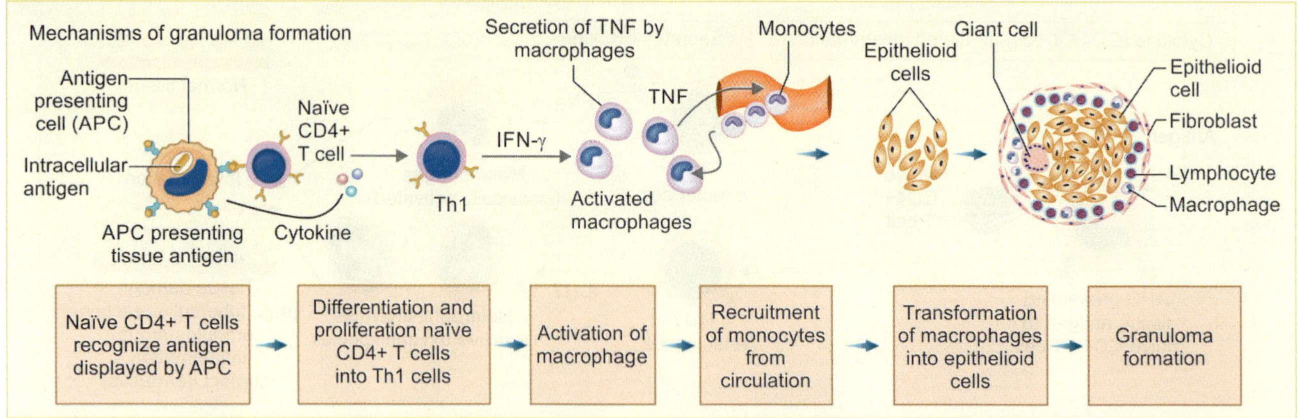

Fig. 6.9: Mechanisms of granuloma formation in cell-mediated (type IV) hypersensitivity reactions.

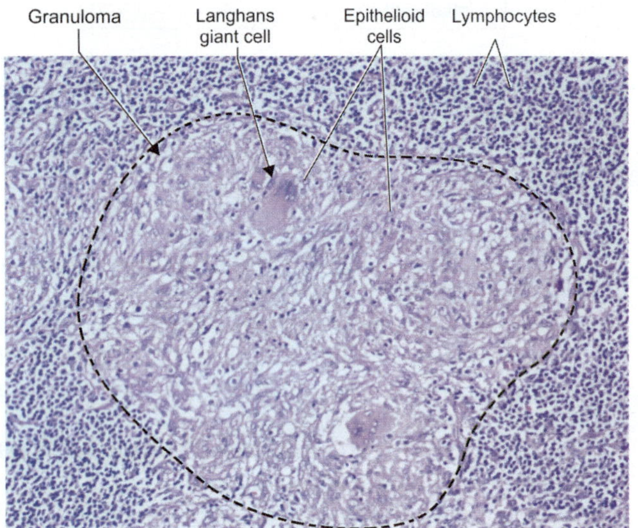

Fig. 6.10: Granulomatous inflammation. Section of a lymph node with granuloma (dotted line). It consists of an aggregate of epithelioid cells surrounded by lymphocytes. The granuloma shows several multinucleate giant cells.

Diseases caused by CD4+ T-cell-mediated inflammation are presented in **Table 6.7**. This hypersensitivity reaction is involved in several **autoimmune diseases** (e.g., rheumatoid arthritis), pathological **reactions to environmental chemicals** (e.g., poison ivy, nickel), and **persistent microbes (e.g., tuberculosis, leprosy)**.

CD8+ T-cell-mediated Cytotoxicity (Fig. 6.11)

It is a type of T-cell-mediated **tissue injury due to CD8+ T lymphocytes** (also called **cytotoxic T lymphocytes** or CTLs). The **CD8+ T-cells kill antigen-bearing target cells.** **Diseases caused:** Destruction of tissues by CTLs may play an important role in some T-cell-mediated diseases. Examples include **type 1 diabetes, transplant rejection** (CTLs directed against cell surface histocompatibility antigens), **killing of virus-infected cells** (e.g., in viral hepatitis), and **some tumor cells**. By killing the infected cells, it eliminates the infection. However, in a few cases, it is responsible for cell damage that accompanies the infection (e.g., in viral hepatitis). CD8+ T-cells also produce cytokines, particularly IFN-γ. These cytokines are involved in inflammatory reactions resembling DTH. For example, following virus infections and exposure to few contact-sensitizing agents.

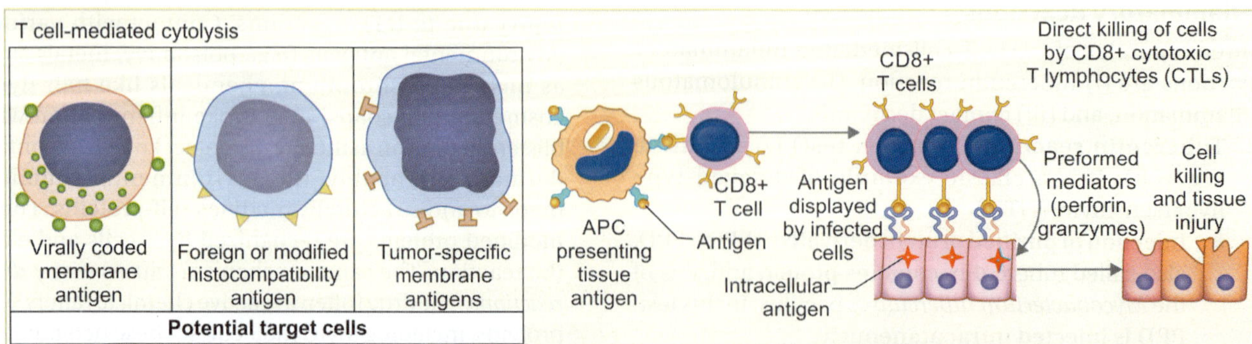

Fig. 6.11: Mechanisms of CD8+ T-cell-mediated (type IV) hypersensitivity reactions. CD8+ cytotoxic T lymphocytes (CTLs) directly kill tissue cells expressing intracellular antigens.

Examples of diseases caused by T-cell mediated (type IV) hypersensitivity are shown in **Table 6.7**.

Salient features and differences between hypersensitivity reactions are presented in **Table 6.8**.

MAJOR HISTOCOMPATIBILITY COMPLEX MOLECULES

PA 9.3a (CC): Describe the HLA system.

Major histocompatibility complex (MHC) is a crucial set of genes and encodes the MHC molecules. It is mainly responsible for the immune system's ability to distinguish between self and non-self-cells and to recognize and respond to foreign substances (e.g., pathogens or antigens).

MHC Gene and Molecules

- **Human leukocyte antigen (HLA) complex:** The **human MHC** is **commonly called the human leukocyte antigen (HLA) complex.** MHC was **named HLA because,** in humans, MHC-encoded proteins were **initially detected on leukocytes by the binding of antibodies. HLA haplotype** is the combination of HLA alleles in each individual. Each individual inherits one set of HLA genes from each parent and thus typically expresses two different molecules for every locus. Each set of maternal and paternal HLA genes is termed an *HLA haplotype*.
- **MHC genes:** The genes that determine the fate of grafted tissues are called MHC genes. Other polymorphic genes that contribute to graft rejection to a lesser degree are called minor histocompatibility genes. **MHC genes** are the **loci of genes** densely packed (clustered) on a **small segment on chromosome 6** (6p21.3). The **MHC gene is highly polymorphic**. Polymorphism means that there are many alleles of each MHC gene at each locus. It results in extreme (high degree) variation in the MHC in the human population (genetic diversity). Each person inherits one set of these alleles that is different from the alleles in most other persons. The possibility of two different individuals having the same combination of MHC molecules is very remote. Therefore, grafts exchanged between individuals are recognized as foreign and attacked by the immune system. **Polymorphism is an important barrier in organ transplantation.** The best-known MHC genes are the HLA class I and class II genes.
- **Major histocompatibility complex molecules:** The **products of the MHC gene are molecules that evoke rejection of transplanted organs.** All human cells have a series of molecules on their surfaces that are recognized by other individuals as foreign antigens. MHC molecules **evoke rejection of transplanted organs** and are responsible for tissue compatibility between individuals. These **major histocompatibility complex (MHC) molecules** were discovered during studies

TABLE 6.7 Examples of T-cell-mediated (type IV) hypersensitivity.

Disease	*Antigen and mechanism*	*Manifestations*
CD4+ T-cell-mediated inflammation		
Rheumatoid arthritis	Collagen ?; citrullinated self-protein? Inflammation mediated by Th17 cytokines	Chronic arthritis, inflammatory destruction of articular cartilage and bone
Inflammatory bowel disease	Enteric bacteria, self-antigen. Inflammation mediated by Th1 and Th17 cytokines	Chronic inflammation of the intestine, ulceration
Contact sensitivity (dermatitis)	Environmental chemicals (e.g., poison ivy). Inflammation mediated by Th1 cytokines	Inflammation of skin and blisters
CD8+ T-cell-mediated inflammation		
Viral infection	Viral antigen. Destruction of virally infected host cells by CD8+ T lymphocytes	Depends on the virus
Rejection of transplant	Foreign (histocompatible transplanted) cells. Direct killing of graft cells by CD8+ T lymphocytes, inflammation	Transplant rejection
Immune response against tumor	Tumor antigen: mutated self-protein, overexpressed or aberrantly expressed self-protein, or oncogenic virus. Destruction of tumor cells by CD8+ T lymphocytes	Varies depending on the tumor and the response
Involves both CD4+ T lymphocytes and CD8+ cytotoxic T lymphocytes		
Type 1 diabetes mellitus	Antigens of pancreatic islet β cells (insulin, glutamic acid decarboxylase, others). T-cell-mediated inflammation (CD4+ T) and destruction of islet cells by CTLs (cytotoxic T lymphocytes)	Insulitis (chronic inflammation in islets), destruction of β-cells; diabetes mellitus
Hashimoto thyroiditis	Thyroglobulin and other thyroid proteins. Destruction of thyroid cells by infiltrating cytotoxic T-cells, and locally released cytokines	Hypothyroidism

TABLE 6.8 Salient features and differences between hypersensitivity reactions.

Features	Type I	Type II	Type III	Type IV
Antigens	Exogenous allergens include Pollen, moulds, mites, drugs, food, etc.	Cell surface or tissue-bound	Soluble exogenous (viruses, bacteria, fungi, parasites) or endogenous autoantigens	Cell/tissue bound
Antibody involved	IgE	IgG and IgM	IgG, IgM, IgA	None
Mediators	From mast cells	Complement	Complement	T lymphocytes, activated macrophages
Time taken for reaction to develop	5–10 min	6–36 hours	4–12 hours	48–72 hours
Pathogenesis	Formation of IgE antibodies and release of mediators from mast cells	• Opsonization and phagocytosis • Complement system activation and inflammation • Antibody-mediated cellular dysfunction	• Circulating immune complex-mediated cell injury. • Local immune complex injury (Arthus reaction)	• CD4+ T-cell-mediated inflammation • CD8+ T-cell-mediated cytotoxicity
Immunopathology	Edema, vasodilatation, mast cell degranulation, eosinophils	Antibody and complement-mediated damage to target cells/ tissue	Acute inflammatory reaction, neutrophils, vasculitis	Perivascular inflammation, mononuclear cells, granulomas, caseating necrosis in tuberculosis
Examples of diseases and conditions produced	• Asthma (extrinsic) • Urticaria/edema • Allergic rhinitis • Food allergies • Anaphylaxis	• Autoimmune hemolytic anemia • Transfusion reactions • Goodpasture syndrome • Acute rheumatic fever • Pernicious anemia	• Autoimmune, e.g., SLE • Glomerulonephritis • Rheumatoid arthritis	• Pulmonary TB • Contact dermatitis • Tuberculin test • Tuberculoid leprosy • Transplant rejection • Reaction against virus-infected cells

on graft rejection and acceptance (tissue, or *"histo,"* compatibility).

- **Normal function of MHC molecules:** To **display peptide** (short chain of amino acids) **for recognition by CD4+ and CD8+ T lymphocytes.** In each individual, T lymphocytes recognize only peptides displayed by that person's MHC molecules. This property of T-cell antigen recognition is called *MHC restriction*. Variations in MHC molecules among individuals elicit strong immune responses. This is the responsible for rejection of the graft.
- **Importance of MHC:** (1) The MHC products are important for immunologic specificity and in organ/tissue transplantation and (2) MHC plays a major role in susceptibility to several autoimmune diseases and HLA is linked to many autoimmune diseases.

Classification of MHC Molecules

MHC gene product is classified based on their structure, cellular distribution, and function into **two main and one minor groups (Fig. 6.12)**. MHC class I and class II gene products are critical for immunologic specificity and transplantation histocompatibility, and they play a major role in susceptibility to several autoimmune diseases.

Class I MHC Molecules

- **Expressed on all nucleated cells and platelets:** The products of MHC class I genes are **expressed on all nucleated cells and platelets** (except erythrocytes/RBCs and trophoblasts).
- **Encoded by three closely linked loci:** These are **designated as *HLA-A*, *HLA-B* and *HLA-C*.**
- **Highly polymorphic** in the population and most highly polymorphic segment known within the human genome.
- **Functions:** Products of the MHC class I gene are integral participants in the **immune response to intracellular infections, tumors, and allografts. Class I molecules interact with CD8+ T lymphocytes during antigen presentation** and are **involved in cytotoxic reactions. CD8+ T lymphocytes** recognize antigens only in the context of self-class I molecules, they are referred to as **class I MHC-restricted.**

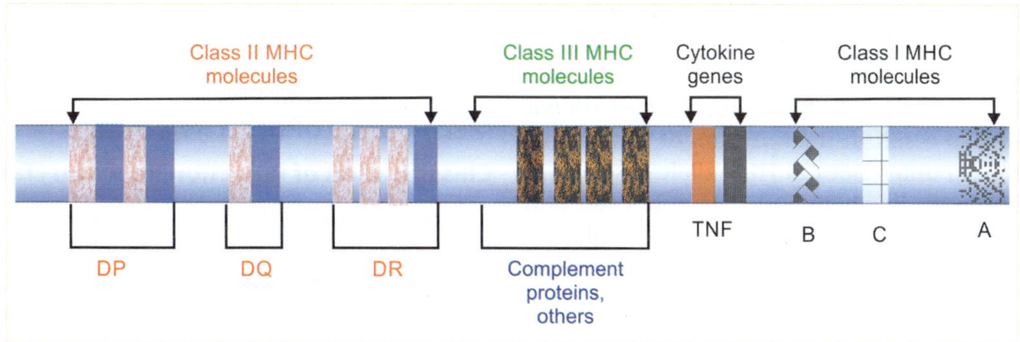

Fig. 6.12: Major histocompatibility complex (human leukocyte antigen complex) showing the location of genes.

Class II MHC Molecules

- **Encoded in a region called *HLA-D*.** It has three sub-regions: ***HLA-DP, HLA-DQ*, and *HLA-DR*.**
- **Expression:** The expression of class II MHC molecules is restricted to a few cell types. They are expressed mainly in **antigen-presenting cells** (APCs) (e.g., dendritic cells), macrophages, and B cells.
- **Function:** This locus contains genes that **encode many proteins involved in antigen processing and presentation**. The **class II-peptide complex is recognized by CD4+ T-cells** (function as helper cells) and this CD4 molecule acts as the co-receptor. Because **CD4+ T-cells can recognize antigens only in the context of self-class II molecules** are referred to as **class II MHC- MHC-restricted.**

Class III MHC Molecules

Their gene **encodes** components of the **complement system, cytokines, tumor necrosis factor (TNF), lymphotoxin,** and some proteins without an apparent role in the immune system.

TABLE 6.9 Association with HLA alleles with diseases.

Disease	*HLA allele*
Class I MHC molecules	
Ankylosing spondylitis	B27
Post-gonococcal arthritis	
Acute anterior uveitis	
Behçet's syndrome	B51
21-hydroxylase deficiency	HLA-BW47
Hereditary hemochromatosis	HLA-A
Class II MHC molecules	
Chronic active hepatitis	DR3
Primary Sjögren syndrome	
Rheumatoid arthritis	DR4
Ulcerative colitis	DR103
Type 1 diabetes	DR3/DR4
Primary biliary cirrhosis	DR8
Graves disease and myasthenia gravis	DR3

HLA and Disease Association (Table 6.9)

Q. Write a short note on diseases associated with HLA.

Some diseases are associated with the inheritance of certain HLA alleles and these diseases can be broadly grouped into:

- **Inflammatory diseases (e.g., ankylosing spondylitis most strikingly associated with HLA-B27).**
- **Autoimmune diseases** (e.g., autoimmune endocrinopathies associated with alleles at the DR locus).
- **Inherited errors of metabolism** [e.g., 21-hydroxylase deficiency (HLA-BW47) and hereditary hemochromatosis (HLA-A)].

IMMUNOLOGY OF TRANSPLANTATION

PA 9.3b (CC): Describe the immune principles involved in transplant and the mechanism of transplant rejection.

Q. Write a short note on transplant rejection.

Transplantation is a **procedure for the replacement of irreparably damaged tissue or organs to restore their lost function**. **A tissue or organ transplanted** is called a **transplant or graft**. An individual from which a transplant is obtained is known as a **donor** and the individual who receives it is called a **recipient**.

Transplant rejection: A **major limitation of transplantation** is the process known as **rejection. In rejection, the recipient's immune system recognizes the graft as being foreign and mounts immunological reactions against it.**

Recognition and Rejection of Allografts

Role of HLA in transplantation: In transplantation, donor **HLA (MHC) molecules** (MHC-encoded antigens) **are the major graft antigens.** They are immunogenic and **are recognized by the recipient as foreign. These antigens stimulate the rejection of transplanted tissues.** Maximum survival of graft occurs when there is a close match of major histocompatibility antigens (HLAs) between recipient and donor. **HLA genes are highly polymorphic**. Therefore, there will be always some differences between the HLA molecules of individuals (except, identical twins; 25% of siblings may also inherit the same HLA alleles). Hence, in practice, an exact HLA match is not possible, except between monozygotic twins.

Rejection: The major antigenic differences between a donor and recipient that result in the rejection of transplants are mainly due to differences in HLA alleles. Rejection is a complex process in which both T lymphocytes and antibodies are produced against graft antigens. Both cell-mediated immunity and circulating antibodies play a role in transplant rejection. They react against and destroy the grafts.

Thus, after organ transplantation, immunosuppressive therapy and vigilant monitoring of graft function are necessary. Present therapeutic advances have greatly improved transplant success rates, even when there is a degree of histoincompatibility.

Recognition of Graft Alloantigens

Allograft is the term used for **a graft from an individual of the same species**. The antigens in the allograft are termed as allogeneic antigens or alloantigens. Both T-cell–mediated and antibody-mediated reactions may be involved in transplant rejection.

Pathways of recognition of graft alloantigens: Following transplantation, the recipient's T cells recognize donor HLA antigens from the graft (alloantigens) by two pathways.

1. **Direct pathway:** In this pathway, the **graft antigens are presented directly to recipient T cells by graft APCs.** This pathway may play a greater role in CTL-mediated acute rejection.
2. **Indirect pathways:** In this pathway, the graft **antigens are taken up by host APCs**, processed (like any other foreign antigen), **and presented to host T cells.** This pathway may be most important in chronic rejection. The production of anti-HLA antibodies occurs via an indirect pathway in which the donor HLA antigens are taken up by host B cells and presented to helper T cells. This results in the production of alloantibodies specific to donor HLA.

Both the above pathways of recognition of alloantigen, **activate CD8+ T-cells and CD4+ T-cells.**

CD8+ T-cells become cytotoxic T-cells (CTLs) and CD4+ T-cells develop into cytokine-producing effector cells, mainly Th1 cells.CD4+ T-cells.

Mechanisms of Graft Rejection

Classification of Rejection Reaction (Table 6.10)

Q. Write a short note on transplant rejection reactions.

Depending on the clinical (**time of occurrence**) and pathologic features, the solid organ transplant rejection reactions are classified as: **(1) hyperacute, (2) acute,** and **(3) chronic**. Each type of rejection is brought out by a particular kind of immune response. However, features usually overlap and create diagnostic ambiguity.

Hyperacute rejection

Q. Write a short note on hyperacute rejection.

- **Time of occurrence: It occurs within minutes or hours after transplantation, so fast that it occurs intraoperatively.**
- **Preformed antibodies:** Hyperacute rejection **is mediated by preformed antibodies specific for antigens on graft endothelial cells. These** preformed antibodies **are present in the circulation before transplantation.** These may be natural IgM antibodies specific for blood group antigens or may be antibodies specific for allogeneic HLA molecules. These antibodies were produced by prior exposure through blood transfusions, pregnancy, or organ transplantation
  - **Multiparous women**, who develop anti-HLA antibodies against paternal antigens that are shed from the fetus.
  - **Prior blood transfusions**, because platelets and white blood cells are rich in HLA antigens.
  - Host has **previously rejected a renal transplant**.
- **Mechanism of damage (Fig. 6.13):** Immediately after the graft is transplanted and blood flow is restored, the antibodies bind to antigens on the graft endothelium. They activate the complement and clotting systems. This causes injury to endothelium, formation of thrombus, and ischemic necrosis of the graft. It results in rapid and irreversible destruction of the graft. Nowadays, all donors and recipients are matched for blood type,

TABLE 6.10 Classification and characteristics of transplant rejection.

Type	*Time*	*Mechanism*	*Pathological findings*
Hyperacute rejection	Minutes to hours	Preformed antibody and complement activation (type II hypersensitivity)	Arteritis, thrombosis, and necrosis
Acute rejection			
Acute cellular rejection	5 days to weeks (30 days) of transplantation	Activated T lymphocytes: CD4+ and CD8+ T-cells (type IV hypersensitivity)	Extensive interstitial mononuclear cell infiltration (CD4+ and CD8+), edema and endothelitis
Acute humoral rejection		Antibody and complement activation	Necrotizing vasculitis, neutrophilic infiltration, and thrombosis
Chronic rejection	Months to years	Immune and non-immune mechanisms	Fibrosis, scarring

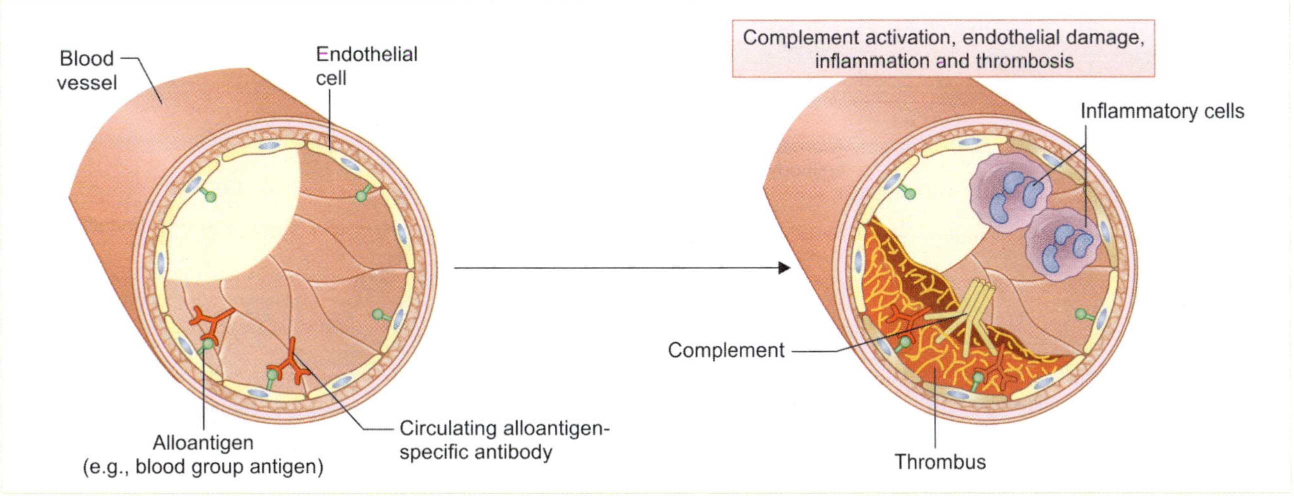

Fig. 6.13: Hyperacute rejection. Immediately after transplantation, a preformed allogenic-specific antibody from the recipient of the graft gets deposited on alloantigen on the endothelium of graft blood vessels. This activates the complement system causes injury to endothelial cells, and produces vascular thrombosis, and ischemic necrosis of the graft.

and potential recipients are tested for antibodies against the cells of the prospective donor, a test called a *cross-match*. Hence, hyperacute rejection is now uncommon. Kidneys were the first solid organs to be transplanted and are the most commonly transplanted organ. Hence, the morphologic changes are discussed mainly in relation to renal transplants. Fortunately, hyperacute rejection is distinctly uncommon with the currently available adequate pretransplantation antibody screening.

MORPHOLOGY

Hyperacute Rejection

Gross: The affected renal **graft rapidly becomes cyanotic, mottled, and flaccid**, and may excrete a few drops of bloody urine (anuria).

Microscopy: All arterioles and arteries show **acute fibrinoid necrosis of their walls** and **narrowing or complete occlusion of their lumens by thrombi. Neutrophils accumulate within arterioles, glomeruli, and peritubular capillaries.** Later, these changes become severe and diffuse. The glomerular capillaries also undergo thrombotic occlusion. In the end, the cortex undergoes necrosis (infarction), and the kidney becomes nonfunctional and has to be removed.

Q. Differences between hyperacute and acute transplant rejection (for answer refer to Table 6.10).

Acute rejection

- **Time of occurrence:** Occurs **within days to weeks** after transplantation. It is the main cause of early graft failure. It also may develop suddenly months or even years later, after tapering or termination of immunosuppression.
- **Mediators: It is mediated by T cells and antibodies that are activated by alloantigens in the graft.**
- **Types:** Depending on the role of T-cells or antibodies, acute rejection can be divided into two types. However, both patterns are present in most rejecting grafts.

Acute cellular (T-cell–mediated) **rejection** (*refer* **online Fig. 6.14**)**:** Graft damage with the destruction of graft cells may be by direct **damage through CD8+ CTLs, or CD4+ cells secrete cytokines and induce inflammation**. T cells may also damage graft vessels, leading to vascular damage. Current immunosuppressive therapy mainly prevents and reduces acute rejection by blocking the activation of alloreactive T-cells.

- **Acute antibody-mediated (vascular or humoral) (Fig. 6.15):** It is mediated by antibodies (anti-donor antibodies) that bind to vascular endothelium. These activities complement through the classical pathway. It induces inflammation and endothelial damage leading to graft failure.

MORPHOLOGY

Acute Rejection

Acute cellular (T-cell–mediated) **rejection:** It may produce two different patterns of injury.

- **Tubulointerstitial pattern:** It is characterized by severe interstitial inflammation and tubular inflammation (tubulitis) associated with focal injury to tubules. The inflammatory infiltrates are composed of activated CD4+ and CD8+ T lymphocytes.
- **Vascular pattern:** It is characterized by inflammation of vessels and sometimes accompanied by necrosis of vessel walls. The involved vessels show swelling of endothelial cells, and at places show lymphocytes between the endothelium and the vessel wall. This finding is termed *endotheliitis* or *intimal arteritis*. Most patients with cellular rejection without accompanying humoral rejection, respond well to immunosuppressive therapy.

Acute antibody-mediated rejection: It mainly shows damage to glomeruli and small blood vessels. Usually, it shows inflammation of glomeruli and peritubular capillaries associated with the deposition of complement products. The activation of the complement system is by the antibody-dependent classical pathway. There may also be focal thrombosis in small vessels.

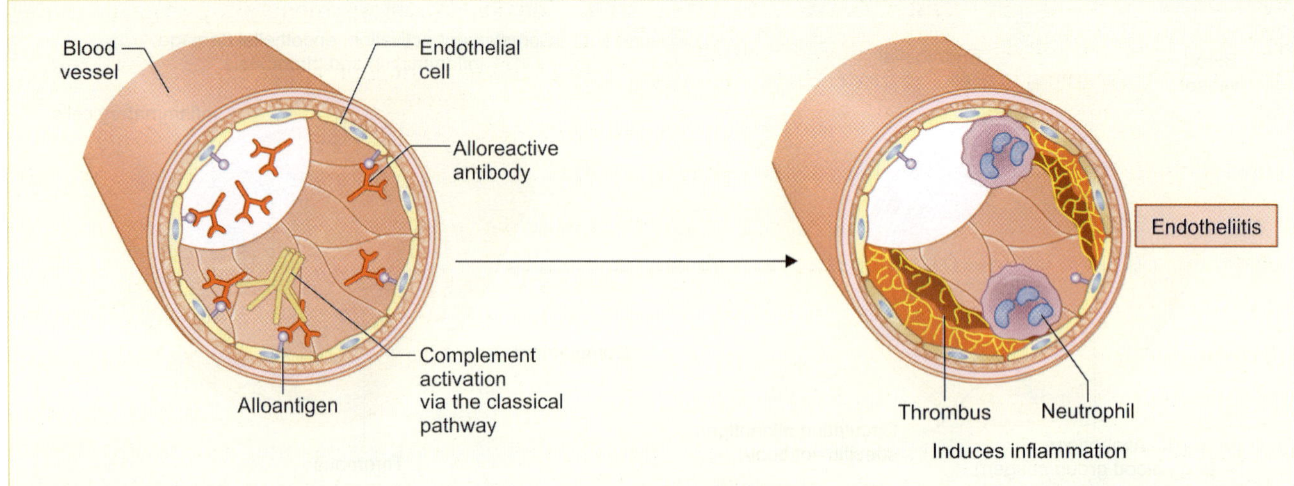

Fig. 6.15: Acute antibody-mediated (humoral) rejection. Graft damage is caused by antibody deposition in vessels which activates the complement system via the classical pathway. This induces inflammation and causes endothelial damage. This leads to failure of the graft. Vessels may also show focal thrombosis.

C4d staining: It is a fragment of complement protein C4. Its deposition in the capillaries of the graft indicates local activation of the classic pathway of the complement system. Thus, C4d staining provides evidence for antibody-mediated (humoral) graft rejection. This is useful for the early detection of vascular rejection. If detected early, acute rejection can be reversed with immunosuppressive therapy.

Chronic rejection

It is also known as **chronic allograft failure.**

- **Time of occurrence: It occurs over months to years after transplantation. It is a slow-growing form of graft damage leading to progressive loss of graft function.**
- **Pathogenesis (Fig. 6.16):** Chronic rejection is characterized by interstitial *fibrosis* and gradual narrowing of the blood vessels of the graft *(graft arteriosclerosis).* Both these lesions are probably due to the reaction of T-cells against graft alloantigens and secretion of cytokines. They stimulate the proliferation of fibroblasts and vascular smooth muscle cells in the graft **(Fig. 6.16).** Alloantibodies also may contribute to chronic rejection. Chronic rejection is refractory to most therapies and is a major cause of graft failure.

MORPHOLOGY

Chronic Rejection

It is dominated by changes in blood vessels. It is associated with **thickening of the intima and vascular occlusion.** Chronically rejecting kidney grafts show **glomerulopathy, with duplication of the glomerular basement membrane.** This is probably secondary to chronic endothelial injury. Other changes include **peritubular capillaritis with multilayering of peritubular capillary basement membranes.** Vascular lesions may lead to interstitial fibrosis and tubular atrophy with loss of renal parenchyma. Usually, interstitial mononuclear cell infiltrates are minimal.

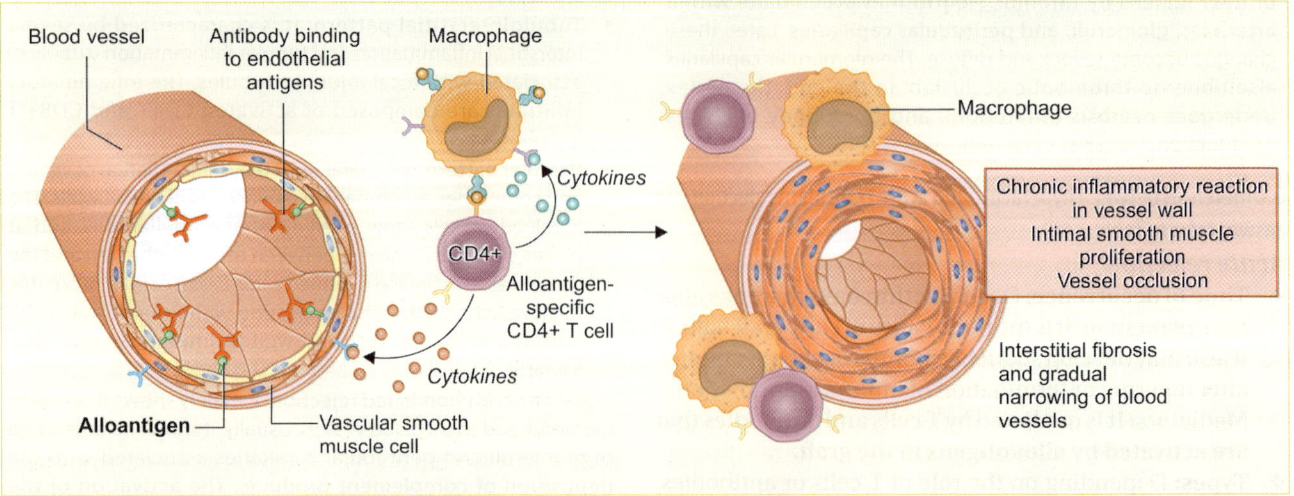

Fig. 6.16: Chronic rejection. Narrowing of graft blood vessels by T-cell cytokines and antibody deposition.

Methods of Increasing Survival of Graft

HLA matching: HLA molecules are the major antigens targeted in transplant rejection. Therefore, HLA matching of the donor and the recipient improves the survival of the graft. HLA matching is more useful for living-related kidney transplants than for other types of organ transplants. The survival of graft improves with increasing number of HLA loci are matched. Due to improvements in immunosuppressive drugs, HLA matching is not done for heart, lung, liver, and islet transplantation. In such transplantation, the recipient usually urgently requires a transplant.

Immunosuppression of the recipient: It is a requirement in all organ transplants, except in identical twins.

- **Complications of immunosuppression:** These are as follows: Suppression of the immune system increases the **susceptibility to opportunistic fungal, viral, and other infections. Reactivation of latent viruses, such as cytomegalovirus (CMV) and polyomavirus**, is frequent in these patients. Immunosuppressed patients are also at increased risk for **developing virus-induced tumors,** such as Epstein-Barr virus (EBV)–associated lymphomas and human papillomavirus (HPV)-induced squamous cell carcinomas.

Transplantation of Hematopoietic Stem Cells

Q. Indications for hematopoietic stem cell (HSC) transplantation.

Historically, **hematopoietic stem cells** (HSCs) were obtained from the bone marrow and were termed bone marrow transplantation. HSCs are usually harvested from **peripheral blood** after they are mobilized from the bone marrow by administration of hematopoietic growth factors, or from the **umbilical cord blood of newborn infants** (a rich source of HSCs). Hematopoietic stem cell (HSC) transplantation is a preferred term.

Definition: Hematopoietic stem cell (HSC) transplantation is a procedure that involves eliminating an individual's hematopoietic and immune system by chemotherapy and/or radiotherapy and replacing them with stem cells either from another individual or with the individual's own hematopoietic stem cells.

Types of hematopoietic stem cell transplant: These are as follows:

- **Autologous** ("from self"): Own HSCs removed, cryopreserved, and re-infused.
- **Allogeneic** ("from different genes"): HSCs obtained from another individual.
- **Syngeneic** ("from same genes"): HSCs obtained from an identical twin.

Sources of hematopoietic stem cells: These include:

- **Bone marrow:** Richest store.
- **Peripheral blood:** Very few HSCs but can be mobilized from bone marrow by administering G-CSF or GM-CSF.
- **Umbilical cord blood:** Easily available and is a rich source.

Indications for HSC transplantation: The main indications are as follows:

- To treat hematologic malignancies (e.g., leukemia, lymphoma, multiple myeloma).
- **Bone marrow failure syndromes,** e.g., aplastic anemia.
- **Disorders caused by inherited HSC defects,** e.g., sickle cell anemia, thalassemia, and primary immunodeficiencies.

Complications of HSC Transplantation

Autologous HSC transplants have fewer immunologic complications but have higher rates of relapse of the disease after transplant. Allogeneic HSC transplants have lower rates of relapse but have more immunologic complications.

Irradiation or chemotherapy for HSC transplantation: In most of the conditions requiring HSC transplantation, the recipient is irradiated or treated with chemotherapy to destroy the immune system (and, sometimes, cancer cells). It also "opens up" niches in the microenvironment of the marrow to promote HSCs, and allows the engraftment of the transplanted HSCs. These treatments usually produce immune deficiency before the transplanted HSCs can generate a functional immune system.

Graft-versus-host Disease

Q. Write a short note on graft-versus-host disease (GVHD). List the organs involved in GVHD.

Graft-versus-host disease (GVHD) is the major complication that follows an allogeneic HSC transplant. This is due to infused donor T lymphocytes (CD4+ and CD8+ T-cells) reacting against the recipient's tissues/organs. **Three conditions are necessary** for the development of GVHD:

1. **An immunocompetent graft** (i.e., one containing T-cells **or their precursors**).
2. **HLA mismatch** (minor or major) **between donor and recipient.**
3. **An immunologically depleted recipient** who cannot mount an immune response to the graft.

When immunosuppressed recipients receive HSC transplantation from allogeneic donors, **the immuno competent T-cells present in the donor HSCs recognize the recipient's HLA antigens (alloantigens) as foreign and attack against it.** This results in the activation of donor CD4+ and CD8+ T-cells. This leads to inflammation and the killing of recipient cells. GVHD can be minimized by careful HLA-matching of the donor and recipient during HSC transplants using DNA sequencing. Rarely, GVHD may occur following transplantation of organs rich in lymphoid cells (e.g., the liver or intestine).

Forms of GVHD: There are two forms acute and chronic.

1. **Acute GVH disease:** It occurs days to weeks after transplantation (before 100 days). Direct cytotoxicity by CD8+ T-cells and cytokines released by the sensitized donor T-cells are responsible for the damage. It often produces epithelial cell necrosis of three primary **target**

organs simultaneously, namely the **liver, skin, and gastrointestinal (GI) tract**.
- Destruction of small bile duct. Presents with jaundice.
- Mucosal ulceration of the gut. It manifests with bloody diarrhea.
- Skin involvement is characterized by lymphocyte infiltration and apoptosis of epidermal cells. It manifests as a rash.

2. **Chronic GVH disease:** It may follow the acute syndrome or may occur insidiously. Patients develop skin lesions with dermal fibrosis. These lesions resemble those of systemic sclerosis and manifestations mimicking other autoimmune disorders.

Other Complications

- **Infections:** Patients are susceptible to a variety of infections (bacterial, viral, and fungal) due to a lack of granulocytes, as well as a lack of a functioning immune system.
- **Organ toxicity:** Damage to the GI tract, liver, and lungs.
- **Immunodeficiency:** It **is a frequent complication of bone marrow transplantation**. The immunodeficiency may be due to prior treatment, preparation for the graft, a delay in the repopulation of the recipient's immune system, and an attack on the host's immune cells by grafted lymphocytes. Immunodeficiency predisposes to infections, particularly infection with cytomegalovirus which can cause fatal pneumonitis.

AUTOIMMUNE DISEASES

PA 9.4 (CC): Define autoimmunity. Enumerate autoimmune disorders.

Definition: Autoimmunity is defined as **immune reactions against self (auto) antigens.** In this **body produces autoantibodies** and **immunologically competent T lymphocytes against self-antigens.**

Autoimmunity is a disturbance in the immunologic tolerance of self-antigens. Normally, the immune system does not strongly recognize the individual's own antigens. Healthy individuals of all ages (particularly the elderly), may produce small quantities of antibodies against their own antigens *(autoantibodies)* without causing any overt autoimmune disease. Therefore, the mere presence of low quantities of autoantibodies does not indicate an autoimmune disease. Autoimmune diseases develop when the immune system reacts against self-antigens to the extent that autoantibodies or autoreactive T cells produce damage to the individual's tissues.

Autoimmune Diseases

Autoimmunity is an important cause of certain diseases in humans. In autoimmune diseases, the immune system fails to discriminate between self and non-self. Autoimmune diseases may be organ-specific or systemic (generalized) **(Table 6.11)**.

- **Organ-specific disease:** The immune responses are directed against one particular organ or cell type. It results in localized tissue damage (e.g., β-cells of pancreatic islets in type 1 diabetes).
- **Systemic or generalized disease:** It is characterized by lesions in many organs [e.g., systemic lupus erythematosus (SLE)]. These are caused by immune complexes and autoantibodies. The lesions mainly affect the connective tissues and blood vessels of involved organs. Therefore, these diseases are often termed ***collagen vascular diseases*** or ***connective tissue diseases***. However, the immunologic reactions are not specifically directed against constituents of connective tissue or blood vessels in these disorders.
- **Involving more than one organ** (e.g., Goodpasture syndrome, in which lung and kidney are involved).

Refer **online** for **discussion on Immunological Tolerance** and **Figure 6.17**.

Q. List autoimmune diseases.

TABLE 6.11 Examples of autoimmune diseases.
DISEASES MEDIATED BY ANTIBODIES
Organ-specific
• Autoimmune hemolytic anemia
• Autoimmune thrombocytopenia
• Autoimmune atrophic gastritis of pernicious anemia
• Goodpasture syndrome
• Myasthenia gravis
• Graves disease
Systemic
• Systemic lupus erythematosus
• ANCA-associated vasculitis
DISEASES MEDIATED BY T-CELLS
Organ-specific
• Type 1 diabetes mellitus
• Multiple sclerosis
• Hashimoto thyroiditis
Systemic
• Rheumatoid arthritis
• Systemic sclerosis (scleroderma)
• Sjögren syndrome
DISEASES PROBABLY AUTOIMMUNE
Organ-specific
• Inflammatory bowel diseases (Crohn disease, ulcerative colitis)
• Primary biliary cholangitis
• Autoimmune (chronic active) hepatitis
Systemic
• Polyarteritis nodosa

(ANCA: antineutrophil cytoplasmic antibody)

Mechanisms of Autoimmunity

Breakdown of self-tolerance and development of autoimmunity may be due to the combined effects of:

(1) susceptibility genes (influence lymphocyte tolerance), and (2) environmental factors (such as infections or tissue injury). They alter the display of and responses to self-antigens.

Genetic Factors

Role of susceptibility genes: Most autoimmune diseases are complex multigenic disorders. Evidence indicates that genetic factors have an important role.

- **Autoimmune diseases run in families:** The incidence is greater in monozygotic than in dizygotic twins.
- **Association with HLA (MHC) genes:** Several autoimmune diseases are linked to the HLA locus. It is usually linked with alleles of HLA-DR and HLA-DQ. The disease-associated MHC alleles may increase susceptibility to autoimmune disease but are not the cause of the disorder.

Environmental Factors

A. **Role of infections** (*refer* **online Figs. 6.18A and B): Various microbes,** such as bacteria, mycoplasmas, and viruses **may trigger autoimmunity by several mechanisms**.
   - **Induction of costimulatory on APCs:** Microbial infections and associated tissue necrosis and inflammation can trigger the expression of costimulatory molecules on APCs. The cytokines produced can activate T cells. This favors the breakdown of T-cell tolerance leading to T cell–mediated tissue injury.
   - **Molecular mimicry: Few viruses and other microbes may express antigens that have the same amino acid sequences as self-antigens.** Immune responses against them may attack self-tissue and this phenomenon is known as molecular mimicry. For example, in **rheumatic heart disease,** antibodies formed against streptococcal bacterial proteins cross-react with cardiac antigens and cause rheumatic carditis.

   The development of autoimmunity may be influenced by the normal gut and skin *microbiome* (the various commensal microbes that live with us in a symbiotic relationship). Probably, different commensal microbes affect the relative proportions of effector and regulatory T cells. They may determine the host's response toward or away from aberrant activation.

B. **Other environmental factors:** The display of tissue antigens may be altered by other environmental factors. These include ultraviolet radiation, cigarette smoking, local tissue injury, and hormones. Ultraviolet (UV) radiation causes cell death and may produce abundant nuclear antigens. Exposure of these antigens to the immune system may elicit pathologic immune responses in lupus. *Smoking* may cause chemical modification of self-antigens and is a risk factor for rheumatoid arthritis. Local tissue injury due to any cause may release normally sequestered self-antigens (such as antigens in the eye and testis) and produce autoimmune responses. Autoimmune disorders are more common in women than in men. This may be due to the effects of hormones on immune cells.

SYSTEMIC LUPUS ERYTHEMATOSUS

PA 9.5 (CC): Define and describe the pathogenesis of systemic lupus erythematosus.

Definition: Systemic lupus erythematosus (SLE) is a chronic autoimmune disease involving multiple organs. It is characterized by the production of various autoantibodies, particularly antinuclear antibodies (ANAs).

Systemic lupus erythematosus (SLE) has **multisystemic involvement.** It can affect every organ in the body but mainly involves the **skin, kidneys, joints, serous membranes, and the heart. Injury is due to the deposition of immune complexes and the binding of antibodies to various cells and tissues.** It shows a **broad spectrum of autoantibodies,** most important is antinuclear antibodies (ANAs).

Etiology

Q. Discuss the etiology and pathogenesis of systemic lupus erythematosus (SLE).

Systemic lupus erythematosus is an **autoimmune disease** in which a fundamental defect is **failure of self-tolerance.** It leads to the production of **many autoantibodies** that **damage the tissue either directly or indirectly by depositing immune complex deposits.** A combination of genetic and environmental factors plays a role in the pathogenesis of SLE.

Genetic Factors

Evidence to support genetic predisposition are:

- **Familial association: Family members** of SLE patients have an **increased risk** of SLE. About 20% of unaffected first-degree relatives may show autoantibodies. It shows a **high rate** of concordance (>25%) in **monozygotic twins** when compared with dizygotic twins (1–3%).
- **HLA association:** Risk is higher with HLA-DR2 or HLA-DR3.
- **Other genetic factors:** These include:
   - **Genetic deficiencies of early complement components (such as C1q, C2, or C4):** It may result in (1) impaired removal of circulating immune complexes by the mononuclear phagocyte system, (2) defective phagocytic clearance of apoptotic cells and (3) failure of B-cell tolerance. If apoptotic cells are not cleared, their nuclear components may elicit immune responses.
   - **Polymorphism in the inhibitory Fc receptor FcγRIIb:** It can lead to inadequate control of B-cell activation.

Environmental Factors

Environmental factors are also involved in the pathogenesis of SLE:

- **Exposure to ultraviolet (UV) radiation:** Exposure to sunlight exacerbates the lesions of the disease. UV irradiation may cause **apoptosis** of host cells and may alter the DNA in such a way that it becomes immunogenic.
- **Sex hormones:** SLE is 10 times greater during the reproductive period (17 through 55 years) **in women** than in men. SLE shows exacerbation during normal menses and pregnancy. It may be related to genes on the X chromosome.
- **Drugs:** These include **hydralazine, procainamide, isoniazid, and D-penicillamine** can produce SLE-like disease. The disease remits after the withdrawal of the drug.
- **Cigarette smoking:** It is associated with the development of SLE.

Immunological Abnormalities

Several immunological abnormalities of **both innate and adaptive immune** systems have been observed in SLE. These may produce persistent and uncontrolled activation of self-reactive lymphocytes.

- **Failure of self-tolerance in B cells:** It may be due to (i) defective receptor editing or (ii) elimination of self-reactive B cells in the bone marrow or (iii) defects in peripheral tolerance mechanisms.
- **CD4+ helper T cells specific for nucleosomal antigens.** These cells also escape tolerance and produce high-affinity pathogenic autoantibodies.
- **Type I interferons:** IFN-α is a type I interferon produced mainly by plasmacytoid DCs. It is produced in abnormally **large amounts** in SLE. It may indirectly produce autoantibodies.
- **Toll-like receptor (TLR) signals** (*refer* **Fig. 3.2**)**:** TLRs that recognize DNA (DNA-recognizing TLR9) and RNA (RNA-recognizing TLR7), produce signals that regulate responses of B cells specific for self-nuclear antigens. These **activated B-cells** specific for nuclear antigens may **produce antinuclear autoantibodies.**

Pathogenesis of SLE (Fig. 6.19)

The exact pathogenesis of SLE is not well known. It is associated with susceptibility genes with failure of self-tolerance. **Genetic abnormalities in B lymphocytes and T lymphocytes are responsible for the failure of self-tolerance** (defective tolerance). It **results in the survival of self-reactive lymphocytes** and they remain functional.

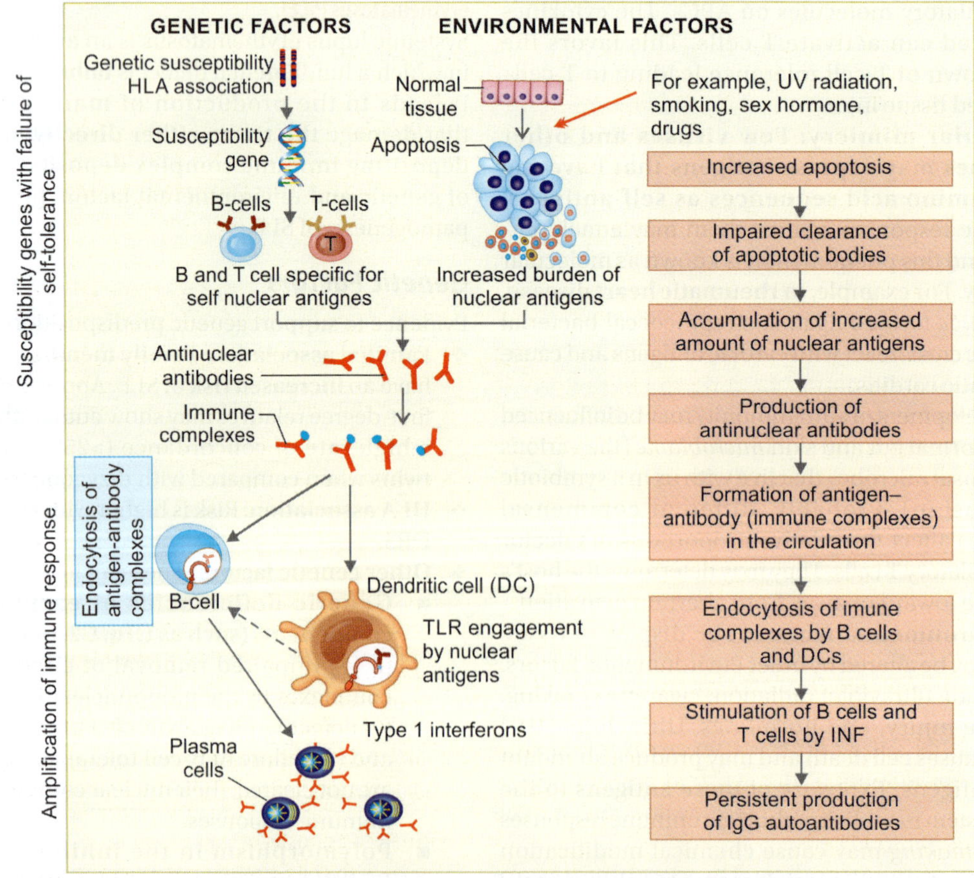

Fig. 6.19: Pathogenesis of systemic lupus erythematosus.

Different steps in the proposed model in the pathogenesis of SLE are as follows:

1. **Increased apoptosis triggered by environmental agents:** UV irradiation and other environmental factors cause the death of cells by **apoptosis.**
2. **Inadequate clearance of apoptotic cells:** It results in the accumulation of a large number of nuclear antigens. It is partly due to defects in complement proteins.
3. **Stimulation of self-reactive B-cells stimulated by nuclear self-antigens. These B cells produce antibodies against the self-antigens.**
4. **Formation of antigen–antibody (immune) complexes** in the circulation.
5. **Endocytosis of immune complexes by B cells and dendritic cells:** The antibody portion of immune complexes binds to Fc receptors on B-cells and dendritic cells (DCs) and the immune complexes may be internalized by endocytosis. In patients with SLE, there are decreased cell membrane C3b receptors. Thus, Fc-receptor-dependent phagocytosis of immune complexes is impaired. So ongoing autoimmunity may be exacerbated by persistent antigenic stimuli.
6. **TLR engagement by nuclear antigens:** Nucleic acid components of immune complexes bind to TLRs of B-cells and DCs.
7. **TLR stimulation of B-cells and DCs:** The binding to TLR has the following actions:
   - They stimulate B-cells to produce more auto-antibodies.
   - Activates dendritic cells (mainly plasmacytoid DCs) to produce interferons and other cytokines. They stimulate B- and T-cells to further amplify immune response and cause more apoptosis.
8. **Persistent production of autoantibodies:** Thus, a cycle of antigen release and immune activation results in the persistent production of high-affinity IgG autoantibodies.
   The antigen-antibody complexes deposit in tissues and induce inflammation leading to characteristic vasculitis, synovitis, and glomerulonephritis. Although the role of T cells in provoking tissue damage is less well understood, some damage is due to cell-mediated immune responses.

The Spectrum of Autoantibodies in SLE

Q. Write a short note on antibodies in systemic lupus erythematosus.

Systemic lupus erythematosus (SLE) is characterized by the production of **several diverse autoantibodies.** Autoantibodies are directed against multiple self-antigens. Some antibodies are against different nuclear and cytoplasmic components of the cell that are not organ-specific. Other antibodies are directed against specific cell surface antigens of blood cells.

Importance of autoantibodies: These antibodies are (1) **useful** for the **diagnosis and management** of patients with SLE and (2) responsible for the **pathogenesis of tissue damage (e.g.,** the immune complex-mediated glomerulonephritis).

Types of Antibodies

Autoantibodies are against plasma proteins (complement components, clotting factors), protein-phospholipid complexes, cell surface antigens (lymphocytes, neutrophils, platelets, erythrocytes), intracellular cytoplasmic components (microfilaments, microtubules, lysosomes, ribosomes, RNA) and nuclear DNA, ribonucleoproteins, and histones.

Antinuclear Antibodies (ANAs)

They are autoantibodies that are directed against various **nuclear self-antigens** including DNA, RNA, and proteins (all together called generic ANAs). ANAS can be grouped into four different categories: antibodies to (1) DNA; (2) histones; (3) nonhistone proteins bound to RNA; and (4) nucleolar antigens **(Table 6.12)**. Diagnostically, ANAs are the most important autoantibodies because the test is positive in >95% of patients. These ANAs are usually detected by indirect immunofluorescence.

Other Autoantibodies

Autoantibodies against blood cells: These may be against (1) red cells, (2) platelets, (3) neutrophils and (4) lymphocytes.

Q. Write a short note on antiphospholipid antibody/syndrome.

Antiphospholipid antibodies (aPL) are detected in 30–40% of SLE patients but they are not specific for SLE.

- The term **antiphospholipid antibody** is misleading because these antibodies react with plasma proteins of

TABLE 6.12 Important antinuclear antibodies and their clinical utility.

Specificity of autoantibody	*Disease associations*
Double-stranded DNA*	Nephritis; specific for SLE
U1-RNP	
Smith (Sm) antigen (core protein of small RNP particles)*	Specific for SLE; do not usually correlate with disease activity or clinical manifestations
Ro (SS-A) nucleoprotein	Congenital heart block; neonatal lupus Not specific for SLE
Phospholipid-protein complexes (anti-PL)	Antiphospholipid syndrome (in ~10% of patients with SLE)
Multiple nuclear antigens ("generic ANAs")	Found in other autoimmune diseases, not specific

* Virtually diagnostic of SLE

Females with child-bearing potential and SLE should be screened for aPL and anti-Ro.

complexes rather than directly with phospholipids. **For this reason, these antibodies were previously termed lupus anticoagulant antibodies.**

- **Types:** Antiphospholipid antibody **includes anticardiolipin antibody and anti-β_2 glycoprotein antibody. Antibodies against phospholipid-β_2-glycoprotein complex** also bind to cardiolipin antigen. Since cardiolipin antigen is used in the serological test for syphilis, SLE patients **may give a false-positive serological reaction for syphilis.**
- **Complications due to aPL:** These autoantibodies can lead to **increased venous and arterial thrombosis and thrombocytopenia, recurrent spontaneous miscarriages,** and **focal cerebral or ocular ischemia.**
- **Two tests that measure different antibodies (anticardiolipin and the lupus anticoagulant):** (1) ELISA for anticardiolipin and (2) a sensitive phospholipid-based activated prothrombin time, such as the dilute Russell viper venom test.

LE Bodies or Hematoxylin Bodies

Q. Write a short note on LE cell and its associated conditions.

LE Bodies

ANAs cannot penetrate intact cells, but if nuclei of the cell are exposed, they can bind to them. In tissues, nuclei of damaged cells react with ANAs, lose their chromatin pattern, and appear homogeneous, to produce **LE bodies or hematoxylin bodies.** Hematoxylin bodies, the pathognomonic light microscopic feature of systemic lupus erythematosus commonly found in renal glomeruli affected with active nephritis. Hematoxylin bodies (hematoxyphilic material) represent DNA deposition in stroma, sinuses and blood vessel walls.

LE Cell (Figs. 6.20A to C and *refer* page 447)

It is related to LE bodies and can be demonstrated in vitro. **Demonstration of LE cells:** The blood sample is agitated to damage the nucleated cells and it releases the nuclei. The nuclei of damaged cells react with ANAs to form a homogenous denatured nuclear material. The LE cell is any phagocytic leukocyte (blood neutrophil or macrophage) that has engulfed this denatured nucleus of an injured cell.

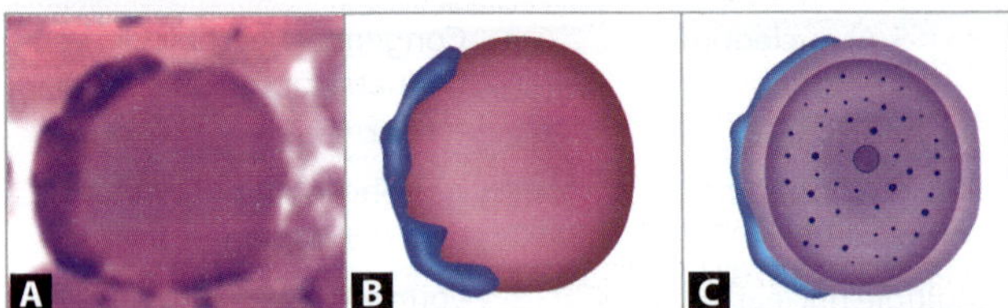

Figs. 6.20A to C: Appearance of LE cell: (A) Leishman stain; (B) diagrammatic; (C) tart cell.

(SLE: subendothelial immune complex deposits give rise to "wire-loop" lesions on light microscopy).

The demonstration of LE cells in vitro was used as a test for SLE. With the advent of new techniques for the detection of ANAs, this test is of only historical interest. Sometimes, LE cells can be found in body fluids such as pericardial or pleural effusions.

Interpretation: LE cell is **positive in about 70% of SLE.** It may **also be positive in conditions such as rheumatoid arthritis, lupoid hepatitis, penicillin sensitivity, etc.**

Mechanisms of Tissue Injury

Autoantibodies mediate tissue injury and produce most of the lesions of SLE.

- **Immune complexes (type III hypersensitivity):** The deposition of **immune complexes** is the most **common cause of tissue injury and most of the systemic lesions.**
- **Type II hypersensitivity: Autoantibodies against cell surface antigens** specific for **RBCs, white cells, and platelets lead to opsonization** of these cells. This promotes their **phagocytosis** and lysis resulting in **cytopenias.**
- **Antiphospholipid antibody syndrome:** Patients with antiphospholipid antibodies are prone to **venous and arterial thromboses.** This syndrome may be associated with **recurrent spontaneous miscarriages and focal cerebral or ocular ischemia.** This combination of clinical features, in association with lupus, is called the *secondary antiphospholipid antibody syndrome.* Some patients develop these autoantibodies and the clinical syndrome without associated SLE. This syndrome is termed the *primary antiphospholipid antibody syndrome.*

MORPHOLOGY

SLE is a systemic autoimmune disease and morphologic changes in SLE are **extremely variable.** The most **characteristic lesions** of SLE are **due to the deposition of immune complexes** in **blood vessels, kidneys, connective tissue, and skin.**

Blood Vessels

Acute necrotizing vasculitis: It affects small arteries and arterioles of any involved tissue. The arteritis leads to **fibrinoid necrosis** in the vessel walls. In **chronic stages,** vessels show fibrous thickening of the wall accompanied by **narrowing of the lumen.**

Kidney

The kidney **involvement is significant in about 50%** of SLE patients and is one of the most important organs involved.

Pathogenesis of glomerulonephritis: Immune complexes composed of **DNA and anti-DNA antibodies** get deposited in the glomeruli and produce inflammation. It leads to the proliferation of cells (endothelial, mesangial, and/or epithelial).

Morphologic classification of lupus nephritis: Six patterns are recognized but none of these are specific for SLE. There is overlap within these patterns and lesions may evolve from one class to another.

1. **Minimal mesangial lupus nephritis (class I):** It is characterized by **immune complex deposition in the mesangium, granular**

deposits of immunoglobulin and complement, and no recognizable structural changes by light microscopy. It is the least common nephritis in SLE.

2. **Mesangial proliferative lupus nephritis (class II):** It is characterized by granular **immune complex deposition in the mesangium** and **mild-to-moderate increase in mesangial cells and mesangial matrix.**
3. **Focal lupus nephritis (class III):** In this less than 50% glomeruli are involved. It is seen in 20–35% of patients. The lesions are **focal and may be segmental** (affecting only a portion of the glomerulus) or **global** (involving the entire glomerulus). Affected glomeruli may show **proliferation of endothelial and mesangial cells, or parietal epithelial cells** (crescent formation), **fibrinoid necrosis, leukocyte infiltration, and eosinophilic deposits or intracapillary thrombi.**
4. **Diffuse lupus nephritis (class IV):** It is the most common and most severe form of nephritis. It occurs in 35–60% of patients. Lesions are diffuse (>50% of glomeruli) and most of the involved glomeruli may show **proliferation of endothelial, mesangial, and epithelial cells.** The proliferation of parietal epithelial cells may produce cellular crescents. **Prominent, subendothelial deposits cause homogeneous thickening of the capillary wall,** which on light microscopy appears as a "**wire-loop**" lesion **(Fig. 6.21).** These **wire loops may be seen in both focal and diffuse proliferative (class III or IV) lupus nephritis.**
5. **Membranous lupus nephritis (class V):** It is seen in 10–15% of patients and is characterized by **diffuse thickening of the capillary walls** similar to idiopathic membranous glomerulonephritis leading to nephrotic syndrome.
6. **Advanced sclerosing lupus nephritis (class VI):** It shows sclerosis of more than 90% of glomeruli.

Interstitium and tubules: They may show changes, but are usually not dominant abnormality.

Immunofluorescence: It shows granular deposits of antibody and complement.

Electron microscopy: It shows electron-dense deposits (immune complexes) in mesangial, intramembranous, subepithelial, or subendothelial locations.

Heart (*refer* page 528)

Any layer of the heart may be involved. **Valvular endocarditis** (Libman–Sacks/**nonbacterial verrucous endocarditis)** appears as **single or multiple 1–3 mm warty deposits on either surface of the leaflets of any heart valves** (*refer* **Fig. 16.34D**).

Skin

It shows a characteristic erythema involving the face along the bridge of the nose and cheeks (the **butterfly rash**) in about 50% of patients.

Clinical Features

- SLE is a **multisystem** disease with extremely **variable clinical presentation.**
- **Age and gender:** It usually occurs in young women between **20 and 30 years,** but may manifest at any age. It predominantly affects **women,** with female-to-male ratio of 9:1.

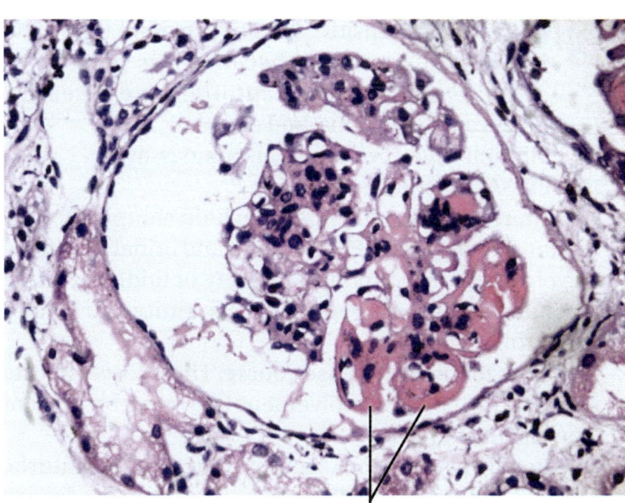

Fig. 6.21: Lupus nephritis showing glomerulus with "wire-loop" lesions due to extensive subendothelial deposition of immune complexes.

BOX 6.3: Major clinical manifestations of systemic lupus erythematosus according to the descending order of frequency.

- Hematologic: Anemia, thrombocytopenia
- Arthritis, arthralgia, or myalgia
- Skin
- Fever
- Fatigue
- Weight loss
- Renal

- **Onset:** Acute or insidious with fever.
- **Typical presentation: Butterfly rash over the face, fever, pain** without deformity in one or more **peripheral joints, pleuritic chest pain, and photosensitivity.** SLE patients are **susceptible to infections,** because of immune dysfunction and treatment with immunosuppressive drugs. Major clinical manifestations of systemic lupus erythematosus according to the descending order of frequency are presented in **Box 6.3.**

Laboratory Findings

Q. Write a short note on laboratory diagnosis of systemic lupus erythematosus (SLE).

- **Purpose:** (1) To establish or rule out the diagnosis, (2) to follow the course of disease, and (3) to identify adverse effects of therapies.
- **Tests for autoantibodies** (*refer* pages 191-2 and **Table 6.12**): ANAs are found in almost all patients, but it is not specific. Various methods of detecting antibodies include:
  - **Indirect immunofluorescence assay (IFA):** They can identify ANAs. Significance of IFA assay are:

- Extremely sensitive (positive in more than 95%)
- Limited specificity because it is positive in patients with other autoimmune diseases, chronic infections, and cancer.
  - Multiplex flow cytometry immunoassay.
  - ELISA (for smith antigen).
- **Standard tests for diagnosis:** Include complete blood count, platelet count, ESR (raised), and urinalysis. Renal involvement may produce a variety of findings. These include hematuria, red cell casts, proteinuria, and nephrotic syndrome.
- **Tests for following disease course:** These tests indicate the status of organ involvement known to be present during SLE flares.
  - **Renal involvement:** Urinalysis may show **hematuria, red cell casts, proteinuria**, or nephrotic syndrome.
  - **Hematologic changes:** Hemoglobin levels (anemia) or platelet counts (thrombocytopenia) and ESR.
  - **Serum levels of creatinine or albumin**.
  - **Decreased complement component levels in serum** such as C3 and C4 are often indicators of enhanced consumption and increased disease activity.

Course: It is variable and unpredictable. It shows remissions and exacerbations.

Cause of death: Renal failure and intercurrent infections.

OTHER AUTOIMMUNE DISORDERS

PA 9.7 (NC): Define and describe the pathogenesis of other common autoimmune diseases.

Rheumatoid Arthritis

Rheumatoid arthritis is an autoimmune disease that mainly affects the joints but also may involve extra-articular tissues (e.g., skin, blood vessels, lungs, and heart). It is discussed on pages 926-8.

Sjögren Syndrome

Sjögren syndrome is a chronic disease characterized by dry eyes (*keratoconjunctivitis sicca* or *xerophthalmia*) and dry mouth (xerostomia). It is due to immunologically mediated destruction of the lacrimal and salivary glands.

Types: It may be primary or secondary.

- **Primary form:** It is an isolated primary disorder also known as the ***sicca syndrome*** (SS).
- **Secondary form:** It occurs in association with another autoimmune disease. It is more common than primary.

Pathogenesis: It is an autoimmune disorder with activation of autoreactive T cells and B cells.

Autoantibodies: Most patients (about 90%) with Sjögren syndrome reveal antibodies against two cytoplasmic ribonucleoprotein (RNA) associated antigens, SS-A (Ro) and SS-B (La).

MORPHOLOGY

Exocrine glands: Lacrimal and salivary glands are the major sites of the disease.

Microscopy: The involved glands show **dense infiltration by lymphocytes (CD4+ helper T cells** and some B cells) which may destroy acini and ducts. As the disease progresses, the affected glands show atrophy and may be replaced by hyalinized fibrotic tissue.

Clinical Features

Gender and age: Sjögren syndrome is most common in females between 50 and 60 years of age.

Symptoms: These are the consequences of a lack of tears and saliva.

- **Eye:** Keratoconjunctivitis produces eye discomfort, blurred vision, burning, and itching. May develop infections and ulcers of the cornea and conjunctivae.
- **Salivary gland:** Xerostomia produces dry mouth (dryness of the buccal mucosa), difficulty in swallowing solid foods, decrease in taste, cracks, and fissures in the mouth.
- **Extraglandular disease:** May develop in one-third of patients. These include synovitis, pulmonary fibrosis, and peripheral neuropathy.

Systemic Sclerosis

Systemic sclerosis or *scleroderma* is an immunologic disorder with evidence of autoimmunity, mainly the production of multiple autoantibodies. It is characterized by excessive fibrosis in multiple tissues and obliterative vascular disease.

The term ***systemic sclerosis*** is preferred because excessive fibrosis is seen in multiple organs. Involvement of skin is the usual presenting manifestation and is found in about 95% of patients. However, visceral involvement (e.g., gastrointestinal tract and skeletal muscles) is responsible for morbidity and mortality. A disease restricted to the skin is called ***localized scleroderma.***

Classification: Based on its course, systemic sclerosis is classified into two groups:

1. **Diffuse systemic sclerosis:** It is characterized by initial extensive involvement of skin, with rapid progression and early visceral involvement.
2. **Limited systemic sclerosis:** It is associated with relatively mild involvement of skin (usually the fingers and face). Involvement of the viscera occurs late and it usually follows a benign course. This presentation also is called **CREST (Calcinosis, Raynaud phenomenon, Esophageal dysmotility, Sclerodactyly, and Telangiectasia) syndrome.**

Pathogenesis: The cause and the pathogenesis of systemic sclerosis are not well understood. The disease likely **results from three interrelated processes namely (i) autoimmune responses** (humoral and cellular immunity),

(ii) vascular damage, and **(iii)** excessive and often progressive **deposition of collagen.**

- **Autoimmunity:** Probably, CD4+ T cells respond to an unidentified antigen and accumulate in the skin. They release cytokines (e.g., IL-13) that activate inflammatory cells and fibroblasts. The production of numerous disease-specific various autoantibodies such as ANAs stimulates fibrosis.
- **Vascular damage:** During the early stage of systemic sclerosis, it shows microvascular disease It is characterized by repeated cycles of endothelial injury with proliferation of endothelial cells and fibrosis in the intima and perivascular region. This in turn produces narrowing of the microvasculature and leads to ischemic injury and scarring.
- **Fibrosis:** It is the characteristic feature of the disease. The fibroblasts of these patients can produce excessive amounts of collagen. Progressive fibrosis and vascular lesions may lead to ischemic damage.

MORPHOLOGY

Sites involved: Most prominently the skin, alimentary tract, musculoskeletal system, and kidney.

Skin: It is characterized by **diffuse fibrosis of the skin and associated atrophy**. Skin shows **edema and perivascular infiltrates by CD4+ T cells** accompanied by swelling and degeneration of collagen fibers (appear eosinophilic). **Capillaries and small arteries** may **show hyaline thickening of the walls** and **partial occlusion**. As the disease progresses **increased fibrosis occurs in the dermis** along with thinning of the epidermis and atrophy of dermal appendages.

Alimentary tract: It is the most commonly (in about 90% of patients) involved internal organ system. It is characterized by progressive atrophy and fibrous replacement of the muscularis at any level of the gut. The mucosa becomes thinned and may ulcerate. The lamina propria and submucosa show excessive collagenization.

Musculoskeletal system: It may be the first manifestation of the disease. Severity may vary from mild polyarthralgias to more severe arthralgias. Inflammation of the synovium (synovitis) is common in the early stages and fibrosis later stages.

Kidneys: Renal involvement may be found in two thirds of patients. The most prominent are the **vascular lesions** characterized by **thickening of the intima of interlobular arteries and afferent arterioles** with luminal narrowing.

Lungs: It may be affected in more than 50% of patients and may manifest **as pulmonary hypertension and interstitial fibrosis.**

Heart: It may be involved in one-third of patients. It may manifest as pericarditis with effusion, patchy myocardial fibrosis, and thickening of intramyocardial arterioles. The changes in the lung may lead to right ventricular hypertrophy and failure (cor pulmonale).

Clinical Features

Age and gender: The peak age of presentation is between 50 and 60 years of age. More frequent in females with a female-to-male ratio of 3:1.

Scleroderma can manifest as two distinct clinical syndromes either as a generalized or diffuse **(progressive systemic)** form and a **limited variant.**

Systemic sclerosis: The most distinguishing clinical features of systemic sclerosis are due to the progressive thickening and fibrosis of the skin and later involvement of specific internal organs.

- **Skin:** Symptoms usually begin with the **Raynaud phenomenon**, characterized by intermittent episodes of ischemia of the fingers (due to vasoconstriction of the arteries and arterioles), marked by triphasic color changes, paresthesias, and pain. Progressive collagen deposition in the skin produces **increasing stiffness** (especially of the hands) and is followed by complete **immobilization of the joints**. "Stone facies" due to tightening of facial skin and restricted motion of the mouth may be seen. Progression of vascular lesions in the fingers can lead to ischemic ulceration of the fingertips.
- **Internal organs:** It involves GIT, respiratory system, heart, and renal system. **These organs show fibrosis.**

Autoantibodies: Almost all patients have ANAs that react with a variety of nuclear antigens. Two ANAs strongly associated with systemic sclerosis are: (i) against DNA topoisomerase I (anti-Scl 70) and (ii) anticentromere antibody.

- **Anti-Scl 70:** It is highly specific and is associated with pulmonary fibrosis and peripheral vascular disease.
- **Anticentromere antibody:** It is associated with CREST syndrome.

Prognosis: For most of the patients, it steadily follows a downhill course over many years.

Inflammatory Myopathies

Inflammatory myopathies are uncommon, probably immunologically mediated, heterogeneous groups of disorders. They are characterized by injury and inflammation of mainly the skeletal muscles. Depending on clinical, morphologic, and immunologic features, three disorders have been described namely: (i) polymyositis, (iii) dermatomyositis, and (III) inclusion body myositis.

Mixed Connective Tissue Disease

As the name suggests, mixed connective tissue disease (MCTD) is a disorder with clinical features of several different disorders such as SLE, systemic sclerosis, and polymyositis. It is more common in females and most are adults (mean age, 37 years).

Laboratory findings: The disease is characterized serologically by a most distinctive ANA directed against an extractable nuclear antigen. These patients have high titers of antibodies to U1 (uridine-rich) ribonucleoprotein (anti-U1-RNP antibody) which is used as the most diagnostic criterion for MCTD. However, their role in the development of any of the characteristic lesions of MCTD is not clear.

Clinical features: Clinical features of MCTD are shared with other diseases. Usually, it presents with synovitis of the fingers, the Raynaud phenomenon, and mild myositis. They respond favorably to corticosteroids, at least in the short term.
Complications: These include pulmonary hypertension, interstitial lung disease, and renal disease.

Polyarteritis Nodosa and Other Vasculitides

Polyarteritis nodosa is an immunologic disease that belongs to a group of disorders characterized by necrotizing inflammation of the walls of blood vessels. It can involve any type of vessel (arteries, arterioles, veins, or capillaries). These vasculitides are discussed in pages 495-8.

IgG4-related Disease

Definition: IgG4-related disease (IgG4-RD) is a newly identified fibroinflammatory disorder characterized by rich infiltration by IgG4 antibody-producing plasma cells and lymphocytes (mainly T cells) in the tissues, associated with fibrosis and obliterative phlebitis.
Diagnostic feature: Increased numbers of IgG4-producing plasma cells in tissue are required for the diagnosis of this disorder. Though this disorder is often associated with elevated serum IgG4 concentrations, it need not be present in all cases.
Organs involved: IgG4-related disease can occur in any organ system. These include the biliary tree, salivary glands, periorbital tissues, lymph nodes, kidneys, lungs, meninges, aorta, prostate, thyroid, breast, pericardium, and skin.
IgG4-RD spectrum: Examples include Mikulicz syndrome (enlargement and fibrosis of salivary and lacrimal glands), Riedel thyroiditis, idiopathic retroperitoneal fibrosis, autoimmune pancreatitis, and inflammatory pseudotumors of the orbit, lungs, and kidneys.
Age group and gender: Usually affects middle-aged and older men.
Pathogenesis: Not known. Though IgG4 production in lesions is a characteristic of the disease, it is not known whether it contributes to the pathology of the disease.

IMMUNODEFICIENCY SYNDROMES

Immunodeficiency is a defect in immunity.
Classification: Immune deficiencies can be divided into **primary (or congenital) and secondary (or acquired) immunodeficiencies and by the host defense defect.** Primary immunodeficiency (PID) disorders due to an intrinsic defect in the immune system. Secondary immunodeficiency states may arise as complications of an underlying condition. The underlying condition includes cancers, infections, malnutrition, or immunosuppression, irradiation, or chemotherapy for cancer and other diseases.

Manifestations of immunodeficiencies: It clinically presents with **increased infections**, which may be newly **acquired or reactivation of latent infections**. Many immunodeficiencies are also associated with autoimmune disorders.

Primary (Congenital) Immunodeficiency

Primary immunodeficiency diseases are inherited genetic disorders. They impair mechanisms of innate immunity (phagocytes, NK cells, or complement) or the humoral and/or cellular arms of adaptive immunity (mediated by B lymphocytes and T lymphocytes, respectively). Classification of primary immune deficiency diseases is presented in **Box 6.4.** Most of them manifest themselves in infancy, between 6 months and 2 years of life. They come to clinical attention because they are susceptible to recurrent infections.

X-linked Agammaglobulinemia

X-linked agammaglobulinemia (XLA), or Bruton disease is one of the more common primary immunodeficiency diseases. It is characterized by **the failure of pre-B cells to differentiate into mature B cells. This leads to the absence of antibodies (gamma globulin) in the blood.**
Etiology: Due to mutations in a cytoplasmic tyrosine kinase gene, called **Bruton tyrosine kinase (*Btk*) gene.** The gene is located on the long arm of the X chromosome at Xq21.22. ***Btk gene*** product is a kinase that is required for the maturation of pre-B-cell to B-cell stage. **Mutation of the *Btk gene* blocks B-cell maturation at pre B-cell stage, there is no production of light chains** and reduced production of immunoglobulin. They have intact T-cell-mediated immunity.

BOX 6.4: Classification of primary immune deficiency diseases.

Deficiencies of the Innate Immune System
- **Phagocytic cells:** Impaired adhesion (leukocyte adhesion deficiency/LAD), impaired killing (chronic granulomatous disease/CGD)
- **Innate immunity receptors and signal transduction:** Defects in toll-like receptor signaling
- **Complement deficiencies:** Classical, alternative, and lectin pathways.

Deficiencies of the Adaptive Immune System
- **Humoral (B lymphocytes):** XL and AR agammaglobulinemia, hyper-IgM syndrome
- **Cellular (T lymphocytes):** DiGeorge syndrome, Wiskott–Aldrich syndrome.

Regulatory Defects
- **Innate immunity:** Severe colitis
- **Adaptive immunity:** Autoimmune lymphoproliferation syndrome (ALPS)

Characteristic features: These include (i) absent or markedly decreased B lymphocytes in the circulation, (ii) decreased serum levels of all classes of immunoglobulin, (iii) underdeveloped germinal centers in lymph nodes, Peyer's patches, the appendix, and tonsils, (iv) absence of plasma cells throughout the body, and (v) normal T-cell mediated immunity.

Clinical manifestation: It is seen in males and does not manifest till about 6 months of age (till maternal immunoglobulins are depleted). Patients are susceptible to infections. They present with recurrent bacterial infections of the respiratory tract, such as acute and chronic pharyngitis, sinusitis, otitis media, bronchitis, and pneumonia. Other infections include viral infections (e.g., echovirus, poliovirus, and coxsackievirus) and *Giardia lamblia*. They have increased susceptibility to autoimmune diseases (e.g., arthritis and dermatomyositis).

DiGeorge Syndrome (Thymic Hypoplasia)

It is caused by a congenital defect in the development of the thymus. It is a T-cell immunodeficiency disorder characterized by the absence of cell-mediated immunity due to low numbers of T lymphocytes in the blood and lymphoid tissues. The T-cell zones of lymphoid organs (paracortical areas of the lymph nodes and the periarteriolar sheaths of the spleen) are depleted.

Etiology: It is due to defective embryologic development of the third and fourth pharyngeal pouches, which normally give rise to the thymus, parathyroid glands, some of the clear cells of the thyroid, the ultimobranchial body and influence conotruncal cardiac development. Patients develop a **variable loss of T-cell mediated immunity** (due to hypoplasia or lack of the thymus), tetany (due to lack of the parathyroids), and congenital defects of the heart and great vessels (due to conotruncal cardiac development). In the absence of a thymus, T-cell maturation is interrupted at the pre-T-cell stage. Most patients with DiGeorge syndrome have a point deletion (**22q11 deletion**) in the long arm of chromosome 22.

Clinical manifestations: It usually presents during infancy with conotruncal congenital heart defects and severe hypocalcemia (due to hypoparathyroidism). Infants are prone to recurrent or chronic viral, bacterial, fungal, and protozoal infections.

Immunodeficiency with Thrombocytopenia and Eczema (Wiskott–Aldrich Syndrome)

It is an X-linked recessive disease characterized by thrombocytopenia, eczema, and a marked susceptibility to recurrent infection, ending in early death.

Etiology: It is caused by **mutations in the WASP gene** encoding the ***Wiskott–Aldrich syndrome protein (WASP)***, which is located at Xp11.23. It leads to reduced levels of WASP. WASP gene mutations affect not only T lymphocytes but also the other lymphocyte subsets, dendritic cells, and platelets.

Clinical manifestations: Typically present with **recurrent bacterial infections, eczema, and bleeding** caused by thrombocytopenia.

Features: The thymus is morphologically normal. In later stages, it shows progressive secondary depletion of T lymphocytes in the peripheral blood and the T-cell zones (paracortical areas) of the lymph nodes, with variable loss of cellular immunity. These patients have an increased risk of developing non-Hodgkin B-cell lymphomas.

BOX 6.5: Causes of secondary (acquired) immunodeficiencies.

- Human immunodeficiency virus infection
- Involvement of bone marrow by cancers (e.g., leukemias)
- Immunosuppression for graft rejection, or to treat autoimmune diseases
- Irradiation and chemotherapy treatments for cancer
- Severe acute malnutrition
- Removal of spleen
- Diabetes and other metabolic diseases

Secondary (Acquired) Immunodeficiencies

The causes of secondary (acquired) immune deficiencies are listed in **Box 6.5**. The secondary immune deficiencies are more common than the primary disorders of genetic origin. The most important secondary immune deficiency disease is AIDS.

ACQUIRED IMMUNODEFICIENCY SYNDROME

PA 9.6 (CC): Define and describe the pathogenesis and pathology of HIV and AIDS.

Definition: Acquired immunodeficiency syndrome (AIDS) is **caused by the retrovirus human immunodeficiency virus** (HIV). It is characterized by **severe immunosuppression that leads to opportunistic infections, secondary neoplasms, and neurologic manifestations. It causes depletion of CD4+ T lymphocytes.**

Route of Transmission

HIV is a relatively weak virus outside of the body. HIV is **found in every bodily fluid** and is broadly disseminated in the body. Since it is present in very low titers in saliva, tears, cerebrospinal fluid, amniotic fluid, and feces; it is not transmitted through these body fluids. Transmission of HIV occurs when there is an **exchange of blood or body fluids containing the virus or virus-infected cells**. There is no animal reservoir for HIV and it cannot persist in aerosols. Hence, HIV **infection does not occur by inhalation, ingestion, or contact with the skin.** It is transmitted by introduction into mucosal tissues or by injection. The **three major routes** of transmission are:

1. **Sexual transmission:** It is the **main and most common route of infection** in more than 75% of cases of HIV.
   - **Homosexual or bisexual men** or **heterosexual contacts:** It may be male-to-male, male-to-female, or female-to-male transmission. **HIV is present in genital fluids** such as vaginal secretions and cervical secretions/cells (in women) and semen (in men). **The risk of sexual transmission of HIV is increased** when there is a **high viral load in the source**, and **coexisting sexually transmitted diseases**, especially those associated with genital ulceration (e.g., syphilis, chancroid, and herpes).
   - **Viral transmission** can occur in two ways: (1) **Direct inoculation of virus or infected cells into the blood vessels** at the site of breach caused by trauma, and (2) **by uptake into the mucosal dendritic cells** (DCs).
2. **Parenteral transmission:** It occurs via blood, blood products, or blood-contaminated needles or syringes. Three groups of individuals are at risk.
   a. **Intravenous drug abusers:** Transmission occurs by **sharing needles and syringes contaminated** with HIV-containing blood.
   b. **Hemophiliacs:** Mainly those who received large amounts of factor VIII and factor IX concentrates before 1985. Now increasing use of recombinant clotting factors have eliminated this mode of transmission.
   c. **Transfusion of blood or blood components:** Recipients of blood transfusion of **HIV-infected whole blood or components** (e.g., platelets, plasma) was one of the modes of transmission. Screening of donor blood and plasma for antibodies to HIV has reduced the risk of this mode of transmission. Because of recently infected individual may be antibody-negative (seronegative), there is a small risk of acquiring AIDS through transfusion of blood. **Organs from HIV- infected donors can also transmit AIDS.**
3. **Perinatal transmission (mother-to-infant transmission): It is the major mode of transmission of AIDS in children.** Transmission of infection can occur by **three routes**:
   a. **In utero:** It is transmitted by transplacental spread.
   b. **Perinatal spread:** During normal vaginal delivery or childbirth (intrapartum) **through an infected birth canal** and in the immediate period (peripartum).
   c. **After birth:** It is transmitted by ingestion of breast milk or from the genital secretions.

Transmission of HIV infection to healthcare workers: There is an extremely small risk of transmission to healthcare professionals, after accidental needle-stick injury or exposure of nonintact skin to infected blood.

Properties of HIV

Acquired immunodeficiency syndrome (AIDS) is caused by HIV, which is a **non-transforming human retrovirus belonging to the lentivirus family**. This subfamily is so named after the Latin word lentus, meaning "slow," because the infection develops gradually. Retroviruses are **single-stranded RNA viruses having an enzyme called reverse transcriptase**, which **prepares a DNA copy of the RNA genome of the virus in the host cell.**

Genetic forms: HIV occurs in **two genetically different but related main forms, HIV-1, and HIV-2.** Both are similar in structure and function but are differentiated from each other by their envelope glycoproteins, point of origin, and latency periods. Many subspecies or strains of HIV also exist because of the rapid rate of HIV virion mutation.

- **HIV-1** is most common in the United States, Europe, and Central Africa. About 10 subtypes of HIV-1 have been identified: group N (YBF30), group O, and group M with 8 subtypes (A, B, C, D, E, F, G, and H). The most common cause of AIDS in India is HIV-1 group M subtype C.
- **HIV-2 is common in West Africa and confined to western and southern India** (found near Goa). HIV-2 is differentiated from HIV-1 by a **longer clinical latency period** from the onset of infection to the development of symptoms. It is possible to have coinfection with both HIV-1 and HIV-2.

Structure of HIV (Fig. 6.22)

Q. Write a short note on the structure of HIV.

HIV-1 is a **spherical enveloped retrovirus** (virus that uses RNA as its genomic material), which is about 90–120 nm in diameter. It consists of a **viral core surrounded by a nucleocapsid cell which in turn is covered by a lipoprotein envelope.**

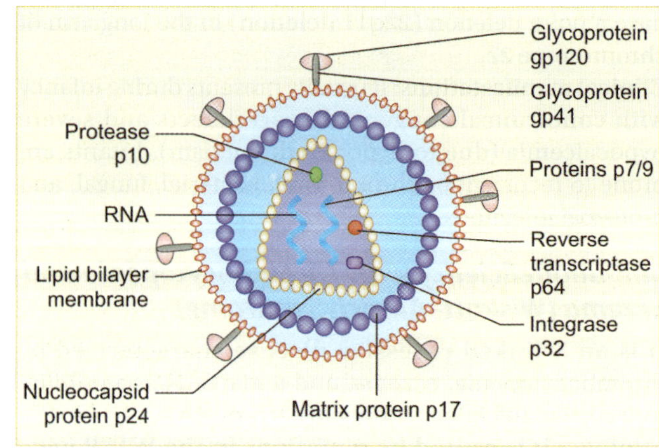

Fig. 6.22: Diagrammatic representation of the structure of the human immune deficiency virus (HIV)-1 virion. The viral particle is covered by a lipid bilayer derived from the host cell and studded with viral glycoproteins gp41 and gp120.

Viral core: It is **electron-dense, and cone-shaped.** It contains:

1. **Major capsid protein *p24*: p24 is the most abundant** viral antigen. This antigen p24 and the antibodies against this are **used for the diagnosis of HIV infection** in enzyme-linked immunosorbent assay (**ELISA**).
2. **Nucleocapsid protein *p7/p9***
3. **Two identical copies of single-stranded viral RNA.**
4. **Three viral enzymes:** These enzymes are very important because they facilitate the conversion of RNA to DNA.
   a. **Protease:** It works as a "molecular scissor" and splits the other viral components and activates the virions.
   b. **Reverse transcriptase:** It is RNA-dependent DNA polymerase which allows the virus to copy RNA into DNA. Thus, it makes a DNA copy (cDNA, provirus) of the virus.
   c. **Integrase:** It integrates the copy of the provirus into the host DNA. **When the virus infects a cell, viral RNA** is not translated, but instead **transcribed by reverse transcriptase into DNA**. The **DNA form of the retroviral genome** is called a **provirus** which can be **integrated into the chromosome of the host cell**.

Matrix protein: The viral core is surrounded by a matrix protein called p17. It is present below the virion lipid envelope.

Lipid envelope: The virus contains a lipoprotein envelope, which **consists of lipids derived from the host cell membrane and two viral glycoproteins. These glycoproteins are essential for HIV infection of cells.** These glycoproteins are: **(1) gp120,** project as knob-like spikes (look like a studded ball) on the surface, and **(2) gp41,** anchoring transmembrane pedicle. Gp120 and gp41 proteins cover the viral particle surface. Gp120 is the most external and distal part of each "stud/knob-like," whereas gp41 is the bridge that holds it onto the virion surface.

HIV Genome

The HIV genome contains two main groups of genes and their products act as antigens. IHIV RNA encodes for nine genes, i.e., 3 standard genes and 6 accessory genes.

Standard genes: The HIV-1 RNA genome **contains three standard retroviral genes**, which are **typical of retroviruses**. These include *gag*, *pol*, and *env* genes. The *gag* gene encodes nucleocapsid proteins. The *pol* gene encodes reverse transcriptase, integrase, and protease (enzymes that are essential for the viral life cycle). The *env* gene encodes the viral envelope protein glycoprotein gp160, which is split into two fragments, gp120 and gp41, by cellular protease.

Accessory genes: HIV contains 6 accessory genes namely *tat*, *rev*, *vif*, *nef*, *vpr*, and *vpu*. These genes **regulate the synthesis (regulatory genes) and assembly of infectious viral particles** and the **pathogenicity of the virus**.

The envelope proteins, especially gp120, show marked variability among viral isolates. It is due to a high frequency of mutation occurring in the *env* gene. This property of the virus makes it difficult to produce gp120 vaccines. Neither a vaccine nor a cure has been developed to date.

Pathogenesis of HIV Infection and AIDS

Q. Write a short note on the pathogenesis of HIV infection and AIDS.

HIV is an extraordinarily successful human pathogen. Infection is transmitted when the virus enters the blood or tissues of an individual.

Major targets: HIV can infect many tissues, but two major targets of HIV infection are:

- **Immune system:** HIV is an RNA retrovirus that causes a defect in cell-mediated immunity that may progress to AIDS. It **mainly infects and subsequently causes loss of CD4+ T-cells. Severe immune deficiency, mainly affecting cell-mediated immunity is the hallmark of AIDS.**
- **Central nervous system (CNS).**

Life Cycle of HIV

Q. Write a short note on the life cycle of HIV.

The life cycle of HIV consists of four main steps, namely: (1) infection of cells by HIV, (2) integration of the provirus into the host cell genome, (3) viral replication, and (4) production and release of infectious virus **(Fig. 6.23)**.

Infection of Cells by HIV (1 in Fig. 6.23)

Portal of entry of initial infection: HIV may enter the body through several portals. The most efficient (except for direct inoculation of blood products) portal of entry is the GI tract. Infants get infected by HIV from their mothers by ingesting blood and cervical mucus during birth, or breast milk during feeding. At the time of exposure to HIV, infection occurs when the virus moves across the epithelium or mucosal membrane of the body.

Tropism of HIV for host cells with CD receptor: Once inside the body, HIV has **selective affinity for host cells with surface CD4 molecule receptors and various chemokine receptors as coreceptors**. The cells with CD4 receptors include **CD4+ T-cells** and other CD4+ cells such as **monocytes/macrophages** and **dendritic cells**. The **HIV envelope contains two glycoproteins, surface gp120** (expressed in all HIV strains) noncovalently attached to a transmembrane protein **and gp41**.

Binding of HIV gp120 to CD4 receptor and coreceptor of the host cell: It is the first and essential step in HIV infection. The binding of HIV to the host cell occurs in the mucosal or other tissue at or near the site of exposure.

- **Binding to CD4 receptor:** Binding occurs between the **CD4 molecule receptor of the host cell to the envelope protein gp120 of HIV**. Binding to CD4 alone is not enough for HIV infection (for the fusion of the virion and host cell). HIV gp120 must also bind to other cell surface molecules (**coreceptors**) for its entry into the host cell. The important coreceptors on the target cells that are necessary for the virus to gain entry into cells are chemokine receptors **(particularly CCR5 and CXCR4)**. The CCR5 must be present for the HIV particles to bind to the CD4+ cells, especially in early infection and CXCR4 is often present in later infection. Chemokines (chemoattractant cytokines that regulate leukocyte trafficking to sites of inflammation) play a significant role in the pathogenesis of HIV disease.

- **Conformational change in HIV with the formation of recognition site on gp120 for the coreceptors: For binding of HIV to coreceptor on the host cell, HIV should undergo a conformational change in gp120.** Binding to CD4 leads to a conformational change (change in shape by refolding) **in HIV. It results in the formation of a new recognition site on gp120 for the coreceptors CCR5 or CXCR4 on the host cell.**
- **Gp120, CD4 binding to chemokine receptor (coreceptor):** A new recognition site on gp120 of HIV binds to **chemokine receptors,** i.e., CCR5 and CXCR4 on the host cell. Chemokine receptors play a role in viral cell entry.
- **Conformational change in gp41 of HIV with exposure to fusion peptide:** The binding of gp120 of HIV to the coreceptors produces conformational changes in gp41. This exposes a hydrophobic region at the tip of gp41 called the fusion peptide.

Penetration of host cell membrane by fusion peptide of gp41: The fusion peptide exposed at the tip of gp41 inserts into the cell membrane of the target (host) cells. The conformational change in gp41 allows **HIV to penetrate the cell membrane of the target cells** (e.g., CD4+ T-cells or macrophages), **leading to the fusion of the virus with the host cell.**

Entry of viral genome into cytoplasm of host cell: After fusion, the virus core containing the HIV genome enters the cytoplasm of the host cell, and infection is produced.

Integration of the Proviral DNA into the Genome of the Host Cell (2 in Fig. 6.23)

Reverse transcription and production of proviral DNA: After the HIV genome enters the cytoplasm (after the internalization of the virus core), **reverse transcription of the RNA genome of the** virus occurs. During this process, a **single-stranded DNA copy is made** from the viral RNA **by reverse transcriptase.** Using this single-stranded DNA as a template, DNA polymerase copies it to make **a second (complementary) DNA strand** and destroys the original RNA strands. Thus, it produces **double-stranded DNA, called proviral DNA** (cDNA). The accuracy of DNA transcription is poor because the reverse transcriptase of HIV lacks an editing function. Hence, reverse transcription frequently creates a huge number of mutations. This tendency to mutate makes HIV resistant to antiviral medications.

Integration of the proviral DNA into the genome of the host cell: Once formed, this new proviral DNA is called provirus or preintegration complexes (PICs). This provirus migrates to the nucleus of the host cell and is actively transported in the nuclear compartment.

- **Episomal form: In quiescent** (unactivated, nondividing) **T-cells, HIV cDNA** may remain in a linear **episomal form in the cytoplasm of infected cells.**
- **Integration of cDNA: In dividing (proliferating) T-cells,** HIV **cDNA circularizes and enters the nucleus. Then it becomes integrated into the genome of the host cell using several host proteins including a viral integrase protein.**

Viral Replication (3 in Fig. 6.23)

After the integration of the provirus into the host DNA, it may remain either latent or productive.

- **Latent infection:** During latent infections, the **provirus remains silent** for months or years. **In these latently infected host cells, completion of the viral life cycle occurs only after these cells are activated. In most CD4+ T cells, virus activation results in the death of the infected cells.** The virus **infection remains latent for long periods in lymphoid tissues.**
- **Productive infection:** Once the proviral DNA is integrated into the host cell's DNA, it may be transcribed. This leads to the expression of viral proteins that are required for the formation of complete viral particles.

Production and Release of Infectious Virus (4 in Fig. 6.23)

The complete **virus particle** forms **buds from the cell membrane** and **releases a new infectious virus.** This productive infection when extensive, leads to the death of infected host cells. **Active viral replication is associated with more infection of cells and progression to AIDS.** The infected cell, or free virus, binds another cell and the cycle repeats.

Dissemination: The virus disseminates to other target cells. This occurs either by the fusion of an infected cell with an uninfected one or by the budding of virions from the membrane of the infected cell.

Mechanism of T-cell Depletion

Direct cytopathic effect: Loss of CD4+ T-cells in HIV is mainly due to the direct cytopathic effects of the replicating virus. The normal CD4+/CD8+ ratio is 2:1. Loss of CD4+ cells in AIDS patients leads to an inversion of the **CD4+/CD8+ ratio to** 0.5 or less.

HIV infection of non-T-cells: HIV can infect non-T-cells such as macrophages and dendritic cells **(mucosal and follicular)**. HIV-1 can multiply in terminally differentiated nondividing macrophages and may be reservoirs of HIV infection. In the late stages of HIV infection, CD4+ T-cell

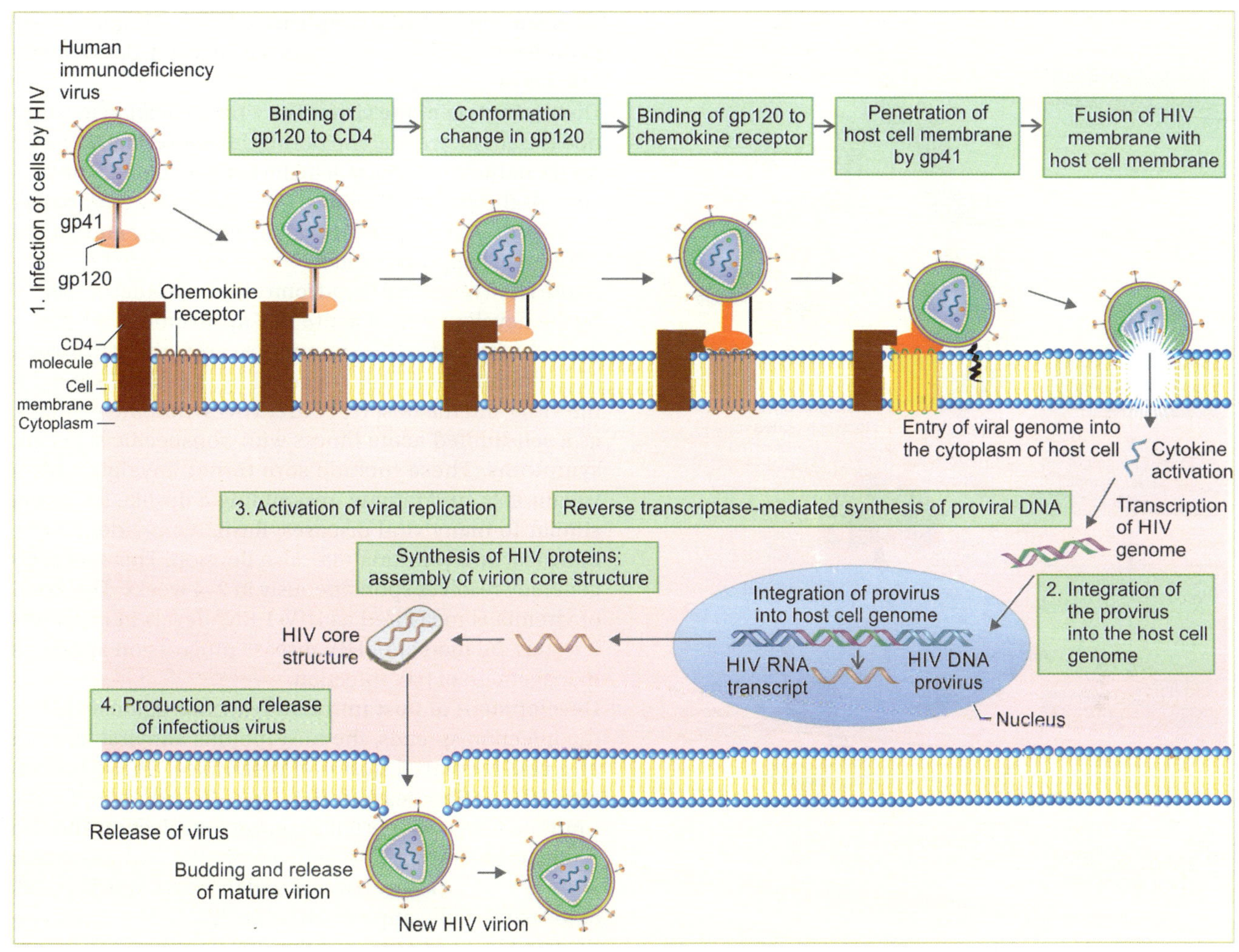

Fig. 6.23: Various molecular steps involved in the life cycle of HIV.

numbers are markedly reduced, and macrophages may be an important site for continued replication of the virus. Follicular dendritic cells (FDCs) in the germinal centers of lymph nodes are also potential reservoirs of HIV.

B Cell function in HIV Infection: HIV cannot infect B cells, but they may show severe abnormalities. These include spontaneous polyclonal activation of B-cells and hypergammaglobulinemia. There is an inability to elicit antibody responses to newly encountered antigens Impaired humoral immunity may lead to disseminated infections caused by capsulated bacteria, such as *S. pneumoniae* and *H. influenzae.*

Pathogenesis of central nervous system involvement: HIV infection also affects the central nervous system. HIV is carried into the brain by infected monocytes. HIV does not infect neurons. The neurologic deficit is caused indirectly by viral products and by soluble factors produced by infected macrophages (e.g., cytokines).

Natural History and Course of HIV Infection (Fig. 6.24)

Q. Write a short note on the natural history of HIV infection.

HIV infection starts as an acute infection. This infection is only partially controlled by the host's immune response. Acute infection progresses to chronic infection of the peripheral lymphoid tissues.

Acute Phase

Primary infection of memory CD4+ T-cells in the mucosal lymphoid tissue: Usually, HIV typically enters the host through mucosal surfaces. In the (acute) early infection, HIV first infects memory CD4+ T-cells (which express coreceptor, CCR5), present in **the mucosal lymphoid tissue** (the largest reservoir of T-cells and where most memory cells are lodged). HIV **causes the death of many of these infected CD4+ cells** resulting in **significant depletion of T-cells**. At this stage, few infected cells can be detected in the blood and other tissues.

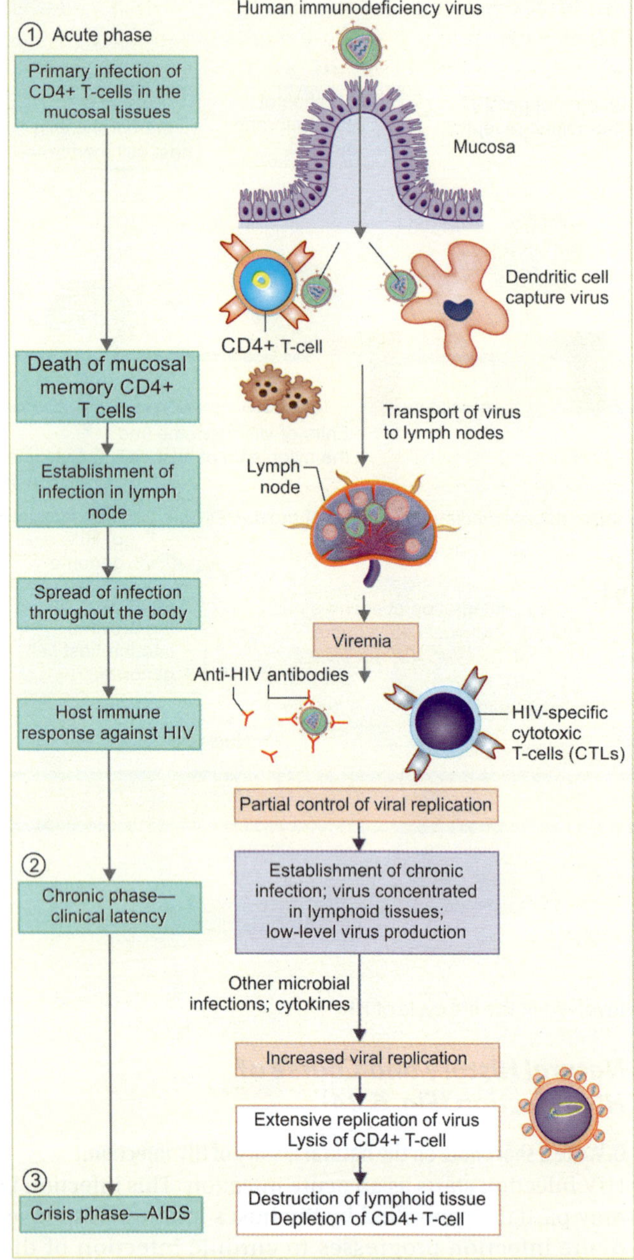

Fig. 6.24: Pathogenesis of HIV infection. (1) Acute phase. The initial infection begins in mucosal tissues. HIV infects mainly memory CD4+ T-cells and dendritic cells. HIV spreads to lymph nodes. Viral replication in lymph nodes leads to viremia and widespread seeding of lymphoid tissue. (2) Chronic phase. The viremia is controlled by the host immune response and the disease enters a phase of clinical latency. During the chronic latency phase, viral replication in both T-cells and macrophages continues. (3) Ultimately, there is a progressive decrease of CD4+ T lymphocytes.

Spread to lymphoid tissue: Dendritic cells in epithelia **at the primary site of virus entry capture the virus** and **migrate to lymphoid tissue** such as **lymph nodes and spleen**. In the lymphoid tissues, **DCs pass HIV on to CD4+ T-cells via direct cell-to-cell contact.**

Viral replication in the lymph node: Viral replication begins in the lymph node and can be detected within days after the first exposure to HIV.

Dissemination of the virus: The viral replication in lymph nodes leads to viremia, and during this period high numbers of HIV particles are present in the patient's blood. The virus spreads throughout the body. The viremia is accompanied by infection of helper T cells, macrophages, and DCs in peripheral lymphoid tissues.

Acute HIV (retroviral) syndrome: Viremia is accompanied by the development of **acute HIV syndrome** in 40–90% of individuals. Acute HIV syndrome occurs within 3 to 6 weeks of initial infection. It is triggered by the initial spread of the virus and the host response. This syndrome manifests as a self-limited acute illness with nonspecific signs and symptoms. These include sore throat, myalgias, fever, weight loss, and fatigue, resembling a flu-like syndrome similar to many viral diseases. Rash, lymphadenopathy, diarrhea, and vomiting may also develop. This syndrome generally resolves spontaneously in 2–4 weeks. The extent of viremia is measured as HIV-1 RNA levels in the blood. It is a useful marker of HIV disease progression and in the management of HIV infection.

Development of host immune response against HIV: As the infection spreads, the host mounts antiviral humoral and cell-mediated immune responses. These include **anti-HIV antibodies** and **HIV- specific cytotoxic T-cells.** Immune responses partially control the infection and viral replication. During this, seroconversion (usually within 3–7 weeks of exposure) occurs and the virus-specific CD8+ cytotoxic T cells appear. HIV-specific CD8+ T cells are detected in the blood when the viral titers begin to fall and these are most likely responsible for the initial control of HIV infection. These immune responses partially control HIV infection and viral production. This results in a drop in viremia to low but detectable levels by about 12 weeks after the initial exposure to HIV.

Chronic Phase

Following the acute phase, HIV infection progresses to the chronic phase **of the disease**. During this chronic phase, the **virus continuously replicates and causes cell destruction in the lymph nodes and spleen.**

Clinical latency period: During this period of the disease, **few or no clinical manifestations of the HIV infection** are present. Hence, this phase of disease is called the *clinical latency period.* The host immune response can handle most infections with opportunistic microbes with no or minimal clinical symptoms.

Progressive decrease of CD4+ T-cells: During this phase, few peripheral blood T cells harbor the virus, but there is **continuous destruction of CD4+ T-cells in the lymphoid tissue.** It is accompanied by a steady **decrease in the number of** CD4+ T cells **in the peripheral blood.** During the early course of the disease, the loss of CD4+ T-cells can be replaced by new T-cells. However, over a period of years, the continuous cycle of viral infection and death of T-cells leads to a steady decrease in the number of CD4+ T-cells both in the lymphoid tissue and in circulation.

HIV-1 RNA levels in the blood: The extent of viremia is measured by estimating the HIV-1 RNA levels in the blood. It is a useful marker of HIV disease progression and is useful in the management of patients with HIV.

Viral set point: The HIV-1 RNA levels (viral load) at the end of the acute phase reflect the equilibrium reached between the virus and the host response. In each patient, viral load may remain stable for several years. This level of steady-state viremia is called the *viral set point.* It predicts the rate of decline of CD4+ T cells and, the progression of HIV disease.

Q. Write a short note on CD count in HIV.

Centers for Disease Control (CDC) classification of HIV infection: The loss of immune containment is associated with declining CD4+ T-cell counts. The Centers for Disease Control and Prevention (CDC) classification of HIV infection divided patients into three groups based on CD4+T cell counts: (i) 500 cells/µL or greater, (ii) 200–499 cells/µL, and (iii) fewer than 200 cells/µL.

AIDS

The final phase of HIV infection is progression to AIDS. It is characterized by a breakdown of host defense, a **sudden increase in viremia, and severe, life-threatening clinical disease.**

Clinical features: The patient presents with a fever of more than 1 month duration, fatigue, weight loss, and diarrhea. After a variable period, the patient develops opportunistic infections, secondary neoplasms, or neurologic diseases (grouped under the rubric *AIDS indicator diseases* or *AIDS-defining illnesses).* With these features, the patient is said to have developed AIDS.

Most untreated (with exceptions) patients with HIV infection **progress to AIDS after a chronic phase lasting from 7 to 10 years**. These exceptions are:

- **Rapid progressors:** In these patients, the middle, **chronic phase is shortened to 2–3 years** after primary infection. These patients **rapidly progress to AIDS**.
- **Long-term nonprogressors:** It is defined as **untreated patients who remain asymptomatic for 10 years or more, with stable CD4+ T-cell counts and low levels of plasma viremia** (usually <500 viral RNA copies/mL).

Elite controllers: About 1% of HIV infected individuals have no detectable plasma virus (<50 to 75 RNA copies/ mL). These are called *elite controllers.* These individuals show evidence of a strong anti-HIV immune response. Some of them have high levels of HIV-specific CD4+ and CD8+ T-cell responses.

Clinical Features of AIDS

Untreated adult patient with AIDS: They present with **fever, weight loss, diarrhea, generalized lymphadenopathy, multiple opportunistic infections**, and **neurologic disease**. Many patients may develop **secondary neoplasms**.

Hematologic manifestations: Patients may develop **anemia, neutropenia, and thrombocytopenia**. These may be due to the infection of hematopoietic progenitor cells by HIV.

Highly active antiretroviral therapy (HAART): In HAART, a combination of three or four drugs that block different steps of the HIV life cycle are used. This has markedly reduced the morbidity and mortality associated with HIV infection.

Opportunistic Infections

Q. Write briefly on opportunistic/fungal infections in AIDS.

Opportunistic infections are infections that occur in individuals with weakened immune system. **In AIDS, most deaths in untreated patients with AIDS are due to opportunistic infections.** Many of these infections are due to the reactivation of latent (inactive) infections. Normally, these latent infections are controlled by a powerful immune system but are not destroyed. This is because the infectious agents have developed to coexist with their hosts. The opportunistic infections found in patients with HIV infection are presented in **Table 6.13**.

Tumors

Q. Write briefly on common neoplasms in HIV patients.

Certain tumors occur with high incidence in patients with AIDS. Main tumors are (i) Kaposi sarcoma, (ii) B-cell lymphoma, (iii) cervical cancer in women, and (iv) anal cancer in men. HIV patients are also more susceptible to tumors (e.g., lung and skin cancers and certain lymphoma) than in the general population. The neoplasms found in patients with HIV infection are presented in **Table 6.14.**

Central Nervous System Disease in AIDS

Q. List the CNS lesions found in AIDS.

Central nervous system (CNS) involvement is a common and important manifestation of AIDS. CNS lesions in AIDS patients are listed in **Box 6.6**.

AIDS, acquired immunodeficiency syndrome; CNS, central nervous system

Diagnosis of HIV Infection or AIDS

Q. Write a short note on laboratory diagnosis of AIDS.

The investigations of a suspected case of HIV/AIDS can be categorized into three groups: (i) tests for establishing HIV infection, (ii) tests for detection of defects in immunity (e.g., CD4+ T-cell count, ratio of CD4+/CD8+ T cells), and (iii) tests for detection of opportunistic infections and secondary neoplasms (FNAC, exfoliative cytology, biopsy). Various laboratory diagnostic test for diagnosis of HIV infection is listed in **Box 6.7**.

Effect of antiretroviral drug therapy on the course of HIV infection: Currently available new drugs target the viral

TABLE 6.13 AIDS-defining opportunistic infections and neoplasms found in patients with HIV infection.

Opportunistic infections	*Organ or site involved or type of damage*	*Comments*
Fungal Infections		
Pneumocystosis	Pneumonia or disseminated infection	About 15–30% of untreated HIV patients develop *pneumonia* caused by the fungus *Pneumocystis jirovecii*
Candidiasis	Esophageal, tracheal, or pulmonary	The most common fungal infection, involves the oral cavity, vagina, and esophagus
Cryptococcosis	Infection of the central nervous system	*Cryptococcosis* occurs in about 10% of AIDS patients mainly meningitis
Coccidioidomycosis	Disseminated	
Histoplasmosis	Disseminated	
Viral Infections		
Cytomegalovirus (CMV)	Retinitis, CNS, pulmonary, and intestinal infections	May cause disseminated disease but more commonly affects the eye and gastrointestinal tract
Herpes simplex virus	Localized or disseminated	Mucocutaneous ulcerations of the mouth, esophagus, external genitalia, and perianal region
Varicella-zoster virus	Localized or disseminated	
*JC virus (*human papova virus)	Central nervous system	Causes progressive multifocal leukoencephalopathy
Protozoal and Helminthic Infections		
Cryptosporidiosis or isosporidiosis	Enteritis	Persistent diarrhea in untreated patients with advanced AIDS is often due to protozoa, such as *Cryptosporidium hominis,* or enteric bacteria
Toxoplasmosis	Pneumonia or CNS infection	*Toxoplasma gondii* frequently invades the CNS and causes encephalitis
Bacterial Infections		
Mycobacteriosis		
Atypical, e.g., *Mycobacterium avium intracellulare*	Disseminated or extrapulmonary	Disseminated infection with *Mycobacterium tuberculosis* and *nontuberculous,* or *atypical, mycobacteria* (mainly *Mycobacterium avium complex).* Many are resistant to multiple anti-mycobacterial drugs
M. tuberculosis	Pulmonary or extrapulmonary	
Nocardiosis	Pneumonia, meningitis, disseminated	
Salmonella infections	Disseminated	

TABLE 6.14 Neoplasms found in patients with HIV infection.

Neoplasms	*Cause—oncogenic virus*	*Comment*
Kaposi sarcoma (KS)	Kaposi sarcoma herpes virus *(human herpesvirus 8 [HHV8])*	Vascular tumor is considered an AIDS-defining malignancy
Non-Hodgkin B-cell lymphoma—primary lymphoma of the brain	Epstein-Barr virus (EBV)	AIDS-defining tumor. Often occurs in extranodal sites, such as the CNS, GI tract, orbit, and lungs
HIV-associated Hodgkin lymphoma	Reed-Sternberg cells are infected with EBV	
Carcinoma of the uterine cervix (cervical cancer) in women	Human papillomavirus (HPV)	*Human papillomavirus* infection is poorly controlled due to immunodeficiency
Anal carcinoma	HPV	

BOX 6.6: CNS lesions in AIDS patients.

- AIDS—dementia complex
- Non-Hodgkin B-cell lymphoma—primary lymphoma of the brain
- Progressive multifocal leukoencephalopathy *(HIV-associated neurocognitive disorder)*
- Meningoencephalitis (tuberculous, cryptococcal)
- Aseptic meningitis or viral meningoencephalitis
- Vacuolar myelopathy
- Peripheral neuropathy
- Demyelinating lesions of the spinal cord

BOX 6.7: Laboratory diagnostic test for diagnosis of HIV infection.

1. **ELISA:** Detects antibodies against viral protein, the **most sensitive** and best screening test for the diagnosis of AIDS.
2. **Western blot:** The **most specific** or **confirmatory test** for HIV.
3. **Direct detection of viral infection:**
   - **p24 antigen capture assay.**
   - **Reverse transcriptase polymerase chain reaction (RT-PCR).**
   - **DNA-PCR.**
   - **Culture of virus from the monocytes and CD4+ T-cells.**

(AIDS: acquired immunodeficiency syndrome; DNA: deoxyribose nucleic acid; ELISA: enzyme-linked immunosorbent assay, HIV: human immunodeficiency virus; PCR: polymerase chain reaction)

reverse transcriptase, protease, integrase enzymes, and other proteins. These drugs have changed the clinical course of AIDS. Antiretroviral therapy has reduced the transmission of HIV, especially from infected mothers to newborns.

MORPHOLOGY

Tissue changes that occur with HIV infection are neither specific nor diagnostic. Common pathologic lesions of AIDS include opportunistic infections, Kaposi sarcoma, and B-cell lymphomas.

Lymph Node

Early stage: Biopsy of enlarged lymph nodes in the early stages of HIV infection shows a marked **hyperplasia of B-cell follicles** that may have a serpiginous shape.

With disease progression: The proliferation of of B-cells decreases and **lymphoid involution** begins. The lymph nodes are depleted of lymphocytes, and the germinal centers disappear or sometimes become hyalinized. In the later stages of AIDS, the lymphoid involution affects the spleen and thymus. They may lack lymphocytes.

Prognosis: The prognosis of AIDS is poor.

AMYLOIDOSIS

PA 3.1 (CC): Describe the pathogenesis and pathology of amyloidosis.

Q. Define amyloidosis.

Definitions: Amyloidosis is a pathologic condition associated with several disorders (a variety of clinical conditions) **in which fibrillar proteins are deposited in the extracellular space of various tissues and organs** of the body. **These deposits produce tissue damage and dysfunction.**

The pathologic fibrillar protein deposited in the extracellular space is termed amyloid.

General Features

- **Amyloidosis occurs in various inherited and inflammatory disorders.**
- **Amyloid deposits cause structural and functional damage to involved tissue and organs.**
- **Improper folding of proteins:** During normal protein synthesis, chaperones in the ER (endoplasmic reticulum) control the proper folding of newly synthesized proteins. These normally folded proteins are soluble. The misfolded proteins undergo proteolysis. **Basically, amyloidosis is a disorder of protein misfolding.** The abnormal fibrils in amyloidosis are produced by the aggregation of misfolded (improperly folded) proteins. **Accumulation of misfolded proteins may be either due to increased production or reduced ability to eliminate them.**
- **Staining characteristics:** The fibrillar deposits of amyloid bind a wide variety of proteoglycans and glycosaminoglycans. It contains charged sugar groups and **has staining characteristics that were thought to resemble starch (amylose** = starch-like**).** Hence, it was called amyloid by the pathologist Rudolf Virchow (1821 to 1902) in 1854. However, these deposits are not related to starch.
- **Usually a systemic (sometimes localized) disease.**

Properties of Amyloid Proteins

Q. Describe the physical and chemical nature of amyloid.

Forms of amyloid: All amyloid has similar morphological and staining properties, but amyloidosis is **not a single disease.** It is **a group of diseases** having **in common the deposition of similar-appearing proteins** in which the protein composition varies (more than 20 different proteins) and the mechanism of formation is different.

Q. Write a short note on the physical and chemical nature of amyloid.

Physical Nature of Amyloid

By electron microscopy, all types of amyloid are composed of nonbranching fibrils of 7–10 nm diameter. X-ray crystallography and infrared spectroscopy show a characteristic **cross-β-pleated sheet conformation.** In this, each fibril is wound around one another (*refer* **online Fig. 6.25**). **Congo-red dye** binds to these fibrils and produces **classic apple-green birefringence** (dichromism). Hence,

Congo-red stain is used to identify amyloid deposits in tissues.

Chemical Nature of Amyloid

Fibrillar proteins bind with a variety of substances. **About 95%** of the amyloid material consists of **fibril proteins. The remaining 5%** consists of **proteoglycans, glycosaminoglycans, serum amyloid P(SAP), etc.**

Biochemical forms of amyloid: It consists of **three major** (most common) **distinct proteins and more than 20 minor forms.**

A. **Major forms:** These are amyloid light chain (**AL**), amyloid associated (**AA**) and β **amyloid (Aβ)**
   1. **Amyloid light chain (AL) protein:** It consists of **complete immunoglobulin** (Ig) **light chains** (mostly λ, rarely κ) or the **amino-terminal fragments of light chains, or both**. These AL proteins are **produced by plasma cells** and associated with some monoclonal B-cell proliferation (e.g., plasma cell tumors).
   2. **AA (amyloid-associated) protein: It is a non-immunoglobulin synthesized by the liver**. It is **derived from** the proteolysis of a larger precursor in the serum called **SAA (serum amyloid-associated)** protein. **Increased synthesis of SAA** protein occurs under the influence of cytokines (e.g., IL-6 and IL-1) **during inflammation** (as part of the acute phase response). Therefore, it is associated with **chronic inflammation** and is called secondary amyloidosis.
   3. **β amyloid (Aβ) protein:** It is **derived by proteolysis of a larger** transmembrane glycoprotein called **amyloid precursor protein (APP)**. It is **found in the cerebral plaques and walls of cerebral blood vessels** of **Alzheimer disease**.

B. **Minor types:**
   1. **Transthyretin (TTR):** It is a **normal serum protein** that **transports thyroxine and retinol. Mutations** in gene encoding TTR **alter its structure and misfolds.** It is **found in** genetically determined disorders called **familial amyloid polyneuropathies. Unmutated TTR is deposited in the heart of aged individuals** (senile systemic amyloidosis).
   2. **β_2-microglobulin:** It is a **normal serum protein** and is a component of MHC class I molecules. Amyloid fibril subunit namely **$A\beta_2m$ is derived from β_2-microglobulin.** This amyloid is found in or around the joints or soft tissues of patients **on long-term hemodialysis.**

Pathogenesis of Amyloidosis (Fig. 6.26)

Q. Write a short note on the pathogenesis of amyloidosis.

Misfolding of Proteins

Amyloidosis is a pathologic condition that results from abnormal folding or misfolding of proteins. These misfolded proteins assume a β-pleated sheet arrangement, aggregate, and deposit as fibrils in extracellular tissues.

- **Normal processing of misfolded proteins:** The intracellular misfolded proteins **are normally degraded in proteosomes (proteases that degrade proteins),** and the **extracellular protein aggregates are taken up and degraded by macrophages.**
- **Failure of quality control mechanism involved in the processing of misfolded protein in amyloidosis:** There is **failure of the above-mentioned quality control mechanism in amyloidosis.** The production of misfolded proteins exceeds the degradation capacity. These misfolded proteins are unstable and self-associated. They accumulate as fibrillar proteins outside cells (in extracellular tissues).

Categories of Proteins in Amyloidosis

Amyloidosis is a disorder due to the abnormal folding of proteins. The proteins that form amyloid belong to two general categories (1) production of abnormal amounts of normal protein, and (2) production of normal amount of mutant protein.

Production of Abnormal Amounts of Normal Protein

- In this category, normal proteins have **an inherent tendency to fold improperly or undergo misfolding.** They self-associate (form clusters with each other using attractive forces), and form fibrils particularly when they are produced in increased amounts.
- **Example:** During inflammation, SAA is synthesized by the liver cells under the influence of cytokines such as IL-6 and IL-1 secreted by activated macrophages, and is degraded by monocyte-derived enzymes. In individuals prone to amyloidosis, there may be defects in the monocyte-derived enzymes with **incomplete breakdown of SAA** and **formation of insoluble AA molecules**. Genetically defective SAA may also be responsible for resistant degradation by macrophages.

Production of the Normal Amount of Mutant Protein

In this category, **the mutant protein is prone to misfolding and subsequent aggregation** to form amyloid. For example, in familial amyloidosis, mutation of the gene encoding TTR leads to alterations in the structure of serum protein TTRs. These mutated proteins are prone to misfolding and aggregate. These are resistant to proteolysis.

Pathological effects of amyloid: Amyloid deposits produce pressure on adjacent normal cells and lead to **atrophy of cells.** Deposition in the blood vessel wall causes (i) narrowing of the lumen and leads to **ischemic damage**, and increased vascular permeability with the **escape of protein out of the vessel.**

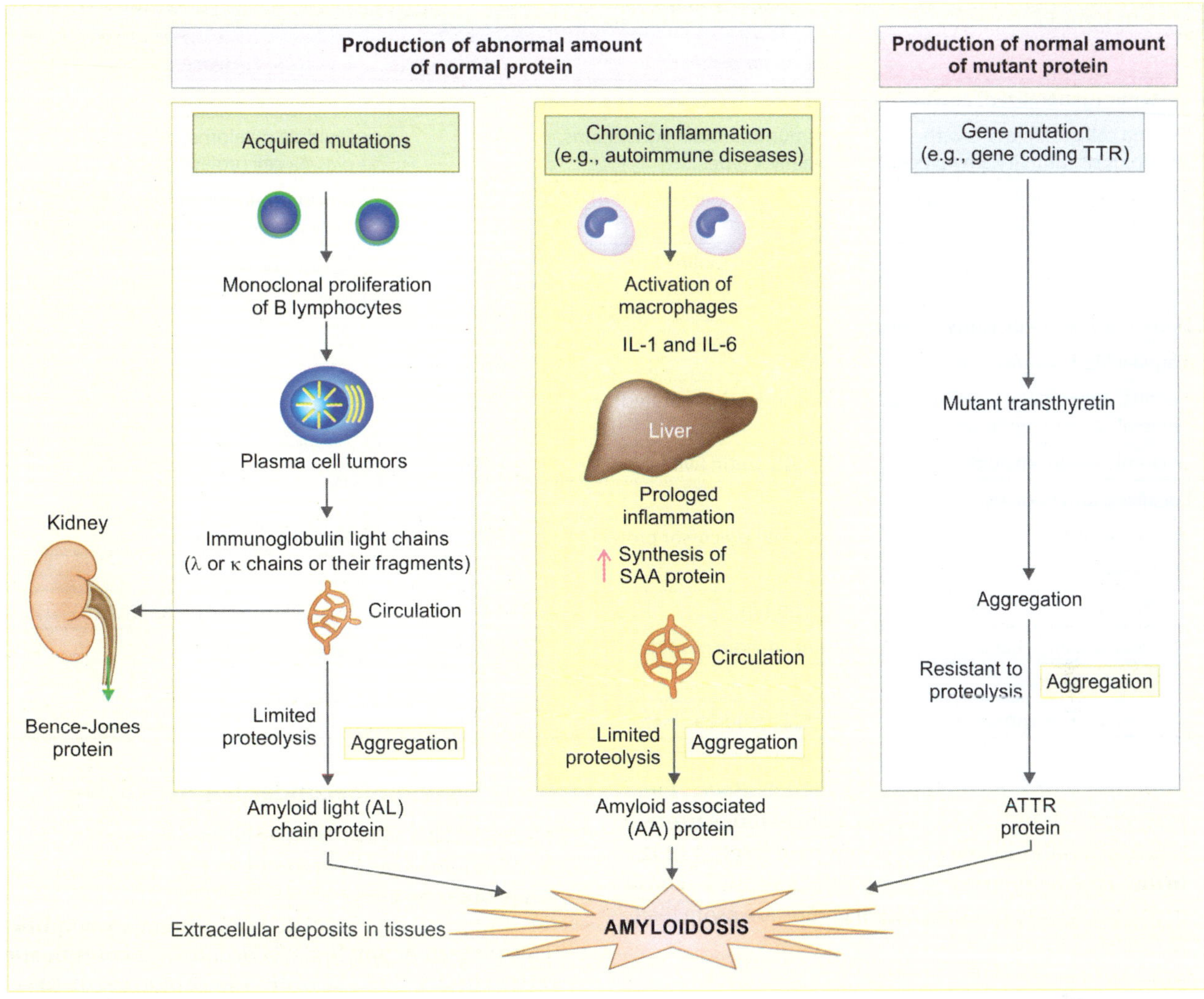

Fig. 6.26: Pathogenesis of amyloidosis. AL protein is seen in association with B lymphocyte and plasma cell proliferation which secrete immunoglobulin light chains that are amyloidogenic. AA protein is seen in a variety of diseases associated with the activation of macrophages, which in turn, leads to the synthesis and release of SAA. The SAA is converted to AA protein. ATTR protein is due to mutant proteins that aggregate and deposit as amyloid.

(SAA: serum amyloid; ATTR: transthyretin).

Classification of Amyloidosis

Q. Classify amyloidosis.

Amyloidosis is classified **depending on biochemical and clinical characteristics (Table 6.15)**

Systemic (Generalized)

Amyloid involves several organs/systems. It may be subclassified into primary or secondary.

Q. Describe the pathology of primary amyloidosis.

Primary amyloidosis: Plasma cell proliferations associated with amyloidosis.

Primary Amyloidosis

It is associated with or without clonal plasma cell proliferation.

Clonal proliferation of plasma cells

In this category, amyloid is of the **AL type** and is usually **systemic in distribution**. It is the **most common form** of amyloidosis.

Multiple myeloma: Primary amyloidosis is caused by a *clonal proliferation of plasma cells*. These cells **produce abnormal immunoglobulin** (Ig) **molecules**. The AL type of systemic amyloidosis occurs in **5–15% of patients with multiple myeloma.**

- **Excessive production of single specific Ig:** Multiple myeloma is a plasma-cell tumor characterized by **excessive synthesis of a single specific Ig** (monoclonal gammopathy) that appears as an **M (myeloma) protein spike on serum electrophoresis.**
- **Excessive synthesis of light chains:** Tumor also **produces free immunoglobulin light chains.** The free,

TABLE 6.15 Classification of amyloidosis.

Type	*Precursor protein*	*Fibril protein*	*Associated disease/s*
A. Systemic (generalized) amyloidosis			
1. Plasma cell proliferation with amyloidosis (primary amyloidosis)	Immunoglobulin light chains, mainly λ type	AL	Multiple myeloma, other monoclonal plasma cell proliferations
2. Reactive systemic amyloidosis (secondary amyloidosis)	Serum amyloid associated (SAA)	AA	Chronic inflammatory process (e.g., rheumatoid arthritis, Crohn disease)
3. Hemodialysis-associated amyloidosis	β_2-microglobulin	$A\beta_2m$	Chronic renal failure
B. Hereditary or familial amyloidosis			
1. Familial Mediterranean fever	SAA	AA	
2. Familial amyloidotic neuropathies (several types); cardiac amyloidosis	Transthyretin (mutated)	ATTR	
3. Systemic senile amyloidosis	Transthyretin (wild-type)	ATTR	
C. Localized amyloidosis			
1. Senile cerebral	Amyloid precursor protein (APP)	Aβ	Alzheimer disease
2. Endocrine			
– Thyroid	Calcitonin	A Cal	Medullary carcinoma
– Islets of Langerhans	Islet amyloid peptide	AIAPP	Type 2 diabetes
– Type 2 diabetes			
3. Isolated atrial amyloidosis	Atrial natriuretic factor	AANF	

unpaired κ or λ light chains (termed as *Bence-Jones protein*) are found in the serum. **Bence–Jones protein** being of small molecular size **can be excreted in the urine**. Free light chains tend to aggregate and deposit in tissues as amyloid. The λ light chains are more likely to deposit as amyloid than κ light chains.

Primary amyloidosis without clonal proliferation of plasma cells

- **No dateable myeloma or B-cell neoplasms:** The majority of patients with AL amyloid do not have multiple myeloma or any other observable B-cell neoplasm. These are termed primary amyloidosis because their clinical features are entirely because of amyloid deposition rather than the formation of tumor masses.
- **Presence of monoclonal Ig and/or free light chains:** Almost all these patients **have monoclonal immunoglobulins or free light chains, or both, in the serum or urine**.
- **Increased plasma cells in bone marrow: Bone marrow** in most of these patients shows an **increase in the number of plasma cells**. Probably, these cells secrete the precursors of AL protein. Thus, these may represent plasma cell dyscrasia characterized by the production of an abnormal protein, instead of the production of tumor masses.

Reactive Systemic (Secondary) Amyloidosis

Q. Write a short note on reactive systemic amyloidosis.

- **Amyloid deposits in systemic in distribution** and is of **AA protein** type.
- **Secondary to an associated inflammatory condition**: This pattern of amyloidosis occurs as a **complication of** (secondary to) **chronic inflammatory** or **tissue-destructive process**. Hence, was previously known as **secondary amyloidosis**. It **complicates or occurs in association with diseases,** such as:
  - **Previously followed chronic inflammatory conditions:** Examples, **tuberculosis, bronchiectasis,** and **chronic osteomyelitis**. Currently, these infections usually resolve with antibiotic treatment. Hence, they less often produce amyloidosis.
  - **Presently complicates autoimmune states:** These include **rheumatoid arthritis (most frequently associated)**, other connective tissue disorders (e.g., ankylosing spondylitis), inflammatory bowel disease (Crohn disease, and ulcerative colitis).
  - **Heroin abusers:** These patients develop chronic skin infections or abscesses due to subcutaneous self-administration of narcotics.
  - **Nonimmunocyte-derived tumors:** Renal cell carcinoma and Hodgkin lymphoma.

Hemodialysis-associated Amyloidosis

Patients with **chronic renal failure on long-term hemodialysis** have high **levels of β_2-microglobulin** in the serum. This is because, in the past, it cannot be filtered through dialysis membranes and gets deposited as amyloid. These patients usually present with symptoms due to the deposition of amyloid in joints, muscles, tendons, or ligaments. One of the common presentations is carpal tunnel syndrome. With new and improved dialysis membrane filters, the incidence of this complication has substantially reduced.

Hereditary or Familial Amyloidosis

Q. Write a short note on heredofamilial amyloidosis.

It constitutes a separate, heterogeneous group, are a rare familial form of amyloidosis, and occurs in certain geographic areas. It has several distinctive patterns of organ involvement.

Familial mediterranean fever (FMF): It is an **autosomal recessive disorder.** It is an "autoinflammatory" syndrome associated with **excessive production of the cytokine IL-1.** It is characterized by recurrent attacks of fever associated with inflammation of serosal surfaces (peritoneum, pleura, and synovial membrane). The **gene for FMF encodes a protein called pyrin** (for its relation to fever), that regulates inflammatory reactions by producing high levels of proinflammatory cytokines IL-1. The amyloid fibril proteins in FMF are of **AA type** probably produced due to recurrent attacks of inflammation.

Others: TTR is a transporter of the hormone thyroxine. A group of autosomal dominant familial disorders show deposition of amyloid made up of fibrils derived from mutant *transthyretin* (TTR). **Familial amyloidotic neuropathies** are characterized by deposition of amyloid in peripheral and autonomic nerves and the fibrils are made up of mutant TTRs. In some cardiac deposits predominate (cardiac amyloidosis).

Localized Amyloidosis

Q. Write a short note on localized amyloidosis.

- **Amyloid deposit may be limited to a single organ (e.g., heart) or tissue:** These deposits may be either grossly visible as nodular masses or detected only by microscopic examination.
- **Sites:** Nodular localized deposits of amyloid may occur in the lung, larynx, skin, and urinary bladder, tongue and region around the eye.
- **Microscopy:** Amyloid deposits may be surrounded by lymphocytes and plasma cells. In some cases, the amyloid is AL protein type and may represent a localized form of plasma cell-derived amyloid.

Endocrine Amyloid

Q. Write a short note on endocrine tumors showing microscopic deposits of amyloid.

Microscopic deposits of localized amyloid may occur in certain endocrine tumors.

- **Endocrine tumors** associated with amyloid: These include **medullary carcinoma of the thyroid** (*refer* pages 880-2 and **Fig. 24.16**), **islet tumors of the pancreas, pheochromocytomas, and undifferentiated carcinomas of the stomach.** The amyloidogenic proteins may be derived from polypeptide hormones (e.g., calcitonin in medullary carcinoma).
- **Endocrine gland: Islets of Langerhans in type II diabetes mellitus** may show deposits of amyloid.

Amyloid of Aging

Q. Write briefly on amyloid of aging.

Several forms of amyloid deposition occur with aging. **Senile systemic amyloidosis is** characterized by the systemic deposition of amyloid in elderly patients usually between 70 and 80 years. The heart is the dominant organ involved and associated with dysfunction of the heart. Hence, this form was previously called *senile cardiac amyloidosis*. They may have symptoms of restrictive cardiomyopathy and develop arrhythmias **The amyloid is derived from the wild-type (normal) TTR molecule.**

PA 3.2 (NC): Identify and describe amyloidosis in a pathology specimen.

MORPHOLOGY

Amyloidosis does not show any consistent or distinctive patterns of organ or tissue distribution in any of the categories. A few generalizations about organ involvement are as follows:

AA amyloidosis secondary to chronic inflammatory disorders: It occurs in the kidneys, liver, spleen, lymph nodes, adrenal glands, thyroid glands, and other tissues.

AL amyloidosis associated with plasma cell proliferations: It more often involves the heart, gastrointestinal tract, respiratory tract, peripheral nerves, skin, and tongue.

Gross

May or may not be apparent grossly. If a large amount accumulates, the affected organs are **enlarged, firm in consistency and have a gray, waxy appearance (Fig. 6.27).**

Cut surface: If the amyloid deposits are large, **painting** the cut surface **with iodine gives a yellow color, which is transformed to blue violet after the application of sulfuric acid** (which acidifies iodine). This method was used for demonstrating cellulose or starch. This staining property was responsible for the coining of the **term amyloid (starch-like). But it is neither starch nor cellulose.**

Microscopy

Q. Write a short note on special stains for amyloid.

The diagnosis of amyloidosis is made based on histopathologic findings.

Hematoxylin and Eosin Stain

- Amyloid deposits are always **extracellular (Figs. 6.28A and B)** and **begin between the cells, usually** closely adjacent to basement membranes. In AL form, perivascular and vascular deposits are common.
- Progressive accumulation of **amyloid produces pressure atrophy of adjacent cells.**

- Amyloid appears as an **amorphous, eosinophilic, hyaline, glassy, extracellular substance.**
- Many other hyaline materials (e.g., collagen, fibrin) also stain eosinophilic with hematoxylin and eosin. Hence, it is necessary to differentiate amyloid from these other hyaline deposits by using special stains.

Staining (Tinctorial) Properties of Amyloid (Box 6.8)

1. **Congo-red stain:** It is the **special stain most commonly used for the diagnosis of amyloidosis.** Amyloid **stains pink or red** with the Congo-red dye **under ordinary light (Fig. 6.29A).** But **more specifically** when viewed **under a polarizing microscope**; amyloid gives **apple-green birefringence (Fig. 6.29B).** Congo-red staining gives a positive reaction with all forms of amyloid and this reaction is due to the cross-β-pleated configuration of amyloid fibrils. Amyloid can be confirmed by electron microscopy and specific type by immunohistochemistry.
2. **Van Gieson stains:** It takes up the khaki color.
3. **Alcian blue:** It imparts blue color to glycosaminoglycans in amyloid.
4. **Periodic acid-Schiff (PAS) reaction:** It stains pink.
5. **Methyl violet and cresyl violet:** These metachromatic stains (belonging to the rosaniline group of basic dyes) give rose pink color to the amyloid deposits whereas the surrounding tissue is colored blue.
6. **Iodine solution** produces a dark, mahogany brown color when poured over the cut surface of the organ involved by amyloidosis. It is **transformed to blue-violet after the application of sulfuric acid.**
7. **Thioflavin T:** It is not specific for amyloid, but amyloid fluoresce when viewed in ultraviolet light.
8. **Immunohistochemical staining:** It can distinguish specific types of amyloid. Immunohistochemistry is best for AA, and TTR-associated amyloid types. But definitive identification, especially of AL amyloid, requires mass spectroscopy or protein sequencing.

MORPHOLOGY OF MAJOR ORGANS INVOLVED

Q. Describe the gross and microscopic features of organs involved in primary/secondary amyloidosis.

Morphology of major organs involved in different forms of amyloidosis is variable.

Kidney

Kidney is the **most common** and the **most serious** form of organ involvement.

Gross (Fig. 6.27): It may be of normal size and color during early stages. In advanced stages, it may be shrunken due to ischemia. Ischemia is caused by the narrowing of vessels due to amyloid deposits within arterial and arteriolar walls.

Microscopy: Most commonly renal amyloid is of light-chain (AL in primary amyloidosis) or AA (in secondary amyloidosis type).

- **Glomeruli:** It is the main site of amyloid deposition **(Figs. 6.28A and B).**
  - First, **focal deposits within** the **mesangial matrix**, accompanied by **diffuse or nodular thickening of the glomerular basement membranes.**
  - **Later,** both the mesangial and basement membrane deposits cause **capillary narrowing.** Progressive accumulation of amyloid results in **obliteration of the capillary lumen** and **glomerulus shows broad ribbons of amyloid.**
- Amyloid may also be deposited in the **peritubular interstitial tissue, walls of the arteries,** and **arterioles.**
- These deposits appear homogenous pink, which when stained with Congo-red and viewed under a polarizing microscope, give rise to characteristic green birefringence.

Spleen

Q. Describe the gross and microscopic appearance of the spleen in amyloid (Sago and Lardaceous spleen).

Gross: Spleen may be **normal in size or may cause moderate to marked splenomegaly** (200–800 g). It may show one of **two distinct patterns of deposition (Figs. 6.30A and B).**

- **Sago spleen:** Amyloid **deposits are mainly limited to the splenic follicles**; they **grossly appear like tapioca/sago granules**; hence known as **sago spleen.** Microscopically, the **amyloid is deposited in the wall of arterioles in the white pulp.**
- **Lardaceous spleen: Amyloid is deposited in the walls of the splenic sinuses and connective tissue framework in the red pulp.** This may result in **moderate to marked enlargement of the spleen.** Fusion of the early deposits gives rise to **large, map-like areas of reddish color on the cut surface.** This resembles pig fat (lardaceous) and is hence called a **lardaceous spleen.** Microscopically, it shows **amyloid deposits in the wall of the sinuses.**

Light microscopy: These deposits appear homogenous pink, which when stained with Congo-red and viewed under a polarizing microscope, give rise to characteristic green birefringence.

Liver

Gross: It may be not apparent grossly or it may cause moderate to marked enlargement. In advanced stages, it appears pale, gray, and waxy.

Microscopy

- Amyloid **first deposits in the space of Disse** and then **progressively encroaches on adjacent hepatic parenchymal cells and sinusoids.**
- Progressive accumulation leads to **pressure atrophy and disappearance of liver cells.** It may lead to total replacement of liver parenchyma.
- It may show deposits in the vessels and Kupffer cells. Liver function is usually preserved even with quite severe involvement.

Heart

Heart may be involved in **any form of systemic amyloidosis (AL type).** It may be the major organ involved in **senile systemic amyloidosis.**

Gross: Heart usually does not show any gross changes, but may be enlarged and firm. Subendocardial deposits may appear as gray-pink-like dew-drop.

Microscopy: Amyloid is **deposited between the muscle fibers and their progressive accumulation causes pressure atrophy of myocardial fibers.** Subendocardial deposits may affect the conduction system and give rise to arrhythmias.

Other Organs

They may be involved in systemic disease and include adrenals, thyroid, and pituitary. Nodular deposits in the tongue may cause

macroglossia. There may be focal or diffuse involvement of the respiratory **tract** from the larynx down to the smallest bronchioles. A distinct form of amyloid occurs in the **brains** of patients with Alzheimer disease. It is present in plaques as well as blood vessels. Amyloidosis of peripheral and autonomic **nerves** is observed in familial amyloidotic neuropathies.

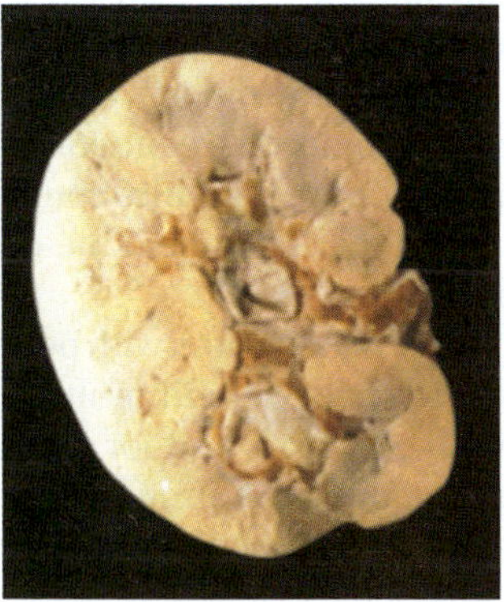

Amyloid

- Congo-red stain gives apple-green birefringence when viewed under a polarizing microscope.
- X-ray crystallography and infrared spectroscopy show characteristic cross β-pleated sheet configuration.
- Electron microscopy shows nonbranching fibrils of indefinite length and 7–10 nm diameter.

Fig. 6.27: Amyloid kidney. Cut section of an amyloid kidney showing waxy appearance.

BOX 6.8: Special stains for amyloid.

1. **Congo-red stain stains pink or red, and under a polarizing microscope** gives **apple-green birefringence.**
2. **Van Gieson stains give** khaki color.
3. **Alcian blue** imparts blue color.
4. **Periodic acid-Schiff (PAS) reaction:** It stains pink.
5. **Methyl violet and cresyl violet:** give rose pink color to the amyloid deposits whereas the surrounding tissue is colored blue.
6. **Iodine solution** produces a dark, mahogany brown color over the cut surface and is **transformed to blue violet after the application of sulfuric acid.**
7. **Thioflavin T:** Amyloid fluoresce when viewed in ultraviolet light.
8. **Immunohistochemical staining:** It can distinguish specific types of amyloid. Immunohistochemistry is best for AA, and TTR- associated amyloid types.

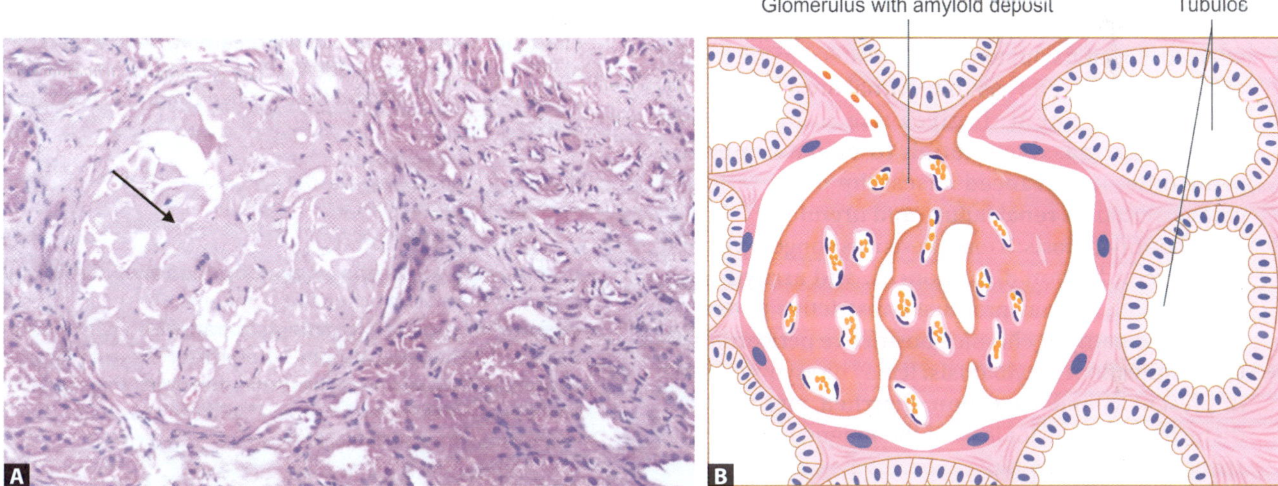

Figs. 6.28A and B: Amyloidosis of the kidney (A) H& E and (B) diagrammatic. Shows pink, amorphous extracellular amyloid deposits in the entire glomerulus.

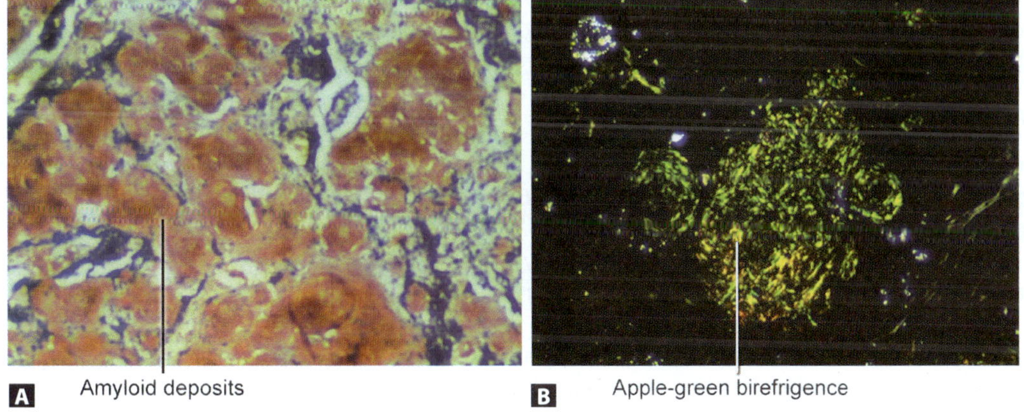

Figs. 6.29A and B: Amyloid deposits in medullary carcinoma of the thyroid: (A) Congo-red stain gives the red color to the amyloid deposits; (B) Congo-red stained section viewed under polarizing microscope gives apple-green birefringence to amyloid deposits.

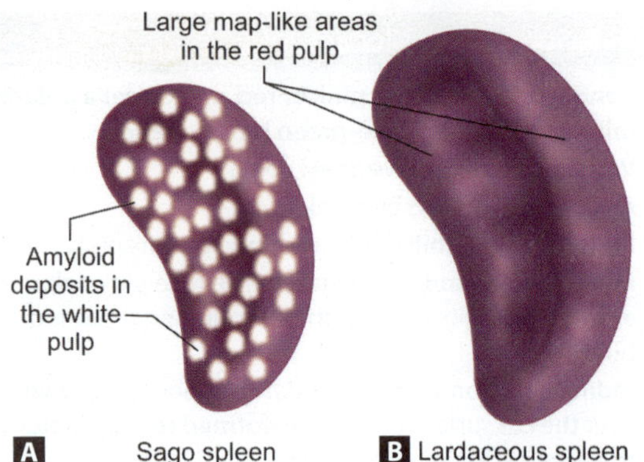

Figs. 6.30A and B: Diagrammatic representation of two distinct patterns of amyloid deposits in spleen.

Clinical Features

- Amyloidosis may not produce any clinical manifestations, or it may produce symptoms related to the sites or organs affected. Clinical manifestations **initially may be nonspecific** (e.g., weakness, weight loss, lightheadedness, or syncope). The symptoms depend on the amount of the deposits and on the sites or organs affected. Specific symptoms appear later and are related to renal, cardiac, and gastrointestinal involvement.
- **Renal involvement:** It gives rise to **proteinuria sometimes massive enough to cause nephrotic syndrome**. In advanced cases, the obliteration of glomeruli causes **renal failure and uremia**.
- **Cardiac amyloidosis:** It may present as **congestive heart failure, conduction disturbances, and arrhythmias**. Occasionally, it may produce a restrictive pattern of cardiomyopathy or chronic constrictive pericarditis.
- **Gastrointestinal amyloidosis:** It may be asymptomatic, or present as **malabsorption, diarrhea, and digestive disturbances**. Amyloidosis of the tongue may hamper speech and swallowing.
- **Vascular amyloidosis:** It causes fragility of vessels and may lead to bleeding, sometimes massive. Bleeding can occur spontaneously or following minor trauma. Sometimes AL amyloid may bind and inactivate factor X (a critical coagulation factor), causing a life-threatening bleeding disorder.

Diagnosis

Q. Write a short note on the diagnosis of amyloidosis.

Diagnosis is based on the **histologic demonstration of** Congo red-positive **amyloid deposits** in tissues.

- **Biopsy:** The most common sites of biopsy are the **kidney** in patients with renal manifestations**, and rectum or gingival tissues** in suspected systemic amyloidosis.
- **Examination of abdominal fat aspirates** stained with Congo-red is quite specific but has low sensitivity. It can be used for the diagnosis of systemic amyloidosis.
- **Serum and urine protein electrophoresis and immunoelectrophoresis:** It is performed in suspected cases of AL amyloidosis. Bone marrow aspirates in these patients may show monoclonal plasmacytosis, even in the absence of multiple myeloma.
- **Scintigraphy with radiolabeled serum amyloid** P (SAP) component: It is a **rapid and specific test** because SAP binds to amyloid deposits and shows their presence. It also gives a measure of the extent of amyloidosis. Hence, can be used to follow up with patients on treatment.
- **Mass spectroscopy:** It is useful for the identification of the protein component of amyloid. It can be done on paraffin-embedded tissues.

Prognosis: Generalized amyloidosis is associated with poor prognosis. Patients with AL amyloidosis without multiple myeloma have a median survival of 2 years and for those with myeloma, the prognosis is poorer. The prognosis of patients with reactive systemic amyloidosis is somewhat better.

SCENARIO-BASED MCQs

1. **A 16-year-old girl has a bee sting. Within 5 minutes she suddenly develops difficulty in breathing, with respiratory stridor from laryngeal edema. She also develops urticaria and swelling of the hand that has bee sting. This reaction is due to:**
   A. Type I hypersensitivity
   B. Type II hypersensitivity
   C. Type III hypersensitivity
   D. Type IV hypersensitivity
2. **In a blood bank, samples are obtained by phlebotomy procedure from two hospitalized patients. These samples are mislabelled. One of the patients is transfused with packed RBCs later that day. Within 1 hour after the transfusion, the patient develops tachycardia, becomes hypotensive, and passes pink-colored urine. The likely possibility that is responsible for the clinical picture is:**
   A. Complement-mediated lysis of red cells
   B. Antigen-antibody complex deposition in glomeruli
   C. Mast cell degranulation with release of histamine
   D. Antibody-dependent cellular cytotoxicity by natural killer cells
3. **A 48-year-old woman met with an automobile accident and requires a blood transfusion. Four hours after the transfusion of blood, she developed a fever with severe back pain. Laboratory investigation shows evidence of intravascular hemolysis. Her blood group is A Rh+. It is discovered that by mistake she is given B Rh+ blood. The mechanism responsible for intravascular hemolysis in this patient is:**
   A. Immediate hypersensitivity
   B. Immune complex disease
   C. Delayed-type hypersensitivity
   D. Antibody-mediated complement fixation
4. **A 9-year-old boy complains of periorbital edema, the passage of cola-colored urine, and throbbing headaches. His mother reveals that he had a "sore throat" 3 weeks ago. Urinalysis shows 3+ hematuria. A renal biopsy shows hypercellular**

glomeruli. The electron microscopic examination of glomeruli shows a subepithelial "humps." The most likely pathogenesis of glomerulonephritis in this patient is:

A. IgE-mediated mast cell degranulation
B. Antineutrophil cytoplasmic autoantibodies
C. Deposition of circulating immune complexes
D. T cell-mediated delayed hypersensitivity reaction

5. **A 35-year-old woman has a sensitivity to body jewelry. She is tested with a skin patch test for nickel compounds. Within 24 to 48 hours, she develops focal erythema and induration of her skin at the site of the test, accompanied by itching and pain. This reaction is an example of:**
   A. Immediate hypersensitivity
   B. Delayed hypersensitivity
   C. Antibody-mediated reaction
   D. Immune complex deposits in skin
6. **An 11-year-old girl develops a fever and chest pain. On enquiry, she complained that she had a sore throat, and fever about 3 weeks back. A throat culture at that time showed group A β-hemolytic *Streptococcus*. At present her anti-streptolysin O titer is raised. The immunologic mechanisms that have most likely led to the chest pain are:**
   A. Antibody-dependent cellular cytotoxicity involving lung parenchyma
   B. Release of sequestered antigens
   C. Mast cell degranulation
   D. Molecular mimicry
7. **A 22-year-old woman complains of malaise; facial erythematous malar skin lesions exacerbated by sunlight exposure; and arthralgias and myalgias for the past 2 months. On physical examination, she has mild pedal edema. Laboratory findings show pancytopenia and serum creatinine 3 mg/dL. Urinalysis shows hematuria and proteinuria. A renal biopsy shows granular deposits of IgG and complement in the mesangium and along the basement membrane.**
   A. Rheumatoid arthritis
   B. Systemic lupus erythematosus
   C. Post-streptococcal glomerulonephritis
   D. Nodular glomerulosclerosis
8. **A 26-year-old woman comes with a history of bouts of joint pain for the past 2 years. On physical examination, there is no joint swelling or deformity. She has a rash on the cheeks and bridge of the nose. Laboratory findings show anemia, leukopenia, polyclonal gammopathy, proteinuria, and hematuria. Of the following the test likely to be useful in the diagnosis of this condition is:**
   A. Serum ANA test
   B. Rheumatoid factor
   C. Anti-streptolysin O titer
   D. Examination of synovial fluid from affected joint
9. **A 45-year-old man complains of fever, cough, and worsening dyspnea for the past few days. On enquiry, he had many sexual partners for the past 10 years. On auscultation of the chest, breath sounds are decreased over all lung fields. A bronchoalveolar lavage and sputum examination showed cysts of *Pneumocystis jirovecii*. Laboratory studies show a WBC count of 8200/mm^3 with 75% segmented neutrophils. The serologic laboratory finding that is most likely to be positive in this patient is:**
   A. Antibodies to HIV
   B. Anti-streptolysin O
   C. Anti-double-stranded DNA antibody
   D. Anti-neutrophil cytoplasmic autoantibody
10. **A 58-year-old man complains of increasing malaise and back pain for the past 3 months. On physical examination, he is afebrile with mild muscle wasting. Urine examination shows no blood, protein, or glucose, but a specific test for Bence-Jones proteins is positive. A radiographic examination of his spine shows multiple rounded lucent lesions. The microscopic appearance of his liver shows pink amorphous material between the hepatocytes. Congo-red stain with polarized light shows apple-green birefringence. Of the following underlying conditions, the most likely to be present in this patient is:**
    A. Rheumatic fever
    B. Multiple myeloma
    C. Tuberculosis of the spine
    D. Acquired immunodeficiency syndrome
11. **A 60-year-old man has complained of chronic arthritis for the past 13 years. Physical examination shows ulnar deviation with bony ankylosis producing swan neck deformities of the fingers. Laboratory studies show markedly elevated levels of C-reactive protein. A rectal biopsy is performed. With H&E staining, the rectal mucosa shows extracellular deposition of amorphous pink material. Amorphous material shows positivity with Congo-red. The most likely precursor to this pink material in the mucosa is:**
    A. Transthyretin
    B. λ light chains
    C. β_2-Microglobulin
    D. Acute-phase reactant

Answers and Explanation

1. **The answer is A: Type I hypersensitivity.** The girl developed a systemic anaphylactic reaction that is due to an immediate type I hypersensitivity reaction. The antigen triggers mast cell-bound IgE with the release of preformed mediators such as histamine. All other options are not correct in this scenario.
2. **The answer is A: Complement-mediated lysis of red cells.** A major transfusion reaction is due to a type II hypersensitivity reaction. The mislabelling has resulted in a mismatched blood transfusion. The patient's serum contains naturally occurring antibodies to the incompatible donor RBCs. These antibodies get attached to the donor RBCs and activate the complement activation. It generates the C5-9 membrane attack complex. This is a major transfusion reaction, and most result from clerical errors. Option (B): Antigen-antibody complex formation with deposition in glomeruli is typical of a type III hypersensitivity reaction. Option (C) Mast cells degranulate with antigen attachment to IgE in type I hypersensitivity reactions. Option (D) Natural killer cell lysis is seen with antibody-mediated diseases.
3. **The answer is D: Antibody-mediated complement fixation causing hemolysis.** It is a type II hypersensitivity reaction mediated by antibodies directed against fixed antigens on red blood cells. In this scenario, preformed antibodies in the patient's serum attached to foreign antigens on the membranes of the red blood cells. The antigen and antibody reaction elicits activation of the complement system. Activated

complement cascade generates a membrane attack complex that leads to the destruction of the target cells (red blood cells). Delayed-type hypersensitivity (choice C) occurs over days and does not involve preformed antibodies. Other options are not correct.

4. **The answer is C: Deposition of circulating immune complexes.** This patient is having postinfectious glomerulonephritis. The glomeruli show deposition of circulating immune complexes that appear as subepithelial humps. This is an example of type III hypersensitivity reactions. Streptoccocal infection in this boy led to the deposition of antigens and antibodies in glomerular basement membranes, resulting in clinical features of nephritic syndrome (e.g., hematuria, oliguria, and hypertension). Post-streptococcal illnesses do not include any of the other choices.
5. **The answer is B: Delayed hypersensitivity.** It is a delayed-type hypersensitivity reaction (type IV hypersensitivity). Many individuals react to nickel, particularly with body-piercing jewelry. Immediate reaction is a type I hypersensitivity brought out by IgE. Other options are not true regarding the type IV reactions.
6. **The answer is D: Molecular mimicry.** Streptococcal M proteins elicit immunologic reactions. The antibodies and cell-mediated immunity cross-react with cardiac glycoproteins, resulting in rheumatic heart disease. It is a type of autoimmunity. The other options are not responses to streptococcal infection. Antibody-dependent cellular cytotoxicity involving lung parenchyma is not a feature of post-streptococcal disease. Release of sequestered antigens can cause autoimmunity but is not in streptococcal pharyngitis. Mast cell degranulation is a type I hypersensitivity reaction involving IgE against allergens.
7. **The answer is B: Systemic lupus erythematosus.** This young woman has classic features of systemic lupus erythematosus (SLE). The erythematous malar facial skin rash known as butterfly rash, and renal failure with proteinuria and hematuria from immune complex deposition in the glomeruli. Rheumatoid arthritis is an autoimmune disease that mainly affects joints. Post-streptococcal glomerulonephritis does not manifest with facial lesions. Nodular glomerulosclerosis is a pathognomonic renal lesion observed in diabetes mellitus and without any immune deposits in the kidney.
8. **Answer is A: Serum ANA test.** This patient is likely to have systemic lupus erythematosus (SLE). Serum ANA test can be positive in other autoimmune diseases but is useful for its diagnosis in consideration of the other features. Rheumatoid factor is useful for the diagnosis of rheumatoid arthritis. Anti-streptolysin O titer is useful for the diagnosis of post-streptococcal glomerulonephritis. Examination of synovial fluid from affected joints may not be useful for SLE patients.
9. **The correct answer is A: Antibodies to HIV.** This patient is likely suffering from HIV. *Pneumocystis jirovecii* pneumonia is a common complication in patients with HIV infection progressing to AIDS. Other options are not true in this case. The anti-streptolysin O (ASO) titer is raised in patients with rheumatic fever. Anti-double-stranded DNA antibody is usually positive in SLE. Anti-neutrophil cytoplasmic autoantibody (C-ANCA or P-ANCA) can be positive in some patients with vasculitis.
10. **The answer is B: Multiple myeloma.** Amyloid gives "apple-green" birefringence when viewed under polarized light after staining with Congo-red. Amyloidosis is most commonly caused by to excessive production of light chains with plasma cell neoplasms such as multiple myeloma (AL amyloid). His spinal lesions are focal collections of neoplastic plasma cells. Chronic inflammatory conditions, such as rheumatic fever, and tuberculosis also may result in amyloidosis (AA amyloid), but not associated with the secretion of light chains in urine (i.e., Bence-Jones proteinuria). The clinical and laboratory findings do not support acquired immunodeficiency syndrome.
11. **The answer is D: Acute-phase reactant.** This patient has rheumatoid arthritis which is one of the chronic inflammatory conditions. It is associated with elevated levels of serum amyloid-associated (SAA) precursor protein. SAA is an acute phase reactant that increases with inflammatory conditions. It forms the major amyloid fibril protein AA. All amyloid shows characteristic "apple green" birefringence when viewed under polarized microscopy after Congo-red staining. Amyloid fibrils in cardiac and heredofamilial forms of amyloidosis are derived from prealbumin transthyretin (TTR). Amyloid derived from light chains in association with multiple myeloma consists of AL fibrils. Amyloid derived from β_2-microglobulin occurs with hemodialysis-associated amyloidosis.

Type I hypersensitivity:
- IgE bound to mast cells
- Activation of Th2 cells

Type II hypersensitivity:
- IgG/IgM mediated
- Mechanism of damage: (1) opsonization and phagocytosis, (2) activation of complement system, and (3) antibody-mediated cellular dysfunction

Type III hypersensitivity:
- Immune complex-mediated

Type IV hypersensitivity:
- Mediated by T lymphocytes
- Mechanism of damage: (1) CD4+ T-cell-mediated inflammation and (2) CD8+ T-cell-mediated cytotoxicity

Neoplasms found in patients with HIV infection:
- Kaposi sarcoma
- Non-Hodgkin B-cell lymphoma—primary lymphoma of the brain
- HIV-associated Hodgkin lymphoma
- Carcinoma of the uterine cervix (cervical cancer) in women
- Anal carcinoma

ABCDE of amyloidosis:
A: Apple green birefringence on Congo red
B: β-pleated sheet conformation on X-ray crystallography and infrared spectroscopy
C: Congo red stain: Amyloid gives apple green birefringence
D: Diverse conditions are associated with amyloidosis
E: Extracellular amyloid deposits between the cells

Spleen in amyloidosis:
- Sago spleen: Amyloid deposits in the white pulp
- Lardaceous spleen: Amyloid deposits in the walls of sinusoids

Neoplasia

CHAPTER OUTLINE

- Nomenclature of Neoplasms
- Characteristics of Benign and Malignant Neoplasms
- Epidemiology of Cancer
- Genetic Lesions in Cancer
- Molecular Basis of Cancer
- Etiology of Cancer: Carcinogenic Agents
- Clinical Aspects of Neoplasia
- Laboratory Diagnosis of Cancer
- Examples of Benign Tumors

INTRODUCTION

Cancer is the second leading cause of death, the first being cardiovascular diseases.

Fundamental Features of Cancer

Genetic disorder: Cancer is a **genetic disorder caused by permanent changes in the cell's DNA**, known as **mutations**.

- **Mutations:** It **may be acquired or inherited**. Acquired mutations may be due to exposure to mutagens or occur spontaneously due to error-prone processes in cells.
- **Epigenetic alterations:** Apart from mutations, cancers frequently show epigenetic alterations such as altered DNA methylation and histone modification.

These genetic and epigenetic abnormalities alter the expression or function of the main genes that regulate fundamental cellular processes. These processes include cell growth, survival, and senescence.

Heritable: The genetic alterations **in cancer cells** are passed down to the daughter tumor cells **upon cell division**. The **cells with mutations have a growth or survival advantage over their neighboring cells.** Thus, cancer cells dominate over normal cells.

- **Clonal**: During the tumor initiation, these selective advantages are granted to a single cell. Thus, individual tumors are *clonal* (i.e., the progeny of one cell).
- **Tumor progression:** As the cancer progresses, it shows proliferation of **genetically distinct subclones** with more aggressive characteristics. This concept is referred to as *tumor progression.*

Cancer hallmarks: Mutations and epigenetic alterations provide the cancer cells with a set of properties. These properties are collectively called *cancer hallmarks.* These properties produce the cellular phenotypes that determine the natural history of cancers and their response to various therapies.

Definition and General Features

PA 7.1a (CC): Define and classify neoplasia.

Q. Define neoplasia.

Neoplasia means "new growth" and a new growth formed is known as a neoplasm (Greek, *neo* = new + *plasma* = thing formed).

Willis definition of neoplasm: "A neoplasm is an abnormal mass of tissue, the growth of which exceeds and is uncoordinated with that of the normal tissues and persists in the same excessive manner after cessation of the stimuli which evoked the change."

In the present era, a **neoplasm can be defined** as a **disorder of cell growth triggered by a series of acquired mutations involving a single cell and its clonal progeny.**

Autonomous growth: In neoplasia, there is **excessive** and **unregulated proliferation** of cells. The neoplastic cells are "transformed" cells that continuously proliferate because they are resistant to normal regulatory mechanisms that control normal cells. Thus, neoplasms have a degree of autonomy, but some important dependencies remain. For example, neoplasms depend on the host for their nutrition and blood supply, and neoplasms derived from hormone-responsive tissues usually require endocrine support.

- **Tumor versus neoplasm:** Most neoplasms occupy space, often called tumors (Gr., swelling). The term "tumor" was originally used for the swelling caused by inflammation, but it is now used synonymously with neoplasm. Oncology (Greek, *oncos* = tumor) is the study of tumors or neoplasms.

- **Differentiation** (*refer* pages 220-3): It refers to the **extent to which the tumor cells resemble the cell of origin**. A tumor may show a variable degree of resemblance to (mimic) its tissue of origin. The differentiation ranges from relatively mature structures that mimic normal tissues (well differentiated) to cells so primitive that the cell of origin cannot be identified (poorly differentiated). It usually allows us to know about tumors' sources and potential behavior.
- **Arise from cells that normally can multiply**: Neoplasms arise from cells that normally can multiply (i.e., cells that maintain a **proliferative capacity**). The mature neurons and cardiac myocytes cannot multiply after birth. Hence, they do not give rise to tumors.

Classification

Q. Classify neoplasia. Discuss the histogenesis and biological behavior of tumors.

Tumors are classified as **benign and malignant, depending on** the **biological behavior** of a tumor.

Benign tumors: These tumors have relatively innocent microscopic and gross characteristics, indicating that they will remain localized.

- **Remain localized without invasion or metastasis.**
- **Well differentiated:** Their cells **closely resemble their tissue of origin**.
- **Excellent prognosis:** It can be cured by surgical removal in most patients and the patient will generally be cured of their disease. However, not all benign tumors are easily excised, and some benign tumors may cause significant morbidity or are even lethal, especially those located near a vital structure or organ. A benign intracranial meningeal tumor (meningioma) may be fatal if it produces pressure on an important brain structure. A pheochromocytoma in the adrenal medulla may trigger a hypertensive crisis.

Malignant tumors: **Cancer is the general term** used **for malignant tumors**. The term "cancer" is derived from the Latin word for *crab*, because similar to a crab's behavior, malignant tumors adhere to any part that they grasp upon normal tissues, firmly.

- **Local invasion:** Malignant tumors invade or infiltrate the adjacent tissues or structures locally.
- **Metastasis:** Cancers **spread to distant sites** (metastasize), where the malignant cells reside, grow, and again invade.
  - **Exception: Basal cell carcinoma** of the skin, which is histologically malignant (i.e., it invades aggressively), but rarely metastasizes to distant sites. **A glioma** is a malignant tumor of the CNS.
- **Prognosis:** Most malignant tumors cause death. Not all cancers follow an aggressive course. Some of the most aggressive cancers are also highly curable. Some malignant tumors (e.g., papillary carcinoma of the thyroid) grow so slowly that they never threaten life.

PA 7.1b (CC): Describe the characteristics of neoplasia including gross, microscopy, biologic, behavior, and spread.

Basic Microscopic Components of Neoplasms

All tumors (both benign and malignant) consist of two basic components: (i) *parenchyma,* and (ii) *stroma.*

1. **Parenchyma:** It is made up of transformed or neoplastic cells. The **nomenclature and biological behavior of tumors** are **based primarily** on the **parenchymal component** of the tumor.
2. **Stroma:** It is the **supporting, non-neoplastic tissue** derived **from the host**.
   - **Components of stroma: Stroma consists of connective tissue, blood vessels, and inflammatory cells** (e.g., macrophages and lymphocytes).
   - **Importance of stroma:** It is **essential to the growth, survival, and replication of tumor cells** since it provides **the blood supply**. The stromal cells and tumor cells carry on a two-way conversation that conditions the behavior and growth pattern of tumor cells.
   - **Inflammatory reaction:** Stroma may show inflammatory reactions in and around the tumors. It may be due to ulceration and secondary infection in the tumors, especially on the surface of the body. This type of inflammatory reaction **may be an acute, chronic, or rarely granulomatous reaction**. Some tumors show inflammatory reactions even in the absence of ulceration. It is due to the **cell-mediated immunologic response of the host against the tumor** in an attempt to destroy the tumor. For example, **lymphocytes in the stroma are seen in seminoma testis, dysgerminoma of ovary, and medullary carcinoma of the breast**.
   - **Tumor consistency depends on the amount of stroma:**
     - **Soft and fleshy:** These tumors have **scanty stroma**.
     - **Desmoplasia (Fig. 7.1 and *refer* Fig. 23.8): Parenchymal tumor cells may stimulate the formation of an abundant collagenous stroma** referred to as desmoplasia. For example, some carcinomas in female breasts have a **stony hard consistency** (or **scirrhous**).

NOMENCLATURE OF NEOPLASMS

Q. Discuss the nomenclature and classification of tumors.

Q. Write a short note on the histogenesis of tumors.

Benign Tumors

Generally, benign tumors are **named by attaching the suffix "oma" to the cell type from which the tumor arises (cell of origin)**.

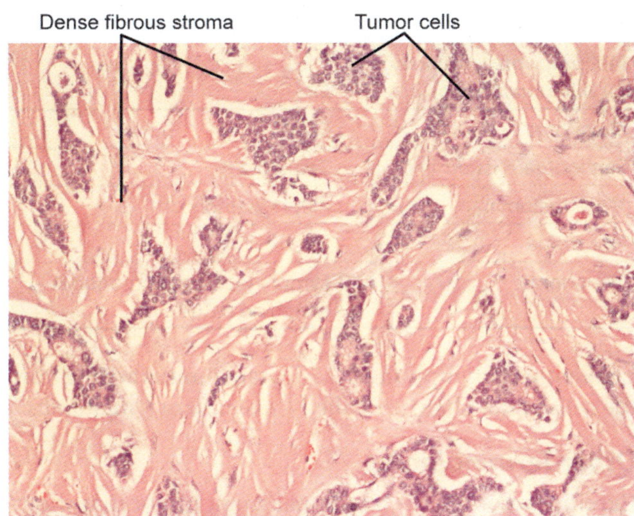

Fig. 7.1: Carcinoma of the breast with abundant stroma separating malignant cells.

Mesenchymal Tumors

The nomenclature of benign mesenchymal tumors usually follows the above nomenclature (**Table 7.1**). For example, a benign cartilaginous tumor is a chondroma, and a tumor of fibroblasts is a fibroma.

Epithelial Tumors (Figs. 7.2A to D)

The nomenclature of benign epithelial tumors is not uniform but more complex. They are classified in different ways: **(i) cell of origin, (ii) microscopic pattern, and (iii) macroscopic architecture.**

TABLE 7.1 Nomenclature of a few benign and malignant mesenchymal tumors.

Cell of origin	*Benign*	*Malignant*
Fibrous tissue	Fibroma	Fibrosarcoma
Fat cell	Lipoma	Liposarcoma
Blood vessel	Hemangioma	Angiosarcoma
Cartilage	Chondroma	Chondrosarcoma
Bone	Osteoma	Osteogenic sarcoma
Smooth muscle	Leiomyoma	Leiomyosarcoma
Skeletal muscle	Rhabdomyoma	Rhabdomyosarcoma

Adenoma (Fig. 7.2A): The term adenoma is applied to **most benign epithelial neoplasms.** This includes those tumors that produce glandlike structures and those without any glandular structures. **Examples:**

- **Adenomas with glandular structures: Tubular adenoma of the colon shows well-formed glandular structures.** Microscopically, **follicular adenoma of the thyroid** usually shows numerous tightly packed small glands.
- **Adenomas without glandular structures: Adrenocortical adenoma** shows a heterogeneous mass of adrenal cortical cells growing as a solid sheet without any glands. It is called adenoma because the cell of origin is the glandular epithelium.

Cystadenoma: It is a benign tumor forming hollow cystic masses, e.g., serous cystadenoma of the ovary **(Fig. 7.2B).**

Papilloma: It is a **benign epithelial neoplasm** that produces microscopic or macroscopic **finger-like, exophytic, or warty projections** from epithelial surfaces, e.g., squamous papilloma **(Figs. 7.2C and 7.27).**

Papillary cystadenoma: It is a tumor that consists of papillary structures that project into cystic spaces, e.g., papillary serous cystadenoma of the ovary **(Fig. 7.2D and** *refer* **Figs. 22.26 and 22.27C).**

Polyp (Fig. 7.3A): It is a mass that grossly produces **visible projection above a mucosal surface and projects into the lumen.** It may be either **benign or malignant.** A polyp may have a stalk (**pedunculated** polyp) or may be without a stalk (**sessile** polyp), e.g., a polyp of the stomach or intestine. However, the term polyp non-neoplastic conditions such as nasal polyps, are inflammatory in origin.

Borderline tumors: The term borderline tumor is used mainly for surface tumors of the ovary (e.g., borderline serous or mucinous or endometrioid tumors). These tumors have **behavior intermediate between benign and malignant tumors.**

Malignant Tumors

They are termed carcinoma or sarcoma depending on the parenchymal cell of origin. The likely malignant macroscopic architecture is shown in **Figure 7.3B.**

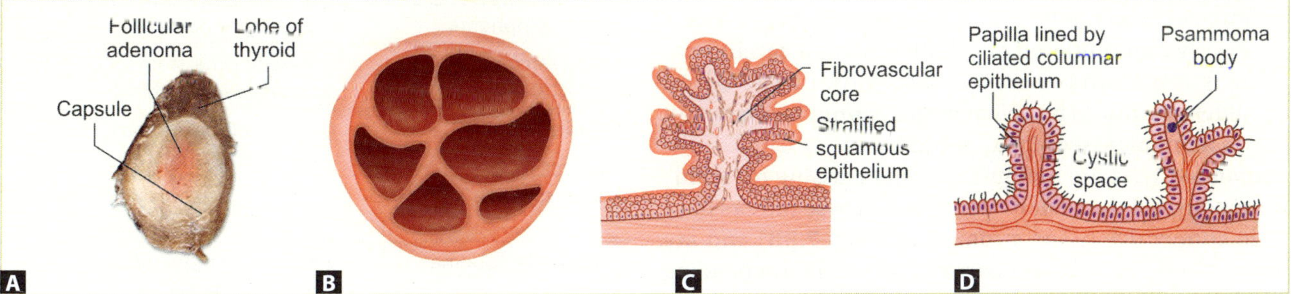

Figs. 7.2A to D: Morphological (gross/microscopic) appearance of some benign epithelial tumors: (A) Gross appearance of follicular adenoma of thyroid; (B) Cut section showing cystadenoma (e.g., mucinous cystadenoma of ovary); (C) Squamous papilloma composed of finger-like projections; (D) Microscopy of papillary cystadenoma of ovary showing a papilla projecting into the cystic cavity.

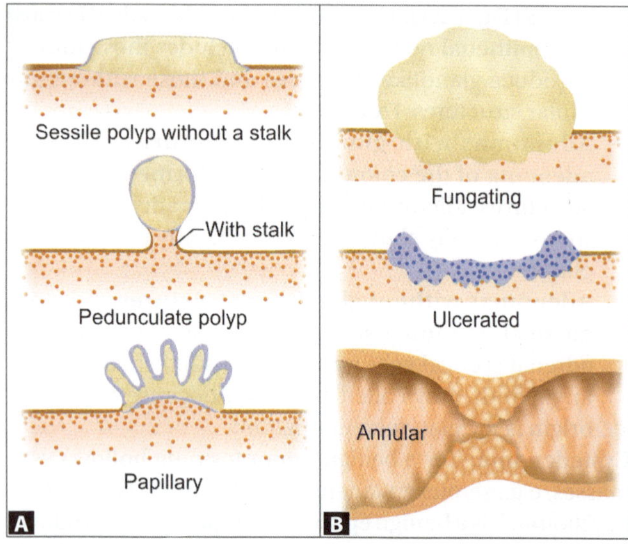

Figs. 7.3A and B: Gross types of tumors: (A) Usually benign growth pattern; (B) Likely to be malignant growth pattern.

TABLE 7.2 Nomenclature of carcinomas.

Germ layer	Tissue/cell	Malignant tumor
Ectoderm	Epidermis	Squamous cell **carcinoma**
Mesoderm	Renal tubules	Adeno**carcinoma**
Endoderm	The lining of the gastrointestinal tract	Adeno**carcinoma**

Carcinomas: These are **malignant neoplasms arising from epithelial cells.** These epithelial cells may be derived from any of the three germ layers **(Table 7.2)** and are called *carcinomas* regardless of the tissue of origin. Thus, malignant epithelial tumors arising in the renal tubular epithelium (mesoderm), the skin (ectoderm), or the lining epithelium of the gastrointestinal tract (endoderm) are all termed carcinomas.

- **Subdivision of carcinomas:** Carcinomas in which the tumor cells grow in a glandular pattern are called *adenocarcinomas,* and tumors composed of squamous cells are called *squamous cell carcinomas.* Sometimes the tissue or organ of origin is specified in the terminology. For example, the designation of renal cell carcinoma indicates carcinoma arising from the kidney.
- **Poorly differentiated or undifferentiated carcinoma:** It is a malignant tumor that shows little or no differentiation. The **cell of origin cannot be made out on light microscopic examination.**

Sarcomas: They are **malignant tumors arising in "solid" mesenchymal tissue** or its derivatives. These tumors have little connective tissue stroma (*refer* **Fig. 7.8B)** and are fleshy (Greek, *sar* = **fleshy**). Sarcomas are named depending on their main cell type. Thus, a malignant neoplasm comprising fatlike cells is a *liposarcoma*, and composed of chondrocyte-like cells is a *chondrosarcoma*.

TABLE 7.3 List of malignant tumors with the suffix "oma".

Inappropriate terminology for malignant tumor	Site
Melanoma	Skin
Seminoma/dysgerminoma	Testis/ovary
Mesothelioma	Pleura, peritoneum
Hepatoma	Liver
Lymphoma	Lymph nodes and extranodal lymphoid tissue

Leukemias or lymphomas: Malignant tumors arising from the cells of the blood are called *leukemias* or *lymphomas.*

Other Terminologies

Carcinosarcoma: It is a rare malignant tumor that shows a **mixture of carcinomatous and sarcomatous elements.**

Inappropriate terminology "oma" for malignant tumors: Some terminology is so varied that tumor names do not specify biological behavior. In certain malignant tumors, the term suffix "oma" is inappropriately used and sounds **like a benign tumor (Table 7.3)**. Hamartomas are not even true neoplasms but disorganized masses composed of multiple structures.

Eponymously named tumors: These tumors are named after the person (eponymous) who first described or recognized the tumor **(Table 7.4)**.

Other Tumors

Mixed Tumor (Fig. 7.4): In both benign or malignant tumors, the neoplastic cells usually resemble each other. This indicates that they originate from a single transformed progenitor cell. However, in some tumors, the tumor cells undergo divergent differentiation. This produces so-called "mixed tumors." These mixed tumors are **clonal, derived from a single germ layer** but the **progenitor cells show divergent differentiation along more than one lineage.** For example, a mixed tumor of the salivary gland (commonly referred to as pleomorphic adenoma) is derived from a

TABLE 7.4 Examples of some eponymously named tumors.

Eponymously named tumors	Cell or tissue of origin
Burkitt lymphoma	B-cell lymphoma
Ewing sarcoma	Mesenchymal stem cell origin and arises in the bone
Grawitz tumor	Renal cell carcinoma arising from renal tubular epithelium
Kaposi sarcoma	Malignant neoplasm of vascular endothelium
Hodgkin lymphoma	Malignant tumor of post-germinal B-cells
Brenner tumor	Benign tumor arising from the surface epithelium of the ovary

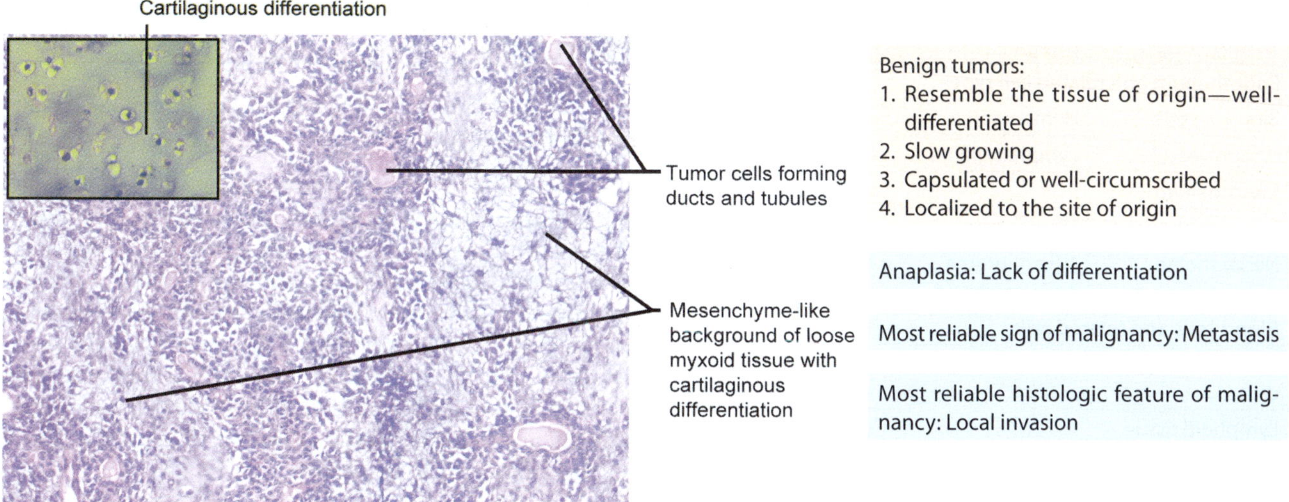

Fig. 7.4: Pleomorphic adenoma showing epithelial cells and myoepithelial cells separated by chondroid matrix. The inset shows cartilage.

single clone (either myoepithelial or ductal reserve cell). It gives rise to two components, namely epithelial and myoepithelial (stromal elements) cells (*refer* pages 592-3). The epithelial components are distributed throughout a fibromyxoid stroma, sometimes containing islands of cartilage.

Q. Write a short note on teratoma.

Teratoma: It is a special type of mixed tumor. It contains recognizable mature or immature cells or tissues derived from more than one germ cell layer, and sometimes all three. Teratoma is **derived from totipotent germ cells**. These totipotent cells are normally located in the **ovary, and testis** and sometimes abnormally present in embryonic rest in midline. These germ cells can **differentiate into any of the cell types** found in the adult body. Thus, teratoma contains recognizable **mature or immature cells** or tissues representative of more than one germ cell layer. These cells or tissues are arranged in a **helter-skelter (haphazard/disorderly) fashion**. The **tissue derivative from various germ cell layers** may include (i) **ectoderm** (e.g., skin, neural tissue, glia), (ii) **mesoderm** (e.g., smooth muscle, cartilage, bone, fat), and (iii) **endoderm** (e.g., respiratory tract epithelium, gut, thyroid), for details *refer* pages 826-8 of Chapter 21 (Male Genital Tract) and pages 826-8 of Chapter 22 (Female Genital Tract).

Q. Write a short note on hamartoma.

Hamartoma: It is a **disorganized mass of benign-appearing cells, in which** the tissue resembles the involved site. It consists of cells that occur naturally in a particular site of origin. It occurs in the lung or the liver. For example, **pulmonary chondroid hamartoma** consists of islands of disorganized, but histologically normal cartilage, bronchi, and vessels. Historically, hamartoma was thought of as a developmental malformation. However, they have clonal chromosomal aberrations that are acquired through somatic mutations. Hence, these are considered unusual benign neoplasms.

Q. Write a short note on choristoma.

Choristoma: It is a congenital anomaly consisting of an **ectopic island of normal tissue (heterotopic** rest, i.e., normal tissue in an abnormal site). For example, the presence of a small nodular mass of normally organized pancreatic tissue in the submucosa of the stomach, duodenum, or small intestine. The designation *-oma*, suggests a neoplasm, but they are usually insignificant.

Embryonal tumors (blastomas): They are the type of tumors that develop only in children (usually below 5 years of age) and microscopically resemble embryonic tissue of the organ in which they arise **(Table 7.5)**.

TABLE 7.5 Different types of embryonal tumors and their site.

Type of embryonal tumor	*Site*
Retinoblastoma	Eye
Nephroblastoma or Wilms tumor	Kidney
Neuroblastoma	Adrenal medulla or nerve ganglia
Hepatoblastoma	Liver

The nomenclature of the more common forms of neoplasia is listed in **Table 7.6**.

TABLE 7.6 Nomenclature of common tumors.

Tissue of origin	*Benign*	*Malignant*
Composed predominantly of single parenchymal cell type		
Tumors of mesenchymal origin		
Connective tissue and derivatives	Fibroma	Fibrosarcoma
	Lipoma	Liposarcoma
	Chondroma	Chondrosarcoma
	Osteoma	Osteogenic sarcoma

(Contd...)

(Contd...)

Tissue of origin	Benign	Malignant
Endothelium and related cell types		
Blood vessels	Hemangioma	Angiosarcoma
Lymph vessels	Lymphangioma	Lymphangiosarcoma
Mesothelium		Mesothelioma
Brain coverings	Meningioma	Invasive meningioma
Nerve sheath	Neurofibroma, neurilemmoma	Malignant peripheral nerve sheath tumor
Blood cells and related cells		
Hematopoietic cells		Leukemia
Lymphoid tissue		Lymphoma
Muscle		
• Smooth muscle	Leiomyoma	Leiomyosarcoma
• Striated muscle	Rhabdomyoma	Rhabdomyosarcoma
Skin tumors of epithelial origin		
Stratified squamous	Squamous cell papilloma	Squamous cell carcinoma
Basal cells of skin or adnexa		Basal cell carcinoma
Tumors of melanocytes	Nevus	Melanoma
Epithelial lining of glands or ducts or organs	Adenoma	Adenocarcinoma
	Papilloma	Papillary carcinoma
	Cystadenoma	Cystadenocarcinoma
	Papillary cystadenoma	Papillary cystadenocarcinoma
Urinary tract epithelium (transitional)	Transitional-cell papilloma	Urothelial carcinoma
Placenta	Hydatidiform mole	Choriocarcinoma
Testis		Seminoma Embryonal carcinoma
Ovary	Serous cystadenoma, mucinous cystadenoma	Serous cystadenocarcinoma, mucinous cystadenocarcinoma
Composed of multiple cell types, derived from the same germ cell layer		
Salivary glands	Pleomorphic adenoma (mixed tumor) of salivary origin	Malignant mixed tumor of salivary gland origin
Renal anlage		Wilms tumor
Composed of multiple cell types derived from more than one germ cell layer		
Totipotential cells in gonads or embryonic rests	Mature teratoma, dermoid cyst	Immature teratoma

CHARACTERISTICS OF BENIGN AND MALIGNANT NEOPLASMS

PA 7.1c (CC): Differentiate between benign from malignant neoplasms.

Q. Describe the characteristics of malignant tumors.

It is **very important to differentiate benign from malignant tumors** mainly because of the different prognostic outcomes. In general, **benign, and malignant tumors can be distinguished based on three fundamental features,** namely: **(1) Differentiation and anaplasia, (2) local invasion, and (3) metastasis**. Generally, rapid growth of tumors also suggests malignancy, but some malignant tumors grow slowly. Hence, the **rate of growth is not a reliable distinguishing feature**.

Differentiation and Anaplasia

Differentiation

Differentiation is defined as the **extent to which neoplastic parenchymal cells resemble** the corresponding **normal parenchymal cells of origin**. This includes both morphological and functional differentiation. Differentiation **determines the grade of the tumor**. The **lack of differentiation is called *anaplasia*.**

Benign Tumors

1. **Well-differentiated:** The neoplastic cell of benign tumors **closely resembles the normal cell of origin and is thus well-differentiated.** It may be not possible to recognize it as a tumor by microscopic examination of individual cells. For example, a lipoma is composed of mature fat cells containing cytoplasmic lipid vacuoles, and a chondroma consists of mature cartilage cells that synthesize cartilaginous matrix (showing morphologic and functional evidence of differentiation).
2. **Mitoses rare:** In well-differentiated benign tumors, mitoses are usually rare. If present they are of normal configuration.

Malignant Neoplasms

Most malignant neoplasms show morphologic changes that indicate their malignant nature.

Show a wide range of differentiation: Most malignant neoplasms show a wide range of differentiation of parenchymal cells. It may vary from **well-differentiated to completely undifferentiated.** Cancers are usually graded either as well, moderately, or poorly differentiated, or numerically often by strict criteria such as grade 1, grade 2, or grade 3.

- **Well-differentiated cancers:** For example, well-differentiated adenocarcinoma of the colon may form normal-appearing glands **(Fig. 7.5)**; and squamous

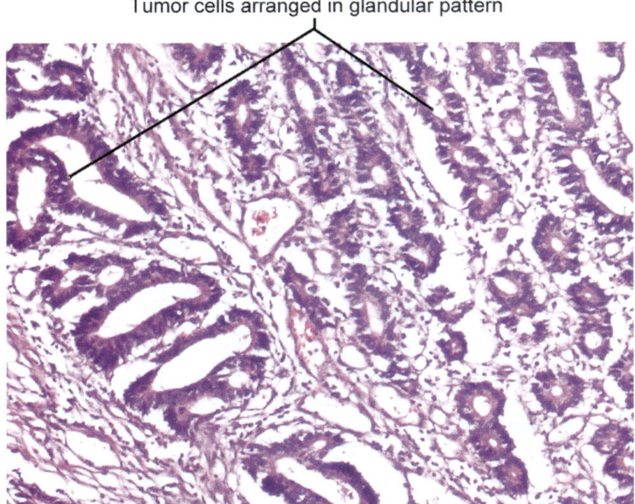

Fig. 7.5: Well-differentiated adenocarcinoma of the colon. It shows cancerous glands that are irregular in shape and size invading the muscular layer of the colon.

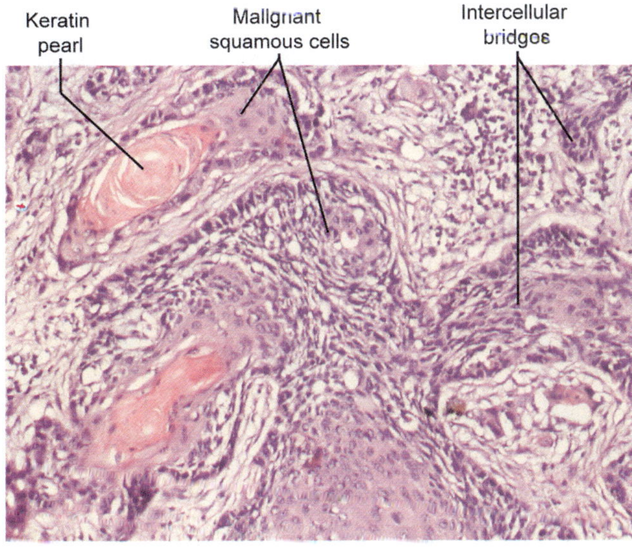

Fig. 7.6: Well-differentiated squamous cell carcinoma of the skin. The tumor consists of cells that are similar to normal squamous epithelial cells, with intercellular bridges and keratin pearls.

cell carcinomas may show cells that appear similar to normal squamous epithelial cells **(Fig. 7.6)**. Well-differentiated tumors may show slight morphologic changes of malignant neoplasms. For example, well-differentiated follicular carcinoma of the thyroid may show normal-appearing thyroid follicles and its malignant nature is revealed only by invasion into adjacent tissues or metastasis.

- **Poorly differentiated tumors:** They consist of **cells** that have **little resemblance to the cell of origin**.
- **Moderately differentiated cancers:** These tumors show differentiation between the well and poorly-differentiated tumors.

Q. Write a short note on anaplasia.

Anaplasia: Anaplasia literally **means "to form backward/ backward formation."** Anaplasia refers to dedifferentiation (**reversal of differentiation of cell to a more primitive level**), or loss/lack of the structural and functional differentiation of normal cells. **Anaplasia (cellular atypia)** is the extent to which a tumor's appearance deviates from that of its normal tissue or cellular counterparts. It is a **characteristic of malignancy**. The degree of anaplasia in a cancer cell correlates with the aggressiveness of the tumor. Thus, the more anaplastic the tumor, the more aggressive it becomes.

Anaplastic neoplasms: Malignant neoplasms composed of undifferentiated cells are called anaplastic tumors.

Microscopic (cytologic) features of anaplasia (Figs. 7.7 and 7.8)

Q. Write a short note on the morphology of malignant cells.

Cytologic evidence of anaplasia **(Box. 7.1)** includes the following:

- **Cellular and nuclear pleomorphism:** It is defined as great **variation in the size and shape of cells and their nuclei**. It is a feature of malignancy. Thus, cells within the same malignant tumor range from large cells (many times larger than the neighbor cells), to extremely small (primitive appearing) cells. **Nuclear shape and size are variable** and may be irregular.
- **Abnormal nuclear morphology:** These include the following:
  - **Extremely hyperchromatic (dark staining) nuclei of tumor cells:** It is **due to abundant chromatin** and **increased amount of DNA per cell** compared to that of a normal cell. Microscopically, these **nuclei stain darkly (hyperchromatic nuclei). Chromatin is coarsely clumped** and distributed along the nuclear membrane.
  - **Unusually prominent single or multiple nucleoli** are usually seen. Nucleoli may become surprisingly large, sometimes as big as the diameter of normal lymphocytes.
- **Increased nuclear-cytoplasmic (N:C) ratio:** In a normal cell, the N: C ratio is 1:4 or 1:6. In a malignant cell, the nuclei are enlarged, become disproportionately large for the cell, and the nuclear-to-cytoplasm ratio may be **increased (Figs. 7.8A and B)** and may reach even up to 1:1.
- **Bizarre cells, including tumor giant cells:** Some tumors may show **bizarre cells and tumor giant cells.** These cells are considerably larger than neighboring cells. They may contain either **a single large polymorphic nucleus or** others may have **two or more large, hyperchromatic nuclei (Figs. 7.8A and B)**.
- **Atypical (abnormal) mitoses:** The presence of mitotic figures **indicates the higher proliferative activity** of the parenchymal cells. Compared to benign and few

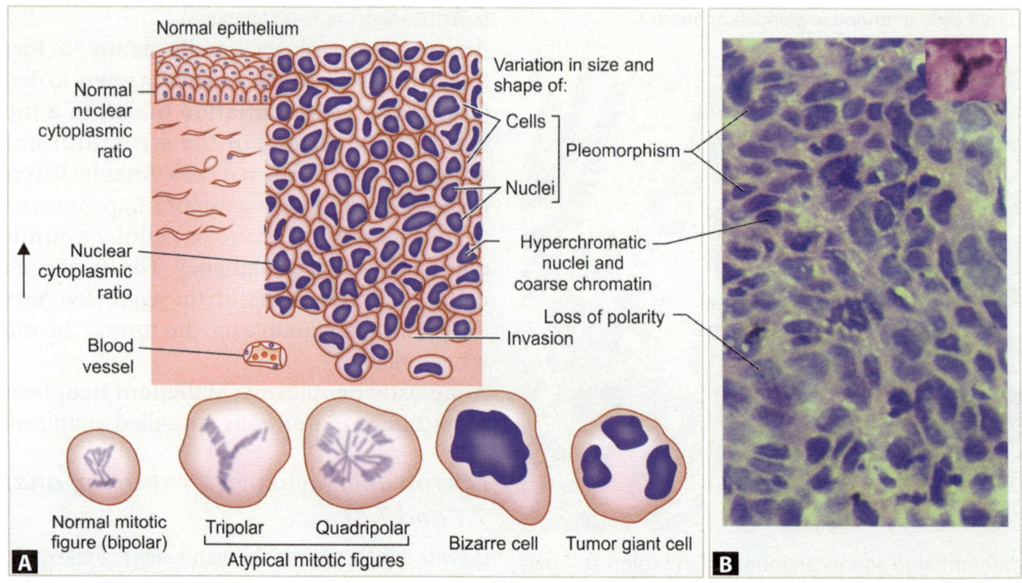

Figs. 7.7A and B: Microscopic features of anaplasia: (A) Diagrammatic; (B) Photomicrograph showing nuclear and cytoplasmic pleomorphism, hyperchromatic nuclei, high nuclear-cytoplasmic ratio, and loss of polarity. The Inset of B shows a tripolar mitotic figure.

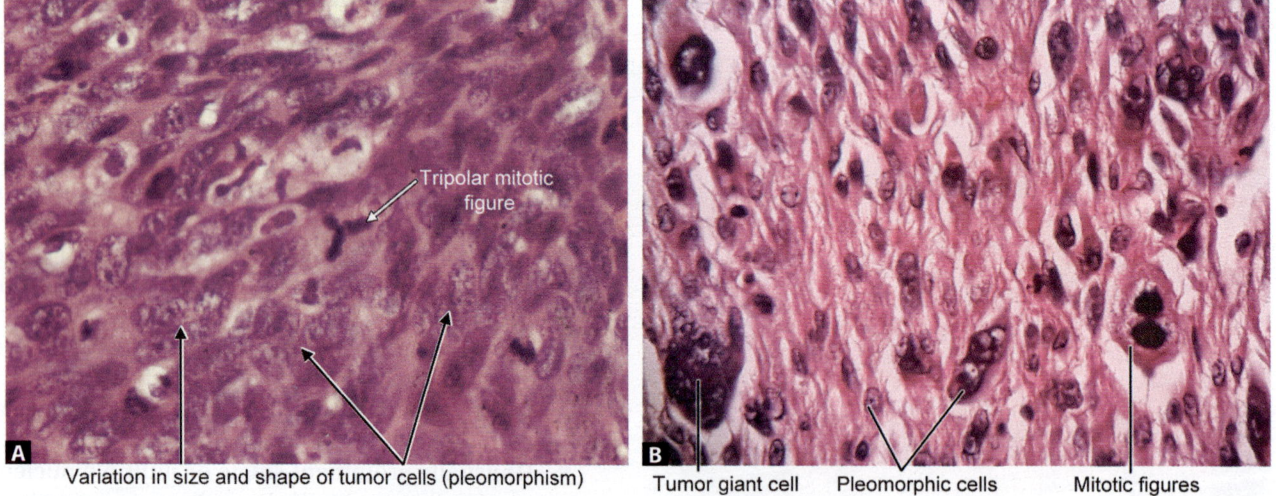

Figs. 7.8A and B: (A) Poorly differentiated carcinoma consisting of tumor cells showing variation in size of cells and nuclei. One tumor cell in the center shows an abnormal tripolar spindle; (B) Sarcoma shows cellular and nuclear pleomorphism, tumor giant cells, and mitotic figures.

BOX 7.1: Microscopic features of anaplasia.

Cellular and nuclear pleomorphism (variation in the size and shape).

Abnormal nuclear morphology
- Extremely hyperchromatic, enlarged nuclei with coarsely clumped chromatin
- Unusually prominent single or multiple nucleoli

High nuclear-cytoplasmic (N: C) ratio

Bizarre cells, including tumor giant cells

Atypical mitoses (mitotic figures)

Loss of polarity

well-differentiated malignant tumors, **undifferentiated tumors usually show abundant (many) mitotic figures (Figs. 7.8A and B)**. Normal mitosis produces bipolar spindles, and one cell divides into two. When the **mitotic spindles are more than two, it is called atypical**. Multiple spindles may produce **tripolar or quadripolar mitotic figures**. The presence of atypical bizarre mitotic figures is **an important morphological feature of malignancy (Figs. 7.8A and B)**.

- **Loss of polarity: The normal orientation of cells to one another** is known as polarity. The anaplastic cells lose the normal polarity and show markedly disturbed orientation (architecture) of tumor cells. The malignant tumor cells grow in sheets, with a loss of normal orientation. Identifiable growth patterns are absent, such as glands (in adenocarcinoma) or stratified squamous architecture (in squamous cell carcinoma).

- **Other features:** These include:
  - **Growth pattern:** This feature is a variably useful determinant of malignancy. Malignant neoplasms usually show disorganized growth. The tumor cells may form sheets of cells, arranged around blood vessels, papillary structures, whorls, rosettes, etc.
  - **Necrosis and apoptosis:** Many rapidly growing malignant tumors undergo large central areas of ischemic necrosis and/or apoptosis. Some malignant tumors show central ischemic necrosis due to impaired blood supply.

Functional Activities

Well-differentiated tumors usually retain the functional characteristics of their normal counterparts. However, **anaplastic tumor cells are less likely to retain their specialized functional activities.** The function may be in the form of secretion and vary depending on the tumor type.

- **Secretion of normal substances:** Examples are as follows:
  - **Hormones: Benign tumors** and even **well-differentiated carcinomas of endocrine glands frequently secrete the hormones** characteristic of their cell of origin (e.g., steroid hormones from an adrenocortical adenoma).
  - **Secretion of normal products of the cell of origin:** For example, **well-differentiated squamous cell carcinomas** produce keratin and form characteristic **epithelial pearls** (*refer* **Fig. 7.6**), and well-differentiated hepatocellular carcinomas secrete bile.
- **Production of fetal proteins:** Some tumors may secrete fetal proteins, **which are not produced by comparable normal cells in the adult.** For example, carcinoembryonic antigen (CEA) by adenocarcinomas of the gastrointestinal tract.
- **Ectopic hormones:** Cancers of nonendocrine origin may produce **substances such as "ectopic hormones" that** are **not indigenous to the tissue of origin** (*refer* **Table 7.17**). For example, lung carcinoma may secrete adrenocorticotropic hormone (ACTH), and parathyroid hormone-like hormones, insulin, glucagon, and others. They produce "paraneoplastic syndromes" (*refer* pages 261-2).

Differences between carcinoma and sarcoma are shown in **Table 7.7**.

Q. Write a short note on the differences between carcinoma and sarcoma.

TABLE 7.7 Differences between carcinoma and sarcoma.

Features	*Carcinoma*	*Sarcoma*
Definition	Malignant tumor of epithelial origin	Malignant tumor of mesenchymal origin
Meaning of the term	"Carcinoma" came from the Greek word "karkinos" which means crab and "oma" which means growth	"Sarcoma" came from the Greek word "sarc" meaning flesh and "oma" which means growth
Site of origin	Mostly from the inside lining of the colon, breast, and lung or prostate	Arise from the musculoskeletal system, such as bones, muscles, and connective tissues
Incidence	More common cancer (more than 90% of cancers)	Less common (less than 1%)
Age	More common in middle and old age	Can occur at any age
Rate of growth	Usually not very rapid	Usually, rapid
Route of spread	Initially lymphatics and later hematogenous	• Spread by satellite nodules • Usually hematogenous and lymphatic spread is rare
Site of metastasis through blood	Liver, lung, brain, bone, and adrenals	May spread to the lungs
Gross appearance	• Varies depends on the subtype (e.g., cauliflower-like in squamous cell carcinoma) • Carcinomas infiltrate all nearby structures (nerves, veins, and muscles)	Fleshy, grow in ball-like masses and tend to push nearby structures such as arteries, nerves, and veins away
Hemorrhage and necrosis	Usually not extensive	May be extensive
Microscopy	The pattern varies and parenchymal cells may be arranged in glands, acini, sheets, cords, or papillae depending on the subtype	Tumor cells are arranged in different patterns depending on the subtype
Radiosensitivity	High	Radioresistance
Prognosis	Depends on the location and stage	Depends on the location and stage
Examples	Carcinoma breast, squamous cell carcinoma of skin and mucus membranes, carcinoma of stomach and colon	Osteosarcoma, chondrosarcoma, liposarcoma

Dysplasia

Q. Write a short note on dysplasia.

Dysplasia refers to disorderly proliferation (growth) and shows abnormal differentiation (cellular growth and maturation) and anaplasia. **The dysplastic epithelium shows a loss of uniformity of individual cells (pleomorphism) and disturbed architectural orientation (loss of polarity).** The **cells show cytological features of malignancy (features of anaplasia—*refer* Box 7.1).**

Sites of dysplasia: Dysplasia mostly occurs in **epithelial tissues.**

- **Squamous epithelium:** Most common sites of dysplastic changes are seen in the **squamous epithelial lining of the uterine cervix (*refer* Figs. 22.3, 22.4 and 22.5 and pages 803-5), respiratory tract, and skin.** Dysplasia is most common in hyperplastic squamous epithelium and in areas of squamous metaplasia, such as in the bronchus or the cervix.
- **Other epithelium:** Dysplasia can occur in epithelium other than squamous epithelium.
    - **Columnar mucosa:** Dysplasia can occur in the columnar mucosal cells of the colon **in ulcerative colitis**
    - Ductal lining cells in the **breast**
    - Metaplastic epithelium of **Barrett esophagus**
    - **Prostate glands:** Prostatic intraepithelial neoplasia
    - **Urothelium** of the bladder

Cytologic features of dysplasia: Dysplasia represents the morphologic expression of a disturbance in growth regulation (*refer* **Box 7.1**). However, unlike cancer cells, dysplastic cells are not entirely autonomous, and with intervention, the cells can revert to normal. In dysplasia, the normal pattern is disturbed and it shows the following changes:

- **Cellular and nuclear pleomorphism** characterized by loss in the uniformity of the individual cells.
- **Abnormally large hyperchromatic nuclei.**
- **High/increased nuclear-to-cytoplasmic ratio.**
- **Increased mitotic activity:** Mitotic figures are normally confined to the basal layer. In dysplasia, mitotic figures are more than in the normal tissue and abnormally located. It may be seen at all levels (instead of only basal cells), including superficial epithelial (surface) cells.
- **Architectural disarray (loss of polarity):** Dysplasia shows the disorderly arrangement of cells from the basal layer to the surface layer. For example, the normal stratified squamous epithelium shows progressive maturation of tall cells in the basal layer to flattened squames on the surface. In dysplasia, the normal progressive maturation may fail in part or entirely. This may lead to the replacement of the epithelium by a disordered mixture of dark basal-appearing cells with hyperchromatic nuclei.

Asymptomatic: In this stage, dysplasias are usually asymptomatic.

Etiologic factors: Like metaplasia, dysplasia may develop as a **response to chronic irritation or prolonged/persistent inflammation.** It may regress or disappear after removal of the inciting stimulus, e.g., dysplasia in bronchial epithelium may regress after cessation of smoking, or dysplasia in the cervix due to human papillomavirus (HPV) may regress following the disappearance of HPV from the cervix. Dysplastic changes may be seen adjacent to foci of invasive carcinoma. In some situations, such as in long-term cigarette smokers and individuals with Barrett esophagus, severe epithelial dysplasia may antedate the appearance of cancer.

Classification, fate, and significance of dysplasia: It can be classified as (1) mild, (2) moderate, and (3) severe dysplasia depending on the thickness of epithelium involved by the dysplastic cells.

- **Mild-to-moderate dysplastic changes**, which do not involve the entire thickness of epithelium **may be reversible** if the cause is removed. The **dysplasia may be a precursor to malignant transformation, but dysplasia need not progress to cancer.**
- **Carcinoma in situ:** When dysplastic changes are marked and involve the entire thickness of the epithelium, it is a preinvasive neoplasm and is termed carcinoma in situ (*refer* below). However, the lesion does not penetrate the basement membrane of the lining epithelium.
- **Carcinoma: Once the dysplastic/tumor cells breach the basement membrane,** the **tumor is said to be invasive,** and carcinoma in situ may take years to become invasive. Most in situ tumors, with time, penetrate the basement membrane and invade the subepithelial stroma.

Metaplasia: It is a reversible change in which one type of differentiated cell is replaced by another type of differentiated cell (*refer* pages 41-2). It is a cellular adaptation that develops in association with tissue damage, repair, and regeneration, e.g., gastroesophageal reflux damages the squamous epithelium of the esophagus which is replaced by glandular (gastric or intestinal) epithelium, columnar epithelium of endocervix is replaced by stratified squamous epithelium. Malignancy may develop in these metaplastic epithelia.

Carcinoma In Situ

Q. Write a short note on carcinoma in situ.

When dysplastic changes are severe and involve the entire thickness of the epithelium, the lesion is termed *carcinoma in situ*. This is a preinvasive stage of cancer and some carcinomas evolve from carcinoma in situ (*refer* pages 803-6 of Chapter 22).

Definition: Carcinoma in situ is defined as:
- A **preinvasive epithelial neoplasm.**
- Shows **all the cytological features of malignancy.**
- **Involves the entire thickness of the epithelium.**
- Remains **confined within the epithelial basement membrane.**

The tumor cells cannot reach the potential routes of metastasis, such as blood vessels and lymphatics until the basement membrane has been breached or invaded.

Local Invasion

Identification of local invasion is an important feature for the diagnosis of malignancy.

Benign Tumors

Remain localized: Most benign tumors **grow as expansile masses** and remain localized to their site of origin. They expand slowly. There is **no infiltration** into adjacent tissue or capsule (if present) and **no metastasis**.

Presence of capsule (Fig. 7.9): It is a rim of compressed fibrous tissue. It consists of an extracellular matrix of the surrounding normal tissue. The extracellular matrix of the capsule is deposited by stromal cells such as fibroblasts. These fibroblasts may be activated by the mechanical stress produced due to the compression of normal tissue by the expanding tumor. **The presence of a capsule creates a tissue plane that makes the tumor discrete, palpable, and movable (nonfixed) mass.** It also helps in the easy excision of tumors by surgical enucleation.

- **Few benign tumors are unencapsulated (not capsulated) but circumscribed:** Not all benign tumors are encapsulated. For example, **leiomyoma of the uterus** is a circumscribed tumor without a capsule. It is separated from the surrounding smooth muscle of myometrium by a zone of compressed and attenuated normal myometrium.
- **Few benign tumors are neither encapsulated nor circumscribed:** These benign tumors are not clearly demarcated and may be difficult to excise. For example, benign vascular neoplasms such as **hemangiomas**. Thus, is pointed out only to emphasize that, although encapsulation is the rule in benign tumors, the lack of a capsule does not indicate that a tumor is malignant.

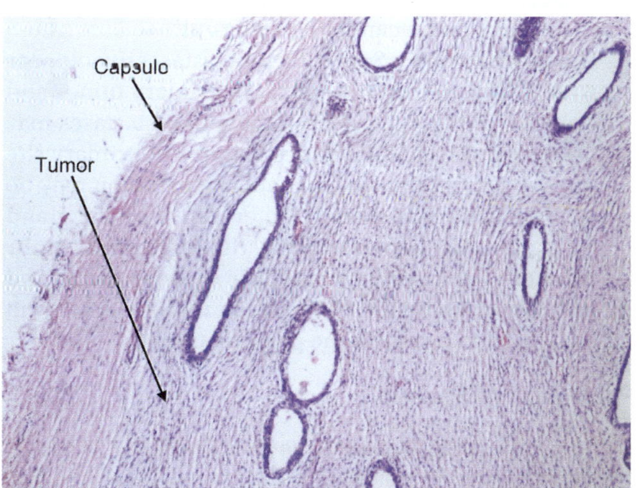

Fig. 7.9: Microscopic appearance of fibroadenoma of the breast with a well-defined fibrous capsule.

Malignant Tumors

Lack of capsule: Malignant tumors are poorly demarcated from the surrounding normal tissue and lack well-defined true capsules. Some malignant tumors are slowly growing (e.g., follicular carcinoma of the thyroid), and appear to be surrounded by a capsule. But careful microscopic examination shows tiny tongues of tumor penetrating the margin and infiltrating adjacent structures.

Local invasion: The two most reliable features that differentiate malignant from benign tumors are **local invasion and metastases.**

- **Invasion of adjacent tissue/organ (Figs. 7.10 and 7.11A):** The cancers may progressively infiltrate, invade, and destroy the surrounding (adjacent) tissues/organs. **Invasiveness is the most reliable microscopic feature that distinguishes cancers from benign tumors.** In some tumors such as follicular thyroid cancer, local invasion is important for a diagnosis of malignancy.

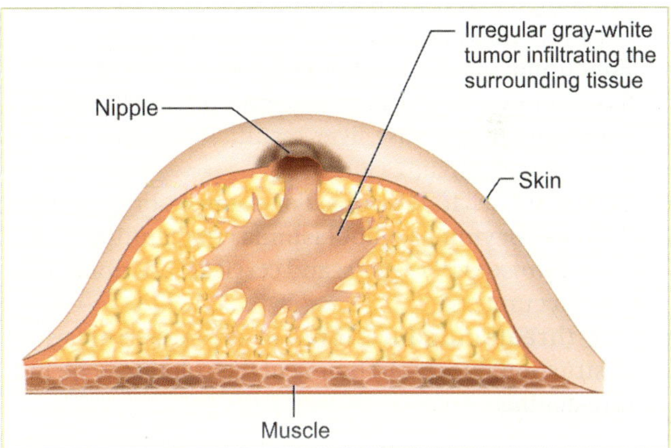

Fig. 7.10: Diagrammatic representation of cut section of an invasive ductal carcinoma of the breast.

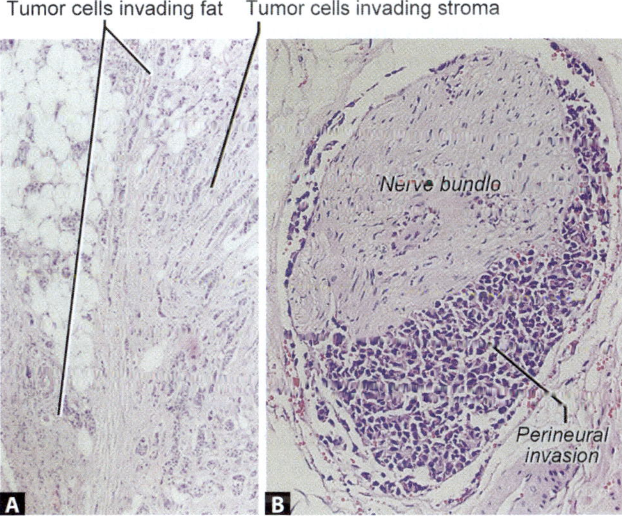

Figs. 7.11A and B: (A) Microscopic appearance of breast carcinoma showing invasion of breast stroma and fat by nests and cords of tumor cells; (B) Perineural invasion in prostatic carcinoma.

- **Invasion into blood vessels and lymphatics:** It helps to identify malignancies.
- **Perineural invasion** [e.g., cancer of prostate and pancreas (**Fig. 7.11B** and *refer* **Fig. 21.18**), adenoid cystic carcinoma of salivary glands].

Q. Write briefly on the pagetoid spread and give an example.

- **Pagetoid infiltration***:* It is an invasion within the epithelium and is seen in Paget's disease of the nipple (*refer* **Figs. 23.15 and 23.16**).
- **Tissues that resist invasion:** They include mature cartilage (e.g., epiphysis) and elastic tissue of arteries.

The consequences of invasion into the organ/tissue of origin are as follows:

- The infiltrative nature of growth, makes its **surgical resection difficult**. Hence, it is necessary to remove a wide margin of surrounding normal tissue during the attempt of complete excision of a malignant tumor. In these resected tumors, pathologists carefully examine the margins to ensure that the resected margins are free of cancer cells *(clean surgical margins).*
- **Functional insufficiency may occur** if much of normal tissue is replaced by cancer. For example, hepatocellular carcinoma may cause liver insufficiency, and ocular tumors may impair vision.
- **Compromise vital regions:** For example, brain tumors (e.g., astrocytomas, glioblastoma) may infiltrate and compromise vital regions, and cervical carcinoma may obstruct ureters.
- **Life-threatening location:** For example, intestinal obstruction due to carcinoma of the colon may be life-threatening.

Rates of Growth

Q. Write a short note on the rate of growth of tumors.

Factors determining the rate of growth: These include:

- **Degree of differentiation: Benign tumors** are well differentiated and **usually grow slowly and most malignant tumors grow more rapidly.**
- **Dependency:** Growth also depends on (i) **adequacy of blood supply, and (ii) in certain tumors on hormonal stimulation**, e.g., uterine leiomyomas may suddenly grow during pregnancy and may undergo atrophy after menopause.
- **Balance between cell production and cell loss:** This in turn is determined by three main factors:
  - **Doubling time of tumor cells:** It is the **time required for the total cell cycle**, i.e., cell to double by mitosis.
  - **Growth fraction:** It is the **proportion of cells in the proliferative or replicative pool** within the tumor.
  - **Rate of tumor cell death:** The rate of growth depends on the balance between cell production and cell loss. When **both the rate of cell production and the rate of cell loss** (by apoptosis) **is high,** it is termed a **high cell turnover.**

Metastasis

Q. Define metastasis and describe its mechanism.

The invasive nature of cancers allows them to penetrate blood vessels, lymphatics, and body cavities. Thus, invasiveness provides an opportunity for the spread of cancer.

Definition: Metastasis is defined by the spread of a tumor to physically discontinuous sites (located in a distant tissue) **with the primary tumor.** It is **one of the characteristic features of malignant tumors.** The **process of spread of a tumor is known as metastasis** and the resulting **secondary deposits are called metastases.**

Significance of metastasis: These are as follows:

- **Indicates tumor is malignant:** Metastases **identify a tumor as malignant** because benign neoplasms never metastasize. **Exceptions** include **two malignant tumors,** which are locally invasive but rarely metastasize.
  - **Basal cell carcinomas of the skin**
  - **Most primary tumors of** the central nervous system **are locally invasive but rarely metastasize.** Examples are **gliomas** (malignant neoplasms of the glial cells).
- Metastases **strongly reduce the possibility of a cure for cancer.**
- Metastatic spread is the most **common cause of cancer death.**

Factors favoring metastasis: Generally, poorly differentiated (anaplastic) tumors, more rapidly growing tumors, and large primary tumors are more likely to metastasize.

Leukemias and lymphomas: These tumors are derived from blood-forming cells that normally can enter the bloodstream. These tumors disseminate at diagnosis and are always malignant.

Morphological Appearance of Metastases

- Microscopically, **metastases resemble the primary tumor**. But occasionally, they may be so anaplastic that their cell of origin cannot be made out.
- **Unknown primary: Sometimes metastases may appear without any clinically detectable primary tumor** and even the microscopic examination of metastases may not reveal the characteristics features of primary site tumor, e.g., metastases from adenocarcinoma may be so anaplastic that there is no evidence of any gland formation. In such situations, **tissue-related tumor markers, electron microscopic examination, and immunohistochemistry** by specific tumor markers will be **helpful to establish the primary tumor.**

Pathways of Spread

Q. Write a short note on different modes/pathways of spread of malignant tumors with examples.

The invasiveness of cancers allows them to penetrate blood vessels, lymphatics, and body cavities. It provides

BOX 7.2: Pathways of spread of malignnat tumors.

- Lymphatic spread
- Hematogenous/blood spread
- Seeding of the body cavities and surfaces
- Direct transplantation

an opportunity for the spread/dissemination of cancers through the following different pathways (**Box 7.2**). Usually, malignant **neoplasms are spread by one of three pathways: (1) lymphatic spread; (2) hematogenous spread; or (3) seeding of the body cavities and surfaces.**

Lymphatic Spread

Q. Write a short note on the lymphatic spread of malignant tumors.

Lymphatic spread is the most common pathway of spread for carcinomas. It is **more typical of carcinomas, whereas sarcomas spread through a hematogenous route.**

- **Regional node involvement:** The walls of lymphatics in the region of cancer are readily invaded by cancer cells and form a continuous growth within the lymphatic channels (lymphatic permeation). Once the tumor cells gain access to the lymphatic vessels, they may detach to form tumor emboli and are carried to the regional draining lymph nodes. In the lymph node, the **tumor emboli** enter through afferent lymphatics at its convex surface and **lodge and grow in the subcapsular sinus. Subsequently, the entire lymph node** may be replaced by the metastatic tumor.
- **Sentinel lymph node:** It is the **first regional lymph node that receives lymph flow from a primary cancer.** During surgery, it can be identified by injecting blue dyes or radiolabelled tracers near the primary cancer. A biopsy of the sentinel lymph node is performed to know the presence or absence of metastatic lesions. Thus, it helps to determine the extent of the spread of the tumor and to plan the treatment.
- **Pattern of lymph node involvement follows the natural routes of lymphatic drainage:** The pattern of lymph node involvement depends on the site of the primary neoplasm and the pathways of local lymphatic drainage Examples are as follows:
  - **Lung carcinomas:** Lung cancer first metastasizes to the regional bronchial lymph nodes and then to the tracheobronchial and hilar nodes.
  - **Breast carcinoma:** Carcinoma of the breast usually arises in the upper outer quadrant and the initial metastases are almost always through lymphatic. Breast cancers in the upper outer quadrant (lateral aspect) of the breast first spread to axillary lymph nodes; medial breast lesions drain through the chest wall to the internal mammary thoracic lymph nodes (along the internal mammary artery), later, tumors at both these sites may spread to the supraclavicular and infraclavicular nodes.

Q. Write a short note on skip and retrograde metastasis.

- **Skip metastasis:** In some cancers, the tumor cells travel in lymphatic channels through the immediately proximal local nodes. But they **bypass this regional lymph node and** get trapped in subsequent lymph nodes **distant from the site of the primary tumor**. This is called "skip metastases." For example, cancers of **abdominal organs such as stomach cancer** may be **first detected by an enlarged supraclavicular node** (this lymph node is called **Virchow's lymph node**).
- **Retrograde metastasis: Tumors spreading against the flow of lymphatics** may cause metastases at unusual sites, e.g., **carcinoma prostate metastasizing to the supraclavicular lymph node.**
- **Lymphatic compartment to vascular compartment:** The cancer cells may also traverse all the lymph nodes and then to the thoracic duct. From here, it can reach the vascular compartment.
- **Enlargement of lymph nodes near primary cancer may be without metastatic deposits:** Though enlargement of regional lymph nodes raises suspicion of metastatic spread, it does not always indicate metastatic deposits. The necrotic cells of the cancer and tumor antigens may elicit immunologic responses in draining nodes. This may lead to reactive hyperplasia *(lymphadenitis)*. Hence, biopsy and histopathological identification of a tumor within an enlarged lymph node is needed to determine whether an enlarged lymph node is involved in cancer.
- **Microscopic pattern of deposits:** Initially, tumor cells are deposited in the marginal sinus and later extend throughout the node. Micrometastases (microscopic involvement of lymph nodes) consist of single tumor cells or very small clusters in lymph nodes.
- **Significance of lymph node metastases: It is of prognostic value**, e.g., in breast cancer, involvement of axillary lymph nodes is very important for assessing prognosis and for the type of therapy. However, all regional nodal enlargements need not be due to metastasis because necrotic products of tumors and antigens may produce sinus histiocytosis in lymph nodes.

Hematogenous Spread

Q. Write a short note on the hematogenous spread of malignant tumors.

Hematogenous spread is usual for sarcomas but is also found in carcinomas. Blood-borne metastasis usually occurs in **osteosarcoma, choriocarcinoma,** and **renal cell carcinoma.**

- **Vessels invaded:** Cancer cells easily invade **capillaries and thin-walled venules**, but thick-walled arterioles and arteries are relatively resistant. With venous invasion, the bloodborne cancer cells usually first get arrested in the capillary bed they come across.

- **Tumors with an affinity for venous invasion:** Few carcinomas tend to grow within veins. However, they may not be accompanied by widespread dissemination.
  - **Renal cell carcinoma:** It can invade the renal vein and grow in a snake-like fashion up the inferior vena cava, sometimes reaching the right side of the heart.
  - **Hepatocellular carcinoma:** It may invade branches of the portal and hepatic vein and grow within the main venous channels.

Pattern of involvement

With venous invasion, the pattern of metastases follows the venous flow.

The target organ for metastasis (*refer* online Fig. 7.12): The liver and lungs are the most common sites of hematogenous spread.

- **Livers: All the blood from the portal area** (portal system) **drains to the liver**. Therefore, it is one of the common sites of blood spread.
- **Lung: All caval blood (both from the inferior and superior vena cava) flows to the lungs.** Tumors that penetrate systemic veins, eventually drain into the vena cava. Hence, the lungs are the other common site for secondaries by hematogenous spread. Through pulmonary veins, cancer cells from the primary lung cancer and metastatic deposits in the lungs may be carried to the left side of the heart. From here the tumor emboli may be carried in systemic circulation to form secondary masses elsewhere in the body.
- **Bone metastasis:** Cancer metastasizing to bone are primary cancers of the **prostate, lung, breast, liver, intestine, kidney, and thyroid**.
  - **Vertebral column: It is a common site.** Cancers arising in organs near the vertebral column (e.g., thyroid and prostate) typically embolize and spread through the paravertebral plexus. Radiograph appearance of bone metastasis may be osteolytic or osteoblastic.
    - **Osteolytic lesion:** It is characterized by radiolucencies (e.g., lung cancer) and may lead to pathological fractures and hypercalcemia.
    - **Osteoblastic lesion:** It is characterized by radiodensities (e.g., prostatic cancer, breast, thyroid) and increased serum alkaline phosphatase due to reactive bone formation.
- **Other common sites: Brain**—most common primary is lung cancer, kidney, and adrenals.
- **Organs relatively resistant:** These include **skeletal muscle and spleen**.

MORPHOLOGY OF METASTATIC DEPOSITS

Gross (Fig. 7.13): It appears as multiple round nodules of varying sizes found throughout the organ.

Microscopy: The metastatic deposits generally resemble the structure of the primary tumor.

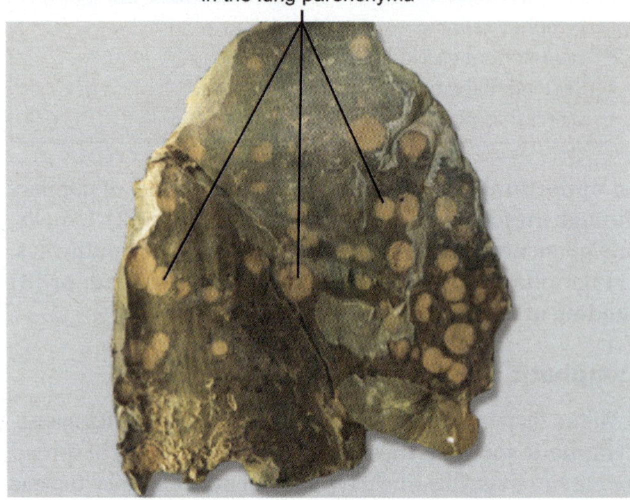

Fig. 7.13: Lung with multiple metastatic cancer.

Spread by Seeding

Q. Write a short note on spread by seeding (transcoelomic spread).

This method of spread may be seeding of body cavities or spread along epithelial surfaces.

Spread by seeding of body cavities: It is a method of spread of malignant tumors that **arise in organs adjacent to body cavities and invade** a body cavity. The malignant cells may exfoliate or shed from the organ surfaces into the body cavities and cytological examination of this fluid may show malignant cells. Body cavities include peritoneal (most common), pleural cavities (common), pericardial (occasionally), joint space and subarachnoid space.

- **Peritoneal cavity: Spread into the peritoneum through seeding may occur in ovarian tumors,** such as primary carcinomas of surface epithelial origin and **malignant GI tract tumors.** They may spread to involve the peritoneal cavity leading to ascites. Sometimes, mucus-secreting carcinoma of the appendix or ovary may spread to a peritoneal cavity that may form a gelatinous neoplastic mass in the peritoneal cavity referred to as *pseudomyxoma peritonei.*
- **Pleural cavity:** Spread by seeding may occur in peripherally situated **lung tumors and may lead to** pleural effusions.
- **Through cerebrospinal fluid:** Neoplasms of the central nervous system, such as a **medulloblastoma or ependymoma**, may penetrate the cerebral ventricles and tumor cells may be carried by the cerebrospinal fluid (CSF). They may implant on the meningeal surfaces surrounding the brain or spinal cord.

Spread along the surfaces: It is **not common**. For example, carcinoma **endometrium may spread to the ovary** (or vice versa) **through the fallopian tube, and carcinoma of the kidney may spread to the lower urinary tract via ureters.**

Direct transplantation: Tumor cells may be directly

Q. Discuss the differences between benign and malignant tumors.

TABLE 7.8 Differences between benign and malignant tumors.

Characteristics	*Benign*	*Malignant*
A. MICROSCOPIC FEATURES		
1. Differentiation/anaplasia	Well-differentiated	Well to poorly differentiated. Anaplasia is characteristic
2. Pleomorphism of cells and nuclei	Usually not seen	Commonly present
3. Nuclear features		
– **Nuclear morphology**	Usually, normal	Usually hyperchromatic, irregular outline, and pleomorphic
– **Nucleoli**	Usually absent	Usual and prominent
– **Mitotic activity**	Rare and if present they are normal bipolar	High and may be abnormal or atypical (tripolar, quadripolar, multipolar)
4. Tumor giant cells	Not seen	May be seen and show nuclear atypia
5. Nuclear cytoplasmic (N: C) ratio	Normal (1:4 to 1:6)	Increased (may be as much as 1:1)
6. Polarity	Maintained	Usually lost
7. Chromosomal abnormality	Not found	Usually seen
B. GROSS FEATURES		
1. Border/capsule	Mostly circumscribed or encapsulated	Usually poorly defined
2. Areas of necrosis and hemorrhage	Rare	Common, often found microscopically
C. CLINICAL FEATURES		
1. Local invasion	Usually well-demarcated without invasion/ infiltration of the surrounding normal tissues	Locally invasive, infiltrates surrounding normal tissue
2. Rate of growth	Usually, slow	Relatively rapid
3. Metastasis	Absent	Frequent
4. Biological behavior/prognosis	Usually, the prognosis is good	Prognosis is poor; usually death due to local invasion or metastatic complications

transplanted (e.g., by surgical instruments like scalpel, needles, or sutures) or implantation by direct contact (e.g., transfer of cancer of the lower lip to the corresponding opposite site in the upper lip). Even though this method is theoretically possible, they are rare.

Differences between benign and malignant tumors are summarized in Table 7.8.

Q. Describe the differences between benign and malignant tumors. Mention the four characteristics of benign neoplasms.

Metastasis is the spread of a tumor to sites that are physically discontinuous with primary.
Metastasis is the process and the resulting secondary deposits are called metastases.
Metastases: First important criteria for malignancy. Some organs or tissues may be unfavorable soil for the growth of tumor deposits (e.g., spleen and skeletal muscle).

EPIDEMIOLOGY OF CANCER

Environmental Factors

Environmental factors are important **risk factors for most cancers. These are as follows:**

Q. Write a short note on diet and cancer.

- **Smoking:** Cigarette smoking (*refer* pages 291-2) is an important factor involved in cancer of the lung, mouth, pharynx, larynx, esophagus, pancreas, and bladder.
- **Diet:** Diet may be a risk factor for carcinoma of the colorectum, prostate, and breast. **Three factors in the diet are probably involved in the development of cancer:**
  - **Exogenous carcinogen in diet:** *Aflatoxin* is involved in the development of hepatocellular carcinomas.
  - **Endogenous synthesis of carcinogens from dietary components:**
    - **Nitrosamines and nitrosamides in the diet:** They can induce gastric cancer.
    - **High animal fat intake:** This along with consumption of red meat and low dietary fiber intake has been implicated in the causation of carcinoma colon.
  - **Lack of protective factors:**
    - **High-fiber diet** may have a protective role in carcinoma colon.

- **Antioxidant:** Fruits and vegetables, consumption of vitamin C and E, β-carotenes, and selenium which have antioxidant properties, have been presumed to have anticarcinogenic effects.
- Epidemiologic studies suggest that a **folate-rich diet** decreases the risk of colorectal cancer.

- **Alcohol abuse:** Alcohol abuse (*refer* pages 292-3) is a risk factor for carcinomas of the oropharynx (excluding lip), larynx, and esophagus, and can produce alcoholic cirrhosis which is a risk factor for hepatocellular carcinoma. Alcohol and tobacco together increase the risk of cancers in the upper airways and digestive tract.
- **Infectious agents:** *Human papillomavirus* (HPV) spreads through sexual contact and is an etiological factor for carcinoma of the cervix as well as some head and neck cancers.
- **Obesity:** It is associated with cancer risk.
- **Reproductive history:** Lifelong cumulative exposure to estrogen stimulation, particularly if unopposed by progesterone, increases the risk for cancers of the endometrium and breast.
- **Carcinogens:** They may be present in food (e.g., grilled meat, high-fat diet, alcohol), water (e.g., arsenic), environment [e.g., ultraviolet (UV) rays, asbestos], drugs medications (e.g., methotrexate), etc.

Acquired Predisposing Conditions

Acquired conditions may predispose to cancer. These include disorders associated with chronic inflammation, immunodeficiency states, and precursor lesions. Cancer risk rises in certain tissues in which there is increased cellular proliferation caused by chronic inflammation or hormonal stimulation **(Table 7.9)**.

TABLE 7.9 Examples of chronic inflammatory states and associated cancers.

Chronic inflammatory state	*Associated cancer*	*Etiology*
Asbestosis, silicosis	Mesothelioma, carcinoma of the lung	Asbestos fibers, silica particles
Reflux esophagitis, Barrett esophagus	Carcinoma of esophagus	Gastric acid
Gastritis/ulcers	Gastric adenocarcinoma, MALT lymphoma	*Helicobacter pylori*
Inflammatory bowel disease (mainly ulcerative colitis)	Colorectal carcinoma	The exact etiological agent is not known
Hepatitis	Hepatocellular carcinoma	Hepatitis B and/or C virus
Chronic cholecystitis	Cancer of gallbladder	Bile acids, bacteria, gallstones
Pancreatitis	Carcinoma of pancreas	Alcohol, germline mutations (e.g., in the trypsinogen gene)
Hashimoto thyroiditis	MALT lymphoma	Autoimmune disorder
Osteomyelitis	Carcinoma in draining sinuses	Bacterial infection
Chronic cystitis	Bladder carcinoma	Schistosomiasis

Precursor Lesions

Q. Write a short note on precancerous or precursor lesions/premalignant neoplasms.

Precursor lesions are **non-neoplastic disorders** and are localized disturbances of epithelial differentiation. Lining epithelial cells in certain locations may develop morphologic changes and these are associated with a **well-defined increased risk of developing cancer**; such lesions are termed precursor lesions. These lesions may develop secondary to chronic inflammation or hormonal disturbances (in endocrine-sensitive tissues) or may occur spontaneously. Recognizing precursor lesions is important because their removal or reversal lowers cancer risk. The most common precursor lesions are as follows:

1. **Squamous metaplasia and dysplasia of bronchial mucosa:** It is observed in chronic smokers (a risk factor for lung carcinoma), intralobular and intraductal carcinoma of the breast, and carcinoma in situ of the cervix.
2. **Endometrial hyperplasia and dysplasia** in women with unopposed estrogen stimulation (a risk factor for endometrial carcinoma): **Chronic atrophic gastritis** of pernicious anemia.
3. **Leukoplakia** (erythroplakia) **of the oral cavity, vulva, and penis:** These may progress to squamous cell carcinoma in the respective sites.
4. **Villous adenoma of the colon:** It is associated with a high risk for progression to colorectal carcinoma.
5. **Barrett esophagus may progress to adenocarcinoma.**
6. **Solar or actinic keratosis of the skin, Bowen's disease of the skin.**
7. **Chronic inflammation (Table 7.9):** Chronic ulcerative colitis (carcinoma colon), cirrhosis of the liver (hepatocellular carcinoma), *H. pylori* gastritis (gastric cancer and lymphoma), chronic irritation from jagged tooth or ill-fitting denture (cancer of the oral cavity) and old burn scar—Marjolin's ulcer (squamous cell carcinoma).
8. Malignant peripheral nerve sheath tumor in patients with **neurofibromatosis.**
9. Congenital abnormalities may predispose to cancer, e.g., the **undescended testis** is more prone to neoplasms than the normally located testis.

BOX 7.3: Precancerous lesions of the gastrointestinal tract.

Esophagus

Barrett esophagus, achalasia, post-ingestion of caustic soda lye (alkaline burn)

Stomach

- *H. pylori*, especially if treated with PPI without eradication of *H. pylori*
- Gastric polyps
- Ménétrier's disease (hypertrophic gastropathy)
- Achlorhydria, pernicious anemia
- Post-gastrectomy, post-vagotomy, post-gastrojejunostomy

Small intestine

Hereditary cancer syndromes, FAP (especially post-cholecystectomy), Peutz-Jeghers syndrome

Colon (large intestine)

- Hereditary cancer syndromes, FAP, Gardner's, HNPCC (Lynch syndrome)
- Inflammatory bowel disease, especially chronic extensive ulcerative colitis
- Sporadic adenomatous polyps, especially villous and tubulovillous polyps

10. **Immunodeficiency states:** Patients with deficits in T-cell immunity have increased risk for cancers mainly those due to oncogenic viruses.

Precancerous/preneoplastic lesions of the GI tract are listed in **Box 7.3**.

Q. Write a short note on preneoplastic (precancerous) conditions/lesions of GIT.

Cancer Incidence

Cancer incidence of common types of cancer is presented in **Table 7.10**. It varies depending on geographic location and other factors.

Cancer Genes

Cancer is a disease caused by mutations that alter the function of a limited subset of genes: There are a total of about 20,000 human genes of which only a few (about hundreds in number) constitute cancer genes. These genes are called cancer genes because **they contribute directly to the malignant behavior of cancer cells.** Tumors are systematically analyzed by genomic sequencing, and these findings strongly support that **cancer is a genetic disease.**

Definition of cancer genes: It can be defined as **genes that are recurrently affected by genetic aberrations in cancers.** This is **probably because these genes directly contribute to the malignant behavior of cancer cells.**

Mutations in cancer genes may be acquired or inherited: Cancer genes are **formed from the mutations of normal genes.** The cause of the **mutations** that are responsible for carcinogenesis **may be either acquired or inherited.**

- **Acquired mutations in cancer genes**: In most cancers, the causative mutations that give rise to cancer genes are acquired during life and may occur spontaneously. Hence, **these mutations are confined only to the cancer cells.** The cause of the acquired mutations includes the action of environmental agents such as **chemicals, radiation, or viruses.**
- **Inherited mutations in cancer genes:** Causative mutations sometimes are inherited in the germ line. Therefore, **these mutations are present in every cell in the body.** The affected individual is at a higher risk of developing cancer. In families with germ-line mutations, these mutations are passed from generation to generation and cancer behaves like an inherited trait.

Classification of cancer genes: Cancer genes can be classified into four major functional classes: (i) oncogenes, (ii) tumor suppressor genes, (iii) genes that regulate apoptosis, and (iv) genes that regulate interactions between tumor cells and host cells (**Box 7.4**).

Oncogenes are discussed on pages 235-9 and tumor suppressor genes on page 239-45.

TABLE 7.10 Most common types of cancers.	
Common location of tumors in descending order according to the incidence	
Males	***Females***
Prostate	Breast
Lung and bronchus	Lung and bronchus
Colon and rectum	Colon and rectum
Urinary bladder	Uterine corpus
Melanoma of the skin	Thyroid
Kidney	Melanoma of skin
Non-Hodgkin lymphoma	Non-Hodgkin lymphoma

Genes that Regulate Apoptosis

Apoptosis is a programmed cell death and **is one of the normal protective mechanisms by which a cell with DNA damage (mutation) undergoes cell death.** Many types of signals such as DNA damage, potent oncoproteins such as MYC, and loss of adhesion to the basement membrane (termed anoikis), can initiate apoptosis.

Genes that regulate apoptosis: They mainly act by increasing the survival of the cells, rather than stimulating the proliferation of cells. In cancer cells, the genes that protect against apoptosis (i.e., anti-apoptotic genes) are

BOX 7.4: Major functional classes of cancer genes.

- Oncogenes
- Tumor suppressor genes
- Genes that regulate apoptosis
- Genes that regulate interactions between tumor cells and host cells

often overexpressed, whereas those that promote apoptosis (i.e., proapoptotic genes) are either underexpressed or functionally inactivated by mutations.

Mutations or abnormalities in the genes that regulate apoptosis: It may result in the accumulation of neoplastic cells due to less death and increased survival of the cells. There may be **gain-of-function mutations in anti-apoptotic genes** (their products suppress apoptosis) **and loss-of-function mutations in proapoptotic genes** (their products promote cell death). The *apoptosis-regulating genes* can behave as **proto-oncogenes** (loss of one copy is enough) or **tumor suppressor genes** (loss of both copies required).

Genes that Regulate Interactions Between Tumor Cells and Host Cells

Genes that regulate interactions between tumor cells and host cells are also recurrently mutated or functionally altered in certain malignant tumors. Important in this group are genes that enhance or inhibit the recognition of tumor cells by the host immune system.

Mutations in Cancer Genes

In most cancers, the specific mutations that form cancer genes are acquired during life, and these mutations are found only in the cancer cells. Sometimes, specific causative mutations are inherited in the germline. Hence, these mutations are present in every cell in the body. These affected individuals are at high risk for particular cancers (**Table 7.11**).

GENETIC LESIONS IN CANCER

TABLE 7.11 Examples of inherited predisposition to cancer.

Inherited predisposition	*Gene(s) involved*
Autosomal Dominant Cancer Syndromes	
Retinoblastoma	*RB*
Li-Fraumeni syndrome (various tumors)	*TP53*
Familial adenomatous polyposis/ colon cancer	*APC*
Breast and ovarian tumors	*BRCA1, BRCA2*
Neurofibromatosis 1 and 2	*NF1, NF2*
Hereditary nonpolyposis colon cancer	*MSH2, MLH1, MSH6*
Melanoma	CDKN2A
Autosomal Recessive Syndromes of Defective DNA Repair	
Xeroderma pigmentosum	Genes involved in nucleotide excision repair
Ataxia-telangiectasia	*ATM*
Bloom syndrome	*BLM*

Genetic changes in cancer may be **minute or large** enough to be identified in a karyotype.

Driver and Passenger Mutations

Driver mutations: These mutations alter the function of cancer genes and thus directly contribute to the development or progression of cancer. These mutations are usually acquired.

Passenger mutations: These are **acquired mutations that do not affect cellular behavior**. Passenger mutations may become driver mutations if selective pressure on the tumor changes (e.g., treatment with an effective therapeutic drug).

Tumor cells may acquire driver mutations by different mechanism.

Point Mutations

Point mutation is characterized by the substitution of a single nucleotide base by a different base in a gene (*refer* page 273). It may change the code in a triplet of bases and lead to the replacement of one amino acid by another in the gene product. **Point mutations in genes can either activate or inactivate the protein products of the affected genes. It depends on the exact position of the point mutation and its consequence.**

Point mutations in proto-oncogenes: Point mutation is a common mechanism of oncogene activation. It can convert proto-oncogenes into oncogenes and usually produce a **gain of function**. For example, point mutations that convert the proto-oncogene ***RAS*** into a cancer gene *RAS* mutations are observed in~85% of pancreatic cancers and 45% of colon cancer, point mutations of ***RET*** in leukemia and ***BRAF*** in melanoma.

Point mutations in tumor suppressor genes: They can reduce or disable the function of the protein product of the gene. The tumor suppressor gene that is most commonly affected by point mutations in cancer is *TP53.*

Gene Rearrangements

Genetic events that lead to gene rearrangements may be by chromosomal translocations, inversions, deletions, or others. Specific gene rearrangements are commonly observed in certain malignant tumors, particularly those of hematopoietic cells and other mesenchymal cells. There are two ways by which gene rearrangements can activate proto-oncogenes: by (i) overexpression or (2) forming a chimeric gene.

Gene rearrangements causing overexpression of proto-oncogenes: Some gene rearrangements lead to overexpression of proto-oncogenes. This is by removing these genes from their normal regulatory elements (leads to loss of normal regulatory control) **and placing them under the control of a highly active promoter or enhancer (promotes proliferation). Examples are as follows:**

- **Burkitt lymphoma:** In more than 90% of *Burkitt lymphoma,* the tumor cells show a balanced reciprocal translocation, usually between chromosomes 8 and 14[**t (8;14) (q24; q32)]**. It leads to overexpression of the *MYC* gene on chromosome 8 by juxtaposition of *MYC* with immunoglobulin heavy chain gene regulatory elements on chromosome 14 (*refer* **Fig. 12.20**). It leads to **uncontrolled cell proliferation** and **inhibition** of apoptosis.
- **Follicular lymphoma:** In this tumor, a balanced reciprocal translocation occurs between chromosomes 14 and 18. It leads to overexpression of the antiapoptotic gene *BCL2* on chromosome 18. It is also driven by immunoglobulin gene regulatory elements as in Burkitt lymphoma.

Oncogenic gene rearrangements produce fusion genes encoding novel chimeric proteins: Reciprocal translocation may lead to chimeric genes. The chimeric protein produced can cause cellular proliferation. A classic example is the Philadelphia (Ph) chromosome in chronic myeloid leukemia. It shows a **balanced reciprocal translocation (seen** in more than 90% of cases) between the long arm of chromosomes 9 and 22, i.e., **t (9;22) (q34;q11.2). The shortened chromosome 22 is termed Philadelphia chromosome** (*refer* **Fig. 12.9**). *ABL* (Abelson murine leukemia virus) proto-oncogene from chromosome 9 **joins** the ***BCR*** (breakpoint cluster region) on chromosome 22 and produces a new **chimeric (fusion) gene called BCR-ABL oncogene. This causes cell division** and **inhibition of apoptosis.**

Deletions

Recurrent deletion of specific regions of chromosomes in cancer cells usually leads to the loss of particular tumor suppressor genes. Chromosomal deletions are more **common in non-hematopoietic solid tumors** and are the second most common structural abnormality found in tumor cells. Deletion is **common with tumor suppressor** genes and causes **loss of particular tumor suppressor gene protein.** Example: **Deletion of RB gene** (involving chromosome 13q14) is associated with **retinoblastoma.** Deletion of chromosome 17p is associated with the loss of *TP53* (the most important tumor suppressor gene).

Gene Amplification

Gene amplification is a chromosomal alteration in which there is an **increased number (several hundred) of gene copies. Proto-oncogenes may be converted to oncogenes by gene amplification**. Gene amplification produces several hundred copies of the proto-oncogene in tumor cells. This leads to **overexpression and hyperactivity of otherwise normal protein** products of the gene. It has been found mainly in **human solid tumors**. Gene amplification

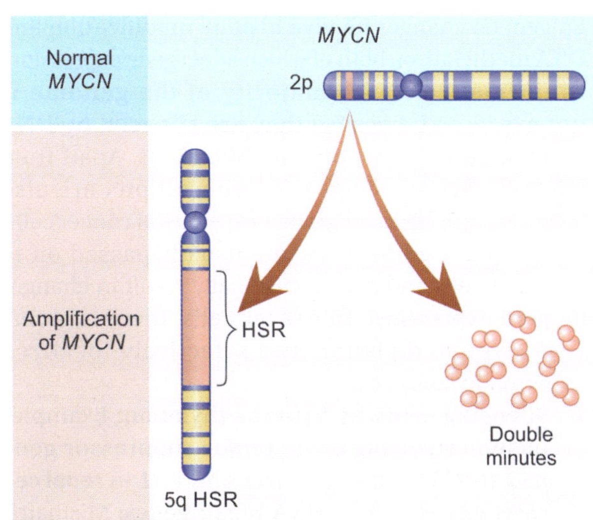

Fig. 7.14: Amplification of the *N-MYC* gene in neuroblastomas. The *MYCN* gene is present normally on chromosome 2p. It becomes amplified and is seen either as extrachromosomal double minutes or as a chromosomally integrated, homogeneous staining region (HSR).

can produce two patterns **(Fig. 7.14)**: (1) **multiple small, extrachromosomal structures** called *double minutes/* dmins and (2) *homogeneously staining regions (HSR).* In **homogeneous staining regions (HSR)** increased copies of the gene are inserted into new chromosomal locations, which may be distant from the normal location of the involved genes. Because regions containing amplified genes do not show normal banding. They give rise to a homogeneous staining pattern in a G-banded karyotype. Examples: (1) **N-MYC gene amplified in neuroblastomas** and associated with poor prognosis. (2) **HER2/Neu (also called ERBB2) amplification in breast cancer.**

Aneuploidy

Aneuploidy is the **presence of chromosome numbers that are not multiple of haploid numbers** (i.e., multiples of 23). It is common in cancers, particularly in carcinomas.

MicroRNAs and Cancer

MicroRNAs (miRNAs) are short, noncoding, single-stranded RNAs. They act as negative regulators of genes and control cell growth, differentiation, and survival. They can also contribute to carcinogenesis by (a) increasing the expression of oncogenes or (2) reducing the expression of tumor suppressor genes.

Epigenetic Modifications and Cancer

Definition: Epigenetics is a **reversible, heritable mechanisms that control gene expression independent of DNA base sequences. It occurs without mutation.** It is unrelated to the gene nucleotide sequence. **Epigenetics is the mechanism that controls gene expression.**

- Epigenetic changes **involve histone modification** and **DNA methylation**, both of which affect gene expression.
- **In normal cells**, the **majority of the genome is not expressed**, because **they are silenced by DNA methylation and histone modifications**. Apart from DNA mutations, epigenetic aberrations are also responsible for the malignant properties of cancer cells.
- Epigenetic modifications are usually passed on to daughter cells and may occasionally result in changes in gene expression. In cancer cells, there is global DNA hypomethylation and selectively localized hypermethylation, e.g.:
    - **Silencing genes by hypermethylation**: Examples include silencing of (1) **tumor suppressor gene *p53*, *BRCA1*** in breast cancer, and ***VHL* in renal cell carcinomas** and (2) **DNA repair genes:** Mismatch repair gene ***MLH1* in colorectal cancer**.
    - **Hypomethylation** can **cause chromosomal instability**, derepression of growth regulatory genes, and overexpression of antiapoptotic genes and induce tumors.
    - **Changes in histones:** Cancer cells may show changes in histones near genes that influence cellular behavior.

Unlike DNA mutations, **epigenetic changes are potentially reversible** by drugs that inhibit DNA-or histone-modifying factors.

MOLECULAR BASIS OF CANCER

PA 7.2 (CC): Describe the molecular basis of cancer.

All cancers exhibit several fundamental changes in cell physiology. These changes are considered the hallmarks of cancer (Box 7.5). Most cancer cells acquire these hallmarks during their development, generally due to mutations in critical genes. Apart from hallmarks, two cancer-enabling factors aid and accelerate the process namely *cancer-promoting inflammation* and *genomic instability*. Conventionally, the gene symbols are italicized but their protein products are not (e.g., *RB* gene and RB protein, *TP53* and p53, *MYC* and MYC).

Q. Enumerate steps of malignant transformation of a cell.

Hallmarks of cancer: Normal cells may undergo malignant transformation by corrupting any one of the normal steps involved in cell proliferation.

Self-sufficiency in Growth Signals

Entry and progress of normal cells through the cell cycle (see below) is highly regulated. However, cancer cells enter and progress through the cell cycle without normal control. **This self-sufficiency in growth in cancer cells is generally due to gain-of-function mutations that convert proto-oncogenes to oncogenes (*refer* page 235).** Oncogenes encode proteins called *oncoproteins*. These oncoproteins promote growth of cells even in the absence of normal growth-promoting signals.

BOX 7.5: Eight hallmarks of cancer.

1. Self-sufficiency in growth signals (by growth-promoting oncogenes)
2. Insensitivity to growth-inhibitory signals (mutated tumor suppressor gene)
3. Altered cellular metabolism *(the Warburg effect)*
4. Evasion of apoptosis (escaping cell death by apoptosis)
5. Limitless replicative potential (immortality) (by telomerase)
6. Sustained angiogenesis (sustained perfusion of cancer)
7. Invasion and metastasis *(cancer dissemination)*
8. Evasion of immune surveillance *(evasion of host immunity)*

Steps in normal cell proliferation (Fig. 7.15): To understand the process by which oncogenes produce inappropriate cell growth, the sequence of events that characterize normal cell proliferation is briefly outlined. Under physiologic conditions, cells follow a controlled proliferation. The signals that lead to cell proliferation involve different sequential steps. These are as follows:

1. **Growth factor binding to its specific receptor** on the cell membrane.
2. **Transient and limited activation of the growth factor receptor**. This activates several signal-transducing proteins on the inner aspect of the cell membrane. Following this signaling, the receptor reverts to its resting state.
3. **Intracellular signal transduction:** Most of the signal-transducing proteins are located on the inner aspect of

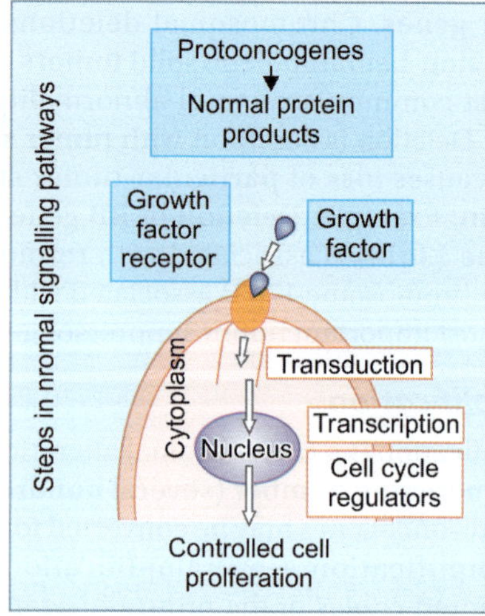

Fig. 7.15: Steps involved in a downstream signaling pathway involved in normal cell proliferation. Normal proto-oncogenes encode different molecules involved in the steps.

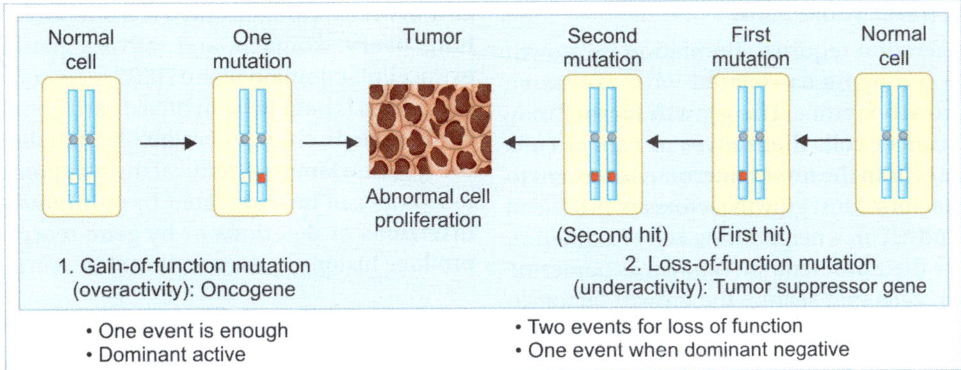

Fig. 7.16: Diagrammatic representation of gain of function (oncogenes) and loss of function (tumor suppressor gene).

the cell membrane. They **receive external signals** and get activated (by binding of growth factor to its growth factor receptors). They **transmit the growth signal across the cytoplasm to the nucleus of the cell** by second messengers or a cascade of signal transduction molecules. The most important signal-transducing protein belongs to the **RAS family and ABL**.

4. **Transcription:** Activation of nuclear regulatory factors initiates and regulates DNA transcription. This results in the synthesis of other cellular components that are required for cell division, such as organelles, membrane components, and ribosomes.
5. **Cell cycle:** Entry and progression of the cell into the cell cycle ultimately results in the division of the cell.

In cancer cells, each one of the above-mentioned five steps is susceptible to undergo deviation from normal.

Q. Define proto-oncogenes and write a short note oncogene. List the different products of oncogenes.

Q. Describe the mechanism of activation of oncogene giving suitable examples.

Oncogenes

Oncogenes are genes that, **when expressed in cells induce tumor formation**. This is by **promoting increased cell growth.**

Proto-oncogenes: These are **normal cellular genes**, which encode several nuclear proteins that **regulate normal cell proliferation, differentiation, and survival**. Proto-oncogenes have multiple roles, but all act at some level in signaling pathways involved in the proliferation of cells.

Oncogenes: Oncogenes are **mutated (altered) or overexpressed versions of normal cellular genes, namely *proto-oncogenes***. Oncogenes **promote autonomous cell growth in cancer cells**. Most oncogenes encode transcription factors that are involved in pro-growth signaling pathways or factors that increase the survival of cells.

Oncoproteins: Oncogenes usually produce increased encoded **gene products (proteins) called oncoproteins (products of oncogenes)** and cause tumors.

- **Gain-of-function mutations (Fig. 7.16):** The mutations in oncogenes are called **"gain-of-function" mutations because they can transform cells even in the presence of a normal copy of the same gene.** Thus, oncogenes **behave like dominant genes** over their normal counterparts, because **mutation of a single allele is sufficient to produce a pro-oncogenic effect. Oncogenes** can **promote cell growth in the absence** of external normal growth-promoting/**mitogenic signals/stimuli.**
- **Oncoprotein production is not under normal regulatory control:** The cells with an oncogene, proliferate without the usual requirement for external signals and are freed from checkpoints and **growth becomes autonomous. Oncoproteins act like accelerators that speed the replication of cells and their DNA. In contrast, tumor suppressors act as brakes that slow or arrest this process.**

Groups of oncogenes: One or more genes that stimulate cell proliferation (multiplication) are usually dysregulated or mutated during oncogenesis. Tumor-driving mutations may occur at any step of the growth factor-induced signal transduction pathway and cell cycle regulation. The oncoproteins that cause cancer cells to proliferate can be grouped according to their role in the signaling pathways (**Box 7.6**).

Those mutations drive cellular proliferation without the normal restraints that match cell numbers to the body's needs.

BOX 7.6: Groups of oncoproteins that lead to self-sufficiency in growth signals.

- Growth factors
- Growth factor receptors
- Signal transduction proteins
- Nuclear transcription factors
- Cell cycle regulators.

Growth Factors (*refer* Table 7.14)

Normal cell proliferation requires stimulation by growth factors. Neoplasm may be associated with **excessive production of growth factors. The growth factors may be produced by cancer cells themselves or cancer cells stimulate stromal cells in the tumor microenvironment to produce growth factors.** Most growth factors are produced by one cell type and act on a neighboring cell of a different type and stimulate their proliferation (known as paracrine action). Normally, cells that secrete the growth factor do not express that factor's receptor. Thus, it prevents its own stimulation. This "rule" is broken in several ways by certain cancers.

The action of growth factors in cancer: These oncoproteins (products of oncogenes) may act in one of two ways: (1) autocrine or (2) paracrine action.

- **Autocrine action**: Some cancer cells synthesize the same growth factors to which they are responsive. For example, in many **glioblastomas** (malignant glial cell tumors) the tumor cells secrete **excess platelet-derived growth factor (PDGF)** and have amplifications of the PDGF receptor gene expression, and many sarcomas secrete transforming growth factor-α (TGF-α) and express its receptor.
- **Paracrine action:** In these tumors, the growth factors are produced by one cell type and act on a neighboring cell and stimulate their proliferation. In some cancers, the tumor cells send signals that stimulate normal cells in the supporting stroma to produce growth factors. These in turn stimulate tumor growth.

Growth Factor Receptors (*refer* Table 7.14)

The next step in growth signaling is growth factor receptors. **Normally, when the growth factor binds to the growth factor receptors, it produces transient dimerization (activity).** Many of these receptors have intrinsic kinase activity when activated by growth factor binding. **Constitutive** (unrestrained) **dimerization of growth factor receptors produces continuous mitogenic signals to the cell, even in the absence of the growth factor. Many growth factor receptors function as oncoproteins when they are mutated or if they are overexpressed.** The mutated receptors are either constitutively active, delivering mitogenic signals to cells even in the absence of growth factors, or are hyperresponsive to growth factors.

Overexpression (*refer* **page 233**) **of growth factor receptor:** An example is **overexpression of the epidermal growth factor (EGF) receptor** family may be due to gene amplification. For example, **ERBB1 is the EGF receptor, which is overexpressed in squamous cell carcinomas of the lung** (80% of cases), **glioblastomas** (50% or more), and **epithelial tumors of the head and neck** (80–100%).

Gene amplification (*refer* **page 233**)**:** The gene encoding an EGF-related receptor, **HER2 (ERBB2) is amplified in about 20% of breast cancers and a few adenocarcinomas of the lung, ovary, stomach, and salivary glands.** Blocking the extracellular domain of the HER2 receptor with anti-HER2 antibodies is beneficial in breast carcinoma.

Other genetic changes are involved in the stimulation of the tyrosine kinase activity of the receptors. Growth factor receptors can be stimulated by **point mutations or small insertions or deletions or by gene rearrangements** that produce fusion genes encoding chimeric receptors.

Signal-transducing Proteins (*refer* Table 7.14)

Different genes encode different components of signaling pathways downstream of growth factor receptors. **Cancer cells usually acquire growth autonomy because of mutations in these different genes.** The signal-transducing proteins couple growth factor receptors to their nuclear targets. These proteins are activated by binding of ligands to growth factor receptors. Two important oncogenic signaling (signal-transducing) molecules are RAS and ABL.

RAS

Function of normal RAS (Fig. 7.17)

RAS proteins (product of the *RAS* gene) are attached to the cytoplasmic aspect of the cell membrane by farnesyl (also the endoplasmic reticulum and Golgi membranes).

- **Regulation of RAS activity**: RAS is a member of a family of small G proteins and it binds guanosine nucleotides [guanosine diphosphate (GDP) and guanosine triphosphate (GTP)]. The activity of RAS is regulated by the relative binding of GDP and GTP. Normally, RAS orderly cycle between a quiescent (inactive) state [RAS proteins bound to guanosine diphosphate (GDP)] and an active (excited) signal transmitting state (RAS is bound to GTP).
- **Activation of RAS:** RAS is inactive when bound to GDP. The binding of growth factors (e.g., EGF, PDGF) to growth factor receptors stimulates cells by exchange of GDP for GTP. This change from inactive GDP to active GTP in turn activates RAS. The active (excited) GTP signal-emitting state is short-lived because an intrinsic enzyme GTPase (guanosine triphosphatase) hydrolyzes GTP to GDP. This releases a phosphate group and returns the GTP to its quiescent GDP-bound state.
- **GAPs:** The GTPase activity of activated RAS is markedly increased by a family of GTPase-activating proteins (GAPs). These GAPs act as molecular brakes and prevent uncontrolled RAS activation by causing hydrolysis of GTP to GDP.
- **Activation of downstream pathways:** Activated RAS stimulates downstream regulators of cell proliferation by several interconnected pathways. These pathways converge on the nucleus and alter the expression of genes that regulate growth, such as MYC.

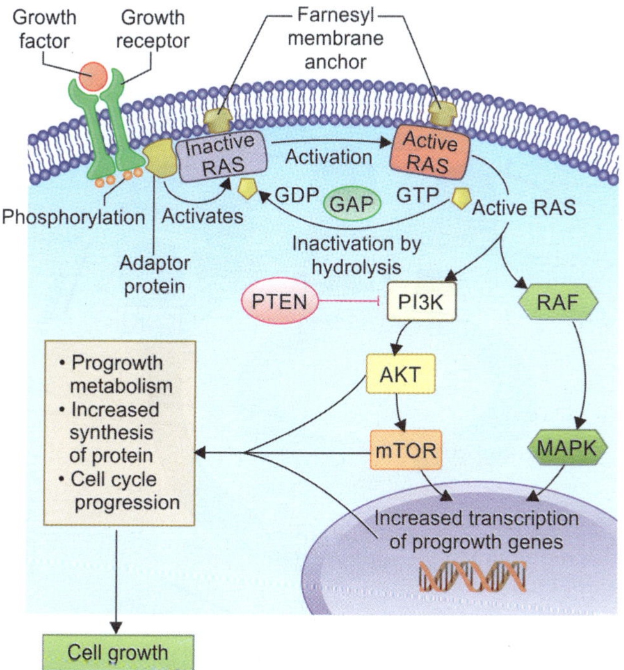

Fig. 7.17: Schematic representation of the mode of action of RAS. RAS is anchored to the cell membrane by the farnesyl moiety and is essential for its action. In a normal cell, when a growth factor binds to the growth factor receptor, inactive (GDP bound) RAS become activated to a GTP bound state. The active GTP state is short-lived because the enzyme GTPase hydrolyses GTP to GDP. Activated RAS in turn transduces proliferative signals to the nucleus along two pathways: (i) the "RAF/MAP kinase pathway" and (ii) the "PI3K/AKT kinase" pathway. GAPs and PTEN (inhibitor of PI3 kinase), act as important brakes on signaling downstream of activated RAS. Growth factor receptors, RAS, PI3K, MYC, and D cyclins are activated by mutations in various cancers.

(GDP: guanosine diphosphate; GTP: guanosine triphosphate; MAPK: mitogen-activated protein kinase; mTOR: mammalian target of rapamycin; PI3K: phosphatidylinositol 3-kinase).

RAS in cancer

Q. Write a short note on the RAS oncogene.

Mutated RAS: *RAS* is the most mutated oncogene in tumors. RAS proto-oncogene can be converted to RAS oncogene. The mutated *RAS* is trapped in its activated GTP-bound form resulting in continuous proliferation of cells. The human genome contains three types of *RAS* genes.

Tumors with RAS mutations (Table 7.12): About 20% of all tumors contain mutated *RAS* genes, and it is more frequent in certain cancers (e.g., pancreatic adenocarcinoma).

TABLE 7.12 Examples of tumors with RAS mutations.

Type of mutated RAS	*Associated tumors*
KRAS	Adenocarcinomas of the colon, lung, and pancreas
HRAS	Bladder and kidney tumors
NRAS	Melanoma, hematopoietic tumors

Type of mutation in RAS: RAS most commonly becomes constitutively activated because of point mutations. This interferes with the breakdown of GTP and RAS stays in the GTP-bound active form. Thus, the cell continuously proliferates. Activated RAS stimulates downstream regulators of proliferation. The mutational activation of the signaling intermediates involved in RAS signaling pathways also mimics the growth-promoting effects of activated RAS. Two main downstream pathways send the signal to the nucleus resulting in cell proliferation. These are: (i) **RAF/ERK/MAP kinase pathway, and (ii) PI3 kinase/AKT (PI3K/AKT) pathway (Fig. 7.17).**

- **BRAF mutations:** BRAF is a serine/threonine protein kinase belonging to the "RAF/ERK/MAP kinase pathway." Similar to activating RAS mutations, BRAF mutations activate transcription factors. BRAF, which is part of the so-called is mutated in more than 60% of **melanomas** and is associated with unregulated cell proliferation.
- **Mutations in kinases of the PI3K family:** Mutations of phosphatidylinositol-3 kinase (PI3 kinase) in the PI3K/AKT pathway also occur with high frequency in some tumor types and are associated with unregulated cell proliferation.

ABL

Several non-receptor tyrosine kinases function as signal-transducing molecules. A well-known ABL product of ***ABL*** is a proto-oncogene and has tyrosine kinase activity.

Translocation of *ABL* gene: In **chronic myelogenous leukemia and certain acute leukemias,** part of the ***ABL*** gene from its normal site on chromosome 9 translocates and fuses with part of the breakpoint cluster region ***(BCR)*** gene on chromosome 22 (*refer* **Fig. 12.9**). It produces a new **chimeric (fusion) gene called *BCR-ABL*, thus converting the *ABL* proto-oncogene into an oncogene.** This fusion gene encodes a BCR-ABL hybrid protein. It contains the ABL tyrosine kinase domain and a BCR domain. The BCR-ABL hybrid protein activates all the signals that are downstream of RAS. This **leads to cell growth. BCR-ABL kinase inhibitors** (imatinib mesylate) **show dramatic clinical response in patients with chronic myeloid leukemia.**

Nuclear Transcription Factors (*refer* Table 7.14)

The signaling through oncoproteins such as RAS or ABL inappropriately and continuously stimulates nuclear transcription factors. These transcription factors bind DNA and regulate the transcription of genes.

Transcription: It is a process in which RNA is synthesized from DNA.

Transcription factors: Transcription factors cause the expression of growth-promoting genes which activate the cell cycle. The transcription factors regulate the expression of growth-promoting genes, such as cyclins.

TABLE 7.13 Examples of tumors with dysregulated MYC.

Tumor	*Mode of MYC dysregulation*
Burkitt lymphoma	(8;14) translocation
Cancers of breast, colon, lung, etc.	*MYC* amplification
Neuroblastoma	*MYCN* gene amplification
Small cell cancers of the lung	*MYCL* gene amplification

Mutation of transcription genes: Tumor may develop due to mutations of transcription genes. The mutation results in oncogenes like ***MYC, MYB, JUN, FOS,*** and ***REL***.

Q. Write a short note on MYC oncogene.

MYC

Normal actions of MYC: MYC is one of the transcription factors encoded by the *MYC* gene expressed in all cells during normal cell proliferation. *MYC* is considered a **master transcriptional regulator of cell growth. MYC** mainly functions by **activating the transcription of several genes involved in cell growth.** These include several growth-promoting genes, such as cyclin-dependent kinases (CDKs).

Mutation of *MYC* gene: It is **most common in human tumors (Table 7.13).**

- **Mode of action: Mutation of *MYC* promotes tumorigenesis by (i) promoting the progression of cells through the cell cycle and (ii) alterations in metabolism that support cell growth.** The metabolic pathways produce the building blocks (e.g., amino acids, lipids, nucleotides) needed for cell growth and division.

Control of the Cell Cycle (*refer* Table 7.14)

The growth-promoting stimuli ultimately lead to the entry of quiescent cells into the cell cycle. The cell cycle (*refer* **pages 91-2 and Fig. 3.20**) is a complex process that regulates cellular proliferation.

Cyclins, Cyclin-dependent Kinases, and Cyclin-dependent Kinase Inhibitors

The cell cycle is regulated by several activators and inhibitors. These include (i) cyclins, (ii) cyclin-dependent kinases (CDKs), and (iii) cyclin-dependent kinase inhibitors.

Normal role of cyclins, cyclin-dependent kinases (CDKs), and cyclin-dependent kinase inhibitors

Q. Write a short note on the role of cyclins in the cell cycle.

Cyclins: These proteins are named so because their levels cyclically rise and fall due to production and degradation respectively. There are more than 15 cyclins of which cyclins D, E, A, and B appear sequentially (one after another) during the cell cycle.

Cyclin-dependent kinases (CDKs): These are cyclin-associated enzymes. CDKs can phosphorylate protein

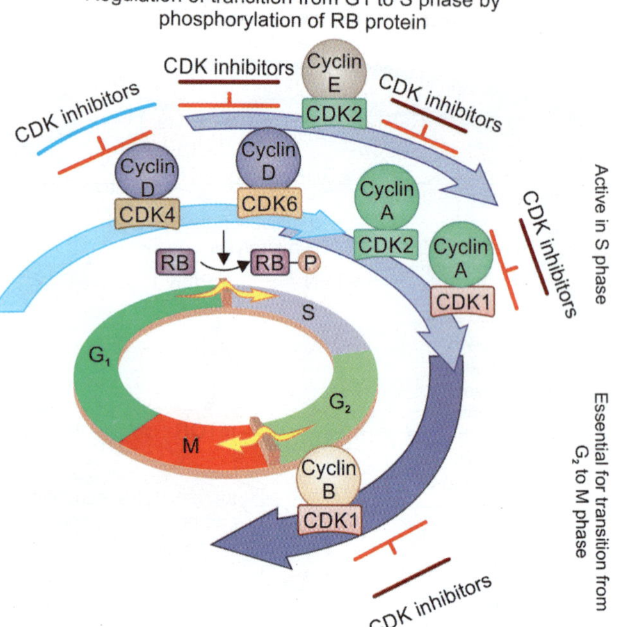

Fig. 7.18: Role of cyclins, CDKs, and CDK inhibitors in regulation of the cell cycle. Cyclin D-CDK4, cyclin D-CDK6, and cyclin E-CDK2 promote the passage of the cell cycle through the G_1-S checkpoint by phosphorylating the RB protein (RB-P). Cyclins active in the S phase are cyclin A-CDK2 and cyclin A-CDK1. The transition from G_2 to M phase is by cyclin B-CDK1. CDK inhibitors can block the activity of CDKs and progression through the cell cycle.

(CDK: cyclin-dependent kinase).

substrates (i.e., kinase activity) and form complexes with specific cyclin partners **(Fig. 7.18)**. The CDK–cyclin complexes promote the progression of the cell cycle following which the cyclin levels decline quickly. Like a relay race, in the cell cycle, each step is regulated by a distinct set of cyclin/CDK complexes. When a set of cyclin/CDK complexes leaves the track, the next set takes over.

Two main checkpoints in the cell cycle: These are sensing mechanisms that sense DNA or chromosomal damage and constitute quality control in the cell cycle. There are two check points **(i) G_1-S checkpoint and (ii) G_2-M checkpoint.** These checkpoints make sure that cells with defective DNA do not go forward in the cell cycle (i.e., they arrest the progression of the cell cycle). If the cells have defective DNA, activation of checkpoint delays the progression of the cell cycle and triggers DNA repair mechanisms. If the genetic defect is too severe to be repaired, the cells either undergo apoptosis or enter a nonreplicative state called *senescence*—mainly via p53-dependent mechanisms.

CDK inhibitors (CDKIs): While cyclins and CDKs drive the cell cycle, **negative control over the cell cycle** is achieved by **silencing the CDKs by their inhibitors (CDKIs).** The job of *CDK inhibitors (CDKIs)* is enforcement of the cell-cycle checkpoints. CDKIs modulate CDK-cyclin complex activity. There are several different CDKIs: (i) one family of CDKIs inhibits multiple CDKs, and (ii) another family of CDKIs inhibits cyclin CDK4 and cyclin CDK6.

Dysregulation of the cell cycle in cancer cells

Loss of normal cell cycle control is central to malignant transformation in many tumors.

Defective CDKI checkpoint proteins: Of two checkpoints namely G_1 -S and G_2 -M checkpoints involved in the **cell cycle, particularly the G1-S checkpoint is likely to be lost in cancer cells.** Once cells pass through the G_1/S checkpoint, the cells usually undergo cell division. The cells with defects in this checkpoint proliferate excessively. Almost all cancers appear to have genetic lesions with defective G_1/S checkpoint. This allows the cells with damaged DNA to continually reenter the S phase and divide. These cells produce mutated daughter cells that can undergo malignant transformation. They belong to two major categories.

1. ***Gain-of-function mutations involving CDK4 or D cyclins:*** These oncogenes **promote G_1/S progression.** Mutations that increase the expression of cyclin D or CDK4 are common in neoplastic transformation.
   - **Overexpression of cyclin D genes:** Cyclin D include D1, D2, and D3 and they undergo mutations in many cancers. These include **cancers of the breast, esophagus, and liver**, a few lymphomas, and plasma cell tumors.
   - **Amplification of the *CDK4* gene:** It occurs in **melanomas, sarcomas, and glioblastomas**.
2. ***Loss-of-function mutations involving CDKIs:*** CDKIs act as tumor suppressors. CDKIs are disabled in many malignant tumors. For example, germline mutations of **CDKN2A** (a gene encoding the CDK inhibitor) are observed in **some familial melanomas**. Acquired deletion or epigenetic silencing of *CDKN2A* occurs in many gliomas, carcinomas, sarcomas, and leukemias.

Apart from the above-mentioned conditions, loss of function mutations in *RB* (a tumor suppressor gene) can disable the G_1 S checkpoint.

Categories of oncogenes and examples of associated tumors are presented in **Table 7.14**.

TABLE 7.14 Categories of oncogenes and examples of associated tumors.

Category of oncogene	*Proto-oncogene*	*Examples of associated tumors*
Growth Factors		
PDGF-β chain	PDGFB	Astrocytoma
FGFs	HST1	Osteosarcoma
	FGF3	Cancer of the stomach, bladder, breast, and melanoma
HGF	HGF	Hepatocellular carcinomas, thyroid cancer
Growth Factor Receptors		
EGF-receptor family	ERBB1 (EGFR)	Adenocarcinoma of lung
ALK receptor	ALK	Adenocarcinoma of the lung, certain lymphomas, neuroblastoma
Receptor for neurotrophic factors	RET	Multiple endocrine neoplasia 2A and B, familial medullary carcinoma thyroid
Receptor for KIT ligand	KIT	Gastrointestinal stromal tumors, seminomas, leukemias
FMS-like tyrosine kinase 3	FLT3	Leukemia
PDGF receptor	PDGFRB	Gliomas, leukemias
Signal Transduction Proteins		
GTP-binding (G) proteins	KRAS	Tumors of the colon, lung, and pancreas
	HRAS	Tumors of the bladder and kidney
	NRAS	Melanomas, hematologic malignancies
RAS signal transduction	BRAF	Melanomas, leukemias, colon carcinoma
Nonreceptor tyrosine kinase	ABL	Chronic myelogenous leukemia, acute lymphoblastic leukemia
JAK/STAT signal transduction	JAK2	Myeloproliferative neoplasms, acute lymphoblastic leukemia
Notch signal transduction	NOTCH1	Leukemias, lymphomas, breast carcinoma
Nuclear Regulatory Proteins/Transcription Factors		
Transcriptional activators	MYC	Burkitt lymphoma
	NMYC	Neuroblastoma
Cell Cycle Regulators		
Cyclins	CCND1 (Cyclin D1)	Mantle cell lymphoma, multiple myeloma, breast, and esophageal cancers
Cyclin-dependent kinase	CDK4	Glioblastoma, melanoma, sarcoma

(CDK: cyclin D kinases; EGF: epidermal growth factor; FGF: fibroblast growth factor; HGF: hepatocyte growth factor; PDGF: platelet-derived growth factor).

Insensitivity to Growth Inhibitory Signals: Tumor Suppressor Genes

Q. Write a short note on tumor suppressor genes and cancers produced by their mutations.

Normal cells and tissues have complex mechanisms that prevent their indefinite proliferative growth. This prevents tumor development. The molecular guardians involved in this protection are called tumor suppressors and the genes that encode these proteins are tumor suppressor genes (TSGs). Cancer cells are generally insensitive to those restrictions.

Tumor Suppressor Genes

Tumor suppressor genes are **genes that normally prevent uncontrolled growth or cell proliferation.** When mutated or lost from a cell, they allow the cells to develop tumors. **Mutations of tumor suppressor genes may be hereditary and spontaneous.**

Loss of Heterozygosity

Both alleles must be activated for tumor formation: Each gene has two alleles. Usually, for the tumor to develop, **both normal alleles of tumor suppressor genes must be inactivated (damaged/mutated).**

- **Heterozygous state:** In this one allele of the tumor suppressor gene is normal and the other allele is inactive. **A heterozygous state (i.e., even the presence of one normal allele)** is **sufficient to protect against cancer.**
- **Loss of heterozygosity leads to cancer (Fig. 7.16): Cancer develops when the cell loses heterozygosity** (known as loss of heterozygosity—**LOH**) **for the normal tumor suppressor gene** by **deletion or somatic mutation**. Tumor can develop when the cell becomes homozygous (both alleles are inactive) for the mutant allele. Thus, mutated tumor suppressor genes usually behave in a recessive fashion. However, sometimes, the loss of a single allele of a tumor suppressor gene can lead to cell proliferation. **When loss of gene function is caused by damage to a single allele, it is called haploinsufficiency.**

Mechanism of action: Most tumor suppressors **inhibit cell growth through one or other mechanism**. Mutations that affect tumor suppressor genes usually cause a "**loss of function**." Some tumor suppressors **prevent cellular transformation** through other mechanisms. These include **altering cell metabolism** (e.g., the serine-threonine kinase STK11) or **maintaining genomic stability** (e.g., the DNA repair factors *BRCA1* and *BRCA2*).

Groups of Tumor Suppressor Genes

Tumor suppressor genes can be categorized into two general groups: (i) genes that act as brakes on cellular proliferation (**governors**) and (ii) genes that sense genomic damage (**guardians**).

Genes that act as brakes on cellular proliferation (governors)

Role of intact tumor suppressor gene: One group of tumor suppressor genes (e.g., ***RB*** **gene**) **are part of a regulatory network.** They act as important brakes on cellular proliferation. They apply **brakes on cell cycle progression and DNA replication.** They recognize genotoxic stress from any source and prevent the proliferation of these cells. Thus, these genes **prevent uncontrolled cell proliferation. The protein product of this tumor suppressor suppresses any of the various hallmarks of cancer.** Tumor suppressor proteins form a network of checkpoints and act as negative growth regulators. As discussed earlier, **oncogenes stimulate the proliferation of cells,** whereas **the protein products of most tumor suppressor genes apply brakes and prevent uncontrolled cell proliferation.** Cells with intact tumor suppressor genes may result in quiescence, or permanent arrest of the cell cycle (oncogene-induced senescence), rather than uncontrolled proliferation. These cells may ultimately undergo apoptosis.

Mutation or loss of tumor suppressor gene: In the cells with mutated (abnormalities) or loss of these groups of tumor suppressor genes, there will be a loss of function of these negative growth regulators (i.e., **failure of growth inhibition). This releases the brake for cellular proliferation, leads to failure of growth inhibition,** and cells are **transformed to develop tumors (neoplasia)**. So, a second mechanism of carcinogenesis results from the failure of the negative growth regulator (growth inhibition), due to deficiency of normal tumor suppressor genes and their products.

Genes that sense genomic damage ("Guardians")

The second group of tumor suppressor genes (e.g., *p53)* sense the genomic damage. Some guardian genes initiate a complex "damage control response" and prevent the proliferation of cells with genetic damage. If the genetic damage is too severe to be repaired, these genes induce apoptosis of those cells.

Insensitivity to growth inhibitory signals: Oncogenes are mutated proto-oncogenes that encode oncoproteins and promote cell growth. **The products of tumor suppressor genes apply brakes to cell proliferation.** The disruption of tumor suppressor genes makes the cells resistant to growth inhibition and mimics the growth-promoting effects of oncogenes.

Normal functions (actions) of tumor suppressor genes: The **products of tumor suppressor genes produce antigrowth signals**. These signals can **prevent cell proliferation** by several complementary mechanisms.

- **Entry of dividing cells to G_0 (quiescence) phase:** The signals may cause dividing cells to enter G_0 (quiescence) phase.
- **Lose replicative potential:** The cells may enter a postmitotic, differentiated pool and lose their replicative capacity.
- **Nonreplicative senescence:** By this mechanism, the cells escape from sustained cell growth. Finally, these cells may undergo death by apoptosis.

Selective examples of tumor suppressor genes are listed in **Box 7.7**.

Q. Write a short note on Knudson's two-hit hypothesis.

Knudson's two-hit hypothesis of oncogenesis: It explains the inherited and sporadic occurrence of an identical tumor. According to Knudson's hypothesis:

BOX 7.7: Selective examples of tumor suppressor genes.

- *RB*
- *p53*
- *PTEN*
- *BRCA 1* and *BRCA 2*
- WT1
- *APC/β*-catenin
- *SMAD 2* and *SMAD 4*
- NF1 and NF2
- TGF-β receptor
- E-cadherin

- **Two mutations (hits),** involving **both alleles** of tumor suppressor gene **are required to produce the tumor.**
- **In familial cases, one mutation (first hit) takes place in the germline,** and the **second hit after birth.**
- In **sporadic cases both mutations** (two hits) **develop after birth.**

Retinoblastoma Gene (RB)

Governor of the Cell Cycle

Q. Write a short note on the role (function) of the retinoblastoma (RB) gene in the cell cycle.

***RB* gene** was the **first discovered tumor suppressor gene.** It is **located on chromosome locus 13q14. *RB* gene is the governor of the cell cycle.** It is a model gene of this family of cancer suppressor genes.

Functions of the normal *RB* gene (Figs. 7.19A and B): The product of the *RB* gene is the **RB** protein. It is a DNA-binding protein expressed in all cells and is a **key negative regulator of the cell cycle.**

- **Active and inactive state of RB protein:** RB protein is present either in an **active hypophosphorylated** state (in quiescent cells) or **inactive hyperphosphorylated** state (in cells passing through the G_1/S cell cycle phase). Signals that promote cell cycle progression lead to the phosphorylation and inactivation of RB, while signals that block cell cycle progression maintain RB in an active hypophosphorylated state.
- **Action of active RB protein:** The cell cycle is tightly controlled by cyclins, and cyclin-dependent kinases (CDKs). Before the replication of DNA commences, the cells must pass through an important G_1 to S checkpoint. **RB protein regulates this G_1/S checkpoint of the cell cycle** thereby playing a crucial role in the cell cycle.

The mechanisms by which RB carries out G_1/S transition (Figs. 7.19A and B): These are as follows:

- **Active state of RB protein inhibits E2F-mediated transcription:** The initiation of **DNA replication (S phase) requires the activity of cyclin E/CDK2 complexes.** Growth inhibitors (e.g., TGF-β, p53) stimulate the synthesis of **CDK inhibitors, which keeps RB in a hypophosphorylated (active form).** E2F are transcription factors required for cell cycle progression. Early in G_1, the **hypophosphorylated, active form of RB binds and inhibits the function of E2F** transcription **factors** in two ways **(Figs. 7.19A and B).**
  1. **Sequestration of E2F factors: Active RB sequesters (isolates) E2F,** and prevents interaction of E2F with transcriptional activators.
  2. **Recruitment of chromatin remodeling factors that inhibit transcription of genes required for the S phase: Active RB recruit enzymes such as histone deacetylases and histone methyltransferases.** These enzymes **inhibit the transcription of genes** whose products are **required for the S phase** of the cell cycle.
- **Inactive state of RB protein and its effects: The inhibitory effect of RB is overcome by mitogenic signals that hyperphosphorylate RB** (RB becomes inactive).
  - **Inactivation of RB by cyclin D-CDK4/6 complexes:** Growth factor (mitogenic) signaling leads to the expression of cyclin D and forms cyclin D-CDK4/6 complexes. The cyclin D-CDK4/6 complexes phosphorylate (hyperphosphorylation) and inactivate RB (i.e., hypophosphorylated RB into inactive hyperphosphorylated RB).
  - **Release of E2F and progression of the cell cycle:** Inactivated RB releases E2F factors to induce the transcription of genes such as cyclin E. It forms cyclin E/CDK complexes and stimulates DNA replication allowing cells to progress through the cell cycle from G_1 to S phase. Once cells enter the S phase, they divide without additional stimulation by the growth factor. During the M phase of the cell cycle, the phosphate groups are removed from RB by phosphatases. This regenerates the active, hypophosphorylated form of RB.

Inactivation of RB Gene

***RB* gene is directly or indirectly inactivated in most cancers.**

Retinoblastoma

RB gene was discovered during the study of an uncommon (rare) **childhood tumor called retinoblastoma** derived from the retina.

Pathogenesis of retinoblastoma (Figs. 7.20A and B): Loss of function of both alleles of the *RB* leads to neoplastic proliferation of the retinal cells. Retinoblastoma may occur either as a hereditary or sporadic form. *Both normal alleles* (an individual inherits two alleles, one from each parent) *of the RB locus must be inactivated* (hence the two hits) for the development of retinoblastoma.

1. **Familial/hereditary retinoblastoma**: It constitutes about 40% of retinoblastoma and two hits occur as follows:

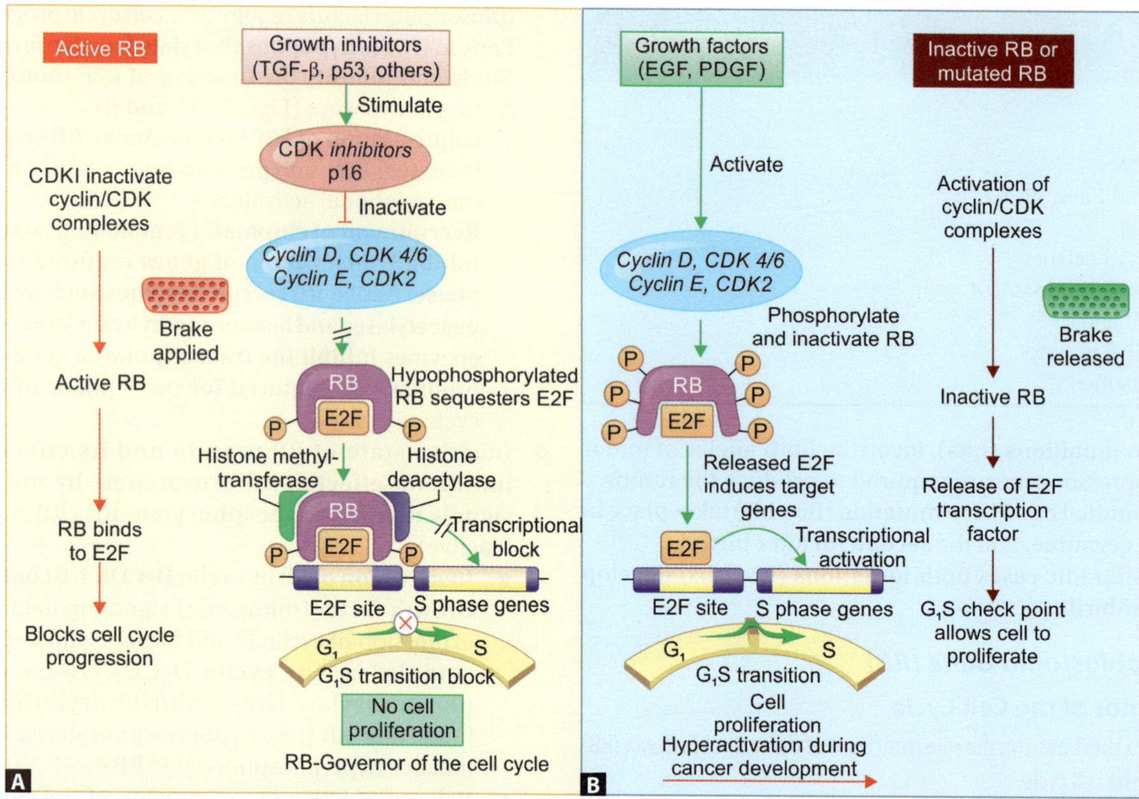

Figs. 7.19A and B: The role of RB in the regulation of the G_1–S checkpoint of the cell cycle: (A) Active RB. Growth inhibitors (e.g., TGF-β, p53) stimulate the synthesis of CDK inhibitors. These inhibitors keep RB in a hypophosphorylated (active) state. Hypophosphorylated RB in complex with E2F transcription factors binds to DNA. Active RB recruits chromatin remodeling factors (histone deacetylases and histone methyltransferases) and inhibits transcription of genes whose products are needed for the S phase of the cell cycle (inhibits progression from the G1-S phase of the cell cycle); (B) Inactive RB. Growth factors bind receptors that transmit signals and activate cyclin-CDK complexes. Cyclin D-CDK4, cyclin D-CDK6, and cyclin E-CDK2 complexes phosphorylate (hyperphosphorylation) RB (inactive RB). Inactive RB releases E2F factors, which then activate the transcription of S-phase genes. Almost all cancer cells show dysregulation of the G_1–S checkpoint. Most commonly it is due to the mutations in genes encoding RB, CDK4, cyclin D, or CDKN2A.

(EGF: epidermal growth factor; PDGF: platelet-derived growth factor; TGF-β: transforming growth factor-β).

- **First hit:** In familial cases, **children inherit one defective copy** (mutated allele) of the ***RB* gene in the germline** (one hit) and the other copy of the *RB* gene is wild-type (a gene that predominates in the natural population). Thus, the child is heterozygous at the *RB* locus). The product of one wild-type (normal) *RB* gene is sufficient to prevent tumors.
- **Second hit: Retinoblastoma develops when** the remaining wild-type *RB* gene/allele is inactivated (mutated) in retinoblasts due to **spontaneous somatic mutation** (second hit). Because only a single germline mutation is sufficient to transmit disease risk in familial retinoblastoma, it is **transmitted as an autosomal dominant trait.**

Patients with **familial retinoblastoma** have also an **increased risk** of developing **osteosarcoma** and other **soft tissue sarcomas.**

2. **Sporadic retinoblastoma:** It forms about 60% of cases. The child has two *wild-type* (normal) *RB* alleles in all somatic cells. To develop retinoblastoma, **both wild-type *RB* alleles must undergo** *functionally inactivation by somatic* **mutation** in a retinoblast. Thus, it **needs two hits.** When a retinal cell loses both wild-type copies of the *RB* gene, it becomes cancerous. Since both alleles must be inactivated, the mutation is recessive. (This contrasts with oncogenes which are dominant and a single mutated allele is sufficient for transformation).

Tumors associated with the inactivation of RB

In most cancers, at least one of four key regulators of **normal cell cycle control is lost.** These are (1) p16 (CDKI), (2) cyclin D, (3) CDK4, and (4) RB. Various **mechanisms** of inactivation of RB are as follows:

1. **Loss-of-function mutations involving both *RB* alleles.** It may be:
   - **Germline mutation,** e.g., in **retinoblastomas** and **osteosarcomas.**
   - **Acquired mutation:** Biallelic loss of the *RB* gene is common in several sporadic tumors, such as

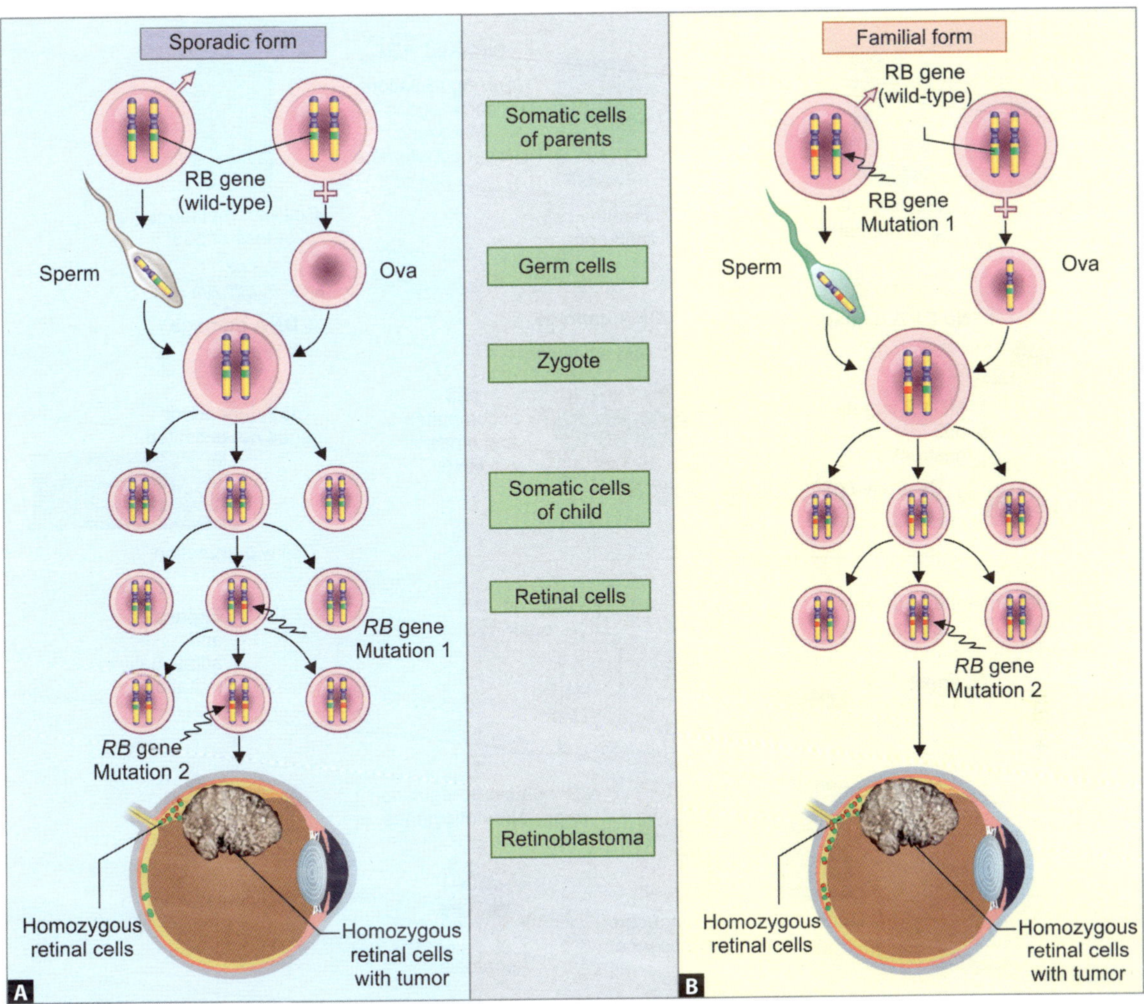

Figs. 7.20A and B: Pathogenesis of retinoblastoma. Loss of function of both alleles of the *RB* locus leads to neoplastic proliferation of the retinal cells. (A) Sporadic form. Initially, all the somatic cells, including retinal cells have two functional copies of *RB*. Hence, both *RB* mutations in the tumor-retinal cell are acquired; (B) Familial form. All somatic cells including nontransformed retinal cells have only one functional copy of *RB*. Thus, all somatic cells inherit one mutant *RB* gene from a carrier parent and require only one additional *RB* mutation in a retinal cell for complete loss of *RB* function.

osteosarcoma, **small-cell carcinomas of the lung, breast cancers, and bladder carcinomas.**

2. **Shifting of the active RB to an inactive RB state.** This may be due to (1) **gain-of-function mutations that upregulate CDK/cyclin D activity** or (2) **loss-of-function mutations that abolish/cancel the activity of CDK inhibitors.**
3. **Direct targeting of RB by viral proteins:** In cancers caused by certain oncogenic viruses, RB is directly targeted by viral oncoproteins. It may occur even without *RB* mutation. For example, the E7 protein of human papillomavirus (HPV) binds to the hypophosphorylated form of RB. This prevents RB from inhibiting the E2F transcription factors. The free E2F causes the progression of the cell cycle and cervical carcinomas (*refer* **Fig. 7.25).** Thus, RB function is lost, and it leads to uncontrolled growth.

TP53

Guardian of the Genome

Q. Write a short note on the *TP53* and its role in neoplasia.

Q. Why *p53* gene is called the "Guardian of genome"?

TP53: It is a **tumor suppressor gene located on the small arm of chromosome 17(17p13.1).** *TP53* functions as **critical gatekeeper genes.** It plays a **main role in maintaining the integrity of the genome** and is thus known as the **guardian of the genome** or **"molecular policeman."**

Suppression of neoplastic transformation by p53 (Fig. 7.21)

The p53 is the protein product of *TP53* and is present in almost all normal tissues. **The p53 protein** is a **transcription factor. In nonstressed, healthy cells, p53 has a short half-life** (20 minutes) because of its association with MDM2

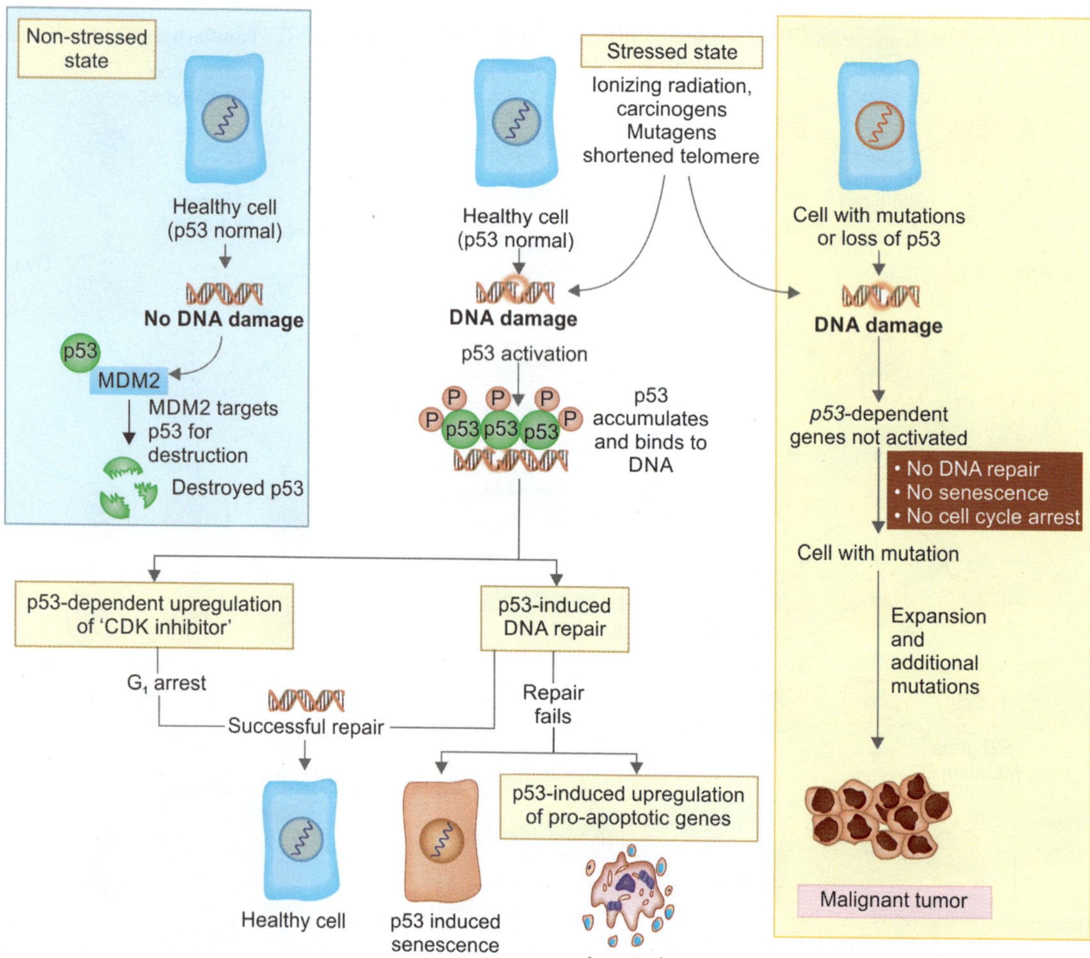

Fig. 7.21: Role of *p53* in maintaining the integrity of the genome. In nonstressed healthy cells, the p53 protein levels are low. This is due to the degradation of p53 by MDM2. When healthy cells suffer DNA damage, it activates p53. This leads to cell cycle arrest in G_1 and p53 induces DNA repair by DNA repair genes. If DNA damage is successfully repaired, the cells proceed with the cell cycle. If DNA repair fails, p53 triggers either apoptosis or senescence. In cells with loss of p53 function or mutations of p53, DNA damage does not induce cell cycle arrest or DNA repair. These genetically damaged cells proliferate to form malignant neoplasms.

(murine double minute). MDM2 is a protein that destroys p53. **In stressed** (e.g., DNA damage, shortened telomeres, hypoxia, and stress caused due to increased pro-growth signaling such as mutations in *RAS* and *MYC* genes) **cells, p53 becomes activated and stimulates the transcription of hundreds of genes.** These genes suppress neoplastic transformation by three mechanisms **(i) quiescence, (ii) senescence, or (iii) apoptosis.** RB is a "sensor" of external signals, whereas p53 monitors internal stress, and directs stressed cells toward one of these pathways:

1. **p53-mediated cell cycle arrest (quiescence) in response to DNA damage: DNA damage**, causes p53-mediated transient, rapid cell cycle arrest late in the G_1 phase. It is caused mainly by p53-dependent transcription of the *CDKN1A* gene (encodes the CDK inhibitor). This CDKI inhibits CDK4/D cyclin complexes and maintains RB in an active, hypophosphorylated state. This blocks the progression of cells from the G_1 phase to the S phase. This cell cycle arrest gives the cells time to repair DNA damage. The p53 protein also induces the expression of DNA damage repair genes. **If DNA damage is successfully repaired,** the p53 undergoes its own destruction. This releases the block in the cell cycle and cells return to a normal state. **If the DNA damage is not repaired,** the cell may enter **p53-induced senescence or undergo p53-directed apoptosis (Fig. 7.21)** (described below). By managing DNA damage responses, p53 plays the main role in maintaining the integrity of the genome. Because of these activities, p53 is called the "**guardian of the genome.**"
2. **p53-induced senescence:** Senescence is a type of permanent cell cycle arrest. Senescence requires activation of p53 and/or RB and expression of CDKIs. Senescence may be stimulated in response to different types of stresses (e.g., unopposed oncogene signaling, hypoxia, and shortened telomeres). The senescent cells are prevented from forming tumors.

3. **p53-induced apoptosis (programmed cell death): Cells with irreversible DNA damage undergo *p53*-** induced apoptosis which is the protective mechanism against the development of cancer. *p53* stimulates transcription of several pro-apoptotic genes (e.g., *BAX* and *PUMA*) resulting in apoptosis of cells via the intrinsic (mitochondrial) pathway.

Inactivation of TP53 and associated tumors

Mutations of *TP53*: The p53 has an **important role in controlling carcinogenesis. Most cancers have mutations in the *TP53* gene. The remaining malignant tumors usually have defects in genes upstream or downstream of *TP53* that impair p53 function.**

Tumors associated with TP53 abnormalities

Acquired mutations of *TP53*: Biallelic abnormalities of the *TP53* gene (loss-of-function mutations) are found in almost every type of malignant tumor. These include the three leading causes of cancer death namely **carcinomas of the lung, colon, and breast.** In most cancers, both *TP53* allele mutations are acquired in somatic cells. Mutations in both alleles lead to loss of the p53 "guardian" function. In these cases, DNA damage goes unrepaired, and mutations become fixed in dividing cells. Thus, the cell undergoes malignant transformation.

Germline mutations in one allele of *TP53*: It is less common. Patients may **inherit one mutated/*TP53* allele and one additional "hit" in the other wild-type (normal) *TP53* allele** will produce malignant tumors. For example, **Li-Fraumeni syndrome** has germline mutations in one *TP53*. Like familial retinoblastoma, inheritance of one mutant *TP53* allele predisposes these individuals to develop malignant tumors. This is because only one additional "hit" is required for the inactivation of the second, wild-type allele. Patients with Li-Fraumeni syndrome usually develop cancer at a younger age, have a greater chance of developing a malignant tumor by age 50, and are more prone to develop multiple primary tumors of varying types (a common feature of familial cancer syndromes). The most common types of tumors are **sarcomas, breast cancer, leukemias, brain tumors, and carcinomas of the adrenal cortex**

Mutations of proteins that regulate p53 function: Loss of p53 function with intact *TP53* occurs in some tumors, such as certain sarcomas. This may occur due to **amplification and overexpression of the *MDM2* gene.** *MDM2* encodes a protein (MDM2 enzyme that ubiquitinylates p53) that degrades p53 leading to a functional deficiency of p53.

Blocking of p53 function: Like RB, the **transforming proteins of many oncogenic DNA viruses bind and degrade** wild-type p53 even without mutation in *TP53*. For example, viral oncoprotein E6 of high-risk human papillomaviruses (HPVs) promotes p53 degradation and causes cervical carcinoma and a subset of squamous cell carcinomas of the head and neck. Some polyomaviruses also bind to p53 and neutralize its protective function. Thus, transforming DNA viruses inactivate the two best-understood tumor suppressors, RB and p53.

Consequences of loss of p53 **function:** These include (i) DNA damage goes unrepaired, (ii) driver mutations accumulate in oncogenes and other cancer genes, and (iii) cells blindly follow a dangerous path leading to malignant transformation.

Therapeutic implications of TP53

- **Wild type versus mutated *TP53*:** Irradiation and chemotherapy used for the treatment of cancer, mediate their effects by causing damage to the DNA and producing apoptosis of tumor cells. Tumors with **wild-type *TP53*** (wild type refers to the most common form of phenotype in nature) alleles are **more susceptible to apoptosis than tumors with mutated *TP53* alleles.** For example, childhood acute lymphoblastic leukemias which have wild-type *TP53* alleles respond to radio and chemotherapy; whereas lung cancers and colorectal cancers with mutated *TP53* alleles are relatively resistant to chemotherapy and irradiation.
- **Consequences of mutated *TP53*:** Tumor cells with mutated p53 **tend to acquire additional mutations** at a high rate and are **resistant to any mono/single therapy** (radiation/conventional chemotherapy/molecularly targeted therapy).

Q. Write a short note on familial syndromes/inherited cancers.

Few tumor suppressor genes and associated familial syndromes and sporadic cancers are presented in **Table 7.15.**

Altered Cellular Metabolism

Cancer cells have different needs than their normal counterpart. Their proliferative rate generally exceeds that of normal cells. They must quickly synthesize the structural components (e.g., protein, lipid, etc.) required for rapid cell growth (that is to sustain their mitotic activity).

Aerobic glycolysis (*Warburg effect*): Cancer cells have a distinctive metabolism. Generally, even with adequate oxygen supply, cancer cells undergo a metabolic switch to **aerobic glycolysis** over oxidative phosphorylation for ATP generation. The distinctive form of cellular metabolism is characterized by the **increased amount of glucose and glutamine uptake and increased conversion of glucose to lactose (fermentation) via the glycolytic pathway.** This *aerobic glycolysis* is also termed the ***Warburg effect.*** It was described in 1930 by Otto Warburg. Aerobic glycolysis ("Warburg metabolism") is not cancer-specific but observed in growing cells and it becomes "fixed" in cancer cells. It is seen because tumor cells have an **M2 isoform of the pyruvate kinase enzyme. Aerobic glycolysis provides metabolic intermediates needed for the synthesis of cellular components in rapidly dividing tumor cells.** These **metabolic intermediates** cannot be met with normal mitochondrial oxidative phosphorylation.

TABLE 7.15 Few tumor suppressor genes and associated familial syndromes and sporadic cancers.

Gene (protein)	*Function*	*Familial syndromes*	*Sporadic cancers*
Inhibitors of mitogenic signaling pathways			
APC (Adenomatous polyposis coli)	Inhibits Wnt signaling	Familial colonic polyps and carcinomas	Carcinomas of the stomach, colon, and pancreas; melanoma
NF1 (Neurofibromin-1)	Inhibits RAS/MAPK signaling	Neurofibromatosis type 1	Neuroblastoma
PTEN (Phosphatase and tensin homologue)	Inhibits of PI3K/AKT signaling	Cowden syndrome	Carcinomas and lymphoid tumors
SMAD2, SMAD4 (SMAD2, SMAD4)	TGF-β signaling pathway	Juvenile polyposis	Carcinoma of the colon and pancreas
Inhibitors of cell cycle progression			
RB (Retinoblastoma protein)	G_1/S transition during cell cycle	Familial retinoblastoma syndrome	Retinoblastoma; osteosarcoma, carcinomas of breast, colon, lung
Inhibitors of "pro-growth" programs of metabolism and angiogenesis			
VHL (Von Hippel–Lindau protein)	Hypoxia-induced transcription factors	Von Hippel–Lindau syndrome	Renal cell carcinoma
Inhibitors of invasion and metastasis			
CDH1 (E-cadherin)	Cell adhesion, inhibition of cell motility	Familial gastric cancer	Gastric carcinoma, lobular carcinoma of the breast
Enablers of genomic stability			
TP53 (*p53* protein)	Cell cycle arrest and apoptosis in response to DNA damage	Li-Fraumeni syndrome	Majority of cancers
DNA repair factors			
BRCA1(Breast cancer-1), *BRCA2* (breast cancer-2)	Repair of double-stranded breaks in DNA	Familial carcinoma of breast and ovary; carcinomas of male breast; chronic lymphocytic leukemia (*BRCA2*)	Rare
Unknown mechanisms			
WT1 (Wilms tumor-1)	Transcription factor	Familial Wilms tumor	Wilms tumor, certain leukemias

Clinical utility: The "glucose-hunger" of tumors is made use for visualization of tumors in **positron emission tomography (PET) scanning.** In PET scanning, patients are injected with ^{18}F-fluorodeoxyglucose (a non-metabolizable derivative of glucose). This is preferentially taken up into tumor cells (and actively dividing normal cells, e.g., bone marrow cells). **Most tumors are PET-positive,** and markedly positive are the rapidly growing tumors.

Autophagy

Autophagy ("self-eating"): It is **a survival (adaptive) mechanism that occurs during a state of severe nutrient deficiency.** In this, the **cells arrest their growth and consume their own organelles, proteins, and membranes as carbon sources for energy production.** This provides nutrients and energy. If this adaptive mechanism fails, the cells die.

Autophagy in cancer: Tumor cells can grow under marginal environmental conditions without triggering autophagy. This suggests that the **pathways that induce autophagy are disrupted in cancer**. The role of autophagy in the development and progression of cancer is complex and represents a double-edged sword. Several autophagy genes (e.g., Beclin-1 and some *Atg* genes) that promote autophagy, act as tumor suppressors and are deleted or mutated in many cancers. Tumor cells may accumulate mutations that derange the pathways that induce autophagy and allow the cancer cells to grow without triggering autophagy. Tumor cells may corrupt the autophagy process to provide nutrients for continued growth and survival. On the other hand, autophagy can protect cancer cells if they are deprived of nutrients or oxygen because of therapy or insufficient blood supply.

Oncometabolism

Oncometabolism is a new group of genetic alterations in oncogenesis in which **mutations occur in enzymes that participate in the Krebs cycle.** One of them being mutations in the enzyme isocitrate dehydrogenase (IDH).

Acquired mutation in IDH: It results in the mutated protein (oncoprotein) that loses its ability to function as an isocitrate dehydrogenase (IDH). This protein acquires a new enzymatic activity that catalyzes the **production of high levels of *oncometabolite* namely 2-hydroxyglutarate (2-HG)**. 2-HG in turn **inhibits several other enzymes** of the **TET family**, including TET2. TET2 regulates DNA methylation (an epigenetic modification that controls normal gene expression). Loss of TET2 activity leads to **abnormal DNA methylation and oncogenesis. Oncogenic IDH mutations** have been found in many cancers (e.g., **cholangiocarcinomas, gliomas, acute myeloid leukemias, and sarcomas**).

Evasion of Cell Death

In normal cells, factors such as genomic instability, and poor adhesion may trigger cell death by apoptosis. **Cancer cells often develop strategies to avoid apoptosis. Tumor cells often contain mutations in genes that regulate apoptosis. This makes the tumor cells resistant to cell death.** Apoptosis is a form of regulated cell death and does not elicit inflammation.

Pathways of apoptosis (*refer* Fig. 2.13): Two pathways lead to apoptosis: The extrinsic pathway, and the intrinsic pathway (*refer* pages 24-7).

1. **Extrinsic (death receptor) pathway:** It is initiated when certain ligands (e.g., CD95L, TNF, FasL) bind to the death receptor expressed on the surface of the plasma membrane.
2. **Intrinsic pathway (mitochondrial pathway):** It is initiated by various stimuli (e.g., loss of growth factors, DNA damage). Activation of the intrinsic pathway leads to increased permeability of the mitochondrial outer membrane, releases cytochrome c, and initiates apoptosis. Integrity of the mitochondrial outer membrane is controlled by: (1) proapoptotic, and (2) antiapoptotic proteins.
   - **Proapoptotic proteins *BAX* and *BAK*** increase mitochondrial permeability and initiate apoptosis.
   - **Antiapoptotic proteins *BCL2*,** and ***BCL-X$_L$*:** Belong to ***BCL2*** family of proteins, inhibit the action of proapoptotic proteins.
   - **Regulator of balance between proapoptotic and antiapoptotic proteins:** It is achieved by **BH3-only proteins** and includes **BAD, BID, and PUMA.**

The **intrinsic pathway of apoptosis is most disabled in cancer.** Cancer cells are subject to several intrinsic stresses that can initiate apoptosis. These include DNA damage, metabolic disturbances due to dysregulated growth, and hypoxia due to insufficient blood supply. These stresses markedly increase when tumors are treated with chemotherapy or radiation therapy, which mainly kill tumor cells by the intrinsic pathway of apoptosis. The cancer cells can develop resistance to intrinsic stresses that induce apoptosis, both before and during therapy. Thus, evasion of apoptosis by cancer cells occurs mainly by acquired mutations and changes in gene expression that disable the intrinsic pathway, or factors that favor cell survival during intrinsic stresses.

Major Mechanism of Evasion of Apoptosis and Associated Tumors

Tumor cells may escape or undergo reduced apoptosis. The major mechanisms involve (i) loss of p53 (a key component of early steps in the intrinsic pathway), and (ii) increased expression of antiapoptotic members of the BCL2 family.

1. **Loss of p53 function**: *TP53* is commonly mutated in cancers. The frequency of *TP53* mutations is higher in tumors that relapse after cytotoxic therapy. Loss of p53 function **prevents the upregulation of a proapoptotic protein called PUMA**. Thus, cells with DNA damage survive.
2. **Overexpression of antiapoptotic proteins: Overexpression of BCL2** is common and this protects tumor cells from undergoing apoptosis. **Follicular lymphoma** is a B-cell tumor that carries a characteristic **(14;18) (q32; q21) translocation**. In this translocation, that fuses the *BCL2* gene (located at 18q21) is transcribed to the transcriptionally active immunoglobulin heavy chain gene (located at 14q32). The result is **excess production of BCL2**. The **antiapoptotic BCL2 protein protects lymphocytes from apoptosis** and increases their survival.

Loss of Replicative Potential (Immortality)

Q. Write briefly on telomerase activity.

Normal cells have limited replicative capacity (cellular senescence). Most normal cells are capable of replication (division or doubling) at most 70 times. After this, the cells lose the capacity to divide (cannot divide) and enter replicative senescence. These cells permanently leave the cell cycle. This is **due to the progressive shortening of telomeres (special structures) at the ends of chromosomes. During each cell division**, a small section of the **telomere** is not duplicated resulting in **progressive shortening**, which is responsible for the limited replicative property of a cell. The shortening of telomeres is prevented by an enzyme called telomerase. Markedly shortened telomeres in normal cells are recognized as double-stranded DNA breaks by the DNA repair machinery. This leads to cell cycle arrest and senescence, mediated by p53 and RB.

Mitotic catastrophe: It is a mode of cell death that results from **premature or inappropriate entry of cells into mitosis. In cells in which p53 or RB are disabled by mutations**, the nonhomologous end-joining pathway system is activated in a final attempt to save the cell. This inappropriately activated repair system joins the shortened ends of two chromosomes. It produces dicentric chromosomes that are pulled apart at anaphase, leading to a new double-stranded DNA break. The repeated bridge-fusion-breakage cycles result in genomic instability. It eventually produces mitotic catastrophe and death by apoptosis.

Cellular Immortalization in Cancer Cells

All cancers contain immortal cells and can multiply indefinitely**. These tumor cells, unlike normal cells, are capable of unlimited (limitless) replication (cellular immortalization).** The ability of tumors to grow indefinitely, the loss of growth control is not enough. Tumor cells must also avoid cellular senescence and mitotic catastrophe.

Telomere maintenance and activation of telomerase: Telomerase is active in normal stem cells, but expressed at very low levels or absent in most somatic cells. With each cell division, their telomeres shorten and telomerase can prevent this shortening of telomeres. Telomere maintenance is seen in almost all types of cancers. In 85–95% of cancers, this telomere maintenance is due to upregulation of the enzyme telomerase. **If a cell manages to reactivate telomerase**, the bridge-fusion-breakage cycles cease, and the **cell can avoid death.** However, repeated bridge-fusion-breakage cycles that precede telomerase activation result in genomic instability. During genomic instability, several mutations may accumulate, leading to the progression towards malignancy. *TERT* encodes a subunit of telomerase. Many tumors with telomerase expression have mutations in the promoter of the gene. These mutations lead to high levels of *TERT* expression.

- **Loss of senescence:** Cancer cells evade the process of senescence and retain the ability to reproduce. The senescence is probably associated with the upregulation of tumor suppressors (e.g., *p53*). These tumor suppressors maintain RB in a hypophosphorylated state that favors cell cycle arrest. RB-dependent G_1/S cell cycle checkpoint is disrupted in almost all cancers by a wide variety of acquired genetic and epigenetic aberrations.
- **Loss of mitotic catastrophe:** Cells resistant to (or escape from) senescence have an increased capacity to replicate. Loss of mitotic catastrophe is observed in cancer cells.

Sustained Angiogenesis

Induction of angiogenesis in cancer: A solid tumor having all the genetic aberrations needed for malignant transformation, requires huge supplies of nutrients and oxygen to grow. They cannot grow beyond 1–2 mm unless it has a blood supply. Thus, an important hallmark of all cancers is its capacity to induce angiogenesis. Tumor cells and their neighbors secrete molecules that stimulate angiogenesis (new blood vessel formation).

Effects of neoangiogenesis: Neoangiogenesis is a process in which new vessels sprout from previously existing capillaries. Neovascularization (neoangiogenesis) has two effects on tumor growth:

1. **Supplies required nutrients and oxygen:** Neovascularization in tumors can effectively supply nutrients and remove wastes.
2. **Newly formed endothelial cells stimulate the growth of adjacent tumor cells:** This is **by secreting growth factors** [e.g., insulin-like growth factors (IGFs) and PDGF].

Abnormal intratumoral vessels: Intratumoral vessels are not normal. They are **dilated and leaky and show a haphazard pattern of connection.** These abnormal features can be seen on angiograms. These **favor metastatic spread.**

Mechanism of Angiogenesis

Under homeostatic conditions, angiogenesis is controlled by a local balance between angiogenesis promoters (factors that favor new blood vessel formation), and inhibitors (those that prevent angiogenesis). In angiogenic tumors, the balance is shifted toward angiogenesis promoters. This may be due to increased local production of angiogenic factors and/or loss of angiogenic inhibitors. Several factors influence this balance:

- **Transcription of proangiogenic VEGFs:** Relative lack of oxygen due to hypoxia triggers angiogenesis through the actions of HIF-1α (an oxygen-sensitive transcription factor) on the transcription of the proangiogenic factor VEGF.
- **Mutations involving tumor suppressors and oncogenes:** In cancers, these mutations tilt the balance in favor of angiogenesis. For example, wild-type p53 stimulates the synthesis of the angiogenesis inhibitor thombospondin-1 and suppresses the expression of proangiogenic molecules such as VEGF. Thus, the loss of p53 favors angiogenesis.
- **Other mechanisms:** The transcription of VEGF also depends on signals from the RAS-MAP kinase pathway. The gain-of-function mutations in RAS or MYC upregulate the production of VEGF. Raised levels of VEGF can be observed in the serum and urine of some cancers. VEGF inhibitors slow the growth of advanced cancer.

Invasion and Metastasis

Q. Discuss the mechanism of invasion and metastasis.

Usually, solid tumor masses do not kill the host by growing large. They kill by metastasizing widely. **Invasion and metastasis are characteristic of malignant tumors. These are the major causes of cancer-related morbidity and mortality.** Invasion-metastatic cascade constitutes the **entire sequence of events from** the beginning of **invasion to** the development of **metastasis.**

Steps: Invasion-metastatic cascade is a **complex multistep process. It involves complex interactions between**

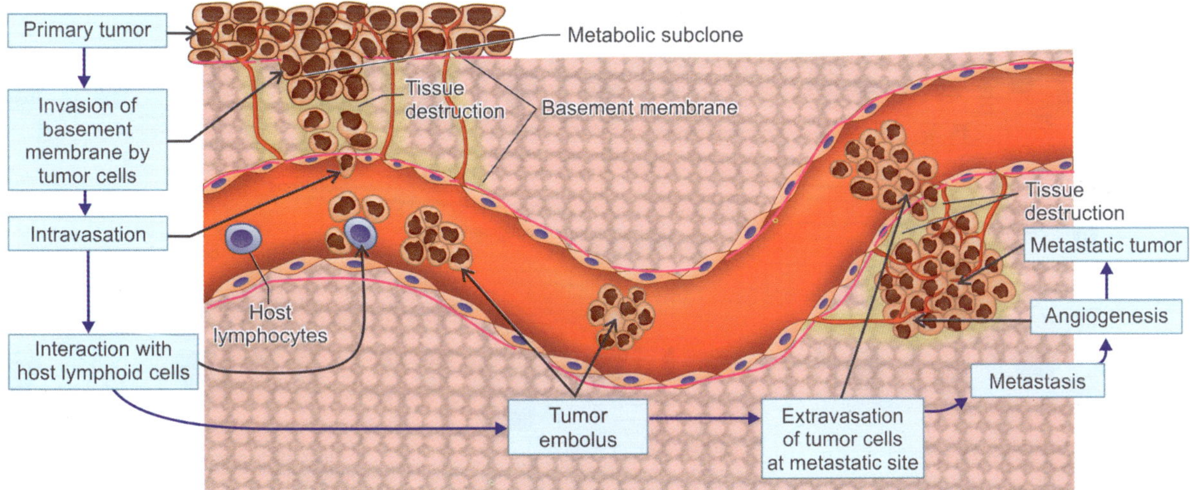

Fig. 7.22: Various steps involved in vascular dissemination and homing of tumor cells during the metastatic cascade.

cancer cells, stromal cells, and the extracellular matrix (ECM). These interactions involve a series of steps. These consist of local invasion, penetration of blood and lymph vessels, transport through the vessels, extravasation from the vessels, formation of micrometastases, and growth of micrometastases into macroscopic tumors **(Fig. 7.22)**.

Phases

The steps in the metastatic cascade can be divided into two main phases, namely: (1) **invasion of the extracellular matrix (ECM)** and (2) **metastasis (vascular dissemination and homing of tumor cells)**.

Invasion of Extracellular Matrix (Figs. 7.23A to F)

Tumor cells interact with ECM at several steps: Tumor cells must interact with two types of ECM: basement membranes and interstitial connective tissue. Both types of ECM are composed of collagens, glycoproteins, and proteoglycans. Tumor cells interact with the ECM at several steps in the metastatic cascade **(Fig. 7.22)**. These are as follows:

- **Breaching of basement membrane:** A carcinoma cell must first break the underlying basement membrane.
- **Travel through the interstitial connective tissue.**
- **Entry into the circulation by penetrating the vascular basement membrane.**

The above process is repeated in reverse order when tumor cell emboli extravasate at a distant site to form a metastatic deposit. Invasion of the ECM is an active process and initiates the metastatic cascade. It consists of several sequential steps.

1. **Loosening of intercellular connections between tumor cells: Normally, cells** are **attached by E-cadherins.** These are adhesive molecules that act as a cement between the cells. The cytoplasmic portions of E-cadherins bind to β-catenin (*refer* **Fig. 18.47**).
   - **Decreased or loss of E-cadherin function:** It is observed in many epithelial cancers (e.g., **adenocarcinomas of the colon and breast**) due to mutational inactivation of E-cadherin genes, or activation of β-catenin gene. This **loosens tumor cells** and the separated cells get **detached from the primary cancer**.
2. **Local degradation (proteolysis) of basement membrane and interstitial connective tissue:** Basement membrane and interstitial connective tissue are extracellular matrix. Their degradation occurs by the following mechanism:
   - **Secretion of degrading enzymes:** Malignant **tumor cells** and **stromal cells** (e.g., fibroblasts and inflammatory cells) **in cancers secrete many proteolytic enzymes** that **degrade ECM**. These enzymes include: **Matrix metalloproteinases (MMPs), cathepsin, and urokinase plasminogen activator (u-PA)**. Overexpression of MMPs and other proteases occurs in several malignant tumors.
3. **Changes in the attachment of tumor cells to ECM proteins:** Normal epithelial cells have receptors (e.g., integrin) for basement membrane components (e.g., laminin and collagen). These receptors are located at the basal surface of the basement membrane and maintain the cells in a polarized, resting, differentiated state. In normal cells, loss of adhesion between the cells causes apoptosis of cells. However, loosened tumor cells are resistant to apoptosis.
   - **Modification of matrix to promote invasion:** In cancer, the matrix itself is also modified to promote invasion and metastasis. For example, local degradation of the basement membrane proteins (collagen IV, laminin) by matrix metalloproteinases (MMP-2 and MMP-9) generates **new and strange** (novel) sites in the basement membrane.
   - **Stimulation of tumor cell migration:** The new sites in the basement membrane attach to receptors on tumor cells and stimulate migration of tumor cells.

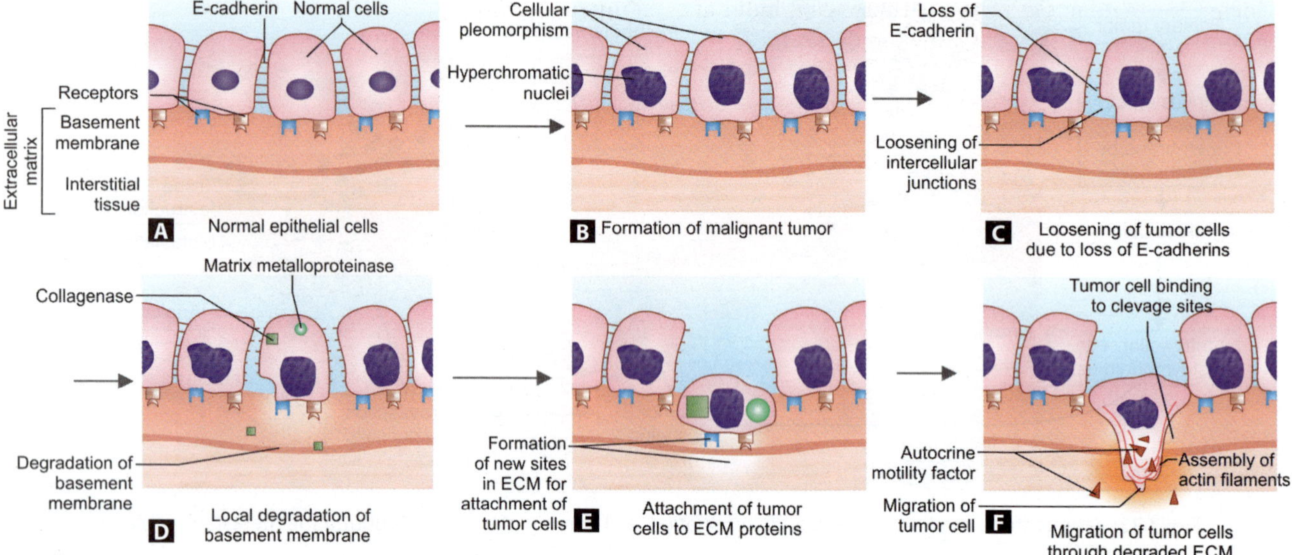

Figs. 7.23A to F: Various steps in the invasion of extracellular matrix in the invasion–metastasis cascades: (A) Normal cells; (B to F) Tumor cells loosen and detach from each other because of reduced adhesiveness. The tumor cells bind components of the extracellular matrix and secrete proteolytic enzymes that degrade the extracellular matrix. With binding to proteolytically generated new binding sites in the ECM, tumor cell migration follows. The tumor cells reach the nearby vessels to start the next phase, namely metastasis.

4. **Locomotion (migration) of tumor cells through degraded ECM:** It is the final, complex, multistep step process in the invasion.
   - **Movement of tumor cells through the degraded basement membranes and proteolyzed ECM: Locomotion** drives the tumor cells **forward through the degraded basement membranes** and zones of proteolysis in the **interstitial connective tissue matrix.**
   - **Locomotion involves many receptors and signaling proteins**. The locomotion is potentiated by tumor cell-derived cytokines, such as **autocrine motility factors** (AMF) and other molecules (assembly of actin filaments in tumor cells).
   - **Migration through interstitial tissue:** The tumor cells invade and traverse through the surrounding interstitial connective tissue and ultimately **reach nearby blood and lymphatic vessels.** Cells gain access to the circulation by penetrating the basement membrane of vessels.

   The stromal cells surrounding tumor cells also participate in reciprocal signaling events.

Metastasis (Vascular Dissemination and Homing of Tumor Cells)

Tumor cells have invasive properties: Following the invasion of surrounding interstitial tissue, **they frequently escape from their sites of origin. These tumor cells enter the circulation** and may spread to distant sites by metastasis. Metastasis is a **multistep process** by which a tumor produces a secondary growth at a distant site or location. It has several steps **(Fig. 7.22)**.

1. **Penetration of vascular or lymphatic channels (intravasation into the lumen of vessels):** Malignant cells penetrate the basement membrane of blood vessels or lymphatic channels and enter the circulation.
2. **Invasion of the circulation:** The blood samples obtained from patients with solid tumors ("liquid biopsies") show millions of tumor cells that daily enter circulation from even small cancers. Therefore, both tumor cells and tumor-derived DNA can be detected in circulation.
3. **Transit through the circulation and formation of tumor emboli:** Most of the tumor cells circulate as single cells. Other cells form tumors by aggregating and adhering to circulating blood elements, particularly platelets. Tumor cells may also bind and activate coagulation factors and form emboli. In the circulation, tumor cells are susceptible to destruction by several mechanisms. These include mechanical shear stress, apoptosis stimulated by loss of adhesion (termed *anoikis*), and innate and adaptive immune defenses.
4. **Arrest within circulating blood or lymph:** It occurs at a distant location away from the primary tumor. At the site of the arrest, tumor cells adhere to endothelial cells.
5. **Exit from the circulation into a new tissue site:** The location at which circulating tumor cells leave the capillaries to form secondary deposits depends on the anatomic location and vascular drainage of the primary tumor and the tropism of particular tumors for specific tissues. Exit occurs through the basement membrane of lymphatics or blood vessels. The site at which circulating tumor cells leave the vessel or lymphatics must repeat the same events involved in the invasion but in reverse order.

6. **Formation of micrometastases:** Tumor cells lodge at a distant new site to form micrometastases.
7. **Angiogenesis.**
8. **Local growth of micrometastases into macroscopic tumors:** If neglected, almost all malignant tumors may eventually produce macroscopic metastases. Most metastases occur in the liver and lung. **The site of metastases is generally related to two factors: the anatomic location and vascular drainage of the primary tumor and the tropism of particular tumors for specific tissues.** Examples of favored sites of metastasis:
   - Prostatic carcinoma to the bone.
   - Bronchogenic carcinomas to the adrenals and the brain.
   - Neuroblastomas to the liver and bones.

Evasion of Immune Surveillance

PA 7.5 (NC): Describe immunology and the immune response to cancer.

Protective immunologic responses against the cancer cells: The immune system distinguishes self from non self (foreign) molecules and is very effective against infectious agents. Paul Ehrlich first suggested that tumor cells also can be recognized as "foreign/nonself" and the immune system can elicit protective immunologic responses against the tumor cells. The immune system may suppress tumor development or **recognize and** destroy the cancer cells.

Immune surveillance: Lewis Thomas and Macfarlane Burnet stated that the **normal function of the immune system is to constantly "scan" the body for any emerging malignant cells and destroy them.** This mechanism was termed immune surveillance.

Principles involved in immune reactions: Several factors may control the outcome of interactions between cancer cells and the host immune system. The basic principles involved are as follows:

- **Expression of a variety of antigens by cancer cells:** These antigens stimulate the host immune system and may have an important role in preventing the appearance of cancers.
- **Immune response may be ineffective in established tumors:** Though the antigens expressed by cancer cells can elicit an immune response, it may be ineffective against established tumors. In some tumors, the immune response may promote cancer growth. This may be due to acquired changes in cancer cells which permit them to escape from anti-tumor responses and may encourage pro-tumor responses.
- **Effective new immunotherapies to reactivate latent host immune responses:** By understanding the mechanisms of immune evasion and "immunomanipulation" by cancer cells, it was possible to invent effective new immunotherapies. These therapies reactivate latent host immune responses.

Tumor Antigens

A tumor antigen is an antigenic substance produced in tumor cells. **Cancer cells express various types of antigens. These may be recognized by the immune system as foreign.** The three main sources (classes) of tumor antigens are (i) products of mutated genes, (ii) overexpressed or aberrantly expressed proteins, and (iii) tumor antigens produced by oncogenic viruses.

1. **Neoantigens (products of mutated genes):** Cancer is a genetic disorder caused by mutations in oncogenes and tumor suppressor genes. Most of these mutations (both driver and passenger mutations) are acquired (caused by mutagenic exposures such as sunlight, and smoking) rather than inherited. These mutations may generate new protein sequences (neoantigens) that the immune system has not come across. Hence, the immune system can recognize them as foreign and react against them.
2. **Unmutated proteins expressed by tumor cells:** They also can stimulate the host immune response.
   - **Self-antigen:** For example, **tyrosinase** is an enzyme involved in the synthesis of melanin and is expressed only in normal melanocytes and melanomas. The immune system can respond against this normal self-antigen.
   - **Cancertestis antigens:** These antigens are encoded by genes that are silent in all adult tissues except germ cells in the testis (hence termed testis antigens). This antigen is present in the testis. Sperm do not express MHC class I molecules. Therefore, this antigen is not expressed on the cell surface in a form that can be recognized by CD8+T cells. These antigens are tumor-specific and can stimulate anti-tumor immune responses.
3. **Viral proteins (tumor antigens produced by oncogenic viruses):** The cells of cancer transformed by oncogenic viruses can express viral proteins. The most powerful viral antigens are proteins produced by cells infected with DNA viruses [e.g., human papillomavirus (HPV) and Epstein-Barr virus (EBV)]. The cytotoxic T lymphocytes (CTLs) can recognize viral antigens and play important roles in surveillance against virus-induced tumors. CTLs can recognize and kill virus-infected cells.

Effective Immune Responses to Tumor Antigens

Death of individual tumor cells initiates immune reactions to cancers: The death of cancer cells is frequent and may occur due to dysregulated growth, metabolic stresses, and hypoxia due to inadequate blood supply. Dead tumor cells release "danger signals" (damage-associated molecular patterns) and they stimulate innate immune cells (resident phagocytes, antigen-presenting cells).

Killing of tumor cells by cytotoxic T lymphocytes: Killing of tumor cells by cytotoxic T lymphocytes specific for tumor antigens is the main immune mechanism of eradication of tumors. The CTLs recognize and kill tumor cells presenting neoantigens.

Immune Evasion by Cancers

The immune system can recognize and destroy cancer cells. When a tumor becomes clinically significant in size, it is composed of cells that are either not recognized by the host immune system or that the tumor cells express factors that suppress the host immunity. **Immune responses may fail to check tumor growth. This may be by evading immune recognition or resisting immune effector mechanisms.**

Cancer immunoediting: The immune system can promote the Darwinian selection of tumor subclones that avoid host immunity or that even manipulate the immune system. The immune system can also promote tumor progression through chronic inflammation, immunoselection of poorly immunogenic variants, and suppressing antitumor immunity. In immunocompetent patients, several mechanisms may avoid the response by the immune system to tumors. These include selective outgrowth of antigen-negative variants, loss or reduced expression of histocompatibility molecules, and immunosuppression mediated by expression of certain factors (e.g., PD-1 ligands) by the tumor cells.

Cytotoxic T-cells

Cytotoxic T-cells (CTLs) are the **most important cells involved in the defense of the host against tumors**. Hence, tumor cells undergo a variety of changes to avoid CTL responses. These alterations include (i) acquired mutations in β2-microglobulin that prevent the assembly of functional MHC class I molecules, and (ii) increased expression of proteins that inhibit CTL function. These proteins activate immune checkpoints which are regulators of the immune system.

Immune checkpoints are inhibitory pathways that are normally important for maintaining self-tolerance. It prevents the immune system from attacking cells indiscriminately. However, some cancers can protect themselves from attack by stimulating immune checkpoint targets. One of the immune checkpoints involves a protein called PD-L1 (programmed cell death ligand 1). PD-L1 ligand is usually expressed on the surface of tumor cells. When the PD-L1 ligand engages itself to its receptor, PD-1, on CTLs, the CTLs become unresponsive and lose their ability to kill tumor cells.

Blocking of checkpoints: The checkpoints can be blocked by using appropriate antibodies. This will shut off antitumor immunity and release the brakes on the immune response. Checkpoint blockade therapies are being used in various solid tumors (melanoma, lung cancer, bladder cancer, and others), and in some hematologic malignancies (e.g., Hodgkin lymphoma). Since these checkpoints are blocked to prevent responses to self-antigens, the patients treated with checkpoint blockade therapy may develop various autoimmune manifestations (e.g., colitis), most of which can be controlled with anti-inflammatory agents.

Chimeric antigen receptors (CARs) and CAR-T-cell therapy: Recently personalized tumor vaccines are prepared against neoantigens identified in the tumors of individual patients. One of the examples of immunotherapy is the development of patient-derived CTLs that are engineered to express CARs. CARs have extracellular and intracellular domains. The extracellular domains consist of antibodies that bind tumor antigens on the surface of tumor cells and intracellular domains which deliver signals that activate CTLs. CAR T-cells kill the tumor cells and are used for treating certain leukemias (e.g., B-cell acute lymphoblastic leukemia). However, CAR T cells can produce serious complications due to cytokines released from the activated CTLs.

Processes that Facilitate Tumor Growth and Spread

Mainly two mechanisms play supporting roles in developing and maintaining many cancers. These are genomic instability and inflammation.

Genomic Instability as an Enabler of Malignancy

Genome instability refers to a high frequency of mutations within the genome of a cell: Most human cancer cells generate random mutations faster than their normal counterparts. This allows tumor cells to progress quickly, to adapt to changing environments, and to be autonomous. We are surrounded by environmental agents that are mutagenic (e.g., chemicals, radiation, sunlight). Thus, DNA is under stress from many environmental agents (exogenous stresses) and internal stresses such as reactive oxygen species (ROS), etc. These stresses can damage cellular DNA. However, cancers are relatively rare outcomes of these stresses. This may be because the cells maintain genomic stability through different mechanisms that detect and repair DNA damage, cause the death of cells with irreparable damage, oncogene-induced senescence, and immune surveillance. *TP53* tumor suppressor gene protects the genome from oncogenic damage, (1) by arresting cell division to provide time for repair of DNA damage caused by environmental mutagens, and (2) by initiating apoptosis in irreparably damaged cells. Genes that repair DNA are called **DNA repair genes which protect the integrity of the genome**.

DNA Repair Genes

- Normally, DNA repair genes repair nonlethal damage in other genes including proto-oncogenes, tumor suppressor genes, and genes that regulate apoptosis. Mutations of these DNA repair genes do not directly transform cells. **Loss-of-function mutations involving DNA repair genes** contribute to carcinogenesis (neoplastic transformation) indirectly by **loss of the ability of the cell to recognize and repair nonlethal genetic damage in other genes**. These affected cells acquire mutations at an accelerated rate, a state referred to as a ***mutator phenotype*** **and it is marked by genomic instability. Individuals with inherited disorders of DNA repair defects are at greatly increased risk of cancer.**

- Genomic instability may be due to either **microsatellite instability** (single or oligo-nucleotide mutations) or more commonly due to **chromosomal instability** leading to aneuploidy (abnormal number of chromosomes in a cell).

Types of DNA repair genes (Flowchart 7.1)

These include (i) mismatch repair, (ii) nucleotide excision repair, homologous recombination, and DNA polymerase proofreading. These are affected by inherited disorders.

Diseases caused by defects in mismatch repair: After DNA replication is complete; **mismatch repair genes act as spell checkers or proofreaders. They excise and replace the mismatched nucleotides**. Defect in these genes, mismatched nucleotide errors gradually accumulate in the genome. These **errors may involve proto-oncogenes and tumor suppressor genes. Hereditary nonpolyposis colon cancer syndrome** is characterized by **familial predisposition to the development of carcinomas of the colon** affecting predominantly the cecum and proximal colon. **It is due to defects in DNA mismatch repair genes.**

- **Microsatellite instability:** One of the characteristics of patients with mismatch-repair defects is microsatellite instability. **Microsatellites are tandem repeats of one to six nucleotides found throughout the genome.** Normally the length of these microsatellites remains constant. In individuals with **HNPCC**, **these satellites are unstable and increase or decrease in length** in tumor cells, creating alleles not found in normal cells of the same patient. Minisatellites are longer tandem repeat units (n = 15–500 nucleotides) also termed a variable number of tandem repeats (VNTR) because the number of repeats in a given minisatellite varies widely among individuals.

Each affected patient inherits one defective copy of a DNA mismatch-repair gene and acquires the second hit of the DNA mismatch repair gene in colonic epithelial cells. Thus, the **mode of inheritance of DNA-repair genes is like tumor suppressor genes.**

Diseases caused by defects in nucleotide excision repair: Example—xeroderma pigmentosum. Xeroderma pigmentosum is an autosomal recessive disorder caused by a defect in DNA repair. It is associated with a markedly increased risk for cancers of sun-exposed skin. Ultraviolet (UV) rays in sunlight cause cross-linking of pyrimidine residues. This DNA damage is repaired by the nucleotide excision repair system.

Diseases caused by defects in the **repair of DNA by homologous recombination:** Recombination is a process in which random crossing over of double-stranded DNA occurs between two parental homologous chromosomes. This occurs through the breakage of homologous DNA molecules and the rejoining of the parts in new combinations. It is a necessary process in meiosis and involves the exchange of genetic information. Recombination also occurs during mitosis at a predictable rate. Exposure to ionizing radiation significantly increases the rate of breakage in chromosomes. Usually, these breakages are accurately repaired by recombination repair genes. Disorders associated with recombination repair genes include **Bloom syndrome, ataxia-telangiectasia, and Fanconi anemia.** ***BRCA1*** **and** ***BRCA2*** **are mutated in familial breast cancer** and both are associated with many proteins involved in the homologous recombination repair pathway.

Genomic instability caused by DNA polymerase mutations: Normally, cellular DNA polymerases act as "proofreaders" and are involved in DNA replication. It has a very low rate of error. Cancers with DNA polymerase mutations (mainly endometrial and colorectal cancers) are the most mutated of all cancers.

Tumor-promoting Inflammation as an Enabler of Malignancy

Inflammatory cells infiltrate most developing solid tumors. These cells secrete factors that favor tumor development and progression.

Chronic inflammatory reaction in infiltrating tumors: Infiltrating cancers stimulate a chronic inflammatory reaction. In advanced cancers, this inflammatory reaction can be severe enough to produce systemic signs and

Flowchart 7.1: Different types of DNA repair gene defects and associated conditions.

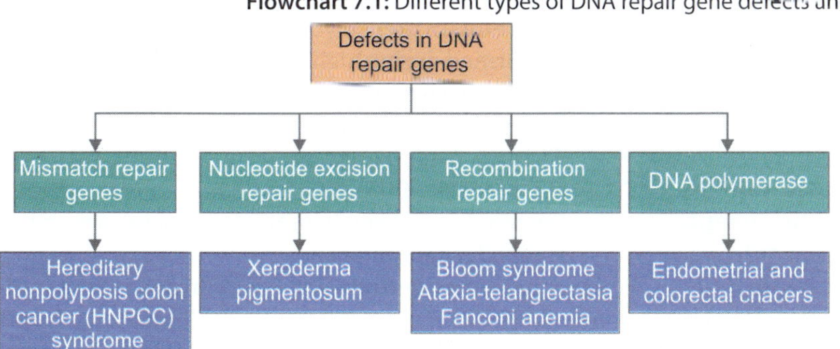

Xeroderma pigmentosum

Defects in the nucleotide excision repair gene are associated with an increased risk of cancer of skin exposed to UV light. UV radiation causes cross-linking of pyrimidine residues, preventing normal DNA replication. Such DNA damage is normally repaired by the nucleotide excision repair system.

symptoms. These include anemia ("anemia of chronic inflammation"), fatigue, and cachexia.

Tumor-promoting inflammation facilitates malignancy: Inflammatory cells can modify the tumor microenvironment and facilitate many of the hallmarks of cancer. These effects may be due to direct interactions between inflammatory cells and tumor cells, or indirect effects of inflammatory cells on other resident stromal cells (particularly fibroblasts and endothelial cells).

Mechanism of cancer-enabling effects of inflammatory cells and resident stromal cells: These are as follows:

- **Release of factors promoting proliferation by infiltrating leukocytes and activated stromal cells** (e.g., EGF).
- **Removal of growth suppressors:** Proteases from inflammatory cells can degrade the adhesion molecules involved in cell–cell, and cell–ECM interactions. This removes a barrier to growth because these interactions normally suppress the growth of epithelial cells.
- **Increased resistance to cell death**.
- **Angiogenesis:** Inflammatory cells release various factors such as VEGF that stimulate angiogenesis.
- **Invasion and metastasis:** Proteases released from macrophages remodel the ECM and facilitate tissue invasion. TNF and EGF may directly stimulate the motility of tumor cells.
- **Evasion of immune destruction:** Several soluble factors released by macrophages and other stromal cells may immunosuppress the tumor microenvironment.

ETIOLOGY OF CANCER: CARCINOGENIC AGENTS

PA 7.3 (CC): Enumerate carcinogens and describe the process of carcinogenesis.

Q. Classify different carcinogenic agents.

Definition: A **carcinogen** is an **agent known or suspected to cause tumors** and such agents are said to be **carcinogenic** (cancer-causing). **Carcinogenic agents cause genetic damage.**

Classes of carcinogenic agents (Flowchart 7.2): They belong to three classes (1) chemicals, (2) microbes, and (3) radiant energy (radiation). They may act singly or in concert or sequentially to produce multiple genetic abnormalities leading to neoplastic transformation.

Flowchart 7.2: Major types of carcinogenic agents.

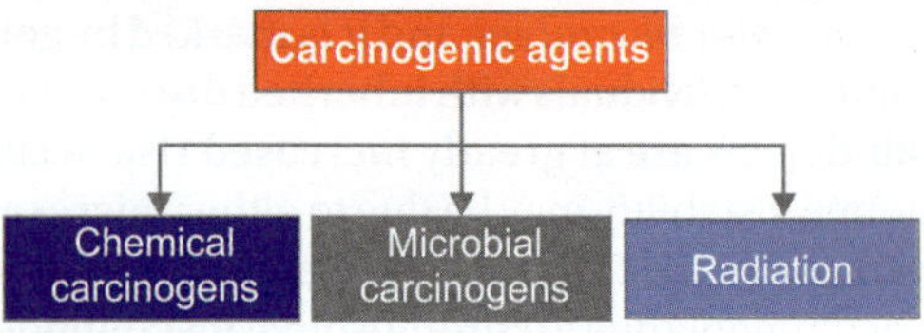

Chemical Carcinogenesis

Q. List major chemical carcinogens and describe in detail chemical carcinogenesis.

Sir Percival Pott (London surgeon) **first related scrotum skin cancer in chimney sweeps to a specific chronic chemical exposure to soot**. Based on this, a rule was made that chimney sweep members must bathe daily, and this public health measure controlled scrotal skin cancer. Japanese investigators (Yamagiva and Ichikawa) experimentally produced skin cancers in rabbits by using coal tar. Subsequently, hundreds of chemical carcinogens were discovered.

Classification of Chemical Carcinogens

Chemical carcinogens may be classified into two categories: Direct-acting and indirect-acting. Major chemical carcinogens are listed in **Box 7.8**.

Direct-acting Agents

Direct-acting chemical agents **do not require metabolic conversion to become carcinogenic**. Most of them are usually **weak carcinogens**. Some of them are used as **chemotherapeutic drugs** (e.g., alkylating agents) to cure, control, or delay the recurrence of some cancers (e.g., leukemia, lymphoma). They are also used for nonneoplastic disorders, such as rheumatoid arthritis.

Alkylating agents: Many chemotherapeutic drugs used to treat cancer (e.g., cyclophosphamide, cisplatin, busulfan) are alkylating agents. Alkylating agents **contain electron-deficient atoms** that **react with electron-rich atoms in DNA.** These drugs not only destroy cancer cells by damaging DNA but also injure normal cells. **Cancers produced** are **solid and hematological malignancies.**

Indirect-acting Agents (Procarcinogens)

Q. Write a short note on polycyclic hydrocarbons.

Indirect-acting carcinogens are chemicals that **require metabolic conversion to produce an active ultimate carcinogen.**

Polycyclic aromatic hydrocarbons: They are the most powerful indirect-acting chemical carcinogens. Examples (**Box 7.8**): Benzo[a]pyrene, dibenzanthracene, and 3-methylcholanthrene.

- **Source:** Originally derived from coal tar and fossil fuels. Other sources include:
  - **Cigarette smoke:** Polycyclic aromatic hydrocarbons are formed during high-temperature combustion of tobacco in cigarette smoking and are responsible for lung cancer in cigarette smokers.
  - **Animal fats:** These may be produced during the process of broiling (exposure to direct heat). Polycyclic aromatic hydrocarbon is also present in smoked meats and fish.
- **Mechanism of action:** Polycyclic hydrocarbons are metabolized by cytochrome P450-dependent mixed function oxidases to **electrophilic** (have electron-

BOX 7.8: Major chemical carcinogens.

DIRECT-ACTING CARCINOGENS

1. *Alkylating Agents*
   - β-Propiolactone
   - Anticancer drugs (cyclophosphamide, chlorambucil, nitrosoureas, etc.)
   - Dimethyl sulfate
   - Diepoxybutane
2. *Acylating Agents*
   - 1-Acetylimidazole
   - Dimethylcarbamoyl chloride

INDIRECT-ACTING CARCINOGENS (PROCARCINOGENS)

1. *Polycyclic and Heterocyclic Aromatic Hydrocarbons*
   - Benz[*a*]anthracene
   - Benzo[*a*]pyrene (active component of soot)
   - Dibenz[*a,h*]anthracene
   - 7,12-Dimethylbenz[*a*]anthracene
   - 3-Methylcholanthrene
2. *Aromatic Amines, Amides and Azo Dyes*
   - 2-Naphthylamine (β-naphthylamine)
   - Benzidine
   - 2-Acetylaminofluorene
   - Dimethylaminoazobenzene (butter yellow)

NATURAL PLANT AND MICROBIAL PRODUCTS

- Aflatoxin B_1
- Griseofulvin
- Betel nuts

OTHERS

- Nitrosamine and amides
- Vinyl chloride
- Metals: Nickel, chromium
- Insecticides, fungicides
- Asbestos

deficient atoms) **epoxides. Epoxides react with proteins and nucleic acids** (DNA, RNA). For example, **polyvinyl chloride** (used in the plastic industry) is metabolized to an epoxide and causes **hepatic angiosarcomas.**

- **Cancers produced:** The specific type of cancer produced depends on the route of administration. It produces cancers in the **skin, soft tissues, lungs, and breast.**

Aromatic amines and azo dyes: They are indirect-acting carcinogens.

- **Source: In the past, aromatic amines** (β-naphthylamine) and azo dyes were used **in the aniline dye and rubber industries. Azo-dyes** were used **for coloring food** (e.g., butter and margarine which give yellow color, and scarlet red for coloring cherries).
- **Mechanisms of action:** They are not carcinogenic at the point of application. Both aromatic amines and azo dyes are mainly metabolized in the liver.
  - The **aromatic amines are converted to active carcinogens in the liver.** However, can be **detoxified immediately by conjugation with glucuronic acid in the liver.**
  - The conjugated metabolite is **excreted in the urine and deconjugated in the urinary tract by the enzyme glucuronidase**. The urothelium is thus exposed to the active carcinogen (reactive hydroxylamine) which may cause bladder cancer.
- **Cancers produced: Bladder cancer** (aromatic amines: β-naphthylamine and benzidine) and **liver tumors** (azo dyes).

Natural Microbial Product

Aflatoxin B_1: Aflatoxin B_1 is a natural product of *Aspergillus flavus*, a mold that grows on improperly stored grains and peanuts.

- **Mechanism of action:** Metabolized to an **epoxide that binds to DNA** and produces **mutations of the *p53* gene.**
- **Cancers produced:** Powerful liver carcinogen that produces **hepatocellular carcinoma.**

Others

- **Nitrosamines**: They are potent carcinogens.
  - **Source: Before the advent of refrigerators,** nitrites were added as **a preservative for meats and other foods.**
  - **Mechanism of action: Nitrites in the food react with amines and amides in the diet.** They are **metabolized by commensal bacteria within the gut** and converted to **carcinogenic nitrosamines.**
  - **Cancers produced:** Mainly **gastrointestinal neoplasms.**
- **Metals:** Compounds like arsenic, nickel, lead, cadmium, cobalt, chromium, and beryllium can produce cancer. Most metal-induced cancers occur due to occupational exposure.
- **Asbestos:** Inhalation of asbestos fibers results in asbestosis, pleural plaques, **mesothelioma,** and **carcinoma of the lung.** Mesothelioma may involve the pleura as well as the peritoneum.

Detection of carcinogenicity of a chemical: Mutagenicity testing of chemicals is done by the **Ames test**. The appearance of frameshift mutations and base-pair substitutions in a culture of **bacteria of a *Salmonella* species** indicates that the chemical tested is carcinogenic.

Mechanism of Action of Chemical Carcinogens

Molecular targets of chemical carcinogens: Most chemical carcinogens are mutagenic. A **mutagen** is an agent, which can **permanently alter the genetic constitution** of a cell.

- **All direct and ultimate carcinogens** (indirect carcinogens) **contain highly reactive electrophilic groups and form chemical adducts with DNA.**
- **Genes affected:** Any gene may be affected but commonly involved are **proto-oncogenes (*RAS*) and tumor suppressor genes** (*p53*). Aflatoxin B_1 produces a characteristic mutation in *TP53*.

Multistep Hypothesis (Fig. 7.24)

Q. Write a short essay on multistep carcinogenesis.

Chemical carcinogenesis is a **multistep process** and is called the **initiation-promotion sequence of chemical carcinogenesis.** Once the tumor process is started, it does not require the continued presence of the carcinogen. **Two major steps involved in chemical carcinogenesis are (i) initiation, and (ii) promotion.**

Q. Differences between initiators and promoters.

Initiation: It is the first important step that develops from exposure of cells to a sufficient dose of a carcinogenic agent (initiator).

- **Permanent DNA damage:** All initiators are highly reactive electrophiles (electron-deficient atoms) and can react with nucleophilic (electron-rich). Initiators **produce permanent (irreversible) alterations or damage to DNA (mutations)** in a cell. If damage is lethal or severe it causes cell death.

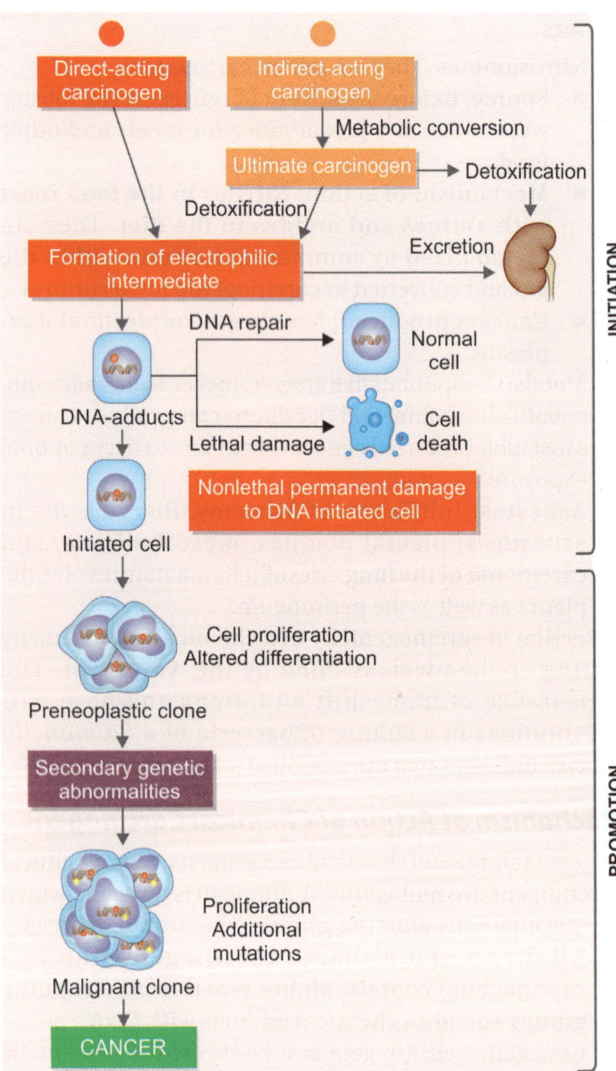

Fig. 7.24: Initiation and promotion of cancer by chemical carcinogens.

Q. Write a short note on promoters in carcinogenesis.

Promotion: Promoters by themselves are nontumorigenic **(noncarcinogenic/not mutagenic) agents. They cannot directly damage DNA (mutation).** The carcinogenicity of some chemicals is increased by subsequent administration of *promoters*. **They produce changes only on the initiated cell. Tumors develop only if the promoter is applied after the initiator** and not in the reverse way. Examples of promoters include **phorbol esters, hormones, phenols, and some drugs.** Some chemicals can act as both initiators and promoters.

- **Repeated or sustained exposure to the promoter** must follow the application of the mutagenic chemical, or *initiator*.
- **Sustained cell proliferation:** Promoters stimulate the initiated (with permanent DNA damage-mutated) **cells to enter the cell cycle leading to cell proliferation.** Unlike initiators, the **cellular changes produced by promoters are reversible.**
- **Neoplastic transformation: Continuous proliferation** of initiated cells **leads to secondary genetic abnormalities.** The tumor growth becomes independent of the initiator or the promoter (i.e., autonomous). **Many accumulated mutations finally immortalize the cells.**
- The result of the different steps is the development of neoplasm, invasion, and metastases.

Examples: The morphologic sequence of hyperplasia, dysplasia, and carcinoma in situ found in the epithelium (e.g., skin, cervix, and colon) indicate multistep carcinogenesis.

Microbial Carcinogenesis

Q. Define, list and classify oncogenic viruses. Explain the mechanism of tumor production by viruses.

Viruses that cause tumors are called oncogenic viruses: Many viruses have been proven to be oncogenic in animals, but only a few have been associated with cancer in humans. **Classification (Flowchart 7.3):** They are mainly classified depending on the genetic material into (1) oncogenic **RNA viruses,** and (2) oncogenic **DNA viruses.** Various viruses implicated in human tumors are listed in **Table 7.16.**

Q. Explain the mechanism involved in tumor production by viruses.

Oncogenic RNA Viruses

Q. Discuss the role of RNA viruses in tumorigenesis.

Human T-cell Leukemia Virus Type 1

Human T-cell leukemia virus type 1 (HTLV-1) is a retrovirus that is firmly involved in the pathogenesis of cancer in humans.

Flowchart 7.3: Classification and types of oncogenic viruses.

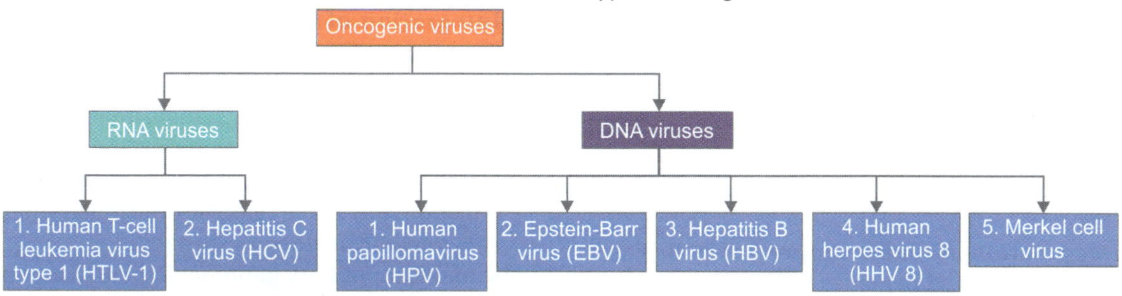

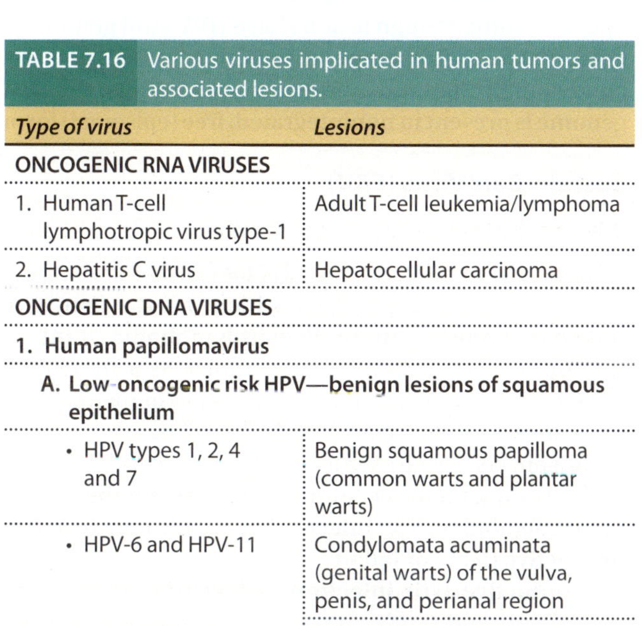

TABLE 7.16 Various viruses implicated in human tumors and associated lesions.

Type of virus	*Lesions*
ONCOGENIC RNA VIRUSES	
1. Human T-cell lymphotropic virus type-1	Adult T-cell leukemia/lymphoma
2. Hepatitis C virus	Hepatocellular carcinoma
ONCOGENIC DNA VIRUSES	
1. Human papillomavirus	
A. Low-oncogenic risk HPV—benign lesions of squamous epithelium	
• HPV types 1, 2, 4 and 7	Benign squamous papilloma (common warts and plantar warts)
• HPV-6 and HPV-11	Condylomata acuminata (genital warts) of the vulva, penis, and perianal region
	Laryngeal papillomas
B. High-oncogenic risk HPV—malignant tumors	
• HPV types 16 and 18	Squamous cell carcinoma of the cervix and anogenital region
	Oropharyngeal cancers (tonsil)
2. Epstein-Barr virus	Burkitt lymphoma (requires cofactor-malaria)
	Nasopharyngeal cancer
3. Hepatitis B virus	Hepatocellular carcinoma
4. Human herpes virus-8	Kaposi's sarcoma
	Pleural effusion lymphoma, multicentric Castleman disease
5. Merkel cell polyomavirus	Merkel cell carcinoma

Mode of infection: The virus is transmitted through infected T-cells by (1) Sexual intercourse, (2) blood products, and (3) breastfeeding.

Mechanism of oncogenesis: It is a **multi-step process, but the exact** steps involved in the development of adult T-cell leukemia/lymphoma are not known. HTLV-1 infects CD4+ T-cells.

- **Major target for neoplastic transformation: CD4+ T-lymphocyte** is the major target for neoplastic transformation (human immunodeficiency virus (HIV), which causes AIDS also targets CD4+ T cells).
- **Tumor caused:** It causes **adult T-cell leukemia/lymphoma (ATLL)**-develops after a long latent period (20–50 years).
- **HTLV-1 genome:** It contains the *gag, pol, env,* and *tax.* **Tax protein** (product of *tax*) is **needed for viral replication and cellular transformation.** Tax protein also activates other genes involved in T-cell proliferation and differentiation. The proliferating CD4+ T-cells are at **increased risk of developing mutations and genomic instability** because of Tax. Accumulation of mutations and chromosomal abnormalities eventually leads to form a monoclonal neoplastic **proliferation of CD4+ T-cell.** HTLV-1 **does not contain oncogene and its genes cannot integrate into the host genome.**

Oncogenic DNA Viruses

Five DNA viruses are strongly associated with cancer in humans. These are: (i) human papillomavirus (HPV), (ii) Epstein-Barr virus (EBV), (iii) Kaposi sarcoma herpesvirus [KSHV, also called human herpesvirus-8 (HHV-8)], (iv) a polyomavirus called Merkel cell virus (associated with Merkel cell carcinoma), and (v) hepatitis B virus (HBV) **(Flowchart 7.3).** HCV is an RNA (not a DNA) virus and found to be associated with cancer.

Human Papillomavirus (HPV)

Q. Write a short note on oncogenesis by human papillomavirus.

- **Types of HPV and associated lesions (Table 7.16):** More than 70 genetically different types of HPV have been identified. They are divided into **low-risk and high-risk HPVs** (*refer* pages 801-2). Low-risk HPVs cause benign lesions and high-risk HPVs cause malignant lesions.
- **Cell infected:** Human papillomaviruses (HPV) infect **only the immature squamous cells** but **its replication occurs in the maturing, nonproliferating squamous cells.** Thus, their full productive life cycle occurs only in squamous cells. The physical state of the virus differs in different lesions.

Q. Write a short note on high-risk human papillomaviruses.

Mode of action (Fig. 7.25)

Oncogenic effects of HPV: It is related to the products of **the two viral genes *E6* and *E7*. Protein products of E6 and E7 (oncoproteins)** are important for the oncogenic effects of HPV.

- **Oncogenic activities of E6:** The E6 protein has following actions:
  - **Degradation of tumor suppressor p53:** The E6 protein binds and degrades p53. E6 from high-risk HPV types has more attraction for p53 than E6 from low-risk HPV types.
  - **Activation (upregulation) of telomerase:** E6 stimulates the expression of TERT (the catalytic subunit of telomerase). This leads to the immortalization of cells.
- **Oncogenic activities of E7 protein:** The E7 protein supplement the effects of E6. All these effects speed up the passage of cells through the G_1 -S cell cycle checkpoint. The E7 protein has the following actions.
  - **Binding and inactivation of RB protein: The E7 protein of HPV binds** to the hypophosphorylated (active) form of **RB protein** and **inactivates RB.** This **releases the E2F transcription factors** (that are normally bound to active RB) and promotes the **progression of the cell cycle**. Similar to E6, E7 proteins from high-risk HPV types have a higher affinity for RB than E7 proteins from low-risk HPV types.
  - **Inactivation of CDK inhibitor (p21) of the cell cycle: This activates the progression of the cell cycle.**
  - **Increase of CDK/cyclin D:** This **activates the progression of the cell cycle.**
- **Combined action of E6 and E7: Both increase cell proliferation, produce genomic instability, immortalization of cells, and resistance to cell death.**
- **Integration of HPV genome into host DNA:** The oncogenic effect of HPVs is also related to the viral integration into the host genome. This integration is essential for malignant transformation. Integration interrupts a negative regulatory region in the viral DNA. This leads to overexpression of the E6 and E7 oncoproteins. These cells with integrated viral genomes show significant genomic instability.

Episomal form of HPV genome: In benign and precursor cervical lesions, the HPV genome is in a nonintegrated episomal form. **Benign lesions have HPV viral genome in episomal form.** In **benign lesions** such as benign warts, condylomata, and most **precancerous lesions**; the **HPV genome is present in nonintegrated, free** (episomal) **form.**

Epstein-Barr Virus (EBV)

Q. Write a short note on the Epstein-Barr virus.

Q. List diseases and cancers produced by the Epstein-Barr virus.

EBV is a human **herpesvirus, which was the first virus linked to a human tumor, Burkitt lymphoma.** It **infects B lymphocytes**. Patients may manifest as a short-lived **infectious mononucleosis** or develop a few human cancers. The **cancers** produced are listed in **Box 7.9.**

Pathogenesis: EB virus infects B lymphocytes by binding to the complement receptor CD21 (CR2) on the surface of the membrane. The **infection of B-cells may be either productive** (lytic) **or latent**.

- **Productive/lytic infection**: It **develops only in a few patients** and results in the death of infected cells and the release of virions. These virions infect other B-cells.
- **Latent infection**: It **occurs in most of the cases.** The virus becomes latent inside the B-cells. These B cells are transformed into immortal B lymphoblastoid cell lines"

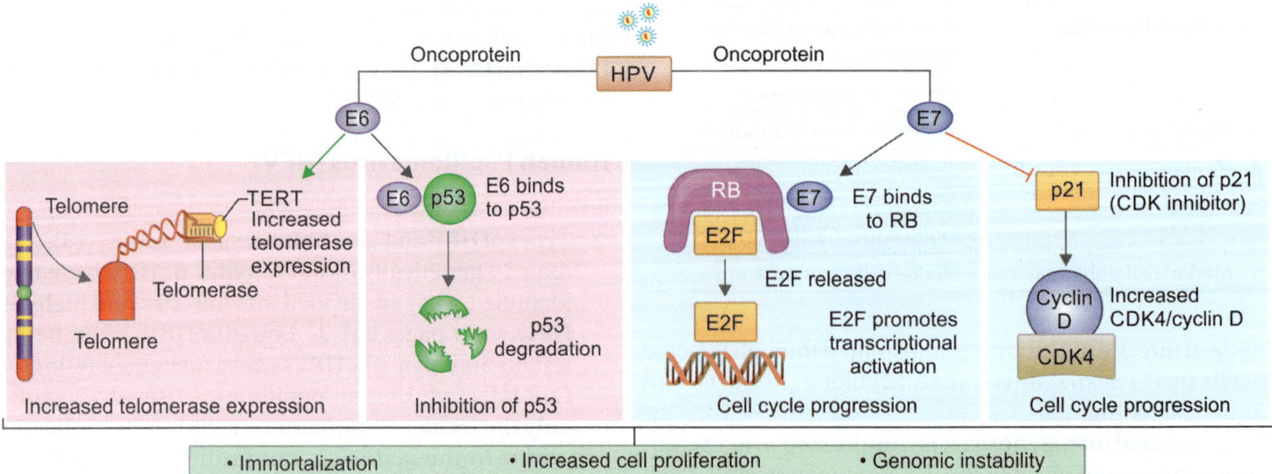

Fig. 7.25: Transforming effects of HPV E6 and E7 proteins on the cell cycle. Both HPV E6 and E7 proteins immortalize cells, protect cells from cell death, and result in increased cell proliferation.

(CDK: cyclin dependent kinase; HPV: human papillomavirus; RB: retinoblastoma; TERT: telomerase reverse transcriptase).

BOX 7.9: List of cancers produced by Epstein-Barr virus.

1. African form of Burkitt lymphoma.
2. B-cell lymphomas in immunosuppressed (e.g., HIV infection or immunosuppressive therapy after organ transplantation).
3. A subset of Hodgkin lymphoma.
4. Nasopharyngeal carcinoma (T-cell tumor).
5. Some gastric carcinomas.
6. Rare forms of T-cell lymphomas and natural killer (NK) cell lymphomas.
7. Very rarely sarcomas (smooth muscle tumors, mainly in immunosuppressed patients).

so that they are capable of proliferation indefinitely. **Immortalization of B lymphocytes is the hallmark of EBV infection. The molecular basis of B-cell immortalization** is related to **two EBV-coded genes** and **viral cytokines.**

1. **LMP1 (latent membrane protein 1):** It is an EBV-encoded gene and **acts as an oncogene** and **promotes** B-cell **proliferation and survival** (prevents apoptosis by activating **Bcl-2**).
2. **EBNA2 (Epstein-Barr nuclear antigens 2):** EBV-encoded protein **stimulates transcription of many** other **host genes**, including genes that drive the cell cycle (e.g., cyclin D) and the *SRC* family of proto-oncogenes.
3. **Viral cytokine (vIL-10):** It is pirated from the host genome, **preventing macrophages and monocytes from activating T-cells and killing virally infected cells.**

African form of Burkitt lymphoma: It is a **B-cell neoplasm** and is the **most common childhood tumor in central Africa** and New Guinea. A morphologically similar lymphoma occurs sporadically throughout the world.

- **Mechanism of endemic Burkitt lymphoma: Normally, EBV infects B-cells and stimulates B-lymphocyte proliferation which is controlled by suppressor T-cells.** The sequence of events in the pathogenesis of endemic African Burkitt lymphoma are:
  - **Accompanying infections** (such as **malaria** or other infections) **impairs immune competence. The absence of an adequate suppressor T-cell response** allows **uncontrolled proliferation of B-cell.**
  - **EBV-infected B-cells expressing LMP-1 are eliminated by the immune system.**
  - **Lymphoma develops** only **when there are chromosomal translocations** that activate the ***c-MYC*** **oncogene** (*refer* **Fig. 12.20**) resulting in **uncontrolled proliferation** of a malignant clone of B lymphocytes.
- **Mechanism of nonendemic Burkitt lymphoma**: All tumors possess the t (8;14) or other translocations that dysregulate c-*MYC*. For details *refer* page 389.

Hepatitis B and C Viruses

HBV is a DNA virus whereas **HCV is an RNA virus**. There is a strong association between chronic infection with HBV and HCV (chronic hepatitis and cirrhosis) with primary **hepatocellular carcinoma**.

Mechanism: The oncogenic effects of both HBV and HCV are **multifactorial.**

- **Immunologically mediated chronic inflammation**: It has a dominant effect and causes **death of the hepatocytes.**
- **Compensatory liver cell regeneration**: It is due to several growth factors and cytokines produced by **activated immune cells of inflammation.**
- **Genomic damage and mutation:** These are due to mediators (e.g., reactive oxygen species) produced by activated immune cells.

  HBV: HBV genome contains a viral regulatory gene known as ***HBx***. Various actions of *HBx* are:
  - Direct or indirect **activation of many transcription factors and signal transduction pathways.**
  - **Inactivation of *p53***
  - **HBV DNA can be integrated within the human genome** and can **cause multiple deletions,** which may harbor unknown tumor suppressor genes.

  HCV: The HCV genome, such as the **HCV core protein**, may **activate many growth-promoting signal transduction pathways** and cause tumors. HCV is associated with **lymphoplasmacytic lymphoma**.

Human Herpes Virus 8 (HHV 8)

It is a **DNA virus**, which **infects the spindle cells of Kaposi sarcoma** and also **lymphocytes.**

Neoplasm produced

- **Kaposi sarcoma:** It is a **vascular neoplasm**, which is the **most common neoplasm, associated with AIDS.** HHV 8 has also been found in Kaposi sarcoma from HIV-negative patients.
- **B-cell lymphoid malignancies**: Two uncommon lymphoid malignancies, namely **primary effusion lymphoma** and **multicentric Castleman disease** are associated with HHV 8.

Mechanism

- **HHV 8 viral genome encodes proteins, which interfere with the *p53* and *RB* tumor suppressor pathways.**
- HHV 8 also **encodes gene products, which downregulate class I major histocompatibility complex (MHC) expression.** The infected cells **escape recognition by cytotoxic T lymphocytes.**

Other Microbial Carcinogens

Bacteria

Helicobacter pylori: Diseases caused by *H. pylori* are: (1) **peptic ulcers, (2) gastric adenocarcinomas, and (3) gastric lymphomas.**

Gastric adenocarcinomas

Mechanism: It is like that of HBV and HCV-induced hepatocellular carcinoma. *H. pylori* causing gastric adenocarcinoma contains **cytotoxin-associated A (*CagA*)** gene that can penetrate gastric epithelial cells, initiate signals, and lead to unregulated growth factor stimulation.
Chronic inflammation: *H. pylori* causes chronic inflammation (chronic gastritis), followed by gastric atrophy, intestinal metaplasia, dysplasia, and ultimately cancer.

Gastric lymphoma

H. pylori produces lymphomas of **B-cell origin** which are called lymphomas of mucosa-associated lymphoid tissue, or **MALTomas**. *H. pylori* is associated with t (11;18) translocation in MALT lymphomas.

Fungi

Fungi may cause cancer by producing toxic substances (mycotoxins). **Aflatoxin B_1** produced by *Aspergillus flavus* is a potent carcinogen responsible for **hepatocellular carcinoma.**

Parasites

Two parasites that can cause tumors are:

1. ***Schistosoma*** is strongly implicated in **carcinoma of the urinary bladder (usually of squamous cell type)**. The ova of the parasite can be found in the affected tissue.
2. ***Clonorchis sinensis*** (Chinese liver fluke) lodges in the bile ducts and produces an inflammatory reaction, epithelial hyperplasia, and sometimes **adenocarcinoma of the bile ducts (cholangiocarcinoma)**.

Hormones

Hormones in the body may act as cofactors in carcinogenesis.

Estrogen

- **Endometrial carcinoma:** It may develop in females with estrogen-secreting **granulosa cell tumors of the ovary** or those receiving exogenous estrogen.
- **Adenocarcinoma of the vagina:** Increased frequency of adenocarcinoma of the vagina is observed in **daughters of mothers who received estrogen during pregnancy**.
- **Abnormal vascularity of tumor: Estrogens can make existing tumors abnormally vascular** (e.g., adenomas and focal nodular hyperplasia).

Androgenic and anabolic steroids: They may cause hepatocellular tumors.

Hormone-dependent Tumors

- **Prostatic carcinoma** usually responds to administration of estrogens or castration.
- **Breast carcinomas** regress following oophorectomy.

Radiation Carcinogenesis

Q. Write a short note on radiation-induced cancers.

Radiation is a **well-known carcinogen**.
Latency: Extremely long latent period is common and **it has a cumulative effect**. Radiation has also **additive or synergistic effects with other** potential **carcinogenic agents**.
Types of radiation: They are divided into two types, namely (1) ultraviolet (UV) rays of sunlight, and (2) ionizing electromagnetic and particulate radiation.

Ultraviolet Rays

They are derived from the sunlight.
Tumors caused: UV radiation derived from the sun can cause **skin cancer,** namely (1) **squamous cell carcinoma,** (2) **basal cell carcinoma,** and (3) **melanoma**. They are more common in parts of the body regularly exposed to sunlight and ultraviolet light (UVL).
Risk factors: The amount of damage incurred depends on:

- **Type of UV rays**
- **Intensity of exposure**
- **Protective mantle of melanin: Melanin** absorbs UV radiation and has a **protective effect.** Skin cancers are more common in fair-skinned people and those living in geographic locations receiving a greater amount of sunlight (e.g., Queensland, Australia, close to the equator).

Pathogenesis

- UV radiation leads to the **formation of pyrimidine dimers in DNA**, which is a type of DNA damage that is responsible for carcinogenicity.
- **DNA damage is repaired by the nucleotide excision repair pathway.**
- With **excessive sun exposure**, the DNA **damage exceeds the capacity of the nucleotide excision repair pathway** and **genomic injury becomes mutagenic and carcinogenic**.

Xeroderma pigmentosum: It is a rare **hereditary autosomal recessive disorder** characterized by **congenital deficiency of nucleotide excision repair DNA**. These individuals **develop skin cancers** (basal cell carcinoma, squamous cell carcinoma, and melanoma) due to impairment in the excision of UV-damaged DNA.

Ionizing Radiation

Electromagnetic (X-rays, γ-rays) and particulate (α particles, β particles, protons, neutrons) radiations are all carcinogenic.

Cancers Produced

- **Medical or occupational exposure**, e.g., **leukemia and skin cancers.**

- **Nuclear plant accidents:** Risk of **lung cancers.**
- **Atomic bomb explosion:** Survivors of the atomic bomb explosion (dropped on Hiroshima and Nagasaki) increased the incidence of **leukemias,** mainly acute and chronic myelogenous leukemia after about 7 years. Subsequently, increased mortality due to **solid tumors** (e.g., breast, colon, thyroid, and lung).
- **Therapeutic radiation:** (1) **papillary carcinoma of the thyroid** follows irradiation of the head and neck and (2) **angiosarcoma of the liver** due to radioactive thorium dioxide used to visualize the arterial tree.

Mechanism: Hydroxyl free radical injury to DNA.

Tissues that are relatively resistant to radiation-induced neoplasia: Skin, bone, and the gastrointestinal tract.

CLINICAL ASPECTS OF NEOPLASIA

PA 7.4 (CC): Describe the effects of the tumor on the host including paraneoplastic syndrome.

Q. Clinical features of malignant tumors.

Both benign and malignant tumors may produce clinical features through their various effects on the host. Usually, malignant tumors are more likely to harm than benign tumors. However, morbidity and mortality may be associated with any tumor, even benign.

Effects of Tumor on the Host

Malignant and benign tumors may cause damage in different ways. These are as follows:

Damage of healthy tissues: This may be due to compression (e.g., adenoma in the ampulla of Vater obstructing the biliary tract) encroachment on adjacent structures.

Endocrine insufficiency may be caused by to destruction of an endocrine gland either due to primary or metastatic cancer. The location of both benign and malignant tumors is essential. For example, a small (1 cm) pituitary adenoma can compress and destroy the surrounding normal gland, causing hypopituitarism.

Ulceration of surfaces leading to bleeding and secondary infections: It may develop in benign or malignant tumors in the skin or mucosa of the GI tract, e.g., melena (blood in the stool) in neoplasms of the gut, hematuria in neoplasms of the urinary tract.

Release of substances: These include hormones and procoagulants. These may produce systemic effects. **Hormonal effects** may be observed both in benign and malignant tumors of endocrine glands, e.g., β-cell adenoma of the pancreas may produce insulin to cause fatal hypoglycemia. Nonendocrine tumors may secrete hormones or hormone-like substances and produce **paraneoplastic syndromes** (explained below).

Alteration of immune function: This may lead to infection and certain paraneoplastic syndromes.

Mechanical obstruction: It may be caused by both benign and malignant tumors. For example, tumor may protrude into the gut lumen and cause intussusception, intestinal obstruction or infarction in the GI tract.

Fever: It is most commonly associated with Hodgkin disease, renal cell carcinoma, and osteogenic sarcoma. Fever may be due to the release of pyrogens by tumor cells or IL-1 produced by inflammatory cells in the stroma of the tumor.

Tumor lysis syndrome: It is a group of metabolic complications that can occur after treatment for leukemias such as **acute lymphoblastic leukemia (ALL), chronic lymphocytic leukemia (CLL); lymphomas such as Burkitt lymphoma,** and uncommonly in solid tumors.

- **Cause:** It is caused by **breakdown products of tumor cells following chemotherapy or glucocorticoids or hormonal agents** (tamoxifen). The killed tumor cells **release intracellular ions and large amounts of metabolic byproducts into the systemic circulation.**
- **Metabolic abnormalities** include:
  - **Hyperuricemia:** Due to increased turnover of nucleic acids. It can cause uric acid precipitation in the kidney resulting in **renal failure.**
  - **Hyperkalemia:** Due to the release of the most abundant intracellular cation potassium.
  - **Hyperphosphatemia:** Due to the release of intracellular phosphate.
  - **Hypocalcemia:** Due to the complexing of calcium with elevated phosphate.
  - **Lactic acidosis.**

Cancer Cachexia (Wasting)

Q. Write a short note on cachexia.

It is defined as **progressive loss of body fat and lean body mass (weight loss), accompanied by severe weakness, anorexia, and anemia developing in patients with cancer.** There may be some correlation between the size and extent of the spread of the cancer and the severity of the cachexia.

Mechanism: It is poorly understood. Cachexia is not due to the nutritional demands of the tumor. It may be due to the action of soluble factors (e.g., cytokines) produced by the tumor and the host, not simply due to reduced food intake. **TNF and other cytokines,** produced by macrophages or the tumor cells themselves may mediate cachexia.

Paraneoplastic Syndromes

Q. Write a short note on paraneoplastic syndrome.

Q. Write a short note on:

- Tumors which produce paraneoplastic syndromes.
- Paraneoplastic syndromes produced by small cell (oat cell) carcinoma of the lung.
- Paraneoplastic syndromes produced by renal cell carcinoma (RCC).

Malignant tumors invade local tissue, produce metastasis, and can produce a variety of products that can stimulate hormonal, hematologic, dermatologic, and neurologic responses. Usually, the symptoms of cancer are due to local effects of the primary tumor mass or its metastases. However, in some patients, cancers produce unknown effects not due to tumor invasion or metastasis. These are collectively called paraneoplastic syndromes.

Definition: Paraneoplastic syndromes are **symptom complexes in cancer patients** that **cannot be explained by local or distant spread of the tumor or by the secretion of hormones typical to the tissue of tumor origin.**

Importance of recognition: Though they occur in 10–15% of patients, it is important because:

1. **They may be the first manifestation** of an **occult neoplasm**.
2. **They may be mistaken for metastatic disease** leading to inappropriate treatment.
3. They may present clinical illness or **may be fatal**.
4. Certain tumor products causing paraneoplastic syndromes may be **useful in monitoring recurrence** in patients who had surgical resections or are undergoing chemotherapy or radiation therapy.

Some paraneoplastic syndromes, their mechanism, and common cancer-causing them are listed in **Table 7.17**.

Types of paraneoplastic syndromes: Paraneoplastic **syndromes** are of multiple types and are associated with many different tumors **(Table 7.17)**. **The most common are hypercalcemia, Cushing syndrome, and nonbacterial thrombotic endocarditis.** The most common neoplasms associated with paraneoplastic syndromes are **lung and breast cancers and hematologic malignancies**. Hypercalcemia in cancer patients is multifactorial, but the most important mechanism of the paraneoplastic syndrome is due to the secretion of a parathyroid hormone-related protein (PTHrP) by tumor cells.

Prognosis

Q. Write a short note on prognostic factors of malignant tumors.

The prognosis of malignant tumors varies and is determined partly by the characteristics of the tumor cells (e.g., growth rate, invasiveness) and partly by the effectiveness of therapy.

Prognostic indices: Prognosis and the treatment of a malignant tumor depend on:

1. **Tumor type:** It is usually identified from the growth pattern of the tumor and its origin by only histopathological examination.
   - **Prognosis depends on the histological type** (e.g., squamous cell carcinoma, melanoma, adenocarcinoma, leiomyosarcoma).
   - Some tumors like lymphomas require further subclassification into Hodgkin and non-Hodgkin lymphoma, each of which is then further subclassified by the cell type.
2. **Grading of malignant tumors** (discussed below)
3. **Staging of tumors** (discussed below).

Grading and Staging of Cancer

These are necessary to predict prognosis and to compare the results of various treatment protocols. For example, the treatment plan and prognosis markedly differ between well-differentiated tumors localized to the organ (e.g., thyroid gland) and anaplastic cancers that invade the surrounding structures (e.g., neck in thyroid carcinoma). The grading is the level of differentiation, and staging is for assessing the extent of the spread of cancer within the patient. **Staging is of greater clinical value than tumor grading.**

Grading of Malignant Tumors

Grading is done by histological examination and is mainly based on the **degree of differentiation** of the tumor cells. In certain cancers, the number of mitoses, the extent of tumor necrosis, and the presence of certain architectural features (e.g., loss of gland formation and replacement by solid sheets of cells) are also used for grading. In general, there is a **correlation between histological grade and biological behavior**. Grading schemes are evolved for each type of malignancy. Generally grading ranges from two categories (low grade and high grade) to five categories. Most grading systems classify tumors into **three or four grades** of increasing malignancy. Low-grade tumors are well-differentiated; high-grade ones tend to be anaplastic.

Shortcomings of grading: (1) Less correlation with behavior: In general, in soft-tissue sarcomas, grading is of less clinical value than staging; **(2) subjective:** Grading is subjective and the degree of differentiation can vary in different areas of the same tumor.

Staging of Tumors

Staging **refers to the extent of the spread of a malignant tumor** and is independent of grading. The **mode of treatment is determined by the stage of a cancer** than by its grade.

Criteria for staging: Staging requires **both histopathological examinations** of the resected tumor and **clinical assessment** of the patient [including additional non-invasive techniques like computed tomography (CT), magnetic resonance imaging (MRI), and positron emission tomography (PET)]. The **criteria used** for staging **vary with different organs**. Commonly the staging of solid cancers is based on:

- **Size and extent of local growth of the primary tumor:** For example, in colorectal cancer, the tumor that has penetrated the muscularis and serosa of the bowel is associated with a poorer prognosis than with a tumor restricted to superficial mucosa/submucosa.

TABLE 7.17 Paraneoplastic syndromes.

Clinical syndromes	*Cause/mechanism*	*Example of associated cancer*
1. Endocrinopathies		
Cushing syndrome	ACTH or ACTH-like substance	Small-cell carcinoma of the lung
Syndrome due to inappropriate antidiuretic hormone secretion (SIADH)	Antidiuretic hormone	Small-cell carcinoma of the lung
Hypercalcemia	Parathyroid hormone-related protein (PTHRP), TGF-α	Squamous cell carcinoma of the lung
		Renal carcinoma, breast carcinoma
Hypoglycemia	Insulin or insulin-like substance	Fibrosarcoma
Polycythemia	Erythropoietin	Renal carcinoma, hepatocellular carcinoma
2. Nerve and muscle syndromes		
Myasthenia	Immunological	Lung carcinoma
Disorders of the central and peripheral nervous systems	Immunological	Breast carcinoma, teratoma
3. Dermatologic disorders		
Acanthosis nigricans	Secretion of epidermal growth factor or other growth factors	Carcinoma of the stomach, lung, and uterus
Dermatomyositis	Immunological	Lung and breast carcinoma
4. Changes in osseous, articular and soft-tissue		
Hypertrophic osteoarthropathy and clubbing of the fingers	Not known	Lung carcinoma
5. Vascular and hematologic changes		
Venous thrombosis (Trousseau syndrome)	Tumor products like mucins which activate clotting	Pancreatic carcinoma
		Lung carcinoma
Nonbacterial thrombotic endocarditis	Hypercoagulability	Advanced cancers
Red cell aplasia	Immunological	Thymoma
6. Renal syndromes		
Nephrotic syndrome	Tumor antigens, immune complexes	Various cancers
7. Amyloidosis		
Primary amyloidosis	Immunological (AL protein)	Multiple myeloma
Secondary amyloidosis	AA protein	Renal cell carcinoma and other solid tumors

(ACTH: adrenocorticotropic hormone; IL: interleukin; TGF: transforming growth factor; TNF: tumor necrosis factor).

- **Extent of spread to regional lymph nodes**: The presence of lymph node metastases indicates poor prognosis than without lymph node involvement.
- **Presence of or absence of blood-borne (distant) metastases**: The presence of blood borne distant metastases is a bad prognostic sign and is a contraindication to surgical intervention other than for palliative measures.

Currently, the major staging system in use is the American Joint Committee on Cancer Staging. This system uses a classification called the *TNM system*. Tumor spread is usually designated more compactly as stage I, II, III, or IV, often with substages.

TNM Systems (Fig. 7.26)

Q. Grading and staging of cancer.

TNM system is the cancer staging system widely used and it varies for each specific form of cancer. Its general principles are:

- T refers to the **primary tumor**. Primary tumor (T) is suffixed by a number that indicates the size of the tumor or local anatomical extent. The number varies according to the organ involved in the tumor. The primary lesion is characterized as **T1 to T4**, based on increasing size and invasion of adjacent structures. T0 indicates an in-situ lesion in which the lesion is still bounded by the basement membrane.

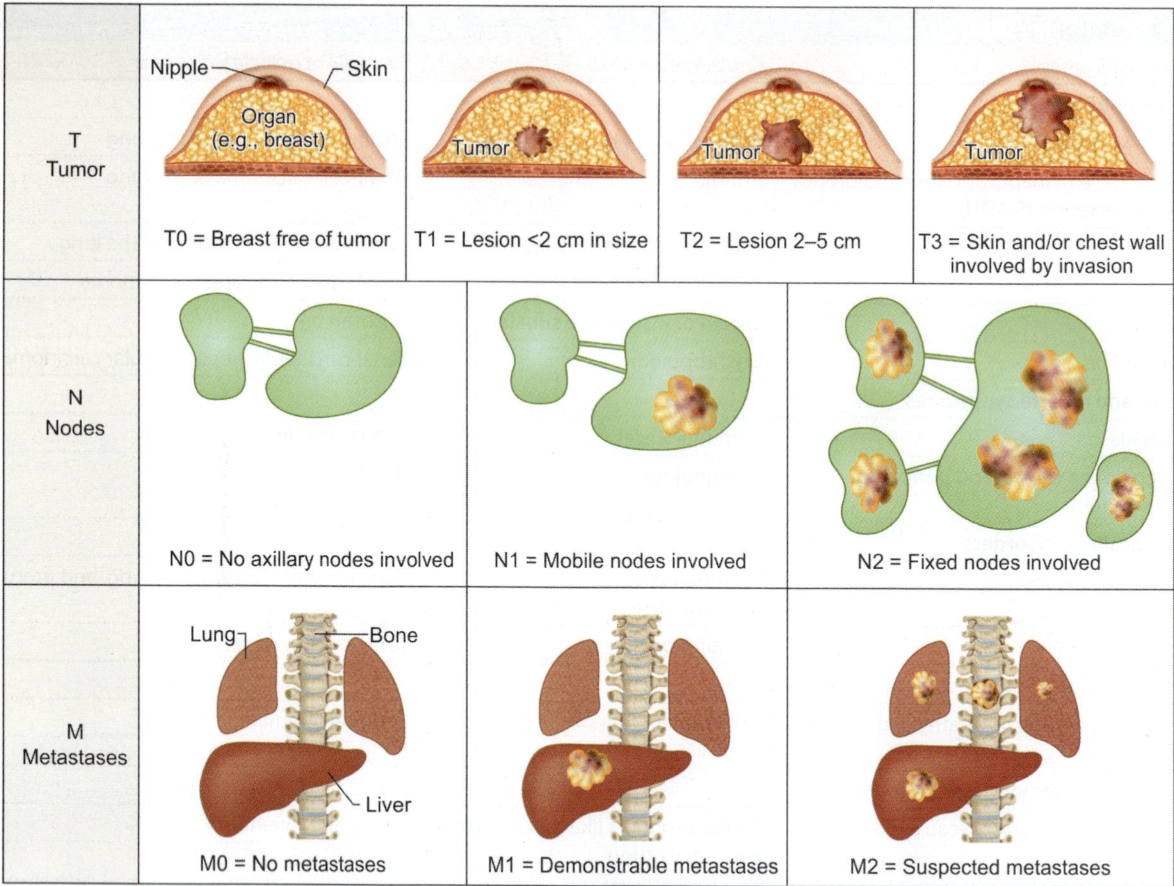

Fig. 7.26: Tumor staging by TNM system (e.g., breast carcinoma). TNM system is just one of many staging systems in current use.

- **N** refers to **lymph node status**. It is suffixed by a number to indicate the number of regional lymph nodes or groups of lymph nodes showing metastases. N0 would mean no nodal involvement. N1 to N3 would denote the involvement of an increasing number and range of nodes.
- **M** refers to the presence and anatomical extent of **distant metastases**. M0 signifies no distant metastases, whereas M1 indicates the presence of metastases.

In modern times, the grading and staging of tumors are being expanded by the addition of molecular characterization.

LABORATORY DIAGNOSIS OF CANCER

Q. Write a short note on laboratory diagnosis of cancer.

Confirmation of lesion as neoplastic usually requires cytological and/or histopathological examination of the suspected organ or tissue. With modernization, laboratory diagnosis of cancer is becoming more complex, more sophisticated, and more specialized. Different laboratory methods available for the diagnosis of malignant tumors are:

Morphological Methods

In most situations, the laboratory diagnosis of the benign-malignant spectrum of neoplasm is not problematic. However, accurate diagnosis may be challenging.

Histopathological Examination

Histopathological diagnosis is based on the microscopic features of neoplasm and by this method of examination, **accurate diagnosis can be made in most cases.** For optimal pathologic diagnosis, it is necessary to have clinical and radiologic data.

- **Clinical data:** It should be provided for accurate pathologic diagnosis. For example, radiation causes changes in the skin or mucosa that mimic changes seen in cancer, and sections taken from the site of a healing fracture can mimic osteosarcoma.
- **Adequate and representative** area of the **specimen** should be sent.
- **Proper fixation**.

Frozen Section

Q. Write a short essay/note on the frozen section and its uses.

In a rapid frozen section, the freshly removed **tissue is hardened rapidly by freezing** (quick-frozen, hence termed frozen section) and **sections are cut by a special instrument** called **freezing microtome or cryostat** (microtome in a refrigerated chamber). It permits histologic evaluation within minutes. **Uses of the frozen section are (Box 7.10):**

- **Rapid diagnosis:** Frozen section is sometimes used for quick histologic diagnosis (direct immediate surgical decisions within minutes) and useful **for determining the nature of a mass/tumor** (benign or malignant) lesion, especially when the **patient is still on the operation table**. It will help to determine whether a lesion is a neoplasm and, if so, whether it is benign or malignant.
- **Evaluation of the margins of an excised cancer** to know whether excision of the neoplasm is complete. If resection margins are inadequate, additional tissue can be removed immediately, without the need for a subsequent operation.
- **Demonstration of fat** mainly in non-neoplastic lesions.
- **To know the lymph node (sentinel/regional) status in a patient with carcinoma.** Knowing the extent of regional tumor metastases may be useful in deciding further surgery.
- **To determine whether additional workup is necessary** for a particular tissue specimen while it is still fresh. For example, if the metastatic tumor found in a lymph node is recognized as a poorly differentiated carcinoma, special fixation and electron microscopy may be needed for proper diagnosis.

Various Techniques for Tissue Sampling (Table 7.18)

Several means are used clinically to sample tumors.

- **Needle biopsy:** It is called as cutting-needle or core-needle or drill biopsy. Using a cutting needle, a core of tissue 1–2 mm wide and 2 cm long is obtained for histologic examinations or special studies that permit evaluation of architectural structure. The tissue obtained is small and interpretation may be difficult.
- **Endoscopy biopsy:** It is performed through endoscopy. Usually performed for lesions in gastrointestinal, respiratory, urinary, and genital tracts.

BOX 7.10: Uses of frozen section.

- Rapid diagnosis
- Evaluation of the margins of an excised cancer
- Demonstration of fat.
- To know the lymph node (sentinel) status in carcinoma.
- To determine whether additional workup is necessary.

TABLE 7.18 Various techniques for obtaining tissue for diagnosis.

Procedure	*Purpose*	*Example*
Histopathological examination		
Core needle biopsy	Performed with direct vision, or guided with ultrasound or CT	Needle biopsy of prostate or liver mass
Endoscopic biopsy	Performed through endoscopy	Gastrointestinal, respiratory, urinary, and genital tracts
Incisional biopsy	Removal of a portion of the lesion	Lymph node biopsy, large tumor
Excisional biopsy	Complete removal, usually with a margin of normal tissue	Full resection (e.g., mastectomy, partial colectomy)
Cytological examination		
Fine needle aspirate	Cells by aspiration for cytologic study	Thyroid, breast mass, salivary gland
Exfoliative cytology	Cells shed from the surface [e.g., from the cervix, sputum (lung), or urine]	Brushings from lung or colon endoscopy

- **Incision biopsy:** In this representative tissue sample is obtained by incising the lesions. Incisional biopsy (along with fine-needle aspiration) is often the method of choice for inoperable lesions, that or too large for excision, or when excision causes functional or cosmetic impairment.
- **Excision biopsy**: In this entire abnormal lesion is surgically removed. It provides generous amounts of tissue for diagnosis and may be surgical therapy for some tumors (e.g., small- to medium-sized breast cancers.

Pitfalls in biopsy interpretation: These include inadequate tissue sampling and artifacts due to the procedure itself (e.g., thermal damage caused by an electrocautery or laser).

Cytological Examination

Cytologic (Papanicolaou) tests are another method for the diagnosis of cancer. It is performed on many tissues and is usually done for identifying neoplastic cells.

Methods of Obtaining Cells

Exfoliative cytology: It is the **study of spontaneously exfoliated (shed) cells** from the lining of an organ into a body cavity. Discussed in detail on pages 307-12.

Fine-needle aspiration cytology (FNAC): It is a minimally invasive approach that involves **aspiration of cells and attendant fluid** from a mass **using a small-bore needle.** The smears are prepared by spreading them out on a slide and stained. These cells are microscopically examined. It is a **widely used, simple,** reliable, useful, **and quick procedure** used most commonly with readily palpable lesions affecting the breast, thyroid gland, lymph nodes, and salivary glands. The current availability of imaging techniques allows the FNAC method for deeper structures, such as the liver, pancreas, and pelvic lymph nodes. FNAC obviates surgery and its attendant risks. For details *refer* pages 313-5.

Liquid-based cytology (thin prep): This is a special technique for the preparation of samples that provides uniform monolayered dispersion of cells on smears.

Tumors Where Cytology is Useful for Diagnosis

Cytology is useful for detecting **carcinomas of the uterine cervix, endometrium, lung, bladder, prostate, and stomach.** It is also used for the identification of tumor cells in **abdominal, pleural, joint, and cerebrospinal fluids.**

Cytological Characteristics of Cancer Cells

Cancer cells have decreased cohesiveness than normal and are readily shed into fluids or secretions. The shed cells are examined for cellular features of **anaplasia**. Cytologically, differentiation can be made between normal, dysplastic, carcinoma in situ, and malignant cells. The cytological method has helped in the early diagnosis and control of cervical cancer.

Disadvantages of Cytological Examination

- **Diagnosis is based on the features of individual cells** or a clump of cells, without supporting evidence of loss of orientation.
- The **invasion** which is diagnostic of malignant tumor under histology **cannot be assessed** by cytology.

Histochemistry and Cytochemistry

These are stains, which identify the chemical nature of cell contents or their products. H&E staining cannot demonstrate certain specific substances/constituents of cells. This requires some special stains. Common histochemical and cytochemical stains useful in the diagnosis of tumors are listed in **Table 7.19**.

TABLE 7.19 Common histochemical and cytochemical stains useful in the diagnosis of tumors.

Chemical substance	*Name of the stain*
Basement membrane/ collagen	Periodic acid-Schiff (PAS), reticulin, Masson trichrome, Van Gieson
Glycogen	PAS with diastase
Mucin	Combined Alcian blue-PAS, and Mucicarmine
Cross-striation	Phosphotungstic acid hematoxylin (PTAH)
Enzymes	Myeloperoxidase, acid phosphatase, alkaline phosphatase

Immunohistochemistry

Q. Write a short note on immunohistochemistry and its role in the diagnosis of tumors.

It is an immunological method of **identifying the antigenic component in the cell or one of its components** by **using specific antibodies.** It is a powerful supplement to routine histologic examination and helps in accurate identification of tissue types. It is widely used in the diagnosis or management of malignant neoplasms.

Uses of Immunohistochemistry

- **To categorize undifferentiated cancers:** Many malignant tumors of diverse origin resemble each other and are difficult to distinguish on routine hematoxylin and eosin (H&E) sections. For example, a few anaplastic carcinomas, lymphomas, melanomas, and sarcomas may histologically look almost similar. They should be accurately diagnosed because of their different modes of treatment and prognosis.
  - In **poorly differentiated carcinoma intermediate filaments** (e.g., cytokeratins) **show positivity (Table 7.20).**
  - **Malignant melanomas when unpigmented** (amelanotic melanoma) appear similar to other poorly differentiated carcinomas. They express **HMB-45** and S-100 proteins but are negative for cytokeratins.
  - **Desmin** is found in neoplasms of **muscle cell origin.**
- **To determine the origin of poorly differentiated metastatic tumors**: It may be determined by using tissue-specific or organ-specific antigens **(Table 7.21).** For example, detection of prostate-specific antigen (PSA) in metastatic tumor deposits, is useful for a definitive diagnosis of a primary tumor in the prostate gland.
- **For prognosis or to select the mode of treatment:** Examples include:

TABLE 7.20 Intermediate filaments and their use in the diagnosis of neoplasms.

Type of intermediate filament	*Normal tissue expression*	*Diagnostic usefulness*
1. Cytokeratin	All epithelial cells	Carcinoma
2. Vimentin	Mesenchymal cells	Sarcoma
3. Desmin	Muscle cells	Tumors of muscle (e.g., rhabdomyosarcoma)
4. Glial fibrillary acid protein (GFAP)	Glial cells	Glial tumors (e.g., astrocytoma)
5. Neurofilament (NF)	Neurons and neural crest derivatives	Neural tumors (e.g., neuroblastoma)

TABLE 7.21 Lineage-associated immunohistochemical markers useful in establishing the origin of a poorly carcinoma.

Lineage-associated markers	*Associated cancer*
Prostate-specific antigen (PSA) and prostate-specific acid phosphatase (PSAP)	Prostatic carcinoma
Carcinoembryonic antigen (CEA)	Colonic carcinoma
Thyroglobulin	Thyroid carcinoma
CA 125	Ovarian cancers
Nuclear receptors for estrogen and progesterone	Carcinoma of breast

- Identification of **hormone** (estrogen/progesterone) **receptors in breast cancer** cells is of **prognostic and therapeutic value**. These cancers respond well to antiestrogen therapy and have a better prognosis.
- Breast cancers with **ERBB2 protein (HER2/neu) positivity have a poor prognosis.**

Immunohistochemical Markers

Q. List tumors in which immunohistochemistry has a diagnostic role.

Apart from the various immunochemical markers mentioned above, other markers useful are as follows:

- **Neuroendocrine tumors** show positivity for cytokeratins like carcinomas, but they can be identified by their contents, namely: **chromogranins** (proteins found in neurosecretory granules), **neuron-specific enolase (NSE)**, and **synaptophysin.**
- **Soft tissue sarcomas:** They show intermediate filament positivity (i) **vimentin, (ii) desmin** (positive in smooth or striated muscle fibers), (iii) **muscle-specific actin** marker for muscle tissue.
- **Neurofilament proteins: Marker for tumors of neurons, neuroblastomas, and ganglioneuroma.**
- **Neuron-specific enolase** in **neuroblastomas**.
- **Glial fibrillary acidic protein** (GFAP), also intermediate filament expressed in **glial cell neoplasms.**
- **Malignant lymphomas:** Generally positive for **leukocyte common antigen** (LCA, CD45). Markers for lymphomas and leukemias are called cluster designations (CDs) and are useful to differentiate T and B lymphocytes, monocytes, and granulocytes and the mature and immature variants of these cells.
- **Vascular tumors** derived from endothelial cells, include benign hemangiomas, and malignant hemangiosarcomas and are positive for factor **VIII-related antigen** or certain lectins.
- **Proliferating cells:** Cells in the cell cycle show positivity for **Ki-67** and proliferating cell nuclear antigen (**PCNA**).

Electron Microscopy

It helps in the **diagnosis of poorly differentiated/ undifferentiated cancers**, that cannot identify the origin by light microscopy, e.g., carcinomas show desmosomes and specialized junctional complexes, structures which are not seen in sarcomas or lymphomas.

Flow Cytometry

Q. Write a short note on modern techniques in tumor diagnosis.

Flow cytometry quantitatively measures various individual cell characteristics, such as membrane antigens and the DNA content of tumor cells. Flow cytometry is useful for the identification and **classification of tumors of T and B lymphocytes** (leukemias and lymphomas) and mononuclear-phagocytic cells. In this method, fluorescently labeled antibodies against cell surface molecules and differentiation antigens are used to identify the type of malignant cells.

Circulating Tumor Cells

Almost all advanced tumors are associated with both intact circulating tumor cells and products derived from tumors (e.g., cell-free circulating tumor DNA). Detection, quantification, and characterization of rare solid tumor cells (e.g., carcinoma, melanoma) circulating in the blood is emerging as a diagnostic modality though presently in the research stage. Few latest devices detect three-dimensional flow cells coated with antibodies specific for tumor cells of interest (e.g., carcinoma cells) in the blood. It will be useful for early diagnosis, to assess the risk of metastasis, and assess the response of tumor cells to therapy. These are detected through sensitive blood tests (so-called *liquid biopsies)* that identify circulating tumor-specific nucleic acid sequences.

Tumor Markers

Q. List tumor markers and write a short note on tumor markers with one example for each.

Q. Write a short note on the carcinoembryonic antigen.

Q. Write a short note on tumor markers for choriocarcinoma.

Q. Write a short note on alpha-fetoprotein.

Tumor markers are **products of malignant tumors** that can be detected in **the cells themselves or in blood and body fluids.**

Types of tumor markers (Table 7.22): These may be associated with enzymes, hormones, oncofetal antigens, specific proteins, mucin and glycoproteins, enzymes, and molecular markers.

Usefulness

Biochemical assays for tumor markers in the blood cannot be used for a definitive diagnosis of cancer. However, they have the following usefulness:

- **Detection of cancer:** They can be used as screening tests. Tumor markers lack the specificity and sensitivity needed for early detection of cancers. For example,

TABLE 7.22 Common tumor markers.

Tumor marker	*Associated tumors*
1. Hormones	
– Human chorionic gonadotropin (hCG)	Trophoblastic tumors, nonseminomatous tumors of testis
– Calcitonin	Medullary carcinoma of the thyroid
– Catecholamine	Pheochromocytoma
– Ectopic hormones	Paraneoplastic syndromes (Table 7.17)
2. Oncofetal Antigens	
– α-fetoprotein (alpha-fetoprotein/AFP)*	Hepatocellular carcinomas, yolk sac tumors, and occasionally embryonal carcinomas
– Carcinoembryonic antigen (CEA)*	Carcinomas of the colon, pancreas, lung, and stomach
3. Mucins and Other Glycoproteins	
– CA-125 (cancer antigen 125)*	Cancers of the fallopian tube, ovary, and colon
– CA-19-9 (cancer antigen 19-9)*	Cancers of the pancreas, gastrointestinal and hepatobiliary tracts, and ovary
4. Isoenzymes	
– Prostatic acid phosphatase (PAP)	Prostate carcinoma
– Neuron-specific enolase (NSE)	Small-cell carcinoma of the lung, neuroblastoma
5. Specific Proteins	
– Immunoglobulins	Multiple myeloma and other gammopathies
– Prostate-specific antigen (PSA)*	Prostate carcinoma
6. New Molecular Markers	
– *p53, APC, RAS* mutants in stool and serum	Carcinoma colon
– *p53* and *RAS* mutants in sputum and serum	Lung cancer

*They can be raised in a variety of non-neoplastic conditions.

PSA is the most common and useful tumor marker used to screen **prostatic adenocarcinoma**. High levels of PSA are found in the blood of prostatic carcinoma patients but it also may be elevated in benign prostatic hyperplasia. However, prostate cancer may be present even when PSA levels are within the normal range. Thus, the PSA has low sensitivity and low specificity, and its use as a screening tool is controversial.

- **Determine the effectiveness of therapy:** They are useful in monitoring disease once the diagnosis is made. These markers disappear once the tumor is successfully resected.
- **Detection of recurrence:** The reappearance of tumor markers indicates the recurrence of the tumor. For example, a PSA assay is useful for detecting residual disease or recurrence following treatment for prostate cancer.

Molecular Diagnosis

Molecular diagnostics are techniques used to analyze biological markers in the genome (sometimes in the proteome). Several molecular techniques are available for the diagnosis of tumors and for predicting their behavior. Two commonly used techniques for molecular diagnosis are the **FISH technique and PCR (polymerase chain reaction) analysis.**

Uses of Molecular Diagnosis

These are as follows:

Diagnosis of Malignancy

- **Monoclonal** (malignant) **versus polyclonal (benign):** Each T cell and B cell has unique antigen receptor gene rearrangements. Polymerase chain reaction (PCR)-based detection of rearranged T-cell receptor or immunoglobulin genes helps to differentiate benign, polyclonal (reactive) proliferations of T-or B-cells from malignant (monoclonal) proliferations.
- **Chromosomal alterations:** Many **hematopoietic neoplasms** (leukemias and lymphomas) and few solid tumors (e.g., Ewing sarcoma) have characteristic translocations that can be detected by FISH technique or by PCR analysis. For example, PCR-based detection of **BCR-ABL transcription** can be used for the diagnosis of **chronic myeloid leukemia.**

Prognosis and Behavior of Cancer

Certain genetic alterations are of prognostic value. They can be detected by routine cytogenetics and also by FISH or PCR assays. Examples of **poor prognostic** features are an **amplification of the N-MYC oncogene in neuroblastoma** and the **amplification of the HER-2/Neu oncogene in breast cancer.**

Detection of Minimal Residual Disease

Minimal residual disease (MRD) is the small number of cancer cells that may be in the body after cancer treatment. PCR can detect minimal residual disease or the onset of relapse in patients who are treated for leukemia or lymphoma. For example, the detection of *BCR-ABL* transcription by PCR assay in patients treated for CML gives a measure of residual disease.

Detection of Hereditary Predisposition to Cancer

Germline mutations in many tumor suppressor genes are associated with increased risk for specific cancers. This will help in prophylactic surgery and counseling of relatives at risk. For example, *BRCA1*, *BRCA2,* and the *RET* proto-oncogene.

For Therapeutic Decision-making

Recent advances have helped to develop therapies that directly target specific mutations (target therapy). Detection of such mutations in a tumor can guide "personalized" therapy. For example, melanomas with the *BRAF* mutation respond well to BRAF inhibitors.

Molecular Profiling of Tumors

Traditional Cancer Typing

Traditionally cancer is diagnosed and classified according to the morphological (histopathology/cytopathology) appearance of the cells and their surrounding tissue. It has limitations such as (i) it relies on a subjective review of the tissue which is dependent on the knowledge and experience of a pathologist, and therefore may not be reproducible, (ii) limited ability to determine the individual recurrence risk of cancer, (iii) insufficient to reflect the complicated underlying molecular events that drive the neoplastic process and (iv) histopathology reports lack or offer very little information regarding the potential drug treatment regime to which cancer will respond. Traditional pathology reports help to determine treatment that leads to better outcomes. However, tumors with identical pathology may have different origins and respond differently to treatment.

Newer Cancer Diagnostics

Until recently, molecular studies of tumors consisted of the analysis of individual genes. Currently, with the advances in technology, an entire genome can be rapidly sequenced, can identify epigenetic modifications (the epigenome), quantitate all the RNAs expressed in a cell population, measure many proteins simultaneously, and detect all the cell's metabolites (the metabolome).

Molecular profiling of tumors is the identification and documentation of the structure of a specific DNA, RNA, or protein molecule. Classification of cancer typing by molecular profile overcomes the limitations of traditional cancer typing. A molecular profile determines the level of gene expression within the cancer by hybridizing the cellular RNA with known genes. However, RNA is prone to degradation and is a more difficult analyte to work with than DNA in clinical practice.

DNA Microarray

Currently, the most common method for large-scale analysis of RNA expression is based on DNA microarrays. A DNA **microarray** (also known as a DNA chip or biochip) is a collection of microscopic DNA spots attached to a solid surface. This provides information on thousands of genes simultaneously. Once the gene expression pattern is determined, this information is compared to the expression profiles of cancers with known outcomes using a predetermined algorithm.

DNA Sequencing

It is the process of determining the precise order of nucleotides within a DNA molecule and is technically simpler than RNA sequencing. **Next-generation sequencing** refers to non-Sanger-based high-throughput DNA sequencing technologies. Millions or billions of DNA strands can be sequenced in parallel, yielding substantially more throughput and minimizing the need for the fragment-cloning methods that are often used in "Next-generation [NextGen] sequencing" (*refer* page 287) which can be readily performed on virtually any tissue specimen. By nextGen sequencing, the process of whole-genome of individual tumors can be completed in as little as a few weeks. The cancer genome sequencing can identify new mutations in various cancers; describe the full, extensive collection of genetic lesions in individual cancers; and the presence of genetic heterogeneity in individual cancers from area to area. It is particularly useful for tumors, such as lung carcinomas, that are genetically diverse and require a "personalized" approach for successful targeted therapy. However, histopathological examination of tumors provides information about important characteristics of cancers, such as anaplasia, invasiveness, and tumor heterogeneity. These cannot be obtained from DNA sequences. Thus, the most accurate diagnosis and assessment of prognosis in cancer can be arrived at by a combination of morphologic and molecular techniques (i.e., molecular profiling of tumors by RNA expression profiling, DNA sequencing, and DNA copy number arrays).

EXAMPLES OF BENIGN TUMORS

Squamous Papilloma

Squamous papilloma is a common benign tumor of squamous epithelium of the skin and mucosa.

It can occur anywhere in the skin and mouth.

Gross: It has exophytic papillary or finger-like projections. The number of papillae varies.

Microscopy (Figs. 7.27A and B): Each papillary (finger-like) projection consists of proliferating squamous epithelia of the epidermis with intact basement membrane and the basal cells. The central region of each papilla is composed of a vascularized connective tissue core.

Lipoma and Schwannoma (Neurilemmoma)

For lipoma *refer* page 936 and schwannoma *refer* page 943.

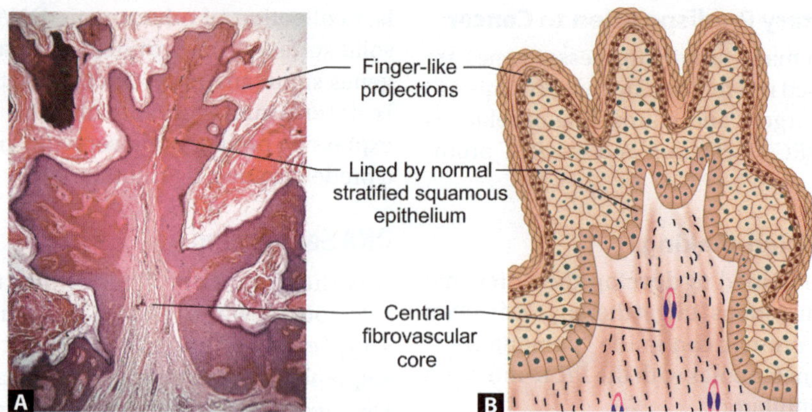

Figs. 7.27A and B: Squamous papilloma: (A) H & E and (B) Diagrammatic. Microscopic appearance of squamous papilloma.

SCENARIO-BASED MCQs

1. A 42-year-old man underwent colonoscopy and a 1 cm, circumscribed, pedunculated mass with a short stalk is found in the upper rectum. His stool was positive for occult blood. The most probable diagnosis of the lesion in the rectum is:

A. Hyperplasia B. Adenoma
C. Adenocarcinoma D. Hamartoma

2. A 45-year-old woman presents with a lump in the right breast. On examination of breast, a 4 cm firm and fixed mass is noted. Excisional biopsy shows malignant cells arranged in solid nests and cords, surrounded by a dense collagenous stroma. A connective tissue stain (trichrome) of the biopsy shows extensive stroma surrounding tumor cells shown in the image. The descriptive term used for this type of stromal change in a tumor is:

A. Papillomatosis B. Comedocarcinoma
C. Desmoplastic change D. Medullary carcinoma

3. A 42-year-old woman notices a lump in her left breast. On physical examination, she has a firm, non-movable, 2 cm mass in the upper outer quadrant of the left breast. An enlarged, firm, non-tender lymph node is detected in the left axilla. A fine-needle aspiration biopsy is performed, and the cytological features are consistent with the clinical diagnosis of carcinoma. A lumpectomy with axillary lymph node dissection is performed. Infiltrating carcinoma is present in two of eight axillary nodes. Reduced expression of the molecules by the tumor cells is most likely responsible for the lymph node metastases. Of the following, the molecules that show reduced expression in primary tumors is:

A. E-cadherin B. ERBB2 (HER-2)
C. Estrogen receptors D. Progesterone receptors

4. A 48-year-old woman complains of a painless lump in her left breast. On examination, left axillary lymph nodes are enlarged. These nodes are painless but firm. The most likely diagnosis of the lesion in her left breast is:

A. Fibroadenoma B. Infiltrating carcinoma
C. Intraductal carcinoma D. Acute mastitis with abscess

5. A 3-year-old child is having difficulty with vision in her right eye. On physical examination, there is leukocoria of the right eye, a feature favoring a mass in the posterior chamber. MR imaging reveals a mass that nearly fills the globe. The child undergoes enucleation of the right eye. Molecular analysis of the neoplastic cells shows the absence of both copies of a gene that is involved in the control of the cell cycle. The gene that has most likely undergone mutation in this neoplasm is:

A. TP53 B. RB
C. BCR-ABL D. RAS

6. A 32-year-old woman comes to the hospital for a history of vaginal bleeding and discharge for the past 5 days. She gives a history of having sex with multiple sexual partners. Gynecologic examination shows an ulcerated lesion at the squamocolumnar junction of the uterine cervix. The cervical Pap smear shows "koilocytic atypia" characterized by perinuclear halos and wrinkled nuclei. A cervical biopsy is performed and a microscopic examination shows an invasive tumor of squamous epithelium, with keratin pearls. Molecular test shows human papillomavirus type 16 (HPV-16) DNA within the tumor cells. In this tumor, the molecular abnormalities most likely related to infection with HPV-16 is:

A. Inability to repair DNA damage
B. Epigenetic silencing of the RB gene
C. Functional inactivation of the RB protein
D. Increased expression of epidermal growth factor receptor

Answers and Explanation

1. **The answer is B: Adenoma.** It is a benign tumor that arises from epithelial surfaces. A hyperplastic colonic lesion is generally smaller and flatter. Though adenocarcinoma may arise from a colonic adenoma, such lesions tend to be larger and more irregular. A hamartoma is a rare benign mass composed of tissues usually found at the site of origin.
2. **The answer is C: Desmoplastic change.** Scirrhous or desmoplastic change indicates dense fibrous stroma. Papillomatosis describes frond-like structures. Comedocarcinoma is an intraductal carcinoma in which necrotic material can be expressed from the ducts. Medullary carcinoma is a soft cellular tumor.
3. **The answer is A: E-cadherin.** First, the tumor cells must become discohesive and detach from the primary site, degrading the basement membrane and interstitial connective tissue. Then it gives rise to metastases. E-cadherin/s is an adhesive molecule

that bind the cells to each other. Reduced expression of these molecules promotes metastases. Expression of estrogen and progesterone receptors are indicative of responsiveness of breast cancer to antihormone therapy. HER-2 is a form of epidermal growth factor receptor and an antibody to this is used for therapy. It is not involved in the spread of tumors.

4. **The answer is B: Infiltrating carcinoma.** Lymphatic spread to regional lymph nodes draining from the primary site is typical of a carcinoma. An intraductal carcinoma does not extend beyond the basement membrane and does not invade and spread to lymph nodes. A fibroadenoma is a benign tumor that cannot invade or metastasize. Acute infection with abscess can spread to the lymph nodes, but the involved lymph nodes are typically associated with pain (a cardinal sign of acute inflammation).
5. **The answer is B: Rb.** The RB gene is a tumor suppressor gene. It shows a two-hit mechanism with the loss of both alleles. About 60% of retinoblastoma are sporadic, and the remaining are familial from. The RB gene controls the G1 to S transition of the cell cycle. The loss of both copies of *RB* gene leads to loss of control of a checkpoint in the cell cycle. Many cancers have a mutation in the TP53 tumor suppressor gene, but this is not typical of childhood ocular neoplasms The BCR-ABL fusion gene occurs in chronic myeloid leukemia Many cancers have the mutation in the *RAS* gene, which acts as an oncogene.
6. **The answer is C: Functional inactivation of the RB protein.** Human papillomavirus (HPV) is a sexually transmissible oncogenic virus. Its oncogenic property is related to two early viral gene products E6 and E7. E7 protein binds to RB protein and degrades it releasing the E2F transcription factor. E6 protein binds to and inactivates the p53 gene product. The silencing of RB is not due to epigenetic modifications. The inability to repair DNA damage is involved in some colon and skin cancers. Increased epidermal growth factor receptor expression is a feature seen in many pulmonary squamous cell carcinomas, and the related ERBB2 (HER2) receptor is seen in some breast carcinomas.

Malignant tumors that does not metastasize:
- Basal cell carcinoma (skin)
- Glioma (CNS)

Pathways of spread of malignant tumors:
- Lymphatic spread
- Hematogenous/blood spread
- Seeding of the body cavities and surfaces
- Direct transplantation

Most common sites of hematogenous metastasis:
- Lung
- Liver
- Bone
- Brain

Most important tumor suppressor genes:
- TP53: p 53 acts at G1 S check point.
- Retinoblastoma (RB) gene: regulates G1-S transition.

p53 (wild type): Non-mutated form is termed wild form.

Human papillomavirus (HPV):
- E6 gene product inhibits TP53 suppressor gene
- E7 gene product inhibits RB suppressor gene

Intraoperative histological examination (frozen section):
- Used to confirm suspected metastasis
- Useful for detecting positive margins after resection
- Cannot be used for immediate definite diagnosis of a cancer.

Exfoliative cytology is useful in the diagnosis of cancers of:
- Cervix
- Endometrium
- Lung
- Bladder

Trousseau phenomenon (Migratory thrombophlebitis) is seen with carcinoma of:
- Pancreas
- Lung
- GIT
- Breast

Parathormone related peptide: Most common hormone producing hypercalcemia in tumors.

The sentinel lymph node: First node in regional lymphatic drainage
that receives lymph flow from the primary tumor. It is useful for:
- Carcinoma of breast
- Malignant melanoma
- Cancer of colon cancer
- Cancer of vulva

Genetic and Pediatric Diseases

CHAPTER OUTLINE

- Basics of Genetics
- Genetic Disorders
- Cytogenetic Abnormalities and Mutations in Childhood
- Tumors and Tumor-Like Lesions of Infancy and Childhood
- Storage Diseases

BASICS OF GENETICS

Genetics is the study, which deals with the **science of genes**, heredity, and its variation in living organisms. Disorders of childhood are usually of genetic origin. Hence, developmental and pediatric diseases are discussed along with genetic diseases.

Genes

Definition: A gene is defined as a **segment of deoxyribonucleic acid (DNA)** which carries genetic information. Gene is the basic **physical and functional unit of heredity**. DNA has also segments that do not contain genes.

The human genome contains more than **19,000 protein-encoding genes comprising 1.5% of the genome. Each** gene varies in size.

Structure of Gene (Fig. 8.1)

Each gene consists of a specific sequence of nucleotides. These genes encode proteins that are the fundamental constituents of cells. These proteins function as enzymes, structural elements, and signaling molecules. **Genes may be silent or active**. When active, the **genes direct the process of protein synthesis**. Genes **use a genetic code** for protein synthesis. The **genetic code** consists of a sequence codeword called **codons.** A codon for an amino acid consists of a sequence of **three nucleotide base pairs** called a **triplet codon. Human genome has about 3.3 billion DNA base pairs.**

Regions of Gene

- **Initiator and stop codons:** The boundaries of a gene are known as **start and stop codons**. The start codon tells when to begin protein production and the stop

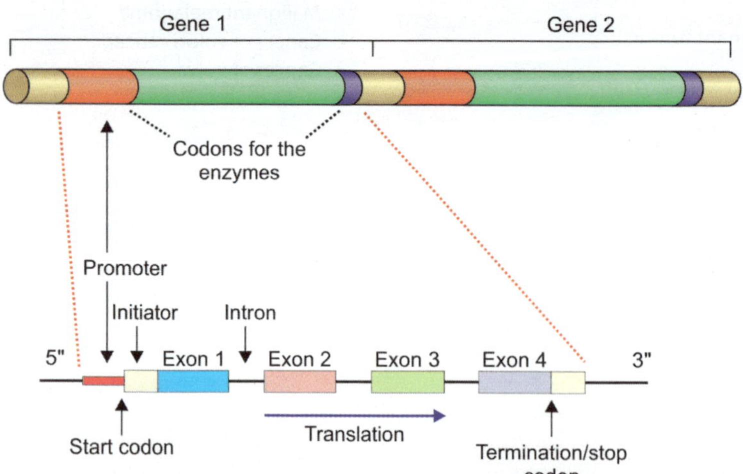

Fig. 8.1: Diagrammatic structure of gene. Start and termination codons mark the limits of the gene. The coding portion of the gene is exons (four in this example), and interspersed with introns.

(termination) codons tells when to end the protein production.

- **Coding region:** The **nucleotide sequence between the start and stop codons is** the core region known as the **coding region**. This region is divided into **two main segments namely—exons and introns**. Most of the genes contain both exons and introns, the number of which varies with different genes.
  - **Exons:** This region **codes for producing a protein**.
  - **Introns:** These are the regions between exons and **do not code for a protein (noncoding region)**.
- **Regulatory regions:** These are also noncoding regions that control gene expression.
  - **Promoters** are regions that bind to transcription factors, either strongly or weakly.
  - **Enhancers** are regions that can enhance the effect of a weak promoter.
  - **Silencers** are regulatory regions that can inhibit transcription.
- **Special structural regions of DNA:** These include *telomeres* (chromosome ends) and *centromeres* (chromosome "tethers").

Nature of Genetic Abnormalities Causing Disease

Many types of genetic abnormalities affect the structure and function of proteins. This may disrupt the cellular homeostasis and produce disease.

Mutations

Definition: A mutation is defined as a **permanent change in the genetic material (DNA) that results in a disease.**

Single-gene disorders result from mutations in a single gene. The term mutation was coined by Müller in 1927.

Causes of gene mutations: These may be spontaneous or induced.

- **Spontaneous mutation:** The majority of mutations occur spontaneously **due to errors in DNA replication and repair**.
- **Induced mutation:** Mutations can be caused due to exposure to mutagenic agents like **chemicals, viruses, and ultraviolet or ionizing radiation.**

Polymorphism: If the **genetic material change/variant does not cause an obvious effect upon phenotype, it is termed as polymorphism.** Polymorphism is a genetic variation that exists in a population with a frequency of >1%. Many *polymorphisms* associated with diseases are in non-protein-coding regions of the genome.

Classification of mutations: Depending on the cell affected, mutations can affect either somatic cells or germ cells.

- **Germ cell mutations:** Mutations that affect the germ cells are transmitted to the progeny/descendants and can produce inherited/hereditary diseases.
- **Somatic cell mutations:** Mutations involving the somatic cells can produce cancers and some congenital malformations. These mutations are not inherited and do not cause hereditary diseases. These are known as de novo mutations.

Structural Chromosomal Mutations

The rearrangement of genetic material causes structural change. Structural mutations may be (1) **visible during karyotyping** (*refer* pages 277-8) or (2) **submicroscopic** (minute/subtle changes). The **submicroscopic gene mutations** can result in **partial or complete deletion of a gene or more often, a single nucleotide base**. A few examples of genetic mutations are discussed below.

Mutations in protein-coding genes

Q. Write a short note on point mutation.

Point mutation is characterized by the **replacement of one nucleotide base by a different nucleotide base within a gene. Most point mutations occur in the coding region of a gene.**

- **Missense mutations:** If point mutations change the genetic code, it may code for a different amino acid and protein.
  - **Conservative missense mutation:** In this type, the substituted amino acid produces **only little change in the function of the protein.**
  - **Nonconservative missense mutation:** In this type, the normal amino acid is replaced by a very different amino acid resulting in a **change in the function of the protein.** For example, sickle cell anemia in which mutation affects the β-globin chain of hemoglobin **(Fig. 8.2)**. In this, a point mutation in the β-globin chain of hemoglobin produces hemoglobin S (HbS), instead of normal hemoglobin.

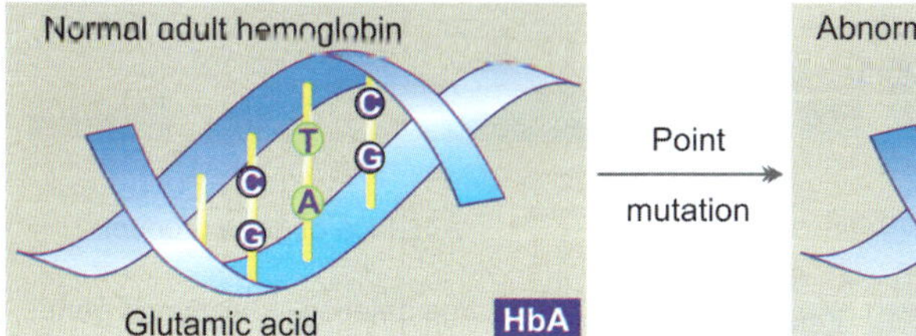

Fig. 8.2: Nonconservative missense point mutation in sickle cell anemia. When adenine replaces thymidine, the amino acid valine replaces glutamic acid in the sixth position of β-globin chain of hemoglobin and gives rise to abnormal sickle hemoglobin.

- **Nonsense mutation (stop codon):** In this type, point mutations creates a stop codon, resulting in a truncated protein or complete failure of protein synthesis. For example, in β-globin chain, a point mutation affecting the codon for glutamine (CAG) creates a stop codon (UAG) if U replaces C **(Fig. 8.3)**. This change leads to premature termination of β-globin gene translation and deficiency of β-globin chains. There is no synthesis of hemoglobin A. It produces a severe form of anemia called β^0-thalassemia.

Frameshift mutation: This may occur due to the **insertion or deletion of one or more nucleotides** in the coding regions. If the number of nucleotide bases inserted or deleted is not a multiple of 3, the code will be changed **(Fig. 8.4A)**. This leads to alterations in the reading frame of the DNA strand; hence they are known as frameshift mutation. If the number of base pairs involved is three or a multiple of three, frameshift does not occur. This may synthesize an abnormal protein lacking or gaining one or more amino acids. When deletions involve a large segment of DNA, the coding region of a gene may be entirely removed **(Fig. 8.4B)**.

Trinucleotide repeat mutation: The **DNA contains several repeat sequences of three nucleotides (trinucleotide)**. When they are repeated directly adjacent to each other (one right after the other), they are known as **tandem repeats (Fig. 8.5)**. When the repetitive trinucleotide sequences reach above a particular threshold, they can expand (amplify) or contract. The amplification is more common. These trinucleotide-repeat mutations are dynamic (i.e., the degree of amplification increases during gametogenesis).

Functional effects of mutations: Mutations in DNA can lead to either a change in the amino acid sequence of a specific protein or may interfere with its synthesis. The consequences vary from those without any functional effect to those which have serious effects.

- **Loss-of-function (LOF) mutations:** These mutations cause the reduction or loss of normal function of a protein.
- **Gain-of-function mutations:** In gain-of-function mutation, the protein function is altered in a manner that results in a change in the original function of the gene.
- **Lethal mutations:** These lead to the death of the fetus.

Alterations in protein-coding genes other than mutations: Apart from alterations in DNA sequence, coding genes also can undergo structural variations. These are copy number changes—*amplifications* or *deletions*—or *translocations*. It may lead to aberrant gain or loss of protein function. Like mutations, structural changes may occur in the germline, or be acquired in somatic tissues. Somatically acquired structural alterations (e.g., amplifications, deletions, and translocations) are often seen in cancers. For example, "Philadelphia chromosome"—translocation t(9;22)

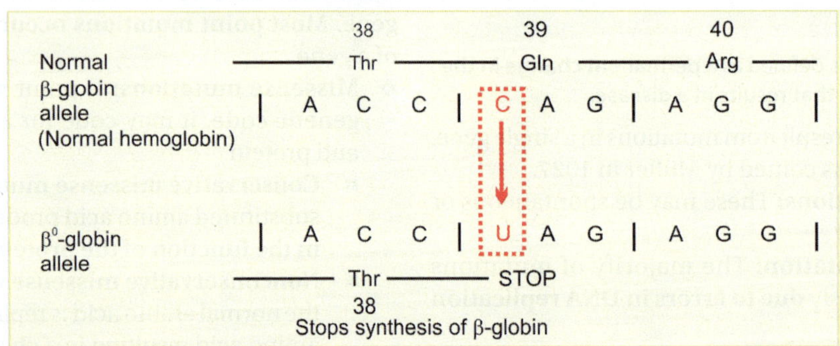

Fig. 8.3: Nonsense point mutation leading to premature chain termination. A point mutation (C replaced by U) in codon 39 changes the glutamine (Gln) codon to a stop codon. This stops the synthesis of protein at amino acid 38.

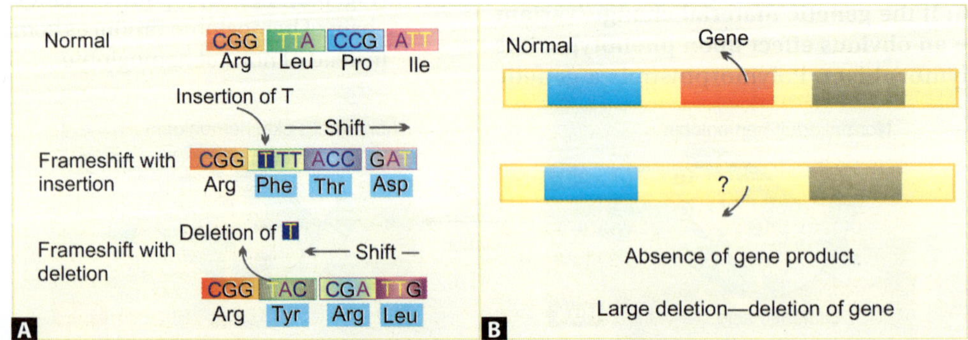

Figs. 8.4A and B: Frameshift mutations: (A) Insertion or deletion of nucleotide bases if not a multiple of 3, the code will be changed; (B) Deletions involving a large segment of DNA in the coding region may entirely remove the gene.

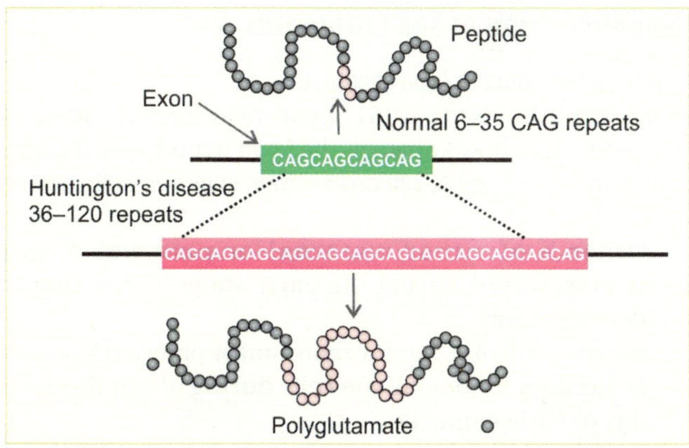

Fig. 8.5: Trinucleotide repeat disorder, e.g., Huntington's disease. It results from the expansion of a CAG triplet repeat from a normal number of 6–35 repeats to greater than 36 repeats. This results in the expansion of a polyglutamine sequence in the corresponding protein.

between the *BCR* and *ABL* genes in chronic myeloid leukemia (*refer* **Fig. 12.9**).

Alterations in non-coding RNAs: There are a very large number of genes that do not encode proteins. The nonencoded products of these genes—so-called "non-coding RNAs (ncRNAs)"—play important regulatory functions [e.g., small RNA molecules called microRNAs (miRNAs) and long non-coding RNAs (lncRNAs)].

Chromosomal Aberrations

A chromosomal aberration (abnormality) is a disorder characterized by a morphological or numerical alteration in single or multiple chromosomes. It may affect autosomes, sex chromosomes, or both.

Classification (Box 8.1): It is classified as (1) numerical chromosomal aberrations and (2) structural chromosomal aberrations. Both may involve either the autosomes or the sex chromosomes.

Numerical Chromosomal Aberrations

Total number of chromosomes may be **either increased or decreased**. The **deviation from the normal number of chromosomes** is called numerical chromosomal aberrations.

Types of Numerical Aberrations

1. **Aneuploidy:** It is defined as a **chromosome number that is not a multiple of 23** (the normal haploid number-n).
   - **Trisomy:** It is a **numerical abnormality with** the presence of **one extra chromosome** (2n + 1). **It may involve either sex chromosomes or autosomes.** For example, **Down's syndrome** (trisomy 21) has three copies of chromosome 21 (47,XX, + 21).
   - **Monosomy:** It is the **numerical abnormality** with the **absence or loss of one chromosome** (2n - 1). It may **involve autosomes or sex chromosomes**. For example, **Turner syndrome** 45,XO instead of normal 46,XX.
2. **Polyploidy:** This term is used when the **chromosome number is a multiple greater than two of the haploid number** (multiples of haploid number 23).
3. **Mosaicism:** It is the presence of **two or more populations of cells with different chromosomal complement in an individual**.

Structural Chromosomal Aberration

Aberration of the structure of one or more chromosomes may **occur during either mitosis or meiosis**. The various structural chromosomal aberrations (*refer* **Box 8.1**) include:

Translocations: It is a structural alteration between two chromosomes in which a **segment of one chromosome gets detached and is transferred to another chromosome**. It can be:

- **Balanced reciprocal translocations (Fig. 8.6A):** It is characterized by single breaks in each of two chromosomes with the exchange of genetic material distal to the break.
- **Robertsonian translocation/centric fusion (Fig. 8.6B):** It is a translocation between two acrocentric chromosomes. The breaks occur close to the centromeres of each chromosome. Transfer of the segments leads to one very large chromosome and one extremely small one. The small one is because of the fusion of short arms of both chromosomes which lack a centromere and are lost in subsequent divisions. This loss is compatible with life, but it may produce abnormal progeny.

Inversion: It involves two breaks within a single chromosome, the affected segment inverts with reattachment of the inverted segment. The genetic material is transferred within the same chromosome. Inversions are usually fully compatible with normal development. Two types of inversions are:

1. **Paracentric inversions (Fig. 8.6C)** result from breaks on the same arm (either the short arm or the long arm) of the chromosome.
2. **Pericentric inversions (Fig. 8.6D)** result from breaks on the opposite sides of the centromere where both the short and long arms are involved.

Isochromosome (Fig. 8.6E): They are formed due to faulty centromere division. Normally, centromeres divide in a plane parallel to the long axis of the chromosome. If a centromere divides in a plane transverse to the long axis, it results in a pair of isochromosomes. One pair consists of two short arms and the other of two long arms.

Ring chromosome (Fig. 8.6F): It is a special form of deletion. Ring chromosomes are formed by a break at both ends of a chromosome with a fusion of the damaged ends. The consequences depend on the amount of genetic material lost due to the break. Loss of a significant amount of genetic material will result in phenotypic abnormalities.

It is expressed as *46,XY,r(14)*. Ring chromosomes do not behave normally in meiosis or mitosis and usually result in serious consequences.

Deletion (Figs. 8.6G and H): It is the loss of a part of a chromosome. It is of two types namely: interstitial (middle) and terminal (rare).

Insertion: It is a form of nonreciprocal translocation in which a fragment of a chromosome is transferred and inserted into a nonhomologous chromosome. Two breaks occur in one chromosome, which releases a chromosomal fragment. This fragment is inserted into another chromosome following one break in the receiving chromosome, to insert this fragment.

Genomic imprinting: All individuals inherit two copies of each autosomal gene. One of these is from maternal and the other is from paternal chromosomes. It was earlier thought that there was no functional difference between the alleles derived from the mother or the father. It is found that different clinical features can result, depending on whether a gene is inherited from the father or mother. These differences are due to an epigenetic process, called **imprinting**. Mostly imprinting selectively inactivates either the maternal or paternal allele. Thus, in ***maternal imprinting***, there is the silencing of the maternal allele, whereas, in ***paternal imprinting***, there is the inactivation of the paternal allele. Imprinting occurs during gametogenesis in the ovum or the sperm, before fertilization, and then is stably transmitted to all somatic cells through mitosis. The pattern of imprinting is maintained to variable degrees in different tissues.

Demonstration of Sex Chromatin

Q. Write a short note on Lyon hypothesis.

Lyon hypothesis: In 1961, Lyon outlined the idea of X-inactivation, now known as the Lyon hypothesis. It states that **only one of the X-chromosomes is genetically active** and:

1. **Other X of either maternal or paternal origin is inactivated** during the early stage of embryonic development.
2. **Inactivation of either the maternal or paternal X** occurs **at random** among all the cells **during about the 16th day of embryonic life.**
3. **Inactivation of the same X-chromosome persists in all the cells derived from each precursor cell.**

Q. Write a short note on Barr body and sex chromatin.

Barr Body and Sex Chromatin

There are two simple methods: (i) Buccal smear for Barr body (sex chromatin), and (ii) leukocytes—nuclear sexing.

Buccal smear for Barr body (Fig. 8.7A): Barr and Bertram in 1949 identified the presence **of tiny dark granules adjacent to the nuclear membrane.** This granule is known as the **Barr body, or X chromatin or sex chromatin.** It represents one inactive and condensed X-chromosome in a female. The inactive X can be seen in the interphase nucleus as a darkly staining small mass in contact with the nuclear membrane.

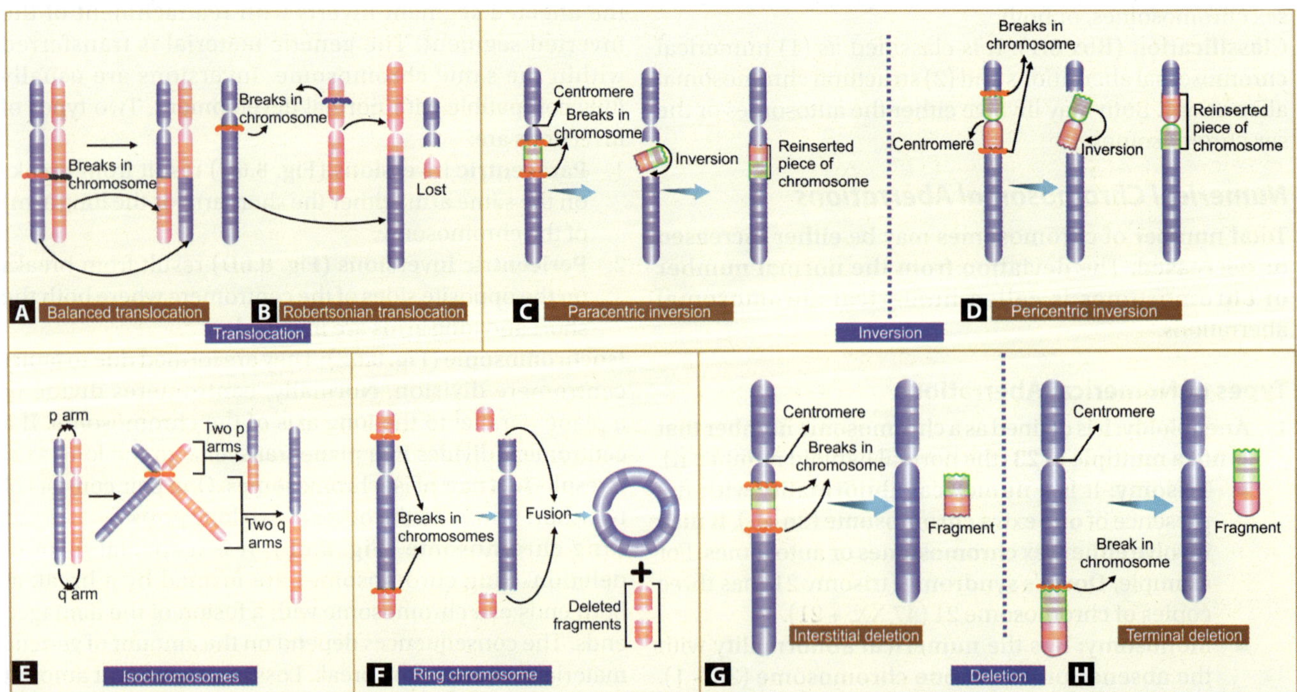

Figs. 8.6A to H: Types of chromosomal rearrangements.

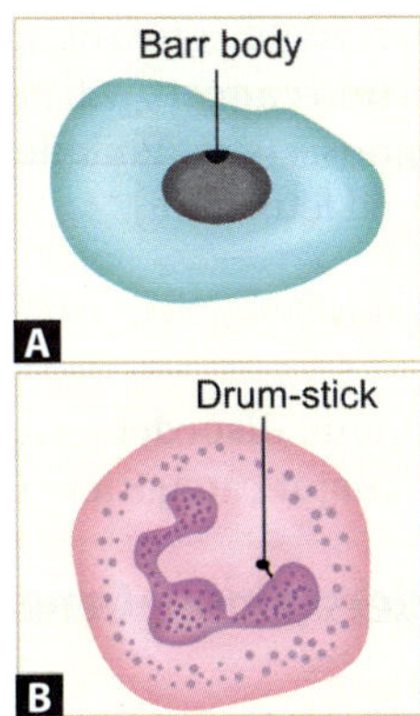

Figs. 8.7A and B: (A) Nuclei of intermediate squamous cell with Barr body; (B) Neutrophil with drumstick.

- The **number of Barr bodies in a cell depends upon the number of X-chromosomes.** It is always one less than the number of X-chromosomes. Thus, normal cells in females (XX) have one Barr body, and the presence of Barr bodies indicates the female genotype. Normal cells in males (XY) have no Barr bodies because they have only one active X chromosome. The XXXY cells have two Barr bodies.
- **Demonstration:** Buccal smears are used for demonstration of Barr body and are prepared with a thin wooden spatula, by scraping the buccal mucosa. Smears are stained by Papanicolaou stain.

Leukocytes—nuclear sexing (Fig. 8.7B): Neutrophils in the peripheral smear may also be examined for nuclear sexing. Abnormalities of sex chromosomes can be diagnosed by nuclear sexing. In a normal female (XX), the **neutrophils in a peripheral smear show a drumstick** which is the counterpart of Barr body in a buccal smear. **Absence of drumstick** is observed in **Turner syndrome** (XO), while **one drumstick** is found in males with **Klinefelter syndrome** (XXY). Irrespective of the number of X chromosomes, the presence of a single Y determines the male sex.

Cytogenetics

Cytogenetics is a branch of genetics that deals with the **study of chromosomes**. Karyotype is one of the basic tools of cytogenetics.

Techniques of cytogenetics: It can be broadly divided into:
- **Conventional cytogenetics:** It is the routine chromosome analysis.
- **Molecular cytogenetics:** Molecular genetics (often called 'DNA technology') is the study of the genetic material at the level of the individual nucleotide bases of DNA.

Karyotyping

Q. Write a short essay/note on karyotyping.

- The **chromosomal constitution of a cell or individual** is known as the **karyotype.** The normal human karyotypes contain 22 pairs of autosomal chromosomes and one pair of sex chromosomes. Normal karyotype for females is denoted as 46,XX, and for males as 46,XY.
- **The study of structural patterns** of the chromosomes in a sample of cells is known as **karyotyping.** This includes both **the number and appearance (photomicrograph) of a complete set of chromosomes.** Karyotyping requires cells to be in a state of division and arresting this cell division at the metaphase of the cell cycle.

Source of chromosome: To produce a karyotype, it is necessary to obtain cells capable of growth and division. Cells for chromosomal study may be obtained either by culture or directly.
- **Culture:** The source may be fibroblast or cells obtained by amniocentesis (amniotic fluid) or peripheral blood. The more commonly used cell for chromosomal study is a **circulating lymphocyte** obtained from the blood sample **cultured in a media.**
- **Direct:** Cells obtained **from bone marrow and chorion villous** biopsy samples may be used without culture.

Staining: There are many staining methods using **specific dyes** to identify individual chromosomes. The most commonly used is **Giemsa stain.**

Classification of Chromosomes in Karyotyping

There are various systems used to study the morphology of the chromosomes.

Denver system of classification: In this system, the chromosomes are grouped from A to G according to the length and position of the centromere of the chromosomes.

Paris system of classification: This is a universally accepted classification. According to this, the chromosomes are identified based on the various banding patterns.

Chromosomal Banding

Banding is a method to **study the structure of a chromosome.** In this method, chromosomes are stained by a special stain (e.g., Giemsa) which binds to specific bands of chromosomes. Each chromosome shows a characteristic banding pattern (light and dark bands) which will help to identify them.

Techniques: Different banding techniques are:
- **G-banding** (G for Giemsa): It is most commonly used and shows a series of light and dark-stained bands **(Fig. 8.8).** Giemsa stain is specific for the phosphate groups of DNA.
- **Q banding** (Quinacrine fluorescent stain).
- **R-banding:** It is the reverse of G-banding (the R stands for "reverse").
- **C-banding** (centromeric): This method stains centromeres.
- **T-banding:** It stains the terminal ends of chromosomes (telomeres).
- **High-resolution banding:** It provides greater sensitivity.

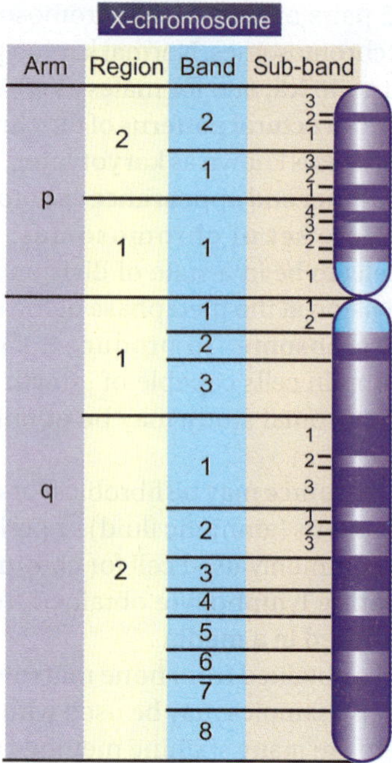

Fig. 8.8: G-banded karyotype (diagrammatic) shows the banding pattern of the X-chromosome with nomenclature of arms, regions, bands, and sub-bands.

Karyotype analysis: Karyotypes are usually described using a standard shorthand format in the following order:

- **Total number of chromosomes**
- **Sex chromosome** constitution
- **Description of abnormalities** in ascending numerical order.
  - **Short arm or long arm:** The short arm of the chromosome is designated "p" (petit) and the long arm "q" (queue).
  - **Region:** Each arm of the chromosome is divided into two or more regions. The regions are numbered (e.g., 1, 2, 3) from the centromere outward.
    - Bands and sub-bands: Each region is further subdivided into bands and sub-bands, and these are ordered numerically as well. This will help for precise localization of the gene.
- **Structural changes in chromosomes**

Examples: The notation *Xp21.2* (read as " X P two one point two") refers to a chromosomal segment located on the short arm of the X-chromosome, in region 2, band 1, and sub-band 2. 3p22.1 is read as "three P two two point one."

Uses of Karyotyping

- **For diagnosis:** Diagnosis of **genetic disorders** including prenatal diagnosis.
- **To detect the cause of repeated abortions:** Many chromosomal aberrations can cause repeated spontaneous abortions and they can be identified by karyotyping.
- **Prognostic value:** Identification of specific chromosomal anomalies **in certain cancers** will help in predicting the course and prognosis (e.g., Philadelphia chromosome in chronic myeloid leukemia).

GENETIC DISORDERS

Classification of genetic disorders: Genetic disorders are classified into three major categories **(Box 8.1)**.

Mendelian Disorders (Single-Gene or Monogenic Disorders)

Q. Give four examples of each for different Mendelian inheritance.

Mendelian disorders result from mutations in a single gene. General features of Mendelian disorders are:

- **Location of defective gene: It is on autosomes (autosomal inheritance) or the sex chromosomes (sex-linked inheritance).**
- **Dominant versus recessive gene: Genes are inherited in pairs**—one gene from each parent. However, the inheritance may not be equal, and **one gene may overpower the other** in its coded characteristic. The **gene that overshadows the other is called the dominant gene; the overshadowed gene is the recessive one.**
- **Homozygote versus heterozygote:** In some autosomal mutations, the disease is partially expressed in the heterozygote and fully expressed in the homozygote, e.g., sickle cell anemia.
- **Codominant inheritance:** Sometimes both of the alleles of a gene pair contribute to the expression of phenotype. It is called codominance, e.g., blood group antigen.

BOX 8.1: Classification of genetic disorders.

A. Single-gene or monogenic disorders/Mendelian disorders
   - Autosomal dominant
   - Autosomal recessive
   - X-linked dominant
   - X-linked recessive

B. Cytogenetic disorders–chromosomal disorders (aberrations/abnormalities)
   - Numerical aberrations aneuploidy (trisomy, monosomy), polyploidy, and mosaicism
   - Structural aberrations
     - Translocations
       - Balanced reciprocal translocations
       - Robertsonian translocations
     - Inversion
     - Isochromosome
     - Ring chromosome
     - Deletions
     - Insertions

C. Complex/multifactorial multigenic/polygenic disorders
   - Diabetes mellitus
   - Hypertension

Autosomal Dominant Pattern of Inheritance

Q. Name autosomal dominant disorders.

General features of autosomal dominant disorders are as follows:

- **Location of mutant gene:** It is on **autosomes**.
- **Required number of defective genes:** Only **one copy**.
- **Sex affected:** Both **males and females** are **equally** affected.
- **Pattern of inheritance:**
  - **Manifests in the heterozygous state. So, every affected** individual **has at least one affected parent.** Normal members of a family do not transmit the disorder to their children.
  - **Risks of transmission to children (offspring): Affected males and females have an equal risk of passing on the disorder to children.**
- **Additional properties:**
  - **Penetrance:** It is the percentage of individuals (with mutation) having clinical symptoms.
    - With **complete penetrance, all individuals show clinical symptoms**
    - With **reduced penetrance,** only **some individuals show disease**
    - In **nonpenetrance,** individuals may **not show any symptoms.**
  - **Variable expressivity** (qualitatively or quantitatively) of disorder is the term used for variable expression among individuals (even within the same family).
  - **Delayed onset:** Symptoms and signs may be delayed and may not appear until adulthood. For example, Huntington's disease.

Table 8.1 shows common autosomal dominant disorders.

TABLE 8.1 Example of autosomal dominant disorders.

System affected with examples
Nervous system • Huntington's disease • Neurofibromatosis • Tuberous sclerosis
Musculoskeletal system • Marfan syndrome • Osteogenesis imperfecta • Achondroplasia
Hematopoietic system • Hereditary spherocytosis • von Willebrand disease
Renal system: Polycystic kidney disease
Gastrointestinal system: Familial polyposis coli
Metabolic disorders: Familial hypercholesterolemia

Autosomal Recessive Pattern of Inheritance

Q. Name autosomal recessive disorders.

Autosomal recessive disorders **constitute the largest group of Mendelian disorders.** General features of autosomal recessive disorders are as follows:

- **Location of mutant gene:** It is on an **autosome.**
- **Required number of defective genes: Symptoms of the disease appear only when** an individual has **two copies** (both alleles at a given gene locus) of the mutant gene (**manifested in the homozygous state**). **When an individual has one mutated gene and one normal gene,** this heterozygous state is called a **carrier.**
- **Pattern of inheritance:** For a child to be at risk, **both parents must be having at least one copy of the mutant gene.** For example, all inborn errors of metabolism.
- **Sex affected: Females and males are equally affected.**
- **Consanguineous marriage:** It is a common predisposing factor.
- **Risks of transmission:** Siblings have a **one in four chance** of having the trait (i.e., the recurrence risk is 25% for each birth).
- **Expression of disease:** It is more uniform than in autosomal dominant disorders.
- **Penetrance: Complete penetrance** is common.
- **Onset:** It frequently manifests early in life.

Examples of autosomal recessive disorders are shown in **Table 8.2.**

TABLE 8.2 Examples of autosomal recessive disorders.

System affected with examples
Inborn errors of metabolism • Phenylketonuria • Galactosemia • Cystic fibrosis • Homocystinuria • Hemochromatosis • Lysosomal storage diseases (*refer* page 285) • Glycogen storage diseases • Wilson disease • α1-antitrypsin deficiency
Hematopoietic system • Sickle cell anemia • Thalassemias
Skeletal system: Alkaptonuria
Nervous system: Friedreich ataxia
Endocrine system: Congenital adrenal hyperplasia

X-linked Pattern of Inheritance

Q. Name sex-linked inherited disorders.

Most of the sex-linked Mendelian disorders are X-linked. Males with mutations involving the Y-linked genes are usually infertile, and hence there is no Y-linked inheritance. **Expression of an X-linked disorder is different in males and females.**

- **Females:** The **clinical expression** of the X-linked disease is **variable,** depending on whether it is dominant or recessive. **Females are rarely affected by X-linked recessive diseases**; however, they are affected by X-linked dominant diseases.

- **Males:** Mutation affecting X-chromosome is **fully expressed** even with one copy, regardless of whether the disorder is dominant or recessive.

X-linked Recessive Traits

General features of X-linked recessive traits are as follows:

- **Location of mutant gene:** It is on the **X-chromosome** and there is **no male-to-male transmission.**
- **Required number of defective genes: One copy** for the manifestation of disease **in males**, but **two copies** are needed **in females.**
- **Sex affected:** Males are more frequently affected than females; daughters of affected males are all asymptomatic carriers. Affected males do not transmit the disorder to their sons.
- **Pattern of inheritance: Transmission is through female carriers** (heterozygous).
- **Risks of transmission to children (offspring):**
  - An affected male does not transmit the disorder to his sons, but all daughters are carriers.
  - Sons of heterozygous women have a 50% chance of receiving the mutant gene.

Examples of X-linked recessive disorders are shown in **Table 8.3.**

X-linked Dominant Disorders

They are very rare, e.g., vitamin D resistance rickets. **General features of X-linked dominant disorders are as follows:**

- **Location of mutant gene:** It is on the X-chromosome and there is no transmission from affected male to son.
- **Required number of defective genes:** One copy of the mutant gene is required for its effect.
  - Often lethal in males and so may be transmitted only in the female line.

TABLE 8.3 Examples of X-linked recessive disorders.

System affected with examples
Blood • Hemophilia A and B • Glucose-6-phosphate dehydrogenase deficiency • Chronic granulomatous disease
Musculoskeletal system: Duchenne muscular dystrophy
Nervous system: Fragile-X syndrome
Metabolic disorders • Diabetes insipidus • Lesch–Nyhan syndrome
Immune systems • Agammaglobulinemia • Wiskott–Aldrich syndrome

  - Often lethal in affected males and they have affected mothers.
  - No carrier state
  - More frequent in females than in males.
- **Risks of transmission to children (offspring):**
  - Transmitted by an affected heterozygous female to 50% of her sons and half of her daughters
  - Transmitted by an affected male parent to all his daughters but none of his sons, if the female parent is unaffected.

Developmental Defects

Definition: Developmental defects are a group of abnormalities that occur during fetal life due to errors in morphogenesis.

Q. Write a short notes on malformations, disruption, and deformities with examples.

- **Congenital anomaly (birth defect/congenital defect/ congenital disorder):** The term congenital means "born with". All types of **structural abnormalities** or defects that are present at birth are termed **congenital anomalies.**
- A **malformation** is a primary (or intrinsic) **structural defect** occurring during the development of an organ or tissue. It may be due to a single gene or chromosomal defect but is more commonly multifactorial in origin. Malformations may involve one organ/system or multiple systems.
  - **Single system defect** (single abnormality): Single abnormalities may have a genetic or non-genetic basis. Examples are congenital heart defects (such as ventricular or atrial septal defects), anencephaly (absence of the brain), cleft lip and/or palate, and neural tube defects.
  - **Multiple malformation syndromes (multiple abnormalities):** These consist of defects in two or more systems and are more likely to be due to chromosomal abnormalities.
  - **Syndrome:** When a **combination of congenital abnormalities** occurs together repeatedly in a consistent pattern due to a single underlying cause, it is termed as "syndrome".
- **Dysmorphology** is the study of **malformations arising from abnormal embryogenesis.**
- **Agenesis** is the complete absence of an organ, e.g., unilateral or bilateral agenesis of the kidney.
- **Aplasia** is the absence/failure of development of an organ or tissue to develop or to function normally, e.g., aplasia of the lung.
- **Hypoplasia** is underdevelopment or incomplete development of an organ or tissue that does not reach the normal adult size, e.g., microglossia.
- **Atresia** refers to incomplete formation of lumen in hollow viscus, e.g., esophageal atresia.
- Dystrophy is a disorder in which an organ or tissue of the body degenerates.

CYTOGENETIC ABNORMALITIES AND MUTATIONS IN CHILDHOOD

PA 11.1 (NC): Describe the pathogenesis and features of common cytogenetic abnormalities and mutations in childhood.

Cytogenetic Disorders Involving Autosomes

Most important is trisomy 21.

Trisomy 21 (Down Syndrome)

Q. Write a short note on Down syndrome.

- Down syndrome was first described by Dr John Langdon Down. It is a **cytogenetic disorder involving autosomes**.
- Most **common chromosomal disorder** and is a **leading cause of mental retardation**.
- About **95%** of these individuals have **trisomy 21 (extra copy of chromosome 21)**, resulting in a **chromosome count of 47** instead of the normal 46.
- **Parents of children with Down syndrome are normal** and have a normal karyotype.

Etiology and Pathogenesis

- **Maternal age: Older mothers** (above 45 years of age) have much **greater risk**.
- **Other factors:** Increased incidence may be associated with exposure of the mother to pesticides, electromagnetic fields, anesthetic drugs, alcohol, and caffeine.

Mechanism of trisomy 21: The **three copies of chromosome 21** in somatic cells cause Down syndrome. It may be due to:

- **Nondisjunction in the first meiotic division of gametogenesis** and is responsible for trisomy 21 **in most (95%) of the patients.**
- **Robertsonian translocation** (*refer* page 275 and **Fig. 8.6B**) of the long arm of chromosome 21 to chromosome 22 or 14 in about 4% of cases.
- **Mosaicism** in about 1% of cases.

Clinical Features

Diagnosis of Down syndrome is **usually apparent at the time of birth** by the infant's **characteristic craniofacial appearance (Fig. 8.9)**. These include flat facial profile, oblique palpebral fissures, and epicanthic folds. The **diagnosis is confirmed by cytogenetic analysis. Characteristic features** appear as the child grows.

- **Mental status:** Children are **mentally retarded with low IQ** (25–50).
- **Craniofacial features:** Diagnostic clinical features are:
  - **Flat face and occiput, with a low-bridged nose, reduced interpupillary distance, and oblique palpebral fissures.**
  - Epicanthal folds of the **eyes impart an oriental appearance** (obsolete term mongolism).
  - Speckled appearance of the iris **(Brushfield spots)**.
  - **Enlarged and malformed ears.**
  - A prominent tongue **(macroglossia)**, which typically **lacks a central fissure** and protrudes through an open mouth.
- *Heart:* **Congenital cardiac anomalies** are responsible for the majority of the deaths in infancy and early childhood. The cardiac defects are:
  - **Septal and AV defect:** These defects include atrial septal defect, ventricular septal defect, and one or more atrioventricular (AV) valves.
  - **Other cardiac anomalies:** Tetralogy of Fallot and Patent ductus arteriosus.
- *Skeleton:* These **children are small** because of shorter bones of the ribs, pelvis, and extremities. The hands are broad and short and show a **Simian crease** (a single transverse crease across the palm). The fifth finger curves inwards.
- *Gastrointestinal tract:* It may show **esophageal/ duodenal stenosis or atresia, imperforate anus, and Hirschsprung disease** (megacolon).
- *Reproductive system:* **Men are sterile** because of spermatogenesis arrest.
- *Immune system:* Affected children are susceptible to serious infections (particularly of the lungs),due to defective immunity.
- *Endocrine system:* **Antithyroid antibodies** may cause hypothyroidism.
- *Hematologic disorders:* They have an increased **risk of both acute lymphoblastic and acute myeloid leukemia.**
- *Atlantoaxial instability:* It is characterized by excessive movement at the junction of the atlas (C1) and axis (C2) vertebrae, due to laxity of either bone or ligament. Neurological symptoms develop when the spinal cord is compressed. Clinically, it may present with easy fatigability, difficulty in walking, abnormal gait, restricted neck mobility, torticollis, etc.

Cytogenetic Disorders Involving Sex Chromosomes

Two important disorders are **Klinefelter syndrome and Turner syndrome.**

Klinefelter Syndrome

Q. Write a short note on Klinefelter syndrome.

It is a **cytogenetic disorder involving sex chromosomes.**

Definition: Klinefelter syndrome (testicular dysgenesis) is **defined by male hypogonadism and is characterized by at least two (may be more) X-chromosomes and one or more Y chromosomes.**

It is the most important genetic disease involving **trisomy of sex chromosomes.** It is an **important** and **most frequent genetic cause of male hypogonadism.** It is associated with **reduced spermatogenesis and male infertility.**

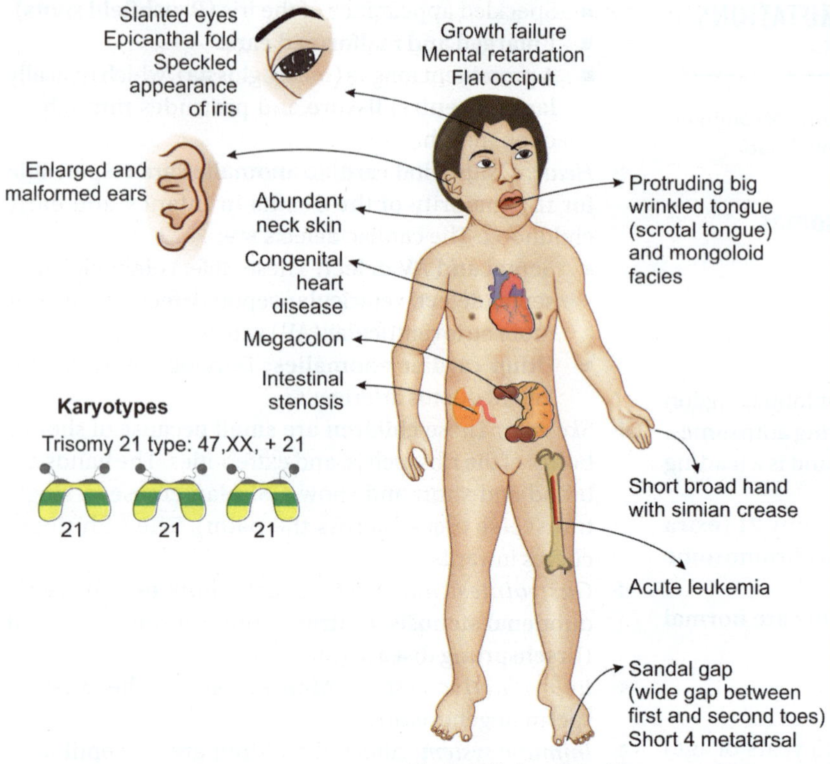

Fig. 8.9: Major clinical features of Down syndrome.

Down syndrome
- Non-disjunction of chromosome 21.
- A most common cause of mental retardation
- Alzheimer disease at a younger age.

Klinefelter's syndrome
- Two or more extra copies of X chromosomes and 1 Y chromosome.
- The classic karyotype of Klinefelter's syndrome is 47,XXY.
- An important genetic cause of male infertility.
- Increased levels of LH and FSH and decreased levels of testosterone.

Turner syndrome
- Webbed neck, streak gonads, and menopause before menarche.
- Primary amenorrhea (menopause before menarche).
- Most common genetic cause of primary amenorrhea.
- Karyotype is 45 X and Barr body is not seen in: Turner syndrome

Pathogenesis

- **47,XXY karyotype: Most of the patients with Klinefelter syndrome have an extra X-chromosome (47,XXY karyotype)**. This results from **nondisjunction of sex chromosomes during the meiotic divisions in one of the parents.**
- A **minority** of them **are mosaic** (e.g., 46,XY/47, XXY) or have more than two X-chromosomes (e.g., 47,XXY/48,XXXY) and one or more Y-chromosomes.
- Regardless of the number of extra X-chromosomes (even up to 4), the Y-chromosome results in a male phenotype.

Clinical Features

The clinical manifestations of Klinefelter syndrome show a wide range of symptoms **(Fig. 8.10)**. It is usually diagnosed after puberty and **hypogonadism is a consistent finding**.

- **Distinctive body constitution:** Patients have increase in length between the soles and the pubic bone. It creates the appearance of an elongated body (**tall and thin**) with relatively long legs (eunuchoid body habitus).
- Mental retardation is uncommon, although average IQ is reduced.
- At puberty, the **testes and penis remain small** with a **lack of secondary male characteristics** (reduced facial, body, and pubic hair).
- Female characteristics include a **high-pitched/deep voice, gynecomastia, and a female pattern of pubic hair.**

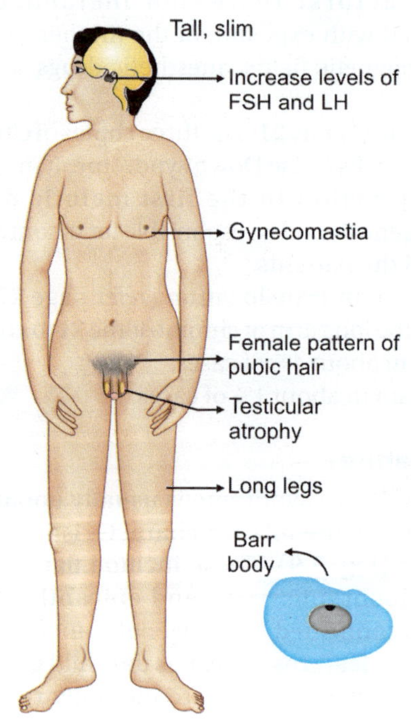

Fig. 8.10: Features of Klinefelter's syndrome.

- **Hypogonadism, reduced levels of testosterone, remarkably high levels of follicle-stimulating hormone (FSH) and luteinizing hormone (LH).**
- **Reduced spermatogenesis with** azoospermia results in **infertility**. The testis may show atrophy of seminiferous

tubules containing pink, hyaline, and collagenous ghosts. Leydig cells may appear prominent.

- **Increased incidence of type 2 diabetes and metabolic syndrome.** Mitral valve prolapse is seen in about 50% of cases.
- **Higher risk for breast cancer, extragonadal germ cell tumors, and autoimmune diseases** such as systemic lupus erythematosus.

Turner Syndrome

Q. Write a short note on Turner syndrome.

It is a **cytogenetic disorder involving sex chromosomes**. Turner syndrome **(Fig. 8.11)** is a spectrum of abnormalities that **results from complete or partial monosomy of the short arm of the X-chromosome** in a **phenotypic female**. It is characterized by hypogonadism and is the most common sex chromosome abnormality in females.

Karyotypic abnormalities: Three types of karyotypic abnormalities are found in Turner syndrome.

Missing of an entire X-chromosome (about 57% of cases): It results in a **45,X karyotype**.

Structural abnormalities of the X-chromosomes (about 14%): These include isochromosomes of the long arm, translocations, and deletions.

Mosaics (about 29%): These patients have 45,X cell population along with one or more karyotypically normal or abnormal cell types. Examples: (1) 45,X/46,XX; (2) 45,X/46,XY.

The molecular pathogenesis of Turner syndrome is not completely understood.

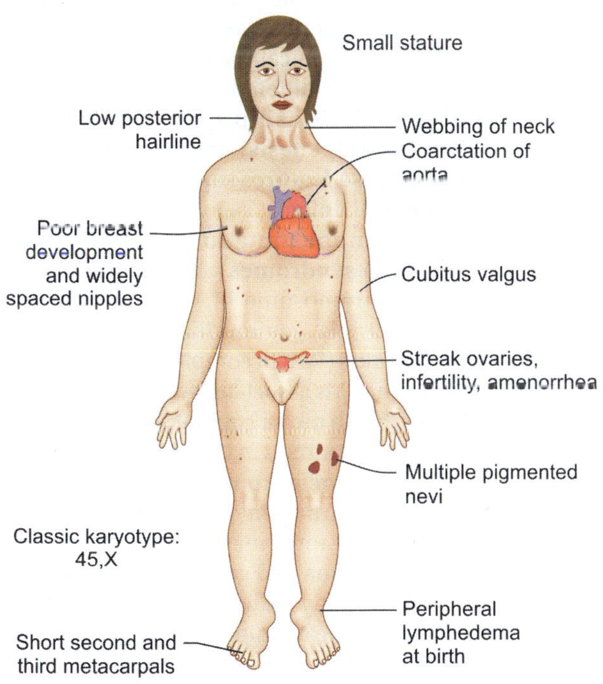

Fig. 8.11: Clinical features of Turner syndrome.

Clinical Features

Turner syndrome is usually **not discovered before puberty**. It presents with **failure to develop normal secondary sex characteristics.** Important diagnostic features are:

- **Growth retardation: Affected adult women have an abnormally short stature** (less than 5 ft tall), **primary amenorrhea, and sterility.** At puberty, normal secondary sex characteristics fail to develop.
- **Webbed neck, low posterior hairline, wide carrying angle of the arms** (cubitus valgus), **broad chest** with **widely spaced nipples,** and hyperconvex fingernails.
- Other features: **Infantile genitalia, inadequate breast development, and little pubic hair.** The **ovaries** are converted to **fibrous streaks.**
- **Pigmented nevi** become prominent as the age advances.
- **Congenital malformations: Cardiovascular anomalies** like congenital heart disease particularly coarctation of the aorta. Also may have horseshoe kidney.
- **Development of autoantibodies:** About 50% show autoantibodies that react with the thyroid gland and 50% of them may develop **hypothyroidism.**

TUMORS AND TUMOR-LIKE LESIONS OF INFANCY AND CHILDHOOD

PA 11.2 (NC): Describe the pathogenesis and pathology of tumor and tumor-like conditions in infancy and childhood.

Tumors in infancy and childhood may be benign or malignant. Benign tumors are more common than malignant tumors. However, **malignant tumors constitute the second most common cause of death in children between the ages of 4 and 14 years** (first being the accidents).

Tumor-like lesions: Two tumor-like lesions in infancy and childhood are:

- **Heterotopia or choristoma:** It is defined as the presence of microscopically normal cells or tissues in abnormal locations (*refer* page 219). Examples include the presence of (i) ectopic pancreatic tissue nodules in the wall of the stomach or small intestine and (ii) a small mass of adrenal cells in the kidney, lungs, ovaries, etc. These are usually of little clinical importance, but may be mistaken as neoplasms.
- **Hamartoma:** It is a jumbled mass consisting of an excessive but focal overgrowth of cells and tissues native/indigenous to the organ in which it occurs (*refer* page 219). The cellular elements are mature and similar to those found in the remainder of the organ. However, they do not have the normal architecture of the surrounding tissue. The distinction between a hamartoma and a benign neoplasm is frequently not clear. For example, hemangiomas, lymphangiomas, rhabdomyomas of the heart, and adenomas of the liver blur the distinction between hamartomas and neoplasms.

Benign Neoplasms

Any benign neoplasm may develop in the pediatric age group. Only hemangiomas, lymphangiomas, and teratomas are discussed below.

Hemangiomas

Hemangiomas are the **most common neoplasms of infancy.**
Histological types: It may be **cavernous or capillary** hemangiomas (*refer* pages 498-9 of Chapter 16 for morphological features).
Sites: Most hemangiomas in children are found in the **skin**, particularly on the face and scalp.
Appearance: They vary in size and appear as **flat to elevated, irregular, red-blue masses.** The flat, larger congenital capillary hemangiomas are called **port-wine stains.** Hemangiomas may enlarge as the child grows, but many a times they **may spontaneously regress**. The majority of superficial hemangiomas have only a cosmetic significance. Rarely, hemangiomas may be the manifestation of a hereditary disorder associated with disease within internal organs (e.g., von Hippel-Lindau syndrome). Few cavernous hemangiomas of CNS can occur in the familial setting and the affected families show mutations in one of three cerebral cavernous malformation (CCM) genes.

Lymphangiomas

They are considered as the lymphatic counterpart of hemangiomas and are also called cystic hygromas. **Unlike hemangiomas,** these lesions do not regress spontaneously and should be resected.

MORPHOLOGY

Site: They are **poorly circumscribed** swellings that are usually present at birth. They may be found on the **skin** but, more commonly, they are seen in the **deeper regions of the head and neck**, axilla, mediastinum, floor of the mouth, and retroperitoneum. They may increase in size after birth and may compress the mediastinal structures or nerve trunks in the axilla.
Microscopy: They may be **unilocular or multilocular**. They show cystic and cavernous spaces lined by endothelial cells and surrounded by lymphoid aggregates. The lumen/ spaces usually contain pale straw-colored fluid.

Teratomas

Teratomas are neoplasms consisting of tissues derived from all three (at least more than two) germ cell layers: ectoderm, endoderm, and mesoderm. They may classified into three types:

1. **Mature teratomas:** Benign, well-differentiated cystic lesions
2. **Immature teratomas:** Lesions of indeterminate potential or
3. **Malignant teratomas:** These are definitely malignant neoplasms usually admixed with another germ cell tumor such as an endodermal sinus tumor.

Age: Most of the benign teratomas are observed in younger infants (4 months of age or younger), whereas children with malignant teratomas are seen in somewhat older.

Sacrococcygeal Teratomas

Sacrococcygeal teratomas are the most common (about 40%) teratomas of childhood. About 10% of sacrococcygeal teratomas may be associated with congenital anomalies such as primarily defects of the hindgut and cloacal region and other midline defects (e.g., meningocele, spina bifida).

MORPHOLOGY

Sacrococcygeal teratomas present as masses near the sacrum and buttocks. About 75% of these tumors are mature teratomas with a benign course. About 12% may be malignant and lethal. The remainder are immature teratomas, and their malignant potential depends on the amount of immature tissue elements present.
Microscopy: Teratomas contain multiple tissues derived from more than one germ cell layer.

Prognosis: About 75% of are mature teratomas have a benign course, and about 12% are malignant. The remainder are immature teratomas, and their malignant behavior depends on the amount of immature tissue elements.

Malignant Neoplasms

Malignant neoplasms in infancy and childhood are uncommon and their distribution is presented in **Table 8.4**. Most common of these include **neoplasms of the hematopoietic system, nervous system, and soft tissues.** This distribution is unlike that in adults, in whom most cancers are of epithelial origin such as carcinomas of the lung, breast, prostate, and GI tract.

Biologically and histologically differ from malignant tumors in adult. Malignant neoplasms developing during infancy and childhood biologically and histologically differ from those in adults. These differences are:

- **Shows a close relationship between abnormal development (teratogenesis) and tumor induction (oncogenesis). These features** suggest that these have a **common stem cell defect.**
- **Prevalence of germline mutations that predispose to cancer (familial syndromes)**. For example, short-arm deletions of chromosome 11, cause Wilms tumor associated with aniridia, genitourinary malformations, and mental retardation (WAGR complex); Loss of the long arm of chromosome 13 is associated with retinoblastoma due to the loss of the Rb tumor suppressor gene. Somatic mutations are more common in cancers in adults.
- **Tendency of malignancies to regress spontaneously or to undergo "differentiation" into mature elements.** For example, neuroblastoma may show a differentiation to ganglioneuroblastoma and ganglioneuroma.

Histologically unique: Many malignant tumors in infancy and childhood have unique histological features.

- **Primitive appearing tumor cells:** They consist of primitive (embryonal) cells rather than pleomorphic-

TABLE 8.4 Common malignant neoplasms of infancy and childhood.

Age: 0–4 Years	5–9 Years	10–14 Years
• Leukemia • Retinoblastoma • Neuroblastoma • Nephroblastoma (Wilms tumor) • Hepatoblastoma • Soft tissue sarcoma (e.g., rhabdomyosarcoma) • CNS tumors • Lymphoma • Teratomas	• Leukemia • Retinoblastoma • Neuroblastoma • Hepatocellular carcinoma • Soft tissue sarcoma • Ewing tumor • Central nervous system (CNS) tumors • Lymphoma • Wilms tumor • Neuroblastoma	• Leukemia • Hepatocellular carcinoma • Soft tissue sarcoma • Osteosarcoma • Thyroid carcinoma • Hodgkin lymphoma

BOX 8.2: List of small, round, blue-cell tumors.

- Neuroblastoma
- Lymphoma
- Rhabdomyosarcoma
- Ewing sarcoma (peripheral neuroectodermal tumor)
- Medulloblastoma
- Retinoblastoma
- Some cases of Wilms tumor

anaplastic microscopic appearance characteristic of malignant tumors in adults. They frequently show features of organogenesis specific to the site of tumor origin.

- **Small, round, blue-cell tumors: Because of the tumor cells have primitive appearance, many childhood tumors have been collectively called small, round, blue-cell tumors (Box 8.2).** These small cells have small, round nuclei and are arranged in sheets.
- **Diagnosis:** These tumors usually show distinctive microscopic features that helps in definitive diagnosis. However, confirmatory molecular studies are becoming increasingly useful, both for diagnosis and prognosis.

Neuroblastoma (*refer* pages 906-7), retinoblastoma (*refer* pages 997-8) and Wilms tumor (*refer* pages 763-4) are the three important tumors.

STORAGE DISEASES

PA 11.3 (NC): Describe the pathogenesis of common storage disorders in infancy and childhood.

Q. Name storage disorders.

- Lysosomal enzymes are used for the intracellular digestion/degradation of many complex biological macromolecules.
- **Deficiency of lysosomal enzymes:** Inherited deficiency of lysosomal enzyme may cause **incomplete catabolism of its normal macromolecular substrate**. This can lead to the **accumulation of the partially degraded insoluble substrate within the lysosomes**. The inherited disorders resulting from mutations in genes that encode lysosomal hydrolases are known as lysosomal storage disorders.

General features of storage disorders are as follows:

- Lysosomal disorders are **transmitted as an autosomal recessive disorder**.
- Usually **detected in infants and young children.**
- **Hepatosplenomegaly** due to the accumulation of insoluble intermediate compounds in the mononuclear phagocytes.
- **CNS involvement** is associated with damage to neurons.

Classification of lysosomal storage disorders: They are classified according to the biochemical nature of the metabolite accumulated within the lysosomes. The subgroups include **glycogenoses, sphingolipidoses (lipidoses), sulfatidoses, and mucopolysaccharidoses (MPSs).**

Niemann–Pick Disease

Q. Write a short note on Niemann-Pick disease and its enzyme deficiency.

Niemann–Pick disease (NPD) is one of the **lysosomal storage disorders (lipidoses)** that are characterized by lysosomal **accumulation of sphingomyelin** due to an **inherited deficiency of sphingomyelinase**.

- Mode of transmission: **Autosomal recessive.**

Classification of Niemann–Pick disease: It is classified into three types:

1. **Type A:** It is a **severe infantile form** with an **almost complete deficiency of sphingomyelinase**. It is characterized by **extensive neurologic involvement, massive visceromegaly,** marked accumulations of **sphingomyelin in the liver and spleen**, and progressive wasting and **death occurring by 3 years of age**.
2. **Type B:** It usually presents with **hepatosplenomegaly** and generally **without the involvement of the central nervous system**. They **usually survive into adulthood**.
3. **Type C:** It is **more common than types A and B**. It is due to **mutations in** two genes namely—***NPC1*** **(Niemann-Pick disease, type *C1*)** and ***NPC2*** **(Niemann-Pick disease, type *C2*)**. It is due to a **primary defect in lipid transport**. Commonly manifests in childhood with ataxia, vertical supranuclear gaze palsy, dysarthria, dystonia, and psychomotor regression.

MORPHOLOGY

Deficiency of sphingomyelinase enzyme blocks degradation of the lipid—sphingomyelin → accumulates inside the lysosomes of cells of the mononuclear phagocyte system.

Organs involved: They show **moderate to marked enlargement.**

- **Brain:** It shows shrunken gyri and widened sulci. Microscopically, the **neurons show vacuolation and ballooning**, which in time leads to cell death and loss of brain substance.
- **Retina:** It shows a **cherry-red spot.**
- **Other organs: Spleen (massively enlarged)**, liver, lymph nodes, bone marrow, tonsils, gastrointestinal tract, and lungs.

Light microscopy:

- **A characteristic storage cell is a macrophage with many, small, uniform vacuoles** (contains sphingomyelin and cholesterol) within the cytoplasm.
- These lipid-laden foam cells are large (20–90 µm in diameter) and frozen sections—vacuoles take up fat stains.

Electron microscopy: The lipid vacuole resembles concentric lamellated myelin figures which are called **"zebra" bodies.**

Tay–Sachs Disease (GM2 Gangliosidosis: Hexosaminidase β-Subunit Deficiency)

- Tay-Sachs disease is inherited as an **autosomal recessive** trait.
- **Most common** form of GM2 gangliosidosis.
- Characterized by genetic **mutations in the *HEXA* gene** on chromosome 15 and a severe **deficiency of** β-subunit **hexosaminidase A** enzymes.
- **Hexosaminidase A enzymes are absent in almost all the tissues.**

MORPHOLOGY

GM2 ganglioside accumulates in many tissues such as the CNS, retina, heart, liver, and spleen.

Special stains: Special stains for fat such as oil red O and Sudan black B stain positive with gangliosides.

Light microscopy:

- **Neurons: Ballooned with many cytoplasmic vacuoles,** each representing a severely distended lysosome filled with gangliosides → followed by destruction of neurons, proliferation of microglia, and accumulation of lipids in phagocytes within the brain substance.
- **Retina:** Ganglion cells in the retina distended with GM2 ganglioside, more prominent at the margins of the macula and give rise to characteristic **cherry-red spot** in the macula. The cherry-red spot is also seen in other storage disorders affecting the neurons.

Electron microscopy: The most prominent features are **prominent lysosomes with whorled configurations which represent onion-skin layers of membranes.**

Clinical Features

- Usually presents between 6 and 10 months of age.
- Clinical features are mainly due to **neuronal involvement in the central and autonomic nervous systems and retina.** Symptoms include progressive motor and mental deterioration, blindness, and increasing dementia.
- Ophthalmoscopy cherry-red spot in the macula.
- Over the span of 1 or 2 years a complete vegetative state is reached. Most children die before 3 years of age.
- **Antenatal diagnosis and carrier detection:** It can be done by enzyme assays and DNA-based analysis.

Gaucher Disease

Q. Write a short essay/note on Gaucher disease.

- **Most common lysosomal storage disorder** due to mutation in the gene that encodes glucocerebrosidase (cleaves glucose residue from ceramide).
- **Autosomal recessive mode of transmission.**
- Due to **deficiency of enzyme glucocerebrosidase → results in accumulation of glucocerebroside,** mainly in **lysosomes of macrophage.**
- **Pathological changes** are both due to:
  - **Accumulation of glucocerebroside**
  - **Activation of macrophages** → secretes cytokines such as IL-1, IL-6, and tumor necrosis factor (TNF).

Q. Write a short note on enzyme deficiency in Gaucher disease.

Clinical subtypes: There are three variants namely:

1. **Type I or the chronic non-neuronopathic form:**
   - **Most common type** (about 99% of cases)
   - **Glucocerebrosides** are stored only **in the mononuclear phagocytes throughout the body** mainly in the **spleen and skeletal system.** It does not involve the brain.
2. **Type II or acute neuronopathic Gaucher disease:**
   - **Infantile acute cerebral pattern**
   - Almost **complete absence of glucocerebrosidase** activity in the tissues → progressive **involvement of CNS → death at an early age.**
3. **Type III:** It is **intermediate between types I and II.**

MORPHOLOGY

Q. Write a short note on the Gaucher cell and its morphology.

Light microscopy: Gaucher cells are the hallmark of this disorder and its characteristics are:

- **Enlarged, phagocytic cells** (sometimes up to 100 µm in diameter) distended **with massive amounts of glucocerebrosides.**
- **Seen throughout the body in virtually all organs,** especially in the **spleen, liver, bone marrow,** lymph nodes, tonsils, thymus, and Peyer's patches.
- **Gaucher cells** have a **fibrillary type of cytoplasm** such as a **crumpled/wrinkled tissue paper (Fig. 8.12)** and one or more dark, eccentrically placed nuclei.
- The **cytoplasm** of Gaucher cells stain intensely **positive with Periodic acid-Schiff.**

Electron microscopy: The fibrillary cytoplasm appears as elongated, distended lysosomes, containing the stored lipid arranged in parallel layers of tubular structures.

Clinical Features

Type I

- Manifests in adult life and follows a progressive course.
- **Spleen is enlarged, sometimes up to 10 kg** and **hypersplenism** may lead to pancytopenia or thrombocytopenia. Hepatomegaly is also seen.

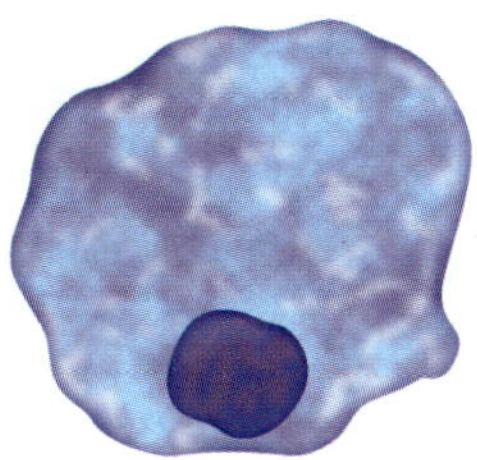

Fig. 8.12: Appearance of Gaucher cells (diagrammatic).

- **Bone marrow: Accumulation of Gaucher cells** produces extensive expansion of the marrow space, bone erosion, focal lytic bone lesions, osteonecrosis, osteopenia, and pathologic fractures.

Types II and III

In patients with CNS involvement, it may produce cerebral dysfunction, convulsions, and progressive mental deterioration. Gaucher cells are seen in the Virchow–Robin spaces.

Molecular Diagnosis of Genetic Disorders

Q. Laboratory diagnosis of genetic diseases.

Genetic disease may be caused by single base substitutions up to gains or losses of entire chromosomes. These can be detected by various genetic tests **(Box 8.3)**.

Polymerase Chain Reaction (PCR)

It is a widely used, powerful tool in the molecular diagnosis of human disease.

Subsequent analysis can be done by different techniques such as **(1) Sanger sequencing, (2) pyrosequencing, (3) single-base primer extension, (4) restriction fragment length analysis, (5) amplicon length analysis, and (6) real-time PCR.**

BOX 8.3: Various tests done for genetic disorders.

TYPE OF TEST

Biochemical Assays
- Quantitative assays for metabolites or electrolytes
- Assay of enzyme activity
- Hemoglobin electrophoresis

Cytogenetic Assays
- Karyotyping
- Fluorescence in situ hybridization (FISH)

"Molecular" Cytogenetic Assays
- Multiplex ligation-dependent probe amplification
- Array-based genomic hybridization
- Next-generation sequencing (NGS)

Genetic Assays
- Allele-specific PCR and related techniques
- Sanger DNA sequencing
- Next-generation sequencing (NGS)

Advantages

- **Wide range of samples:** PCR allows analysis of DNA from any cellular source containing nuclei.
- **Small quantity required:** PCR needs a very small quantity of genetic material and can amplify DNA from even a single cell.
- **Sensitivity:** It has remarkable sensitivity.
- **Rapid:** It produces DNA fragments in a matter of hours.

Disadvantages

- It requires knowledge of the nucleotide sequence of the target DNA fragment.
- It can amplify DNA fragments usually up to 1 kb.

Molecular Analysis of Genomic Alterations

Genetic lesions with large deletions, duplications, or more complex rearrangements cannot easily be assayed by standard PCR methods. Such genomic alterations can be studied by hybridization-based techniques.

1. **Fluorescence in situ hybridization (FISH):** Uses DNA probes that detect and localize sequences specific to particular chromosomal regions.
2. **Multiplex ligation-dependent probe amplification (MLPA):** Blends DNA hybridization, DNA ligation, and PCR amplification to detect deletions and duplications of a genome of any size. It detects genetic alterations that are too large to be detected by PCR and too small to be identified by FISH. It can either be performed on dividing cells (metaphase chromosomes) or nondividing cells (interphase nuclei) making it much more versatile than traditional karyotyping.
3. **Southern blotting:** Detects changes in the structure of specific loci.
4. **Cytogenomic array technology: It detects genomic abnormalities without prior knowledge** in contrast to FISH which needs prior knowledge of the one or few specific chromosomal regions suspected of being altered in the test sample.

Next-Generation Sequencing

- **Next-generation sequencing (NGS) consists of several newer DNA sequencing technologies that can produce large amounts of sequence data in a massively parallel manner.**
- NGS can perform previously impossible analyses at extremely low relative cost.
- **Advantage:** Any DNA from almost any source can be used and is well suited to heterogeneous DNA samples. NGS is useful for detecting genetic anomalies of essentially any size scale ranging from SNPs (single nucleotide polymorphisms—SNPs are pronounced "snips") to very large rearrangements including aneuploidy.

CHAPTER 9

Environmental and Nutritional Diseases

Chapter Outline

- Environmental Pollution
- Effects of Tobacco
- Effects of Alcohol
- Malnutrition
- Obesity
- Common Vitamin Deficiencies

ENVIRONMENTAL POLLUTION

Environmental diseases are disorders caused by exposure to chemical or physical agents in the ambient, workplace, and personal environments. These include nutritional diseases.

PA 12.1a (NC): Enumerate and describe the pathogenesis of disorders caused by air pollution.

Air Pollution

Air pollution is responsible for a **significant cause of morbidity and mortality**, especially among individuals with pre-existing lung or heart disease. The air that we breathe also contains many potential causes of disease. Airborne microorganisms are responsible for major morbidity and death; one example being COVID-19 from 2019 to 2021. More widespread are the air pollutants which include chemical and particulate pollutants. Air pollutants may be found in both outdoor and indoor air.

Outdoor Air Pollution

The outdoor air surrounding us is contaminated with a mixture of gaseous and particulate pollutants. The most important air pollutants are generated by the burning of fossil fuels and industrial and agricultural processes. The main pollutants causing disease are listed in **Box 9.1**.

BOX 9.1: Main outdoor air pollutant.

1. Ozone
2. Nitrogen dioxide
3. Sulfur dioxide (SO_2)
4. Carbon monoxide (CO)
5. Acid aerosols
6. Particulates (solid particles and liquid droplets in the air), especially carbon particles.

Organs affected: The **lungs** are the most common organ affected by air pollution. But it can affect many organ systems.

Ozone: Tropospheric **ozone** (i.e., ozone near the ground as opposed to in the upper atmosphere) is a gas mainly formed by the action of sunlight on nitrogen oxides (NO_2). Most of the nitrogen oxides (refer to below) are released by automobile exhaust. Together with oxides and fine particulate matter, ozone forms smog (derived from the words *smoke* and *fog*). Ozone is one of the **most common and strong oxidant air pollutants**. Its **toxicity is due to the production of free radicals**, which damage the cells lining the respiratory tract and the alveoli (which produce cough and dyspnea) during acute exposure. Healthy individuals can tolerate low levels of ozone. However, they harm the lung function in patients with asthma or emphysema. Chronic exposure to ozone in smog can cause **deterioration in pulmonary function** and is associated with a slight increase in mortality.

Sulfur dioxide (SO_2), particles, and acid aerosols: SO_2 is mainly derived from burning fossil fuels, especially by coal- and oil-fired power plants and industrial processes burning these fuels. Sulfur dioxide is highly irritative and may be oxidized to sulfuric acid. **Acute exposure produces bronchoconstriction and inflammation of the respiratory tract. Particles** particularly of **size <10 µm in diameter can reach the alveoli** and are responsible for morbidity and death. In the alveoli, they are phagocytosed by macrophages and neutrophils, release mediators, and produce an inflammatory reaction. In contrast, larger particles are less dangerous because they are removed from the nose or are trapped by the mucociliary action in the upper respiratory tract.

Carbon monoxide: It is a nonirritating, colorless, tasteless, odorless gas. It is generated during the incomplete combustion (oxidation) of organic substances (carbonaceous materials). The **sources of CO include automotive engines**

(exhaust), home oil burners, industries using fossil fuels, and cigarette smoke.** The low levels of CO usually found in the air may produce impaired respiratory function but are not usually life-threatening. However, individuals working in confined environments with high exposure to fumes (e.g., tunnel and underground garage workers), may develop chronic poisoning. CO can also be an **important cause of accidental and suicidal death**. Treatment of such acute CO poisoning (e.g., those who attempt suicide or are trapped in fires) consists mainly of the administration of 100% oxygen. Carboxyhemoglobin concentrations under 10% are common in smokers and usually do not produce symptoms. CO is a systemic asphyxiant with an affinity for hemoglobin that is 200 times more than that of oxygen. CO binding to hemoglobin forms carboxyhemoglobin and prevents oxygen transport. The oxygen from carboxyhemoglobin does not dissociate as readily as in oxyhemoglobin. This produces hypoxia that in turn leads to central nervous system (CNS) depression. Systemic hypoxia develops when the hemoglobin is 20–30% saturated with CO, and unconsciousness and death occur with 60–70% saturation. **In fatal CO poisoning**, the **skin shows a characteristic cherry-red color** due to carboxyhemoglobin in the superficial capillaries. The diagnosis of CO poisoning depends on the detection of high levels of carboxyhemoglobin in the blood.

Indoor Air Pollution

In the modern world there is increased potential for pollution of the indoor air. The most common pollutant is **tobacco smoke** and others include CO, nitrogen dioxide (already discussed above under outdoor pollutants), and asbestos (*refer* pages 572-4). A few of the other indoor pollutants are briefly presented here.

Smoke from burning of organic materials: They contain **various oxides of nitrogen and carbon particulates.** These are irritants that predispose to **lung infections** and also may contain **carcinogenic polycyclic aromatic hydrocarbons.** It is produced by burning carbon-containing material, such as wood, dung, or charcoal in homes for cooking, heating, and light.

Radon: It is **a radioactive gas derived from uranium.** It is present in soil and homes. Radon **exposure in uranium miners** (especially in smokers) can cause **lung cancer.** However, low-level chronic exposures in nonsmokers' home are less likely to increase the risk of lung cancer.

Bioaerosols: These may contain pathogenic microbiologic agents. They can cause **Legionnaires' disease, viral pneumonia, and the common cold.** They may also contain allergens derived from pet dander, dust mites, fungi, and molds that can cause **rhinitis, eye irritation, and even asthma.**

Metals as Environmental Pollutants

The various heavy metals that can produce harmful effects in humans include **lead, mercury, arsenic, and cadmium.**

Lead

Lead is a readily absorbed, heavy metal commonly found in the environment of industrialized countries.

Source: Exposure to lead occurs **through contaminated air, food, and water.** The major sources of lead in the environment were house paints and gasoline (a mixture of volatile, flammable liquid hydrocarbons derived from petroleum and used as fuel). Now, the use of lead-based paints and leaded gas has been greatly decreased. Currently, the main sources of lead in the environment include **mines, foundries, batteries, and spray paints,** all of which are occupational hazards. The flaking lead paint in older houses, lead pipes, and soil contamination also contain lead.

Pathophysiology: Lead is absorbed through the lungs or gastrointestinal tract, with 80–85% taken up by developing teeth and bone. It **binds to sulfhydryl groups in proteins, interferes with calcium metabolism,** and stays in these sites for 20–30 years. Once in the blood, it circulates and is excreted by the kidneys. Around 5–10% remains in the blood, while the rest is distributed in soft tissues. Lead easily crosses the blood-brain barrier, affecting the brain, liver, kidneys, and bone marrow. It interferes with zinc-dependent enzymes and calcium metabolism, causing **hematologic, skeletal, neurologic, GI, and renal toxicities.** In bones, teeth, nails, and hair, it forms a harmful, tightly bound lead pool.

The major clinical and pathologic features of lead poisoning are shown (*refer* **online Fig. 9.1**).

Laboratory diagnosis: For a definitive diagnosis of lead poisoning, intoxication, elevated blood lead, and red cell-free protoporphyrin levels (>50 μg/dL) or raised blood levels of zinc-protoporphyrin or its product is required. In milder cases of lead exposure, anemia may be the only obvious abnormality.

Treatment: Lead poisoning is treated with chelating agents namely ethylenediaminetetraacetic acid (EDTA), either alone or in combination with dimercaprol (BAL). Usually, hematologic and renal manifestations of lead intoxication are reversible whereas the alterations in the CNS are usually irreversible.

Mercury

Mercury binds to sulfhydryl groups (like lead) in certain proteins with high affinity.

Main organs damaged: The kidney is the main target of the toxicity of inorganic mercury and the CNS (brain) is damaged by organic mercury. It can also **damage the GI tract.**

Source: These are as follows:

1. **Inorganic mercury:** It has been used by humans since prehistoric times as a pigment in cave paintings, a cosmetic, a remedy for syphilis, and a component of diuretics. It is used as a medicine in homeopathy.

2. **Organic mercury (derived from living matter):** It has been the main source of exposure in recent years. Organic mercury is present in contaminated fish and dental amalgams that release mercury vapors. Mercury used in gold mining, or fertilizer and plastics factories, is discharged into and contaminates the rivers. Inorganic mercury from industrial wastes can be converted to highly neurotoxic organic compounds (e.g., methyl mercury) by bacteria in bays and oceans. Methyl mercury is taken by carnivorous fish (e.g., swordfish, shark, tuna, pike, and bluefish). Consumption of such fish contaminated with mercury can produce mercury poisoning. The main source of mercury at present time is contaminated fish.

Neurotoxicity: Children exposed in utero showed **delayed developmental milestones** and abnormal reflexes, cerebral palsy, deafness, blindness, and major CNS defects. The developing brain is susceptible to methyl mercury. It **can affect the motor, sensory, cognitive, and behavioral functions of the brain. It may lead to cerebral and cerebellar atrophy.**

Nephrotoxicity: In the kidneys, mercury can produce **acute tubular necrosis (proximal tubular necrosis) and renal failure.**

GIT: Almost 90% of the ingested organic mercurial compounds are readily taken up in the GI tract because of their lipid solubility. Ingested mercury can damage the gut and cause **ulcerations and bloody diarrhea**.

Arsenic

The toxic properties of arsenic are well known. **Arsenic interferes with several aspects of cellular metabolism. It produces its toxic effects mainly in the GI tract, nervous system, skin, and heart.**

Sources: Arsenic was used as a poison by skilled practitioners in Italy. Arsenic compounds have been used as **insecticides, herbicides, weed killers, other agricultural products, and wood preservatives**. Arsenicals may also be found naturally in soil and ground water (in countries, such as Bangladesh, Chile, and China) because of naturally occurring arsenic-rich rock formations, from coal burning, or the use of arsenical pesticides. It may contaminate the environment by the mining and smelting industries. Arsenic is present in **Chinese and Indian herbal medicine as well as homeopathic medicine.**

Toxic effects: These include:

- **Acute arsenic poisoning** is almost always due to accidental or homicidal ingestion. Ingestion of large quantities of arsenic causes **severe abdominal pain, diarrhea; cardiac arrhythmias, shock, and respiratory distress syndrome**; and acute encephalopathy. GI, cardiovascular, and CNS toxicity may be severe and cause death. These effects may be due to the interference with mitochondrial oxidative phosphorylation.
- **Chronic exposure to arsenic:** Chronic arsenic intoxication affects many organ systems (e.g., gastrointestinal, cardiovascular, and hematologic systems). It produces nonspecific symptoms such as malaise and fatigue. **Cancers of the skin, respiratory tract** (lung carcinoma), and **gastrointestinal tract** may develop due to industrial and agricultural exposure. Arsenic produces hyperpigmentation and hyperkeratosis of the skin. This may be followed by the development of **basal and squamous cell carcinomas** (but not melanomas). A symmetrical sensorimotor polyneuropathy can also develop. Arsenic-induced skin tumors occur on palms and soles and may be multiple. Arsenic can cause encephalopathy and peripheral neuropathy (paresthesias, motor palsies, and painful neuritis).

Other Metals

Cadmium: It is a plasticizer and a pigment and is relatively a modern toxic agent. It is used in manufacturing alloys, producing rechargeable nickel-cadmium batteries, and electroplating other metals (e.g., automobile parts and musical instruments). Cadmium oxide fumes are released during the welding of steel parts previously plated with a cadmium anticorrosive. Cadmium can contaminate soil and plants directly or through fertilizers and irrigation water. The main routes of exposure are ingestion and inhalation. Both plant- and animal-derived foodstuffs may contain substantial amounts of cadmium.

- **Effects**: **Cadmium is mainly toxic to the kidneys and the lungs.** To a lesser extent, it may affect the skeletal and vascular system. They may **generate increased production of ROS.** It accumulates in the human body with a half-life of over 20 years. It is rarely recycled.
  - **Short-term cadmium inhalation**: It irritates the respiratory tract and causes pulmonary edema.
  - **Chronic cadmium exposure:** It can lead to obstructive lung disease (emphysema) and renal toxicity. In the kidney, initially, it produces proteinuria due to tubular damage (rather than glomerular damage) that may progress to end-stage renal disease. Cadmium can cause skeletal abnormalities due to loss of calcium loss.

Chromium (Cr): It is used in several industries, such as metal plating and some types of manufacturing. Chronic exposure is highly genotoxic and increases the **risk of lung cancer** and other tumors.

Nickel: It is used in electronics, coins, steel alloys, batteries, and food processing. The most frequent effect of exposure to nickel is contact dermatitis ("nickel itch") which can develop due to contact with metals containing nickel, such as coins and costume jewelery. Exposure to nickel increases the risk of **lung cancer and cancer of the nasal cavities**.

EFFECTS OF TOBACCO

PA 12.1b (CC): Enumerate and describe the pathogenesis of disorders caused by tobacco.

Q. Write a short note on the effects of tobacco.

Tobacco is the most common exogenous cause of cancers in humans. It is **responsible for about 90% of lung cancers. Smoking tobacco is the single largest preventable cause of human death**. Apart from death due to various types of cancers, tobacco can cause deaths from cardiovascular and metabolic diseases, deaths from nonmalignant lung diseases, and perinatal deaths.

Types of tobacco: Tobacco may be used either for **smoking** or as **smokeless tobacco**.

- **Smoking:** It is the main culprit and may be used in the form of **cigarettes, beedi, cigars, pipe smoking, or reverse smoking** (smoking a cheroot with the burning end inside the mouth is practiced in certain regions of India). Regular marijuana use has also been associated with oropharyngeal cancer. Life expectancy is reduced by cigarette smoking and **overall mortality is proportional to the amount (dose-dependent) and duration of smoking** commonly quantitated as "pack-years." Tobacco smoking not only produces personal risk, but passive tobacco inhalation from the environment (**"second-hand smoke"**) can also cause lung cancer in nonsmokers. Cessation of smoking greatly decreases the risk of death from lung cancer.
- **Smokeless tobacco:** It is also harmful to health and is an **important cause of oral cancer**. It may be used in its various forms such as **chewing tobacco or snuff.** Betel quid/pan is a type of tobacco chewing that contains several ingredients, such as areca nut, slaked lime, and tobacco which are wrapped in a betel leaf. It is commonly used in India and Southeast Asia and is associated with a marked increase in oral cancer. **Betel quid appears to be the major carcinogen**. However, it may also be related to slaked lime and the areca nut. Other methods of tobacco consumption include snuff dipping and tobacco chewing.

Oral cancers are found on the **buccal and gingival** surfaces in the sites **where tobacco products** are held in **contact** with the mucosa for long periods.

Constituents of tobacco smoke: Tobacco contains more than 2,000 substances (potentially noxious) and more than 60 have been identified as carcinogens and few of them along with the type of injury produced by these agents are listed in **Table 9.1**.

- **Nicotine:** It is an alkaloid present in tobacco leaves. It does not directly cause tobacco-related diseases, but is strongly addictive and is responsible for tobacco addiction. Nicotine binds to nicotinic acetylcholine receptors in the brain and releases catecholamines from sympathetic neurons. This is responsible for the acute ill effects of smoking namely an increase in heart rate, blood pressure, cardiac contractility, and output.
- **Tobacco products and smoking:** Any irritating smoked product increases the risk for tumors of the oral cavity. Nicotine in tobacco and other tobacco leaf components causes cancer. **Carcinogens in tobacco can act as initiators, as well as promoters.** Risk increases with the amount and duration of tobacco use.

TABLE 9.1 Effects of major constituents of tobacco smoke.

Constituent of tobacco smoke	*Effect(s)*
Cigarette, tar	Carcinogenesis
Polycyclic aromatic hydrocarbons	
Benzopyrene	
Nitrosamine	
Nicotine	Release catecholamine, causes depression, and promotes tumor
Phenol	Promotes tumor and irritates the mucosa
Carbon monoxide (CO)	Impaired oxygen transport and use
Formaldehyde	Toxic to cilia and irritates mucosa
Oxides of nitrogen	

Diseases Caused

Q. Write a short note on diseases caused and cancers associated with smoking.

Respiratory system: The most common diseases caused by cigarette smoking involve the respiratory system mainly the lungs. These include **chronic bronchitis, emphysema, chronic obstructive pulmonary disease, and lung cancer.**

- **Direct irritant effect on the tracheobronchial mucosa:** Contents in **tobacco smoke directly irritate the tracheobronchial mucosa**, producing inflammation and increased production of mucus (bronchitis) Cigarette smoke also recruits leukocytes to the lung and increases the local production of elastase. This injures lung tissue leading to emphysema. Children living along with adult smokers are susceptible to increased respiratory illnesses and asthma.
- **Lung cancer:** Components of cigarette smoke, mainly **polycyclic aromatic hydrocarbons and nitrosamines** are directly involved in the **development of lung cancer** in humans (*refer* page 575). Cytochrome P-450 phase I enzymes (CYPs) and phase II enzymes increase the water solubility of the carcinogens, thereby helping in their excretion. However, few intermediates produced by CYPs are electrophilic and combine with DNA to form DNA adducts. If DNA adducts persist, they can cause mutations in oncogenes and tumor suppressors.

The **risk of developing lung cancer depends on the intensity of exposure and is usually expressed in terms of the number of "pack years"** (e.g., one pack daily for 20 years is equal to 20 pack years) **or cigarettes smoked per day and duration of the smoking habit**. Smoking also increases the risk of other carcinogens (e.g., asbestos, uranium). In nonsmokers, passive environmental smoke inhalation is also associated with a risk of lung cancer than those who are not exposed to passive smoke. The risk of lung cancer declines after one quits smoking.

- **Cancers of other systems:** These are as follows:
  - **Oral cancers:** Smokeless tobacco along with alcohol consumption is an important cause of oral cancer (*refer* page 590). These include **cancers of the lip, tongue, and buccal mucosa**. All forms of tobacco use—cigarette, cigar and pipe smoking, and tobacco chewing are associated with oral cancer.
  - **Other cancers:** Cigarette smoking is associated with **cancers of the esophagus, larynx, pancreas, bladder, kidney, cervix, bone marrow** (some forms of leukemia), colon, and liver. Tobacco consumption interacts with alcohol in multiplying the risk of oral, laryngeal, and esophageal cancer.

Nonmalignant lesions of other systems: Apart from lung cancer, tobacco smoking is a risk factor for many other nonmalignant disorders of many organ systems.

- **Atherosclerosis and myocardial infarction** (*refer* pages 479 and 512)**:** Cigarette smoking is a major risk factor, for atherosclerosis and its major complication is myocardial infarction. Smoking is a risk factor for **atherosclerotic peripheral vascular disease** and **cerebrovascular disease** (ischemic stroke, intracranial hemorrhage). If smoking is combined with other risk factors, such as hypertension (elevated blood pressure) and hypercholesterolemia (raised blood cholesterol levels), this multiplies the risk of atherosclerosis and myocardial infarction. Cigarette smoking is a strong risk factor for **atherosclerotic aortic aneurysms**.
- **Buerger disease:** It is an inflammatory and occlusive disease of the lower leg vasculature that occurs almost only in heavy smokers.
- **Peptic ulcer disease** (*refer* page 600).
- **Maternal smoking:** Increases the **risk of spontaneous abortions and preterm births** and results in **intrauterine growth retardation** (fetal tobacco syndrome).
- **Type II diabetes mellitus:** It may develop in smokers. It may be due to nicotine-related insulin resistance and beta cell apoptosis, increased central obesity, and altered metabolism of estrogens and androgens in smokers.
- The **course of tuberculosis** is **more severe** in smokers.

Diseases linked to smoking are depicted in **Table 9.2** (*refer* **online Fig. 9.2)**.

E-cigarette (vape): It is a device that simulates tobacco smoking. In this, an aerosol of nicotine and other components is inhaled as vapor. Probably, the risk of cardiopulmonary disease and cancer is lower than with conventional tobacco cigarettes. However, the use of e-cigarettes may cause a form of acute lung injury related to compounds in the vaping fluid. It usually presents with dyspnea, cough, and GI symptoms. Changes in the lung vary from organizing pneumonia to diffuse alveolar damage.

TABLE 9.2 Various cancer and non-neoplastic diseases associated with smoking .

Cancers	*Non-neoplastic diseases*
• Lung cancer • Cancers of the lip, tongue, and buccal mucosa • Laryngeal cancer • Cancer of the esophagus • Bladder cancer • Carcinoma of the kidney • Pancreatic cancer • Cancer of the uterine cervix • AML (acute myeloid leukemia) • Colon and rectum cancers • Liver cancers • Breast cancer • Ovarian tumors	• Chronic bronchitis and emphysema • Peptic ulcers • Diabetes mellitus type II • Tuberculosis • Asthma • Impaired immune function • Seropositive rheumatoid arthritis • Osteoporosis • Thyroid diseases • Ocular diseases, particularly macular degeneration and cataracts • Brain development may be impaired by nicotine in adolescent smokers

EFFECTS OF ALCOHOL

PA 12.1c (CC): Enumerate and describe the pathogenesis of disorders caused by alcohol.

Alcohol (ethanol) consumption in moderation is not harmful. However, **excessive amounts of alcohol can cause marked physical and psychological damage.** Alcohol abuse (improper/bad use) is hazardous. Alcohol can cause acute and chronic toxic effects.

Chronic alcoholism: It is defined as the **regular intake of sufficient alcohol to injure an individual socially, psychologically, or physically**. It may lead to death either directly or due to accidents caused by drunken driving alcohol-related homicides and suicides, and as a consequence of cirrhosis of the liver. Alcoholism is more common in men, but the number of female alcoholics is gradually increasing.

Metabolism of Alcohol

Absorption and distribution: After consumption, ethanol is directly absorbed in the stomach and small intestine. Then ethanol gets distributed to all the tissues and fluids of the body. The ethanol levels in tissues and body fluids are directly proportional to its level in the blood. Less than 10% of the alcohol is excreted directly in the urine, sweat, and breath.

Alcohol level in blood: The amount of **alcohol exhaled is proportional to its level in the blood**. The breath test used by traffic police for drunken driving is based on alcohol exhaled. When the alcohol level reaches 200 mg/dL, drowsiness develops, 300 mg/dL level stupor, and with more than this level, coma with respiratory arrest may develop.
Factors affecting alcohol levels in blood: Apart from the amount of alcohol consumed many other factors also affect the alcohol levels in the blood. These include such as sex, age, medications, rate of consumption, and **rate of metabolism**. Chronic alcoholics develop tolerance to alcohol and they metabolize alcohol at a higher rate than normal. Hence, chronic alcoholics show lower peak levels of alcohol than others for the same amount of alcohol consumed.
Metabolism of alcohol in the liver (*refer* **Fig. 19.14**): Discussed on pages 664-6. Blood alcohol is metabolized to acetaldehyde in the liver by alcohol dehydrogenase (in the cytosol of hepatocytes). The most important toxic effects of ethanol metabolism are as follows:

- **Depletion of nicotinamide adenine dinucleotide (NAD^+):** Alcohol dehydrogenase breaks down alcohol and reduces NAD^+ and elevates NADH (the reduced form of NAD^+). NAD^+ is required for hepatic fatty acid oxidation. Depletion of NAD^+ with excess alcohol intake can lead to fat accumulation in the liver. The increase in the NADH/NAD^+ ratio also can lead to lactic acidosis.
- **Acetaldehyde toxicity:** Metabolism of alcohol produces acetaldehyde, causing acute effects.
- **Generation of ROS:** Ethanol metabolism by CYP2E1 generates reactive oxygen species (ROS) that damage cell membranes via lipid peroxidation, contributing to cellular injury.
- **Endotoxin release:** Alcohol may prompt the release of endotoxin from gram-negative bacteria present in the intestinal flora. This endotoxin stimulates the release of tumor necrosis factor (TNF) and other cytokines from macrophages and Kupffer cells in the liver. They may produce injury to liver cells.

Acute Alcoholism

It produces its effects mainly on the CNS. It may also produce reversible **hepatic and gastric damage**. Acute alcohol intoxication may cause fatalities from motor vehicle accidents.

- **Central nervous system:** In the CNS, alcohol is a depressant. In a normal individual, intellectual **behavioral changes** can be observed at low alcohol concentrations (below 50 mg/dL). Levels above 80 mg/dL are usually associated with **slower reaction times and gross incoordination**. Most individuals become comatose at levels above 300 mg/dL, and at concentrations above 400 mg/dL, death from respiratory **arrest**/failure is common.
- **Liver:** Even moderate intake of alcohol produces an **accumulation of multiple fat droplets in the cytoplasm** of hepatocytes (fatty change or hepatic steatosis—*refer* pages 44 and 669).
- **Gastric damage:** It may induce **acute gastritis and ulceration**.

Chronic Alcoholism (Table 9.3 and Refer Online Figs. 9.3 and 9.4)

Q. Write a short note on diseases and cancers associated with chronic alcoholism.

Chronic alcoholics usually develop CNS tolerance to alcohol and may easily tolerate blood alcohol levels of 100–200 mg/dL. **Most alcohol-related disorders are due to the toxic effects of alcohol itself.** Chronic alcoholism can affect any organs and tissues, but the main effects are found in the liver and stomach. Chronic alcoholics have significant morbidity and shortened life span. This is mainly due to liver, GI tract, CNS, cardiovascular system, and pancreas damage.

MALNUTRITION

PA 12.2 (CC): Describe the pathogenesis of disorders caused by protein-calorie (severe acute) malnutrition and starvation.

Introduction

A healthy diet: It provides sufficient carbohydrates, fats, and proteins. These are needed to support the daily metabolic needs of the body. Adequate amounts of vitamins and minerals are necessary because they act as coenzymes or hormones, or as important structural components (e.g., calcium, phosphate).
Malnutrition: Lack of proper nutrition is called malnutrition. It may be primary or secondary.

- **Primary malnutrition:** In this type, one or all the components of a healthy diet are missing from the diet. Common causes include poverty, ignorance, chronic excess alcohol use, acute and chronic illnesses, self-imposed dietary restrictions, etc.
- **Secondary, or conditional, malnutrition:** In this, the dietary intake of nutrients is adequate. Malnutrition occurs due to malabsorption of nutrients, impaired use or storage, excess losses, or increased requirements. The causes of secondary malnutrition belong to three general and overlapping categories: gastrointestinal diseases, chronic wasting diseases, and acute critical illness.

Severe Acute Malnutrition

World Health Organization (WHO) definition: Severe acute malnutrition (SAM) is defined as a state characterized by a weight-to-height ratio that is 3 standard deviations below the median growth standard, visible wasting, or the presence of nutritional edema.

SAM, previously called protein-energy malnutrition (PEM) or protein-calorie malnutrition. **SAM** is a serious,

TABLE 9.3 Chronic alcoholism and associated diseases (main effects).

The organ or system affected	*Associated diseases*
Liver	Fatty liver, alcoholic hepatitis, cirrhosis, and an increased risk of hepatocellular carcinoma
GI tract	Massive bleeding from gastritis, peptic/gastric ulcer, or esophageal varices (a complication of cirrhosis), reflux esophagitis. Violent retching may cause tears at the esophageal–gastric junction (Mallory–Weiss syndrome). Impaired small intestinal absorption
CNS	Thiamine deficiency resulting in peripheral neuropathies and the Wernicke-Korsakoff syndrome (due to nutritional thiamine deficiency), cerebral atrophy, cerebellar degeneration, and optic neuropathy
CVS	Dilated congestive cardiomyopathy (alcoholic cardiomyopathy), arrhythmias, and increased incidence of hypertension
Pancreas	Increased risk of acute and chronic pancreatitis
Effects on the fetus	Consumption during pregnancy can cause fetal alcohol syndrome
Carcinogenesis	Increased incidence of cancers of the oral cavity, esophagus, liver, and, possibly, breast in females
Malnutrition and deficiencies of B vitamins	Inhibits the active transport of amino acids, thiamine, and vitamin B12
Hemopoietic dysfunction	Megaloblastic anemia, hemolytic anemia. Transient thrombocytopenia after acute alcohol intoxication
Endocrine system	Feminization, loss of libido and potency, gynecomastia, and testicular atrophy in male alcoholics
Bone	Osteoporosis and aseptic necrosis of bone
Immune system	Prone to many infections (particularly pneumonia) with micro-organisms that are unusual in the general population (e.g., *Haemophilus influenzae*)

often lethal disease and usually affects children of low-income countries.

Range of syndrome: SAM includes a range of clinical syndromes that result from an inadequate intake of dietary protein and calories to meet the body's requirements. The two ends of the spectrum of SAM are **(i)** ***marasmus*** **and (ii)** ***kwashiorkor***.

Protein compartments: From a functional view, the body has two protein compartments: **(i) the somatic compartment** (consisting of proteins in skeletal muscles), and **(ii) the visceral compartment** (protein stores in visceral organs, primarily the liver). These two compartments are regulated differently. The somatic compartment is more severely affected in marasmus and the visceral compartment is reduced more severely in kwashiorkor.

Diagnosis of SAM: SAM may be mild moderate or severe. When severe, SAM can be easily diagnosed.

1. **Comparing body weight and height against standard tables**: In mild to moderate forms, the diagnosis is made by comparing body weight for a given height against standard tables. Other helpful parameters are fat stores, muscle mass, and levels of certain serum proteins.
2. **Reduced skinfold thickness**: The skinfold thickness includes skin and subcutaneous tissue. It is reduced with loss of body fat.
3. **Reduced midarm circumference**: The reduction of somatic protein decreases muscle mass and circumference. It is estimated by measuring the circumference in the midarm and is reduced in SAM.
4. **Reduced visceral protein compartment:** Estimation of the adequacy of the visceral protein compartment is by measuring serum proteins (e.g., albumin, transferrin).

Role of the gut microbiome in the pathogenesis of SAM: The microbial flora of children with SAM seems to be different when compared with the gut microbiome of properly nourished children. Thus, the alterations in the microbiome may be involved in its causation and also the consequence of SAM.

Marasmus

Q. Write short note on marasmus.

Marasmus is the childhood form of global starvation—that is, a deficiency of all elements of the diet. It develops **due to a diet that is severely lacking in calories.**

Depletion of somatic protein compartment: Marasmus is characterized by growth retardation and loss of muscle mass due to catabolism and depletion of the somatic protein compartment. This is an adaptive response to provide the body with amino acids as a source of energy.

Marginal depletion of visceral protein compartment: The visceral protein compartment is more important for survival. It is depleted only marginally. Therefore, *serum levels of albumin are normal or only slightly reduced.*

Mobilization of subcutaneous fat: Apart from muscle proteins, subcutaneous fat is also mobilized and used as fuel. Production of leptin (discussed below on pages 297) is low. This may stimulate the hypothalamic-pituitary-adrenal axis to produce high levels of cortisol leading to lipolysis.

Manifestations

Emaciation with obvious muscle wasting and loss of body fat: Losses of muscle and subcutaneous fat lead to emaciation of the extremities. It leads to reduced body weight and subcutaneous fat, a protuberant abdomen, muscle wasting, and a wrinkled face. The child appears like a "shrunken old person." Visceral organs such as the heart and liver, show wasting and increased lipofuscin pigment. There marasmus is growth failure. No **edema.**

Large head: The head appears too large for the body.

Other features: These include **anemia,** features of **multivitamin deficiencies**, and evidence of **immune deficiency**, particularly of T cell-mediated immunity. The child usually suffers from frequent infections, which forces additional stress on a weakened body. Diarrhea occurs frequently.

Kwashiorkor

Inadequate protein intake: Kwashiorkor develops due to an inadequate protein intake with reasonable caloric (energy) intake. **Thus, the deficiency of protein in the diet is relatively greater than the reduction in total calories.** It is the **most common form of SAM in children.**

Causes

Early weaning with subsequent exclusive carbohydrate diet: Kwashiorkor occurs in children who have been weaned early and subsequently fed, almost exclusively, a carbohydrate diet. The term kwashiorkor is from the Ga language in Ghana and describes the illness in a child who is weaned when another baby is born.

Other causes: Less severe forms may develop in individuals with chronic diarrheal states. In these persons, the protein is not absorbed, or there is chronic loss of protein (e.g., protein-losing enteropathies, the nephrotic syndrome, or the aftermath of extensive burns).

Rare causes: Resulting from fad diets (promotes fast weight loss without scientific evidence) or replacement of milk with rice-based beverages.

Manifestations (Fig. 9.5)

Generalized or dependent edema: Unlike in marasmus, kwashiorkor is associated with marked protein deprivation is associated with severe loss of the visceral protein compartment. This produces hypoalbuminemia leading to **generalized or dependent edema**. Edema is not a characteristic feature of marasmus.

Weight loss: In severe kwashiorkor, the weight is usually 60–80% of normal. However, true weight loss is masked

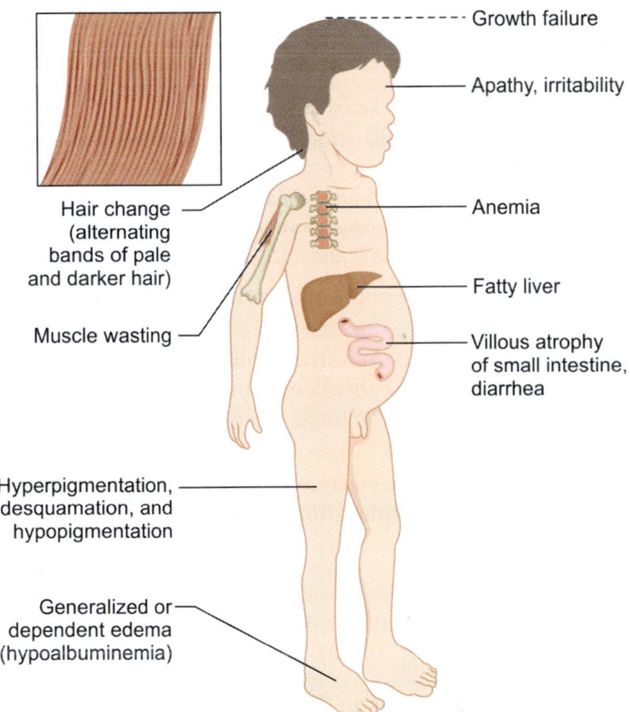

Fig. 9.5: Manifestations of kwashiorkor.

due to increased retention of fluid (edema). In contrast with marasmus, **subcutaneous fat and muscle mass are relatively spared.**

Skin lesions: These are characteristic in children with kwashiorkor. These lesions consist of **alternating zones of hyperpigmentation,** desquamation, **and hypopigmentation, producing a "flaky (peeling/scaly) paint" appearance.** The face, extremities, and perineum appear dry and hyperkeratotic.

Hair changes: These include **loss of color or alternating bands of pale and darker** hair (sandy or reddish color). They show straightening, with fine texture, and loss of firm attachment to the scalp. In severe cases, characteristic linear depigmentation of the hair ("flag sign") is observed.

Q. Write a short note on the flag sign.

Other features: The other features that differentiate kwashiorkor from marasmus are as follows:

- **Fatty liver: The liver is enlarged and shows steatosis (fatty liver)** due to reduced synthesis of the carrier protein component (apoprotein) of lipoproteins.
- **General features: Development of apathy (lack of interest), listlessness, and loss of appetite.**
- **Viscera: Usually atrophic.**
- **Vitamin deficiencies: The intestinal villous atrophy may impair nutrient and vitamin absorption.**
- **Defects in immunity and secondary infections.**

Marasmus and kwashiorkor are considered as two ends of a spectrum, and they show considerable overlap.

MORPHOLOGY OF SAM

- Growth failure.
- Peripheral edema in kwashiorkor.
- Loss of body fat and atrophy of muscle more marked in marasmus.
- **Bone marrow:** It may be hypoplastic in both kwashiorkor and marasmus. It is mainly due to a decrease in red cell precursors. It is usually hypochromic and microcytic due to iron deficiency.

Differences between kwashiorkor and marasmus are listed in **Table 9.4**.

Cachexia: SAM is a common complication that develops in patients with AIDS or advanced cancers. In these settings, it is called cachexia. Cachexia occurs most commonly in patients with cancers of gastrointestinal, pancreatic, and lung. It is characterized by extreme weight loss, fatigue, muscle atrophy, anemia, anorexia, and edema.

Starvation

Definition: Starvation is a state of overall deprivation of nutrients. The causes of starvation are listed in **Box 9.2**.

Metabolic Changes in Starvation

Starvation is a gradual process in which there is a decrease in the metabolic rate as storage carbohydrate reserves are metabolized.

1. **Glucose:** A normal body has glucose stores that are sufficient only for one day's metabolic needs. During fasting, insulin-independent tissues, such as the brain, blood cells, and renal medulla continue to utilize glucose. However, insulin-dependent tissues like muscle do not utilize glucose. To maintain normal blood glucose levels, there will be the release of glycogen stores from the liver. When the liver glycogen stores are depleted (within a few days), the supply of glucose released into the blood decreases. Subsequently, hepatic gluconeogenesis from other sources, such as the breakdown of proteins takes place.
2. **Proteins:** Protein stores and the triglycerides of adipose tissue have enough energy for about 3 months. In starvation, the proteins are broken down to release amino acids and these amino acids are utilized as fuel for hepatic gluconeogenesis. Protein is used for energy using gluconeogenesis because certain tissues prefer glucose as an energy source. The use of protein for gluconeogenesis produces a negative nitrogen balance.
3. **Fats:** When insulin levels decline during fasting, triglycerides of adipose tissue are broken down to form glycerol and free fatty acids. The fatty acids are converted into ketone bodies in the liver and they are used for energy use in place of glucose by most organs including the brain. As starvation continues, overall energy needs are reduced by slowing metabolism. The tissues that usually need glucose for energy adapt by using ketone bodies produced from fat. Eventually, lipolysis of stored fat provides the source of required energy and the use of protein as an energy source decreases. Through this adaptive response, the body strives to conserve lean body mass. Overall, there will be a reduction and depletion of the body's protein. Fasting (voluntary starving) is not associated with high mortality unless it is prolonged. Starvation can continue till a stage when all the body fat stores are exhausted. After the exhaustion of fat stores death will occur.

TABLE 9.4 Differences between kwashiorkor and marasmus.

Feature	*Kwashiorkor*	*Marasmus*
Definition	Inadequate protein intake with reasonable caloric (energy) intake	Inadequate intake of both protein and calories
Age	Children 6 months to 3 years	Infants under 1 year
Growth failure	Present	Present
Edema	Localized or generalized	Absent
Liver	Enlarged fatty	Not enlarged

BOX 9.2: Causes of starvation.

- Deliberate fasting (religious or political)
- Famine conditions (country or community)
- **Secondary undernutrition:** Due to chronic wasting illness/ diseases (e.g., infections, inflammatory conditions, liver disease), cancer (*refer* page 261)

BOX 9.3: Infections associated with starvation.

- Gastroenteritis and gram-negative sepsis
- Respiratory infections, e.g., bronchopneumonia
- Viral diseases, e.g., measles, herpes simplex
- Tuberculosis
- Streptococcal and staphylococcal skin infections
- Helminthic infestations

Manifestations: The starved patient has lax, dry skin, wasted muscles, and atrophy of internal organs. In chronic starvation, the patient is susceptible to infections **(Box 9.3)**.

Laboratory findings: Characteristic findings in starvation include decreased serum glucose levels and urinary nitrogen excretion, along with elevation in the levels of ketone bodies (with ketonuria) and free fatty acids.

OBESITY

PA 12.3 (CC): Describe the pathogenesis of obesity and its consequences.

Q. Write a short note on obesity.

Definition: Obesity is defined as an accumulation of excess body fat (adipose tissue) that is of sufficient magnitude to impair health.

TABLE 9.5 Classification of overweight and obesity by body mass index.

	BMI Kg/m²
Normal	18.5–24.9
Overweight	25.0–29.9
Obesity—Class I	30.0–34.9
Obesity—Class II	35.0–39.9
Extreme obesity—Class III	≥40

BOX 9.4: Diseases associated with obesity and excess body weight.

- Type 2 diabetes
- Dyslipidemias
- Cardiovascular disease
- Hypertension
- Cancer

Prevalence of obesity: Obesity is a major health problem in higher-income countries and an emerging health problem in lower-income countries, such as India.

Classification of overweight and obesity by body mass index is presented in **Table 9.5**. Diseases associated with obesity and excess body weight are listed in **Box 9.4**.

Types of obesity: The distribution of the stored fat is important in obesity and according to body fat distribution obesity is divided into:

- **Central ('abdominal', 'visceral', 'android' or 'apple-shaped') obesity:** This type of obesity shows the increased accumulation of fat in the trunk and the abdominal cavity/intra-abdominal (in the mesentery and around viscera). It is associated with a greater risk for several diseases (e.g., Type 2 diabetes, metabolic syndrome, and cardiovascular disease) than generalized obesity.
- **Generalized' ('gynoid' or 'pear-shaped') obesity:** This type is characterized by excess accumulation of fat diffusely in the subcutaneous tissue.

Body mass index (BMI): It is calculated as (weight in kilograms)/(height in meters)^2 or kg/m^2. It is used for the initial assessment of health. Healthy BMI ranges from 18.5 to 25 kg/m^2 (varies according to country and population). Persons with BMI more than 30 kg/m^2 are classified as obese and those with BMI between 25 kg/m^2 and 30 kg/m^2 are considered overweight.

Pathogenesis

The **etiology** and **pathogenesis of obesity** are complex and **incompletely understood. Genetic, environmental, and psychological factors may be involved in its development.**

Energy balance between consumption and expenditure: These are the two **sides of the energy equation**. They are **finely regulated by neural and hormonal (humoral) mechanisms** and maintain the body weight within a narrow range for many years. This fine **energy balance is controlled by an internal setpoint (lipostat)**. This senses the quantity of energy stores (adipose tissue) and appropriately regulates food intake as well as energy expenditure.

Obesity genes: Several "obesity genes" encode molecular components of the physiologic system that regulates energy balance. **The main player in energy homeostasis** is the ***LEP* gene and its product, *leptin*** (discussed below).

Energy imbalance in obesity: Accumulation of fat in obesity can be considered to be the result of an **energy imbalance between intake** (consumption) **and expenditure.**

Neurohumoral Mechanisms

The neurohumoral **(neural and humoral)** mechanisms that regulate energy balance and body weight can be divided into three components (i) a peripheral or afferent system, (ii) a central processing system, and (iii) an efferent system **(Fig. 9.6)**.

Peripheral or Afferent System

The peripheral or afferent system generates signals from various sites and provides signals to the central processing system in the brain. The main components of this system are (i) leptin produced by fat cells, (ii) ghrelin from the stomach, (iii) peptide YY (PYY) and glucagon-like peptide 1 (GLP-1) from the ileum and colon, and (iv) insulin from the pancreas.

Leptin (Greek term leptos, meaning 'thin.'): It is a member of the cytokine family, **secreted by adipocytes**. It regulates both sides of the energy equation namely (i) intake of food and (ii) expenditure of energy. The **net effect of leptin is to reduce food intake and to increase the expenditure of energy.** Leptin stimulates the POMC/CART pathway **(Fig. 9.6)** and inhibits the NPY/AgRP pathway and **appetite is suppressed** (anorexigenic). Increased leptin **stimulates physical activity**, heat **production** (thermogenesis), and **energy expenditure**.

Ghrelin: It is produced by the **oxyntic cells of the fundus of the stomach** and in the **arcuate nucleus of the hypothalamus.** Ghrelin **increases food intake** (orexigenic effect) and **stimulates appetite** by activating the central appetite-stimulating NPY/AgRP pathway.

Peptide YY (PYY) and glucagon-like peptide 1 (GLP-1): They are **secreted by the endocrine cells** (L-cells) in the ileum and colon. They **reduce appetite.**

Insulin: It is **secreted by β-cells of the pancreas** and acts centrally to **activate the appetite-suppressing pathway**.

Central Processing System

It resides in the arcuate nucleus of the hypothalamus. It integrates neurohumoral peripheral afferent signals and generates efferent signals.

First-order neurons: The efferent signals are transmitted by a pair of first-order neurons:

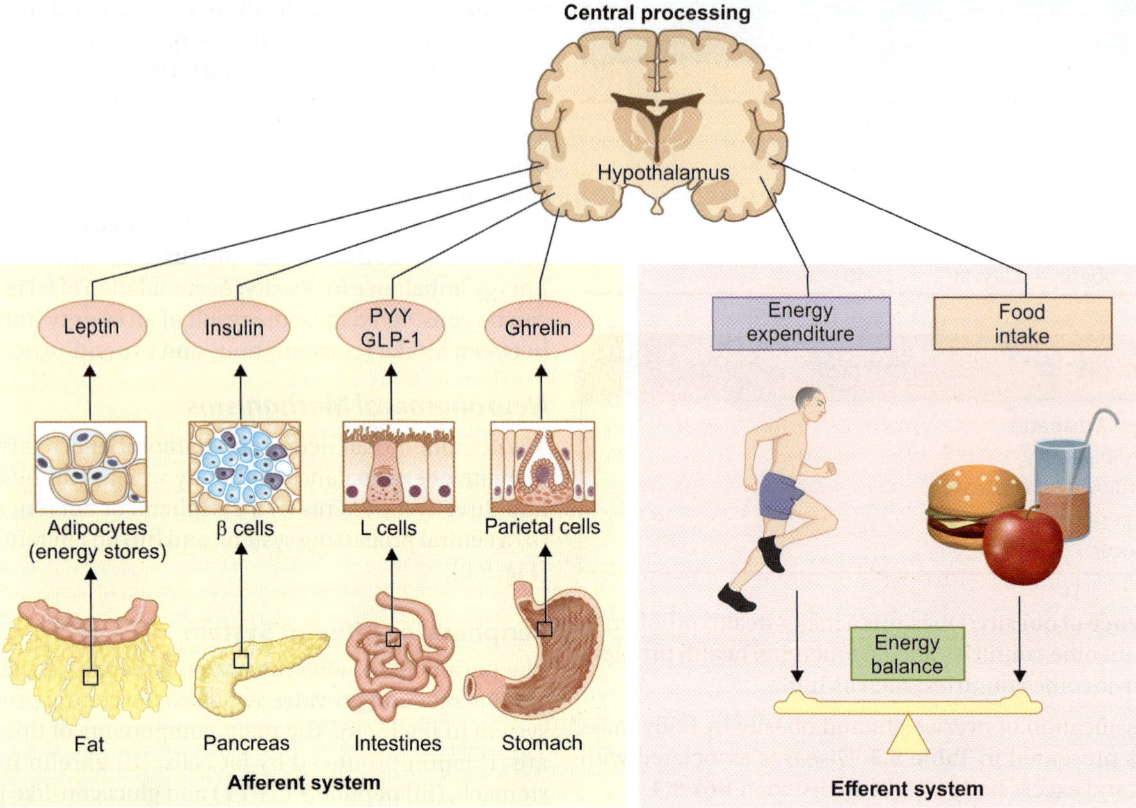

Fig. 9.6: Simplified schematic representation of regulation of energy balance. The peripheral afferent system influences the activity of the hypothalamus, which is the central regulator of appetite and satiety. Signals from the hypothalamus in turn act on the peripheral efferent system (food intake and energy expenditure).
(GLP-1: glucagon-like peptide-1; PYY: peptide YY).

1. **Appetite-suppressing**: POMC (proopiomelanocortin) and CART (cocaine- and amphetamine-regulated transcript) neurons; and
2. **Appetite-stimulating**: NPY (neuropeptide Y) and AgRP (agouti-related peptide) neurons.

Second-order neurons: The first-order neurons communicate with a pair of second-order neurons. These are:

1. Neurons that have α melanocortin stimulating hormone (α-MSH) receptors 3 and 4 (MC3/4R) and receive signals from first-order POMC/CART neurons
2. Neurons that have Y1 and Y5 receptors and receive signals from first-order NPY/AgRP neurons.

Efferent System

It consists of signals produced by second-order neurons. It is organized along two pathways, (i) catabolic (downstream of MC3/4R) and (ii) anabolic (downstream of Y1 and Y5 receptors). These pathways control food intake and energy expenditure.

Clinical Consequences of Obesity (Complications of Obesity) (Box 9.5)

Q. Write a short note on important diseases associated with obesity.

Obesity (particularly central obesity) is associated with the following consequences.

BOX 9.5: Major clinical consequences of obesity.

- Increased morbidity and mortality.
- Metabolic syndrome
- Metabolic complications
  - Insulin resistance, hyperinsulinemia, and 2 diabetes mellitus
  - Obesity-related hypertension
  - Hypertriglyceridemia and low HDL cholesterol levels
- Higher incidence of gallstones especially cholesterol gallstones
- Nonalcoholic fatty liver disease
- Osteoarthritis
- Obstructive sleep apnea and right-sided heart failure.
- Elevated markers of inflammation.
- Increased risk of cancer

Morbidity and mortality: Obesity (particularly central obesity) has many adverse effects on health and is associated with an increase in mortality and morbidity. Obese individuals are at risk of early death, mainly from type 2 diabetes, and cardiovascular, and cerebrovascular disease.

Metabolic syndrome: Central obesity is linked to metabolic syndrome. This syndrome is characterized by abnormalities of glucose and lipid metabolism, hypertension, and systemic inflammation.

Metabolic complications of obesity: Central obesity or upper body fat distribution is associated with increased concentration of FFA which can produce several metabolic complications of obesity.

- **Insulin resistance, hyperinsulinemia, and Type 2 diabetes mellitus***:* Insulin resistance is the decrease/failure of target (peripheral) tissues to insulin action. Central/upper body/visceral obesity is found in more than 80% of patients with type 2 diabetes mellitus.
- **Obesity-related hypertension:** Insulin resistance and hyperinsulinemia may be associated with hypertension.
- **Hypertriglyceridemia and low HDL cholesterol levels:** Obese individuals generally have hypertriglyceridemia and low HDL cholesterol levels. They increase the risk of coronary artery disease.

Gallstones: Higher incidence of gallstones especially cholesterol gallstones.

Nonalcoholic fatty liver disease: Currently called metabolic dysfunction-associated steatotic liver disease (MASLD). It is commonly associated with obesity and type 2 diabetes. It can progress to cirrhosis and has an increased risk of liver cancer.

Osteoarthritis: Marked obesity predisposes to degenerative joint disease (osteoarthritis) and also gout.

Obstructive sleep apnea: It may lead to right-sided heart failure. Hypoventilation syndrome is a respiratory abnormality in very obese persons.

Elevated markers of inflammation: CRP and proinflammatory cytokines like TNF, are often elevated in obese individuals, particularly those with central obesity.

Increased risk of cancer: Increased incidence of certain cancers is observed in the overweight. These include cancers of the esophagus, thyroid, colon, and kidney in men and cancers of the esophagus, endometrium, gallbladder, and kidney in women.

COMMON VITAMIN DEFICIENCIES

Vitamins are vital organic substances required in limited amounts with key roles in certain metabolic pathways.

Categories: Thirteen vitamins are necessary for health and are categorized as follows:

- **Fat-soluble vitamins:** These include A, D, E and K. Fat-soluble vitamins are stored in the body, but their absorption may be poor in fat malabsorption disorders or disturbances of digestive functions.
- **Water-soluble vitamins:** All other vitamins (vitamins of the B complex group and vitamin C).

Vitamin A

Vitamin A is part of the family of retinoids which is present in food and the body as esters combined with long-chain fatty acids. Vitamin A is a generic name for a group of compounds that include *retinol, retinal,* and *retinoic acid.*

Functions: Vitamin A has several metabolic roles. The main functions of vitamin A in humans are as follows:

- **Maintenance of normal vision in reduced light:** The visual process involves vitamin A-containing pigments.
- **Potentiating the differentiation of specialized epithelial cells:** Vitamin A is involved in the orderly differentiation of mucus-secreting column epithelium. In vitamin A deficiency, mucus-secreting cells are replaced by keratin-producing cells and this process is known as **squamous metaplasia**.
- **Metabolic effects of retinoids:** Retinoids inhibit adipogenesis and stimulate the breakdown of lipids.
- **Increases resistance to infections.** Vitamin A is required for optimal immune function and it increases resistance to infections. Retinoids, β-carotene, and some related carotenoids act as photoprotective and antioxidant agents.

Deficiency States

Q. Write a short note on vitamin A deficiency.

Causes: Due to poor nutrition or as a secondary deficiency because of malabsorption of fats (e.g., celiac disease, Crohn disease, and ulcerative colitis, and Bariatric surgery).

Effects of Vitamin A Deficiency (Fig. 9.7)

Effects on the eye: These are as follows:

- **Night blindness:** Vitamin A is a component of rhodopsin and other visual pigments. Hence, vitamin A deficiency manifests as impaired vision, particularly in reduced light *(night blindness).*
- **Xerophthalmia:** Vitamin A deficiency produces **epithelial metaplasia** and **keratinization**. In the eyes, it produces keratinization of the cornea—**xerophthalmia** (dry eye). Initially, it produces dryness of the conjunctiva (**xerosis conjunctivae**) because of the replacement of the normal lacrimal and mucus-secreting epithelium by keratinized epithelium.
- **Bitot spots: keratomalacia and irreversible blindness:** Subsequently, a buildup of keratin debris in **small opaque plaques** (**Bitot spots**), which may progress to erosion of the corneal surface, softening and destruction of the cornea (**keratomalacia**), scarring, and **irreversible blindness.**

Squamous metaplasia of other epithelia: The epithelium lining the upper respiratory passage and urinary tract also undergoes **squamous metaplasia**.

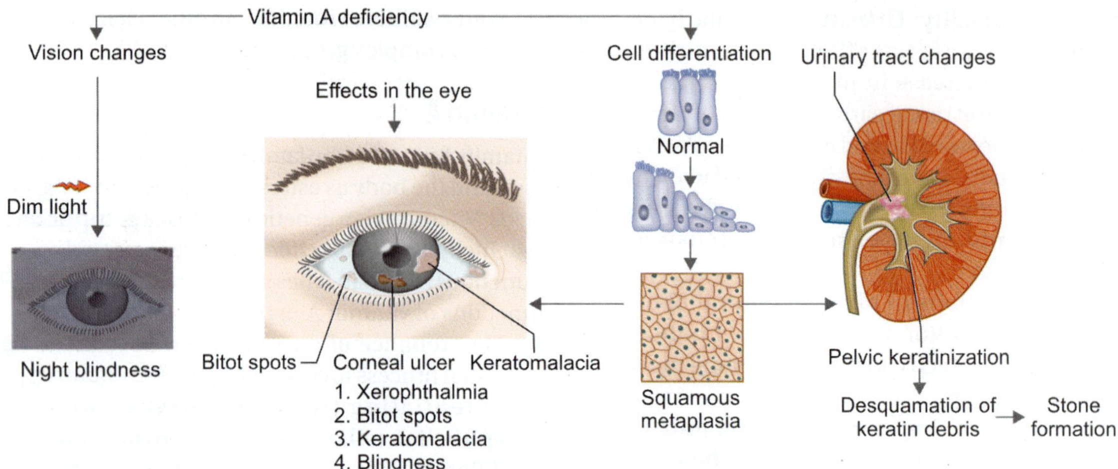

Fig. 9.7: Pathological effects of vitamin A deficiency.

Secondary pulmonary infections may develop due to loss of the mucociliary epithelium (due to metaplasia) of the airways.

Renal and urinary bladder stones: The desquamation of keratin debris in the urinary tract can lead to the formation of **renal and urinary bladder stones.**

Follicular or popular dermatosis (in the skin).

Immune deficiency: It is responsible for higher mortality rates from common infections, such as measles, pneumonia, and infectious diarrhea.

Vitamin D

Vitamin D is a **fat-soluble vitamin.**

Functions

1. **Maintenance of adequate plasma levels of calcium and phosphorus:** The main functions of vitamin D on calcium and phosphorus homeostasis are as follows:
   - **Stimulates intestinal absorption of calcium.**
   - **Stimulates calcium reabsorption in the kidney.**
   - **Regulation of PTH synthesis by chief cells.**
2. **Bone mineralization and resorption.**
3. **Neuromuscular transmission**
4. **Antiproliferative effects.**
5. **Immunomodulatory:** Vitamin D is involved in the innate and adaptive immune system.

Deficiency

Q. Write a short note on vitamin D deficiency.

Causes

- Impaired cutaneous production due to **limited exposure to sunlight.**
- **Dietary absence:** Diets deficient in calcium and vitamin D.
- **Malabsorption.**

Milder forms of vitamin D deficiency also called **vitamin D insufficiency**, lead to an increased risk of bone loss and hip fractures in older adults.

Skeletal Effects of Vitamin D Deficiency

Q. Write a short note on rickets and their clinical features.

Vitamin D deficiency causes rickets in children and osteomalacia in adults. The basic defect in both rickets and osteomalacia is an excess of unmineralized bone matrix.

MORPHOLOGY

Rickets in Children (Figs. 9.8A and B)

In children, before the closure of epiphyses, vitamin D deficiency causes retardation of growth associated with an **expansion of the growth plate** known as **rickets.** In vitamin D deficiency, hypophosphatemia due to secondary hyperparathyroidism is responsible for the development of the **rachitic** (related to rickets) **growth plate. Gross skeletal changes in rickets:** It depends on the **severity and duration of the vitamin D deficiency** and the **stresses** to which individual bones are subjected.

During the nonambulatory stage of infancy

During this stage, the head and chest are subjected to the greatest stresses.

Head: The changes are as follows:

- **Craniotabes:** The **softened occipital bones become flattened.** The **parietal bones buckle inward** by pressure; with the release of the pressure, **elastic recoil snaps the bones back into their original positions** (craniotabes). The **skull appears square and box-like.** Cranial bones show delayed closure of anterior fontanelle.
- **Frontal bossing:** Excess of osteoid produces **frontal bossing** and a **squared appearance of the head.**

Q. Write a short note on rachitic rosary.

Chest: The changes are as follows:

- **Rachitic rosary: Overgrowth of cartilage or osteoid tissue at the costochondral junction** causes deformation of the chest producing characteristic nodularity of the junctions. This is termed **"rachitic rosary** (string of beads)."

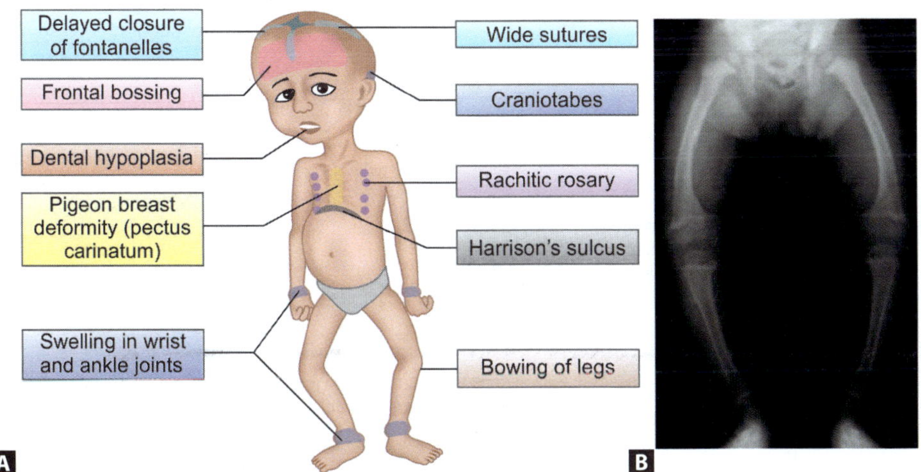

Figs. 9.8A and B: (A) Features of rickets; (B) X-ray of rickets showing splaying of epiphyses and bow legs.

- **Pigeon breast/chest deformity:** The weakened metaphyseal areas of the ribs are subject to the pull of the respiratory muscles. This causes them to bend inward. It creates **anterior protrusion of the sternum** producing **pigeon breast deformity** (pectus carinatum).
- **Harrison's sulcus/groove:** It is due to the indrawing of ribs at the margin of the diaphragm on inspiration.

During the Ambulatory Stage

When an ambulating child develops rickets, skeletal deformities affect the spine, pelvis, and lower extremity long bones.

- **Lumbar lordosis:** It is characterized by excessively curving affecting the lumbar spine, and pelvis.
- **Bowing of the legs (Fig. 9.8B):** Due to the skeletal defects involving the tibia.

Osteomalacia in Adults (Levell 2)

Q. Write a short note on osteomalacia.

Bone changes: Vitamin D deficiency in adults is **accompanied by hypocalcemia and hypophosphatemia** which result in **impaired** (hypo/under/inadequately) **mineralization of bone matrix** proteins, a condition known as osteomalacia. This hypomineralized bone matrix is biomechanically inferior (weak) to normal bone. This **bone is prone to bowing of weight-bearing extremities** and **gross skeletal fractures or microfractures** which are most likely to affect vertebral bodies and femoral necks.

Proximal myopathy: It is observed both in children and in adults with severe vitamin D deficiency. It rapidly resolves by vitamin D treatment.

Hypocalcemic tetany: Calcium is required for normal neural excitation and the relaxation of muscles. Hypocalcemic tetany is a **convulsive state** caused by an insufficient extracellular concentration of ionized calcium.

Nonskeletal Effects of Vitamin D

Vitamin D receptors are also present in various cells and tissues that are not involved in calcium and phosphorus homeostasis. Many cells, such as macrophages, keratinocytes, and tissues, such as the breast, prostate, and colon can produce 1,25-dihydroxyvitamin D.

Low levels of 1,25-dihydroxyvitamin D (<20 ng/mL) may **increase the incidence of cancers of colon, prostate, and breast cancers**, but whether vitamin D supplements can reduce cancer risk is not known.

Vitamin C (Ascorbic Acid)

It is a **water-soluble vitamin.**

Functions

- **Hydroxylation of procollagen: Ascorbic acid** is necessary for the formation of collagen from procollagen. It is involved in the hydroxylation of proline and lysine in procollagen to hydroxyproline and hydroxylysine in mature collagen. Inadequately hydroxylated procollagen has no tensile strength, is more soluble, and are more vulnerable to enzymatic degradation. Collagen in blood vessels is particularly affected and predisposes to hemorrhages in scurvy.
- **Antioxidant properties:** Ascorbic acid is the most active powerful reducing agent controlling the redox potential within cells. Vitamin C can scavenge free radicals directly and can act indirectly by regenerating the antioxidant form of vitamin E.
- **Promotes absorption of nonheme iron.**

Deficiency

Causes: Ascorbic acid is present in abundance in many foods. Hence, its deficiency is rare. Rarely, it may occur as a secondary deficiency, particularly among older persons who live alone, and chronic alcoholics.

Effects of Deficiency (Fig. 9.9)

Q. Write a short note on scurvy and its pathological findings.

Scurvy: It is caused due to vitamin C deficiency. It is characterized by:

- **Bone disease:** More common in growing children. It shows the **deranged formation of an osteoid matrix.**

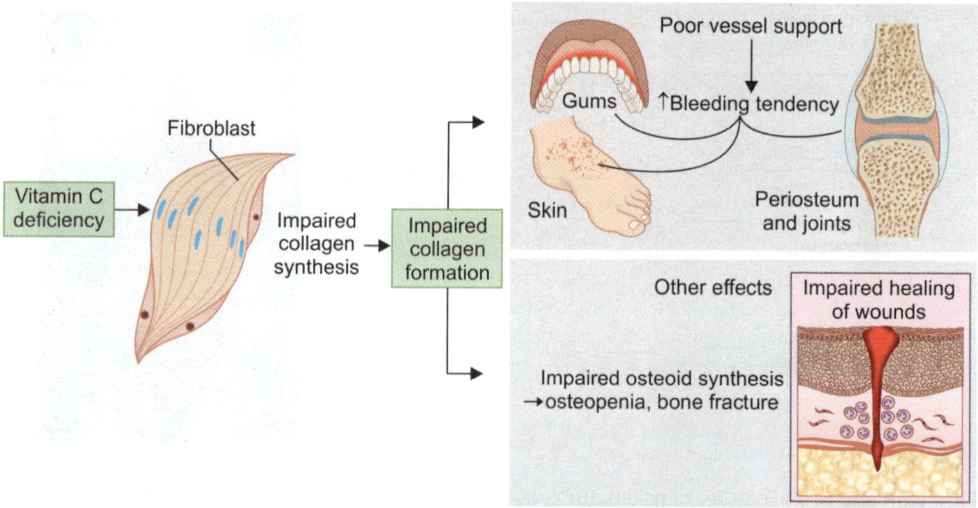

Fig. 9.9: Major consequences of impaired formation of collagen due to vitamin C deficiency.

- **Hemorrhages:** Marked tendency to bleed into the skin (petechiae, ecchymoses, perifollicular hemorrhages), bleeding into muscles, joints, and underneath the peritoneum.
- **Gums**: **Inflamed and bleeding** gums.
- **Delayed wound healing**.
- **Anemia.**

Vitamin E

Vitamin E is a collective name for 8 stereoisomers of tocopherols and tocotrienols. The most important dietary form is α-tocopherol.

Functions

- **Antioxidant:** It prevents oxidation of low-density lipoproteins (LDLs) and polyunsaturated fatty acids in cell membranes by free radicals. Other antioxidants (e.g., vitamin C, glutathione) and enzymes maintain vitamin E in a reduced state. Acts in conjunction with other antioxidants, such as selenium.
- It **helps maintain cell membrane structure**.
- **Anti-inflammatory:** Vitamin E also inhibits prostaglandin synthesis and the activities of protein kinase C and phospholipase A_2.
- **Immune systems**
- It affects DNA synthesis and cell signaling.

Deficiency

- Dietary deficiency of vitamin E is very rare.
- Vitamin E deficiency is seen only in premature infants and in severe and prolonged malabsorption diseases, such as celiac disease, or after small-intestinal resection.
- It can cause **mild hemolytic anemias, ataxia, and visual scotomas.**

Vitamin K

Forms of vitamin K: There are two natural forms: Vitamin K_1 (phylloquinone) derived from vegetables (green leafy vegetables, such as kale and spinach) and animal sources (liver), and vitamin K_2 (menaquinone) which is synthesized by bacterial flora in the colon and hepatic tissue. Phylloquinone can be converted to menaquinone in some organs.

Function

Coagulation: Vitamin K is necessary for the production of four of the coagulation factors II, VII, IX, and X. Thus, it is involved in the coagulation process.

Deficiency

Causes

In adults: The causes are as follows:

- **Chronic small-intestinal disease** (e.g., celiac disease, Crohn's disease).
- **Obstruction of biliary tracts:** In obstructive jaundice, dietary vitamin K is not absorbed and it is necessary to administer the vitamin in parenteral form before surgery.
- After small-bowel resection.
- **Broad-spectrum antibiotics:** They can precipitate vitamin K deficiency by reducing gut bacteria that synthesize menaquinones, and by inhibiting the metabolism of vitamin K.
- **Warfarin and related anticoagulants:** Warfarin-type drugs prevent the conversion of vitamin K to its active hydroquinone form.

Deficiency in newborns: It is because of (1) low-fat stores, (2) low breast milk levels of vitamin K, (3) sterility of the infantile intestinal tract, (4) liver immaturity, and (5) poor placental transport.

Effects of Deficiency

- Vitamin K deficiency leads to **delayed coagulation and bleeding**. Hence, the symptoms of vitamin K deficiency are due to hemorrhage.
- **Newborn:** In breastfed newborns, it may cause **hemorrhagic disease of the newborn**. Intracranial, gastrointestinal, and skin bleeding can occur in vitamin K-deficient infants 1–7 days after birth. Thus, vitamin K (1 mg IM) is given routinely to newborn babies to prevent hemorrhagic disease.

Thiamine (Vitamin B_1)

Thiamine was the first B complex vitamin identified and is referred to as vitamin B_1.

Functions: Thiamine functions as a coenzyme in many reactions. Inadequate thiamin results in inadequate adenosine triphosphate synthesis and abnormal carbohydrate metabolism, respectively. May have an additional role in neuronal conduction.

Deficiency

Causes

- Most dietary deficiency of thiamine is due to **poor dietary intake**. Alcoholism, chronic renal dialysis, and chronic illnesses, such as cancer are common precipitant factors. High carbohydrate intake increases the need for B_1. Alcohol interferes with the absorption of thiamine and with the synthesis of thiamine pyrophosphate.
- Women with **prolonged hyperemesis gravidarum** can develop thiamine deficiency. Maternal thiamine deficiency can lead to infantile beriberi in breastfed children.
- Anorexia.
- **Other causes:** It occurs in patients (i) with overall poor nutritional status on parenteral glucose, (ii) after bariatric bypass surgery, and (iii) those on chronic diuretic therapy due to increased urinary thiamine losses.

Effects of Deficiency

Mild deficiency: Thiamine deficiency in its early stage is characterized by irritability, decrease in short-term memory, anorexia, fatigue, and headaches.

More severe deficiency—beriberi: Prolonged thiamine deficiency causes beriberi. It is classically categorized as **wet or dry or a combination of two**. It is the classic deficiency syndrome observed **in individuals consuming a polished rice** diet. It shows combinations of peripheral neuropathy, cardiovascular dysfunction, and cerebral dysfunction.

- **Peripheral neuropathy: Dry beriberi** presents with a symmetric peripheral neuropathy of the motor and sensory systems with diminished reflexes. Patients complain of pain and paresthesia associated with diminished reflexes. The neuropathy affects the legs most markedly, and these patients have difficulty rising from a squatting position.
- **Cardiovascular dysfunction ("wet beriberi"): Wet beriberi** presents primarily with cardiovascular symptoms. It is associated with congestive heart failure and low peripheral vascular resistance.
- **Cerebrovascular dysfunction:**
  - ***Wernicke's encephalopathy:*** Acute appearance of nystagmus, ophthalmoplegia, ataxia, and psychotic symptoms. The acute symptoms are reversible when treated with thiamine. However, if untreated, they may be followed by a prolonged and largely irreversible condition, called Korsakoff syndrome.
  - ***Korsakoff syndrome:*** Characterized clinically by hallucinations, disturbances of short-term memory, and confabulation. The syndrome is common in chronic alcoholics but may also be seen with thiamine deficiency resulting from gastric disorders including carcinoma, chronic gastritis, or persistent vomiting.

Riboflavin (Vitamin B_2)

It is **important for the metabolism of fat, carbohydrate, and protein**. It also plays a role in drug and steroid metabolism including detoxification reactions. Serves as a coenzyme for a diverse array of biochemical reactions and as an electron donor. The primary coenzymatic forms of riboflavin are flavin mononucleotide (FMN) and flavin adenine dinucleotide (FAD) and are known as *flavoenzymes* (e.g., succinic acid dehydrogenase, monoamine oxidase, glutathione reductase).

Deficiency

Causes: Almost always due to dietary deficiency and is usually seen in conjunction with deficiencies of other B vitamins.

Effects of deficiency: Nonspecific and mainly manifests as **lesions of the mucocutaneous surfaces of the mouth and skin**. These include **hyperemia and edema of nasopharyngeal mucosa, cheilosis, angular stomatitis, glossitis, and seborrheic dermatitis.** Other lesions include corneal vascularization, normochromic-normocytic anemia, and personality changes.

Niacin (Vitamin B_3)

Q. Write a short note on niacin deficiency.

The term ***niacin*** **refers to nicotinic acid** and the corresponding amide, nicotinamide, and their biologically active derivatives. Nicotinic acid and nicotinamide **serve as precursors of two coenzymes, nicotinamide adenine dinucleotide (NAD) and NAD phosphate (NADP)** which are important in numerous **oxidation and reduction reactions.** NAD and NADP are active in adenine diphosphate–ribose transfer reactions involved in DNA repair and calcium mobilization.

Deficiency

Pellagra

Niacin deficiency causes **pellagra.** It is found mostly in populations in which corn is the major source of energy in parts of China, Africa, and India.

- **Early symptoms:** Loss of appetite, generalized weakness and irritability, abdominal pain, and vomiting.
- **Early signs:** Bright red glossitis, stomatitis, vaginitis, esophagitis, vertigo and burning dysesthesias.
- **Advanced stages:** Characteristic skin rash develops that is pigmented and scaling that develops in skin areas exposed to sunlight. This rash is known as **Casal's necklace** because it forms a ring around the neck.
- **Four Ds: D**iarrhea (in part due to proctitis and in part due to malabsorption), **d**epression, seizures and **d**ementia (or associated symptoms of anxiety or insomnia) leading to **d**eath and **d**ermatitis are part of the pellagra syndrome.

Pyridoxine (Vitamin B_6)

- *Vitamin* B_6 refers to several derivatives of pyridine including pyridoxine (PN), pyridoxal (PL), and pyridoxamine (PM), which are interconvertible in the body. The coenzymatic forms are pyridoxal-5-phosphate (PSP) and pyridoxamine-5-phosphate (PMP). 5'-pyridoxal phosphate (PLP) is a cofactor for more than 100 enzymes involved in amino acid metabolism.
- Vitamin B_6 is also involved in the synthesis of heme and many neurotransmitters and the metabolism of glycogen, lipids, steroids, sphingoid bases, and several vitamins, including the synthesis of niacin from tryptophan.

Deficiency

- Deficiency is usually seen in conjunction with other water-soluble vitamin deficiencies.
- Certain medications, such as isoniazid, cycloserine, penicillamine, L-dopa, ethanol, and theophylline can inhibit B_6 metabolism. Pyridoxine should be given concurrently with isoniazid to avoid neuropathy. Because vitamin B_6 interferes with the action of L-dopa, it should not be given with this drug.

Effects of Deficiency

- **Stomatitis, angular cheilosis, glossitis, irritability, depression, and confusion** occur in moderate to severe depletion.
- **Microcytic hypochromic** anemia is due to diminished hemoglobin synthesis since it is the first enzyme involved in heme biosynthesis. It may also produce normochromic-normocytic anemia.
- **In infants: Diarrhea, seizures/convulsions and anemia.**
- **Severe vitamin B_6 deficiency: Peripheral neuropathy** and abnormal electroencephalograms.

Vitamin B_{12}

A group of closely related cobalamin compounds.

Functions

Vitamin B_{12} is indirectly **required for DNA synthesis** in various metabolic steps and its deficiency impairs DNA synthesis. The two active coenzyme forms are deoxyadenosylcobalamin and methylcobalamin.

- Methylcobalamin is the main form of vitamin B_{12} in plasma and is an essential coenzyme for the conversion of homocysteine to methionine and the formation of tetrahydrofolate (THF) from methyl THF.
- Vitamin B_{12} is also required for the conversion of methylmalonyl-CoA to succinylmalonyl-CoA.

Deficiency

Causes (*Refer* Table 11.15)

- Dietary inadequacy is a rare cause of deficiency except in strict vegetarians.
- Mostly due to loss of intestinal absorption. These include pernicious anemia, pancreatic insufficiency, atrophic gastritis, small bowel bacterial overgrowth, or ileal disease. Effects of deficiency
- **Hematological changes: Megaloblastic anemia** (*refer* page 337) and megaloblastic changes in other epithelia.
- **Neurologic complications: Demyelination of peripheral nerves,** posterior and lateral columns of the spinal cord, and nerves within the brain. Altered mentation, depression, and psychoses occur.

Folic Acid

Folates are a group of related pterin compounds. The fully oxidized form is called folic acid which is not found in nature but is the pharmacologic form of the vitamin.

Functions: All folate functions relate to its ability to transfer one-carbon groups. The active form of folic acid is tetrahydrofolate (THF) which is the biological "middleman" involved in metabolic processes that synthesize DNA.

Causes of deficiency (*refer* **Table 11.15**).

Effects of deficiency: Megaloblastic anemia (*refer* page 337), and diarrhea.

Vitamins and their principal clinical manifestations are summarized in **Table 9.6.**

TABLE 9.6 Vitamins and their principal clinical manifestations.

Vitamin	*Manifestations*
Water-soluble	
Vitamin B_1(thiamine)	Beriberi (dry or wet): Neuropathy, muscle weakness and wasting, cardiomegaly, edema, ophthalmoplegia, confabulation, Wernicke syndrome, Korsakoff syndrome
Vitamin B_2 (riboflavin)	Magenta tongue (glossitis), angular stomatitis, seborrhea, cheilosis, seborrheic dermatitis, and corneal vascularization
Niacin	Pellagra: Pigmented rash of sun-exposed areas, bright-red tongue, diarrhea, apathy, memory loss, disorientation ("four Ds" depression, dementia, diarrhea and dermatitis.
Vitamin B_6 (pyridoxine)	Cheilosis, glossitis, dermatitis, peripheral neuropathy, depression, confusion, anemia
Folate	Megaloblastic anemia, atrophic glossitis, neural tube defects
Vitamin B_{12}	Megaloblastic anemia, loss of vibratory and position sense, abnormal gait, dementia
Vitamin C	Scurvy: Petechiae, ecchymosis, inflamed and bleeding gums, joint effusion, poor wound healing, fatigue
Fat-soluble	
Vitamin A	Xerophthalmia, night blindness, Bitot spots, follicular hyperkeratosis, vulnerability to infection, particularly measles, squamous metaplasia
Vitamin D	Rickets in children: Skeletal deformation, rachitic rosary, bowed legs Osteomalacia in adults
Vitamin E	Peripheral neuropathy, spinocerebellar ataxia, skeletal muscle atrophy, retinopathy, hemolytic anemia in premature infants
Vitamin K	Elevated prothrombin time, bleeding diathesis

SCENARIO-BASED MCQs

1. **A 65-year-old man living in a city with very poor air quality came to the medical outpatient for worsening cough over the past 8 months. He has an history of heavy smoking of cigarettes for the last 20 years. He gives a history of an episode of hemoptysis one week back. A chest X-ray shows a 4 cm infiltrative, perihilar mass in the right lung. Of the following airborne agents, the most likely to be associated with these findings is:**
   A. Nicotine
   B. Carbon monoxide
   C. Nitrous oxide compounds
   D. Polycyclic aromatic hydrocarbons
2. **A 4-year-old child is brought to hospital with the complaint of recurrent upper respiratory infections for the past 3 months. On examination, the child is having 55% of height and the 40% of weight compared with normal standard. Physical examination reveals generalized edema, ascites, muscle wasting, and areas of desquamating skin over the trunk and extremities. The laboratory investigation in this child is likely to show:**
   A. Hypocalcemia B. Hypoalbuminemia
   C. Abetalipoproteinemia D. Megaloblastic anemia
3. **A starving, 4-year-old, boy is brought to pediatric outpatient. He presents with apathy, generalized edema, and an enlarged fatty liver. The pediatrician observes that despite generalized growth failure, subcutaneous fat is preserved. The most probable diagnosis is:**
   A. Scurvy B. Beriberi
   C. Kwashiorkor D. Marasmus

Answers and Explanation

1. **The answer is D: Polycyclic aromatic hydrocarbons.** The X-ray finding of an infiltrative perihilar mass suggests lung cancer.
   Polycyclic hydrocarbons in tobacco smoke are the main chemical carcinogen that contributors to the development of lung cancer. The cigarette smoke contains nicotine and it has a stimulant effect on the central nervous system. But it does not play a major role in the development of cancer. The levels of carbon monoxide are increased in smokers, but this does not promote cancer. Nitrous oxide compounds are found in smog, but does not increase the risk of lung cancer.
2. **The answer is B: Hypoalbuminemia.** The clinical features and findings are consistent with kwashiorkor. It is one of the severe acute malnutrition disorders predominantly due to decreased protein in the diet. Hypoalbuminemia is characteristic of this condition. Hypocalcemia can occur due to vitamin D deficiency. Abetalipoproteinemia is a rare disorder and causes deficiency of vitamin E. Megaloblastic anemia is due to deficiencies of vitamin B_{12} or folate.
3. **The answer is D: Marasmus.** It is one of the severe acute malnutrition disorders due to deficiency of all elements of the diet. The pathological changes include decreased body weight, diminished subcutaneous fat, a protuberant abdomen, muscle wasting, and a wrinkled face. Generally, the child appears as a "shrunken old person." No edema is present. Kwashiorkor (choice C) results from deficiency of protein in the diet. Choices A, and B result from deficiencies of vitamin C and vitamin B_1 respectively.

CHAPTER 10

Basic Diagnostic Cytology

Chapter Outline

- Diagnostic Role of Cytology
- Methods for Obtaining Specimens
- Techniques in Exfoliative Cytology
- Fine Needle Aspiration Cytology
- FNAC Appearance of Some Common Lesions
- Other Cytology Techniques

INTRODUCTION

Biopsy was used as the main diagnostic method in pathology for over a century. **Cytology is a branch of science that deals with the study of cells and/or tissue fragments** and **cytopathology is a branch of pathology that deals with the study and diagnosis of disease at the cellular level.** In 1920, **Dr George N Papanicolaou** introduced cytology as a method of diagnosis by obtaining cells naturally shed off (exfoliated) into cervical and vaginal secretion. Subsequently, the use of cytological examination was extended to cells that shed off into other body cavities. Later, similar to *bone marrow aspiration* for the diagnosis of hematopoietic diseases, **fine needle aspiration cytology (FNAC)** was used for the diagnosis of solid lesions. Though FNAC was started in the 1930s in the US, it was in the 1960s that it was used mainly in Scandinavian countries of Europe and later it spread to the rest of the world.

Branches of diagnostic cytology: Diagnostic cytology consists of the interpretation of cells from the human body. It has two branches (i) exfoliative and (ii) interventional.

1. **Exfoliative cytology:** In this, cells that exfoliate (desquamate) spontaneously from epithelial surfaces are examined.
2. **Interventional cytology:** In this, cells are obtained from various organs/tissues by different clinical procedures.

Histopathology versus cytopathology: In surgical pathology, the diagnosis is based on changes in tissue architecture. In contrast to surgical pathology, cytopathology deals primarily with **morphology observed in single cells or small groups of cells without regard to stroma**. The pathologist who deals with and reports cytological material is called a cytopathologist.

DIAGNOSTIC ROLE OF CYTOLOGY

PA 8.1 (CC): Describe the diagnostic role of cytology and its application in clinical care.

Applications of Cytology

Q. Write a short note on the application of cytology and its diagnostic role.

Cytopathology has numerous applications. It is usually **used for screening, diagnosing, and management of lesions that may represent cancer or its precursors.** Advantages include **cost-effectiveness, rapid turnaround time, and a diagnosis with minimal patient risk.** Cytopathology is also helpful in other conditions.

The most important applications of cytopathology are:

1. **Diagnosis and management of cancer:** In oncology, diagnosis is essential for proper management of a cancer patient. Cytology can be used for both diagnosis and management in oncology.
   a. **For diagnosis:**
      - Cytopathology is a **valuable adjunct to histopathology for the diagnosis** of benign, dysplastic, and malignant lesions. For example, imprint smears for the diagnosis of lymphomas.
      - **Provides a preliminary diagnosis of cancer** which can be confirmed by histopathology. For example, the detection of malignant cells in ascitic fluid in a patient with an ovarian tumor.
      - **Primary method of diagnosis:** For example, the detection of malignant cells in an FNAC of the breast is considered sufficient for planning the management and may avoid the need for diagnostic surgical biopsy.
      - **Detection of premalignant lesions:** Used for the early detection and diagnosis of clinically silent carcinoma in situ. For example, carcinoma in situ in the uterine cervix.
      - **For rapid diagnosis:** It helps in starting the treatment at the earliest in life-threatening conditions. For example, mediastinal lymphoma causes respiratory distress.

- **Ancillary techniques:** Immunocytochemistry and molecular studies (flow cytometry, PCR, genomics, etc) can be performed on cytologic material or cell blocks.

b. **Management of cancer:** Cytology has the following uses:
   - Cytopathology may help **in assessing response to therapy:** For example, cervical smears examination after radiotherapy in carcinoma cervix.
   - **Follow-up** of previously diagnosed cancer. For example, detection of metastasis or recurrence of cancer.

2. **Diagnosis of benign neoplasms:** Cytopathology **helps to distinguish between benign and malignant neoplasms.** For example, to distinguish fibroadenoma of the breast from carcinoma.
3. **Intraoperative consultation:** Intraoperative cytology is the procedure by which the cells are obtained during operation. **It complements the histopathological diagnosis.** For example, imprint smears along with frozen sections for breast tumors or resection margins. **Various** intraoperative cytological **techniques include:**
   a. **Touch (imprint) cytology:** Smears are prepared by forcefully pressing the clean glass slide to the cut surface of the organ. Discussed on page 315.
   b. **Scrape cytology:** Smears are prepared from material obtained by scraping the cut surface of the biopsy specimen with a clean scalpel.
   c. **Crush preparation (crush cytology):** Small fragments of fresh unfixed surgical tissue are crushed between two slides. This technique is mainly used in neuropathology.
4. **Diagnosis of specific infections:** A variety of bacterial, viral, protozoal, and fungal infections can be diagnosed by cytopathology. For example, tubercle bacilli in lymph node aspirates, herpetic inclusions and trichomonas in cervico-vaginal smears, and fungal hyphae in touch preparations from draining sinuses.
5. **Diagnosis of non-neoplastic and inflammatory lesions:** It helps in the diagnosis of conditions that do not routinely require surgical intervention. For example, Hashimoto's thyroiditis.
6. **Cytogenetics:** Cytological specimens can be used for chromosomal studies including tissue cultures and for demonstrating sex-chromatin (e.g., buccal smear for Barr body).
7. **Assessment of hormonal status in females:** Vaginal smears reflect changes in female sex hormonal levels, e.g., to confirm the onset of menopause.
8. **Identification of a cell of origin:** The cytoplasmic characteristics may help in identifying the cell of origin **in malignant tumors**, e.g., keratinization in squamous cell carcinoma, mucin in mucin secreting adenocarcinoma, melanin pigment in malignant melanoma.
9. **Others:** It is useful for DNA cytometry and DNA ploidy analysis.

METHODS FOR OBTAINING SPECIMENS

PA 8.2 (CC): Describe the basis of exfoliative cytology including the technique and stains used.

Two categories of methods are involved in diagnostic cytology to obtain cells for microscopic examination namely—exfoliative and interventional.

Exfoliative Cytology

Q. Write a short note on exfoliative cytology.

Exfoliative cytology (*refer* page 265) is the **study of spontaneously/naturally exfoliated (shed) cells from the epithelial lining of an organ into a body cavity or body fluids** such as **urine, sputum**, etc. The rate of exfoliation is increased in disease states and yields a larger number of cells for study.

Abrasive cytology: Apart from exfoliation, cells for study may also be obtained by **scraping, brushing, or washing** various mucosal surfaces. In abrasive cytology, viable cells are artificially obtained by **abrasive techniques** from the surface of an organ. The instrument used to obtain the cells includes a **scraper or spatula** (cervical, oral cavity-buccal smear for sex chromatin) and a cytological brush (bronchial, gastrointestinal tract). The cells may also be obtained by **washing or lavage** (peritoneal, bronchoalveolar), where a small amount of saline or similar solution is instilled into the target organ and aspirated. The cells obtained by abrasive technique do not show degenerative changes or necrosis, in contrast to that of exfoliative cytology. **When the cells are collected with an instrument, the cells are either rinsed into a preservative solution or simply directly spread onto slides.**

Q. Write a short note on various sites of collections of exfoliative cells.

Various sources of exfoliated cells used in cytopathology are listed in **Box 10.1**.

Gynecologic Exfoliative Cytology

This involves microscopic examination of cells exfoliated from the female genital tract and the smears from the female genital tract have been **traditionally known as 'Pap smears' (Papanicolaou smear)**. There are different methods of obtaining exfoliated cells and smears are prepared from the material obtained.

- **Lateral vaginal smears (LVS):** The material is obtained by scraping the upper third of the lateral walls of the vagina and is ideal for hormonal assessment.
- **Vaginal 'pool' or 'vault' smears:** The material is obtained by scraping or aspiration from the posterior fornix of the vagina and used for the detection of endometrial and ovarian cancer.

BOX 10.1: Sources of exfoliated cells.

The surface of the mucosal or epithelial lining

Cells may be shed naturally or obtained by artificial exfoliation

1. Gynecologic exfoliative cytology (female genital tract):
   - Lateral vaginal smears (LVS)
   - Vaginal 'pool' smears
   - Cervical smears
   - Combined (fast) smears
   - Triple smears (CVE)
   - Endocervical/endometrial aspiration
2. Non-gynecologic exfoliative cytology:
   - Respiratory tract
     - Sputum
     - Bronchial washings/brushing/bronchoalveolar lavage (BAL) by bronchoscopy
   - Gastrointestinal tract: Endoscopic lavage/brushing
   - Urinary tract
     - Urinary sediment (in voided urine)
     - Bladder washings
     - Retrograde catheterization
     - Prostatic massage (secretions)
   - Other samples: Buccal smears (for sex chromatin) by scrapping

Body fluids

Usually, cells are shed naturally into body fluids:

- Effusions: Pleural, peritoneal, pericardial
- Cerebrospinal fluid (CSF)
- Synovial fluid
- Seminal fluid (semen)
- Amniotic fluid
- Hydrocele fluid
- Nipple discharge

- **Cervical smears:** The material obtained by Ayre's spatula (*refer* **Fig. 10.1**) from the portio of the cervix is ideal for the detection of intraepithelial lesions (*refer* pages 800-3) and carcinoma of the uterine cervix.
- **Combined (Fast) smears:** The material is obtained by a combination of vaginal pool and cervical scrapings. They are recommended for routine population screening for cervical cancers and endometrial cancers.
- **Triple (cervical-vaginal-endocervical or CVE) smears:** These smears contain three distinct samples representing the ectocervix, vagina, and endocervix on three separate areas of the same slide. Though they are recommended for routine screening and help in the localization of lesions (if present) but are difficult to prepare.
- **Endocervical and endometrial smears:** They are prepared by aspirating the contents of the endocervical canal and endometrial cavity respectively.

Applications of Pap Smear

Pap smears in gynecological sites may be used for hormonal evaluation, and identification of non-neoplastic, benign, and malignant tumors.

Hormonal evaluation

Assessment of hormonal status is carried out on smears from the lateral vaginal wall. However, vaginal 'pool' or fast smears may also be used.

Nonspecific (benign) cellular changes

In cervicovaginal cytopathology, reporting is done using The Bethesda system (TBS) so that uniformity is maintained in the evaluation.

Nonspecific inflammatory changes are commonly observed in gynecological smears and these changes may reflect acute or chronic inflammatory process.

Specific inflammatory changes: They may be seen with a variety of infectious agents and their detection helps to identify these agents as the cause of the disease.

- **Bacteria:** *N. gonorrhoeae* (a gram-negative, intracellular, diplococcus) and *Gardnerella vaginalis* (a gram-negative bacteria).
- **Virus:** *Human papillomavirus (HPV)* is a sexually-transmitted infection and the smears from HPV-infected individuals show aggregates of rounded to oval squamous cells with 'koilocytotic changes' (*refer* **page 803 and Fig. 22.4B**). Genital infection by *herpes simplex virus (HSV)* can affect the squamous epithelium of the vulva, vagina, and cervix. HSV-infected cells show enlarged nuclei with watery, 'ground-glass' chromatin, multinucleation with internuclear molding, and intranuclear acidophilic inclusions.
- **Fungus:** Moniliasis (infection by *Candida albicans)* is a common fungal infection and associated with diabetes, pregnancy, and the use of antibacterial agents (which alter the vaginal flora). In the smears, Candida (*refer* page 118) may appear in two forms namely—the *yeast form* (unicellular) appears as round to oval budding organisms within conspicuous capsules, and the *fungal form* (pseudohyphae) as thin, elongated, pseudo septate, bamboo-like filaments.
- **Parasites:** *Trichomonas vaginalis* is a protozoan, which appears in the background as a fuzzy, gray-green, round, or elliptical structure 8–20 μm in size, containing a small vesicular nucleus. *Entamoeba histolytica* in trophozoite form appears in Pap smears as basophilic, round to oval structures, 15 to 20 μm in size, with ingested RBCs.

Neoplastic epithelial cell abnormalities

Detection of carcinoma of the uterine cervix and its precursor lesions is considered the most important

TABLE 10.1 The Bethesda system (TBS) of reporting squamous cell abnormalities.

Squamous cell abnormalities	*Salient features*
Atypical squamous cells of undetermined significance (ASCUS)	Cellular changes falling short of intraepithelial lesion
Low-grade squamous intraepithelial lesion (LSIL)	Includes CIN-I and cellular changes associated with HPV infection
High-grade squamous intraepithelial lesion (HSIL)	Includes CIN grade II, III, and CIS.
Squamous cell carcinoma	Frank features of carcinoma with tumor diathesis (dirty, necrotic background)

(CIN: cervical intraepithelial neoplasm; CIS: carcinoma in situ; HPV: human papillomavirus)

application of exfoliative cytology in the female genital tract. These include:

- **Pre-invasive and invasive squamous cell abnormalities:** Pre-invasive intraepithelial neoplastic process of the uterine cervix usually precedes the fully-developed invasive squamous cell carcinoma and can be detected by cytologic examination. Classification of cervical precancerous lesions and cervical cancer screening are discussed on pages 803-4, and page 807 respectively. **The Bethesda system** (TBS) divides squamous cell abnormalities into four categories and its reporting of squamous cell abnormalities is presented in **Table 10.1.**
- **Glandular cell abnormalities:** They can be detected in the smears and The Bethesda system is also used for glandular abnormalities.

Automation in Cervical Cytology

Presently, automated devices such as PapNet for primary screening are available in the market. Automation can perform routine pre-screening of many Pap smears, reduce the workload of cytopathologists, and also provide quality assurance. It can be applied to both conventional Pap smears and *Thin-Preps.*

Non-gynecologic Exfoliative Cytology

Respiratory Tract

Cellular material from the respiratory tract may be obtained by different techniques. Exfoliated cells (sputum) by spontaneous expectoration:

- Cells obtained by **bronchial wash and by abrasive techniques [brush, bronchoalveolar lavage (BAL)].**
- **Fine needle aspiration cytology:** Either by transbronchial needle aspiration (TBNA) or ultrasound-guided fine needle aspiration cytology (USG FNAC).

Sputum (sampling of exfoliated cells)

Sputum contains mucus admixed with exfoliated cells from the entire respiratory tract. By examining the morphology of these cells, it is possible to identify the underlying pathological process. Sputum is the most commonly examined sample from the respiratory system and is easy to collect and examine. Sputum is collected in the early morning and produced by a spontaneous deep cough to bring up material from small airways and alveoli. If the patient is not able to produce sputum, then expectoration (cough reflex) can be artificially induced by 20 minutes of aerosol-inhalation of cough-stimulating substances [e.g., the vapor of 15% NaCl (hypertonic saline) and 20% propylene glycol heated at 37°C]. Sputum should be collected in a clean container and should be kept in a petri dish on a white background. It is recommended to examine fresh sputum samples. If any tissue fragment or blood-mixed material is present, it should be taken and multiple smears should be prepared. However, if it cannot be examined immediately, the sputum sample can be collected in 70% ethyl alcohol solution as a fixative. Both alcohol-fixed and air-dried smears should be kept for staining.

- **Advantages:** Easy to obtain/collect the sample; simple, non-invasive; its cellular content is representative of the entire respiratory tract.
- **Disadvantages:** A large number of cells have to be scrutinized; not possible to locate the exact localization of the lesion within the respiratory tract and considerable degeneration of the cells develops.

Bronchial specimens

- **Bronchial aspirate and wash:** Using a bronchoscope, the bronchial secretion can be aspirated directly. For bronchial wash, 3–5 mL of balanced salt solution or normal saline is introduced through the bronchoscope, and the fluid is re-aspirated. The fluid is centrifuged and multiple smears are prepared and stained.
- **Bronchial brush:** Using a fiberoptic bronchoscope, the lesion is localized/directly visualized and the brush is applied to the lesion through the instrument. Multiple smears are prepared and fixed in 95% ethanol or the brush is rinsed in a collection solution by the clinician and sent to the laboratory. Since the direct visualization of the lesion is possible, the bronchial brush gives excellent diagnostic cellular yield.
- **Bronchoalveolar lavage:** Bronchoalveolar lavage (BAL) is a powerful cytological technique in pulmonary medicine. BAL should be performed before performing any other techniques such as bronchial wash/brush or biopsy. First, 20 mL of normal saline is flushed through a bronchoscope in the desired segment of the lung. Then through gentle suction and lavage specimen is collected.

Gastrointestinal Tract

Cytology plays a significant role in the diagnosis of various lesions of the gastrointestinal tract (GIT) mainly due to efficient, improved technology of the sampling method and visualization techniques. Various endoscopic procedures that can be performed in GIT include esophagoscopy, gastroscopy, duodenoscopy, colonoscopy, sigmoidoscopy, and endoscopic retrograde cholangiopancreatography (ERCP).

The common techniques used in the GI tract include **endoscopic brush cytology, salvage cytology, endoscopic FNAC, endoscopic ultrasound-guided (EUS) FNAC, balloon technique, and FNAC by endoscopic retrograde cholangiopancreatography**.

Lesions in the oral cavity may be sampled by scraping the surface with wooden and metal tongue depressors.

Urinary Tract

Urinary cytology is considered as a useful adjunct to the cystoscopy. It is an inexpensive, rapid, and highly reliable technique for screening for cancer of the lower urinary tract. The major advantage of urine cytology is that it helps to detect malignant lesions that are either not visible by cystoscopy or difficult to see on cystoscopy.

Specimen collection technique for urine is mainly of three types:

1. Voided urine specimen
2. Catheterized urine specimen
3. Bladder wash, ureter wash, urethral wash, and brush cytology

Voided urine specimen: It is the specimen of choice for screening in patients with specific symptoms such as hematuria. The urine sample should be collected 3–4 hours after the last micturition. It is better to avoid the first morning voided urine sample because it shows a considerable amount of degeneration in the cells due to prolonged stagnation. Fresh randomly voided urine samples should be collected in a clean container and should be sent to a laboratory immediately for processing to avoid cellular degenerative changes. About 50 mL of urine is sufficient for cytological examination. The urine is centrifuged and the sediment is examined.

Catheterized urine: Catheterized urine sample yields better cellularity and shows less degenerative changes. It is used for follow-up of patients with neoplastic lesions of the lower urinary tract.

Bladder wash (irrigation) and brush cytology: Bladder wash and brush are indicated in cases of suspected urothelial neoplasm or follow-up of a case of known neoplastic lesion. This technique gives good cellularity and better preservation of the cells.

Processing of urine sample

The urine sample should be processed immediately. The processing methods include:

- **Simple centrifugation:** About 50 mL of urine is centrifuged for 10 minutes at 1,200 RPM (revolution/rounds per minute). From the sediment, multiple smears are prepared and these are fixed in alcohol and stained.
- **Cytocentrifugation:** When the amount of urine is less than 50 mL, it can be processed by cytocentrifugation.
- **Liquid-based technique**: In this technique, the cytological material is filtered or processed through a machine, such as ThinPrep Processor (Cytyc Corp, Boxborough, MA) or SurePath PREP system (TriPath Imaging, Inc, Burlington, NC). LBC technique gives better morphology, cell preservation, and better cellularity. However, it is an expensive technique.
- **Cell block:** If the urine sample shows any fleshy tissue, a cell block preparation can be done.

Body Fluids

Body fluids may be divided into two types:

1. Effusions in body cavities
2. Other body fluids (usually of small volume)

Effusions

Excessive accumulation of fluid in any of the three body cavities (pleural, pericardial, and peritoneal) is termed an "effusion". Effusion is always a pathological process. An effusion in the peritoneal cavity is also called an ascites. Effusion can be transuded or exudate (Differences between transudate and exudate are presented in **Table 3.3**).

This differentiation is important because malignant effusions are invariably exudates with a protein content greater than 3 g/dL. The effusion samples are obtained mainly to identify malignant cells and wherever possible for their classification. In benign effusions, cytological findings are mostly non-specific.

Cerebrospinal Fluid (CSF)

CSF examination is important both in non-neoplastic and neoplastic diseases of central nervous system (CNS).

Samples are obtained by lumbar puncture. It is discussed on pages 465-7 and *refer* **Table 27.2**.

Components in Routine Cytology

Different components/steps involved in routine cytology laboratory techniques are:

- **Specimen collection:** Unlike histopathology, the specimen collection is different in cytology.
- **Fixation:** Different fixatives are used for various cytology samples.
- **Processing:** The processing of the cytology sample is different. It mainly depends on the type of sample and facilities available in the laboratory.
- **Staining:** The common stains used in the cytology laboratory are Papanicolaou's and May-Grunwald-Giemsa (MGG) stain.

TECHNIQUES IN EXFOLIATIVE CYTOLOGY

Sample Collection

The common types of samples received in the cytology laboratory are presented in **Box 10.1**.

Cervical Cytology

The cervical cytology sample is usually collected by the gynecologist or the trained nurse. The sample should be adequate with optimal cellularity.

Collection of Samples

Q. Write a short note on cervical cytology and its uses.

- Keep the patient in the dorsolithotomy position and clean the vagina with a wet swab with water.
- Open the vagina by introducing a speculum to visualize the cervix.
- For the *conventional smear*
  - Insert the *Ayre's* spatula **(Fig. 10.1)** within the vagina so that the tip of the spatula fits with the contour of the cervix (i.e., the longer limb of the spatula should fit into the external os).
  - Rotate the spatula in a complete round turn (through 360°) to sample the entire cervix. Gently withdraw the spatula.
  - Spread the sample on the spatula on the glass slide so that the smears are thin and uniform.
  - Immediately immerse the slides and fix the smears in the 95% ethyl alcohol fixative in a Coplin's jar to prevent artifacts in cells caused by drying.
- For **liquid-based cytology** *(LBC) preparation:* LBC is a special technique used for the preparation of both gynecologic and non-gynecologic samples. The smears will show monolayered dispersion of cells without overlapping or clumping and will not contain background material or debris. There are two types of LBC systems commercially available namely—ThinPrep and SurePath.
  - For LBC, use a cervix brush. Introduce the central part of the broom into the endocervical canal so that the shorter bristles of the broom touch the ectocervix.
  - Rotate the broom four to five times in a clockwise direction.
  - Withdraw the broom and place it (or rinse it) in the fixative solution in a vial provided by the manufacturer.

Vaginal Smear

The cytology sample is obtained by scraping the lateral walls of the upper third of the vagina (at the level of the cervical external os) with the flat surface of a wooden tongue depressor or spatula and smearing the material directly onto labeled slides.

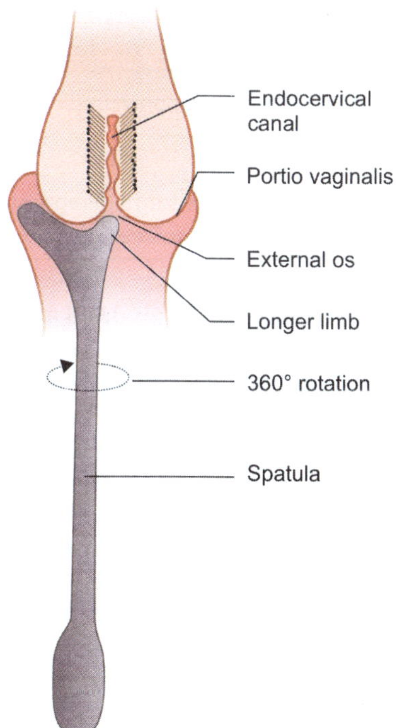

Fig. 10.1: Method of obtaining cervical smear with Ayre's spatula.

Endometrial Aspiration Smear

It is obtained by using a sterile cannula and a syringe and the endometrial sample is aspirated.

Collections of samples from respiratory, gastrointestinal, urinary tract, and cerebrospinal fluid are discussed on pages 465-7 of Chapter 15.

Fixation and Fixatives

1. **Routine fixatives:** Similar to histopathology, all cytological material for examination must be properly fixed so that the morphological details of cells are preserved. Smears prepared (either at the bedside or in the laboratory) from fluid samples should be immediately placed in a 95% ethanol fixative without allowing them to dry before fixation. Drying distorts cells and produces staining artifacts in the cytoplasm. Smears should be transported to the laboratory in the fixative preferably in a screw-capped Coplin jar. Routinely used cytological fixatives for Papanicolaou's and hematoxylin stains are listed in **Box 10.2**. **Methods of fixation:** It varies depending on the type of staining used. Different methods of fixation of cytological smears are:
   - **Wet fixation:** Cytological smears are fixed immediately (when smears are wet). Usually, smears prepared from exfoliated cells are immersed immediately in a fixative without allowing them to dry. This is called wet-fixation. These smears are then stained with Papanicolaou (Pap) or hematoxylin and eosin (H&E) stains.

BOX 10.2: Routinely used cytological fixatives for Papanicolaou's and hematoxylin stains.

- 95% ethyl alcohol (most commonly used)
- 100% methanol
- Denatured alcohol
- Methanol-based preservative for ThinPrep system
- Ethanol-based preservative for SurePath system

- **Dry fixation:** Smears are air dried and fixed in 95% alcohol (ethanol) for 5 minutes (for May-Grunwald-Giemsa stain). When Romanowsky stain is used, exfoliative cytology smears are air-dried and then stained. In Romanowsky staining, fixation is performed during the staining procedure itself.
- **Spray fixation (coating fixative):** In this method, the cytological smears are immediately fixed with a spray fixative (*refer* below). This type of fixative usually contains alcohol (e.g., hair spray).

2. **Coating fixatives:** Coating or spray fixatives are applied as aerosol sprays or with a dropper to the surface of freshly prepared cytological smears. These are commercially available (e.g., cytospray). However, as an alternative a standard hairspray with a high alcohol content may also be used. The components of spray fixatives usually include ethanol or isopropyl alcohol along with polyethylene glycol (carbowax). Within a few seconds, the smear is dried and carbowax in the spray fixative covers over the slide and prevents the shrinkage of the cell.
   Use: It is used for cervical smears but should be used for smears prepared from fluid specimens and smears with blood.
3. **Special purpose fixatives:** These include Carnoy's fixative (for hemorrhagic fluid), 10% neutral buffered formalin (for cell block materials), etc.
4. **Preservation of fluid samples:** Fluid samples should be submitted to the laboratory in a fresh state for immediate processing. If a delay is expected in dispatch to the laboratory or in processing, the sample is collected in a suitable preservative for 'prefixation' so that cellular morphology is preserved. The best preservative for general use is 50% ethanol in volumes equal to that of the fluid sample. Pericardial, pleural, and peritoneal fluids may be pre-fixed with an equal volume of 10% formalin if ethanol is not available.

Processing of Samples in the Laboratory

The commonly used processing techniques include (i) direct smear, (ii) centrifuge, (iii) cytocentrifuge, (iv) liquid-based preparation, and (v) cell block.

Prepared smears: If the smears are prepared at the bedside and wet-fixed in ethanol, they need no further processing in the laboratory before staining.

Processing of sputum (direct smear): Pour the received sputum sample into a Petri dish kept on a black background. Carefully inspect for any tissue fragments (solid particles) or gray-white substance or bloody material. Pick up the tissue fragments with clean forceps or wooden applicator sticks and place them on clean glass slides. Strands of ropy mucus are also selected (exfoliated cells adhere to mucus strands). Prepare the smears on the clean glass slide by crushing the particles/mucus and evenly spreading the material. Four such smears are prepared and immediately placed in 95% ethanol for fixation.

Processing of fluid: Urine, body fluids, and lavage—if large volumes of fluid are received, they are allowed to stand in the refrigerator for half to one hour. Then, all except the bottom 200 mL is discarded. The retained bottom fluid is then processed. In specimens showing large amounts of blood, RBCs may be lysed by adding 1 mL of glacial acetic acid for every 50 mL of specimen. Commonly employed techniques for processing fluids are as under:

- **Centrifuge:** If the fluid is of moderate amount (50–100 mL), it should be processed by centrifugation (e.g., effusion fluid, turbid urine, etc.). The fluid sample is poured into clean, air-tight 50 mL centrifuge tubes and centrifuged at 1,500 rounds per minute (RPM) for 10 minutes. Discard the supernatant liquid and prepare multiple smears from the sediments.
- **Cytocentrifuge and membrane filter preparations:** These methods are most useful for small volume (0.5–1 mL) fluids of low cell content (e.g., CSF).
- **Cell block technique:** The cell block technique employs the retrieval of small tissue fragments in the sediment and they are processed to form a paraffin block.

Staining of Smears

Three staining procedures commonly used in cytology are: **Papanicolaou and H&E stains are used for wet-fixed smears** while **Romanowsky stains are used for air-dried smears**.

1. **Papanicolaou stain:** It is the best method used for routine cytological smears (wet smears). In this technique, three solutions are used namely—one nuclear stain (Harris' hematoxylin) and two cytoplasmic counter-stains (Orange G or OG-6, and eosin-azure or EA-65 or EA-50). Nuclear stain gives a basophilic color to the nucleus whereas two cytoplasmic stains give orange and cyanophilic tints to cytoplasm respectively.
2. **Hematoxylin and eosin (H&E) stain:** It is essentially similar to that used for histological sections. Harris' hematoxylin is the nuclear stain, and eosin is the cytoplasmic counterstain.
3. **Romanowsky stains:** They are commonly used in hematology and may be used for cytological smear preparations. Leishman's, May-Grünwald-Giemsa (MGG), and Wright's stains are most commonly used.

FINE NEEDLE ASPIRATION CYTOLOGY

Q. Write a short note on fine needle aspiration cytology (FNAC) and FNAB (fine needle aspiration biopsy).

Fine needle aspiration cytology is also termed fine needle aspiration biopsy (FNAB) or Aspiration Biopsy Cytology (ABC). FNAC is aspiration of cells from tissue an fluid by using a thin needle and a syringe. In exfoliative cytology, the cytological samples are obtained/smears are prepared and sent to the pathologist by the clinician and the cytopathologist interprets them. In contrast, in FNAC, the cytopathologist often performs the clinical examination of the patient and performs the procedure. Presently, FNAC is a popular and effective technique for rapid tissue diagnosis.

Q. Write a short note on applications and advantages of FNAC.

A. **Applications of FNAC:** FNAC procedure can be performed in any organ of the body or any tissue or swelling. FNAC is most often used for diagnosis readily or assessment of **palpable superficial mass lesions**. These include mass in the **breast, enlarged lymph nodes, enlarged thyroid, superficial soft tissue masses, and salivary gland masses**. Presently due to imaging techniques (ultrasound or CT-guided), FNAC can be done on intra-abdominal/pelvic organs (e.g., liver, pancreas, pelvic lymph node), retroperitoneum, prostate, and lung masses.

B. **Advantages of FNAC:** Various advantages of FNAC are listed in **Box 10.3**.

Method of Aspiration

FNAC of Superficial Lesions

Routinely, transcutaneous FNAC of palpable masses is performed without any anesthesia. It is generally advisable to perform FNAC by the cytopathologist.

- The syringe with the attached needle is properly fitted to the pistol handle. The swelling/mass is immobilized by holding it between the two fingers of the operator. The overlying skin is cleaned with an alcohol/antiseptic pad.
- The needle is gently and swiftly introduced into the mass. The needle is moved into and from within the mass with gentle negative suction by gentle retraction of the plunger of the syringe. Aspiration is terminated by releasing the suction with the release of the plunger to stop the suction. The cellular material within the needle is adequate for diagnostic purposes.
- At the end of the FNAC, the needle is withdrawn sharply. Then the needle is rapidly detached from the syringe and the plunger is retracted to get enough air within the syringe. The needle is reattached and the air is pushed to eject the aspirated material in the syringe onto one end of the glass slide.
- Following withdrawal of the needle from the mass, firm pressure should be applied to the site of FNAC for 2–3 minutes to prevent hematoma formation.

Contraindications of FNAC are listed in **Box 10.4**.

Complications of FNAC are presented in **Box 10.5**.

Fine needle sampling (FNS) is done without using any syringe. In this, there is no artificial negative suction is applied, and the material gets aspirated into the needle with the help of negative capillary pressure.

FNAC of Deep-seated Lesions

Fine needle aspiration cytology of the deep-seated masses/lesions is almost similar to that of FNAC of superficial masses/lesions. FNAC of deep-seated lesions needs radiological guidance and clinical details before performing FNAC of radiologically guided lesions. Depending on the clinical case, the radiologists decide the mode of FNAC of deep-seated lesions. The guidance used is ultrasonography (USG), computerized tomography (CT), or fluoroscopy. The advantages of USG-guided FNAC are that it is easy to perform, less expensive, and rapid technique. Computerized tomography-guided FNAC is useful for a small lesion that needs precise localization. However, it is a time-consuming and expensive procedure. The needle used for USG and CT-guided FNAC is longer. Local anesthesia is required for

BOX 10.3: Advantages of FNAC.

- Simple and less invasive technique
- Outpatient (OPD) procedure and requires no hospitalization
- Rapid, safe, and least painful. Reports are available in a matter of hours
- No anesthesia required
- Economical and cost-effective procedure and does not require major equipment
- Wide area of sampling and multiple attempts is possible without inconvenience
- High sensitivity and specificity
- Avoids the need for tissue biopsy in case of inoperable malignancy or infective conditions (extremely reliable and useful)
- Almost all the ancillary techniques can be done on material obtained by FNAC

BOX 10.4: Contraindications of FNAC.

- Hemophilia or other coagulation disorders
- Aneurysm of blood vessels
- Hydatid cyst

BOX 10.5: Complications of FNAC.

- Hematoma
- Infraction of lymph node and thyroid
- Accidental rupture of aneurysm or spleen
- Surgical emphysema
- Anaphylaxis in hydatid cyst
- Biliary peritonitis and perforation of bowel
- Needle tract seedling of cancer cells (if a thick bore needle is used for the procedure)

radiological-guided FNAC. The rest of the procedure is the same as that of superficial FNAC described above.

Preparation of Smears

The material obtained is pushed on the clean glass slide a little away from the corner. Smear is prepared by gently pressing another clean glass slide over the material and moving the upper slide over the lower slide so that there is a uniform spreading of the material. Multiple smears are prepared and both **air-dried** and **wet-fixed** (alcohol-fixed) smears should be kept for staining.

Fixation: Air-dried smears are used for May-Grünwald-Giemsa (MGG) staining. For routine Pap staining wet fixation is done using 95% ethanol, methanol, or isopropyl alcohol. The wet-fixed smears need at least 30 minutes of fixation. Commercially available spray fixatives can also be used as an alternative to wet fixation.

Staining of the Smear

- **Air-dried smear:** These smears are stained by MGG, Romanowsky stain, or Diff-Quik stain. Romanowsky stain consists of a mixture of methylene blue and Azure A, B, or C.
- **Wet fixed smear:** This alcohol (95% ethanol, methanol, or isopropyl alcohol) fixed smear is stained either by Pap stain or hematoxylin and eosin stain.
- **Rapid staining:** Diff-Quick stain is a commercially available stain used for rapid staining which stains the smear within 2 minutes. Rapid Pap stain can also be done within 3 minutes.

Application of Ancillary Studies on Cytologic Materials

Almost all ancillary studies (e.g., immunocytochemistry, flow cytometry, and molecular biology) can be applied to cytologic materials.

Special and Ancillary Techniques

All the ancillary techniques used in histopathology can also be performed on FNAC samples. Most routinely performed include cell block for immunocytochemistry and flow cytometry for immunophenotyping. Various special and ancillary techniques are as follows:

- **Special stains:** These are performed on wet-fixed smears. The special stains used in cytology include alcian blue, mucicarmine, and PAS (for mucin and carbohydrates); methyl violet or Congo red (for amyloid); and bacterial and fungal stains (for microbial agents).
- **Microbiological studies:** FNAC material may also be used for cultures such as viral, fungal, mycobacterial, and bacterial cultures. When there is a clinical suspicion of infection, usually an additional aspirate is obtained and it is delivered into a sterile culture tube.
- **Cell block:** Aspirated material may be centrifuged and the cell button obtained can processed similar to histopathology and paraffin blocks can be prepared. The sections can also be used for ancillary techniques.
- **Immunocytochemistry:** Immunocytochemical stains can be performed on smears or cell block sections by using a panel of antibodies similar to immunohistochemistry.
- **Image analysis and morphometry:** They determine the cellular parameters such as nuclear-cytoplasmic (N/C) ratio, nuclear area, shape and size of nuclei and nucleoli, etc. This will help quantitation and cytodiagnosis.
- **Flow cytometry:** This is helpful in the determination of ploidy status and S phase fraction of tumor cells, thereby enhancing the diagnostic and prognostic information.
- **Electron microscopic (ultrastructural) studies:** These can also be performed on FNAC materials**.**
- **Molecular techniques:** They help in the detection of oncogenes like *ERBB-2* in breast cancer, and *BCL-2* in lymphomas, DNA sequence analysis, gene expression profiling, and fluorescence in situ hybridization (FISH) can all be performed on FNAC material.

FNAC APPEARANCE OF SOME COMMON LESIONS

PA 8.3 (CC): Observe diagnostic cytology and its staining and interpret the specimen.

Granulomatous (Tuberculous) Lymphadenitis (Fig. 10.2)

- Smears are cellular and composed of epithelioid cells in cohesive clusters forming granulomas.
- Epithelioid cells have elongated (oblong/slipper-shaped) nuclei and abundant pale cytoplasm.
- Multinucleated Langhans type of giant cells may be seen.
- The background shows lymphocytes and eosinophilic granular caseous necrotic material.
- Ziehl-Neelsen stain for acid-fast bacilli may show positivity for the tubercle bacilli.

Pleomorphic Adenoma (Fig. 10.3)

- Epithelial cells in clusters, sheets and singly scattered.
- Regular ovoid nuclei with bland nuclear chromatin and well-defined cytoplasm.
- Fibrillary chondromyxoid ground substance.
- Spindle-shaped cells seen in stromal matrix.

Fibroadenoma Breast (Fig. 10.4)

- Moderately cellular smears
- Large, branching monolayered sheets of uniform benign ductal epithelial cells having **antler horn** configuration.
- Numerous single bare bipolar nuclei of benign type.
- Fragments of loose fibromyxoid stroma.

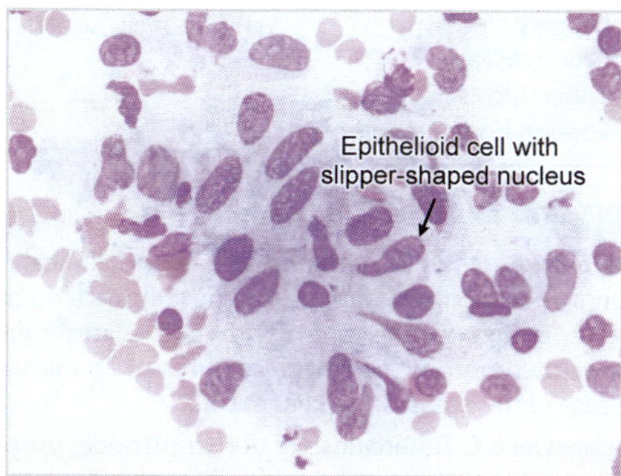

Fig. 10.2: Tuberculous lymph node aspirate with granuloma composed of epithelioid cells showing slipper-shaped nuclei and abundant pale cytoplasm.

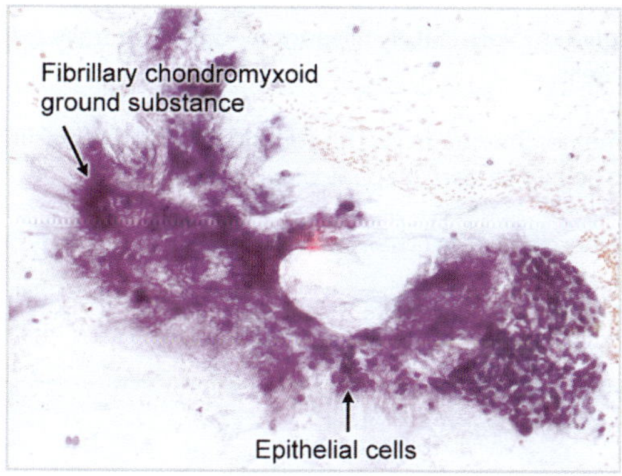

Fig. 10.3: FNAC of pleomorphic adenoma of salivary gland composed of sheets of epithelial cells in a fibrillary myxoid stroma.

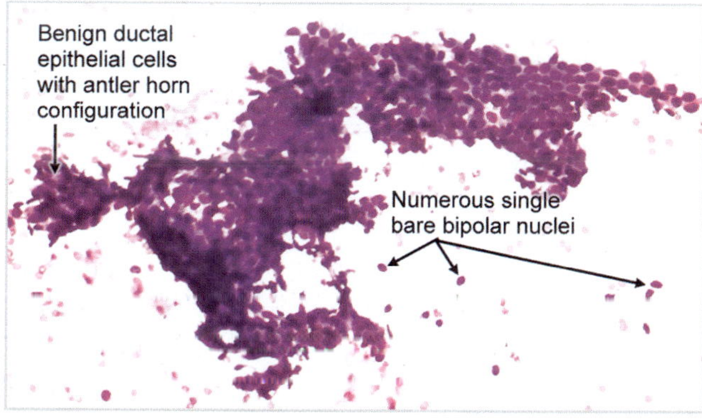

Fig. 10.4: FNAC breast of fibroadenoma consisting of monolayered sheets of benign ductal cells with antler horn configuration.

Infiltrating Duct Carcinoma Breast (Fig. 10.5)

- Highly cellular smear consisting of clusters of loosely cohesive malignant cells of variable size and shape.
- High nuclear cytoplasmic ratio; nuclei are enlarged, and hyperchromatic with irregular nuclear membranes.
- Absence of single bare nuclei of benign type.
- The background may show necrosis.

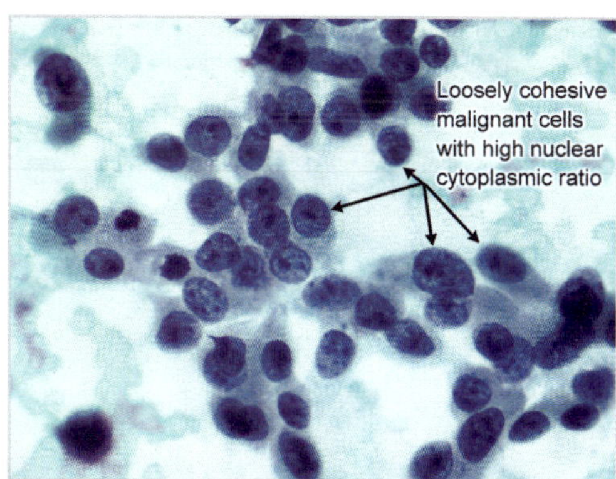

Fig. 10.5: FNAC breast showing malignant cells in infiltrating duct carcinoma.

OTHER CYTOLOGY TECHNIQUES

Imprint Cytology

In imprint cytology, cells are obtained by touch preparations from cut surfaces of fresh unfixed surgically excised mass. Imprint smears can also be obtained from draining sinuses or ulcerated areas. For surgically resected specimens (e.g., lymph nodes), first the specimen is bisected or sliced. Then smears are prepared by gently touching or pressing freshly exposed surface (without smearing) onto a glass slide. Imprint smears cannot be prepared from specimens that are fixed. Imprint smears may be wet-fixed or air-dried and stained accordingly. The advantage of the imprint smear is that the cell distribution recapitulates tissue architecture to some extent, thereby aiding in interpretation. Imprint cytology is used for the intraoperative diagnosis of malignancy as a complement to frozen-section, and is also valuable as an adjunct to histopathology in the typing of lymphomas.

Crush Smear Cytology

In crush smear cytology, the tissue particles are crushed to prepare smears. This is used in the diagnosis of brain tumors.

Biopsy Sediment Cytology

In biopsy sediment cytology, the smears are prepared from sediment obtained by centrifugation of fixatives/fluids in which surgical biopsy specimens are received by the laboratory. This method may be useful in the rapid diagnosis of bone tumors because histological sections of bone need many days for processing due to the necessity of decalcification.

The cytologic appearance of exfoliated malignant cells in ascitic fluid is shown in **Figure 10.6**.

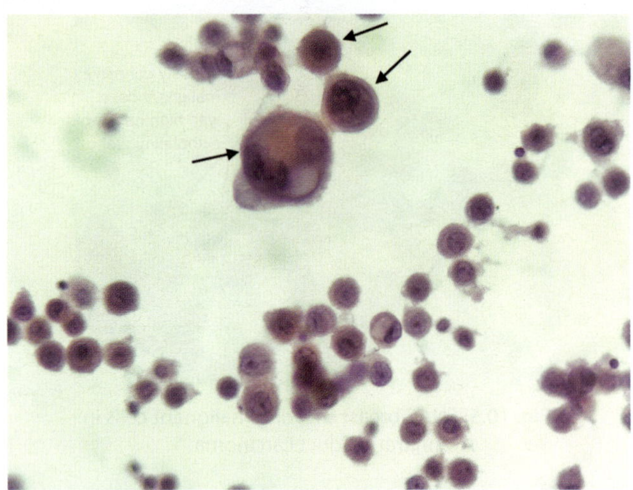

Fig. 10.6: Ascitic fluid positive for malignant cells (adenocarcinoma). It shows malignant cells (arrows). The background shows a large number of reactive mesothelial cells and lymphocytes (Papanicolaou stain).

SCENARIO-BASED MCQs

1. **A 19-year-old girl presents with a breast lump in the upper outer quadrant. On examination, the lump is painless and freely mobile. She underwent FNAC. It shows monolayered sheets of benign ductal cells with antler horn configuration. The probable diagnosis is:**
   A. Lipoma
   B. Fibroadenoma
   C. Carcinoma of the breast
   D. Paget disease
2. **A 32-year-old female presents with a swelling in the right side of her neck. She also complains of low-grade fever with evening rise and loss of weight for the last 5 months. On examination, multiple matted lymph nodes are noted. FNAC shows granuloma composed of epithelioid cells showing slipper-shaped nuclei and abundant pale cytoplasm. Probable cytological diagnosis is:**
   A. Leprosy
   B. Crohn disease
   C. Tuberculosis
   D. Foreign body granuloma

Answers and Explanation

1. **The answer is B: Fibroadenoma.** Age and clinical findings along with cytological features suggest fibroadenoma of the breast. Lipoma consists of mature adipocytes. Carcinoma shows pleomorphic cells with features of anaplasia. Paget disease of the breast shows Paget cells.
2. **The answer is C: Tuberculosis of the lymph node.** The presence of granuloma suggests tuberculosis. Though granuloma can be observed in the other three options, they have specific features and sites. Tuberculoid leprosy usually involves the skin, Crohn disease involves mesenteric lymph nodes and the GI tract, and foreign body granuloma shows granuloma with foreign bodies.

Exfoliative cytology: Study of spontaneously/naturally exfoliated (shed) cells.

Pap smears: Smears from the female genital are traditionally known as 'Pap smears' (Papanicolaou smear).

The Bethesda system (TBS): used for reporting cytology smears.

Commonly used cytological stains:
1. Papanicolaou's
2. May–Grunwald–Giemsa (MGG) stain
3. Hematoxylin Eosin.

FNAC is aspiration of cells from tissue an fluid by using a thin needle and a syringe.

FNAC
- Simple and less invasive technique
  - Outpatient (OPD) procedure
  - Rapid, safe, and least painful.
- Reports are available in a matter of hours
  - No anesthesia required

Hematology, Transfusion and Clinical Pathology

Section Outline

11. Introduction to Hematology and Disorders of Red Blood Cell
12. Disorders of White Blood Cells, Lymph Nodes, and Spleen
13. Bleeding Disorders: Hemorrhagic Diathesis
14. Blood Banking and Transfusion
15. Clinical Pathology

Introduction to Hematology and Disorders of Red Blood Cell

Chapter Outline

- Normal Hematopoiesis
- Anticoagulants

Red Blood Cell Disorders
- Anemia

Anemias of Impaired Red Cell Production
- Iron Deficiency Anemia
- Megaloblastic Anemia
- Aplastic Anemia

Increased Red Cell Destruction (Hemolytic Anemias)
- Hemolytic Anemias
- Hereditary Spherocytosis
- Glucose-6-phosphate Dehydrogenase Deficiency
- Hereditary Defects in Hemoglobin
- Thalassemia
  - β-Thalassemia Major
  - β-Thalassemia Minor/Trait
  - α-Thalassemia
- Sickle Cell Anemia
- Sickle Cell Trait
- Immunohemolytic Anemias

Anemia of Blood Loss
- Approach to the Diagnosis of Hemolytic Anemia

INTRODUCTION

Hematology is the **study of normal and pathologic aspects of blood and blood cells.**

The hematopoietic (hemopoietic) system consists of all organs and tissues involved in hematopoiesis.

Components of the Hematopoietic System

The components of the hematopoietic system are divided into **myeloid tissue and lymphoid tissue.** The pluripotent **hematopoietic stem cell (HSC)** is the progenitor of all the cells in the blood and gives rise to cells of both myeloid and lymphoid systems.

The Myeloid Tissue

Myeloid tissue **consists of bone marrow** (medullary cavity) **and the cells derived from it.**

Cells derived from bone marrow: These include:

1. **Red blood cells** (RBCs/erythrocytes)
2. **White blood cells** (WBCs/leukocytes, except lymphocytes): It consists of:
   - **Granulocytes: Neutrophils, eosinophils, and basophils** are collectively called granulocytes because of their different types of cytoplasmic granules. However, the term **granulocyte is often referred to only neutrophils.**
   - **Monocytes**
   - **Lymphocytes** (even though included under WBCs; they are lymphoid derived).
3. **Platelets** (thrombocytes)

The Lymphoid Tissue

The lymphoid tissue **consists of the thymus, lymph nodes, and spleen**. The **common lymphoid progenitor cell gives rise to B, T, and natural killer (NK) cell precursors.** They mature to form respective lymphoid cells.

The above division of hematopoietic elements as myeloid and lymphoid tissue is mainly for understanding their pathology. It is not always possible to distinguish between the diseases affecting them.

Functions of Blood Cells

The formed elements of blood are red cells, white cells, and platelets. The main functions of blood cells are presented in **Table 11.1**.

TABLE 11.1 Main functions of formed elements of blood.

Type of blood cell	*Main function*
Red blood cells	Delivery of oxygen to tissues
White blood cells	Defense against infectious organisms
Lymphocytes	Immune regulation
Platelets	Hemostasis

NORMAL HEMATOPOIESIS

PA 13.1 (CC): Describe hematopoiesis and extramedullary hematopoiesis.

Hematopoiesis (hemopoiesis) is the continuous, regulated process of blood cell production or formation.

Sites of hematopoiesis: The sites of hematopoiesis during various phases of life are different **(Table 11.2)**.

Terminology used in hematopoiesis: The meaning of the terms used concerning hematopoiesis is shown in **Table 11.3.**

Normal Development of Blood Cells

The hematopoietic system is a hierarchy of cells in which pluripotent hematopoietic stem cells (HSCs) proliferate and differentiate. After several steps, HSCs finally give rise to mature blood cells **(Fig. 11.1)**.

Q. Write a short note on the contents of bone marrow.

Normal erythropoiesis: Erythropoiesis is the process by which marrow hematopoietic stem cells pass through several stages, proliferate, differentiate, and mature to form red blood cells The various stages of erythropoiesis are shown in **Figure 11.2. Mature RBCs** are anucleate cells measuring 7–8 µm diameter, **similar in size to small lymphocyte nuclei**. RBCs are round, biconcave disks with reddish, eosinophilic cytoplasm, and centers paler than their outer rims. **The pale center** comprises roughly **one-third of the total diameter of the cell**. The average **life span of red blood cells is 120 days.**

Myelopoiesis (granulopoiesis): It results in the production of neutrophils, eosinophils, basophils and monocytes. The various stages in myelopoiesis are shown in **Figure 11.3**.

Megakaryopoiesis (thrombopoiesis): It is the process of platelet formation. The various stages of megakaryopoiesis are shown in **Figure 11.4**.

TABLE 11.2 Different sites of hematopoiesis during various phases of life.

Phase	*Period*	*Site*
The yolk sac (mesoblastic) phase	First 3 months of gestation	Yolk sac
Hepatic phase	4–9 months of gestation	Liver (chief site till birth), spleen (minor site)
The medullary (myeloid) phase	By 3rd week after birth up to puberty	Bone marrow throughout the skeleton
	Adults	Active marrow is limited to the ends of long bones and flat bones

TABLE 11.3 Different terminologies used in hematopoiesis.

Terminology	
Pluripotent	Ability to generate all mature hematopoietic cells
Multipotent	Ability to produce a limited range of differentiated cell lineages appropriate to their location
Unipotent	Restricted ability to differentiate and generate one specific cell type

Q. Write a short note on erythropoietin.

Regulation of hematopoiesis: It is regulated by hematopoietic growth factors, cytokines, and hormones. The main factors are:

- **Erythropoiesis**: Erythropoiesis is regulated by **erythropoietin (EPO).** EPO is a glycosylated protein synthesized mainly by the kidney and a minor part from the liver. EPO production is increased in response to hypoxia/reduced oxygen tension (e.g., due to anemia, or lung disease). *Erythropoietin* acts on the erythroid precursors through **EPO receptors present on erythroid precursors.** This stimulates proerythroblast to proliferate and differentiate to produce RBCs.
- **Myelopoiesis**: It is regulated by various growth factors and cytokines, the most important being **granulocyte-macrophage colony-stimulating factor (GM-CSF)** and **granulocyte colony-stimulating factor (G-CSF).**
- **Thrombopoiesis**: It is regulated by cytokines and growth factors, the most important being **thrombopoietin (TPO),** which is synthesized in the liver.

Compensatory hyperplasia: Anemia is associated with a decrease in tissue oxygen tension. Except for anemia caused by chronic renal failure or chronic inflammation, tissue hypoxia induced by anemia triggers increased production of the growth factor *erythropoietin* from specialized cells in the kidney. Erythropoietin causes a compensatory hyperplasia of erythroid precursors in the bone marrow. This results in the replacement of the fatty marrow by hematopoietic tissue.

Extramedullary hematopoiesis: Normally, the cells of the myeloid lineage arise in the central bone marrow (medullary cavity). In severe anemia, the increased demand for blood cells is not met with compensatory hyperactivity of marrow alone. This induces **hematopoietic islands to appear in the secondary hematopoietic organs such as the liver and spleen** (resulting in hepatosplenomegaly) and even in **lymph nodes**. This appearance of hematopoietic tissue in secondary hematopoietic organs (arising outside the marrow elsewhere in the body) is termed *extramedullary hematopoiesis* **(agnogenic myeloid metaplasia)**. The causes of extramedullary hemopoiesis are severe anemia (as in thalassemia major, sickle cell anemia) and bone marrow disorders (e.g., myelofibrosis).

Various cells and components in normal adult bone marrow (age 18–70 years) are presented in **Table 11.4**.

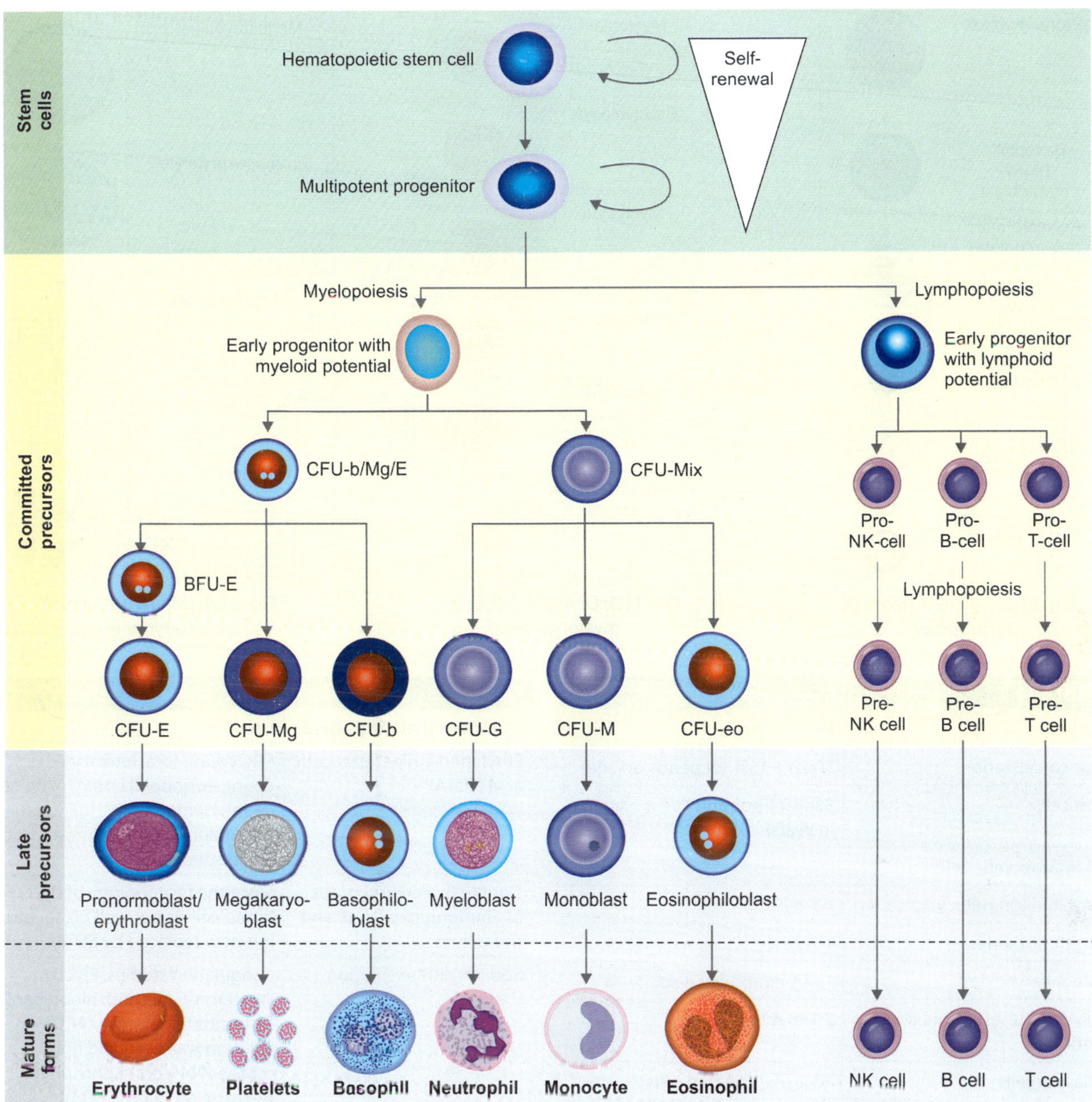

Fig. 11.1: Different stages of hematopoiesis.

(Baso: basophil; BFU: burst forming unit; CFU: colony forming unit; E: erythrocyte; Eo: eosinophil; G: granulocyte; M: macrophage; Mg: megakaryocyte; NK: natural killer).

ANTICOAGULANTS

PA 13.2 (CC): Describe the role of anticoagulants in hematology.

Q. Write a short on various types of anticoagulants used in hematology. Mention their mode of action. List the uses of trisodium citrate.

Blood coagulates when withdrawn from the vessel and anticoagulants are used to prevent blood from clotting. Commonly used anticoagulants are listed in **Table 11.5**.

Calcium Chelating Agents

Most of the anticoagulants used in the laboratory act by binding calcium as an insoluble salt or soluble but unionized salt. Since calcium is essential for many of the steps in the clotting mechanism, the chelation of calcium prevents clotting.

Ethylenediaminetetraacetic Acid

Commonly disodium or tripotassium salts of ethylenediaminetetraacetic acid (EDTA) are used in the laboratory.

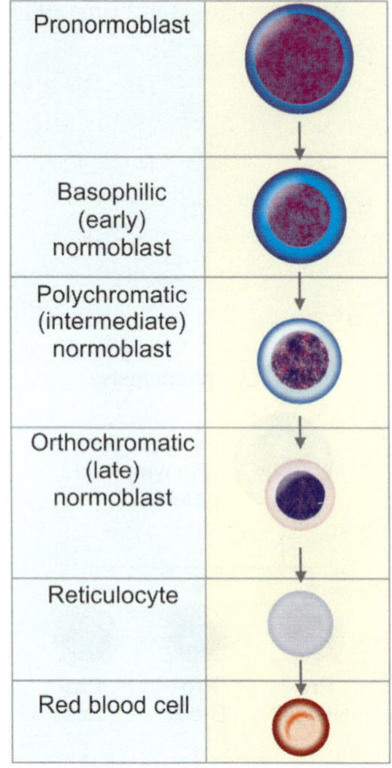

Fig. 11.2: Different stages of erythropoiesis.

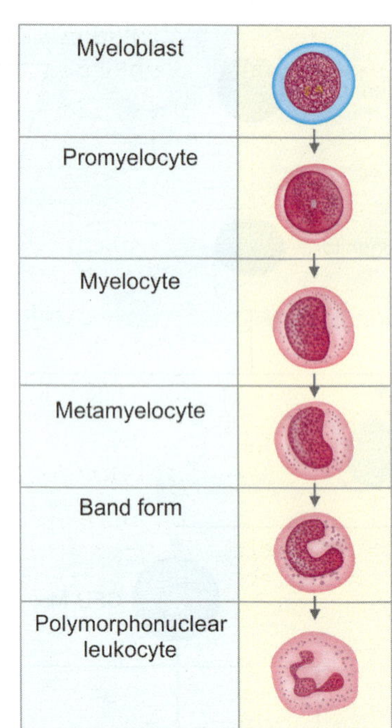

Fig. 11.3: Different stages of myelopoiesis.

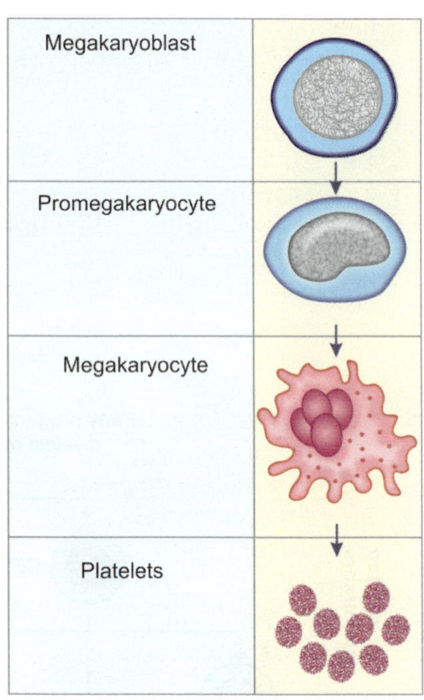

Fig. 11.4: Different stages of megakaryopoiesis.

TABLE 11.4 Contents of normal adult bone marrow.

Cell type	*Percentage*
Fat-to-cell ratio	50:50 ± 15% (depends on age)
Fat cells	35–65% (roughly % fat = age in years)
Hematopoietic cells	
Myeloid (granulocytic) series	40–65%
Erythroid series	10–20%
Megakaryocytes	1–4/high-power field
Myeloid-to-erythroid (M: E) ratio	2:1 to 4:1
Plasma cells	<3% of nucleated cells
Lymphocytes	<20% of nucleated cells
Other contents of marrow: Vessels, nerves, reticuloendothelial cells, and stroma	

Mode of action: They bind and **remove free calcium ions from the blood** by chelation, thereby preventing coagulation.

Advantages: Ethylenediaminetetraacetic acid (DIA) **preserves the morphology** of the blood cells even up to 3 hours and cell counts to 12 hours after collection of the blood. Therefore, it is the **anticoagulant of choice** for all cell counts and peripheral smears. Tripotassium salts of EDTA are more soluble and are preferred for cell counters than that of less soluble sodium salt. EDTA is used in solid form at a concentration of 2 mg/mL of blood.

TABLE 11.5 Commonly used anticoagulants.

I. Calcium chelating agents	Uses
Ethylenediaminetetraacetic acid (EDTA)	RBC count, total leukocyte count, eosinophil count, platelet count. Hemoglobin, HbF (fetal hemoglobin) estimation, and Hb electrophoresis
Double oxalate (mixtures of ammonium oxalate and potassium oxalate)	Since the morphology of the blood cells is not well preserved, it is now replaced by EDTA
Sodium citrate solution	Coagulation studies, ESR by Westergren method, blood bank [acid citrate dextrose (ACD) solution was used and now replaced by citrate phosphate dextrose adenine (CPDA)]
Sodium fluoride	Estimation of blood sugar
II. Heparin	Osmotic fragility test, red cell enzyme studies [e.g., G6PD and PK (pyruvate kinase) deficiency], electrolyte estimation, arterial blood gas analysis

Disadvantages: It is more expensive than oxalate, but this is usually outweighed by the advantages. It is **not suitable for coagulation studies.**

Alterations Induced by EDTA

Peripheral smear

- **RBC:** Red cells **may assume the spherocytic or macrocytic form** and show **crenation.**

- **WBC:**
  - **Neutrophils:** Morphologic changes take place in the neutrophils within 30 minutes of blood collection. **Neutrophils show separation of nuclear lobes**, and **vacuoles, and loss of granules in the cytoplasm**.
  - **Monocytes and lymphocytes:** They show **irregular lobulation of the nucleus** and **vacuoles in the cytoplasm.**
- **Platelets:** They **swell and disintegrate** and a false decrease in their count may be observed.

Hematological tests

- **Hematocrit/PCV and mean cell volume: Increased** due to swelling of cells.
- **Osmotic fragility: Increased**
- **Total WBC count and platelet count: Progressively decreased.**

Uses

- **Cell counts:** RBC count, total leukocyte count, eosinophil count, platelet count, reticulocyte count.
- **Hemoglobin, HbF estimation, hematocrit, and Hb electrophoresis.**
- Peripheral smear

Oxalate

Q. Write a short note on the double oxalate mixture.

- **Potassium oxalate:** Most often **used for chemical analysis. Shrinks RBCs** and is therefore not recommended for packed cell volume (PCV), erythrocyte sedimentation rate (ESR), or peripheral smear.
- **Ammonium oxalate:** It causes **swelling of RBCs** and is therefore not used for PCV, ESR, or peripheral smear.
- **Double oxalate:** To balance the swelling effect of ammonium oxalate and the shrinking effect of potassium oxalate, the two are combined in a **mixture in the ratio of 3 parts of ammonium oxalate to 2 parts of potassium oxalate.** Morphology of the blood cells is not well preserved; hence it has now been replaced by EDTA. As it is toxic, it is **not used as an anticoagulant for blood transfusion**. It is used in a concentration of 2 mg/mL of blood.

Sodium Citrate

Mode of action: Sodium citrate **binds with calcium ions** in the blood to form a soluble calcium citrate complex thus preventing coagulation of blood.
Disadvantages: Since it is **used as a liquid** which results in dilution of cellular elements, it is **not suitable for cell counts, Hb**, etc.

Uses

- **Coagulation studies:** Either 3.8% trisodium citrate pentahydrate or 3.2% trisodium citrate dihydrate solution is used for coagulation studies. One part of the anticoagulant is mixed with 9 parts of blood (1:9, i.e., ratio of 0.5:4.5 mL); thus, there is less plasma dilution.
- **ESR by Westergren method:** In the Westergren method of ESR estimation, **1 part of 3.8% sodium citrate is mixed with 4 parts of blood (e.g., 0.4 mL citrate and 1.6 mL blood)**, thus maintaining a **ratio of 1:4 between citrate and blood.**
- **Blood bank:** Acid citrate dextrose solution (ACD solution) was used as an anticoagulant in blood banking. This has been replaced by **citrate phosphate dextrose adenine (CPDA).**

Sodium Fluoride

Sodium fluoride acts as an **antiglycolytic agent** which inhibits the use of glucose by blood cells. Thus, it maintains stable levels of glucose.
Use: It is used for the **estimation of blood sugar.**

Heparin

Mode of action: Heparin acts as an anticoagulant by **preventing the conversion of prothrombin to thrombin.**

Uses

It is used **when almost instantaneous anticoagulation is required** and to prevent any chances of hemolysis after the blood is drawn. The syringe is heparinized by taking 1 drop of heparin to wet the inner surface of the syringe and the blood is collected.

- **Osmotic fragility test** done for diagnosis of spherocytosis.
- **Red cell enzyme studies**, such as G6PD and PK deficiency.
- **Electrolyte estimation.**
- **Arterial blood gas analysis.**

Disadvantages of Heparin

- **Expensive.**
- **Causes clumping of platelets and leukocytes**, so it is not used for automated cell counters.
- **Gives bluish discoloration to the background of peripheral blood smears.**
- **Prevents coagulation for only a limited period** and its effect slowly disappears as the heparin is metabolized or neutralized in the blood.

Blood Sample

Type of Blood Sample

Q. Write a short note on the method of obtaining plasma and serum.

1. **Whole blood:** It is used for **complete hemogram** (hemoglobin, ESR, platelet count, reticulocyte count, and peripheral smear evaluation), osmotic fragility test, estimation of HbF, Hb electrophoresis, Coombs test, and for biochemical investigations, such as blood glucose.

2. **Serum:** It is obtained by **allowing the blood to clot** in a tube or a vial (without adding any anticoagulant). It is **used for the estimation of bilirubin, creatinine, uric acid, proteins, albumin, globulin, and albumin/globulin (A/G) ratio, serum enzyme levels** [e.g., alkaline phosphatase, acid phosphatase, aspartate (AST/SGOT) and alanine aminotransferase (ALT/SGPT)], **serum electrophoresis of proteins, lipoproteins, and immunoglobulins**.
3. **Plasma:** It is obtained by **centrifugation of the anticoagulated blood**. Red blood cells form the sediment and the supernatant is the plasma. It is **used for coagulation studies** [prothrombin time (PT), activated partial thromboplastin time (APTT), thrombin time], assay of various coagulation factors (e.g., factor VIII, IX), assay of FDP and D-dimer (in disseminated intravascular coagulation), confirmation of hemoglobinemia where plasma is colored red (e.g., PNH).

Collection of Blood

Venous blood for the tests is collected by (i) syringe or (ii) vacuum tubes.

Q. Write short note on vacutainer.

Vacutainer: These are **vacuum tubes** that have a colored top **(Table 11.6 and Fig. 11.5)**. They are used in most laboratories and have replaced the collection of blood with syringes. It is very essential to use appropriate vacuum tubes with the proper ratio of anticoagulant and blood for specific tests.

Capillary blood: May be collected either from the finger or heel pricks using a sterile disposable lancet/needle.

Arterial blood: Is usually required for blood gas analysis and is collected from the femoral artery by disposable needle and syringe.

Complications Encountered During Blood Collection

Q. Write a short note on complications of venipuncture.

- **Ecchymosis** and **hematoma** at the site of puncture.

TABLE 11.6 Types of commonly used vacuum tubes, their color, content, and uses.

Color of the top	*Anticoagulant*	*Uses*
Red	No chemicals—plain	Serum for various studies
Purple or lavender	EDTA	Routine hematological tests
Light blue	Sodium citrate 3.2%	Coagulation studies
Gray	Sodium fluoride	For glucose estimation
Green	Heparin	Osmotic fragility test, red cell enzyme study
Black	Citrate	Erythrocyte sedimentation rate

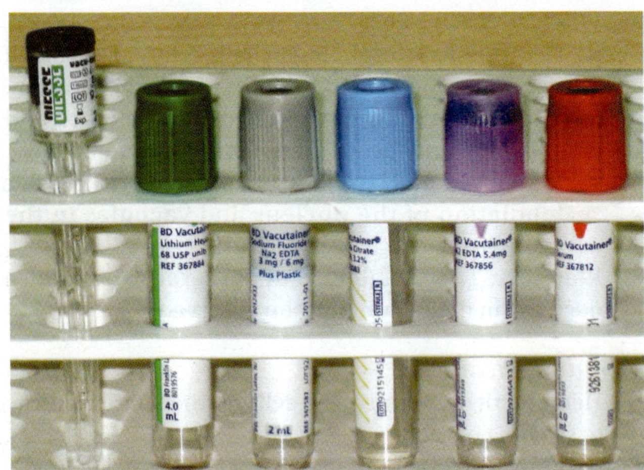

Fig. 11.5: Different types of vacuum tubes.

- **Syncope or fainting.**
- **Failure to get blood** because the needle might not have entered the vessel. In obese individuals, it is often difficult to locate the vein.
- **Hemolysis of blood sample** due to narrow bore of needle, quick withdrawal of blood with excessive suction, or contamination of syringe by water. A hemolyzed blood sample is not suitable for testing.

RED BLOOD CELL DISORDERS

A common disorder of red cells is anemia or, less commonly, *polycythemia* (an increase in red cells, also known as *erythrocytosis*).

ANEMIA

PA 13.3 (CC): Define and classify anemia.

Definition

Q. Define anemia.

Anemia is defined as a **reduction of the total circulating red cell mass below normal limits.** It **results in a reduction of the oxygen-transporting capacity of blood** and, if severe, leads **to tissue hypoxia.**

Anemia is diagnosed by a **decrease below the normal limit** (below the reference level for the age and sex of the individual) of **hemoglobin concentration, erythrocyte (RBC) count, or hematocrit/HCT** (ratio of packed red cells to total blood volume). WHO criteria for anemia for adult males Hb <13 g/dL and adult females Hb <12 g/dL.

Q. Classify anemia/give the etiological classification of anemia.

Anemia may be **absolute** (decreased RBC mass), or **relative** (associated with a higher plasma volume). Anemia is conventionally used for absolute anemia.

Classification of Anemia

Anemia can be classified according to the morphology of RBCs in anemia and its etiology.

1. **Morphological classification (Table 11.7):** It is based on:
   - **Red cell size** (normocytic, microcytic, or macrocytic), and
   - **Degree of hemoglobinization** (normochromic or hypochromic).
2. **Etiological classification:** The etiological classification of anemia is presented in **Box 11.1**.

Q. Etiological classification of anemia.

Anemia can be due to (1) bleeding (blood loss), (2) decreased (impaired) red cell production, or (3) increased red cell destruction (hemolysis). These mechanisms are used for classifying anemia.

Classification of severity of anemia is presented in **Box 11.2**

Clinical Features of Anemia

Irrespective of the cause, anemia when severe, presents with certain clinical features. The symptoms depend on four main factors:

1. **Speed of onset of anemia:** Rapidly progressive anemia causes more symptoms than that of gradual onset. This is because there is less time for adaptation in the cardiovascular system.
2. **Severity of anemia:** Mild anemia produces no symptoms compared to significant symptoms in severe anemia.
3. **Age of the patient:** Young patients can tolerate anemia better than the elderly.
4. **Underlying pathogenic mechanism:** The illness/disease that caused the anemia produces symptoms related to the disease. For example, iron deficiency anemia due to gynecologic disorders may produce vaginal bleeding.

In anemia, the lowered oxygen content of the circulating blood leads to tissue hypoxia. General clinical features are either due to tissue hypoxia or compensatory mechanisms **(Fig. 11.6)**.

1. **Due to tissue hypoxia:**
   - *Nonspecific symptoms:* Weakness, malaise, and easy fatigability due to hypoxia of muscles.
   - *Dyspnea on mild exertion:* It is due to the lowered oxygen content of the circulating blood.
   - *Pallor:* Patients appear pale due to a deficiency of red-colored hemoglobin which is better appreciated in the conjunctiva, mucous membrane of the tongue, and nail beds. Pallor associated with icterus is suggestive of hemolytic anemia.
   - *CNS:* Patients with severe anemia may complain of headache, vertigo, tinnitus, and lack of concentration.
2. **Due to compensatory mechanisms:**
   - *Cardiac features:* Dyspnea on mild exertion, palpitation, tachycardia, and cardiac murmur occur due to compensatory mechanisms. The resulting increase in the cardiac output may cause congestive cardiac failure.

Investigation of Anemia

PA 13.4 (CC): Enumerate and describe the investigation of anemia.

The general scheme of investigation of anemia is listed in **Box 11.3**.

Complete Blood Counts (Hemogram) (Table 11.8)

Q. Write a short note on complete blood counts (CBC) (hemogram).

Various parameters obtained in automated cell counters are listed in **Table 11.9**.

TABLE 11.7 Morphological classification of anemia.

Type of anemia	*Microcytic hypochromic*	*Normocytic normochromic*	*Macrocytic*
Size of RBCs	Smaller than normal	Normal	Larger than normal
Central pallor in RBCs	More than 1/3	Normal	Normal
Mean corpuscular volume (MCV)	Reduced (<80 fL)	Normal (82–98 fL)	Increased (>100 fL)
Mean corpuscular hemoglobin concentration (MCHC)	Reduced (<30 g/dL)	Normal (31–36 g/dL)	Normal (31–36 g/dL)
Examples	Iron deficiency anemia, thalassemia, sideroblastic anemia	During blood loss, anemia of chronic diseases, anemia due to bone marrow failure	Deficiency of vitamin B_{12} and folic acid
Morphology of RBC	RBC smaller than normal; Central pallor more than 1/3	RBC normal	RBC larger

BOX 11.1: Etiological classification of anemia (according to underlying mechanism).

1. **Blood Loss**
   - **Acute:** Trauma
   - **Chronic:** Lesions of the gastrointestinal tract (e.g., carcinoma colon), gynecological disorders
2. **Impaired Red Cell Production**
   - Disturbed proliferation and maturation of erythroblasts
     - Defective DNA synthesis: Megaloblastic anemias due to deficiency or impaired utilization of vitamin B_{12} and folic acid
     - Defective hemoglobin synthesis
       - Deficient heme synthesis: Iron deficiency, sideroblastic anemias
       - Deficient globin synthesis: Thalassemia
     - Others
       - Anemia of renal failure (erythropoietin deficiency)
       - Anemia of chronic disease (iron sequestration, relative erythropoietin deficiency)
       - Anemia of endocrine disorders
   - Disturbed proliferation and differentiation of stem cells: aplastic anemia, pure red cell aplasia
   - Marrow replacement: primary hematopoietic neoplasms (acute leukemia, myelodysplastic syndromes)
   - Marrow infiltration (myelophthisic anemia): metastatic neoplasms, granulomatous disease
3. **Increased Red Cell Destruction (Hemolytic Anemias)**
   - **Intrinsic (intracorpuscular) abnormalities:**
     - **Hereditary**
       - ***Red cell membrane abnormalities:*** Hereditary spherocytosis, hereditary elliptocytosis
       - ***Enzyme deficiencies***
         a. **Hexose monophosphate shunt enzyme deficiencies:** G6PD deficiency
         b. **Glycolytic enzyme deficiencies:** Pyruvate kinase deficiency, hexokinase deficiency
       - ***Disorders of hemoglobin synthesis***
         a. Deficient globin synthesis: Thalassemia syndromes
         b. Structurally abnormal globin synthesis (hemoglobinopathies): Sickle cell anemia
     - Acquired
       - ***Membrane defect:*** Paroxysmal nocturnal hemoglobinuria
   - Extrinsic (extracorpuscular) abnormalities
     - **Antibody-mediated**
       - **Isohemagglutinins:** Hemolytic disease (Rh disease) of the newborn, transfusion reactions
       - **Autoantibodies:** Idiopathic (primary), drug-associated, autoimmune diseases, e.g., systemic lupus erythematosus
     - **Mechanical trauma to red cells**
       - **Microangiopathic hemolytic anemias:** Hemolytic uremic syndrome, disseminated intravascular coagulation, thrombotic thrombocytopenic purpura
       - **Dysfunctional cardiac valves**
     - **Infections of red cells:** Malaria, babesiosis
     - **Toxic or chemical injury:** Clostridial sepsis, snake venom, lead poisoning
     - **Membrane lipid abnormalities:** Abetalipoproteinemia, severe hepatocellular liver disease
     - **Sequestration:** Hypersplenism

(G6PD: glucose-6-phosphate dehydrogenase; PK: pyruvate kinase)

BOX 11.2: Severity of anemia.

- Mild anemia: Hb 9.1–10.5 g/dL
- Moderate anemia: Hb 6.0–9.0 g/dL
- Severe anemia: Hb less than 6.0 g/dL

Q. Write a short note on various parameters obtained in automated cell counters.

Red Cell Indices

Q. Write a short note on red cell indices.

Features that can provide etiologic clues to the etiology of anemia include the size, color, and shape of the red cells. These are detected by visual inspection of peripheral smears and are expressed quantitatively using the red cell indices. Red cell indices are useful in morphological characterization and diagnosis of anemias. They are either directly measured or automatically calculated by specialized instruments in clinical laboratories (automated cell counters). Red cell indices include:

Q. Write a short note on mean corpuscular volume.

1. **Mean corpuscular volume (MCV):** MCV **signifies the average volume of the RBC** and is expressed in femtoliters (fL) (cubic microns). It is **used for classification and differential diagnosis of anemias. Normal range: 82–98 fL.** Microcytic anemia has MCV <80 fL and macrocytic anemia have MCV >100 fL.

$$MCV = \frac{PCV \times 1,000}{RBC\ count\ in\ millions} = 0.45 \times 1,000/5 = 90\ fL$$

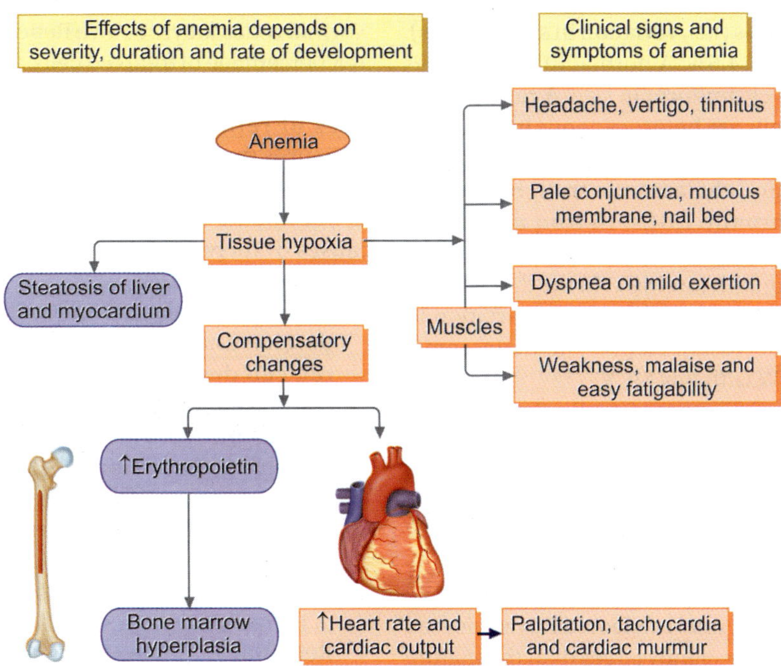

Fig. 11.6: Clinical features and effects of anemia.

BOX 11.3: General scheme of investigation of anemia.

Routine investigations

- Estimation of hemoglobin and packed cell volume (hematocrit) (*refer* Ch 15)
- Complete blood counts (CBC): RBC, WBC, and platelet counts
- Peripheral smear examination (*refer* pages 440-3)
- Red cell indices
- Reticulocyte count
- Erythrocyte sedimentation rate (*refer* pages 445-7)
- Bone marrow examination (*refer* pages 477-8 of Chapter 15)
- Special investigations: Depends on the type of anemia (*refer* individual types of anemia)

TABLE 11.8 Complete blood counts.

• Hemoglobin	• Reticulocyte count
• Total leukocyte count	• Peripheral blood smear
• RBC count	• RBC morphology
• Platelet count	• Platelets morphology
• Differential leukocyte count	• Hemoparasites
• Hematocrit (HCT)/packed cell volume (PCV)	• Any abnormal/atypical cell

2. **Mean corpuscular hemoglobin:** Mean corpuscular hemoglobin (MCH) **indicates the average amount (mass) of Hb (weight) per RBC** and is expressed as picograms (1 pg = 10^{-12} g). It is of limited value in the differential diagnosis of anemias. **Normal range: 27–32 pg.** MCH <26 pg is seen in microcytic anemia and MCH >33 pg is seen in macrocytic anemia.

TABLE 11.9 Various parameters obtained in automated cell counters.

Hemoglobin Absolute values: • Mean corpuscular volume (MCV) • Mean corpuscular hemoglobin (MCH) • Mean corpuscular hemoglobin concentration (MCHC) • Red cell distribution width (RDW)	• Mean platelet volume (MPV) • Hematocrit (Hct)/packed cell volume (PCV) • Total leukocyte count • RBC count • Platelet count • Reticulocyte count • Differential leukocyte count (3 part or 5 part)

$$MCH = \frac{Hb\ (in\ g/L)}{RBC\ (in\ millions/\mu L)} = 15 \times 10/5 = 30\ pg$$

Q. Write a short note on mean corpuscular hemoglobin concentration.

3. **Mean corpuscular hemoglobin concentration (MCHC):** MCHC indicates the **average hemoglobin concentration in the RBC** in a given volume of packed red cells (i.e., **taking volume into account**). It is expressed as grams/deciliter (dL). Earlier it was expressed as a percentage (%). It is a better indicator of hypochromasia than MCH. Normal range: 31–35 g/dL. MCHC <31 g/dL is seen in hypochromic RBCs such as iron deficiency anemia (IDA) and thalassemia. MCHC >36 g/dL is an indication of hyperchromic RBCs. MCHC = Hb (in g/dL)/PCV = 15/0.45 = 33 g/dL

Q. What is RDW? What is its significance?

4. **Red cell distribution width (RDW):** It is the coefficient of variation of red cell volume. RDW is a **quantitative**

measure of anisocytosis (i.e., variation in size of RBCs). Normal RDW is 11.5–14.5%. A normal RDW indicates that RBCs are relatively uniform in size. **A raised RDW indicates that red cells are heterogeneous in size and/or shape.** RDW is **useful for differentiating anemia due to iron deficiency and thalassemia trait, both show microcytic hypochromic RBCs. In iron deficiency anemia**, there is a wide variation in the size of RBCs, and RDW increases along with low MCV. In the thalassemia trait, the red cells do not show significant variation in size (uniform microcytosis). Hence, the thalassemia trait has normal RDW with low MCV.

RDW = (Standard deviation÷ mean cell volume) × 100

Reticulocyte Count

Q. Write a short essay on reticulocyte, its morphology, staining method, normal values, and its importance/utility.

Q. List the conditions in which reticulocyte count is increased.

Reticulocytes are **immature, non-nucleated RBCs** released from bone marrow. They are slightly larger than the mature RBCs. They continue to synthesize hemoglobin after the loss of the nucleus.

Methods of Reticulocyte Count

1. **Visual method: Staining in a living state** is known as **supravital staining.** Reticulocytes contain ribosomes and RNA and can be stained by supravital stains in the live and unfixed state. When blood is briefly incubated in supravital stains, such as **new methylene blue or brilliant cresyl blue** solution, the RNA is precipitated **(Fig. 11.7)** as a dye-ribonucleoprotein complex. On microscopy, the complex appears as a dark blue network (reticulum or filamentous strand or granular material). Reticulocytes stain ***polychromatic*** with Romanowsky stains and hence, the term ***"polychromatophil"*** is used to indicate their presence in peripheral smear.
2. **Automated method.**

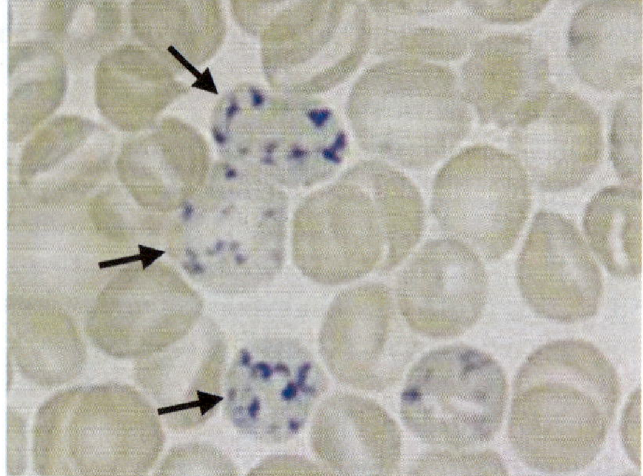

Fig. 11.7: Smear shows reticulocyte (arrows) with blue filamentous/granular material (new methylene blue).

Normal reticulocyte count: Reticulocyte count is expressed as a percentage of total red cells. Normal is 0.5– 2.5% and in newborns (cord blood) it is 1–7.0%.

Uses of reticulocyte count: The reticulocyte count **measures the capacity of bone marrow to produce RBCs.** So, it is of use in differential diagnosis of anemia as well as to estimate the degree of effective erythropoiesis. **The causes of increased and reduced reticulocyte count** are listed in **Table 11.10.**

- **Reticulocytosis**: In well-nourished individuals who develop **anemia due to acute bleeding or increased red cell destruction** (hemolysis), the compensatory response by bone marrow can increase the red cell production by 5–8 times more than normal. This marrow response is characterized by the appearance of increased numbers of newly formed red cells *(reticulocytes)* in the peripheral blood. Following therapy for anemia, the reticulocyte production starts increasing from around the 3rd day and reaches a maximum on the 6th/7th day of therapy.
- **Reticulocytopenia**: **Anemia caused due to decreased red cell production** (regenerative anemia) is associated with subnormal reticulocyte counts (reticulocytopenia).

Special Investigation

Depending on the differential diagnosis of anemia, several other blood tests may be necessary to evaluate anemia. These include the following:

- **Serum iron indices**: These include serum iron levels, total iron-binding capacity, transferrin saturation, and ferritin concentrations. This investigation will help to **distinguish among microcytic anemia** caused by iron deficiency, chronic inflammation, or thalassemia.
- **Serum and red cell folate and vitamin B_{12} concentrations:** These are low in megaloblastic anemia caused by folate and vitamin B_{12} deficiency respectively.
- **Hemoglobin electrophoresis:** It is used to detect abnormal hemoglobin such as HbS, HbF, etc.
- **Plasma unconjugated bilirubin, haptoglobin, and lactate dehydrogenase levels;** Their levels are abnormal in **hemolytic anemia.**

TABLE 11.10 Causes of increased and reduced reticulocyte count.

Causes of increased reticulocyte count (reticulocytosis)	*Causes of reduced reticulocyte count (reticulocytopenia)*
• Hemolytic anemias • Hemolytic crisis • Following hemorrhage (bleeding) • Following treatment in iron/folic acid/vitamin B_{12} deficiency anemias. Highest counts are found on the 6th/7th day of treatment and indicate marrow response to hematinic	Due to decreased erythropoietic activity • Aplastic anemia • Aplastic crisis due to parvovirus (hereditary spherocytosis and sickle cell disease) • Pure red cell aplasia • Fanconi anemia • Myelofibrosis

- **Antihuman globulin (AHG) test (Coombs test):** This test is used to detect antibodies or complement bound to red cells in suspected cases of antibody-mediated hemolytic anemia.

Bone Marrow Examination

Tests done on the peripheral blood are usually sufficient to establish the cause of anemia in many types of anemia. But, when anemia is accompanied by thrombocytopenia and/or granulocytopenia, it is more likely to be associated with marrow aplasia or infiltration. In such cases, a marrow examination is usually necessary. It is discussed on pages 447-9.

Reference ranges for various parameters of red blood cells are presented in **Table 11.11**.

TABLE 11.11 Reference ranges for red blood cells.

Parameter	*Reference value*
RBC count	
Males	4.5–5.5 × 10^{12}/L (Mean 5.0 × 10^{12}/L)
Females	3.8–4.8 × 10^{12}/L (mean 4.3 × 10^{12}/L)
RBC diameter	6.7–7.7 µm (mean 7.2 µm)
RBC indices (absolute values)	
Mean corpuscular volume (MCV)	82–100 fL
Mean corpuscular hemoglobin (MCH)	27–32 pg
Mean corpuscular hemoglobin concentration (MCHC)	31–35 g/dL
Red cell distribution width (RDW)	**11.5–14.5%.**
RBC lifespan	120 days
Hemoglobin (Hb)	
Adult hemoglobin (HbA)	95–98%
Males	13.0–17.0 g/dL
Females	12.0–15.0 g/dL
Hemoglobin A_2 (HbA_2)	1.5–3.5%
Hemoglobin, fetal (HbF) in adults	<0–2%
HbF, children under 6 months	<5%
Reticulocytes	
Adults	0.5–2.5%
Infants	2–6%
Newborn (cord blood)	1–7%
Hematocrit (PCV)	
Males	38–47%
Females	36–46%
Infants (cord blood)	45–70%
Ferritin (serum)	
Males	20–300 ng/mL
Females	15–200 ng/mL
Folate (serum)	3–20 µg/L
Iron, total (serum)	50–150 µg/dL
Total iron binding capacity (TIBC)	310–340 µg/dL
Iron saturation	20–45%
Osmotic fragility	
Slight hemolysis	At 0.45 to 0.39 g/dL NaCl
Complete hemolysis	At 0.33 to 0.36 g/dL NaCl
Mean corpuscular fragility	0.4–0.45 g/dL NaCl
Transferrin saturation	
Male	25–56%
Female	14–51%
Vitamin B_{12} (serum)	
Body stores	10–12 mg
Daily requirement	2–3 µg
Serum level	280–1,000 pg/mL
Autohemolysis test (whole blood)	0.4–4.50%
Autohemolysis test with glucose (whole blood)	0.3–0.7%

ANEMIAS OF IMPAIRED RED CELL PRODUCTION

Most of the anemias due to deceased erythropoiesis include those caused by an inadequate dietary supply of nutrients, particularly iron, vitamin B_{12}, and folic acid. Other anemias of this type are listed in **Box 11.1**.

IRON DEFICIENCY ANEMIA

Iron is required for the synthesis of normal heme of hemoglobin. Its deficiency leads to decreased erythropoiesis and anemia. Iron deficiency anemia (IDA) is the **most common nutritional disorder in the world.** IDA produces **clinical signs and symptoms that are mostly due to anemia.** About 10% of people living in higher-resource countries and 25–50% of those in lower-resource countries are anemic, and in both settings, the most frequent cause is iron deficiency. The factors responsible for iron deficiency differ in various populations and are best understood in the context of iron metabolism.

Iron Metabolism

PA 14.1 (CC): Describe iron metabolism.

Distribution of Iron

Iron is an essential metal present in the human body. The total body iron content is divided into functional and storage compartments **(Table 11.12)**. Iron in the body is extensively recycled between the functional and storage pools.

- **Functional:** Approximately **80% of the functional iron is present in hemoglobin**. The remaining functional iron is found in myoglobin and iron-containing enzymes (catalase, cytochromes, and peroxidases).
- **Storage:** The storage pool contains 15–20% of total body iron. Free iron is highly toxic because it can result in tissue damage due to its capacity to form free radicals. Therefore, iron is bound to protein and stored in the body in two forms namely—**ferritin** and **hemosiderin**. The storage iron can be readily mobilized whenever there is an increase in the requirements of iron, as may occur after blood loss. Two-thirds of the iron is stored as ferritin and one-thirds as hemosiderin.
  - **Ferritin** is a protein-iron complex (apoferritin + iron) found in all tissues but particularly in the liver, spleen, bone marrow, and skeletal muscles. Very small amounts of ferritin circulate in the serum, the value normally being 15–300 µg/L. **Serum ferritin levels reflect the iron stores**. Serum ferritin level is usually below 12 µg/L in iron deficiency and it is very high (as high as 5,000 µg/L may be observed) in conditions associated with iron overload. Ferritin is water-soluble and not visible by light microscopy.
  - **Hemosiderin** is an aggregate of iron and protein that is found in the reticuloendothelial cells of bone marrow, spleen, and liver. Hemosiderin **appears as golden yellow granules in the cytoplasm of the cells** when stained with routine hematoxylin and eosin. When treated with **Prussian blue (Perl's) stain, hemosiderin takes up a blue-black color** due to the iron reacting with potassium ferrocyanide of Perl's stain. In iron-overload, most of the iron is stored in the cells as hemosiderin.

TABLE 11.12 Iron distribution in healthy young adults (in mg).

Pool	*Men in mg*	*Women in mg*
Total	3,450	2,450
Functional (~80% of total body iron)		
Hemoglobin	2,000–2,500	1,750
Myoglobin and iron-containing enzymes (e.g., catalase, cytochromes)	350–400	300
Storage (15–20% of body iron)		
Ferritin-bound iron, and hemosiderin. Mainly in macrophages (liver, spleen, and bone marrow) and in skeletal muscle cells	500–1,000	400
Transport: Transferrin in plasma	120 µg/dL	100 µg/dL

Daily requirements: The daily requirement in adult males is **5–10 mg/day and in females 20 mg/day**.

Dietary sources: The diet contains iron either in the form of **heme** contained in animal products **and/or nonheme** iron in vegetables.

Iron Absorption

Site of absorption: Iron is absorbed from the **duodenum** and **proximal jejunum.** Iron balance is maintained mainly by regulating the dietary absorption of iron.

Molecular Aspect of Iron Absorption (Fig. 11.8)

About 20% of heme and 1–2% of nonheme iron are absorbable.

- **Nonheme iron:** Iron in nonheme form is mostly in the Fe^{3+} (ferric) state and is **reduced to Fe^{2+} (ferrous) iron by duodenal cytochrome B (it is ferric reductase)**. Ferrous (Fe^{2+}) iron is then transported across the brush border of the cytoplasmic membrane of the enterocyte (duodenal or jejunal epithelial cells) by **divalent metal transporter 1 (DMT1).**
- **Heme iron:** The **absorption** of heme iron is **better than nonheme**. Heme iron is moved across the brush border of the cytoplasmic membrane of the enterocyte through **heme transporters** into the cytoplasm.

Iron (heme or nonheme) that enters the cytoplasm of the enterocyte may be either transported to the blood or stored as mucosal iron (incorporated into cytoplasmic ferritin). Fe^{2+} iron destined for transport from cytoplasm to the circulation is carried out by **ferroportin-1**. This process is coupled by the iron oxidase like **hephaestin** (which is expressed predominantly in the enterocyte) which oxidizes Fe^{2+} iron to Fe^{3+} form.

Note: Both DMT1 and ferroportin are also involved in iron transport in other tissues and are distributed widely in the body.

Transport of Iron

Iron is transported in plasma by the iron transport protein **transferrin**, which is synthesized in the liver. The major function of plasma transferrin is to deliver iron to erythroid precursors for the synthesis of hemoglobin. In normal individuals, transferrin is about 33% saturated with iron, with an average serum iron level of 120 µg/dL in men and 100 µg/dL in women. Thus, the total iron-binding capacity of serum is in the range of 310–340 µg/dL.

Iron Excretion

Iron metabolism is unique as it is very efficiently utilized and reutilized by the body. There is no physiologically regulated mechanism for iron excretion and 1–2 mg per day is lost by the shedding of epithelial cells of the GI tract, skin epithelial cells (by sweat), and renal tubules.

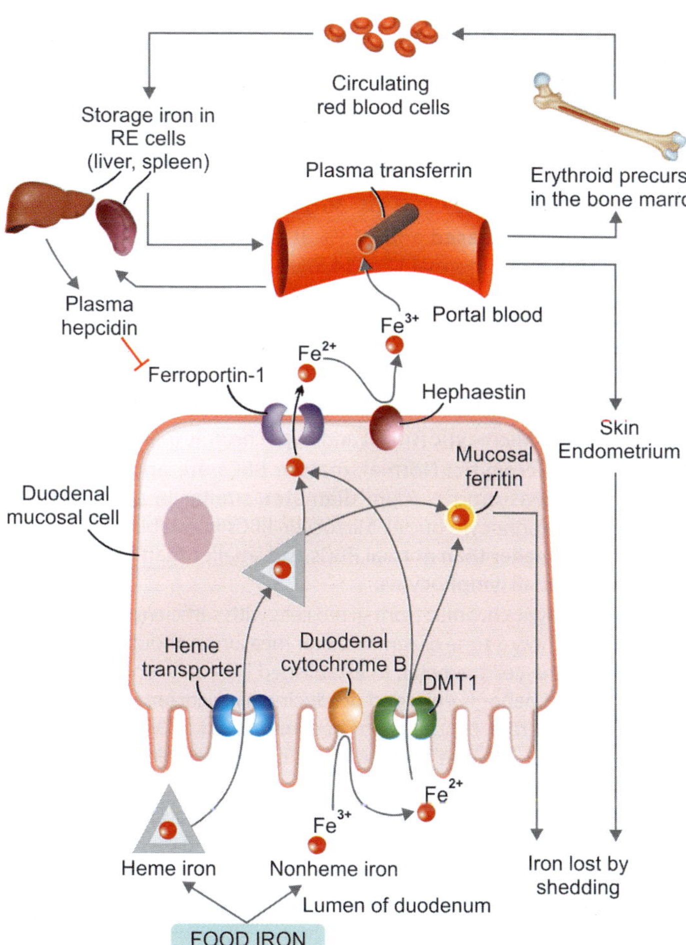

Fig. 11.8: Metabolism and regulation of iron absorption. Duodenal epithelial cell uptake of heme and nonheme iron. When the iron storage sites of the body are full of iron and erythropoietic activity is normal, plasma hepcidin balances iron uptake and loss. Hepcidin maintains iron hemostasis by downregulating ferroportin and limiting iron uptake.

(DMT1: divalent metal transporter 1; RE: reticuloendothelial)

Regulation of Iron Balance

Iron is essential for cellular metabolism; at the same time, excess of it is highly toxic. Therefore, the total body iron stores must be properly regulated. Iron balance is mainly achieved by regulating the absorption of iron in the diet. As body stores decrease, the absorption of iron rises and vice versa.

Role of Hepcidin

Q. Write a short note on the role of hepcidin in iron hemostasis.

Hepcidin is a small peptide secreted by the liver in an iron-dependent fashion. It is the **central regulator of iron homeostasis and controls iron absorption and storage.** It creates a feedback loop that maintains iron stores within a physiologic range. Hepcidin negatively regulates ferroportin. Hepcidin can bind to ferroportin (which exports iron from cells) and **inhibits iron transfer from the enterocyte to plasma**. The absorption of dietary iron from the duodenum is determined by the plasma level of hepcidin.

Adequate iron stores: When the body has adequate stores of iron, the hepatocytes will **increase production of hepcidin**. When hepcidin levels rise **leading to inactivation of ferroportin** and iron gets stored within enterocytes forming mucosal ferritin and is shed with the cells. The rise in plasma iron levels stimulates hepcidin production and reduces iron absorption.

Reduced body iron: When the body iron begins to drop, the liver decreases hepcidin production and increases iron absorption. The ferroportin becomes active and able to transport iron into the blood.

Alterations in the production of hepcidin are a common feature observed in disorders of iron metabolism.

Etiology of Iron Deficiency Anemia (Box 11.4)

PA 14.2a (CC): Describe the etiology of microcytic hypochromic (iron deficiency) anemia.

Q. Discuss the causes (etiology/etiopathogenesis) of iron deficiency anemia.

1. **Dietary deficiency/lack:** Low intake of iron is the **most common cause** of iron deficiency. Deficiency is observed in infants fed exclusively milk, elderly with improper diet and poor dentition, low socioeconomic sections, and predominantly vegetarians (contains poorly absorbable inorganic iron). Infants who consume large amounts of cow's milk are susceptible to developing IDA. Dietary deficiency is the most common cause of IDA in developing nations.
2. **Impaired iron absorption**: Malabsorption of iron may occur in patients with celiac disease, various forms of gastritis, or after gastrectomy.
3. **Increased iron demands:** It may not be met by normal dietary intake and occur during pregnancy and infancy.
4. **Chronic blood loss:** It is an important cause of iron deficiency anemia in developed nations. The most common sites of **bleeding are the gastrointestinal tract** (e.g., chronic gastrointestinal blood loss due to peptic ulcers, colon cancer, hemorrhoids) and the **female genital tract** (e.g., menorrhagia, metrorrhagia, endometrial cancer). In a well-nourished individual, microcytic hypochromic anemia is not a disease but a symptom of another underlying disorder (e.g., colon cancer leading to chronic blood loss).

Pathogenesis of Iron Deficiency Anemia

Iron deficiency anemia (IDA) is due to a deficiency of iron causing **defective heme synthesis**. Irrespective

BOX 11.4: Causes of iron deficiency anemia.

1. **Dietary deficiency/lack**
   - Milk-fed infants
   - Elderly with improper diet and poor dentition
   - Low socioeconomic sections
   - Vegetarians (contains poorly absorbable inorganic iron)
2. **Impaired absorption**
   - Total/partial gastrectomy
   - Intestinal absorption is impaired in sprue, other causes of intestinal steatorrhea and chronic diarrhea
   - Specific items in the diet, like phytates of cereals, tannates, carbonates, oxalates, phosphates, and drugs can impair iron absorption
3. **Increased demand/requirement**
   - Growing infants, children, and adolescents
   - Pregnancy and lactation
4. **Chronic blood loss: Due to bleeding from the**
   - Gastrointestinal tract (e.g., peptic ulcers, gastric carcinoma, colonic carcinoma, hemorrhoids, hookworm infestation, or nonsteroidal anti-inflammatory drugs)
   - Urinary tract (e.g., renal or bladder tumors)
   - Genital tract (e.g., menorrhagia, uterine cancer)
   - Respiratory tract (e.g., hemoptysis)

of the cause, iron deficiency develops insidiously and is divided into three stages **(Flowchart 11.1)**

Laboratory Findings

PA 14.2b (CC): Describe the investigations, and differential diagnosis of microcytic hypochromic anemia.

Q. Discuss the laboratory findings/investigations in iron deficiency anemia.

Q. Describe the peripheral blood picture and bone marrow findings in iron deficiency anemia.

PA 14.3 (CC): Identify and describe the peripheral smear in microcytic anemia.

Flowchart 11.1: Various stages of iron deficiency anemia.

Stage 1 (Depletion of iron stores)
Iron is adequate to maintain normal hemoglobin levels
Only serum ferritin decreased
Absence of stainable iron in bone marrow

↓

Stage 2 (Iron deficient erythropoiesis)
Decrease of serum iron
No anemia (Hb, MCV, and MCH within normal range).
Bone marrow shows iron-deficient erythropoiesis

↓

Stage 3 (Iron deficiency anemia)
Low serum iron, serum ferritin. Impaired hemoglobin production.
Morphologically, **first reduction in the size (microcytic) and later an increase in the central pallor (hypochromia) of RBCs**

Peripheral Blood

- **Hemoglobin and hematocrit (PCV): Decreased**
- **Red cell indices: MCV, MCH, and MCHC are reduced in IDA.**
  - ↓ **MCV:** <80 fL (normal 82–98 fL)
  - ↓ **MCH:** <25 pg (normal 27–32 pg)
  - ↓ **MCHC:** <27 g/dL (31–36 g/dL)
- **RDW: Increased** and >15%. It is the **earliest sign of iron deficiency** (normal 11.5–14.5%).

Q. Write a short note on peripheral smear findings in iron deficiency anemia.

Peripheral Smear (Figs. 11.9A and B)

- **RBCs: Microcytic** (small) and **hypochromic** (pale).
  - **Microcytic:** Normal, mature RBCs are anucleate cells measuring 7–8 µm diameter, similar in size to small lymphocyte nuclei. Microcytic RBCs in established IDA are **smaller than normal RBCs and smaller than the nuclei of small lymphocytes.**
  - **Hypochromic:** Normal red cells with sufficient hemoglobin show a zone of central pallor measuring about one-third of the cell diameter. In established iron deficiency, **the zone of pallor is enlarged producing hypochromasia**. In severe anemia, central pallor becomes 2/3rd to 3/4th of the cell and only the peripheral rim of hemoglobin is seen (ring/pessary cells).
  - **Moderate anisocytosis** (variation in size) and **poikilocytosis** (variation in shape). Some of the RBCs are very thin and oval and are called pencil/cigar-shaped cells.
- **WBCs: Normal**; eosinophilia may be seen in hookworm infestation.
- **Platelets: Normal**. In anemia associated with hemorrhage, platelets are increased.

Reticulocyte count: It is 1–2% in untreated patients and is **low for the degree of anemia.**

Bone Marrow

- **Cellularity:** Moderately **hypercellular**.
- **Myeloid-to-erythroid (M:E) ratio:** Varies from 2:1 to 1:2 (normal 2:1 to 4:1).
- **Erythropoiesis:** Iron deficiency causes defects in RBC production and the marrow shows **erythroid hyperplasia**. It shows **micronormoblastic maturation**. However, blood reticulocytosis does not occur.
- **Myelopoiesis:** Normal.
- **Megakaryopoiesis:** Normal.
- **Absence of bone marrow iron:** Bone marrow aspiration to assess iron stores is a **"Gold standard"** test. It shows a **negative Prussian blue reaction**. It is a reliable but more invasive method (compared to serum ferritin) for estimating iron stores.

Serum Iron Profile

Table 11.13 shows the serum iron profile in iron deficiency anemia.

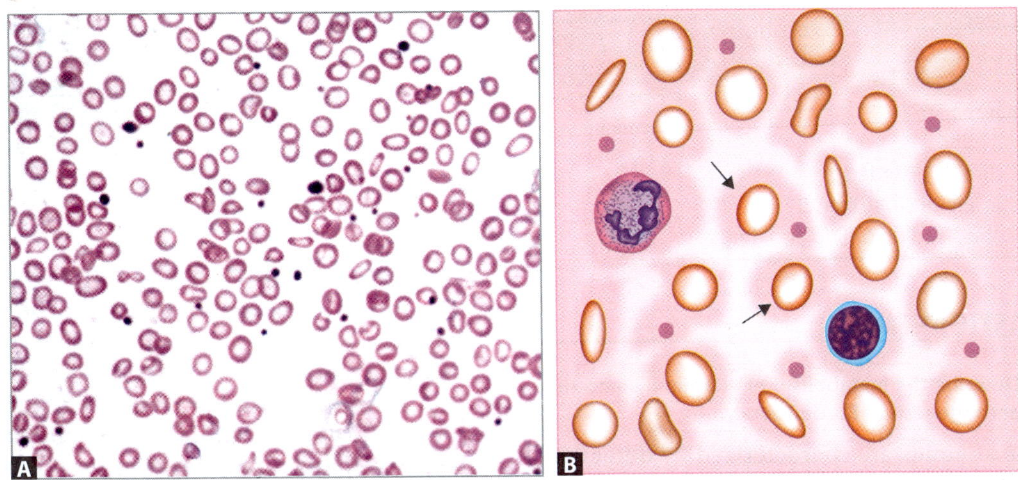

Figs. 11.9A and B: (A) Leishman stain; (B) Diagrammatic. Peripheral blood smear showing microcytic hypochromic red blood cells. Red blood cells (RBCs) are significantly smaller than the nucleus of a small lymphocyte, and they have increased central pallor (normal central pallor is about one-third of the RBC diameter).

TABLE 11.13 Serum iron profile in iron deficiency anemia.

	Normal range	*Value in IDA*	*Observation*
Serum ferritin*	15–300 µg/L	<15 µg/L	↓ All three parameters are reduced
Serum iron	50–150 µg/dL	10–15 µg/dL	
Serum transferrin saturation**	30–40%	<15%	
Total plasma iron-binding capacity (TIBC)	310–340 µg/dL	350–450 µg/dL	↑ All three parameters are increased
Serum transferrin receptor (TFR)	0.57–2.8 µg/L	3.5–7.1 µg/L	
Red cell protoporphyrin	30–50 µg/dL	>200 µg/dL	

*Serum ferritin is mainly derived from the storage pool of iron. Hence, its level is usually a good representative measure of iron stores.
**Normally, transferrin is about 33% saturated with iron. Its serum iron levels are about 120 µg/dL in men and 100 µg/dL in women. Thus, the normal total iron-binding capacity of serum is 300–350 µg/dL.

Reticulocyte Hemoglobin

Reticulocyte hemoglobin measures the amount of Hb in 1–2-day-old red cells. It is an **early sensitive indicator of iron deficiency**. Its normal range is 29–33 pg. It is **decreased in IDA**.

Clinical Features of IDA

Q. Describe the various clinical features of iron deficiency anemia.

Nonspecific and related to both severity and the cause of the anemia (e.g., gastrointestinal disease)

- **Onset:** Insidious.
- **Nonspecific symptoms: Fatigue, palpitations, breathlessness**, weakness, and irritability.
- **Pharyngeal/esophageal webs** formed cause dysphagia.
- **Patterson-Kelly or Plummer-Vinson syndrome:**
  - Microcytic hypochromic anemia
  - Atrophic glossitis
  - Esophageal webs
- **Congestive heart failure in severe** anemia.
- **Central nervous system: Pica**-unusual craving for substances with no nutritional value such as clay or chalk.

Craving for ice (pagophagia) **specific to iron deficiency**. Pica may be the cause rather than the effect of IDA.

Physical Findings

Diminished tissue enzymes cause characteristic epithelial changes of iron deficiency anemia.

- **Angular stomatitis and glossitis**
- **Chronic atrophic gastritis**
- **Koilonychia** (spoon nails): It is a physical finding seen in iron deficiency. First fingernails become thin and flat-paronychia, then brittle and finally spoon-shaped.

Causes of Microcytic Hypochromic Anemia (Box 11.5 and Table 11.14)

PA 14.2c (CC): Differential diagnosis of microcytic hypochromic anemia.

Q. Enumerate the causes of microcytic hypochromic anemia.

Various differentiating features of microcytic hypochromic anemias are presented in **Table 11.14**.

BOX 11.5: Various causes of microcytic hypochromic anemia.

- Iron deficiency anemia
- Thalassemia minor
- Anemia of chronic disorders
- Sideroblastic anemia (rare cause)
- Others: Alcohol, lead poisoning and drugs

MEGALOBLASTIC ANEMIA

PA 15.1 (CC): Describe the metabolism of vitamin B_{12} and the etiology and pathogenesis of B_{12} deficiency.

Megaloblastic anemias are characterized by **defective/** impaired **DNA (thymidine) synthesis. It results in an imbalance in cell growth** and shows **distinct megaloblasts in the bone marrow.** Megaloblastic anemias are common among anemias due to impaired red cell production.

Metabolism of Vitamin B_{12} and Folic Acid

Metabolism of vitamin B_{12} (cobalamin) and folic acid are closely related and **both are essential for normal DNA synthesis and nuclear maturation.** Other disorders may be associated with macrocytosis but megaloblastic hematopoiesis is most commonly **due to deficiency of vitamin B_{12} or folic acid.**

Vitamin B_{12} Metabolism

Source of vitamin B_{12}: Humans are totally dependent on animal products in the diet for vitamin B_{12} requirements. **Vitamin B_{12} is not present in food from vegetable sources.** Therefore, strict vegetarians do not get an adequate quantity of vitamin B_{12}. A balanced diet (not rigid vegetarian!) contains significantly large amounts of vitamin B_{12}, which accumulates in the body (liver) and is enough for several years. Due to this adequate storage, if there is any dietary deficiency or malabsorption of vitamin B_{12}, its clinical manifestations appear only after about 2–4 years. Vitamin B_{12} is a complex compound known as cobalamin and the daily requirement is about 2–3 µg.

Absorption, Transport, and Storage (Fig. 11.10)

- **Vitamin B_{12} is bound to binding proteins in food:** Vitamin B_{12} in food is usually in coenzyme form and bound to binding proteins in the diet.
- **Pepsin in the stomach releases vitamin B_{12} from binding protein and binds with haptocorrin:** In the stomach, pepsin releases vitamin B_{12} from binding protein in the food. **Released vitamin B_{12} binds to** salivary protein **haptocorrin** (secreted in salivary juices) and **forms haptocorrin-B_{12} complexes.**
- **Intrinsic factor secreted by the parietal cells of the fundic mucosa:** The intrinsic factor (IF)is a special protein produced by the parietal (oxyntic) cells of the fundic mucosa). The intrinsic factor is also called the Castle intrinsic factor. The haptocorrin-B_{12} complexes leave the stomach along with an unbound **intrinsic factor** (IF).
- **Release vitamin B_{12} from haptocorrin and formation of the IF- vitamin B_{12} complex:** As the haptocorrin-B_{12} complexes pass into the second part of the duodenum, pancreatic proteases release vitamin B_{12} from haptocorrin. The released vitamin B_{12} then associates with the intrinsic factor and forms the IF-B_{12} complex.
- **Endocytosis of IF vitamin B_{12} complex by ileal enterocytes via cubilin receptor:** The stable IF-vitamin B_{12} complex from the duodenum is transported to the

TABLE 11.14 Various differentiating features of microcytic hypochromic anemias.

	Iron deficiency anemia	*Thalassemia trait (minor)*	*Anemia of chronic disease*	*Sideroblastic anemia*
RBCs in peripheral blood smear	Microcytic hypochromic	Microcytic hypochromic with target cells	Normal/microcytic hypochromic	Variable
Mean corpuscular volume (MCV)	Reduced	Very low for the degree of anemia	Low normal or normal	Low in inherited type but often raised in acquired type
Serum iron (normal 60–170 µg/dL)	Reduced (<30 µg/dL)	Normal to high	Reduced (<50 µg/dL)	Raised
Serum TIBC (total iron binding capacity) (normal 300–350 µg/dL)	Raised (>350 µg/dL)	Normal	Reduced (<300 µg/dL)	Normal
Serum ferritin (normal 15–300 µg/dL)	Reduced (<15 µg/dL)	Normal (50–300 µg/dL)	Normal or raised (30–200 µg/L)	Raised
Serum soluble transferrin receptors	Increased	Normal or raised	Normal	Normal or raised
Iron in marrow	Absent	Present	Present	Present
Iron in erythroblasts	Absent	Present	Absent or reduced	Ring forms
Hemoglobin A_2 (normal <3%)	Reduced	Increased	Normal	Reduced

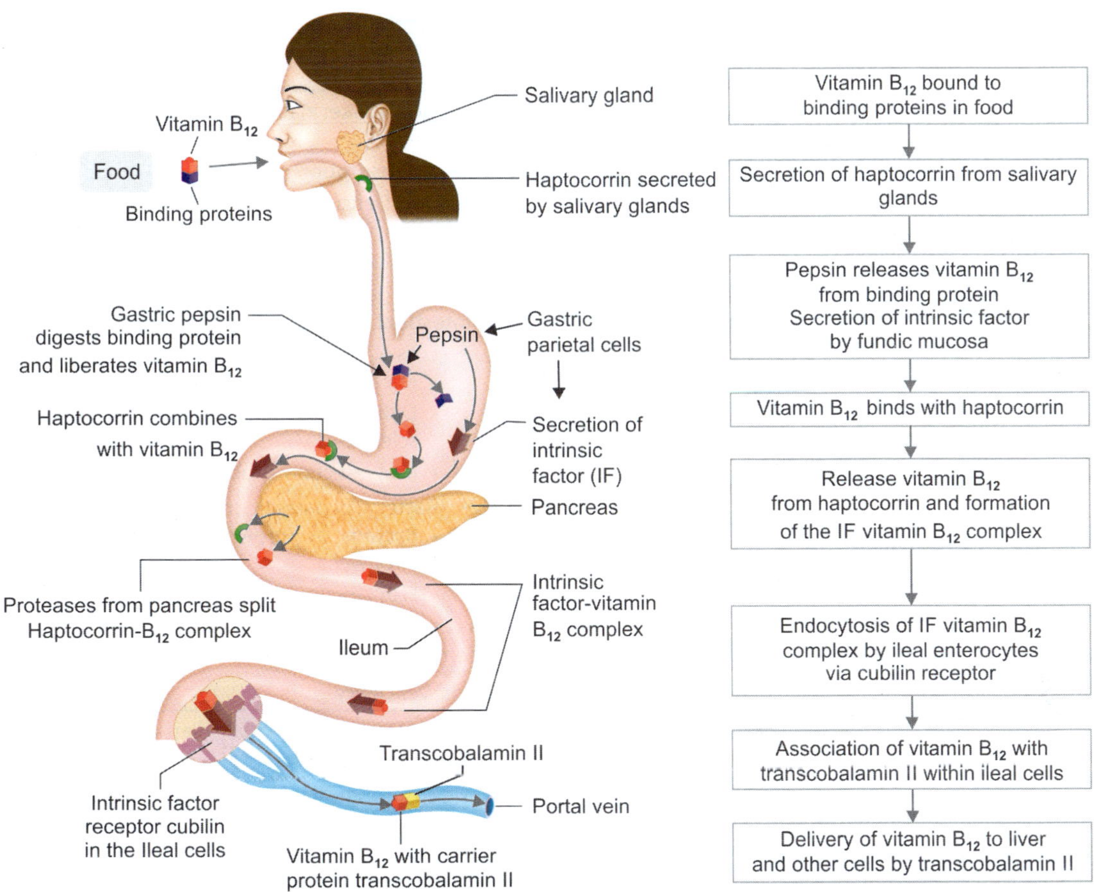

Fig. 11.10: Mechanism of vitamin B_{12} absorption.

ileum, where it is endocytosed by ileal enterocytes. These ileal enterocytes express a receptor for the intrinsic factor on their surfaces. These receptors are called **cubilin**.

- **Association of vitamin B_{12} with transcobalamin II within ileal cells:** Within the ileal epithelium, vitamin B_{12} combines with a major carrier protein, transcobalamin II, and is secreted into the blood.
- **Delivery of vitamin B_{12} to the liver and other cells by transcobalamin II:** Transcobalamin II delivers vitamin B_{12} to the liver and other cells of the body, including rapidly proliferating cells in the bone marrow and mucosal lining of the gastrointestinal tract.

Role of Vitamin B_{12}

Vitamin B_{12} is indirectly **required for DNA synthesis in various metabolic steps and its deficiency impairs DNA synthesis.** Vitamin B_{12} is **also required for the conversion of methylmalonyl CoA to succinyl malonyl CoA.** Deficiency of vitamin B_{12} causes increased levels of methylmalonic acid in plasma and urine. This results in the formation of abnormal fatty acids which get incorporated into neuronal lipids. Consequently, this predisposes to myelin breakdown and is probably responsible for **neurologic complications** of vitamin B_{12} deficiency.

Folic Acid Metabolism

Humans are entirely dependent on dietary sources for their folic acid requirement. The daily requirement is 50–200 mg. Green vegetables, yeast, legumes, fruits, and animal proteins are the richest sources and most normal diets contain sufficient amounts of folic acid. The folic acid in these foods is largely in the form of polyglutamate. Polyglutamates are sensitive to heat (thermolabile); boiling, steaming frying, and cooking destroy most of the folic acid. Intestinal conjugases split the polyglutamate into monoglutamates that are readily absorbed in the proximal jejunum. During intestinal absorption, they are modified to 5 methyl tetrahydrofolates, the normal transport form of folic acid.

Role of Folic Acid (FA)

The active form of folic acid is tetrahydrofolate (THF) which is the biological "middleman" involved in metabolic processes that synthesize DNA. The various reactions in which folic acid plays a main role are:

- **Synthesis of purine (required for DNA and RNA).**
- **Conversion of homocysteine to methionine, a reaction also requiring vitamin B_{12}.**
- **Conversion of deoxyuridine monophosphate (dUMP) to deoxythymidine monophosphate (dTMP):** 5,10-methylene THF polyglutamate is required for conversion of dUMP to dTMP and DNA, a rate-limiting step in pyrimidine synthesis.
- **Metabolism of histidine**: Histidine is metabolized to formiminoglutamic acid (FIGLU) which combines with THF to form glutamic acid. In folic acid deficiency, this reaction cannot take place and therefore FIGLU accumulates and is excreted as such in the urine. This is used as a test to measure folic acid deficiency.

Q. Discuss the causes and pathogenesis of megaloblastic anemia.

Causes of Megaloblastic Anemia

Table 11.15 shows the causes of megaloblastic anemia. One of the causes of vitamin B_{12} deficiency is deficiency of intrinsic factor which occurs in pernicious anemia.

Pathogenesis (Refer Online Flowchart 11.2)

Impaired DNA synthesis: Vitamin B_{12} and folate are both required for thymidine synthesis. Thymidine is **one of the building blocks of DNA** and is required for DNA replication. Megaloblastic anemia is commonly due to a deficiency of **vitamin B_{12} (cyanocobalamin) or folic acid. This leads to inadequate biosynthesis of thymidine.**

Delayed maturation of the nucleus: Thymidine deficiency (due to vitamin B_{12} and folic acid deficiency) produces **abnormalities in all rapidly dividing cells throughout the body** (including skin, gastrointestinal tract, and bone marrow). The most severely affected is the hematopoietic marrow. In these cells, the **nuclear maturation** due to impaired synthesis of thymidine characteristically **lags behind the cytoplasmic maturation** and results in **abnormally large** nucleated **erythroid precursors** named **megaloblasts.**

Cytoplasm matures normally: The RBCs derived from erythroid precursors are larger than normal and are called **macrocytes.**

Ineffective erythropoiesis: Many red cell progenitors with defective DNA synthesis, trigger a DNA damage response leading to apoptosis *(ineffective hematopoiesis)*. The megaloblast precursors undergo intramedullary destruction resulting in anemia. In "ineffective erythropoiesis," the marrow is hypercellular but, the reticulocyte count is low and the patient has anemia.

Also affects granulopoiesis and megakaryopoiesis: Granulocytes and platelet precursors are also affected (although not as severely) in megaloblastic anemia. Most patients present with pancytopenia (anemia, thrombocytopenia, and granulocytopenia).

TABLE 11.15 Causes of megaloblastic anemia.

Vitamin B_{12} Deficiency
1. **Decreased intake:** Inadequate diet, "pure vegetarians" (vegans)
2. **Impaired absorption**
– **Gastric:** Deficiency of gastric acid or pepsin or intrinsic factor
◆ Pernicious anemia
◆ Post-gastrectomy
– **Intestinal**
◆ Loss of absorptive surface
• Malabsorption syndromes
• Diffuse intestinal disease, e.g., lymphoma, systemic sclerosis
• Ileal resection, Crohn disease
◆ Bacterial or parasitic competition for vitamin B_{12}
• Bacterial overgrowth in blind loops and diverticula of bowel
• Fish tapeworm infestation (*Diphyllobothrium latum*)
3. **Increased demand:** Pregnancy, hyperthyroidism, disseminated cancer
Folic Acid Deficiency
1. **Decreased intake:** Inadequate diet—alcoholism, malnutrition
2. **Impaired absorption**
– Malabsorption states: Nontropical and tropical sprue
– Diffuse infiltrative diseases of the small intestine (e.g., lymphoma)
– Drugs: Anticonvulsant phenytoin and oral contraceptives
3. **Increased loss:** Hemodialysis
4. **Increased demand:** Pregnancy, infancy, disseminated cancer, markedly increased hematopoiesis
5. **Impaired utilization:** Folic acid antagonists, such as methotrexate

Pernicious Anemia

Q. Discuss the etiopathogenesis and morphology of pernicious anemia.

Definition: Pernicious anemia (PA) is an autoimmune disease due to a **deficiency of intrinsic factors** causing **impaired absorption of vitamin B_{12}** and megaloblastic anemia.

Rare in India. A genetic predisposition is suspected.

Age: Older age—**fifth to eighth decades** of life.

Sex: Females are more involved than males (F: M is 1.5:1).

Etiopathogenesis of Pernicious Anemia (Refer Online Flowchart 11.3)

- Pernicious anemia is an **autoimmune** disease due to the destruction of the gastric mucosa.
- **Chronic atrophic gastritis**: Stomach shows **damage to parietal cells** and **dense infiltration by lymphocytes and plasma cells. This produces chronic atrophic gastritis and** failure **of the production of intrinsic factor**.

- **Presence of autoantibodies: Two major types** of autoantibodies in PA are as follows:
  - **Anti-intrinsic factor (IF) antibody**
    - **Type I (blocking) antibody:** Blocks the binding of vitamin B_{12} to IF. Present in 50–75% of the cases.
    - **Type II (binding) antibody:** Attaches to the IF–vitamin B_{12} complex and prevents its binding to receptors in the ileum. Present in about 40% of patients.
  - **Parietal cell (Type III) antibody:** Neither specific for PA nor other autoimmune disorders. It is found in 90% of patients.

MORPHOLOGY OF PERNICIOUS ANEMIA

Alimentary System

- **Atrophic glossitis:** Tongue shiny, glazed, and beefy.
- **Stomach shows diffuse chronic atrophic gastritis:** There is impaired secretion of hydrochloric acid, pepsin, and intrinsic factor. Microscopically, it shows **atrophy of the glands, with loss of both chief cells and parietal cells.** The nuclei of mucosal cells look like that of megaloblasts. There is dense infiltration by lymphocytes and plasma cells. It also shows intestinal metaplasia. Atrophic gastritis may predispose to carcinoma stomach.

Central Nervous System

Involvement of CNS is found in 75% of cases.

- **Demyelination in the dorsal and lateral tracts:** Subacute combined degeneration.
- **Peripheral neuropathy.**

Laboratory Findings of Megaloblastic Anemia

PA 15.2 (CC): Describe laboratory investigations of macrocytic anemia.

Q. Write a short note on the laboratory findings in megaloblastic anemia.

Q. Write a short note on laboratory findings in pernicious anemia.

Blood findings in vitamin B_{12} (including pernicious anemia) and/or folic acid deficiency are similar.

Peripheral Blood

- **Hemoglobin and hematocrit (PCV): Reduced and in severe anemia it may be** *as* low as 2–3 g/dL.
- **Red cell indices**
  - **MCV: It is increased and above 100 fL** (normal 82–98 fL)
  - **MCH: Increased** (normal 27–32 pg)
  - **Normal MCHC** (31–36 g/dL)

Q. Write a short note on the peripheral smear findings in megaloblastic anemia.

Q. Write a short note on the macropolycyte/oval macrocyte.

PA 15.3 (CC): Identify and describe the peripheral blood picture of macrocytic anemia.

PERIPHERAL SMEAR (FIGS. 11.11A AND B)

Pancytopenia: Moderate to severe deficiency shows **pancytopenia** (decreased RBCs, WBCs, and platelets. It is the most common cause of pancytopenia in India.

- **RBCs:**
  - **Macro-ovalocytes:** RBCs are **macrocytic (large) and oval (egg-shaped macro-ovalocytes)** and these are **diagnostic.**
  - **Lack of central pallor:** Most **macrocytes** are well hemoglobinized and **lack the central pallor.**
  - **Anisopoikilocytosis:** Red cells show **marked variation in size and shape.**
  - **Evidence of dyserythropoiesis: Basophilic stippling, Cabot ring** (acidophilic), and **Howell Jolly bodies** (nuclear remnants).
- **WBCs:**
  - **Decreased WBC count** (leukopenia) usually of neutrophils.
  - **Hypersegmented neutrophils:** Normal neutrophils contain three or four nuclear lobes. Hypersegmented neutrophils have **6–10 nuclear segments (more than five nuclear lobes).**

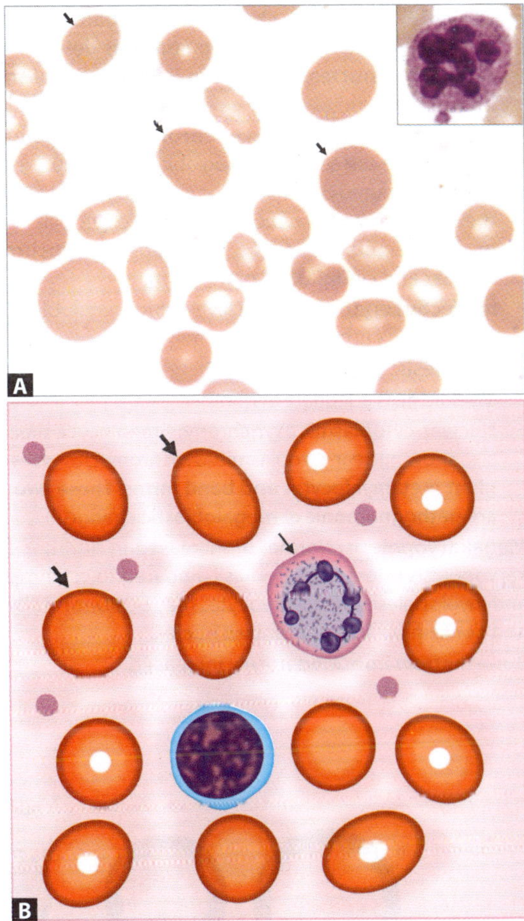

Figs. 11.11A and B: Peripheral blood smear in megaloblastic anemia. (A) Leishman stain shows macro-ovalocytes (arrows) and hypersegmented neutrophils (inset); (B) Diagrammatic appearance showing macroovalocytes (thick arrows) and hypersegmented neutrophils (thin arrow).

The **first and specific morphological sign (earliest change) of megaloblastic anemia.** It appears before the onset of anemia. These neutrophils are **also larger than normal (macropolys).**

- **Platelets: Decreased** (thrombocytopenia) and usually platelets are between 60,000–1,00,000/μL.

Reticulocyte count: In megaloblastic anemia due to vitamin B_{12} deficiency, reticulocyte count may be normal or low. High reticulocyte count is seen on the 7th day following vitamin B_{12} therapy.

Q. Write a short note on megaloblast.

BONE MARROW

- **Cellularity:** Moderately to **markedly hypercellular.**
- **M: E ratio:** Due to marked erythroid hyperplasia, the **M: E ratio is reversed** ranging from 1:1 to 1:6 (normal 2:1 to 4:1).
- **Erythropoiesis: Megaloblastic type (Figs. 11.12 and 11.13).** Different stages of the megaloblastic type of erythropoiesis are presented in **Figure 11.12.**
  - **Megaloblasts:** These are **large, abnormal counterparts of normal normoblasts** (normal erythroid progenitors).
  - **Delicate, sieve-like chromatin**: Megaloblasts have **open sieve-like nuclear chromatin.** This **delicate, finely reticulated nuclear chromatin** is indicative of nuclear immaturity.
  - **Nuclear-cytoplasmic asynchrony:** As megaloblasts differentiate and acquire hemoglobin, the nucleus retains its finely distributed chromatin. The chromatin fails to undergo the clumping typical of normoblasts. The cytoplasm shows normal hemoglobinization. This leads to **asynchrony of nuclear and cytoplasmic maturation.**
  - **Ineffective erythropoiesis:** Developing megaloblasts die in the marrow (intramedullary hemolysis).
- **Myelopoiesis:**
  - Myeloid cells adequate in number.
  - **Nuclear-cytoplasmic asynchrony:** Granulocytic precursors also show nuclear-cytoplasmic asynchrony. This gives rise to **giant metamyelocytes and band forms. These two forms are pathognomonic of megaloblastic change.**
- **Megakaryopoiesis:** Normal or increased in number. Megakaryopoiesis is less disturbed as compared to erythropoiesis and myelopoiesis. Megakaryocytes **may be abnormally large and contain bizarre multilobed nuclei.**
- **Bone marrow iron: Moderately increased.**

The differences between normoblasts and megaloblasts are shown in **Table 11.16.**

Q. List the differences between normoblasts and megaloblasts.

Biochemical Tests for Megaloblastic Anemia

Common for Both Vitamin B_{12} and Folic Acid Deficiency

- **Serum homocysteine:** Increased.
- **Serum bilirubin:** Mild increase (1–3 mg/dL) due to the hemolytic component and causes mild jaundice.
- **Serum iron and ferritin:** Usually elevated.
- **Plasma lactate dehydrogenase (LDH):** Increased
- Serum vitamin B_{12}/folate decreased.

Diagnostic Tests for Vitamin B_{12} Deficiency

- **Serum vitamin B_{12} levels:** Decreased.
- **Serum methylmalonic acid:** Increased.
- **Urinary excretion of methylmalonic acid:** Increased.
- **Schilling test** for vitamin B_{12} absorption (*refer below*).

Deoxyuridine suppression test: It is a sensitive measure of deficiency of 5,10-methylene THF, which occurs in both folic acid and vitamin B_{12} deficiency.

Specific Diagnostic Tests for Pernicious Anemia

Q. What is the Schilling test?

- **Schilling test for vitamin B_{12} absorption: Abnormal.** Diagnostic of PA but now very infrequently performed. The Schilling test was used historically to determine the cause of vitamin B_{12} deficiency. This test involved measuring radiolabeled vitamin B_{12} absorption, with or without intrinsic factor (IF), along with urinary B_{12}. **Helps in distinguishing megaloblastic anemia due to IF deficiency (pernicious anemia) from other causes of vitamin B_{12} deficiency.**
- **Serum antibodies to intrinsic factors** are highly specific for pernicious anemia
- **Achlorhydria** with histamine/pentagastrin stimulation.
- Severe **deficiency of the intrinsic factor.**

Specific Tests for Folic Acid Deficiency

- **Serum folic acid levels:** Decreased.
- **FIGLU in urine: Excessively excreted.**

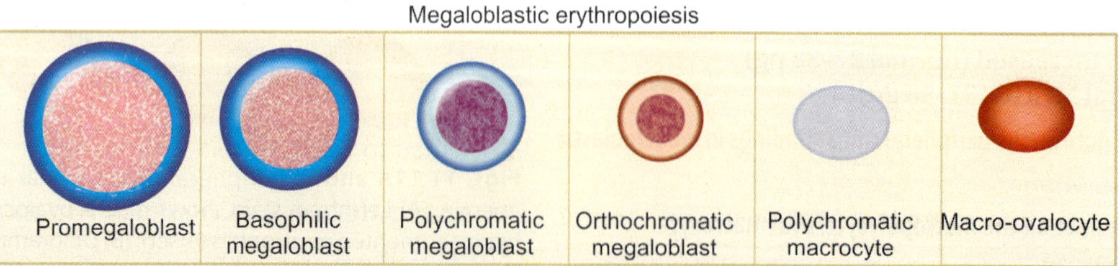

Fig. 11.12: Different stages of megaloblastic type of erythropoiesis (compare with **Fig. 11.2** that shows normal erythropoiesis).

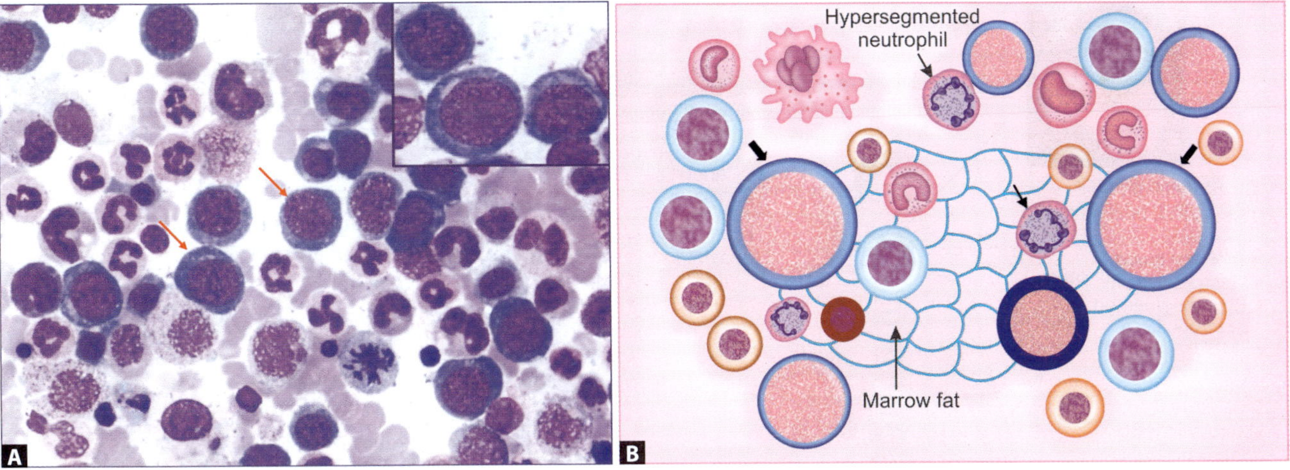

Figs. 11.13A and B: Bone marrow aspirate of megaloblastic anemia: (A) Leishman stain shows megaloblastic precursors (arrows) in varying stages of maturation. The inset shows early megaloblast; (B) Diagrammatic picture of bone marrow aspirates showing megaloblastic precursors (thick arrows) in varying stages of maturation.

TABLE 11.16 Differences between normoblasts and megaloblasts.

Characteristics	*Normoblast*	*Megaloblast*
Cell size	Normal	Larger than the corresponding normoblast
Nuclear chromatin	Normal	Open sieve-like
Nuclear maturation	Normal	Lags behind cytoplasmic maturation
Mitosis	Normal	Increased and abnormal
Maturation in bone marrow	Normal (late > intermediate > early normoblast)	Increased proportion of more primitive erythroid cells (late < intermediate < early megaloblast)
Evidence of dyserythropoiesis	Absent	Present (irregular nuclei, Howell Jolly bodies)
Myelopoiesis	Normal	Shows giant metamyelocytes
Found in	Normal bone marrow	Bone marrow of megaloblastic anemia

Clinical Features of Megaloblastic Anemia

Q. Mention the various clinical features of megaloblastic anemia.

The clinical features of vitamin B_{12} deficiency anemia and pernicious anemia **(Fig. 11.14)** are:

- **Onset: Insidious** and progresses slowly.
- **Classic triad of presentation: Weakness, sore throat, and paresthesia.**
- **Tongue:** Painful red **"beefy"** tongue.
- **PA patients sometimes have a lemon-yellow color** owing to a combination of pallor and mild jaundice caused by excess breakdown of hemoglobin.
- **Neurological manifestations.**

Q. Write a short note on the effects of vitamin B_{12} deficiency on the nervous system.

- **Bilateral peripheral neuropathy:** Glove and sock distribution of **numbness or paresthesia.**
  - **Demyelination of spinal cord: Subacute combined demyelination/degeneration of dorsal and lateral tracts—ataxia**, uncoordinated gait, impairment of vibration, and position sense.
- **Atherosclerosis:** Serum homocysteine level is raised and is a **risk factor for atherosclerosis** and thrombosis.

Macrocytic Anemia

Q. What is macrocytic anemia? List the causes of macrocytic anemia.

PA 15.4 (NC): Enumerate the differences and describe the etiology and distinguishing features of megaloblastic and non-megaloblastic macrocytic anemia.

Macrocytic anemia: It is characterized by the **presence of abnormally large RBCs in the peripheral blood**. This is usually recognized by the automated blood cell counter and confirmed on examination of the peripheral blood smear. **Categories:** Based on the examination of the bone marrow, macrocytic anemia can be divided into two categories **(i) megaloblastic and (ii) nonmegaloblastic**. This division is important and frequently helps in determining the etiology of the anemia. The causes of megaloblastic anemia are presented in **Table 11.15.**

Nonmegaloblastic Causes of Macrocytic Anemia

Box 11.6 shows the etiology of nonmegaloblastic macrocytic anemia.

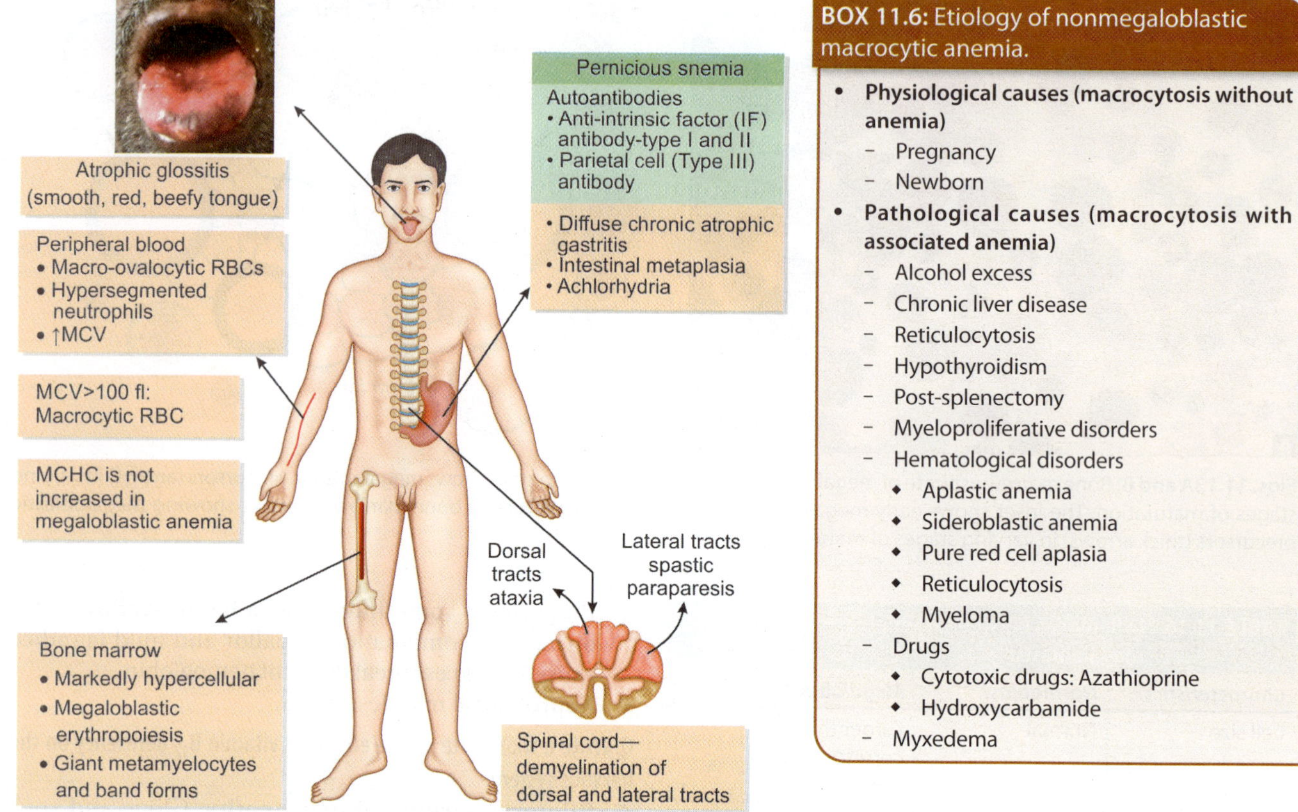

BOX 11.6: Etiology of nonmegaloblastic macrocytic anemia.

- **Physiological causes (macrocytosis without anemia)**
  - Pregnancy
  - Newborn
- **Pathological causes (macrocytosis with associated anemia)**
  - Alcohol excess
  - Chronic liver disease
  - Reticulocytosis
  - Hypothyroidism
  - Post-splenectomy
  - Myeloproliferative disorders
  - Hematological disorders
    - Aplastic anemia
    - Sideroblastic anemia
    - Pure red cell aplasia
    - Reticulocytosis
    - Myeloma
  - Drugs
    - Cytotoxic drugs: Azathioprine
    - Hydroxycarbamide
  - Myxedema

Fig. 11.14: Clinical features and laboratory findings in megaloblastic anemia including pernicious anemia.

Investigation of Macrocytosis

The evaluation of macrocytosis needs a systemic approach and consists of a comprehensive history and physical examination followed by appropriate laboratory investigations. Laboratory studies include a complete blood count, a peripheral blood smear, and a reticulocyte count. In certain cases, it may be necessary to perform a bone marrow examination.

Peripheral blood smear: Examination of the peripheral smear is important for the determination of the etiology of macrocytosis.

- The presence of **macro-ovalocytes having an MCV >115 fL**, anisocytosis, poikilocytosis, and **hypersegmented neutrophils** suggests **megaloblastic anemia** due to a nutritional deficiency (i.e., vitamin B_{12} or folate deficiency).
- **Round macrocytes** are commonly seen in **many chronic disorders**.
- **Round target-appearing macrocytes** are characteristic of **liver diseases** such as hepatitis, obstructive jaundice, and acute and chronic alcoholism with liver disease.

Reticulocyte count: Its interpretations are as follows:

- **Hemolysis or an acute bleed**: The presence of **increased polychromasia** of the macrocytes on the peripheral smear and a **reticulocyte count of >10%** should raise suspicion of hemolysis or an acute bleed.
- **Increased erythropoiesis**: The **large polychromatophilic RBCs** on the peripheral smear represent reticulocytes, immature RBCs that are larger than mature RBCs. Their presence indicates increased erythropoiesis or RBC production and, if present in increased numbers, can raise MCV.

Bone marrow examination: Its interpretations are as follows:

- **Megaloblastic marrow: Macrocytosis associated with megaloblastic marrow is usually associated with anemia due to ineffective erythropoiesis** (*refer* to bone marrow findings in megaloblastic anemia on page 338).
- **Nonmegaloblastic marrow:** Nonmegaloblastic macrocytic anemia does not show any megaloblasts in the marrow.

Other investigations: They depend on the probable cause of nonmegaloblastic macrocytic anemia.

Salient laboratory findings in megaloblastic anemia are presented (*refer* **online Box 11.7).**

Dimorphic Anemia

- A mixture of microcytic hypochromic and macrocytic RBCs is termed a dimorphic picture and occurs in combined vitamin B_{12}/folic acid and iron deficiency.
- Peripheral smear shows two populations of RBCs namely—macro-ovalocytes and microcytic hypochromic **(Fig. 11.15)**.

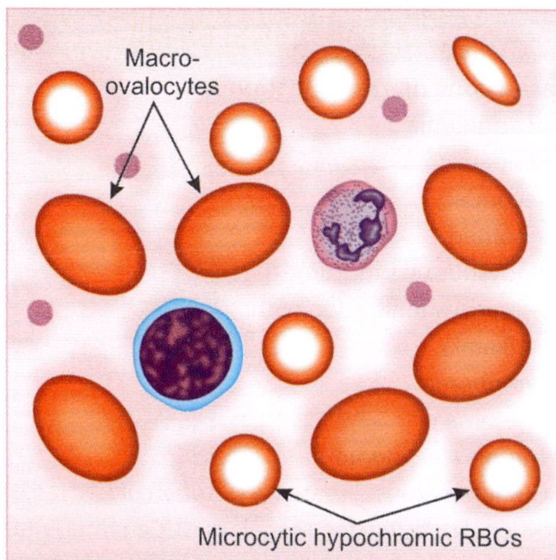

Fig. 11.15: Diagrammatic peripheral blood smear of dimorphic anemia showing macro-ovalocytes and microcytes.

APLASTIC ANEMIA

PA 17.1 (NC): Enumerate the etiology, pathogenesis, and findings in aplastic anemia.

Q. Write a short note on aplastic anemia.

Definition: Aplastic anemia is a disorder in which there is **suppression of multipotent myeloid stem cells.** This leads to **bone marrow failure and pancytopenia** (anemia, neutropenia, and thrombocytopenia). The **bone marrow is markedly hypocellular** (less than 30% cellularity).

Etiology

Q. Write a short note on the causes of aplastic anemia.

The most common causes associated with aplastic anemia are shown in **Box 11.8.**

BOX 11.8: Common causes of aplastic anemia.

Acquired

Idiopathic: Acquired stem cell defects, immune-mediated

Secondary

- **Chemical agents:**
  - **Dose-related:** Alkylating agents, benzene, chloramphenicol
  - **Idiosyncratic:** Chloramphenicol, phenylbutazone, carbamazepine
- **Physical agents:** Whole-body Irradiation
- **Viral infections:** Hepatitis virus, Epstein-Barr virus, cytomegalovirus, herpes zoster (varicella-zoster), HIV

Inherited

- Fanconi anemia
- Telomerase defects

5 "I"s

1. Idiopathic
2. Idiosyncratic
3. Irradiation
4. Infections
5. Inherited

Pathogenesis (Fig. 11.16)

The exact pathogenesis of aplastic anemia is not known and probably involves several mechanisms. Two major mechanisms may be involved (i) an extrinsic, immune-mediated suppression of marrow progenitors, and (ii) an intrinsic abnormality of stem cells.

Extrinsic, immune-mediated suppression of marrow progenitors: Stem cells may first be antigenically altered by exposure to drugs, infectious agents, or other unidentified environmental agents. This causes a cellular immune response with the activation of T cells. The activated Th1 cells produce cytokines such as interferon-γ (IFN-γ) and TNF. These cytokines suppress and kill hematopoietic progenitors (stem cells).

Intrinsic abnormality of stem cells: According to this, the aplastic anemia results from a fundamental stem cell abnormality. Some marrow insult (or a predisposition to DNA damage) probably produces sufficient injury to stem cells This may limit the proliferative and differentiation capacity of stem cells. If the damage is severe, it results in aplastic anemia. About **5–10% of patients with aplastic anemia have inherited defects in telomerase** (needed for the maintenance and stability of chromosomes). Defects in the telomerase lead to premature senescence of hematopoietic stem cells. These genetically altered stem

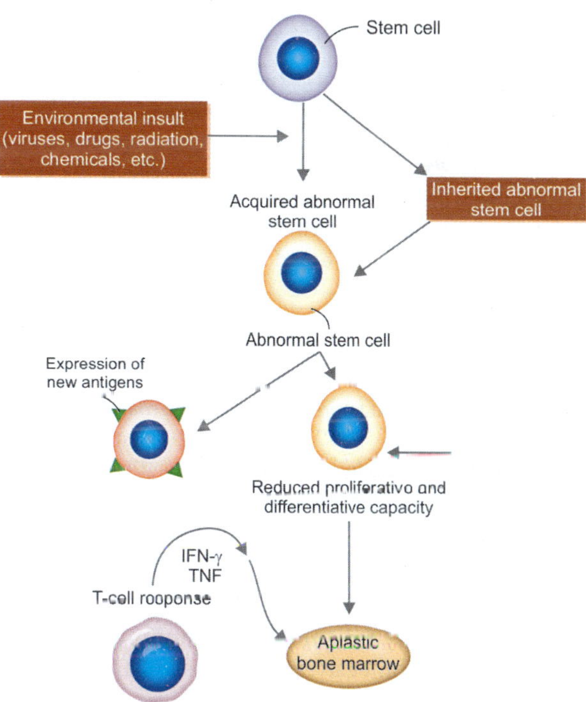

Fig. 11.16: Pathogenesis of aplastic anemia. Damage to stem cells may be by extrinsic agents or an inherited abnormality. These abnormal stem cells can produce progeny expressing neoantigens that induce an autoimmune reaction, or give rise to a clonal population with reduced proliferative capacity.

cells (e.g., those with abnormal telomeres) also might express "neoantigens." T cells can attack these cells.

In both the above-mentioned mechanisms, the stem cells are genetically altered and may express "neoantigens" that could act as targets for a T-cell attack.

Clinical Features

Any age of both sexes. Symptoms are due to pancytopenia and include the following:

- **Anemia:** Slowly progressive development of weakness, pallor, and dyspnea due to anemia.
- **Neutropenia:** Frequent (mucocutaneous bacterial infections) or fatal infections due to neutropenia.
- **Thrombocytopenia:** Bleeding manifestations in the form of petechiae, bruises, and ecchymoses due to thrombocytopenia.

Laboratory Findings

Peripheral Blood

- **Hemoglobin: Reduced**
- **Packed cell volume (PCV): Reduced**
- **Reticulocyte count: Markedly decreased (less than** <1%) and is a **characteristic feature**.
- **Pancytopenia: Decreased red cells, neutrophils (absolute neutrophil count reduced), and platelets.**

Q. Write a short note on peripheral smear in aplastic anemia.

PERIPHERAL SMEAR

Pancytopenia: All the blood cells are decreased

- **RBCs: Normocytic normochromic anemia.**
- **WBCs: Total leukocyte count decreased. Neutrophils are markedly diminished** and neutropenia reflects the severity of aplasia. Initial stages, lymphocytes are normal in number as the disease progresses their count decreases.
- **Platelets:** Count is **decreased.**

BONE MARROW

Bone marrow elements are replaced by fat and aspiration usually yields dry tap or diluted with blood.

Marrow aplasia—best appreciated in a **bone marrow (trephine) biopsy**

- **Cellularity:** Marked **hypocellularity.**
- **Hematopoiesis: Deficiency of all erythroid, myeloid, and megakaryocytic precursors.**
- **Other cells: Lymphocytes and plasma cells are prominent and are relatively increased.**

No splenomegaly (absence of splenomegaly): In the presence of splenomegaly, the diagnosis of aplastic anemia should not be made.

Diagnosis: Diagnosis is made with **peripheral blood** and **bone marrow biopsy findings.**

Differential diagnosis: Aplastic anemia should be distinguished from other causes of pancytopenia **(Box 11.9).**

BOX 11.9: Causes of pancytopenia.

Decreased bone marrow function

- Aplastic anemia
  - Idiopathic
  - Secondary
  - Inherited
- Myelodysplastic syndromes
- Bone marrow infiltration with:
  - Leukemia
  - Lymphoma
  - Myeloma
  - Tumors (carcinoma)
  - Granulomatous diseases (e.g., tuberculosis, sarcoidosis)
- Nutritional deficiencies: Megaloblastic anemia (vitamin B12 and folic acid deficiency)
- Paroxysmal nocturnal hemoglobinuria
- Myelofibrosis (rare)
- Hemophagocytic syndrome

Increased peripheral destruction: Hypersplenism

Pancytopenia

Q. Write a short note on pancytopenia.

Definition. Pancytopenia is defined as a condition in which there is a reduction in the number of red and white blood cells, as well as platelets.

Prognosis of aplastic anemia: Unpredictable.

INCREASED RED CELL DESTRUCTION (HEMOLYTIC ANEMIAS)

PA 16.1 (CC): Define and classify hemolytic anemia.

Q. Define and classify hemolytic anemia.

Definition: Hemolytic anemias are a diverse group of disorders characterized by an increase in the rate of red cell destruction (hemolysis/premature elimination from circulation).

Consequences: The red cell life span of normal RBCs is about 120 days. The consequences of hemolysis (premature destruction of RBCs) are as follows:

- **Anemia:** In hemolytic anemia RBC life span is shortened, often markedly. It results in anemia. **Morphological features of RBC destruction** include the presence of **microspherocytes*, elliptocytes, red cell fragments**, etc., in the peripheral blood. Red cell survival is **shortened** and can be detected by the 51Crlabeled method.
- **Erythroid hyperplasia and reticulocytosis:** These are hallmarks of hemolytic anemias. Anemia and resultant tissue hypoxia stimulate increased erythropoietin (EPO) release from the kidney. Increased erythropoietin

produces **compensatory erythroid hyperplasia in the bone marrow**. Bone marrow hyperplasia leads to **increased** production of reticulocytes and the **peripheral blood shows reticulocytosis**.

- **Expansion of marrow space**: X-ray of the bone shows expansion of marrow space especially in tubular bones and skull. Mostly found in hereditary hemolytic anemias like **thalassemia and sickle cell anemia**.

- **Extramedullary hematopoiesis**: In severe hemolytic anemias, **when marrow erythroid hyperplasia is not able to improve moderate to severe anemia**, extramedullary hematopoiesis develops in the **liver, spleen, and lymph nodes**.
- **Other laboratory findings associated with hemolysis**: These include **increased LDH** (particularly isoenzyme 1) and **unconjugated (indirect) bilirubin, decreased haptoglobin, free (extracellular) hemoglobin in the blood and urine, increased urobilinogen, and urine hemosiderin**.

Classification of Hemolytic Anemias (Box 11.10)

Q. Enumerate the causes of hemolytic anemia.

Q. List the differences between extravascular hemolysis and intravascular hemolysis.

There are several ways to classify hemolytic anemias. It depends on:

Source of defect causing hemolysis: Whether the pathogenic red cell defect is **intrinsic (intracorpuscular) or extrinsic (extracorpuscular)**.

Mode of onset: Hereditary and acquired disorders.

Underlying mechanisms of hemolysis.

Location of hemolysis: A clinically useful approach is to classify according to whether hemolysis is primarily extravascular or intravascular. In **most hemolytic anemias red cell destruction is extravascular**.

- **Extravascular hemolysis:** It is caused by factors "extrinsic" to the RBC (e.g., immune, mechanical, thermal, and osmotic causes). It is **due to defects that increase the destruction of red cells by phagocytes. This particularly occurs in the spleen.** Features that are relatively specific for extravascular hemolysis (as compared to intravascular hemolysis) are as follows:
  - **Hyperbilirubinemia and jaundice**: These are due to the degradation of hemoglobin in macrophages (especially in the spleen).
  - **Splenomegaly**: It shows varying degrees of *splenomegaly* due to "work hyperplasia" of phagocytes in the spleen.
  - **Pigment stones:** If long-standing hemolytic anemia, the patient has an increased risk of developing *cholelithiasis*. These are *bilirubin-rich gallstones* (pigment stones).
- **Intravascular hemolysis:** In this type of hemolysis, **RBCs are destroyed while circulating**. It **is characterized by injuries to red cells that are so severe that they rupture within the circulation.** The causes of intravascular (extrinsic abnormalities) hemolysis are presented in **Box 11.10**.

Features that distinguish intravascular hemolysis from extravascular hemolysis are as follows:

- **Hemoglobinemia, hemoglobinuria, and hemosiderinuria:** In intravascular hemolysis, the **hemoglobin is released into the circulation (hemoglobinemia).** Free **hemoglobin in the plasma combines with a plasma protein called haptoglobin. This leads to a marked decrease in serum haptoglobin levels**. A small amount **of hemoglobin is excreted in the urine (hemoglobinuria)**. This hemoglobin in urine is partly resorbed by renal tubular cells and is converted into hemosiderin. The **hemosiderin is passed in the urine (hemosiderinuria)** when renal tubular cells are shed.

BOX 11.10: Classification, and causes of hemolytic anemia.

Intrinsic (Intracorpuscular) Abnormalities

- **Hereditary (inherited)**
  - **Red cell membrane abnormalities:** Hereditary spherocytosis, hereditary elliptocytosis
  - **Enzyme deficiencies**
    a. **Hexose monophosphate shunt enzyme deficiencies:** G6PD deficiency
    b. **Glycolytic enzyme deficiencies:** Pyruvate kinase deficiency, hexokinase deficiency
  - **Disorders of hemoglobin synthesis**
    a. **Deficient globin synthesis:** Thalassemia syndromes
    b. **Structurally abnormal globin synthesis (hemoglobinopathies):** Sickle cell anemia
- **Acquired**
  - **Membrane defect*:** Paroxysmal nocturnal hemoglobinuria (deficiency of phosphatidylinositol-linked glycoproteins)

Extrinsic (Extracorpuscular) Abnormalities

- **Antibody-mediated (immunohemolytic anemias)**
  - **Isohemagglutinins:** Hemolytic disease (Rh disease) of the newborn, transfusion reactions*
  - **Autoantibodies*:** Idiopathic (primary), drug-associated, autoimmune diseases (e.g., systemic lupus erythematosus)
- **Mechanical trauma to red cells (Fragmentation syndrome)***
  - **Microangiopathic hemolytic anemias:** Hemolytic uremic syndrome, disseminated intravascular coagulation, thrombotic thrombocytopenic purpura
  - **Dysfunctional cardiac valves** (turbulence created by a defective heart valve)
- **Infections of red cells*:** Malaria, babesiosis and COVID-19.

(G6PD: glucose-6-phosphate dehydrogenase).

* Intravascular hemolysis

TABLE 11.17 Differences between extravascular and intravascular hemolysis.

Characteristics	*Extravascular hemolysis*	*Intravascular hemolysis*
Site of hemolysis	RE system (spleen, bone marrow)	Within circulation
Splenomegaly	Usual	Uncommon
Laboratory findings		
• Serum bilirubin (unconjugated)	Moderately raised	Mildly raised
• Serum haptoglobin	Normal	Decreased and is characteristic of intravascular hemolysis
• Hemoglobinemia	Not seen	Positive
• Lactate dehydrogenase	Mildly raised	Moderately raised
Urine		
Hemoglobinuria (hemoglobin in the urine)	Absent	Present
Hemosiderinuria (hemosiderin in the urine)	Absent	Present
Examples of hemolytic anemia	Thalassemia, sickle cell anemia	G6PD deficiency, PNH

(RE: reticuloendothelial; G6PD: glucose-6-phosphate dehydrogenase; PNH: paroxysmal nocturnal hemoglobinuria).

- **Loss of iron: Persistent intravascular hemolysis may lead to iron deficiency.** By contrast, in extravascular hemolysis, iron recycling by phagocytes is very efficient. Hence, **iron deficiency is not a feature of extravascular hemolytic anemias.**

The differences between the extravascular hemolysis and intravascular hemolysis are listed in **Table 11.17**.

Laboratory Findings in Hemolytic Anemias

PA 16.2 (CC): Describe the pathogenesis, clinical features, and hematologic indices of hemolytic anemia.

Q. Write a short note on laboratory findings in hemolytic anemias.

Peripheral Blood

PA 16.5 (CC): Describe the peripheral blood picture in different hemolytic anemias.

Decreased hemoglobin: Hemoglobin is decreased and varies with the type and duration of hemolytic anemia.

Markedly increased reticulocyte count.

PA 16.6 (CC): Perform and show how to prepare a peripheral blood smear (*refer* pages 440-1) and identify hemolytic anemia from it. The procedure requires certification.

Q. Write a short note on the peripheral blood picture of hemolytic anemias.

PERIPHERAL SMEAR

It is the **most important investigation in hemolytic anemia.** The following findings alone or in combination suggest hemolysis:

- **Red blood cells (RBCs)**
  - **Markedly increased reticulocyte count:** These reticulocytes appear as large **polychromatophilic red blood cells** in the peripheral blood.
  - **Nucleated red cells:** Moderate to marked hemolysis results in the appearance of **nucleated red cells, mostly late normoblasts.**
  - **Red cell morphology**: It provides a clue to the underlying hemolytic disorders like **spherocyte, sickle cell, target cell, acanthocyte, schistocyte, malarial parasite, etc.**
- **White blood cells: Neutrophilia with a shift to left** (increase in the percentage of immature/young neutrophils in the circulating blood) and the presence of metamyelocytes and myelocytes are seen in active hemolysis.
- **Platelets:** In acute hemolysis, there is **thrombocytosis** with numerous large platelets.

BONE MARROW

Bone marrow examination is **usually not necessary for the diagnosis** of hemolytic anemia.

- **Cellularity:** Due to **erythroid hyperplasia, the overall cellularity** of the bone marrow is **increased.**
- **Erythropoiesis:** Anemia with tissue hypoxia stimulates increased production of erythropoietin, which causes erythroid hyperplasia in bone marrow. **Erythroid hyperplasia is the morphological hallmark** of various hemolytic anemias and is characterized by the **increased number of erythroid precursors (normoblasts) in the marrow.**
- **M: E ratio:** The myeloid-erythroid ratio is **decreased with a reversal ranging from 1:1 to 1:6.**

HEREDITARY SPHEROCYTOSIS

Q. Discuss the etiology and diagnosis of hereditary spherocytosis.

Definition: Hereditary spherocytosis (HS) is a rare **hemolytic anemia** resulting from an **inherited defect in the red cell membrane.** It **leads to the formation of spherocytes. These RBCs are nondeformable cells that are highly susceptible to sequestration and destruction in the spleen.**

Q. Describe the etiopathogenesis/molecular pathology of hereditary spherocytosis.

Normal structure of the RBC membrane (Fig. 11.17A): The membrane skeleton of RBC consists of a network of proteins. These proteins stabilize the lipid bilayer of the red cell. The major membrane skeleton protein is **spectrin**. It is a long, flexible that self-associates at one end with another spectrin and binds short **actin filaments** at its other end. These contacts produce a two-dimensional meshwork. This meshwork is connected to the intrinsic membrane **proteins band 3 and glycophorin A** via **linker proteins namely ankyrin and band 4.1.**

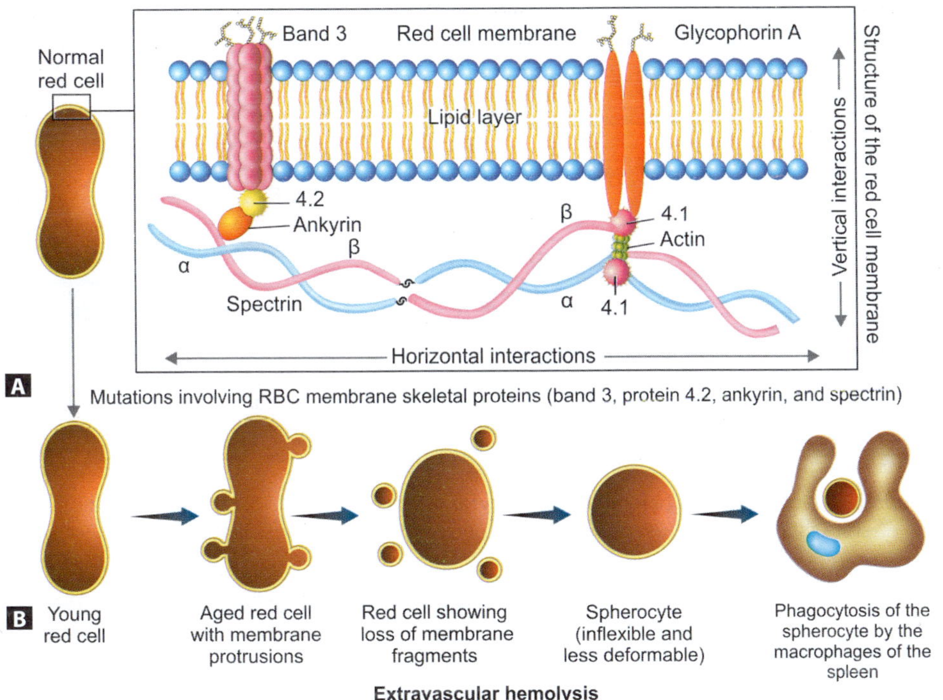

Figs. 11.17A and B: Pathogenesis of hereditary spherocytosis. (A) Shows normal red cell membrane with the relationship of the major red cell membrane skeleton proteins. Mutations in spectrin, ankyrin, band 4.2, and band 3 weaken the association between the membrane skeleton and the plasma membrane. This causes red cells to shed membrane vesicles (fragments) into the circulation. These RBCs are transformed into spherocytes (B). The spherocytes are inflexible and nondeformable. Hence, they are trapped in the spleen and are phagocytosed by macrophages.

Pathogenesis (Figs. 11.18A and B)

- HS is usually transmitted as an **autosomal dominant** disorder.
- **RBC membrane protein defect: Hereditary spherocytosis is caused by inherited** (intrinsic) **defects in the** RBC **membrane skeleton.** It is caused by various **mutations, most common mutations involve band 3, protein 4.2, ankyrin, or spectrin (Fig. 11.17B).**
- **Spherical RBCs:** The mutations in RBC membrane proteins weaken interactions between the membrane skeleton and intrinsic red cell membrane proteins. This destabilizes the lipid bilayer of red cells. Young RBCs in hereditary spherocytosis are normal in shape. But **as they age, RBCs shed membrane vesicles (fragments) into the circulation.** During this process, a small amount of cytoplasm is lost. As the time progresses, the **RBCs assume a spherical shape (spherocytes).**
- **Extravascular hemolysis: Spherocytes are rigid, inflexible, and less deformable.** They get trapped in the spleen leading to **premature destruction** of spherocytes. **Splenectomy is beneficial in HS, and this indicates the important role of the spleen in hereditary spherocytosis. Splenectomy corrects anemia, but the red cell defect and spherocytes persist.**

Laboratory Findings

Q. Write a short note on laboratory findings in hereditary spherocytosis.

Peripheral Blood

- **Decreased hemoglobin:** The level depends on the degree of hemolysis.
- **Red cell indices**
  - **MCV: Reduced** (normal 82–98 fL)
  - **MCHC: Raised and >35 g/dL** (normal 31–36 g/dL).
- **Reticulocyte count: Increased**

Q. Write a short note on spherocyte.

PERIPHERAL SMEAR

Peripheral smear examination is very important for diagnosis (**Figs. 11.18A and B**).

- **RBCs:**
  - **Spherocytes** are **most distinctive but not pathognomonic.** Spherocytes are **small, dark staining** (hyperchromic) **RBCs without any central pallor.**
  - **Reticulocytosis:** The anemia due to excessive red cell destruction leads to compensatory hyperplasia of red cell progenitors in the marrow. This causes an increase in red cell production marked by reticulocytosis.
- **WBCs:** Total leukocyte count (TLC) **increased.**
- **Platelets:** Normal.

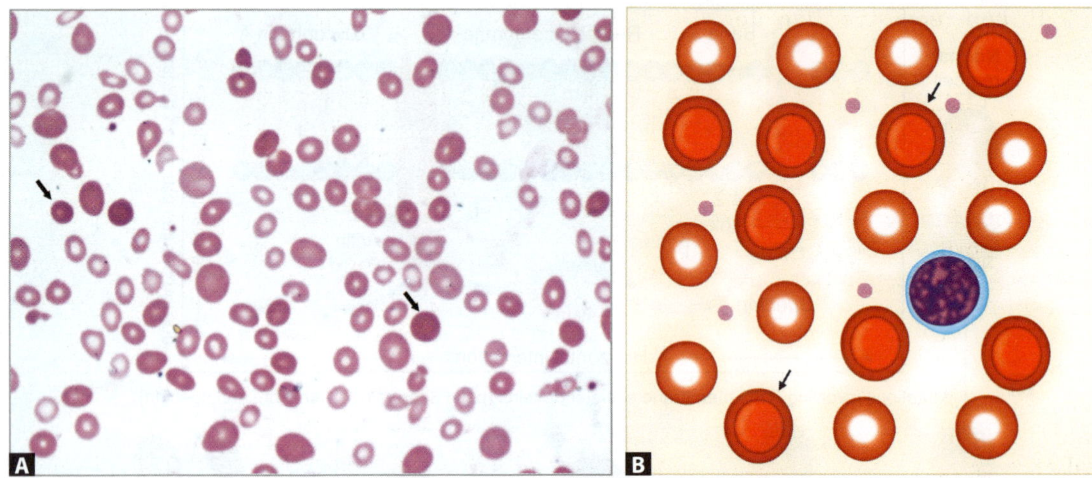

Figs. 11.18A and B: Peripheral blood smear of hereditary spherocytosis: (A) Leishman stain; (B) Diagrammatic. The peripheral blood smear shows numerous spherocytes (arrows) and anisocytosis (variation in size).

BONE MARROW

- **Cellularity: Markedly hypercellular**
- **M:E ratio:** Increased and may be 8:1.
- **Erythropoiesis: Erythroid hyperplasia**
- **Myelopoiesis:** Normal
- **Megakaryopoiesis:** Normal.

Autohemolysis Test

In this test, blood is incubated at 37°C for 48 hours and the amount of hemolysis is noted. Hereditary spherocytes show a **marked increase in spontaneous autohemolysis** (10–15% of red cells compared to normal which is less than 4%) and may be partially corrected by the addition of glucose.

Direct Antiglobulin (Coomb's) Test

It is **negative** and helps to distinguish from acquired immunohemolytic anemia where it is positive (for details, *refer* pages 359-60).

Biochemical Findings

- **Mildly raised serum bilirubin.**
- **Increased urine urobilinogen.**
- **Decreased serum haptoglobin.**

Osmotic Fragility Test

Osmotic fragility (for details, *refer pages* 449-50): Red cells in hereditary spherocytosis show increased osmotic fragility (**shift of the curve to the right**) when placed in hypotonic salt solutions (*refer* **Figs. 15.10 and 15.11**). This can help to establish the diagnosis.

Clinical Features

- **Age:** Anytime from the **neonatal** period **to adulthood**.
- **Family history:** Most (75%) are inherited as **autosomal dominant trait**.

BOX 11.11: Causes of spherocytes in peripheral smears.

- Hereditary spherocytosis
- Autoimmune hemolytic anemia
- ABO hemolytic disease of the newborn
- Hypersplenism
- Hemolytic transfusion reaction
- Burns.

- **Characteristic features: These consist of anemia, splenomegaly, and jaundice.**
  - **Anemia:** Mild to moderate
  - **Jaundice: Intermittent attacks**, precipitated by pregnancy, fatigue, or infection.
  - **Splenomegaly:** It is more common and prominent in hereditary spherocytosis than in other hemolytic anemia. The weight of the spleen is usually between 500 g and 1,000 g (normal, 150–200 g).
- **Gallstones (cholelithiasis): Pigment** gallstones occur in 40–50% of patients with hereditary spherocytosis.
- **Aplastic crises:** The course of HS is usually stable but may develop recurrent *aplastic crises.*
  - **These may be triggered by an acute parvovirus infection.**

Causes of spherocytes in peripheral smears are listed in **Box 11.11**.

Q. Causes of spherocytes in peripheral smears.

GLUCOSE-6-PHOSPHATE DEHYDROGENASE (G6PD) DEFICIENCY

Q. Write a short note on G6PD deficiency.

- G6PD deficiency is due to **red cell enzyme defects**.
- In G6PD deficiency, **RBCs are susceptible to oxidative injury** by free radicals. There are different subtypes.

- It is an **X-linked recessive disorder** and its **full expression is seen only in males.**

Pathogenesis

Reduced glutathione (GSH) in normal RBCs protects them against oxidant injury by the breakdown of compounds such as H_2O_2 to H_2O. The **housekeeping enzyme, G6PD is required for normal GSH.** In G6PD deficiency, oxidants can cause primarily **intravascular hemolysis.**

- In G6PD deficiency, there is decreased synthesis of **reduced glutathione.**
- **RBCs, when exposed to oxidant stress** (during infections, exposure to drugs such as primaquine, sulfonamides, nitrofurantoin, phenacetin, aspirin or chemicals, fava beans) **accumulate H_2O_2.** It damages the RBC membrane causing **hemolysis.**
- Hemolyzed red cells **liberate hemoglobin.**
- **The hemoglobin is oxidized** by oxidants leading to the formation of **methemoglobin, which** forms **Heinz bodies (Fig. 11.19)** in the cytoplasm of RBCs.
- Heinz bodies are removed from the RBC membrane by macrophages in the spleen and **bite cells** are produced. These bite cells are removed via **erythrophagocytosis in the spleen.**

Clinical Presentation

G6PD deficiency manifests in several distinct clinical patterns. Usually present as self-limited **(transient) acute episodes of intravascular hemolytic anemia** following exposure to oxidative stress. G6PD deficiency has a protective effect against *Plasmodium falciparum* malaria.

Laboratory Findings

Peripheral Blood

- **Hemoglobin: Decreased**
- **Reticulocyte count: Increased**

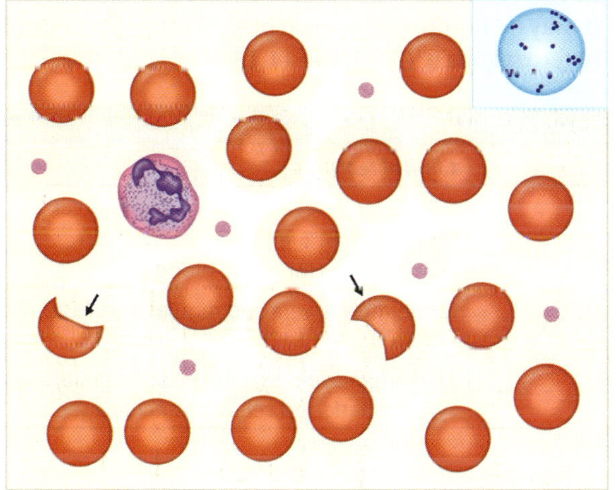

Fig. 11.19: Peripheral blood smear in G6PD deficiency with "bite cells" (arrows). The inset shows Heinz bodies (supravital stain).

PERIPHERAL SMEAR

- **RBCs:** Moderate anisopoikilocytosis with **polychromatophilia, microspherocytes,** and **bite cells (Fig. 11.19). Heinz bodies are identified with a supravital stain** and are best seen during active hemolysis.
- **WBCs:** Mild leukocytosis.
- **Platelets: Normal.**

Self-limited hemolysis: Primarily, the **old red cells are hemolyzed,** hence hemolysis is self-limited.

Others

Urine: Hemoglobinuria will be found **during hemolysis** and may last for about 1–6 days.

RBC enzyme analysis: Tests for G6PD deficiency are positive and should be assessed a few weeks after the acute hemolytic episode.

Conditions protecting against malaria are listed (*refer* **online Box 11.12**).

HEREDITARY DEFECTS IN HEMOGLOBIN

Classification of Hereditary Defects in Hemoglobin

Q. Classify hereditary disorders of hemoglobin.

Hemoglobin defects may be quantitative (reduced production of normal hemoglobin) or qualitative (production of abnormal hemoglobin).

Quantitative defect: Genetic mutations in the globin loci (e.g., thalassemia) may quantitatively reduce the synthesis of α-*globin* or β-*globin* chain. It leads to a net reduction of hemoglobin.

Qualitative defect: Genetic mutations in the α-*globin or* β-*globin* locus may produce abnormal hemoglobin (e.g., sickle cell anemia). The abnormal hemoglobin may be functionally normal, but its physical or physiologic properties differ from normal hemoglobin. The term **hemoglobinopathy is usually used for a qualitative hereditary disorder of hemoglobin. Hemoglobinopathies** are a group of hereditary disorders caused due to inherited mutations producing **structural abnormalities in hemoglobin.** One example is **sickle cell disease (SCD)** is a group of hereditary disorders of hemoglobin characterized by the production of **defective hemoglobin called sickle hemoglobin (HbS).** On low oxygen tension or deoxygenation, RBC with **HbS becomes sickle-shaped.** HbS is produced due to a **qualitative defect in hemoglobin production** caused by a mutation in the β-globin gene.

THALASSEMIA

PA 16.3b (CC): Describe the pathogenesis, features, hematologic indices, and peripheral blood picture of thalassemia.

Q. Classify thalassemia.

Q. Write a short note on the molecular pathogenesis of β-thalassemia.

Q. Describe the laboratory findings in β-thalassemia major.

A thalassemia is a group of **inherited (congenital) disorders caused by deficient globin chain synthesis due to mutations in globin genes.** It is characterized by **decreased or absence of synthesis of either α or β-globin chain** of adult hemoglobin, HbA ($\alpha_2\beta_2$).

Normal hemoglobin and its variants: Normal hemoglobin contains four globin chains: two α- and two non–α-chains. Based on the nature of the non–α-chains, there are three normal hemoglobin variants.

- **Adult hemoglobin (HbA):** It constitutes 95–98% of hemoglobin in adults. It is a tetramer composed of two α chains and two β chains ($\alpha_2\beta_2$). The α chains are encoded by two α-globin genes on chromosome 16, and the β chains are encoded by a single β-globin gene on chromosome 11.
- **Hemoglobin A2 (HBA2):** It consists of two α chains and two δ chains ($\alpha_2\ \delta_2$).
- **Fetal hemoglobin (HbF):** It is present in small amounts and consists of two α chains and two γ chains ($\alpha_2\gamma_2$).

Normal adult cell contains 96% HbA ($\alpha_2\beta_2$), 3% HbA_2 ($\alpha_2\delta_2$) and 1% HbF ($\alpha_2\gamma_2$).

Anemia and hemolysis: Consequences of decreased synthesis of one globin chain are:

- **Deficient hemoglobin formation**
- **Hemolysis**: The excess of unpaired normal globin chain forms intracellular precipitates causes damage to red cells and leads to hemolysis.

Classification

Thalassemia is mainly classified depending on the affected globin chain as:

- **β-Thalassemia syndromes: Impaired synthesis of β-chains** of globin.
- **α-Thalassemia syndromes: Impaired synthesis of** α-chains of globin.
- **Miscellaneous thalassemia syndromes.**

The basic defect is usually a "quantitative abnormality" with reduced or absent production of the respective globin chains (i.e., reduced levels of β-globin in β-thalassemia or α-globin in α-thalassemia). Normal adult hemoglobin contains α- and β-chains paired to form hemoglobin tetramers. The lack of one type of globin chain leads to unpaired normal globin chains in RBCs. In β-thalassemia, excess normal α-chains form an unstable structure that precipitates at the RBC membrane. This makes the RBCs very fragile, and they are destroyed within the bone marrow.

β-Thalassemia

- **Autosomal recessive** hereditary disorder.
- **Diminished synthesis** of **β-globin chains** and **normal synthesis of a-chains.**

Molecular Pathology

β-globin chains are encoded by a single gene.

Mutations: Different types of **mutations in the β-globin gene** can occur in β-thalassemia. More than 100 different causative mutations can occur in the **β-globin gene**, majority consist of single-base changes. Point mutations leading to aberrant RNA splicing are the most common cause of β-thalassemia. These mutations fall into two categories:

1. β^0: In this, there is no production of β-globin chains.
2. β^+: In this, there is reduced (but detectable) β-globin synthesis.

Table 11.18 shows the clinical and genetic classification of β-thalassemias.

β-THALASSEMIA MAJOR

- β-thalassemia major (also called Mediterranean or Cooley's anemia) is a **hereditary hemolytic anemia** due to the **absence of synthesis of the β-globin** chain of hemoglobin. The **synthesis of the α-globin** chain **is not affected.**
- It may be homozygous form of β^0/β^0 or β^+/β^+ or double heterozygous β^0/β^+ **(Table 11.18).**

TABLE 11.18 Clinical and genetic classification of β-thalassemias.

Clinical syndromes	*Genotype*	*Clinical features*
β-thalassemia major (inherit any two β^0 and β^+ alleles)	Homozygous (β^0/β^0, β^+/β^+) or double heterozygous (β^0/β^+)	Severe form, severe anemia, and regular transfusion required. High level of HbF in the blood
β-thalassemia intermedia (inherit at least one β^+ allele)	Variable (β^0/β^+, β^+/β^+, β^0/β, β^+/β)	Moderately severe and regular transfusion not required
β-thalassemia minor/β-thalassemia trait (one abnormal allele)	Heterozygous (β°/β β^+/β)	Mild anemia and asymptomatic or mildly symptomatic, red cell abnormalities seen

β^0 = Total absence of β-globin synthesis

β^+ = Markedly reduced or diminished β-globin synthesis

β = Normal β-globin synthesis.

- Most common in Mediterranean countries, parts of Africa, and South East Asia.
- **Hemolytic anemia** is of **severe degree**.

Pathophysiology of β-thalassemia Major (Fig. 11.20)

Q. Describe the pathophysiology/pathogenesis of β-thalassemia major.

Mechanism of Severe Hemolytic Anemia

In β-thalassemia, there is a defective synthesis of β-globin. It produces anemia through two mechanisms:

1. **Inadequate HbA formation: The absence of the β-globin chain** results in the **absence of synthesis of HbA** ($\alpha_2\beta_2$). This produces **RBCs that are poorly hemoglobinized (hypochromic) and small (microcytic).**
2. **Accumulation of unpaired (free) α-globin chains damaging membranes: They form toxic precipitates that severely damage the membranes of red cells and erythroid precursors.**
   - **Extravascular hemolysis:** RBCs with α-chain inclusions are removed by macrophages of the spleen (extravascular hemolysis).
   - **Ineffective erythropoiesis: Unpaired and excess α-chains aggregate** into insoluble precipitates and **damage the membrane of erythroid precursors**. Many erythroid precursors are badly damaged. They fail to mature and die by **apoptosis** in the bone marrow. This phenomenon is termed *ineffective erythropoiesis*. Few red cells are produced and they have a shortened life span.

Consequences of Ineffective Erythropoiesis

- **Changes in bone marrow: Marked erythroid hyperplasia.**

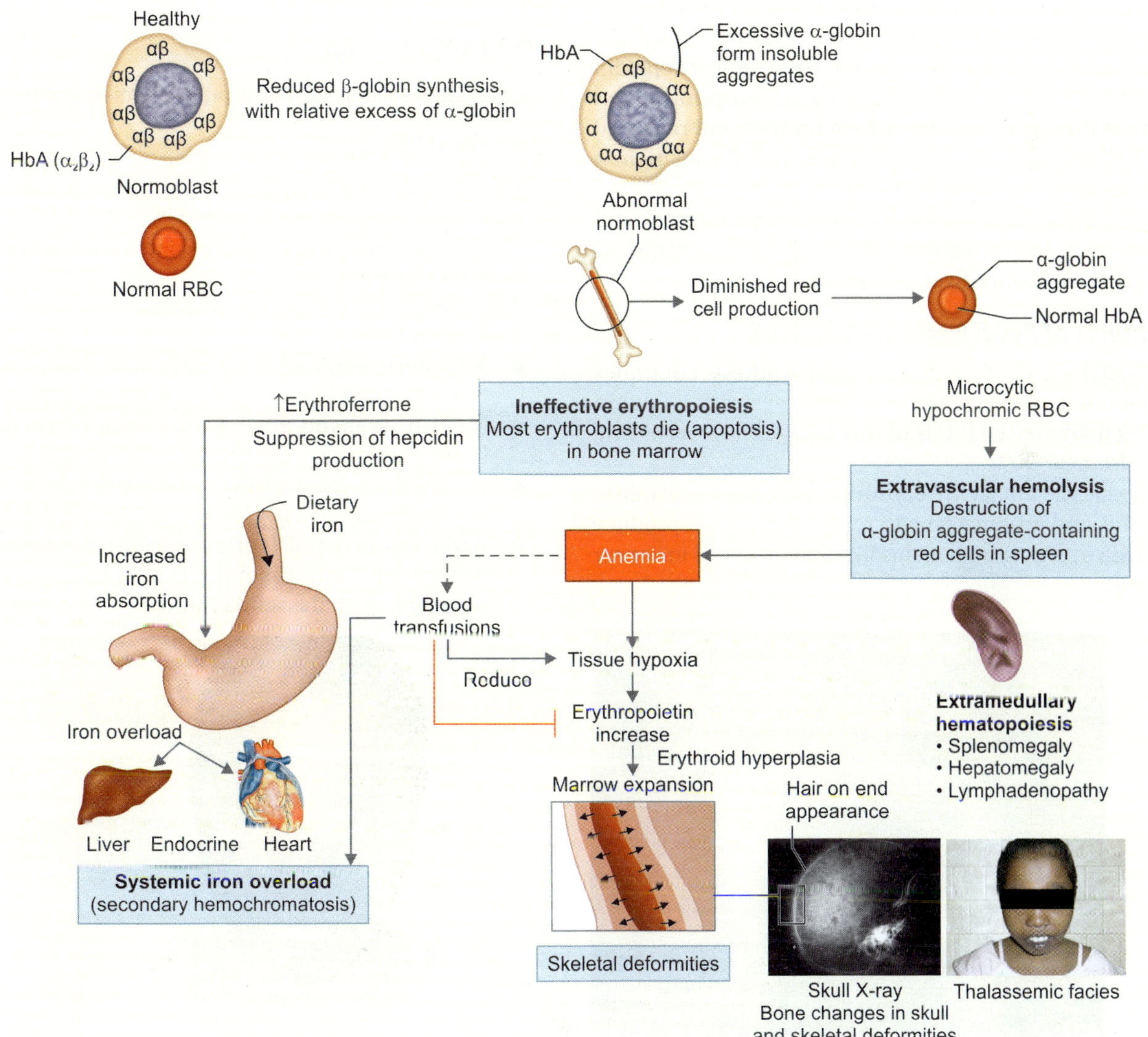

Fig. 11.20: Pathogenesis of β-thalassemia major and its consequence.

- **Changes in bone:** The expanded erythropoietic marrow may completely fill the intramedullary space of the bones, invade the bony cortex, and impair bone growth. These lead to **skeletal deformities**.
  - **Skull X-ray: Hair-on-end (crew-cut) appearance (Fig. 11.21A)** due to new bone formation. The diploe (the spongy layer between the inner and outer compact layers of the skull) widens due to increased erythropoiesis. It expands bone marrow giving this classical X-ray appearance.
  - **Typical facies: Thalassemic (chipmunk face) face (Fig. 11.21B)**—prominent forehead, cheekbones, and upper jaw.
- **Extramedullary hematopoiesis:** In the **liver and spleen it leads to hepatosplenomegaly.**

Iron Overload and its Consequences

Iron overload: Ineffective hematopoiesis with an expanded pool of erythroblasts secretes a hormone called *erythroferrone.* This hormone circulates to the liver and suppresses the release of hepcidin. **Suppression of hepcidin synthesis** is associated with an **excessive absorption of iron from the diet**. This together with **hemolysis and repeated transfusions** (the usual mode of treatment) leads to *iron overload.*

Hemosiderosis: Iron overload produces **hemosiderosis** and **secondary hemochromatosis.** It damages the parenchyma of organs (e.g., **heart**, **liver,** and **pancreas).**

Synthesis of Fetal Hemoglobin (HbF)

In β-thalassemia, the γ-globin chain synthesis continues even 6 months after birth and combines with α-globin leading to **increased levels of HbF** ($\alpha_2\gamma_2$). The level of HbF varies from 30–90%.

Cachexia: The ineffective erythropoietic precursors utilize nutrients and produce growth retardation. It can produce **cachexia** in untreated patients like that observed in cancer patients.

Clinical Features

- **Age: Infants develop moderate to severe anemia,** 6–9 months after birth.
- **Growth and development:** Untreated/untransfused children **fail to thrive** and die within 4–5 years of age.
- **Bone changes:** Those who survive longer develop distortion of skull and facial bones. **X-ray skull shows a hair-on-end appearance (Fig. 11.21A)** and the face shows a characteristic **thalassemic (chipmunk) face (Fig. 11.21B)**.
- **Marked splenomegaly:** Up to 1,500 grams due to hyperplasia and extramedullary hematopoiesis.
- **Extramedullary hemopoiesis: Liver and lymph nodes** may show **extramedullary hematopoiesis.**
- **Iron overload:** Multiple blood transfusions may lead to iron overload and result in **hemosiderosis and secondary hemochromatosis** (heart, liver, and pancreas).

Laboratory Findings

Q. Mention the laboratory findings in β-thalassemia major.

Peripheral Blood

- **Markedly reduced hemoglobin** (ranges from 3–8 g/dL) **and hematocrit** (ranges from 8–23%).
- **RBC count increased/normal** (in contrast to iron deficiency anemia).
- **Reticulocyte count increased** in the range of 5–15%.
- **Red cell indices:**
  - **MCV decreased** and in the range of **50–70 fL** (normal range 82–98 fL).
  - **MCH decreased** and in the range of **12–20 pg** (normal range 27–32 pg).
  - **MCHC decreased** and in the range of **22–32 g/dL** (normal range 31–35 g/dL).
  - **RDW is elevated** (reflecting anisocytosis) in **untreated β-thalassemia major**, but it is often **normal in β-thalassemia minor.**

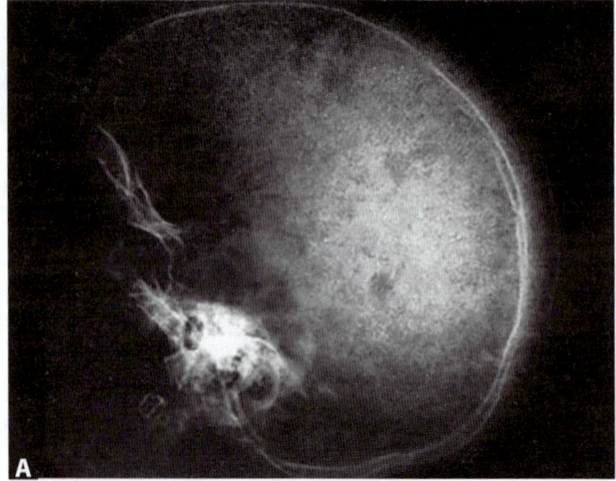

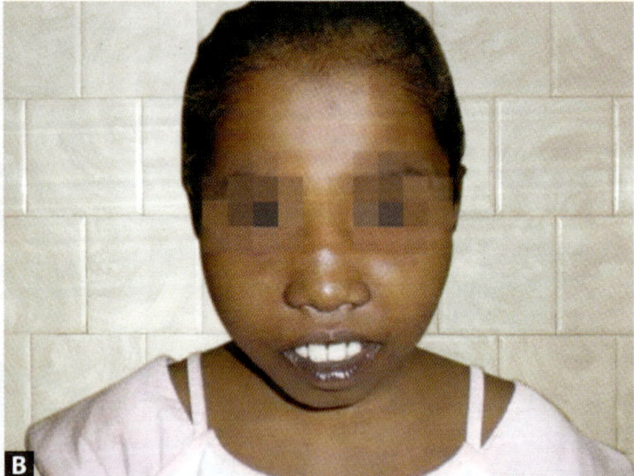

Figs. 11.21A and B: (A) X-ray of the skull (lateral view) in β-thalassemia showing hair-on-end (crew-cut) appearance due to new bone formation; (B) The appearance of the typical thalassemic face: Chipmunk face.

PERIPHERAL SMEAR

Q. Write a short note on peripheral smear findings in β-thalassemia major.

Q. Write about the target cell and its appearance.

RBCs:

- **Microcytic hypochromic anemia:** RBCs are small (microcytic) and pale (hypochromic), but **regular in shape.**
- **Anisocytosis and poikilocytosis:** RBCs show **moderate to marked variation in size (anisocytosis) and shape (poikilocytosis).**
- **Target cells:** Many **target cells (Figs. 11.22A and B)** are seen. The target cell is morphologically abnormal RBC. These cells have an increased surface area-to-volume ratio that allows the cytoplasm to collect in a central dark red "puddle" (small, shallow pool of liquid that has spread on the ground). In the target cell hemoglobin is redistributed in such a way that only the **periphery and central region of RBC appear hemoglobinized** and it resembles a target. These target cells can be seen in other conditions also **(Box 11.13).**
- **Basophilic stippling is constantly seen.**
- **Nucleated RBCs** (mainly late normoblasts) in variable numbers (5–40%).

WBCs: Leukocytosis with mild left shift.

Platelets: Normal.

BONE MARROW

- **Cellularity: Markedly hypercellular.**
- **Myeloid-to-erythroid (M:E) ratio: Reversed to 1:1 to 1:5 depending upon the degree of erythroid hyperplasia.**
- **Erythropoiesis: Normoblastic with marked erythroid hyperplasia.**
- **Myelopoiesis:** Normal.
- **Megakaryopoiesis:** Normal.
- **Bone marrow iron: Markedly increased** due to increased dietary absorption, hemolysis, and repeated transfusions.

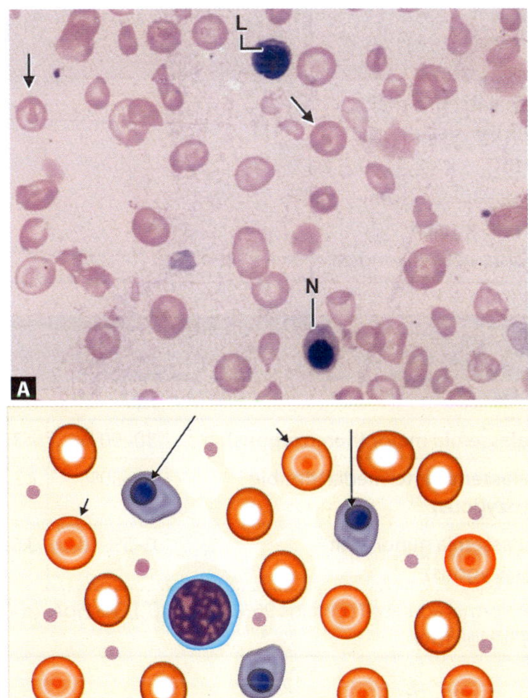

Figs. 11.22A and B: Peripheral blood smear in β-thalassemia: (A) Leishman stain showing target cells (arrows). Smear also shows microcytic hypochromic RBCs, one lymphocyte (L) and one nucleated RBC (N); (B) Diagrammatic appearance showing target cells (short arrows) and nucleated red cells (long arrows). One lymphocyte is shown in the center. The size of RBCs is less than lymphocytes indicating that RBCs are microcytic.

Biochemical Findings

Increased bilirubin—mainly of unconjugated type.
Increased urine urobilinogen.
Markedly reduced serum haptoglobin.
Increased serum iron status: Serum iron, serum ferritin [usually >1,000 μg/L (normal 15–300 μg/L)], and **transferrin saturation** [55–90% (normal 30–40%)] are **markedly increased.**
Total iron-binding capacity (TIBC): Reduced to 250–300 μg% (normal 310–340 μg%).

Special Tests

Fetal hemoglobin (HbF) ($\alpha_2\gamma_2$) **increased** to 30–90% (normal range 0–1%). In the RBCs, HbF can be demonstrated by acid elution test. RBCs containing HbA appear as ghost cells whereas HbF containing RBCs are well stained.

Hemoglobin electrophoresis (Table 11.19):

- β^+ **thalassemia** (β^+/β^+ or β^0/β^+ genotypes): Demonstrates bands of **both HbA and HbF.**
- β° **thalassemia** (β^0/β^0 genotype): Since no β-chains are formed, there is **no HbA. Major hemoglobin is HbF (>90%) with normal or low HbA_2.**

High-performance liquid chromatography (HPLC): HbF is increased (30–90%). HPLC measures various fractions of hemoglobin (Hb) and is used **for confirmation of diagnosis.**
Prenatal diagnosis by **molecular analysis of DNA.**
Estimation of globin chains: Normally, α: β ratio is 1:1. Lack of β-chain alters this ratio to 5–30:1.
Diagnosis of β-thalassemia major: It can be strongly suspected based on clinical features. Hb electrophoresis shows a severe reduction or absence of HbA and increased levels of HbF.

β-THALASSEMIA MINOR/TRAIT

More common than β-thalassemia major. Most patients are heterozygous for the thalassemic gene. **Usually, asymptomatic,** and anemia is mild.

Laboratory Findings in β-Thalassemia Minor

- **Peripheral blood: Microcytosis, hypochromia,** basophilic stippling, and target cells.
- **Bone marrow: Mild erythroid hyperplasia.**

BOX 11.13: Conditions with target cells in peripheral smear.

- Thalassemia major
- Sickle cell anemia
- HbC
- Post-splenectomy
- Liver disease
- Obstructive jaundice.

TABLE 11.19 Hemoglobin (Hb) F and HbA_2 percentage in β-thalassemia syndromes.

Type	*HbF*	*HbA_2*
β-Thalassemia major (homozygous)	30–90%	<3.5%
β-Thalassemia intermedia (double heterozygous)	10–30%	<3.5%
β-Thalassemia minor/trait (heterozygous)	0–5%	3.6–8%

Note: Normal adult cell contains 96% HbA ($\alpha_2\beta_2$), 3% HbA_2 ($\alpha_2\delta_2$) and 1% HbF ($\alpha_2\gamma_2$).

- **Hemoglobin electrophoresis:** Increase in HbA_2 ($\alpha_2\delta_2$) to 4–8% of the total hemoglobin (normal 2.5 ± 0.3%). HbF levels may be normal or slightly increased **(Table 11.19)**.
- **NESTROF test** (naked eye single tube red cell osmotic fragility test): **Positive (*refer* online Fig. 11.23).**
  - In NESTROF test, 0.02 mL of the patient's blood is added to 5 mL of 0.35% saline in a test tube.
  - After half an hour white paper with a dark black line is held behind the tube.
  - The microcytic hypochromic RBCs of thalassemia minor are more resistant to lysis than normocytic normochromic RBCs.
  - Hence, the black line on the paper is not clearly visible through the test tube compared to normal cells.
  - This test is used as a screening test for thalassemia. However, this test is also positive for α-thalassemia trait, sickle cell trait, and iron deficiency anemia.
- **Estimation of HbA_2:** HPLC is used for accurate estimation. HbA_2 estimation is diagnostic and the level ranges from 4–8%.

β-thalassemia intermedia: It is a clinical entity intermediate between thalassemia trait and thalassemia major.

β–thalassemia trait/minor should be differentiated from iron deficiency anemia. Treatment with iron in β-thalassemia worsens the iron load and its consequences. Differences between iron deficiency anemia and β-thalassemia major are presented in **Table 11.20.**

α-THALASSEMIA

Inherited disorders are characterized by **reduced or absent synthesis of α-globin chains.** It is an autosomal recessive disorder.

TABLE 11.20 Differences between iron deficiency anemia and β-thalassemia minor/trait.

Character	*Iron deficiency anemia*	*β-thalassemia minor*
Etiology	Deficiency of iron	Reduced synthesis of β-chain
Laboratory findings		
Peripheral smear—RBCs	Microcytic hypochromic	Microcytic hypochromic
Serum iron profile		
• Serum ferritin	Reduced <15 µg/L	Normal/slightly increased
• Serum iron	Reduced	Normal
• TIBC	Increased	Normal
• Transferrin saturation %	<15%	30–40%
HbA_2 level	Normal or decreased (2.5 ± 0.3%)	Increased (4–8%)
RBC count	<5 million/cu mm	>5 million/cu mm
RDW	Increased	Normal

(RDW: red cell distribution width; TIBC: total iron-binding capacity).

Molecular pathology: In contrast to a single gene coding β-globin chain, each α-globin chain is encoded by two genes. **Deletion of α-gene is the most common cause** of reduced α-chain synthesis.

Clinical syndromes: Four genes control α-chain synthesis. The severity of α-thalassemia varies greatly depending on the number of α-globin genes deleted (*refer* **online Fig. 11.24**). Each of the four α-globin genes normally contributes 25% of the total α-globin chains.

SICKLE CELL ANEMIA

PA 16.3c (CC): Describe the pathogenesis, features, hematologic indices, and peripheral blood picture of sickle cell anemia.

Sickle cell disease is a hemoglobinopathy that includes: Sickle cell anemia (SS) and sickle cell trait (AS). **Sickle cell anemia is a homozygous state in which both the β-globin chains are abnormal/defective (HbS and HbS)** and sickle cell trait (AS) is a heterozygous state with one defective gene (for HbS) while the other gene is normal (for HbA). Sickle cell anemia is discussed below followed by sickle cell trait.

Features

- Sickle cell anemia is the classical hemoglobinopathy. It is a **homozygous state (SS) caused by a mutation in β-globin that produces sickle hemoglobin (HbS).**
- **HbS constitutes more than 70% of hemoglobin in their RBCs with no HbA. HbS is protective against falciparum malaria.**

- It is an **autosomal recessive disorder that manifests early in life**.

Pathogenesis (Fig. 11.25)

Q. Discuss the pathogenesis of sickle cell anemia.

Normal hemoglobin: It is composed of two pairs of similar globin chains. A normal adult red cell contains 96% HbA ($\alpha_2\beta_2$), 3% HbA2 ($\alpha_2\delta_2$), and 1% fetal Hb (HbF, $\alpha_2\gamma_2$).

Production of abnormal sickle hemoglobin (HbS): Sickle cell anemia is characterized by the presence of an abnormal hemoglobin called sickle hemoglobin (HbS). HbS is responsible for the characteristics of the disease.

Missense point mutation: In HbS, there is **a single amino acid substitution in the β-globin chain of hemoglobin. This results in** the **substitution of glutamic acid by valine in the 6th position of the β-globin (Fig. 11.25)**. It **results in a tendency for deoxygenated HbS to** alter the solubility or stability of the hemoglobin. It leads to hemolytic anemia.

Sickle cell anemia: In these patients, **HbA is completely replaced by HbS**. In heterozygous carriers, namely sickle cell trait only about half of hemoglobin is replaced by HbS. HbS differs from HbA by having a valine instead of a glutamate (glutamic acid) at the 6th amino acid position in β-globin.

Molecular Basis of Sickling (Fig. 11.25)

Q. Write a short note on irreversible sickle cells.

Sickling during low O_2 tension or deoxygenation: During low O_2 tension or deoxygenation, **HbS molecules undergo aggregation and polymerization**.

- If deoxygenation continues, the **aggregated HbS** molecules **form long needle-like fibers** (or pseudo-crystalline structures known as **tactoids**) within RBCs.
- The **tactoids grow** in length beyond the diameter of RBCs and **distort RBC shape**.
- **RBC becomes elongated and assumes** a **shape** such as a **sickle** (or crescent moon or holly-leaf or boat) and **predisposes to stasis and vascular occlusion**.

Factors affecting sickling are listed in **Table 11.21**.

Reversal of sickling: Initially, the sickling of red cells is reversible on reoxygenation or **when** the **oxygen tension returns** to normal. The **sickled red cell returns to its normal shape**. However, the RBC membrane is distorted during each episode of sickling. Structural changes in the RBC membrane cause the entry of calcium, which activates an ion channel resulting in the loss of potassium and water. This injures the membrane skeleton.

Irreversibly sickled cells (ISC) and hemolysis: With time, **recurrent sickling** causes cumulative red cell membrane damage, and these RBCs become **more rigid**

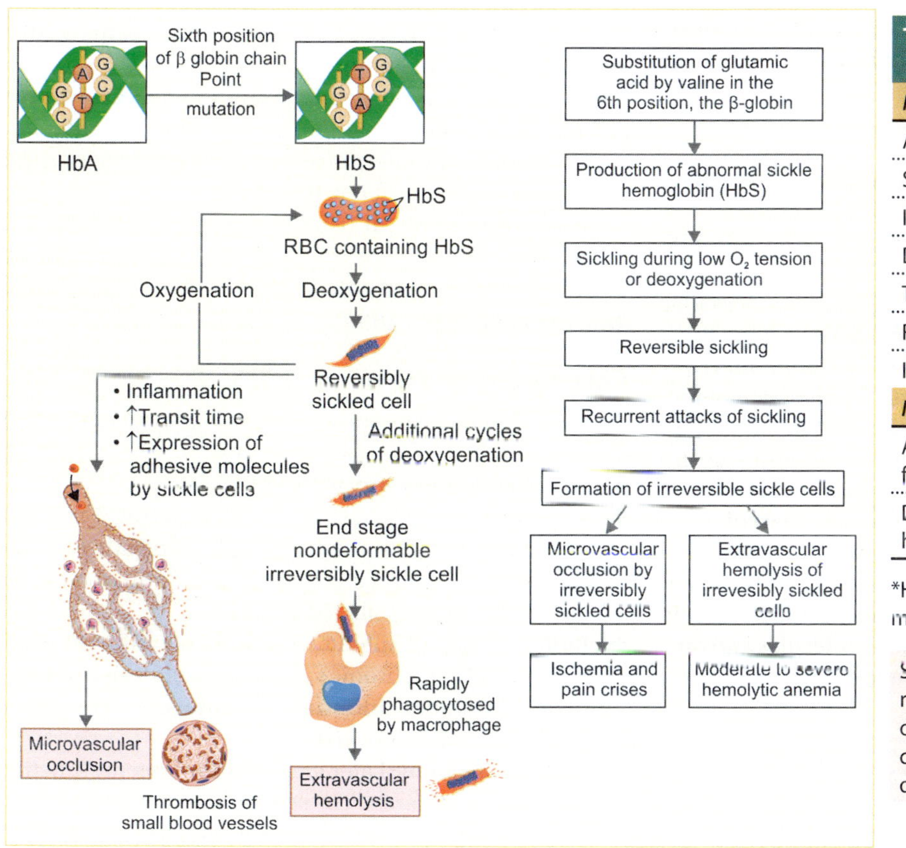

Fig. 11.25: Pathogenesis of sickle cell anemia.

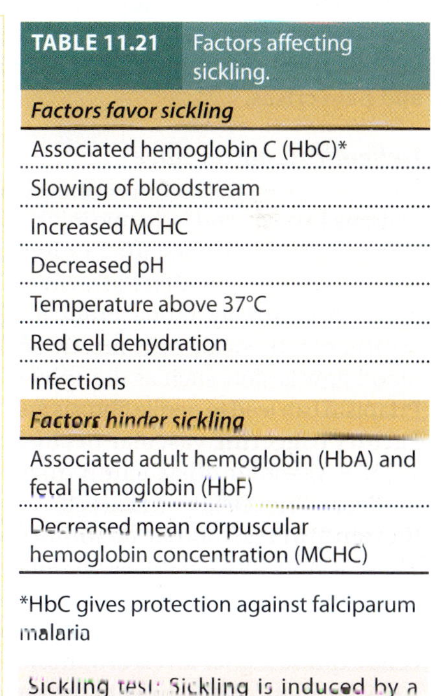

TABLE 11.21 Factors affecting sickling.

Factors favor sickling
Associated hemoglobin C (HbC)*
Slowing of bloodstream
Increased MCHC
Decreased pH
Temperature above 37°C
Red cell dehydration
Infections
Factors hinder sickling
Associated adult hemoglobin (HbA) and fetal hemoglobin (HbF)
Decreased mean corpuscular hemoglobin concentration (MCHC)

*HbC gives protection against falciparum malaria

Sickling test: Sickling is induced by a reducing agent such as 2% metabisulfite or dithionite to blood. However, this test cannot differentiate between sickle cell disease and sickle cell trait.

and nondeformable and are termed irreversibly sickled cells (ISC). These ISCs are **susceptible to hemolysis.**

Pathologic Consequence of Sickling

Two major pathologic consequences of the sickling of red cells are (i) chronic moderately severe hemolytic anemia and (ii) vascular obstructions.

Chronic Hemolytic Anemia

The inflexibility of sickled cells is susceptible to destruction (hemolysis) during passage through the spleen. This leads to extravascular hemolysis resulting in hemolytic anemia.

Moderate to severe hemolytic anemia: The red cell membrane damage in sickle cell anemia leads to lifelong hemolysis (mainly extravascular). This causes chronic **moderate to severe hemolytic anemia.** The mean life span of RBCs in sickle cell anemia is about 20 days (one-sixth of a normal RBC life span of 120 days). The degree or severity of the hemolysis correlates with the percentage of irreversibly sickled cells that are present in the blood.

Raised unconjugated bilirubin and pigment gallstones: Chronic hemolysis raises the unconjugated (indirect) bilirubin and predisposes to pigment bilirubin gallstones (cholelithiasis) and cholecystitis.

Vascular Obstructions

Sickle cells are **rigid and form aggregates.** The aggregated irreversibly sickle cells **block** the small blood **vessels.** Vascular obstruction **produces ischemic tissue damage and pain crises.**

Ischemic tissue damage

The rigid sickled RBCs obstruct the microcirculation, leading to tissue hypoxia and ischemic injury in many organs.

Organs affected: **Vascular congestion, thrombosis, and infarction** can affect any organ. These include the bones, liver, kidney, retina, brain, lung, and skin. Vascular obstruction by sickle cells mostly affects tissues in which blood flow is slow such as the **spleen, and bone marrow**. Priapism can lead to penile fibrosis and erectile dysfunction.

Factors triggering vascular occlusion by red cells (Fig. 11.25): Vascular obstruction does not depend on the number of irreversibly sickled cells. It is **triggered by factors that tend to arrest and sickle within the microvasculature**. These factors include **infection, inflammation** (slows the blood flow and increases the adhesion of leukocytes and red cells to endothelium), **dehydration, and acidosis. Sickle cells express higher levels of adhesion** molecules and thus **become abnormally sticky to the endothelium**.

Pain crises

Q. Write a short note on crises in sickle cell anemia.

Four types of crises can occur in sickle cell anemia. These are (i) vaso-occlusive, (ii) hemolytic, (iii) aplastic, and (iv) sequestration crisis.

Vaso-occlusive crisis (sickling/pain/painful/infarctive crisis): It is the **most common type.** Blockage of microcirculation by sickled red cells **produces hypoxic injury and infarction.** It is **characteristically associated with pain.**

- **Bone:** Manifest as the **hand-foot syndrome, dactylitis of the bones of the hands or feet**, or both. Hand-foot syndrome results from infarction of bones in the hands and feet. It is the **most common presenting symptom in young children.**
- **Lung**: In **acute chest syndrome,** sluggish blood flow in an inflamed lung (e.g., an area of pneumonia) leads to sickling within hypoxemic pulmonary beds. This increases the dysfunction of the lung. This further worsens pulmonary and systemic hypoxemia, sickling, and vaso-occlusion. Acute chest syndrome may also occur due to fat emboli originating from infarcted bone.
- **Stroke:** It may occur in patients with acute chest syndrome. Stroke and acute chest syndrome are the two leading causes of ischemia-related death in sickle cell anemia.
- **Proliferative retinopathy**: It is due to vaso-occlusions in the eye and can lead to loss of visual acuity and blindness.
- **Spleen**: **Acute abdominal pain due to infarcts of abdominal viscera** caused by occlusion of vessels. Recurrent splenic infarction results in autosplenectomy.

Hemolytic crisis: It is a rare type and presents with a **marked increase in hemolysis.**

Aplastic crisis: It is **caused by a sudden decrease in red cell production accompanied by reticulocytopenia.** It is usually triggered by infection of erythroblasts by parvovirus B19. Although severe, it is self-limited.

Sequestration crisis: It usually occurs in children. It is characterized by **sudden trapping of blood in the spleen or liver.** It causes rapid enlargement of these organs and a drop in hematocrit leading to hypovolemic shock.

Chronic Organ Damage

Particularly seen in the spleen, bones, kidneys, heart, lungs, brain, and skin.

Spleen: The changes vary with age.

- **Moderate splenomegaly: Children after 6 months of life** present with moderate splenomegaly (splenic weight up to 500 g). It is due to congestion of red pulp caused by trapped sickled red cells.
- **Reduced size of spleen with multiple infarcts**: After 5–6 years of age, chronic splenic red cell stasis produces hypoxic damage and **multiple infarcts**. The spleen **gradually reduces in size**.
- **Autosplenectomy:** Later, gradual **loss of splenic function** secondary to infarcts. The spleen becomes fibrosed and results in a process referred to as **autosplenectomy**.

Extremities: Skin ulcers over the lower extremities.

Increased Susceptibility to Infections

Pneumonia: Common infections are **pneumonia due to *Pneumococcus, and* meningitis due to *Streptococcus pneumoniae*.**

Osteomyelitis: Patients are also predisposed to bacterial osteomyelitis. The increased frequency of osteomyelitis is due to bone infarcts, in which bacteria become seeded. The most common causative organisms are encapsulated bacteria and gram-negative organisms, particularly *E. coli* and *Salmonella* (*Salmonella typhimurium*).

Septicemia and meningitis: These are the most common causes of death in children.

Causes of Susceptibility to Infections

- **Hypofunction of the spleen**: In children, it is due to **congestion and poor blood flow,** and in adults due to **multiple infarcts** and resultant **autosplenectomy**.
- **Defects in the alternative complement pathway:** Impairs opsonization of encapsulated bacteria such as pneumococci and *Haemophilus influenzae.*

Clinical Features (Fig. 11.26)

Symptoms appear after 6 months of age: The presence of **HbF in the first 6 months** of life has a **protective** role. Hence, it is **usually asymptomatic until 6 months of age** when the shift from HbF (HbF disappears) to HbS is complete.

Hemolytic anemia and vaso-occlusive crises: Sickle cell disease presents with features of chronic hemolytic anemia and superimposed vaso-occlusive crises. Chronic hemolysis raised bilirubin levels in the blood.

- **Infants and children** present with acute problems like **severe infection, acute chest syndrome, splenic sequestration, and stroke.**
- **Chronic hypoxia:** Its consequences are:
  - **Generalized impairment of growth and development in children.**
  - **Chronic organ damage in adults.**

Various effects of vascular occlusion and hemolysis in sickle cell anemia are depicted in **Figure 11.26.**

Laboratory Findings in Sickle Cell Anemia

Q. Mention laboratory findings (diagnosis) of sickle cell anemia.

Peripheral Blood

- **Decreased hemoglobin:** Anemia is moderate to severe with hemoglobin ranging from 5 to 10 g/dL.
- **Decreased hematocrit (PCV):** Most patients have hematocrits of 18–30% (normal range, 38–48%).
- **Low ESR: This is because sickle cells cannot form rouleaux.**

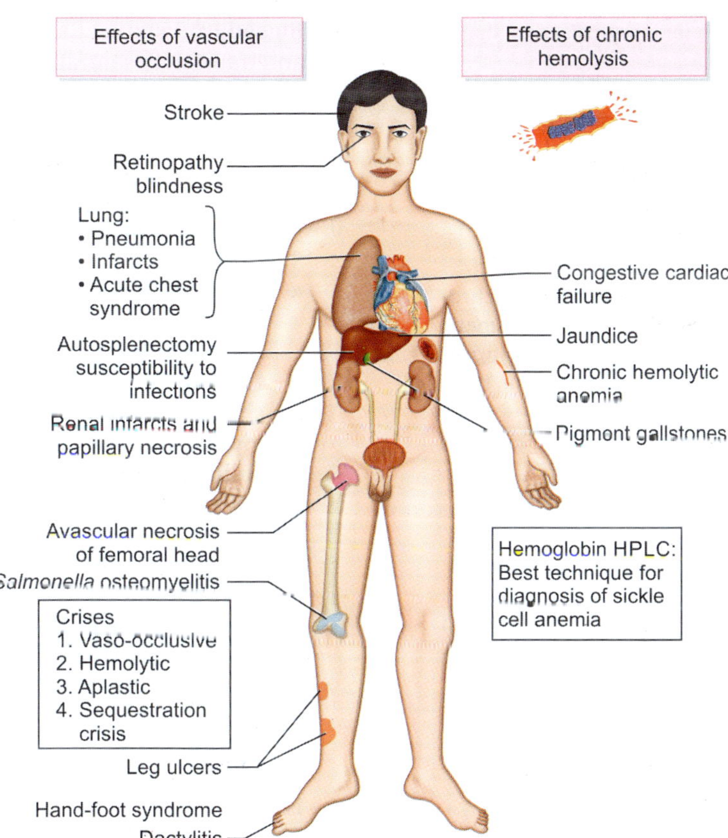

Fig. 11.26: Various effects of vascular occlusion and hemolysis in sickle cell anemia.

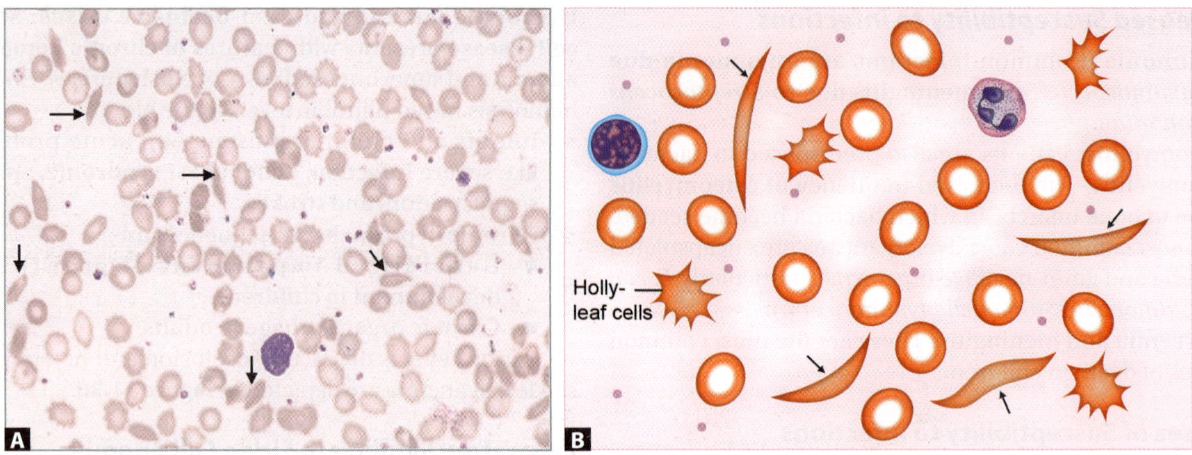

Figs. 11.27A and B: (A) Leishman stain (B) Diagrammatic. Peripheral blood smear with sickle cells (arrows).

- **Increased reticulocyte count:** Chronic hemolysis is associated with increased reticulocyte count. It ranges from 3–10%.

PERIPHERAL SMEAR

Q. Write a short note on peripheral smear findings in sickle cell anemia.

RBCs: It shows the following features:

- **RBCs are normocytic normochromic to mildly hypochromic.**
- **Anisopoikilocytosis:** RBCs show a moderate to severe degree of variation in size (anisocytosis) and shape (poikilocytosis).
- **Sickle cells: Characteristic cells are** the irreversibly **sickle cells.** They appear as **long (elongated), curved (spindled or boat-shaped) cells** with pointed ends **(Figs. 11.27A and B).** Their number varies.
- **Target cells:** It may also be seen due to red cell dehydration. Also, may find **ovalocytes.**
- **Increased reticulocytes (reticulocytosis) with few nucleated RBCs: Reticulocytosis produces polychromatophilia in the peripheral smear.** The **polychromatic cells are reticulocytes (immature red cells) that appear as blue, bluish-gray, or purple cells** among the pink-colored normal red blood cells.

WBCs: Mildly increased with a shift to left (the bands or stabs forms are increased).

Platelets: Mildly increased.

BONE MARROW

Cellularity: Hypercellular.

Erythropoiesis: Compensatory normoblastic erythroid hyperplasia, which expands the marrow and causes resorption of bone and secondary new bone formation.

Myelopoiesis: Normal.

Megakaryopoiesis: Normal.

Iron stores: Usually increased.

"Crewcut" appearance in radiographs: The cellular proliferation in the marrow usually produces resorption of and secondary new bone formation. This results in prominent cheekbones and changes in the skull resembling a "crewcut" in radiographs.

Extramedullary hematopoiesis: It may appear in the liver and spleen.

Serum Findings

- **Raised serum bilirubin:** Chronic hemolysis leads to increased breakdown of heme to bilirubin. This causes raised serum bilirubin and predisposes to pigment gallstones.
- **Raised iron status:** Raised serum iron, serum ferritin, and transferrin saturation.
- **Reduced serum haptoglobin.**
- **Increased urobilinogen in urine.**

Diagnostic (Confirmatory) Tests

Q. Write a short note on the sickling test.

- **Sickling test**
  - **Principle: Sickling is induced by** adding a reducing (oxygen-consuming) agent like **2% sodium metabisulfite or sodium dithionite to the blood sample. Red cells with HbS become sickle in shape (Fig. 11.28) and holly leaf** appearance. It is **diagnostic** of sickle cell anemia.
- **Solubility test for hemoglobin S:** This is performed by adding the anticoagulated blood to the reducing reagent solution (consisting of phosphate buffer, saponin, and sodium dithionate). RBCs are hemolyzed and if HbS is present, it will be reduced by dithionate. HbS forms tactoids and refracts light. The solution appears turbid whereas normal Hb gives a clear solution.
- **Hemoglobin electrophoresis:** HbS is slow-moving compared to HbA and HbF. Electrophoretic analysis shows that 80–95% of total hemoglobin is HbS. HbF and HbA2 make up the remaining hemoglobin. HbA is absent.
- **Estimation of HbF:** In the homozygous state constitutes about 5–8% of total hemoglobin.

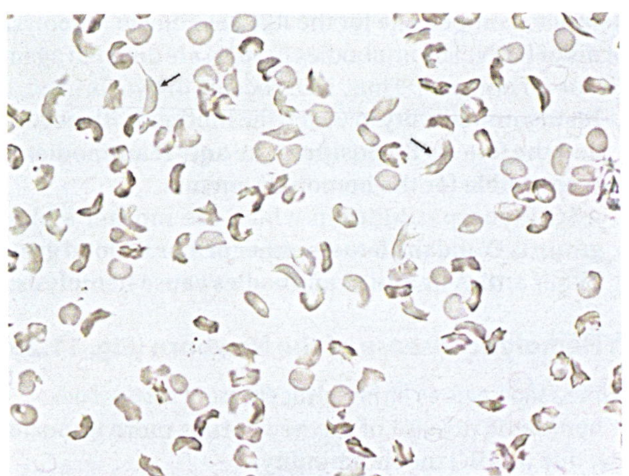

Fig. 11.28: Sickling test. Sickled red cells (arrows) induced by reducing agent (2% sodium metabisulfite).

- **High-performance liquid chromatography:** Useful for confirmation of diagnosis.

Prenatal diagnosis: It is by **analysis of fetal DNA obtained by amniocentesis or chorionic villous biopsy,** to detect the point mutations.

SICKLE CELL TRAIT

Heterozygous state for the hemoglobin S mutation and shows both HbA and HbS (HbA and HbS). One defective gene (from one parent with HbS) and while the other gene is normal (HbA).

Pathogenesis

In the sickle cell trait, approximately 40% (varies from 25–40%) of hemoglobin is HbS and the remainder is HbA. The hemoglobin A in RBCs interacts only weakly with deoxygenated HbS. Thus, HbA reduces or prevents hemoglobin S polymerization and the red cells have little tendency to sickle. However, RBCs may sickle under extreme conditions (e.g., flight at high altitude in unpressurized aircraft, deep sea diving).

Clinical features: Usually, asymptomatic. Normal growth and development, lifespan, and life expectancy.

Laboratory Findings

Peripheral Blood

Hemoglobin: Normal or mildly decreased.

PERIPHERAL SMEAR

RBCs: Normocytic normochromic picture with very few target cells and a mild degree of anisopoikilocytosis.

WBCs: Normal.

Platelets: Normal.

BONE MARROW

Hypercellular because of a compensatory normoblastic erythroid hyperplasia.

Diagnostic Tests

- **Hb electrophoresis:** Demonstrates two bands of HbS and HbA.
- **Sickling test:** Sickling test is positive.
- **High-performance liquid chromatography:** Useful for confirmation of diagnosis.

Abnormal Hemoglobins

Q. List the abnormal hemoglobins.

These include HbS, HbC, HbD-Punjab, HbE, Hb Barts, HbH, Hb Portland, HbO-Arab, etc.

IMMUNOHEMOLYTIC ANEMIAS

PA 16.4 (CC): Describe the etiology pathogenesis, hematologic indices, and peripheral blood picture of acquired hemolytic anemia.

Immunohemolytic anemias are caused due to **premature RBC destruction** (hemolysis) of RBCs mediated **by antibodies** that **bind to antigens on the red cell membrane.** The RBCs themselves are intrinsically normal but are targets for immune-mediated attack. The antibodies may be either alloantibodies or auto-antibodies, and the hemolysis may be extravascular or intravascular. Alloantibodies with respect to RBC are produced following exposure to foreign red blood cell antigens (non-self antigens) and autoantibodies are against self-antigens.

Classification of immunohemolytic anemias: Immunohemolytic anemia is uncommon. It is classified based on (1) the nature of the antibody and (2) the presence of predisposing conditions **(Box 11.14)**.

BOX 11.14: Classification of immunohemolytic anemias.

Alloimmune hemolytic anemia
- Hemolytic disease of the newborn
- Hemolytic transfusion reactions: Mismatched blood transfusion

Autoimmune hemolytic anemia
- **Warm antibody type (IgG antibodies active at 37°C)**
  - Primary (idiopathic)
  - Secondary: B-cell neoplasms (e.g., chronic lymphocytic leukemia), autoimmune disorders (e.g., systemic lupus erythematosus), drugs (e.g., α-methyldopa, penicillin, quinidine)
- **Cold antibody type (IgM antibodies active at 4–18°C)**
  - Acute: *Mycoplasma* infection, infectious mononucleosis
  - Chronic: Idiopathic, B-cell lymphoid neoplasms (e.g., lymphoplasmacytic lymphoma)
- **Cold hemolysin type (IgG antibodies active below 37°C—Donath-Landsteiner antibodies)**

Alloimmune Hemolytic Anemia

In these anemias, alloantibodies are produced against foreign antigens not present in an individual's red blood cell. Alloantibodies are present either in the serum or bound to red cells.

Hemolytic Disease of the Newborn

Q. Write a short note on the hemolytic disease of newborns.

Affects fetus and newborn: Hemolytic disease of the newborn (HDN) is alloimmune hemolytic anemia developing in the fetus and newborn baby. Hemolysis is extravascular.

Incompatibility of blood types between a mother and her developing fetus: The mother lacks an antigen present on fetal RBCs. HDN develops when the maternal IgG alloantibodies against the blood group of the fetus pass from mother to fetus through the placenta. This causes hemolysis of fetal RBCs.

Erythroblastosis in peripheral blood smears of the fetus: Erythroblasts [synonym normoblasts (RBC precursors)] are released from the bone marrow of a developing fetus in an attempt to compensate for the RBC loss due to hemolysis.

Forms of HDN: The antibodies in HDN are directed against ABO or Rh antigens. Thus, HDN occurs in two forms:

1. **Rh incompatibility** in which the **mother is Rh negative and the fetus is Rh positive**. The **anti-D antibodies** are **responsible for the hemolytic anemia.**
2. **ABO incompatibility** in which the **mother's blood group is O and the fetus is either of A or B blood group.** Either **anti-A or anti-B antibodies cause hemolysis.**

Rh Hemolytic Disease of the Newborn (Fig. 11.29)

Q. Write a short note on Rh hemolytic disease of the newborn.

Rh hemolytic disease of the newborn is **more important than due to ABO incompatibility.**

Pathogenesis

- **Rh-negative mother with Rh-positive fetus**: It occurs when the **mother is Rh (D antigen) negative and the fetus is Rh positive.**
- **Sensitization occurs during previous pregnancy or transfusion:** Sensitization occurs when fetal Rh-positive RBCs enter the blood circulation of Rh-negative

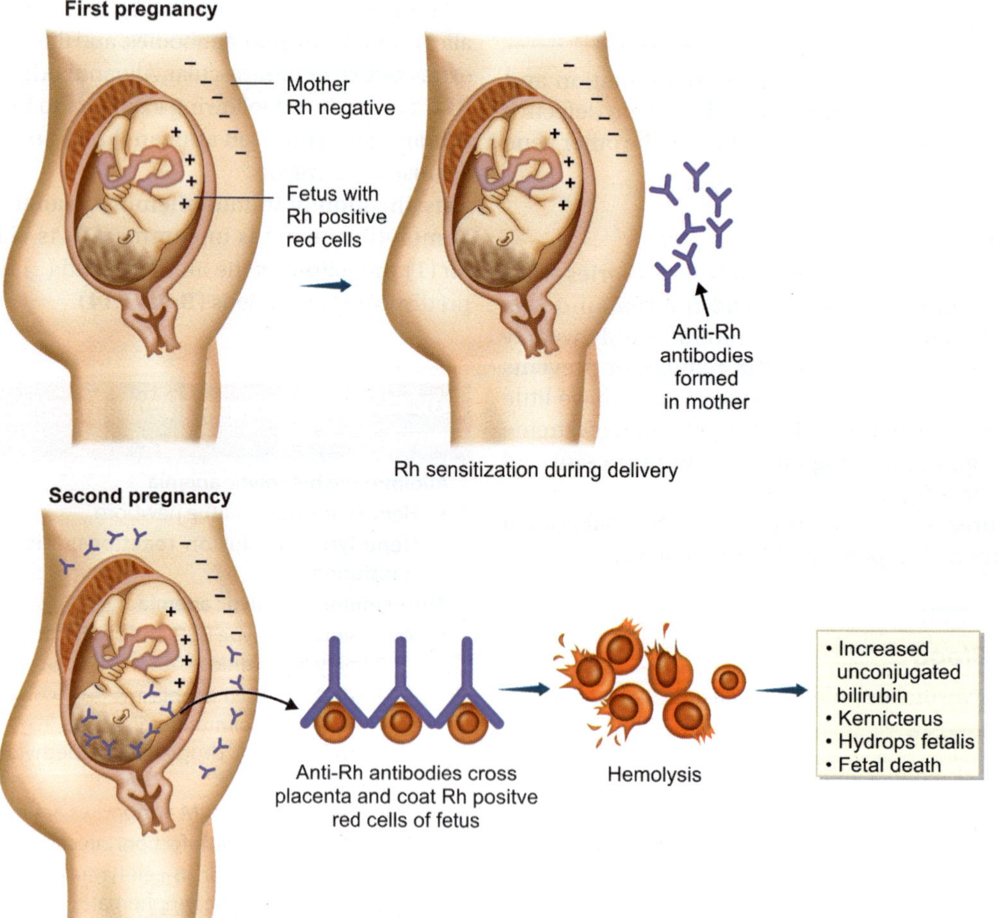

Fig. 11.29: Pathogenesis of Rh hemolytic disease of the newborn.

mothers. Rh-negative mother develops **anti-Rh antibodies. Sensitization occurs** only at the time of **delivery of a previous pregnancy/ during miscarriage or transfusions.** So, it **does not manifest in the first pregnancy.**

- **Destruction of fetal red cells in subsequent pregnancy:** In the subsequent pregnancy, **anti-Rh antibodies present in mother circulation cross the placenta and coat the Rh-positive fetal red cells.** These anti-Rh antibodies cause **immune destruction of fetal red cells and result in severe hemolytic anemia** leading to **jaundice** in the newborn. The fetus may develop cardiac failure—**hydrops fetalis** (immune type). Hydrops fetalis is a fatal condition, characterized by left and right-sided heart failure producing generalized edema and may result in death.

Clinicopathological features

- **Jaundice at birth:** The affected infants may have jaundice at birth. When the disease is severe, the levels of **unconjugated bilirubin** in the blood are **high** and bilirubin can **pass the blood-brain barrier**.
- **Kernicterus:** The unconjugated bilirubin is deposited in the **central nervous system** (especially the basal ganglia) producing **neurological damage** and is known as **kernicterus** (yellow coloration of the cerebellum and basal ganglia due to bilirubin deposition). It can cause the **death** of the infant.

Prevention of Rh HDN: By the prophylactic removal of fetal cells entering the maternal circulation before sensitization develops, by **injecting anti-D** into the **Rh D negative mother.**

Laboratory findings

Peripheral blood: Hemoglobin is decreased and reticulocyte count is increased.

PERIPHERAL SMEAR

RBCs: Normocytic normochromic anemia with **numerous nucleated RBCs, polychromatophils,** and few spherocytes.

WBCs: Normal.

Platelets: Normal.

Antiglobulin test (Coombs test): Antibodies in the mother and baby are detected by the Coombs test **(Fig. 11.30).**

- **Indirect Coombs test: It is done using the mother's serum to detect ant-Rh antibodies.**
- **Direct Coombs test:** It is performed **on fetal RBCs** to detect anti-Rh antibodies bound to RBCs.

Serum findings: These are as follows:

- **Increased serum bilirubin.**
- **Increased lactate hydrogenase (LDH).**
- **Decreased haptoglobin.**

ABO Hemolytic Disease of the Newborn

It is less severe. No prior exposure through pregnancy or transfusion is required for hemolysis to develop. The fetus may be affected in the first pregnancy of a **mother with blood group O. The fetus is either of the A or B blood group.** The naturally occurring IgG antibodies to A (**anti-A**) or B (**anti-B**) from maternal blood cross the placenta and enter the fetal circulation. These maternal **anti-A or anti-B antibodies react** with A and B antigens present in **fetal red cells, fluids, and tissues.** This results in the consumption of a major portion of the maternal IgG and the small portion that is left combines with fetal red cells causing **only mild hemolysis.**

Antiglobulin (Coombs) Test

Q. Write a short note on Coombs (antiglobulin) test.

The antiglobulin test is useful to detect the presence of incomplete antibody (IgG) and/or complement on the RBC membrane.

Principle

- **RBCs coated with incomplete antibody (IgG) or C3 complement do not cause agglutination of RBCs.**
- Coombs reagent contains antibodies (antiglobulins) against human IgG/IgM/complement.
- If the RBCs coated by incomplete antibody or complement, are **treated with Coombs reagent**, the antiglobulins in the reagent will **induce agglutination** of such RBCs.

Types of antiglobulin test (Fig. 11.30)

- **Direct** (Coombs) **antiglobulin test (DAT)**
- **Indirect** (Coombs) **antiglobulin test (IAT)**

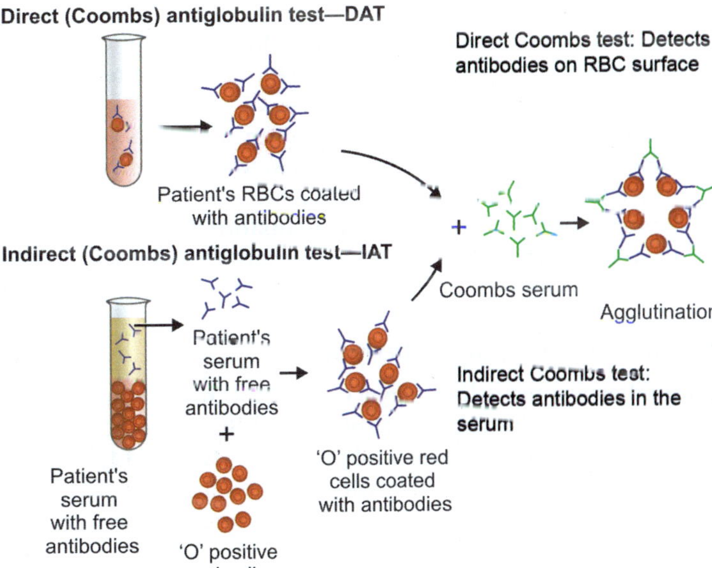

Fig. 11.30: Direct and indirect methods of antiglobulin test (Coombs test).

Q. Write a short note on the direct Coombs (antiglobulin) test, its procedure, and conditions in which it is positive.

Direct antiglobulin test (Fig. 11.30): Direct antiglobulin test (DAT) or direct Coombs test **detects antibodies** (IgG) and/or complement coated **on the surface of the patient's RBC** membrane. This is done by **using the patient's red cells.**

- Patient's RBCs are taken in a test tube and washed three times in normal saline.
- Coombs (antiglobulin) reagent is added and observed for agglutination.
- Agglutination or clumping of the patient's red cells indicates the presence of antibodies (human immunoglobulin) or complement on the RBC membrane. The test is interpreted as a positive DAT.

Uses of direct antiglobulin test: These are as follows:

- **Hemolytic disease of the newborn** (HDN), in which direct Coombs test is performed on the newborn baby's red cells from the cord blood. This test will be positive.
- **Autoimmune hemolytic** (immunohemolytic) **anemia:** To demonstrate in vivo attachment of antibodies to red cells.
- **Drug-induced red cell sensitization.**
- **Investigation of hemolytic transfusion reaction.**

Indirect antiglobulin test (Fig. 11.30)

Indirect antiglobulin test (IAT) or indirect Coombs test **detects the presence of incomplete antibodies (IgG) and/or complement in the patient's serum.** It assesses the ability of the patient's serum to agglutinate test red cells bearing defined surface determinants.

- The patient's serum is taken and the "O" Rh-positive cell suspension of any normal individual is added.
- "O" Rh positive RBCs are coated with (IgG) anti-Rh antibodies (if present) in the patient's serum.
- Add Coombs (antiglobulin) reagent and examine for agglutination.
- Agglutination of RBCs indicates the presence of antibodies in the patient's serum and the test is reported as positive for indirect antiglobulin test.

Uses of indirect antiglobulin test: These are as follows:

- **Hemolytic disease of the newborn:** Mother's serum is tested to detect anti-Rh antibodies.
- **Cross-matching for blood transfusion:** To detect incompatibility of the recipient's serum with the donor's cells.

Autoimmune Hemolytic Anemia

Antibodies against self-antigens on the RBC membrane cause premature destruction of RBCs. Anti-RBC antibodies can be divided into three general categories **(Box 11.14).** Interaction of the autoantibody with the red cell antigen is **dependent on the temperature, i.e., warm, or cold type.**

Warm Antibody Immunohemolytic Anemia

- Most common type (50–70%).
- **Idiopathic** (primary) or **secondary** to drug exposure or predisposing disease.
- **IgG** type antibodies combine with RBC antigen at 37°C—**warm antibody.**
- **Direct antiglobulin test:** DAT (Coombs test) **positive** in 90–95% of cases.
- **LE cell test: Positive** in SLE with secondary autoimmune hemolytic anemia (AIHA).

Cold Antibody Immunohemolytic Anemia

- Caused by **cold agglutinins.**
- Mediated by IgM antibodies optimally active below 30°C.
- Occurs as a complication of infections (e.g., infectious mononucleosis, *Mycoplasma* infections) and lymphoid neoplasms.

Cold Hemolysins Type (Donath–Landsteiner Antibodies)

- Autoantibodies directed against the P antigen system on red cells.
- Responsible for a rare disorder known as **paroxysmal cold hemoglobinuria.**
- **Direct antiglobulin test** is usually **negative.**

Fragmentation Syndrome

The **RBCs subjected to trauma** (physical or mechanical) in the circulation can undergo **fragmentation** and result in **intravascular hemolysis** leading to hemolytic anemias. These are known as fragmentation syndrome.

Q. Write a short note on microangiopathic hemolytic anemia.

Classification: According to the site of hemolysis it is classified as:

- **Macroangiopathic** (large vessels) **hemolytic anemia:** They are also known as cardiac hemolytic anemias the red cell trauma is from an abnormal vascular surface (e.g., prosthetic heart valve, synthetic vascular graft).
- **Microangiopathic hemolytic anemia (MAHA) occurs in capillaries** due to abnormal narrowing of the lumen (e.g., disseminated intravascular coagulation).

Q. Write a short note on peripheral blood picture in microangiopathic hemolytic anemia.

Laboratory findings: They are similar in both macro- and microangiopathic hemolytic anemias.

Hemoglobin: Decreased. Anemia is mild to moderate.

PERIPHERAL SMEAR

RBCs: Show **fragmented red blood cells (known as schistocytes), polychromasia,** with or without nucleated red blood cells, and microspherocytes. The **fragmented red cells** assume different shapes like **"triangular cells," "burr cells," and "helmet cells" and are the hallmark of diagnosis** of this group of hemolytic anemias.

WBCs: Count within normal limits or increased.

Platelets: Thrombocytopenia is often seen.

Paroxysmal Nocturnal Hemoglobinuria (PNH)

Q. Write a short note on paroxysmal nocturnal hemoglobinuria.

It is **rare** and is the only hemolytic anemia-acquired mutation in the hematopoietic stem cell.

Etiology and pathogenesis: Acquired mutations in the phosphatidylinositol glycan-group A (PIGA) gene in **the hematopoietic stem cell.** PIGA gene mutation causes **deficient synthesis of GPI-linked proteins** in blood cells and loss of anchor for decay-accelerating factor (DAF). Normally, DAF is responsible for complement degradation. RBCs are abnormally sensitive to **complement-mediated intravascular hemolysis.**

Clinical Features

- **Intravascular hemolysis:** Hemoglobin in acidic urine is converted into acid hematin and **results in dark brown urine.**
- **Thrombosis:** In the hepatic, portal, or cerebral veins.

Laboratory Findings

- **Ham's acidified serum test and sucrose hemolysis test:** The patient's RBCs undergo lysis when incubated with acidified serum (Ham test) or sugar (sucrose hemolysis test).
- **Flow cytometry:** Detects RBC deficient in GPI-linked proteins (CD55 and CD59) and is useful for diagnosis of PNH.

ANEMIAS OF BLOOD LOSS

Acute blood loss (hemorrhage): Causes **loss of intravascular volume** and if massive can lead to **hypovolemic shock** and death. **Bleeding** may be **external** (e.g., open fracture, knife wound) or **internal** (e.g., ruptured spleen, ruptured abdominal aneurysm).

BOX 11.15: Parasites causing anemia.

- *Plasmodium*: *falciparum, vivax, ovale, malariae*
- *Diphyllobothrium latum* (megaloblastic)
- *Leishmania donovani*
- *Ancylostoma duodenale* (iron deficiency)
- *Necator americanus*
- *Taenia solium*

PERIPHERAL SMEAR

RBCs: Normocytic normochromic anemia. Polychromasia during the recovery phase due to **increased reticulocytes.**

WBCs: Leukocytosis.

Platelets: Increased in number (thrombocytosis) **during recovery** phase.

Chronic blood loss: Produces anemia when the rate of blood loss exceeds the regenerative capacity of the bone marrow or when iron reserves are depleted which results in **iron deficiency anemia.**

Parasites causing anemia are listed in **Box 11.15.**

Q. Write a short note on parasites causing anemia.

APPROACH TO THE DIAGNOSIS OF HEMOLYTIC ANEMIA

It is a three-step process:

1. Diagnosis of anemia as hemolytic **(Flowchart 11.4).**
2. Determine the cause of the hemolysis **(Flowchart 11.5)**
   - Acquired
   - Hereditary
3. Confirmation of the disease by specific test **(Box 11.16).**

Flowchart 11.4: Steps involved in the diagnosis of hemolytic anemia.

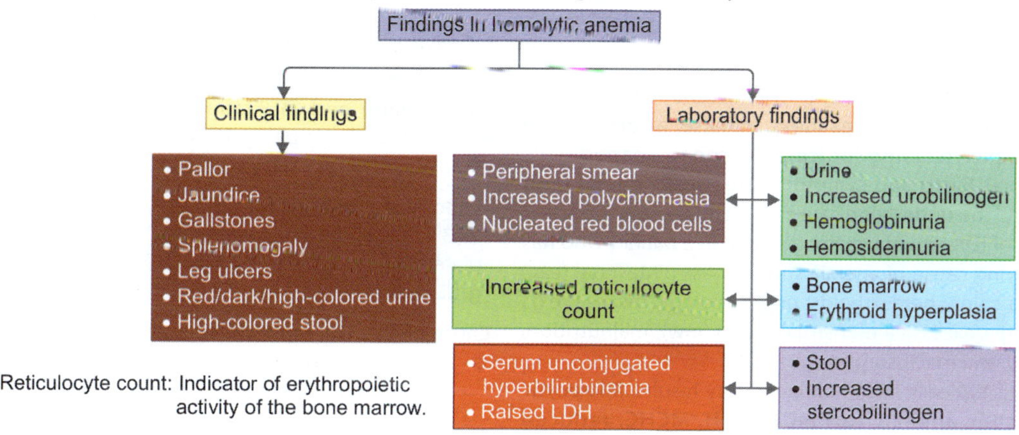

Flowchart 11.5: Steps involved in identifying the causes of hemolytic anemias.

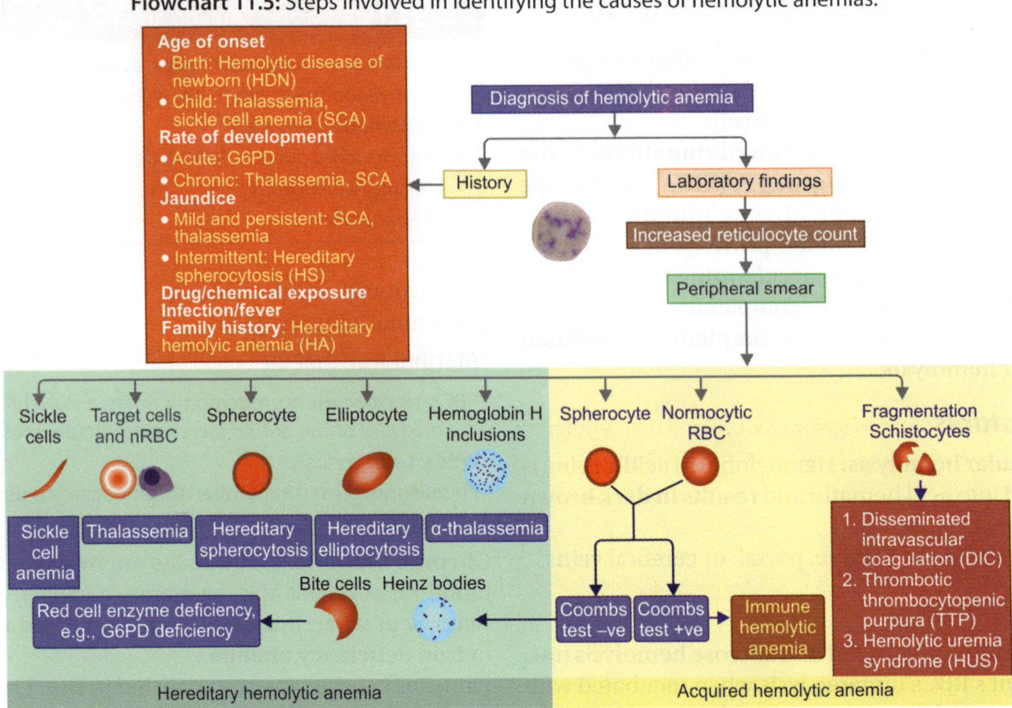

BOX 11.16: Confirmation of hemolytic anemia by special tests.

1. ***Osmotic fragility test***
2. Autohemolysis test
3. Hemoglobin electrophoresis
4. Estimation of HbF, HbA_2
5. ***Sickling test***
6. Screening test for G6PD
7. High-performance liquid chromatography (HPLC)

CLINICAL SCENARIOS FOR ESSAY QUESTIONS

Iron Deficiency Anemia

- History strongly indicative of **iron deficiency (IDA):** A **pale patient with tiredness, weakness, malaise, a sore tongue** (glossitis), pica **(craving for ice),** and **spoon-shaped nails** (koilonychia). **Signs and symptoms are** usually **due** to both **anemia** and the **underlying cause** of anemia.
- Diagnosis of **IDA** would be strengthened in a patient who has an underlying cause of anemia such as gastrointestinal (e.g., carcinoma colon, hemorrhoids) or gynecologic disease (e.g., menorrhagia/excessive menstrual blood flow), malnutrition, pregnancy, and malabsorption.
- Diagnosis is typically based on laboratory results. **Microcytic hypochromic anemia, low MCV, MCH, MCHC, reduced serum ferritin,** and other serum profiles were observed in IDA **(Table 11.13).**

Case 1

History: A 28-year-old **pregnant** lady comes to the hospital with complaints of weakness, easy fatigability, and breathlessness of 4 months duration. She is a **laborer** of low economic status and used to **eat clay.** On examination, she is pale and has **spoon-shaped (koilonychia) nails.**

Case 2

History: A 20-year-old girl complains of weakness, easy fatigability, and breathlessness of 6 months duration. She also complains of **heavy menstrual bleeding** every month. On examination, she is pale and had **spoon-shaped (flattened) brittle nails** and **cheilosis.**

Case 3

History: A 73-year-old male complains of increasing weakness, malaise, and easy fatigability for the past 10 months. On examination, he is pale without hepatosplenomegaly. He also complains of a **black tarry stool** (stool for occult blood was positive).

Laboratory findings for cases 1, 2, 3: Hb 9.1 g/dL, hematocrit 27.3%, RBC count 3 million/cu mm, WBC count 6,700/cu mm, and platelet count 4,20,000/cu mm. **MCV 70 fL, MCH 26 pg, MCHC 28 g/dL,** and **RDW 18.**

Cause of IDA: The causes of iron deficiency:
- Case 1 is probably due to **inadequate intake** (due to low socioeconomic status) or increased demand for iron during pregnancy.
- Case 2 is caused by **chronic blood loss**, due to **excessive menstrual flow.**

- Case 3 is due to **chronic blood loss** through the **gastrointestinal tract**. The black tarry stool indicates that the patient has occult bleeding probably from GI tract malignancy.

Megaloblastic Anemia

- History strongly indicative of **megaloblastic anemia** (vitamin B_{12} deficiency and/or pernicious anemia): **Middle-aged, pure vegetarian, pale patient** with prematurely gray hair, **severe glossitis** and **stomatitis, and a smooth painful tongue, significant neuropathy** and difficulty in walking, uncoordinated gait, **impairment of vibration sense and position sense tingling a and numbness** with delirium/dementia.
- Patients with megaloblastic anemia due to folic acid/folate deficiency present with symptoms of anemia or of the underlying cause.
- Peripheral smear with **macro-ovalocytes, hypersegmented neutrophils, raised MCV, and bone marrow with megaloblasts** are features of **megaloblastic anemia**.

Case 4

History: A 34-year-old male, **pure vegetarian**, executive complains of anorexia, premature graying of hair, weight loss, and **tingling and numbness in fingers and toes.** On examination, he is pale and anemic. The **tongue** is **shiny** and has a **glazed appearance** (glossitis).

Laboratory findings: Hb 9 g/dL, WBC count 3,800/cu mm, platelet count 60,000/cu mm, RBC count 2.5 million/cu mm. **MCV is 104 fL**, MCH 32 pg and MCHC is 32 g/dL.

Case 5

History: A 45-year-old female complains of **tiredness, mild breathlessness while climbing steps**, and **tingling and numbness.** On examination, she is pale, has a **raspberry-red tongue**, and shows **numbness and paresthesia**. Biochemical investigation reveals a **normal serum iron profile.**

Laboratory findings: Hb 8.2 g/dL, WBC count 4,800/cu mm, platelet count 1,20,000/cu mm, **MCV is 108 fL**, MCH 33 pg and MCHC is 32 g/dL. Peripheral smear and bone marrow examination confirm the clinical diagnosis. The patient is further subjected to gastric biopsy and shows **atrophic gastritis.** Other tests including serological tests is done.

Case 6

History: A 50-year-old male complains of **loss of appetite, increasing fatigue**, tingling, and **numbness of both lower limbs** and difficulty in walking for the past 10 months. On physical examination, he is pale and his tongue was beefy red.

Laboratory findings: Hb 9.2 g/dL, hematocrit 27.9%, **MCV 132 fL**, platelet count 242,000/cu mm, and WBC count 7,590/cu mm. Peripheral smear shows **macro-ovalocytes** and **hypersegmented neutrophils.**

Hereditary Spherocytosis

History strongly indicative of chronic extravascular hemolysis, usually but not always **hereditary spherocytosis**: Normal patient presenting with **pallor, mild jaundice, an enlarged spleen (classic triad**), and a family history of a relative who had been "cured" of the same problem by splenectomy. Also, family history of **pigment gallstones** in a young person. Peripheral smear with **spherocytes and raised osmotic fragility** test are features of HS.

Case 7

History: A 24-year-old woman complains of chronic fatigue since childhood and mild icterus. On examination, she is **anemic, jaundiced, and has moderate splenomegaly**. Her mother had similar complaints and has multiple **pigment gallstones.**

Case 8

History: A 15-year-old girl presents with weakness and fatigue. On examination, her sclera shows mild jaundice and mild splenomegaly. **Family history** indicated that her father had recurrent gallstones.

Laboratory findings for cases 7 and 8: Hb 11.1 g/dL, RBC count 3.6 million/cu mm. WBC count 6,800/cu mm and platelet count 1,75,000/cu mm. MCV is 78 fL, MCH is 32 pg and MCHC is 38 g/dL. In a laboratory test, her **RBCs lyse at a higher concentration of saline (osmotic fragility test)** compared to normal patients.

Thalassemia Major

History strongly indicative of thalassemia major: Short stature, failure to thrive, severe pallor, jaundice, maxillary over-growth (bossing), **frontal bossing**, sallow complexion, and splenomegaly.

Laboratory findings of microcytic hypochromic anemia with **many target cells, reduced MCV, MCH, and MCHC, and increased serum iron** are features of thalassemia major.

Case 9

History: An **11-month-old male child** was brought to the pediatric outpatient by his parents who complained that the child was **failing to thrive**. On examination, jaundice, **pallor,** and a **palpable spleen** were detected.

Laboratory findings: Hb 7.8 g/dL, hematocrit 23.4%, **MCV 66 fL,** platelet count 1,75,000/cu mm, and WBC count 8,200/cu mm. His **serum ferritin was 3,250 ng/mL.** Peripheral examination showed **microcytic hypochromic anemia** with many **target cells.** A bone marrow aspiration was performed and revealed a myeloid: erythroid ratio of 1:4, and increased iron stores.

Sickle Cell Anemia

- **History strongly indicative of sickle cell anemia: Recurrent episodes of vaso-occlusion** in connective and musculoskeletal structures anywhere in the body producing ischemia and manifesting as **acute pain, tenderness, and fever.** The child may show generalized impairment of growth and development. **Adults** manifest with **chronic organ damage.**
- Presence of **sickle cells** in the peripheral smear, **a positive sickling test,** along with a demonstration of HbS by **hemoglobin electrophoresis** and **HPLC** is diagnostic of **sickle cell anemia.**

Case 10

History: A 10-year-old boy complains of **severe pain** in the **chest, abdomen, and bones.** On enquiry, his mother revealed that he had **several episodes** of severe abdominal and back pain since early childhood. Physical examination shows **anemia, jaundice, and leg ulcer.**

Laboratory findings: Hb 11.0 g/dL, RBC count 3.2 million/cu mm, WBC count 8,800/cu mm and platelet count 1,95,000/cu mm. Peripheral smear examination, **hemoglobin electrophoresis, and HPLC** confirm the diagnosis.

SCENARIO-BASED MCQs

1. **A 35-year-old woman presents with upper abdominal pain, weakness, and fatigue for the last 2-month. Physical examination shows marked pallor. Laboratory examinations show microcytic, hypochromic anemia (hemoglobin of 7.5 g/dL) and mild thrombocytosis. Gastroscopy is performed and reveals a mucosal defect in the antrum measuring 1.5 cm in diameter. The pathogenesis of anemia in this patient is:**
   A. Impaired heme synthesis
   B. Defective globin chain synthesis
   C. Poor absorption of vitamin B_{12}
   D. Synthesis of structurally abnormal hemoglobin molecules
2. **A 41-year-old woman has had abdominal pain and intermittent diarrhea for the past 3 months. On physical examination, she is pale and afebrile. A stool sample is positive for occult blood. A colonoscopy is performed, and biopsy specimens are taken from the terminal ileum and colon. It shows microscopic features of Crohn disease. She does not respond to medical therapy, and part of the colon and terminal ileum is removed. Laboratory tests show hemoglobin of 9.8 g/dL, hematocrit of 30.8%, RBC count of 2.64 million/μL, MCV of 118 fL, platelet count of 348,000/mm^3, and WBC count of 8,200/mm^3. The reticulocyte count is 0.3%. The above findings favor the diagnosis of:**
   A. Hemolytic anemia
   B. Chronic blood loss
   C. Vitamin B_{12} deficiency
   D. Anemia of chronic disease
3. **The mother of a 3-year-old boy brings him to pediatric outpatient for a poor appetite and underweight for his age and height. On physical examination, hepatosplenomegaly is detected. The hemoglobin concentration is 5.6 g/dL, and the peripheral blood smear shows microcytic and severely hypochromic RBCs. The total serum iron level is normal, and the reticulocyte count is 11%. A radiograph of the skull shows deformities of maxillofacial bones and expanded marrow spaces. The most likely cause of this child's condition is:**
   A. Deficiency of iron
   B. Qualitative defect of β-globin chain
   C. Destruction of RBCs due to anti-Rh antibodies.
   D. Imbalance in the production of α-globin and β-globin chain
4. **A 10-year-old boy complains of sudden onset severe abdominal pain accompanied by cramping chest pain, non-productive cough, and fever. On physical examination, he has diffuse abdominal tenderness without any masses or organomegaly. Laboratory findings: Hematocrit is 22%. The peripheral blood smear shows crescent-shaped RBCs. A chest X-ray shows bilateral pulmonary infiltrates. The most likely cause of his pulmonary condition is:**
   A. Autosplenectomy
   B. Myocardial infarction
   C. Vaso-occlusive crisis
   D. Pulmonary tuberculosis

Answers and Explanation

1. **The answer is A: Impaired heme synthesis.** The presence of a peptic ulcer is the cause of gastrointestinal bleeding and is the cause of anemia. Chronic blood loss results in iron deficiency that impairs heme synthesis and leads to impaired hemoglobin production and anemia. Defective globin chain synthesis (choice B) and synthesis of structurally abnormal hemoglobin molecules (choice D) are hemoglobinopathies. Poor absorption of vitamin B_{12} (choice C) causes macrocytic anemia.
2. **The answer is C: Vitamin B_{12} deficiency.** The high MCV of 118 fL (normal range 82–98 fL) indicates severe macrocytosis. The two common causes of such anemia are vitamin B_{12} and folate deficiency. These are megaloblastic anemia and show characteristic megaloblastic precursors in the bone marrow. The vitamin B_{12} form complexes with intrinsic factors secreted by the stomach. This complex is absorbed in the terminal ileum. In this patient, the terminal ileum is removed and it can cause vitamin B_{12} deficiency. The findings do not fit into any hemolytic anemia. Chronic blood loss and iron deficiency are associated with microcytic hypochromic anemia. Anemia of chronic disease is usually a normocytic anemia.
3. **The answer is D: Imbalance in the production of α-globin and β-globin chains.** This child is suffering from β-thalassemia major. In this condition is due to severe reduction in the synthesis of β-globin chains without normal synthesis of α-globin. The free, unpaired α-globin chains form aggregates that precipitate within normoblasts and these normoblasts undergo apoptosis. The premature destruction of RBC precursors in the bone marrow is called "ineffective erythropoiesis." A deficiency of iron causes microcytic hypochromic anemia, but it is associated with reduced iron levels. Qualitative defect of the β-globin chain produces usually sickle cell anemia. Destruction of RBCs due to anti-Rh antibodies occurs in the newborn in hemolytic disease of the newborn. But features do not favor this.
4. **The answer is C: Vaso-occlusive crisis.** The crescent-shaped RBCs (sickled RBCs) are characteristic of sickle cell anemia. The sickled RBCs undergo hemolysis (mainly vascular, in the spleen), and can also cause microvascular occlusions anywhere in the body leading to ischemia and severe pain. Most commonly vaso-occlusion occurs in bone, lungs, liver, and brain. Vascular occlusions in the lungs produce "acute chest syndrome." Abdominal pain is another common manifestation. Autosplenectomy occurs in sickle cell anemia and can predispose to pneumonia. However, it is not responsible for acute chest syndrome. Myocardial infarction is associated with crushing retrosternal pain and it usually does not manifest at the age of 10 years. Pulmonary tuberculosis can produce chest pain, but crescentic cells are not seen in peripheral blood.

Disorders of White Blood Cell, Lymph Node, and Spleen

Chapter Outline

Non-neoplastic Disorders of White Cells
- Quantitative Disorders of Leukocytes
- Qualitative Disorders of Leukocytes
- Infectious Mononucleosis (Glandular Fever)

Neoplastic Proliferations of White Cells
- Acute Leukemia
- Acute Lymphoblastic Leukemia/Lymphoma
- Acute Myeloid Leukemia
- Myeloproliferative Neoplasms
- Chronic Myeloid Leukemia
- Polycythemia or Erythrocytosis

Lymph Node and Spleen
- Lymph Node
- Non-Hodgkin Lymphomas
- Hodgkin Lymphomas
- Splenomegaly
- Plasma Cell Neoplasms

NON-NEOPLASTIC DISORDERS OF WHITE CELLS

QUANTITATIVE DISORDERS OF LEUKOCYTES

PA 18.1 (CC): Enumerate and describe the causes of leukocytosis, leukopenia, lymphocytosis, and leukemoid reactions.

Disorders of white cells can be deficiencies (leukopenias) or proliferation. Proliferations of leukocytes may be reactive or neoplastic. Reactive proliferation of white blood cells commonly occurs as a response to microbial infections. Neoplastic disorders are less common and are more dangerous.

The normal range of differential leukocyte count (DLC) in an adult is presented in **Table 12.1**.

TABLE 12.1 Normal range of different leukocytes in an adult.

Type of white blood cell	*Normal range*
Neutrophils	40–70% (2.0–7.0 × 10^9/L)
Lymphocytes	20–40% (1.0–3.0 × 10^9/L)
Monocytes	2–10% (0.2–1.0 × 10^9/L)
Eosinophils	1–6% (0.02–0.5 × 10^9/L)
Basophils	Less than 1% (0.02–0.1 × 10^9/L)

Leukocytosis

Q. Define leukocytosis and list its causes.

Definition: An increase in the total number of leukocytes (white cells) in the blood to more than 11,000/cu mm (11 × 10^9/L).

Leukocytosis may be reactive or neoplastic.

Reactive leukocytosis: It is **common in various inflammatory conditions** caused by microbial and nonmicrobial agents.

Classification of reactive leukocytosis: Leukocytosis is relatively nonspecific and can be classified according to the particular white cell series that is affected: (i) neutrophilic leukocytosis, (ii) eosinophilic leukocytosis (eosinophilia), (iii) basophilic leukocytosis (basophilia), (iv) monocytosis, and (v) lymphocytosis.

Causes: Common causes of leukocytosis are shown in **Box 12.1**.

Leukopenia

Q. Write a short note on leukopenia.

Definition: Leukopenia is defined as a total leukocyte count below 4,000/cu mm (4 × 10^9/L).

Causes: Common causes of leukopenia are shown in **Box 12.2**. Leukopenia is **most commonly due to a decrease in granulocytes** (the most numerous circulating white cells). Lymphopenia is less common. Lymphopenia can occur in rare congenital immunodeficiency diseases, advanced human immunodeficiency virus (HIV) infection, and treatment with high doses of corticosteroids.

BOX 12.1: Common causes of leukocytosis.

Reactive leukocytosis
- Infections
  - Bacterial
  - Viral infections (e.g., infectious mononucleosis)
- Leukemoid reactions:
  - Infections
- Physiological
  - Pregnancy
  - Exercise

Neoplastic leukocytosis
- Leukemia
  - Acute leukemia: Acute myeloid, acute lymphoid leukemia, etc.
  - Chronic: Chronic lymphocytic leukemia and chronic myeloid leukemia

BOX 12.2: Common causes of leukopenia.

- Typhoid and paratyphoid
- Anemia
  - Aplastic anemia
  - Megaloblastic anemia
- Hypersplenism
- Drugs including cytotoxic drugs
- Radiation
- Rarely leukemia

BOX 12.3: Major causes of neutrophilia.

Secondary causes
1. **Pathological:**
   - **Acute bacterial and fungal infections**
     - Localized: **Pyogenic microorganisms** causing infections, e.g., pneumonia, pyogenic meningitis, cellulitis, diphtheria, abscess, tonsillitis, etc.
     - Generalized: Septicemia, acute rheumatic fever
   - **Immunologic/inflammatory conditions**: Immunologic (e.g., rheumatoid arthritis, rheumatic fever, vasculitis) Inflammatory conditions (e.g., acute appendicitis),
   - **Tissue necrosis**: Burns, trauma, myocardial infarction, gangrene, neoplasms (tumor necrosis)
   - **Acute stress or hypoxic states**: Following hemorrhage, hemolysis, and surgery
   - **Metabolic:** Uremia, acidosis, gout
   - **Medications:** Granulocyte colony-stimulating factor (G-CSF), glucocorticoids
   - Miscellaneous: Eclampsia, steroid therapy
2. **Physiological:**
   - Exercise (shift from marginating pool to circulating pool), newborns, extremes of temperature, pain, emotional stress, and during obstetric labor

Primary causes

Myeloproliferative neoplasms
- Chronic myeloid leukemia
- Polycythemia vera

Disorders of Neutrophils

Q. Define neutrophilia and mention its causes.

Neutrophilia (Fig. 12.1)

Definition: Neutrophilia is defined as an absolute neutrophil count above 8,000/cu mm (8 × 10^9/L). Differential count shows more than 70% neutrophils and is usually accompanied by leukocytosis (15–30 × 10^9/L). Hence termed **neutrophilic leukocytosis.**

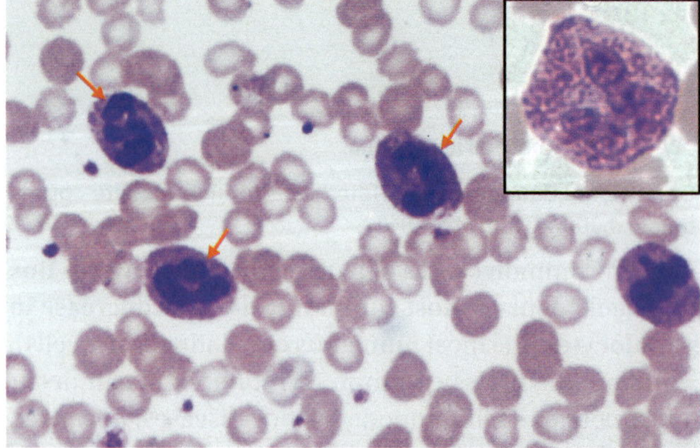

Fig. 12.1: Peripheral smear showing neutrophilia (arrows) with toxic granulation (inset).

Causes of neutrophilia: Neutrophilia can be primary (occurring in myeloproliferative neoplasm) or secondary **(Box 12.3)**. Acute bacterial infections usually produce leukocytosis with neutrophilia and an **increased number of band forms (a left shift)**. In bacterial infections, the neutrophils can contain **toxic granulations** (prominent dark blue granulation of the cytoplasm and are primary granules). Dohle bodies are small round to oval structures seen in the cytoplasm, and can also be observed in bacterial infections.

Leukemoid Reaction

Q. Write a short note on the leukemoid reaction.

Definition. Non-neoplastic (benign) leukocytic proliferation characterized by a **moderately increased total leukocyte count that rarely exceeds 50 × 10^9/L with few immature white cells** (like band forms, metamyelocytes, and myelocytes).

It is characterized by a reactive increase in the white blood cells and the blood picture closely resembles various types of leukemia.

Types of leukemoid reactions: Leukemoid reactions may be **myeloid or lymphoid type.** Various causes are presented in **Box 12.4.**

The blood picture of lymphoid leukemoid reaction shows leukocytosis (not exceeding 100,000/μL) and mostly mature lymphocytes resembling the blood picture of chronic lymphocytic leukemia.

BOX 12.4: Types and various causes of leukemoid reactions.

Myeloid leukemoid reaction*
- **Severe bacterial infections** (e.g., staphylococcal pneumonia, endocarditis, meningitis, septicemia).
- **Intoxications** (e.g., eclampsia, severe burns, mercury poisoning).
- **Malignancy** (e.g., multiple myeloma, Hodgkin lymphoma, bone marrow metastasis).
- Severe hemorrhage and hemolysis.

Lymphoid leukemoid reaction
- Infections:
  - **Viral** (e.g., infectious mononucleosis, cytomegaloviral infections)
  - **Bacterial:** Tuberculosis, whooping cough.
- Malignancy.

* Should be differentiated from chronic myelocytic/myeloid leukemia (**Table 12.2**).

Q. Tabulate the differences between leukemia and leukemoid reaction.

Neutropenia/Agranulocytosis

Q. Write a short note on agranulocytosis.

Definition:

Neutropenia: It is the reduction in the absolute neutrophil count (total WBC count × % segmented neutrophils and band forms) below 1.5 × 10^9/L (1,500/cu mm).

Agranulocytosis: It is a severe neutropenia and neutrophil count is below 0.5 × 10^9/L. These patients are highly susceptible to severe potentially fatal bacterial and fungal infections.

Etiology

The causes of neutropenia are described in **Box 12.5**.

Pathogenesis

The mechanisms that produce neutropenia can be divided into two major categories:

Decreased production of granulocytes

Marrow hypoplasia: It occurs transiently during cancer chemotherapy and chronically in aplastic anemia.

Severe replacement of the marrow by tumor: For example, leukemia.

Selective suppression of neutrophil production: In certain conditions, there may be selective suppression of granulopoiesis without the involvement of other blood lineages. It may be caused by certain drugs or by neoplastic proliferations of cytotoxic T cells and natural killer (NK) cells (so-called "large granular lymphocytic leukemia").

Increased destruction of granulocytes

Increased destruction may be due to **immune-mediated injury** (triggered by drugs) or **severe bacterial, fungal, or rickettsial infections. Splenomegaly** can also lead to

TABLE 12.2 Differences between leukemoid reaction and chronic myeloid leukemia.

	Leukemoid reaction	*Chronic myeloid leukemia*
Clinical features	Features of the causative disease (e.g., infection, stress, chronic inflammation, and certain neoplasms)	Splenomegaly (often massive) and bone pain are common
Peripheral blood findings		
WBC		
• Total WBC count	Moderately increased, rarely exceeds 50 × 10^9/L	Markedly increased and usually more than 50 × 10^9/L
• Differential leukocyte count	Shift to the left with a few immature forms (<5%). Toxic granulation and Dohle bodies in neutrophils	Shift to the left with numerous immature forms. Myelocyte and neutrophil peak
• Eosinophilia and basophilia	Variable	Present
• Leukocyte alkaline phosphatase (LAP) score	Increased	Decreased
RBC		
• Anemia	Usually minimal or absent	Severe and progressive
Platelets		
• Number	Variable	Normal or increased
Extramedullary myeloid tumors	Absent	Present
Philadelphia chromosome	Absent	Present
Response to therapy	Resolution	No resolution

BOX 12.5: Causes of neutropenia.

Decreased Production of Granulocytes
- **Marrow hypoplasia:** During cancer chemotherapy and aplastic anemia
- **Severe replacement of the marrow by tumor:** Leukemia, metastatic tumors, granulomatous disorders
- **Selective suppression of neutrophil production:** Drugs and chemicals (e.g., sulfonamides, analgesics, arsenicals), ionizing radiation

Increased Destruction of Granulocytes
- **Immune-mediated injury**: Drugs, autoimmune disorders (e.g., systemic lupus erythematosus)
- **Severe bacterial, fungal, or rickettsial infections**
  - Bacterial (e.g., typhoid, paratyphoid, septicemia)
  - Viral (e.g., influenza, infectious mononucleosis, hepatitis, measles)
  - Rickettsial (e.g., scrub typhus)
  - Protozoal (e.g., malaria, kala-azar)
- **Splenomegaly:** Splenic sequestration may be associated with pancytopenia

the sequestration and rapid removal of neutrophils from circulation.

Eosinophilia (Fig. 12.2)

Q. Write a short note on eosinophilia—definition and its causes.

Definition: Eosinophilia (eosinophilic leukocytosis) is defined as an eosinophil count of more than 450/cu mm (0.45×10^9/L).

The causes of eosinophilia are presented in **Table 12.3**.

Basophilia

Q. Write a short note on basophilia and its causes.

Normally basophils **(Fig. 12.3A)** are less than 1% of WBCs in peripheral blood. Basophilia (basophilic leukocytosis)

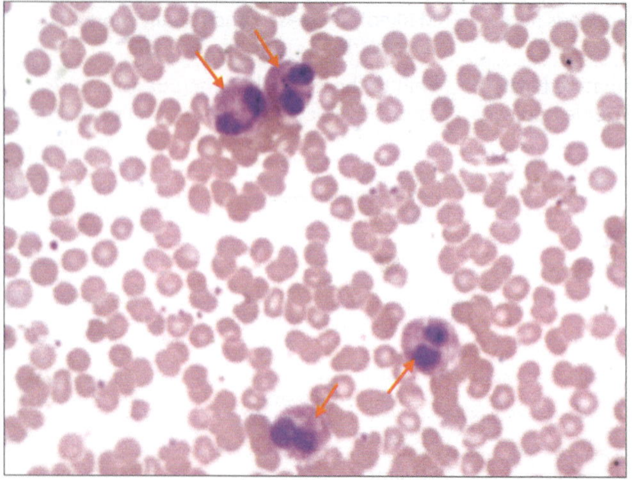

Fig. 12.2: Peripheral smear showing eosinophilia (arrow).

TABLE 12.3 Causes of eosinophilia.

1. **Allergic/atopic conditions**
   - Asthma
   - Hay fever
   - Allergic rhinitis
   - Allergic skin diseases (e.g., pemphigus, dermatitis herpetiformis)
   - Drug reactions
2. **Parasitic infestations (with tissue invasion)**
   - Roundworm infestation
   - Filariasis
   - Hookworm infestation
3. **Fungal infections** (e.g., coccidioidomycosis)
4. **Skin diseases**
   - Dermatitis (eczema)
   - Scabies
5. **Hematological diseases**
   - Chronic myeloid leukemia
   - Hodgkin lymphoma
   - Eosinophilic leukemia
   - Polycythemia
   - Some non-Hodgkin lymphomas
   - Acute myelomonocytic leukemia
6. **Miscellaneous**
   - Tropical eosinophilia
   - *Löeffler's* syndrome
   - Eosinophilic granuloma
   - Pulmonary eosinophilia
   - Hypereosinophilic syndrome
   - Collagen-vascular disorders
   - Some vasculitides

are rare. The causes of basophilia myeloproliferative neoplasms such as **chronic myeloid leukemia**, immediate hypersensitivity reactions, mastocytosis, viral infections (e.g., smallpox, chickenpox), etc.

Monocytosis (Box 12.6)

Q. Write a short note on monocytosis and its causes.

Definition: Monocytosis is defined as the presence of more than 10% of a differential count or an absolute monocyte **(Fig. 12.3B)** count exceeding 500/cu mm (0.5×10^9/L).

Lymphocytosis

Q. Write a short note on lymphocytosis and its causes.

Definition: Lymphocytosis is defined as a lymphocyte (Fig. 12.3C) count of more than 4,000/cu mm (4×10^9/L) in adults and more than 8,000/cu mm (8×10^9/L) in children.

Common causes of lymphocytosis are listed in **Box 12.7**. In many disorders, it accompanies monocytosis.

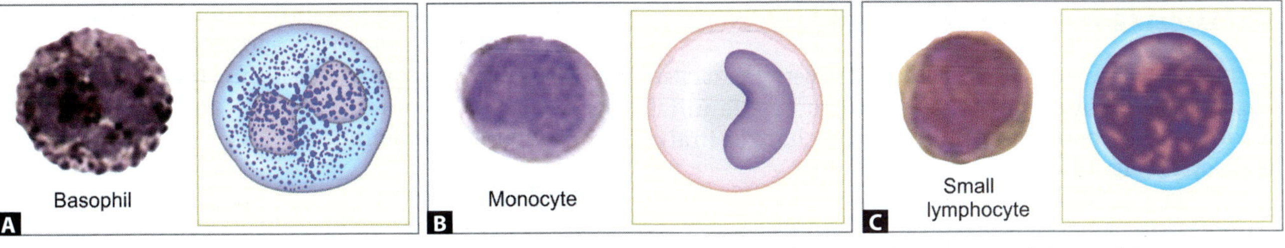

Figs. 12.3A to C: Appearance of cells in peripheral smear (right half of A to C—diagrammatic): (A) Basophil; (B) Monocyte; (C) Lymphocyte.

BOX 12.6: Causes of monocytosis.

1. **Infections**
   - Bacterial: Tuberculosis, bacterial endocarditis, brucellosis
   - Protozoal: Malaria, kala-azar
   - Spirochetal: Syphilis
   - Rickettsial: Typhus, Rocky Mountain fever
   - Recovery phase of neutropenia and acute infections
2. **Inflammatory diseases**
   - Inflammatory bowel disease: Ulcerative colitis, Crohn disease
   - Autoimmune diseases: Systemic lupus erythematosus, rheumatoid arthritis
   - Sarcoidosis
3. **Hematologic malignancies**
   - Acute monocytic, myelomonocytic, and myelocytic leukemias
   - Chronic myelomonocytic leukemia
   - Hodgkin lymphoma
   - Multiple myeloma

BOX 12.7: Causes of lymphocytosis.

1. **Acute infections**
   - Viral infections: Hepatitis A, cytomegalovirus, Epstein-Barr virus (infectious mononucleosis), mumps, measles, chickenpox
   - *Bordetella pertussis*
   - Toxoplasmosis
2. **Chronic infections/Inflammatory diseases**
   - Tuberculosis
   - Syphilis
   - Brucellosis
   - Inflammatory bowel disease: Crohn disease and ulcerative colitis
3. **Hematologic malignancies**
   - Acute lymphoblastic leukemia
   - Chronic lymphocytic leukemia
   - Non-Hodgkin lymphoma with spillover
   - Adult T-cell leukemia/lymphoma
   - Hairy cell leukemia

BOX 12.8: Causes of lymphocytopenia.

1. **Increased destruction**
   - Corticosteroids
   - Cytotoxic drugs
   - Radiation
2. **Decreased production**
   - Aplastic anemia
   - Advanced malignancy: Hodgkin lymphoma
   - Infections: AIDS, miliary tuberculosis
3. **Increased loss via GI tract**
   - Obstruction to intestinal lymphatic drainage (e.g., tumor)
   - Congestive heart failure

Lymphocytopenia

Definition: Lymphocytopenia is defined as lymphocyte counts below 1,500/cu mm (1×10^9/L) in adults and below 3,000/cu mm (3×10^9/L) in children.

Some of the important causes of lymphocytopenia are listed in **Box 12.8**.

Leukoerythroblastic Reaction/Blood Picture

Q. Write a short note on leukoerythroblastic reaction/blood picture and its causes.

Definition: It is the presence of immature white blood cells (myelocytes, metamyelocytes, and promyelocytes) as well as nucleated RBCs in the peripheral blood.

Causes of leukoerythroblastic reaction are listed in **Box 12.9**.

BOX 12.9: Causes of leukoerythroblastic reaction.

- **Infectious diseases:** Miliary tuberculosis
- **Bone metastasis.** For example, carcinoma of the lung, breast, prostate, gastrointestinal tract)
- **Hematological conditions:** Myelofibrosis, severe hemolysis (e.g., erythroblastosis fetalis), multiple myeloma, lymphoma
- **Storage disorders:** Gaucher's disease, Niemann–Pick disease.

QUALITATIVE DISORDERS OF LEUKOCYTES

Q. Write a short note on qualitative/functional disorders of leukocytes.

Qualitative disorders of leukocytes are rare familial disorders that manifest as morphologic changes in the leukocytes **(Fig. 12.4)**.

INFECTIOUS MONONUCLEOSIS (GLANDULAR FEVER)

Q. Write a short note on infectious mononucleosis.

Definition: Infectious mononucleosis is an acute, benign, self-limiting lymphoproliferative disorder **caused by Epstein-Barr virus** (EBV). It is a **disease of adolescents and young adults.**

- **Incubation period:** 4–8 weeks.
- **Mode of transmission: Oropharyngeal secretions (kissing)** through direct oral contact, hence the nickname kissing disease.

Pathogenesis

- **EBV infects B lymphocytes** by binding to **CD21 (CR2) receptor.**
- Viral infection begins in the submucosal lymphoid tissues of the nasopharynx and oropharynx.
- Virus remains dormant inside the B-cells.
- B-cells are **"immortalized"** and are capable of **proliferation indefinitely.**

Clinical Features

- **Age:** Young adults among upper socioeconomic classes in developed nations and children of low socioeconomic status.
- **Signs and symptoms: Classical triad**
  1. Fever
  2. Pharyngitis (sore throat)
  3. Generalized lymphadenopathy.

Laboratory Finding

Q. Mention the laboratory findings in infectious mononucleosis.

- **Lymphocytosis: Total leukocyte count is increased** (12,000–25,000 cells/cu mm) and shows **absolute lymphocytosis (activated CD8+ cells).**
- **Atypical lymphocytosis (mononuclear cells): These are CD8+ subsets (cytotoxic) of T-cells** and not the virus-infected B-cells. EBV infects B-cells but the

Qualitative abnormality	Mode of inheritance	Characteristic morphology	Functional abnormalities	Appearance of leukocyte
Pelger–Huet anomaly	Autosomal dominant	Lack of neutrophil nuclear segmentation beyond 2 lobes	Normal	
Alder–Reilly anomaly	Autosomal recessive	**Large lilac inclusions** in cytoplasm of all leukocytes	Normal	
May–Hegglin anomaly	Autosomal dominant	**Large basophilic inclusions** in all leukocytes. Giant platelets and thrombocytopenia	Abnormal bleeding due to thrombocytopenia	
Chediak–Higashi anomaly	Autosomal recessive	• **Large gray blue granules in cytoplasm** of monocytes and granulocytes • Defective lysosomal granules	• Poor chemotaxis • Increased susceptibility to pyogenic infections • Bleeding tendency	
Chronic granulomatous disease of childhood (CGD)	X-linked autosomal recessive	Normal appearance but defective function	• Deficient NADPH oxidase, with absent H_2O_2 production • Phagocytosis and killing of organisms is impaired	

Fig. 12.4: Various quantitative disorders of leukocytes.

Main causes of leukemoid reaction:
- Infections
- Hemorrhage
- Drugs (glucocorticoids)
- Malignancies
- Down syndrome.

Differential leukocyte count (DLC) is one of the routine, useful, and important investigations

- Dengue fever is caused by the flavivirus transmitted by fresh-water mosquitoes (*Aedes aegypti*).
- Peripheral smear shows transformed lymphocytes and thrombocytopenia

peripheral blood shows CD8+ T-cells, which appear as atypical lymphocytes.

- **Serological tests:**
  - **Demonstration of heterophile antibodies:**
    - Paul Bunnell test is characteristically positive.
    - Monospot test is a sensitive slide test.
  - **Demonstration of specific antibodies against EBV antigens:** The demonstration of specific antibodies to EBV is the most specific test for infectious mononucleosis.
    - Antibody against viral capsid antigens (anti-VCA).
    - Antibodies to Epstein-Barr nuclear antigen (EBNA).

NEOPLASTIC PROLIFERATIONS OF WHITE CELLS

Neoplasms of white cells are the **most important disorders**. Almost all these tumors are malignant. But, show a wide range of behaviors, ranging from indolent to the most aggressive cancers. Hematologic malignancies can occur at all ages.

ACUTE LEUKEMIA

PA 18.2a (CC): Describe the etiology, genetics, pathogenesis, classification, features, and hematologic features of acute leukemia.

Leukemias are **malignant disorders characterized by the proliferation of hemopoietic cells**.

Q. Define leukemia.

Definition: Acute leukemias are a **diverse group of malignant tumors characterized by neoplastic proliferations of immature hematopoietic cells.** The immature neoplastic cells are referred to as blasts. These **blast cells constitute more than 20% of the nucleated cells in the peripheral blood/bone marrow (WHO criteria).**

The neoplastic blast cells often replace normal marrow elements, leading to symptoms related to marrow failure. The proliferating neoplastic blast cells fail to mature. The **peripheral blood shows abnormal numbers and forms of immature white blood cells. Aleukemic/subleukemic leukemia** is characterized by **very few/no blasts in the peripheral blood.**

Groups of acute leukemia: Most acute leukemia can be subclassified into two major groups acute lymphoblastic leukemia (ALL) and acute myeloid leukemia (AML). ALL is further divided into B-ALL and T-ALL.

Etiology

Q. Write a short note on the etiology of leukemias.

Risk factors **(Box 12.10)** involved in the pathogenesis of leukemia may cause mutations in the protooncogenes and tumor suppressor genes.

BOX 12.10: Risk factors for acute leukemia.

Environmental Factors

- **Ionizing radiation**
- **Drugs:**
  - Alkylating agents—nitrogen mustard, chlorambucil, etc.
  - AML occurs in myeloma patients treated with melphalan
  - Leukemia follows chemotherapy for lung and ovarian cancer
- **Chemicals:** Benzene (used in the paint industry, plastic glues, etc.)

Genetic Disorders

Example: Down syndrome (ALL or AML), Fanconi anemia (AML), ataxia telangiectasia (ALL, NHL)

Acquired Disorders

- **PNH and aplastic anemia** may transform into acute leukemia
- AML may develop **de novo or secondary to myelodysplastic syndrome** (MDS)

Pathogenesis

Driver mutations: The most common driver mutations in all types of acute leukemia are gene rearrangements and point substitutions.

Transcription factor mutations: The driver mutations interfere with the function of transcription factors that regulate normal hematopoietic stem cell differentiation. These mutations usually affect gene products that regulate the lineage to which the leukemia belongs. For example, B-ALL contains mutations affecting the transcription factor PAX5. This PAX5 is specifically needed for the differentiation of early B cell progenitors.

Complementary recurrent driver mutations: Transcription factor mutations alone are not enough for the development of acute leukemia. It undergoes different complementary recurrent driver mutations. Several of these mutations affect signaling molecules like tyrosine kinases and RAS. These increase the proliferation of tumor cells and their survival.

Epigenetic alterations: Other mutations may involve factors that regulate chromatin-associated proteins such as histones. This suggests that epigenetic alterations are also important in the development of acute leukemias.

Examples of Driver Mutation

***BCR-ABL* in B-ALL:** Rearrangements is a broad term that consists of a range of structural genomic alterations leading to gene fusions. In BCR-ABL, there is rearrangements of the *ABL* gene on chromosome 9 and the *BCR* gene on chromosome 22. It is usually produced by a balanced (9;22) translocation and forms the Philadelphia chromosome (or Ph chromosome, named after the city where it was discovered). This gene rearrangement forms a *BCR-ABL* fusion (chimeric) gene that encodes a constitutively active tyrosine kinase. This in turn activates all the pathways that lie downstream of growth factor receptors. About 5% of childhood B-ALL and 25% of adult B-ALL are associated with *BCR-ABL* fusion genes. This gene is also found in chronic myeloid leukemia (*refer* page 379 and **Fig. 12.9**). Patients with *BCR-ABL* + B-ALLs respond to tyrosine kinase inhibitors.

***PML-RARA* in acute promyelocytic leukemia:** Acute promyelocytic leukemia is a subtype of AML. It is almost always associated with the presence of rearrangements involving the *PML* gene on chromosome 15 and the *RARA* gene on chromosome 17. It is usually formed by a balanced (15;17) translocation. *RARA* encodes the retinoic acid receptor. The chimeric (fusion) *PML-RARA* gene encodes a fusion protein that blocks myeloid differentiation at the promyelocytic stage. Probably in part, it inhibits the function of normal retinoic acid receptors. All-trans retinoic acid (ATRA) is an analog of vitamin A, prevents this block, and allows the neoplastic promyelocytes to differentiate rapidly into neutrophils. Because neutrophils die after an average life span of a day or so, ATRA treatment produces "death by differentiation."

***IDH1 and IDH2* mutations in AML:** *IDH* genes that encode isoforms of isocitrate dehydrogenase (IDH), which is a metabolic enzyme. About 10% of AMLs have mutations in either *IDH1* or *IDH2.* Mutant forms of IDH contribute to transformation by creating the oncometabolite 2-hydroxyglutarate. Inhibitors of mutated IDH1 and IDH2 can induce the differentiation of IDH-mutated AMLs.

Classification of Acute Leukemia

Q. Classify acute leukemia.

Traditional classification depending on the microscopic appearance of the involved cell and the course of leukemias is presented in **Box 12.11**. It is no longer used but is mentioned here for the sake of beginner students in pathology.

FAB Classification of Acute Leukemias

The first French, American, and British (FAB) classification (1976) was **based on the (1) morphological and (2) cytochemical characteristics of blast cells. Revised FAB classification (Box 12.12)** includes (1) morphology and cytochemistry of blast cells, (2) immunophenotyping (technique that uses specific antibodies to detect specific protein expression within a cell population), (3) cytogenetics (looking for changes in the chromosomes), and (4) molecular genetics (study of structure and function of genes at the molecular level).

BOX 12.11: Traditional (conventional) classification of leukemia.

- **Acute leukemia**
  - Acute myelogenous/myeloblastic/myeloid leukemia (AML)
  - Acute lymphoblastic leukemia (ALL)
- **Chronic leukemia**
  - Chronic myeloid leukemia (CML)
  - Chronic lymphocytic leukemia (CLL)

BOX 12.12: Revised French, American, and British (FAB) classification of acute leukemias.

Acute Lymphoid Leukemia

L1	Small homogenous cells with inconspicuous nucleoli
L2	Large cells with variable size and 1–2 nucleoli
L3	Large, homogeneous cells with finely stippled chromatin and prominent nucleoli. The cytoplasm is basophilic and vacuolated

Acute Myeloid Leukemia

M0	Minimally differentiated AML
M1	AML without maturation
M2	AML with maturation
M3	Promyelocytic leukemia
M4	Myelomonocytic leukemia
M5	Monocytic leukemia
M6	Erythroleukemia
M7	Megakaryocytic leukemia

AML M2 is the most common type of AML. AML M3 is associated with disseminated intravascular coagulation (DIC). AML M7 is the most common type of AML in Down syndrome.

WHO Classification (2022) of Acute Leukemia (Boxes 12.13–12.15)

Q. Classify acute leukemia as per WHO guidelines.

According to WHO (2022) classification, acute leukemias are classified as (1) acute myeloid leukemias, and (2) acute lymphoblastic leukemia. An outline of the WHO (2022) classification of acute leukemia is presented in **Box 12.13 (also *refer* Boxes 12.14 and 12.15).**

Cytochemistry in Leukemia

Q. Write a short note on cytochemistry in acute leukemia.

Cytochemistry is the study of chemical elements found in the cytoplasm of the cells. The chemical element in the cell may be an enzyme (e.g., myeloperoxidase) or a non-enzymatic substance (e.g., lipids and glycogen). They are

BOX 12.13: Outline of WHO (2022) classification of acute leukemia.

Acute Myeloid Leukemia (AML)
- Acute myeloid leukemia with defining genetic abnormalities
- Acute myeloid leukemia, defined by differentiation

Acute Lymphoblastic Leukemia (ALL)
- **B-cell neoplasms**
  - **Precursor B-cell neoplasms**
    - B-lymphoblastic leukemias/lymphomas
  - **Mature B-cell neoplasms**
- **T-cell neoplasms**
  - **Precursor T-cell neoplasms**
    - T-lymphoblastic leukemia/lymphoma
  - **Mature T-cell and NK-cell neoplasms**
    - Mature T-cell and NK-cell leukemias

used to characterize the blast cells as myeloid or lymphoid in acute leukemias.

Myeloperoxidase (MPO): It is an enzyme present in the primary granules of **mature and immature** cells of **myeloid series** (*refer* **Fig. 12.8B**). Leukemic myeloblasts are positive (AML M1, M2, M3, and M4 blasts and Auer rods); and lymphoblasts and normoblasts are negative. Thus, useful in differentiating AML from ALL.

Sudan Black B (SBB): It stains lipids and phospholipids present in the granules of the cells of the **myeloid series** (*refer* **Figs. 12.8C and D**). The granules take up a black color. The staining patterns in MPO and SBB are similar. It is useful in the differentiation of AML from ALL.

Periodic acid-Schiff (PAS) stain: It is **useful for diagnosing ALLs**, and erythroid and megakaryocytic (M6 and M7) types of acute myeloid leukemia. The periodic acid oxidizes glycogen, mucoproteins, and other high molecular weight (HMW) carbohydrates present in the cells to aldehydes. These aldehydes react with colorless Schiff reagent and take bright-red pink (*magenta*) color. The staining pattern may be fine and diffuse, coarse, and granular (block positivity), or a mixture of both patterns. It is useful for differentiating AML from ALL. **Myeloblasts are negative and lymphoblasts show blocks of PAS-positive (Figs. 12.5 inset and 12.6B) material in the cytoplasm.** Block positivity in lymphoblasts is observed in most of the ALL L1 cases.

Neutrophil alkaline phosphatase: Alkaline phosphatase is an enzyme located in the specific (secondary) or tertiary granules present in the cytoplasm of mature neutrophils, with some activity in metamyelocytes. The positive reaction gives rise to a blue and granular appearance in the cytoplasmic granules. Normal NAP/LAP score: 40–100. **LAP increased** in **leukemoid reaction and polycythemia rubra vera. LAP decreased** in **chronic myeloid leukemia.**

ACUTE LYMPHOBLASTIC LEUKEMIA/LYMPHOMA

Definition: Acute lymphoblastic leukemia/lymphoma [ALL/lymphoblastic lymphoma (LBL)] is a group of neoplasms consisting of **lymphoblasts.**

WHO (2022) Classification of Acute Lymphoblastic Leukemia/Lymphoma (Box 12.14)

Lymphoblastic leukemias/lymphomas are grouped by their lineage. Lymphoblast is an immature, precursor B (pre-B) or T (pre-T) lymphocyte. By immunophenotype, **ALL may be further divided into B-cell and T-cell types** of ALL. B-cell lymphoid proliferations and lymphomas represent the most common lymphoid neoplasms.

- **B-cell (B-cell acute lymphoblastic leukemia, or B-ALL)**
  1. **Childhood leukemia:** B-ALL is the most common childhood leukemia. Its peak incidence is between **2 and 10 years of age**. It constitutes about 85% of all ALL. These are tumors of precursor B cells.

BOX 12.14: WHO (2022) classification of B and T-cell leukemia/lymphoma.

B-CELL NEOPLASMS

Precursor B-cell neoplasms
- B-lymphoblastic leukemia/lymphoma
- B-lymphoblastic leukemia/lymphoma with high hyperdiploidy
- B-lymphoblastic leukemia/lymphoma with hypodiploidy
- B-lymphoblastic leukemia/lymphoma with iAMP21
- B-lymphoblastic leukemia/lymphoma with cancer is BCR::ABL1 fusion
- B-lymphoblastic leukemia/lymphoma with BCR::ABL1-like features
- B-lymphoblastic leukemia/lymphoma with KMT2A rearrangement
- B-lymphoblastic leukemia/lymphoma with ETV6::RUNX1 fusion
- B-lymphoblastic leukemia/lymphoma with ETV6::RUNX1-like features
- B-lymphoblastic leukemia/lymphoma with TCF3::PBX1 fusion
- B-lymphoblastic leukemia/lymphoma with IGH::IL3 fusion
- B-lymphoblastic leukemia/lymphoma with TCF3::HLF fusion
- B-lymphoblastic leukemia/lymphoma with other defined genetic alterations
- B-lymphoblastic leukemia/lymphoma, NOS

Mature B-cell neoplasms
- Pre-neoplastic and neoplastic small lymphocytic proliferations
  - Chronic lymphocytic leukemia/small lymphocytic lymphoma
- Splenic B-cell lymphomas and leukemias
  - Hairy cell leukemia

T-CELL NEOPLASM

Precursor T-cell neoplasms
- T-lymphoblastic leukemia/lymphoma
  - T-lymphoblastic leukemia/lymphoma, NOS
  - Early T-precursor lymphoblastic leukemia/lymphoma

Mature T-cell and NK-cell neoplasms
- Mature T-cell and NK-cell leukemias
  - Adult T cell leukemia/lymphoma
  - Sezary syndrome

2. **Always arises within bone marrow:** It almost always arises within the marrow and replaces normal marrow elements.
3. **Symptoms of bone marrow failure:** Replacement of marrow elements produces **symptoms related to anemia** (weakness, fatigue), **thrombocytopenia** [petechiae (small bleeds into the skin and mucosal membranes)], and **neutropenia** (infection).
4. **Leukemia versus lymphoma:**
   - **B-lymphoblastic leukemias (or B-ALL): They present with bone marrow and blood involvement by lymphoblast.**

- **B-lymphoblastic lymphomas: They present with extramedullary disease (e.g., lymph nodes, thymus, skin).**

- **T-cell (T-cell acute lymphoblastic leukemia, or T-ALL)**
  - **During adolescence:** T-ALL most commonly presents during adolescence. It constitutes about 15% of all ALL. It accounts for 15% of childhood ALL.
  - **Involves thymus and bone marrow:** T-ALL usually involves the thymus and the bone marrow.
  - **Symptoms of bone marrow failure and mediastinal mass:** These tumors develop symptoms of marrow failure and more than 50% present with mediastinal masses due to thymic involvement.
  - **Malignant T-cells are immature** T-cells. It may present as T-cell acute lymphoblastic leukemia (T-ALL) or T-cell lymphoblastic lymphoma (T-LBL). Like precursor B-ALL, the decision to call the tumor leukemia or lymphoma is often inconsistent.

Typically, ALL is characterized by a **complete maturation arrest at the early stages of B- or T-cell differentiation.** Hence, in ALL, **blasts are the major tumor cell population in involved tissues.**

Molecular Pathogenesis

Chromosomal (nonrandom karyotypic) abnormalities are found in about 90% of ALLs.

B-ALL

- **Numerical abnormality:** Hyperploidy (more than 50 chromosomes/cell) in B-ALL and hypoploidy.
- **Structural abnormality:** These include the following:
  - A (12;21) translocation involving the *ETV6* and *RUNX1* genes in B-ALL.
  - A (9;22) balanced translocation involving the *ABL* and *BCR* genes (Philadelphia chromosome). occur in about 25% of adult pre–B-cell tumors.

T-ALL

Pre–T-cell tumors are associated with different chromosomal aberrations. These include the following:

- **Translocations involving the T-cell receptor loci** and certain transcription factor genes.
- **Mutations that inactivate tumor suppressor genes:** Examples, tumor suppressor gene *PTEN* (leading to increased pro-growth signaling) and *CDKN2A* (encodes a negative regulator of the cell cycle and a positive regulator of p53).

Clinical Features

Age: ALL is the most common hematological malignancy of **children**. Most common between **1 and 5 years** of age and between **30 and 40 years.**

Sex: Slight male preponderance.

Onset: Acute leukemia is an aggressive disease with **abrupt onset.**

Symptoms

- **Bone marrow failure:**
  - **Anemia:** Causes **fatigue, and weakness.**
  - **Neutropenia: Infections** by bacteria or opportunistic fungi. Develop sore throat and respiratory infections.
  - **Thrombocytopenia: Bleeding** into the skin and mucosa in the form of purpura or ecchymoses.

  Bone pain and **sternal tenderness:** Due to marrow expansion and infiltration of the subperiosteum.
- **Extramedullary infiltration:**
  - **Lymphadenopathy: About** 75% of patients, usually involve **cervical lymph nodes.**
  - **Hepatosplenomegaly:** Splenomegaly is more common than hepatomegaly.
- **Mediastinal thymic mass:** More common in T-ALL. It may be accompanied by *compression of large vessels and airways in the mediastinum.*
- **CNS involvement:** Spread into the meninges causes leukemic meningitis ALL (pre-B). It may produce headache, vomiting, and nerve palsies.
- **Testicular enlargement** due to leukemic infiltration.

Laboratory Findings

Q. Describe the laboratory diagnosis (including peripheral smear, bone marrow finding, and special stains) of acute lymphoblastic leukemia (ALL).

Peripheral Blood

- **Total WBC count: Markedly raised** ranging from 20 × 10^9/L to 100 × 10^9/L (i.e., 20,000 to 1,00,000/cu mm)
- **Platelet count: Reduced** (thrombocytopenia).
- **Hemoglobin: Decreased** and may be as low as 3 g/dL.

Q. Write a short note on peripheral smear findings in acute lymphoblastic leukemia.

PERIPHERAL SMEAR (FIGS. 12.5 AND 12.6)

RBCs: Normocytic normochromic anemia.

WBCs: Total count **markedly increased** and **20% or more lymphoblasts.** The lymphoblasts of B-ALL and T-ALL are similar morphologically. **Morphologic features of lymphoblasts are as follows:**

- **Size: Larger than small lymphocyte**
- **High N: C (nuclear-cytoplasmic) ratio**
- **Nucleus:** Nucleus with **condensed, delicate, finely stippled chromatin. The nucleoli are either absent or small inconspicuous.**
- **Cytoplasm: Scant to moderate agranular basophilic cytoplasm.**

Platelets: Thrombocytopenia.

Cytochemistry of Lymphoblasts

- **PAS (periodic acid-Schiff):** Cytoplasmic aggregates of PAS-positive **[Figs. 12.5 (inset) and 12.6B]** material **(block positivity).**

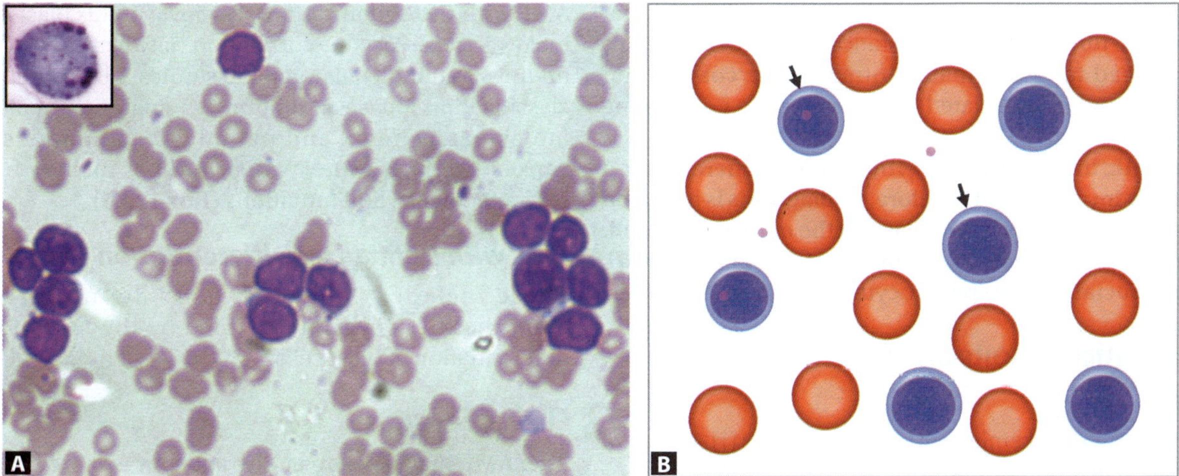

Figs. 12.5A and B: Peripheral blood smears in acute lymphoblastic leukemia: (A) Peripheral smear shows several lymphoblasts. Inset shows lymphoblast with block positivity with PAS stain; (B) The diagrammatic appearance of peripheral blood smear in acute lymphoblastic leukemia shows lymphoblasts (arrows).

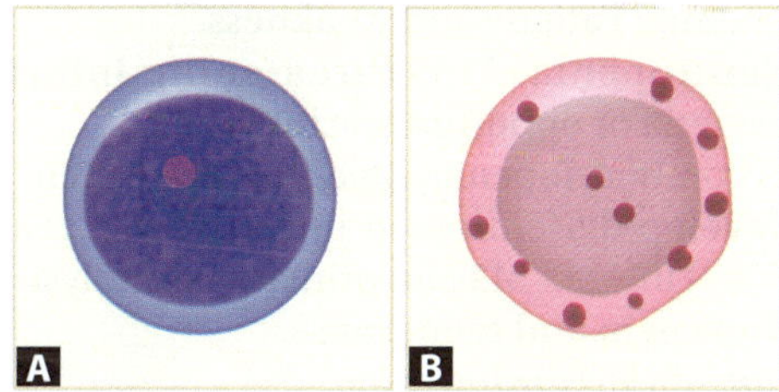

Figs. 12.6A and B: (A) Diagrammatic appearance of lymphoblast: (B) Periodic acid Schiff (PAS) stain showing lymphoblast with block positivity (diagrammatic).

- **Myeloperoxidase (MPO) negative.**
- **Sudan Black B negative.**
- **Nonspecific esterase negative**

BONE MARROW

- **Cellularity:** Markedly **hypercellular** due to the proliferation of blasts.
- **Erythropoiesis and myelopoiesis: Reduced.**
- **Megakaryopoiesis:** Megakaryocytes **gradually decrease.**
- **Blasts: Constitute 20–100% of the marrow cells.**

Immunophenotyping: Definitive diagnosis depends on stains performed with antibodies specific for B, and T markers, usually by flow cytometry.

- **Terminal-deoxynucleotidyl-transferase (TdT):** It is an enzyme specifically expressed in pre-B and pre-T cells. It is a sensitive but not entirely specific marker of ALL.
- Immature B-cells stain positive for pan B cell markers CD19 and CD10 (CALLA—common ALL antigen).
- Precursor T ALL cells are positive for CD2, CD5 and CD8.

Biochemical Findings

- **Serum uric acid: Raised** due to the destruction of leukemic cells **during chemotherapy** leading to hyperuricemia.

TABLE 12.4 Factors involved in prognosis of childhood ALL.

Worse prognosis	*Favorable prognosis*
Age younger than 2 years	Age between 2 and 10 years
Presentation in adulthood	A low white cell count
Peripheral blood blast counts greater than 100,000/cu mm	Hyperdiploidy

- **LDH: Raised**, because of increased turnover of leukemic cells.

CSF Examination

To know/rule out CNS involvement.

More than 80% of children with B-ALL and T-ALL are cured with the presently available therapy.

Prognosis in childhood ALL: Prognostic features are outlined in **Table 12.4.**

ACUTE MYELOID LEUKEMIA

Q. Classify acute myeloid leukemia (AML) as per WHO guidelines. Add a note on laboratory findings in a case of acute promyelocytic leukemia.

Definition: AML is a **neoplasm of hematopoietic progenitors** characterized by **proliferation resulting in the accumulation of immature myeloblasts in the marrow.**

General features of acute myeloid leukemia (AML): These are as follows:

- **Any age:** AML can occur throughout life. **Most common in individuals older than 60 years of age.**
- **Most often arises from a preexisting myeloid neoplasm:** Unlike ALL, AML usually arises from a preexisting myeloid neoplasm (either a **myeloproliferative neoplasm or a myelodysplastic syndrome**).
- **Symptoms of bone marrow failure:** Like ALL, most symptoms of AML are due to marrow failure. Some

specific subtypes of AML are composed of cells that release thromboplastic substances into the blood. This can lead to disseminated intravascular coagulation (DIC) and its associated complications (e.g., bleeding complications).

In AML, in contrast to ALL, the block in differentiation is usually incomplete. Therefore, its diagnosis is based on the presence of at least 20% blasts in the marrow or blood. However, this diagnostic requirement is relaxed in AML types associated with specific cytogenetic abnormalities.

Classification of Acute Myeloid Leukemia (AML) (Box 12.15)

Acute myeloid leukemia (AML) is classified as (i) AML *with defining genetic abnormalities* and (ii)AML *with defined by differentiation.* A diagnosis of AML requires at least 20% myeloblasts in the blood or bone marrow. However, this diagnostic requirement is relaxed in AML types associated with specific cytogenetic abnormalities.

AML with Defining Genetic Abnormalities

The present WHO classification has **eliminated the 20% blast requirement for AML types with defining genetic abnormalities** (except **AML with *BCR::ABL1* fusion and AML with *CEBPA* mutation**). Removal of this blast cut-off makes it necessary for correlation between morphologic findings and molecular genetic studies. The overall AML classification focuses attention to integration of clinical, molecular/genetic, and pathologic parameters. The various *defining genetic abnormalities* include fusion, rearrangements, and mutations **(Box 12.15)**.

BOX 12.15: WHO (2022) classification of acute myeloid leukemia.

Acute myeloid leukemia with defining genetic abnormalities
- Acute promyelocytic leukemia with PML::RARA fusion
- Acute myeloid leukemia with RUNX1::RUNX1T1 fusion
- Acute myeloid leukemia with CBFB::MYH11 fusion
- Acute myeloid leukemia with DEK::NUP214 fusion
- Acute myeloid leukemia with RBM15::MRTFA fusion
- Acute myeloid leukemia with BCR::ABL1 fusion
- Acute myeloid leukemia with KMT2A rearrangement
- Acute myeloid leukemia with MECOM rearrangement
- Acute myeloid leukemia with NUP98 rearrangement
- Acute myeloid leukemia with NPM1 mutation
- Acute myeloid leukemia with CEBPA mutation
- Acute myeloid leukemia, myelodysplasia-related
- Acute myeloid leukemia with other defined genetic alterations

Acute myeloid leukemia, defined by differentiation
- Acute myeloid leukemia with minimal differentiation
- Acute myeloid leukemia without maturation
- Acute myeloid leukemia with maturation
- Acute basophilic leukemia
- Acute myelomonocytic leukemia
- Acute monocytic leukemia
- Acute erythroid leukemia
- Acute megakaryoblastic leukemia

Myeloid sarcoma
- Myeloid sarcoma

AML with Defined by Differentiation

These include AML which lacks defining genetic abnormalities. They are defined by the morphologic differentiation of blast cells.

Clinical Features

Age: AML may develop at **any age**, but is more **common in adults**.

Onset: Acute leukemias are **abrupt in onset**.

Symptoms*:* Related to depressed marrow function.

- *Bone marrow failure*:
  - Anemia: **Fatigue and weakness.**
  - Neutropenia: **Life-threatening infections** by bacteria or opportunistic fungi.
  - Thrombocytopenia: **Bleeding,** the patient may also develop disseminated intravascular coagulation (DIC) in AML M3 and primary fibrinolysis.
  - **Bone pain and tenderness.**
- *Extramedullary infiltration:*
  - **Gingival hypertrophy (M4 and M5) due to infiltration of gums** and **infiltration of skin** (leukemia cutis).
  - **Hepatosplenomegaly: Usually more than in ALL.**

Laboratory Findings

Q. Describe the laboratory diagnosis of acute myeloid leukemia (AML).

Peripheral Blood

- **Total WBC count: Markedly raised,** ranging from 20 × 10^9/L to 100 × 10^9/L (i.e., 20,000 to 1,00,000/cu mm).
- **Hemoglobin:** Decreased and ranges from 5 g/dL to 9 g/dL.

Q. Write a short note on peripheral smear findings in AML.

Q. Write a short note on Auer rods.

PERIPHERAL SMEAR (FIGS. 12.7 AND 12.8A)

RBCs: Normocytic normochromic type of anemia.

WBCs: Total WBC **count markedly increased.**

- **Differential count: More than 20% myeloid blasts.** May show more than one type of blast or blast with hybrid features. **The morphology of myeloblasts is as follows:**
  - **Size: Medium to large, 3 to 5 times larger than** the diameter of a **small lymphocyte.**
  - **High N: C (nuclear cytoplasmic) ratio.**
  - **Nuclei: Round or slightly irregular nuclei and immature fine nuclear chromatin with 2–4** variably **prominent (distinct) nucleoli.**

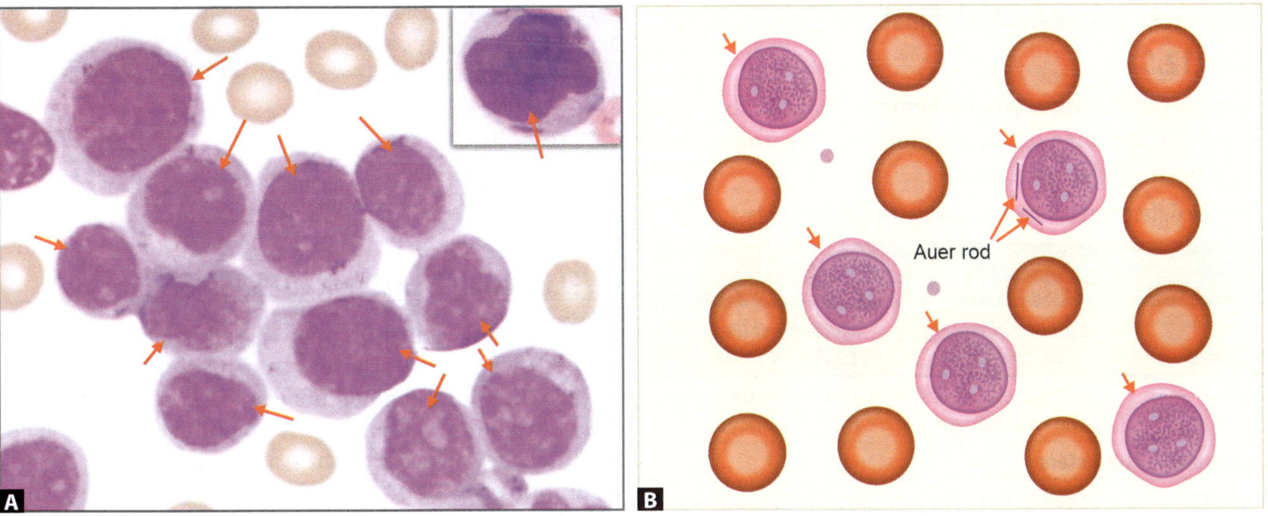

Figs. 12.7A and B: Peripheral smear in AML with myeloblasts: (A) Leishman stain shows myeloblasts (arrows). The inset shows the myeloblast with an Auer rod (arrow); (B) The diagrammatic appearance shows myeloblasts (short arrows). One myeloblast with two Auer rods (long arrows) is also seen.

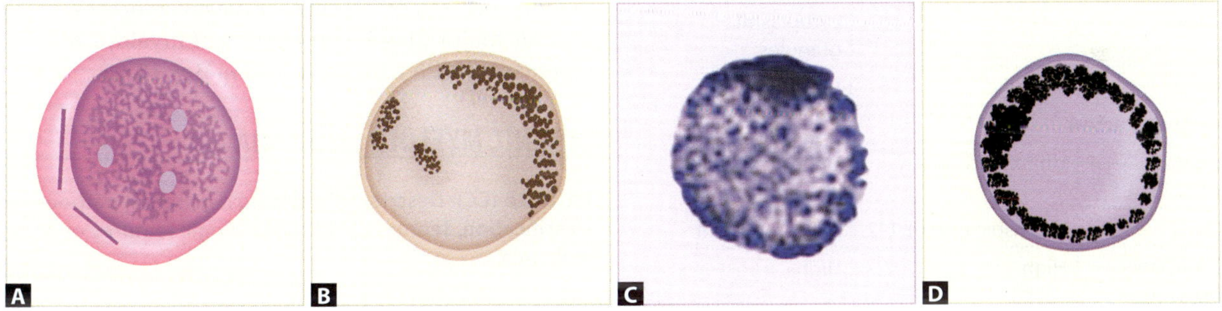

Figs. 12.8A to D: (A) Diagrammatic appearance of myeloblast; (B) Myeloblast stained positively with myeloperoxidase (diagrammatic); (C) Myeloblast stained positively with Sudan Black; (D) Diagrammatic appearance of Sudan Black.

- **Cytoplasm: Moderate amounts of cytoplasm and more than that of lymphoblasts.** It shows a **variable number of azurophilic, peroxidase-positive granules.**
- **Auer rods:** These are **slender, eosinophilic, needle-like, peroxidase positive structures (inclusions) in** the cytoplasm of **myeloblasts (M2 and M3 subtype).** These are **coalesced primary (azurophilic) granules.** The presence of **Auer rods is pathognomonic** and **definitive evidence of myeloid differentiation.**

Platelets: Moderate to severe thrombocytopenia and cause bleeding from skin and mucosa.

Cytochemical stains for myeloblasts: These are helpful in classifying AML.

Q. Write a short note on special stains in AML.

- **Myeloperoxidase: Positive (Fig. 12.8B)**
- **Sudan black** (lipids): **Positive (Figs. 12.8C and D)**
- **PAS: Negative.**
- Nonspecific esterase positive in M4 and M5 of FAB classification.

Q. Describe the bone marrow findings in AML including special stains.

BONE MARROW

Cellularity: Markedly **hypercellular.**

Erythropoiesis: Markedly suppressed.

Myelopoiesis: Typically, **myeloblasts progressively accumulate in the marrow. These myeloblasts cannot differentiate and mature further** (suppression of myeloid maturation). They displace normal hematopoietic cells and **suppress normal hematopoiesis.** The **myeloblasts constitute more than 20% of marrow cells.**

Megakaryopoiesis: Gradually decreased.

Accurate WHO classification of AML: It requires immunophenotyping by flow cytometry, chromosomal analysis (cytogenetic studies), and molecular studies.

- **Immunophenotyping:** Diagnosis of AML is confirmed by using stains for myeloid-specific antigens. For example, CD13, CD15, CD33, and CD117 (c-kit).
- **Cytogenetics:** Very important in the WHO classification of AML (*refer* **Box 12.15**).

Differences between Myeloblast and Lymphoblast (Table 12.5)

It is important to differentiate between lymphoblast and myeloblast because of the difference in treatment and prognosis of AML and ALL.

Q. List the differences between myeloblast and lymphoblast.

TABLE 12.5 Differences between lymphoblast and myeloblast based on morphology and cytochemistry.

Features	*Lymphoblast (Figs. 12.5, and 12.6A)*	*Myeloblast (Figs. 12.7, and 12.8A)*
Size	2–3 times the size of the lymphocyte	3–5 times the size of the lymphocyte
Cytoplasmic characters		
Amount	Scanty (less cytoplasm than myeloblast)	Scanty to moderate (more cytoplasm than lymphoblast)
Color	Blue	Gray
Cytoplasmic granules	Agranular	May have cytoplasmic granules
Auer rod	Negative	Positive
Nuclear characters		
Nuclear chromatin	Uniform, coarse	Uniform, fine
Nucleoli	Inconspicuous or 1–2	3–5, prominent
N: C (nuclear-cytoplasmic) ratio	High	High
Accompanying cells	Lymphocytes	Promyelocytes, myelocytes, metamyelocytes, band forms, and neutrophils
Cytochemistry		
Myeloperoxidase	Negative	Positive
Sudan Black	Negative	Positive
PAS	Block positivity	Negative
Nonspecific esterase	Negative	Positive in M4 and M5

Myeloid sarcoma: It is a solid tumor mass consisting of myeloid blasts (myeloblasts or monoblasts) with or without maturation occurring at extramedullary sites. This entity is sometimes called a chloroma (because of its greenish color), granulocytic sarcoma, extramedullary myeloid tumor, or monoblastic sarcoma. Myeloid sarcoma is frequent in the skin, lymph nodes, GI tract, bone, soft tissue, and testis. **Microscopically shows myeloblasts** with or without features of promyelocytic or neutrophilic maturation.

BOX 12.16: Major diagnostic entities of myeloproliferative neoplasms.

- Chronic myeloid leukemia
- Polycythemia vera
- Essential thrombocythemia
- Primary myelofibrosis.

MYELOPROLIFERATIVE NEOPLASMS

Hematopoietic pluripotent stem cells have self-renewal capability and give rise to either myeloid or lymphoid lineage. They further differentiate into various mature blood cells. The mature cells include red blood cells, lymphocytes, granulocytes, megakaryocytes, and macrophages.

Definition of myeloproliferative neoplasms (MPNs): MPNs are clonal HSC disorders with abnormal (unregulated) and increased proliferation of one or more terminal differentiated myeloid cell lines (lineages). in the peripheral blood. These terminally differentiated myeloid cells are granulocytes, red blood cells, or megakaryocytes.

Four major diagnostic entities **of myeloproliferative neoplasms (MPN)** are presented in **Box 12.16.**

CHRONIC MYELOID LEUKEMIA

PA 18.2b (CC): Describe the etiology, genetics, pathogenesis classification, features, and hematologic features of chronic leukemia.

Q. Discuss peripheral blood smear, bone marrow, biochemical findings, and the characteristic chromosomal abnormality associated with chronic myeloid leukemia.

Definition: Chronic myelogenous leukemia (CML) is a **myeloproliferative neoplasm (MPN)** characterized by **overproduction of cells of the myeloid series** (leukocytosis) with **prominent granulocytes in blood and bone marrow.** It harbors the **BCR::ABL1 gene** and associated with marked **splenomegaly.**

Risk factor: Exposure to ionizing radiation and benzene.

Pathogenesis

Q. Write a short note on the Philadelphia chromosome.

CML is distinguished from other myeloproliferative neoplasms by the presence of the **Chimeric *BCR-ABL1* gene.**

Chimeric BCR-ABL1 Gene

The chimeric *BCR-ABL1* gene is formed from **portions of the *BCR*** (breakpoint cluster region) **gene on chromosome 22 and the *ABL*** (named after the Abelson murine leukemia virus) **gene on chromosome 9. ABL1** is a proto-oncogene. The **chimeric (fusion) gene is called BCR-ABL1, thus**

converting the ABL1 proto-oncogene into an oncogene. The product of the fusion gene plays a central role in the development of CML. The gene produces a constitutively active BCR-ABL tyrosine kinase. The term chimeric is a mythical animal formed from parts of various animals.

Cells with the *BCR-ABL* fusion gene: This fusion gene is present in **granulocytic, erythroid, megakaryocytic, and B-cell precursors**, and in some cases also in T-cell precursors. It indicates that CML arises from a transformed hematopoietic stem cell.

Philadelphia (Ph) Chromosome (Fig. 12.9)

- **In 95% of CML, the chimeric *BCR-ABL1* gene** forms the Philadelphia (Ph) chromosome.
- **Balanced reciprocal translocation:** In about 95% of CML, the *BCR-ABL* gene is formed by a balanced (9;22) translocation that moves *ABL* from the long arm chromosome 9 to a position on the long arm of chromosome 22 adjacent to *BCR,* i.e., **t(9; 22) (q 34; q 12.2)**. It increases the length of chromosome 9 and the shortening of 22. This **shortened chromosome 22** is known as the **Philadelphia chromosome (Fig. 12.9)**.

Other mechanisms of the BCR-ABL fusion gene: In the remaining 5% of cases, a *BCR-ABL* fusion gene is formed by cytogenetic **rearrangements involving more than two chromosomes.**

Mode of action of *BCR-ABL* gene: This gene encodes a fusion protein consisting of portions of BCR and the tyrosine kinase domain of ABL.

- **Constitutive signals generated by BCR-ABL:** The growth and survival of normal myeloid progenitors depend on signals produced by growth factors and their receptors. **BCR-ABL protein in CML generates constitutive signals that mimic the effects of growth factor receptor activation, such as activation of RAS. This greatly decreases the growth factor dependence of CML progenitors.**
- **BCR-ABL does not inhibit differentiation:** Thus, **during the early course** of the disease, there is **excessive production of relatively normal blood cells,** particularly granulocytes and platelets.

Clinical Features

- **Age: Usually occurs in adults between 30 and 60 years** of age. The peak incidence is in the fourth (between 30 and 39) and fifth decades (between 40 and 49) of life.
- **Sex:** Males are slightly more affected than females.
- **Onset:** The onset of CML is **insidious.**

Symptoms:

- **Nonspecific symptoms:** The initial symptoms are usually nonspecific such as easy fatigability, weakness, weight loss, and anorexia.
- **Fullness of abdomen (dragging sensation** in the abdomen) **due to splenomegaly:** Sometimes this may be the first symptom. Splenomegaly is moderate to severe and is a characteristic feature in the majority (80–90%) of patients. The splenomegaly is caused by leukemic infiltration and extramedullary hematopoiesis.
- **Hepatomegaly:** Mild or moderate seen in 60–70% of cases.

Differential diagnosis: Occasionally, CML must be distinguished as a **leukemoid reaction** (*refer* **Table 12.2**). Leukemoid reaction is characterized by marked elevation of the granulocyte count. It occurs in response to infection, stress, chronic inflammation, and certain neoplasms. CML shows the presence of the *BCR-ABL* fusion gene, which can be tested by karyotyping, fluorescence in situ hybridization (FISH), or PCR assay.

Natural History of Chronic Myeloid Leukemia

Three different phases: The natural history of CML is divided into three phases (1) chronic phase (CP), (2) accelerated phase, and (3) blast phase (BP).

Chronic Stable (Indolent) Phase (CP)

The natural history of CML initially shows a slow progression. Most are diagnosed in this phase. It lasts for 2–6 years. Even without treatment, the median survival is 3 years. In the chronic phase (CP), the neoplastic cells are mostly confined to the blood, bone marrow, spleen, and liver. If not treated, it progresses gradually to the accelerated phase or abruptly to the blast phase.

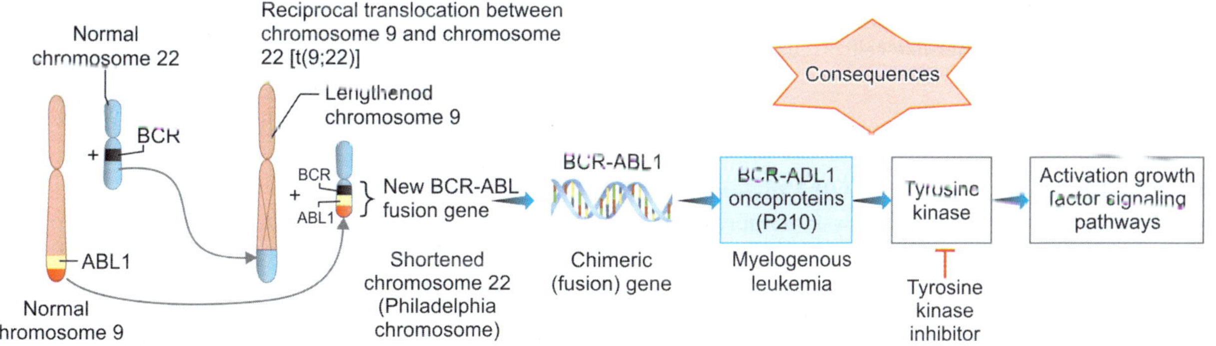

Fig. 12.9: Balanced reciprocal translocation between the long arm of chromosome 9 and chromosome 22 resulting in shortened chromosome 22 known as the Philadelphia chromosome.

Laboratory Findings

Q. Write a short note on laboratory findings/peripheral smear in chronic myeloid leukemia (CML).

Peripheral Blood

The peripheral blood findings are highly characteristic.
Hemoglobin: Usually less than 11 g/dL.
WBC count: The leukocyte count **is raised, often more than 100,000 cells/μL (100 × 10^9/L).**

PERIPHERAL SMEAR

RBCs: Normocytic normochromic anemia

WBCs:

- **Marked leukocytosis** (12–600 × 10^9/L): Total **leukocyte count** usually **exceeds 100 × 10^9/L (1,00,000/cu mm).**
- **Shift to the left (shift to immaturity):** The granulocytes at all stages of development (neutrophils, metamyelocytes, myelocytes, promyelocytes, and occasional myeloblasts) are seen.
- **Predominant cells** are **neutrophils and immature granulocytic progenitors, particularly myelocytes.** The preponderance of myelocytes in CML is called a **myelocyte bulge (Figs. 12.10A and B).**
- **Blasts** are usually less than **10%** of the circulating WBCs.
- **Basophilia and eosinophilia: Both basophils** and **eosinophils** are also usually increased in number.
- **Decreased NAP/LAP score:** NAP score in CML is decreased below 20 (normal score range is 40–100). Helpful in differentiating CML from leukemoid reaction (*refer* **Table 12.2**).

Platelets: They range from normal (150–450 × 10^9/L) to more than 1,000 × 10^9/L. Up to 50% have **thrombocytosis.**

BONE MARROW

- **Cellularity:** The bone marrow is markedly **hypercellular** due to increased numbers of maturing granulocytic (**myeloid hyperplasia**) and megakaryocytic precursors.
- **M: E ratio:** Often exceeds **20:1.**
- **Erythropoiesis: Shows diminished erythropoiesis** as the disease progresses.
- **Myelopoiesis: Shows marked hyperplasia. Blast** cells are usually **less than 10%.** Basophils, eosinophils, and their precursors are usually found.
- **Megakaryopoiesis:** Megakaryocytes are either **normal or increased. Dwarf megakaryocytes.**
- **Sea-blue histiocytes (Gaucher-like cells/Pseudo-Gaucher cells)** are seen.

Biochemical findings: Uric acid serum and serum LDH are raised.
Philadelphia chromosome and ***BCR-ABL1 fusion gene demonstrated*** either by chromosomal analysis or **fluorescent in situ hybridization (FISH)** or PCR-based tests.
Spleen: It is **enlarged.** The red pulp of the spleen resembles bone marrow because of the presence of extensive **extramedullary hematopoiesis.** This extensive proliferation often compromises the local blood supply. This can produce **splenic infarcts.**

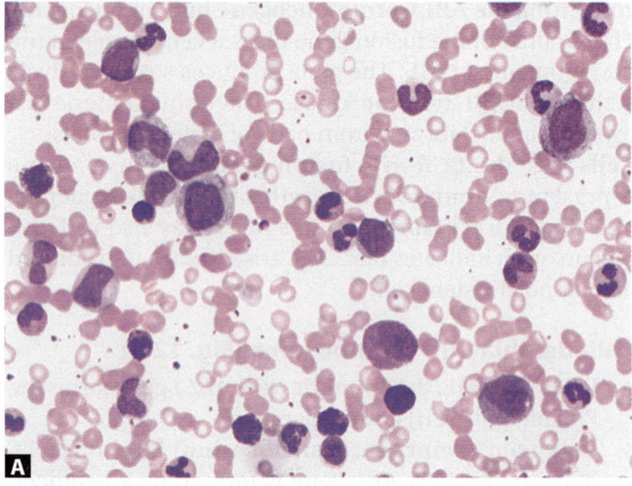

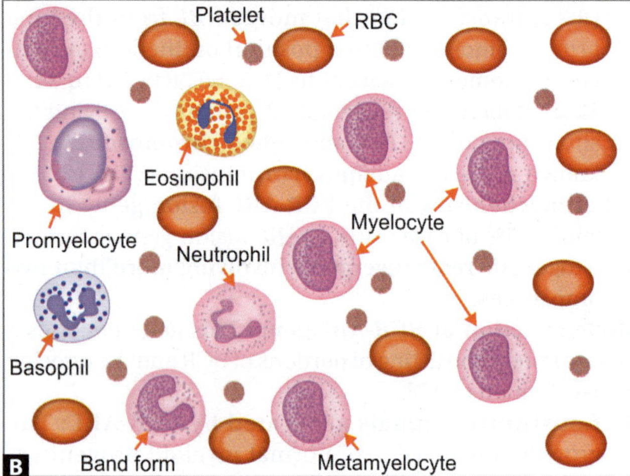

Figs. 12.10A and B: Peripheral blood picture in chronic/stable phase of chronic myeloid leukemia. It shows granulocytic forms at various stages of differentiation: (A) Leishman stain (myelocytes with arrows); (B) Diagrammatic.

Accelerated Phase (AP)

After a variable period, about 50% of CML cases enter an accelerated phase. This phase is **more aggressive** and lasts for a few months. It **shows increasing anemia** and **new thrombocytopenia** (less than 100 × 10^9/L). **Myeloblasts are 10–19%** in the blood or bone marrow. It shows **striking basophilia** (20% or more). Bone marrow shows **megakaryocyte proliferation in sheets** or clusters in association with fibrosis. There is **persistent or increasing splenomegaly** unresponsive to therapy.

Blast Phase (Crisis) (BP)

In about 50% of CML cases, a blast crisis occurs abruptly, without an accelerated phase. In the blast phase (BP), the blasts can infiltrate any extramedullary site (e.g., spleen, liver, lymph nodes, skin, and soft tissue). The blood picture resembles acute leukemia (blast crisis) and has a poor prognosis. Peripheral smear shows **20% or more blasts.** These blasts **may be either myeloblast** (70% cases) **or**

lymphoblast (30% cases). Myeloblast does not contain Auer rods. **Thrombocytopenia** causes bleeding episodes.

POLYCYTHEMIA OR ERYTHROCYTOSIS

Polycythemia is characterized by an **increase in the RBC mass**, usually with a corresponding increase in hemoglobin level. The increase in red cells can be absolute or relative. **Pathophysiologic classification of polycythemia** is given in **Box 12.17**.

Polycythemia Vera

Q. Write a short note on polycythemia vera.

Definition: Polycythemia vera (PV) is an **acquired** clonal **myeloproliferative neoplasm** arising from the malignant transformation of the **hematopoietic stem cells**. It is characterized by:

- **Erythrocytosis is frequently accompanied by leukocytosis, and/or thrombocytosis.**
- **Increased risk of hemorrhage and thrombosis** (venous and arterial).
- **Strongly associated with activating mutations in the tyrosine kinase JAK2 (Janus kinase 2).**

Pathogenesis

- **Normal function of JAK 2:** Normally, a tyrosine kinase protein called JAK2 (Janus 2 kinase) acts in the signaling pathways downstream of the **erythropoietin receptors of hematopoietic cells**. The activation of signaling pathways causes hematopoietic cells to replicate.
- **Acquired somatic mutations in JAK2:** It markedly **lowers the dependence of hematopoietic cells on growth factors** for growth and survival. This leads to excessive proliferation of erythroid, granulocytic, and megakaryocytic elements (panmyelosis). However, most clinical signs and symptoms are due to an absolute increase in red cell mass.

BOX 12.17: Pathophysiologic classification of polycythemia.

ABSOLUTE

Primary (low erythropoietin level)
- Polycythemia vera

Secondary (high erythropoietin level)
- Physiologically appropriate
  - Compensatory
  - Lung disease
  - Living in high-altitude
  - Cyanotic heart disease (tetralogy of Fallot)
- Physiologically inappropriate (with increased erythropoietin)
  - Paraneoplastic: Erythropoietin-secreting tumors (e.g., renal cell carcinoma, uterine leiomyoma, hepatocellular carcinoma)

RELATIVE

Reduced plasma volume
- Hemoconcentration (dehydration due to diarrhea, vomiting)
- Gaisböck's syndrome (spurious polycythemia)

Polycythemia vera versus relative polycythemia: Relative polycythemia results from hemoconcentration. Polycythemia vera is associated with low levels of serum erythropoietin and causes the growth factor-independent proliferation of the neoplastic clone.

Clinical Features

- Polycythemia vera appears insidiously, usually in **late middle age** (median age at onset is 60 years).
- Plethora (fullness) and cyanosis, headache, dizziness, and visual problems result from vascular disturbances in the brain and retina.
- **Thrombotic episodes** [e.g., deep venous thrombosis, myocardial infarction, thrombosis of hepatic veins (producing Budd-Chiari syndrome)] and hemorrhagic tendencies occur in about 0% of patients.

Laboratory Findings

Peripheral Blood

- **Hemoglobin: Increased** and are more than 18.5 g/dL in men and 16.5 g/dL in women.
- **Hematocrit: Increased** and about 60% or more (*refer* **Fig. 15.7D**, page 445).
- **Red cell count: Increased** and range from **6 to 10 million/cu mm (6×10^{12}/L)**.
- **White cell count: Increased** as high as 50,000 cells/cu mm.
- **Platelet count: Often more than 400,000/cu mm**. The platelets are functionally abnormal in most cases.

PERIPHERAL SMEAR

RBCs: Normocytic normochromic picture

WBCs: Mild to moderate leukocytosis. Neutrophils are morphologically normal. **Basophils** often **increased (basophilia).** **NAP** (LAP) score is **increased** to 150–300 (Normal 40–100).

Platelets: Abnormally large and **functionally defective.** There is moderate thrombocytosis.

BONE MARROW

Hypercellular due to **hyperplasia of all elements** (trilineage hyperplasia/panmyelosis) namely erythroid, myeloid, and megakaryocytic series with a **prominence of erythroid precursors** in the bone marrow.

Bone marrow biopsy shows increased reticulin fibers and fibrosis as the disease progresses.

Other Findings

- **Extramedullary hematopoiesis** in the **liver and spleen** that causes **hepatosplenomegaly**.
- **Arterial oxygen saturation (pO_2):** Normal (75–100 mm Hg) and is useful for **differentiating it from secondary** polycythemia.

- **Erythropoietin levels: Decreased** in contrast to secondary polycythemia.
- **Serum vitamin B_{12} and uric acid: Increased** indicating increased cell turnover.
- ***JAK2 V617F* mutation:** Can be demonstrated.

Chronic lymphocytic leukemia/small lymphocytic lymphoma is discussed on page 384-6. Features of essential thrombocythemia and primary myelofibrosis is presented online.

LYMPH NODE AND SPLEEN

LYMPH NODE

Normal Structure (Fig. 12.11)

The lymph nodes are bean-shaped or oval structures and are part of the lymphatic network throughout the body. Each lymph node is covered by a connective tissue called a capsule. Afferent lymphatics carrying lymph from the region drained by the lymph node enter the convex surface of the capsule. They drain into the peripheral subcapsular sinus and travel to the lymph node. They form a single efferent lymphatic vessel and leave the lymph node at the concavity (hilum).

The parenchyma of the lymph node is divided into a peripheral (outer) cortex and a central medulla. The cortex consists of many rounded aggregates of lymphocytes called lymphoid follicles. Each follicle consists of a pale-staining germinal center surrounded by small dark-staining lymphocytes called the mantle zone. The deeper region of the cortex or paracortex consists of a zone between the peripheral cortex and the inner medulla.

The medulla is mainly composed of cords of plasma cells and some lymphocytes.

Lymphadenopathy

PA 19.1 (CC): Enumerate the causes and describe the differentiating features of lymphadenopathy.

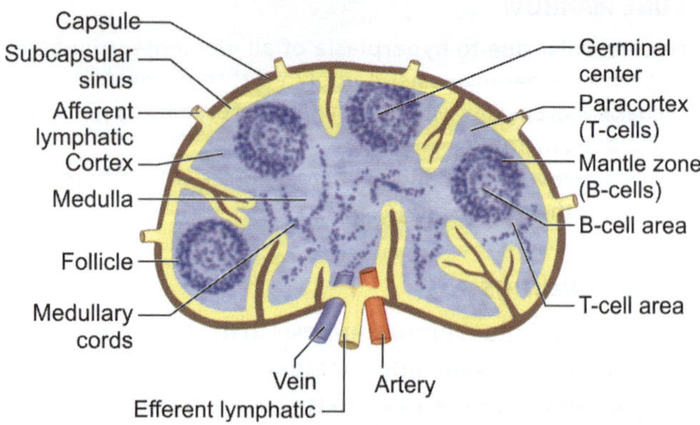

Fig. 12.11: Diagrammatic representation of the normal structure of a lymph node.

Definition: Enlargement of the lymph nodes is called lymphadenopathy.

Significance: It is a **common clinical finding.** It **may be an incidental finding** during an examination of the patient for various reasons, or it **may be a presenting sign or symptom of the patient's illness.** Hence, it is necessary to differentiate whether the lymphadenopathy is a normal finding or needs further study (e.g., fine needle aspiration, biopsy). It is common to observe soft, flat, palpable submandibular nodes (less than 1 cm) in healthy children and young adults. Palpable inguinal nodes of up to 2 cm usually are considered normal in healthy adults. Hence, these normal nodes do not require further evaluation. In contrast, if the node(s) appear to be abnormal, it requires a more precise diagnosis.

Causes of Lymphadenopathy

Q. Enumerate the causes of lymphadenopathy.

Lymphadenopathy may develop in many primary or secondary disorders **(Box 12.18)**. Most of these disorders are infrequent causes of lymphadenopathy. In more than two-thirds of cases cause of lymphadenopathy is nonspecific or is due to upper respiratory diseases (viral or bacterial) and less than 1% have a malignancy. Thus, most patients with lymphadenopathy have nonspecific etiology and require only a few diagnostic tests.

BOX 12.18: Causes of lymphadenopathy.

- **Infectious**
  - **Bacterial:** Streptococci, staphylococci, cat-scratch disease, chancroid, tuberculosis, primary and secondary syphilis, leprosy
  - **Viral:** Infectious mononucleosis syndromes* [Epstein-Barr virus (EBV), cytomegalovirus (CMV), human immunodeficiency virus (HIV)]*
  - **Fungal:** Histoplasmosis, coccidioidomycosis
  - **Chlamydial:** Lymphogranuloma venereum, trachoma
  - **Parasitic:** Filariasis, toxoplasmosis, leishmaniasis, trypanosomiasis
  - **Rickettsial:** Scrub typhus, Q fever
- **Malignancy (neoplastic)**
  - **Primary hematological:** Hodgkin's lymphoma, non-Hodgkin's lymphomas*, acute or chronic lymphocytic leukemia*
  - **Metastatic (secondary):** From numerous primary sites (e.g., lung, breast, thyroid, stomach, melanoma)
- **Immunological**
  - **Autoimmune diseases:** Rheumatoid arthritis*, systemic lupus erythematosus (SLE)*
  - Drug hypersensitivity*: Diphenyl hydantoin, hydralazine
- **Others**
  - Castleman's disease (giant lymph node hyperplasia)*
  - Sarcoidosis*, amyloidosis*
  - Dermatopathic lymphadenitis
  - Histiocytic necrotizing lymphadenitis (Kikuchi's disease)*

* Most likely associated with generalized lymphadenopathy.

Differentiating features of lymphadenopathy are presented online.

Laboratory investigation

The laboratory investigation for lymphadenopathy depends on the etiology suspected from the patient's history and physical findings. About 50% of patients do not require laboratory studies.

Complete blood count: The initial investigation required is a complete blood count (CBC) [to detect neutrophilia in pyogenic infection, EBV or CMV mononucleosis, immune cytopenias in illnesses such as SLE, evidence of hematological disease (acute or chronic leukemias, lymphoma with a leukemic component)].

Other laboratory tests: These include measurement of **erythrocyte sedimentation rate** (ESR), throat culture (if suspected infection of the throat), and **serologic studies** (to demonstrate antibodies specific to components of EBV, CMV, HIV, etc.). If SLE is suspected, antinuclear and anti-DNA antibody studies.

Radiological: A **chest X-ray** to detect the presence of a pulmonary infiltrate or mediastinal lymphadenopathy. It suggests tuberculosis, lymphoma, primary lung cancer, or metastatic cancer and requires further investigation. Imaging techniques (CT, MRI, ultrasound, color Doppler ultrasonography) may be used to differentiate benign from malignant lymph nodes (especially in patients with cancer in the head and neck region).

FNAC of lymph node: Fine-needle aspiration of lymph node should not be performed as the first diagnostic procedure unless for the diagnosis of certain infections (e.g., tuberculosis) or metastatic tumors (e.g., secondaries from carcinoma of the upper respiratory tract). Most diagnoses (e.g., lymphoma) need more tissue than obtained by aspiration and may delay a definitive diagnosis.

Biopsy of lymph node: Most lymphadenopathy does not require a biopsy. However, it is a valuable diagnostic tool. If the patient's history and physical findings suggest a benign condition, careful follow-up for 2–4 weeks is suggested. If the patient's history and physical findings suggest a malignancy, a cutting needle or excision biopsy of a representative node is indicated for a histological diagnosis. Examples include the presence of a solitary, hard, nontender cervical node in an older patient who uses tobacco; supraclavicular lymphadenopathy; and solitary or generalized firm, movable adenopathy suggestive of lymphoma.

Refer **online for lymphadenitis (acute and chronic) and for Figures 12.12 and 12.13.**

Tuberculous Lymphadenitis

PA 19.2 (CC): Describe the pathogenesis and pathology of tuberculous lymphadenitis.

Lymph nodes are the **most common extrapulmonary site of tuberculosis.** For the pathogenesis of tuberculosis *refer* pages 560-3.

The regions involved: Most commonly it involves the lymph nodes of the **cervical and mediastinal region, followed by axillary and inguinal.** Sometimes, more than one region may be involved.

Type of infection: Tuberculous lymphadenitis **may occur as a part of primary infection or spread from contiguous sites or reactivation.**

- **Cervical lymphadenitis:** The primary focus in the pharynx and tonsils will produce enlargement of the cervical lymph node.
- **Supraclavicular lymphadenopathy:** It is usually due to the spread of mediastinal disease.

Clinical presentation: Lymphadenitis is the most frequent presentation of extrapulmonary tuberculosis, usually occurring in the cervical region.

- **Matted lymph nodes**: The **involved nodes are usually painless and initially mobile. Later they become matted together due to periadenitis.**
- **Collar-stud' abscess and sinus formation:** When caseation and liquefaction occur, the swelling becomes fluctuant. The caseous material may be discharged through the skin with the formation of a 'collar-stud' abscess and sinus formation ("scrofula"). The abscess is called a cold abscess because it is not associated with erythema, heat, or tenderness. About 50% of patients do not show constitutional features, such as fevers or night sweats.

Tuberculin test: It is usually strongly positive.

PA 19.3 (CC): Identify and describe the features of tuberculous lymphadenitis in a gross and microscopic specimen.

MORPHOLOGY

Gross (Fig. 12.14)

The lymph nodes are **enlarged and matted** together **because of periadenitis** (inflammation of the capsule of the lymph node and surrounding structures). The **cut surface** in the tuberculous areas shows **characteristic map-like areas** which are **yellowish, granular, opaque, soft necrotic material that resembles dry cheese.**

Microscopy (Figs. 12.15A to C)

It shows tuberculous granuloma. Granuloma in tuberculosis is called a tubercle. The tubercle may show the central area of caseous necrosis (caseating granuloma/soft tubercle) or may not show caseation (noncaseating tubercles/hard tubercle). Individual tubercles are identified only by microscopic examination. When multiple granulomas coalesce, they may be grossly identified. Caseating granuloma consists of:

- Central area of caseous necrosis
- Surrounded by epithelioid cells (modified macrophages), some of which may fuse to form multinucleate giant cells. The giant cells may be Langhans type (nuclei arranged in a horse-shoe pattern) or foreign body type (nuclei in the center).
- The epithelioid cells are surrounded by a rim of lymphocytes.
- These granulomas are usually enclosed within fibroblasts.

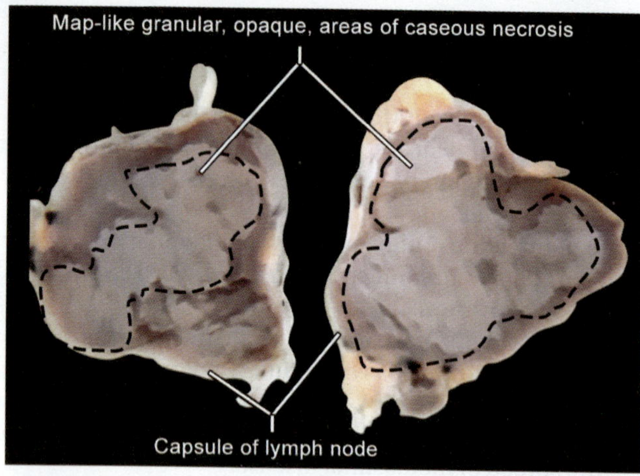

Fig. 12.14: Tuberculous lymphadenitis: Cut section of a lymph node shows opaque areas of caseous necrosis (within dotted line).

NON-HODGKIN LYMPHOMAS

PA 19.4a (CC): Describe and discuss the pathogenesis, and pathology of non-Hodgkin's lymphoma.

Introduction

Lymphoid tumor cells: The non-Hodgkin lymphomas (NHLs) and chronic lymphoid leukemias are composed of **tumor cells that resemble stages of mature lymphocytic differentiation.**

Manifestations: Their clinical presentation and behavior vary widely.

- **Leukemias:** Some characteristically **involve the bone marrow and the peripheral blood** and manifest as *leukemias.*
- **Lymphoma:** Other tumors tend to **produce masses in lymph nodes or other tissue** and present as *lymphomas.* Lymphomas **mostly affect lymph nodes, but any tissue or organ** may be involved. These tissues or organs are called **extranodal lymphoma**. These sites include the GI tract, thyroid, liver, skin, lungs, and brain. If lymphoma cells are present in the blood and/or bone marrow, the tumor is "leukemic."

These lymphoid tumors have overlapping clinical behavior. Hence, their diagnosis is based on the morphologic and molecular characteristics of the tumor cells. It is most important to identify the kind of tumor of cells rather than the site where the tumor cells reside. All lymphomas are malignant and show a wide spectrum of clinical behavior. Some follow an indolent clinical course (and may not even require treatment), while others are very aggressive (and can cause death in a short time, if untreated).

Classification of Lymphoid Neoplasms (Box 12.19)

Lymphomas are clonal lymphocytic malignancies. They may be B-cell, T-cell, and NK-cell type lymphomas. These may be derived from precursor cells (immature cells or lymphoblasts) or derived from mature effector cells (mature). **The majority (80–85%) of lymphoid neoplasms are of mature B-cell origin** and the remaining (15–20%) are of T-cell/NK cell type. Cell type and its antigens detected by monoclonal antibodies are presented in **Table 12.6**. Selected examples are discussed below. Hodgkin lymphoma (HL) is classified separately from non-Hodgkin lymphoma (NHL).

Q. Name mature B-cell neoplasms.

Mature B-cell Neoplasms

Mature B-cell neoplasms are clonal proliferations of differentiated B-cells (**Box 12.19**). Mature B-cell lymphomas are the most common lymphomas and represent over 90% of lymphoid neoplasms. Most mature B-cell lymphomas occur in older adults (age 65 or more).

Chronic Lymphocytic Leukemia/Small Lymphocytic Lymphoma

PA 18.2c (CC): Describe the etiology, genetics, pathogenesis classification, features, and hematologic features of chronic leukemia.

Q. Write a short note on chronic lymphocytic leukemia.

Definition: Chronic lymphocytic leukemia **(CLL)/small lymphocytic lymphoma (SLL) is a B-cell lymphoma comprising monomorphic small mature B-cells.**

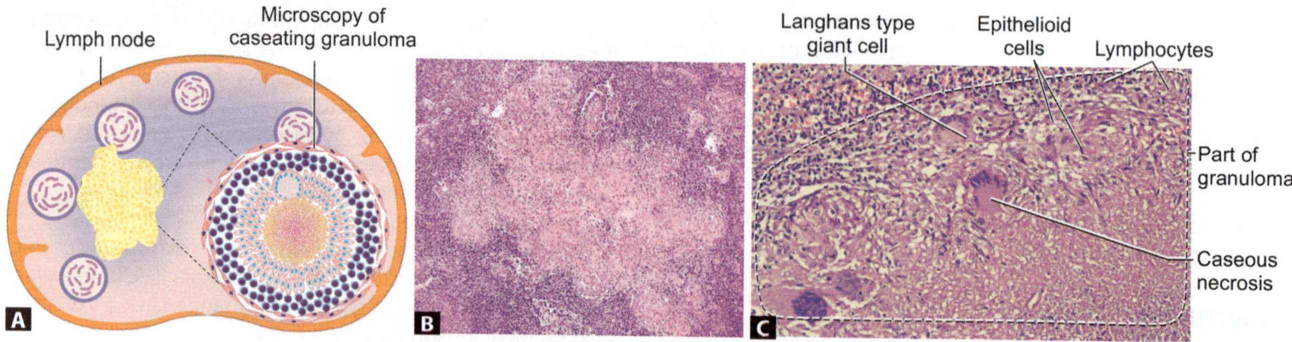

Figs. 12.15A to C: (A) Diagrammatic representation of lymph node with granulomatous inflammation; (B) Microscopy shows granuloma without caseous necrosis; (C) Microscopy shows granuloma with caseous necrosis.

BOX 12.19: WHO (2022) classification (Abridged) of B, T, and NK cell neoplasms.

B-CELL NEOPLASMS

Precursor B-cell neoplasms (*refer* **Box 12.14**)

Mature B-cell neoplasms

- Pre-neoplastic and neoplastic small lymphocytic proliferations
  - Chronic lymphocytic leukemia/small lymphocytic lymphoma
- Follicular lymphoma
- Large B-cell lymphomas
  - Diffuse large B-cell lymphoma
- Burkitt lymphoma
  - Burkitt lymphoma
- Marginal zone lymphoma
- Splenic B-cell lymphomas and leukemias
  - Hairy cell leukemia
- Mantle cell lymphoma
- Lymphoplasmacytic lymphoma
- Cutaneous follicle center lymphoma
- Transformations of indolent B-cell lymphomas
- KSHV/HHV8-associated B-cell lymphoid proliferations and lymphomas
- Lymphoid proliferations and lymphomas associated with immune deficiency and dysregulation

T-CELL NEOPLASMS

Precursor T-cell neoplasms

- T-lymphoblastic leukemia/lymphoma
  - T-lymphoblastic leukemia/lymphoma, NOS
  - Early T-precursor lymphoblastic leukemia/lymphoma

Mature T-cell and NK-cell neoplasms

- Mature T-cell and NK-cell leukemias
  - Sezary syndrome
- Primary cutaneous T-cell lymphoid proliferations and lymphomas
  - Mycosis fungoides
- Intestinal T-cell and NK-cell lymphoid proliferations and lymphomas
- Hepatosplenic T-cell lymphoma
- Anaplastic large cell lymphoma
  - ALK-positive anaplastic large-cell lymphoma
  - ALK-negative anaplastic large-cell lymphoma
- Nodal T-follicular helper (TFH) cell lymphoma
- Other peripheral T-cell lymphomas
- EBV-positive NK-cell and T-cell lymphomas
- EBV-positive T-cell and NK-cell lymphoid proliferations and lymphomas of childhood

They are essentially identical and **differ only in the extent of peripheral blood involvement and presentations.** CLL/SLL tumor cells coexpress **CD5 and CD23.**

- **Chronic lymphocytic leukemia**: A **peripheral blood** diagnosis of CLL requires a **B-cell count of more than 5,000 cells/cu mm** (>5 × 10^9/L), with the characteristic morphology and immunophenotype. No nodal, splenic, or extramedullary involvement.

TABLE 12.6 Cell type and its antigens detected by monoclonal antibodies.

Cell type	*Antigen detected*
T-cell	CD1, CD3, CD4, CD5, CD8
B-cell	CD10, CD19, CD20, CD21, CD23, CD79a
Monocyte or macrophage	CD11c, CD13, CD14, CD15, CD33, CD64
NK cell	CD16, CD56
Stem cell and progenitor cell	CD34
Activation marker	CD30
All leukocytes	CD45 (LCA)

(CD: cluster designation; NK: natural killer; LCA: leukocyte common antigen)

- **Small lymphocytic lymphoma tumor:** A tissue-based diagnosis of SLL requires organ enlargement (e.g., lymphadenopathy >15 mm) and its infiltration by the monomorphic neoplastic B-cells. The name **SLL is used for cases with <5 × 10^9/L circulating B cells and nodal (lymph nodes), splenic, or other extramedullary involvement.**

Pathogenesis

BCL2 **overexpression with increased tumor cell survival: CLL/SLL is a slowly growing tumor characterized by increased tumor cell survival than the proliferation of tumor cell.** There is inhibition of apoptosis in CLL/SLL cells. Thus, the tumor cells contain high levels of BCL2 (a protein that inhibits apoptosis).

Immune dysregulation of normal B cells: CLL/SLL also causes immune dysregulation, particularly of normal B cells.

- **Hypogammaglobulinemia:** Immune dysregulation often causes hypogammaglobulinemia in more than 50% of the patients, usually late in the course. It leads to an increased susceptibility to bacterial infections.
- **Autoimmune hemolytic anemia:** Paradoxically, about 15% of patients develop **warm autoantibodies against their own red cells** (autoimmune hemolytic anemia, warm antibody type) **or platelets** (autoimmune thrombocytopenia).

Clinical Features

Age: CLL/SLL occurs between **50 and 60 years** of age.

Sex: More in males than in females (2:1).

Symptoms: These are as follows:

- **Asymptomatic:** When first detected, CLL/SLL is usually asymptomatic in about 25–30%
- **Nonspecific symptoms:** The most common signs and symptoms are nonspecific. These include fatigue, loss of weight, and anorexia.
- **Generalized lymphadenopathy** and hepatosplenomegaly: It is observed in 50–60% of patients.

- **Immunological defects** either as **immune deficiency or autoimmunity.**

Laboratory Findings

Peripheral blood

Q. Write a short note on peripheral blood picture in chronic lymphocytic leukemia.

- **Hemoglobin: Decreased** and usually below 13 g/dL.
- **Total leukocyte count is increased (20–50 × 10^9/L).** The leukocyte count may be increased only slightly in SLL.

PERIPHERAL SMEAR (FIGS. 12.16A AND B)

RBCs: Normocytic normochromic anemia.

WBCs:

- **Absolute lymphocytosis:** Differential leukocyte count shows an absolute lymphocytosis and constitutes **more than 50% of the white cells.** Variable numbers of larger activated lymphocytes may also be seen.
- **Mature-looking lymphocytes:** These are small with scant cytoplasm. Their **nuclei** are round with clumped coarse chromatin **(" soccer ball"/block-type chromatin).** Nucleoli absent.
- **Smudge cells or basket cells** (fragile leukemic cells): The circulating lymphocytes are fragile. During the preparation of peripheral smears, many lymphocytes are disrupted. This produces characteristic smudge cells.

Platelets: Initially **normal** count and later may be decreased.

BONE MARROW

Cellularity: Hypercellular marrow due to infiltration by mature lymphocytes. **Lymphocytes constitute more than 30% of the nucleated cells** of the bone marrow cells—a diagnostic feature of CLL.

Erythropoiesis: Normal.

Myelopoiesis: Normal.

Megakaryopoiesis: Normal.

Lymphocytic infiltrate: As the disease advances, neoplastic lymphocytes replace the normal erythroid, myeloid, and megakaryocytic series in the bone marrow resulting in anemia, neutropenia, and thrombocytopenia.

Immunophenotype

Tumor cells express the pan-B cell markers CD19 and CD20. CD5+ and CD23+ are distinctly positive in CLL.

Lymph node

- **Loss of normal architecture:** The involved lymph nodes are effaced by sheets of small lymphocytes.
- **Diffusely infiltration by monomorphic lymphocytes:** The lymph node is diffusely infiltrated by monomorphic, small, resting, round lymphocytes. Lymphocytes have scanty cytoplasm and round nuclei with coarse chromatin.
- **Proliferation centers:** Scattered within lymphocytes are ill-defined foci of larger, actively dividing lymphocytes. These small, nodular foci of mitotically active cells are called **proliferation centers or pseudo-follicles, or growth centers.** These are **pathognomonic** for CLL/SLL.

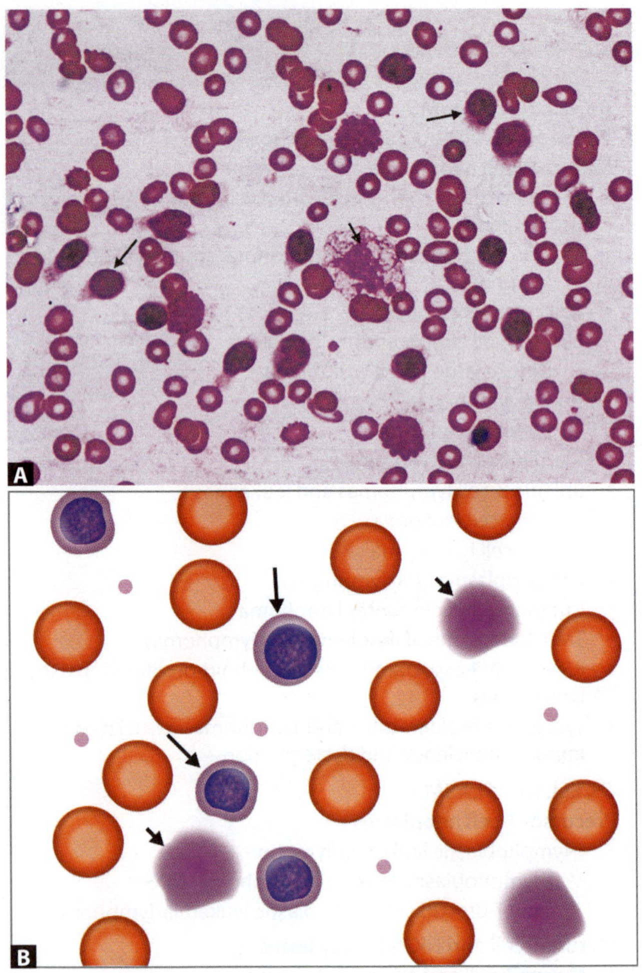

Figs. 12.16A and B: Peripheral blood smear (A, Leishman stain and B, diagrammatic) in chronic lymphocytic leukemia showing numerous small lymphocytes (long arrows) and few smudge cells (short arrow).

Course and prognosis: These are highly variable and depend on the disease stage and genetic findings. **Median survival rate is 4–6 years.** A small percentage of tumors transform into aggressive tumors resembling diffuse large B-cell lymphoma *(Richter transformation).* The median survival after transformation is less than 1 year.

Follicular Lymphoma

Q. Write a short note on follicular lymphoma.

Definition: Follicular lymphoma (FL) is a **neoplasm of mature germinal center (GC) B-cells with varying proportions of centrocytes (CC) and centroblasts** (CB) or large transformed cells. It shows a **follicular growth pattern** (at least partially).

Pathogenesis

Q. Write a short note on the pathogenesis of follicular lymphoma.

BCL2 **rearrangement*:* Follicular lymphoma is strongly associated with chromosomal translocations involving** ***BCL2*****.** It is characterized by a **(14;18) translocation** rearrangement involving the *IGH* locus on chromosome

14 and the *BCL2* gene on chromosome 18. This causes **overexpression of *BCL2* which acts as an antiapoptotic factor and promotes the survival of follicular lymphoma cells**. Normal germinal centers contain numerous B cells that undergo apoptosis. In follicular lymphoma, there are no apoptotic cells.

MORPHOLOGY

Q. Write a short essay on the morphology of follicular center cell lymphoma.

Gross

- Involves **lymph nodes**, spleen, and bone marrow.
- **The architecture** of the lymph node is **lost**; frequently the tumor infiltrates the perinodal tissue **(Fig. 12.17)**. The cut surface of lymph nodes involved in FL may show a vaguely nodular pattern.

Microscopy

- **Follicular (nodular) growth pattern**: The **neoplastic follicles** are organoid structures that are **poorly defined (Figs. 12.18A and B)**. The **size and shape of follicles considerably varies** from case to case. It must have at least a partially follicular (nodular) architecture for its diagnosis. Neoplastic follicles usually show a back-to-back arrangement with little intervening paracortex.
- **Cellular composition:** It consists of a mix of **two types of neoplastic B cells: small centrocytes with variable numbers of large centroblasts.**
  - **Centrocytes** (small cleaved cells)
    - **Size:** Centrocytes (CCs) are **slightly larger than small (resting) lymphocytes.**
    - **Cleaved nucleus:** These cells have **angulated, elongated, twisted, or cleaved nuclei** with prominent indentations and linear infoldings. The **chromatin is less dense than those of small lymphocytes.** Nucleoli are inconspicuous.
    - **Cytoplasm:** It is **scant, pale, and barely visible** in routinely stained sections.
  - **Centroblasts** (large noncleaved cells): In most tumors, centroblasts are a minor component of cells.
    - **Size:** Centroblasts (CBs) are large cells usually **3 times the size of normal lymphocytes.**
    - **Nucleus:** They have **round or oval nuclei with open nuclear (vesicular) chromatin** and **multiple (1 to 3) peripherally located (at the nuclear membrane) nucleoli.**
    - **Cytoplasm:** It is usually **visible (moderate amount) and lightly amphophilic (basophilic with Giemsa stain).**

Grading: FL can be graded as FL1, 2, 3A, and 3B based on the quantification of absolute numbers of centroblasts/transformed cells in 10 consecutive high-power fields.

Immunophenotype

Expresses B-cell antigens (CD19, CD20 [pan-B cell markers], CD22, CD79a, PAX-5) and surface immunoglobulin. They also express germinal center-associated markers CD10 (CALLA), and *BCL2* protein.

Cytogenetics and Molecular Genetics

t(14; 18) (q32;q21), with *IgH* and *BCL2* as partner genes, leads to constitutive overexpression of *BCL2* protein.

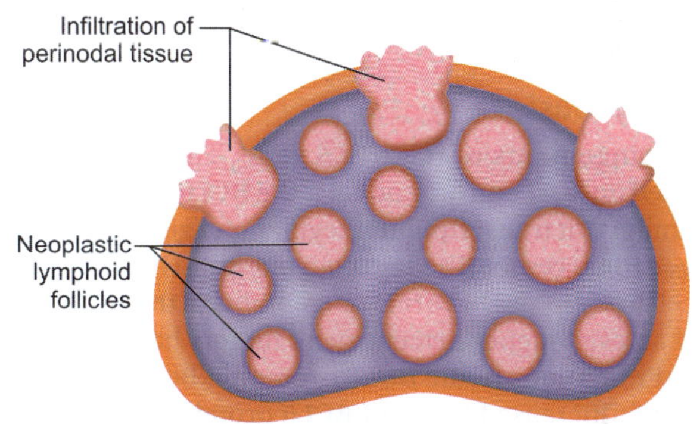

Fig. 12.17: Follicular lymphoma: (A) Diagrammatic. Neoplastic follicles are seen in both the cortex, medulla of lymph node, and infiltration of the perinodal tissue.

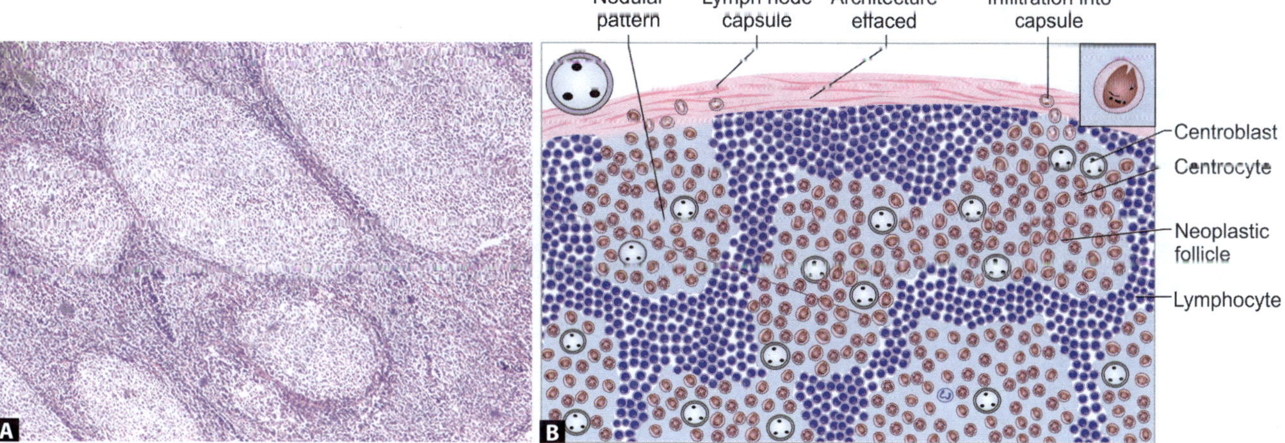

Figs. 12.18A and B: Follicular lymphoma: (A) The normal lymph node architecture is replaced by malignant lymphoid follicles in a back-to-back pattern; (B) The diagrammatic appearance of one follicle in follicular lymphoma is composed of centrocytes and centroblasts. Left inset shows centroblast and right inset shows centrocyte.

Clinical Features

- Follicular lymphoma mainly occurs in adults older than 50 years of age. Peak in the **sixth and seventh decades**.
- **Most patients develop generalized, painless lymphadenopathy**. The bone marrow is involved at the time of diagnosis in about 80–85% of cases.

Prognosis: Most cases follow an indolent clinical course. Overall median survival is 7–9 years.

Diffuse Large B-Cell Lymphoma (DLBCL)

It is the most common type of NHL in adults. Diffuse large B-cell lymphoma **is an aggressive** neoplasm of large B-cell with a **diffuse growth pattern**. It accounts for about 20–35% of adult NHLs and 60–70% of aggressive lymphoid neoplasms.

Large B cells with a diffuse growth pattern: Diffuse large B-cell lymphoma consists of medium-sized to large B cells with a diffuse growth pattern.

The heterogeneous group of aggressive NHLs: DLBCL is a heterogeneous entity with several subtypes. Their heterogeneity is evident at the morphologic, molecular, immunophenotypic, genetic, and clinical levels. They share an aggressive natural history.

Pathogenesis

Rearrangements of the *BCL6* gene: The *BCL6* gene is located on 3q27 and its product is the **BCL6 protein**. This is an important **transcriptional regulator of gene expression in germinal center B cells.** About one-third of diffuse large B-cell lymphomas have **rearrangements of the *BCL6* gene**, and an even higher percentage of tumors have **activating point mutations in the *BCL6* promoter.** Both aberrations result in **increased levels of BCL6 protein**. It leads to the neoplastic proliferation of germinal center B cells.

A translocation involving the *BCL2* gene: Another 30% of DLBCL have a (14;18) translocation involving the *BCL2* gene. It results in overexpression of BCL2 protein. Some of these tumors may be "transformed" follicular lymphomas.

Others: The remaining DLBCLs have other diverse driver mutations (e.g., translocations involving the *MYC* gene).

MORPHOLOGY

Site affected: DLBCL most often involves **lymph nodes**. But, **extranodal sites, especially the GI tract**, may be involved.

Gross

Involved lymph nodes are enlarged. On the cut section, it has a homogeneous, whitish, and fleshy appearance. The presence of grey areas of necrosis and adhesion to surrounding soft tissue indicates extra-capsular spread.

Microscopy (Figs. 12.19A and B)

- **Partial or total effacement of architecture: Loss of architecture is seen in involved** lymph nodes or extranodal sites.
- **Diffuse growth pattern**: The tumor cells show a **diffuse growth pattern** or vaguely nodular pattern.
- **Neoplastic B-cells:**
  - **Size:** The neoplastic B cells are **large**, round, or oval Their size is at least 3 **to 4 times the size** of a **small resting lymphocyte.**
  - **Nucleus:** The tumor cells have **round or oval nuclear contours.** Their **size is equal to or larger than the nucleus of a macrophage** or more than twice the size of a small lymphocyte nucleus. The nucleus shows **dispersed chromatin and several distinct nucleoli.** The mitotic rate is usually high.
  - **Cytoplasm:** Tumor cells have a moderate amount of pale or basophilic cytoplasm.

Diagnosis of DLBCL: It requires ancillary studies to exclude other diseases with similar morphologic features.

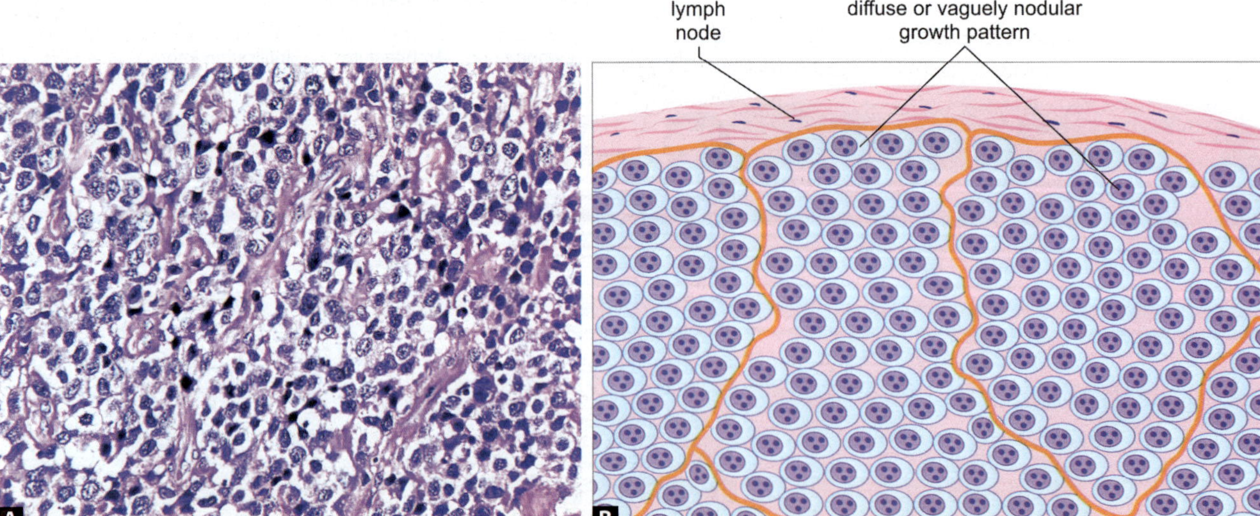

Figs. 12.19A and B: (A) H&E, and (B) Diagrammatic. Diffuse large B-cell lymphoma showing sheets of large lymphoma cells with prominent nucleoli.

Immunophenotype

- These tumors express the pan-B cell markers such as **CD19, CD20, CD22, and CD79a.**
- Also, variably express **germinal center markers** like CD10, MYC, and *BCL6*.
- Negative for TdT.

Cytogenetics and Molecular Profile

- **Translocation of *BCL2* gene:** t(14; 18) translocation
- **Mutations of the *BCL6* gene.**

Special subtypes: Large B-cell lymphoma consists of several clinicopathologic subtypes. For example, (1) ALK-positive large B-cell lymphoma, (2) EBV-positive diffuse large B-cell lymphomas, and (3) primary mediastinal large B-cell lymphoma.

Clinical Features

- **Age and gender:** It can occur at any age. More common between **65 and 70 years** of age, with slight **male** preponderance.
- Present with **rapidly enlarging** mass at single or multiple **nodal or extranodal sites.**

Prognosis: These tumors are highly aggressive, proliferative, and rapidly fatal if untreated. They and sensitive to chemotherapeutic agents that target rapidly dividing cells. Most (60–80%) patients achieve complete remissions.

Burkitt Lymphoma

Q. Write a short note on Burkitt lymphoma.

Definition: Burkitt lymphoma (BL) is a **mature aggressive B-cell neoplasm of germinal center B-cell phenotype.** It is composed of **medium-sized, monomorphic lymphoid cells.** These cells have basophilic **vacuolated cytoplasm and a nucleus with multiple small nucleoli.** They have a high proliferation index and an *IG::MYC* rearrangement.

Subtypes

Traditional Subtypes

Extranodal sites: BL usually arises at extranodal sites.

1. **Endemic (African) Burkitt lymphoma (BL):** Occurs in Africa, and affects **children and adolescents. Associated with Epstein-Barr virus infection and malaria.** They usually occur in the jaws (**mandible, maxilla), and other facial bones**. They may also occur as an **abdominal tumor** involving the bowel, retroperitoneum, and ovaries.
2. **Sporadic (nonendemic) BL:** Occurs in **children or young adults.** It commonly involves the **abdomen, soft tissues of the orbit, Waldeyer ring, gingiva, thyroid gland, ovaries, testis, and breast.**
3. **Immunodeficiency-associated (HIV) BL:** They are more common in the **lymph nodes** but may also occur in the extranodal sites.

Age: Endemic and sporadic BL occurs mainly in children and young adults.

Recommended by WHO

Molecular data suggest that the presence or absence of EBV correlates better with biological behavior.

1. EBV-associated BL
2. EBV-negative BL

Pathogenesis

Risk Factors

- **Mixed *P. falciparum* infection:** Children exposed to this infection have a higher risk for BL.
- **Immunodeficiency** such as HIV can be a risk factor.
- **Epstein-Barr virus:** Recent evidence suggests that EBV plays an initiating role in oncogenesis in BL.

Molecular Pathogenesis

Overexpression of the MYC transcription factor (Fig. 12.20)

MYC (c-MYC): It is a **proto-oncogene** and is a **master regulator of Warburg metabolism** (aerobic glycolysis). The Warburg metabolism is a hallmark of cancer and is associated with rapid cell growth.

Translocations of *MYC* gene: Burkitt lymphoma shows a high association with translocations involving the *MYC* gene on chromosome 8. It results in overexpression of the MYC transcription factor. Because MYC is a master regulator of Warburg metabolism, its overexpression leads to the fastest growth of tumor cells. **Burkitt lymphoma is one of the fastest-growing human tumors.**

- ***IG::MYC* translocation:** This is the most common translocation in which the *MYC* from chromosome 8 fuses with the IGH gene on chromosome 14, i.e., **t(8:14) (q24; q32).** The MYC translocation is highly characteristic of BL, it is not limited to BL, and other diagnostic features are required to confirm the diagnosis.
- **Uncontrolled cell proliferation: Translocations of the *MYC* gene,** convert **proto-oncogene into *MYC*** oncogene, which leads to **overexpression of MYC protein** (oncoprotein). This causes **uncontrolled cell proliferation.**

MORPHOLOGY

Gross

It usually produces a **bulky mass** of tumors with adjacent lymph nodes and surrounding tissue. The **cut surface has a fish-flesh appearance with focal areas of necrosis and hemorrhage.** In tumors involving the jaw, shows a tumor of the maxilla or mandible with large areas of necrosis and destruction.

Microscopy

Q. Write a short note on the microscopy of Burkitt lymphoma.

Burkitt lymphomas, **irrespective of the categories**, are **histologically similar.**

Loss of architecture and diffuse growth pattern: Tumors involving nodes show **loss of architecture.** Involved tissues show **diffuse** infiltrate of **lymphoid cells (Figs. 12.21A and B).**

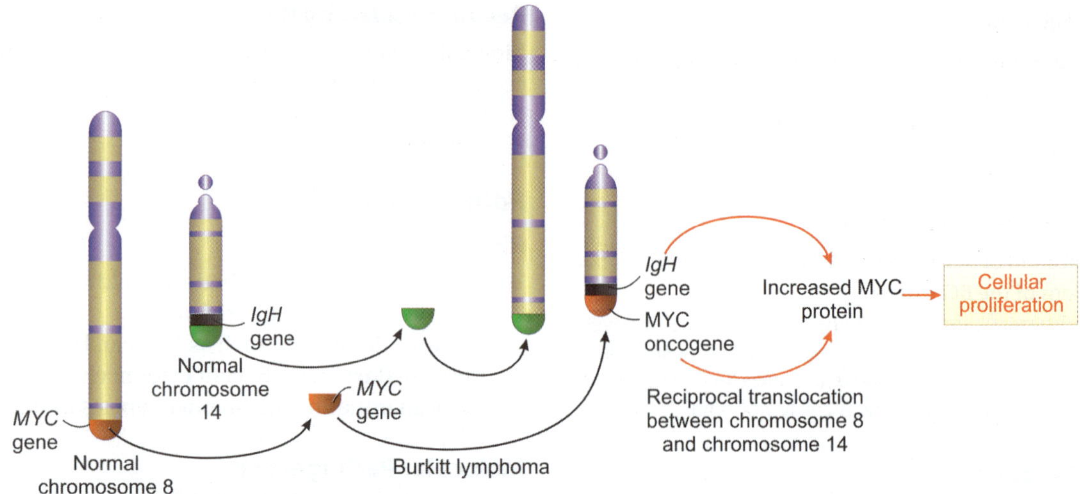

Fig. 12.20: Chromosomal translocation and activated MYC oncogene in Burkitt lymphoma.

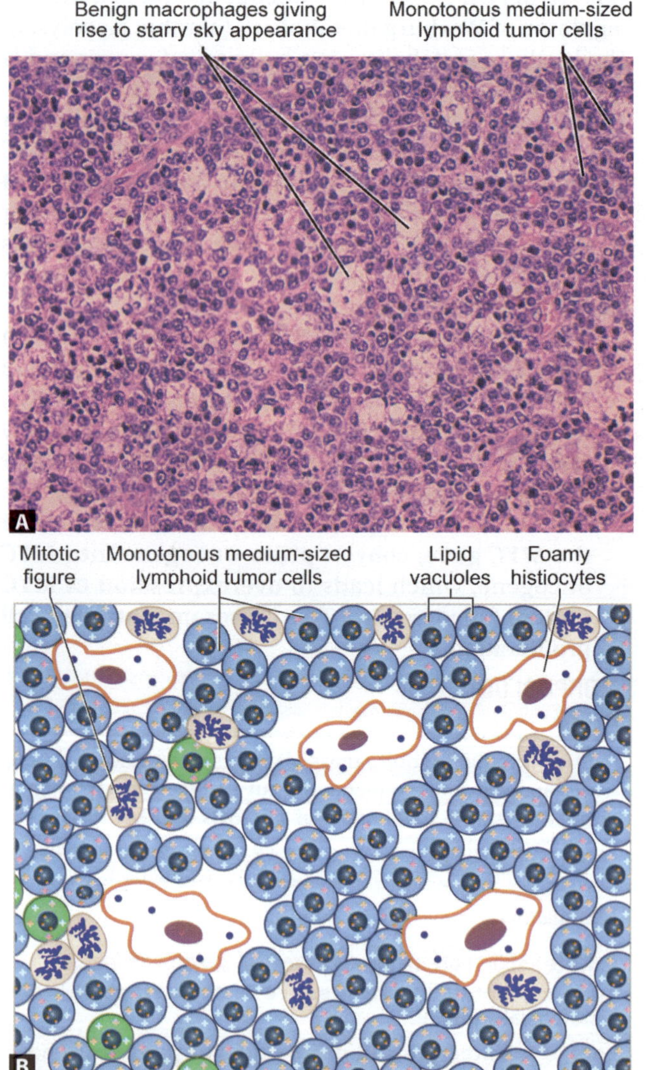

Figs. 12.21A and B: (A) H&E; (B) Diagrammatic. Burkitt lymphoma is composed of medium-sized lymphoid cells admixed with benign macrophages giving a "starry sky" appearance.

Features of neoplastic lymphoid cells:

- **Medium-sized lymphoid cells: The cells are monotonous and are medium-sized (intermediate in size).**
- **Round to oval nuclei:** Tumor cells have **round or oval nuclei** having **finely clumped and dispersed chromatin.** It shows **multiple (2–5) basophilic paracentrally located nucleoli.**
- **Basophilic or amphophilic cytoplasm:** Tumor cells have a **moderate amount of deeply basophilic cytoplasm** with squared-off cytoplasmic borders. The cytoplasm contains **multiple, small, round lipid-filled** (clear) **vacuoles** (appreciated on aspirate or imprint smears). which stain positive with oil red O. Amphophilic means stains with both the basic and the acidic dyes without any special affinity for either of these stains.
  - **Numerous mitotic figures and apoptosis:** EBV is present in almost all cases of endemic BL but in less than 30% of sporadic and immunodeficiency-related BL.

Starry sky pattern: Tumor cells undergo **apoptosis** and nuclear remnants of these apoptotic cells are phagocytosed and **cleared by benign macrophages.** The **sprinkling of these tangible-body macrophages** in the **background of cohesive blue lymphoid cells.** These benign macrophages often are surrounded by a clear space, creating a classic—though not specific **"starry sky"** appearance **(Figs. 12.21A and B).**

Immunophenotype

Strong expression of surface **IgM.**

Positive for common pan B-cell markers CD19, CD20, CD79a, CD22, and PAX5.

Positive for germinal center B-cell markers CD10 and *BCL6*.

BCL2 negative: BL does not express TdT, and this helps in distinguishing these tumors from precursor B-cell acute lymphoblastic leukemia/lymphoma.

Poor prognostic factors: Burkitt lymphoma is **highly aggressive lymphoma.** However, it responds well to very intensive chemotherapy regimens, and the majority of patients are cured.

Mantle Cell Lymphoma

Mantle cell lymphoma is a neoplasm composed of cells resembling the naïve B cells found in the mantle zones of normal lymphoid follicles (*refer* **Fig. 12.11**). It usually occurs in men older than 50 years of age.

Pathogenesis: Mantle cell lymphoma **has an (11;14) translocation that fuses the cyclin D1 gene to the IgH locus.** This results in overexpression of cyclin D1. This in turn stimulates growth by promoting the progression of cells from the G_1 phase to the S phase of the cell cycle by stimulating hyperphosphorylation of Rb.

MORPHOLOGY

The tumor **cells of mantle cell lymphoma are usually slightly larger than normal lymphocytes.** They have an irregular nucleus, inconspicuous nucleoli, and scant cytoplasm. In most cases, it involves the bone marrow and the peripheral blood in about 20% of cases.

Mantle cell lymphoma is moderately aggressive and incurable. The median survival is 6–7 years.

Miscellaneous Lymphoid Neoplasms

Among the many other forms of lymphoid neoplasms, several with distinctive or clinically important features merit brief discussion.

Hairy Cell Leukemia

Definition: Hairy cell leukemia is an uncommon, inactive neoplasm of small mature B cells having abundant cytoplasm with fine **hair-like cytoplasmic projections** (hence the name **hairy cell leukemia**) when viewed under the **phase-contrast microscope.**

Pathogenesis: Almost all cases are associated with activating mutations in the serine/threonine kinase BRAF. This mutation is also seen in several other cancers.

MORPHOLOGY

Presence of fine, hairlike cytoplasmic projections: Tumor cells are morphologically distinctive, characterized by the presence of fine, hairlike cytoplasmic projections. **Hairy cells** may be seen in the marrow and they have a **"fried egg" or "honeycomb"** appearance.

Immunophenotype: The tumor cells express B-cell markers (CD20), surface immunoglobulin, and CD11c and CD103. CD11c and CD 103 are not present in most other B-cell tumors and are useful for their diagnosis.

Clinical features: It affects **middle-aged to elderly men,** with a male-to-female ratio of 5:1. It presents with **massive splenomegaly** and **pancytopenia.**

Mycosis Fungoides and Sézary Syndrome

These tumors are neoplasms of CD4+ T cells. Mycosis fungoides and Sézary syndrome **occur in the skin. These tumors are often referred to as cutaneous T-cell lymphoma.**

Mycosis Fungoides

Mycosis fungoides is **cutaneous T-cell lymphoma** that usually manifests as a nonspecific erythrodermic rash. Mycosis fungoides has three stages: (i) patch stage, (ii) plaque stage, and (iii) tumor stage.

It may progress to a plaque phase and then to a tumor phase. With disease progression, it may spread to nodes and viscera.

- Lymphoid cells with **irregular nuclear outlines.**
- Limited to **skin.**

Age: Most are adults or elderly.

MORPHOLOGY

In mycosis fungoides, the **epidermis (epidermotropism) and upper dermis** are infiltrated by neoplastic T-cells. They may form groups in the epidermis forming **Pautrier's microabscess.** The neoplastic T-cells have **convoluted (cerebriform) nuclear contours** produced by the infoldings of the nuclear membrane.

Sézary Syndrome

Sézary syndrome is a clinical variant and is a rare disease. It is characterized by (i) **generalized exfoliative erythroderma, and (ii) the presence of characteristic Sézary cells (tumor cells)** in the skin, lymph nodes, and peripheral blood.

Prognosis: Aggressive disease and most die of opportunistic infections.

Adult T-cell Leukemia/Lymphoma

Adult T-cell leukemia/lymphoma **is a neoplasm of CD4+ T cells. It is caused by a retrovirus, human T-cell leukemia virus type 1 (HTLV-1).** It is commonly associated with skin lesions, lymphadenopathy, hepatosplenomegaly, hypercalcemia, and lymphocytosis. Most of these tumors are very aggressive and respond poorly to treatment. The median survival time is about 8 months.

Peripheral T-cell Lymphoma (PTCL)

It is a heterogeneous group of lymphomas and constitutes about 10% of adult NHLs. They mainly involve lymph nodes. They occur during the fifth to seventh decade and present with generalized lymphadenopathy. These are aggressive tumors that respond poorly to therapy.

Characteristics of the more common non-Hodgkin lymphomas, lymphoid leukemias, and plasma cell tumors are presented (*refer* **online Table 12.7**).

HODGKIN LYMPHOMAS

PA 19.4b (CC): Describe and discuss the pathogenesis, and pathology of Hodgkin's lymphoma.

Definition: Malignant lymphoid neoplasms with the following characteristics:

- **Minority** (1–3%) **of specific neoplastic cells** (Hodgkin cells and **Reed-Sternberg cells**).
- **Majority background of reactive non-neoplastic cells.**

BOX 12.20: Distinctive features of Hodgkin lymphoma in contrast to non-Hodgkin lymphoma.

1. Distinctive neoplastic **Reed-Sternberg giant (RS) cells.**
2. **Strong, but ineffective, host immune response** to the Reed-Sternberg cells. This results in only a small fraction of the tumor mass of RS cells.
3. Typically **spreads in a stepwise fashion.** HL arises in a single lymph node or chain of lymph nodes and spreads to anatomically contiguous nodes in a stepwise pattern.

Both non-Hodgkin and Hodgkin lymphomas most commonly arise in lymphoid tissues. The majority occurs in **young** adults. However, Hodgkin lymphoma has several features compared to non-Hodgkin lymphoma **(Box 12.20)**.

Classification (Box 12.21)

Q. Classify and discuss Hodgkin lymphoma.

Hodgkin lymphoma (HL) has five subtypes. It is broadly divided into two types: classic Hodgkin lymphoma (CHL), and nodular lymphocyte predominant type **(Box 12.21)**. They differ in clinical features, behavior, morphology, and immunophenotype (*refer* **online Table 12.8**). The classic HL are (1) nodular sclerosis, (2) mixed cellularity, (3) lymphocyte rich, and (4) lymphocyte depletion. In the classic type, four subtypes are included together because the RS cells in these shares certain morphologic and immunophenotypic features. CHL are CD15 and CD30 positive. They fail to express CD45 (leukocyte common antigen) and B-cell and T-cell markers. The nodular lymphocyte predominant type is separated from CHL because of the expression of germinal center B-cell markers in the Reed-Sternberg cells. They are CD15 and CD30 negative. They epress B-cell markers CD20+, and CD 45+.

Pathogenesis

The pathogenesis of HL is complex and not fully understood.

Cell of origin is germinal center B cell: Hodgkin lymphoma is a neoplasm that arises from germinal center B cells.

EBV infection and HL: EBV is present in the RS cells in around 70% of cases of the mixed-cellularity subtype Hodgkin lymphoma and in a few other classic forms of Hodgkin lymphoma. It indicates the role of EBV. In each case, the integration site of the EBV genome in all RS cells is identical. This suggests that EBV infection precedes (and therefore may be related to) transformation and clonal expansion. Thus, EBV infection is probably one of several steps involved in the development of tumors, particularly of the mixed-cellularity subtype.

BOX 12.21: WHO classification (2016) of Hodgkin lymphoma.

- **Classical Hodgkin lymphoma (CHL)**
  - **Nodular sclerosis classical Hodgkin lymphoma (NSCHL)**
  - **Mixed cellularity classical Hodgkin lymphoma (MCCHL)***
  - **Lymphocyte-rich classical Hodgkin lymphoma (LRCHL)***
  - **Lymphocyte depleted classical Hodgkin lymphoma (LDCHL)***
- **Nodular lymphocyte predominant Hodgkin lymphoma (NLPHL)**

*May be associated with EBV.

Activation of nuclear factor (NF-κB) common event in classical HL. It **turns on genes that promote the growth and survival of Reed-Sternberg cells**. This can occur by several mechanisms:

- **EBV+ tumor cells**: They express latent membrane protein-1 (LMP-1), a protein encoded by the EBV genome. It transmits signals that up-regulate NF-κB.
- **EBV– tumor cells:** In these tumors, activation of NF-κB may occur due to acquired loss-of-function mutations in IκB or TNF-α-induced protein 3. Both are negative regulators of NF-κB.

Activation of NF-κB rescues the "crippled" germinal center B cells from undergoing apoptosis.

Cytokine causing accumulation of reactive inflammatory cell infiltrate: Several cytokines secreted generate the characteristic inflammatory cell infiltrate. Some of these cytokines are secreted by RS cells. These include **IL-5 (a chemoattractant for eosinophils); transforming growth factor-β (a fibrogenic factor); and IL-13 (may stimulate RS cell growth through an autocrine mechanism)**. The inflammatory cells that infiltrate the tumor do not act as innocent observers. They produce additional factors that help the growth and survival of RS cells and further produce the tissue reaction.

Escapes of HL from the host immune response: Hodgkin lymphoma is one important example of a tumor that escapes from the host immune response**.** This is achieved **by the expression of proteins that inhibit T-cell activation.**

PA 19.5 (CC): Identify and describe the features of Hodgkin's lymphoma in a gross and microscopic specimen.

Reed-Sternberg (RS) Cell and its Variants

Q. Write a short note on the RS cell and its variants. Mention the types of Hodgkin lymphoma where they are seen.

Reed-Sternberg (RS) Cells

These are neoplastic cells **pathognomonic of Hodgkin lymphoma** and they are **necessary for the diagnosis of HL.** These RS cells **represent a minority of the neoplastic cells**.

Large cells: RS cell is a very large cell (15–45 µm in diameter) and at least **four to five times the size of background lymphocytes**.

Large nuclei with prominent eosinophilic nucleoli: RS cells have large nuclei with **exceptionally prominent (large) eosinophilic centrally placed** nucleoli surrounded by a **perinuclear halo**. The typical RS cell has **at least two nuclei** but can have a multilobate (having several lobes) nucleus.

Particularly characteristic are RS cells with **two mirror-image nuclei or nuclear lobes, each containing a large (inclusion-like) acidophilic (eosinophilic) nucleolus surrounded by a clear zone (perinuclear halo).** This produces an **"owl-eye" appearance**.

Abundant slightly eosinophilic cytoplasm: RS cells have abundant, usually slightly eosinophilic, cytoplasm.

Appearance and description of diagnostic Reed-Sternberg cells and their variants are shown in **Figure 12.22.**

Variants of Reed-Sternberg (RS) Cells

Hodgkin cell: It has a round nucleus with a prominent nucleolus.

Lacunar cell: It is characteristic of **nodular sclerosis classical Hodgkin lymphoma (NSCHL).** Its characteristics are described below under NSCHL.

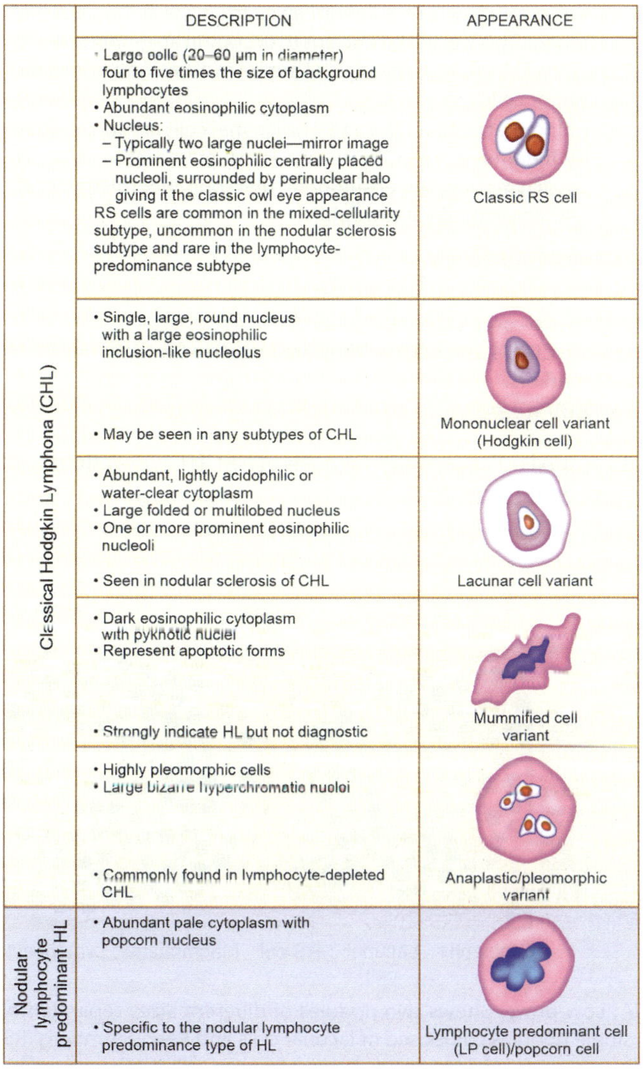

	DESCRIPTION	APPEARANCE
Classical Hodgkin Lymphoma (CHL)	• Large cells (20–60 μm in diameter) four to five times the size of background lymphocytes • Abundant eosinophilic cytoplasm • Nucleus: – Typically two large nuclei—mirror image – Prominent eosinophilic centrally placed nucleoli, surrounded by perinuclear halo giving it the classic owl eye appearance RS cells are common in the mixed-cellularity subtype, uncommon in the nodular sclerosis subtype and rare in the lymphocyte-predominance subtype	Classic RS cell
	• Single, large, round nucleus with a large eosinophilic inclusion-like nucleolus • May be seen in any subtypes of CHL	Mononuclear cell variant (Hodgkin cell)
	• Abundant, lightly acidophilic or water-clear cytoplasm • Large folded or multilobed nucleus • One or more prominent eosinophilic nucleoli • Seen in nodular sclerosis of CHL	Lacunar cell variant
	• Dark eosinophilic cytoplasm with pyknotic nuclei • Represent apoptotic forms • Strongly indicate HL but not diagnostic	Mummified cell variant
	• Highly pleomorphic cells • Large bizarre hyperchromatic nuclei • Commonly found in lymphocyte-depleted CHL	Anaplastic/pleomorphic variant
Nodular lymphocyte predominant HL	• Abundant pale cytoplasm with popcorn nucleus • Specific to the nodular lymphocyte predominance type of HL	Lymphocyte predominant cell (LP cell)/popcorn cell

Fig. 12.22: Diagrammatic appearances and characteristic features of Reed-Sternberg cells and their variants.

Mummified cell: It is a common finding in HL. It has a dense cytoplasm and pyknotic nuclei. It represents apoptotic forms.

Lymphocyte predominant (LP) cell: It was previously termed lymphohistiocytic (L&H) variant RS cell. It has a **delicate multilobed nucleus resembling popped corn ("popcorn cell")**. It is seen in **nodular lymphocytic predominant HL.** Its immunophenotype is different from classic Hodgkin lymphoma.

In the affected lymph node of HL, RS cells may constitute 0.1–10% of the number of cells in the infiltrate. In almost every case, it is **possible to find the classic RS cell,** but they are **usually not as numerous as the mononuclear Hodgkin cells.**

Immunophenotype: RS cells of CHL **express the CD30 lymphoid activation marker, and the CD15 macrophage/monocyte marker in most cases.** Unlike non-Hodgkin lymphoma cells, RS cells of CHL do **not usually express the pan-leukocyte marker CD45** (i.e., negative for CD45), B-cell antigens CD20 and CD79a, T-cell antigens (CD2, CD3), or histiocyte antigens (CD68, CD163).

The Cellular Microenvironment

The neoplastic RS cells are surrounded by a non-neoplastic cellular microenvironment. It varies with the subtype and EBV status of HL.

Reactive lymphocytes: In most cases, the background lymphocytes are T cells.

Other cells: Lymphocyte is accompanied by variable numbers of **eosinophils, histiocytes, neutrophils, and plasma cells.** Various types of cells found in Hodgkin lymphoma are listed in **Table 12.9.**

Classic Hodgkin Lymphoma

Q. Describe the gross and microscopic features of subtypes of Hodgkin lymphoma. Compare their prognosis.

Classic Hodgking lymphoma (CHL) is defined by the **presence of mononuclear Hodgkin cells and bi- or multinucleated Reed Sternberg cells within a characteristic non-neoplastic cellular microenvironment.** HL usually involves **lymph nodes. The involved lymph**

TABLE 12.9 Types of cells found in Hodgkin lymphoma.

Neoplastic cells	*Non-neoplastic cells*
• Reed-Sternberg cells (classical) • Variants – Mononuclear – Lacunar – Mummified – Anaplastic/pleomorphic • Lymphocyte predominant (LP) cell/popcorn	• Reactive lymphocytes • Macrophages/histiocytes • Granulocytes – Eosinophils – Neutrophils • Plasma cells

HL: The majority are non-neoplastic cells and the minority are neoplastic cells.

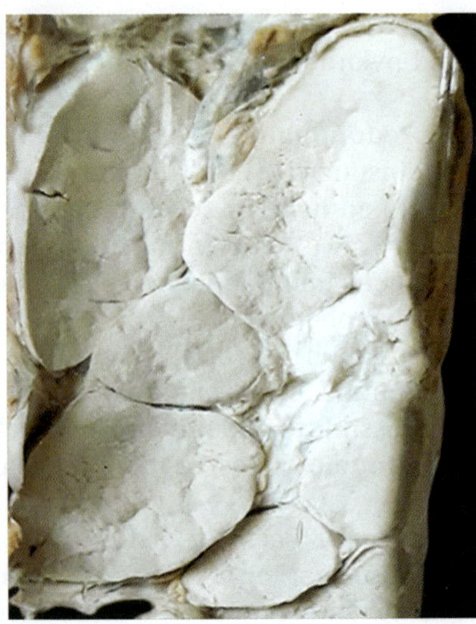

Fig. 12.23: Hodgkin lymphoma showing enlarged, encapsulated lymph nodes with fish flesh appearance on the cut surface.

nodes are enlarged, encapsulated with fish flesh appearance on the cut surface (Fig. 12.23). Classical Hodgkin lymphoma (CHL) accounts for 95% of Hodgkin lymphomas and has four subtypes. They are discussed below.

Nodular Sclerosis Classical Hodgkin Lymphoma (NSCHL)

Q. Write a short note on nodular sclerosis HL.

Most common type of HL: Nodular sclerosis Hodgkin lymphoma is a subtype of CHL and is the **most common form** constituting **40–70%** of cases of HL.

Age and gender: Most patients are adolescents or young adults between **20 and 30 years of age.** It has an **equal** frequency in **males and females.**

Site affected: It involves the **lower cervical, supraclavicular, and mediastinal lymph nodes.**

MORPHOLOGY

Microscopy of NSCHL (Figs. 12.24A to C)

- **Collagen (sclerotic) bands surrounding nodules:** It shows **broad collagen** (sclerotic) bands that extend from the capsule and divide the lymphoid tissue into **circumscribed cellular nodules of varying sizes and shapes.** It causes **loss of lymph node architecture.** The fibrosis may be scant or abundant. Thus, **collagen bands surround one to several nodules.** Capsule of the lymph node also shows fibrosis.
- **Nodules contain RS cells and the reactive infiltrate: The nodules consist of lacunar cells, typical RS cells, and Hodgkin cells.**
- **Presence of lacunar cells (Inset of Fig. 12.24B):** Lacunar cell is a **variant of Reed-Sternberg cells** and are characteristic of this subtype. It has a **single multilobate (multiple lobes) nucleus with multiple small nucleoli.** It contains **abundant, pale-staining cytoplasm.** In sections of formalin-fixed tissue, the cytoplasm is usually torn away from the cell border and retract. This leaves the nucleus to occupy in an empty space (a holes or lacune). Necrosis is common in areas with numerous tumor cells.
- **Inflammatory background:** The lacunar cells are **surrounded by inflammatory infiltrate** consisting of numerous reactive **small lymphocytes, eosinophils, macrophages (histiocytes), and occasionally neutrophils.**

Immunophenotype

- The immunophenotype of the lacunar variant is identical to that of other RS cells found in classic subtypes. These cells are **CD15+ and CD30+. They are negative for CD45 and T cell markers.**
- **EBV negative.**

Prognosis: The overall prognosis of NSCHL is **excellent** with a cure rate of 80–85%.

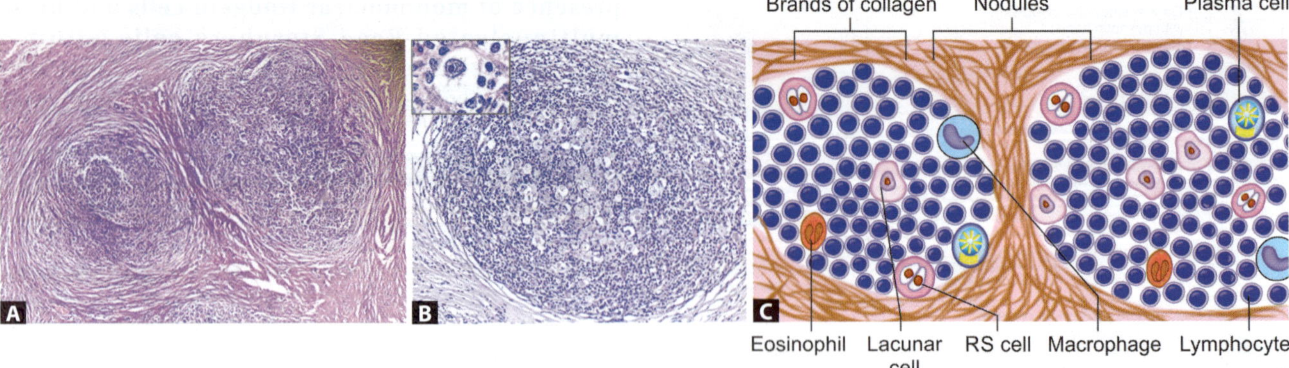

Figs. 12.24A to C: Nodular sclerosis classical Hodgkin lymphoma: (A) Low power shows two nodules of different sizes separated by well-defined bands of pink, acellular collagen; (B) High power shows single nodules composed of lacunar cells and Reed-Sternberg (RS) cells within the background of lymphocytes, eosinophils, plasma cells, and macrophages. Inset shows a lacunar cell; (C) Diagrammatic appearance showing 4 nodules of varying sizes separated by collagen fibers. Also seen are in each nodule.

Mixed Cellularity Classical Hodgkin Lymphoma (MCCHL)

Q. Write a short note on mixed cellularity HL.

Second common subtype: Mixed-cellularity Hodgkin lymphoma is the second common subtype constituting 20–25% of cases. It is the most common form of Hodgkin lymphoma in patients older than 50 years of age.

Gender and age: More common in males. It is present in **older age**, with **systemic symptoms** (such as night sweats and weight loss) and **advanced tumor stage**.

Strongly associated with EBV and involves **peripheral lymph nodes**.

MORPHOLOGY

Microscopy of MCCHL (Figs. 12.25A and B)

- Lymph node **architecture is diffusely effaced** (obliterated).
- **Plenty of Reed-Sternberg cells and Hodgkin cells:** Compared to other CHL subtypes, it frequently shows bi- or multinucleated RS cells. These RS cells are diffusely scattered.
- **Inflammatory background:** It shows a mixed (heterogeneous) inflammatory infiltrate comprising of **small lymphocytes, and benign macrophages (histiocytes), eosinophils (sometimes numerous), and plasma cells.**

Immunophenotype: RS cells are CD15+, CD30+ and EBV+ (about 70%).

Prognosis: MCCHL is more likely to be disseminated and associated with systemic manifestations. Overall prognosis is **very good**.

Lymphocyte-rich Classical Hodgkin Lymphoma (LRCHL)

- Subtype of classical Hodgkin lymphoma with **scattered Hodgkin and RS cells**.
- **Uncommon**—about 5% of classical HL.
- More in **elderly** patients, associated with **EBV in 40%** of cases.
- Involves **peripheral lymph nodes**.

MORPHOLOGY

Microscopy of LRCHL

- **Growth patterns:** May show two patterns (i) **nodular** (common) and (ii) **diffuse** (rare)
- **Only a few Reed-Sternberg cells and Hodgkin cells.**
- **Background: Abundant reactive small lymphocytes.**

Immunophenotype: RS cells are CD15+ and CD30+. CD45-, and CD20-.

Prognosis: LRCHL has a good to excellent prognosis.

Lymphocyte-depleted Classical Hodgkin Lymphoma (LDCHL)

A subtype of classical Hodgkin lymphoma **rich in Hodgkin and RS cells** in a background depleted in non-neoplastic lymphocytes.

- **Rarest**—less than 2% of cases
- Predominantly in **older, HIV-positive patients**, often **EBV-associated** (over 90%)
- Predominantly **retroperitoneal lymph nodes, abdominal organs, and bone marrow.**
- It is strongly associated with EBV.

MORPHOLOGY

Microscopy of LDCHL

- **Plenty of RS cells** or their **anaplastic/pleomorphic variants.**
- **Histological types**
  - **Reticular: Numerous Hodgkin and RS cells** with depletion of lymphocytes.
  - **Diffuse sclerosis/fibrosis:** Hypocellular infiltrate containing bizarre RS cells with fine fibrosis.
- **Background: Paucity (scarcity) of lymphocytes.**

Immunophenotype: RS cells are CD15+ and CD30+; the majority are EBV+.

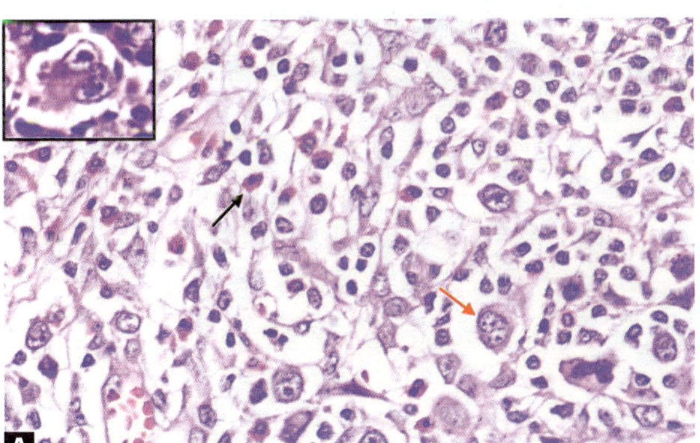

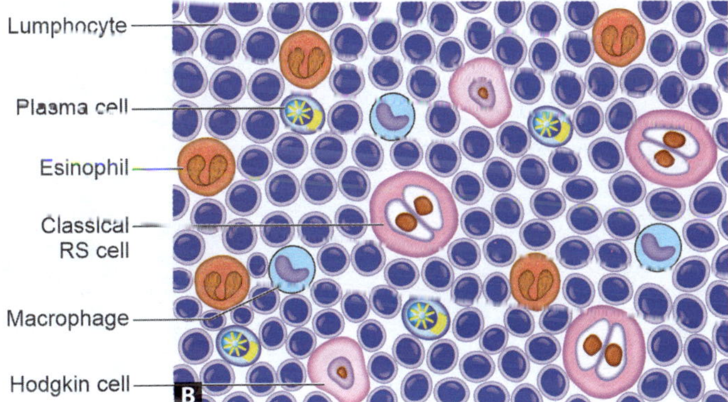

Figs. 12.25A and B: Mixed cellularity classical Hodgkin lymphoma: (A) Shows classical diagnostic binucleate Reed-Sternberg (RS) cell (red arrow), and surrounded by a mixed cellular population consisting of lymphocytes, eosinophils (black arrow), plasma cells, and histiocytes (macrophages). The inset shows a classic binucleate RS cell; (B) Diagrammatic appearance.

Nodular Lymphocyte Predominant Hodgkin Lymphoma

Q. Write a short essay on nodular lymphocyte predominant Hodgkin lymphoma (NLPHL).

- **Uncommon**—5% of all Hodgkin lymphomas.
- **Not associated** with **EBV**.
- Majority males, usually **30–50 years** of age.
- Involves mainly **cervical or axillary lymph nodes.**

MORPHOLOGY

Microscopy of NLPHL (Figs. 12.26A and B)

- **Partial or complete loss of lymph node architecture.**
- **Nodular and/or diffuse infiltrate** of **abundant small lymphocytes** with **histiocytes** and **scattered neoplastic LP cells**. Neutrophils and eosinophils are absent.
- **Lymphocyte predominant cells** (LP cells)/"popcorn" cells **(Fig. 12.26)**: These are specific to NLPHL. They are large with relatively abundant, pale cytoplasm. They have a single large delicate **multilobulated** nucleus **or folded nuclei** resembling the bubbly outlines of popcorn kernels. LP cells have one or more **inconspicuous nucleoli.**
- **Hodgkin and RS cells are not found.**

Immunophenotype: LP cells express B-related markers. They are CD20+, CD 45+ and CD15-, C30- and EBV–ve. Express BCL6.

Prognosis: NLPHL is more likely to recur than the classical subtypes, but the prognosis is excellent.

Laboratory Findings

PERIPHERAL SMEAR

RBCs: Normocytic normochromic anemia.

WBCs: Leukocytosis occurs in 1/3rd of the patients. Eosinophilia is frequent.

Platelets*:* Normal or increased.

ESR*:* Raised.

Bone marrow: It is involved in the later stages.

Fine Needle Aspiration Cytology (FNAC)

It shows RS cells/its variants against a background of inflammatory cells (depending on the subtype).

Spread: Mainly by contiguity (lymph node close to the affected node). **First nodal disease, then splenic disease, hepatic disease, and finally marrow involvement and extranodal disease.**

Clinical Features

Hodgkin lymphoma, like NHL, usually presents as a painless enlargement of lymph nodes (lymphadenopathy). **Extranodal involvement is uncommon.**

Staging of Hodgkin Lymphoma

After the diagnosis of HL, staging is used to guide therapy and determine prognosis. The clinical staging of Hodgkin lymphoma is discussed in **Table 12.10**.

"B symptoms": These systemic/constitutional symptoms include fever, weight loss, and night sweats. Pel-Ebstein fever is characterized by alternating bouts of fever followed by remissions. Younger patients with more favorable subtypes usually present with stage I or stage II. They are free of these "B symptoms." Patients with advanced disease (stages III and IV) are more likely to manifest with B symptoms and as pruritus and anemia.

All stages are further divided depending on the absence (A) or presence (B) of the following systemic symptoms and signs: significant fever, night sweats, and unexplained loss of more than 10% of normal body weight.

Prognosis: It is **very good even for those with advanced disease.** The 5-year survival rate for those with stage I-A or

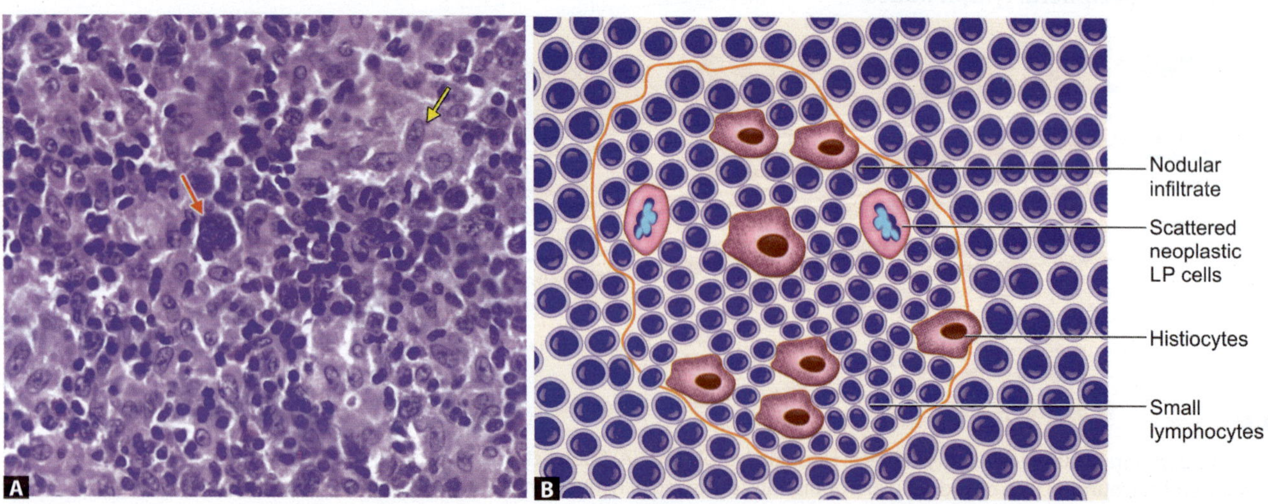

Figs. 12.26A and B: (A) H&E; (B) Diagrammatic. Nodular lymphocyte predominant Hodgkin lymphoma with 'popcorn' cells (arrow in Fig. 12.26A) in a background of reactive lymphocytes and histocytes (yellow arrow).

TABLE 12.10 Clinical staging of Hodgkin lymphomas (Ann Arbor staging classification).

Stage	*Definition*
I	Involvement of a single lymph node region (I) or involvement of a single extralymphatic organ or tissue (I_E)
II	Involvement of two or more lymph node regions on the same side of the diaphragm alone (II) or with involvement of limited contiguous extralymphatic organs or tissue (II_E)
III	Involvement of lymph node regions on both sides of the diaphragm (III), which may include the spleen (III_S), limited contiguous extralymphatic organ or site (III_E), or both (III_{ES}).
IV	Multiple or disseminated foci of involvement of one or more extralymphatic organs or tissues with or without lymphatic involvement

E, involvement of a single extranodal site, or contiguous or proximal to known nodal site of disease.

II-A disease is more than 90%. For advanced disease (stage IV-A or IV-B), the overall 5-year disease-free survival rate is around 50%.

A summary of various subtypes of Hodgkin lymphoma is presented (*refer* **online Table 12.11**).

PA 19. 4c (CC): Differentiating features of Hodgkin's and non-Hodgkin's lymphoma.

Q. List the differences between HL and NHL.

HL differs from NHL in several respects and their main differences are shown in **Table 12.12**.

TABLE 12.12 Differences between Hodgkin and non-Hodgkin lymphomas.

Sl. No.	*Characteristics*	*Hodgkin lymphoma*	*Non-Hodgkin lymphoma*
1.	Site of involvement	Arises in a single node or chain of nodes (cervical, mediastinal, para-aortic)	Mainly involves multiple peripheral nodes
2.	Pattern of spread	Orderly spread by contiguity in a predictable fashion	Noncontiguous spread in an unpredictable fashion
3.	Mesenteric nodes and Waldeyer ring	Rarely involved	Commonly involved
4.	Extranodal involvement	Uncommon	Common
5.	Characteristic of neoplastic cells	Neoplastic cells—Hodgkin or Reed-Sternberg cells form minor tumor cell mass (1–5%)	Neoplastic cells form the major tumor cell mass

SPLENOMEGALY

PA 19.6 (CC): Enumerate and differentiate the causes of splenomegaly.

The spleen is rarely the primary site of disease. Enlargement of the spleen is called splenomegaly and occurs in a wide variety of systemic diseases (secondary involvement). The main causes of splenomegaly are listed in **Box 12.22**. Splenomegaly may be grouped into three degrees namely mild, moderate, and massive.

PA 19.7 (CC): Identify and describe the gross specimen of an enlarged spleen.

Mild Splenomegaly (Weight <500 g)

Its causes include acute splenitis; acute splenic congestion; infectious mononucleosis, bacterial endocarditis, acute malaria, and other disorders (e.g., septicemia, chronic venous congestion of spleen in congestive heart failure, systemic lupus erythematosus, rheumatoid arthritis, intra-abdominal infections, typhoid fever, and thalassemia minor).

BOX 12.22: Main causes of splenomegaly.

Infections: Nonspecific splenitis of various blood-borne infections (particularly infectious endocarditis)
- Acute: Infectious mononucleosis, typhoid fever, brucellosis, bacterial septicemia
- Subacute: Subacute bacterial endocarditis
- Chronic: Tuberculosis, malaria, syphilis, kala-azar, leishmaniasis

Immunologic inflammatory disorders
- Rheumatoid arthritis
- Systemic lupus erythematosus
- Sarcoidosis

Non-neoplastic hematological disorders
- Hemolytic anemias: Thalassemia major, hemoglobinopathies
- Immune thrombocytopenia

Congestive states related to portal hypertension
- Cirrhosis of the liver
- Splenic or portal vein thrombosis or stenosis
- Right-sided cardiac failure

Primary or metastatic neoplasm
- Lymphohematogenous neoplasms: Leukemia, Hodgkin lymphoma, non-Hodgkin lymphomas and lymphocytic leukemias, myeloproliferative disorders, multiple myeloma
- Primary neoplasms (e.g., hemangiosarcoma) and cysts of spleen
- Metastatic neoplasm: Sarcoma, carcinoma

Storage diseases
- Gaucher disease
- Niemann–Pick disease
- Mucopolysaccharidoses

Miscellaneous disorders
- Amyloidosis

Moderate Splenomegaly (Weight 500–1,000 g)

Causes of moderate splenomegaly include chronic congestive splenomegaly (portal hypertension or splenic vein obstruction), acute leukemias, disorders with extravascular hemolysis (hereditary spherocytosis, thalassemia major, autoimmune hemolytic anemia), amyloidosis, Niemann–Pick disease, many infections (e.g., infective endocarditis, tuberculosis, and typhoid), sarcoidosis; metastatic carcinoma or sarcoma.

Massive Splenomegaly (Weight >1,000 g)

Q. Write a short note on the causes of massive splenomegaly.

A spleen is considered as massively enlarged when its lower pole is within the pelvis, or which has crossed the midline into the right lower or right upper abdominal quadrants. Its causes are listed in **Box 12.23**.

Hypersplenism: It is characterized by the excessive removal of red blood cells, granulocytes, or platelets from the circulation. A chronically enlarged spleen usually removes excessive numbers of one or more of the formed elements of blood. This may lead to anemia, leukopenia, or thrombocytopenia. Platelets are more susceptible to sequestration in the red pulp. Hence, thrombocytopenia is more common and severe in patients with splenomegaly compared to anemia or neutropenia. Hypersplenism is characterized by splenomegaly, cytopenia(s), normal or hyperplastic bone marrow, and a response to splenectomy.

Laboratory Assessment

Complete blood count: The CBC may show cytopenia of one or more blood cell types. This suggests hypersplenism.

- **RBC count:** It may be normal, decreased (thalassemia major syndromes, SLE, cirrhosis with portal hypertension), or increased (polycythemia vera).
- **WBC count:** It may be normal, decreased (congestive splenomegaly, leukemias), or increased (infections or inflammatory disease, myeloproliferative disorders).
- **Platelet count:** It may be normal, decreased due to increased sequestration or destruction of platelets in an enlarged spleen (congestive splenomegaly, Gaucher's disease, immune thrombocytopenia), or increased in the myeloproliferative disorders such as polycythemia vera.

Other laboratory studies: It depends on the differential diagnosis of the underlying illness responsible for splenomegaly.

BOX 12.23: Causes of massively enlarged spleen (massive splenomegaly).

- Chronic myeloid leukemia
- Myelofibrosis (primary or secondary to polycythemia vera or essential thrombocytosis)
- Hyper-reactive malarial splenomegaly syndrome (tropical splenomegaly syndrome)
- Gaucher's disease
- Lymphoma (mantle cell lymphoma, marginal B-cell lymphoma), hairy cell leukemia
- Infectious diseases (e.g., chronic malaria), kala-azar (visceral leishmaniasis)
- Beta-thalassemia major
- AIDS with *Mycobacterium avium* complex
- Splenic cysts
- Leukemias: Chronic lymphocytic leukemia, hairy cell leukemia
- Others: Sarcoidosis, autoimmune hemolytic anemia

PLASMA CELL NEOPLASMS

Plasma cell neoplasms are **B-cell proliferations containing neoplastic plasma cells.**

Q. Write a short note on M proteins.

Characteristics of plasma cell neoplasms: These are as follows:

Secretion of a single type of immunoglobulin or its fragments: These neoplastic (**monoclonal, single clone**) plasma cells **almost always secrete a complete single type of (monoclonal) immunoglobulin (Ig) or immunoglobulin (Ig) fragments (immunoglobulin light chains).** The abnormal immunoglobulins associated with plasma cell neoplasm are termed monoclonal gammopathy, dysproteinemia (excessive, synthesis of immunoglobulin (Ig) or light chains), and paraproteinemia (presence of monoclonal immunoglobulin or light chain in serum).

- **M proteins in serum:** The monoclonal (single type) immunoglobulins secreted into the blood by these tumors are referred to as an *M protein* (or M component, originally called myeloma protein). It is detected as a **monoclonal spike on electrophoresis.** These complete M proteins have high molecular weights (160 kilodaltons or more), and they are restricted to the plasma and extracellular fluid. In the absence of glomerular damage, they are **not excreted in the urine.**
- **Bence-Jones (BJ) proteins in urine:** Neoplastic plasma cells often synthesize excess immunoglobulin light chains along with complete immunoglobulins. The free light chains have less molecular weight (approximately 25 kilodaltons). These **free light chains** pass through glomeruli into the urinary space. They are excreted in the urine and referred to as **Bence-Jones (BJ) proteins.**

These secretions of monoclonal plasma cells serve as tumor markers and usually produce pathologic effects.

WHO (2022) classification of plasma cell neoplasms is presented in **Box 12.24**.

Plasma Cell Myeloma/Multiple Myeloma

PA 20.1 (CC): Describe the features of plasma cell myeloma.

BOX 12.24: WHO (2022) classification of plasma cell neoplasms.

- Plasmacytoma
- Plasma cell myeloma/multiple myeloma
- Plasma cell neoplasms with associated paraneoplastic syndrome

WHO Definitions

Plasma cell myeloma: It is a **bone marrow-based, multifocal neoplastic proliferation of plasma cells.**

Multiple myeloma: It is defined by the **combination of plasma cell myeloma,** usually **associated with** a **serum and/or urine monoclonal immunoglobulin,** and

- Either **evidence of organ damage** related to the disease or
- **In the absence of organ damage, laboratory or imaging findings** that **suggest a high risk of developing end-organ damage within 2 years.**

Multiple myeloma is the **most important plasma cell neoplasm (monoclonal gammopathy).** It is one of the most common lymphoid malignancies. **It produces multifocal (multiple) destructive tumor masses in the bone (lytic or "punched out" radiographically) distributed throughout the skeleton, most commonly in the vertebral column, ribs, skull, pelvis, and femurs.**

Age and gender: The median age at diagnosis of multiple myeloma is 70 years. It is more common in males.

Organs involved: Multiple myeloma **mainly involves the bone marrow**. It is usually associated with **multiple lytic lesions throughout the skeletal system.**

Type of M protein produced by myeloma cells: The most frequent is **IgG (60%),** followed by **IgA (20–25%).** Rarely, it may produce IgM, IgD, or IgE M proteins. In the remaining cases, the myeloma cells secrete only κ or λ light chains.

Risk factors: These include genetic predisposition, exposure to ionizing radiation, and exposure to chemicals like benzene, herbicides, and insecticides. Other risk factors are chronic antigenic stimulation associated with chronic infections (HIV and chronic osteomyelitis) and chronic inflammatory disorders (e.g., rheumatoid arthritis).

Pathogenesis

Chromosomal translocations involving the IGH locus on chromosome 14 **with dysregulation of cyclin D: Myeloma often has chromosomal translocations with fusion of the IgH locus on chromosome 14 to oncogenes such as the cyclin D1 and cyclin D3 genes.** This dysregulated D cyclins and increases the proliferation of cells. The cytokine interleukin-6 (IL-6) produced by fibroblasts and macrophages in the bone marrow stroma also causes the proliferation of myeloma cells.

Laboratory Findings

Q. Write a short note on the laboratory diagnosis of multiple myeloma.

Peripheral Blood

- **Hemoglobin: Decreased** and ranges from 6 g/dL to 10 g/dL.
- **ESR: High** and is due to high gamma globulin (immunoglobulin) and rouleaux formation.
- **Bleeding time: Increased.**

PERIPHERAL SMEAR

- **RBCs: Normocytic normochromic anemia,** red blood cells show **rouleaux formation** due to increased immunoglobulins.
- **WBCs: Normal.**
- **Platelets: Normal.**

BONE MARROW

Q. Write a short note on the morphology of plasma cells in multiple myeloma.

Q. Write a short note on bone marrow findings in multiple myeloma.

Cellularity: Plasma cells are **more than 30% of cells in bone marrow:** The marrow is **hypercellular** due to an **increased number of plasma cells (myeloma cells, i.e., malignant plasma cells) (Figs. 12.27A and B).** The presence of **more than 30% plasma cells in the bone marrow is diagnostic.** They may predominantly consist of **normal-appearing plasma cells, plasmablasts** with vesicular nuclear chromatin and a prominent single nucleolus, or **bizarre, multinucleated cells.**

Morphological features of plasma cells (Figs. 12.27A and B): The morphology of cells in the bone marrow **varies from mature-looking relatively normal plasma cells to immature, plasmablastic, and pleomorphic variants.**

- **Mature plasma cells:** They are **oval-shaped** with an **eccentric nucleus. The nuclei have a spoke wheel or clockface chromatin without nucleolus.** They contain **abundant basophilic cytoplasm with a perinuclear hof (clearing)** due to the prominent Golgi apparatus.
- **Immature forms of plasma cells (myeloma cells):** They have (i) **more dispersed nuclear chromatin, (ii) a higher nuclear/cytoplasmic ratio, (iii) a prominent nucleolus, and (iv)** cytoplasmic inclusions **(Russell bodies)** containing immunoglobulin. It includes **multinucleated and multilobate forms.** Nuclear immaturity and pleomorphism rarely occur in reactive plasma cells and these features are reliable indicators of malignancy. The cytoplasm of myeloma cells has abundant endoplasmic reticulum. These cells are usually uninucleated or may show binucleation. **Plasmablasts** have vesicular nuclear chromatin and a prominent single nucleolus, and pleomorphic variants are **bizarre with multinucleation.**
- **Other cytologic variants:** The bone marrow of myeloma may contain cytologic variants resulting from dysregulated synthesis and secretion of Ig. This may lead to intracellular accumulation of intact or partially degraded (condensed or crystallized) proteins. Such variants include:
  - **Mott cells** (Morula cells) (upper right corner inset of **Fig. 12.27A**) have multiple pale bluish-white, grape-like cytoplasmic accumulations.
  - **Flame cells** (left corner inset of **Fig. 12.27A**) with fiery red cytoplasm (vermilion staining) that contain glycogen-rich IgA.

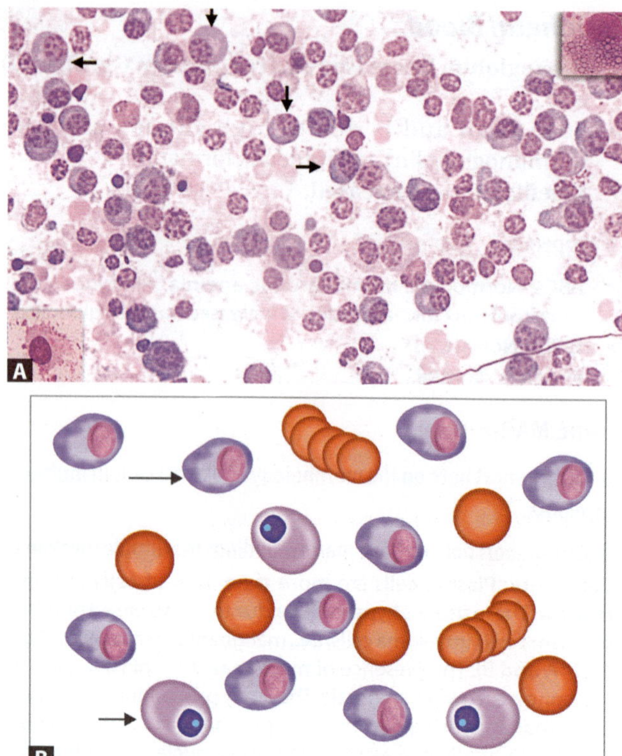

Figs. 12.27A and B: Bone marrow aspirate in multiple myeloma: (A) Leishman stain shows numerous myeloma plasma cells (arrows). Inset shows flame cell (left lower corner) and mott cell (right upper corner); (B) Diagrammatic appearance showing plasmablasts (short arrow) and plasma cells (long arrow).

- Cells containing other inclusions, including fibrils, crystalline rods, and globules. The globular inclusions are termed **Russell bodies** (if cytoplasmic) or **Dutcher bodies** (if nuclear).

Erythropoiesis: Diminished and is normoblastic.

Myelopoiesis: Normal.

Megakaryopoiesis: Normal.

Serum Findings

- **Serum β_2 microglobulin: Prognostic marker** and **high values signify poor prognosis.**
- **Hypercalcemia**
- **Renal function tests: Blood urea, serum creatinine, and uric acid levels** are **raised** with renal involvement.
- **Serum albumin:** Decreases in advanced stages of the disease.

Electrophoretic Studies on Serum and Urine (Figs. 12.28A and B)

Q. Write a short note on urinary findings in multiple myeloma.

Q. Write a short note on Bence-Jones protein and its demonstration.

- **Increased levels of immunoglobulins**: Blood shows raised levels of **monoclonal immunoglobulins**. Immunoglobulin may be **IgG** (most common)/IgD/IgA/IgE type. It produces **monoclonal spikes** in 80–90% of cases.

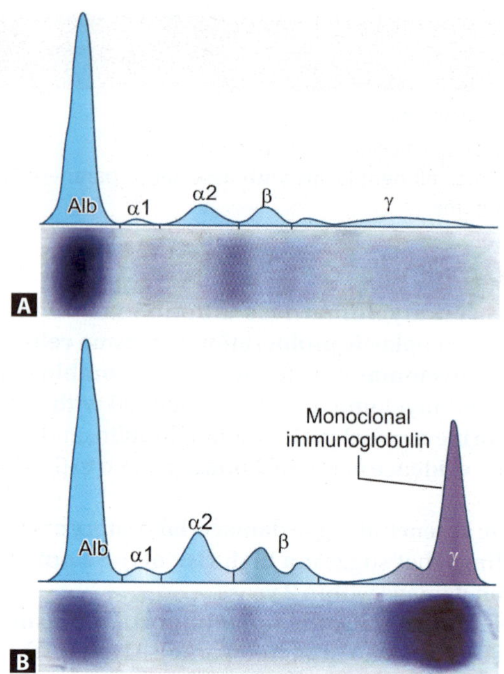

Figs. 12.28A and B: Serum electrophoresis: (A) Shows a normal pattern; (B) Shows monoclonal immunoglobulin ("M Band") in multiple myeloma.

- **Light chains** or **Bence-Jones (BJ) proteins** in the urine may be seen in 60–80% of cases. BJ protein may be of κ or λ type of light chain.

Untoward Effects of Multiple Myeloma

Multiple myeloma produces untoward effects on the **skeleton, the immune system, and the kidney**. These are responsible for morbidity and mortality.

Resorption of bone: The major pathologic feature of multiple myeloma is the resorption of bone. It usually produces **multifocal destructive skeletal lesions.** They commonly involve the vertebral column, ribs, skull, pelvis, femur, clavicle, and scapula. The lesions arise in the medullary cavity, erode cancellous bone, and progressively destroy the bone cortex. On gross examination, the bone defects are filled with soft gelatinous, fish flesh, and hemorrhagic tissue. Bone resorption is caused by factors produced by neoplastic plasma cells. Myeloma-derived factors upregulate the expression of the receptor activator of NF-κB ligand (RANKL) by bone marrow stromal cells. This in turn activates osteoclasts. Other factors released from tumor cells also inhibit osteoblast function. All these result in **increased bone resorption**. Bone destruction leads to **hypercalcemia and pathologic fractures** (most frequent in the vertebral column or femur). The destructive bone lesions usually appear as **punched-out** (lytic lesions) **defects** 1–4 cm in diameter **(Fig. 12.29).**

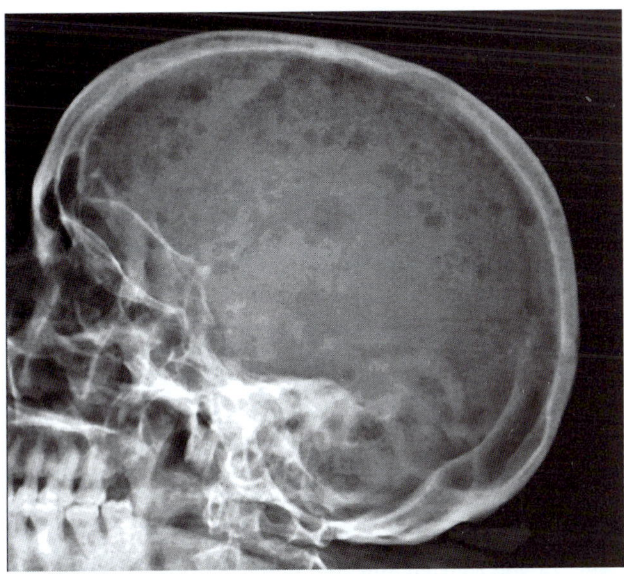

Fig. 12.29: Radiograph of the skull, lateral view. Skull bone showing multiple, sharply punched-out bone defects (lytic lesions).

Defects in humoral immunity: Myeloma causes defects in humoral immunity. Myeloma cells compromise the function of normal B cells. The plasma shows raised levels of immunoglobulin due to M protein. However, the production of functional antibodies is usually severely decreased. Thus, these patients are susceptible to bacterial infections.

Renal dysfunction: It is due to several pathologic effects of myeloma and these may occur alone or in combination.

- **Obstructive proteinaceous casts (myeloma kidney):** The proteinaceous casts are often formed in the distal convoluted tubules and the collecting ducts. These obstruct and damage the renal tubules. The casts consist of mainly Bence-Jones proteins and variable amounts of complete immunoglobulin, proteins secreted from tubular epithelium, and albumin.
- **Light chain deposition:** These may be deposited in the glomeruli or the interstitium, either as amyloid or linear deposits. **Amyloidosis** of the AL type may lead to **nephrotic syndrome** and renal damage.
- **Hypercalcemia:** Bone resorption leads to hypercalcemia. This may lead to dehydration and renal stones. Hypercalcemia may also cause **metastatic calcification in the kidney.**
- **Increased incidence of bacterial pyelonephritis:** It is partly due to hypogammaglobulinemia. Patients are prone to acute and chronic pyelonephritis.

Clinical Manifestations (Flowchart 12.1)

Onset: Insidious.

Age and sex: Affects old age between 50 and 60 years with slight male preponderance.

The **clinical features** of multiple myeloma are:

1. **Due to tumor cells causing bone lesions: Resorption of bone** results in pathologic fractures, chronic bone pain, and tenderness. It leads to **hypercalcemia. Pallor due to** anemia and result in weakness and fatigue.
2. **Production of M-proteins (increased immunoglobulins): Bleeding tendency, coagulation abnormalities, and amyloidosis** of the AL type.
3. **Humoral immune deficiency:** Predisposes to recurrent bacterial infections.
4. **Renal disease:** Renal failure, infections, or nephrotic syndrome.

Flowchart 12.1: Clinical features and laboratory findings in myeloma.

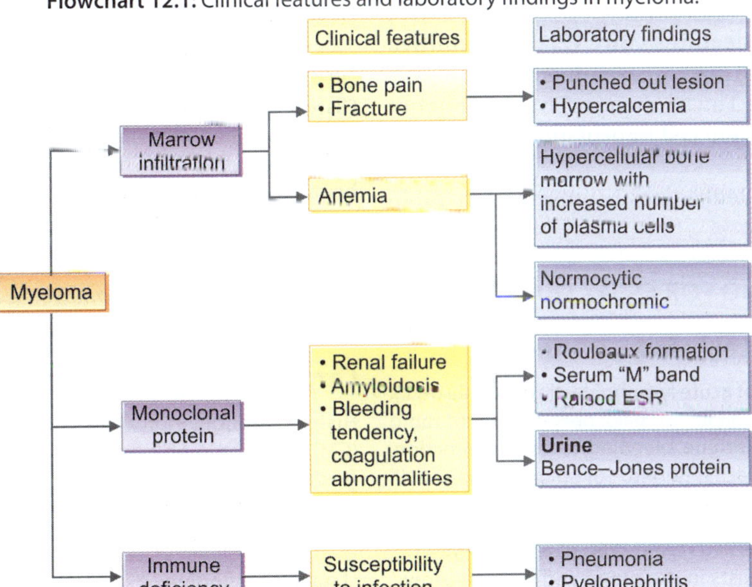

(ESR: erythrocyte sedimentation rate).

BOX 12.25: Criteria for diagnosis of myeloma (WHO 2022).

- Demonstration of clonal plasma cells in the bone marrow using flow cytometry or immunohistochemistry.
- Demonstration of one or more myeloma-defining criteria (SLIM-CRAB)
  1. MRI showing more than 1 focal lesion, and/or
  2. Serum free light chain ratio >100, and/or
  3. Bone marrow plasma cell percentage >60%, and/or
  4. Anemia, and/or
  5. Hypercalcemia, and/or
  6. Lytic lesions and/or osteoporosis with compression fracture demonstrated by low-dose CT or skeletal X-ray, and/or
  7. Renal impairment

TABLE 12.13 Reference range for leukocytes.

Component (specimen)	*Reference value*
Differential leukocyte count (DLC)	
• P (polymorphs or neutrophils)	40–70% (2,000–7,500/µL)
• L (lymphocytes)	20–40% (1,500–4,000/µL)
• M (monocytes)	2–10% (200–800/µL)
• E (eosinophils)	1–6% (40–450/µL)
• B (basophils)	<1% (10–100/µL)
Total leukocyte count (TLC)	
• Adults	4,000–11,000/µL
• Infants (full term, at birth)	10,000–25,000/µL
• Infants (1 year)	6,000–16,000/µL

Diagnosis: It requires a combination of laboratory, radiologic, and clinical features **(Box 12.25)**. Definitive diagnosis requires a bone marrow examination.

Prognosis: It is variable. The median survival is for about 5 years. Hematopoietic stem cell transplantation prolongs life but is not curative.

Reference range for leukocytes is presented in **Table 12.13**.

CLINICAL SCENARIO FOR ESSAY QUESTIONS

Acute Lymphoblastic Leukemia

History strongly indicative of acute lymphoblastic leukemia (ALL): Child (**1–6 years** of age)/adult (30–40 years) presenting with **rapid onset** (few weeks) of **pallor, fatigue, bleeding, fever, and infection**. Presence of **lymphadenopathy**, hepato- or splenomegaly, CNS disease, testicular enlargement.

Laboratory findings of marked raised WBC count, presence of **more than 20% lymphoblasts in the blood and bone marrow, blasts + with PAS** (block positivity), and TdT + are features of **acute lymphoblastic leukemia.**

Case 1

History: A **6-year-old** boy presents with fatigue, **bone pain, weakness,** and a low-grade fever of 1-week duration. Physical examination shows anemia, **sternal bone tenderness, and lymphadenopathy.**

Case 2

History: A **5-year-old** boy complains of sudden onset of fever, tiredness, and pallor. On examination, there are many **enlarged cervical lymph nodes**, hepatosplenomegaly, **bone tenderness, and petechial hemorrhages** on the skin.

Case 3

History: A **4-year-old** boy is becoming increasingly lethargic for the past 1 month. On examination, he has fever, **ecchymoses** on the skin of his lower legs and shoulder, generalized lymphadenopathy, and tenderness on palpation of long bones.

Laboratory findings of cases 1 to 3: Hb 8 g/dL, hematocrit 24%, **WBC 18,200 cells/cu mm,** and **platelet count of 90,000/cu mm**. Serum LDH is markedly increased. **The peripheral blood smear** shows **abnormal cells,** which are **PAS-positive.** A **bone marrow** examination shows 100% cellularity with **replacement by primitive cells.** These abnormal primitive cells have scanty cytoplasm and large nuclei with indistinct nucleoli.

Following a blood smear examination, the child is admitted to the medical oncology ward.

Acute Myeloblastic Leukemia

History strongly indicative acute myeloblastic leukemia (AML): Adult presenting with **rapid onset** (few weeks) of **pallor, fatigue, bleeding, fever, and infection.**

Laboratory findings of marked raised WBC count, presence of **more than 20% myeloblasts in the blood and bone marrow, presence of Auer rods** (not seen in all subtypes), **blasts + with MPO and Sudan Black B** are features of **acute myeloblastic leukemia.**

Case 4

History: A **45-year-old** man presents with **fatigue, episodes of epistaxis, bleeding from gums,** and low-grade fever of 1-week duration. Physical examination reveals a temperature of 37.4°C and **hepatosplenomegaly.**

Laboratory findings of very high WBC count with **myeloid precursors, neutrophils, and myelocyte peak, low LAP, and presence of Ph chromosome are diagnostic of chronic myelogenous leukemia.**

Chronic Myelogenous Leukemia

History strongly indicative of chronic myelogenous leukemia (CML): Patient in **fifth and sixth decades of life** presenting with gradual development of **fatigue, weakness, weight loss, anorexia** and fullness of abdomen, early satiety and left upper quadrant pain or mass (due to **splenomegaly**).

Laboratory findings: Hb 7 g/dL, **WBC count 51,000/cu mm,** and **platelet count 80,000/cu mm. The peripheral blood smear** shows abnormal large cells with **Auer rods.**

Case 5

History: A **50-year-old** male comes to the hospital with complaints of generalized weakness, weight loss, easy fatigability, **abdominal discomfort, and dragging sensation in the left hypochondrium** for the last 8 months. On examination, he is pale and has marked **splenomegaly.**

Laboratory findings: Hb 11.9 g/dL, hematocrit 36%, **WBC count 1,20,000/cu mm**, platelet count 4,12,000/cu mm. Peripheral smear examination shows a characteristic blood picture **with myeloid precursors, neutrophils, and myelocyte peak** confirming the clinical diagnosis. **The leukocyte alkaline phosphatase (LAP) score is low**. Chromosomal analysis shows t(9:22) positivity. He is admitted to the oncology department for treatment.

SCENARIO-BASED MCQs

1. **A 40-year-old woman has a cough and fever for the last 1 week. On physical examination, she is febrile and has diffuse crackles heard in all lung fields on auscultation. A chest radiograph shows bilateral extensive infiltrates. CBC shows hemoglobin, 14.1 g/dL; hematocrit, 43%; MCV, 89 fL; platelet count, 240,000/cu mm; and WBC count, 56,000/cu mm. Differential count shows 62% segmented neutrophils, 15% bands, 8% metamyelocytes, 4% myelocytes, 1% blasts, 8% lymphocytes, and 2% monocytes. A bone marrow aspiration shows normal maturation of myeloid cells. The most probable diagnosis is:**
   A. Acute myeloid leukemia
   B. Leukemoid reaction
   C. Chronic myelogenous leukemia
   D. Chronic lymphocytic leukemia
2. **A 10-year-old boy complains of discomfort in the chest for the past 5 days. On physical examination, he has generalized lymphadenopathy. A chest radiograph shows is widening of the mediastinum and all lung fields are clear. A chest CT scan shows a 9 cm mass in the anterior mediastinum. A biopsy is performed on the mediastinal mass. Microscopic examination shows loss of architecture and contains lymphoid cells with lobulated nuclei having delicate, finely stippled, nuclear chromatin. They have scant cytoplasm, and many mitotic figures are seen. The oncologist advises the parents that chemotherapy can be curative in most of such cases. The most likely diagnosis is:**
   A. Burkitt lymphoma
   B. Hodgkin lymphoma
   C. Follicular lymphoma
   D. Lymphoblastic lymphoma
3. **A 60-year-old man comes with complaints of increasing fatigue for the past 6 months. On physical examination, shows nontender axillary and cervical lymphadenopathy, without any hepatosplenomegaly. The CBC shows hemoglobin, 9.6 g/dL; hematocrit, 29%; MCV, 90 fL; platelet count, 115,000/cu mm; and WBC count, 35,000/cu mm. His peripheral blood smear shows a monotonous population of small, round, mature-looking lymphocytes forming more than 80% of WBCs with smudge cells. The most likely diagnosis is:**
   A. Chronic myeloid leukemia
   B. Chronic lymphocytic leukemia
   C. Leukemoid reaction
   D. Acute lymphoblastic leukemia
4. **A 4-year-old boy presents with fatigue, weakness, and bone pain. Two days back he developed large ecchymoses on the thigh and shoulder. CBC shows hemoglobin, 9.1 g/dL; hematocrit, 28.0%; MCV, 96 cu mm; platelet count, 45,000/cu mm; and WBC count, 14,100/cu mm. The peripheral blood smear shows blasts. These blasts are negative for myeloperoxidase but show block PAS-positivity. The most likely diagnosis is:**
   A. Acute myeloid leukemia
   B. Acute lymphoblastic leukemia
   C. Chronic lymphocytic leukemia
   D. Chronic myelogenous leukemia
5. **A 68-year-old man complains of an increasing number and size of lumps over his body in the past 6 months. On examination, there is firm, nontender inguinal, axillary, and cervical lymphadenopathy. A biopsy of a cervical node shows nodular aggregates of small, cleaved lymphoid cells and larger cells with open nuclear chromatin, several nucleoli, and moderate amounts of cytoplasm. Karyotyping of these lymphoid cells shows the presence of t(14;18). The most probable diagnosis is:**
   A. Follicular lymphoma
   B. Large cell lymphoma
   C. Tuberculous lymphadenitis
   D. Hodgkin lymphoma, nodular sclerosis type
6. **An 11-year-old boy was brought to the hospital for increasing abdominal distention and pain for the past 3 days. Physical examination of the abdomen shows lower abdominal tenderness and reduced bowel sounds. An abdominal CT scan shows a mass in the region of the ileocecal valve which measures 7 cm in diameter. Surgery was performed and the mass was removed. Microscopically, the resected mass shows sheets of intermediate-sized lymphoid cells. They have nuclei with coarse chromatin, several nucleoli, and many mitotic figures. Many macrophages containing nuclear and cytoplasmic debris are also seen. Cytogenetic analysis of the tumor cells shows a t(8;14) karyotype. The most probable diagnosis is:**
   A. Burkitt lymphoma
   B. Follicular lymphoma
   C. Diffuse large B-cell lymphoma
   D. Acute lymphoblastic leukemia/lymphoma
7. **An 8-year-old boy from Africa came for pain and swelling on the left side of his face over the past 8 months. Physical examination shows a large, nontender mass involving the mandible, and deforms the left side of his face. There is no lymphadenopathy or splenomegaly, and he is afebrile. Microscopic examination of the biopsy of the mass shows intermediate-sized lymphocytes with a high mitotic rate. A chromosome analysis shows a 46,XY, t(8;14) karyotype in these cells. The hemoglobin concentration is 12.8 g/dL, the platelet count is 264,000/cu mm and the WBC count is 6,200/cu mm. Of the following viruses, the most likely causally related to the development of lesions In the jaw is:**
   A. HIV B. Cytomegalovirus
   C. Epstein-Barr virus D. Human papillomavirus
8. **A 65-year-old woman complains of increasing back pain for 1 month. On physical examination, there is tenderness over the lower back without any kyphosis or scoliosis. A radiograph of the skull shows multiple 0.5- to 1.5-cm lytic lesions with a rounded soap bubble appearance. A bone**

marrow aspiration shows hypercellularity with more than 30% mature and immature plasma cells. These showed a perinuclear hof (clearing). The laboratory findings that are most likely to be seen in this patient are:

A. Hypogammaglobulinemia
B. WBC count of 3,94,000/cu mm
C. Bence-Jones proteins in the urine
D. Decreased serum alkaline phosphatase level

9. **A 26-year-old man has lumps in his neck that have been enlarging for the past 6 months. Physical examination shows a group of enlarged, nontender right cervical lymph nodes. A biopsy of one of the lymph nodes is performed. Microscopically, it shows macrophages, lymphocytes, neutrophils, eosinophils, and a few plasma cells. The lesion shows large cells with multiple nuclei or a single nucleus with multiple nuclear lobes scattered. They have a large inclusion-like nucleolus in the lesion. These cells are CD15+ and CD30+. The most likely cell of origin with infectious agent for these large cells is:**

A. B lymphocyte, Epstein-Barr virus
B. CD4+ cell, human T lymphotropic virus
C. Macrophage, human immunodeficiency virus
D. Endothelial cell, Kaposi sarcoma herpesvirus

10. **A 34-year-old woman presents with generalized fatigue and night sweats for the past 3 months. Physical examination reveals nontender right cervical lymphadenopathy. A biopsy of one lymph node is performed. Microscopic examination shows a pattern of thick bands of fibrous connective tissue separating nodules of varying sizes. The nodules consist of lymphocytes, plasma cells, eosinophils, macrophages, and occasional large multinucleated Reed-Sternberg (RS) cells. These RS cells had vacuolated cytoplasm with prominent nucleoli. The most likely subtype of this patient's disease is:**

A. Lymphocyte rich B. Mixed cellularity
C. Nodular sclerosis D. Lymphocyte depletion

11. **A 74-year-old man complains of recurrent fevers and a 7-kg loss of weight over the past 6 months. Physical examination shows splenomegaly. An abdominal CT scan shows an enlargement of the mesenteric lymph node. A lymph node biopsy is performed. It shows effacement of the nodal architecture and small lymphocytes, plasma cells, eosinophils, and macrophages. The additional cell types that stain positively for CD15 and CD30 are most likely to be found in this disease are:**

A. Mast cell B. Myeloblast
C. Epithelioid cell D. Reed-Sternberg cell

12. **A 31-year-old man complains of multiple nosebleeds and bleeding gums for the past 1 month. On examination, he has multiple ecchymoses in the skin. Laboratory studies show hemoglobin, 8.2 g/dL; hematocrit, 25.2%; platelet count, 13,000/cu mm; and WBC count, 52,100/cu mm. Differential count shows 5% segmented neutrophils, 5% bands, 2% myelocytes, 82% blasts, 4% lymphocytes, and 2% monocytes. Peripheral smear shows the blasts with delicate nuclear chromatin and with fine azurophilic granules in the cytoplasm. These blasts are myeloperoxidase and Sudan black positive. The morphologic findings that are most probably present on his peripheral blood smear are:**

A. Sickle cells B. Auer rods
C. Heinz bodies D. Toxic granulations

13. **A 47-year-old man comes with complaints of gradual weight loss and weakness, anorexia, easy fatigability, and dragging pain in the left hypochondrium for 7 months. On physical examination, marked splenomegaly is detected. CBC shows hemoglobin, 12.9 g/dL; hematocrit, 37.8%; MCV, 92 fL; platelet count, 4,10,000/cu mm; and WBC count, 1,68,000/cu mm. The peripheral blood smear shows granulocytes at all stages of development (neutrophils, metamyelocytes, myelocytes, promyelocytes, and occasional myeloblasts) and basophils. LAP score is decreased. Karyotypic analysis shows the Ph1 chromosome. The most likely diagnosis is:**

A. Acute myeloid leukemia
B. Acute lymphoblastic leukemia
C. Chronic lymphocytic leukemia
D. Chronic myelogenous leukemia

Answers and Explanation

1. **The answer is B: Leukemoid reaction.** Marked leukocytosis and immature myeloid cells in the peripheral blood can occur as an exaggerated response to infection (leukemoid reaction) or in chronic myelogenous leukemia (CML). Bone marrow aspirate showing normal maturation of myeloid cells rules out CML. A leukocyte alkaline phosphatase (LAP) score is high in the more differentiated cell population of reactive leukocytosis, whereas in CML, the LAP score is low. The Philadelphia chromosome is present in most patients with CML and is absent in leukemoid reactions. The blast count of 1% rules out acute myeloid leukemia in which the blasts are more than 20%. Chronic lymphocytic leukemia shows lymphocytosis with smudge cells.
2. **The answer is D: Lymphoblastic lymphoma.** The age and the mediastinal location of the mass are classical of a lymphoblastic lymphoma involving the thymus. This lesion is within the spectrum of acute lymphoblastic leukemia or lymphoma (ALL). Burkitt lymphoma is a B-cell lymphoma that also occurs in adolescents, but usually is present in the jaw or abdomen. Hodgkin lymphoma does occur in the mediastinum, but it involves mediastinal nodes, not the thymus. The microscopic feature of Hodgkin lymphoma includes the presence of Reed-Sternberg cells. Follicular lymphomas are B-cell tumors usually seen in older patients, and they do not involve the thymus.
3. **The answer is B: Chronic lymphocytic leukemia.** The clinical history and the peripheral blood smear are characteristic of chronic lymphocytic leukemia (CLL). CLL is a clonal B-cell neoplasm. The tissue component of CLL is small lymphocytic lymphoma (SLL). The clinical features and peripheral smear findings do not fit all other options.
4. **The answer is B: Acute lymphoblastic leukemia.** The clinical and blood findings are characteristic of childhood acute lymphoblastic leukemia. The proliferation of blasts causes the rapid expansion of the marrow and can lead to bone pain and tenderness. Laboratory features supporting the diagnosis of acute leukemia are anemia, thrombocytopenia, and the presence of blasts in the peripheral blood and bone marrow. Anemia and thrombocytopenia are due to the suppression of normal hematopoiesis by the leukemic cells in the marrow. Acute myeloid leukemia is a disease of young to middle-aged adults, and the myeloblasts will be peroxidase positive. Chronic lymphocytic leukemia is a disease of older adults, and peripheral blood shows many small circulating mature lymphocytes.

Chronic myelogenous leukemia is a disease of adults, and the WBC count is severely increased.

5. **The answer is A: Follicular lymphoma.** It is the most common type of non-Hodgkin lymphoma among adults. It equally affects both men and women. The neoplastic B cells mimic a follicular center cell and produce a nodular or follicular pattern. The t(14;18) translocation is characteristic and overexpresses the BCL2 gene. These cells are resistant to apoptosis. The tuberculous lymphadenitis shows characteristic granulomas. In large-cell lymphoma, the lymphoid cells are large and non-cleaved. In Hodgkin lymphoma, few Reed-Sternberg cells, are surrounded by a reactive lymphoid cell.
6. **The answer is A: Burkitt lymphoma.** It can occur as sporadic (in young individuals), endemic form in Africa (in children), and in association with HIV infection. All are associated with translocations of the MYC gene on chromosome 8. The tumor cells in African form and HIV-infected patients are latently infected with Epstein-Barr virus (EBV), but sporadic cases are negative for EBV. Diffuse large-cell lymphomas and follicular lymphomas are most common in adults. Both do not have the t(8;14) translocation. Acute lymphoblastic lymphomas can occur in boys this age, but the mass is in the mediastinum.
7. **The answer is C: Epstein-Barr virus.** The endemic African type of Burkitt lymphoma is a B-cell lymphoma that usually occurs in the maxilla or mandible of the jaw. It is related to Epstein-Barr virus infection. HIV infection can be a risk factor for non-Hodgkin lymphomas, but most of these are either diffuse large B-cell lymphomas or small noncleaved Burkitt-like lymphomas. Cytomegalovirus infection usually occurs in immunocompromised patients and can be a congenital infection. It is not a direct cause of neoplasia. Human papillomavirus infection leads to squamous dysplasias and carcinomas, most commonly in the cervix.
8. **The answer is C: Bence Jones proteins in the urine.** The characteristic punched-out bone lesions of multiple myeloma seen on radiographs are caused by to destruction of bone. Myeloma produces hypergammaglobulinemia and not hypogammaglobulinemia. Myeloma is not accompanied by increased leukocyte count (leukocytosis). Patients with bone destruction and remodeling can have hypercalcemia and an increased serum alkaline phosphatase level.
9. **The answer is A: B lymphocyte, Epstein-Barr virus.** The large cells seen on microscopy are Reed-Sternberg cells. Reed-Sternberg cells are of B-cell origin, and in many cases, it accompanies Epstein-Barr virus (EBV) infection. The other listed options are not part of the pathogenesis for Hodgkin lymphoma.
10. **The answer is C: Nodular sclerosis.** The bands of fibrosis and vacuolated RS cells namely lacunar cells are seen in the nodular sclerosis type of Hodgkin lymphoma. The findings do not fit with the other forms of Hodgkin lymphoma.
11. **The answer is D: Reed-Sternberg cell.** The features suggest Hodgkin lymphoma (HL), a mixed cellularity type. It often affects older men. The Reed-Sternberg cells and variants stain with CD15. These cells also express CD30. In HL, Reed-Sternberg cells form a relatively small percentage of the tumor mass. Most of the cell population consists of reactive cells such as lymphocytes, plasma cells, macrophages, and eosinophils. Mast cells are not numerous in HL and they are seen in type I hypersensitivity reactions. Myeloblasts are numerous in acute myelogenous leukemia. Epithelioid cells are seen in granulomatous inflammatory reactions.
12. **The answer is B: Auer rods.** In acute myelogenous leukemia (AML), myeloblasts infiltrate the marrow and reduce normal hematopoiesis. This is responsible for anemia and marked thrombocytopenia. The Auer rods are condensations of the azurophilic granules that can be seen in myeloblast. Sickling of RBCs is seen in sickle cell anemia, which is not related to leukemia. Heinz bodies are seen in G6PD deficiency and are precipitates of denatured globin. Toxic granules are seen in neutrophils in infections.
13. **The answer is D: Chronic myelogenous leukemia.** This is a classic history of chronic myelogenous leukemia (CML). The peripheral smear shows different stages of myeloid differentiation and the Philadelphia chromosome confirms the diagnosis. Acute myeloid leukemia (choice A) and acute lymphoblastic leukemia (choice B) are clonal expansion of myeloblasts, and lymphoblasts respectively. Features do not fit for the diagnosis of chronic lymphocytic leukemia.

Lymphoblast staining positively with PAS and (TdT)

Myeloblast stains positively with Sudan black B, myeloperoxidase (MPO) and Nonspecific esterase (NSE).

According to WHO classification: Blasts should be >20% in bone marrow for diagnosis of acute leukemia.

Aleukemic leukemia: Diagnosed by the presence of >20% blasts in the bone marrow.

Biophenotypic acute leukemia: Acute leukemia with a single blast cells population showing markers of two different lineage.

Bilinear acute leukemia is acute leukemia with two different blast cells population.

Alkaline phosphatase is specific for neutrophils and is called as NAP/LAP

LAP score is increased in leukemoid reaction.

Hodgkin lymphoma:
- Characteristically shows Reed-Sternberg (RS) cells.
- Painless lymphadenopathy
- Pel Ebstein fever.

Multiple myeloma is a plasma cell neoplasm. It secretes excessive amount of immunoglobulin, and light chains.

Most important prognostic factor of multiple myeloma: Serum β2-microglobulin.

Bleeding Disorders: Hemorrhagic Diathesis

CHAPTER OUTLINE

- Normal Hemostasis
- Bleeding Disorders
- Bleeding Disorders Caused by Vessel Wall Abnormalities
- Bleeding Disorders Due to Reduced Number of Platelets: Thrombocytopenia
- Coagulation Disorders
- Disseminated Intravascular Coagulation

NORMAL HEMOSTASIS

PA 21.1 (CC): Describe normal hemostasis.

- Hemostasis is the **body's response to vascular damage/ injury** (for details *refer* pages 145-7 and **Fig. 5.14**).
- Includes several sequences of events at the site of vascular injury. They are as follows:
  - **Primary hemostatic plug: Platelet adheres** to subendothelial structures at the site of injury. The **platelets change their shape** and **release granule contents.** The released contents cause platelet **aggregation and form a primary hemostatic plug.**
  - **Secondary hemostatic plug: Exposure of tissue factor** at the site of vascular injury **activates the extrinsic coagulation system. The fibrin formed develops into a secondary hemostatic plug.**

BLEEDING DISORDERS

Q. Define bleeding disorders.

Bleeding disorders (hemorrhagic disorders/hemorrhagic diathesis) are characterized clinically by an **abnormal tendency to bleed (hemorrhage) due to failure of hemostasis**. Bleeding may appear spontaneously or follow an inciting event (e.g., trauma or surgery).

Terminologies Used in Bleeding Disorders

Petechiae (Fig. 13.1A): They are **small (1-2 mm in diameter), red to purple hemorrhagic spots** in the skin, mucous membranes (e.g., conjunctiva), or serosal surfaces. They result from blood leaking through the intact endothelial lining of capillaries. Petechiae are pinpoint hemorrhages seen most **commonly found with low platelet counts (thrombocytopenia) or defective platelet function** or loss of vascular wall support (e.g., vitamin C deficiency).

Q. Define purpura.

Purpura (Fig. 13.1B): The term purpura means purple. They are **slightly larger (>3 mm) than petechiae**, but <1 cm in diameter. Palpable purpura suggests vasculitis (e.g., Henoch-Schönlein purpura). The causes are **thrombocytopenia, increased vascular fragility, and vasculitis** (inflammation of vessels). **Purpura may be classified as nonthrombocytopenic (vascular)** purpura **(Box 13.2)** and **thrombocytopenic (Box 13.3)**.

Ecchymoses/bruises: They are larger (1-2 cm) and result from **blood escaping through the endothelium into intact subcutaneous tissue.** They result from trauma or hemostatic disorder and usually **do not produce significant swelling as in hematoma**. Extravasated RBCs in the lesions are phagocytosed and degraded by macrophages and release the hemoglobin which gives rise to red-blue color. The pigment from heme is converted into biliverdin and then to bilirubin (blue-green color) and iron from red cells forms hemosiderin (golden-brown color). These changes are responsible for the characteristic color changes in ecchymoses. A good example of an ecchymosis is a "black eye (*refer* **Table 5.3**)."

Hematoma: It is **swelling formed when blood leaks from a vessel and collects within a tissue**. The swelling results from a large area of hemorrhage in subcutaneous tissue or muscle. It is blue or purple and slightly raised.

Classification of Bleeding Disorders

Q. Classify bleeding disorders.

Bleeding disorders may be due to: diseases of blood vessels, platelet disorders, and coagulation disorders **(Box 13.1)**. They may occur alone or in combination.

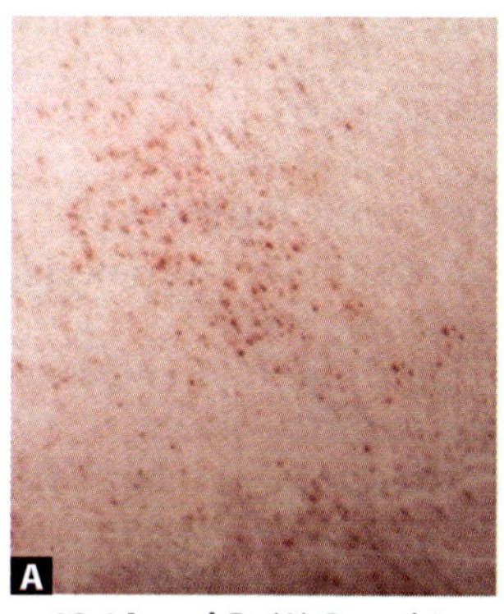
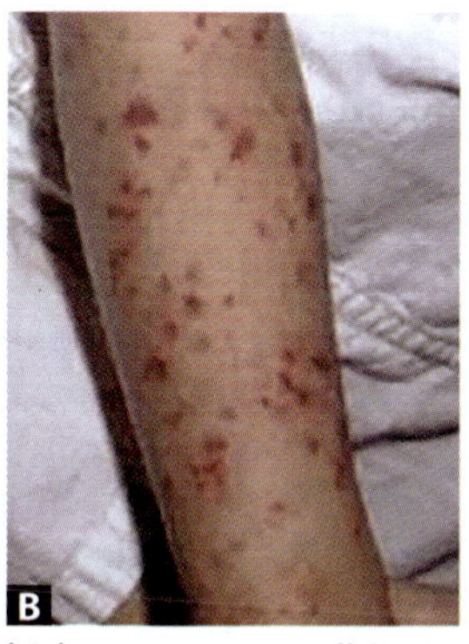

Figs. 13.1A and B: (A) Petechiae which appear as small (1–2 mm in diameter), red to purple hemorrhagic spots in the skin, mucous membranes or serosal surfaces; (B) Purpura—slightly larger (>3 mm) than petechiae.

BOX 13.1: Broad classification of bleeding disorders.

Bleeding disorders

1. **Vessel wall abnormalities (Box 13.2)**
2. **Platelet abnormalities (Box 13.3)**
3. **Defects in the coagulation system (Box 13.4)**

BOX 13.2: Classification of bleeding disorders caused by vessel wall abnormalities (nonthrombocytopenic purpura).

Acquired disorders

1. Due to a decreased amount of connective tissue
   - Senile purpura
   - Scurvy
   - Cushing syndrome and steroid therapy (glucocorticoid excess)
2. Due to vasculitis
   - Henoch–Schönlein purpura: Characterized by hypersensitivity vasculitis and palpable purpura
   - Infections: Meningococcemia, other forms of septicemia, infective endocarditis, and several of the rickettsioses.
   - Drug reactions
3. Associated with plasma cell neoplasms
   - Amyloidosis
4. Miscellaneous
   - Simple easy bruising

Congenital/inherited disorders

- Hereditary hemorrhagic telangiectasia
- Ehlers–Danlos syndrome
- Marfan syndrome

BLEEDING DISORDERS CAUSED BY VESSEL WALL ABNORMALITIES

PA 21.2a (CC): Classify and describe the etiology, pathogenesis, and pathology of vascular bleeding disorders.

Vascular purpura (**nonthrombocytopenic purpura**) is a group of **disorders of blood vessels** that result in **bleeding.** They should be distinguished from bleeding disorders due to abnormalities of platelets. **Classification of bleeding disorders caused by vessel wall abnormalities** is presented in **Box 13.2.** Bleeding may be due to *vascular fragility* and occur with vitamin C deficiency (scurvy), amyloidosis affecting blood vessels, chronic use of glucocorticoid, rare inherited disorders of the connective tissues, and a large number of infectious and hypersensitivity vasculitides. Bleeding purely due to vascular fragility is characterized by the "spontaneous" appearance of petechiae, purpura, and ecchymoses in the skin and mucous membranes (particularly the gingivae). This may result from minor trauma. In most cases, platelet count, and laboratory tests of coagulation (PT, PTT) are normal. A few are discussed below:

- **Senile purpura**: It is due to an age-related atrophy of supporting connective tissues. Senile purpura is associated with superficial, sharply demarcated, purpuric spots (purple or red bruises in light skin). They develop on the forearms and other sun-exposed areas.
- **Scurvy**: Deficiency of vitamin C causes scurvy. It impairs collagen synthesis and leads to purpura. It is characterized by perifollicular hemorrhages.
- **Henoch–Schönlein purpura**: It is an allergic vascular disease that results from immunologic damage to blood vessel walls. In children, this purpura usually follows viral infections and is self-limited. In adults, it is caused by exposure to various drugs and may be chronic. Henoch–Schönlein purpura is characterized by leukocytoclastic vasculitis, with perivascular infiltration of neutrophils and eosinophils. It shows fibrinoid necrosis of vessel walls, and platelet plugs within the vascular lumens.

BLEEDING DISORDERS DUE TO REDUCED NUMBER OF PLATELETS: THROMBOCYTOPENIA

PA 21.2b (CC): Classify and describe the etiology, pathogenesis, and pathology of platelet disorders.

Thrombocytopenia

Definition: Thrombocytopenia is defined as a **decrease in the platelet count below** the lower limit of **150,000/cu mm** (150 × 10^9/L).

Deficiencies of platelets (thrombocytopenia) are an important cause of bleeding. The bleeding disorder may also occur due to qualitative defects in platelet function.

Clinical features of thrombocytopenia: These include (i) cutaneous bleeding appears as **pinpoint hemorrhages (petechiae) and ecchymoses**, (ii) **mucosal bleeding** (bleeding from gastrointestinal tract particularly gingival

BOX 13.3: Causes of thrombocytopenia.

1. **Decreased production of platelets**
   - Generalized bone marrow dysfunction
     - Aplastic anemia: Congenital and acquired
     - Bone marrow infiltration: Leukemia, disseminated cancer, granulomatous disease
   - Selective impairment of platelet production
     - Drug-induced: Alcohol, thiazides, cytotoxic drugs
     - Infections: Measles, human immunodeficiency virus (HIV) infection
   - Ineffective megakaryopoiesis
     - Megaloblastic anemia due to vitamin B_{12}, and folic acid deficiency
2. **Increased platelet destruction (decreased platelet survival)**
   - Immunological destruction
     - Autoimmune: Immune thrombocytopenic purpura (ITP), systemic lupus erythematosus
     - Alloimmune: Post-transfusion or pregnancy or neonatal
     - Drug-induced: Quinidine, heparin, sulfa compounds
     - Infections: HIV infection, infectious mononucleosis, dengue fever, cytomegalovirus infection
   - Nonimmunological destruction
     - Disseminated intravascular coagulation (DIC)
     - Thrombotic thrombocytopenic purpura (TTP)
     - Hemolytic uremic syndrome (HUS)
     - Microangioathic hemolytic anemias
3. **Sequestration (abnormal platelet distribution, or pooling)**
   - Hypersplenism and hypothermia.
4. **Dilutional:** Multiple transfusions (e.g., for massive blood loss)

bleeding; epistaxis; menorrhagia; and bleeding from urinary tracts), and (iii) **intracranial bleed** (subarachnoid and intracerebral hemorrhage) rare but serious.

Severity of bleeding: It depends on platelet count.

- **Post-traumatic** bleeding occurs when the platelet **count is 20,000–50,000/cu mm**.
- **Spontaneous** bleeding develops when the platelet count falls **below 20,000/cu mm**.
- **Intracranial** bleeding occurs when the platelet count is **<10,000/cu mm.**

Causes of Thrombocytopenia (Box 13.3)

Q. Write a short note on the causes of thrombocytopenia.

Immune Thrombocytopenic Purpura

PA 21.2c (CC): Describe the etiology, pathogenesis, and pathology of ITP.

Q. Describe the etiology, pathogenesis, clinical features, and laboratory findings/hematological features of immune/idiopathic thrombocytopenic purpura.

Immune thrombocytopenic purpura (ITP) is the **most common form of thrombocytopenia.**

Subtypes

ITP includes two clinical subtypes.

Acute Immune Thrombocytopenic Purpura

- It is a **self-limited** disease. **Sudden onset with petechiae, gum bleeding, epistaxis,** and mild fever.
- **Age and gender:** It occurs mostly **in children between 2–4 years of age.** It affects both sexes equally.
- Presents **1–3 weeks after viral** (measles, rubella, EBV) **infection.** It is likely to be caused by virus-induced changes in platelet antigens that elicit autoantibodies. Complement bound at the surface of these antibody-coated platelets lyse them in the blood or mediate their phagocytosis and are destroyed by splenic and hepatic macrophage.
- **Platelet count is decreased**, sometimes even below 10,000/cu mm (10×10^9/L).
- Recovery within 6 months in 80% of cases.

Chronic Immune Thrombocytopenic Purpura

- Chronic ITP is relatively common.
- **Age and gender**: It occurs between the ages of 20 and 40 years. Most often affects women (F: M = 3:1).

Pathogenesis of chronic ITP (Fig. 13.2)

Autoimmune disorder: Chronic ITP is an autoimmune disorder (type II hypersensitivity reaction). It is characterized by the formation of **antiplatelet antibodies**, directed **against platelet membrane glycoproteins IIb/IIIa or Ib/IX complexes.** These antiplatelet antibodies are found in about 80% of patients with chronic ITP. They are of the **IgG type.** These IgG antiplatelet antibodies act as opsonins and coat the platelets.

Importance of spleen: It is the **important site of production antiplatelet antibodies**. It is also the **major site of destruction of the IgG-coated platelets** thereby resulting in thrombocytopenia. Splenomegaly is not a feature of uncomplicated chronic ITP. However, splenectomy normalizes the platelet count and induces complete remission of ITP in more than two-thirds of patients.

Clinical features of chronic ITP

- **Insidious onset**: The onset of chronic ITP is insidious.
- **Presentation**: These include petechiae, easy bruising, **mucosal bleeding,** epistaxis, gum bleeding, **menorrhagia** in females, and hemorrhage after minor trauma. Splenomegaly and lymphadenopathy are uncommon and, in their presence, one should consider a diagnosis other than ITP.
- It is usually treated by immunosuppressive agents and, in some cases, splenectomy.

Laboratory Findings in ITP

Q. Write a short note on laboratory findings in ITP.

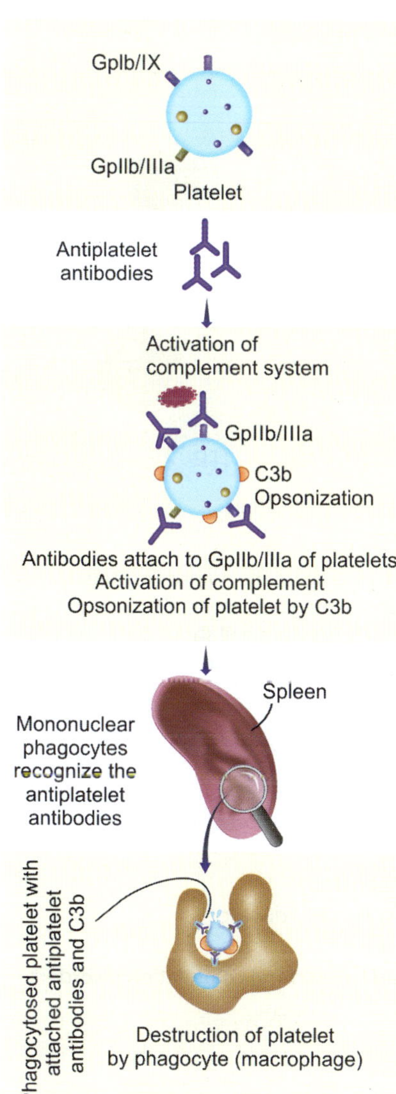

Fig. 13.2: Pathogenesis of chronic immune thrombocytopenic purpura. It is a type II hypersensitivity reaction characterized by complement-dependent opsonization and phagocytosis. The antibody (usually IgG type) binds to antigens on the platelets (most often IIb/IIIa or Ib/IX of platelets). Activation of complements produces opsonin C3b. Opsonization of platelets by antibodies and complement leads to the ingestion of platelets by phagocytes in the spleen. This results in the destruction of platelets.

Peripheral Blood

- **Platelet count: Markedly reduced** below 80,000/cu mm (80×10^9/L).
- **Hemoglobin:** Ranges from 7–12 g/dL.

PERIPHERAL SMEAR

- **Platelets: Markedly reduced** (thrombocytopenia). It shows many **abnormally large-sized platelets (megathrombocytes/ giant platelets)** owing to the rapid release of young platelets by bone marrow actively engaged in platelet production.
- **RBCs: Chronic blood loss** (e.g., menorrhagia) due to ITP may **lead to microcytic hypochromic anemia.**
- **WBCs:** Normal

Q. Write a short note on bone marrow changes in ITP.

BONE MARROW

- **Cellularity: Hypercellular**
- **Megakaryopoiesis:**
  - **Moderate increase in number (Figs. 13.3A and B)** of both **immature and mature** forms of **megakaryocytes.** Decreased megakaryocytes—against the diagnosis of ITP.
  - **Immature megakaryocytes predominate: They have large nonlobulated single nuclei and basophilic less granular cytoplasm.**
- **Erythropoiesis:**
  - **Prolonged bleeding** may cause anemia leading to **normoblastic erythroid hyperplasia.**
  - Constant bleeding leads to **iron deficiency** and **micronormoblastic erythroid hyperplasia.**
- **Myelopoiesis:** Normal.
- **Storage iron:** Severe and chronic bleeding causes iron deficiency with reduced iron stores.

Bleeding time (BT): Prolonged, but prothrombin time (PT) and partial thromboplastin time (PTT) are normal.

- **Tourniquet test: Positive.**
- **Clotting time (CT): Normal.**
- **PT and APTT normal.**
- **Tests for platelet autoantibodies: Platelets carry detectable IgG in more than 80% of patients with chronic ITP.**
- **Spleen:** Normal size.

Qualitative Platelet Disorders

Q. Write a short note on qualitative/functional disorders of platelets.

Classification of platelet functional (qualitative) disorders is presented in **Figure 13.4** and **Box 13.4**.

COAGULATION DISORDERS

Coagulation disorders may be due to congenital or acquired deficiencies of clotting factors. It may be a quantitative or qualitative disorder of the coagulation factors. Acquired deficiencies are most common and usually involve several factors simultaneously. For example, vitamin K is required for the synthesis of prothrombin and clotting factors VII, IX, and X. Therefore, vitamin K deficiency causes a severe coagulation defect. The liver is involved in the synthesis of several coagulation factors and the removal of activated coagulation factors from the circulation. Thus, diseases of liver parenchyma are common causes of complex hemorrhagic diatheses. Classification of coagulation disorders is discussed in **Box 13.5**.

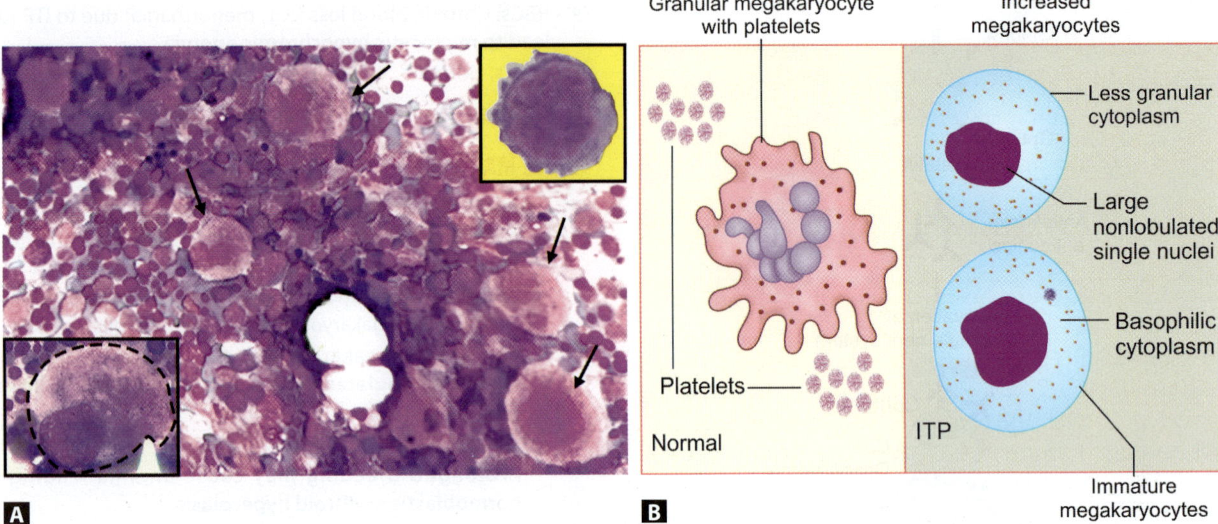

Figs. 13.3A and B: Bone marrow aspirate in ITP: (A) Leishman stain shows a moderate increase in the number of megakaryocytes (arrows), left lower inset shows a hypolobated megakaryocyte, right upper inset shows a normal megakaryocyte; (B) Diagrammatic appearance. The left half shows a normal megakaryocyte having a single nucleus with multiple lobes. The right half shows bone marrow in ITP. It shows an increased number of immature megakaryocytes. They have basophilic, less granular cytoplasm and large nonlobated single nuclei.

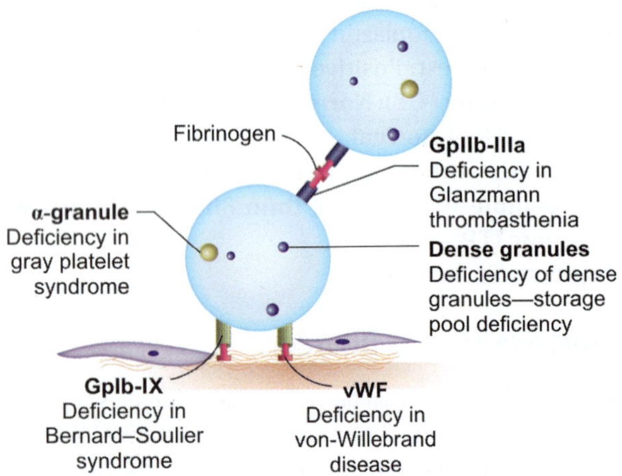

Fig. 13.4: Functional disorders of platelet.

BOX 13.4: Classification of platelet functional (qualitative) disorders.

A. Hereditary
1. ***Disorders of platelet adhesion:*** Bernard–Soulier syndrome
2. ***Disorders of platelet secretion:*** Storage pool deficiency
3. ***Disorders of platelet aggregation:*** Glanzmann thrombasthenia

B. Acquired
1. ***Drugs:*** Aspirin, nonsteroidal anti-inflammatory drugs (NSAIDs), dipyridamole, sulfinpyrazone
2. ***Renal failure:*** Uremia
3. ***Hematologic malignancies:*** Myeloproliferative neoplasms and myelodysplastic syndromes

BOX 13.5: Classification of coagulation disorders.

A. Hereditary coagulation disorders
1. Hemophilia A
2. Hemophilia B
3. von Willebrand disease
4. Others

B. Acquired (secondary) coagulation disorders
1. Vitamin K deficiency
2. Liver disease
3. Others

Hereditary Coagulation Disorders

Hereditary deficiencies are usually, due to a deficiency of a single coagulation factor. Hemophilia A (a deficiency of factor VIII) and hemophilia B (Christmas disease, a deficiency of factor IX) are X-linked diseases. Hereditary deficiencies of other factors are transmitted as autosomal recessive disorders. Three inherited deficiencies namely von Willebrand disease, hemophilia A, and hemophilia B are discussed below.

Deficiencies of Factor VIII–von Willebrand Factor Complex

Hemophilia A and von Willebrand disease are caused by qualitative or quantitative defects involving the factor VIII–vWF complex. As background for subsequent discussion of these disorders, it is useful to review the structure and function of these two proteins.

Factor VIII–vWF Complex

Factor VIII–vWF complex has two components: Plasma **factor VIII and von Willebrand factor (vWF). vWF protects factor VIII** and is important for its stability. Most factor VIII is synthesized in the liver, and the major source of plasma vWF is endothelial cells.

Various sites of vWF: It is found in the following sites:
- In the plasma (associated with factor VIII)
- In platelet granules
- In endothelial cells (within vesicles called Weibel-Palade bodies in the cytoplasm)
- In the subendothelium (binds to collagen).

Functions of vWF: These are as follows:
- **Subendothelial vWF promotes the adhesion of platelets to damaged blood vessel walls:** The subendothelial vWF is exposed whenever there is trauma or injury to endothelial cells. This subendothelial vWF facilitates the adhesion of platelets to damaged blood vessel walls. It is a crucial step in the formation of a hemostatic plug. Inadequate platelet adhesion is responsible for bleeding tendency in von Willebrand disease.
- **Plasma vWF stabilizes factor VIII:** vWF stabilizes factor VIII. Thus, a deficiency of vWF leads to a secondary deficiency of factor VIII.

Hemophilia

PA 21.2d (CC): Classify and describe the etiology, pathogenesis, and pathology of hemophilias.

Q. Write a short note on hemophilia.

Features of hemophilias: These are as follows:
- **Classic hemophilia is two distinct diseases** hemophilia **A (factor VIII deficiency) and B (factor IX deficiency).** They are **similar in both clinical and pathological features,** the **difference** being **in the deficient factor.**
- Both are **sex-linked recessive disorders** resulting in an inherited deficiency of the clotting factor or synthesis of a defective clotting factor.
- Highlight of the disease is its dissemination of hemophilia throughout Europe's royal families by Queen Victoria's daughters.
- **Males are affected** and **females are carriers.**

Hemophilia A (Factor VIII Deficiency)

Q. Write a short essay/note on hemophilia A.
- **Most common hereditary disease that causes serious bleeding.**
- **X-linked recessive disorders** (70% of cases) caused by **reduced factor VIII activity.** About 30% of hemophiliacs may be due to acquired mutations.
- **Reduced amount or activity of factor VIII** is associated with **life-threatening bleeding**
- Bleeding is due to both inadequate coagulation and inappropriate clot removal (fibrinolysis).

Mode of Inheritance (Fig. 13.5)

- **X-linked recessive disease. Genes** for factor VIII are located **on the long arm of the X chromosome.** It does not manifest when there is a normal copy of the X chromosome.
- It **primarily affects males. Males** with a defective/mutant factor VIII gene (*hemophiliac* gene) on their single X chromosome (X_H) **suffer** from hemophilia.
- **Heterozygous females are carriers** and do not express the full clinical disease because of the **paired normal X-chromosome.**
- However, females with two copies of the defective X_H chromosome may rarely suffer from hemophilia.

Molecular genetics: Causative mutations of the factor VIII gene **at the tip of the long arm of the X chromosome (Xq28)** include deletions, inversions, point mutations, and insertions.

Clinical Features

Clinical severity **depends on the level of factor VIII activity with a normal range expressed as a percentage (Table 13.1).** Severe hemophilia A has marked deficiencies of factor VIII (less than 1% residual factor VIII activity). Common clinical presentations include:
- Tendency toward **easy bruising and hemorrhage after trauma or operative procedures.**
- **Hemorrhage into joints and soft tissues:** They present with frequent and **spontaneous hemorrhage into the joints** (hemarthrosis). It may lead to progressive deformities that can be crippling. Also, develop hemorrhage into **soft tissues.**

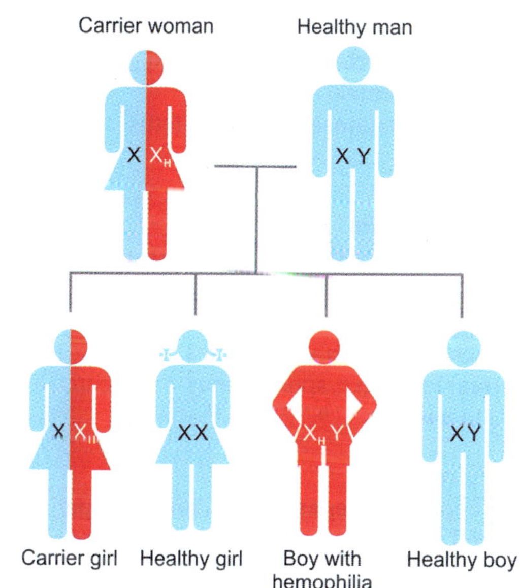

Fig. 13.5: Mode of inheritance in hemophilia.

TABLE 13.1 Factor VIII level and clinical severity in hemophilia A.

Clinical severity	*Level of factor VIII activity in percentage**	*Clinical features*
Mild	>6	In the mildest form, it may be unnoticed. Bleeding develops after trauma only
Moderate	2–5	Bleeding after trauma including dental and other surgical trauma. Easy bruising
Severe	<1	Frequent and spontaneous hemorrhage into joints (hemarthrosis) and soft tissues

*Normal range for factor VIII: 45–158 IU/dL.

- **Prolonged bleeding following trauma:** Hematuria, intestinal obstruction, and respiratory obstruction may occur with bleeding into the respective organs.
- **Petechiae are characteristically absent.**

Laboratory Findings

- **Bleeding time: Normal**
- **Clotting time: Prolonged,** but is not a sensitive test
- **Platelet count: Normal**
- **Prothrombin time: Normal**
- **Prolonged activated partial thromboplastin time (APTT): APTT is prolonged** (normal 30–40 seconds). It is corrected by mixing the patient's plasma with normal plasma (which contains normal factor VIII activity).
- **Factor VIII assay: Essential for the diagnosis** and to assess the levels and severity of disease.
- **Fibrinogen assay:** Normal
- **FDP (fibrin and fibrinogen-degradation products):** Negative
- **Detection of carriers:** By DNA markers.
  - To detect female carriers
  - Prenatal diagnosis of affected fetuses.

Complications

Due to hemophilia

- **Deforming arthritis and contractures:** This is due to repeated bleeding into the joints. Organization and fibrosis of intramuscular hematomas leading to contractures of involved muscles.
- **Anemia:** Excessive, spontaneous, or repeated bleeding leads to anemia.

Due to therapy

- **Viral hepatitis: Hepatitis B, C, and D** in patients who received multiple transfusions of FFP/cryoprecipitate.
- **AIDS:** In individuals who received fresh frozen plasma (FFP) or cryoprecipitate, when screening tests for HIV were not available.
- **Factor VIII inhibitors**: It makes further management difficult.

Causes of death in hemophilia: Intracranial hemorrhage and prolonged bleeding.

Treatment of hemophilia: These include factor VIII concentrate and recombinant factor VIII.

Hemophilia B (Christmas Disease, Factor IX Deficiency)

Q. Write a short note on Christmas disease.

Clinically indistinguishable from hemophilia A, but is much less common. It is an **X-linked recessive** disorder with **variable clinical severity** due to deficiency of factor IX. An assay of factor IX should be done to diagnose Christmas disease (named after the first patient). Usually milder than hemophilia A.

Laboratory Findings

These findings are similar to hemophilia A.

- **Bleeding time:** Normal
- **Clotting time: Prolonged**
- **Platelet count:** Normal
- **Prothrombin time:** Normal
- **Prolonged APTT: Increased** (normal 30–40 seconds)
- **Factor IX assay:** The diagnosis is made using specific assays of factor IX that are **decreased.**

von Willebrand Disease (vWD)

Q. Write a short note on von Willebrand disease, its clinical features, and laboratory investigations.

- vWD is the **most common inherited bleeding disorder.**
- Most cases are transmitted as **autosomal dominant disorders** caused by mutations in the vWF gene.

Categories

vWD has a variable clinical picture with more than 20 variants. These variants can be grouped into two major categories:

1. **Quantitative deficiency of vWF** characterized by **decreased circulating vWF.**
   - **Type I:** Transmitted as an autosomal dominant. **Most common variant of von Willebrand disease,** and forms about 75% of all cases. It is a mild disorder with a reduced quantity of circulating vWF. It also shows a measurable but clinically insignificant reduction in the levels of factor VIII.
   - **Type III:** It is an autosomal recessive, severe disorder. It is the least common type.
2. **Qualitative defects in vWF** are characterized by **qualitative defects** in the circulating vWF.
   - **Type II:** It is transmitted as an autosomal dominant disorder with functional deficiency of vWF. It accounts for 25% of vWD and has several subtypes.

Defects in von Willebrand disease: The patients with vWD have compound defects:

1. **Defect in platelet function:** In most cases, the platelet defect produces clinical findings.

2. **Coagulation defect:** vWD also has a deficiency of factor VIII. However, it is usually not severe to produce symptoms.

Clinical Features

- Most cases are of **mild bleeding.** Common symptoms:
  - **Spontaneous bleeding** from mucous membranes (e.g., epistaxis)
  - **Excessive bleeding** from wounds or menorrhagia.
- In severe cases, like hemophilia A.
- It is **commonly underrecognized.** This is because its clinical manifestations are quite mild and **diagnosis requires sophisticated tests.**

Laboratory Findings

- **Platelet count:** Normal
- **Bleeding time: Prolonged**
- **Clotting time: Prolonged**
- **Tourniquet test (Hess test): Positive due to defect in platelet adhesion.**
- **APTT: Prolonged APTT**
- **PT: Normal**
- **Special tests for diagnosis of vWD**
  - **vWF assay:** Plasma level of active vWF is **decreased**
  - **Platelet function test:** Defective **ristocetin**-induced platelet **aggregation test** is **diagnostic of vWF.**

TABLE 13.2 Summary of laboratory tests in hereditary coagulation disorders.

	Hemophilia A	*Hemophilia B*	*von Willebrand disease*
Bleeding time	N	N	Increased
APTT	Increased	Increased	Increased
Factor VIII levels	Decreased	N	Low or normal
Factor IX levels	N	Decreased	N
vWF levels	N	N	Decreased

(N: normal; APTT: activated partial thromboplastin time; vWF: von Willebrand factor)

Laboratory tests in hereditary coagulation disorders are summarized in **Table 13.2.**

Bleeding due to coagulation disorders must be distinguished from those due to platelet/vascular disorders **(Table 13.3).** The details of the tests are discussed on pages 416-9.

PA 21.3 (CC): Differentiate platelets from clotting disorders based on the clinical and hematologic features.

TABLE 13.3 Distinguishing clinical and hematologic features in platelet/vascular and coagulation disorders.

Characteristics	*Platelet/vascular disorders*	*Coagulation disorders*
Clinical features		
Onset	Spontaneous and develops immediately after trauma/surgery	Delayed bleeding after trauma/surgery
Type of lesion	Petechiae, ecchymoses	Hematomas
Sites of bleeding	Skin, mucous membrane	Deep tissues
Mucous membrane	Common from nose, mouth, gastrointestinal and genitourinary tracts	Uncommon except from gastrointestinal or genitourinary tract
Into the joint	Absent	Common in severe factor deficiencies
Into the muscle	Occurs following trauma	Spontaneous
Clinical examples	Thrombocytopenia, platelet defects, von Willebrand disease, scurvy	Factor deficiency, liver disease, acquired inhibitors
Hematologic features		
Platelet count	Reduced/normal in platelet disorders and normal in vascular disorders	Normal
Clot retraction test	Absent or reduced	Reduced or absent in fibrinogen deficiency (congenital or acquired)
Capillary fragility test (Hess/ tourniquet test)	Positive	Negative
Bleeding time	Prolonged	Normal
Coagulation or clotting time	Normal	Prolonged
Prothrombin time	Normal	Prolonged
Activated partial thromboplastin time (APTT)	Normal	Prolonged

Acquired Coagulation Disorders

Q. Write a short note on acquired coagulation disorders and their causes.

Acquired coagulation factor abnormalities are usually characterized by multiple clotting abnormalities.

Vitamin K Deficiency

Vitamin K is important for the activity of four clotting factors: Prothrombin, factor VII, factor IX, and factor X. In neonates, low levels of vitamin K levels may produce life-threatening hemorrhage during the first week of life known as ***hemorrhagic disease of the newborn.*** Parenteral vitamin K therapy is rapidly effective. Vitamin K is discussed in detail on pages 302-3.

Diagnosis of Vitamin K Deficiency

PA 21.5 (CC): Diagnosis of vitamin K deficiency.

Vitamin K deficiency leads to **delayed coagulation and bleeding** and is usually discovered when unexpected or excessive bleeding occurs. Vitamin K-dependent coagulation factors: II, VII, IX, and X (also protein C).

Prothrombin time: It is the main laboratory test done to investigate the bleeding. Vitamin K deficiency should be suspected as the cause for bleeding when the prothrombin time is prolonged (increased) but other coagulation studies are normal. If bleeding is suspected due to vitamin K deficiency, then **vitamin K should be administered parenterally**. If the bleeding stops and the PT returns to normal, then it can be assumed that vitamin K deficiency is the cause. Of the vitamin K-dependent clotting factors, factor VII (extrinsic pathway) has the shortest half-life. Thus, the prothrombin time is the first to be prolonged. Ultimately, the APTT also will be prolonged as clotting factors in the intrinsic pathway become deficient.

Other coagulation tests: They may be performed in patients with excessive bleeding. These include APTT, thrombin time, platelet count, platelet function tests, coagulation factor tests, fibrinogen, von Willebrand factor, and d-dimer. Measurements of the level of vitamin K in the blood are not routine tests and are usually not done to determine its deficiency.

Liver Disease

Liver synthesizes all the clotting factors and severe liver disease is associated with a hemorrhagic diathesis.

Other Causes

Disseminated intravascular coagulation involves a deficiency of several coagulation factors.

DISSEMINATED INTRAVASCULAR COAGULATION

PA 21.4 (CC): Define and describe disseminated intravascular coagulation (DIC), its laboratory findings, and its diagnosis.

Q. Write a short essay on etiology, pathogenesis, clinical features, and laboratory investigations/diagnosis disseminated intravascular coagulation.

Definition: Disseminated intravascular coagulation (DIC) is a **widespread disorder with a combination of thrombosis and hemorrhage.**

Etiology

DIC is caused by the systemic activation of coagulation. It forms thrombi throughout the microcirculation. It leads to the consumption of platelets and coagulation factors and, secondarily it activates fibrinolysis. Thus, DIC can produce either tissue hypoxia and microinfarcts caused by multiple microthrombi or a bleeding disorder due to pathologic activation of fibrinolysis and depletion of the components required for hemostasis (*consumptive coagulopathy*). DIC develops as a secondary complication of a variety of disorders **(Box 13.6)**. Therefore, DIC causes bleeding more commonly than all the congenital coagulation disorders combined.

Pathogenesis (Fig. 13.6)

Disseminated intravascular coagulation is a disorder that shows the **combination of (i) thrombosis and (ii) hemorrhage.**

BOX 13.6: Major disorders associated with disseminated intravascular coagulation.

Obstetric complications
- Abruptio placentae
- Retained nonviable (dead) fetus
- Septic abortion
- Amniotic fluid embolism
- Toxemia and pre-eclampsia

Infections
- Sepsis (gram-negative and gram-positive)
- Meningococcemia and other bacteria
- Fungi (histoplasmosis, aspergillosis), viruses, Rocky Mountain spotted fever, malaria

Neoplasms
- Carcinomas of the pancreas, prostate, lung, and stomach
- Acute promyelocytic leukemia

Massive tissue injury
- Traumatic
- Burns
- Extensive surgery
- Fat embolism

Vascular disorders: Aortic aneurysm, giant hemangioma

Immunologic reactions
- Transfusion reactions
- Transplant rejection

Respiratory distress syndrome

Miscellaneous: Snakebite, liver disease, acute intravascular hemolysis, shock, heatstroke, hypersensitivity, vasculitis

DIC: Sepsis, obstetric complications, major trauma (especially to the brain), and certain cancers are the major triggers.

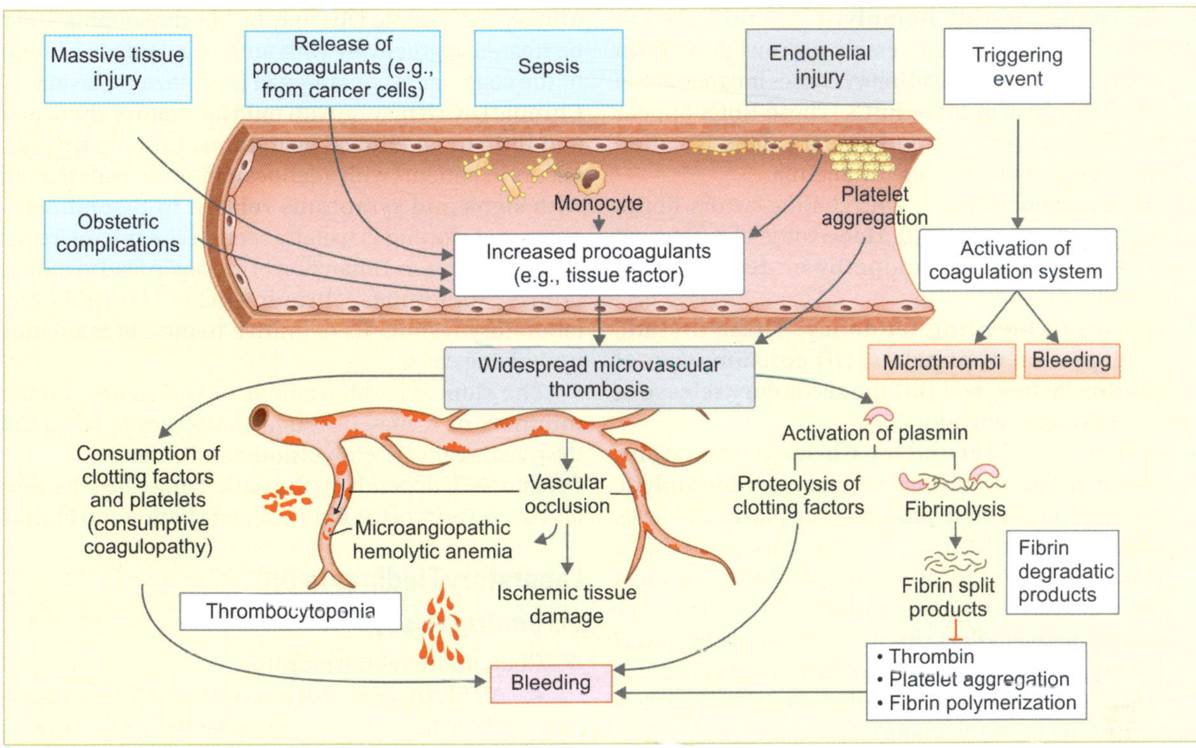

Fig. 13.6: Pathogenesis of microvascular thrombosis, ischemic tissue damage, and bleeding in disseminated intravascular coagulation.

Thrombi/Clot Formation

Normal clotting (coagulation): It can be initiated by either the extrinsic pathway or the intrinsic pathway.

- **Extrinsic pathway**: It is triggered by the release of tissue factor (tissue thromboplastin).
- **Intrinsic pathway**: It involves the activation of factor XII by surface contact, collagen, or negatively charged substances.
- **Common pathway**: Both extrinsic and intrinsic pathways form thrombin.

Limitation of clotting: Normally clotting is limited by the following mechanisms:

1. Rapid clearance of activated clotting factors by the liver
2. **Action of endogenous anticoagulants** (e.g., protein C)
3. Accompanying **activation of fibrinolytic factors.**

Mechanism of Thrombi Formation

Triggering factors of the thrombotic process

Major triggering factors that initiate the thrombotic process of DIC are either **(i) the release of procoagulants into the circulation** or **(ii) widespread endothelial cell damage.**

- **Release of procoagulant (thromboplastic) substances into the circulation:** Thromboplastin substances can be released into the circulation from various sources. The source of thromboplastic/procoagulant substances in the majority is **tissue factor.** For example, placenta in obstetric complications, cancer cells (particularly acute promyelocytic leukemia and adenocarcinomas), and bacterial sepsis (microbial endotoxins or exotoxins) stimulate the expression of tissue factors on monocytes. **Tissue factor activates the** coagulation system.
- **Widespread severe endothelial injury: It releases tissue factor** and **exposes the thrombogenic subendothelial collagen**. The causes of widespread endothelial injury are as follows:
    - Deposition of antigen-antibody complexes, e.g., in systemic lupus erythematosus.
    - Extremes of temperature, e.g., after heat stroke or burn injury.
    - Infections e.g., meningococci, rickettsiae.
    - Consequence of the systemic inflammatory response syndrome: It is triggered by sepsis and other systemic insults.

Consequences of DIC

The two consequences of DIC irrespective of its cause are:

1. **Widespread fibrin deposition within the microcirculation**: Both procoagulant substances (tissue factor) and endothelial injury activate the coagulation system resulting in fibrin-platelet **thrombi formation** in the microvasculature.
    - **Ischemia:** Thrombi obstruct the microvasculature and lead to ischemia in the more severely affected or vulnerable organs. Microvascular thrombi produce **microinfarcts or large areas of infarction** and multiorgan failure.

- **Microangiopathic hemolytic anemia**: As the red cells pass through vessels narrowed by fibrin thrombi, the mechanical injury causes fragmentation and hemolysis of these RBCs. These RBCs appear as schistocytes in blood smears. This is called microangiopathic hemolytic anemia.

2. **Bleeding tendency**: During DIC, clotting factors, fibrin, and platelets are consumed. Hence, it is also referred to as **consumptive coagulopathy** or **defibrination syndrome.**
   - **Causes of bleeding tendency**: These include **(i) depletion of platelets, (ii) consumption of clotting factors, and (iii) the secondary release of plasminogen activators.**
   - **Activation of secondary fibrinolytic system: Fibrin-thrombi activate the secondary fibrinolytic system** and generate **plasmin.** The plasmin cleaves fibrinogen and fibrin. It generates fibrin split products (FSPs) [or fibrin degradation products (FDP)]. FSPs are potent anticoagulants and have an antiplatelet effect (inhibit platelet aggregation) leading to bleeding. Plasmin also cleaves factors V and VIII, thereby reducing their activity. All these contribute to the bleeding tendency.

MORPHOLOGY

Microthrombi and its Consequences

In DIC, microthrombi usually occur in the arterioles and capillaries of the kidneys, adrenals, brain, and heart.

Kidney: The glomeruli show small fibrin thrombi. The microvascular occlusions by microthrombi produce small infarcts in the renal cortex. In severe cases, it may lead to bilateral renal cortical necrosis.

Adrenal glands: Involvement of the adrenal glands can cause the **Waterhouse-Friderichsen syndrome.**

Brain heart and the anterior pituitary: In these organs, microinfarcts are usually surrounded by microscopic or gross foci of hemorrhage. DIC may cause **Sheehan postpartum pituitary necrosis.**

Bleeding tendency associated with DIC

It manifests as hemorrhages near foci of infarction, diffuse petechiae, and ecchymoses on the skin, serosal linings of the body cavities, epicardium, endocardium, lungs, and mucosal lining of the urinary tract.

Clinical Features

The clinical manifestations of DIC depend on the balance between clotting and bleeding tendencies. Clinical presentation of DIC can be acute or chronic. It is **serious, often acute DIC**: It is likely to be **uncontrollable** and to be associated with **marked coagulation test abnormalities.** Generally, acute DIC (e.g., that associated with obstetric complications) is **dominated by bleeding**. Most commonly DIC manifests as petechiae, ecchymoses on the skin, or bleeding from mucous membranes or at venipuncture sites. In severe DIC, severe hemorrhage may occur in the gut or urinary tract. Acute DIC may be life-threatening and must be treated aggressively with anticoagulants (e.g., heparin) or the coagulants contained in fresh frozen plasma.

Chronic DIC: It may be with **mild laboratory abnormalities** and **little to no clinical symptoms.** Chronic DIC (e.g., as occurs in patients with adenocarcinoma) tends to manifest with **signs and symptoms related to thrombosis.** The abnormal clotting is usually seen in the microcirculation. Tissue hypoxia and infarction of the organ lead to multiorgan failure. Sometimes, chronic DIC is identified only by laboratory testing. Its definitive treatment is treating the underlying cause.

The clinical manifestations of DIC in general may be minimal, or it may produce shock, acute renal failure, dyspnea, cyanosis, convulsions, and coma.

Prognosis: It depends on the underlying causative disorder and the severity of the intravascular clotting and fibrinolysis.

Laboratory Findings in DIC

Screening Assays

- **Coagulation abnormalities:**
  - **APTT: Increased** due to consumption and inhibition of the function of clotting factors and fibrinogen.
  - **Prothrombin time: Prolonged.**
  - **Thrombin time (TT): Increased** because of decreased fibrinogen.
  - **Fibrinogen:** Decreased.
- **Bleeding time: Increased** due to decreased platelet count.
- **Platelet count: Decreased** due to utilization of platelets in microthrombi leading to depletion.
- **Peripheral smear: Microangiopathic hemolytic anemia with schistocytes.**

Confirmatory Tests

Fibrinolysis abnormalities:

- **Fibrin degradation/split products (FDP/FSP):** Secondary fibrinolysis results in the **generation of FDPs,** which can be measured by latex agglutination. Thus, fibrin split products are increased in the plasma.
- **D-dimer test:** It is **specific for diagnosing DIC.**

A summary of screening tests for bleeding disorders is presented in **Table 13.4.**

Laboratory Evaluation of Bleeding Disorders

Q. Discuss laboratory diagnosis in a case of bleeding disorder.

The clinical laboratory evaluation is an integral part of the diagnosis and management of patients with bleeding disorders. Laboratory tests for bleeding disorders depend on the component that is involved **(Table 13.5).**

Most bleeding disorders are caused by one of three defects: (i) a defect in platelet number or function, (ii) a defect in platelet-vessel wall interactions (i.e., an abnormality in the adhesive interactions between

TABLE 13.4 Summary of screening tests for bleeding disorders.

Investigation	*Normal range*	*The main causes of abnormal test*
Blood count and film	Show the number and morphology of platelets and any blood disorder	Platelet disorders, leukemia, or lymphoma
Platelet count	150–450 × 10^9/L	Thrombocytopenia
Bleeding time (template method)	2–9 minutes	Platelet disorders • Thrombocytopenia • Abnormal platelet function Deficiency of von Willebrand factor Vascular abnormalities
Prothrombin time (PT)	11–16 seconds	Deficiency or inhibitors of factors II (prothrombin) V, VII, or X or fibrinogen (I). Others e.g., heparin, warfarin
Activated plasma thromboplastin time (APTT)	30–40 seconds	• Deficiency or inhibitors of prekallikrein; high molecular weight kininogen; factors II, V, VIII, IX, X, XI, XII or fibrinogen (I) • Treatment with heparin, warfarin • Antibodies against clotting factors • Lupus anticoagulant
Thrombin time	15–19 seconds	Hypofibrinogenemia, disseminated intravascular coagulation (DIC)

platelets and the vessel wall) or (iii) a defect or deficiency in coagulation factor. The diagnosis of bleeding disorders requires various tests (**Table 13.6**) which include screening tests done in all patients with a history of bleeding, followed by specific tests to identify the exact nature of the disorder. The approach to bleeding disorder is shown in **Flowchart 13.1**.

TABLE 13.5 Laboratory tests for hemostatic disorders depending on the component involved.

Platelet component	*Plate-vessel wall interaction*	*Coagulation component*
• Platelet count • Platelet aggregation test • Clot retraction test	• Capillary fragility test (Tourniquet test) • Bleeding time	• Prothrombin time (PT)* • Activated partial thromboplastin time (APTT)* • Fibrinogen* • Thrombin time* • D-dimers* • Prothrombin consumption time • Factor assay

*Along with platelet count are the screening coagulation tests.

TABLE 13.6 Laboratory tests in bleeding disorders.

Screening tests	*Accessory tests*	*Others*
• Platelet count • Bleeding time • Prothrombin time (PT) • Activated partial thromboplastin time (APTT) • Peripheral smear	• Capillary fragility test (Tourniquet test) • Clot retraction test	• Prothrombin consumption time • Factor assay

Tests for Platelet Component

Platelet Count

Platelet count is performed on anticoagulated blood either manually or by electronic particle counters.

- **Normal range of platelet count:** 1,50,000–4,50,000 platelets/cu mm.
- **Causes** of thrombocytopenia (*refer* **Box 13.3**).

Platelet Aggregation

Principle: These tests measure the ability of platelets to aggregate in response to agents that produce aggregation like thrombin

Usefulness: It forms the basis for **qualitative tests of the von Willebrand factor**. They are used for the **classification of congenital qualitative disorders of platelets.**

Flowchart 13.1: Approach to bleeding disorder.

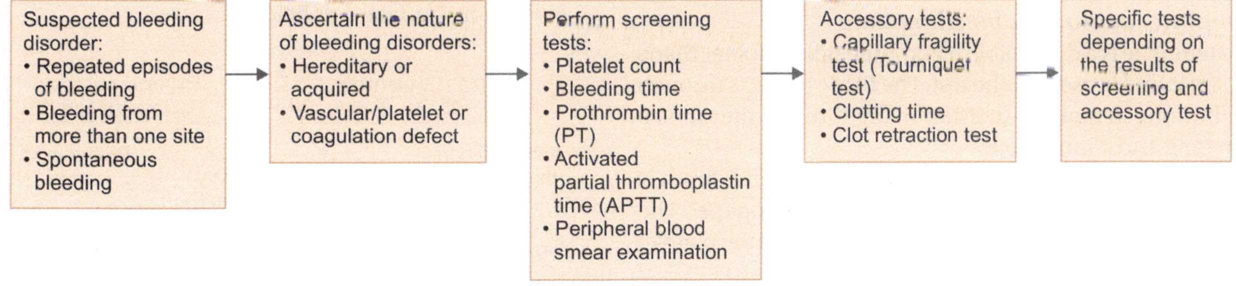

Clot Retraction Test

After the coagulation of blood, the clot undergoes contraction and starts retracting within one hour. This is due to the action of thrombosthenin (a substance released from platelets).

Normal value: Normal clot retraction shows 50% retraction in 2–4 hours. The serum is completely separated at the end of 24 hours. A normal clot is firm, rubbery, elastic, and not easily broken. Subsequently, the fibrin clot dissolves due to fibrinolysis and the RBCs sink to the bottom.

Interpretation: Clot retraction is **dependent on normal platelet number, platelet function, concentration of fibrinogen, and the activity of the fibrinolytic pathway. Absent or reduced clot retraction is seen in:**

- Thrombocytopenia.
- Thrombasthenia
- Fibrinogen deficiency (congenital or acquired).

Tests for Platelet and Vascular Component

Capillary Fragility Test (Hess Test/Tourniquet Test)

Q. Write a short essay/note on the capillary fragility test (Hess test/Tourniquet test).

Principle: Capillary fragility test **measures the ability of capillaries to withstand the increased stress.**

Procedure: The sphygmomanometer cuff is tied to the upper arm above the elbow and the cuff is inflated to 80 mm for 5 minutes. Release the pressure after 5 minutes. The number of petechiae present in a circle of 5 cm diameter on the flexor aspect of the forearm (below the bend of the elbow) is noted.

- **Normal:** 0–5 petechiae.
- **Interpretation:** A positive test is indicated by more than 10 petechiae and is found in:
  - **Vessel wall abnormalities:** Vascular purpura, scurvy.
  - **Platelet disorders**: Thrombocytopenia, defective platelet function.

Bleeding Time

Principle: Bleeding time (BT) is used as a screening test for disorders of platelet-vessel wall interactions. It measures the time required for bleeding to stop after a standardized superficial cut of the skin capillary bed.

Methods: Duke's method (obsolete), Ivy's method, and template method (method of choice).

Template method for bleeding time

The template is a disposable blade fitted onto a holder made of plastic and is used for the test. The blade projects through the bottom so that the incision made through the slit is 9 mm long and 1 mm deep.

Principle: A small skin cut of a standard size and depth is made and the oozing blood is wiped with a filter paper. The bleeding stops when the capillaries contract and the platelet plug seals the vessel.

Normal range: 2–9 minutes.

Uses: Tests for bleeding time are prone to problems of reproducibility, sensitivity, and specificity. Though, it is one of the screening tests, it is not recommended as a routine preoperative screening test. This test evaluates the defects of primary hemostasis. Thus, bleeding time measures the platelet-vessel wall interactions (integrity of capillary and platelet function).

Note: The bleeding time usually is not prolonged in patients with coagulation factor deficiencies.

Interpretation: Prolonged bleeding time is found in:

- **Platelet disorders:**
  - **Quantitative:** Thrombocytopenia. If the platelet count is below 50,000/mm^3, BT should not be performed as bleeding may be difficult to stop.
  - **Qualitative:** von Willebrand disease, Bernard–Soulier syndrome, Glanzmann's thrombasthenia.
- **Primary vascular disorders:** Ehlers–Danlos syndrome.
- **Platelet-vessel wall interactions:** von Willebrand disease.
- **Others:** Afibrinogenemia, severe hypofibrinogenemia, uremia, aspirin.

Tests for Coagulation Component

Complete blood count and peripheral blood smear examination are important in case of any hemostatic disorder. It can provide useful information. For example, fragmented red cells in DIC, leukemic cells, and thrombocytopenia. Various coagulation factors involved in intrinsic, extrinsic, and common pathways of coagulation are mentioned in **Figure 13.7**.

Coagulation or Clotting Time (Lee–White Method)

Principle: It measures the time taken for the fresh blood to clot. **Normal** clotting time **is 4–11 minutes.**

Disadvantages

- **Not a sensitive test:** It is one of the oldest tests and is not sensitive as it fails to detect mild/moderate coagulant defects. Hence, it is obsolete now and not recommended as a screening test. PTT is a more sensitive test for assessment of the coagulation cascade. Clotting time is prolonged only with severe deficiency of factor VIII, IX, or fibrinogen (afibrinogenemia) and in heparin therapy.
- **Misleading:** Normal value may be obtained in mild-to-moderately severe hemophilia A and B and it does not exclude major factor deficiency.

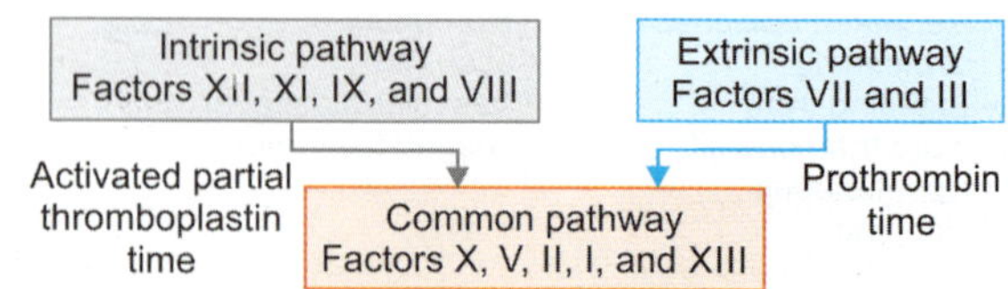

Fig. 13.7: Various coagulation factors involved in intrinsic, extrinsic, and common pathways of coagulation.

Prothrombin Time

Q. Write a short note on prothrombin time (PT) and its normal range.

Principle: Prothrombin time (PT) is the **time taken by citrated patient plasma to clot after the addition of a PT reagent that contains tissue thromboplastin** (consists of tissue factor and phospholipid) **and calcium chloride ($CaCl_2$).**

Normal range: 11–16 seconds.

Reporting of prothrombin time: Prothrombin time may be reported in different ways:

- Patient PT and control PT in seconds.
- Ratio of patient PT to control PT.

Q. Write a short note on INR.

International normalized ratio (INR): Due to the inherent variation in the sensitivity of thromboplastin reagents, it is advisable to report the PT in INR. It provides a uniform scale despite using different sources of thromboplastin. WHO recommended that each thromboplastin should have an ISI (International sensitivity index) value. INR is calculated using the formula: INR = (PT patient in seconds/PT normal plasma in seconds) ISI.

Interpretation of prothrombin time

It tests extrinsic and common pathways of the coagulation system (Fig. 13.7).

- **Screening test to evaluate coagulation disorders:** It measures coagulation factors VII. It also measures factors I, II, V, and X. Deficiency of any one of these factors leads to prolongation of PT. It should be used along with PTT.
- **To monitor oral anticoagulant therapy:** PT is prolonged during administration of oral anticoagulants like coumarin.
- **To evaluate liver function:** PT is prolonged in liver disease. Liver disease can result in a deficiency of the coagulation factors. Hence, **PT should be performed before a liver biopsy** and prolonged PT is a contraindication for liver biopsy.
- Prolonged PT is seen in **vitamin K deficiency**: Obstructive jaundice, hemorrhagic disease of the newborn.
- PT is also prolonged in **disseminated intravascular coagulation (DIC).**

Activated Partial Thromboplastin Time (Partial Thromboplastin Time)

Q. Write a short note on activated plasma thromboplastin time (APTT) and its normal range.

Principle: Activated partial thromboplastin time (APTT) is the time taken for citrated plasma to clot in the presence of a contact activator (e.g., ellagic acid, silica, kaolin), phospholipid, and calcium.

Normal range: 23–35 seconds.

Reporting: The patient's value is always to be reported with the control values in seconds. A prolongation of the patient value >8 seconds of the control value is considered abnormal.

Interpretation

Activated partial thromboplastin time (APTT) is a measure of the ***intrinsic*** and ***common coagulation pathways*** *(***Fig. 13.7***).*

- **Best single screening test for coagulation disorders.** This test is abnormal with deficiencies of II, V, VIII, IX, X, XI, and XII. Prolonged APTT is observed in inherited coagulation disorders—deficiency of factor II, V, VIII, IX, X, XI, XII.
- **Prolonged APTT:** APTT is used for screening hemophilia A and B; and von Willebrand disease. In these diseases, APTT is prolonged.
- For detecting coagulation inhibitors.
- For monitoring anticoagulant therapy like heparin. It is prolonged after oral anticoagulant therapy.
- Common causes of prolonged APTT are disseminated intravascular coagulation, heparin therapy, vitamin K deficiency, and liver disease.

APTT Mixing Study

APTT mixing study involves equal parts of patient plasma and normal pooled plasma (NPP). A circulating inhibitor is suspected when there is an incomplete correction of prolonged APTT, and a factor deficiency is suspected when there is complete correction of the prolonged APTT.

Thrombin Time

Thrombin time (TT) is not a commonly used test because of its limited use in laboratory assessment of most bleeding disorders. The most common causes of prolonged TT are heparin, hypofibrinogenemia, and dysfibrinogenemia.

Reference range for platelet coagulation are presented in **Table 13.7.**

CASE SCENARIO FOR ESSAY QUESTIONS

Immune Thrombocytopenic Purpura (ITP)

History strongly indicative of acute immune thrombocytopenic purpura: Sudden development of bruising, petechiae, and **mucocutaneous bleeding** in a **child following a bacterial or nonspecific viral** (upper respiratory or gastrointestinal) **infection** without features of acute leukemia (such as anemia and bone tenderness).

Laboratory findings of markedly reduced platelet count and **megakaryocytic hyperplasia with immature megakaryocytes.** The bone marrow favors the diagnosis of **acute immune thrombocytopenic purpura.**

TABLE 13.7 Reference range for platelets and coagulation.

Component (specimen)	*Reference value*
Bleeding time (BT)	
• Ivy's method	2–7 minutes
• Template method	2–9 minutes
Clot retraction time (clotted blood)	
• Qualitative	Visible in 60 minutes (complete in <24 hours)
• Quantitative	48–64% (55%)
Clotting time (CT)	
• Lee and White method	4–11 minutes
• D-dimer (plasma)	220–740 ng/mL
• Fibrinogen (plasma)	200–400 mg/dL
• Fibrin split (or degradation) products (FSP or FDP)	<10 µg/mL
• Partial thromboplastin time with kaolin (PTTK) or activated partial thromboplastin time (APTT/aAPTT)	30–40 second
• Platelet count	150,000–450,000/µL
• Prothrombin time (PT) (Quick's one stage method)	11–16 second
• Thrombin time (TT)	15–19 seconds (control ± 2 sec)

Case

History: A **14-year**-old male comes to the OPD with **petechial rashes of 2 days** duration. He has no history of bleeding in the past. He had an attack of **viral infection 3 weeks before** this complaint.

Laboratory findings: Hb 14.5 g/dL, hematocrit 45%, RBC count 5.1 million/cu mm. WBC count 7,200/cu mm and **platelet count 75,000/cu mm**. MCV is 85 fL, MCH is 32 pg and MCHC is 31 g/dL and RDW is 14.

SCENARIO-BASED MCQs

1. **A 7-year-old boy has come to the hospital for prominent bruises on his extremities over the past week. On physical examination, there are ecchymoses and petechiae on his arms and legs. Laboratory studies show hemoglobin, 13.5 g/dL; hematocrit, 41.3%; MCV, 93 fL, platelet count, 12,500/cu mm; and WBC count, 7,720/cu mm. The bone marrow shows an increased number of megakaryocytes. He had virus pneumonia 3 weeks back. His condition improves with corticosteroid therapy and the platelet count returns to normal. The abnormalities that are responsible for his bleeding tendency are:**
   A. Vitamin C deficiency
   B. Bone marrow failure
   C. Antiplatelet antibodies
   D. Dysfunction of glycoprotein IIb/IIIa
2. **A 34-year-old woman comes with a complaint of excessively heavy menstrual flow for the past 4 months. She also has found increasing numbers of pinpoint hemorrhages on her lower extremities in the past one month. Physical examination does not show organomegaly or lymphadenopathy. CBC shows hemoglobin of 13.2 g/dL, hematocrit of 39.5%, MCV of 91 Fl, platelet count of 15,000/cu mm, and WBC count of 6,950/cu mm. A bone marrow aspiration shows a marked increase in megakaryocytes. The prothrombin and partial thromboplastin times are within the reference range. On admission to the hospital, she has melena and is given a transfusion of platelets. However, her platelet count does not increase. The most likely cause for her bleeding tendency is:**
   A. Defective platelet-endothelial interactions
   B. Excessive loss of platelets in menstrual blood
   C. Abnormal production of platelets by megakaryocytes
   D. Destruction of antibody-coated platelets by the spleen
3. **A 27-year-old woman in the 24th week of pregnancy has felt no fetal movement for the past 3 days. She has not given birth even after three weeks. She suddenly develops dyspnea with cyanosis. On physical examination, her pulse is 106/min, and her blood pressure is 80/40 mm Hg. There are large ecchymoses seen over the skin of the entire body. A stool sample is positive for occult blood. Laboratory studies show decreased platelet count, an elevated prothrombin time, and partial thromboplastin time. The plasma fibrinogen is markedly reduced, and fibrin split products are seen. The probable cause of her bleeding diathesis is:**
   A. Increased vascular fragility
   B. Defects in platelet aggregation
   C. Reduced production of platelets
   D. Consumption of coagulation factors
4. **A 10-year-old boy was brought to outpatient for worsening joint mobility involving his arms and legs, particularly his knees and ankles, for the past 6 years. He has been receiving treatment for this condition. His grandfather had a similar condition and died at the age of 25 years. Family history indicates that other male relatives have similar problems. On physical examination, he has no petechiae or purpura. Laboratory studies show normal prothrombin time and elevated partial thromboplastin time. Hemoglobin is 12.2 g/dL, platelet count is 2,35,200/cu mm, and WBC count is 7,200/cu mm. His platelet function studies are normal. The most probable inheritance pattern for his condition is:**
   A. X-linked recessive
   B. Autosomal recessive
   C. X-linked dominant
   D. Autosomal dominant

Answers and Explanation

1. **The answer is C: Antiplatelet antibodies.** Both acute immune thrombocytopenic purpura (ITP) and chronic ITP are caused by antiplatelet autoantibodies. But the acute ITP usually develops in children after a viral disease. Scurvy caused by vitamin C deficiency is associated with increased capillary fragility and ecchymoses but does not produce thrombocytopenia. In the bone marrow failure, all cell lines should be reduced.

Dysfunction/deficiency glycoprotein IIb/IIIa is seen with Glanzmann thrombasthenia and chronic ITP.

2. **The answer is D: Destruction of antibody-coated platelets by the spleen.** The bleeding tendency is caused by a low platelet count. Most probably, she has chronic immune thrombocytopenic purpura (ITP). In ITP, the platelets are coated with antibodies to platelet membrane glycoproteins IIb-IIIa or Ib-IX. These antibodies coat both the patient's platelets as well as transfused platelets. These platelets are destroyed in the spleen. Platelet functions are normal in ITP. Abnormal platelet-endothelial interactions cause thrombosis. There is neither excessive loss of platelets in menstrual blood nor a defect in the production of platelets.
3. **The answer is D: Consumption of coagulation factors.** The features that suggest the development of disseminated intravascular coagulation (DIC) are the presence of thrombocytopenia, increased prothrombin and partial thromboplastin times, fibrin split products, and low fibrinogen concentration. The most likely cause of DIC is a retained dead fetus. The thromboplastins are released from the retained dead fetus. The thromboplastins cause widespread microvascular thrombosis and consume clotting factors and platelets. There is no damage to the endothelium or the vascular wall. There is no defect in platelet function and platelet production is normal. The platelets are consumed by widespread thrombosis of small vessels.
4. **The answer is A: X-linked recessive.** His condition is hemophilia A. It is monitored with factor VIII activity. Hemophilia A and hemophilia B are X-linked recessive inherited conditions, so males are mainly affected. Hemophilia B due to factor IX deficiency also presents with similar findings, but it is much less common. Transfusion of factor VIII helps to prevent joint and soft-tissue hemorrhage. Mucocutaneous bleeding is more common in platelet disorders and von Willebrand disease. In hemophilia, bleeding occurs in joints and soft tissues. The prothrombin time (PT) is normal, and partial thromboplastin time (PTT) is prolonged. Other options are not true in this case.

Immune thrombocytopenic purpura:
- Autoimmune disorder due to antiplatelet antibodies
- Platelets are markedly reduced
- Bone marrow shows increased megakaryocytes (precursors's of platelets)

Hemophilia:
- A due to factor VIII deficiency
- B due to factor IX deficiency

Hemophilia A:
- X-linked recessive disease.
- Males are sufferers and females are carriers
- Prolonged activated partial thromboplastin time

Disseminated intravascular coagulation (DIC):
- Widespread disorder with a combination of thrombosis and hemorrhage.
- Increased: APTT, PT, BT, D-dimer. D-dimer test is a specific diagnostic test
- Decreased: Platelets, fibrinogen

Blood Banking and Transfusion

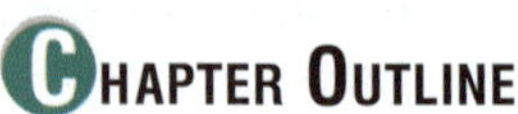

- Blood Group System
- Transfusion Medicine

BLOOD GROUP SYSTEM

PA 22.1 (CC): Classify and describe blood group systems (ABO and Rh).

Q. Write a short note on blood grouping/methods of blood grouping.

Karl Landsteiner in 1900 first described the existence of major human blood groups. More than 400 red blood cell antigens have been identified, most of which are inherited in a Mendelian dominant fashion and only a few are clinically important.

Classification of blood groups (Box 14.1): The term *blood group* is used to well-defined system of red blood cell antigens which are inherited characteristics. The blood group antigens form more than 20 genetically determined blood group systems.

- **Major blood group systems:** The two most important blood group systems are: (1) ABO and, (2) Rhesus (Rh) systems.
- **Minor blood group systems:** There are several minor and clinically less important blood group systems **(Box 14.1)**. These are weak antigens.

BOX 14.1: Blood groups systems.

Major blood group systems
- ABO system
- Rhesus (Rh) system

Other blood group systems
- Lewis system
- P system
- Kell and Duffy system
- I system
- MNS system
- Duffy system
- Kidd system
- Lutheran system
- Yt system
- Dombrok system
- Colton system
- Diego system

ABO Blood Group System

Q. Write a short note on the ABO blood group.

ABO blood group system consists of 3 major allelic genes: A, B, and O. These are located on the long arm of chromosome 9. These three genes control the synthesis of blood group antigens A and B.

ABO Antigens

According to the ABO blood group system, there are four different kinds of blood groups: **A, B, AB, or O**. The antigen on red cells may be A/B/AB or no antigen at all. There are **two subgroups in group A, namely A1 and A2**. A and B antigens are inherited as per the Mendelian laws. Everyone inherits two ABO genes, one from each parent and these genes determine the ABO antigens on their red blood cells. The absence of both antigens, A, and B on the red cells is seen in blood group O.

ABO Antibodies

Natural ABO antibodies: The serum of individuals (who have not been previously transfused) who lack the corresponding red cell antigen contains naturally occurring antibodies. These antibodies are against red cell A (anti-A)/B (anti-B)/AB (anti-AB) antigens. These are of IgM type and do not cross the placental barrier. Group A has two subgroups namely A1 and A2, and similarly, AB has two subgroups namely A1B and A2B. But these are not of major significance.

Acquired ABO antibodies: An individual lacking a particular antigen may develop an antibody after (acquired) exposure to red blood cells carrying the corresponding antigen. Exposure occurs due to parenteral introduction of red cell antigens. This may develop during:

- **Transfusion of red cells:** These acquired antibodies cause a hemolytic transfusion reaction.
- **Pregnancy:** Passage of fetal red cells (having paternal antigens foreign to the mother) into the maternal circulation during pregnancy may result in mainly IgG-type antibodies. They can cross the placental barrier

resulting in hemolytic disease of the newborn. The most important acquired *antibody* is anti-D which is a major cause of hemolytic disease of the newborn.

H Genes and H Antigens

The expression of A and B antigens is dependent on the presence of H gene. Most of the individuals are homozygous for the H gene. The sequence of events in the formation of A and B red cell antigens are:

- A and B red cell antigens are glycoproteins and their formation starts with a basic precursor substance **(Fig. 14.1)**.
- Basic precursor substance is first converted into H substance (by transferase) under the influence of the H gene.
- H substance is partially converted under the influence of A and B genes (and specific transferase) into A and B antigens. Some of the H substance remains unconverted.
- Since, O group individuals do not have A and B genes, neither A nor B antigen is formed and these have only H substance (H substance remains unchanged).

Note: A, B, and H antigens may be detected in the saliva and other body fluids also. Such individuals are called **secretors,** while the remaining without them are **nonsecretors.**

Bombay Blood Group

Q. Write a short note on the Bombay blood group.

- In 1952, Bhende, Bhatia, and Deshpande discovered a new blood group known as the Bombay blood group (phenotype Oh). **These individuals lack the H gene and therefore, the basic precursor substance cannot be converted into an H substance. This in turn results in failure to form A or B antigen.**
- When their blood sample is tested for routine ABO grouping, they will be labeled as blood group O. However, their serum contains anti-A, anti-B, and anti-H antibodies. These individuals, therefore, should be transfused with only the Bombay blood group.

Landsteiner's Rule (Law)

It exists **only in the ABO system.**

- **Corresponding antigens and antibodies cannot normally coexist in the same individual's RBCs.**
  - Individuals with group A who have A antigen on their RBCs will not normally have anti-A antibodies in their serum.
  - Individuals with group B who have B antigen on their RBCs will not normally have anti-B antibodies in their serum.
  - Individuals with group AB with AB antigens on their RBCs will not normally have anti-A and anti-B antibodies in their serum.
- In the ABO system (unlike other blood group systems), **if an individual lacks A or B antigen on the red cell, the corresponding antibody will be found in the serum.** These are the so-called isoantibodies (naturally occurring) usually of IgM type. These antibodies can cause intravascular hemolysis if incompatible blood is transfused.
  - Adults lacking group A antigen will have an anti-A antibody in their sera.
  - Adults lacking group B antigen will have an anti-B antibody in their sera.
  - Adults lacking group both A and B antigens (O group) will have anti-A or anti-B antibodies.

ABO Grouping Technique

- ABO grouping is of two types namely (i) forward (cell) typing in which antigens on RBCs are detected and (ii) reverse (serum) typing in which antibodies in the serum/plasma are detected.
- ABO grouping is performed by making a 2% saline suspension of red cells and adding anti-A, anti-B, and anti-AB sera.

Methods: The different methods available are as follows: Slide or tile technique, tube technique, microplate method, microtyping system, and automated or semiautomated method.

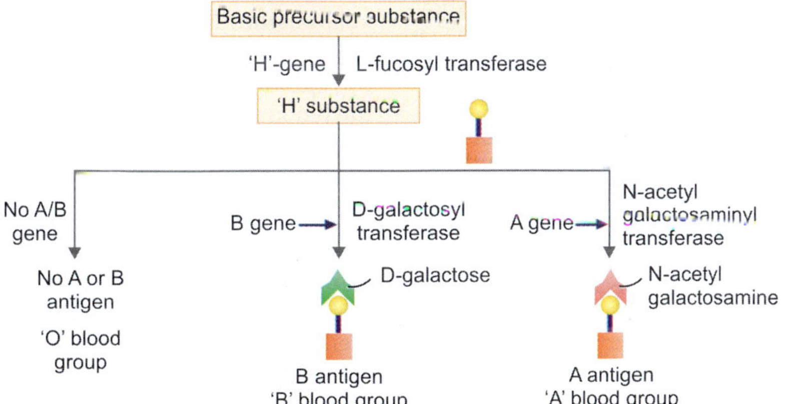

Fig. 14.1: Role of H gene in the formation of A and B antigens.

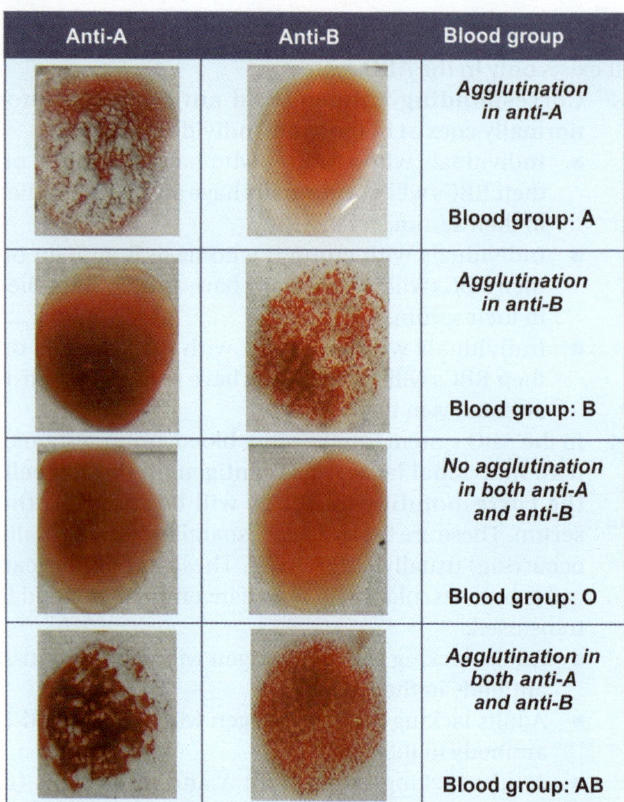

Fig. 14.2: Interpretation of blood group by slide method.

Slide or Tile Technique

Take a slide/white tile and mark it anti-A, anti-B, and anti-AB. Put one drop each of anti-A, anti-B, and anti-AB sera on the market slide. Add one drop of washed 2% red cell suspension to each antiserum. Mix each one separately with clean applicator sticks and spread the mixture over an area of 2 cm. Rock the slide gently and look for "agglutination" within 5 minutes.

Interpretation (Fig. 14.2): Blood group A, B, AB, or O is interpreted depending on the agglutination in the antisera.

Controls: Each blood group test should preferably have controls, both positive and negative.

- **Positive control:** This is run by performing the above techniques by using cells of known groups A, B, AB, and O. This is especially useful for testing the potency of antisera.
- **Negative control:** Run the above tests by adding saline instead of antisera. If agglutination develops, it indicates autoagglutination or pseudoagglutination.

Note:

- A group has two subgroups namely A_1 and A_2 which can be differentiated by using anti-A_1 lectin.
- Presence of H substance can be detected by anti-H.

Rh Blood Group System

Q. Write a short note on the Rh factor and Rh blood grouping.

Rh blood group system is the second system of clinical significance in transfusion medicine. This is a complete system of antigens which are labeled as D, d, C, c, E, and e. The D antigen is highly immunogenic. Cc and Ee antigens are weak antigens and therefore, the risk of sensitization to these antigens is less than the risk of sensitization to D.

Rh (D) System

Rh Antigens

- ***Rh positive (+ve):*** Individuals who have D antigen on the red cell surface are Rh positive (+). This may be present as a homozygous (DD) or heterozygous (Dd) state.
- ***Rh negative (–ve):*** Individuals who lack the D antigens are called Rh-negative.

Rh Antibodies

- In contrast to the ABO system, there are no naturally occurring antibodies against Rh antigens in Rh-negative individuals.
- Acquired (immune) antibodies: Rh antibodies develop after exposure to Rh antigens following transfusion (Rh +ve blood given to Rh –ve patients). They can be **detected by the antiglobulin test** (Coombs test).

Clinical Significance

- **Rh incompatibility between donor and recipient** results in **hemolytic transfusion reactions.**
- **Rh incompatibility between mother and fetus** results in **hemolytic disease of the newborn** (HDN).

Rh (D) Typing Techniques

Methods: The different methods available are—the slide or tile technique, tube technique, microplate method, microtyping system, and automated or semi-automated method.

Slide or Tile Techniques

Place one drop of anti-Rh (D) reagent (should be monoclonal IgM type) on a slide/white tile. Add 1 drop of 2% red cell suspension. Mix them using a clean applicator stick. Observe for agglutination after 2 minutes.

Interpretation: The presence of agglutination indicates that the blood sample is Rh +ve.

Controls: Known Rh +ve and Rh –ve samples should be run as a positive and negative control.

Other Methods of ABO Grouping and Rh Typing

These include tube technique, microplate method, microtyping system, and automated or semi-automated method **(Box 14.2)**. In test tube method procedure is similar to the slide method except that it is performed in a test tube.

Microplate method: It is ideal for testing many blood samples and has replaced the test tube method in many laboratories.

BOX 14.2: Various methods for ABO blood grouping and Rh typing.

Manual methods
- Traditional methods: Slide or tile technique
- Tube technique
- Microplate method
- Column agglutination technique
  - Gel technology (ID Micro Typing System)
  - Glass microbead technology
- Solid phase red cell adherence assay
- Erythrocytes magnetized technology

Automated or semiautomated method

Molecular blood grouping and genotyping

Microplates are polystyrene plates having 96 small wells. It saves time and cost.

Microtyping system (MTS) (Gel card) (Fig. 14.3): It is a gel-based technology in which plastic cards contain microtubes filled with buffered dextran gel. The gel contains sodium azide (preservative) and group-specific antisera (anti-A, anti-B, anti-AB, anti-D) or antiglobulin (for the Coombs test). These constituents are incorporated into the gel at the time of manufacture.

Both the above methods are used for blood grouping.

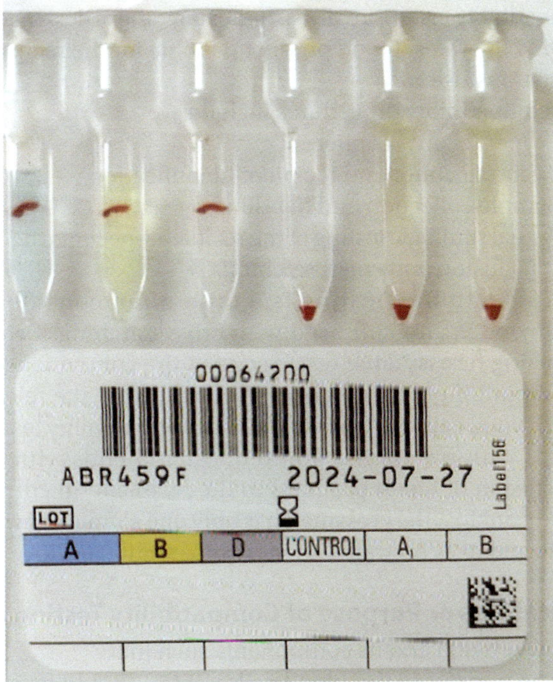

Fig. 14.3: Gel card method of blood grouping. The first three tubes show agglutination in A, B Rh serum. Agglutinated RBCs are floating on the top of the gel card. The blood group is AB Rh positive. The right 3 tubes are controlled in which there is no agglutination. The RBCs are settled at the bottom of the gel card.

Q. Write a short answer on the importance of the blood group.

Importance of blood grouping: Blood grouping is important **before blood transfusion, for pregnant women** (for Rh incompatibility between Rh +ve and Rh –ve mother) and is also of **medicolegal value**.

TRANSFUSION MEDICINE

Transfusion medicine comprises blood and blood component transfusion. Blood cannot be synthesized artificially. So, the source of blood is from a healthy human donor.

Blood Transfusion

Blood transfusion is the **process of transferring blood/ blood products from a donor into the circulating system of the recipient.** It is important to properly collect the blood from a donor, prepare its components (if required) store blood/components in a proper way, and transfuse in such a way as to avoid any risks or hazards.

Sequential steps for blood transfusion: These are as follows:

- **Blood donor selection**
- **Collection of blood by phlebotomy.**
- **Storage of blood bag**
- **Predonation check-up:**
  - **Testing of donor blood for ABO-Rh grouping, and infectious organisms** (HBV, HBsAg, HCV, syphilis, and malaria).
  - **Blood grouping (ABO-Rh) of the recipient.**
- **Pre-transfusion compatibility testing** of donor and recipient: These include the following:
  - **Antibody screening** of the patient's serum to detect the presence of clinically significant antibodies.
  - **Cross-matching** the patient's serum against donor red cells to confirm donor-recipient compatibility.
- **Supervision of blood transfusion:** Observe for any transfusion reactions.

Donor Selection

Q. Criteria for selection of blood donor.

Donor selection is based on medical history and a few routine physical examinations (weight, blood pressure, temperature, hemoglobin) are done to know whether the donor is suitable for donating blood.

- **Donor should be healthy with hemoglobin more than 12.5 g/dL** and free of infectious diseases. There are three types of donors namely voluntary (should be encouraged), replacement, and professional.
- **Age:** Donors should be between 18–65 years of age.
- **Weight:** Should be >45 kg.
- **Blood pressure should be normal** and not a diabetic on insulin or uncontrollable sugar levels.

- The time interval between each blood donation should be 3 months.
- No skin disease at the phlebotomy site.
- It is important to know whether the patient has a history of diseases like hepatitis, AIDS, or syphilis and if so, blood should not be obtained from them.

Collection of Blood

Blood is collected under aseptic conditions using a sterile, plastic bag with an anticoagulant **(Figs. 14.4A and B)**. The **anticoagulant used is CPD-A**. Mix the blood and anticoagulant gently and periodically during its collection.

Q. Write a short answer on anticoagulants used in blood banks.

Anticoagulants used: The different anticoagulants-preservative solutions available are as follows:

- Citrate phosphate dextrose (CPD).
- Citrate phosphate dextrose adenine-1 (CPDA-1)
- Acid citrate dextrose (ACD) is not used nowadays.

Q. Write a short answer on the functions of each component of CPDA-1.

The functions of various chemicals used in blood collection bags are mentioned in **Table 14.1**.

Storage of blood: Blood is stored in a **refrigerator at 2–6°C.**

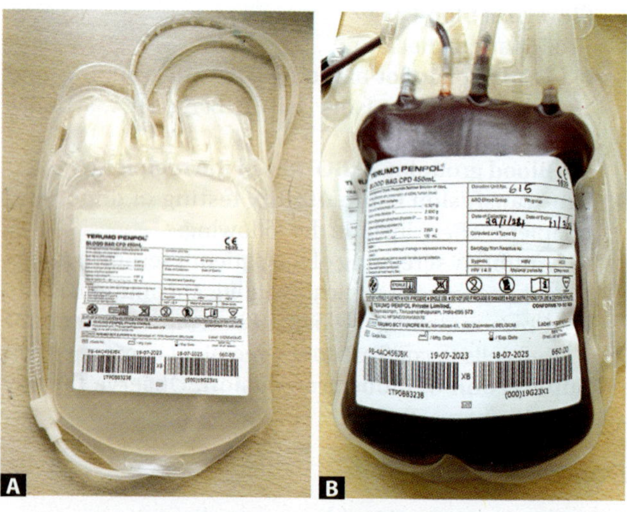

Figs. 14.4A and B: (A) Sterile, plastic bag with an anticoagulant for collection of blood; (B) Blood bag with collected blood.

TABLE 14.1 Functions of various chemicals used in anticoagulant-preservative solution.

Chemical used	*Function*
Citrate	Prevents clotting by chelating calcium
Sodium biphosphate	Buffers the end product of glycolysis (lactic acid) and maintains pH
Dextrose	Needed for ATP generation by glycolysis is required for the viability of red cells
Adenine	Substrate for red cell synthesis of ATP

Predonation Check-up

Q. Write a short answer on screening of blood donors.

Donor blood: The following tests are routinely carried out on the donor's blood:

- ABO and Rh grouping.
- Tests for:
  - **HBsAg, anti-HCV, anti-HIV-1 and HIV-2,** and serum alanine aminotransferase (ALT).
  - **Malaria and syphilis.**

Recipient blood: The recipient's ABO and Rh grouping are also carried out.

Pretransfusion and Compatibility Testing

PA 22.2 (CC): Enumerate the indications, describe the principles, and enumerate and demonstrate the steps of compatibility testing.

Q. Write a short answer on screening of the blood unit before transfusion (pretransfusion tests).

Introduction: Before transfusion of any blood or its components, it is essential to know whether they are compatible with the recipient's blood. This is achieved by performing a set of procedures (serologic and nonserologic protocols) known as **pretransfusion testing** also referred to as **compatibility testing**. Compatibility testing is an entire quality process **composed of many procedures**. The compatibility testing involves many steps and is designed to provide the safest blood product possible for the recipient of the transfusion.

The compatibility procedures include:

- Proper record keeping,
- Accurate donor and recipient identification,
- Sample collection and handling,
- Actual serologic testing of the recipient specimen before transfusion and crossmatching.

Compatibility testing is a term often considered synonymous and confused with crossmatching. **Crossmatching (crossmatch test) is one of the components of a compatibility test that is performed** before the release of red blood cells for transfusion. The compatibility testing begins with the transfusion request and ends with the transfusion of blood products to the recipient. In current blood banking, the crossmatch is only one element of what is referred to as pretransfusion (compatibility) testing.

Indications or Purpose of Compatibility Testing

To select blood and its components such that:

- The transfused red blood cells (RBCs) should have an acceptable survival rate when transfused.
- There should not be significant destruction of the recipient's own red cells, i.e., prevent an immune-mediated hemolytic transfusion reaction. There should be no adverse reactions from transfused blood.

A list of compatibility tests is presented in **Box 14.3**.

BOX 14.3: Pretransfusion testing protocol (steps).

- Recipient blood sample collection: Accurate identification of patient (recipient), proper sample collection, labeling and handling
- Review of patient's past blood bank history and records (if done earlier).
- Pretransfusion testing of recipient's and donor blood specimen
  - ABO grouping and Rh typing
  - Antibody screening test of recipient's and donor's serum
- Crossmatch: Crossmatch of recipient's sample with donor units:
  - Selection of crossmatch procedure (serologic or non-serologic)
  - Selection of blood for transfusion
  - Performance of a crossmatch: Recipient serum with donor red blood cells
- Proper labeling of blood or blood components of the donor before use with the recipient's identifying information and issue

Crossmatching (Crossmatch Testing)

Q. Write a short answer on crossmatching.

The term crossmatch is a crossway mixing of donor and recipient blood components. In **crossmatching, the serum or plasma from the recipient is mixed with red cells from the donor**. A crossmatch is only one part of pretransfusion (compatibility) testing and is very important before any blood transfusion.

Principle: Crossmatching should be carried out to ensure that there are no antibodies in the patient's serum that will react with the donor's cells when transfused. Crossmatching is routinely done only with donor products containing red cells, hence must be performed for red cell transfusions. **Hemolysis or agglutination at any phase or step** of the crossmatch process **indicates that the antibodies present in the recipient** interact with donor red cell antigens and a mismatch between donor and recipient. A crossmatch is considered as compatible when there is neither agglutination nor hemolysis in testing and the donor unit is acceptable for transfusion purposes. A cross-match is considered incompatible when there is the presence of either agglutination or hemolysis.

The importance of crossmatching is as follows:

- It is the **final check of ABO compatibility** between donor and recipient.
- **Detects the presence of any clinically significant, unexpected antibodies in the recipient's serum** that may react with the donor's cells, thereby preventing any transfusion reaction.
- A thorough crossmatching is performed with the recipient's serum and the donor's red cells.

Types: The crossmatching procedure may be divided into two major parts, namely, (i) major and (ii) minor crossmatching **(Table 14.2)**. The **various crossmatch techniques** are listed in **Box 14.4**.

TABLE 14.2 Types of crossmatches.

Type of crossmatch	*Donor's*	*Recipient's (patient's)*
Major crossmatch	Red cells	Serum
Minor crossmatch	Serum	Red cells

BOX 14.4: Crossmatch techniques.

- **Serological crossmatch**
  - Immediate spin (IS) technique
  - Saline room temperature technique
  - Albumin/low ionic strength solution (LISS) addition technique at 37°C
  - Indirect antiglobulin technique (using gel card)
- **Nonserological crossmatch**: Computer/electronic crossmatch

Serological Crossmatch Techniques

Major serological crossmatch test consists of testing the patient's (recipient's) serum with donor RBCs **(Table 14.2)**. The routinely used two serological methods are—(i) an **immediate-spin (IS) crossmatch**, and, (ii) an **indirect antiglobulin test (IAT) crossmatch**. In both these serologic crossmatch procedures, the recipient's serum or plasma is tested with the red cells from the donor unit.

Principles of serological testing: The pretransfusion testing is performed to detect in vitro red cell antigen and antibody reactions by observing for either agglutination or hemolysis. Only one serological method namely immediate-spin (IS) crossmatch is discussed here.

Immediate-spin Crossmatch (Fig. 14.5)

This is the simplest serologic test to detect most ABO incompatibility in which the **recipient's serum or plasma is mixed with the donor's red cell suspensions and centrifuging immediately** (i.e., immediate spin). Then observe it for agglutination. **Absence of hemolysis or agglutination indicates ABO compatibility**. This serologic test is used to detect ABO incompatibility and is enough to rule out any ABO grouping error. In this method, there should not be any delay in the centrifugation step or reading the reaction.

Advantages: IS crossmatch procedure requires less turn-around time, workload, and reagent cost compared to full AHG crossmatch.

Disadvantages: This method **does not detect all ABO incompatibilities** and is inadequate for the detection of clinically significant IgG-type of antibodies.

Procedure for immediate-spin crossmatch (Fig. 14.5)

- Take two drops of the patient's serum/plasma in a prelabeled glass test tube.

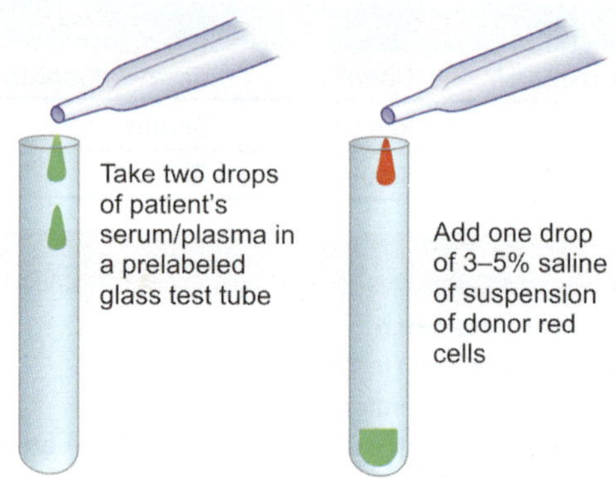

Fig. 14.5: Immediate spin crossmatch. Patient/recipient serum is crossmatched with donor red cells and it is called a major crossmatch. In minor crossmatch, the donor's serum is crossmatched with the patient's/recipient's red cells. Antibody screen testing on donor samples has replaced the minor crossmatch.

- Add one drop of 3–5% saline of suspension of donor red cells. Cells usually are washed once to remove any anticoagulant or plasma protein that may interfere with the testing.
- Mix the contents and incubate for 5–10 minutes for the IS method or 45–60 minutes for the saline room temperature technique.
- Immediately centrifuge the tube at 1,000 rpm for 1 minute (IS method). In the case of the saline room temperature technique, centrifugation is optional.
- Gently dislodge the cell button and examine the tube for the presence or absence of hemolysis or agglutination. This procedure is known as the abbreviated or IS crossmatch.

Interpretation

- **Positive test:** If hemolysis or agglutination is present at this stage, the test is considered as reactive/positive. It indicates that the unit selected may be **ABO incompatible** and the unit is **not considered acceptable for transfusion** (crossmatch is incompatible).
- **Negative test:** If there is **no hemolysis or agglutination,** the test is considered nonreactive/negative and the **unit is considered acceptable for transfusion** (compatible).

It is always necessary to monitor the recipient during and after transfusion so that any complications can be dealt with accordingly. **Presently indirect antiglobulin technique** (by gel card technology) is used in blood banks.

Blood Components

PA 22.4 (CC): Enumerate blood components and describe their clinical uses.

Q. Write a short note on blood components.

It is possible to separate different components of blood from a single unit of whole blood. These components can be used individually to help more than one patient for many purposes. Thus, red cells can be transfused to an anemic patient and plasma to a burn patient. This also ensures that only the required components are transfused.

Flowchart 14.1: Blood components.

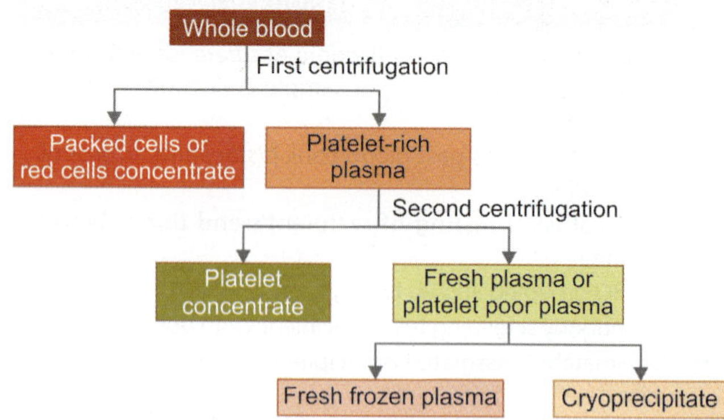

The various blood components **(Flowchart 14.1)** are as follows:

- Red cells concentrate or packed red blood cells (PRBCs)
- Platelet concentrates
- Plasma
- Fresh frozen plasma (FFP)
- Cryoprecipitate

The main uses of various blood components are presented in **Table 14.3**.

Preparation of Blood Components

1. **Centrifugation:**
   - Separation of components from the original whole blood unit is performed by using a centrifuge.
   - **PRP (platelet-rich plasma) is separated from whole blood by "light spin" centrifugation and the platelets are concentrated by "heavy spin" centrifugation** [light spin (short time and low RPM) and heavy spin (longer spin, high RPM and concentrates component)].
2. **Apheresis:**
   - Whole blood can also be separated into components using apheresis.

TABLE 14.3 Main uses of various blood components.

Various blood components	*Main uses*
Red cell concentrates packed red blood cells (PRBCs)	To restore tissue oxygenation
Platelets [platelet rich plasma (PRP), platelet concentrates]	To treat bleeding due to thrombocytopenia
Fresh frozen plasma (FFP)	Coagulation factor deficiencies
Cryoprecipitate	As a source of fibrinogen
Factor VIII and von Willebrand factor	Deficiency of factor VIII and von Willebrand factor
Specific factor concentrates	Specific factor deficiency

- Apheresis is the process of removing normal (from a donor) or abnormal (from patient) blood constituents from circulating blood.
- The whole blood is removed from the donor/patient and passed through an apparatus that separates out one (or more) particular blood constituent.
- Then the desired (or unwanted) components are retained and the remaining constituents are returned to the donor/patient's circulation.

Red Cells Concentrate or Packed Red Blood Cells

It is the red blood cells remaining after the removal of most of the plasma from whole blood.

Indications for use of PRBCs (Box 14.5): RBCs in the blood contain hemoglobin which transports oxygen to the tissues. They are used to raise the oxygen-carrying capacity of blood. Transfusion of PRBCs increases the mass of circulating red cells in conditions where there is impaired tissue oxygenation due to acute or chronic blood loss (e.g., hemorrhage, anemia). It is used in normovolemic patients with anemia without cardiac disease. In the packed red cell unit, the hematocrit is between 55% and 65%. Since the volume is only 200 mL; there is less risk of volume overload. One unit of packed RBCs may raise hemoglobin by 1 g/dL. Packed red cells are obtained by **centrifugation or sedimentation** of the whole blood and the plasma is transferred to another bag.

Platelet Concentrate

Q. Write a short answer on platelet concentrate.

Platelet concentrate may be obtained from a single donor or pooled plasma. Each unit of platelets can raise platelet count by 5,000 to 10,000/cu mm. Platelets can also be obtained from a single donor by platelet apheresis. Indications for platelet concentrate transfusion are listed in **Box 14.6**.

Fresh Frozen Plasma

Q. Write a short answer on fresh frozen plasma.

BOX 14.5: Indications for use of packed red blood cells.

Anemia
- Hemolytic anemia especially in aplastic crisis
  - β-thalassemia major
  - Sickle cell anemia in sequestration crisis
- Hypoplastic anemia: Aplastic anemia and anemia of chronic renal disease
- Severe anemia of any cause to reduce the chances of circulatory overload
- Hypovolemia due to hemorrhage (trauma)
- Blood loss during surgery: Patients undergoing cardiac, orthopedic, and other surgeries
- Other causes: Oncology patients undergoing chemotherapy or radiation therapy, end-stage renal disease, premature infants, and neonates

BOX 14.6: Indications for platelet concentrate.

Bleeding due to:
- Thrombocytopenia, when platelet count is less than 20,000/mm^3
  - Chemotherapy, radiation therapy or drug-induced
  - Leukemia
  - Marrow infiltration, e.g., leukemia, carcinoma
  - Dilutional (e.g., massive transfusion with stored blood)
  - Hypoplastic anemia
  - Viral disease associated (e.g., dengue)
- Abnormal platelet function
- Disseminated intravascular coagulation (DIC)
- Recipients of hematopoietic progenitor cell transplants for a period after transplant
- Patients with postoperative bleeding
- Organ transplant patients (e.g., liver transplant)

BOX 14.7: Indications for fresh frozen plasma.

- Patients on anticoagulant drug therapy (Coumarin)
- Antithrombin deficiency
- Coagulopathy of liver diseases
- Vitamin K deficiency
- Microangiopathic hemolytic anemia including thrombotic thrombocytopenic purpura (TTP), hemolytic uremic syndrome and hemolysis, elevated liver enzymes, and a low platelet count (HELLP) syndrome
- Disseminated intravascular coagulation (DIC)

Fresh frozen plasma (FFP) is prepared by freezing the plasma. FFP is plasma separated from whole blood (along with anticoagulant, placed at –18°C or lower (frozen) within 6–8 hours after collection. It contains plasma proteins and all coagulation factors that include albumin, protein C and S, antithrombin, and von Willebrand factor. It is indicated for the replacement of coagulation factors in acquired coagulation factor deficiencies **(Box 14.7)**. Each unit of FFP raises coagulation factors by about 2%.

Cryoprecipitate

Q. Write a short answer on cryoprecipitate.

Cryoprecipitated antihemophilic factor (AHF) is **also known as cryoprecipitate or simply CRYO.** It is the **cold insoluble portion of plasma that precipitates or remains after FFP is thawed** (melted) between 1 and 6°C refrigerator temperatures. Cryoprecipitate is a source of insoluble plasma proteins, fibrinogen, factor VIII, and vWF.

Indications for cryoprecipitate: Patients who need fibrinogen, factor VIII, and vWF. Transfusion of a single unit of cryoprecipitate provides about 80 IU of factor VIII. Transfusion of a single unit of cryoprecipitate yields about 80 IU of factor VIII.

TABLE 14.4 Blood products that can and cannot transmit HIV.

Blood products that can transmit HIV	*Blood products which cannot transmit HIV*
Whole blood, packed RBCs, platelets, leukocytes, and plasma	Hyperimmune gamma globulin, hepatitis B immunoglobulin, plasma-derived hepatitis B vaccine, and Rho immunoglobulin

Blood products that can and cannot transmit HIV are listed in **Table 14.4.**

Transfusion-transmitted Diseases

PA 22.5 (CC): Enumerate and describe infections transmitted by blood transfusion.

Blood is a lifesaving resource and blood components should be tested so that it makes them extremely safe and reduces the risk to minimum of the likelihood of a transfusion-transmitted disease (TTD). TTD is the infectious complication of blood transfusion. A variety of infectious agents including bacteria, viruses, parasites **(Table 14.5)**, and prion pathogens can be effectively transmitted through blood transfusions. If they are not detected in the testing process, it can cause harm and even death.

Screening Blood Donors for Transfusion-transmitted Infections

Donor Testing

Once a donor passes the medical screen and donor questionnaire, the serologic tests should be performed for the TTD. Routine screening of donor's blood in India is presented in **Table 14.6.** Performing these tests can make blood transfusion safer than ever before.

Apart from the transfusion-transmitted diseases listed in **Table 14.5,** many other organisms may also be transmitted by transfusion. However, tests for these organisms are not routinely performed in the blood screening process. These include other viruses, such as Epstein-Barr virus (EBV), cytomegalovirus (CMV), parvovirus B19, bacteria (presently the leading cause of death from transfusion), parasites, such as *Babesia microti* and *Trypanosoma cruzi*, malaria, and prion diseases.

Presently performed test methods are extremely sensitive. Hence, confirmatory tests are used only to detect false positives. These tests depend on the disease to be confirmed and include polymerase chain reaction (PCR), Western blot (WB), radioimmunoprecipitation assay (RIPA), and recombinant immunoblot assay (RIBA).

It is important to select a safe donor to provide a safer donation. The safest donors are regular, voluntary, and nonremunerated. Blood for donation should be screened for TTDs.

Test samples: Most of the assays use either serum or plasma. The instructions with the assay must be followed strictly.

TABLE 14.5 Transfusion-transmitted infectious (TTI) agents.

Viral	*Bacterial*	*Parasitic*
Common		
• Human immunodeficiency virus (HIV) • Hepatitis B virus (HBV) • Hepatitis C virus (HCV)	• *Treponema pallidum* (syphilis) is not common nowadays	• *Plasmodium* species (malaria)
Other less common TTIs		
• Epstein-Barr virus (EBV) • Cytomegalovirus (CMV) • Human T lymphotrophic virus-1 (HTLV-1) • Human T lymphotrophic virus-2 (HTLV-2) • West Nile virus • Parvovirus B_{19} (B19V) • Dengue virus (few cases reported)	• Brucella	• *Babesia* species • *Toxoplasma gondii* • *Trypanosome cruzi* (Chaga's disease) • *Leishmania* species
Others: Prion		

TABLE 14.6 Routine serological tests and screening methods used for testing donor blood in India.

Transfusion-transmitted diseases	*Required serological tests*	*Screening method*
Human immunodeficiency virus (HIV)	Antibodies to human immunodeficiency virus (anti-HIV 1/2 RNA) and p24 antigen	ELISA, particulate agglutination, simple rapid assays
Hepatitis B virus	Hepatitis B surface antigen (HBsAg), antibody to hepatitis B core antigen (anti-HBc)	ELISA, simple rapid assays
Hepatitis C virus	Antibody to hepatitis C virus (anti-HCV), HCV RNA	ELISA, simple rapid assays
Syphilis	Nonspecific antibody: Serological tests for syphilis (STS)	VDRL or RPR
Malaria	Trophozoite/ gametocyte	Microscopy or QBC

(ELISA: enzyme-linked immunosorbent assay; VDRL: venereal diseases research laboratory test; RPR: rapid plasma reagin; QBC: quantitative buffy coat)

Mandatory Screening Tests

The five tests that are mandatory as per the Food and Drug Administration (FDA) for the donated blood units are **HBsAg, HIV Ab, HCV Ab, VDRL, and malarial parasites.**

Nucleic acid testing (NAT) or nucleic acid amplification test (NAAT)

Nucleic acid test (NAT) is a general term used for molecular-based methods of screening for infectious agents. A nucleic acid test is a method useful to detect a particular genetic material (nucleic acid) of a virus or bacteria that acts as a pathogen in blood, tissue, urine, etc. The NAT differs from these conventional tests in that it detects genetic materials rather than antigens or antibodies. It detects very low numbers/levels of RNA or DNA of the pathogens (e.g., HIV, HBV, HCV) in the bloodstream before the appearance of antibodies. It detects infection earlier than conventional methods thereby narrowing the window period.

Transfusion Reactions

PA 22.6a (CC): Describe transfusion reactions.

Q. Write a short note on transfusion reactions.

Safety measures are usually taken at all steps of the blood collection, donor unit processing, pretransfusion testing, and patient monitoring. Despite careful precaution and preventive measures, unfavorable adverse effects, such as noninfectious complications of transfusions occur (about 2–4% of cases) and are not always preventable. These adverse effects of blood transfusion are also known as **blood transfusion reactions or simply transfusion reactions**. Most of these reactions are minor and transient.

Definition: An **adverse transfusion reaction** is defined as **any adverse event** (undesirable response/effect or complications related to transfusion) **that occurs in a patient during or after the transfusion** of whole blood, blood components, or human-derived plasma products.

Classification (Box 14.8): Transfusion reactions may range from relatively mild to severe and at times can be fatal. It can be categorized into different types.

According to the time interval between transfusion and the presentation of adverse effects, transfusion reactions can be classified as:

- **Acute (immediate) and delayed transfusion reaction**
  - **Acute transfusion reaction:** It is a transfusion reaction with **signs or symptoms occurring during or shortly after transfusion** (within 24 hours of transfusion).
  - **Delayed transfusion reaction:** It is a transfusion reaction with signs or **symptoms presenting after 24 hours of transfusion.**
- **According to the pathophysiology/mechanism** it may be further classified into:
  - **Infectious and noninfectious** complications **(Box 14.8)**. Noninfectious complications of transfusions are a greater risk to patients than infectious diseases.
  - **Immune versus nonimmune:** Immunologic transfusion reactions may be against red blood cells (hemolytic reactions), leucocytes, platelets, or immunoglobulins. Nonimmune transfusion reactions are presented in **Box 14.8.**

BOX 14.8: Transfusion reaction (complications of blood transfusion).

NONINFECTIOUS COMPLICATIONS

Immediate (acute) reactions

- ***Immunological***
  - Acute hemolytic transfusion reactions (AHTRs)
  - Acute nonhemolytic transfusion reactions
    - Febrile nonhemolytic transfusion reaction (FNHTR)
    - Allergic reaction
    - Anaphylactic
    - Transfusion-related acute lung injury (TRALI)
- ***Nonimmunological***
  - Nonimmune mediated hemolysis
  - Transfusion-associated circulatory overload (TACO)
  - Hypotension
  - Transfusion-associated sepsis (TAS)
  - Metabolic complications (hyperkalemia, hypokalemia, hypocalcemia, hypothermia)
  - Air embolism
  - Physical hemolysis

Delayed reactions

- ***Immunological***
  - Delayed hemolytic transfusion reactions (DHTRs)
  - Transfusion-associated graft versus host disease
  - Post-transfusion purpura
  - HLA alloimmunization
- ***Nonimmunological***
  - Iron overload-transfusion hemosiderosis
  - Citrate toxicity
  - Thrombophlebitis

INFECTIOUS COMPLICATIONS (TRANSFUSION-TRANSMITTED DISEASES)

A few of the diseases transmitted by transfusion are:

- Hepatitis (HBV, HCV, and HDV)
- HIV (AIDS)
- Malaria
- Cytomegalovirus
- Syphilis

Immediate/Acute Transfusion Reactions

Definition: *Acute transfusion reaction* is defined as a reaction in which signs and symptoms occur within 24 hours of a transfusion.

Acute Hemolytic Transfusion Reaction

Q. Write a short note on acute hemolytic transfusion reactions.

A hemolytic transfusion reaction is characterized by the destruction of transfused red cells in the recipient. It results in intravascular or extravascular hemolysis or a combination of both. Hemolytic reactions are classified as acute or delayed, and both types may stem from immune or nonimmune causes.

Definition: Acute hemolytic transfusion reaction (AHTR) is characterized by **rapid destruction of red cells** (i.e., acute hemolysis) with **symptoms developing immediately after or within 24 hours** of transfusion of red cells. The **hemolysis may be due to immune or nonimmune mechanisms.**

Immediate immune-mediated reactions

The severity of symptoms in acute hemolytic reactions ***depends*** on the amount and rate of incompatible blood transfused. As **little as 10 mL of incompatible blood can cause rapid hemolysis.**

Pathophysiology: It is due to the transfusion of ABO-incompatible red cells (Flowchart 14.2). The hemolysis is due to the **interaction of preformed antibodies in the recipient with the donor red cell antigens**. The most severe reactions are associated with transfusion of red cells that have ABO incompatibility with the recipient. It involves naturally occurring IgM antibodies, anti-A, and anti-B. These antibodies bind blood group antigens A or B on red cells and rapidly induce complement-mediated destruction of red blood cells, intravascular hemolysis, and hemoglobinuria.

Signs and symptoms: AHTR ranges in severity from fever to death. The patient typically develops **fever with chills,** nausea, vomiting, diarrhea, pain, dyspnea (chest tightness), tachycardia, hypotension, bleeding, and hemoglobinuria.

Flowchart 14.2: Sequence of events in immune-mediated acute hemolytic transfusion reaction (AHTR).

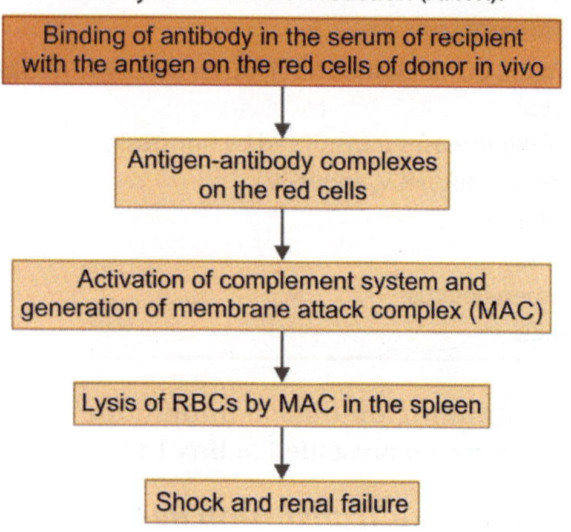

In severe cases, it may rapidly progress to DIC, shock, renal failure, and death.

Causes of immune-mediated acute hemolytic transfusion reaction: These are as follows:

- **Clerical error:** Most common cause of AHTRs is ABO incompatibility due to a clerical error.
- **Technical error: Errors in blood grouping** of recipient or donor, **improper technique a failure to detect weak antibodies.**

Acute transfusion reactions can be divided according to one of three key presenting symptoms: Fever, allergic, and pulmonary **(Flowchart 14.3).**

Acute Nonhemolytic Transfusion Reactions

Febrile nonhemolytic transfusion reactions

Definition: Febrile nonhemolytic transfusion reaction (FNHTR) is defined as a rise in body temperature of 1°C to 37°C or greater. It is an acute nonthreatening complication of transfusion and occurs during or shortly after transfusion (up to 4 hours after transfusion).

Signs and symptoms: FNHTR is a **common adverse effect of transfusion**. Apart from **fever,** these are usually accompanied by **chills or rigors**. It occurs within 6 hours of a transfusion of red cells or platelets. These reactions may be due to inflammatory mediators derived from donor leukocytes. Symptoms respond to antipyretics and are short-lived.

Allergic and Anaphylactic Transfusion Reactions

Definition: It is a **type I IgE-mediated hypersensitivity reaction** against proteins (allergens) present in the donor blood.

Allergic transfusion reactions (ATRs/ALTRs) are acute, immune complications of transfusion. Allergic reactions are the **most common type of transfusion reaction** that **occurs with the transfusion of blood products containing a plasma component.** They **can occur with any type of blood component** including autologous RBCs. **Severe, fatal, allergic reactions may develop when blood products containing certain antigens are given to previously sensitized recipients.**

Presenting symptoms: ATLR can present with a variety of symptoms that can range from minor urticarial effects to fulminant anaphylactic shock and death. Usually, **symptoms occur within minutes** after the transfusion is started.

Flowchart 14.3: Division of acute transfusion reactions according to one of three key presenting symptoms: Fever, allergic, and pulmonary and its causes.

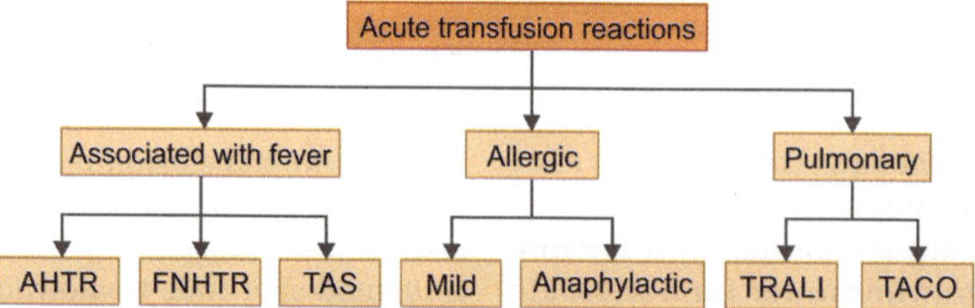

(AHTR: acute hemolytic transfusion reaction; FNHTR: febrile nonhemolytic transfusion reaction; TACO: transfusion-associated circulatory overload; TAS: transfusion-associated sepsis; TRALI: transfusion-related acute lung injury).

Mild allergic reactions (urticarial response) to transfusion are common. **Cutaneous symptoms** include pruritus (itching), urticaria (wheals, hives anywhere in the body), erythema, and cutaneous flushing. **Severe reactions (anaphylactoid or anaphylactic response) are rare.**

The reaction is triggered by IgG antibodies that recognize IgA in the infused blood product. Fortunately, most patients with IgA deficiency do not develop such antibodies, and severe reactions are rare, occurring in 1 in 20,000 to 1 in 50,000 transfusions. *Urticarial allergic reactions* may be triggered by the presence of an allergen in the donated blood product that is recognized by IgE antibodies in the recipient. These are more common, occurring in 1–3% of transfusions, but they are generally mild.

Transfusion-related acute lung injury

Q. Transfusion-related acute lung injury.

Transfusion-related acute lung injury (TRALI) is an acute, severe, frequently life-threatening, or fatal transfusion reaction. It presents with acute respiratory distress and severe hypoxemia usually during or within 6 hours of transfusion in the absence of other causes of acute lung injury.

Pathogenesis of TRALI: The exact pathogenesis is not fully understood. Probably **factors in a transfused blood product trigger the activation of neutrophils in the lung microvasculature.** Currently, favored is a "two-hit" hypothesis.

- **First hit (priming event):** The neutrophils of the recipient are primed for activation by the recipient's underlying clinical condition. This "priming" first hit has many causes, such as smoking, sepsis, and shock. These lead to the sequestration of neutrophils.
- **Second hit:** The second hit involves the activation of primed neutrophils by a factor present in the transfused blood product. The "second hit" is by an antibody in the transfused blood product that recognizes antigens expressed on neutrophils. The most common antibodies associated with TRALI are those that bind MHC class I antigens. These antibodies are usually found in multiparous women and are generated in response to paternal MHC antigens expressed by the fetus.

Symptoms: It presents dramatically with **dyspnea, hypoxemia, tachycardia**, nonproductive cough, fever, hypotension, and cyanosis. Characteristically, there are **no abnormal breath sounds**. A **chest X-ray** usually shows bilateral **pulmonary edema**. This syndrome is the **leading cause of transfusion-associated mortality.** The treatment is mainly supportive.

Nonimmunological Acute Transfusion Reactions

Nonimmune-mediated Hemolysis

Nonimmune hemolysis can also develop following transfusion. It develops **without the presence/involvement of any antibodies**. Most frequently, it **presents as asymptomatic hemoglobinuria**.

Causes of nonimmune-mediated red cell hemolysis

1. **Exposure of red cells to extreme temperatures** (>50°C or <0°C).
2. **Mechanical or chemical damage with destruction of red cells.**
3. **Simultaneous infusion of unapproved incompatible solutions.**
4. **Bacterially contaminated blood products**: If they are transfused, they may cause hemolysis.
5. **Intrinsic red cell defect:** For example, sickle cell disease, thermal burns, glucose-6-phosphate dehydrogenase deficiency, and paroxysmal nocturnal hemoglobinuria.

Clinical signs: These include **hemoglobinemia and hemoglobinuria**. Hyperkalemia may be found in patients with renal failure. Fever may also occur.

Complications: The main complications of nonimmune hemolysis are **renal failure and cardiac arrhythmia** due to hyperkalemia.

Transfusion-associated Circulatory Overload

Transfusion-associated circulatory overload (TACO) is an **acute, common, nonimmune, and preventable transfusion reaction** (complication of transfusion). It presents as congestive heart failure during or shortly after transfusion. It is **the leading cause of transfusion-related death.**

Risk factors: Volume overload should be anticipated in at-risk patients and should be prevented. The risk of developing TACO is observed in the following:

- **Pre-existing disease:** Patients with **pre-existing heart disease, diminished cardiac reserves, end-stage renal disease, pulmonary disease, chronic anemia,** and those who are **very young or very old**, even with a small transfusion volume can produce TACO.
- **Rapid or massive transfusion** of blood.
- **Age:** Patients older than 70 years and infants.

Signs and symptoms: It presents with respiratory distress and hypoxemia within 6–12 hours of transfusion. Signs and symptoms include dyspnea, cough, orthopnea, cyanosis, tachycardia, chest tightness, elevated blood pressure (hypertension), pulmonary edema, distention of jugular veins, elevated central venous pressure, pedal edema, and headache. TACO is also **associated with increased morbidity and mortality**. Treatment is cessation of transfusions and initiation of supportive measures.

Delayed Reactions

Immunological

Delayed hemolytic transfusion reactions

Definition: Delayed hemolytic transfusion reactions (DHTRs) also called delayed serologic/hemolytic transfusion reactions (DSHTRs) are defined as the detection of "new" red cell antibodies at least 24 hours after transfusion of the offending unit. It is an anamnestic response after transfusion with no signs of hemolysis.

Acute hemolytic transfusion reactions are usually associated with the transfusion of ABO-incompatible red cells. In contrast, in DHTRs, the symptoms appear after 24 hours and are caused due to a secondary immune response. The **recipient has been immunized (primary immune response/sensitized) after red cell exposure from either a prior blood transfusion or pregnancy**.

Normally, clinically significant antibodies are detected during pretransfusion testing. However, it may not be detected because of (i) the antibody levels below the detectable levels, (ii) missed in error, (iii) less sensitivity of the test, and (iv) rarely an antibody to a low-frequency antigen which is not demonstrated on the screening cells. These are usually caused by IgG antibodies. These are associated with a positive direct Coombs test and laboratory features of hemolysis (e.g., low haptoglobin and elevated LDH).

Time of development: Most patients develop DHTRs within the first 2 weeks after the transfusion. However, clinical DHTR may be recognized more than 6 weeks later.

Clinical presentation: DHTR are generally mild and may be overlooked. They tend to be much less severe than AHTRs. **A characteristic feature is the development of fever and unexpected anemia** (unexplained or unexpected fall/drop in hemoglobin or hematocrit) days or weeks after transfusion of an RBC component.

Transfusion-associated graft-versus-host disease

Definition: Transfusion-associated graft-versus-host disease (TA-GVHD) is a delayed immune transfusion reaction due to an immunologic attack by viable donor T lymphocytes present in the transfused blood component against the transfusion recipient.

TA-GVHD is a rare but highly lethal (90% mortality rate) complication of transfusion.

Time of manifestation: TA-GVHD usually manifests 2–30 days (usually 10–12 days) after transfusion.

Characteristic findings: The presenting symptoms features include a **maculopapular rash** (usually pruritic, typically starting centrally and extending to the extremities), watery diarrhea (accompanied by bloody stools and abdominal pain), fever, nausea, elevated liver function tests, and pancytopenia (due to marrow failure). These symptoms occur following a transfusion of a nonirradiated cellular blood component.

Delayed Nonimmunological Iron Overload (Transfusion Hemosiderosis)

Definition: Iron overload is a delayed, nonimmune complication of transfusion. It presents with multiorgan (i.e., liver, heart, endocrine organs) damage secondary to excessive accumulation of iron.

Pathophysiology: Hemosiderosis is a condition characterized by the accumulation of excess iron in macrophages in various tissues. Iron overload, also called transfusion hemosiderosis, is a potential complication seen in patients with persistent hemolysis (e.g., thalassemia sickle cell disease) receiving long-term transfusions (who receive multiple transfusions over a period of few years). The excess iron gets deposited (accumulates) in reticuloendothelial cells of the spleen, bone marrow, liver, heart, pancreas, and endocrine glands. It causes greater morbidity than the underlying anemia.

Prevention: The accumulation of toxic levels of iron stores can be prevented or reduced using iron chelators, therapeutic phlebotomy, or red cell exchange transfusion.

Infectious Complications (refer Box 14.8)

Few infectious diseases can be transmitted by transfusion of contaminated blood. Almost any infectious agent can be transmitted through blood products. The most common are bacterial and viral infections. Significant bacterial contamination (sufficient to produce symptoms) is much more common in platelet preparations than in red cell preparations. This is because platelets (unlike red cells) are stored at room temperature and favor the growth of bacterial contaminants.

Infections that can be transmitted through transfusion: These include hepatitis (HBV, HCV), syphilis, malaria, HIV, CMV infection, toxoplasmosis, infectious mononucleosis, brucellosis, and babesiosis. Their incidence increases in patients who receive multiple transfusions. These conditions include hemophilias, thalassemia major, acute leukemias, acute severe hemorrhage, etc. Advances in donor selection, donor screening, and infectious disease testing have reduced the incidence of this transmission by blood products. Now every unit of blood is screened for HIV, HBV, syphilis, and the presence of malarial parasites.

Symptoms: It presents with fever, chills, and hypotension and resemble those of transfusion reactions.

Investigation (Work-up) of Suspected Adverse Transfusion Reactions

PA 22.6b (CC): Enumerate the steps in the investigation of a transfusion reaction.

Q. Investigation (work-up) of suspected adverse transfusion reactions.

It is very essential to *stop the transfusion* if the patient's symptoms and signs suggest a possibility of a transfusion reaction. Clinical signs and symptoms of a transfusion reaction are listed in **Box 14.9**. Initial steps (actions to be taken) in the management of acute transfusion reactions are listed in **Box 14.10**. Steps to be followed when the transfusion is discontinued are listed in **Box 14.11**.

Laboratory investigation

The transfusion laboratory will perform relevant investigations. To rule out hemolysis from the differential diagnosis, the screening tests should be performed as listed in **Box 14.12**.

BOX 14.9: Clinical signs that suggest a transfusion reaction.

- Fever >1°C increase or >38°C, chills, and rigors
- Hypotension or hypertension
- **Respiratory:** Wheezing, coughing, dyspnea, cyanosis
- **Cutaneous:** Urticaria, rash, flushing, edema
- **Pain:** Abdominal, chest, flank or back, infusion site
- Nausea or vomiting
- **Renal:** Oliguria or anuria
- Jaundice or hemoglobinuria
- Abnormal bleeding

BOX 14.10: Initial steps to follow if there is suspicion of adverse reaction.

- **Prompt recognition of an adverse transfusion reaction**
- **Stop the transfusion**
- **Keep IV open with saline:** Maintain an intravenous line (for administration with blood) with normal saline
- **Notify immediately** to the blood center/bank and the patient's physician
- **Monitor/record vital signs**
- **Evaluate the patient** by attending physician to determine clinical intervention and potential medical management

BOX 14.11: Steps to be followed when the transfusion is discontinued.

- Perform clerical checks for any errors
- Visual check for hemolysis at bedside
- Collect post-transfusion sample:
  - Post-transfusion blood sample
  - Post-transfusion urine sample
- Return of the blood bag to blood center/bank

BOX 14.12: Initial standard laboratory investigation of a suspected transfusion reaction.

- Perform clerical check of the component bag, label, and patient sample
- Visual check for hemolysis in the blood center/bank: If hemolysis is established only in the post-transfusion sample, it indicates a hemolytic transfusion reaction
- Laboratory investigation:
  - Confirmation of post-transfusion ABO-Rh
  - Post-transfusion direct antiglobulin test (DAT)

The sample collected following a mismatched blood transfusion and the tests performed are presented in **Table 14.7.**

The hemoglobin (visual hemolysis) and antiglobulin tests are useful for screening purposes. If immune hemolytic reaction is suspected further testing/investigation is necessary.

TABLE 14.7 Sample collected following a mismatched blood transfusion and the tests performed.

Donor sample	*Post-transfusion blood sample*	*Post-transfusion urine sample*
Blood group and Rh typing	Direct antiglobulin test (DAT)	Occult blood
Crossmatching	Repeat grouping and crossmatching	Methemoglobin
Antibody screening	Serum bilirubin	Microscopy: RBC

Autologous Blood Donation and Transfusion

PA 22.7 (CC): Enumerate the indications and describe the principles and procedure of autologous transfusion.

Q. Write a short note on autologous transfusion.

A voluntary donation of blood for use by the general patient population is termed allogeneic. **Autologous transfusion is transfusion to a patient of their own blood.** The advantages, disadvantages, and contraindications of autologous blood transfusion are given in **Boxes 14.13 to 14.15** respectively.

The patient must not suffer from a disease that would put them at risk from this procedure. They may not be able to tolerate phlebotomy.

BOX 14.13: Advantages of autologous blood transfusion.

- **Prevents:**
  - Transfusion-transmitted diseases. Compared to allogeneic, it prevents the transmission of bloodborne pathogens
  - Red cell alloimmunization: It may be useful in patients having antibodies to very common RBC antigens and where compatible allogeneic components are not available
  - Some adverse transfusion reactions (e.g., hemolytic, febrile allergic reactions)
- **Provides:**
  - Compatible blood for patients with alloantibodies and rare blood groups
  - Reassurance to patients concerned about blood risks
- **Supplements the blood supply**

BOX 14.14: Disadvantages of autologous blood transfusion.

- Does not affect:
  - Risk of bacterial contamination
  - Risk of ABO incompatibility error
- More expensive/costly than allogeneic blood
- Results in wastage of blood, if not transfused
- Increases prevalence of adverse reactions to autologous donation. Patients are prone to develop perioperative anemia.

BOX 14.15: Contraindications for autologous blood transfusion.

- Evidence of infection and risk of bacteremia. Bacterial contamination is the most serious consequence of autologous transfusion
- Cardiovascular contraindications:
  - Scheduled surgery to correct aortic stenosis
  - Unstable angina
  - Severe left main coronary artery disease
  - Recent (within 6 months of donations) myocardial infarction or cerebrovascular accident
  - Patients with significant cardiac or pulmonary disease
  - Cyanotic heart disease
- Uncontrolled hypertension
- Active seizure disorder
- Hemoglobin concentration: Should not be significantly anemic (Hb level not <11.0 g/dL)

Preliminary Steps

1. **Age:** No minimum or maximum age limits. Each case must be evaluated individually. The lower age limit is determined by the capacity of the child to understand and cooperate.
2. **Volume of blood to be collected:** It depends on the age and weight of the patient. Volume should not exceed 10.5 mL/kg of the donor's body weight.
3. **Examination:** Medical interview and examination should be structured to the special needs of donor patients. Any contraindication **(Box 14.15)** to autologous transfusion should be ruled out.
4. **Serologic testing:** ABO and Rh typing must be determined on all units. Antibody screening and crossmatch are optional if only autologous units are ordered for transfusion. Screening for blood-transmissible disease is required for the first unit collected from the donor in 30 days.
5. **Labeling:** The unit should be clearly marked for "**autologous use only**" and carry the statement autologous donor. Units should be clearly labeled with the name and age of the patient-donor, identification number, name of collection center, name of hospital, date of collection and expiry, ABO and Rh group, and signature of patient-donor.

Pretransfusion Testing

The patient's blood sample should be tested for ABO and Rh grouping. It is optional to test for unexpected antibodies and crossmatching. The blood unit must be retested to confirm the ABO and Rh group using a sample obtained from a segment of tubing attached to the bag.

Types of autologous transfusion: They are given in **Box 14.16**.

BOX 14.16: Types of autologous transfusion.

- Preoperative collection
- Perioperative blood collection:
  - Acute normovolemic hemodilution (ANH)
  - Intraoperative blood collection
  - Postoperative collection

Preoperative Collection

In this procedure, the blood is drawn and stored before anticipated need. Patients suitable for preoperative collection are stable patients scheduled for surgical procedures in which blood transfusion is likely.

Collection schedule: Usually, a weekly schedule is used. Two or three units of blood may be collected several weeks before surgery by autologous donation. There should be sufficient interval from donation to surgery. The last collection should be done not before 72 hours of the scheduled surgery and preferably be longer. This period helps for the recovery of a substantial portion of the collected red cell mass and adequate volume repletion. During this period, iron supplementation may be needed. Erythropoietin stimulation can be used as an adjunct to autologous donation. It is to be noted that there is no indication of single-unit autologous transfusion in an adult. Indications for preoperative autologous collections are listed in **Box 14.17**.

Perioperative Blood Collection

In perioperative blood collection, the blood is collected either during or after surgery.

Acute Normovolemic Hemodilution (ANH)

In this type, one or more units of blood are collected before starting/beginning the surgery. To maintain the circulatory blood volume, it is replaced simultaneously with a colloid or crystalloid solution. Hematocrit is allowed to come down to 25–30%. The blood collected is reinfused either during or after surgery. The blood units are reinfused in the reverse order of collection. Thus, the first unit collected and therefore, the last unit transfused has the highest hematocrit and concentration of coagulation factors and platelets.

Indications: It is useful in cardiac surgery because:

- Due to hemodilution there is reduced loss of red cells. This is because the whole blood shed during surgery is having a low hematocrit.

BOX 14.17: Indications for preoperative autologous collections.

Preoperative autologous collections:

- Major orthopedic procedures
- Vascular surgery, cardiac or thoracic surgery
- Radical prostatectomy

- The blood collected by ANH is stored at room temperature and is returned to the patient within 8 hours of collection. Thus, there is little deterioration of platelets or coagulation factors which results in the preservation of hemostasis.

Intraoperative Collection

In this type, bloodshed from the surgical (operative) field is recovered by circulatory devices. The shed blood is processed by machines called shell savers and then infused/transfused into the same patient.

Indications: This type of autologous transfusion is useful in:
- Cardiovascular surgery
- Ruptured:
  - Spleen or liver
  - Ectopic pregnancy
  - Aneurysm
- Traumatic penetrating injuries

Contraindications

- When procoagulant materials (e.g., topical collagen) are applied to the surgical field, it may result in systemic activation of coagulation.
- Malignancy
- Contamination of blood with fecal matter, urine, bile, etc.

Postoperative Collection

In this type, blood is collected from drainage devices and reinfused to the patient with or without processing. Postoperative shed blood may be collected into sterile canisters and reinfused after passing through a microaggregate filter. Postoperatively recovered blood is dilute, partially hemolyzed, and may contain high concentrations of cytokines. Hence, a maximum of 1,400 mL of unprocessed blood can be reinfused within 6 hours of initiating collection.

Bombay group: Lack the H gene

Blood transfusion: Anticoagulant used for collecting blood is Citrate phosphate dextrose adenine (CPD-A)

Major cross-match: Donor red cells and recipient's serum
Minor cross-match: Recipient red cells and donor's serum

Blood components:
- Red cells concentrate or packed red blood cells (PRBCs)
- Platelet concentrates
- Plasma
- Fresh frozen plasma (FFP)
- Cryoprecipitate

Main transfusion transmitted diseases:
- HIV
- HBV
- HCV
- Syphilis
- Malaria

Transfusion reactions (complications of transfusion):
- Immediate: Immunological, nonimmunological
- Delayed: Immunological, nonimmunological

Transfusion-related acute lung injury (TRALI): Acute, severe, frequently life-threatening, or fatal transfusion reaction

Stop the transfusion if the patient's symptoms and signs suggest a possibility of a transfusion reaction.

Autologous transfusion: Transfusion to a patient of their own blood.

Apheresis: Process of removing normal (from a donor) or abnormal (from patient) blood constituents from circulating blood.

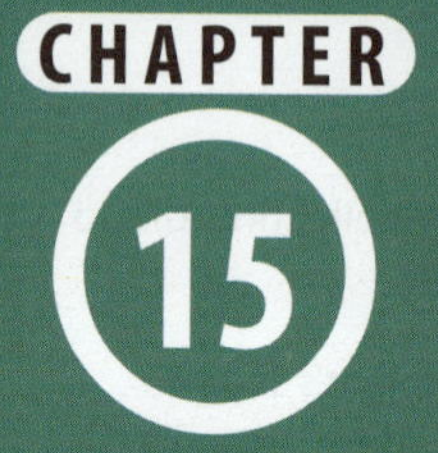

Clinical Pathology

CHAPTER OUTLINE

- Hemoglobin Estimation
- Peripheral Blood Smear
- Hematocrit (Packed Cell Volume)
- Erythrocyte Sedimentation Rate
- LE Cell Test
- Bone Marrow Examination
- Osmotic Fragility Test
- Urine Analysis
- Body Fluids
- Peritoneal Fluid
- Cerebrospinal Fluid Examination
- Semen Analysis
- Thyroid Function Tests
- Renal Function Tests
- Liver Function Tests
- Sputum Examination
- Laboratory Values of Clinical Importance

HEMOGLOBIN ESTIMATION

One of the important features of anemia is a reduction in the red cell mass. Red cell mass can be estimated by measuring hemoglobin (Hb). Indications for hemoglobin estimation are listed in **Box 15.1**.

Methods of Hemoglobin Estimation

Q. Write a short note on methods of hemoglobin estimation.

There are several methods for Hb estimation utilizing different principles **(Table 15.1)**. The **commonly used** methods include the colorimetric method namely Sahli's (outdated but still used in some places) and **cyanmethemoglobin method**.

Sahli's Method or Acid Hematin Method

This was the most popular colorimetric method. Since, it is used in some places, it is described here.

BOX 15.1: Indications for hemoglobin estimation.

- Anemia
  - To determine the presence of anemia
  - To assess its severity
  - To assess response to therapy
- Screening for polycythemia
- For estimation of red cell indices namely mean cell hemoglobin (MCV) and mean cell hemoglobin concentration (MCHC)
- Selections of blood donors

TABLE 15.1 Methods of hemoglobin estimation.

Method	*Principle*
Colorimetric method	
1. Visual colorimetric method; Sahli's method or acid hematin method, alkaline hematin method	These methods are based on measuring the color of hemoglobin or a hemoglobin derivative in the blood either visually or by photocolorimetry
2. Photoelectric method: Cyanmethemoglobin (HiCN) method, oxyhemoglobin method	
3. Haldane method	
Physical (specific gravity) method	Specific gravity
Chemical method	The iron content of hemoglobin
Gasometric method	Oxygen combining capacity of hemoglobin
Cell counter/autoanalyzer	RBCs are lysed by the lysate and color is matched against inbuilt standard color. Most use cyanide-free biodegradable reagent

Principle: When blood is added to N/10 HCl, **hemoglobin becomes acid hematin.** The **resulting brown color of acid hematin is matched against the standard brown color of the comparator.** The intensity of the brown color depends on the amount of acid hematin produced, which in turn, depends on the amount of hemoglobin in the blood sample.

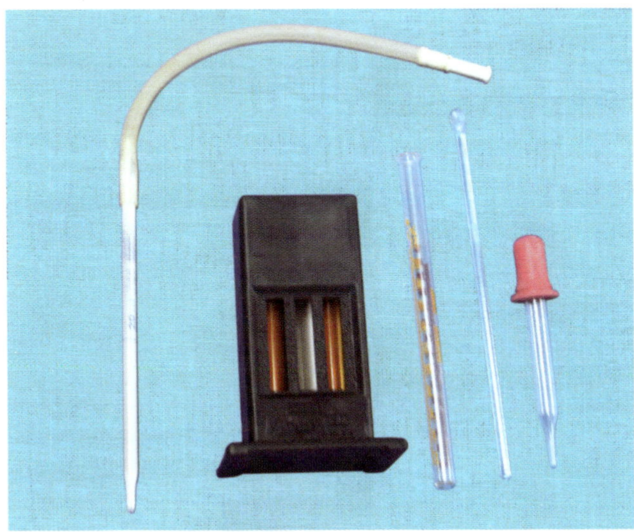

Fig. 15.1: Sahli's hemoglobinometer consisting of Hb pipette, comparator, round tube, glass rod, and dropper.

Apparatus (Fig. 15.1)

- Hemoglobin (Sahli's) pipette which has one mark of 0.02 mL (20 cu mm).
- A comparator that has a flat surface and a standard brown color.
- A square/round tube with markings of hemoglobin percentage (100% = 14.5 g/dL) on one side and hemoglobin (in grams) on the other side.
- Glass rod for mixing the blood in the square/round tube.
- A dropper (pipette) to take and transfer N/10 HCl and distilled water into the square tube.

Reagents: (1) N/10 hydrochloric acid (HCl) and (2) distilled water.

Technique

- Take N/10 HCl with a dropper into the hemoglobinometer tube up to the lowest mark of 2 grams.
- Draw blood exactly up to 20 cu mm (0.02 mL) mark of the Hb pipette and wipe off the excess blood at the nozzle of the pipette with moist cotton or absorbent paper or gauze. Specimen of blood required may be taken either from a finger prick or an EDTA vial.
- Blood in the Hb pipette is blown into the square or round tube of the hemoglobinometer containing N/10 HCl. Ensure that the entire blood inside the Hb pipette is transferred to the tube.
- With the help of a glass rod, mix the acid hematin.
- Wait for 10 minutes for the acid to act on the RBCs which causes lysis of RBCs liberating hemoglobin. The acid converts Hb to acid hematin (about 95% of Hb is converted at the end of 10 minutes, 98% of the color develops at the end of 20 minutes and the maximum color is reached after about 1 hour).
- Match the color of the solution in the tube with that of the comparator by holding it against the natural light or fluorescent tube light.
- Observe the following which interfere with matching and give the wrong reading:
  - Remove the glass rod from the solution in the tube.
  - Keep the tube inside the comparator in such a way that the markings do not interfere with the matching exercise.
- If the solution in the tube is darker, add distilled water drop by drop with a dropper and stir the solution with a glass rod. This process is continued till the color of the solution exactly matches the color of the comparator.
- Take the tube out and remove the glass rod. Take the reading of the lower meniscus.
- Hemoglobin is recorded as g/dL (or g%) and not as percentage figures of the graduated tube.

Advantages of the method: Simple, cheap, and easy method.

Disadvantages of the method: Apart from the technical errors, it is **not an accurate method.** Hydrochloric acid **does not convert all types of hemoglobins** (like carboxyhemoglobin, methemoglobin, sulfhemoglobin, and fetal hemoglobin—HbF) into acid hematin. Thus, the Hb value obtained may be slightly lower than the actual Hb. **Non-hemoglobin substances** such as protein, lipid, and cell stroma **interfere** with the color of blood diluted with acid and hence give false results.

Cyanmethemoglobin Method

Cyanmethemoglobin [hemiglobin cyanide (HiCN)] method is the most accurate, convenient, readily available, and preferred method for the estimation of hemoglobin concentration. It is the standard method used in most of the centers. The advantages of this method are its convenience and a readily available, stable standard solution.

Principle: Blood is diluted in a stable standard solution of **potassium ferricyanide and potassium cyanide. Hemoglobin is first oxidized to methemoglobin** (Hi) by the potassium ferricyanide. The cyanide ions (CN^-) of potassium cyanide convert **methemoglobin (Hi) to stable cyanmethemoglobin** (HiCN). The cyanmethemoglobin has a broad absorption, the maximum being at a wavelength of 540 nm. Thus, the color of this solution is compared against a standard HiCN solution of known Hb value in a spectrophotometer or photoelectric colorimeter at 540 nm.

Apparatus: A photoelectric colorimeter with a green filter or spectrophotometer at a wavelength of 540 nm is used. Other equipment required are Sahli's pipette (mark of 20 mm) and a 5 mL pipette.

Reagents: The diluent is a **detergent-modified Drabkin solution**, the composition of which is shown in **Table 15.2**.

Drabkin solution should be clear and pale yellow and when measured in the photoelectric colorimeter should give zero reading at 540 nm against water blank. The detergent enhances the lysis of RBCs and decreases turbidity due to the precipitation of proteins.

TABLE 15.2 Constituents of Drabkin solution (pH 7.0–7.4).

Constituents	*Quantity*
Potassium ferricyanide	0.20 g
Potassium cyanide (KCN)	0.05 g
Potassium dihydrogen phosphate (anhydrous)	0.14 mg
Non-ionic detergent (*Sterox SE*)	0.5 mL
Distilled water to	1,000 mL

Q. Write a short note on the advantages of the cyanmethemoglobin method of hemoglobin estimation.

Advantages of the cyanmethemoglobin method: They are as follows:

- The Hb value obtained is **accurate** since **almost all forms of hemoglobin** (hemoglobin, oxyhemoglobin, methemoglobin, carboxyhemoglobin, but not sulphemoglobin) **are converted into cyanmethemoglobin.**
- Being a colorimetric method, there is a direct comparison with the HiCN standard. Thus, **visual error** during matching the color like in Sahli's method is **eliminated.**
- Cyanmethemoglobin is a stable compound and **color does not change with time.** So, readings can be made at the operator's convenience, and **delay in taking readings does not alter the value.**
- **Easy** to perform the test.
- The **standard is stable** and certified cyanmethemoglobin standards are available.
- **Reagents are readily available.**

The normal range for hemoglobin: Adult males 13–17 g/dL, adult females 12–15 g/dL, and newborns 14–19 g/dL.

Low hemoglobin values are found in anemias and high values in polycythemia.

Automated Analyzer (Cell Counter)

These instruments measure not only hemoglobin but also various parameters like cell counts, PCV, and absolute values (MCV, MCH, and MCHC).

PERIPHERAL BLOOD SMEAR

PA 13.5 (CC): Perform, identify, and describe the peripheral blood picture in anemia (*refer* **Ch 12**).

Preparation of Blood Smear (Fig. 15.2)

- A drop of blood is placed on a clean grease-free glass slide 1 cm away from one end.
- Take a spreader (either another slide or a narrower piece of slide with a smooth edge) and place its smooth edge over the drop of blood to spread the blood along its edge.
- Place the slide at about 30–40° angle and make the smear with a smooth (not jerky) forward movement. The resulting ideal smear should be about 2.5–3.5 cm in length.
- Allow it to dry at room temperature and label.

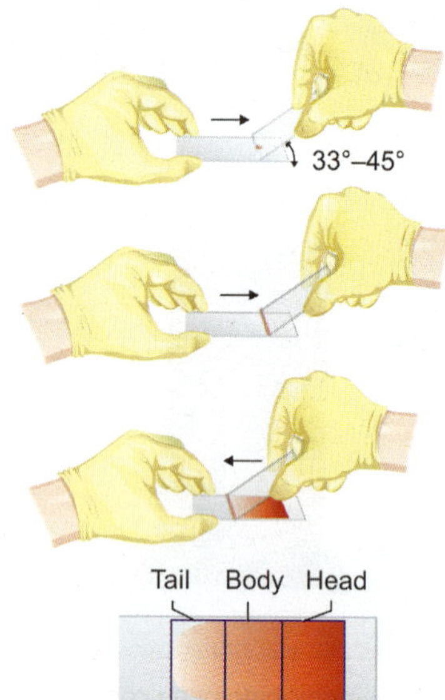

Fig. 15.2: Different steps in the preparation of peripheral blood smear and appearance of a well-made smear.

Features of a well-made peripheral smear are as follows:

- **Length**: Smear should be 2/3 to 3/4 of the length of the slide.
- **Shape**: The smear should be either tongue or finger-shaped (smooth without any irregularities or holes).
- **Well-made smear has three parts** namely, head, body, and tail.

Sources of error: The presence of grease on the slide causes blank oval areas in the smear. If the spreader edge is not smooth, the tail of the smear shows ragged edges and most of the neutrophils accumulate in the tail end. The rest of the smear shows a paucity of neutrophils, a process termed as tailing of the smear. This results in erroneous differential counts.

Stains for Blood Smear

Blood cells contain cellular structures that vary in their reaction (pH), some are acidic and others are basic. The aniline dyes used in staining blood smears are of two general classes: Basic dyes, such as methylene blue, and acidic dyes, such as eosin.

Q. Write a short essay on Romanowsky stains.

Romanowsky stains: All stains that are made of **combinations of acidic (eosin) and basic dyes (methylene blue)** are called **Romanowsky stains (Box 15.2).** The action of these stains depends on compounds formed by the interaction of methylene blue and eosin. Methylene blue on oxidation produces colored compounds called **azures** that can combine with eosin. Oxidation is achieved during maturation/chemical treatment of the stain. The azures are responsible for different shades of staining in the smears (i.e., RBCs—pink, granules of eosinophils—red-

BOX 15.2: Romanowsky group of stains.

- **Leishman stain** contains **acetone-free methyl alcohol which acts as a fixative.** Since acetone destroys the cells, methyl alcohol should be free from acetone.
- **Giemsa stain**
- **Wright stain**
- **Jenner stain**
- **Jenner–Giemsa stain**

orange, granules of basophils—bluish-black, granules of neutrophils—lilac).

- Nuclei and structures in the blood which are stained by the basic dyes are called basophilic.
- Structures that take up only acidic dyes are called acidophilic or eosinophilic.

The differences between the various Romanowsky stains are mainly in the proportion of the reagents and their preparation.

Fixation of blood smears: The blood smears should be fixed within 4 hours for good staining. Blood films are 'fixed' by **acetone-free methyl alcohol** which is present in most of the commonly used stains, namely **Leishman or Wright, or Giemsa stains.** It can also be fixed by dipping the slide 8–10 times in a coplin jar with methyl alcohol.

Procedure of Staining

Staining of the smears is carried out using *Romanowsky stains* which stain red cells, white cells, platelets, and parasites.

Leishman Stain

- Keep the peripheral smear on the staining rack.
- **Pour the undiluted stain** on the slide with a dropper so that the stain covers the entire upper surface of the slide.
- Wait for **2 minutes** for the methyl alcohol to **fix the smear**. Then pour double the amount of buffer water on the slide. Gently mix using a dropper.
- Wait for another **0–10 minutes** (time depends on the batch of stain) for **staining**. Look for greenish metallic scum to appear.
- Displace the stain by pouring running water from one side of the slide so that the stain scum is drained off the slide and no more stain is left on the slide.
  - **Precaution:** Do not discard the stain from a slide by just tilting it, since it will result in stain precipitates over the smear.
- Remove the slide from the staining rack and keep it slanting to dry it up.
- Examine the slide under a microscope.

Giemsa Stain

- Peripheral smear prepared is fixed by dipping 8–10 times in a Coplin jar containing methanol.
- Allow the slide to dry.
- Pour the diluted stain (1 in 10) and wait for 20–30 minutes.
- Wash the slide (as in staining by Leishman) and dry it.

Note: The amount of dilution and time for Leishman and Giemsa staining varies with each batch of stain.

Automated Slide Stainer

Automated slide stainers are also available for routine hematology slides. This stainer is a compact instrument with microprocessor control for flexibility in staining applications. Many slides can be stained uniformly in minutes.

Examination of a Peripheral Blood Smear

Q. Write a short essay on the importance of peripheral smear examination.

Importance of peripheral smear examination: Peripheral smear **(peripheral blood film)** is the most important, valuable, and frequently asked investigation in the hematology laboratory. A **well-prepared peripheral smear** usually has **three parts** namely, **head, body, and tail**. The best area of the smear to study the morphology of cells is the body, where the cells are well separated and touch one another without overlapping. Apply a thin layer of oil over the smear which makes the appearance of cells very clear. First look under low power, followed by high power and oil immersion. Observe the **quality of the film and the uniformity of staining**. Systematically observe the (i) **red blood cells,** (ii) **white blood cells (**number and distribution), (iii) **platelets** (number and distribution), (iv) **hemoparasites** (such as malaria, microfilaria), and (v) **any abnormal cells.**

Red Blood Cells

Q. Write a short note on poikilocytosis, anisocytosis, macrocyte, and target cell. (Ans. *refer* Figs. 15.3 and 15.4)

Select an area (best between the tail and body of the smear) suitable for examination of red cells in the thin area of the smear **where the red cells are evenly placed and just touch each other.** Look for the number, distribution, and staining of the red cells, and the degree of rouleaux formation if present. Red cells are examined for (1) size, (2) shape, (3) color, (4) inclusions and (5) other abnormalities.

- **Size:** In the peripheral smear, the size of the red blood cells is **compared with that of a small lymphocyte which has a size of about 7–8 µm**. The red cells are called microcytic if smaller than a small lymphocyte and macrocytic if larger than 9 µm. The appearance of **size variation (anisocytosis)** and conditions responsible for these variations are shown in **Figure 15.3**.
- **Shape: Variations in red cell shape (poikilocytosis)** and conditions responsible for these variations are shown in **Figure 15.4.**

Term and description	Appearance	Condition
Normocyte* Normal RBC is biconcave, 7.2 μm in diameter		• Normal RBC • Normocytic normochromic anemia
Microcyte* RBCs smaller than normal and less than 6 μm in diameter		• Iron deficiency anemia • Thalassemia
Macro-ovalocyte* Larger than normal, more than 9 μm in diameter and also oval		Megaloblastic anemia due to vitamin B12 and folic acid deficiency
Anisocytosis Variation in size		Severe anemia of any type

Fig. 15.3: Variation in size of red blood cells and associated conditions.

* In the peripheral smear, **the size of the RBC is compared with a small lymphocyte** that has the same size as that of a normal RBC. Accordingly, it is termed microcyte (smaller than lymphocyte), macrocyte (larger than lymphocyte), and normocyte (size same as small lymphocyte).

- **Color:** Variations in red cell color are depicted in **Figure 15.5.** Sometimes red cells appear to be hyperchromic without a central area of pallor. This is not actually due to an increase in the concentration of hemoglobin in the cell, but due to a change in cell shape and an increase in the thickness of the cell membrane in macrocytes. **Polychromatophilia or polychromasia is a blue-gray tint to the red cells.** It is a combination of the affinity of Hb for acid stains and the basic stains. These are the **young red cells that have been in the blood for 1–2 days.**
- **Inclusions in the red cells:** Look for any inclusions in red blood cells. Inclusions in red blood cells and associated conditions are presented in **Figure 15.6**.
- **Nucleated red blood cells (NRBCs):** These are **normoblasts and represent precursors of nonnucleated mature red cells in the blood.** Normally, normoblasts are present only in the bone marrow. They **appear in the circulating blood only in disease (e.g., hemolytic anemia).**
- **Other abnormalities:** For example, **rouleaux formation.**

White Blood Cells

White cells (leukocytes) are examined for the following features:

- **Number:** Note whether the number is decreased, normal, or increased.

Term and description	Appearance	Condition
Normal • Biconcave, flattened on smear		Normal
Poikilocytosis • Variation in shape		Severe anemia
Spherocytes • Smaller and stain darker without any central pallor		• Hereditary spherocytosis • Autoimmune hemolytic anemia
Target cells or leptocytes • Only the periphery and the central regions of the cell appear hemoglobinized		• Thalassemia • Sickle cell anemia • Hemolytic anemia • Post-splenectomy • Liver disease
Sickle cells • Thin, elongated, slightly curved and have shape of a sickle		• Sickle cell anemia
Bite cells • Pairs of spicules		• G6PD deficiency
Schistocytes (fragmented cells) • Small, irregular shaped, triangular or speculated cells		• Microangiopathic hemolytic anemia (e.g., DIC, TTP)
Acanthocytes • RBCs with few spicules of uneven (irregular) length and shape		• Abetalipoproteinemia • Liver disease
Echinocyte/Burr cell • Very small irregular shrunken cells with pointed projections. Resemblance to the small thorny 'burrs'		• Uremia
Elliptocyte or ovalocyte • Oval in shape		• Hereditary ovalocytosis • Hemolytic anemia
Pencil-shaped cells • Elongated thin cells (exaggerated ovalocytes)		• Iron deficiency anemia
Teardrop and pear-shaped cells • These abnormal RBCs have a teardrop or pear-like shape		• Myelofibrosis • Marrow infiltration
Stomatocytes • Red cells with a slit-like area of central pallor		• Hereditary stomatocytosis • Liver disease

Fig. 15.4: Variation in shape of red blood cells and associated conditions.

- **Assessment of approximate total white cell count:** Observe at least 10 high power fields in the thick portion of the smear where red blood cells overlap. Estimate the approximate number of WBCs/high power filed. Each WBC/high power field is approximately equivalent to 2,000 WBC/cu mm.
- **Abnormal or immature forms.**
- **Predominant cell type:** This is determined by performing the differential white cell count. At least

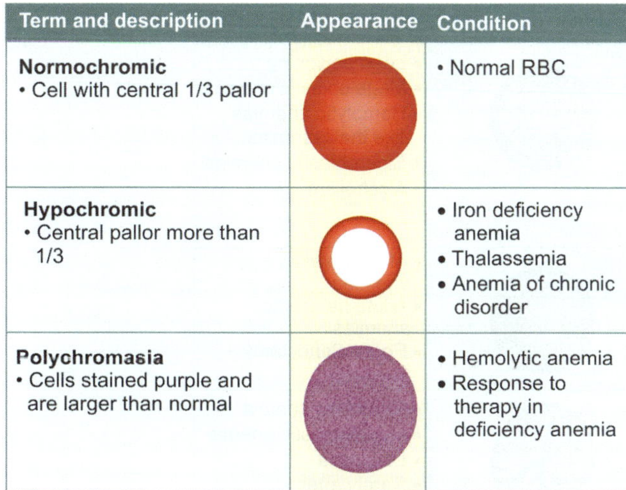

Term and description	Appearance	Condition
Normochromic • Cell with central 1/3 pallor		• Normal RBC
Hypochromic • Central pallor more than 1/3		• Iron deficiency anemia • Thalassemia • Anemia of chronic disorder
Polychromasia • Cells stained purple and are larger than normal		• Hemolytic anemia • Response to therapy in deficiency anemia

Fig. 15.5: Variation in color of red blood cells.

100 white cells should be counted. For a normal range of differential leukocyte count, *refer* **Table 12.13**.

Platelets

Platelets are round or oval, 2–4 μm in diameter, and separated from one another. The platelet count may be estimated from blood smears. On average, when the platelet count is normal, about one platelet is found per 10 to 30 red cells. At 1000× magnification, this is equivalent to about 7 to 20 platelets per oil immersion field. A single platelet under oil immersion is equivalent to 15,000–20,000 platelets/cu mm. They are examined for the following features under oil immersion.

- **Number:** Normal/increased/decreased.
- **Form:** Note the size and shape.
- **Aggregation:** Smears made from finger-prick show aggregation of platelets or platelet clumps.

Hemoparasites

Q. Write a short essay on hemoparasites.

Hemoparasites include (i) malarial parasites, (ii) microfilaria, (iii) trypanosomes, (iv) *Leishmania donovani*, and (v) babesiosis.

1. **Malaria** (*refer* **pages 122-24 and Fig. 4.12):** Malarial parasites can be demonstrated in the peripheral smear; the most common are *Plasmodium vivax* and *Plasmodium falciparum*.
    - ***Plasmodium vivax:*** In the peripheral blood the trophozoites, schizonts and rarely gametocytes of plasmodium vivax may be found.
    - ***Plasmodium falciparum:*** In falciparum infections usually only ring stage and gametocytes may be demonstrated.
2. **Filariasis:** *Microfilaria* (*refer* **Fig. 5.4B**) can also be demonstrated in peripheral blood.
3. **Trypanosomes:** These are motile flagellate protozoa.
4. ***Leishmania donovani*** **(LD):** It causes **kala-azar.** Amastigote forms known as LD bodies can be found in the reticuloendothelial cells of the bone marrow, spleen, and buffy coat preparations of peripheral blood.
5. **Babesiosis:** It is a malaria-like parasitic disease caused by babesia.

Any Abnormal Cells

For example, myeloblast, and lymphoblast.

Reporting of peripheral smear: The format for peripheral smear reporting is shown in **Table 15.3.**

Q. Write a short note on abnormalities in the shape of red blood cells.

Peripheral smear provides the following information:

- **Red cell morphology:** Morphological features (size, shape) of RBCs are important for the diagnosis of anemias and other hematologic disorders **(Figs. 15.3 to 15.6)**.
- **WBC disorders and differential leukocyte count (DLC):** Quantitative and qualitative changes in WBCs help diagnose both hematologic and nonhematologic disorders.
- **Platelet number and morphology**: These features are useful in diagnosing bleeding disorders.
- **Cross-checks the CBC parameters:** It helps in cross-checking the CBC parameters derived from automated cell counters.
- Detection of **blood parasites** (hemoparasites).

HEMATOCRIT (PACKED CELL VOLUME)

Q. Write a short note on the definition, methods, and significance of PCV/hematocrit.

Definition: Hematocrit (Hct) or **packed cell volume (PCV)** is the **ratio of the volume of red cells to that of the whole blood.**

Hematocrit indicates the relative volume of red cells and plasma (e.g., in anemia red cells are reduced with a corresponding reduction in the hematocrit).

Methods of measurement of Hct/PCV

- **Directly by centrifugation with:**
    - **Macromethods** using Wintrobe tube.
    - **Micromethods** using a capillary tube: A capillary Hct tube about 7 cm long and a bore of about 1 mm is used. Microhematocrit centrifuge is used for Hct estimation.
- **Indirect measurement:**
    - **Automated analyzer:** The product of the mean corpuscular volume (MCV) times RBC count in automated instruments

Wintrobe Method

Q. Write a short note on the Wintrobe PCV tube and its uses.

Wintrobe tube (Fig. 15.7A): It is a special thick-walled glass tube measuring **11 cm in length** and an **internal diameter**

Term	Description	Appearance	Condition
Basophilic stippling (punctate basophilia)	Red cells contain small, blue black inclusions and represent precipitated ribosomal RNA		• Lead poisoning • Megaloblastic anemias • Hemolytic anemias like thalassemias • Sideroblastic anemias • Alcoholism
Howell–Jolly bodies	Small, round densely staining dark blue particles and represent nuclear remnants		• Megaloblastic anemias • Acute hemolytic anemias • Post-splenectomy state
Cabot rings	Rings or 'figure of eight' shaped and are probably remnants of the nuclear membrane		• Hemolytic anemia • Megaloblastic anemia • Leukemia • Rarely after splenectomy
Pappenheimer bodies/siderotic granules (RBCs with Pappenheimer bodies are called siderocytes)	Aggregates of ferritin and appear pale blue, but are easily demonstrable with Perl's stain (Prussian blue reaction)		• Sideroblastic anemias • Megaloblastic anemias • Hemolytic anemias • Post-splenectomy
Hemoglobin H inclusions	Free β chains in red cells. Small, regular, multiple and diffusely distributed (golf ball like appearance). Stained by supravital stains		α-thalassemias
Heinz bodies	Refractive, single or multiple rounded inclusions of denatured globin detected by supravital stains		• Intake/exposure to oxidizing drugs or chemicals • G6PD deficiency • Unstable hemoglobin disease
Hemoglobin C crystals	Crystallization of hemoglobin C		Splenectomy in homozygous hemoglobin C

Fig. 15.6: Inclusions in red blood cells and associated conditions.
(RBCs: red blood cells; RNA: ribonucleic acid; G6PD: glucose-6-phosphate dehydrogenase)

of 2.5 mm, with a capacity of 1 mL. This is calibrated at 1 mm intervals up to 105–110 mm. It has bold markings in ascending order from the top as 0, 10, 20, 30,...100 for **ESR determination** and descending order from the top as 100, 90, 80,...10, 0 for **PCV estimation.**

Anticoagulants used: Ethylenediaminetetraacetic acid (EDTA), or dried heparin (double oxalate not used).

Principle: Anticoagulated whole blood is centrifuged at a standard speed. RBCs which are heavier than white cells, platelets, and plasma, sediment at the bottom, and the volume of red cell mass denote the hematocrit.

Normal range for PCV: Hematocrit is expressed as a percentage (conventional) (e.g., 45%) or as a decimal fraction (SI units) (e.g., 0.45). It is useful for evaluating absolute values like MCV and MCHC.

Causes of increased PCV: Polycythemia vera rubra and secondary polycythemia. Decreased PCV is seen in **anemia.**

Uses of Wintrobe Tube and Hematocrit

- **For estimation of hematocrit** which is useful for the following:
  - **Anemia:** To determine the presence of anemia, to assess its severity, and to assess response to therapy.
  - Presence or absence of **polycythemia.**
  - **Checking the accuracy of hemoglobin value** (Hb in g/dL × 3 = hematocrit).

TABLE 15.3 Format for reporting peripheral blood smear.

1. RBCs: Comment on the following features	
– Size	Normocytic (normal), microcytic, or macrocytic (predominant feature to be mentioned)
– Chromasia	Normochromic (normal), hypochromic, absence of central pallor
– Anisocytosis	Present (slight/marked) or absent
– Poikilocytosis	Present (slight/marked) or absent
– Other abnormalities	Spherocytosis, sickle cells, target cells, etc.
– Polychromatophilia	Present or absent
– Nucleated red cells	Normoblasts—per 100 leukocytes
2. WBCs: Comment on total WBC count as normal/increased/decreased	
– Differential count (on 100 cells)	
– Type of WBC (percentage)	Neutrophils, eosinophils, basophils, lymphocytes, monocytes, immature leukocytes (specify different cells)
3. Platelets	Approximate judgment on adequate/increased/reduced
4. Hemoparasites	

(RBCs: red blood cells; WBCs: white blood cells)

- PCV which is also required **to determine** the **red cell indices** namely mean cell volume (MCV) and mean cell hemoglobin concentration (MCHC).

Q. What is a buffy coat? Mention its importance.

- **The buffy coat** is the red-gray layer between the red cells and the plasma and is **obtained by hematocrit.** It includes platelets and leukocytes. **Buffy coat** gives an approximate indication of the number of WBCs (normally 0.1 mm of this layer = 1,000 WBC/cu mm). Uses of the buffy coat are as follows:
    - Thickness of the **buffy coat increases with marked leukocytosis**, as in CML, CLL, and acute leukemias. An absent or minimal buffy coat implies leukopenia.
    - In subleukemic leukemia, a smear made from the buffy coat has a greater concentration of WBCs, and identification of abnormal cells is easier.
    - Lupus erythematous (LE) cell tests.
- **ESR estimation:** However, the Westergren method is preferred as it is more accurate.

ERYTHROCYTE SEDIMENTATION RATE

Q. Write a short note on normal values, indications, anticoagulants used, stages, and factors affecting erythrocyte sedimentation rate.

Erythrocyte sedimentation rate (ESR) estimation is a commonly used **nonspecific test** in routine clinical practice. ESR is a useful but **nonspecific marker of underlying inflammation**. However, other high-sensitivity inflammatory markers (e.g., C-reactive protein) are presently used to detect or monitor disease (e.g., cardiovascular disease and metabolic syndrome).

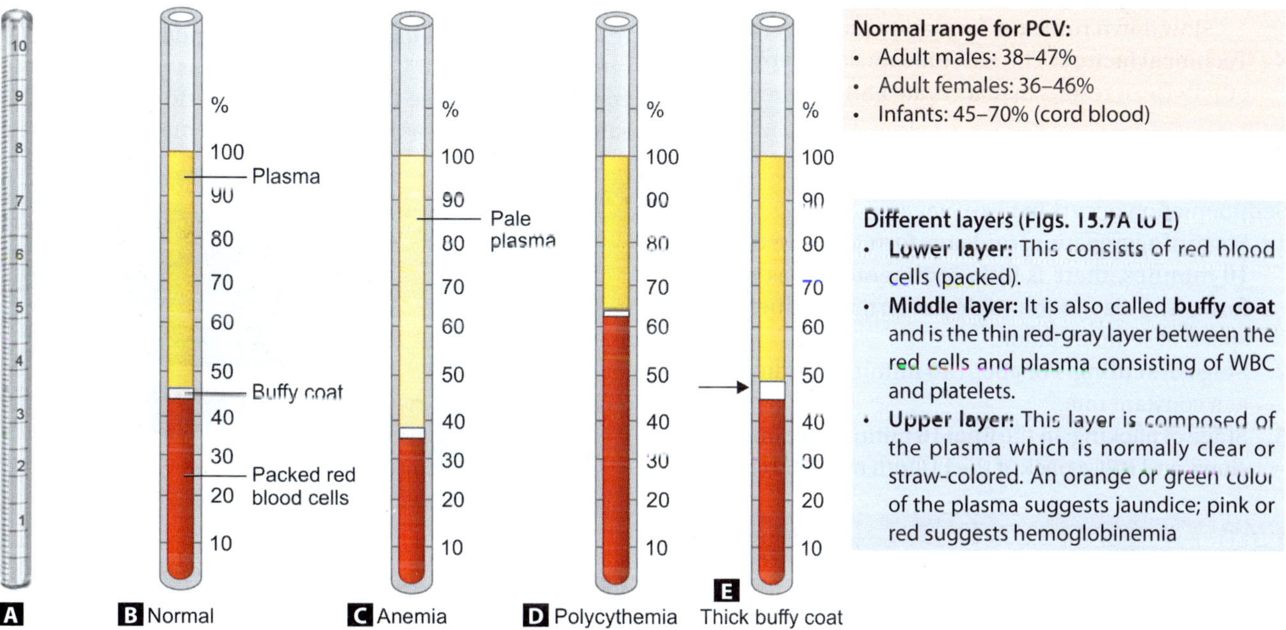

Figs. 15.7A to E: (A) Wintrobe tube; (B to E): Diagrammatic appearance of different columns after the blood is centrifuged in (B) normal; (C) anemia; (D) polycythemia vera; and (E) thick buffy coat.

Principle: When well-mixed anticoagulated blood is placed in a vertical tube and is allowed to stand, RBCs settle towards the bottom of the tube. The length of fall of RBCs from the top of the column in plasma over 1 hour is called the ESR. The length of the RBC column is expressed in millimeters. RBCs have a net negative charge on their surface (zeta potential is the physical property exhibited by RBC in plasm suspension) and tend to repel each other. The repulsive forces are partially or totally counteracted if there is an increase in the positively charged plasma proteins.

Factors Affecting ESR (Box 15.3)

- **Plasma factors:** An **accelerated ESR** is favored by elevated levels of **fibrinogen, globulins, and cholesterol** [which decrease the negative charge of RBCs (zeta potential) that tends to keep them apart]. The decreased zeta potential favors the rouleaux formation, which sediments more rapidly than single red blood cells. The **albumin and lecithin retard ESR.**
- **Red cell factors:** The sedimentation rate is directly proportional to the weight of the cell aggregates and inversely proportional to the surface area.
  - **Size of RBCs: Microcytes sediment more slowly than macrocytes**, which have decreased surface area/volume ratios.
  - **Rouleaux formation:** Rouleaux also has a decreased surface area/plasma volume ratio, **accelerating the ESR.**
  - **Anemia increases the ESR** by changing the erythrocyte/plasma ratio that favors rouleaux formation. **Polycythemia decreases ESR.**
  - **Shape of RBCs:** Red cells with an **abnormal or irregular shape**, such as **sickle cells or spherocytes, slow down rouleaux formation and lower the ESR.**
- **Technical factors:** The ESR tube must be kept vertical; otherwise, it results in inaccurate ESR.

Stages of ESR

Sedimentation occurs in three stages:

1. **Stage of aggregation/rouleaux formation:** In the **initial 10 minutes**, there is **little sedimentation** as rouleaux form. The size of the rouleaux formed influences the speed of sedimentation.
2. **Stage of settling:** For about **40 minutes**, settling occurs at a constant rate.
3. **Stage of packing:** In the **final 10 minutes** sedimentation slows and RBCs pack at the bottom of the tube.

BOX 15.3: Factors that affect ESR.

Factors that increase ESR: Old age, pregnancy, anemia, macrocytosis, raised fibrinogen

Factors that decrease ESR: Microcytosis, polycythemia, marked leukocytosis, low fibrinogen.

Methods

The commonly employed methods are as follows: **Westergren, Wintrobe, automated micro-ESR method, and ESR STAT Plus.**

Westergren Method

Q. Write a short note on Westergren pipette.

The Westergren method is widely used because the method is very simple.

Westergren pipette (tube) (Fig. 15.8A): It is a straight glass pipet **(open at both ends)** 30 cm in length, internal diameter (bore) of 2.55 mm and calibrated in millimeters from 0–200. The capacity of the tube is about 1 mL. The tube is vertically placed on the Westergren rack.

Anticoagulant used: 3.8% trisodium citrate.

Procedure

The ratio of blood and anticoagulant: Two mL of whole blood in 0.5 mL of 3.8% trisodium citrate (or 1.6 mL of blood + 0.4 mL of citrate). **Blood to anticoagulant ratio should be 4:1.**

Fill the Westergren pipette: A Westergren pipette is filled to the 0 mark. It is placed exactly vertically in the rack at room temperature without vibration or exposure to direct sunlight.

Record the reading exactly after 60 minutes: The distance from the 0 mark to the top of the column of red cells is recorded in millimeters as the ESR value at the end of the exact 60 minutes.

Modified Westergren Method

A modification of the Westergren method gives the same results. However, it **uses blood anticoagulated with EDTA** rather than with 3.8% sodium citrate. This method is more convenient because the ESR can be performed from the same tube of blood as is used for other hematologic studies.

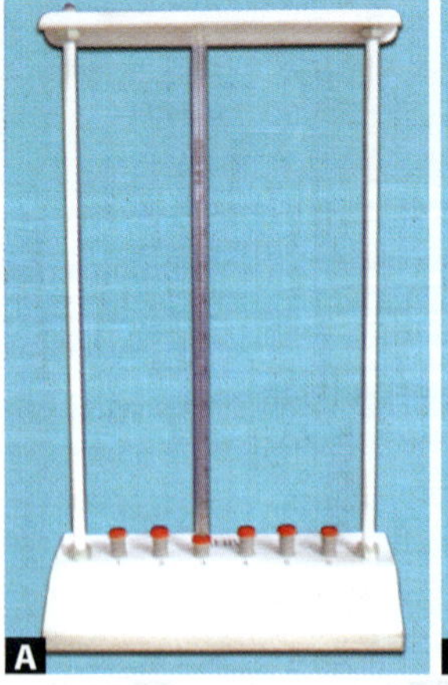

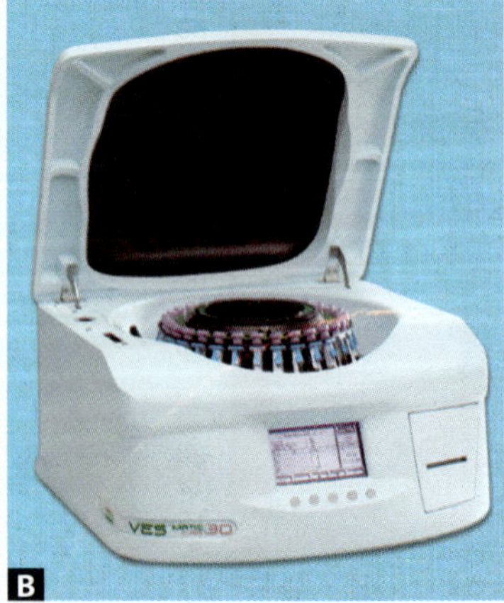

Figs. 15.8A and B: (A) Westergren pipette placed vertically in the rack for ESR (erythrocyte sedimentation rate); (B) VES-MATIC 20 instrument for automated measurement of ESR.

Procedure: Two mL (milliliters) of well-mixed EDTA blood is diluted with 0.5 mL of 3.8% sodium citrate or with 0.5 mL of 0.85% sodium chloride.

Alternative Methods and Technologies to Measure ESR

The VES-MATIC 20 instrument (Fig. 15.8B): It is a bench-top **completely automated analyser** for measuring the ESR in 20 blood samples. The **blood is collected in special cuvets** and is carefully mixed by the instrument. Then the samples are left to sediment for a certain period. The **tubes are at an 18-degree slant** with respect to the vertical axis. This accelerates the sedimentation. The **results are obtained in only 25 minutes comparable with those of Westergren at the first hour**. The optoelectrical sensors automatically read the erythrocyte sedimentation level.

The micro-ESR method: It is used in **pediatric patients**. In the micro-ESR method, 0.2 mL blood is filled into a plastic disposable tube 230 mm long with a 1-mm internal bore. The capillary blood values correlate well with venous blood micro-ESR and Westergren ESR values. Another method of micro-ESR is by using whole blood to completely fill a 75-mm heparinized microhematocrit capillary tube.

ESR stat plus: It is another instrument used to measure ESR. It is a centrifugation-based method. The blood sample is placed in the centrifuge, and an infrared laser tracks the erythrocyte-plasma interface. It makes multiple measurements and from these measurements, a linear portion of the sedimentation curve is identified. This is used by the software algorithm to determine the ESR. This method requires only smaller volumes of blood than the Westergren method and is faster. The disadvantage is the poor correlation with the reference Westergren method, especially in the 0 to 20 mm/hour range.

Indications for ESR estimation (Box 15.4).

Reference values for erythrocyte sedimentation rate (Table 15.4).

The causes of increased ESR are listed in Table 15.5. Causes of decreased ESR are (i) Polycythemia vera, (ii) sickle cell disease, and (iii) hypofibrinogenemia.

BOX 15.4: Indications for ESR.

- Suspicion of infectious, inflammatory, or neoplastic conditions
- To monitor disease activity (e.g., rheumatic fever, tuberculosis)
- As a diagnostic criterion (e.g., temporal arteritis)
- Prognostic value in Hodgkin lymphoma without systemic symptoms (ESR less than 10 mm/hour excellent survival rate)

Note: Normal ESR cannot be used to exclude these diagnostic possibilities.

TABLE 15.4 The upper limits of reference values for erythrocyte sedimentation rate.

Westergren		
Age	*Men*	*Women*
Below 50 years	15 mm/hour	20 mm/hour
Above 50 years	20 mm/hour	30 mm/hour
Above 85 years	30 mm/hour	42 mm/hour
Children	10 mm/hour	
Wintrobe, 1st hour	9 mm/hour	20 mm/hour

TABLE 15.5 Causes of increased ESR.

Markedly increased in:	**Moderately increased** in:
• Multiple myeloma • Macroglobulinemia • Hyperfibrinogenemia	• Infective diseases like tuberculosis • Chronic inflammatory diseases • Rheumatic fever, osteomyelitis • Autoimmune diseases: Rheumatoid arthritis, SLE, etc. • Neoplasia

LE CELL TEST

Q. Write a short note on the LE cell.

In autoimmune diseases (e.g., SLE, rheumatoid arthritis), a variety of antibodies are found. One of them is an antinuclear antibody (ANA) which cannot penetrate intact cells. ANAs can react with nuclei of damaged cells and convert nuclear chromatin into homogeneous material. In vivo, ANAs act on the nuclei of damaged cells and denature them into homogeneous material. This nuclear material is phagocytosed in the presence of complement by phagocytic leukocytes (neutrophils or macrophages). The LE cell (*refer* **Figs. 6.20A and B**) is any **phagocytic leukocyte** (neutrophil or macrophage) **that has engulfed the denatured nucleus of an injured cell. In the tissue, they are known as LE bodies or hematoxylin bodies.**

Tart cell: LE cell must be differentiated from a tart cell (*refer* **Fig. 6.20C**). It is a monocyte/neutrophil containing a phagocytosed nucleus of another cell. The nuclear material is not homogeneous and it retains its chromatin pattern. It may be found in healthy individuals.

Significance: LE cells may be demonstrated in **SLE, rheumatoid arthritis**, other **autoimmune disorders, hepatitis, and penicillin sensitivity.**

BONE MARROW EXAMINATION

PA 17.2 (NC): Enumerate the indications and describe the findings in bone marrow aspiration and biopsy.

The bone marrow examination **assesses the semiquantitative and qualitative state of hematopoiesis.** It helps in the diagnosis of several hereditary and acquired benign and malignant diseases. Bone marrow examination is essentially done to confirm or rule out a hematologic disorder. It also helps in the evaluation of non-hematological disorders (e.g., metastasis). Bone marrow may be obtained by:

- **Aspiration:** Bone marrow aspiration is a simple, easy, and safe procedure.
- **Trephine biopsy** is indicated in conditions where the aspiration either fails to yield marrow or to confirm some of the diseases (where biopsy findings are diagnostic).

Bone Marrow Aspiration

Q. Write a short essay on bone marrow aspiration study.

Bone marrow needles: Needles commonly employed for the aspirations of the marrow are the Salah needle **(Fig. 15.9A)** and the Klima needle.

The usual sites for bone marrow aspiration are listed in **Box 15.5**.

Q. Write a short note on indications for bone marrow aspiration.

Indications for bone marrow aspiration are listed in **Box 15.6. Contraindications for bone marrow aspiration: hemophilia, and congenital hemorrhagic disorders**.

Q. Write a short answer on the causes of dry tap in bone marrow aspiration.

Dry tap: During aspiration, if the marrow is not obtained it is called a dry tap. Dry tap is common in: **(i) hairy cell leukemia, and (ii) myelofibrosis** (marrow has been replaced by fibrous tissue).

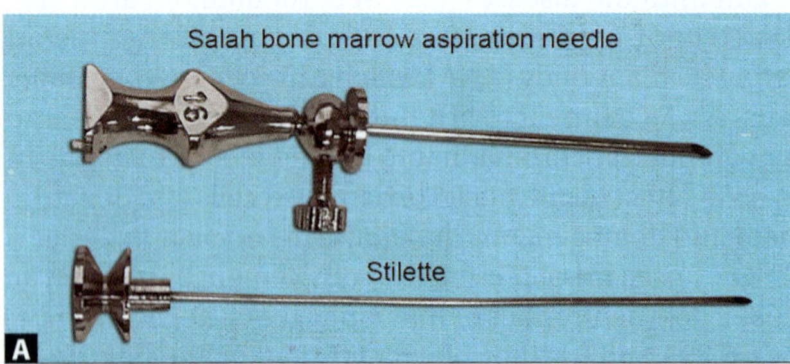

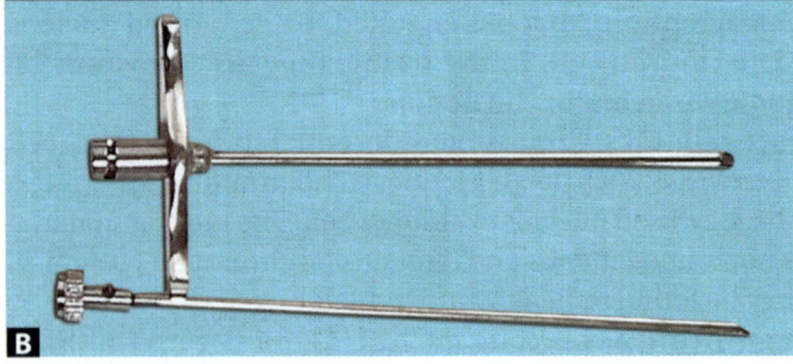

Figs. 15.9A and B: (A) Salah bone marrow aspiration needle with stilette; (B) Jamshidi trephine biopsy needle.

BOX 15.5: Usual sites for bone marrow aspiration.

- Posterior iliac crest (preferred site)
- Posterior superior iliac spine
- Sternum
- Anterior superior iliac spine
- Spinous process of lumbar vertebra.

In **infants**, the upper end of the tibia is the ideal site for marrow aspirate.

BOX 15.6: Indications for bone marrow aspiration.

Diagnostic

- **Primary hematolymphoid disorders**
  - **Red cell disorders:** Nutritional anemia (e.g., megaloblastic anemia), pure red cell aplasia
  - **White cell disorders:** Subleukemic/aleukemic leukemia, diagnosis, and classification of acute leukemias
  - **Megakaryocytic disorders:** ITP and other thrombocytopenias
  - **Myeloproliferative neoplasms:** Polycythemia vera, chronic myeloid leukemia, idiopathic thrombocythemia
  - **Myelodysplastic syndromes**
  - **Plasma cell neoplasms:** Multiple myeloma, Waldenström macroglobulinemia
- **Systemic diseases: Storage disorders** (e.g., Gaucher, Niemann–Pick disease)
- **Staging of lymphoid malignancies and solid tumors:** Lymphoma, metastatic deposits (e.g., carcinoma prostate, breast, lung, kidney)
- **Detection of infection and/or source of pyrexia of unknown origin (PUO)**
  - **Parasitic disorders:** Kala-azar
  - **Fungal disorders:** Histoplasma
  - **Mycobacterial infection**
- **Iron store**
- **Miscellaneous disorders:** Pancytopenia or unexplained cytopenias, PUO

Post-treatment follow-up: To know the response to therapy and follow-up in cases of leukemia, aplastic anemia, and agranulocytosis

Therapeutic: Hematopoietic stem cell (formerly called bone marrow) transplant

Complications of bone marrow aspiration and/or biopsy are **(i) local infection, (ii) hemorrhage, and (iii) cardiac tamponade or mediastinitis.**

Special studies: In certain situations, an additional bone marrow aspirate specimen is collected for ancillary testing. These include **flow cytometry analysis, karyotype, and fluorescent in situ hybridization (FISH) assays and molecular studies.**

The format for bone marrow smear reporting is shown in **Box 15.7**.

Bone Marrow Trephine Biopsy

Marrow trephine biopsy is performed by one of the trephine biopsy needles like the Jamshidi needle **(Fig. 15.9B)**, Westerman–Jensen needle or Islam needle. The biopsy obtained consists of a core of bone with marrow. These are excellent for morphological evaluation as well as for special stains. Trephine biopsy tissue is decalcified and processed like other histopathological tissue containing bone. Sections are stained with hematoxylin and eosin stain,

BOX 15.7: The format for evaluation of bone marrow smear.

- **Cellularity:** It is expressed as the ratio of the volume of hematopoietic cells to the total volume of the marrow space (cells plus fat and other stromal elements). It may be normocellular, hypocellular, or hypercellular. Cellularity of marrow should be correlated with the age of the patient.
- **M: E ratio:** The ratio of total myeloid (total granulocytes) and erythroid cells (total normoblasts). It is normally 2:1 to 4:1.
- **Erythropoiesis:** Erythroid precursors are examined for the:
  - Marrow response: Normal/increased/decreased
  - Maturation: Normoblastic/megaloblastic/micronormoblastic
  - Dyserythropoiesis.
- **Myelopoiesis:** It is examined for:
  - Marrow response: Normal/increased/decreased
  - Maturation arrest
  - Morphological abnormalities: Hypergranular/absent granules
  - Abnormal cells/blasts.
- **Megakaryopoiesis:** They are examined for:
  - Number
  - Morphology.
- **Lymphocytes:** Normal/increased/abnormal.
- **Plasma cells:** Normal/increased.
- **Others:** Metastatic tumor cells, parasites (malaria, Leishmania donovani) and fungus or any other abnormal cells.
- **Iron stores**
  - Iron stores are evaluated by Prussian blue reaction (Perl's stain).
  - Iron stores are commented as normal/increased/decreased or nil.
- **Cytochemistry/special stains.**

reticulin stain, and Masson's trichrome stain (for fibrous tissue). Immunocytochemical staining can be performed especially for acute leukemias. Bone marrow biopsy provides information about the bone marrow architecture, whereas cellular details are better appreciated on the bone marrow aspirate smears.

Sites of trephine biopsy: These include the **posterior superior iliac spine (most used site), anterior superior iliac spine, and spinous process of vertebra.**

Indications for Trephine Biopsy (Box 15.8)

Q. Write a short note on indications for bone marrow trephine biopsy.

Findings in bone marrow aspiration/biopsy of RBC disorders, WBC disorders, and hemostatic disorders are discussed in Chapters 11, 12, and 13 respectively.

OSMOTIC FRAGILITY TEST (OFT)

Q. Write a short note on the osmotic fragility test.

The normal red cell membrane is unstretchable and is freely permeable to water. RBCs are not lysed in normal

BOX 15.8: Indications for trephine biopsy.

- Aplastic anemia
- Myeloproliferative neoplasms—to study reticulin fibrosis in myelofibrosis
- Myelodysplastic syndromes
- Pre- and post-hematopoietic stem cell (bone marrow) transplantation
- Pyrexia of unknown origin (granuloma of tuberculosis)
- Bone morphology in chronic renal failure, osteoporosis, and osteomalacia
- Staging
  - Lymphoma
  - To detect metastasis in cancer patients
- Acquired immune deficiency syndrome (AIDS)

buffered (pH 7) saline solution (9 g/L NaCl). The osmotic fragility test **measures the ability of RBCs to withstand lysis when suspended in buffered solutions of various concentrations of sodium chloride** (NaCl). The pattern of lysis helps to determine whether the shape of RBCs is normal or abnormal. **Spherocytes and stomatocytes hemolyze with higher concentrations of NaCl compared to normal red blood cells.**

Principle

- In the osmotic fragility test, red cells (small volumes of blood) are suspended in a series of tubes containing buffered hypotonic solutions of NaCl (large excess of buffered saline), varying from 0.9% to 0.0% (**Figs. 15.10A and B**). The hypotonic solutions mean the strength of the saline solution is decreased below normal saline (normal saline strength is 0.9%).
- The tubes are incubated at room temperature for 30 minutes, and then centrifuged. The percent hemolysis in the supernatant solutions of each tube is measured and plotted for each NaCl concentration.
- In hypotonic saline, the volume of red blood cells progressively increases till a "critical hemolytic volume" is reached. The red cell membrane ruptures and liberates hemoglobin into the supernatant solution at this critical point. The ability of normal RBCs to withstand hypotonic solution lies in its biconcave shape which allows considerable water to enter the RBC before it stretches enough to break or lyse.
- Incubation of blood overnight at 37°C makes the osmotic fragility test (OFT) more sensitive.

Interpretation

Normal: Lysis of fresh RBCs begins at 0.5% of NaCl solution and is complete at 0.3%. It may be normal in patients with mild HS.

Increased Osmotic Fragility

If RBCs are spherocytic (more spherical) with a decreased surface/volume ratio, they have a limited capacity to expand in hypotonic solutions. The loss of membrane in spherocytes causes a reduction in their surface area. The spherocytes cannot expand as much as normal biconcave

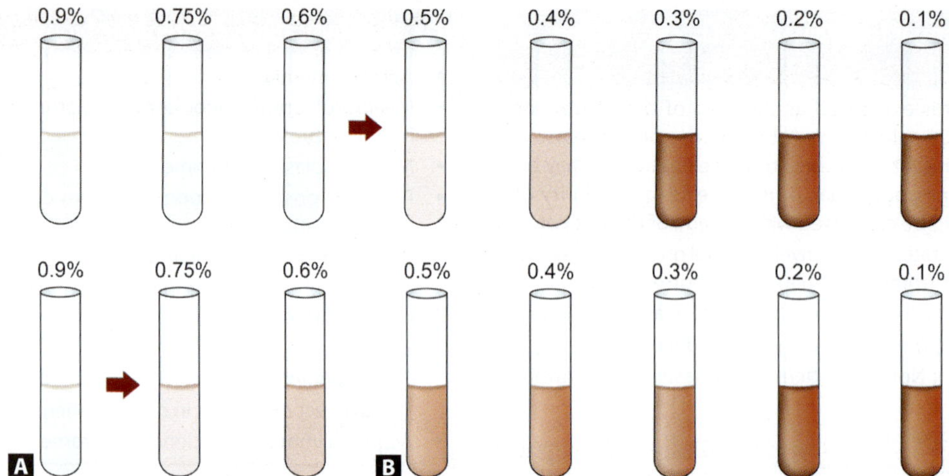

Figs. 15.10A and B: (A) Normal osmotic fragility of fresh RBCs in which hemolysis begins at 0.5% and completes at 0.3%; (B) Abnormal hemolysis begins even at mild dilution (0.75%) in hereditary spherocytosis. (Note: Only a few different concentrations of NaCl solutions are shown).

RBCs and there is a decrease in the critical hemolytic volume. When the strength of the saline solution is decreased (hypotonic) **spherocytic red cells** (which do not have normal biconcave shape) will begin to **hemolyze** early **at a higher concentration of NaCl than do normal biconcave red cells.** The sooner hemolysis occurs, the greater the osmotic fragility of the cells. They are said to have increased osmotic fragility. They show a **shift to the right** of the normal range in the graph **(Fig. 15.11)**. Increased osmotic fragility indicates that the red cells are spherocytic. **Conditions with increased osmotic fragility**: It is observed in **hereditary spherocytosis (hemolysis begins at 0.6 to 0.8% compared to normal 0.5% of NaCl solution), hereditary elliptocytosis,** and other **conditions associated with spherocytosis, like in autoimmune hemolytic anemia, ABO hemolytic disease of newborn and burns.**

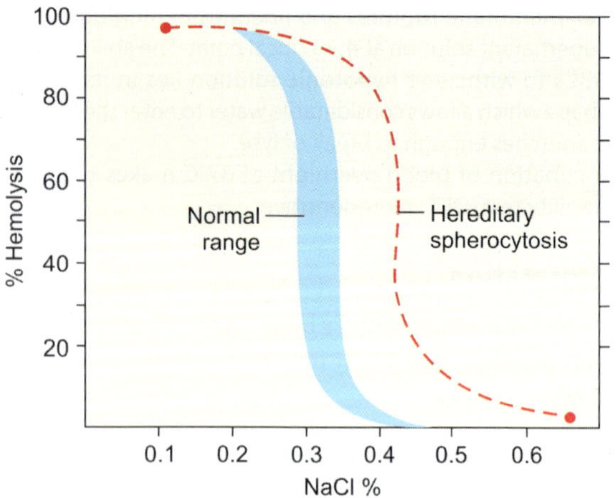

Fig. 15.11: Osmotic fragility test. Normal curve (blue) and increased osmotic fragility in hereditary spherocytosis.

Decreased Osmotic Fragility

Red cells that are hypochromic and flatter have an increased capacity to expand in hypotonic solutions. They lyse at a lower concentration than normal cells. Thus, these red cells have decreased osmotic fragility. The graph shows the **shift to the left** of the normal range and indicates that the red cells are flattened or hypochromic. This type of RBC has an increased surface/volume ratio.

Conditions with decreased osmotic fragility: It is found in **iron deficiency, thalassemia (target cells have increased surface volume), sickle cell anemia, liver disease, and reticulocytosis.**

Use: For the diagnosis of spherocytosis. However, it is time-consuming and, tedious, and cannot distinguish between the causes of spherocytosis. This test may be negative if there are only a few spherocytes in the peripheral blood. The sensitivity of the test can be increased by incubation the red cells at 37°C for 24 hours before performing the test. This test is termed an osmotic fragility test after incubation.

URINE ANALYSIS

PA 23.1 (CC): Describe abnormal urinary findings in disease states and identify and describe common urinary abnormalities in a clinical specimen.

Many different diseases show abnormalities in the urine. Urine analysis (urinalysis) reflects the state of function of the kidneys and urinary tract. It provides information about metabolic or systemic (nonrenal) disorders. Therefore, urine examination is an important laboratory investigation that should precede all other invasive/noninvasive diagnostic investigations for renal function.

Methods of Collection

Q. Write a short note on urine sample collection.

- **First voided morning urine**: It is the most concentrated and is often the best specimen for routine analysis. Some tests may require a 12- or 24-hour urine sample.
- **Midstream specimen:** This is used for all types of urine examination. After voiding the first half of the urine into the toilet, a part of the next voided urine is collected as a midstream sample.
- **Clean-catch specimen:** This is the method of collection for culture and sensitivity of urine. The external genitalia are cleaned with soap and water and the specimen is collected as mentioned in the midstream sample.
- **Catheter specimen:** It is used for culture and sensitivity in bed-ridden patients or patients with urinary tract obstruction.
- **Collection from infants:** It is usually collected by a clean plastic bag attached around the genitalia. For bacteriological examination urine is aspirated from the bladder by needle.

Preservation of Urine

Q. Write a short note on preservatives for urine collection.

The urine sample should be **examined within 2 hours** of collection. **If delay is likely to occur, it should be preserved** by one of the following methods:

- Refrigeration without any preservative
- Use of preservatives like **toluene** (add a few drops to form a thin layer on the urine surface), **concentrated HCl** (in the ratio of 1 mL for 125 mL of urine), **thymol, and formaldehyde** (add 1 drop for 15 mL of urine—preserves cells and casts).

Examination of urine: Basic urine examination consists of (i) physical (gross) examination, (ii) chemical examination, and (iii) microscopic examination.

Physical/Gross Examination

Q. Write a short note on the physical examination of urine.

Volume

Q. Write a short answer on the volume of urine.

Q. Write a short answer on oliguria.

A healthy adult excretes about **600–2,000 mL of urine in 24 hours**. In infants, the volume is 300–600 mL/day. The volume of urine is measured by collecting 24-hour urine samples in a measuring cylinder.

- **Polyuria:** It is defined as increased urine output of **more than 2 liters in 24 hours**. Its causes include physiological (e.g., increased fluid intake/polydipsia) or pathological [e.g., **diabetes mellitus with hyperglycemia, chronic renal failure** (functioning renal tissue is diminished and the ability to concentrate urine is gradually lost), **diuretic therapy, diabetes insipidus, primary aldosteronism**].
- **Oliguria:** It is decreased **urinary output of less than 500 mL in 24 hours**. Its causes include **restricted intake of fluid, excessive loss of fluid** (e.g., in hemorrhage, burns, dehydration, and shock) **renal diseases** (e.g., acute glomerulonephritis, nephrotic syndrome, acute tubular necrosis as in shock, burns, crush syndrome, incompatible blood transfusion and heavy metal poisoning) and Addison's disease.
- **Anuria:** It is the **near-complete suppression of urine formation**. There is markedly diminished urine output, usually **less than 125 mL in 24 hours**. Causes include **renal ischemia, renal tumors, and renal stones**.

Color (Table 15.6)

Normal urine is **straw/yellow/amber-colored** due to the presence of urochrome pigment, the excretion of which is generally proportional to the metabolic rate. It is increased during fever, thyrotoxicosis, and starvation.

Q. Write a short note on chyluria.

Chyluria is a rare condition in which the **urine contains lymph. Obstruction to lymph flow** and rupture of lymphatic vessels into the renal pelvis, ureters, bladder, or urethra may be associated with chyluria. The causes include **filariasis** (*Wuchereria bancrofti*), **abdominal lymphadenopathy, and tumors**. The amount of lymph determines the color of urine which may range from clear to opaque or milky. It contains fatty material which can be extracted from urine using an equal volume of ether or chloroform.

Lipiduria: In **nephrotic syndrome**, urine shows fat globules which are triglycerides (neutral fat) and cholesterol. It may

TABLE 15.6 Conditions associated with color changes in urine.

Color	Condition
Colorless	Dilute urine as in polyuria (e.g., diabetes mellitus, diabetes insipidus)
Dark brown	Oliguria
Red or red-brown (smoky)	Red blood cells (hematuria), hemoglobinuria, myoglobinuria
Yellow-brown or green-brown	Bile pigments mainly bilirubin
Orange-red or orange-brown	Urobilinogen is colorless but is converted in the presence of light and low pH to urobilin, which is dark yellow to orange
Cola colored	Intravascular hemolysis, rhabdomyolysis
Dark-brown colored on standing	Alkaptonuria (presence of homogentisic acid), melanin
Milky	Pus (pyuria/many neutrophils), lipiduria, or chyle (chyluria)
Cloudy	Various cellular elements (e.g., leukocytes, RBCs, epithelial cells, spermatozoa), bacterial growth

TABLE 15.7 Examples of characteristic urine odors associated with amino acid disorders.

Amino acid disorder	*Urine odor*
Cystinuria	Rotten eggs
Ketoacidosis	Sweet, fruity
Phenylketonuria	Mousy, musty
Trimethylaminuria	Rotting fish
Tyrosinemia	Rancid

also be observed in patients with skeletal trauma with fractures of major long bones or the pelvis.

Odor

Urine normally has a **faint, aromatic odor** of an undetermined source. Extensive bacterial overgrowth in the urine can produce an ammoniacal, fetid odor. Characteristic urine odors associated with a few amino acid disorders are presented in **Table 15.7.** Lack of odor in urine from patients with acute renal failure suggests acute tubular necrosis (ATN) rather than prerenal failure.

Specific Gravity

Q. Write a short answer on the specific gravity of urine including normal values and methods of estimation.

The specific gravity of urine is **used as a measure of the concentrating power of the kidney**. It indicates the relative proportions of dissolved solid components to the total volume of the urine (reflects the density of the specimen). Specific gravity depends on the number, density, and weight of the solute particles in the urine. Most of the specific gravity of normal urine is due to urea (20%), sodium chloride (25%), sulfate, and phosphate. In normal adults, the specific gravity is **1.016 to 1.022** over 24 hours. However, normal kidneys can produce urine with a specific gravity that ranges from 1.003 to 1.035. **Specific gravity provides information about the renal status and hydration.**

Methods

Specific gravity (SG) is measured by: (i) reagent strip (dipstick), (ii) urinometer, (iii) refractometer, and (iv) falling drop method. The urinometer and refractometer methods are more accurate as compared to the dipstick method.

Reagent strip

This is an indirect method of measuring specific gravity. The reagent area has three main ingredients: **polyelectrolyte, indicator substance, and buffer**.

Principle: This method is based on the pKa (acid dissociation constant) change of pretreated polyelectrolytes in relation to the ionic concentration of the urine. When the ionic concentration is high, the pKa and pH are decreased. The indicator substance (bromothymol blue) then changes color relative to ionic concentration. This is then translated to specific gravity values.

Inference: The results of this method should be used with caution. This is because it is not affected by the substances that raise the specific gravity such as glucose, protein, or radiographic contrast material.

Urinometer

The urinometer (**Fig. 15.12**) is a specialized hydrometer adapted to directly measure the specific gravity of urine. It consists of a weighted glass cylinder that floats in urine and has a calibrated stem to measure specific gravity at a given temperature. The scale in many urinometers is read in small divisions from 1.000 to 1060. The temperature influences the specific gravity. The **urinometer is usually calibrated in the range of 15–20°C** (depending on the manufacturer). It should be checked each day by measuring the specific gravity of distilled water. If the urinometer does not give a reading of 1.000, an appropriate temperature correction must be applied to all readings taken with that urinometer.

- **Temperature correction:** For **every 3°C rise** in room temperature beyond the calibrated temperature (15°C), **add 0.001** to the recorded reading; and **subtract 0.001** for every 3°C fall in temperature.
- **Correction for protein and sugar present in urine:** Subtract 0.003 for every 1 g/dL of protein and 0.004 for every 1 g/dL of glucose.

Procedure: The urinometer vessel (cylinder) is filled three-fourths full with urine (the minimum volume required is about 15 mL). The urinometer is inserted into the vessel containing urine with a spinning motion. Make sure that it is floating freely without touching the sides or the bottom of the cylinder. Avoid bubbles on the surface, which masks the meniscus. Take the reading of the bottom of the meniscus.

Refractometer method

It is an indirect method based on the refractive index of urine and has the advantage of requiring only a few drops of urine.

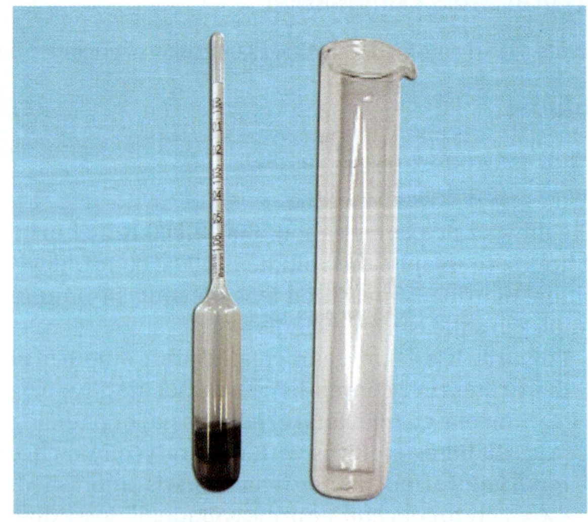

Fig. 15.12: Urinometer for specific gravity measurement.

Q. Write a short answer on the causes of increased and decreased specific gravity of urine.

Causes of increased specific gravity: Glycosuria (e.g., diabetes mellitus), **proteinuria** (e.g., nephrotic syndrome), **dehydration** (e.g., restricted fluid intake, diarrhea, vomiting, fever, and excessive sweating).

Q. Write a short answer on hyposthenuria.

Hyposthenuria (decreased specific gravity): Hyposthenuria is the **secretion of urine of low specific gravity (less than 1.007)** due to the inability of the kidney to concentrate the urine normally. It is closely related to isosthenuria in which the urine has a relatively low specific gravity, though not necessarily equal to that of plasma. Therefore, unlike isosthenuria, this condition is not associated with renal failure as the kidney tubules have altered the glomerular filtrate. Hyposthenuria indicates that the kidney can dilute the urine but is unable to concentrate, i.e., proximal renal tubule and loop of Henle function are retained but the tubules are unresponsive to ADH, either from a primary ADH deficiency (central diabetes insipidus) or lack of responsiveness of renal tubules to ADH due to renal tubular disease or inhibitors of ADH (nephrogenic diabetes insipidus).

- **Causes of hyposthenuria: Excessive fluid intake, diabetes insipidus, and end-stage kidney** (e.g., chronic glomerulonephritis, chronic pyelonephritis, bilateral polycystic kidneys, and hypertension).

Q. Write a short answer on the low fixed specific gravity of urine and its importance.

Isosthenuria (fixed specific gravity): When the **specific gravity of urine is low and fixed at 1.010**, this is known as isosthenuria. In this condition, the urine whose specific gravity (concentration) is neither greater (more concentrated) nor less (more dilute) than that of protein-free plasma (1.008–1.012). It is **indicative of severe renal damage** (chronic renal failure) with **disturbance of both the concentrating and diluting abilities of the kidney**. It reflects damage to the kidney's tubules or the renal medulla.

Chemical Examination

Nowadays, reagent strips are the primary method used for the chemical examination of urine. A basic chemical examination consists of a dipstick analysis for sugar, blood, white blood cells, and other substances. The reading of the strips is traditionally done manually. Automated instruments are now available that will aspirate a precise amount of urine, deposit it on the dipstick, and read the chemical reactions on the reagent strip. These systems give accurate results and are not prone to some of the inconsistencies that occur when done manually. This avoids human errors such as reading at the exact time of the reactions and visual discrimination of different shades of color reactions.

Urine pH

Normal urine is **usually acidic**. However, urinary pH ranges from 4.6 to 8 (if pH is <7 = acidic, if pH is 7.0 = neutral, and if pH is >7.0 = alkaline). Urinary pH is measured as given below.

Litmus paper technique: The reaction of urine is determined with blue and red litmus paper. The urine when examined must be fresh as it turns alkaline on standing due to bacterial decomposition. **Acidic urine turns blue litmus paper red. Alkaline urine turns red litmus paper blue**. Both blue and red litmus papers turn reddish purple when the urine is faintly on the acid side (pH 7.0) or neutral.

Reagent strip: It uses a double indicator system consisting of methyl red and bromothymol blue in the reagent strips. They give a range of orange, green, and blue colors as the pH rises. This allows estimation of pH values within the range of 5 to 9.

Causes of alkaline and acidic urine are shown in **Table 15.8**.

Protein in Urine

Q. What is proteinuria? Name the methods of its detection.

Normally, the daily excretion of protein in the urine is up to 150 mg. Normally, plasma proteins with a molecular weight of less than 50,000–60,000 pass through the glomerular basement membrane and are reabsorbed by cells of the proximal tubules. Only very small amounts of albumin (molecular weight 69,000) are filtered. **Tamm-Horsfall glycoprotein (uromucoid) is secreted by distal tubular cells and cells of the ascending loop of Henle.** These Tamm-Horsfall glycoproteins constitute one-third or more of the total normal protein loss.

Proteinuria: It is the **presence of detectable protein in the urine**. The presence of an abnormal amount of protein in urine is an important indicator of renal disease (particularly glomerular injury). If urine is turbid, filter or centrifuge it before testing.

TABLE 15.8 Causes of alkaline and acidic urine.

Alkaline urine	*Acidic urine*
• Metabolic and respiratory alkalosis • Phosphaturia • Severe vomiting • Infection with ammonia producing urea splitting bacteria like *Proteus* • Potassium deficiency • Hyperaldosteronism • Intake of fruits of the citrus family (orange) • Intake of bicarbonates	• High protein diet • Febrile illness • Ketonuria (e.g. diabetes mellitus, starvation) • Leukemia • Urinary tract infection by *Escherichia coli* • Starvation • Severe diarrhea • Diabetes mellitus • Respiratory disease

BOX 15.9: Tests for protein.

- Reagent strip method
- Heat and acetic acid test
- Sulfosalicylic acid test
- Heller's test

Q. Write a short answers on tests for proteinuria.

Various methods of detection of protein in urine are presented in **Box 15.9**. The reagent strip method is sensitive to albumin while acid precipitation methods detect all proteins.

Reagent Strip Method

Principle: The test is based on the protein error of pH indicators. Proteins carry a charge at physiologic pH, and their presence will elicit a pH change. Thus, any color change in the indicator is due to protein. The reagent strip is impregnated with an indicator tetrabromophenol blue, or tetrachlorophenol-tetrabromosulfophthalein buffered to pH 3.0. At this pH, it is yellow in the absence of protein. If urine contains protein (which will elicit a pH change), it forms a complex with the indicator turning its color to variable shades of green or bluish-green depending on the type and concentration of protein present. The color change occurs within 30–60 seconds following urine application. Results may be read in a "plus" system as negative, trace, and 1+ to 4+. They can detect 5–20 mg of albumin per deciliter.

Heat and Acetic Acid Test

Principle: Heat-induced coagulation of proteins and precipitation. Coagulation can be further enhanced when drops of acetic acid are added.

- **Procedure:** Take a 5 mL test tube and fill 2/3rd with urine. Acidify by adding a few drops of 3% acetic acid if the urine is alkaline. Boil the upper portion for 2 minutes (the **lower part acts as a control**). If precipitation or turbidity appears, add a few drops of 3% acetic acid.
- **Interpretation:** If turbidity or precipitation disappears after the addition of acetic acid, it is due to phosphates; if it persists after the addition of acetic acid, then it is due to proteins. The test is semiquantitative and can be graded from traces to 4+ depending upon the amount of protein.

Acetic Acid Test for Bence-Jones Protein

Procedure: Take 5 mL of clear urine in a test tube and 1 mL of acetate buffer. Heat the urine in a water bath with a thermometer inside. At 40°C, **Bence-Jones proteins start precipitating till 58°C when the precipitation is complete. If urine is heated beyond 60°C, Bence-Jones proteins dissolve in the urine and reappear on cooling at 60°C.** However, the best method for the detection of Bence-Jones protein in urine is by protein electrophoresis.

Sulfosalicylic Acid Test

Q. Write a short answer on a sulfosalicylic acid test.

- This test **detects all types of proteins** (albumin, globulin, glycoproteins, and Bence–Jones proteins).

Principle: Cold precipitation of proteins by a strong acid. More sensitive and reliable than heat and acetic acid tests.

- **Procedure:** Take 2.5 mL of urine in a small test tube. Slowly pour 2.5 mL of 3% sulfosalicylic acid. Wait for 10 minutes.
- **Interpretation:** The presence of a **cloudy precipitate** indicates the presence of proteins in urine. However, it also precipitates mucus and Bence–Jones proteins.

Heller's Test

Principle: Cold precipitation of proteins by a strong acid.

- **Procedure:** Take 5 mL of urine in a test tube and add a few drops of concentrated nitric acid.
- **Interpretation:** The presence of proteins is indicated by a **white ring** at the junction of urine and acid.
- **Precaution:** Filter urine if turbid as it interferes with the final reading.

Quantitative Estimation of Proteins in Urine

Q. Write a short answer on Esbach's albuminometer.

Protein excretion in a 24-hour urine sample is required in suspected cases of nephrotic syndrome (>3.5 g/24 hours) and orthostatic/postural proteinuria. This may be carried out by Esbach's albuminometer **(Fig. 15.13)** method.

Principle: Cold precipitation of proteins by a strong acid.

Procedure: Fill the albuminometer with urine up to the mark U. Add Esbach's reagent (contains picric acid

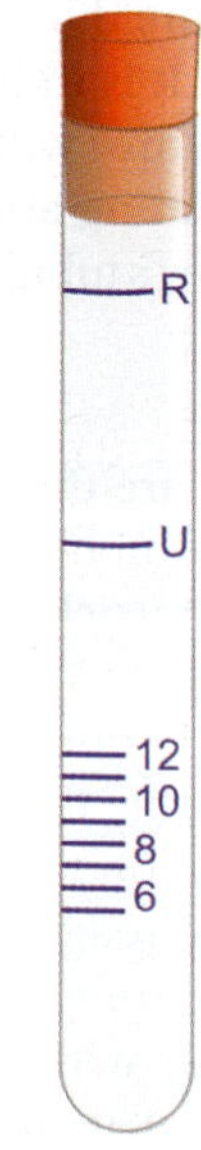

Fig. 15.13: Esbach's albuminometer used for quantitative measurement of proteins in urine.

and citric acid) up to the mark R. Stopper the Esbach's albuminometer, mix, and allow it to stand for 24 hours. Take the reading from the level of precipitation in the albuminometer and divide the value by 10 to get the percentage of total proteins.

Categories of Proteinuria

- **Proteinuria quantification:** Classified depending on the amount of protein in the urine as **heavy** (>4 g/day), **moderate** (1–4 g/day), and **mild** (<1 g/day) proteinuria.
- **Qualitative categories of proteinuria:** Classified depending on the structure involved as (i) **renal** (glomerular causes/pattern, tubular cause/pattern), (ii) **prerenal,** and (iii) **postrenal.**

Types of glomerular proteinuria

Q. Write a short note on selective proteinuria.

- **Selective proteinuria:** In this type, only intermediate-sized (<100 kDa) proteins (such as albumin, and transferrin) leak through the glomerulus.
- **Nonselective proteinuria:** It is characterized by leakage of a range of different proteins including larger proteins (e.g., immunoglobulins) through the glomerulus.

Causes of Proteinuria (Box 15.10)

Q. Write a short note on the causes of proteinuria.

Bence-Jones proteins (*refer* **page 398**): These are light chains of immunoglobulins, secreted in **multiple myeloma.** It may also be found in macroglobulinemia and lymphoma. Bence-Jones proteins **precipitate at temperatures between 40°C and 60°C, and redissolve near 100°C. It reappears on cooling to 40–60°C.**

Microalbuminuria

Screening tests for urine protein are not sensitive enough to detect very small quantities of protein. **Microalbuminuria is the presence of albumin in urine above the normal level but below the detectable range of conventional methods.** It is defined as the **persistent elevation of the urinary albumin excretion of 20–200 mg/L** (or 20–200 μg/min) in an **early morning urine sample.** It indicates early and possibly reversible glomerular damage. Microalbuminuria is measured by immunologic means using antibodies to the proteins, nephelometric methods, immunoassay, protein strip electrophoresis, or high-performance liquid chromatography (HPLC).

Causes of microalbuminuria

- **Diabetes mellitus:** In diabetic patients, the presence of microalbuminuria is associated with **increased cardiovascular mortality** and is a risk factor for **renal mortality.** Early detection can predict the development of renal complications in diabetics.
- **Essential hypertension:** In hypertensive patients, microalbuminuria **predicts cardiovascular morbidity and mortality.**

BOX 15.10: Causes and amount of proteinuria.

1. **Renal**
   - A. **Glomerular damage:** Due to increased permeability of the glomerular capillary wall
     - **Heavy proteinuria:** Nephrotic syndrome
     - **Moderate to heavy:** Acute rapidly progressive glomerulonephritis, chronic glomerulonephritis, malignant hypertension, SLE
     - **Mild to moderate:** Acute glomerulonephritis, nephrosclerosis
   - B. **Tubular damage:** Inability to absorb low molecular weight proteins by tubules
     - **Moderate:** Heavy metal and vitamin D intoxication
     - **Mild:** Acute and chronic pyelonephritis, acute tubular necrosis, polycystic kidney disease, hypokalemia
2. **Prerenal**
   - A. **Overflow proteinuria:** This develops due to the overflow of excess levels of protein in the circulation. This protein in the urine may be hemoglobin, myoglobin, or immunoglobulin
     - **Immunoglobulin: Moderate proteinuria** in plasma cell dyscrasias (Bence-Jones protein-light chain of immunoglobulin)
     - **Hemoglobin:** In intravascular hemolysis
     - **Myoglobin:** In skeletal muscle trauma
     - **Lysozyme:** Acute myeloid leukemia M4 or M5
   - B. **Hemodynamic proteinuria:** Due to alteration of blood flow through glomeruli
     - **Mild asymptomatic proteinuria:** After excessive exercise, postural (orthostatic) albuminuria, congestive cardiac failure, high fever, exposure to cold, dehydration
3. **Postrenal:** Inflammatory or neoplastic lesions of the renal pelvis, ureter, bladder, prostate, or urethra

Glucose and Other Sugars in Urine

Reducing substances are those compounds that **reduce cupric ions (from copper sulfate in Benedict's reagent) in an alkaline solution to cuprous ions (cuprous oxide).** Such substances may be sugar or nonsugar.

- **Sugar:** These include glucose, fructose, galactose, lactose, pentose, maltose, and sucrose. Sucrose gives negative results with Benedict's test and glucose oxidase. Special tests are required to differentiate the sugar occurring in urine.
- **Nonsugar:** These include **ascorbic acid**, uric acid, urates, glucuronides, chloroform, formaldehyde, **salicylates, streptomycin, phenol, PAS,** homogentisic acid (alkaptonuria), and creatinine.

Glucose: Blood glucose level varies between 70 and 120 mg/dL. This may increase to 120–160 mg/dL after a meal. Normally, all the glucose in the blood is filtered through the glomerulus and reabsorbed at proximal tubules. If the renal threshold (the lowest blood glucose level that will result in glycosuria) is exceeded (usually greater than 180–200 mg/dL), the excess glucose will not be reabsorbed into the blood and will be eliminated in the urine as in

BOX 15.11: Tests for reducing substances in urine.

- Reagent strip method
- Benedict qualitative test

cases of diabetes mellitus. The presence of detectable amounts of **glucose in urine** is termed **glycosuria.**

Q. Write a short note on the test for the detection of glycosuria.

Tests for reducing substances are discussed in **Box 15.11.**

Reagent Strip

Principle: The reagent strip (diastix/multistix/dipstix) method is based on a **specific glucose oxidase and peroxidase method,** a double sequential enzyme reaction. The strips contain (i) glucose oxidase, (ii) peroxidase, and (iii) a chromogen. The reagent strips differ only in the chromogen used. Thus, chromogen is O-toluidine in clinistix or potassium iodide in multistix/diastix. The method is specific to glucose. It does not produce any reaction with lactose, galactose, fructose, or reducing metabolites of drugs. Glucose present in the urine is oxidized by atmospheric oxygen in the presence of glucose oxidase to gluconic acid and hydrogen peroxide. The hydrogen peroxide, in the presence of peroxidase, oxidizes the reduced chromogen present in the dipstick to various shades of purple (oxidized chromogen). The color change depends on the amount of glucose present in the urine. Thus, it is a semiquantitative method and the results are reported as approximate grams per deciliter.

The chemistry of reagent strips is as follows:

$$\text{Glucose} + O_2 \xrightarrow{\text{Glucose oxidase}} \text{Gluconic acid} + H_2O_2$$

$$H_2O_2 + \text{Chromogen} \xrightarrow{\text{Peroxidase}} \text{Oxidized chromogen} + H_2O$$

Benedict Qualitative Test (Semiquantitative)

Q. Write a short note on the principle of the Benedict test.

The qualitative Benedict method is the copper reduction method is a sensitive test for the detection of reducing substances in urine. This test detects the presence of reducing substances in urine and is not specific for glucose.

Principle: The copper sulfate present in Benedict's reagent reacts with the **reducing substances** in the urine. This **converts cupric sulfate in the reagent to cuprous oxide** in hot alkaline media. Thus, this test is based on the reduction of cupric ions in Benedict's solution to cuprous ions. In the absence of reducing substances in urine, the color of the reagent remains blue.

The chemistry of Benedict reagent is as follows:

$$\text{Copper sulfate } (CuSO_4) \xrightarrow[\text{Reducing substance in urine}]{\text{Hot alkaline solution, Heat}} \text{Cuprous oxide } (Cu_2O \text{ (red)}) + \text{Water } (H_2O)$$

Procedure: Take **5 mL of Benedict's** (qualitative) reagent in a test tube. Boil to exclude the presence of reducing substance in the reagent. Add **8 drops (0.5 mL) of protein-free urine.** Boil the mixture for 5 minutes and allow to cool. The **ratio** of 5 mL of Benedict's reagent and 8 drops (0.5 mL) of urine **is important because it is a semiquantitative test.** Note the color of the precipitate which is cuprous oxide formed due to the reduction of cupric sulfate of Benedict's reagent.

Interpretation: The change of color from blue to green, yellow, and orange/red depends on the amount of sugar present.

Cause of Glycosuria (Box 15.12)

Q. Write a short note on the causes of glycosuria.

The substances that may give a positive reaction with Benedict's test but negative with glucose oxidase strips are nonsugar substances, such as ascorbic acid, glucuronic acid, homogentisic acid, salicylates, phenylketonuria, and tyrosinemia.

Renal glycosuria: Renal glycosuria is a benign condition due to a **reduced renal threshold for glucose** (180 mg/dL). It is unrelated to diabetes and not accompanied by the classical symptoms of diabetes. Therefore, it should not be mistaken as diabetes mellitus.

Alimentary glycosuria: In certain individuals, blood **glucose levels** may **rapidly increase after meals resulting in its spillover into urine.** This condition is known as alimentary (lag storage) glycosuria. It may be seen in some normal individuals and some patients with hepatic diseases, hyperthyroidism, and peptic ulcer.

Fructosuria: Presence of fructose in urine. It is detected by Seliwanoff's test. *Causes* include a high intake of fruits like grapes and oranges.

BOX 15.12: Causes of glycosuria.

Glycosuria with hyperglycemia

- Endocrine disorders
  - **Diabetes mellitus**
  - Acromegaly
  - Cushing's syndrome
  - Hyperthyroidism
  - Hyperadrenocorticism
  - Functioning α- or β-cell pancreatic tumors
  - Pheochromocytoma
  - Pancreatic disease with loss of functioning islet cells: For example, carcinoma, pancreatitis, and cystic fibrosis
- Non-endocrine diseases
  - Increased intracranial tension (brain tumor or hemorrhage)
  - Liver disorders
  - Drugs: Corticosteroids, adrenocorticotrophic hormones, thiazides
  - Alimentary glycosuria

Glycosuria without hyperglycemia

- Renal glycosuria
- Pregnancy

Lactosuria: Presence of lactose in urine. It is detected by Rubner's test. *Causes*—suckling infants and nursing mothers.

Pentosuria: Presence of pentose in urine. It is detected by Bial's test. *Cause*—ingestion of fruits.

Ketone Bodies

Q. Write a short note on ketone bodies found in urine and tests for its detection.

In cases of defective carbohydrate metabolism or absorption, or when an insufficient amount of carbohydrates is present in the diet, the fat is used as a source of energy. **When increased quantities of fat are metabolized, there is increased production of ketone bodies** (products of incomplete fat metabolism) which begin to accumulate in the blood (ketonemia) and are subsequently excreted in the urine (ketonuria).

Ketone bodies: In ketonuria, the three main metabolically related ketone bodies are found in the urine. These include **(i) acetoacetic (diacetic) acid (approximately 20%), (ii) acetone (around 2%), and β-hydroxybutyric acid (3-hydroxybutyrate) (about 78%).** If urine is left at room temperature, acetone is irreversibly formed from acetoacetic acid, while β-hydroxybutyric acid is formed reversibly from acetoacetic acid.

$$\text{Acetoacetic acid} \xrightarrow{-CO_2} \text{Acetone}$$

$$\text{Acetoacetic acid} \xleftrightarrow{+2H} \beta\text{-hydroxybutyric acid}$$

Tests for ketone bodies are listed in **Box 15.13**.

Reagent Strip

Principle: This method is based on a **nitroprusside** (sodium nitroferricyanide) **reaction for ketones.** The reagent strip contains sodium nitroferricyanide and glycine (buffer). They react with acetoacetic acid in the alkaline medium to form a violet dye. A positive result is indicated by a color change from beige to violet, which is read at 60 seconds. Reagent strips without alkali react to acetoacetic acid and not to acetone. However, acetone can be detected if glycine is incorporated into it.

Rothera's Test

Q. Write a short note on Rothera's test.

Principle: Acetoacetic acid (diacetic acid) **and acetone react with sodium nitroprusside** in the presence of an alkali to form a **purple color compound.**

BOX 15.13: Tests for ketone bodies

- **Reagent strip (nitroprusside):** Detects acetoacetic acid and acetone
- **Rothera's (nitroprusside) test:** Detects acetoacetic acid and acetone
- **Gerhardt's (ferric chloride) test:** Detects acetoacetic acid
- **Hart's test:** Detects β-hydroxybutyric acid

Procedure: Take 4 mL of urine in a test tube. Add a few crystals of sodium nitroprusside and saturate the urine with ammonium sulfate by mixing vigorously. Overlay with a few drops of liquor ammonia along the wall of the tube.

Interpretation: The development of a **purple ring** indicates the presence of **acetoacetic acid/acetone** or both. A brown or red color is of no significance.

Gerhardt's Test (Ferric Chloride Test)

This is neither a very specific nor a sensitive test. The test **detects acetoacetic acid.**

Principle: Acetoacetic acid reacts with ferric chloride to give a deep red color.

Hart's Test

This test detects β-**hydroxybutyric acid**, which the above two tests fail to detect. β-hydroxybutyric acid is usually accompanied by acetoacetic acid.

Principle: β-hydroxybutyric acid is converted into acetone which **reacts with sodium nitroprusside and liquor ammonia** to give purple red color.

Causes of Ketonuria (Box 15.14)

Q. Write a short note on the causes of ketonuria. List the nondiabetic causes.

Tests for Blood, Hemoglobin, Hemosiderin, and Myoglobin in Urine

Q. Write a short notes on tests for blood in urine.

Hematuria: It is defined as the **presence of an abnormal number of red cells in the urine,** e.g., **renal stones, or renal cell carcinoma.** It is relatively common.

Hemoglobinuria: It is characterized by the **presence of free hemoglobin in solution in urine,** e.g., **intravascular hemolysis.** Hemoglobinuria is uncommon.

BOX 15.14: Causes of ketonuria.

Diabetic ketonuria
- **Diabetic ketoacidosis:** Ketonemia and ketonuria are commonly seen in uncontrolled diabetes mellitus

Nondiabetic ketonuria
- Starvation
- Prolonged vomiting or diarrhea
- Infants and children
  - Prolonged febrile illness
  - Toxic states accompanied by vomiting or diarrhea
  - Glycogen storage disorders (von Gierke's disease)
- Hyperemesis of pregnancy
- Cachexia

Lactic acidosis
- Shock, diabetes mellitus, renal failure, liver disease, infection, and drugs (e.g., phenformin and salicylate poisoning)

BOX 15.15: Tests for blood.

- Reagent strip
- Orthotoluidine test
- Benzidine test

Hemosiderinuria: It is the presence of **hemosiderin in urine.** Hemosiderin occurs 2–3 days after an acute hemolytic episode that causes hemoglobinuria.

Myoglobinuria: Presence of **myoglobin in urine**, e.g., crush injury to muscle, strenuous exercise. It is rare.

The tests for blood detect hematuria, hemoglobinuria, or myoglobinuria (**Box 15.15**).

Reagent Strip

Very small amounts of hemoglobin/RBCs are detected by the dipstick method.

Principle: The test is based on the **release of oxygen from peroxide in the reagent strip by the peroxidase-like activity of heme present in hemoglobin, lysed RBCs, or myoglobin.** The liberated oxygen changes the color of the chromogen. The reagent area is impregnated with a buffered mixture of organic peroxide and chromogen. The chromogen is orthotoluidine or tetramethylbenzidine.

$$\text{Organic peroxide} \xrightarrow{\text{Peroxidase from Hb}} H_2O + O$$

$$O + \text{chromogen} \xrightarrow{\text{Orthotoludine}} \text{Oxidized (colored compound)}$$

Heme in the urine catalyzes the oxidation of tetramethylbenzidine (chromogen) to produce a green color. The strip is read at 60 seconds following application of urine.

Orthotoluidine Test

Principle: Peroxidase-like activity of heme present in hemoglobin **liberates oxygen from hydrogen peroxide** in the reagent. The liberated **oxygen changes the color of orthotoluidine.**

- **Interpretation:** The appearance of blue or green color indicates the presence of blood.

Benzidine Test

Q. Write a short answer on the principle of the benzidine test.

Principle: The test depends upon the ability of **heme compounds** derived from hemoglobin to **catalyze the oxidation of benzidine by hydrogen peroxide.**

- **Procedure:** Dissolve a small amount (knife-point full) of benzidine in 2 mL of glacial acetic acid and add an equal volume of 3% hydrogen peroxide. From this, take 2 mL in another test tube and add 2 mL of previously boiled and cooled urine, and mix.
- **Control for the test:** If the test is negative, add a drop of blood to the above test tube. It should give a blue color.

This is to confirm the potency of reagents, especially hydrogen peroxide, and exclude a false negative reaction.

- **Interpretation:** The appearance of **blue color** indicates the presence of blood.
- **Precaution:** The presence of hypochlorite (bleach) and microbial peroxidase can cause false-positive results. **Benzidine is carcinogenic.**

Causes of Hematuria

Q. Write a short note on the causes of hematuria.

Hematuria may be **gross or microscopic**. Gross hematuria is the presence of an increased number of red blood cells in urine and visible to the naked eye. Urine is red-colored in severe hematuria and smoky in mild hematuria. Microscopic hematuria is defined as the presence of three or more red blood cells per high-powered field. RBCs are demonstrable in urinary sediment. The causes of hematuria are shown in **Box 15.16**.

Hemoglobinuria

Hemoglobin is too large to pass through the glomerular filter. **Free hemoglobin is liberated following hemolysis and binds to plasma haptoglobin.** Once this binding capacity is saturated, the free hemoglobin will pass through the glomerulus. If the renal threshold is exceeded the hemoglobin can pass into the urine which becomes cola colored.

Interpretation: If the supernatant is colored pink, it indicates hemoglobinuria.

BOX 15.16: Causes of hematuria.

Renal diseases
- **Glomerular causes**
  - **Acute glomerulonephritis**
  - Renal infarct
  - Bacterial endocarditis with kidney involvement
  - Malignant hypertension
- **Nonglomerular causes**
  - Polycystic kidneys
  - **Renal cell carcinoma**
  - **Renal stones (nephrolithiasis)**
  - **Trauma (including renal biopsy)**
  - Renal tuberculosis
  - Hydronephrosis

Lower urinary tract/prostatic diseases
- **Bladder stones (lithiasis)**
- Cystitis
- Urethritis
- **Carcinoma bladder**
- Carcinoma prostate

Blood disorders
- Bleeding disorders—coagulation disorders, severe thrombocytopenia
- Acute leukemia
- Sickle cell disease

Miscellaneous
- Instrumentation of urinary tract

Note: Hemoglobin is precipitated when the urine is 80% saturated with ammonium sulfate but myoglobin is not.

Causes of hemoglobinuria: Any cause of hemolysis may cause hemoglobinuria and the **presence of hemoglobinuria indicates significant intravascular hemolysis**. These include **paroxysmal nocturnal hemoglobinuria (PNH), paroxysmal cold hemoglobinuria (PCH), incompatible blood transfusion, severe burns, autoimmune hemolytic anemia (AIHA), march hemoglobinuria,** snake bite, blackwater fever (falciparum malaria).

Bilirubin (Bile Pigment)

Q. Write a short note on bile pigments in urine.

Tests for bilirubin in urine provide information concerning metabolic or systemic disorders, especially **liver function. Bilirubin is a breakdown product of hemoglobin.** It is formed in the reticuloendothelial cells of the spleen, liver, and bone marrow. Initially, bilirubin is carried in the blood linked to albumin. This is called unconjugated bilirubin (or indirect bilirubin). This unconjugated bilirubin is water-insoluble and therefore cannot pass through the glomerular barrier of the kidney. Unconjugated bilirubin is transported to the liver, where it is conjugated with glucuronic acid to form bilirubin glucuronide. This conjugated bilirubin (direct bilirubin) is water soluble and can pass through the glomerulus of the kidney into the urine. Normally, conjugated bilirubin is excreted in the bile into the duodenum. **Urine in adults, normally contains only a small amount and is not detected by the usual testing methods.** Bilirubinuria causes yellow-brown to greenish-brown urine and forms yellow foam on shaking. Bilirubin is found only in freshly voided urine which upon standing is oxidized to biliverdin. Tests for bilirubin are listed in **Box 15.17**.

Reagent Strip

Principle: The test is **based on a diazo reaction.** Bilirubin in the urine couples with a diazotized dichloronaniline (content of strip) in a strongly acidic medium to form a colored compound namely azobilirubin. Urine must be fresh because bilirubin glucuronide (conjugated) in urine quickly hydrolyzes to less reactive free bilirubin.

Fouchet's Test

Principle: Fouchet's reagent contains **trichloroacetic acid and ferric chloride.** In an acidic medium ferric chloride oxidizes **bilirubin** to produce a dark green colored **biliverdin.**

Procedure: Take 10 mL of urine in a test tube and add 3 mL of 10% barium chloride solution. Mix the two and filter the mixture through a filter paper. Bilirubin along with barium salt remains on filter paper. Add a few drops of Fouchet's reagent onto the filter paper.

Interpretation: Green or blue color indicates bilirubinuria.

BOX 15.17: Tests for bilirubin.

- Reagent strip
- Fouchet's test

Causes of Bilirubinuria

- **Obstructive jaundice:** Bilirubinuria is **not seen in normal subjects.** Unconjugated bilirubin is not excreted in the urine (e.g., hemolytic anemia) but conjugated bilirubinuria occurs only when there is raised serum conjugated bilirubin (e.g., obstructive jaundice). Obstruction to bile outflow from the liver may be intrahepatic or extrahepatic. The urine shows bilirubin without urobilinogen. Bilirubin is of conjugated type. Causes of extrahepatic obstruction include gallstones in the common bile duct and carcinoma of the head of the pancreas.
- **Hepatocellular jaundice:** In acute viral hepatitis, bilirubin appears in the urine before the jaundice is clinically apparent. In a patient with pyrexia of unknown origin, bilirubinuria indicates hepatitis. In individuals taking potentially hepatotoxic drugs or toxins, bilirubinuria may be an early indication of cholestasis or liver damage.
- **Hemolytic jaundice: Bilirubin is absent in urine.** This is because in hemolytic anemia the hyperbilirubinemia is due to unconjugated bilirubin which is not water insoluble. Hence, not excreted in the urine.

Urobilinogen in Urine

Q. Write a short note on urobilinogen in urine.

Conjugated bilirubin from the liver reaches the duodenum through the bile. The conjugated bilirubin is not absorbed from the small intestine but passes on into the colon. In the colon, bacteria hydrolyze the conjugate and liberate free bilirubin. The free bilirubin is then reduced to urobilinogen and stercobilinogen. Up to 50% of the urobilinogen is reabsorbed into the portal circulation and is reexcreted into the bile. Most of the remaining urobilinogen is excreted in feces as colored urobilins or stercobilin. A small amount (1–2 mg/dL) of urobilinogen is excreted in the urines and is insufficient to cause a significant positive reaction. Whenever the liver is unable to efficiently remove the reabsorbed urobilinogen from the portal circulation (e.g., liver diseases, hemolytic anemia) more urobilinogen than normal is routed through the kidney and hence, excreted in the urine. Tests for urobilinogen are listed in **Box 15.18**.

Reagent Strip

Principle: This test is based on the Ehrlich aldehyde test. The strip is coated with p-amino benzaldehyde with a color enhancer. It reacts with urobilinogen in a strongly acidic medium to produce a pink-red-colored compound. The color is matched with the color chart on the container of the reagent strip.

BOX 15.18: Tests for urobilinogen.

- **Reagent strip**
- Ehrlich test

BOX 15.19: Causes of increased and reduced urobilinogen in urine.

Causes of increased urobilinogen in urine

- **Hemolytic anemias (without bilirubin in urine):** Thalassemia, sickle cell anemia, hereditary spherocytosis.
- **Liver diseases:** Preicteric phase of infective hepatitis, drugs or toxic hepatitis, alcoholic liver disease, cirrhosis.

Causes of decreased/absent urobilinogen in urine

- In obstructive jaundice with complete biliary obstruction, bilirubin does not reach the intestine. Hence, it is not converted into urobilinogen and urobilinogen disappears from the urine

Ehrlich Aldehyde Test

Principle: Ehrlich's reagent reacts with urobilinogen and forms a pink-colored aldehyde complex.

Procedure: Take 2.5 mL of urine in a test tube. Add 2.5 mL of Ehrlich's aldehyde reagent (paradimethyl amino benzaldehyde). Mix well by inversion. Add 10 mL of saturated sodium acetate solution and mix.

Interpretation: Pink to cherry red color indicates the presence of urobilinogen.

Causes of increased and reduced urobilinogen in urine are listed in **Box 15.19**.

Q. Write a short note on urobilinogen in urine or jaundice.

Bile Salts

Q. Write a short note on bile salts in urine and test for its detection.

Bile salts are composed of a mixture of bile acids and glycine or taurine. Two important bile salts are sodium and potassium salts of glycocholate and taurocholate. Normally, bile salts are not present in urine.

Hay's Sulfur Test

Q. Write a short note on Hay's sulfur test.

Principle: Bile salts have the unusual property of **lowering the surface tension of urine** markedly even when present in small concentrations. This property is made use of in Hay's test.

Interpretation: Sulfur powder sinks to the bottom of the test tube in the presence of bile salts in urine.

Causes: Hepatocellular and obstructive jaundice.

Multistix Reagent Strips for Urine Testing

Reagent strips have single/multiple discrete cellulose squares which are impregnated with reagents for testing glucose, protein, pH, specific gravity, hemoglobin, ketone bodies, bilirubin, and urobilinogen. There are single test strips, e.g., diastix for glucose and multistix for multiple tests **(Fig. 15.14)**.

Automated urinalysis: Fully automated urine analyzers provided with automatic functions are presently available, e.g., Uriplus.

Microscopic Examination

Q. Write a short note on the microscopic examination of urine.

Microscopic examination of urinary deposits or sediment is an essential part of urine examination. It may be necessary in many cases. This examination is done to detect **3 Cs** namely: (i) **cellular elements**, (ii) **casts, and (iii) crystals**. The microscopic examination of the urine is usually done manually. However, several automated instruments can perform this analysis.

Cells

The cells include blood cells (red cells and white cells), and **epithelial cells** (renal, transitional, and squamous). They are expressed as the number of cells per low-power or high-power field.

Blood Cells

1. **Red blood cells (RBCs):** The presence of RBCs (more than 2/hpf) in the urine indicates bleeding at any point in the urinary system from the glomerulus to the urethra. In **glomerular diseases**, the urine shows **red cells with cellular protrusions or fragmentation,** and are named as **dysmorphic** (distorted morphology) red blood cells.
2. **White blood cells (WBCs):** An increased number of WBCs (mainly neutrophils more than 5/hpf) in urine is known as **pyuria**. It is indicative of a **urinary tract infection.** The causative organism of infection may be identified by bacteriological examination. When accompanied by **leukocyte casts** or mixed leukocyte–epithelial cell casts, increased urinary leukocytes are indicative of **renal origin.**

Causes of pus cells in urine (pyuria): Pyelonephritis, urethritis, cystitis, urinary tract infection (UTI).

Glitter cell is a **swollen neutrophil with its cytoplasmic granules showing constant Brownian motion**. This results in a shining or glittering appearance of the cell. Causes of glitter cells include dilute or hypotonic urine, chronic pyelonephritis, and lower urinary tract infections.

Epithelial Cells

These are derived from the urinary tract (transitional and renal) or genital tract (squamous). A few (0–2/hpf) transitional cells from the bladder may be present in normal urine and squamous cells from the vulva and vagina usually contaminate a routine specimen from women. **Malignant cells** may be seen in tumors of the urinary bladder.

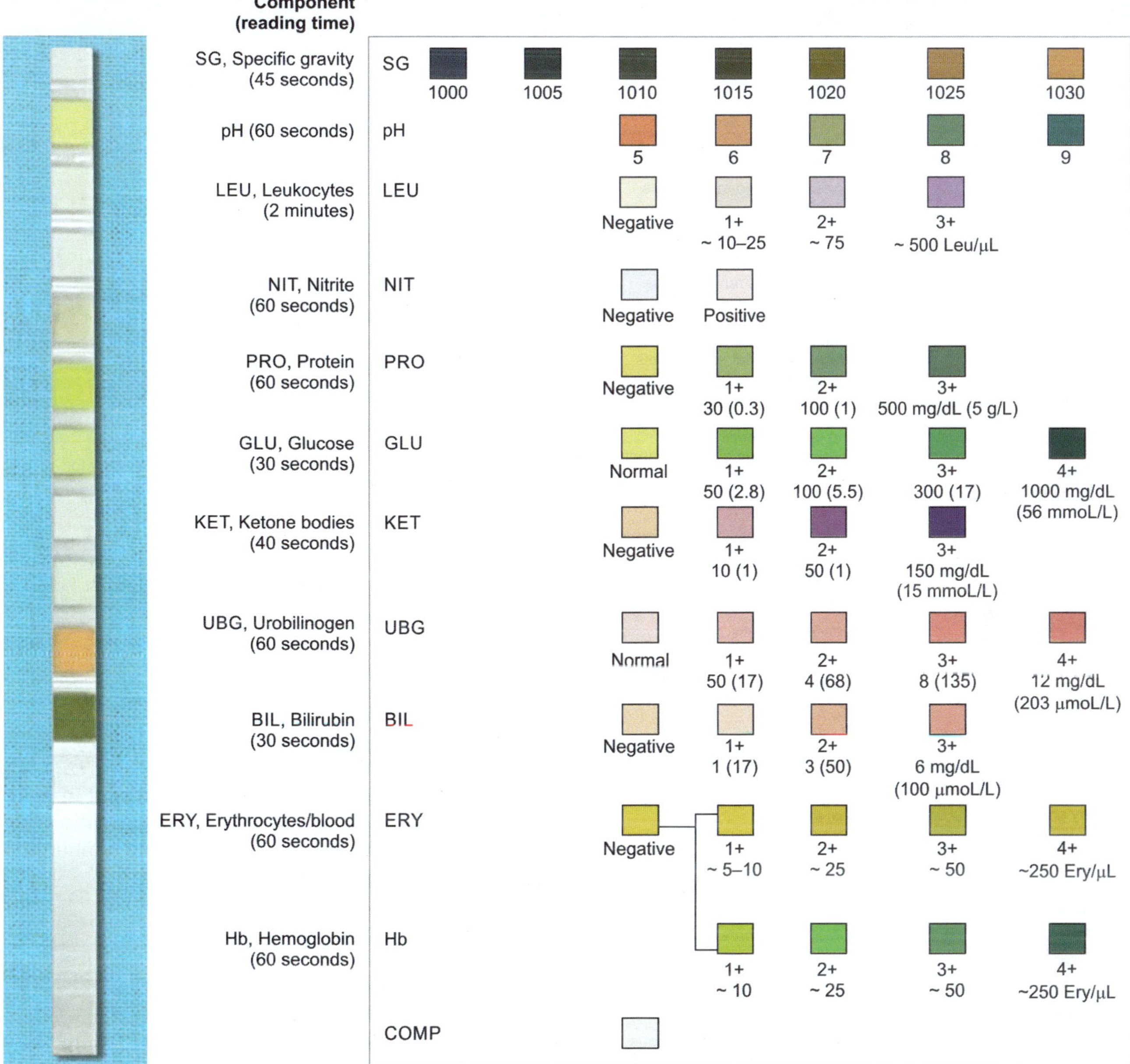

Fig. 15.14: Multistix reagent strip (the reading time varies depending on the manufacturer and the content)

Casts (Box 15.20 and Fig. 15.15)

Q. Write a short note on urinary casts and crystals.

Casts are **formed only in the kidney** and are **indicative of renal disease.** They are formed by the solidification of **Tamm Horsfall protein**, a glycoprotein secreted in the distal convoluted tubules and collecting tubules. These proteins form a fibrillar meshwork (basic matrix) and can trap any elements including cells, cell fragments, or granular material. **Casts** are cylindrical structures with **parallel sides** and rounded ends. They vary in size, shape, and appearance. **Cylindroids** probably represent abortive casts. They have one tapering end while the other end is round and the sides are not parallel. The casts may be with or without inclusions **(Box 15.20)**.

BOX 15.20: Classification of casts.

- **Matrix:** Hyaline, waxy
- **Cells:** RBCs and their remnants, leukocytes (neutrophils, lymphocytes), renal tubular epithelial cells, mixed cells (RBCs, neutrophils, and renal tubular cells)
- **Inclusions:** Granules (proteins, cell debris), fat globules/droplets (triglycerides, cholesterol esters),
- **Pigments:** Hemoglobin, myoglobin, bilirubin, hemosiderin granules

Crystals (Fig. 15.16)

These are not usually present in urine. Crystals of oxalates, urates, and cystine are present in patients with a history

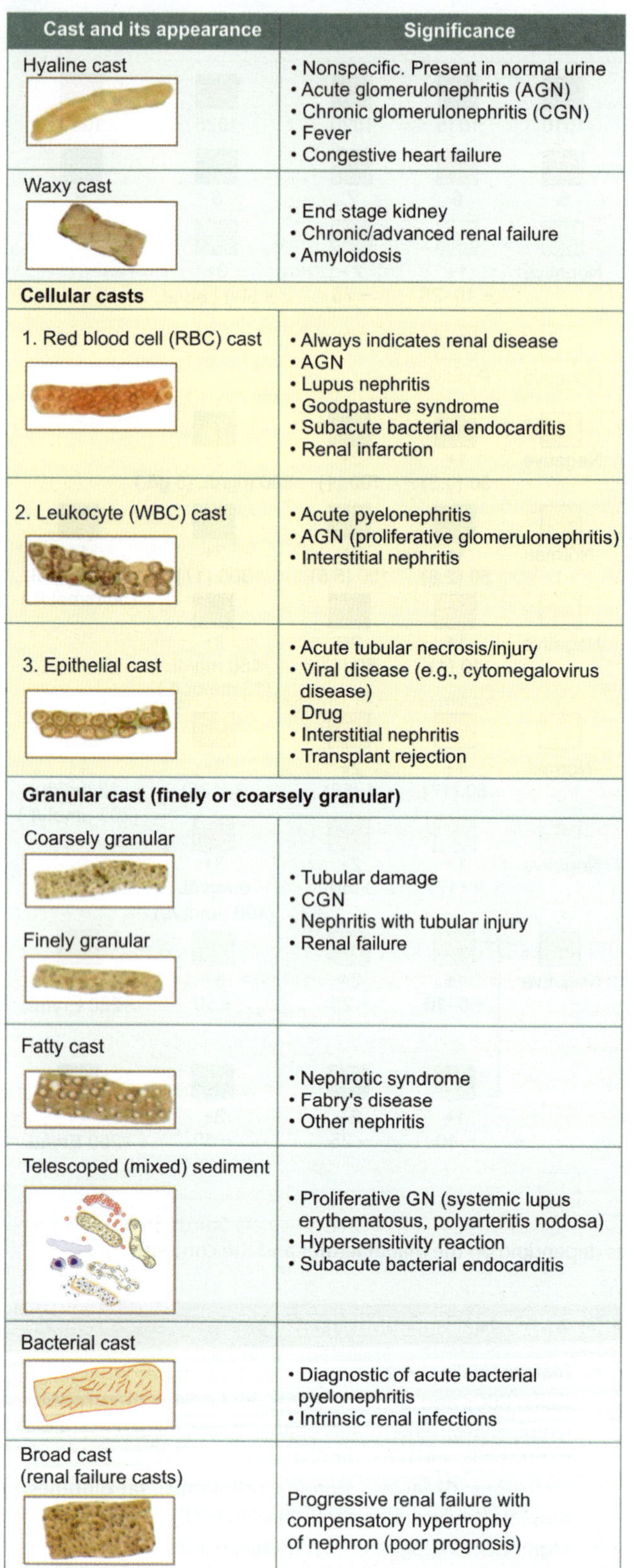

Cast and its appearance	Significance
Hyaline cast	• Nonspecific. Present in normal urine • Acute glomerulonephritis (AGN) • Chronic glomerulonephritis (CGN) • Fever • Congestive heart failure
Waxy cast	• End stage kidney • Chronic/advanced renal failure • Amyloidosis
Cellular casts	
1. Red blood cell (RBC) cast	• Always indicates renal disease • AGN • Lupus nephritis • Goodpasture syndrome • Subacute bacterial endocarditis • Renal infarction
2. Leukocyte (WBC) cast	• Acute pyelonephritis • AGN (proliferative glomerulonephritis) • Interstitial nephritis
3. Epithelial cast	• Acute tubular necrosis/injury • Viral disease (e.g., cytomegalovirus disease) • Drug • Interstitial nephritis • Transplant rejection
Granular cast (finely or coarsely granular)	
Coarsely granular Finely granular	• Tubular damage • CGN • Nephritis with tubular injury • Renal failure
Fatty cast	• Nephrotic syndrome • Fabry's disease • Other nephritis
Telescoped (mixed) sediment	• Proliferative GN (systemic lupus erythematosus, polyarteritis nodosa) • Hypersensitivity reaction • Subacute bacterial endocarditis
Bacterial cast	• Diagnostic of acute bacterial pyelonephritis • Intrinsic renal infections
Broad cast (renal failure casts)	Progressive renal failure with compensatory hypertrophy of nephron (poor prognosis)

Fig. 15.15: Urinary casts and their significance.

Crystal in normal acidic urine	Condition
Amorphous urates	• Normal acidic urine • Concentrated urine as in fever and dehydration
Crystalline urates (sodium, potassium and ammonium)	Normal acidic urine
Crystalline uric acid	• Normal acidic urine • Post-chemotherapy for lymphoma and leukemia
Calcium oxalate	• Normal acidic urine • Large numbers in severe chronic renal disease or ethylene glycol or methoxyflurane toxicity/poisoning • Nephrolithiasis

Fig. 15.16: Urinary crystals and their significance.

of renal stone, while urates alone are present in *gout*. Oxalates, urates, and cystine are present in acidic urine while phosphates, calcium carbonates, and ammonium urates are present in alkaline urine.

BODY FLUIDS

PA 23.2a (CC): Describe abnormal findings in body fluids in various disease states.

Body fluids are lubricating fluids present within the body cavities. Normally, a small amount of fluid is present within the body cavities which keep the surfaces moist and lubricated so that the movement of the adjacent or the opposing membrane surfaces occurs with minimal friction. An increase in the volume of the fluid in these cavities is known as **effusion**. The commonly examined body fluids in the laboratory include **pleural, pericardial, peritoneal, and synovial fluid.**

Specimen collection: The body fluid is collected in a clean, dry container under aseptic precautions and a traumatically to avoid mixing with fresh blood. The fluid is collected in the following three sterile test tubes:

1. **Chemical examination:** Fluoride tube.
2. **Microscopic examination:** EDTA tube.

3. **Bacteriological examination:** Plain tube (without anticoagulant).

They should be examined as early as possible to prevent chemical changes, growth of bacteria, and disintegration of cells.

Pleural Fluid

Causes of pleural effusion: Nonspecific inflammatory pleural effusion is more common than specific effusion. Various causes of pleural effusion are presented in **Table 15.9**.

Examination of Pleural Fluid

It consists of:
- Physical examination (volume, color, and appearance)
- Chemical examination
- Cell counts (microscopic examination)
- Microbiological examination
- Cytological examination

Physical Examination

Note: Volume, color, and appearance (it applies also to pericardial and peritoneal fluid).

Color: Pleural, pericardial, and ascitic (peritoneal) fluids are usually clear and straw-colored.
- Uniform **blood-stained fluid suggests malignancy** involving the organs/tissues surrounding the respective body cavity.
- **Turbid** fluid may be due to high cell count or high protein content.
- **Chylous** with a milky appearance usually indicates high lipid content due to lymphatic obstruction.

Appearance: The effusion may be broadly divided into **transudate** and **exudate**. It is important to differentiate whether the fluid is a transudate or exudate (*refer* **Table 3.3**).
- **Transudate** is usually seen in all body cavities with diseases like heart failure and hypoalbuminemic conditions (e.g., nephrotic syndrome). Cirrhosis results in prominent ascites, but may also cause pleural effusion. Transudates are clear, pale yellow, or straw-colored and do not clot on standing. Transudates are mostly due to circulatory disturbances.
- **Exudate usually suggests infection or malignancy**. Exudates are opaque or turbid due to increased proteins, leukocytes, or the presence of malignant cells. They may clot on standing due to high fibrinogen content. Frank pus with a putrid odor appears in empyema. Exudates can be produced due to: (i) inflammatory processes, (ii) primary and metastatic tumors in serous membranes or serous cavities, or (iii) following a trauma, surgery, or other invasive diagnostic procedures.
- **Bloody or hemorrhagic fluid:** It indicates traumatic tap or malignancy.
- **Milky or chylous fluid:** It is characterized by the accumulation of a milky or chylous fluid. It usually develops due to obstruction of the lymphatic duct (due to injury, carcinoma, or lymphoma). It characteristic shows a triglyceride level >110 mg/dL. Microscopically it shows lymphocytosis and fat droplets that stain positive with fat stains such as Sudan III.
- **Viscous fluid:** It is seen in mesothelioma.

TABLE 15.9 Causes of pleural effusion.

Transudate	*Exudate*
Congestive cardiac failure	**Infections: Bacterial pneumonia, tuberculosis**
Cirrhosis of liver	Pulmonary infarction
Hypoproteinemia	Autoimmune disorders: Systemic lupus erythematosus, rheumatoid arthritis
Pulmonary embolism	**Malignancy: Secondaries from carcinoma lung, breast**, etc., mesothelioma and lymphoma
	Others: Acute pancreatitis, trauma to chest wall

Common causes are highlighted in bold words.

Chemical Examination

Protein estimation: This helps to differentiate transudate from exudate. It is essential to differentiate exudates and transudates. Exudates have at least one of these criteria **[Light's criteria, i.e., (i) pleural fluid protein/serum protein ratio >0.5, (ii) pleural fluid LDH/serum LDH ratio >0.6 and (iii) pleural fluid LDH above 2/3rds of the upper limit of normal for serum LDH]**. There is a direct relation between levels of lactate dehydrogenase in pleural fluid and with degree of pleural inflammation. Transudates do not have any of these criteria.
- **Exudate:** If the fluid is an exudate, further investigations are required. These include **cell counts, cytological examination, estimation of glucose**, test for tuberculosis, Gram smear, and culture.
- **Transudates:** They are usually seen in congestive cardiac failure and cirrhosis.

Glucose estimation: Low glucose in the body fluids usually suggests bacterial infection (**empyema,** including tuberculosis), malignancy, or nonspecific inflammation.

Cell Counts (Microscopic Examination)

Total leukocyte count: It should be performed on all body fluids. ***Cell count*** is done similarly to total WBC count using an improved Neubauer chamber. Normally, a few mesothelial cells (lining cells of body cavities) and lymphocytes are seen. **Differential WBC count:** Centrifuge the body fluid and from the sediment prepare the smears (at least 2). **Stains** employed include: (1) **Leishman's stain:** Stain one smear with Leishman's stain and count 100 cells and express the differential count and (2) **Gram's stain/**

acid-fast stain. These stains are useful in suspected cases of infective/tubercular infections respectively.

- **Neutrophils:** Very high leukocyte count (>50,000/μL) with predominance of neutrophils suggests effusion complication bacterial pneumonia (usually empyema).
- **Lymphocytes:** The presence of many small, mature lymphocytes with few mesothelial cells suggests tuberculosis.
- **Hemorrhagic pleural fluids** having more than 100,000 red cells/μL are seen in pulmonary infarction, malignancy, or traumatic tap.

Transudate and Exudate

- **Transudates:** Usually leukocytes are <1,000/μL and are mostly small, mature lymphocytes.
- **Exudate:** Predominance of neutrophils (>50%) indicates an acute process (e.g., bacterial pneumonia), whereas predominance of lymphocytes indicates a chronic process (e.g., tuberculosis, malignancy).

Microbiological Examination

- **Gram's smear and culture:** It should be done on exudates (especially on purulent, blood-stained, or cloudy fluids). Culture is done to identify the organism in cases of effusion due to infections.
- **Ziehl–Neelsen stain:** Useful for tuberculous pleural effusions. If culture for tubercle bacilli is negative in a suspected case of tuberculosis, polymerase chain reaction for mycobacterial DNA or increased level of adenosine deaminase (released in pleural fluid from activated lymphocytes) will be useful for establishing the diagnosis.

Cytological Examination

Procedure: The pleural fluid is centrifuged; smears are made from the sediment and fixed immediately in absolute alcohol. The smears are stained by Papanicolaou stain. Hematoxylin and eosin stain or Giemsa may also be used. Cytospin is a better alternative for making smears.

The common malignancies that metastasize to pleura are carcinoma of the lung and breast and lymphoma. Pleural effusion is produced due to obstruction of lymphatics by tumor cells. Usually, effusion is blood-tinged or hemorrhagic.

Pleural fluid findings in malignant pleural effusion

Q. Pleural fluid findings in malignant pleural effusion.

- **Often hemorrhagic**, with a high erythrocyte count (>100,000/mm^3).
- Shows the characteristics of exudates such as **high protein content** (>3.0 g/dL), high LDH levels (>200 IU/L), low glucose levels (<60 mg/dL), and **a total leukocyte count exceeding 1,000/mL.**
- **Predominant cells are lymphocytes (>50%).**

TABLE 15.10 Pleural fluid findings in common pleural effusion.

Causes	*Appearance*	*Cells*	*Special studies*
Exudate			
Tuberculosis	Straw-colored	5,000–10,000/μL mostly lymphocytes and few mesothelial cells	Ziehl–Neelsen stain; culture; polymerase chain reaction
Effusion in bacterial pneumonia	Turbid	5,000–40,000/μL mostly neutrophils	Gram stain; culture
Empyema	Purulent	>25,000/μL; mostly neutrophils	Gram stain; culture; low pH; low glucose
Malignancy	Bloody	Lymphocytes, malignant cells	Cytology, pleural biopsy
Transudate			
Congestive heart failure	Clear	Few mesothelial cells	Nil

- Cytological examination may show **malignant cells**. The smears are stained by Papanicolaou stain.

Hematoxylin and eosin stain or Giemsa may also be used. Cytospin is a better alternative for making smears.

Pleural biopsy: Percutaneous needle biopsy of the parietal pleura is indicated if the examination of exudative pleural effusion does not yield a specific diagnosis. It is done when there is suspicion of tuberculosis or malignancy.

Pleural fluid findings in common pleural effusion are discussed in **Table 15.10.**

PERITONEAL FLUID

PA 23.2b (CC): Describe abnormal findings in body fluids in various disease states.

Excessive (pathological) accumulation of fluid in the peritoneal cavity is termed ascites, and the accumulated fluid is called ascitic fluid.

Causes of ascites: The causes of ascites are presented in **Table 15.11.**

TABLE 15.11 Causes of ascites.

Transudate	*Exudate*
Cirrhosis of liver	Bacterial peritonitis (primary or secondary)
Congestive cardiac failure	Tuberculosis
Hypoproteinemia	Malignancy: Lymphoma, hepatocellular carcinoma, metastatic carcinoma (e.g., ovary, colon)
	Others: Abdominal injury, biliary peritonitis (rupture of the gallbladder), pancreatitis, etc.

Examination of Ascitic Fluid

Steps and physical examination are the same as those for pleural fluid as mentioned above.

Chemical Examination

- **Proteins:** In ascitic fluid, the traditional division of fluid as transudate or exudate depending upon its protein content alone is not always sufficient. It is **better to use an albumin gradient** (calculated as serum albumin minus ascitic fluid albumin).
- **Lactate dehydrogenase:** It is raised in **spontaneous bacterial peritonitis** (i.e., without any obvious source of infection), **secondary bacterial peritonitis** (i.e., with identifiable source of infection), and **metastatic carcinoma** to peritoneum.
- **Amylase:** Normally, amylase levels in ascitic fluid are similar to serum amylase. If the amylase level in ascetic fluid is three times more than serum amylase, the cause of ascites is most likely to be due to pancreatic disease (e.g., acute pancreatitis).
- **Bilirubin:** If the bilirubin in ascitic fluid is more than 6.0 mg/dL and if the ascitic fluid bilirubin/serum bilirubin ratio is more than 1.0, it suggests perforation of the biliary tract (biliary peritonitis). The ascitic fluid will be bile-stained.

Cell Counts (Microscopic Examination)

Cell count is performed to distinguish ascites due to cirrhosis from those due to spontaneous bacterial peritonitis. If the total leukocyte count >500/μL and absolute neutrophil count >250/μL, it favors the diagnosis of spontaneous bacterial peritonitis.

Microbiological Examination

- **Gram stain**: It is positive in about ¼ of cases of spontaneous bacterial peritonitis.
- **Culture and sensitivity.**
- **Ziehl-Neelsen stain** for tuberculous bacilli.

Laparoscopic biopsy is more useful for the diagnosis of tuberculous peritonitis.

Cytological Examination

The procedure is the same as that for pleural effusion. Malignant cells can be found in malignant ascites.

Pericardial effusion and hemopericardium are discussed on page 535.

CEREBROSPINAL FLUID EXAMINATION

PA 23.2c (CC): Describe abnormal findings in body fluids in various disease states.

Cerebrospinal fluid (CSF) is formed within the ventricles and circulates in the subarachnoid space (between the arachnoid and pia matter) and the ventricles. The total volume of CSF in adults ranges from 90–150 mL. It is a medium for the transfer of substances from the brain and spinal cord into the blood.

Importance of CSF examination: Analysis of the CSF is of diagnostic importance in conditions like **meningitis or primary/metastatic tumor of CNS with CSF involvement.**

Collection of CSF: CSF is usually obtained by lumbar puncture (LP) using an LP needle under strict aseptic conditions.

Lumbar puncture needle (Figs. 15.17A and B): The needle measures 10–12 cm in length. In children, a shorter needle is used. It has a needle and a stilette. The stilette has a pin that fits into the slot of the head of the needle and helps to keep the needle patent.

Sites of CSF collection: It may be obtained by lumbar, cisternal, or lateral cervical puncture or through ventricular cannulas or shunts.

- **Lumbar puncture:** In **adults,** CSF is normally collected in the midline of the lower back in the **3rd lumbar space** and in **children in the 4th lumbar space.**
- **Cisternal puncture:** It is done in spinal cord block, vertebral deformity, or infections in the tissues where lumbar puncture is usually done.
- **Ventricular puncture:** It is performed in infants who have open fontanella.

Method of Collection

The amount of CSF normally collected is 6–8 mL. The CSF specimen is usually divided into three or four serially collected sterile tubes: Tube 1 is for the estimation of protein and glucose (chemical examination) and serology (immunology), tube 2 is used for the preparation of smears to stain with the Gram stain or other stains and for culture and sensitivity (microbiological examination), tube 3 is for cell counts and differential counts (cytological study), and tube 4 (if indicated) for special tests, such as the

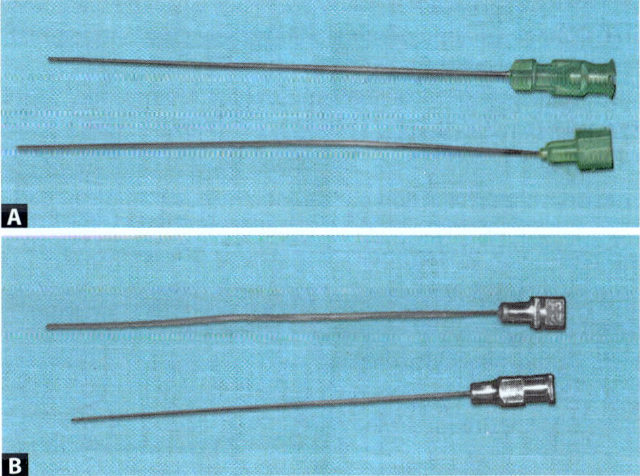

Figs. 15.17A and B: Lumbar puncture needles with stilette [(A) disposable needle with green plastic hub].

cryptococcal antigen, serologic test for syphilis, molecular tests or other serologic studies and cytology.

Q. Write a short note on indications for lumbar puncture.

Indications and contraindications for lumbar puncture are listed in **Box 15.21** and **Box 15.22 respectively**.

Complications of lumbar puncture are listed in **Box 15.23**.

Examination of CSF

Physical Examination

CSF Pressure

The normal CSF pressure in adults is 90–180 mm of water in the lateral position, while in infants and children, it ranges from 10 to 100 mm of water reaching the adult level by 6–8 years.

- **Causes of raised CSF pressure: Meningitis, cerebral edema, mass lesions in the brain,** etc.
- **Causes of decreased CSF pressure***:* Dehydration, circulatory collapse, etc.

BOX 15.21: Indications for lumbar puncture.

Diagnostic indications

- Infection
  - Meningeal infection:
    - Bacterial
      - Pyogenic
      - Tuberculosis
      - Syphilitic: To differentiate general paresis of insane, tabes dorsalis, and meningeal syphilis
    - Viral
    - Fungal
  - Encephalitis
- Subarachnoid hemorrhage
- Primary or metastatic malignancy (e.g., acute leukemia, lymphoma)
- Demyelinating diseases: Multiple sclerosis and subacute sclerosing panencephalitis (SSPE), Guillain–Barre syndrome
- Spinal canal blockage leading to elevated intracranial tension (spinal cord tumors)
- For injecting the radio-opaque dye for myelography

Therapeutic indications

- Spinal anesthesia
- Intrathecal injection of chemotherapeutic drugs for CNS prophylaxis/relapse of ALL, lymphomas

BOX 15.22: Contraindications for lumbar puncture.

- Raised intracranial pressure
- Local infective lesion
- Disseminated sclerosis
- Brain tumor
- Cardiorespiratory compromise
- Bleeding diathesis which is not been corrected

BOX 15.23: Complications of lumbar puncture.

- Herniation of cerebellum through the foramen magnum due to raised intracranial pressure
- Hematoma, either extradural or subdural
- Introduction of infection by the LP needle through the infected skin or subcutaneous tissue
- Post-puncture headache
- Failure to obtain CSF (dry tap)

Color and Appearance

- Normal CSF is clear, colorless, and watery.
- Turbidity of CSF is due to pus cells (white blood cells) or RBCs.
- **Xanthochromia** (yellow CSF): This term commonly refers to a pale pink to yellow color in the supernatant of centrifuged CSF. For the detection of xanthochromia, the CSF should be centrifuged and the supernatant fluid should be compared with a tube of distilled water. Xanthochromic CSF appears pink, orange, or yellow. This color is due to the lysis of RBC and hemoglobin breakdown. It results from (i) Old hemorrhage, (ii) obstructive jaundice, (iii) excess of protein, (iv) Froin syndrome (complete spinal block, xanthochromia, elevated protein, and hypercoagulated CSF).

Differentiation of subarachnoid hemorrhage from a traumatic puncture: The presence of blood in CSF may be due to trauma during lumbar puncture or subarachnoid hemorrhage.

- In traumatic tap, the first few drops are hemorrhagic, and subsequent ones are clear, while in subarachnoid hemorrhage blood is uniformly mixed with CSF.
- After centrifugation, the supernatant fluid is clear with a traumatic tap, whereas the supernatant appears xanthochromic (a faint pink, orange, or yellow color caused by the release of hemoglobin from hemolyzed red blood cells) in subarachnoid hemorrhage.
- **Xanthochromia with microscopic evidence of erythrophagocytosis, or hemosiderin-laden macrophages indicate a subarachnoid bleed.** RBC lysis begins within 1–2 hours after a traumatic tap. Thus, rapid evaluation is necessary to avoid false-positive results.

Clot Formation

Normal CSF does not clot. When the blood-brain barrier is disturbed, fibrinogen appears in CSF. Fibrinogen gets converted to fibrin and forms a clot.

Causes of fibrin clot

- Meningitis: In **tuberculous meningitis, the clot is fine, delicate, and typically described as a cob-web appearance.** In purulent meningitis, a large clot is formed.
- Tumors of CNS.
- Polyneuritis.

Microscopic Examination

Total Cell Count

Normal CSF usually contains no cells, although a cell counts of 0–5 lymphocytes/L is considered normal. An **increased cell count** is known as **pleocytosis.** Total cell count should be done immediately on undiluted CSF, since after a few hours, pus cells stick to each other and the sides of the tube or degenerate. Cell counts are performed in a manual counting chamber, either in a Fuchs-Rosenthal or an improved Neubauer chamber.

Significance: Neutrophils are increased in acute pyogenic meningitis. Lymphocytes are increased in viral, syphilitic, tuberculous, and fungal meningitis.

Increased cell count should always be confirmed by bacterial or serological tests. India-ink preparation is used for the diagnosis of cryptococcal meningitis. In tuberculous meningitis, acid-fast stain can detect tuberculous bacilli.

Chemical Analysis

Proteins are elevated in meningitis and glucose level is reduced due to utilization by the microbes. These changes are more marked in pyogenic meningitis.

Chloride reduction in tuberculous meningitis is due to general chloride deficiency because of dehydration rather than any specific effect of mycobacteria.

Refer **Table 27.2** for CSF changes in various meningitis. Interpretation of CSF findings with clinical scenario are presented on pages 964-6 of Chapter 27.

SEMEN ANALYSIS

PA 23.3a (CC): Describe and interpret the abnormalities in semen analysis.

Q. Write a short note on semen analysis.

Semen (seminal fluid) consists of spermatozoa (sperms) and the fluid part. About 40% of cases of infertility are due to abnormalities in semen and therefore, semen analysis is the first test to be performed while investigating for infertility. **The defect** of sperms may be **quantitative** (absence of sperms, lack of enough sperms) or **qualitative.**

Indications for semen analysis are listed in **Box 15.24**.

BOX 15.24: Indications for semen analysis.

- Assessment of fertility/infertility
- To monitor the success of surgical procedures, such as varicocelectomy and vasectomy
- Determine the suitability of donor semen for artificial insemination
- Medicolegal purpose: In alleged rape cases, vaginal pool smears are examined to detect sperms
- For selection of assisted reproductive technology (e.g., in vitro fertilization, gamete intrafallopian transfer technique)

Collection of the Sample

Q. Write a short note on a collection of semen for analysis.

The patient is asked to collect the semen by masturbation after a minimum of 2 days and a maximum of 7 days of sexual abstinence (2–7 days of ejaculatory abstinence). The specimen should be collected in a clean, dry, wide-mouthed plastic/glass container. Collection of condom samples is not advisable because they often contain spermicidal agents which impair sperm motility.

Examination of Semen

Q. Write a short notes on various tests/parameters of the semen with normal range.

Physical Examination

- **Liquefaction:** Immediately after ejaculation, the semen is normally a semisolid coagulated mass. At room temperature, the semen usually begins to liquefy (become thinner) within a few minutes and completely liquefies within 15 minutes. Within 30 minutes it becomes more homogeneous and watery. Failure to liquefy may be due to inadequate prostate secretion.
- **Semen viscosity:** Fresh semen is viscid and the viscosity can be estimated by gently aspirating semen into a wide-bore (approximately 1.5 mm diameter) plastic disposable pipette, allowing the semen to drop by gravity. Normal semen falls drop by drop and if viscosity is abnormal, the drop will form a thread more than 2 cm long. Normal viscosity is important since the increase in viscosity affects sperm motility.
- **Appearance:** Freshly ejaculated semen is an opaque, white-gray, and viscid fluid. After liquefaction, it has a homogeneous gray-opalescent appearance. Semen may have red-brown color when red blood cells are present (hemospermia) or yellow in patients with jaundice or ingestion of certain vitamins or drugs. The yellow hue appearance is associated with pyospermia; a rust color is due to small bleeding in the seminal vesicle.
- **Semen volume:** Normal volume >1.4 mL. First sample is weighed and then volume is calculated by assuming the density of semen to be 1 g/mL. Low semen volume may be due to obstruction of the ejaculatory duct, congenital bilateral absence of the vas deferens, or can also be due to difficulty in collection. High semen volume may be due to active exudation in cases of inflammatory lesions of the accessory organs.
- **Semen pH:** Alkaline and ranges from 7.2–8 (>7.2). The pH should be measured after liquefaction, preferably after 30 minutes.

Microscopic Examination

Q. Write a short note on the microscopic examination of semen.

- **Sperm aggregation or agglutination:** The adherence either of immotile spermatozoa to each other or of motile spermatozoa to mucus strands, nonsperm cells, or debris is considered to be nonspecific aggregation and should be noted. **Agglutination** refers to **motile spermatozoa sticking to each other,** head-to-head, tail-to-tail, or in a mixed way. Any motile spermatozoa that stick to each other by their heads, tails, or midpieces should be recorded.

- **Cellular elements other than spermatozoa:** During microscopic examination, a search should be made for the presence of cells other than spermatozoa. Some of these cells may be clinically relevant, which includes epithelial cells from the genitourinary tract and "round cells" (leukocytes and immature germ cells).
- **Assessment of sperm motility:** Motility of the sperms helps in the penetration of cervical mucus and migration of the sperms into the fallopian tube. In normal semen, 42 (40–43)% of sperms should be motile (rapidly progressive and slowly progressive). This is assessed by placing a drop of liquefied semen on a clean glass slide with a coverslip placed over it and examining it under a microscope. According to the WHO (2021), the **motility of each spermatozoon (plural is spermatozoa) is categorized as rapidly progressive (29–31%), and slow-progressive (1%)**. A rapidly progressive spermatozoon moves >5 head-lengths per second. Immotile sperms may be 54 (50–56)%.
- **Sperm vitality:** It is important to know whether immotile spermatozoa are alive or dead. Normally, 54 (50–56)% of live forms are observed. The vitality of the spermatozoa is estimated by identifying those with an intact cell membrane and is especially important for samples with less than about 40% progressively motile spermatozoa. The percentage of live spermatozoa is assessed either by dye exclusion or by hypotonic swelling.

Q. Write a short note on sperm count.

- **Total sperm count:** Sperm count is carried out in an improved Neubauer chamber using a Thoma pipette in a dilution of 1 in 20 (as for total leukocyte count) using semen diluting fluid.
  - **Normal range of sperm count:** >39 million/ejaculate.
  - **Aspermia:** No semen.
  - **Azoospermia:** No spermatozoa in the ejaculate.
  - **Oligospermia:** Total number of spermatozoa below the lower reference limit.
- **Sperm morphology (Fig. 15.18):** Smear prepared from semen is fixed and stained with Papanicolaou stain to identify the morphological features. Normal spermatozoa have a head, neck, middle piece (midpiece), principal piece, and endpiece. Since the endpiece is difficult to see under a light microscope, the spermatozoa can be considered to consist of a head (and neck) and a tail (midpiece and principal piece). Normally, >4% of sperms have normal morphology. For a spermatozoon to be considered normal, both its head and tail must be morphologically normal. All other forms should be considered as abnormal.

Q. Write a short answer on abnormal forms of sperm.

Classification of abnormal sperm morphology (Fig. 15.18): During morphological examination all major parts of spermatozoa should be assessed, abnormal spermatozoa usually have a lower fertilizing capacity. The abnormalities in morphology can be classified as:

1. **Head defects:**
   - **Abnormal size:** Large or small head.
   - **Abnormal shape:** Pointed/tapered, round, pyriform, amorphous.
   - **Acrosomal defects:** Vacuolated acrosomal region, abnormality of acrosomal areas.
   - **Abnormal number:** Double-headed.
2. **Neck and midpiece defects:**
   - Sharply bent neck.
   - Asymmetrical insertion of the midpiece into the head.
   - Thick or thin or irregular midpiece.
3. **Tail (principal) piece defects:** These abnormalities include short or bent or coiled or double tail.

Tests for Antibody Coating of Spermatozoa

The agglutination of spermatozoa may be the result of the anti-sperm antibodies (ASAs) or other factors present in the semen. ASAs in the semen belong to IgA and IgG types and they may also be found in sperm-free fluids (seminal plasma, blood serum, and cervical mucus).

Tests for antibodies on spermatozoa ("direct tests"): Two direct tests include the mixed antiglobulin reaction (MAR) test and the immunobead (IB) test.

Tests for antisperm antibodies in sperm-free fluids ("indirect" tests).

THYROID FUNCTION TESTS

PA 23.3b (CC): Describe and interpret the abnormalities in thyroid function tests.

Q. Write a short essay on thyroid function tests.

Thyroid function tests (TFTs) are a collective term for tests used to check the function of the thyroid gland. Various tests and their significance are mentioned in **Table 15.12.**

Indications

Screening for Thyroid Dysfunction

Thyroid function tests are performed to screen patients suspected of having thyroid disease. The indications for screening include:

- Neonates for congenital hypothyroidism
- Patients with autoimmune disease
- Individuals with a strong family history of thyroid diseases
- Patient with suspected hyperthyroidism/hypothyroidism

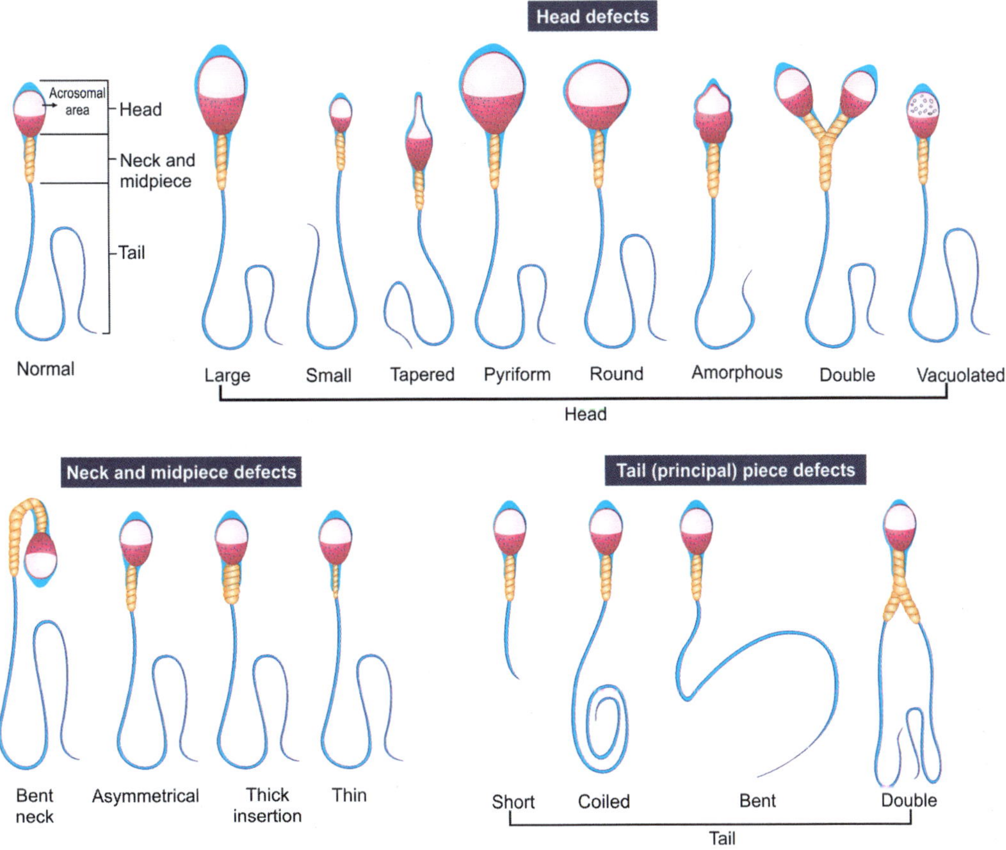

Fig. 15.18: Sperm morphology of both normal and abnormal forms.

TABLE 15.12 Thyroid function tests.

Test	*Significance*
Serum thyroid hormones (normal values)	
• Thyroid-stimulating hormone/ thyrotrophin (TSH 0.4–5.0 µU/mL)	Increased in primary hypothyroidism, Hashimoto thyroiditis. Decreased in hyperthyroidism
• Thyroid hormone levels: Free thyroxine (FT4) (5.4– 11.7 µg/dL), triiodothyronine (T3) (77–135 ng/dL)	Increased in hyperthyroidism and decreased in hypothyroidism
• Thyrotrophin-releasing hormone (TRH) stimulation test (0.4–5.0 µU/mL)	In primary hypothyroidism an exaggerated prolonged rise of already increased TSH levels is observed. In secondary hyperthyroidism (pituitary), there will be no rise in the decreased TSH level
• Thyroglobulin (Tg)	Increased in well-differentiated thyroid carcinoma and hyperthyroidism. Decreased following total thyroidectomy or destruction of thyroid by radiation
• Calcitonin level	Used for diagnosis of primary/recurrence of medullary carcinoma of thyroid or metastases after the removal of the primary. Increased in some paraneoplastic syndromes (e.g., carcinoma of the lung), hypercalcemia of any cause, and C cell hyperplasia
Thyroid autoantibody tests	
• Antimicrosomal antibody • Antithyroid peroxidase antibody (TPOAb) • Antithyroglobulin antibody (TgAb) • TSH receptor antibody (TRAb)	Diagnosis and monitoring of autoimmune thyroid diseases, Hashimoto thyroiditis: Antimicrosomal or antithyroid peroxidase antibodies, Graves' disease: Anti-TSH receptor antibodies
Radioactive iodine uptake (RAIU) ***(10–35% in 24 hours)***	Increased in Graves' disease, toxic multinodular goiter and adenoma, and early thyroiditis. Decreased in hypothyroidism, late thyroiditis

- Conditions linked to thyroid diseases such as atrial fibrillation or anxiety disorder

Surveillance

- Women with a history of postpartum thyroiditis.
- Post-neck irradiation.
- Post-destructive treatment (radioiodine or surgical) for thyrotoxicosis.

Monitoring

One of the common reasons for assessing thyroid function is to monitor therapy.

- Monitoring treatment of **hyperthyroidism** with antithyroid drugs.
- Patients with primary **hypothyroidism** who are taking thyroxine hormone replacement therapy.

Serum Thyroid Hormones

Thyroid-stimulating Hormone/Thyrotrophin

Thyroid-stimulating hormone (TSH) is secreted by the anterior pituitary gland. It increases the production and release of thyroxine (T_3 and T_4) from the thyroid. Its secretion is inhibited by high levels of T_3 and T_4. It is stimulated by high levels of TRH and low levels of T_3 and T_4.

Use (Box 15.25): To assess true metabolic status. It is the most important test to assess function and monitor thyroid hormone replacement therapy.
- **Increased:** Thyroid failure is characterized by a decrease in the level of T_3 and T_4 with increased TSH.
  - Primary hypothyroidism
  - Hashimoto thyroiditis.
- **Decreased:** In hyperthyroidism, the TSH level is suppressed and may be undetectable.

Thyroid Hormone Levels

- **FT_4 (Free thyroxine):** It is produced only by the thyroid gland. It travels in plasma bound to protein or in free form. It is converted to T_3 (active) and RT_3 (inactive) peripherally in blood and tissues.
- **T_3 (Triiodothyronine):** T_4 is converted to T_3 in the peripheral tissue. Most of it is transported in plasma bound to protein and only 0.3% is in free form.

Use: Its level reflects secretory activity.

- **Increased in hyperthyroidism**
- **Decreased in hypothyroidism.**

BOX 15.25: Uses of TSH estimation.

- Screening for thyroid function
- Screening of hypothyroidism in newborn
- Diagnosis of hypo- and hyperthyroidism
- Monitor thyroid hormone replacement therapy

Thyrotrophin-releasing Hormone Stimulation Test

Thyrotrophin-releasing hormone (TRH) is secreted by hypothalamus, which stimulates the release of TSH from the pituitary. TRH secretion is inhibited by high levels of T_3 and T_4 and stimulated by low levels of T_3 and T_4. Serum TSH is measured before and after the intravenous administration of TRH.

Use (Box 15.25): To differentiate two forms (whether due to tumor or not) of thyrotrophin-induced hyperthyroidism.
- In primary hypothyroidism an exaggerated prolonged rise of already increased TSH level is observed.
- In secondary hyperthyroidism (pituitary), there will be no rise in the decreased TSH level.

Thyroglobulin

Thyroglobulin (Tg) is secreted by thyroid follicular cells and is involved in iodination and synthesis of thyroid hormones.

Use: To predict the outcome of therapy for hyperthyroidism.
- **Increased:** Well-differentiated thyroid carcinoma, hyperthyroidism
- **Decreased:** Total thyroidectomy or destruction of thyroid by radiation.

Calcitonin Level

It is secreted by the parafollicular C cells of the thyroid. It decreases the bone-resorption by osteoclasts and causes decreased serum calcium.

Use: Diagnosis of primary/recurrence of medullary carcinoma of thyroid or metastases after the removal of the primary. **Increased in:**
- Some paraneoplastic syndromes (e.g., carcinoma of the lung)
- Hypercalcemia of any cause
- C cell hyperplasia.

Thyroid Autoantibody Tests

The different types of thyroid autoantibodies responsible for the autoimmune thyroid disorders are:

- Antimicrosomal antibody.
- **Antithyroid peroxidase (TPO) antibody (TPOAb):** They are involved in the tissue destructive process associated with hypothyroidism in Hashimoto and atrophic thyroiditis.
- Antithyroglobulin (Tg) antibody.
- **TSH receptor (TR) antibody (TRAb):** These antibodies were previously known as thyroid-stimulating immunoglobulin (TSI) or long-acting thyroid stimulators (LATS). Laboratory assessment of antithyroid peroxidase antibodies is replacing the antimicrosomal and anti-thyroglobulin antibodies. Uses of thyroid autoantibodies measurement are listed in **Box 15.26**.

BOX 15.26: Uses of thyroid autoantibodies measurement.

- **Diagnosis and monitoring of autoimmune thyroid diseases**
- **Hashimoto thyroiditis:** Antimicrosomal or antithyroid peroxidase antibodies
- **Graves' disease:** Anti-TSH receptor antibodies

Radioactive Iodine Uptake (Box 15.27)

T_4 contains high iodine and the thyroid gland must take- up a large amount of iodine from the circulating blood for the synthesis of T_4. The iodine uptake activity of the thyroid can be measured by administering orally a low dose of radioactive iodine (or technetium) and the radioactivity over the thyroid is measured at specified intervals. The amount of radioactivity that is taken up by the thyroid gland is known as radioactive iodine uptake (RAIU). Normal uptake ranges from 10 to 35% in 24 hours. A very high RAIU is seen in hyperthyroidism, while a low RAIU is seen in hypothyroidism.

Contraindication: RAIU is contraindicated in children and during pregnancy/lactation.

BOX 15.27: Use of RAIU.

- Evaluation of hyperthyroidism
- Differentiate Graves from toxic goiter
- Function of a thyroid nodule as hot or cold.

Increased: Graves disease, toxic multinodular goiter and adenoma, and early thyroiditis.

Decreased: Hypothyroidism, late thyroiditis.

BOX 15.28: Use of thyroid scintiscanning.

- Differential diagnosis of high RAIU thyrotoxicosis
  - Uniform or diffuse increase in uptake in Graves' disease
  - Multiple discrete areas of increased uptake in toxic multinodular goiter
  - Single area of increased uptake in adenoma.
- Evaluation of solitary nodule of thyroid
  - Hyperfunctioning: Hot nodule
  - Non-functioning: Cold nodule (~20% are malignant).

Thyroid Scintiscanning (Box 15.28)

In addition to the radioactive iodine uptake, an isotype (99mTc-pertechnetate) can be administered and its distribution within the thyroid gland is assessed by a gamma counter.

Common thyroid function tests in normal and pathological conditions are shown in **Table 15.13.**

RENAL FUNCTION TESTS

PA 23.3c (CC): Describe and interpret the abnormalities in renal function tests.

Q. Name renal function tests.

- **Urine analysis** (both routine and microscopic *refer* pages 450-462).
- **Blood chemistry:** Impaired renal function causes elevation of end-products of protein metabolism which is known as **azotemia.** These include:
  - Blood urea (normal range 20–40 mg/dL).
  - Blood urea nitrogen (BUN): Normal range 10–20 mg/dL.
  - Creatinine (normal range 0.6–1.2 mg/dL).
- **Renal clearance tests.**
- **Concentration and dilution tests.**

Blood Chemistry

Impaired renal function causes elevation of end-products of protein metabolism which is known as **azotemia.** These include:

- Blood urea (normal range 20–40 mg/dL).
- Blood urea nitrogen (BUN): Normal range 10–20 mg/dL. Causes of raised blood urea nitrogen (BUN) are listed in **Box 15.29.**
- Creatinine (normal range 0.6–1.2 mg/dL). The causes of raised serum creatinine are listed in **Box 15.30.**

Renal Clearance Tests

These tests measure the **glomerular function** and renal blood flow.

- Glomerular filtration rate (GFR) is the rate at which fluid passes into the nephron after filtration and it measures renal excretory function. The rate of glomerular filtration is measured by the capacity of the kidneys to clear

TABLE 15.13 Common thyroid function tests in normal and pathological states.

Thyroid functional state	*TSH*	*Free T_4*	*T_3*	*Tg*
Euthyroid	Normal	Normal	Normal	Normal
Hyperthyroidism-Graves' disease	Decreased or undetectable	Increased	Increased	Increased
Hypothyroidism	Increased	Decreased	Decreased	Normal or decreased
Hashimoto thyroiditis hypothyroidism	High	Normal or decreased	Normal or decreased	Normal or decreased

(T_3: triiodothyronine; T_4: thyroxine; Tg: thyroglobulin; TSH: thyroid stimulating hormone)

BOX 15.29: Causes of raised blood urea nitrogen (BUN).

- **Prerenal azotemia:** Congestive cardiac failure, shock, depletion of salt and water
- **Renal azotemia:** Impaired kidney function
- **Postrenal azotemia:** Obstructive lesions of the urinary tract
- **Increased production of urea:** High protein diet, increased catabolism of proteins (e.g., trauma, burns)

BOX 15.30: Causes of raised serum creatinine.

- Azotemia, e.g., prerenal, renal and postrenal
- Large amount of consumption of meat
- Active acromegaly and gigantism

waste products or foreign materials (inulin, mannitol, creatinine, and urea) from the blood into the urine.

- Clearance of a solute from plasma into the urine equals GFR if the solute is freely filtered through the glomerulus and neither secreted into nor absorbed from the renal tubules.
- From the determination of blood concentration of the test material and the quantity eliminated in the urine, "clearance" can be calculated and is expressed in terms of milliliters of blood cleared per unit time.

The various tests are:

Inulin clearance test: Inulin is ideal for the measurement of GFR because it is neither secreted nor reabsorbed by the tubule. Mannitol can also be used.

Creatinine clearance: Creatinine is normally released into the plasma by muscle metabolism and is filtered through the glomerulus. Normally, the clearance of endogenous creatinine approximates the glomerular filtration rate. It is an easy and routinely employed method for GFR estimation.

The urea clearance test: It is less sensitive.

Concentration/Dilution Tests

These tests are used to evaluate the tubular function. The ability of the nephron to concentrate or dilute urine is dependent on the tubular cells in the renal medulla as well as antidiuretic hormone (ADH).

Urine-specific gravity: It is a measure of the capacity of the tubules to reabsorb water, thus concentrating the urine (*refer* pages 452-3). In chronic tubular damage, it remains fixed at 1.010. If the patient's urine contains no sugar or protein and has a specific gravity of 1.025 or higher, a concentration test is unnecessary.

Concentration test: In this test, an artificial deprivation of fluid is induced in a patient for more than 20 hours. With normal tubular function, water is selectively absorbed and urine will have a high solute concentration with a specific gravity of 1025 or more. With tubular damage, the specific gravity remains constant irrespective of water deprivation.

Dilution test: In this test, excessive fluid is given to the patient which will result in a lower solute concentration in a normal individual. The resulting specific gravity will be 1.003 or less. In tubular damage, the specific gravity remains constant irrespective of excessive water intake.

BOX 15.31: Indications for renal biopsy.

- Nephrotic syndrome/glomerular proteinuria in adults
- Nephrotic syndrome in children with atypical presentation/not responding to treatment (steroids)
- Chronic renal failure with normal-sized kidney
- Unexplained acute renal failure
- Differential diagnosis of acute nephritic syndrome
- Isolated hematuria/non-nephrotic proteinuria
- Unexplained renal insufficiency when kidney dimensions are near normal on ultrasonography
- Impaired functioning of renal transplant
- Asymptomatic hematuria when other diagnostic tests cannot detect the cause
- Involvement of kidney in systemic diseases (e.g., systemic lupus erythematosus, amyloidosis)

TABLE 15.14 Contraindications and complications of renal biopsy.

Contraindications	*Complications*
• Coagulation disorders • Thrombocytopenia • Uncontrolled hypertension • Solitary kidney • Rena neoplasms to avoid spread along the needle track • Large and multiple renal cysts • Acute urinary tract infections • Urinary tract obstructions • Kidney <60% predicted size	• Pain • Infection • Bleeding into the urine • Bleeding around kidney • Arteriovenous fistula • Accidental biopsy of other organs or perforation of organs such as liver, spleen • Rarely death

Renal Biopsy

It is used to establish the nature and extent of renal disease. Biopsy is performed transcutaneously with ultrasound guidance. Biopsy material is examined under light microscopy (fixed in neutral buffered formaldehyde), electron microscopy (fixed in glutaraldehyde), and by immunofluorescence (tested for IgG, IgA, IgM, C3, fibrin, and κ and λ light chains by using appropriate antibodies). Indications, for renal biopsy are presented in **Box 15.31** and contraindications and complications of renal biopsy are presented in **Table 15.14**.

Refer **online Table 15.15.**

LIVER FUNCTION TESTS

PA 23.3d (CC): Describe and interpret the abnormalities in liver function tests.

Q. Name liver function tests.

Liver function tests (LFTs) are groups of laboratory tests designed to give information about the state of a patient's

BOX 15.32: Liver function tests.

A. **Tests for excretory functions**
   - Bilirubin metabolism:
     - Serum bilirubin estimation
     - Bilirubin in feces
     - Bilirubin and urobilinogen in urine
   - Bromosulfophthalein (BSP) excretion
   - Bile acids (bile salts)

B. **Tests of liver cell injury**
   - Enzymes that detect hepatocellular injury
     - Transaminases (aminotransferases): Serum aspartate transaminases (AST), serum alanine transaminases (ALT), AST/ALT ratio
     - Lactate dehydrogenase (LDH)
   - Enzymes that detect cholestasis
     - Serum alkaline phosphatase
     - γ-glutamyl transpeptidase
     - 5′-Nucleotidase

C. **Tests of metabolism and biosynthesis**
   - Proteins secreted into the blood
     - Serum proteins: Albumin, globulin, and albumin: globulin (A: G) ratio
     - Clotting factors: Prothrombin time
   - Hepatocyte metabolism: Serum ammonia
   - Lipid and lipoprotein metabolism
   - Carbohydrate metabolism

D. **Immunological tests**

E. **Ancillary diagnostic test:** Alpha-fetoprotein (AFP)

liver (**Box 15.32**). Because of multiple and complex functions of the liver, it is necessary to perform several tests for an accurate diagnosis, to assess the severity of the disease and its prognosis.

Tests for Excretory Functions

Bilirubin Metabolism

Serum Bilirubin Estimation

It is not a sensitive test for liver dysfunction and may not reflect the degree of liver damage.

Normal values: Total serum bilirubin in adults is <1 mg/dL of which conjugated bilirubin is less than 0.25 mg/dL. ***van den Bergh reaction***: Bilirubin estimation is based on **van den Bergh diazo reaction** by spectrophotometric method. Diazo reagent consists of diazotized sulfanilic acid which forms a conjugated azo compound with the porphyrin rings of bilirubin.

- **Direct van den Bergh reaction**: Water-soluble conjugated bilirubin gives direct van den Bergh reaction with diazo reagent within one minute.
- **Indirect van den Bergh reaction**: Alcohol-soluble unconjugated bilirubin gives a positive result with indirect van den Bergh reaction.

Refer to **Box 19.1** for causes of hyperbilirubinemia.

Bilirubin in Feces

Significance: Absence of fecal excretion of the pigment is seen **in obstructive jaundice** which gives rise to clay-colored stool.

Bilirubin and urobilinogen in urine are discussed on pages 459-60.

Bromosulfthalein Excretion

Bromosulfthalein (BSP) is a dye that follows the same routes of binding, conjugation, and excretion as that of bilirubin. BSP is intravenously injected and venous blood after 45 minutes is tested for the percentage of injected dye remaining in the blood. Nowadays, this test is not done due to the availability of enzyme estimations which are better indicators of hepatic dysfunction. The BSP excretion test is **valuable only in the diagnosis of Dubin-Johnson syndrome.**

Bile Acids (Bile Salts)

Primary bile acids (cholic acid and chenodeoxycholic acid) are formed from cholesterol in the hepatocytes. These bile acids are secreted in the bile. In the gut, they undergo deconjugation by the colonic bacteria and produce secondary bile acids (deoxycholic acid and lithocholic acid). About 90% of these bile acids are reabsorbed through **enterohepatic circulation** and reach the liver. About 10% are excreted in the feces.

Significance: Raised blood **levels of bile acids produce itching** (pruritus). Serum bile acids are **raised in hepatobiliary diseases with cholestasis.** Their presence in the urine can be detected by Hay's sulfur test (*refer* page 460).

Tests of Liver Cell Injury

Estimation of serum enzymes is the most sensitive and useful test for diagnosis of various types of liver (both hepatocellular and cholestatic) injury.

Enzymes that Detect Hepatocellular Injury

Transaminases (Aminotransferases)

Hepatocellular damage/necrosis is assessed mainly by the estimation of transaminases (**Table 15.16**).

TABLE 15.16 Common cause of elevated serum transaminases.

Degree	*Serum levels*	*Common causes*
Mild	<100 U/L	Chronic hepatitis C, hemochromatosis, fatty liver (steatosis)
Moderate	100–300 U/L	Apart from the above, it may be found in alcoholic hepatitis, autoimmune hepatitis, Wilson disease
Severe	>300 U/L	Acute viral hepatitis, drug toxicity, toxins

Serum aspartate transaminase (AST): This was formerly known as glutamic oxaloacetic transaminase (SGOT). It is a **mitochondrial enzyme found in the heart, liver, skeletal muscle, and kidney** and is liberated into the blood whenever there is damage to the parenchymal cells. Thus, AST may rise in acute necrosis or ischemia of other organs apart from liver cell injury. Normal serum level is 0.20–0.65 μkat/L (12–38 U/L).

Serum alanine transaminase (ALT): This was formerly called glutamic pyruvic transaminase or SGPT. It is a **cytosolic enzyme** mainly **found in the liver**. Thus, serum ALT is fairly specific for liver tissue and is of greater value in assessing liver cell injury. Normal serum level is 0.12–0.70 μkat/L (7–41 U/L).

AST/ALT ratio: It is usually of little value except if the ratio is >3 (with ALT <300 U/L), which is suggestive of **alcoholic** hepatitis.

- **Significance of transaminase estimations are** (i) early diagnosis of viral hepatitis, (ii) alcoholic liver disease, and (iii) cirrhosis.

Lactate Dehydrogenase (LDH)

It occurs in the cytoplasm of all cells, the highest concentration being found in the liver, heart, skeletal muscle, kidney, and RBCs. Thus, it is not specific to liver diseases.

Significance
- Marked increase in metastatic carcinoma to the liver.
- Moderate increase in cirrhosis, obstructive jaundice, and acute viral hepatitis.

Enzymes that Detect Cholestasis

Serum alkaline phosphatase: It is produced by many tissues (bone, liver, intestine, and placenta) and is excreted in the bile. Normal serum alkaline phosphatase (range in adults 33–96 U/L) is mainly derived from bone.

Significance
- **Increased** levels can be found in **diseases of bone, and liver and pregnancy**
- In the absence of bone disease and pregnancy, an **elevated** serum alkaline phosphatase level (3–10 times normal) indicates **biliary tract obstruction**
- Mild-to-moderate increase is observed in parenchymal liver diseases (hepatitis, cirrhosis, and hepatic metastasis)

A combination of serum transaminases and alkaline phosphatase is very useful in the diagnosis of injury to liver cells.

γ-glutamyl transpeptidase (γ-GT): The liver is the primary source of the serum enzyme, γ-GT. Its serum level parallels serum alkaline phosphatase. So, it is used to confirm that raised serum alkaline phosphatase is due to **hepatobiliary disease**. It is also raised in patients with **alcohol abuse** even without liver disease.

5′-nucleotidase: It is also a phosphatase derived from the liver. It is useful to distinguish alkaline phosphatase of hepatic origin from that of bone.

Tests of Metabolism and Biosynthesis

The liver is the main site of synthesis of amino acids and plasma proteins, lipids, and lipoproteins, carbohydrates, and vitamins.

Plasma Protein Synthesis

Hepatocytes synthesize several proteins including albumin, fibrinogen, prothrombin, alpha-l-antitrypsin, and acute-phase reactant proteins. Levels of these plasma proteins are reduced in extensive liver damage. Estimation of the following will be useful in the diagnosis of liver disorders:

Serum proteins: Routinely done estimations are:
- **Total** serum **proteins** (normal 6.7–8.6 g/dL)
- **Serum albumin** (normal 3.5–5.5 g/dL) is produced solely by the liver.
- **Serum globulin** (normal 2–3.5 g/dL)
- **Albumin/globulin** (A/G) **ratio** (normal 1.5–3:1).

They are evaluated by serum/immunoelectrophoresis. Previously, thymol turbidity and flocculation tests were used for their estimation.

Significance: **Hypoalbuminemia** develops with chronic inflammatory disorders such as **cirrhosis** and **chronic hepatitis.**

Clotting factors: Both prothrombin time and partial thromboplastin time, reflect the activities of various clotting factors. They are prolonged in hepatocellular disease.

Prothrombin time: It depends on the hepatic synthesis of clotting factors and intestinal uptake of vitamin K (fat-soluble vitamin).

- **Prolonged prothrombin time: Obstruction of the bile duct** and intrahepatic cholestasis, which result in vitamin K deficiency due to impaired lipid absorption, are associated with prolonged prothrombin time. With parenteral administration of vitamin K, prothrombin time will return to normal, if the prolongation is due to obstruction. If there is no improvement in prothrombin time, it indicates severe hepatocellular disease.

Serum Ammonia

Ammonia can be metabolized only in the liver and is derived mainly from amino acid (received from the diet and tissue breakdown) and nucleic acid metabolism. Ammonia is a toxic substance ultimately converted into nontoxic urea which is readily excreted. **Increased blood level of ammonia** is found when most of the liver is destroyed as in **acute fulminant hepatitis**, **cirrhosis,** and **hepatic encephalopathy**. The elevated levels are due to the inability of the severely damaged liver to convert ammonia to urea.

Serum Gamma Globulins (Immunoglobulins)

Increased in most forms of **chronic liver disease.**

- IgA is raised in cirrhosis.
- IgG is markedly raised in chronic active hepatitis.
- IgM is markedly increased in primary biliary cirrhosis.

Lipid and Lipoprotein Metabolism

The liver synthesizes cholesterol and cholesterol esters, phospholipids, and triglycerides. These lipids are insoluble in water and are carried in circulation as high-density lipoproteins (HDL), low-density lipoproteins (LDL), and very low-density lipoproteins (VLDL).

Total serum cholesterol (Normal <200 mg/dL)

- Raised in cholestasis, probably due to retention of cholesterol which is normally excreted in the bile.
- Decreased in acute and chronic diffuse liver diseases and malnutrition.

Carbohydrate Metabolism

The liver also plays a central role in carbohydrate metabolism. Blood glucose level is reduced in fulminant hepatitis. Impaired glucose tolerance and relative insulin resistance are found in chronic liver disease.

Immunologic Tests

Diseases of the liver may be associated with various immunological abnormalities.

Specific Antigens/Antibodies

- **Hepatitis B surface antigen (HBsAg), hepatitis B core antibody (anti-HBc), hepatitis Be antigen (HBeAg)** in hepatitis B infection.
- Antibodies to *Entamoeba histolytica* can be demonstrated in amoebic liver abscesses.

Ancillary Diagnostic Tests

Alpha-Fetoprotein

It is a α-globulin found in fetal blood. It originates in the fetal liver, GI tract, and yolk sac. It is one of the tumor markers for hepatocellular carcinoma, but not a specific marker, as it may be found in non-neoplastic and other neoplastic conditions.

The reference range of liver function tests is shown (*refer* **online Table 15.17**).

FNAC and/or Liver Biopsy

Liver Biopsy

Percutaneous needle biopsy of the liver through an intercostal approach is done under local anesthesia. It is a simple, safe procedure for the assessment of liver histology for the diagnosis of various liver disorders.

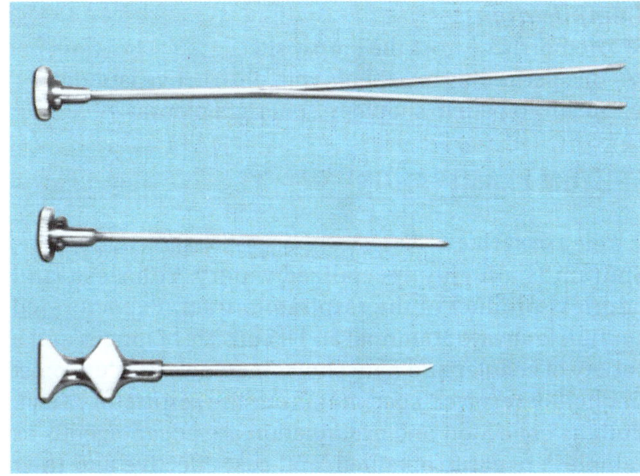

Fig. 15.19: Vim Silverman's needle showing prongs—split needle, stilette, and cannula (top to bottom).

Before the biopsy: Prothrombin time (PT) should be performed before liver biopsy. If it is high, the patient should be given parenteral vitamin K and the test should be repeated. If PT is prolonged by more than 3 seconds than the control, it is a contraindication for liver biopsy.

Needle: Vim Silverman's needle is used for liver biopsy (**Fig. 15.19**).

Indications for liver biopsy

Q. Indications for liver biopsy.

- Unexplained hepatomegaly, splenomegaly, jaundice.
- Cirrhosis of the liver, to assess the type, etiology, and activity of the disease process.
- **Chronic hepatitis:** For identifying, grading inflammatory activity, staging, and evaluation of the course.
- **Pyrexia of unknown origin (PUO):** A liver biopsy may be helpful in the diagnosis of miliary tuberculosis, sarcoidosis, or malignancy.
- **Idiopathic hemochromatosis:** To determine iron stores in the liver.

Contraindications

Q. Contraindications for liver biopsy.

- Congenital coagulation disorders, e.g., hemophilia A and B.
- PT prolonged by more than 3 seconds over control.
- Obstructive jaundice: Liver biopsy may cause leakage of bile from the liver into the peritoneum causing severe and fatal bile peritonitis.
- Massive ascites.
- Patients with severe cough where diaphragm movements cannot be controlled.
- Uncooperative patients.
- Hydatid cyst liver: } These are relative contraindications
- Hemangioma liver }

Complications

- Hemorrhage from the biopsy site.
- Bile peritonitis in patients with obstructive jaundice.
- Referred pain to shoulder from right pleura.

SPUTUM EXAMINATION

Q. Write a short note on the sputum examination and its importance.

Sputum is a highly specialized watery, colorless, and odorless product of the respiratory tract. Expectorated sputum is always abnormal and it consists of mucus and a variety of cellular and noncellular materials. It is the most frequently received specimen from the respiratory tract. Both its collection and examination are advantageous as samples are easily obtained, and cost-effective and their cellular content is representative of the entire respiratory tract.

Indications for Sputum Examination

Q. Write a short answer on indications for sputum examination.

- Smear and culture **identification of causative organisms** in suspected infection (e.g., pneumonia, tuberculosis).
- Cytological examination for **malignant cells, viral inclusions, and asbestosis.**

Sputum Collection

The patient is instructed to cough up to get the sputum proper and the same is collected in a wide-mouthed sterile, glass/plastic container with a screw cap.

In those patients who cannot produce sputum spontaneously by deep coughing, a specimen of sputum may be induced. This is done by inhalation of appropriate solvents which are aerosolized to stimulate sputum production.

An early morning sputum sample is preferred for routine examination and a 24-hour sample for the demonstration of tubercle bacilli by concentration method.

Examination of Sputum

Sputum examination consists of (i) physical examination, (ii) microscopic examination, and (iii) culture study.

Physical Examination

- **Quantity:**
  - In bronchiectasis, a large amount of purulent sputum is coughed out.
  - Large amount of watery sputum with pink tinge suggests pulmonary edema.
- **Appearance/color:** Colors of sputum vary in different pathological conditions.
- **Odor or smell:** Foul-smelling sputum is observed in bronchiectasis and lung abscesses and is due to anaerobic bacterial infections.

Microscopic Examination

Staining of sputum: Two to three smears are made on a clean dry glass slide and are stained with:

- Leishman stain or Wright stain for differential count.
- Other stains (depending on the clinical/pathological features).
  - Gram stain for microorganisms.
  - Ziehl–Neelsen stain for acid-fast tubercle bacilli.
  - Special stains for fungi.
- Papanicolaou stain for study of malignant cells.

Cells

Normal sputum consists of a few neutrophils, a few lymphocytes, carbon-laden macrophages, occasional eosinophils, and red cells. Various types of cells seen in sputum and their significance are shown in **Table 15.18**.

Refer online for laboratory values of clinical importance; and reference values of the clinical chemistry of blood **(Table 15.19)**, and the lipid profile **(Table 15.20)**. Various important bodies and their associated conditions are presented in **Table 15.21**, important cells in various lesions are presented in **Table 15.22** and pathognomonic structures in diseases are presented in **Table 15.23**.

TABLE 15.18 Types of cells in sputum and their significance.

Type of cell	*Significance*
Pus cells (neutrophils)	Numerous pus cells indicate pyogenic infection of the respiratory tract
Eosinophils	Increased eosinophils are seen in asthma and parasitic infections of the lungs
Lymphocytes	Increased lymphocytes are seen in early pulmonary tuberculosis
Red blood cells	If increased, indicate hemorrhage (bleeding) into the lungs or the bronchi
Heart failure cells (hemosiderin-laden macrophages)	• Chronic venous congestion of the lungs • Pulmonary infarction and pulmonary hemorrhage
Anthracotic pigment-laden cells (carbon-laden)	Increased in coal workers' pneumoconiosis and those who live in smoky polluted atmosphere

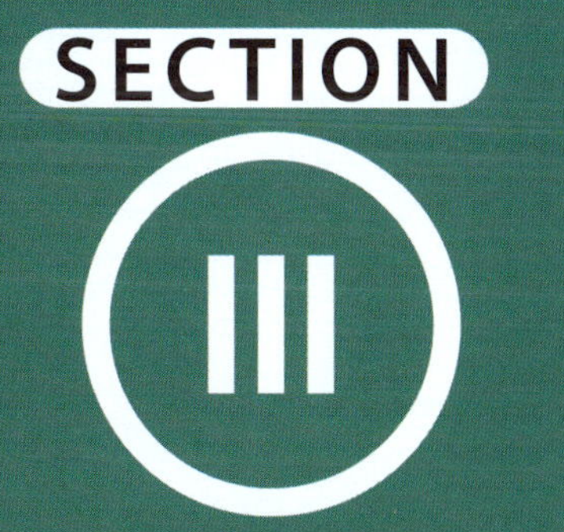

Systemic Pathology

Section Outline

16. Cardiovascular Disorders
17. Respiratory Disorders
18. Oral Cavity and Gastrointestinal Tract
19. Hepatobiliary and Pancreatic Disorders
20. Kidney and Urinary Tract Disorders
21. Male Genital Tract Disorders
22. Female Genital Tract Disorders
23. Breast Disorders
24. Endocrine Disorders
25. Bones, Joints, and Soft Tissue Tumors
26. Skin Disorders
27. Disorders of the Central Nervous System and Eye

CHAPTER 16

Cardiovascular Disorders

CHAPTER OUTLINE

Vascular Disorders
- Arteriosclerosis
- Atherosclerosis
- Aneurysms and Dissection
- Hypertensive Vascular Disease
- Vasculitis
- Vascular Tumors

Heart Disorders
- Heart Failure
- Rheumatic Fever and Rheumatic Heart Disease
- Ischemic Heart Disease
- Myocardial Infarction
- Infective Endocarditis
- Noninfected Vegetations
- Cardiomyopathy
- Pericarditis and Pericardial Effusion
- Congenital Heart Disease
- Cardiac Myxoma

VASCULAR DISORDERS

ARTERIOSCLEROSIS

PA 27.1 (CC): Distinguish arteriosclerosis from atherosclerosis. Describe the pathogenesis and pathology of various causes and types of arteriosclerosis.

Arteriosclerosis (hardening of the arteries) is the general term for thickening and loss of arterial wall elasticity. There are four patterns, each with different clinical and pathological consequences.

Arteriolosclerosis: It is a generalized progressive arterial disease in which sclerosis affects small arteries and arterioles. It is associated with wall stiffening and localized luminal narrowing. They may cause downstream ischemic injury. There are two variants, namely hyaline and hyperplastic arteriolosclerosis. They were discussed under hypertension (*refer* page 494).

Mönckeberg medial sclerosis (*refer* Fig. 2.32A): It is characterized by the deposition of calcium in large- and medium-sized muscular arteries typically starting along the internal elastic membrane. Usually seen in old age (above 50 years). The calcifications do not affect the lumen of the vessel and also blood flow. Hence, they are usually not clinically significant.

Fibromuscular intimal hyperplasia: It is a nonatherosclerotic disease observed in muscular arteries larger than arterioles. It is rich in vascular smooth muscle cells (SMCs) and extracellular matrix (ECM). It usually follows inflammation (e.g., in a healed arteritis, transplant-associated arteriopathy) or mechanical injury (e.g., associated with stents or balloon angioplasty). It is often considered as a healing response to injury. This can lead to significant stenosis of the involved vessel. Fibromuscular intimal hyperplasia underlies in-stent restenosis and is the major factor limiting solid-organ transplants' long-term survival.

Atherosclerosis: It is the most frequent and important disease of the intima.

ATHEROSCLEROSIS

Q. Define atherosclerosis.

Definition: Atherosclerosis is **primarily a progressive disease of intima** involving **large- and medium-sized elastic and muscular arteries.** It is characterized by focal lipid-rich intimal lesions called **atheromas** (atheromatous, atherosclerotic, fibrous, or fibrofatty plaques).

Atherosclerosis is the vascular response to endothelial injury.

Epidemiology: Atherosclerosis is involved in the pathogenesis of coronary, cerebral, and peripheral vascular disease. It is one of the major causes of morbidity and mortality. Atherosclerosis is a worldwide disease seen in both developed and developing countries. Atherosclerotic lesions in the intima may **reduce or block the lumen of the involved vessel** and **can rupture to cause sudden occlusion**. Coronary artery disease is an important manifestation of atherosclerosis and atherosclerosis mortality usually reflects deaths caused by ischemic heart disease. Atherosclerosis of the aorta and carotid arteries (stroke) are also responsible for significant morbidity and mortality.

Risk Factors for Atherosclerosis

Q. Write a short note on risk factors for atherosclerosis.

The probability of development of atherosclerosis depends on the combination of acquired (e.g., cholesterol levels, smoking, hypertension, diabetes), inherited [e.g., low-density lipoprotein (LDL) receptor gene mutations], and gender- and age-associated risk factors. Risk factors for atherosclerosis and ischemic heart disease were identified through several studies most important being the **Framingham Heart Study and Atherosclerosis Risk in Communities Study.** Risk roughly increases with the increase in a number of risk factors. For example, two factors increase risk about four-fold, and three (i.e., hyperlipidemia, hypertension, and smoking), increase risk by a factor of seven.

Classification of risk factors: The risk factors may be broadly classified as modifiable, nonmodifiable (constitutional and less controllable), and additional **(Table 16.1)**.

Modifiable Risk Factors in Ischemic Heart Disease (IHD)

These are **four** in number namely: (1) hyperlipidemia, (2) hypertension, (3) cigarette smoking, and (4) diabetes.

1. Hyperlipidemia

An increase in the serum lipids mainly cholesterol (**hypercholesterolemia**) is a major modifiable risk factor. Hypercholesterolemia can initiate atherosclerotic lesions even in the absence of other risk factors. The major components of lipids in the blood are:

- **Low-density lipoprotein (LDL)** known as **"bad cholesterol"** is one of the components of serum lipid and its **higher level** is associated with an **increased risk of atherosclerosis**. LDL delivers cholesterol to peripheral tissues.
- **High-density lipoprotein (HDL)** known as **"good cholesterol"** and its **higher levels are associated with decreased risk**.
  - HDL mobilizes cholesterol from the periphery (including atheroma) and excretes it through bile in the liver.
  - Exercise and moderate consumption of ethanol raise HDL levels, whereas obesity and smoking lower it.
- **Serum cholesterol level:** Normal range is 140–240 mg/dL. Serum cholesterol is **strongly related to the dietary intake of saturated fat** (in the absence of genetic disorders of lipid metabolism). The risk of atherosclerosis increases with increasing serum cholesterol concentrations and lowering serum cholesterol concentrations reduces the risk. The risk of atherosclerosis can be reduced by lowering LDL or total plasma cholesterol, and/or raising serum HDL. This can be achieved either by dietary modification or by treatment with cholesterol-lowering drugs.
  - **A diet that raises blood cholesterol:**
    - **A diet high in cholesterol and saturated fats** (e.g., egg yolks, animal fats, and butter). Transunsaturated fats are produced by the artificial hydrogenation of polyunsaturated oils (used in baked goods and margarine).
  - **A diet that lowers blood cholesterol:** Diets low in cholesterol and/or with higher ratios of **polyunsaturated fats.**
    - **Omega-3 fatty acids** (high in fish and fish oils).
  - **Cholesterol-lowering drug:** Statins are used to lower circulating cholesterol levels. They inhibit hydroxymethylglutaryl coenzyme A (HMG-CoA) reductase. This is the rate-limiting enzyme involved in cholesterol biosynthesis in the liver.
  - It is found that approaches that exclusively raise HDL are not effective in reducing the risk of atherosclerosis. The contribution of most dietary fats to atherosclerosis is now viewed as minimal.

Disorders associated with hypercholesterolemia: Nephrotic syndrome, alcoholism, hypothyroidism, and diabetes mellitus.

TABLE 16.1 Risk factors for atherosclerosis.

A. Modifiable major risk factors	
• Hyperlipidemia • Hypertension	• Cigarette smoking • Diabetes mellitus
B. Nonmodifiable (constitutional) risk factors	
• Inherited causes (e.g., familial hypercholesterolemia) • Family history	• Increasing age • Male gender
C. Additional risk factors	
• Inflammation • CRP level • Hyperhomocystinemia • Metabolic syndrome • Lipoprotein (a)	• Raised procoagulant levels • Inadequate physical activity • Stressful lifestyle • Obesity • Alcohol

2. Hypertension

It is one of the major risk factors.

- The incidence of atherosclerosis increases as BP rises, and this excess risk **is related to both systolic and diastolic levels of blood pressure.**
- Control of hypertension with antihypertensive therapy reduces the risk of myocardial infarction and stroke.
- Chronic hypertension causes left ventricular hypertrophy (LVH) by increasing oxygen demand. It contributes to myocardial ischemia and is also a surrogate marker for cardiovascular risk.

3. Cigarette Smoking

It is the **most important avoidable cause** of atherosclerosis. Atherosclerosis is **more severe and extensive among smokers than in nonsmokers.** This may be the reason for the increased incidence and severity of atherosclerosis in men compared to women. **There is a strong dose-linked relationship between cigarette smoking and ischemic heart disease. Cessation of smoking reduces the risk.**

4. Diabetes Mellitus

It is a potent risk factor for atherosclerosis. Diabetes is associated with hypercholesterolemia and increases the risk of atherosclerosis. The incidence of myocardial infarction and other atherosclerotic vascular diseases (strokes, gangrene of the lower extremities) is higher in diabetics than in non-diabetics.

Nonmodifiable/Constitutional Risk Factors

- **Genetics: A family history of atherosclerosis** is the most important independent risk factor. Mendelian disorders, such as **familial hypercholesterolemia** are strongly associated with atherosclerosis, but they are responsible for only a small percentage of cases. The well-established familial predisposition to atherosclerosis and ischemic heart disease is usually polygenic. This is related to the small effects of many shared alleles common to a family or population.
- **Age***:* Age is the most powerful independent risk factor and has a dominant influence. The development of atheromatous plaque is a progressive process. Clinical manifestation of atherosclerosis is usually observed after middle age and the lesions progressively rise with each decade. One of the important clinical manifestations of atherosclerosis is ischemic heart disease (IHD) and increased incidence (~five times) of myocardial infarction (one of the IHDs) is observed between the ages of 40 to 60. Death rates from ischemic heart disease rise with each decade of life even during advanced age.
  - **Clonal hematopoiesis of indeterminate potential (CHIP):** With aging, it is observed that there is a tendency for outgrowth of a single clone of hematopoietic stem cells (HSCs) due to one somatic mutation in HSCs. This clone of HSCs is called clonal hematopoiesis of indeterminate potential (CHIP). The mutations confer a proliferative advantage. Many of these affect DNA modifications and transcriptional regulation. Ultimately, these can influence the risk of developing hematologic malignancies. Emerging evidence suggests that individuals with CHIP have an increased risk for atherosclerotic cardiovascular disease. The CHIP mutations that affect cellular proliferation (e.g., *TET2*) can also be involved in the inflammatory response of mononuclear cells and thereby influence atherogenesis.
- **Gender: Premenopausal women have a lower incidence** of atherosclerosis-related diseases compared to males of the same age group. Thus, myocardial infarction and other complications of atherosclerosis are uncommon in premenopausal women unless they have other risk factors such as diabetes, hyperlipidemia, or severe hypertension. However, **after menopause, this sex difference in atherosclerosis-related diseases disappears.** This may be due to the protective role of estrogen. Hormone replacement therapy has no role in the prevention of coronary heart disease. On the contrary, postmenopausal estrogen therapy may actually increase cardiovascular risk in some older women.

Additional Risk Factors

It is found that about 20% of all cardiovascular events occur in individuals without any major risk factors (e.g., hypertension, hyperlipidemia, cigarette smoking, or diabetes). Also, more than 75% of cardiovascular events develop in previously healthy women with LDL cholesterol levels below 160 mg/dL. This points out that other factors are contributory.

- **Inflammation:** It plays a role in atherogenesis and may be a risk factor. Inflammation is observed during all stages of atherogenesis and is closely associated with the formation and rupture of atherosclerotic plaque. Inflammation has been increasingly recognized to play a significant causal role in ischemic heart disease. Hence, assessment of systemic inflammation can be used for risk assessment. One of the circulating markers of inflammation that correlates with ischemic heart disease is *C-reactive protein (CRP).*
- **C-reactive protein** (CRP) **level:** CRP is an acute phase reactant produced mainly in the liver. It is a marker of systemic inflammation and **predicts the risk** of atherosclerosis-related diseases. Though CRP is not causally related to the development of atherosclerosis or its sequelae, plasma CRP levels are a strong, independent marker to predict the risk for myocardial infarction, stroke, peripheral arterial disease, and sudden cardiac death, even in healthy individuals. CRP levels are usually lowered when other risk reduction measures are implemented. These include cessation of smoking, weight loss, exercise, and administration of statin.

Herpes virus, *cytomegalovirus*, and *Chlamydia pneumoniae* have been found in atheromatous plaques. These infections may be responsible for local inflammatory reactions.

Hyperhomocysteinemia: It is a rare autosomal recessive inborn error and results in elevated circulating homocysteine. It is associated with premature and severe atherosclerosis.

Metabolic syndrome: It is associated with central obesity, insulin resistance, hypertension, dyslipidemia (elevated triglycerides and reduced HDL), hypercoagulability, and a pro-inflammatory state. It is a known risk factor for atherosclerosis.

Increased lipoprotein (a) [Lp(a)] levels: It is an altered form of LDL and is associated with increased risk. Lp(a) has structural similarity to plasminogen. It competes with plasminogen in clots and decreases the ability to form and clear clots. Increased Lp(a) levels are associated with a higher risk of atherosclerosis, independent of total cholesterol or LDL levels.

Raised procoagulant levels: These procoagulants include, thrombin (procoagulant and proinflammatory action), platelet activation, and raised fibrinogen. These are associated with increased risk.

Inadequate physical activity: Lack of exercise doubles the risk.

Clonal hematopoiesis: It is defined as the presence of a major clone of cells in the bone marrow that have acquired somatic driver mutations (*refer* page 481) in one or more oncogenes or tumor suppressor genes. It is found that many older individuals have clonal hematopoiesis and typically have normal blood counts despite mutations. It is observed that clonal hematopoiesis is strongly associated with an increased risk of death from cardiovascular disease. This may be due to alterations in the function of innate immune cells derived from mutated hematopoietic stem cells.

Stressful lifestyle: Certain personalities associated with a competitive, stressful life ("type A" personality) are associated with an increased risk of coronary disease.

Obesity: It is often associated with hypertension, diabetes mellitus, hypertriglyceridemia, decreased HDL, and physical inactivity.

Alcohol consumption: It is **associated with reduced rates of coronary artery disease**.

Pathogenesis of Atherosclerosis

Q. Write a short note on the pathogenesis of atherosclerosis. Discuss the role of lipid and endothelial injury in its pathogenesis.

There are several theories proposed for the pathogenesis of atherosclerosis and a few of them are:

- **Insudation hypothesis:** According to this, the focal accumulation of lipids in a vessel wall is due to insudation (transport) of plasma lipoproteins across an intact endothelium.
- **Encrustation hypothesis:** This hypothesis states that small mural thrombi are formed at the site of endothelial damage. These thrombi become organized and form plaque.
- **Monoclonal hypothesis:** The monoclonal concept postulates that a single clone (monoclonal) of smooth muscle migrates from the underlying media into the intima and then proliferates. The stimulus for monoclonal proliferation may be metabolites of cholesterol.
- **Response-to-injury hypothesis:** This is the currently favored hypothesis.

Response-to-Injury Hypothesis (Figs. 16.1A to E)

Q. Write a short note on the reaction-to-injury hypothesis of atherogenesis.

According to this theory, **atherosclerosis develops as a chronic inflammatory** (and healing) **response of the arterial wall to the endothelial injury**. Probably **accumulation of cholesterol crystals and free fatty acids in macrophages and other cells initiates inflammation.** It is thought that chronic inflammation is responsible for both the initiation and progression of atherosclerotic lesions. The **sequence of pathogenic events (Figs. 16.1A to E)** is as follows:

Endothelial Injury and Dysfunction

Early lesions in atherosclerosis begin at sites of intact, but dysfunctional endothelium. Normal endothelium maintains blood vessel (vascular) tone, regulates hemostasis, acts as a barrier to toxic materials, and controls inflammation. With endothelial dysfunction, these normal functions of endothelium become defective.

- **Triggers of endothelial injury or dysfunction:** The two most important triggers of endothelial dysfunction are hemodynamic disturbances and hypercholesterolemia.
  - **Hemodynamic disturbances:** Plaques develop in regions having disturbed blood flow such as the origin or ostia of vessels, branching points of vessels, and along the posterior wall of the abdominal aorta.
  - **Risk factors: Hyperlipidemia, hypertension, toxins from cigarette smoke,** and **advanced glycation end products** in **diabetes** can **produce endothelial injury/dysfunction**. Common lipoprotein abnormalities include (1) increased LDL cholesterol levels; (2) decreased HDL cholesterol levels; and (3) increased levels of lipoprotein(a). The cholesterol and cholesterol esters are the predominant lipids in atheromatous plaques.
  - **Others: Homocysteine, immune complexes**, and **infectious agents**.
- **Effect of endothelial injury or dysfunction that favors the development of atherosclerosis:** These include the following:
  - **Increased vascular permeability**
  - **Increased leukocyte (mainly monocyte) adhesion** to endothelium
  - **Platelet adhesion and increased tendency for thrombus formation**
  - **Movement of low-density lipoproteins (LDLs) across the endothelium into the intima.**

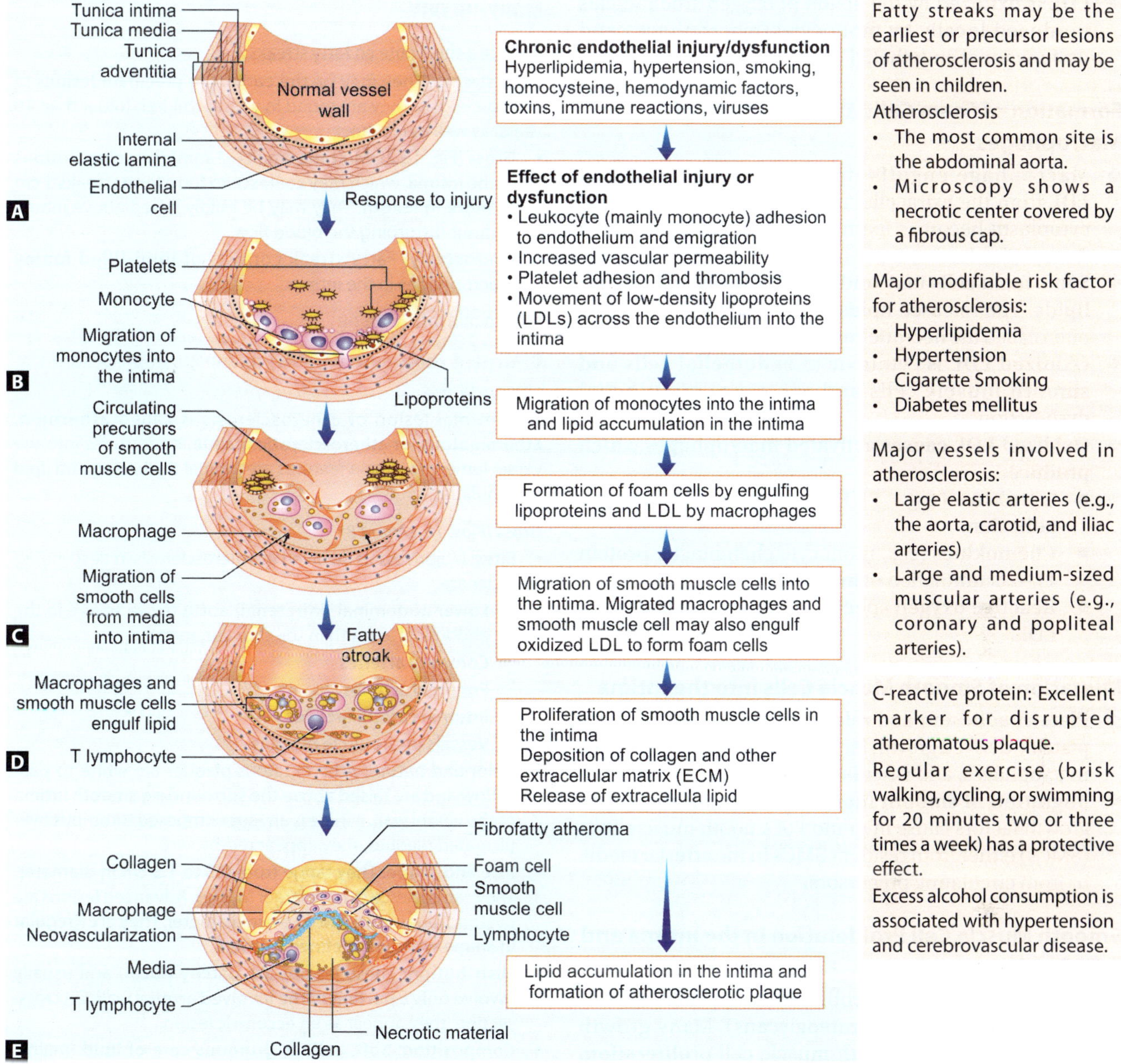

Fatty streaks may be the earliest or precursor lesions of atherosclerosis and may be seen in children.

Atherosclerosis
- The most common site is the abdominal aorta.
- Microscopy shows a necrotic center covered by a fibrous cap.

Major modifiable risk factor for atherosclerosis:
- Hyperlipidemia
- Hypertension
- Cigarette Smoking
- Diabetes mellitus

Major vessels involved in atherosclerosis:
- Large elastic arteries (e.g., the aorta, carotid, and iliac arteries)
- Large and medium-sized muscular arteries (e.g., coronary and popliteal arteries).

C-reactive protein: Excellent marker for disrupted atheromatous plaque.

Regular exercise (brisk walking, cycling, or swimming for 20 minutes two or three times a week) has a protective effect.

Excess alcohol consumption is associated with hypertension and cerebrovascular disease.

Figs. 16.1A to E: Various steps in response to injury hypothesis of atherogenesis: (A) Normal vessel wall; (B) Endothelial injury/dysfunction with the adhesion of monocytes and platelets; (C) Migration of monocytes and smooth muscle cells (from media or circulating precursor) into the arterial intima. Monocytes are transformed into macrophages and become activated; (D) Macrophages and smooth muscle cells engulf modified lipoproteins and oxidized LDL to form foam cells; (E) The intima's smooth muscles proliferate, produce an extracellular matrix, and develop into fibrofatty (atheromatous) plaque.

Monocyte Adhesion to the Endothelium and Migration into the Intima

- The **leukocytes,** which adhere at the site of endothelial injury/dysfunction, are **mainly monocytes and T lymphocytes.** Accumulation of leukocytes **initiates the atheroma formation.** Chronic inflammation is involved in the initiation, progression, and complications of atherosclerotic lesions.
- Locally produced **chemokines allow penetration of the endothelial layer by monocytes and lymphocytes.** The **monocytes migrate into the intima** where they are **transformed into macrophages.**

Lipid Accumulation in the Intima

- Endothelial dysfunction also allows **penetration of endothelium by lipoproteins (mainly LDL)** from blood. This causes the **accumulation of LDLs and cholesterol within the intima** of the vessel.

- **LDL is oxidized** by the action of oxygen-free radicals produced locally by monocytes/macrophages and dysfunctional endothelial cells.

Formation of Foam Cells and Activation of Macrophages

- **Macrophage engulfs lipoproteins** and **oxidized LDL** from the extracellular space in the intima. Their cytoplasm becomes foamy and these cells are called **foam cells.**
- Some **foam cells may undergo apoptosis** and **release lipids.** The released lipids form the lipid-rich center, often called the **necrotic core in atheromatous plaques.**
- **Oxidized LDL is cytotoxic to endothelial cells and smooth muscle** cells and can cause endothelial dysfunction.
- **Oxidized LDL causes activated macrophages which produce:**
  - **Cytokine** (e.g., TNF)—**increases leukocyte adhesion.**
  - **Chemokines** (e.g., monocyte chemotactic protein 1)—accumulation of monocytes.
  - **Reactive oxygen species**—aggravate oxidation of LDL.

Migration of Smooth Muscle Cells into the Intima

- **Platelet adhesion and release of growth factors** (e.g., platelet-derived growth factor) from activated platelets, macrophages, and vascular wall cells.
- **Migration of smooth muscle cells into intima**: The growth factors cause migration of smooth muscle cells (SMCs) either from resident SMCs in the arterial media or from circulating precursors.

Smooth Muscle Cell Proliferation in the Intima and ECM Production

- Smooth muscle cells proliferate and produce ECM (mainly collagen and proteoglycans). Many **growth factors** can **cause smooth muscle cell proliferation.** These include PDGF, fibroblast growth factor (FGF), and transforming growth factor-α (TGF-α).
- Smooth muscle cells **may also engulf oxidized LDL and form foam cells.**

Lipid Accumulation

- Occurs both **intracellularly** (within macrophages and smooth muscle cells) and **extracellularly.**
- **Extracellular lipid** is derived **from insudation** from the vessel lumen (mainly in the presence of hypercholesterolemia) and also from **necrotic foam cells.**
- Cholesterol in the plaque is also due to an **imbalance between influx and efflux.** High-density lipoprotein (HDL) probably transfers cholesterol from these lesions and leads to its excretion by the liver.

MORPHOLOGY

Q. Write a short note on fatty streaks.

Fatty streaks: They may be the earliest or precursor lesions of atherosclerosis. They are found in young children (older than 10 years) as well as in adults.

- **Gross (Fig. 16.2): Multiple small (~1 mm) flat yellow lesions in the intima,** which **may coalesce to form long streaks 1 cm or more in length.** They may be mildly raised above intima without disturbing the blood flow.
- **Microscopy:** Fatty streak consists of **lipid-filled foamy macrophages** in the intima.

Atherosclerotic Plaque

Q. Write a short note on gross and microscopic features of atherosclerosis.

The intimal lesion of atherosclerosis is called **atheroma, atheromatous, or atherosclerotic plaque.** It protrudes into the vessel lumen. The main features are intimal thickening and lipid accumulation.

Gross (Figs. 16.3A and B)

- **Sites:** Major vessels involved in atherosclerosis in descending order are:
  - **Lower abdominal (infrarenal) aorta** (more severe in the abdominal aorta than the thoracic aorta)
  - **Coronary arteries**
  - **Popliteal arteries**
  - **Internal carotid arteries**
  - **Vessels of the circle of Willis.**
- **Color and nature:** Atheromatous plaques are **white to pale yellow and are raised above the surrounding smooth intima of the vessel wall.** If there is any superimposed thrombus over ulcerated plaques, they appear red-brown.
- **Size and shape:** They range **from 0.3 to 1.5 cm in diameter.** They can coalesce to form larger masses. **Advanced lesions** are oval and range from **8 to 12 cm in diameter. They are irregular in shape with well-defined borders.**
- **Distribution:** These lesions are **patchy (focal)** and usually **involve only a portion of the involved arterial wall.** On cross-section, they appear as an **eccentric** lesion.
- **Composition: Soft, yellow, grumous core of lipid** (mainly cholesterol and cholesterol esters) **covered by a white fibrous cap.**

Microscopy (Figs. 16.4A to C, Fig. 16.5 and Fig. 16.1E)

Components: Atherosclerotic plaques occur in the intima and consist of three main components in varying proportions in different lesions:

1. **Cells:** These include variable numbers of **smooth muscle cells, macrophages, and T-cells.**
2. **Extracellular matrix (ECM):** These include **collagen, elastic fibers, and proteoglycans.**
3. **Lipid:** These include **both intracellular and extracellular lipids.**

Regions: Three components occur in three regions in varying proportions and configurations in different lesions.

1. **Superficial fibrous cap:** Typically, the atheromatous plaque has a superficial fibrous cap composed of **smooth muscle cells and collagen.**

2. **Necrotic core:** It is seen deep to the fibrous cap and contains:
   - **Lipid:** Typical atheroma contains **abundant lipids, mainly cholesterol and cholesterol esters.** The extracellular cholesterol usually forms crystalline aggregates that are washed out during routine tissue processing. This is seen as empty needle-shaped cleft-like spaces termed "cholesterol clefts."
   - **Necrotic debris** from dead cells. This necrotic center may undergo dystrophic calcification.
   - **Foam cells** (lipid-laden macrophages and smooth muscle cells).
   - **Others:** Fibrin, organized thrombus, and other plasma proteins.
3. **Shoulder:** It is the peripheral region beneath and to the side of the cap. It is more cellular and contains macrophages, smooth muscle cells, and T-cells.

Neovascularization (proliferating small blood vessels): It may be seen at the periphery of the lesions near the shoulder.

Tunica media: The tunica media deep to the plaque may be thinned and show fibrosis secondary to smooth muscle atrophy and loss.

Q. Write a short note on complications of atherosclerosis.

Complicated plaques (Box 16.1 and Fig. 16.6): Atherosclerotic plaques can undergo the following clinically important changes:

1. **Rupture, ulceration, erosion, or fissuring of the surface of atheromatous plaques:** Plaque protrudes into the lumen and can disturb the blood flow and can produce a turbulent flow of blood. This can damage the endothelium and cause rupture, ulceration, erosion, or fissuring of the intimal surface of plaques.
2. **Thrombosis and embolism:** Ulceration/erosion/rupture of endothelial surface exposes the blood to highly thrombogenic subendothelial collagen. It favors **thrombus formation** and can partially or completely occlude the lumen (depending on the size of the lumen) and lead to ischemia. The thrombus may become organized or fragment to form thromboemboli.
3. **Atheroembolism:** Plaque rupture releases atherosclerotic debris into the bloodstream resulting in atheroemboli.
4. **Hemorrhage into the plaque:** It may occur due to rupture of the fibrous cap of the plaque or the thin-walled vessels formed due to neovascularization.
5. **Aneurysm formation:** Atherosclerosis even though an intimal disease may cause pressure or ischemic atrophy of the underlying media. It may also damage the elastic tissue and cause weakening of the wall and result in aneurysmal dilation. This aneurysm may rupture.
6. **Calcification:** It may occur in the central necrotic area of the plaque (dystrophic calcification).

Complications and major clinical consequences of atherosclerosis are presented in **Figure 16.6.**

Four major clinical consequences of atherosclerosis are listed in **Box 16.2 and Figure 16.6.**

Clinicopathologic Manifestations of Atherosclerosis

Q. Briefly mention the sites and clinical significance of atherosclerosis.

Atherosclerotic lesions are usually responsible for the following clinicopathologic manifestations **(Fig. 16.6).**

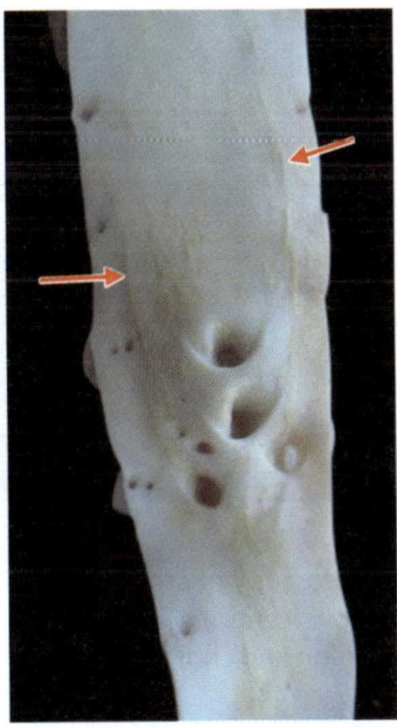

Fig. 16.2: Fatty streaks in the aorta appear as long streaks (arrows).

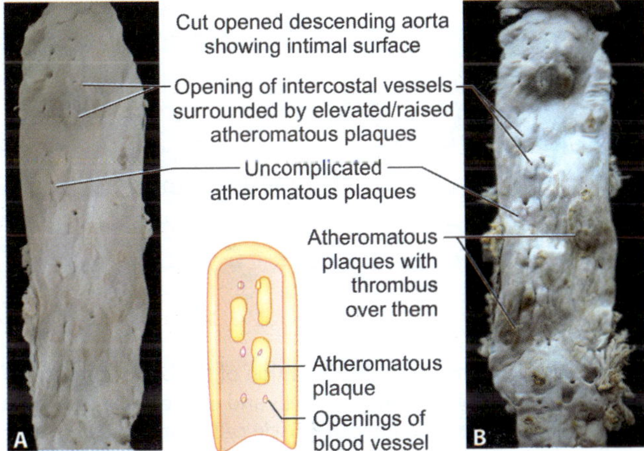

Figs. 16.3A and B: Atheromatous plaques on the intimal surface of the aorta.

Atherosclerotic Stenosis

Critical stenosis: Atherosclerotic plaques reduce the size of the lumen of the involved vessel. **When reduction of the lumen is sufficiently severe it may lead to tissue ischemia** and this lesion is termed as **critical stenosis.**

Consequences: The effects of vascular stenosis depend on arterial supply and the metabolic demand of the affected tissue. In small arteries, it may reduce blood flow leading to ischemic injury. In the coronary artery atherosclerotic lesion when producing a 70% decrease in luminal cross-sectional area, the patient may develop chest pain with exertion (*stable angina*; *refer* page 512). In other site, diminished arterial blood flow can cause ischemia of the bowel (mesenteric occlusion), sudden cardiac death, chronic ischemic heart disease, ischemic encephalopathy, and intermittent claudication (diminished perfusion of the extremities).

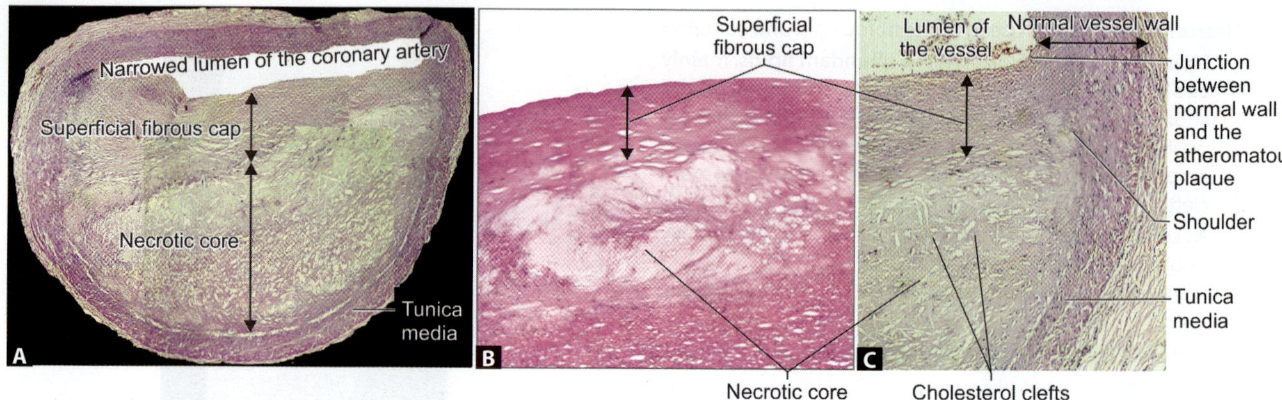

Figs. 16.4A to C: Microscopy of atheromatous plaque: (A) Scanner view of coronary atherosclerosis causing more than 90% narrowing of the lumen; (B) Shows central necrotic core and superficial fibrous cap; (C) Shows junction between the vessel wall and atheromatous plaque, shoulder region and cholesterol clefts in the necrotic core.

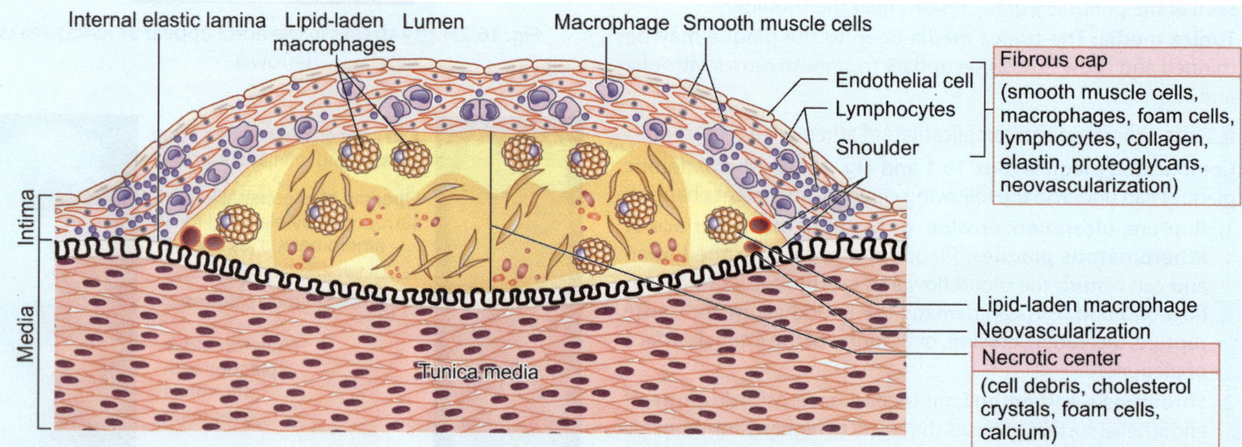

Fig. 16.5: Diagrammatic representation of the basic structure of an atherosclerotic plaque. Atherosclerosis is an intimal-based process involving a complex interplay of cells and extracellular matrix. In a fully developed plaque, the central necrotic core contains lipid-filled macrophages, necrotic smooth muscle cell debris, and cholesterol clefts. The superficial "fibrous" cap comprises mainly smooth muscle cells, which produce collagen, small amounts of elastin, and glycosaminoglycans. There are also macrophages and T lymphocytes. In an uncomplicated plaque, the endothelium over the surface of the fibrous cap usually appears intact. Atherosclerotic plaques can have secondary effects on the underlying tunica media, including a reduction in smooth muscle cells.

BOX 16.1: Major changes that produce complicated atherosclerotic plaques.

1. Rupture, ulceration, erosion, or fissuring (acute plaque change)
2. Thrombosis and embolism
3. Atheroembolism
4. Hemorrhage into the plaque
5. Aneurysm
6. Calcification

BOX 16.2: Major clinical consequences of atherosclerosis.

1. Myocardial infarction (heart attack)
2. Cerebral infarction (stroke)
3. Aortic aneurysms
4. Peripheral vascular disease (gangrene of the legs)

Acute Plaque Change

Atheromatous plaques causing myocardial infarction and other acute coronary syndromes are often asymptomatic. **Acute plaque change** (*refer* page 511 and **Fig. 16.23**) is the **sudden change/event occurring in an atheromatous plaque.** The composition of plaques is dynamic and it decides the risk of rupture. Acute plaque changes are of three categories: (1) **Rupture, ulceration, or erosion** of the luminal surface of atheromatous plaques. It exposes highly thrombogenic substances and favors thrombus formation; (2) **Hemorrhage into a plaque**. Rupture of the surface fibrous cap or of the thin-walled vessels of neovascularization can cause intraplaque hemorrhage. This can produce hematoma and rapid plaque expansion or plaque rupture; (3) **Atheroembolism.** The ruptured plaque

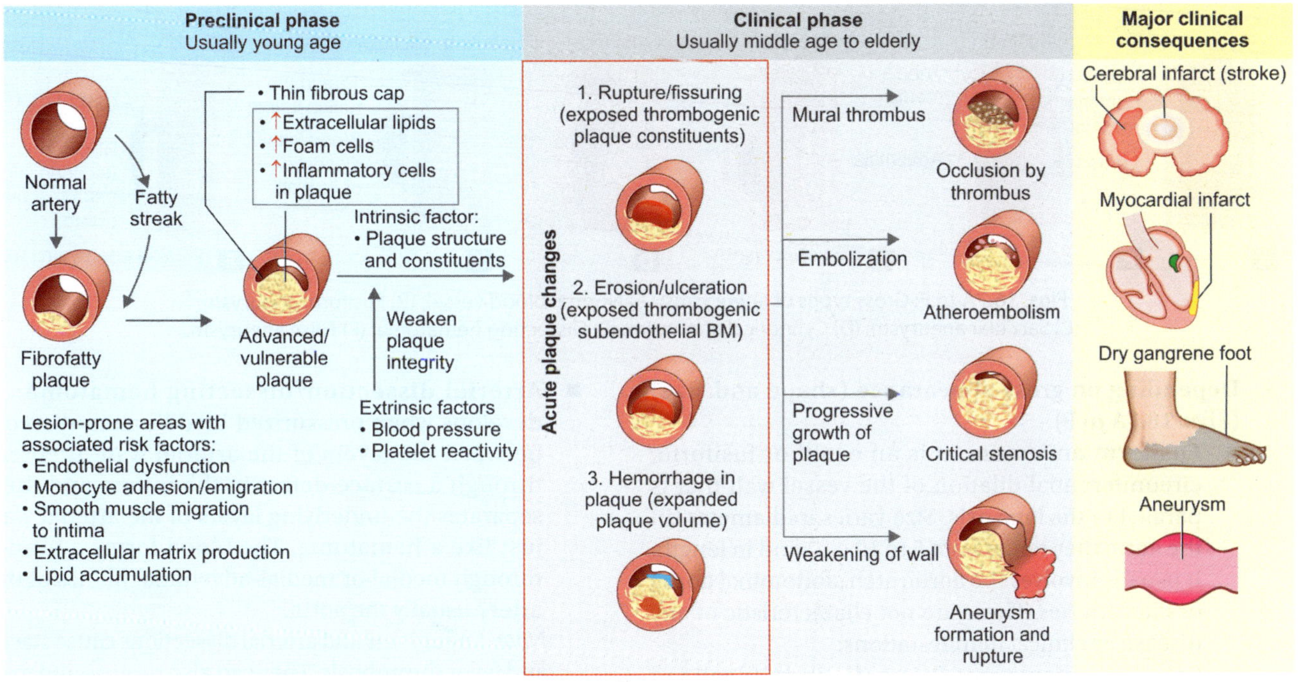

Fig. 16.6: Complications and major clinical consequences of atherosclerosis.

can produce microemboli by releasing the atheromatous plaque contents (debris) into the blood.

Vulnerable plaques are more likely to undergo rupture. These are plaques that have: (1) a necrotic center with large areas of foam cells and extracellular lipids, (2) thin fibrous caps or contain few smooth muscle cells, or (3) clusters of inflammatory cells.

Mechanical strength and stability of plaque:

- **Intrinsic factors:** The mechanical strength and stability of plaque depends mainly on the collagen in the fibrous cap. The balance between the synthesis of collagen against its degradation decides the integrity of the fibrous cap integrity.
  - **Collagen synthesis:** It is mainly by smooth muscle cells and loss of these cells reduces the integrity and strength of fibrous cap.
  - **Collagen degradation:** Generally inflammatory cells in the plaque increase in collagen degradation and reduce collagen synthesis. This reduces the mechanical strength and integrity of the fibrous cap. Statins reduce circulating cholesterol levels and also stabilize plaques by reducing inflammation in plaque.
- **Extrinsic factors:** Also contribute to plaque changes.
  - Adrenergic stimulation raises systemic blood pressure or induces local vasoconstriction and increases the physical stresses on a given plaque.
  - Emotional stress can also contribute to plaque disruption.

Thrombosis

Partial or total thrombosis over a disrupted plaque is observed in acute coronary syndromes. Mural thrombi in a coronary artery can undergo embolization.

Vasoconstriction

Vasoconstriction reduces the size of the arterial lumen and increases the local mechanical forces. This can disrupt plaque.

ANEURYSMS AND DISSECTION

PA 27.2 (CC): Describe the etiology, dynamics, pathology types, and complications of aneurysms including aortic aneurysms.

Q. Define aneurysm.

Definition: An aneurysm is defined as a congenital or acquired, localized, abnormal, permanent dilation of a blood vessel or the heart.

Classification

Q. Write a short note on the aneurysm.

Aneurysms are classified by origin, location, gross appearance, the composition of the vessel wall, and etiology.

1. **Origin:** It can be congenital or acquired.
2. **Location:** It refers to the type of vascular system involved.
   - **Artery** and the specific region involved (e.g., abdominal aorta, popliteal artery)
   - **Vein**
   - **Heart.**

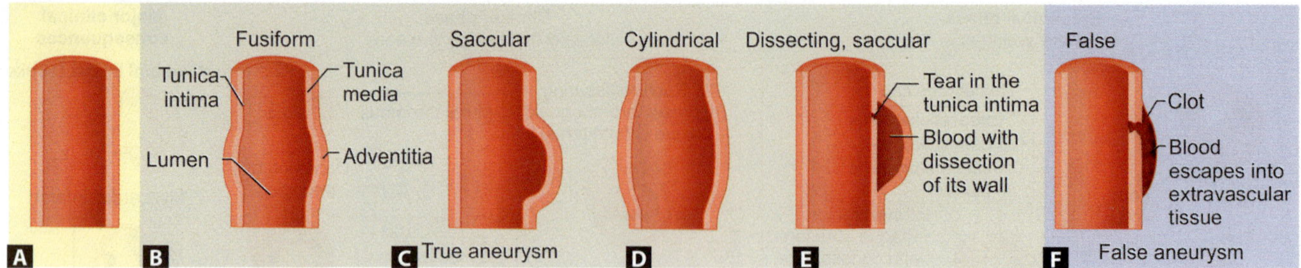

Figs. 16.7A to F: Gross types of aneurysms: (A) Normal blood vessel; (B) Fusiform aneurysm; (C) Saccular aneurysm; (D) Cylindrical aneurysm; (E) Dissecting hematoma; (F) False aneurysm.

3. **Depending on gross appearance (shape and size) (Figs. 16.7A to F)**
   - **Fusiform aneurysm:** It is an ovoid or fusiform, circumferential dilation of the vessel wall that is parallel to the long axis. Size varies in diameter (in the aorta they range from 5 to 10 cm) and in length. It usually involves the aortic arch, abdominal aorta, or iliac arteries. These are not characteristic of any disease or clinical manifestations.
   - **Saccular aneurysm:** It is a distinct, localized spherical outpouching from the portion of the vessel wall. Its size in intracranial vessels varies from 2 to 20 mm in diameter and in the aorta vary from 5 to 10 cm in diameter. Its lumen may contain a thrombus.
   - **Cylindrical aneurysm:** It has parallel dilatation.
   - **Cirsoid aneurysm**: It is the dilatation of a group of blood vessels due to congenital malformations with arteriovenous (AV) shunting (direct communication between an artery and vein). "Cirsoid" means resembling a varix (abnormally dilated and lengthened vessel). It is a synonym with racemose (racemose meaning like a bunch of grapes).
4. **Depending on the composition of the wall of the aneurysm**
   - **A true aneurysm** is **composed of all the layers of the thinned arterial wall** (intima, media, and adventitia) **or thinned ventricular wall of the heart**. Examples: Atherosclerotic, syphilitic, and congenital vascular aneurysms, and ventricular aneurysms that complicate transmural myocardial infarctions.
   - **A false aneurysm** (pseudoaneurysm) is a defect in the vascular wall with the formation of an extravascular hematoma (blood-filled space forms around a blood vessel). It may freely communicate with the intravascular space (**pulsating hematoma**). It usually develops after a traumatic rupture or a perforating injury. Examples: Rupture of the left ventricle, which complicates myocardial infarction (and is enclosed by a pericardial adhesion), hematoma that follows trauma to the artery, or leak at the sutured junction of a vascular graft with a natural artery.
   - **Arterial dissection/dissecting hematoma:** It develops when pressurized blood enters/dissects between the layers of the arterial wall. It enters through a surface defect in the intima and then separates the underlying layers of the arterial wall just like a hematoma. The blood forms a tunnel through medial or medial-adventitial planes of the artery usually the aorta.

   Note: Aneurysms and arterial dissections cause stasis, and favor thrombosis. They can also rupture and may be fatal.

Q. List the causes of aneurysm.

5. **Depending on the etiology**
   - Atherosclerotic aneurysm
   - Syphilitic aneurysm
   - Dissecting hematoma
   - Mycotic aneurysm
   - Berry aneurysm.

Predisposition Factors

The three most important causes of aortic aneurysms are atherosclerosis, hypertension, and smoking.

1. **Atherosclerosis:** It predisposes to aneurysms and more importantly predisposing factor involved in the development of aneurysms in the abdominal aorta.
2. **Hypertension:** It is the most common etiological factor that predisposes to aneurysms of the ascending aorta.
3. **Other pathological conditions and risk factors that weaken vessel walls and lead to aneurysms are:**
   - **Advanced age**
   - **Smoking** (mainly abdominal aortic aneurysms)
   - **Trauma**
   - **Vasculitis**
   - **Congenital defects** (e.g., fibromuscular dysplasia and berry aneurysms in the circle of Willis)
   - **Tertiary syphilis**
   - **Infections (mycotic aneurysms):** The term **mycotic** (*refer* pages 490 and 155) **is a misnomer** and does not indicate that the infection is due to fungus and is usually **bacterial**. The source of infection may be:
     - Septic embolus: Usually occurs as a complication of infective endocarditis

- Extension of an adjacent suppurative process into the vessel wall
- Direct infection of the wall of the artery by circulating microorganisms.

Pathogenesis

The imbalance between the synthesis and degradation of the ECM (*refer* online Fig. 18.8): Normally, the walls of the arteries constantly remodel. This is by synthesizing, degrading, and repairing damage to their ECM constituents. The remodeling maintains the structural and functional integrity of the artery. Aneurysms develop when there is a **weakening of the medial wall of the vessels.** The weakening of the media is due to an imbalance between the synthesis and degradation of the ECM. This will cause defects in the structure or function of the connective tissue within the vascular wall. It may occur both in inherited or acquired forms of aneurysm. Various defects are discussed below.

Inadequate or Abnormal Synthesis of Connective Tissue

Abnormal transforming growth factor-β (TGF-β) signaling: TGF-β regulates proliferation of SMC (smooth muscle cell) and synthesis of connective tissue matrix. Mutations in TGF-β receptors or downstream signaling pathways may lead to **defects in the synthesis of elastin and collagen.** Excessive activity of TGF-β alters the remodeling of vascular walls, mainly that of the ascending aorta. This can lead to reduced ECM content and integrity of the aorta resulting in aneurysmal dilation.

- **Marfan syndrome:** It is characterized by an **inherited defect** in the synthesis of an **extracellular** scaffolding **glycoprotein** called **fibrillin-1.** Fibrillin is abundant in the aorta and it controls the availability of transforming growth factor (TGF)-β. Reduced or altered forms of fibrillin-1 lead to increased availability of TGF-β in the aortic wall. Increased TGF-β signaling, causes inflammation, harms the development of vascular smooth muscle, and increases the activity of metalloproteases. All these results in progressive loss of elastic tissue and extracellular matrix leading to the weakening of the aortic wall. The aorta subsequently dilates resulting in an aneurysm.

Excessive Connective Tissue Degradation by Inflammation-associated Release of Matrix Metalloproteases (MMP)

Transmural inflammation of the vessel wall in atherosclerotic aneurysms increases the amounts of elastolytic MMPs produced by macrophages.

Loss of SMCs or Change in SMC Synthetic Phenotype

Weakening of the vessel wall may be due to the **loss of smooth muscle cells** (SMCs) in the vessel wall. Ischemia of the wall of the aorta can lead to loss of SMC. Examples include:

- **Atherosclerosis:** In atherosclerosis, the thickening of the intima increases the distance for the oxygen and nutrients from the lumen to diffuse into the **inner media.** This results in ischemia of the inner media.
- **Systemic hypertension:** It can produce significant **narrowing of the vasa vasorum lumen** (e.g., in the aorta) and can produce **ischemia of the outer media.** Ischemia causes loss of SMC loss and produces "degenerative changes" in the aorta. These changes include fibrosis (replacement of elastic tissue), inadequate production of ECM by SMCs, and excessive accumulation of amorphous proteoglycans. Microscopically, these changes are together known as *cystic medial degeneration* (but there is no true cyst formation). Such changes are nonspecific. They may occur whenever there is a defect in the synthesis of ECM. These include inherited disorders (e.g., Marfan syndrome) and acquired conditions (e.g., scurvy).
- **Tertiary syphilis:** It is a rare cause of aneurysm of the thoracic aorta. Treponemas have an affinity for vasa vasorum of mainly thoracic aorta. In **tertiary syphilis,** it produces **obliterative endarteritis in the vasa vasorum** of the thoracic aorta and causes ischemia of the aortic media resulting in aortic aneurysms (syphilitic mesoaortitis).

Abdominal Aortic Aneurysm

Atherosclerotic aneurysms most commonly affect the abdominal aorta and common iliac arteries. Less commonly, it occurs in the aortic arch and descending thoracic aorta.
Gender and age: Abdominal aortic aneurysm **(AAA)** is more common **in men, in smokers,** and rare before the age of 50 years.

Causes

Atherosclerotic AAA: It is a **major cause.** Atherosclerotic plaque in the intima reduces the diffusion of nutrients and waste from the vessel's lumen into the arterial wall. This causes **weakness and thinning of the arterial wall.** The inflammatory cell infiltrates mainly macrophages present in the plaque secrete matrix metalloproteinases (MMP) and cause **excessive degradation of ECM.**
Inflammatory AAA: They constitute about 5–10% of all AAAs. They usually occur in younger patients. They often present with back pain and elevated inflammatory markers [e.g., erythrocyte sedimentation rate (ESR)]. It probably represents a localized immune response in the abdominal aortic wall. In most patients, there is no inflammation in other arteries cases.

- **Immunoglobulin G4-related disease (IgG4-RD):** IgG4-RD is a disorder characterized by (in most cases) high circulating levels of IgG4, storiform fibrosis, and IgG4-positive infiltrating plasma cells in involved tissues. It may involve many organs, including the pancreas, thyroid, and other vascular sites, such as the ascending aorta and heart vessels.

Mycotic (infectious) AAAs: These aneurysms develop in the arteries when the **wall of the vessel becomes infected by the lodging of circulating microorganisms.** They may develop in the aortic wall or cerebral vessels during septicemia (e.g., bacteremia from bacterial endocarditis or primary *Salmonella* gastroenteritis). The suppuration produced by microorganisms further destroys the media and can lead to rapid dilation, rupture, and bleeding.

MORPHOLOGY

Atherosclerotic AAAs

Gross

- **Site:** Aneurysm is **usually** observed **below the origin of renal arteries** and **above the bifurcation of the abdominal aorta.**
- **Appearance:**
  - **Shape: Saccular or fusiform.**
  - **Size:** Diameter usually more than 3 cm, and usually less than 5.5 cm. Length may be up to 25 cm.
  - **Wall of the aorta:** Intimal surface shows severe **complicated atherosclerosis** with **destruction and thinning** of the underlying **aortic media.**
  - **Lumen:** It frequently shows a bland, laminated, poorly organized **mural thrombus.**
  - **Extension:** Occasionally, aneurysm may affect the renal and superior or inferior mesenteric arteries. AAAs may be associated with smaller aneurysms involving the iliac arteries.

Inflammatory AAA

- **Dense lymphoplasmacytic inflammation: Inflammatory AAAs** are characterized by dense lymphoplasmacytic (i.e., lymphocytes and plasma cells) inflammation with many macrophages. There may even be giant cells.
- **Dense periaortic fibrosis:** They show dense periaortic scarring that can extend into the anterior retroperitoneum.
- **IgG4-related disease (IgG4-RD):** It a subset of inflammatory AAAs that shows IgG4-positive infiltrating plasma cells in the affected aorta.

Mycotic AAA

- The involved vessels show suppuration with the destruction of the vessel wall.

Clinical Features

Most patients with AAAs are entirely asymptomatic.

Abdominal mass: Most AAAs are discovered incidentally on physical examination as an abdominal mass (often palpably pulsating) that simulates a tumor. It may be detected during radiological examination for some other reason.

Expansion: Most (80%) abdominal aneurysms expand each year. Some patients may develop abdominal pain, due to the expansion of the aneurysm.

Ischemia: Sudden peripheral artery occlusion by an embolus from a mural thrombus in the AAA presents as sudden lower limb ischemia.

Complications

Various complications and their clinical manifestations are as follows:

- **Rupture:** Aneurysm may rupture into the **peritoneal cavity or retroperitoneal tissues**. This may lead to massive, potentially fatal hemorrhage.
- **Obstruction of a branch vessel:** It can **lead to** downstream **ischemia** of tissues supplied by the obstructed vessel, e.g., iliac (leg), renal (kidney), mesenteric (gastrointestinal tract), or vertebral arteries (spinal cord).
- **Embolism:** Atherosclerotic plaque or mural thrombus may fragment to form emboli.
- **Compression of an adjacent structure:** For example, compression of a ureter or erosion of vertebrae.

Prognosis: Operative mortality for unruptured aneurysms is about 5%. However, in case of emergency surgery after rupture, the mortality rate will be >50%. Because atherosclerosis is a systemic disease, a patient with an AAA will likely have atherosclerosis in other vascular beds. So, there is a significantly increased risk of ischemic heart disease and stroke.

Thoracic Aortic Aneurysms

Causes: Hypertension (most common cause), Marfan syndrome, other disorders associated with mutations in TGF-β signaling pathways, and inflammatory conditions [aortitis, syphilis (not observed nowadays)].

Clinical presentation: Symptoms depend on the encroached structure **(Table 16.2)**. Other symptoms include aortic valve dilation and valvular insufficiency; narrowing of the coronary ostia causes myocardial ischemia; rupture of an aneurysm (fatal). Syphilitic aneurysms may lead to heart failure due to aortic valvular incompetence.

Syphilitic Aneurysm

Q. Write a short note on syphilitic aneurysm aortitis.

TABLE 16.2 Clinical presentations in thoracic aortic aneurysm.

Encroached structures	*Symptoms*
Encroachment or erosion of bone (i.e., ribs and vertebral bodies)	Chest pain
Compression of a coronary artery	Myocardial ischemia
Valvular insufficiency	Heart failure
Lungs and airways	Respiratory difficulties
Compression of the esophagus	Respiratory or feeding difficulties
Irritation of or pressure on the recurrent laryngeal nerves	Hoarseness and persistent cough

MORPHOLOGY

Syphilis causes aortitis and aneurysms. Mainly affects the ascending aorta (*refer* page 113).

Gross: Aorta shows depressed medial scars that cause **roughening of the intimal surface.** This produces a **tree bark appearance on the intima.** The continuing pressure of the blood forces on the weakened wall of the ascending aorta and aortic arch produces a **saccular (mostly) aneurysm (Fig. 16.7C).** This may rupture.

Microscopy: It shows **endarteritis and periarteritis of vasa vasorum.** These vessels divide in the adventitia and penetrate the outer and middle thirds of the aorta. Lymphocytes, plasma cells, and macrophages surround these vessels. Obliterative endarteritis (obliteration of the vasa vasorum) causes focal necrosis and scarring of the media. This disrupts and disorganizes elastic lamellae. The aorta shows medial scars.

Aortic Dissection

Q. Write a short note on dissecting aneurysm/hematoma/aortic dissection.

Definition: Aortic dissection develops when **blood from the aortic lumen enters the aortic wall.** Blood travels along and splits the layers of the media to form a blood-filled channel within the aortic wall.

Aortic dissection may or may not be associated with aortic dilation. **The older term "dissecting aneurysm" is replaced by aortic dissection.** It is fatal if the dissection ruptures through the adventitia resulting in hemorrhages into adjacent spaces.

Etiology

It occurs mainly in age two groups: (1) men between **40 and 60 years with hypertension** or (2) **younger** patients **with connective tissue disease** of the aorta (e.g., **Marfan syndrome**).

- **Iatrogenic:** It may develop as a complication of **arterial cannulations** during diagnostic catheterization or cardiopulmonary bypass.
- **During or after pregnancy:** It can develop during or after the third trimester of pregnancy. It may be due to vascular remodeling induced by hormones and the hemodynamic stresses occurring during the perinatal period.

Pathogenesis

Hypertension: It is the **major risk factor.** Aortas of hypertensive patients show narrowing of the vasa vasora, degenerative changes in ECM of the medial wall, and loss of medial smooth muscle cells (SMCs).

Inherited or acquired connective tissue disorders: In these connective tissue disorders, there may be defects in the synthesis or degradation of ECM in the aorta. Examples include **Marfan syndrome, Ehlers-Danlos syndrome, type IV, vitamin C deficiency, and defects in copper metabolism.**

Intimal tear and dissection: An aortic dissection usually starts with a tear in the intima. Regardless of the underlying etiology, the trigger for the intimal tear and initial intramural aortic hemorrhage (medial dissection) is usually unknown. More than 95% of the patients have a transverse tear in the intima and internal tunica media. Probably spontaneous laceration of the intima (i.e., intimal tear) allows the blood to flow under systemic pressure from the lumen to enter and dissect the media. This leads to a progression of the hematoma.

MORPHOLOGY

An aortic dissection is usually initiated with a tear in the aortic intima.

Site of intimal tear: In most patients with spontaneous dissections, the intimal tear is in the **ascending aorta**, usually within 10 cm of the aortic valve.

Characteristic of tear: Typically, intimal tears are (1) **transverse or oblique**, (2) 1–5 cm in length, and (3) sharp with jagged edges.

The extent of involvement: It can extend proximally (retrograde) along the aorta toward the heart and distally, sometimes into the iliac and femoral arteries. It can also involve coronary arteries, great neck vessels, and renal, mesenteric, or iliac arteries.

Spread of dissection in the aortic wall: The dissecting hematoma characteristically spreads between lamellar units of the outer third of the media or between media and adventitial layers.

The fate (complications) of aortic dissection: It can rupture through the tunica adventitia and may result in:

- **Massive hemorrhage** into the thoracic or abdominal cavities, mediastinum, pleural space, and retroperitoneum.
- **Cardiac tamponade:** Dissection may retrogradely rupture and produce hemorrhage into the pericardial sac.
- **Double-barreled aorta:** In some fortunate instances, the **dissecting hematoma may re-enter the lumen of the aorta through a second distal intimal tear.** This creates a new false vascular channel called a **"double-barreled aorta."** The re-entry site produces communication of the aorta with a major artery, most often the iliac artery. It prevents fatal extra-aortic hemorrhage. Over time, such false channels can become endothelialized and be recognized as chronic dissections.

Microscopy: Most cases do not show any identifiable changes in the aortic wall. The most frequent microscopic feature is **medial degeneration.** The characteristic features of medial degeneration are (1) fragmentation and loss of elastic fibers, (2) a decrease in the number and size of smooth muscle cells, and (3) accumulation of mucoid ECM. There will not be any inflammation.

Classification (Fig. 16.9)

In aortic dissections, the morbidity and mortality depend on the part of the aorta that is involved. The most dangerous complications occur when the dissections occur between the aortic valve and the distal arch. Accordingly, aortic dissections can be classified into two types: type A or type B.

1. **Type A dissections:** In this type, **proximal lesions** involve **either the ascending and descending aorta or only the ascending aorta** (types I and II of the DeBakey *classification*). It is more common but dangerous. Dr Michael DeBakey is a pioneer in vascular surgery.

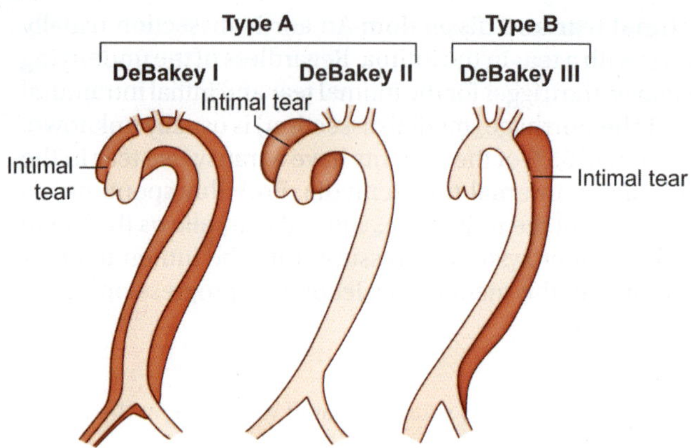

Fig. 16.9: Classification of aortic dissections. Type A (proximal) involves the ascending aorta (DeBakey I and II), and Type B (distal or DeBakey III) dissections arise beyond the subclavian artery.

2. **Type B dissections:** They have **distal lesions,** which **do not involve the ascending part of the aorta** and usually begin **distal to the subclavian artery** (DeBakey type III).

Classical Symptoms

Sudden onset of severe tearing pain. It usually begins in the anterior chest and radiates to the back between the scapulae. As the dissection progresses, the pain moves downward. Pain may be confused with and **misdiagnosed as that of myocardial infarction.** Loss of one or more arterial pulses is common. Hypertension is a frequent finding, and the development of hypotension is an ominous sign and suggests aortic rupture.

Cause of Death

- **Rupture of the dissection** outward and bleeding into the pericardial, pleural, or peritoneal cavities.
- **Retrograde dissection** into the aortic root can cause aortic valvular insufficiency, cardiac tamponade, and myocardial infarction.
- **Dissection** may also extend **into the great arteries of the neck** or into the coronary (causes myocardial infarction), renal, mesenteric, spinal arteries (causes transverse myelitis), or iliac arteries, causing critical vascular obstruction and ischemic damage.

HYPERTENSIVE VASCULAR DISEASE

Hypertension is a common disorder and maintenance of blood pressure is important to prevent untoward consequences. Low blood pressure (hypotension) can cause inadequate perfusion of organs leading to tissue dysfunction or death. High blood pressure (hypertension) can cause end-organ damage and is one of the major risk factors for atherosclerosis. The prevalence and vulnerability to complications of hypertension increase with age.

Definition: Hypertension is a **resting systolic pressure of 130 mm Hg or greater or a diastolic pressure of 80 mm Hg or greater.**

Causes of Hypertension (Box 16.3)

Primary Hypertension

The terms **idiopathic, essential, and benign** are used for this form of hypertension. It constitutes about 95% of cases. It is an insidious condition called benign or essential hypertension. The term essential or benign is used because the gradual age-associated rise in blood pressure was considered "essential" for normal perfusion of end organs such as the brain. However, the rise in blood pressure is neither essential nor benign. It is best called primary hypertension because it is generally without any identifiable cause (idiopathic).

Consequences of Primary Hypertension

Individuals with primary hypertension can usually have long life unless there is a complication (e.g., myocardial infarction, stroke).

- **Risk factor:** Hypertension is one of the major modifiable risk factors for **atherosclerosis.**
- **Lesions/diseases produced:** It is associated with an **increased risk for stroke and atherosclerotic coronary heart disease (ischemic heart disease).** It can also cause **cardiac hypertrophy** (left ventricle) and **congestive heart failure** (hypertensive heart disease),

BOX 16.3: Types and major causes of hypertension (systolic and diastolic).

PRIMARY/ESSENTIAL HYPERTENSION (~ 95% of cases)

SECONDARY HYPERTENSION

Renal
- Acute glomerulonephritis
- Chronic renal disease
- Polycystic kidney disease
- Renal artery stenosis (renovascular hypertension)
- Renin-producing tumors
- Obstructive uropathy

Endocrine
- Adrenal disorders: Cushing syndrome, primary aldosteronism
- Pheochromocytoma
- Exogenous hormones: Glucocorticoids, estrogen
- Pregnancy-induced: Pre-eclampsia/eclampsia
- Others: Hypothyroidism (myxedema), hyperthyroidism (thyrotoxicosis), hypercalcemia, acromegaly

Cardiovascular
- Coarctation of the aorta
- Polyarteritis nodosa
- Increased cardiac output
- Increased intravascular volume

Neurologic
- Psychogenic
- Increased intracranial pressure
- Obstructive sleep apnea
- Acute stress, e.g., surgery

aortic dissection, multi-infarct dementia, subarachnoid hemorrhage, hypertensive encephalopathy, retinal ischemia/infarction and renal failure.

- **Malignant (severe) hypertension:** Approximately 5% of patients with hypertension present with rapidly rising blood pressure. It is characterized by a **systolic pressure above 180 mm Hg or diastolic pressure above 120 mm Hg.** If they are not treated, it leads to death within 1 to 2 years. This has been termed **"malignant" (or severe) hypertension** because it is frequently associated with severe morbidity and mortality (e.g., due to **renal failure and retinal hemorrhages, with or without papilledema**). Most commonly malignant hypertension develops in patients with long-standing preexisting primary, less severe (so-called "benign") hypertension. But it can arise de novo (from the beginning itself).

Secondary Hypertension

It forms about 5% of cases, and there is an identifiable cause. These include **(Box 16.3)** renal (e.g., most forms of chronic renal disease) or adrenal [e.g., the primary elevation of aldosterone levels (primary aldosteronism), Cushing syndrome, pheochromocytoma] disease, renal artery stenosis, diabetes mellitus, hyperthyroidism, coarctation of the aorta and renin-secreting tumors or other identifiable causes.

Regulation of Blood Pressure

Normal blood pressure is essential for survival; it causes damage when it increases continuously above the normal range.

Factors Determining Blood Pressure

- The major factors include age, sex, body mass index, and diet, particularly sodium intake, exertion, emotional state, and others.
- Blood pressure depends on two hemodynamic variables, namely **cardiac output** and **peripheral vascular resistance (Fig. 16.10)**. These two, in turn, are influenced by many genetic, environmental, and demographic factors.
  - **Cardiac output:** It depends on stroke volume and heart rate. Stroke volume in turn is influenced by sodium homeostasis. Heart rate and contractility of the myocardium (affects stroke volume) are regulated by the adrenergic systems (also effects on vascular tone).
  - **Peripheral vascular resistance:** It is determined by functional and anatomic changes in small arteries and arterioles. The vascular tone depends on the balance between vasoconstrictors and vasodilators. Blood pressure is also influenced by tissue pH and hypoxia.

Role of Kidney

The kidneys **play an important role in the regulation of blood pressure.**

- **Renin-angiotensin system:** The kidney influences both peripheral vascular resistance and sodium homeostasis (thereby blood volume) through the renin-angiotensin system.
  - **Renin:** Whenever there is a fall in blood pressure, renin is secreted by the juxtaglomerular cells of the kidney and released into the blood circulation.

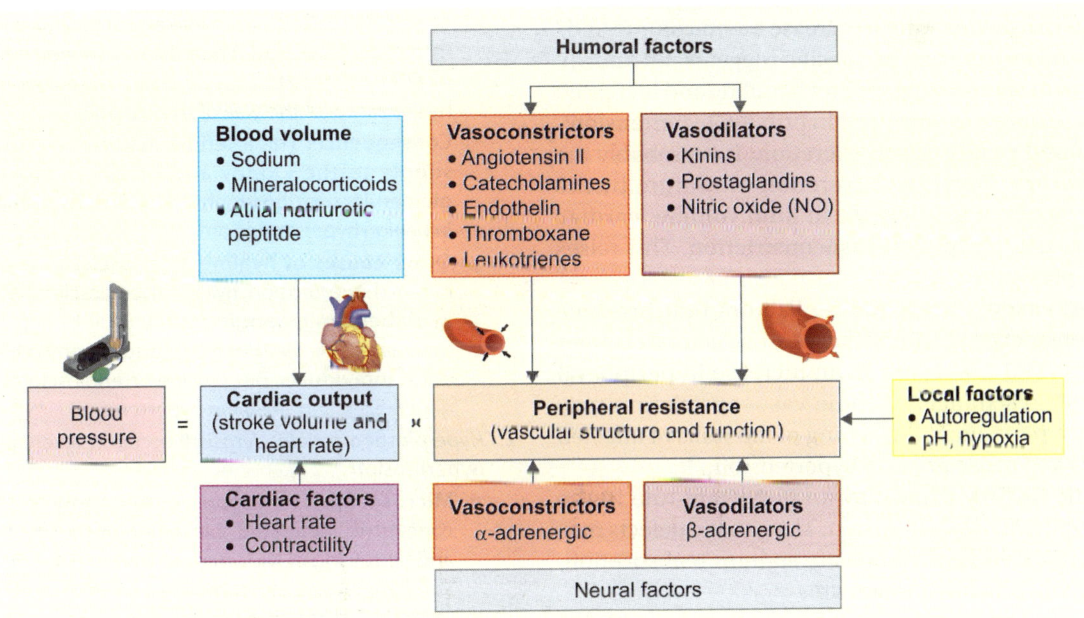

Fig. 16.10: Factors regulating blood pressure. It depends on cardiac output (e.g., blood volume and myocardial contractility) and peripheral resistance (neural and humoral). Local factors also affect blood pressure.

It **cleaves plasma angiotensinogen to angiotensin I**, which is then converted **to angiotensin II** by angiotensin-converting enzyme.
- **Angiotensin II:** It raises blood pressure by **increasing both peripheral resistance** (direct action on vascular smooth muscle cells and causes vasoconstriction) **and blood volume** (by stimulating secretion of aldosterone by the adrenal zona glomerulosa, and increased reabsorption of sodium in distal tubules).

- **Antihypertensive substances:** The kidney also produces substances that cause vasodilatation and have antihypertensive effects. These include prostaglandins and nitric oxide (NO). They counterbalance the vasoconstriction produced by angiotensin II.
- **Sodium homeostasis and blood volume:**
  - **When blood volume is reduced,** the glomerular filtration rate falls leading to increased reabsorption of sodium by proximal tubules of the kidney. This conserves sodium and expands blood volume.
  - **When blood volume is increased,** natriuretic factors (natriuretic peptides) are secreted by the atrial and ventricular myocardium. They inhibit sodium reabsorption in distal tubules and cause excretion of sodium and diuresis. Natriuretic peptides also cause vasodilation and may be considered endogenous inhibitors of the renin-angiotensin system.

Pathogenesis of Hypertension

Mechanisms of Primary Hypertension

Q. Write a short note on the pathogenesis of hypertension.

Primary hypertension is a **complex** and **multifactorial disorder**. It results from the interaction of genetic and environmental factors, which increase blood volume and/or peripheral resistance. The specific trigger is not known. Probably both altered renal sodium handling and increased vascular resistance are involved in primary hypertension:

- **Decreased renal sodium excretion:** It is probably the **key feature**. Decreased excretion of sodium by the kidney leads to an **increase in fluid volume, cardiac output, and peripheral vasoconstriction.** This raises blood pressure.
- **Raised vascular resistance:** Factors that produce vasoconstriction or stimuli that cause structural changes in the vessel wall result in an increase in peripheral vascular resistance. Chronic vasoconstriction may produce permanent thickening of the walls of affected vessels and cause primary hypertension.
- **Genetic factors:** They play an important role in the development of hypertension. The genetic defects may be in aldosterone metabolism, sodium reabsorption, and smooth muscle cell growth.
- **Environmental factors:** These include stress, obesity, smoking, lack of physical activity, and heavy intake of sodium salt.

Pathogenesis of Secondary Hypertension

- **Mechanism of renovascular hypertension:** Renal artery stenosis decreases glomerular flow and pressure in the afferent arteriole of the glomerulus. It stimulates renin secretion and the production of angiotensin II. This causes vasoconstriction and increased peripheral resistance. Renal artery stenosis also increases sodium reabsorption and increases blood volume through the aldosterone mechanism.
- **Primary hyperaldosteronism:** It is one of the most common causes of secondary hypertension.

MORPHOLOGY

Q. Write a short note on vascular pathology in hypertension.

Large and Medium Vessel Disease: Atherosclerosis

- Hypertension is one of the **major modifiable risk factors** for **atherogenesis.**
- Causes **degenerative changes in the walls** of large and medium arteries.
- Predisposes to (1) **Aortic dissection** and (2) **Cerebrovascular hemorrhage.**

Small Vessel Diseases

Two forms can occur in hypertension: (1) Hyaline arteriolosclerosis, and (2) hyperplastic arteriolosclerosis.

1. ***Hyaline arteriolosclerosis:*** It is seen in the arterioles in patients with primary hypertension.
   - **Microscopy:** It shows the **thickening of the wall of the arterioles due to the deposition of homogeneous, pink hyaline material.** It **narrows their lumen (Figs. 16.11A and B).**
   - **Mechanism**: Chronic hemodynamic stress due to hypertension produced by hypertension injures the endothelial cells. It causes **leakage of plasma components into the vessel wall. There is also increased synthesis of ECM by smooth muscle cells.** These changes lead to hyalinization of the wall of the arteriole.
   - **Consequence:** The arteriolar narrowing impairs blood supply to the kidney and produces **ischemia and glomerular scarring (nephrosclerosis).** The kidney changes in benign hypertension are called **benign nephrosclerosis.**
   - **Other causes of hyaline arteriosclerosis**: Apart from benign hypertension, hyaline arteriolosclerosis is also seen in **diabetic microangiography** (due to hyperglycemia-associated EC dysfunction), and **normotensive older adult individuals.** But hyaline arteriolosclerosis is more generalized and severe in hypertension.
2. ***Hyperplastic arteriolosclerosis:*** It occurs in **severe (malignant) hypertension.**
   - **Microscopy:** The blood vessels show **"onion-skin," concentric, laminated thickening of the arteriolar walls** and narrowing of the arteriolar lumen **(Figs. 16.11C to E).** The laminations are composed of SMCs and thickened, reduplicated basement membrane. Blood vessels may also show **fibrinoid necrosis** of the vessel wall **(necrotizing arteriolitis)**, particularly in the kidney.

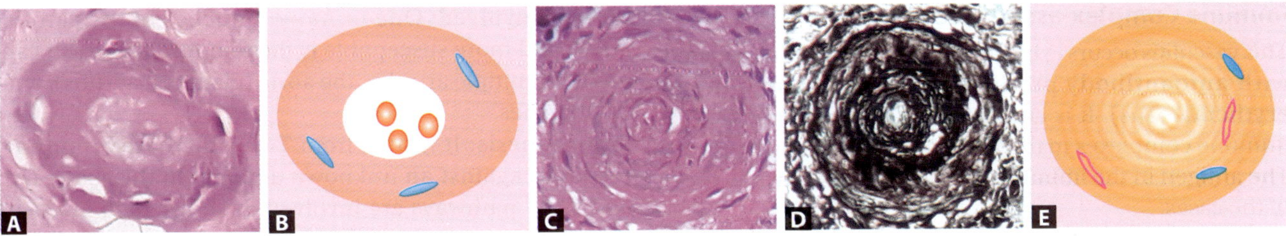

Figs. 16.11A to E: Vascular changes (in renal blood vessels) in hypertension: [A (H&E) and B (diagrammatic)] Hyaline arteriolosclerosis in benign hypertension: The arteriolar wall is thickened, hyalinized, and the lumen is narrowed; [C (H&E), D (PAS-methenamine) and E (Diagrammatic)] Hyperplastic arteriolosclerosis in malignant hypertension: shows onion-skinning with obliteration of arteriolar lumen.

VASCULITIS

Vasculitis is a general term used for inflammation of the vessel wall. The lumen of the involved vessel is usually narrowed and may lead to ischemia of the tissues supplied.

Definition: Vasculitis is a **heterogeneous group** of disorders **characterized by inflammation and damage of the blood vessels.**

General Characteristics

- **Primary or secondary:** Vasculitis may be a primary or secondary component of another primary disease.
- **Vessel involved:** It can involve **any type, size, and location** of blood vessels. Mostly, involve small vessels (arterioles to capillaries to venules).
- **Organ involved:** Vasculitis may be **restricted to one organ** (e.g., skin), or **may involve many organ systems.**

Classification

Vasculitis may be classified in many ways: (1) According to the size of the vessel involved **(Table 16.3)**, (2) the role of immune complexes, and the presence of specific autoantibodies, (3) granuloma formation, and (4) organ specificity.

Pathogenesis of Vasculitis

The two most common pathogenic mechanisms are:

1. Immune-mediated inflammation (noninfectious vasculitis).
2. Direct invasion of vascular walls by infectious pathogens (infectious vasculitis): Infections may also indirectly produce immune-mediated vasculitis (e.g., by forming immune complexes or triggering cross-reactivity).

It is important to distinguish between infectious and immunologic mechanisms. This is because immunosuppressive therapy is useful in immune-mediated vasculitis but can worsen infectious vasculitis.

Noninfectious Vasculitis

Mechanism: The main immunological changes of noninfectious vasculitis are: (1) immune complex deposition, (2) antineutrophil cytoplasmic antibodies, (3) antiendothelial cell antibodies, and (4) autoreactive T-cells.

TABLE 16.3 Classification of vasculitis according to blood vessels involved.

Examples	*Organs/vessels involved*	*Microscopic features*
Predominantly involving large vessels (aorta and large branches to extremities, head, and neck)		
• Giant cell (temporal) arteritis	Temporal artery and aorta. Patients older than age 50	Granulomatous inflammation with giant cells
• Takayasu's arteritis	Aorta, aortic arch and major branches, and pulmonary arteries Patients younger than age 50	Granulomatous with some giant cells and fibrosis in chronic stages
Predominantly involving medium vessels (visceral arteries and their branches)		
• Polyarteritis nodosa (PAN)	Skin, peripheral nerve, GI tract, and renal, etc. Spares pulmonary vessels	Fibrinoid necrosis, with mixed cellular infiltrate
• Kawasaki disease	Arteritis with mucocutaneous lymph node syndrome. Usually occurs in children	Similar to PAN, fibrinoid necrosis is less prominent
Predominantly involving small vessels (arterioles, venules, and capillaries)		
• Granulomatosis with polyangiitis*	Upper respiratory tract, lungs, kidneys, skin, and eyes	Necrotizing or granulomatous (or both); mixed cellular infiltrate
• Churg-Strauss syndrome	Upper respiratory tract, lungs, heart, peripheral nerves	Necrotizing or granulomatous (or both); prominent eosinophils
• Microscopic polyangiitis	Necrotizing glomerulonephritis and pulmonary capillaries	Leukocytoclastic with occasional eosinophils

* Formerly called as Wegener's granulomatosis

Immune Complex-associated Vasculitis

This vasculitis occurs in **immunologic disorders associated with autoantibody production (e.g., systemic lupus erythematosus).** It is characterized by the deposition of immune complexes in the vessel walls (*refer* pages 174-8). The antigen in the immune complex is not known in most of the cases.

Causes of immune-mediated vasculitis

- **Systemic immunological diseases:** For example, **systemic lupus erythematosus** (SLE) and **polyarteritis nodosa**.
- **Drug hypersensitivity vasculitis:** Drugs themselves may be foreign proteins (e.g., streptokinase) or they bind to serum proteins (e.g., penicillin) and behave like antigens.
- **Vasculitis secondary to viral infections:** Viral proteins may form immune complexes. Examples:
  - **Hepatitis B virus (HBV) associated polyarteritis nodosa** (PAN).
  - **Cryoglobulinemic vasculitis is strongly associated with hepatitis C virus (HCV) infection.**

Antineutrophil Cytoplasmic Antibodies

Antineutrophil cytoplasmic antibodies (ANCAs) are heterogeneous groups of **autoantibodies directed against** (mainly enzymes) **in the cytoplasmic granules of neutrophils and lysosomes of monocytes.** Two important ANCAs are:

1. **Anti-proteinase-3 (PR3-ANCA):** PR3 is a constituent of neutrophil azurophilic granule. It shares homology with many microbial peptides and antibodies against microbial peptides may form PR3-ANCAs. They are associated with **granulomatosis with polyangiitis**. PR3-ANCA was previously called c-ANCA.
2. **Anti-myeloperoxidase (MPO-ANCA):** MPO is a lysosomal enzyme normally involved in producing oxygen-free radicals. MPO-ANCAs can be produced by drugs (e.g., propylthiouracil). They are associated with **microscopic polyangiitis and eosinophilic granulomatosis with polyangiitis** (*Churg-Strauss syndrome*). MPO-ANCA was previously called p-ANCA.

Antiendothelial Cell Antibodies and Autoreactive T-cells

Antibodies to ECs cause certain vasculitides (plural of vasculitis) (e.g., Kawasaki disease). Autoreactive T-cells cause injury in some types of vasculitis characterized by the presence of granulomas.

A few examples of vasculitis are considered here.

Giant Cell (Temporal) Arteritis

Definition: Giant cell (temporal/cranial) arteritis is a **chronic inflammatory condition,** typically characterized by **granulomatous inflammation of medium- and large-sized arteries in the head.**

Vessels involved: One or more branches of the carotid artery and more susceptible is the **temporal artery.** It can involve multiple arteries, the aorta (giant cell aortitis), and its branches.

Pathogenesis: It results from **T-cell-mediated immune response against an unknown antigen.** In this, both Th1 and Th17 pathways are involved. It shows high levels of IFN-γ and IL-17 in the walls of affected vessels.

MORPHOLOGY

Gross

The **lesions are patchy.** An involved segment of the artery shows **nodular thickening of the intima** and occasional thromboses. **It reduces the size of the lumen and produces ischemia in the distal region.**

Microscopy (Figs. 16.12A and B)

- **Granulomatous inflammation:** Most of the cases show granulomatous lesions within the **inner tunica media** centered on the internal elastic lamina. It shows **T lymphocytes and macrophages,** along with multinucleated giant cells (either Langhans type or foreign body type).
- **Loss of smooth muscle cells and fragmentation of internal elastic lamina:** This is due to inflammation of the vascular wall.
- **Segmental distribution of inflammation** with segments of relatively normal arteries between the lesions. Lesions at different stages are seen within the same artery.
- **Intimal thickening, medial thinning and scarring, and adventitial fibrosis:** These are seen in the healed stage.

Clinical Features

- Usually manifest **after the age of 50.**
- **Fever, anemia, fatigue, headache** (most severe along the course of the superficial temporal artery), and weight loss.
- Ocular symptoms develop if the ophthalmic artery is involved (about 50% of cases). These symptoms may range from diplopia to complete vision loss.
- On palpation, **the involved artery is tender, thickened, or nodular.**

Diagnosis: It is confirmed by a **biopsy and microscopic examination of the involved (e.g., temporal) artery.** Responds well to corticosteroids and anti-TNF therapy.

Polyarteritis Nodosa

Definition: Polyarteritis nodosa **(PAN)** is a **systemic, necrotizing vasculitis of small and medium-sized muscular arteries.** It characteristically affects the **renal and visceral arteries.**

Vessels involved: It affects small to medium-sized arteries. Thus, it affects vessels of the **kidneys (glomeruli are spared), heart, liver, and gastrointestinal tract.** It **spares the smallest blood vessels** (arterioles, venules, and capillaries). **PAN does not involve pulmonary arteries.**

Etiology: About one-third of cases have chronic hepatitis B infection. It forms **HBsAg-HbsAb (immune) complexes** which get deposited in affected vessels. Less commonly it

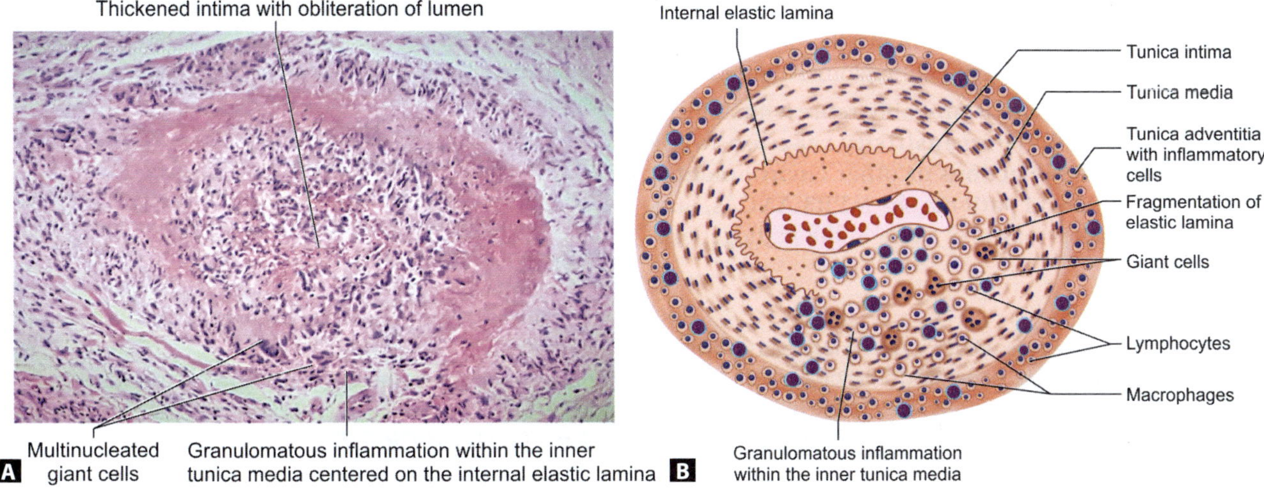

Figs. 16.12A and B: Microscopic features: (A) H & E staining; (B) Diagrammatic representation of giant cell arteritis.

occurs with Hepatitis C. In the remaining cases, the cause is unknown. It is not associated with ANCAs.

MORPHOLOGY

Gross

It causes nodular lesions involving part of the vessel wall mainly **at the points of arterial branching. Thrombosis** and **aneurysms** may be seen.

Microscopy (Fig. 16.13)

Segmental transmural necrotizing inflammation of small to medium-sized arteries: Lesions are **segmental** (involve only part of the vessel circumference) at branch points of arteries.

Acute phase: It is characterized by the following changes:

- **Transmural mixed inflammation of the arterial wall: The infiltrate consists of polymorphonuclear neutrophils** and **mononuclear cells.**
- **Fibrinoid necrosis and luminal thrombosis:** It may produce infarction of the tissues supplied by the involved vessel.
- **Aneurysm** (up to 1 cm in size) may rupture and produce hemorrhage.
- **Older lesions: Fibrous thickening of the vessel wall** that further occludes the vessel lumen. All stages of activity (from early acute to late older lesions) coexist in different vessels or within the same vessel.

Consequences of vasculitis: Thrombosis and impaired perfusion lead to ulcerations, infarcts, ischemic atrophy, or hemorrhages in the distribution of affected vessels. The inflammatory process also **weakens the wall of the artery** leading to **aneurysms or rupture.**

Clinical Features

- Usually occurs in **young adults.**
- Nonspecific symptoms are malaise, fever, and weight loss.
- Specific complaints are due to **ischemia and infarction of affected tissues and organs.**
- **Renal involvement manifests as hypertension** (usually developing rapidly), renal insufficiency, or hemorrhage due to microaneurysms.

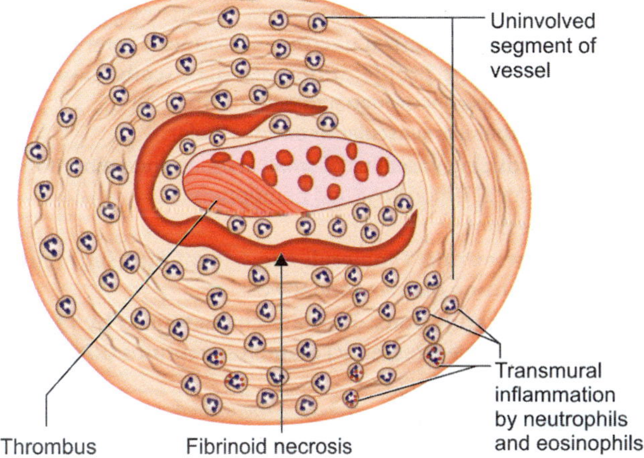

Fig. 16.13: Microscopic features (diagrammatic) of acute phase of polyarteritis nodosa.

- Gastrointestinal tract involvement is present with abdominal pain and melena (bloody stool).

Prognosis: It is fatal, if not treated. Immunosuppression produces remissions or cures in about 90% of patients. Renal arterial involvement is a major cause of death.

Granulomatosis with Polyangiitis

Granulomatosis with polyangiitis (previously called Wegener granulomatosis) is an **ANCA-positive necrotizing vasculitis.** It is characterized by the following triad:

1. **Necrotizing granulomas:** They occur **in the upper respiratory tract** (ear, nose, sinuses, throat) or **the lower respiratory tract** (lung), or both. It may present as chronic sinusitis and mucosal ulcerations of the nasopharynx.
2. **Necrotizing or granulomatous vasculitis:** It affects **small to medium-sized vessels** (e.g., capillaries, venules, arterioles, and arteries). It is most prominent in the lungs and upper airways. But may occur in other

sites. It may present with persistent pneumonitis and bilateral nodular and cavitary infiltrates.

3. **Focal necrotizing, often crescentic, glomerulonephritis.**

Pathogenesis: Not clear. It probably represents a form of **T-cell-mediated hypersensitivity reaction to an exogenous inhaled infectious or other environmental antigen. About 95% of patients show PR3-ANCAs,** and these autoantibodies may play a role in the pathogenesis of this disease.

MORPHOLOGY

It mainly involves three organs but may be widespread involving any organ such as eyes, skin, kidney, and other organs (e.g., heart).

1. **Upper respiratory tract lesions**: They range from **granulomatous sinusitis to ulcerative lesions** in the **nose, palate, or pharynx.**
2. **Lower respiratory tract:** The lung shows **multiple, bilateral, nodules with central cavity.** Microscopically, it is characterized by:
   - **Necrotizing granulomas**: They consist of **geographic patterns of central necrosis** surrounded by a zone of **fibroblastic proliferation with giant cells,** similar to mycobacterial or fungal infections. The granulomas may be **either intravascular or extravascular.**
   - **Necrotizing vasculitis of small arteries and veins.** It may produce hemorrhage and hemoptysis.
3. **Renal lesions:**
   - **Early lesions:** Glomeruli show **focal and segmental necrotizing glomerulonephritis.**
   - **Advanced lesions:** They are characterized by **rapidly progressive (crescentic) glomerulonephritis (RPGN).**

Clinical Features

Age and gender: It usually present during the **fourth to fifth decade. Males** are affected more often than females.

Classic presentations: It presents with bilateral pneumonitis, cavitary nodules (95%), chronic sinusitis (90%), mucosal ulcerations of the nasopharynx (75%), and renal disease (80%).

Course: If not treated, it is usually rapidly fatal and the majority die within 1 year.

VASCULAR TUMORS

Q. Write a short note on tumors of blood vessels (vascular tumors).

Tumors of blood vessels are classified as benign, intermediate-grade, and malignant **(Box 16.4)**.

BOX 16.4: Classification of vascular tumors.

Benign neoplasms, developmental and acquired conditions
- Hemangioma: Capillary hemangioma, cavernous hemangioma, pyogenic granuloma

Intermediate-grade neoplasms
- Kaposi sarcoma
- Hemangioendothelioma

Malignant neoplasms
- Angiosarcoma
- Epithelioid hemangioendothelioma

Hemangioma

Q. Write a short note on hemangioma.

Hemangiomas are **very common benign tumors of blood vessels** and form about 7% of all benign tumors in infancy and childhood. Most of these lesions are present from birth and increase in size as the child grows. Most may regress spontaneously.

Types of hemangioma: Capillary and cavernous.

Capillary Hemangioma

- **Most common type of hemangioma.**
- **Sites:** Most commonly in the **skin, subcutaneous tissues, and mucous membranes of the oral cavities and lips.** It may also occur in **internal organs (e.g., the liver, spleen, and kidneys).**

MORPHOLOGY

Gross

- Bright red to blue in color.
- Size varies from a few millimeters to several centimeters in diameter.
- May be level with the surface of the skin or slightly raised. The skin overlying it is usually intact.

Microscopy (Figs. 16.14A and B)

- **Unencapsulated** lesion.
- Composed of **aggregates of closely packed, thin-walled vascular channels.** The size and structure of these **vascular channels resemble normal capillaries.**
- **Capillaries are lined by flattened endothelium and their lumen is usually filled with blood.** The lumens may contain partially or completely organized thrombus.
- The vessels are separated by scant connective tissue stroma.

Cavernous Hemangioma

It consists of **large, dilated vascular channels;** compared with small vascular spaces in capillary hemangiomas.

MORPHOLOGY

Gross

- It appears as red-blue, soft, spongy masses and measure 1–2 cm in diameter.
- More frequently involve deep structures. They are found in the skin, on the mucosal surfaces, and in visceral organs, such as the liver, spleen, and pancreas.

Microscopy (Figs. 16.15A and B)

- It consists of sharply defined **unencapsulated** mass.
- It is composed of **large, cavernous blood-filled vascular spaces,** separated by a moderate amount of connective tissue stroma. Intravascular thrombosis and dystrophic calcification are common.

Aggregates of closely packed, thin-walled vascular channels

Capillaries are lined by flattened endothelium and their lumen is usually filled with blood

Figs. 16.14A and B: Microscopic appearance of capillary hemangioma: (A) Photomicrograph; (B) Diagrammatic.

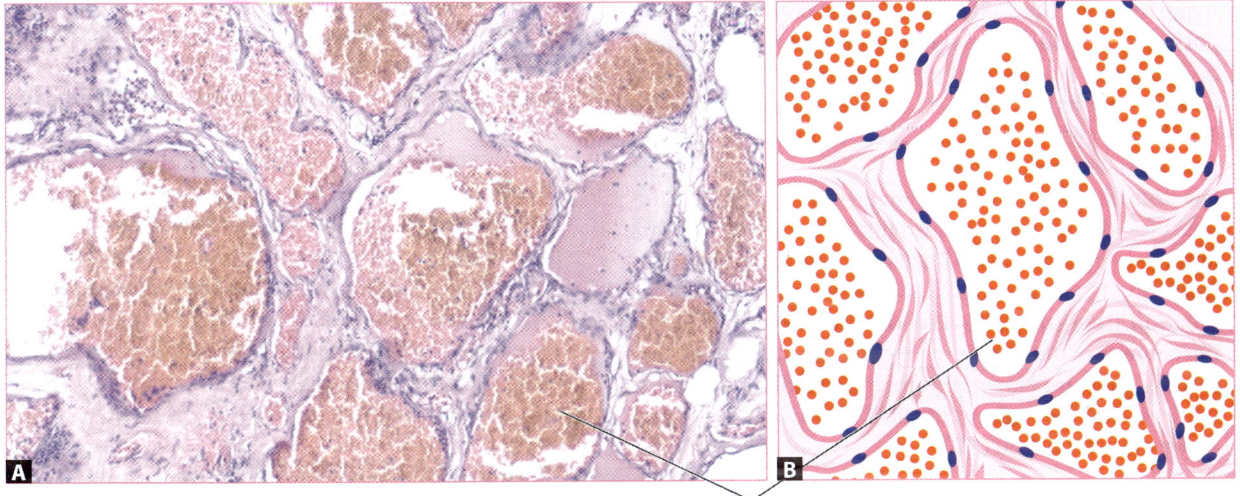

Figs. 16.15A and B: Microscopic appearance of cavernous hemangioma: (A) Photomicrograph; (B) Diagrammatic.

HEART DISORDERS

HEART FAILURE

PA 27.3 (CC): Describe the etiology, types, stages, pathophysiology, pathology, and complications of heart failure.

Heart failure is often **termed congestive heart failure (CHF).** It is a common **end stage of many forms of** chronic **heart disease.** It is usually a progressive condition and has a poor prognosis.

Definition: Heart failure (HF) is defined as a condition in which the **heart cannot generate an adequate cardiac output to meet the metabolic demands of tissues** (low-output failure) **or can do so only at higher-than-normal filling pressures.**

High-output failure: In a few cases, heart failure is due to markedly increased tissue demands, as in hyperthyroidism, or decreased oxygen-carrying capacity, as in anemia.

Onset is gradual (chronic) or acute: Chronic is more common than acute heart failure.

- **Chronic heart failure:** In most cases, CHF develops gradually and insidiously. It occurs due to progressive effects of chronic work overload (e.g., valvular heart disease or hypertension) or increasing loss of myocardial function [e.g., after myocardial infarction (MI) with heart damage].
- **Acute heart failure**: In some cases, the onset of CHF is sometimes abrupt (acute/sudden). It develops with a large myocardial infarct, acute valve dysfunction, rupture of a cardiac valve, or acute hemodynamic stresses, such as fluid overload.

BOX 16.5: Causes of heart failure.

Common causes
- Coronary heart disease (CHD)
- Hypertension (HTN)

Less common causes
- Dilated cardiomyopathy
- Congenital heart defects
- Valvular disorder/dysfunction (e.g., due to endocarditis)
- Respiratory diseases
- Anemia (decreased oxygen-carrying capacity)
- Hyperthyroidism (due to greatly increased tissue demands.

Etiology (Box 16.5)

Heart failure may occur due to any of the cause that decreases the ability of the ventricle to fill with (diastolic failure) **or eject blood** (systolic failure).

- **Systolic failure**: The decreased ability to eject blood results from inadequate myocardial contractile function. It usually occurs in **ischemic heart disease or hypertension.** The inadequate cardiac output and tissue perfusion are called forward failure. It is accompanied by increased congestion or pooling of the blood in the venous circulation, which is, termed backward failure. The backward failure may cause pulmonary edema, peripheral edema, or both.
- **Diastolic failure**: It is characterized by an inability of the heart to adequately relax and fill. These types of heart failure are called **heart failure with preserved ejection fraction**. These are associated with **left ventricular ejection fraction ≥50%. Ejection fraction (EF) is the percentage of blood volume ejected from the ventricle during systole.** Normally during systole, ventricles contract and eject **about 60–80%** of the blood in them at the end of diastole **(EF)**.

Pathophysiology of Heart Failure

Homeostatic Mechanisms in Heart Failure

The cardiovascular system develops several homeostatic mechanisms to compensate for reduced myocardial contractility or increased hemodynamic burden in heart failure. These compensatory mechanisms maintain arterial pressure and organ perfusion. This produces characteristic signs and symptoms of heart failure. Because of the heart's capacity to compensate, congestive heart failure is usually tolerated for years. These mechanisms include:

Frank–Starling mechanism (also known as **Starling's law**): It states that as a larger volume of blood flows into the ventricle (i.e., increased filling volumes), the blood will cause increased stretching of the cardiac myofiber. This produces dilation of the walls of the heart (thereby increasing actin-myosin cross-bridge formation), causing a greater expansion during diastole. These lengthened stretched myofibers contract more forcibly, thereby increasing cardiac output. Thus, the quantity of blood that is pumped into the aorta also increases during systole. **The stages of heart failure** are as follows:

- **Compensated heart failure:** If the dilated ventricle is capable of maintaining the cardiac output by the compensatory changes, the patient is said to be in compensated heart failure.
- **Decompensated heart failure:** The ventricular dilatation produced is at the expense of increased wall tension. This increases the oxygen required by an already-compromised myocardium. With time, the failing myocardial muscle is not able to eject sufficient blood to meet the needs of the body, and the patient develops decompensated heart failure.

Activation of Neurohumoral Systems

The activated neurohumoral system increases the heart function and/or regulates filling volumes and pressures.

- **Release of norepinephrine:** Norepinephrine is a neurotransmitter released by adrenergic cardiac nerves of the autonomic nervous system. Norepinephrine **increases heart rate, myocardial contractility, and vascular resistance.**
- **Activation of the renin-angiotensin-aldosterone system:** Reduced perfusion of the kidney in heart failure activates the renin-angiotensin-aldosterone system as a compensatory mechanism. It leads to the **retention of salt and water, with the expansion of the interstitial and intravascular fluid volumes** (increases circulatory volume) and **increases vascular tone**. This turn **increases the existing pulmonary edema.**
- **Release of atrial natriuretic peptide:** It balances the renin-angiotensin-aldosterone system through diuresis and relaxation of vascular smooth muscle.

Myocardial Structural Changes

Hypertrophy of cardiac muscles: It occurs as a compensatory response to increased mechanical work. Ventricular remodeling is the term used for the molecular, cellular, and structural changes that are observed in the ventricle as a response to injury or altered ventricular loading.

Functional changes: Cardiac hypertrophy is associated with an increase in oxygen consumption by the heart. Hence, the hypertrophied heart is susceptible to ischemia.

Left-sided Heart Failure (LHF)

Heart failure can involve mainly the left or right side of the heart or may affect both sides.

In left-sided heart failure, the left ventricle cannot efficiently eject blood into the aorta. This causes blood to back up into the lungs ("blood builds up behind the failed heart") producing pulmonary congestion (edema).

Etiology: The common causes of left-sided cardiac failure are listed in **Box 16.6**.

BOX 16.6: Common causes of left-sided heart failure.

- Ischemic heart disease (IHD)—most common cause
- Systemic hypertension
- Mitral or aortic valvular disease
- Primary diseases of the myocardium (e.g., amyloidosis, myocarditis).

The pathophysiology of LHF is presented in Flowchart 16.1 and Figure 16.16.

The clinical and morphologic effects of left-sided CHF are due to passive congestion (in the pulmonary circulation), stasis of blood in the left-sided chambers, and inadequate perfusion of tissues.

Flowchart 16.1: Pathophysiology of LHF.

Left heart failure (LHF)—ineffective pumping of the blood from the left ventricle

↓

Compensatory mechanism
Increase of left atrial and pulmonary venous pressures
Escape of fluid the pulmonary capillaries into interstitial and alveolar spaces

↓

Passive pulmonary congestion and edema. Rupture of capillaries and relase of RBCs. Iron from ruptured RBCs phagocytosed by alveolar macrophages

↓

Hemosiderin-laden macrophages (so-called heart failure cells) in alveoli

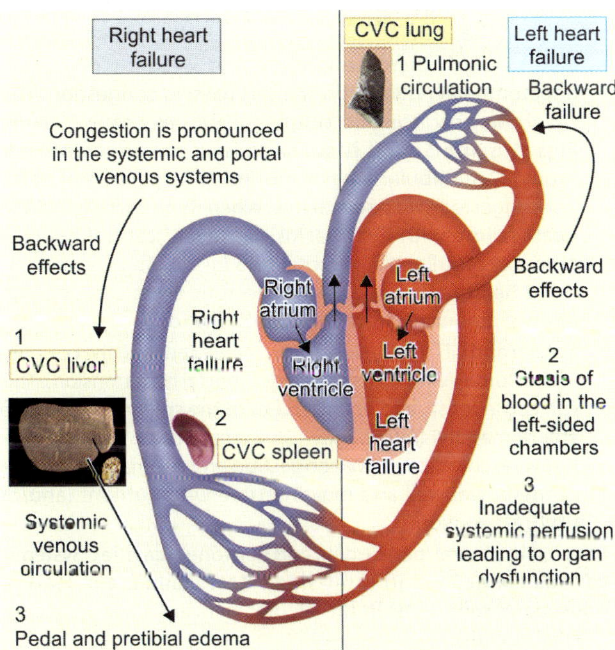

Fig. 16.16: Pathophysiology and effects on pulmonary circulations and systemic in left and right heart failure.
(CVC: chronic venous congestion).

- **Passive congestion (blood backing up in the pulmonary circulation)** (*refer* chronic venous congestion of the lung on pages 135-6).
- **Inadequate systemic perfusion leading to organ dysfunction.**
- **Stasis of blood in the left-sided chambers.**

MORPHOLOGY

Heart

Gross: It depends on the disease process responsible for LHF [e.g., myocardial infarction or valvular deformities (valvular stenosis or regurgitation)]. The **left ventricle is usually hypertrophied and can be dilated** (except in failure due to mitral valve stenosis or restrictive cardiomyopathies). Left ventricular dilation can result in mitral insufficiency and dilatation (enlargement) of the left atrium.

Microscopy: These changes are nonspecific and consist of **hypertrophy of myocyte and variable degrees of interstitial fibrosis.**

Lungs

Gross: Due to pulmonary congestion and edema, the lungs become heavy and boggy. Lungs exude a frothy pink transudate (edema) on the cut surface.

Microscopy: These include:

- Perivascular and interstitial edema and is responsible for the characteristic Kerley B and C lines observed on chest X-rays in patients with CHF.
- Progressive edema of alveolar septa.
- **Accumulation of edema fluid in the alveolar spaces.**
- In chronic heart failure, few red cells and plasma proteins escape from the leaky capillaries into alveolar spaces. These RBCs are phagocytosed and digested by macrophages. Subsequent breakdown of red cells and hemoglobin leads to the liberation of hemosiderin within macrophages. These **hemosiderin-laden alveolar macrophages** (also known as heart failure cells). These heart failure cells tell-tale signs (reflect) of previous episodes of pulmonary edema (*refer* **Fig. 5.7**).

Clinical Features and Complications

Symptoms during early left-sided heart failure are a consequence of pulmonary congestion and edema and may be minimal.

Dyspnea (breathlessness or shortness of breath): It occurs **early and most significant** (cardinal) symptom in the progression of left-sided heart failure. Difficulty breathing may be exacerbated by activity (**dyspnea on exertion**) or lying down (**orthopnea and paroxysmal nocturnal dyspnea**). Initially, there may be cough and dyspnea only on exertion. As heart failure progresses, worsening pulmonary edema may cause **orthopnea** [dyspnea when supine (supine position increases venous return from the lower extremities and also elevates the diaphragm), relieved by sitting or standing (hence patients usually sleep in a semi-seated position)] or **paroxysmal nocturnal dyspnea** (dyspnea usually occurring at night and is a dramatic form of breathlessness, awakening patients from sleep with feelings of suffocation) and dyspnea at rest.

Respiratory system: Cough results from bronchial irritation associated with transudation of fluid into air spaces. **Fine ráles** are abnormal sounds at the base of the lungs caused by the opening of edematous pulmonary alveoli and movement of air through partially fluid-filled alveoli.

Cardiovascular system: Cardiomegaly (an enlarged heart), **tachycardia, a third heart sound (S3)**. With progressive dilatation of left ventricles, the outward displacement of papillary muscles causes mitral regurgitation and a systolic murmur. Subsequent chronic dilation of the left atrium can cause atrial fibrillation. **Atrial fibrillation** causes stasis of the blood (especially in the atrial appendage) and favors the **formation of thrombi** which can fragment and **form emboli**. These emboli can produce **strokes and infarction** in other organs.

Prerenal azotemia: Diminished cardiac output leads to reduced renal perfusion. This stimulates the renin-angiotensin-aldosterone axis, increasing intravascular volume and pressure. Unfortunately, these compensatory mechanisms in heart failure, exacerbate pulmonary edema. With further progression, prerenal azotemia may develop.

Hypoxic encephalopathy: It may occur due to reduced cerebral perfusion. It is characterized by symptoms such as irritability, diminished cognition, and restlessness. This can progress to a stupor and coma.

Treatment: Initially, correct the underlying cause (e.g., a valvular defect). Others include salt restriction or drugs that decrease volume overload (e.g., diuretics), increase myocardial contractility ("positive inotropes"), or reduce afterload (adrenergic blockade or inhibitors of angiotensin-converting enzymes).

Right-sided Heart Failure

Right heart failure (RHF) is defined as the inability of the right ventricle to effectively pump venous blood into the lungs. Thus, RHF cannot provide adequate blood flow into the pulmonary circulation at normal central venous pressure.

Causes (Box 16.7): The right and left ventricles function in series. In RHF, blood builds up in the systemic venous system (vena cava and its tributaries).

- **All the causes of LHF: Right-sided heart failure is usually the result of left-sided heart failure.** Any increase in pressure in the pulmonary circulation produced by left ventricular failure automatically increases the workload (burden) on the right side of the heart (mainly the right ventricle). Thus, the etiology of right-sided heart failure includes all the causes of left-sided failure and **is usually the consequence of left-sided heart failure.**
- **Corpulmonale:** Isolated right-sided heart failure is rare and usually develops **in association with** one of a variety of **disorders of the lungs**; hence it is termed **cor pulmonale.** Corpulmonale occurs with diseases of lung parenchyma (e.g., emphysema, chronic bronchitis). It may develop secondary to disorders that affect the pulmonary vasculature (e.g., primary pulmonary hypertension, recurrent pulmonary thromboembolism), or conditions that cause pulmonary vasoconstriction (obstructive sleep apnea). In cor pulmonale, myocardial hypertrophy and dilation are usually restricted and confined to the right ventricle and atrium. However, bulging of the ventricular septum can occur to the left side and reduce cardiac output by causing outflow tract obstruction.

BOX 16.7: Causes of right-sided heart failure.

- Cor pulmonale
- Right-sided valvular heart disease
- Right-sided disease of the myocardium
- Pulmonary hypertension

Morphologic and clinical effects in isolated right-sided heart failure differ from those of left-sided heart failure. It produces usually marked congestion in the systemic and portal venous systems **(Fig. 16.16)** and pulmonary congestion is minimal.

MORPHOLOGY

Heart: Similar to left heart failure, the morphology of the heart depends on the cause. Isolated right heart failure caused by lung disease, in most cases, shows only hypertrophy and dilation of the right atrium and ventricle.

Liver and portal system: Congestion of the hepatic and portal vessels may produce morphological changes in the liver, the spleen, and the GI tract.

- **Liver:** Usually increased in size and weight (congestive hepatomegaly) due to prominent passive congestion. The cut shows characteristic "**nutmeg liver**" (*refer* page 136 and **Figs. 5.8 and 5.9**). It is characterized by congested red-brown centrilobular areas surrounded by peripheral paler, noncongested liver parenchyma. When there is also left-sided heart failure with hypoperfusion, severe central hypoxia produces centrilobular necrosis. In long-standing severe right-sided heart failure, the central necrotic areas can undergo fibrosis, producing so-called **cardiac cirrhosis.**
- **Spleen and GIT:** Right-sided heart failure can raise the pressure in the portal vein and its tributaries (portal hypertension). This can cause tense, and enlargement of the spleen (**congestive splenomegaly**) (*refer* pages 136-7, and **Figs. 5.10, and 5.11**). If severe, chronic passive congestion and edema can develop in the bowel wall and may interfere with nutrient (and/or drug) absorption.

Effusion in pleural, pericardial, and peritoneal cavities: Systemic venous congestion in right-sided heart failure can lead to transudates (effusions) in the pleural, pericardial, or peritoneal cavities (ascites).

Subcutaneous tissues: Edema of dependent portions of the body [mainly ankle (pedal) and pretibial edema] is a hallmark of right-sided heart failure. In chronically bedridden patients, the edema is mainly found in the presacral region. Generalized massive edema (anasarca) can also develop.

Clinical Features and Complications

Isolated/pure right-sided heart failure usually does not produce respiratory symptoms. The **clinical features are due to systemic and portal venous congestion**. These include **enlargement of the liver and spleen, peripheral edema, pleural effusion, and ascites.** Venous congestion and hypoxia of the kidneys and brain due to right-sided heart failure can produce similar changes to that of hypoperfusion of left-sided heart failure. Renal congestion is more severe with right-sided than left-sided heart failure and leads to greater fluid retention and peripheral edema. As CHF progresses, patients may develop cyanosis and acidosis. In many patients, biventricular CHF with symptoms due to both right-sided and left-sided heart failure are observed.

RHEUMATIC FEVER AND RHEUMATIC HEART DISEASE

PA 27.4 (CC): Describe the etiology, pathophysiology, pathology, gross and microscopic features, criteria, and complications of rheumatic fever.

Q. Define rheumatic fever. Describe etiopathogenesis, pathology, and complications of rheumatic heart disease.

Definition: Rheumatic fever (RF) is an **acute, post-streptococcal, immune-mediated, multisystem inflammatory disease.** It occurs a few weeks after an episode of group A streptococcal infections (usually pharyngitis, and occasionally infections at other sites, such as skin).

Incidence

- **Age group:** It is most common in **children between 5 and 15 years.**
- **Sex:** Both sexes are equally affected.
- **Socioeconomic conditions:** Incidence and mortality rates of RF and RHD have markedly decreased over the past century, due to improved socioeconomic conditions and rapid diagnosis and treatment of streptococcal pharyngitis.
- **Poor economy and overcrowding:** It is a predisposing factor in developing countries.

Major phases: Two major phases of rheumatic disease are:
1. **Acute rheumatic fever:** It frequently manifests as **acute rheumatic carditis.**
2. **Rheumatic heart disease:** It is the cardiac manifestation of rheumatic fever. Acute rheumatic carditis of **acute rheumatic fever may progress to chronic rheumatic heart disease** (RHD).

Etiology and Pathogenesis (Fig. 16.17 and Flowchart 16.2)

Q. Describe the etiopathogenesis and pathology of rheumatic heart disease.

The pathogenesis of acute RF involves the triad, namely (1) infection by a rheumatogenic strain of group A β-hemolytic *Streptococcus*, (2) an abnormal host immune response, and (3) a genetically susceptible host.

Infection by Group A β-hemolytic Streptococcus

Poststreptococcal disease: Acute rheumatic fever (ARF) is a poststreptococcal disease. It develops only after a **latent period of 2–6 weeks after an episode of** pharyngeal infection (pharyngitis or tonsillitis) by **group A β-hemolytic *Streptococcus*.** Streptococcal skin infections usually do not progress to ARF. It occurs most often in children.

Abnormal Host Immune Response

Molecular mimicry and cross-reactivity: These are the most widely accepted theories of RF pathogenesis.

- Streptococcal infection introduces streptococcal antigens into the body. **It activates antibody- and T-cell-mediated immune responses targeted against group A streptococcal antigen.** The major streptococcal antigens are present on the M protein which structurally resembles domains present in myosin as well as other cardiac proteins. The **immune response** is a **cross-reaction against host proteins.**
- **Evidence of immunologic mechanism:** Time is needed for the host immune system to generate an immune response. Thus, the evidence for the immunologic mechanism that brings out RF is (1) the characteristic 2–3-week latent period in symptom onset after infection and (2) streptococci are completely absent from the lesions in rheumatic fever. **Pharyngeal cultures** for streptococci are **negative** at the time the acute rheumatic fever. The immune response includes both antibody and cell-mediated responses.
- **Antibody-mediated reactions (type II hypersensitivity reaction): B lymphocytes may produce antibodies against various antigenic components of the *Streptococcus*.** One antibody is directed against the M proteins of streptococci. This antibody can recognize the M proteins within the myocardium and glycoproteins of the valves in the heart. Thus, these antibodies seem to cross-react with certain similar self-antigens in the myocardial cells (cardiac sarcolemma) and glycoproteins of the valves in the heart (**molecular mimicry**). This may be the mechanism for pancarditis in acute rheumatic fever.
- **T-cell-mediated reactions (type IV hypersensitivity reaction): CD4+ T cells** are also activated by streptococcal antigens. Cytokine is produced by the stimulated T-cells and leads to the activation of macrophages (e.g., macrophages are seen within Aschoff bodies).
- **Mechanism of damage to heart tissue:** Both antibody- and T-cell-mediated reactions in combination cross-react with self-proteins in the heart and may damage the heart tissue.

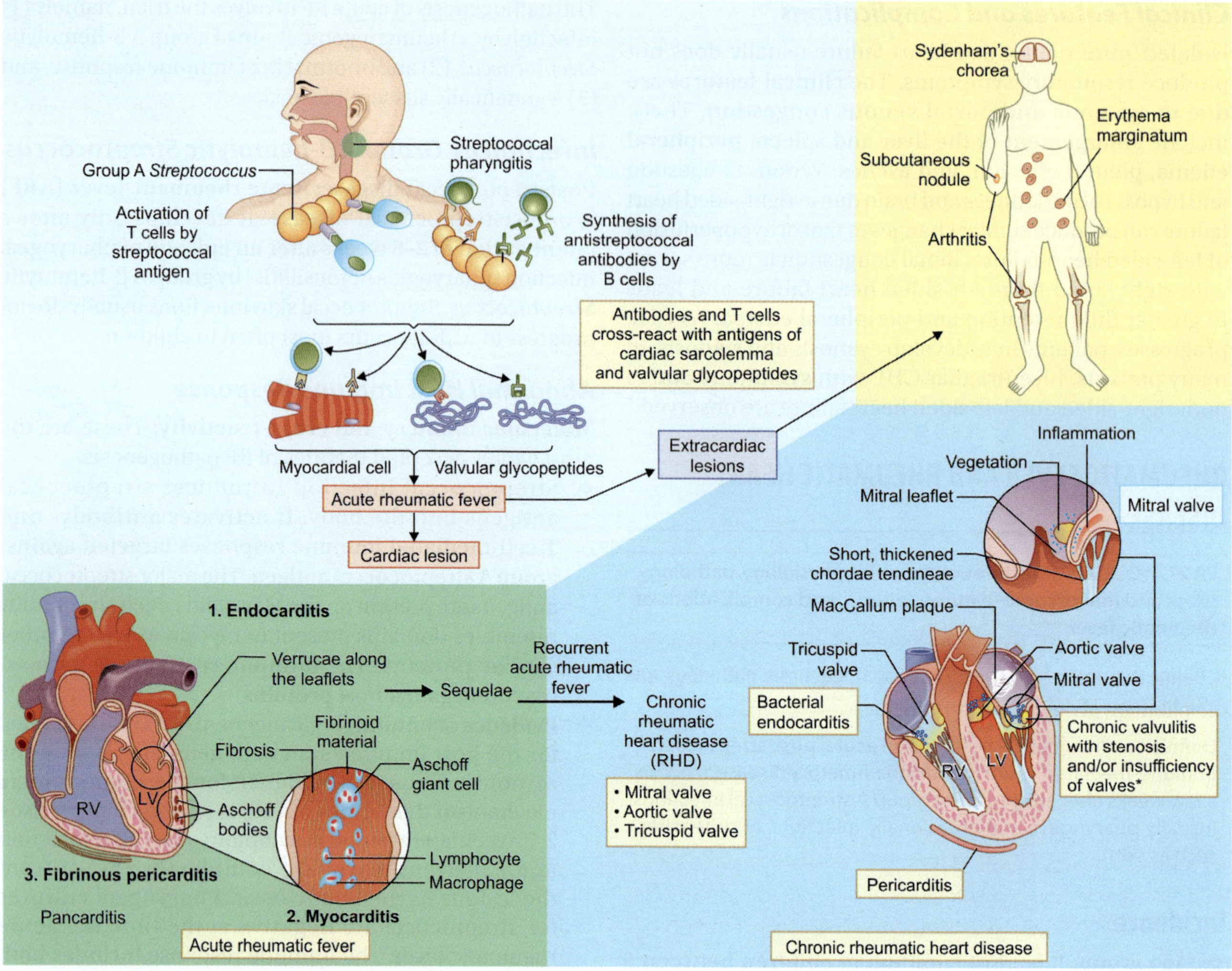

Fig. 16.17: Pathogenesis and sequelae of acute rheumatic fever. Pharyngitis by β-hemolytic streptococci activates both humoral and cellular immunity. The antibodies produced against various antigenic components of the *Streptococcus* can cross-react with cardiac antigens. The result is pancarditis (endocarditis, myocarditis, and pericarditis). Extracardiac lesions include polyarthritis, erythema marginatum, subcutaneous nodules, and Sydenham's chorea. If untreated, recurrent acute rheumatic carditis can progress to chronic rheumatic heart disease.
* Valves affected include mitral, aortic and tricuspid.
(LV: left ventricle; RV: right ventricle)

Flowchart 16.2: Pathogenesis of acute rheumatic fever.

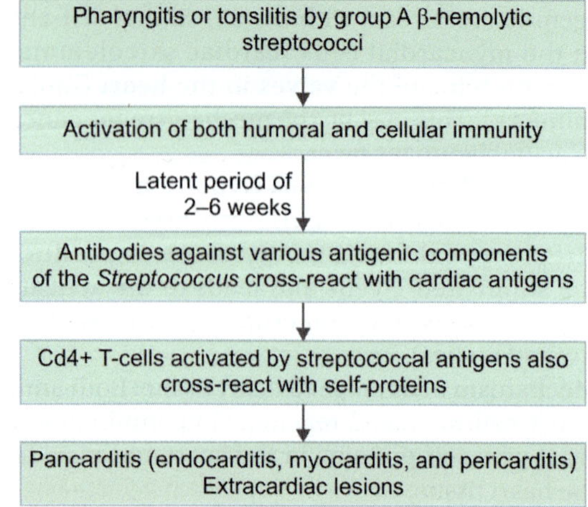

Genetic Susceptibility

It remains unknown why only a small number (about 3%) of infected patients with the offending *Streptococcus* develop RF. A genetic susceptibility is likely involved in the development of cross-reactive immune responses.

MORPHOLOGY

During **acute rheumatic fever**, focal inflammatory lesions are produced in various tissues. These lesions of rheumatic fever can be broadly divided into **cardiac and extracardiac lesions.**

Cardiac Lesions

Q. Write a short note on the morphology of the heart in acute rheumatic heart disease (rheumatic carditis).

Cardiac lesions may be acute rheumatic carditis and chronic rheumatic heart disease.

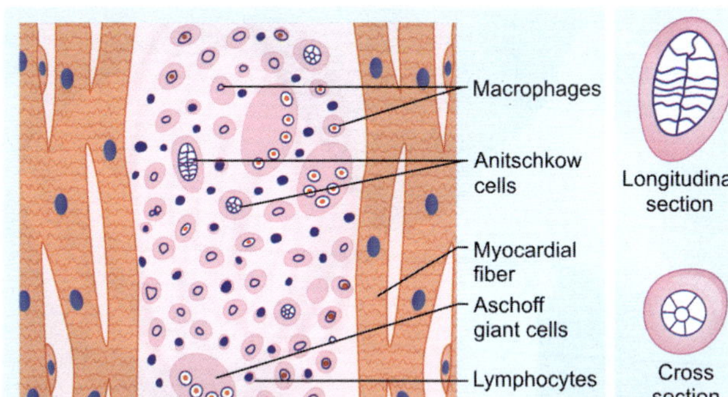

Figs. 16.18A and B: Schematic representation of Aschoff body: (A) Aschoff body in pathognomonic intermediate phase; (B) Longitudinal and cross-sectional view of Anitschkow cells.

Q. Write a short note on Aschoff bodies (Aschoff nodule).

Aschoff Body (Figs. 16.18A and B)

Distinctive or **characteristic lesions** of acute rheumatic fever in the heart are called as **Aschoff body.** It develops several weeks after the symptoms of ARF.

- **Shape:** It is **spheroidal or fusiform.**
- **Size:** It measures about 1–2 mm.
- **Location:** During acute RF, diffuse inflammation and Aschoff bodies may be found in any of the three layers (in the **perivascular interstitial region of the heart**). Aschoff bodies are observed in the peri-vascular interstitial region of the heart.

Formation of Aschoff Body

Its formation consists of three phases.

1. **Early (exudative) phase:** It consists of a perivascular focus of swollen **eosinophilic collagen** surrounded by **lymphocytes, plasma cells, and macrophages.**
2. **Intermediate (granulomatous) phase:** This phase is **pathognomonic of rheumatic myocarditis.** It is a **granulomatous lesion**, with a **central fibrinoid focus** associated with **lymphocytes** (primarily T-cells), **macrophages**, Anitschkow cells (pathognomonic for RF), and occasional plasma cells. **Anitschkow cells are plump activated macrophages**, that have **abundant cytoplasm.** They have central round-to-ovoid nuclei. The chromatin of the nucleus is condensed into a **central, slender, wavy ribbon.** The **chromatin of nuclei resembles a caterpillar** when **cut longitudinally** (hence known as **"caterpillar cells"**). **On cross-section**, these nuclei have an **owl-eye appearance.** Few Anitschkow cells may fuse and become **multinucleated** (with 2–4 nuclei) and these are termed **Aschoff giant cells** (the cytoplasm fuses and nuclei remain intact within fused cytoplasm).
3. **Late (healed or final) phase:** Aschoff body is replaced by a nodule of **scar tissue.**

Acute Rheumatic Heart Disease

It is characterized by **pancarditis,** involving all three layers of the heart (**endocardium, myocardium, and pericardium**).

1. Endocarditis (Fig. 16.19)

Inflammation of the endocardium (valvular/mural) is known as endocarditis. It **may involve valvular** (valvular endocarditis) **or mural endocardium** (mural endocarditis).

Valvular endocarditis

- During acute rheumatic carditis, **valve leaflets become inflamed and edematous.**
- All four valves may be affected, but **left-sided valves (mitral and aortic)** are **more injured than right-sided valves** (tricuspid and pulmonary).
- **Inflammatory damage** causes **focal loss of endothelium** and **fibrinoid deposits along the lines of closure of the valve leaflets** or **the tendinous cords.**
- Fibrin deposits along the lines of closure form **small (1–2 mm) nodular or warty vegetations, called verrucae.** These verrucae are **firmly attached** and do not get dislodged. This contrasts with friable detachable vegetations of infective endocarditis. Thus, RHD is one of the causes of vegetative valve disease.

Mural endocarditis

Inflammation of the mural endocardium is less prominent than valvular lesions and the most common is **MacCallum plaque.**

- Inflammation of the mural endocardium and the left-sided valves usually produces fibrinoid necrosis within the cusps or tendinous cords.

Q. Write briefly on the MacCallum plaque.

MacCallum plaques (Figs. 16.17 and 16.19)

These are **subendocardial lesions,** which appear as **irregular, wrinkled, map-like thickenings** in the mural endocardium.

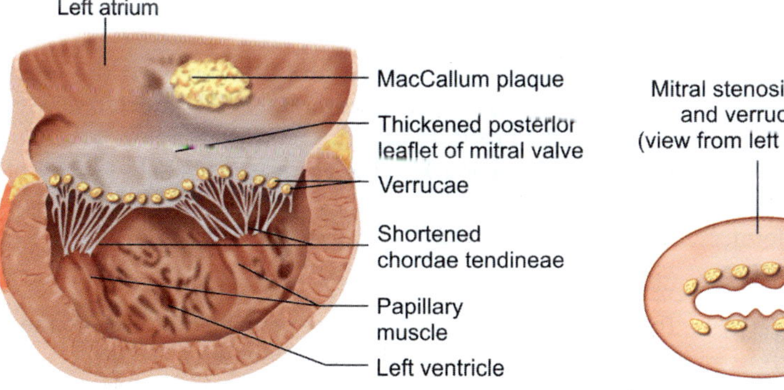

Fig. 16.19: Gross appearance of mitral valve and left atrium in RHD.

Acute rheumatic fever

The mitral valve is more commonly involved and responsible for 99% of cases of acquired mitral stenosis.

Recurrent rheumatic fever is the most common cause of mitral stenosis.

Verrucae are small, warty, firmly attached vegetations along the lines of closure of valve leaflets/tendinous cords.

MacCallum plaques are irregular, wrinkled, map-like thickening seen in the posterior wall of the left atrium in chronic rheumatic heart disease.

Anitschkow cells are pathognomonic for RF.

Usually seen in the **posterior wall of the left atrium** (in chronic RHD and not in acute rheumatic fever), just **above the posterior leaflet of the mitral valve.** These may be formed due to damage induced by chronic regurgitation of blood. **MacCallum plaques or patches** are **more often seen in chronic RHD.** Subendocardial lesions are probably aggravated or exacerbated by regurgitant jets (damage) due to mitral regurgitation during the acute stage and mitral stenosis during the chronic stage. **Microscopically,** they may show **multiple Aschoff bodies.**

2. Pericarditis

Inflammation of the pericardium is known as pericarditis. During acute RF, irregular deposits of fibrin are found on both visceral and parietal surfaces of the pericardium causing **fibrinous pericarditis.**

- This fibrinous pericarditis, grossly resembles the shaggy surfaces of two slices of buttered bread that have been gently pulled apart. Hence, they are commonly called as **bread-and-butter pericarditis (Fig. 16.20).**
- Clinically, it gives a friction rub and may be associated with serofibrinous effusion.

3. Myocarditis

Inflammation of the myocardium is known as myocarditis. **Nonspecific** myocarditis during acute RF may cause dilation of the heart. Microscopically, the myocardium may show **lymphocytes and macrophages or Aschoff bodies.**

- Few patients may die due to myocarditis.

Extracardiac Lesions (Fig. 16.17)

Q. Write a short note on extracardiac lesions of rheumatic fever.

Migratory polyarthritis: It is the **usual presentation** in acute rheumatic fever and is accompanied by fever. Polyarthritis involves more than one joint; migratory means moving from one joint to another over hours or days. In RF, **one large joint becomes painful (or tender), hot, red, and swollen,** which **then subsides, and another joint gets involved over a period.** They resolve spontaneously without any residual disability. Hence, the old dictum **"RF licks the joint but bites the heart."**

Subcutaneous nodules: These are usually seen in children than in adults. The nodules are oval to **spheroidal, painless,** and measure **about 0.5–2 cm** in diameter. They are beneath the skin, overlying bony prominences attached to tendons or ligaments. They are usually located at the **extensor aspect of the wrist, elbows, ankles, or knees.** Microscopically, they appear like a giant Aschoff body.

Erythema marginatum: It is the classic rash of ARF. The skin lesion begins as **pink circular macules** that clear centrally, leaving a serpiginous, spreading edge. They are **nonitchy,** showing a characteristic **bathing suit pattern** of distribution. Thus, it usually occurs on the trunk, sometimes on the limbs, but almost never on the face.

Sydenham's chorea or Saint Vitus' dance: It is found mainly in females. It is a neurologic disorder with **involuntary rapid, jerky, purposeless movements of trunks and extremities** (choreiform movements). It particularly affects the head (causing characteristic rapid tongue movements) and the upper limbs.

Other organs: Rheumatic fever also may involve other organs like the lungs, pleura, and arteries.

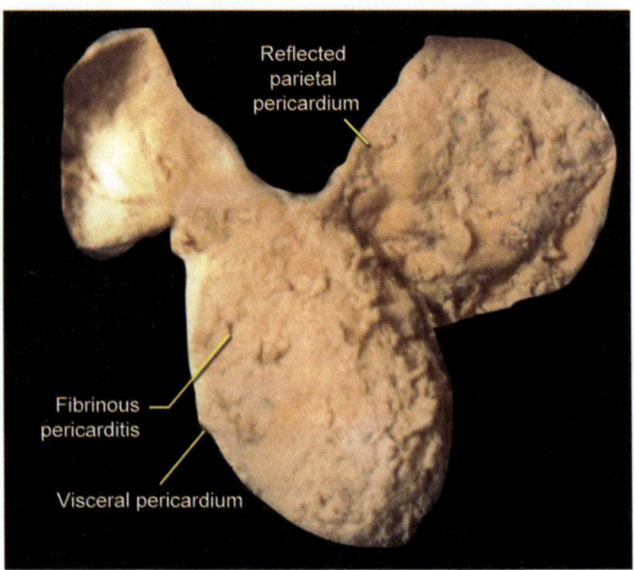

Fig. 16.20: Fibrinous pericarditis developing in rheumatic fever.

Chronic Rheumatic Heart Disease

Q. Morphology of heart in chronic rheumatic heart disease (sequelae of rheumatic fever).

The inflammation of acute rheumatic fever may subside before treatment, leaving behind damage to the heart valves. **Repeated attacks of acute rheumatic fever** cause chronic changes in the organs involved. The myocarditis and pericarditis usually resolve without any sequelae. However, the acute endocarditis, mainly the valvulitis-induced damage, is cumulative. **With each attack of rheumatic fever, the damage progresses** and often produces **long-term structural (valvular inflammation and subsequent scarring) and functional alterations of the valves.** The valvular disease mainly produces deforming fibrotic **mitral stenosis** and is the principal/key feature of chronic RHD. Rheumatic heart disease is mainly the major cause of acquired mitral stenosis. Aschoff bodies are replaced by fibrous scars and these are rare in chronic rheumatic heart disease.

MORPHOLOGY

Valves Affected

- **Mitral valve (Figs. 16.21A and B) alone:** It is the **most commonly (65–70% of cases) and severely affected** valve in chronic rheumatic disease.
- **Mitral valve along with the aortic valve** in another 25% of cases.
- **Tricuspid and pulmonary valves are rarely involved.**

Changes in the Affected Valves

The valve cusps and leaflets become permanently thickened and retracted in chronic rheumatic heart disease.

Changes in Mitral Valve **(Figs. 16.21A and B):**

- **Thickening of valve leaflet**: It is due to fibrosis following inflammation of the valve leaflets.
- **Fusion of commissures:** Healing of rheumatic lesions along the lines of closure leads to the formation of fibrous adhesions (bridging of) valvular commissures. It results in a rigid and partially fused stenotic valve.
- **Severe stenosis of a valve:** In severe chronic rheumatic mitral valve disease, the valve orifice becomes reduced to a fixed narrow opening that has the characteristic appearance of a **fish-mouth (or "buttonhole"**) when viewed from the atrial aspect **(Figs. 16.21A and B).**
- **Shortening, thickening, and fusion of the chordae tendineae.**

Consequences of mitral stenosis:

- **Left atrium progressively dilates** favor **mural thrombi** in the appendage or along the wall.
- **Thrombi can dislodge** and **embolize.**
- **Chronic venous congestion in the lungs.**
- **Pulmonary hypertension, right ventricular hypertrophy, and right-sided heart failure.** The left ventricle is normal in isolated pure mitral stenosis.
- **Clinical features**: Dyspnea and hemoptysis with rust-colored sputum (heart failure cells).

Mitral incompetence: Mitral valves may also be regurgitant. Chronic mitral regurgitation produces a "jet" of blood directed at the posterior aspect of the left atrium. This spring of backflow damages the endocardium of the left atrium. It produces focal rough, wrinkled endocardium called "MacCallum plaques or patches" (*refer* pages 505-6).

Changes in Other Valves

Aortic valve (Fig. 16.21B): This is the **second most involved valve** in rheumatic heart disease. Diffuse fibrous thickening of the cusps and fusion of the commissures cause **aortic stenosis.** The cusps may become calcified as the patient ages, resulting in **stenosis and insufficiency.**

Tricuspid valve (Fig. 16.21B): In cases of recurrent RF, the tricuspid valve may be deformed, always in association with mitral and aortic lesions.

Pulmonary valve: It is rarely affected.

Complications of Chronic Rheumatic Heart Disease

Q. Describe the complications of rheumatic heart disease.

1. **Infective endocarditis:** The **damaged valves** of rheumatic heart **disease provide a site for the deposition of bacteria.** Bacterial endocarditis follows episodes of bacteremia that occur in conditions such as during dental procedures.
2. **Mural thrombi:** They may be formed in **atrial or ventricular chambers.** Rarely, a large thrombus in the left atrial appendage may act as a ball valve and may obstruct the orifice of the mitral valve.
3. **Thromboemboli:** Mural thrombi may dislodge and form thromboemboli leading to **infarcts in various organs.**
4. **Congestive heart failure:** It is associated with the involvement of both mitral and aortic valves.
5. **Adhesive pericarditis:** It follows the fibrinous pericarditis developed during acute attack.
6. **Arrhythmias** (particularly atrial fibrillation): It is observed in mitral stenosis.

Clinical Features

Age: Rheumatic fever is usually seen in **children between 5 and 15 years of age.**

Carditis: It is the **main clinical manifestation.** The clinical signs of carditis include pericardial friction rubs, weak heart sounds, tachycardia, and arrhythmias. Myocarditis may be severe to cause cardiac dilation and produce functional mitral insufficiency and CHF.

Pulmonary artery
Aorta
Right atrium
Dilated left atrium
Stenosed mitral valve with fish-mouth appearance
A

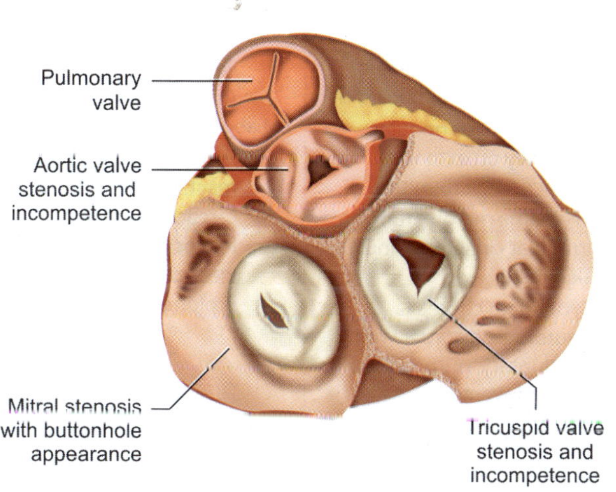

Figs. 16.21A and B: Rheumatic valvular disease viewed from the atrial surface: (A) Mitral stenosis with buttonhole deformity and dilated left atrium developed as a complication of chronic RHD; (B) Multivalvular rheumatic disease affects the mitral, tricuspid, and aortic valve (diagrammatic).

Arthritis: First attacks in adults, predominantly manifest as arthritis.

Symptoms: They begin **2–3 weeks after streptococcal infection** in all age groups. **Typical presentation: Fever and migratory polyarthritis**: one large joint after another becomes painful and swollen for days, followed by spontaneous resolution without any residual disability.

Q. Write a short note on modified Jones criteria for diagnosis of rheumatic fever.

Jones criteria: There is no specific test for RF. Presently diagnosis is based on revised Jones criteria **(Table 16.4)**.

Laboratory Findings

There is **no specific serological test** for rheumatic fever.

- **Serological tests: Pharyngeal cultures** for streptococci are **negative** by the time the illness begins. The antibodies to one or more streptococcal enzymes can be detected in the sera of most patients with RF. These include:
  - **Antistreptolysin O (ASO)**
  - **DNase B**
  - **Antihyaluronidase.**
- **Acute phase reactants**
  - **C-reactive protein (CRP) is usually present during the active stage of rheumatic fever.**
  - **Raised ESR**

Course

- **Recovery: Most acute attacks subside** within 4–6 weeks.

TABLE 16.4 Revised Jones criteria for the diagnosis of rheumatic fever

Major manifestations	*Minor manifestations*
1. Migrating polyarthritis of the large joints 2. Pancarditis (myocarditis, pericarditis, or endocarditis) 3. Subcutaneous nodules (typically on extensor surfaces of extremities) 4. Erythema marginatum (an irregular circinate/annular skin rash) 5. Sydenham chorea (a neurologic disorder with involuntary, purposeless, rapid movements)	1. Clinical (nonspecific signs and symptoms) – Fever – Arthralgias 2. Laboratory – Elevated acute-phase reactants (raised ESR, C-reactive protein, leukocytosis) – Electrocardiogram: Prolonged P-R interval

The diagnosis of acute rheumatic fever is made based on serologic evidence of previous streptococcal infection in conjunction with:

- Two or more of the *Jones criteria*
- Minor criteria can help support the diagnosis

(Formerly the criteria for diagnosis was the presence of two major manifestations, or one major and two minor manifestations)

- **Recurrence:** After an initial attack, patients are increasingly susceptible to reactivation of disease with subsequent streptococcal infections. With each recurrence, carditis is likely to worsen. Usually, the clinical evidence of chronic rheumatic carditis may be seen years or even decades after the initial attack of rheumatic fever.

Prognosis: Long-term prognosis has improved the outlook due to surgical repair or prosthetic replacement of diseased valves.

SCENARIO-BASED ESSAY QUESTION

Q. A 10-year-old child was brought to the hospital by his mother with complaints of migrating/shifting joint pain and swelling of the involved joint. On enquiry, the child had an upper respiratory tract infection (sore throat) and fever 3 weeks back. On examination, a subcutaneous nodule was found on the extensor aspect of the right elbow. On auscultation, the heart sounds were weak with tachycardia.

a. **What is your probable diagnosis? (Answer: Rheumatic fever with rheumatic heart disease)**
b. **Discuss the etiopathogenesis of the condition** *(refer pages 503-4)*.
c. **Describe the morphological features of the main organ involved in this disease** *(refer pages 504-6)*.
d. **List the complications of this condition** *(refer page 507)*.

ISCHEMIC HEART DISEASE

PA 27.5a (CC): Describe the epidemiology, risk factors, etiology, pathophysiology, pathology, presentations, gross and microscopic features, diagnostic tests, and complications of ischemic heart disease.

Definition: Ischemic heart disease (IHD) is a broad term for a group of **closely-related distinct diseases resulting from ischemia of the myocardium.** Myocardial ischemia **occurs due to an imbalance between the blood supply to** a portion of **the myocardium** (perfusion) **and the demand for oxygen and nutrition.**

Ischemic heart disease is the most common and single largest cause of mortality.

Myocardial ischemia: Ischemia is the inadequate blood supply to a tissue or organ. The heart is an aerobic organ. The cardiac myocytes (myocardium) produce adenosine triphosphate (ATP provides energy) almost exclusively through mitochondrial oxidative phosphorylation. ATP is essential for myocardial contraction and myocardial cells cannot store much energy in the form of ATP. **The myocardium (cardiac muscle) cannot be sustained without oxygen**. Hence, **cardiac function depends on the continuous flow of oxygenated blood through the coronary arteries for the aerobic synthesis of ATP**. Ischemia reduces the tissue's oxygen supply, thereby decreasing the production of ATP. Ischemia also reduces the supply of nutrients and removes metabolic wastes from the involved tissue.

Consequences of myocardial ischemia: The consequences of myocardial ischemia are as follows:

1. **Angina pectoris:**
   - **Stable angina**: It develops due to an increased demand for oxygen by the myocardium that exceeds the ability of coronary arteries with fixed (pre-existing) stenoses to increase oxygen delivery. Usually, it is not associated with plaque disruption.
   - **Unstable angina**: It is caused by acute plaque change associated with thrombosis and/or vasoconstriction. It leads to incomplete or transient reductions in coronary blood flow.
2. **Myocardial infarction**: It usually results from the acute plaque change that causes sudden thrombotic occlusion of the coronary lumen. The severity or duration of ischemia is sufficient to cause death of myocardial fibers.
3. **Chronic IHD with CHF:** This is characterized by progressive cardiac decompensation. It occurs after acute MI or secondary to the multiple ischemic episodes, that leads to mechanical pump failure.
4. **Sudden cardiac death**: It may be due to regional myocardial ischemia that produces ventricular arrhythmia. It may be the result of fixed stenosis or acute plaque change.

The list of diseases included under ischemic heart disease is presented in **Box 16.8**.

Acute coronary syndrome: It is a term used for any of the three catastrophic manifestations of IHD: (i) unstable angina, (ii) myocardial infarction (MI), and (iii) sudden cardiac death (SCD).

Etiology

Ischemic heart disease is caused by an imbalance between the demand and supply of oxygenated blood to the myocardium.

Inadequate (Impaired) Coronary Blood Flow

Coronary arterial occlusion is the main cause of myocardial ischemia.

Coronary atherosclerosis: Coronary arteries are small muscular arteries with a prominent internal elastic lamina and they deliver blood to the myocardium. In >90% of patients, reduced blood flow to the myocardium is due to **obstructive (occlusive) atherosclerotic lesions in the epicardial coronary arteries.** Atherosclerosis narrows one or more of the epicardial coronary arteries and reduces the coronary blood flow. Hence, IHD is **often called coronary artery disease (CAD)** or **coronary heart disease.**

BOX 16.8: List of ischemic heart diseases.

1. Angina pectoris (ischemia is less severe to cause frank necrosis)
   - Stable angina
   - Prinzmetal or variant angina
   - Unstable angina*
2. Myocardial infarction (ischemia causes the necrosis of heart muscle)*
3. Chronic IHD with heart failure
4. Sudden cardiac death due to fatal ventricular arrhythmia*

*These are fatal manifestations of IHD and are termed acute coronary syndrome.

BOX 16.9: Causes of ischemic heart disease.

1. Inadequate (Impaired) Coronary Blood Flow

Atherosclerosis of coronary arteries *(more than 90% of cases)*

Nonatheromatous causes

- Coronary emboli
- Coronary vasospasm
- Diminished blood volume, e.g., hypotension, shock
- Diminished blood oxygenation, e.g., pneumonia, congestive heart failure
- Diminished blood oxygen-carrying capacity, e.g., anemia, carbon monoxide poisoning
- Others: Arteritis (e.g., periarteritis nodosa), aortic dissection aneurysm, syphilitic aortitis, anomalous origin of coronary artery

2. Increased Myocardial Demand

- Increased heart rate (tachycardia)
- Hypertension
- Myocardial hypertrophy
- Hyperthyroidism

Other causes of coronary artery occlusion (non-atheromatous causes): In about 10% of cases, MI occurs without atherosclerosis of the coronary vessels. These causes are listed in **Box 16.9.**

Increased Myocardial Demand

It occurs with **myocardial hypertrophy**, increased heart rate (**tachycardia**), **increased physical activity, emotional stress,** etc.

Pathogenesis of Ischemic Heart Disease

IHD develops due to inadequate coronary perfusion relative to myocardial demand. In most patients, it is due to coronary atherosclerosis. In most patients, IHD is due to either or both mechanisms, namely (1) chronic vascular occlusion and (2) acute plaque change.

Chronic Vascular Occlusion

Preexisting ("fixed") atherosclerotic occlusion of the coronary arteries: The epicardial coronary arteries can narrow due to chronic, progressive atherosclerosis. The following features are involved in coronary artery disease.

Degree (Extent) and Severity of Atherosclerotic Occlusion

Atherosclerosis reduces the lumen of the coronary arteries, and **abnormal narrowing of the lumen is called stenosis.**

The degree of coronary lumen **obstruction of preexisting ("fixed") atherosclerotic lesions** is important in IHD.

- **Fixed obstructions less than 70%:** It is usually **asymptomatic**, even with exertion.
- **Fixed obstruction of more than 70% (critical stenosis):** A fixed (preexisting) atherosclerotic lesion in coronary arteries reducing more than **70% of vascular cross-sectional area** is called "**critical stenosis.**" It is considered the threshold for symptomatic **ischemia precipitated by exercise** (i.e., increased demand). It characteristically manifests as chest pain with certain levels of exertion. The patient is said to have **exertional (stable) angina.** With this degree of obstruction, compensatory coronary arterial vasodilation is no longer sufficient to meet even moderate increases in myocardial demand.
- **Fixed obstruction of 90% and above: Obstruction of 90% of the cross-sectional area** of the coronary lumen usually leads to **inadequate coronary blood flow**, with symptoms **even at rest**. Any further, even a minimal decrease in the stenotic orifice will dramatically reduce coronary flow and cause myocardial ischemia at rest or with minimal stress. This is one of the forms of **unstable angina.**

Number of Coronaries Affected

Blood supply to the heart is through three major coronary epicardial arteries, namely (1) the left anterior descending (LAD), (2) the left circumflex (LCX), and (3) the right coronary artery (RCA). The narrowing may involve a **single, two, or all three major coronary epicardial arteries.** In >90% of cases with IHD, **atherosclerosis** involves **one or two or all epicardial coronary arteries.**

Number and Location of Atheromatous Plaque in Coronaries

Clinically significant **atherosclerotic plaques predominately** occur within the **first several centimeters of the LAD and LCX** at the site of origin from the aorta and along the entire length of the RCA.

Rate of Development of Occlusion

Normal coronary arteries act as end arteries. If **obstruction of the coronary lumen occurs slowly** over years, it allows time for the **formation of collateral circulation** to **prevent infarction.** These collaterals enable alternate channels to perfuse myocardium at risk even with high-grade stenosis. These can protect against MI, even if the original vessel becomes completely occluded. In **acute** coronary **blockage, there is no time for collateral flow** to develop**, and it may cause infarction.**

Structure of Atheromatous Plaque

Plaques can be divided into stable and vulnerable (unstable) plaques.

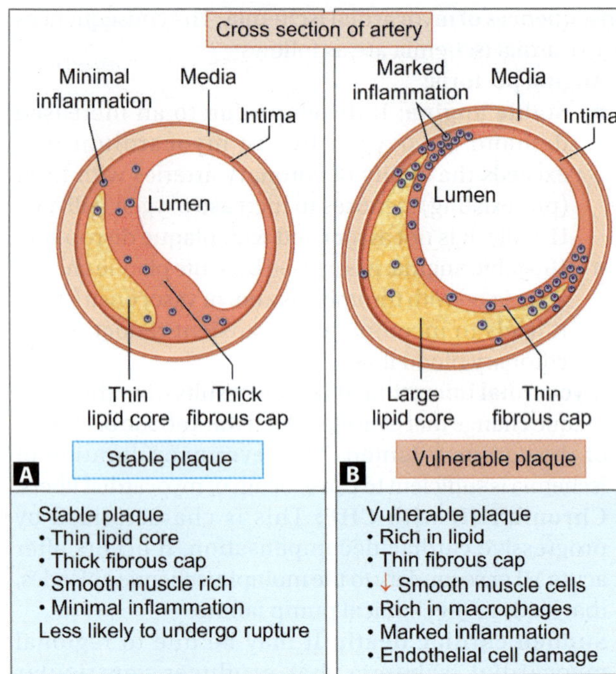

Figs. 16.22A and B: Diagrammatic appearance of stable and vulnerable atherosclerotic plaque: (A) Stable plaques have thick, dense collagenous fibrous caps with minimal inflammation and an underlying lipid core; (B) Vulnerable plaques have thin fibrous caps, large central lipid cores, and increased inflammation.

- **Stable plaques (Fig. 16.22A):** They have **dense collagenous and thick fibrous caps** with **minimal inflammation** and **negligible underlying atheromatous necrotic core.** These are **less likely to undergo rupture.**
- **Vulnerable plaque (Fig. 16.22B):** They have a **large atheromatous core with many foam cells** and **abundant extracellular lipids.** The overlying **fibrous cap is thin** with few smooth muscle cells or groups of inflammatory cells and **increased inflammation.** These are **likely to undergo rupture.** Collagen is produced by smooth muscle cells and degraded by the metalloproteases secreted by macrophages. Therefore, atherosclerotic plaques with a reduced number of smooth muscle cells or large numbers of inflammatory cells are susceptible to rupture.

Vasoconstriction

It can reduce the diameter of the coronary lumen, and also increase the local mechanical shear forces, and can disrupt the plaque. Vasoconstriction in atherosclerotic plaques can be due to (i) circulating adrenergic agonists, (ii) locally released platelet contents, (iii) imbalance between relaxing factors (e.g., nitric oxide) and contracting factors (e.g., endothelin) in the endothelial cell, and (iv) mediators released from perivascular inflammatory cells.

Acute Plaque Change (Fig. 16.23)

The risk of developing IHD depends partly on the number, distribution, structure, and degree of obstruction by atheromatous plaques. However, these factors and fixed stenosis cannot be the sole mechanism of IHD. In such situations, IHD is associated with acute plaque changes. **Acute plaque changes with superimposed thrombosis and/or vasospasm** may produce IHD.

Acute plaque change: It is the sudden morphologic **change (event) occurring in an atheromatous plaque. Acute plaque change occurs, especially in acute coronary syndromes** (unstable angina, myocardial infarction, and sudden cardiac death). **The term acute coronary syndrome** is used for a range of **conditions associated with sudden, reduced blood flow to the heart.**

Nature of acute plaque changes: These **acute plaque changes convert partially occlusive** atherosclerotic **plaque to produce sudden ischemia.** Acute plaque changes are divided into:

1. **Rupture, superficial erosion, ulceration, fissuring of plaque:** They expose highly thrombogenic subendothelial basement membrane favoring sudden **thrombus formation leading to sudden occlusion of the lumen.** Mural thrombi can also embolize. Fissures usually occur at the junction of the fibrous cap and the adjacent normal (plaque-free) arterial segment. In this region, the mechanical stresses are highest and the fibrous cap is thinnest.
2. **Deep hemorrhage into the central core of atheromatous plaque:** It increases the plaque size and may cause sudden **occlusion of the lumen.**

Factors that trigger acute plaque change: These may be intrinsic or extrinsic factors.

- **Intrinsic:** Plaque composition and structure (namely **vulnerable plaque**).
- **Extrinsic:** Blood pressure and platelet reactivity which induces total thrombotic occlusion of already narrowed coronary artery by atheromatous plaque.

Angina Pectoris

Definition: Angina pectoris (literally, "chest pain") clinically present as **paroxysmal** and **recurrent attacks of substernal or precordial chest discomfort or pain.** It is due to **transient** (15 seconds to 15 minutes), **reversible myocardial ischemia** that is insufficient to cause necrosis of myocardial cells.

Variants of Angina Pectoris

Angina is a consequence of the ischemia-induced release of adenosine, bradykinin, and other molecules. These molecules stimulate autonomic nerves. Three variants are (i) stable, (ii) Prinzmetal angina (vasospastic or variant angina), or (iii) unstable angina.

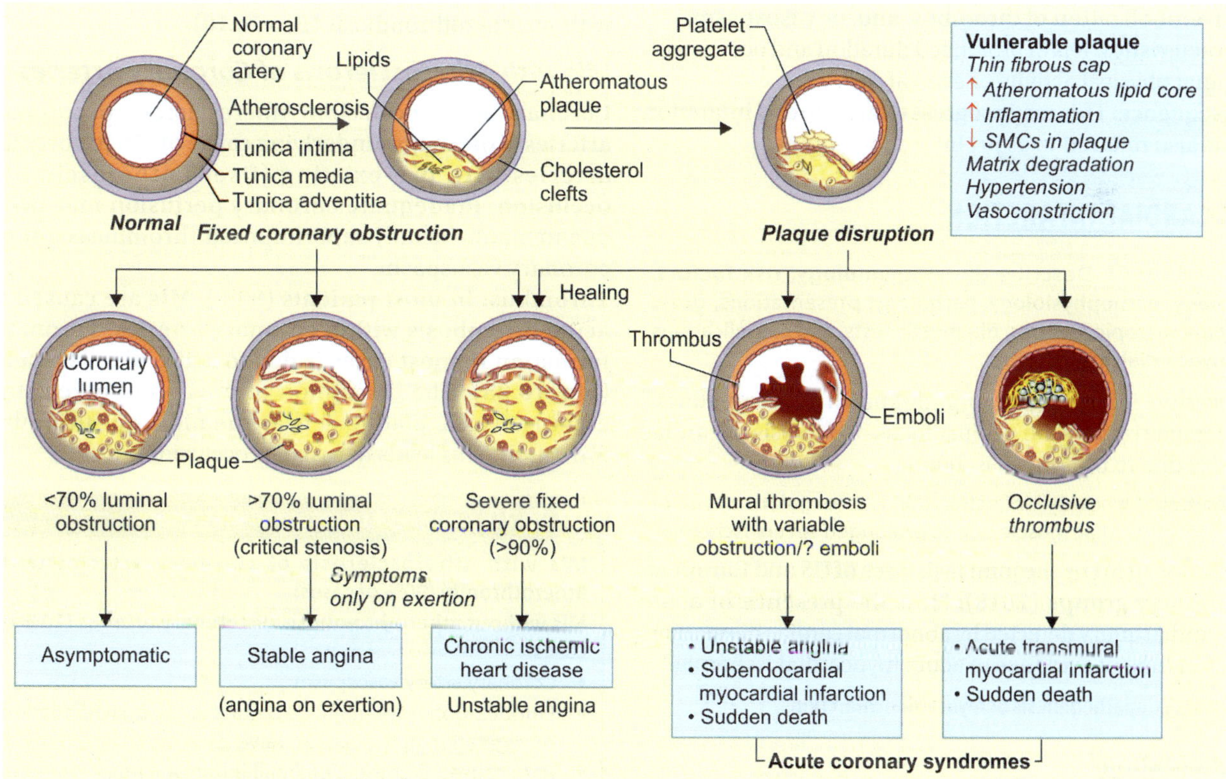

Fig. 16.23: Sequential changes in coronary artery atherosclerosis causing occlusion of the lumen in ischemic heart disease and leading to various acute coronary syndromes.

Typical or Stable Angina

It is the **most common form**. The characteristics of discomfort are as follows:

- **Site:** The discomfort is **crushing or squeezing substernal sensation**. It **may radiate** down the left arm, the left jaw, and the epigastrium (referred pain).
- **Duration:** It ranges from **1–15 minutes**.
- **Nature: Pain is relieved by rest** (which decreases demand) or **by sublingual nitroglycerin**, a strong vasodilator (which increases perfusion).

Cause: Coronary atherosclerosis is the cause and occurs with certain levels of exertion. It develops when myocardial oxygen demand increases due to **increased physical activity or emotional excitement**.

Prinzmetal or Variant Angina

It is an **uncommon atypical form** of angina.

Cause: It can be caused by to **spasm of a coronary artery having atherosclerosis** (vasospastic angina). It is **not related to physical activity, heart rate, or blood pressure.**

Characteristics: It **occurs at rest** and responds promptly to vasodilators such as nitroglycerin and calcium channel blockers.

Unstable or Crescendo Angina

Cause: It is caused by the plaque **disruption (rupture) of an atherosclerotic plaque** complicated by **thrombosis or distal embolization of thrombus, and/or vasospasm.**

Characteristics: It is of prolonged duration and occurs with minimal physical activity or even at rest.

Consequence: This may progress to myocardial infarction and is also referred to as **preinfarction angina.**

MYOCARDIAL INFARCTION

PA 27.5b (CC): Describe the epidemiology, risk factors, etiology, pathophysiology, pathology, presentations, gross and microscopic features, diagnostic tests, and complications of myocardial infarction.

Myocardial infarction, commonly known as "heart attack," is characterized by the distinct focus of necrosis of cardiac muscle due to prolonged ischemia.

Definition: Myocardial infarction (MI) is a **coagulative type of necrosis of cardiac muscle due to prolonged severe ischemia.**

Definition of MI by the joint task force of US and European Cardiology groups (2018): "It is the presence of acute myocardial injury detected by abnormal cardiac biomarkers in the setting of evidence of acute myocardial ischemia."

Q. Discuss etiopathogenesis of myocardial infarction.

Epidemiology

Following are the **risk factors involved in the development of ischemic heart disease including MI.**

Race: Any race can be affected by MI. Whites are affected more than Blacks. Indians also have a high risk of IHD.

Age: Myocardial infarctions (MIs) can occur at **any age**. About 10% of MIs develop in individuals under 40 years of age, and **45% occur in people below 65 years of age**. Its frequency rises progressively with increasing age. It can develop at a younger age in patients with increasing major risk factors of atherosclerosis (hyperlipidemia, hypertension, diabetes, and cigarette smoking).

Gender: Middle-aged males have a significantly higher risk than females in the same age group. Females are usually protected against the occurrence of MI during their reproductive period. However, **after menopause**, there is a decline in estrogen production, and the risk of MI is **similar to that of males**. The protective effect may be due to estrogen.

Risk factors of atherosclerosis: The major underlying cause of IHD is atherosclerosis of coronaries. Refer to risk factors for atherosclerosis (*refer* pages 480-2).

Other risk factors: These include **obesity, family history, use of oral contraceptives, sedentary life, and type A" personality** (aggressive, time-conscious, executive-type individuals).

Etiology

The etiology of MI is the same as that of ischemic heart disease (*refer* pages 509-11 and **Box 16. 9** above). It may be broadly divided into MI with atherothrombosis and MI without atherothrombosis **(Box 16.10)**.

MIs with Atherosclerosis of Coronary Arteries

Coronary artery occlusion: Atherosclerosis of coronary arteries is the major underlying cause of MI. In **coronary arteries with pre-existing (fixed) atherosclerotic occlusion, inadequate coronary perfusion** may occur due to a **new (acute) superimposed thrombosis and/or coronary vasospasm.**

Thrombus: In **most patients (90%), MIs are caused by acute thrombosis within coronary arteries. Thrombus formation in most cases is due to acute plaque change (Fig. 16.23).** The disruption or erosion of preexisting atherosclerotic plaque acts as the nidus for thrombus formation. This leads to vascular occlusion.

BOX 16.10: Causes of myocardial infarctions

MIs with atherosclerosis of coronary arteries with atherothrombi (90% of cases)

MIs without atherothrombosis of coronary arteries (10% of cases)

- Coronary artery vasospasm
- Embolization from mural thrombi (e.g., in atrial fibrillation) or vegetation in the cardiac valve
- Rare causes: Disorders of small intramyocardial arterioles, e.g., vasculitis, amyloid deposition, or stasis, as in sickle cell disease.

Increased myocardial demand: Occasionally, in infarcts limited to the innermost (subendocardial) myocardium, thrombi or emboli are not present. In these patients, severe fixed coronary atherosclerosis leads to marginal perfusion of the heart. The endomyocardium of the heart is most distal to the epicardial vessels. Therefore, a prolonged period of increased demand by the myocardium (e.g., due to tachycardia or hypertension) can cause ischemic necrosis of the endomyocardium.

MIs without Atherothrombosis

In **10% of MIs**, transmural infarction occurs in the absence of occlusive atherosclerotic vascular disease. These infarcts mostly occur due to **coronary artery vasospasm or embolization from mural thrombi** (e.g., in the setting of atrial fibrillation) **or vegetation in the cardiac valve.**

Rare causes: Myocardial ischemia without detectable atherosclerosis or thromboembolic disease may be due to disorders of small intramyocardial arterioles (e.g., vasculitis, amyloid deposition, or stasis, as in sickle cell disease).

Pathogenesis of MI

Coronary Artery Occlusion

In coronary arteries with preexisting (fixed) atherosclerotic occlusion, inadequate coronary perfusion may occur due to a new superimposed thrombosis and/or coronary vasospasm. In most patients, MIs are caused by acute thrombosis within coronary arteries.

The sequence of events in most MIs with atherothrombosis (Flowchart 16.3): These are as follows:

1. **Erosion or sudden disruption of an atheromatous plaque:** An atheromatous plaque is eroded or suddenly disrupted by endothelial injury, intraplaque hemorrhage, or mechanical forces (*refer* **acute plaque change on pages 486 above). Acute plaque change: It is the sudden change/event occurring in an atheromatous plaque (*refer* page 486).** The erosion or disruption of plaque exposes subendothelial collagen and necrotic plaque contents to the blood.
2. **Activation of platelets and formation of microthrombi:** At the site of exposure of subendothelial collagen, circulating platelets passing by the surface of the ruptured plaque adhere, aggregate, and get activated. These activated platelets release thromboxane A_2, adenosine diphosphate (ADP), and serotonin. The released molecules cause further aggregation of platelets and vasospasm. Thus, the process of formation of microthrombi begins on the atheromatous plaque.
3. **Activation of coagulation pathway:** Release of tissue factor and other mechanisms activate the coagulation system. This further favors the growth of the thrombus and increases its size.
4. **Complete occlusion of coronary lumen:** Within minutes, the thrombus can progress and completely occlude the lumen of the coronary artery. Thrombosis develops suddenly and may partially or completely obstruct the artery and cause acute ischemia. Thus, the formation of a thrombus plays an important role in coronary obstruction, and this is the basis of the prophylactic use of antithrombotics, such as aspirin. Studies indicate that the long-term use of small doses of aspirin reduces mortality from IHD.

Flowchart 16.3: Pathogenies of MI with coronary atherosclerosis.

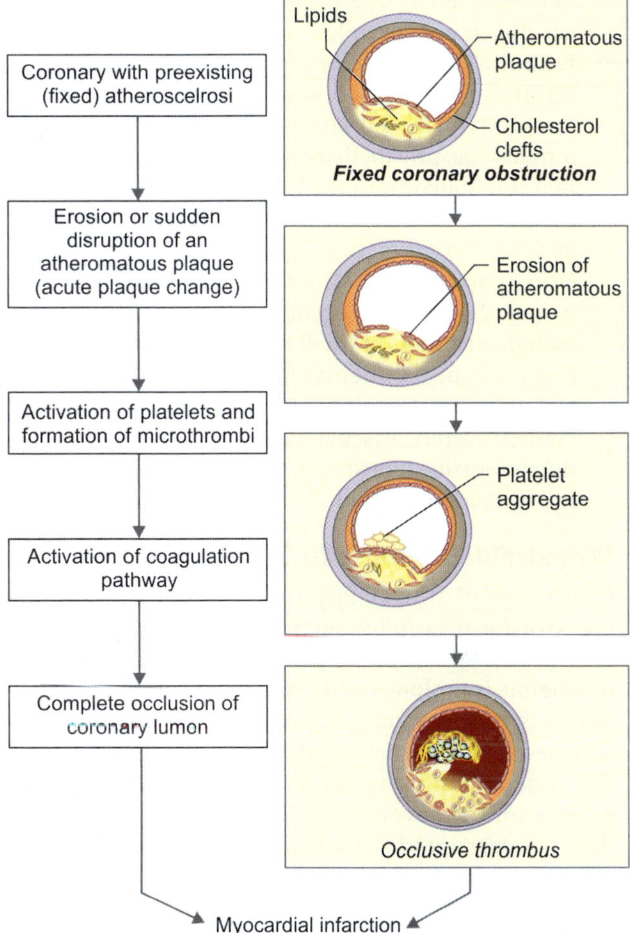

5. **Myocardial necrosis:** Complete occlusion results in **ischemic coagulative necrosis of the area supplied** by the coronary artery. The anatomic area supplied by that artery is called the area at risk.

The sequence of events in a few MIs without athero-thrombosis: In about 10% of patients, MI (transmural infarction) can also occur without coronary atherosclerosis. In such cases, other mechanisms may be involved in reducing the blood flow in coronary arteries. These are as follows:

- **Vasospasm:** It may occur in coronary arteries with or without atherosclerosis, probably associated with platelet aggregation. Activated platelets (release vasoactive products such as serotonin and thromboxane), endothelial cells, and inflammatory cells release mediators and cause vasospasm. Vasospasms may also occur due to the ingestion of drugs (e.g., cocaine or ephedrine).

- **Emboli:** The source of emboli may be from the left atrium in association with atrial fibrillation, mural thrombus on the left side of the heart, vegetations of IE, intracardiac prosthetic material, or paradoxical emboli that originated from the right side of the heart or the peripheral veins passed through a patent foramen ovale and into the coronary arteries.
- **Other rare causes:** MI without atherothrombosis of coronary arteries can occur in several conditions. These include disorders of small intramural coronary arteries (e.g., vasculitis), hematologic diseases (e.g., sickle cell disease), deposition of amyloid in the wall of the coronary artery, vascular dissection, marked LVH (e.g., due to aortic stenosis), or lowered systemic BP (e.g., hypotension in shock).

Myocardial Response to Ischemia

Obstruction of the coronary artery reduces blood flow to a region of the myocardium supplied by that particular vessel. It causes ischemia and rapid myocardial dysfunction, and if ischemia is prolonged, ultimately, it leads to coagulative necrosis of the involved myocyte. The anatomic area supplied by the particular artery is called the area at risk. The outcome of ischemia in the myocardium depends mainly on the severity and length of time that blood flow is interrupted. It also depends on the availability and adequacy of collateral blood flow and the relative workload. These myocardial responses include **functional, biochemical, and morphological changes**. Myocardial response to ischemia can be divided into reversible and irreversible damage/injury.

Reversible Injury

These changes are potentially reversible and include the following:

Biochemical changes: The early biochemical change that occurs in myocardial ischemia is the stopping **of aerobic metabolism** within seconds. This leads to **decreased production of** ATP (adenosine triphosphate) and accumulation of toxic metabolites [e.g., lactic acid (lactate)].

Functional disturbances: Myocardial function depends on the supply of oxygen and nutrients. Within a minute (<2 minutes) or so of the onset of severe ischemia, there is a loss of myocardial contractility (diminished systolic contraction). It can precipitate acute heart failure.

Morphological changes: These are seen at the ultrastructural level and include myofibrillar relaxation, depletion of glycogen, and swelling of cells and mitochondria. They also develop within a few minutes. These early changes of ischemic injury are probably reversible, but if ischemia persists for 20–40 minutes, it leads to irreversible damage and coagulative necrosis of myocytes. Hence, rapid diagnosis in acute MI and early coronary intervention is necessary to establish reperfusion and restore as much "at risk" myocardium within this period.

Irreversible Injury

Irreversible injury to myocytes develops only after prolonged, severe myocardial ischemia of more than 20–40 minutes.

Biochemical changes: The earliest change is the **leakage of intracellular macromolecules out of necrotic cells** into the blood. These macromolecules include **myoglobin, lactate dehydrogenase (LDH), creatine kinase (CK), and troponins I and T.** The leakage of these intracellular myocardial proteins into the circulation is utilized as a sensitive, early biochemical marker for the diagnosis of irreversible damage to myocytes as well as the management of MI.

Functional disturbances: It can produce arrhythmias. Arrhythmia is an irregular heartbeat (loss of rhythm).

Morphological changes: Coagulative necrosis of cardiac muscle fibers is usually complete within 6 hours of the onset of myocardial ischemia. An infarct fully develops in 3–6 hours. Irreversible injury of ischemic myocytes first begins in the subendocardial zone. The progression of ischemic necrosis in the myocardium is summarized in **Figure 16.24**.

Classification of Myocardial Infarct

Q. Classify myocardial infarction.

A. **Depending on the thickness of the myocardium involved: Based on the size of the involved** vessel and the degree of collateral circulation, myocardial infarcts may show one of the following patterns:
   - **Transmural infarct:** Most myocardial infarcts are transmural (**1 to 3 in Fig. 16.25**).
     - **Involves full thickness of myocardium:** It is the **ischemic necrosis of the entire (full) thickness of the ventricular wall**. However, a narrow rim (approximately 0.1 mm) of the viable subendocardial myocardium is preserved due to diffusion of oxygen and nutrients from the ventricular lumen. and **infarction of the atria is rare.**
     - **Cause:** Usually caused by occlusion of epicardial vessels due to **chronic coronary atherosclerosis**, and **acute plaque change**, with **superimposed occlusive thrombosis.**
   - **Subendocardial (nontransmural) infarct (4 to 6 in Fig. 16.25).**
     - **Involves the inner one-third of the myocardium:** In this, ischemic necrosis is limited to the **inner one-third of the myocardium.**
     - **Cause:** It occurs due to **plaque disruption** followed by a **coronary thrombus that is lysed** spontaneously or therapeutically before the necrosis becomes transmural. The subendocardial

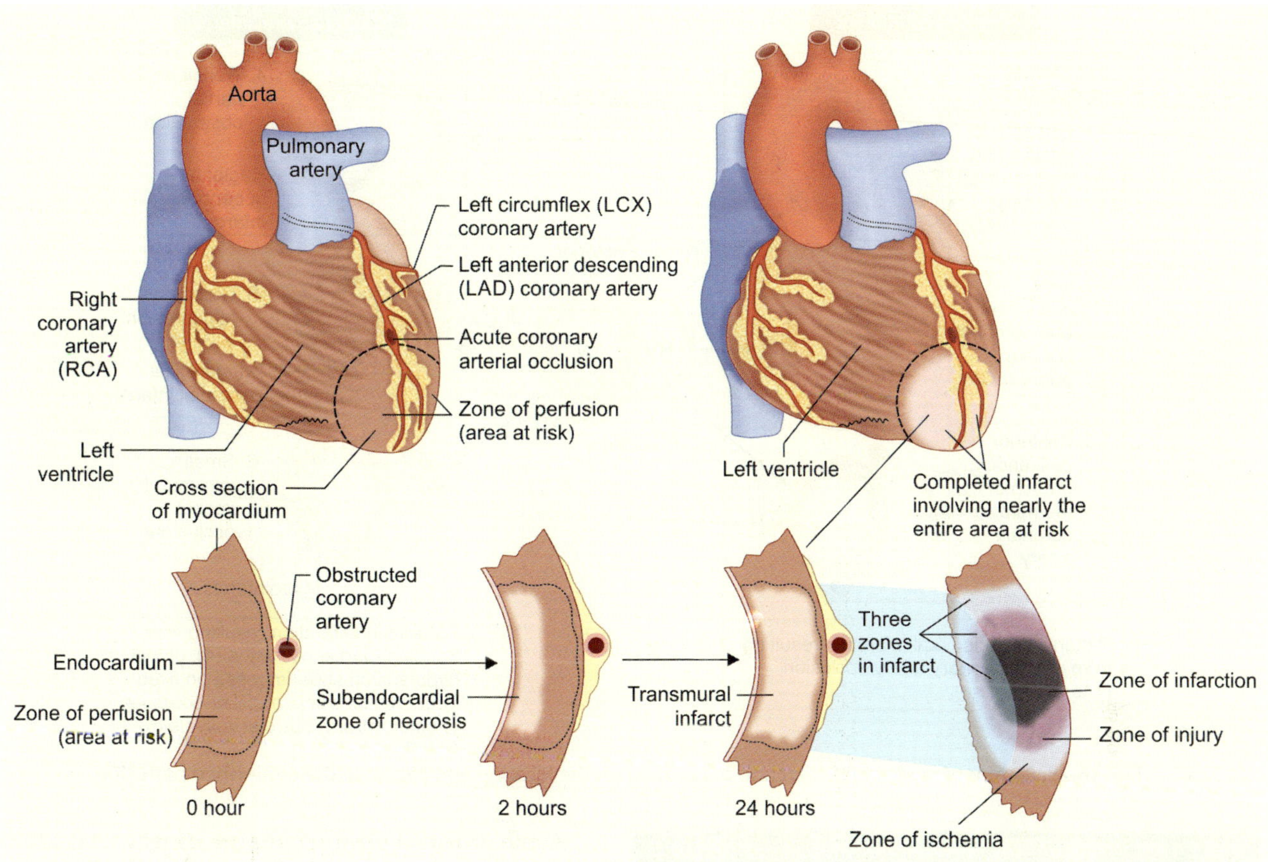

Fig. 16.24: Schematic representation of the progression of myocardial necrosis following occlusion of coronary artery (in this left anterior descending branch is depicted with occlusion. The area of the occluded vessel "at risk" myocardium is shaded). Necrosis begins in a small subendocardial zone of the myocardium. A very narrow zone of myocardium immediately below the endocardium is spared from necrosis because it can obtain oxygen and nutrition by diffusion from the ventricle. There are three zones at the area at risk, namely the central zone of infarction (which shows both coagulative necrosis and apoptosis), the middle zone of injury, and an outer zone of ischemia (reversibly injured cells that are marginally perfused by collaterals).

region is most susceptible to hypoperfusion and hypoxia. Thus, when there is severe coronary artery disease, transient reduction in oxygen delivery (as from hypotension with severe reduction in systemic blood pressure, anemia, or pneumonia) or increases in oxygen demand (as with tachycardia or hypertension) can cause subendocardial ischemic injury.

- **Microscopic infarcts**
  - **Cause:** They develop with the occlusion of small vessels. They may occur in conditions such as vasculitis, embolization of vegetations from cardiac valve or mural thrombi, or spasm of the vessel due to raised catecholamines (e.g., during extreme emotional stress, tumors such as pheochromocytoma).

B. **Depending on the age of the infarct:** Infarct may be classified as recent (fresh) or old (healed).

C. **Depending on the anatomic region involved:** Infarct may be classified as anterior, posterior, lateral, septal, and their combination like posterolateral.

D. **Depending on the electrocardiographic changes:**
- **ST elevated myocardial infarct (STEMI)** found in the transmural infarct. ECG may have negative Q waves with loss of R wave amplitude.
- **Non-ST elevated myocardial infarct (NSTEMI)** found in subendocardial infarct.
- **Electrocardiographically silent** with nonspecific changes in **microinfarctions** (depending on the extent and location of the vascular involvement).

Differences between transmural and subendocardial infarcts are listed in **Table 16.5**.

Patterns of Infarction (Fig. 16.25)

The location, size, and morphologic features of an acute myocardial infarct depend on factors such as (i) size and distribution of the involved coronary artery, (ii) rate of development and duration of the coronary occlusion, (iii) metabolic demands of the affected myocardium (e.g., blood pressure and heart rate) and (iv) extent of collateral blood supply.

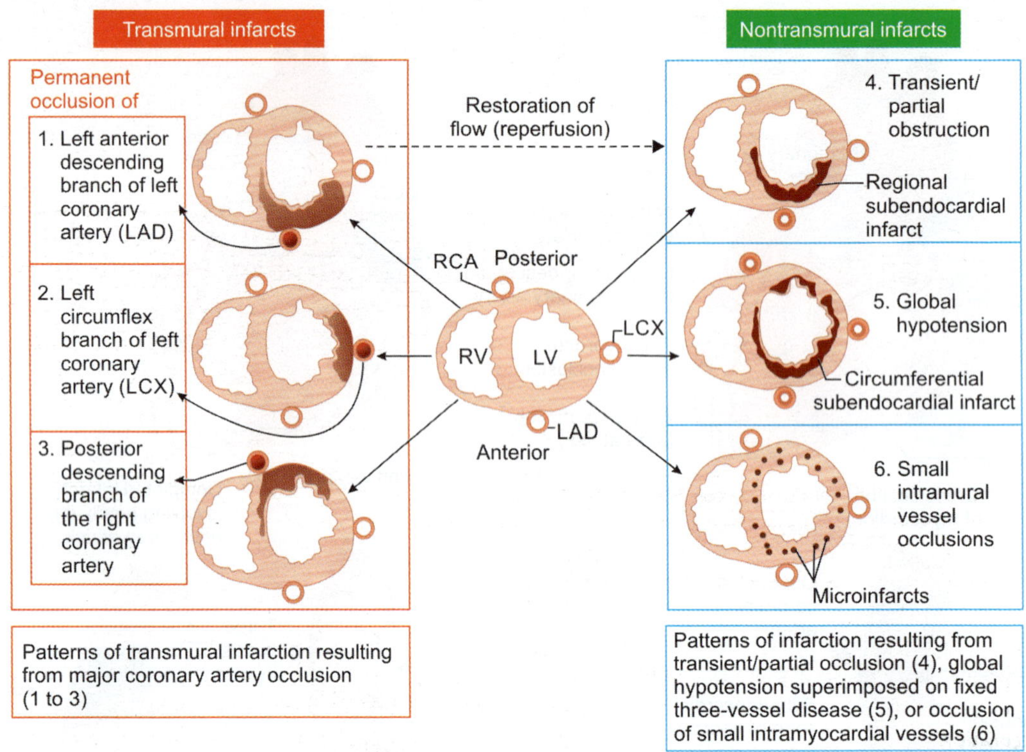

Fig. 16.25: Pattern of myocardial infarction depending on the location and nature of the diminished perfusion.

TABLE 16.5 Differences between transmural and subendocardial infarct.

Characteristics	*Transmural infarcts*	*Subendocardial infarcts*
Nature of lesion	Unifocal and solid	Multifocal and patchy
Distribution	Specific coronary artery	Circumferential
Thrombus in the coronary artery	Common	Rare
Shock	Often causes shock	Often results from hypotension or shock
Pericarditis	Common	Absent
Cardiac aneurysm	May develop	Does not develop
Electrocardiography changes	Elevation of ST segment® ST elevation myocardial infarcts (STEMIs)	Non-ST elevation myocardial infarcts

Acute occlusion of the proximal left anterior descending (LAD) artery: It is seen in 40–50% of all MIs. Regions affected by infarct are:

- **Anterior wall of the left ventricle**
- **Anterior two-thirds of the ventricular septum**
- **Most of the heart apex.**

Acute proximal obstructions are usually fatal whereas more distal occlusion may produce infarction of only the apex.

Acute occlusion of the proximal left circumflex (LCX) artery: The occlusion of the proximal LCX occurs in 15–20% of MIs. Regions affected by infarct are:

- **Lateral wall of the left ventricle**

Proximal right coronary artery (RCA) occlusion: It is responsible for 30–40% of MIs. Regions affected by infarct are:

- **Much of the right ventricle.**

Posterior descending artery occlusion: The posterior descending artery can arise from either the RCA (in 90% of individuals) or the LCX. Regions affected by infarct are:

- **Posterior third of the interventricular septum and the posterior left ventricle.**

Atherosclerosis mainly affects epicardial vessels. Though significant atherosclerosis or thrombosis of penetrating intramyocardial branches of coronary arteries is rare, they may be affected by vasculitis, vasospasm, or embolization.

MORPHOLOGY

Q. Describe the morphology/sequential changes seen in myocardial infarction.

General features:

Region affected

Left ventricle and interventricular septum: Most transmural infarcts (involve 50% or more of the ventricle) affect at **least a portion of the left ventricle** and/or **interventricular septum.**

TABLE 16.6	Sequence of morphologic changes in myocardial infarction.	
Duration	*Gross changes*	*Light microscopic changes*
Reversible injury		
0–½ hour	None	None (electron microscope—relaxation of myofibrils; loss of glycogen and swelling of mitochondria)
Irreversible injury		
½–4 hours	None	Usually, no changes but may show waviness of fibers at the border (electron microscopy: mitochondrial amorphous densities)
4–12 hours	Occasionally dark mottling	Early coagulative necrosis
12–24 hours	Dark mottling	Coagulative necrosis; pyknotic nuclei; increased eosinophilia of cytoplasm; contraction band necrosis at margins; beginning of neutrophilic infiltrate
1–3 days	Mottling with yellow-tan center	Coagulation necrosis, loss of nuclei and striations; increased interstitial infiltration of neutrophils
3–7 days	Hyperemic border; central yellow-tan	The disintegration of dead myocardial cells, with disintegrating neutrophils; phagocytosis of dead cells by macrophages at the border of the infarct
7–10 days	Maximally yellow-tan and soft	Phagocytosis of dead cells; formation of granulation tissue at margins
10–14 days	Red-gray depressed infarct borders	Well-established granulation tissue and collagen deposition
2–8 weeks	Gray-white scar, progressive from the border toward the center of the infarct	Increased collagen deposition and decreased cellularity
>2 months	Scarring complete	Dense collagenous scar tissue

Right ventricle: About 15–30% of MI, that **involve the posterior or posteroseptal wall also extends to involve the right ventricle.**
Isolated infarction of the right ventricle: It occurs only in 1 to 3% of cases.

Almost all transmural infarcts involve at least a portion of the left ventricle (free wall of the ventricle and ventricular septum). A narrow rim (about 0.1 mm) of viable subendocardial myocardium is preserved by diffusion of oxygen and nutrients from the ventricular lumen. The frequencies of involvement of each of the three main coronary arterial trunks and the sites of myocardial lesions are discussed on pages 514-6 above and depicted in **Figure 16.25.**

The gross and microscopic appearance of a myocardial infarct depends on the time between the development of a myocardial infarct and death. The affected myocardium undergoes a progressive sequence of morphologic changes of ischemic coagulative necrosis. This is followed by inflammation and repair that is similar to responses to injury in other tissues. Myocardial necrosis forms scars without any significant regeneration of myocardial fibers.

Gross (Table 16.6)

Q. Describe the morphological changes occurring in myocardial infarction.

Myocardial infarcts less than 12 hours old: They do not show any identifiable/apparent gross changes.

- **Triphenyl tetrazolium chloride:** Infarcts more than 3 hours old can be visualized by **vital histochemical stains,** such as triphenyl tetrazolium chloride. Lactate dehydrogenase (LDH) is an enzyme that leaks out of damaged myocardial cells in the area of ischemic necrosis.
  - **Infarcted areas unstained:** When the affected myocardium is exposed to this stain, the **infarcted area is unstained (pale) due to loss of LDH.**
  - **Noninfarcted myocardium appears brick-red:** Healthy myocardium with preserved LDH activity stains brown-red color.
  - **Old scars of infarcts appear white and glistening.**

By 12–24 hours (Fig. 16.26): Infarct is grossly identifiable. Appears **pale reddish-blue area** (discoloration due to stagnated, trapped blood). It progressively becomes **sharply defined, yellow-tan, and soft area.**

After 3–7 days: It appears mottled (blotched/smudged) with a **central pale, yellowish, necrotic region** with a **well-demarcated border** of the **hyperemic zone** (due to granulation tissue).

By 10–14 days: Appears **soft and rimmed by a hyperemic zone** of highly vascularized granulation tissue.

After 2 weeks: Older, healed infarcts appear **firm, pale gray, and contracted** and develop into a **fibrous scar.**

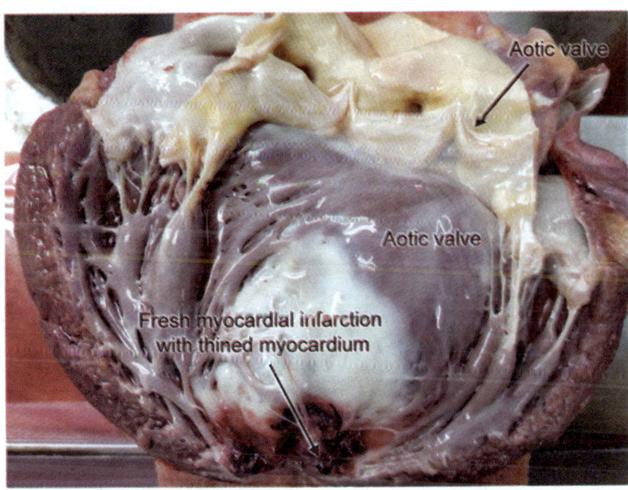

Fig. 16.26: Myocardial infarct at the apex of the heart. The lumen of the ventricle contains a blood clot.

Microscopy (Figs. 16.27A to F and Table 16.6)

Q. Write a short note on microscopic assessment of the age of myocardial infarction.

The myocardial infarct microscopically also undergoes a characteristic sequence of changes.

First 6 hours

Earliest changes can be detected only by electron microscopy (ultrastructural changes)

- **Reversible injury (0–1½ hours): Relaxation of myofibrils, loss of glycogen, and mitochondrial swelling.**
- **Irreversible injury** (½–6 hours): Develops after 30–60 minutes of ischemia. The changes include **mitochondrial amorphous matrix densities, focal disruption of the sarcolemma, and clumping and margination of nuclear chromatin.**

6–12 hours

Coagulative necrosis begins and can be detected. The infarcted area also shows edema and hemorrhage. Other changes include:

- **Wavy fibers:** They represent noncontractile, stretched, buckled dead myofibrils at the periphery of the infarct.
- **Vacuolization of the myocardial cell (myocytolysis):** It is characterized by large vacuolar spaces within the myocardial cell (probably water). These changes are due to sublethal ischemia. These myocytes are viable but contract poorly.

12–24 hours (Figs. 16.18B and F)

Characteristic changes of **coagulation necrosis** appear. These changes include (1) **preserved cell outlines of myocardial cells,** (2) **deeply eosinophilic cytoplasm,** and (3) **pyknotic nuclei.**

1–2 days

- **Acute inflammatory reaction:** Necrotic myocardium elicits acute inflammation. It **is** characterized by the accumulation of polymorphonuclear leukocytes **(Fig. 16.27C) at the periphery/ borders of the infarct.**
- **Continuation of coagulation necrosis of myocardial fibers: Nuclei of myocardial fibers disappear,** and **striations become less prominent. Margins show contraction band necrosis.**

3–7 days

- **Appearance of macrophages:** The polymorphonuclear leukocytes are replaced by macrophages. **Macrophages phagocytose** and remove the necrotic myocardial cells and neutrophil fragments at the border of the infarct.

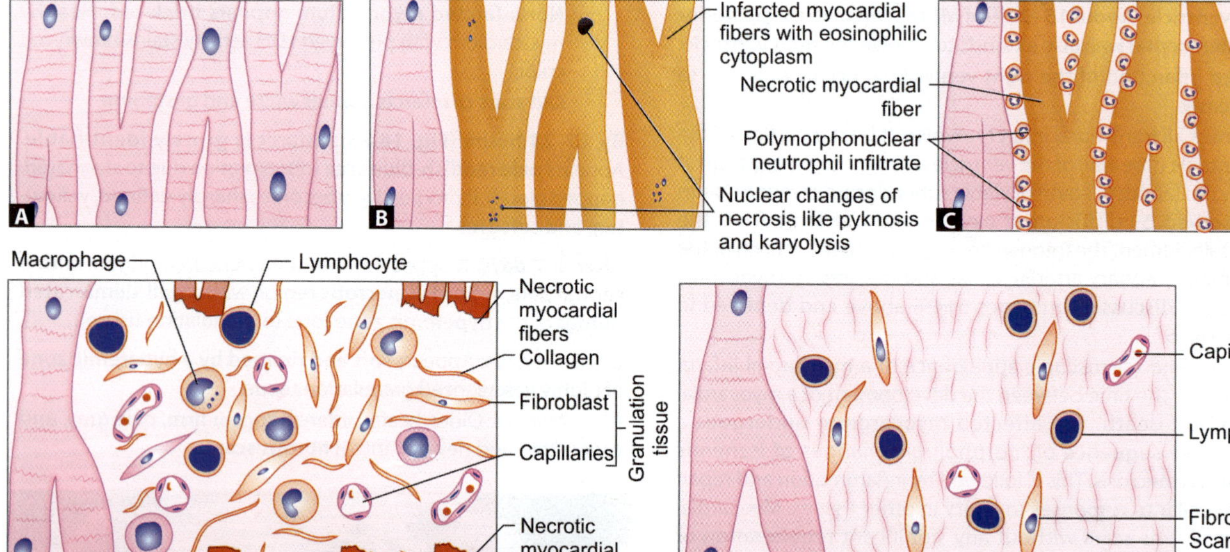

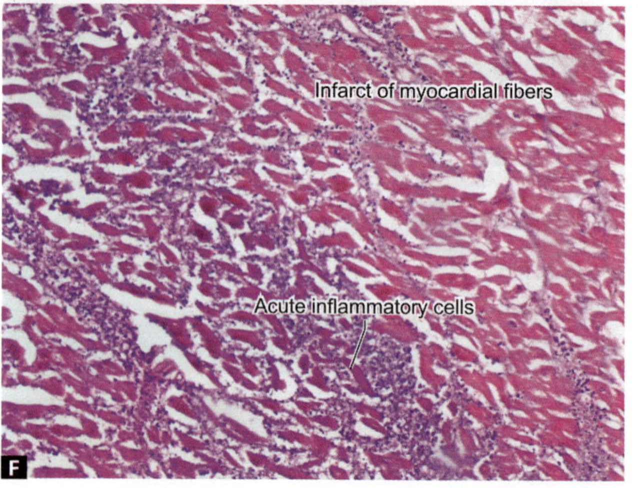

Figs. 16.27A to F: Microscopic changes observed during the development of a myocardial infarct: (A) Normal myocardium; (B) After about 12–18 hours, the infarcted myocardium shows myocardial fibers with eosinophilia; (C) About 24 hours after the onset of infarction, polymorphonuclear neutrophils infiltrate at the periphery of the infarcted area; (D) After about 3 weeks, the infarcted area consists of granulation tissue infiltrated by lymphocytes and macrophages; (E) After 3 months or more, the infarcted region is replaced by collagenous tissue; (F) Photomicrograph of acute myocardial infarction showing coagulative necrosis with acute inflammatory infiltrate.

- **Granulation tissue:** Appears **at the periphery of the infarct,** and gradually replaces the infracted zone, and extends toward the center.

1–2 weeks

The process of healing starts from its margins toward its center which is responsible for most advanced healing at the periphery. During healing, there is migration of inflammatory cells and ingrowth of new vessels from the margins of the infarct.

- **Well-established highly vascularized granulation tissue**: It consists of proliferating capillaries and fibroblasts.
- **Fibroblasts proliferate** and **collagen deposition** proceeds.

2–8 weeks (Fig. 16.18D)

Increased collagen deposition and less cellularity: In most cases, scarring occurs by the end of the sixth week. However, the extent of repair depends on the size of the original area of infarct and the ability of the host tissues to heal.

>2 months (Fig. 16.18E)

Dense collagenous **scar**. In a completely healed infarct, it is not possible to determine its age.

The sequences of the morphologic changes in acute MI and subsequent healing are summarized in **Table 16.6**.

Reperfusion and its Effects on MI

The ischemic myocardium can be rescued by restoring the myocardial blood flow as quickly as possible. Hence, the proverb "time is myocardium."

- **Methods of reperfusion:** It may be by dissolving the thrombus using thrombolytic drugs (tissue plasminogen activator) or angioplasty/stent placement, or coronary artery bypass graft (CABG) surgery.
- **Benefits and outcome of reperfusion:** It depends on the rapidity of restoration. Reperfusion within 20 minutes of the onset of ischemia may completely prevent necrosis. Ischemia-reperfusion injury is discussed on page 37.

MORPHOLOGY OF REPERFUSED INFARCT

Gross

The reperfused infarcted area is **hemorrhagic** because the microvasculature is injured during ischemia and leaks with the restoration of blood flow.

Microscopy

- **Accelerates acute inflammatory responses:** Neutrophils accumulate more rapidly but also disappear more rapidly.
- **Contraction band necrosis:** It is **one of the characteristic features.** They appear as thick, irregular, transverse, intensely eosinophilic intracellular bands in necrotic myocardial cells.

Mediators of reperfusion injury: These include the following:

- Mitochondrial dysfunction promotes apoptosis.
- Myocyte hypercontracture-cytoskeletal damage and cell death.
- Free radicals (reactive oxygen species)-damage to the myocytes.
- Leukocyte aggregation-occlude the microvasculature
- Platelet and complement activation-microvascular injury.

Diagnosis of Myocardial Infraction

It is based on (1) clinical symptoms, (2) electrocardiographic changes, and (3) laboratory findings.

Clinical Symptoms

Chest pain: The classic feature of MI is severe, crushing substernal (retrosternal) chest pain (or pressure). It may radiate to the neck, jaw, epigastrium, or left arm. In contrast to angina pectoris, the pain of MI usually lasts several minutes to hours and is not relieved by nitroglycerin or rest. Other features are:

- **Rapid, weak pulse.**
- **Profuse sweating (diaphoresis) and nausea.**
- **Dyspnea due to impaired contraction** of the ischemic myocardium and the resultant pulmonary congestion and edema.
- **Cardiogenic shock**: If MI is massive MIs with involvement of more than 40% of the left ventricle, cardiogenic shock develops.
- **Arrhythmias**: It is common and caused by electrical abnormalities in the ischemic myocardium and conduction system. Sudden cardiac death from a fatal arrhythmia is responsible for most MI-related deaths occurring before hospitalization.
- **May be entirely asymptomatic**: Up to 25% of MIs are entirely asymptomatic. Such "silent" infarcts are common in diabetic patients with autonomic neuropathy (preventing perception of pain) and in older adults.

Electrocardiographic Changes

Electrocardiographic (ECG) changes in myocardial infarction **(Figs. 16.28A to D)** are important for the diagnosis. These changes include Q waves, changes in the ST segment (elevated ST segment), and inverted T waves. Based on ECG changes, MIs are classified into two categories, ST elevated MI *(STEMI)* and non-ST-elevated MI *(NSTEMI)*.

STEMI: It is due to complete occlusion of a coronary artery and indicates the transmural infarct. They require urgent coronary artery thrombolysis or stent placement.

NSTEMI: It is not associated with complete coronary artery occlusion or full-thickness infarction. It may be managed conservatively.

Laboratory Findings

Q. Laboratory diagnosis (diagnostic tests) of myocardial infarction.

Q. Write a short note on enzyme changes in myocardial infarction/ biochemical markers for myocardial infarction.

Laboratory findings in MI are mainly, due to the **leakage of normal intracellular proteins from the injured (necrotic)**

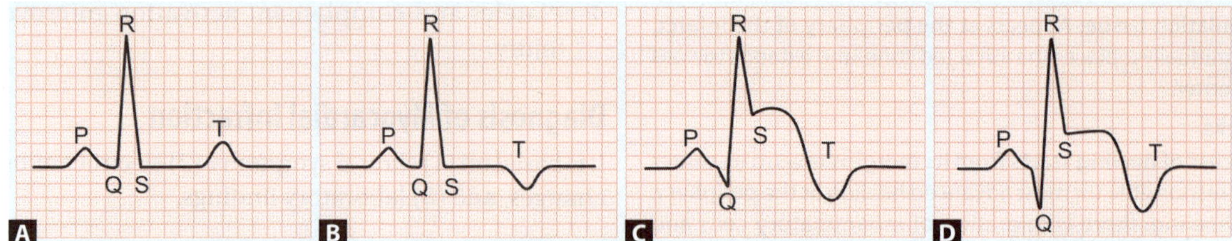

Figs. 16.28A to D: (A) Normal electrocardiogram (ECG). (B to D) ECG changes in myocardial infarction (B) T-wave inversion; (C) ST-segment elevation, deep T wave; and (D) Prominent Q wave indicating more severe myocardial damage.

myocardial cells through the damaged cell membrane into the blood circulation. Measuring their blood levels is useful for diagnosis. These molecules include creatine kinase (CK; specifically, the myocardial isoform, CK-MB) cardiac troponins T and I (TnT, TnI), myoglobin, and lactate dehydrogenase.

1. **Creatine kinase (CK):** It is a **nonspecific enzyme marker** and it is present in the brain, myocardium, and skeletal muscle. It has two isoforms designated "M" and "B". **MB heterodimers chiefly in cardiac** muscle (lesser amounts in skeletal muscle). This biomarker of myocardial injury is now tested less frequently.
   - **MB form of creatine kinase (CK-MB)** is **sensitive but not specific** because it is also raised with a skeletal muscle injury.
   - CK-MB levels **rise within 2–4 hours** of the onset of MI, **peak at 24 hours**, and return to **normal within 72 hours.**
2. **Cardiac troponins:** These are proteins involved in heart muscle contraction. **Increased plasma levels establish the diagnosis of myocardial infarction.**
   - **Cardiac-specific proteins are of two types: Troponins I (TnI) and T (TnT) and** are normally not found in the circulation. They are the **most sensitive and specific markers** of myocardial infarction. Their levels begin to **rise at 2–4 hours** and **peak at 48 hours**. The elevated troponin levels may **remain for 7–10 days** after acute MI.
   - The persistence of raised levels of troponin helps in the diagnosis of an acute MI long after CK-MB levels have returned to normal.
3. **Lactate dehydrogenase (LDH): It is not a specific marker**. It **starts rising** after **24–48 hours**. It remains **for many days** and **returns to normal in 7–14 days.**
4. **Myoglobin:** It is an oxygen-carrying respiratory protein found only in skeletal and cardiac muscle. It is the **earliest marker of MI**, the level rises within 1–3 hours, **peaks in about 8–12 hours,** and **returns to normal in about 24–36 hours.**

Various laboratory markers of MI are presented in **Table 16.7** and **Figure 16.29.**

Consequences and Complications of Myocardial Infarction

Q. Mention the complications of myocardial infarction.

The risk of complications depends on (1) infarct size, (2) location, and (3) thickness of the myocardium involved (subendocardial or transmural). Of the multiple complications of acute MI, three are potentially lethal: (a) rupture of the left ventricular free wall, (b) rupture of the interventricular septum, and (c) acute mitral regurgitation due to papillary muscle necrosis. Almost 75% of MI patients

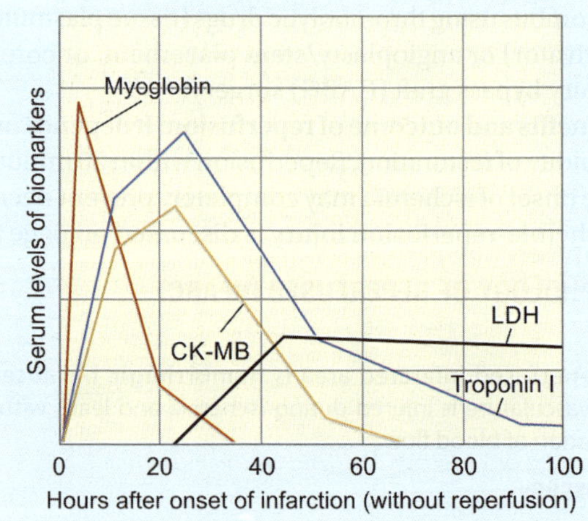

Fig. 16.29: Time course of various serum biomarkers after acute myocardial infarction. Troponin (I and T) and creatine kinase-MB isoenzyme (CK-MB) are the most specific biomarkers. Myoglobin is an early marker but not very specific. Lactate dehydrogenase (LDH) is also not a specific biomarker.

TABLE 16.7 Laboratory markers of myocardial infarction.

Marker	*Onset*	*Peak*	*Normalization*	*Significance*
Troponins T & I	2–4 hours	48 hours	7–10 days	Most sensitive and specific marker
CK-MB	2–4 hours	24 hours	72 hours	Sensitive but not specific
LDH	24–48 hours	Many days	7–14 days	Not specific marker
Myoglobin	1–3 hours	8–12 hours	24–36 hours	Earliest marker

BOX 16.11: Complications of myocardial infarction (MI).

1. Contractile dysfunction: Left ventricular failure and cardiogenic shock
2. Papillary muscle dysfunction
3. Right ventricular infarction
4. Myocardial rupture
5. Arrhythmias
6. Pericarditis (early and delayed type)
7. Dilatation of ventricular chamber
8. Mural thrombus and embolism
9. Ventricular aneurysm
10. Progressive late heart failure
11. Reinfarction

develop one or more of these complications **(Box 16.11)**. These complications are as follows:

1. **Contractile dysfunction:** It produces contractile functional abnormalities of the left ventricle and is roughly proportional to the size of the infarct.
   - **Mild dysfunction:** It may produce **left ventricular failure** resulting **in pulmonary edema.**
   - **Cardiogenic shock:** Severe "pump failure" occurs with a **large infarct** (>40% of the left ventricle) **causing cardiogenic shock** that is **fatal**.
2. **Papillary muscle dysfunction: Ischemia may produce poorly contractile** papillary muscles. This may lead to postinfarct mitral regurgitation. Later, papillary muscle fibrosis and shortening or ventricular dilation can also lead to insufficiency of the mitral valve.
3. **Right ventricular infarction**: Isolated right ventricular infarction is unusual and occurs in only 1–3% of MIs. Occlusions of RCA produce infarction of the posterior septal wall and posterior left ventricle. The right ventricle may be affected due to the extension of any of these infarctions. In either situation, right-sided heart failure is common. This leads to blood pooling in the venous circulation, resulting in systemic hypotension.
4. **Myocardial rupture**: It occurs as a complication in only 1–5% of MIs. But when it occurs, it is often fatal. Rupture may occur in different regions of the heart.
   - **Rupture of the ventricular free wall (Fig. 16.30A):** It is the most common type of rupture and usually leads to rapidly **fatal hemopericardium and cardiac tamponade**. Rupture of the free wall develops in transmural infarcts.
   - **Rupture of the ventricular septum (Fig. 16.30B):** It is less common. It creates acute ventricular septal defect (VSD) with left-to-right shunting.
   - **Rupture of papillary muscle (Fig. 16.30C):** It is the least common and leads to acute severe mitral regurgitation (discussed above).

   Myocardial rupture can occur at any time within 3 weeks of MI. However, it occurs most **commonly within 3–7 days after transmural** infarction when the infarct wall is weakest.
5. **Arrhythmias:** Almost most MI patients develop **abnormal cardiac rhythm causing** myocardial irritability and/or conduction disturbances leading to arrhythmias. These include **sinus bradycardia, tachycardia, ventricular tachycardia, and ventricular fibrillation.** In inferoseptal infarcts, **partial or complete heart block may occur.**
6. **Pericarditis:** It may be an early or delayed type.
   - **Early pericarditis:** A transmural myocardial infarct can involve the pericardium causing **fibrinous or fibrinohemorrhagic** pericarditis **(Fig. 16.30D).** Usually develops on the **second or third day.**
   - **Delayed form of pericarditis (postmyocardial infarction syndrome**/Dressler syndrome): It is rare and develops 2–10 weeks after infarction—**probably immunologically mediated.**
7. **Dilatation of ventricular chamber:** The area of the infarct being a weak region may be disproportionately stretched leading to dilation of the infarct region (especially with anteroseptal infarcts) not severe enough to cause an aneurysm described below.
8. **Mural thrombosis and embolism (Figs. 16.30E):** Infarct causes local abnormality in myocardial contractility (causing stasis) and endocardial damage (creating a thrombogenic surface) and favors **mural thrombosis. This may lead to** left-sided **thromboembolism**. They may also develop **within ventricular aneurysms.**
9. **Ventricular aneurysm (Figs. 16.30F):** After acute transmural infarction, the affected ventricular wall may bulge outward during systole resulting in a ventricular aneurysm. It develops as a late complication of large transmural infarcts.
10. **Progressive late heart failure (chronic IHD):** Usually develops due to the functional decompensation of hypertrophied noninfarcted myocardium.
11. **Reinfarction (Fig. 16.30G)**: It is the acute MI that occurs within 28 days of a previous MI. In many, it represents an extension or enlargement of the earlier infarct. In the present era, it is often caused by stent thrombosis.

SCENARIO-BASED ESSAY QUESTION

Q. A 56-year-old diabetic, hypertensive male was rushed to the hospital following the sudden onset of an episode of crushing substernal/central chest pain of 4 hours duration that radiated to the left arm. It was accompanied by profuse sweating. Serial measurements showed elevated CK-MB levels. He receives advanced life support measures. His course was marked by intractable cardiogenic shock and he died 4 days later.

a. What is your probable diagnosis? (Answer: Acute myocardial infarction).
b. What are the laboratory investigations that will help in arriving at the diagnosis? *(refer pages 519-20).*
c. What are the microscopic findings expected in the heart? *(refer pages 518-19).*
d. What are the complications of this condition? *(refer pages 520-1).*

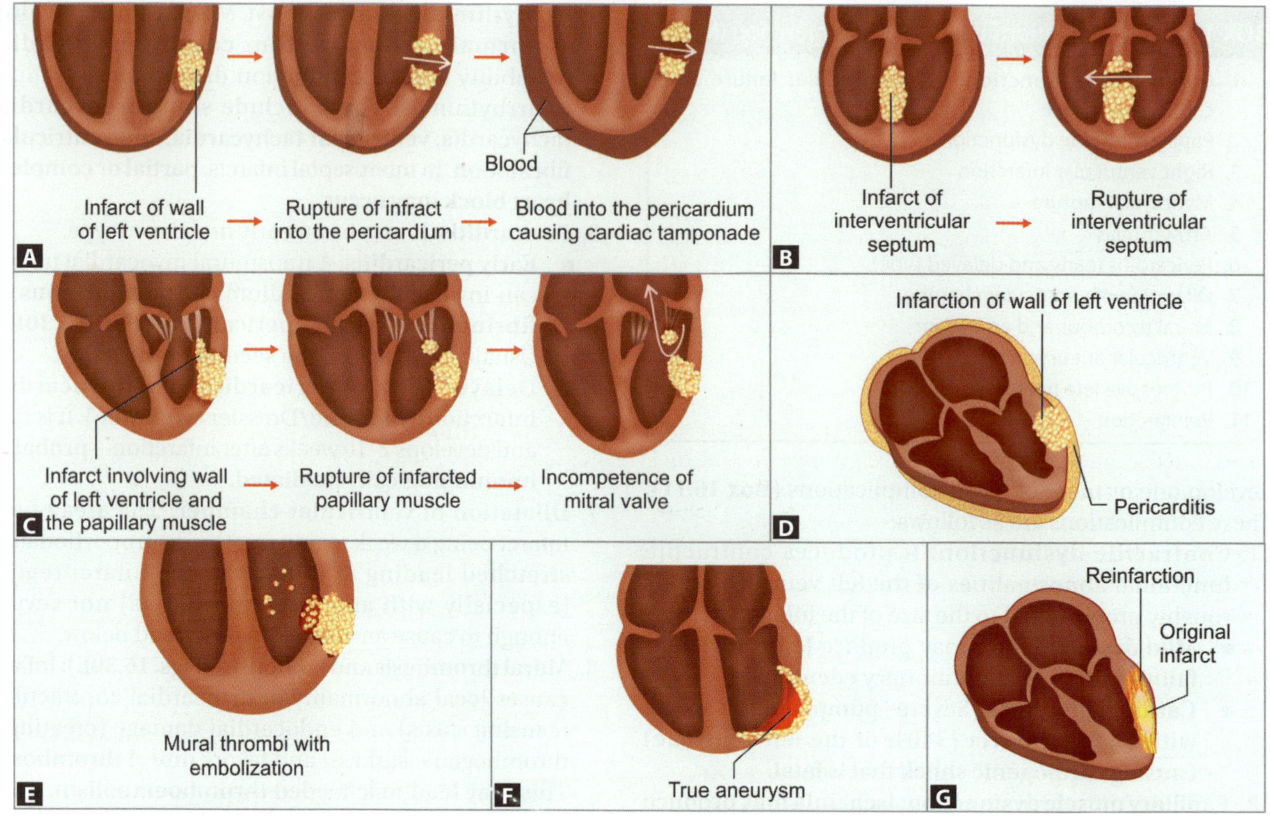

Figs. 16.30A to G: Various complications of myocardial infarction.

Chronic Ischemic Heart Disease

It is **also called ischemic cardiomyopathy.** It is a progressive heart failure developing because of ischemic damage of the myocardium.

Sudden Cardiac Death

Definition: Sudden cardiac death (SCD) is an unexpected death from cardiac causes in individuals without symptomatic heart disease or within 1 hour of the onset of symptoms.

Cause: Usually due to fatal arrhythmia (e.g., asystole, ventricular fibrillation) occurring in IHD. **Acute myocardial ischemia is the most common cause of fatal arrhythmias.** Usually associated with coronary atherosclerosis.

Interpret Abnormalities in Cardiac Function Testing

PA 27.8 (CC): Interpret abnormalities in cardiac function testing in acute coronary syndromes.

Case 1

A 58-year-old male has developed angina on exertion for the last 4 years. One year back, he underwent a coronary angiogram and it showed 75% stenosis of the left circumflex coronary artery and 50% stenosis of the right coronary artery. He complains that there has been increased frequency and severity of attacks of angina for the past 20 days, and pain develops even when lying in bed or taking rest.

Physical examination: His blood pressure is 122/80 mm Hg, and his pulse is 84/minute with irregular beats.

Investigation: ECG shows elevated ST segment.

Laboratory findings: Postprandial blood glucose is 190 mg/dL, serum creatinine is 1.2 mg/dL (Biological reference interval 0.8–1.2 mg/dL), troponin I is 0.02 ng/mL (Biological reference interval is 0–0.04 ng/mL).

Interpretation

A history of angina on exertion for the last 4 years suggests stable (typical) angina. Previous coronary angiogram showed 75% stenosis of the left circumflex coronary artery and 50% stenosis of the right coronary artery. Presently, there has been increased frequency and severity of attacks of angina for the past 20 days. The pain develops even when lying in bed or taking rest. This indicates that recently he developed unstable (crescendo) angina, which is manifested by increased frequency and severity of the attacks and angina at rest. Marked occlusion of the coronary artery prevents adequate perfusion of the heart when myocardial demand is increased during exertion.

ECG findings: The elevation ST segment suggests that acute coronary syndrome developed with myocardial ischemia.

Laboratory findings: The absence of troponin I (cardiac enzyme) elevation suggests that infarction has not yet developed.

In most patients, unstable angina is induced by disruption/fissuring of an atherosclerotic plaque followed by a superimposed mural thrombus and possibly distal embolization of the thrombus, vasospasm, or both. It may progress to myocardial infarction (MI).

Final diagnosis: Stable angina progressing to unstable angina.

Case 2

A 50-year-old male, known diabetic and hypertensive complains of crushing substernal chest pain after arriving at his office. Over the next 6 hours, the chest pain persisted and began to radiate to his left arm and shoulder. He became diaphoretic and developed shortness of breath. He is admitted to the hospital.

Physical examination: His blood pressure is 170/110 mm Hg.

Investigation: ECG showed elevated ST segment.

Laboratory findings: Random blood sugar is 210 mg/dL, total creatine kinase level is 286 U/L (Biological reference interval is 22–198 U/L), creatine kinase-MB (CK-MB fraction) is 8.10 ng/mL (Biological reference interval is 0–2.37 ng/mL), troponin I is 7.43 ng/mL (Biological reference interval is 0–0.04 ng/mL).

Interpretation

A 50-year-old male, known diabetic and hypertensive, crushing substernal chest for 6 hours that persisted and began to radiate to his left arm and shoulder, and diaphoretic, shortness of breath are features suggest acute myocardial infarction.

ECG findings: The elevation ST segment suggests that acute coronary syndrome developed with myocardial ischemia.

Laboratory findings: CK-MB offers a marker for myocardial injury in the first 24–48 hours. In this case, the patient visited the physician within 24 hours of the MI, and the CK- MB levels were raised. The Troponin I levels were raised.

Diagnosis: Acute Myocardial infarction detected within 24 hours of infraction.

Case 3

A 52-year-old male, known diabetic and hypertensive complains of pain in the retrosternal region, left shoulder, and arm for the last 10 hours. Over the next 6 hours, he developed shortness of breath, which persisted for 3 days. On day 3, he visited the cardiology department in the hospital. He is admitted to the cardiology ward.

Physical examination: His blood pressure is 162/102 mm Hg.

Investigation: ECG showed elevated ST segment.

Laboratory findings: Random blood sugar is 220 mg/dL, total creatine kinase level is 186 U/L (Biological reference interval is 22–198 U/L), creatine kinase-MB (CK-MB fraction) is 0.08 ng/mL (Biological reference interval is 0–2.37 ng/mL), troponin I is 6.83 ng/mL (Biological reference interval is 0–0.04 ng/mL).

Interpretation

A 52-year-old male, known diabetic and hypertensive; pain in the retrosternal region, left shoulder, and arm for the last 10 hours, and shortness of breath over the next 6 hours which persisted for 3 days indicates the development of MI 3 days back.

ECG findings: The elevation ST segment suggests that acute coronary syndrome developed with myocardial ischemia.

Laboratory findings: CK-MB offers more specificity, but not more sensitivity. When he visited the physician on day 3, the CK levels had returned to normal. Troponin I levels were raised.

This patient had an MI on the day of the retrosternal pain. He visited the physician on day 3, the CK levels had returned to normal, but troponin I levels were raised. Elevated troponin levels may remain for 7–10 days after acute MI.

Diagnosis: Acute myocardial infarction with changes in enzyme levels after 3 days of onset of infarction.

INFECTIVE ENDOCARDITIS

PA 27.6 (CC): Describe the etiology, pathophysiology, pathology, gross and microscopic features, diagnosis, and complications of infective endocarditis.

Definition: Infective endocarditis (IE) is defined as a microbial infection, **of the heart valves or the mural endocardium.** It results in the focal area of colonization or invasion by microbial agents **and leads to the formation of vegetation. These vegetations are composed of thrombotic debris and organisms and are usually associated with the destruction of the underlying cardiac tissues.**

General Features

Sites of colonization by microbial agents: These include the following:

1. **Heart valves**
2. Mural endocardium
3. Congenital defect (e.g., patent ductus arteriosus or coarctation of the aorta)
4. Other less common sites: (i) aorta, (ii) aneurysmal sacs, (iii) other blood vessels, and (iv) prosthetic devices.

Lesions produced: Vegetations are lesions seen at the site of colonization or invasion. They are composed of thrombotic debris and organisms. **Destruction** of the underlying cardiac tissues/site of colonization is often observed.

Microbes responsible: These include:

- **Bacteria** in most of the cases and produces bacterial endocarditis.

- **Other microbes:** Fungi, *Chlamydia, Rickettsiae* (agents of Q fever), and other microorganisms.

It is important to promptly diagnose IE, identify the causative agent, and provide effective treatment to limit morbidity and mortality.

Classification

A. According to the Clinical Course (Table 16.8)

Infective endocarditis is classified based on the severity of the clinical course as **acute or subacute** endocarditis. The clinical course depends on the virulence of the infecting microorganism and whether any underlying cardiac disease is present.

Acute infective endocarditis: The characteristic features are:

- **Acute** onset and is a rapidly progressing, destructive infection.
- Infection of **previously normal heart** or cardiac valve.
- Caused by highly virulent (suppurative) organisms. Mainly by *Staphylococcus aureus* and *S. pyogenes.*
- **Affected valve is rapidly destroyed** by necrotizing, ulcerative valvular lesions.
- **Capable of seeding** (developing infection at) **extracardiac sites** (due to seeding into other sites by infective emboli).
- Infections may be difficult to cure with antibiotics alone and may need surgery.
- **If untreated, it progresses to death within 6 weeks in many patients**, due to complications like acute heart failure or overwhelming sepsis.

Subacute infective endocarditis: The characteristic features are as follows:

- **Insidious** in onset.
- It **involves structurally abnormal/deformed valves** (e.g., rheumatic heart disease or congenital heart disease).
- **It is caused by organisms of lower virulence** (e.g., ***Streptococcus viridans* or *Staphylococcus epidermidis***).
- The lesions are **less destructive.**
- Accompanied by a **prolonged course of weeks to months** and typically survive for 6 months or more.
- It is most often cured with antibiotics alone.
- **Infectious complications** (due to seeding into other sites by infective emboli) are **uncommon.**

Note: A clear picture between acute and subacute endocarditis may not always be observed, and many cases fall along the spectrum between the two forms.

Differences between acute and subacute endocarditis are listed in **Table 16.8.**

B. According to Anatomic Location and Causative Microbes

The clinical presentations described above are unusual today because of advances in antimicrobial therapy. So, IE is now classified according to the anatomical location and the offending organism, e.g., infective endocarditis of the mitral valve due to *Staphylococcus aureus.*

Etiology

Q. Describe the etiology and pathogenesis of infective endocarditis.

Causative Organism

Many organisms can cause endocarditis, most originate from the normal flora of the body surfaces and enter into the bloodstream in a variety of different ways. More than 80% of IE is caused by streptococci and staphylococci.

- ***Staphylococcus aureus:*** It is a **virulent organism** commonly found on the skin. It can infect either **healthy or deformed** valves. It is responsible for 20–30% of cases of IE. It is the major organism responsible for IE in **intravenous drug abusers.**
- ***Streptococcus viridans:*** It is a less virulent organism present in the **normal flora of the oral cavity**. It most commonly (50–60% of cases) causes endocarditis of previously **damaged** or **abnormal valves.**
- **Other bacteria commensals in the oral** cavity:
  - HACEK group (*Haemophilus, Actinobacillus, Cardiobacterium, Eikenella,* and *Kingella*)
  - Enterococci: They enter the bloodstream mainly from the genitourinary tract.
- **Other agents:** These include gram-negative bacilli and fungi.

Culture-negative endocarditis: They constitute 10–15% of cases in which no organism can be isolated from the blood.

TABLE 16.8 Differences between acute and subacute endocarditis.

Characteristic	*Acute infective endocarditis*	*Subacute infective endocarditis*
Onset	Acute	Insidious
Condition of valve	Infection of normal heart/cardiac valve	Infection of structurally abnormal/deformed valves
Virulence of organisms	Highly virulent (suppurative)	Low virulent
Lesions	The affected valve is rapidly destroyed	Less destructive
Clinical features	Clinical features of acute infection	Clinical features of complications
Course	Death within 6 weeks	The protracted course of weeks
Complications	Acute heart failure or overwhelming sepsis	Infectious complications are uncommon

Prosthetic valve endocarditis: If develops within 1–2 months after surgical implantation, it is usually caused by microbes in skin flora (*S. aureus* and *S. epidermidis*), and infections 1 year or after surgery are usually caused due to streptococci and *S. aureus.*

Predisposing Factors

Three main factors that may predispose to IE are: (1) conditions that lead to bacteremia, (2) underlying heart disease, and (3) impaired host defense mechanism.

1. **Conditions with bacteremia or fungemia:** The most important predisposing factors leading to the development of endocarditis are conditions that lead to bacteremia.
   Sources of infection: The source may be an obvious infection elsewhere (e.g., a dental or surgical procedure, a contaminated needle in intravenous drug users), or may be minor breaks in the epithelial barriers of the gut, oral cavity, or skin. In patients with abnormal valves, or with known bacteremia, the risk of developing IE can be reduced by giving antibiotic prophylaxis.
2. **Underlying heart disease:** IE may involve either normal or damaged heart/valve. IE on previously normal valves develops usually with highly virulent organisms. Underlying heart disease is one of the predisposing factors for IE. These diseases include:
   - **Congenital heart disease:** Unrepaired and repaired congenital defects—most common predisposing condition (e.g., valvular or septal defect).
   - **Acquired heart disease: These include the following**
     - **Chronic rheumatic heart disease** (mitral valve in over 85% of cases, and the aortic valve is involved in 50%).
     - **Mitral valve prolapse** (MVP) in adults.
     - **Degenerative calcific valvular diseases** (mainly in the elderly).
   - **Iatrogenic:**
     - Artificial (prosthetic) valves
     - Indwelling vascular catheters.
3. **Impaired host defense mechanism:** It may occur in:
   - Diabetes mellitus
   - Malignancies: Leukemia and lymphomas
   - Cytotoxic therapy
   - Neutropenia
   - Pregnancy.

Prevention of IE in patients with predisposing risk factors is by prophylaxis with antibiotics.

Pathogenesis

The mechanism by which virulent organisms infect apparently normal valves is poorly understood. The probable sequence of events **(Fig. 16.31)**, which occur with the infection of a damaged valve by less-virulent organisms is as follows:

1. **Endocardial damage and denudation:** The development of infective endocarditis follows a predictable sequence. Endothelial damage is a common predisposing factor for the development of endocarditis. This may result from turbulent blood flow (e.g., as in valvular regurgitation), or micro-abrasion (e.g., as in injection of drug abuse). A damaged valve or a congenital defect creates abnormal high-velocity blood flow at the center and turbulent flow at the periphery causing endocardial damage and denudation of endothelial surfaces.
2. **Formation of sterile thrombus:** Damaged endothelial surface exposes the extracellular matrix, and attracts focal deposition of platelets and fibrin. The aggregation of platelets and fibrin forms small sterile vegetations (sterile thrombi).
3. **Adherence of the microorganisms:** By transient bacteremia, microorganisms gain access to the circulation. The microorganisms adhere and deposit onto the sterile thrombi/vegetations (infection of thrombi).
4. **Proliferation of microorganisms within vegetations:** On the deposited microorganisms, further platelets and fibrin are laid down, which separates them from the bloodstream. Microorganisms proliferate within the vegetation and form colonies. Once infected, these vegetations enlarge and the microorganism is protected from host defense mechanisms.
5. **Formation of emboli:** The vegetation may get detached and form infective emboli causing the spread of infection to visceral organs and the brain.

MORPHOLOGY

Q. Describe the morphology of (heart in) infective endocarditis.

Gross (Figs. 16.32 and 16.33)

Valves affected: Aortic and mitral valves (most common) and **valves of the right heart (especially tricuspid) in intravenous drug abusers.**

Q. Write a short note on the morphology of vegetations in infective endocarditis.

Vegetations: These are the **hallmark/pathognomonic of IE** which has the following features:

- **Appearance: Friable, bulky, potentially destructive vegetations** (less destructive in subacute than in acute endocarditis).
- **Number:** They may be **single or multiple** and may involve **one or more than one valve.**
- **Size:** Lesions **vary in size** from a small, superficial deposit to bulky, exuberant vegetation.
- **Sites:** Vegetations form on:
  - **Atrial side of the atrioventricular valves.**
  - **Ventricular side of the semilunar valves.**
  - **Points of closure of the leaflets or cusps.**
- **Changes in the involved valve: Edema and inflammation** and in severe cases, leaflets may perforate causing regurgitation.

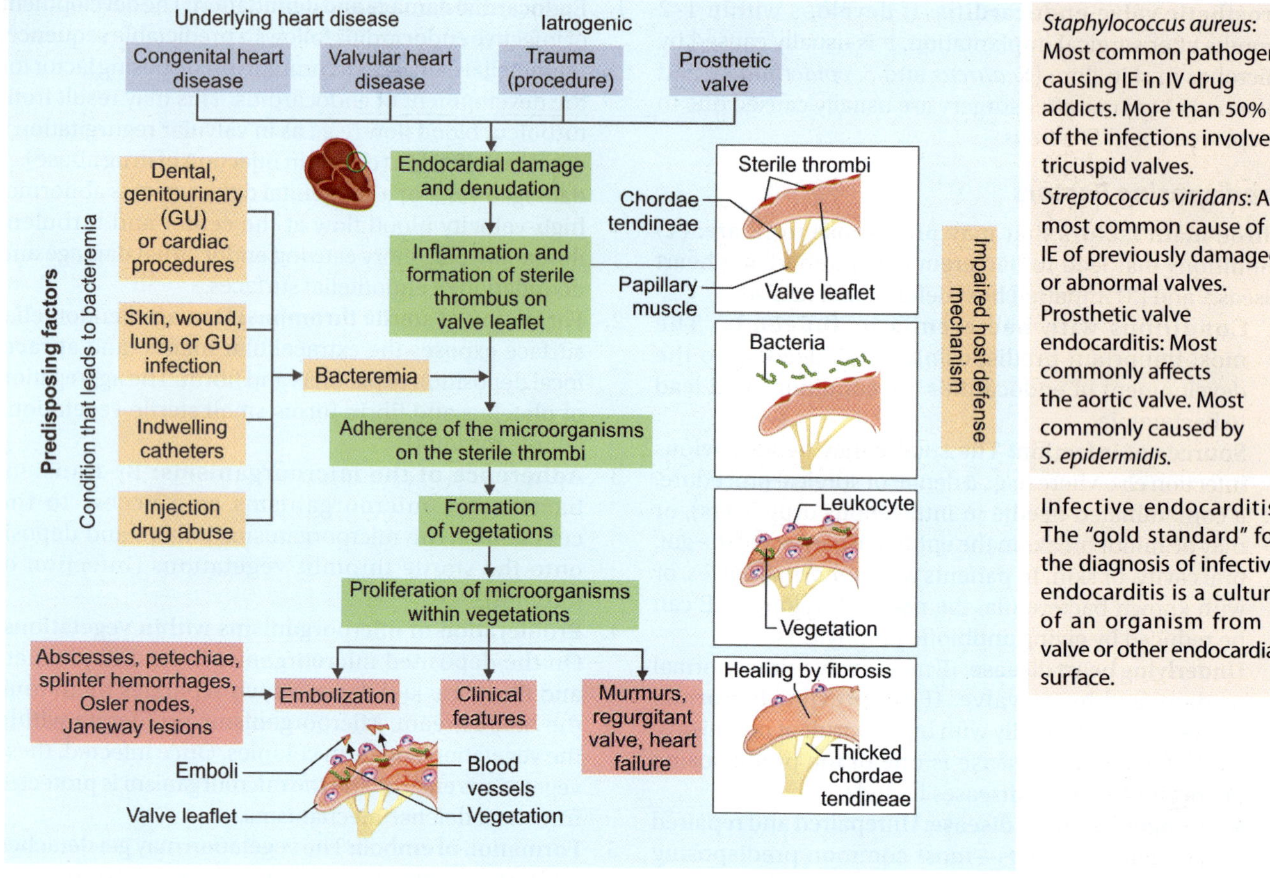

Staphylococcus aureus: Most common pathogen causing IE in IV drug addicts. More than 50% of the infections involve tricuspid valves.

Streptococcus viridans: A most common cause of IE of previously damaged or abnormal valves.

Prosthetic valve endocarditis: Most commonly affects the aortic valve. Most commonly caused by *S. epidermidis.*

Infective endocarditis: The "gold standard" for the diagnosis of infective endocarditis is a culture of an organism from a valve or other endocardial surface.

Fig. 16.31: Pathogenesis of vegetation on a valve leaflet in infective endocarditis (mainly subacute infective endocarditis).

- **Spread:** The infective process may spread locally from valves. They may involve valve rings or adjacent mural endocardium and chordae tendineae.

Microscopy

- Vegetations are composed of platelets, fibrin, cell debris, inflammatory cells, and masses of bacteria or other organisms.
- **Vegetations of subacute IE** may show granulation tissue at their bases indicative of healing. Later it may show fibrosis, calcification, and chronic inflammatory infiltrate.

Complications of Infective Endocarditis

Q. Describe the complications of infective endocarditis.

These may be divided into cardiac and extracardiac (**Box 16.12**).

Cardiac Complications

These are **due to direct valvular damage** and the **consequences of local invasion.** The infection may spread locally from the valve into the valve ring, adjacent mural endocardium, or chordae tendineae.

- **Ring abscess:** Vegetations may erode the **underlying myocardium** and produce an **abscess** which is known as ring abscess.
- **Perforation and rupture:** May involve valve leaflets, aorta, or interventricular septa (depending on the site of infection).
- **Others**: These include **myocardial abscess, suppurative pericarditis**, and **valvular dysfunction** (stenosis or insufficiency).

Extracardiac Complications

Q. List the extracardiac complications of subacute bacterial endocarditis.

Vegetations are usually friable and likely to break, detach, and cause embolism.

1. **Embolic complications (due to septic emboli):** Emboli contain large numbers of virulent organisms. **Abscesses develop at the sites of arrest of the emboli.**
   - **Septic emboli from the left side of the heart:** They enter the systemic circulation and its consequences are:
     - **Septic infarcts** (e.g., spleen, kidney, or brain)
     - **Mycotic aneurysms**
     - **Small emboli (microthromboemboli) may produce tiny hemorrhagic lesions namely: (1) splinter or nail bed hemorrhages** and **(2) Janeway lesions** which are small

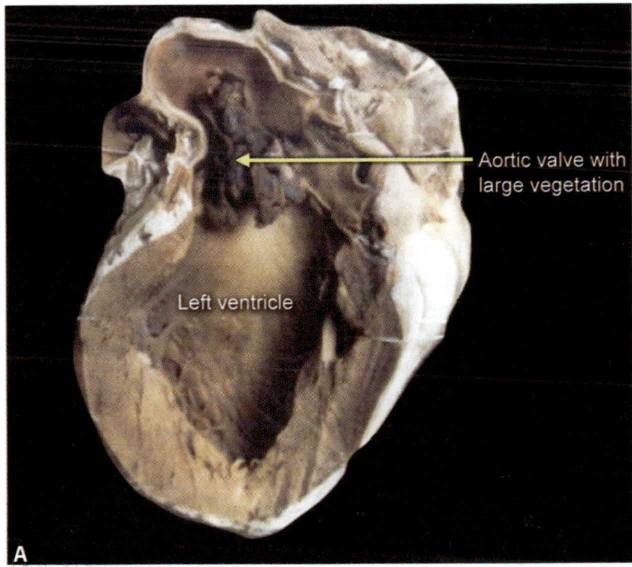

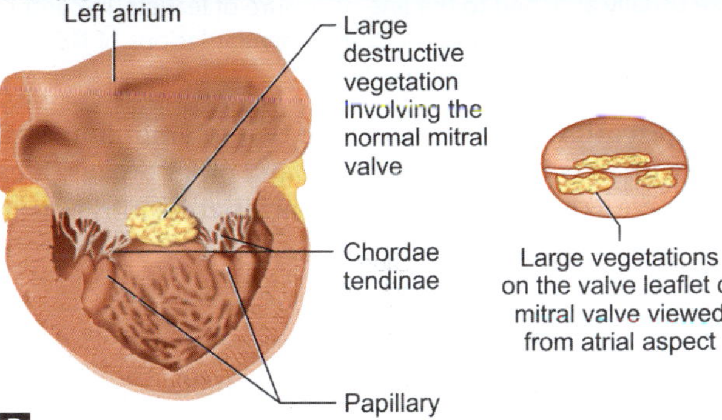

Figs. 16.32A and B: Acute bacterial endocarditis: (A) The aortic valve shows large friable vegetations; (B) The mitral valve shows large friable vegetations (diagrammatic).

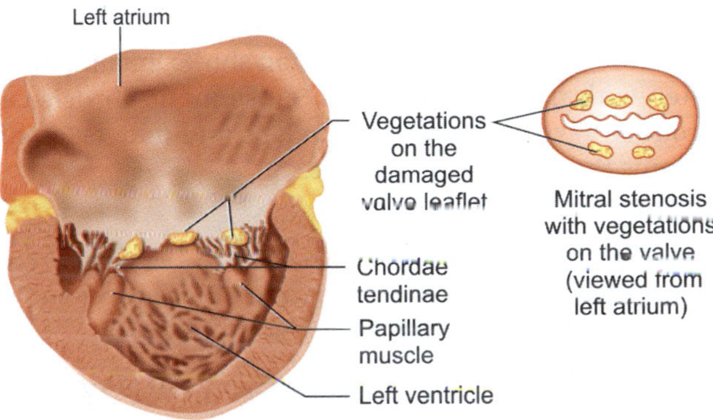

Fig. 16.33: Subacute bacterial endocarditis. The mitral valve shows vegetation.

erythematous or hemorrhagic painless, macular, lesions **on the palms or soles.**

- **Septic emboli from the right side of the heart:** They enter pulmonary circulation and lead to **pulmonary abscess.**

BOX 16.12: Complications of infective endocarditis.

Cardiac complications
- Ring abscess
- Perforation and rupture of the affected valve
- Others: These include myocardial abscess, suppurative pericarditis, and valvular dysfunction (stenosis or insufficiency).

Extracardiac complications
- Embolic complications
  - Abscess at the site of arrest
  - Septic infarcts (e.g., spleen, kidney, or brain)
  - Mycotic aneurysms
  - Splinter or subungual hemorrhages and Janeway lesions
  - Pulmonary abscess
- Immune complex mechanisms
  - Focal segmental glomerulonephritis
  - Osler nodes
  - Roth spots are retinal hemorrhages

2. **Immunological phenomena:** A hallmark of infective endocarditis is sustained high-grade bacteremia. This stimulates both the humoral and cellular immune systems.
   - **Focal segmental glomerulonephritis develops due to the deposition of antigen-antibody complexes** in glomeruli. Grossly, the **outer surface of the kidney** develops a **flea-bitten** appearance due to patchy hemorrhagic foci involving the glomeruli.
   - **Osler nodes** are small, **tender subcutaneous nodules in the pulp of the digits** and persist for hours to several days.
   - **Roth spots** are **retinal hemorrhages** with white or pale centers composed of fibrin.

Clinical Features

Symptoms: These include
- **Fever** is the most common feature of IE. However, in subacute endocarditis (particularly in older adults), fever may be absent, and it may manifest with nonspecific fatigue, weight loss, and a flu-like syndrome. Splenomegaly is common in subacute endocarditis.
- Acute IE develops rapidly presenting with fever, chills, weakness, and lassitude.

Clinical examination: Murmurs may be heard either due to a new valvular defect or a pre-existing cardiac disease.

Diagnostic Criteria for Infective Endocarditis (Box 16.13)

Modified Duke criteria used for diagnosis of suspected infective endocarditis (IE). It requires either pathologic or clinical criteria. If clinical criteria are used, the criteria are as follows:

BOX 16.13: Criteria for diagnosis of infective endocarditis.

Pathologic Criteria

- Demonstration of microorganisms by culture or histologic examination in:
  - Vegetation
  - Embolus from a vegetation
  - Intracardiac abscess
- Histological confirmation of active endocarditis in vegetation or intracardiac abscess.

Clinical Criteria

Major

- Blood culture(s) positive for a characteristic organism or persistently positive for an unusual organism
- Echocardiographic identification of a valve-related or implant-related oscillating mass or abscess, or partial separation of artificial valve
- New valvular regurgitation

Minor

- Predisposition: Predisposing heart lesion or intravenous drug use
- Fever ≥38°C (100.4°F)
- Vascular phenomena: Arterial petechiae, subungual/splinter hemorrhages, emboli, septic pulmonary infarcts, mycotic aneurysm, intracranial hemorrhage, conjunctival hemorrhages, Janeway lesions
- Immunological phenomena: Focal segmental glomerulonephritis, Osler nodes, Roth spots
- Microbiologic evidence, including a single culture positive but not meeting a major criterion, or for an unusual organism that can cause infective endocarditis

- Definite endocarditis, two major, or one major + three minor, or five minor criteria are required for diagnosis.
- Possible endocarditis = One major and one minor, or three minor criteria.

Earlier diagnosis and effective treatment prevent complications.

Prognosis: It depends on the infecting organism and whether or not complications develop.

SCENARIO-BASED ESSAY QUESTION

Q. A 17-year-old male complained of palpitation and joint pains for a one-year duration. Joint pain was a migrating/fleeting type involving multiple major joints and was associated with redness and swelling. About 15 days back he developed a low-grade fever, sometimes accompanied by chills and dyspnea. He is not an IV drug addict. On examination, there was mild pedal edema. On auscultation of the heart, mid diastolic murmur was heard in the mitral region.

a. **What is the probable diagnosis? (Ans: Rheumatic heart disease and mitral stenosis with superimposed subacute infective endocarditis).**
b. **Discuss the etiopathogenesis and the cardiac lesions of the condition *(refer pages 525-6)*.**
c. **List the complications *(refer pages 526-7)*.**

NONINFECTED VEGETATIONS

Nonbacterial Thrombotic Endocarditis

Nonbacterial thrombotic endocarditis (NBTE) is characterized by the deposition of sterile thrombi on heart valves.

Etiology: NBTE occurs in patients with an underlying hypercoagulable state. Examples of these states are chronic disseminated intravascular coagulation, hyperestrogenic states, and in association with underlying malignancy such as mucinous adenocarcinomas. Though NBTE can develop in healthy individuals, it is usually associated with general debility or wasting. Hence, NBTE is **also called marantic endocarditis.**

MORPHOLOGY

The vegetations are small (1–5 mm in diameter), **sterile/bland, and usually occur on previously normal valves (Fig. 16.33).** They are usually attached to the line of closure of leaflets. In contrast to infective endocarditis, the sterile valvular lesions of NBTE **do not destroy the underlying valve.**

Complications: NBTE may give rise to emboli and can cause infarcts in the brain, heart, and other organs. It can also serve as a potential nidus for bacterial colonization and lead to infective endocarditis.

Libman–Sacks Endocarditis

Q. Write a short note on Libman–Sacks endocarditis.

Endocarditis in systemic lupus erythematosus (*refer* page 193) is called Libman-Sacks endocarditis. It is characterized by the presence of sterile vegetations on the valves of patients with systemic lupus erythematosus. It develops in about 10% of SLE patients. The **vegetations probably develop as a consequence of immune complex deposition.** The valve adjacent to the vegetation shows inflammation, often with fibrinoid necrosis. Subsequent fibrosis can produce severe deformity of valves and may resemble chronic rheumatic heart disease.

MORPHOLOGY

The vegetation is small or medium-sized. The **vegetation can occur anywhere on the valve surface, on the cords, or on the atrial or ventricular endocardium (Figs. 16.34A to D).**

Characteristic features of four major types of vegetative endocarditis are presented in **Table 16.9.**

CARDIOMYOPATHY

PA 27.9 (NC): Classify and describe the etiology, types, pathophysiology, pathology, gross and microscopic features, diagnosis, and complications of cardiomyopathies.

Q. Define cardiomyopathy.

The term cardiomyopathy literally means "heart muscle disease".

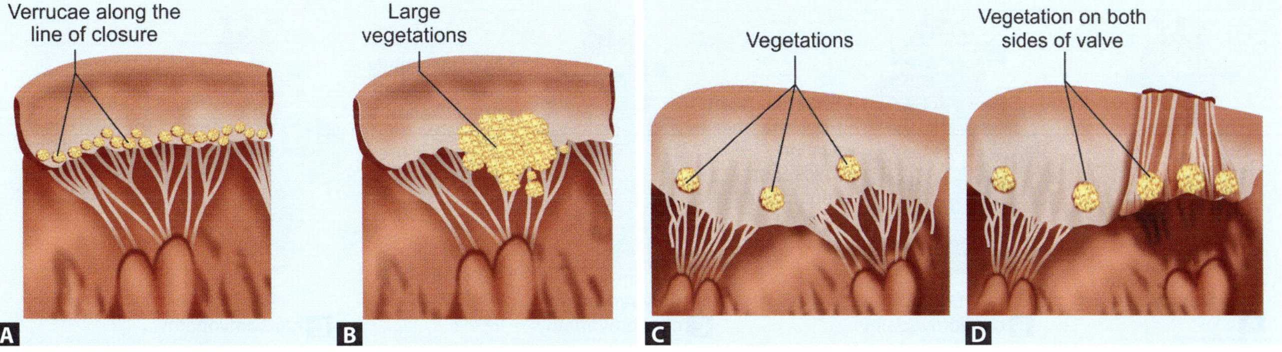

Figs. 16.34A to D: Schematic comparison of the four major types of endocardial vegetations: (A) Vegetations in rheumatic heart disease (RHD) of acute rheumatic fever appear as small, warty verrucae along the lines of closure of the valve leaflets; (B) In infective endocarditis (IE), the vegetations are large, and irregular and develop on the valve cusps and can extend onto the chordae; (C) NBTE shows small, bland vegetation, usually attached at the line of closure. They may be single or multiple; (D) Libman–Sacks endocarditis (LSE) is characterized by small- or medium-sized vegetation on either or both sides of the valve leaflets.

TABLE 16.9 Characteristic features of four major types of vegetative endocarditis.

Type of endocarditis	*Morphological feature*
1. Rheumatic endocarditis	Small, warty vegetations along the line of closure of valve leaflets
2. Infective endocarditis (IE)	Large, irregular on-valve cusps that can extend onto the chordae tendineae
3. Nonbacterial thrombotic endocarditis (NBTE)	Small, bland vegetation is usually attached to the line of closure of valve leaflets
4. Libman-Sacks endocarditis in SLE	Small or medium-sized vegetation on either side of the valve leaflets

Definition: Cardiomyopathies are a **heterogeneous group of cardiac diseases due to intrinsic myocardial dysfunction** (affecting the mechanical and/or electrical function) **in the absence of any other disease.**

Cardiomyopathy term should be restricted to the conditions which primarily affect the myocardium. It **does not include dysfunction of the heart due to other structural heart diseases** such as coronary artery disease, chronic myocardial dysfunction secondary to congenital or acquired valve disease, severe hypertension, or pericardial abnormalities.

Classification

Q. Classify cardiomyopathy

Cardiomyopathies are a diverse group. It can be classified according to a variety of criteria.

Based on Etiology

It is classified as primary or secondary.

Primary cardiomyopathy: In this type, the disease is mainly confined to the myocardium. It may be genetic or acquired. The genetic causes can lead to myocardial dysfunction.

Secondary cardiomyopathy: This consists of myocardial disease (cardiac manifestation) as a part (component) of the generalized systemic or multiorgan disorder. These disorders are as follows:

- Inflammatory disorders (e.g., myocarditis)
- Immunologic diseases (e.g., sarcoidosis, amyloidosis, systemic connective tissue disease)
- Systemic metabolic disorders (e.g., hemochromatosis)
- Muscular dystrophies
- Genetic disorders of myocardial fibers. They can be genetic/inherited or have
- Idiopathic (unknown etiology)

Based on Clinical, Functional, and Pathological Patterns

Three time-honored clinical, functional, and pathologic patterns are **(Figs. 16.35A to D)**:

1. **Dilated cardiomyopathy** (DCM) (including arrhythmogenic right ventricular cardiomyopathy): Most common (~90%)
2. **Hypertrophic cardiomyopathy** (HCM)
3. **Restrictive cardiomyopathy** is the least common

Dilated Cardiomyopathy

Dilated cardiomyopathy (DCM) **is characterized morphologically by progressive cardiac dilation and functionally by contractile** (systolic) **dysfunction.** The clinicopathologic patterns are similar irrespective of the cause.

Etiopathogenesis

At the time of diagnosis, dilated cardiomyopathy presents with end-stage disease marked by heart failure secondary to poor myocardial contractility. It does not reveal any specific pathologic features. Dilated cardiomyopathy can be an inherited abnormality or caused by environmental exposures.

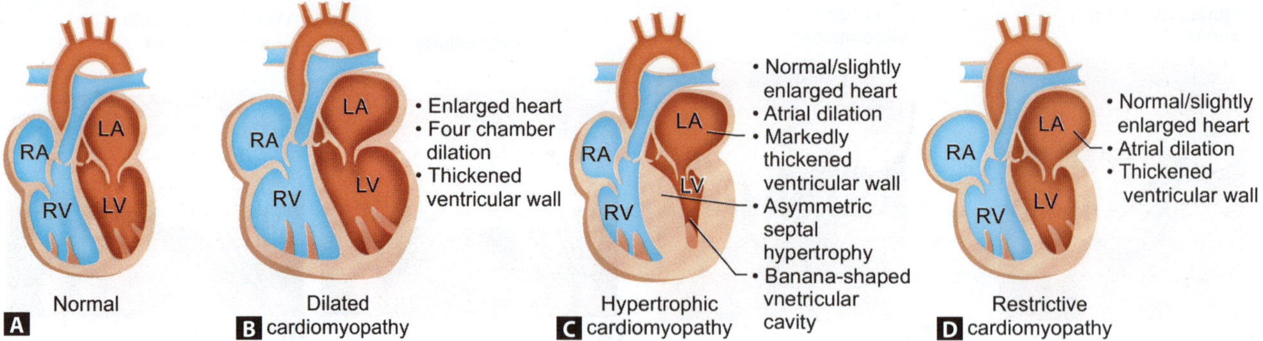

Figs. 16.35A to D: Three major morphologic patterns of cardiomyopathy: (A) Normal; (B) Dilated cardiomyopathy; (C) Hypertrophic cardiomyopathy; (D) Restrictive cardiomyopathy.

(AO: aorta; LA: left atrium; LV: left ventricle; RA: right atrium; RV: right ventricle).

Genetic Causes

DCM is hereditary in about 20–50% of cases. More than 50 genes are mutated in DCM. The main mode of inheritance is **autosomal dominant pattern**. Most are caused by **loss of function mutations of cytoskeletal proteins or proteins that link the sarcomere to the cytoskeleton.** X-linked DCM is most frequently associated with mutations in dystrophin. This is a cell membrane protein that physically binds the intracellular cytoskeleton to the extracellular matrix (ECM).

Non-genetic Causes

- **Infection:** It may occur with infection by adenovirus, parvovirus B-19, and human herpesvirus 6.
- **Alcohol or exposure to other toxins:** Alcohol abuse is strongly associated with the DCM. Alcohol and its metabolites especially acetaldehyde are directly toxic to the myocardium. Chronic alcohol use can produce thiamine deficiency and can result in beriberi heart disease. DCM can also occur after exposure to toxic agents, such as cobalt, and particularly doxorubicin, a chemotherapeutic drug.
- **Pregnancy** (peripartum cardiomyopathy).
- **Iron overload**: In the heart, it may occur either due to hereditary hemochromatosis or from multiple transfusions.

MORPHOLOGY

Gross

- **Heart:** It is characteristically **enlarged, heavy** (2–3 times the normal weight), and **flabby,** with **dilation of all chambers (Fig. 16.35B).**
- **Thickness of dilated ventricles**: It may be **less than, equal to, or greater than normal.**
- **Mural thrombi:** They are usually seen at the apex of the left ventricle and may be a source of thromboemboli.
- **Absence of secondary causes of cardiac dilation**: By definition, the secondary causes that lead to cardiac dilation such as valvular (mitral or tricuspid regurgitation) and vascular lesions (e.g., atherosclerotic coronary artery disease) are absent.

Microscopy

Microscopic features of DCM are nonspecific and **usually do not point to a specific etiology.**

- **Hypertrophy of myocytes:** Most myocytes show **hypertrophy** with enlarged nuclei. Many myocytes are thinned, stretched, and irregular.
- **Interstitial and endocardial fibrosis:** It is of variable degree. Scattered areas of replacement fibrosis; which indicates previous myocyte ischemic necrosis due to hypoperfusion.
- **DCM secondary to iron overload:** They show marked accumulation of intramyocardial hemosiderin. This pigment can be demonstrated by staining with Prussian blue (Perls stain) that imparts a blue color to hemosiderin.

Clinical Features

Age: DCM can occur at any age, but is most common between the ages of **20 and 50 years.**

Initial presentation: It usually presents with slowly progressive **signs and symptoms of CHF**. These include dyspnea, easy fatigability, and poor exertional capacity.

At the end stage: The main **defect in DCM is ineffective contraction.** Thus, in this stage, the cardiac ejection fraction usually is less than 25% (normal is 50–65%). It is common to find secondary mitral regurgitation and abnormal cardiac rhythms. Embolism from intracardiac (mural) thrombi can also occur.

Diagnosis

- **ECHO:** Shows an ejection fraction (EF) <45% (normal >55%).
- **Chest X-ray:** Global enlargement of the heart.

Prognosis: About 50% of patients die within 2 years and about 25% survive longer than 5 years. Death is usually due to progressive cardiac failure or arrhythmia.

Treatment: The only definitive treatment is cardiac transplantation.

Arrhythmogenic Right Ventricular Cardiomyopathy

Arrhythmogenic right ventricular cardiomyopathy (ARVC) **is an autosomal dominant disorder. Manifestations:** It **manifests with right-sided heart failure** (right ventricular failure) **and rhythm disturbances** (such as ventricular tachycardia or fibrillation). It **can cause sudden cardiac death.** It may be responsible for sudden deaths in about 10% of athletes.

Etiology: It is mainly due to **mutations involving genes encoding desmosomal junctional proteins** at the intercalated disk (e.g., plakoglobin), and proteins that interact with the desmosome (e.g., the intermediate filament desmin). The myocyte death in ARVC is due to detachment of desmosomes, particularly during strenuous exercise.

MORPHOLOGY

The wall of the right ventricle is severely thinned due to the replacement of myocytes by fat and fibrous tissue.

Hypertrophic Cardiomyopathy

Hypertrophic cardiomyopathy (HCM) is a **genetic disorder characterized by inappropriate myocardial hypertrophy and defective diastolic filling.** In about one-third of patients, there is **intermittent ventricular outflow obstruction.** It is the leading cause of left ventricular hypertrophy that cannot be explained by other clinical or pathologic causes.

The **heart in HCM is thick-walled, heavy, and hypercontractile.** This is in contrast to the flabby, poorly contractile heart in DCM. In HCM, the myocardium does not relax and therefore shows primary diastolic dysfunction and usually, there is preservation of systolic function. HCM has to be clinically distinguished from disorders causing ventricular stiffness (e.g., amyloid deposition Fabry disease) and ventricular hypertrophy (e.g., aortic stenosis and hypertension).

Etiopathogenesis

Genetic causes: In **most cases of HCM,** there are **missense mutations in one of several genes encoding sarcomeric proteins that form the contractile apparatus.** In most cases of HCM, the transmission pattern **is autosomal dominant, with variable expression/penetrance.** Of the different sarcomeric proteins mutated, three are most frequently involved and are responsible for 70–80% of HCM. These mutated sarcomere proteins include gene encoding for (i) β-myosin heavy chain (β-MHC), (ii) **myosin-binding protein** C (MYBP-C), and (iii) **troponin** T. The prognosis of HCM varies and is strongly correlated with specific mutations.

MORPHOLOGY

Gross

The **heart is always enlarged** and shows **massive myocardial hypertrophy** (the extent of hypertrophy varies in different genetic mutations) **without dilatation of ventricles dilation (Fig. 16.35C).**

- **Asymmetric septal hypertrophy:** Classical features is disproportionate thickening of the ventricular septum relative to the left ventricle free wall (with a ratio of septum to free wall greater than 3:1). Though the entire septum may show marked hypertrophy, it is usually most marked in the subaortic region.
- **Changes in the ventricular wall:** The left **ventricular wall is thick, and its cavity is small.** On the longitudinal section, the normally round-to-ovoid left ventricular cavity may be compressed to assume a **"banana-like" (sometimes only slit) configuration.** This is due to the bulging of the interventricular septum into the lumen.
- **Endocardial mural plaque:** The thickened, hypertrophied interventricular septum bulges into the left ventricular outflow tract early in ventricular systole. This obstructs the aortic outflow tract and may produce an endocardial mural plaque in the outflow tract.
- **Atria:** Both atria are commonly dilated.

Microscopy

The characteristic microscopic features of myocardium in HCM are:

- **Marked hypertrophy of myocytes.**
- **Myofiber disarray: Haphazard myocyte and myofiber** (contractile elements in sarcomeres) **disarray,** which is most extensive in the interventricular septum. **Normally** the myocytes are arranged parallelly into muscle bundles. The myofiber disarray is characterized by oblique and often perpendicular orientations of adjacent hypertrophic myocytes.
- **Interstitial and replacement fibrosis.**

Clinical Features

Age: It can present at any age and usually manifests during the post-pubertal period.

Clinical symptoms: In HCM, there is massive left ventricular hypertrophy associated paradoxically with markedly reduced stroke volume. The **reduced stroke volume is due to impaired diastolic filling and overall smaller chamber size.** The patient may present with exertional dyspnea due to reduced cardiac output and a secondary increase in pulmonary venous pressure. It is associated with a *harsh systolic ejection murmur* on auscultation. Even in the absence of coronary artery disease, the patient may develop focal myocardial ischemia (with angina). This ischemia is due to massive hypertrophy, high left ventricular chamber pressures, and thick-walled intramural arteries.

Complications: These include atrial fibrillation (with formation of mural thrombus leading to embolization stroke), ventricular fibrillation (leading to sudden cardiac death), infectious endocarditis of the mitral valve, and intractable congestive heart failure (CHF). HCM is an important cause of sudden cardiac death (especially in athletes younger than 35 years).

Treatment: In most patient's pharmacologic intervention (e.g., β-adrenergic blockade) to decrease heart rate and contractility can be helpful. Reduction of the septal myocardial mass by surgical excision may relieve the outflow tract obstruction and may be beneficial.

Restrictive Cardiomyopathy

It is the least common type of cardiomyopathy. Restrictive cardiomyopathy **is a group of diseases characterized by impaired ventricular filling during diastole** (the ventricular wall is **stiffer**), **while contractile** (systolic) **function is normal.**

Etiopathogenesis: It may be idiopathic or may be associated with systemic diseases that affect the myocardium. The various causes are as follows:

- **Amyloidosis:** It is characterized by the deposition of extracellular proteins with β-pleated sheet configuration in the interstitial tissues (*refer* page 225).
- **Endomyocardial fibrosis:** It is mainly seen in children and young adults in Africa and other tropical areas. It is characterized by dense diffuse fibrosis of the endocardium and subendocardium of the ventricles. The fibrous tissue severely reduces the volume of affected chambers. Endomyocardial fibrosis may be due to nutritional deficiencies and/or inflammation related to helminthic infections (e.g., hypereosinophilia). It is the most common form of restrictive cardiomyopathy.
- **Loeffler endomyocarditis:** It is also associated with endocardial fibrosis with the formation of large mural thrombi similar to those found in tropical disease mentioned above. However, it has no geographic or population predilection. In addition, it shows peripheral hypereosinophilia and tissue infiltration by eosinophils.
- **Endocardial fibroelastosis:** It is an uncommon heart disease characterized by fibroelastic thickening of the left ventricular endocardium. It is most common during the first 2 years of life. Endocardial fibroelastosis may be a common morphologic endpoint of several different disorders such as viral infections (e.g., intrauterine exposure to mumps) or mutations in the gene for tafazzin (affects mitochondrial inner membrane integrity). Diffuse involvement can lead to cardiac decompensation and death.
- **Other causes** include radiation fibrosis, sarcoidosis, metastatic carcinoma, or products/metabolites of inborn errors of metabolism (e.g., hemochromatosis).

MORPHOLOGY

Gross (Fig. 16.35D)

The **morphologic features are not distinctive.** The **ventricles are almost of normal size** or only slightly enlarged. The myocardium is firm and noncompliant and the ventricular cavities are not dilated. Dilatation of both atria is commonly found as a consequence of restricted ventricular filling and pressure overloads.

Microscopy

It shows **variable degrees of patchy or diffuse interstitial fibrosis.** An endomyocardial biopsy can reveal a specific etiology.

PA 27.10 (NC): Describe the etiology, pathophysiology, pathology features, and complications of syphilis on the cardiovascular system (*refer* pages 113 and 491).

PERICARDITIS AND PERICARDIAL EFFUSION

PA 27.7 (CC): Describe the etiology, pathophysiology, pathology, gross and microscopic features, diagnosis, and complications of pericarditis and pericardial effusion.

Pericardial diseases are usually associated with a pathologic process in other parts of the heart or surrounding structures or are secondary to a systemic disorder. Isolated pericardial disease is unusual. The most important pericardial diseases cause the accumulation of fluid (pericardial effusions), inflammation (pericarditis), inflammatory conditions, fibrous constriction, or a combination of these processes. Normally, the pericardial sac contains less than 50 mL of thin, clear, straw-colored fluid.

Pericarditis

Definition: Pericarditis is the inflammation (or infiltration by cancer) of the pericardium encasing the heart (epicardial surface, parietal surface).

Etiology: It can be primary or secondary. The major causes of pericarditis are listed in **Box 16.14**.

- **Primary pericarditis** is **very rare**. It may be due to viral infection and produces acute pericarditis. Tuberculosis and fungi produce chronic pericarditis.
- **Secondary pericarditis** is the **most common type**. It can occur secondary to various disorders. Uremia is the most common systemic disorder associated with pericarditis.

Classification of pericarditis: It may be classified as **acute or chronic pericarditis (Box 16.15)**:

Acute Pericarditis

It is the most frequent type of pericarditis. Depending on the morphological features (gross and microscopic characteristics) of the pericardial surfaces and fluid, it can be divided into several types **(Box 16.14)**. Most cases of acute pericarditis are of uncertain etiology.

BOX 16.14: Causes of pericarditis.

- **Infectious agents:** Viruses, pyogenic bacteria, tuberculosis, fungi, parasites
- **Presumably immunologically mediated:** Rheumatic fever, systemic lupus erythematosus, postmyocardial infarction (Dressler) syndrome
- **Miscellaneous:** Acute myocardial infarction, uremia, metastatic malignancies, radiation to the mediastinum, infectious processes involving other thoracic structures (e.g., pneumonia or pleuritis).

BOX 16.15: Classification of pericarditis.

Acute pericarditis
- Serous pericarditis
- Fibrinous and serofibrinous pericarditis
- Purulent or suppurative pericarditis
- Hemorrhagic pericarditis

Chronic pericarditis
- Tuberculous (caseous) pericarditis
- Chronic constrictive pericarditis
- Chronic or healed pericarditis
- Adhesive mediastinopericarditis

Clinical features of acute pericarditis: It presents with atypical chest pain (not related to exertion and worse in recumbency), and a prominent friction rub. When acute pericarditis is accompanied by significant fluid in the pericardial cavity, it can cause **cardiac tamponade**, which leads to declining cardiac output and consequent shock.

Serous Pericarditis

It may be accompanied by serous effusion.

Etiology: It is caused by:
- Non-infectious inflammatory diseases, e.g., rheumatic fever, and SLE
- Uremia
- Infectious processes involving other contiguous thoracic structures near the pericardium (e.g., pneumonia or bacteria pleuritis).
- Rarely viral infection elsewhere (e.g., upper respiratory tract infection, pneumonia, parotitis) may antedate the pericarditis and may be the primary focus of infection.
- Very rarely viral pericarditis can develop as a primary infection along with *myopericarditis* in young adults.
- Tumors can produce serous pericarditis by lymphatic invasion or direct contiguous extension into the pericardium.

MORPHOLOGY

Microscopy

Serous pericarditis may show mild inflammatory infiltration of neutrophils and lymphocytes in the epipericardial fat. Pericarditis associated with metastatic malignancies may also show neoplastic cells. Usually, it resolves and very rarely it may undergo organization causing fibrous adhesions of the pericardium.

Fibrinous and Serofibrinous Pericarditis

It is the most common type of pericarditis and the pericardial cavity shows serous fluid mixed with a variable amount of fibrinous exudate.

Etiology: Common causes of fibrinous and serofibrinous pericarditis are listed in **Box 16.16**.

BOX 16.16: Common causes of fibrinous and serofibrinous pericarditis.

- Acute myocardial infarction (MI)
- Postinfarction (Dressler) syndrome (the autoimmune type that develops days-weeks after an MI)
- Uremia
- Chest radiation
- Rheumatic fever, SLE
- Trauma
- Following routine cardiac surgery

MORPHOLOGY

Fibrinous pericarditis: Normal smooth, glistening pericardial surfaces are replaced by dull, fine granular roughening with fibrin-rich exudate. It produces an irregular, shaggy appearance **(Figs. 16.20 and 16.36)** on the pericardial surface ("bread and butter" pericarditis). Effusion fluid is fibrinous and usually rich in protein, and the pericardium contains mainly mononuclear inflammatory cells.

Serofibrinous pericarditis: It shows the accumulation of larger amounts of yellow to brown turbid fluid, containing leukocytes, RBCs, and fibrin.

Outcome: Fibrin may be lysed and inflammation may resolve or can become organized.

Clinical features: Fibrinous pericarditis presents with pain (sharp, pleuritic, and position-dependent) and fever. The rough inflamed pericardial surfaces produce a characteristic loud pericardial friction rub on auscultation.

Purulent or Suppurative Pericarditis

It is usually accompanied by purulent exudate that resembles pus (full of neutrophils) in the pericardial cavity.

Etiology: It is due to infection caused by microbial (pyogenic bacteria) invasion of the pericardial space. The various routes of infection are as follows:

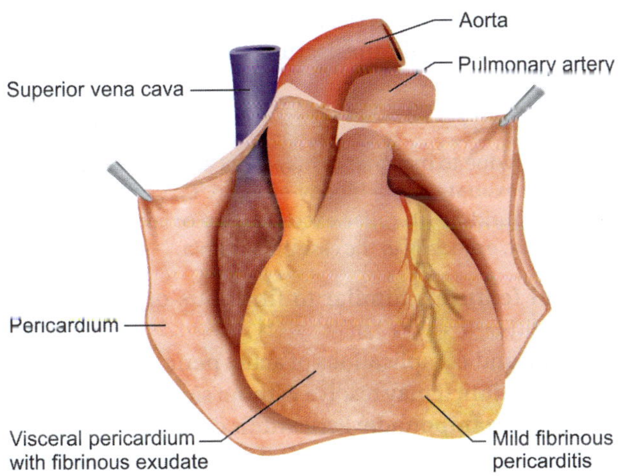

Fig. 16.36: Fibrinous pericarditis (diagrammatic).

- Direct extension of infections from neighboring structures: Examples include empyema of the pleural cavity, lobar pneumonia, mediastinal infections, etc.
- Blood spread
- Lymphatic extension
- Direct infection during cardiotomy

MORPHOLOGY

Gross

The serosal surfaces of the pericardium appear red, granular, and covered with exudate. The exudate may range from a thin cloudy fluid to frank pus. The amount of exudate may be up to 400–500 mL.

Microscopy

The pericardium shows acute inflammatory infiltrate and may extend into surrounding structures to produce mediastinopericarditis.

Outcome: Complete resolution is uncommon and organization by scarring is the usual outcome. The intense inflammatory response and the scarring may lead to constrictive pericarditis.

Clinical features: During the active phase, they are similar to fibrinous pericarditis. However, frank infection can produce more marked systemic symptoms such as fever and rigors.

Hemorrhagic Pericarditis

This type of pericarditis shows an exudate composed of blood mixed with a fibrinous or suppurative effusion.

Etiology: Its causes include:

- **The spread of a malignant neoplasm** to the pericardial space is the most common cause. Cytologic examination of pericardial fluid removed through a pericardial tap often shows neoplastic cells. The most common tumors that involve the pericardium and cause malignant pericardial effusions are breast and lung carcinomas.
- **Other causes:** Bacterial infections in patients suffering from bleeding diathesis, tuberculosis, and following cardiac surgery.

MORPHOLOGY

Pericarditis due to malignancy may show an exuberant, shaggy fibrinous exudate and a bloody effusion. Metastases may be grossly found as irregular excrescences or may be grossly inapparent, especially in the case of leukemia.

Clinical features: Similar to fibrinous or suppurative pericarditis.

Outcome and complications of acute pericarditis:

- **Resolution:** It may resolve without significant sequelae
- **Cardiac tamponade:** Pericarditis can cause immediate hemodynamic complications if there is an accumulation of a large amount of effusion resulting in cardiac tamponade.
- **Progression to chronic fibrosing pericarditis.**

Chronic Pericarditis

Various types of chronic pericarditis are listed in **Box 16.11.**

Tuberculous (Caseous Pericarditis)

Etiology: Caseous pericarditis unless otherwise proved is due to tuberculosis. Very rarely, fungal infections may produce a similar reaction. Pericardial involvement in tuberculosis may occur by direct spread from tuberculous foci within the tracheobronchial nodes.

MORPHOLOGY

Gross

The exudate is caseous or blood-stained and tubercles may be observed on the pericardial surface.

Microscopy

It shows a typical tuberculous granuloma. Granuloma consists of central caseous necrosis surrounded by epithelioid cells, Langhan's giant cells, and lymphocytes (*refer* **Figs. 2.8, 3.17, and 17.19**). They are surrounded by fibrous tissue.

Complications: Caseous pericarditis may progress to a disabling, fibrocalcific, chronic constrictive pericarditis.

Chronic Constrictive Pericarditis

In chronic pericarditis, if delicate adhesions or dense, fibrotic scars occur, it can cause obliteration of the pericardial space. When this process is severe, the heart may be completely encased by dense, fibrous, or fibrocalcific scars. In such cases, the heart cannot expand normally during diastole and there will be a reduction in the cardiac output. This condition is called constrictive pericarditis. These features resemble those of a restrictive cardiomyopathy.

Definition: Chronic constrictive pericarditis is a chronic fibrosing disease of the pericardium (scarring of the pericardial sac) that compresses the heart and limits the ability of the chambers in the heart to fill with blood (i.e., restricts the inflow of blood to the heart).

Etiology: Causes include prior radiation therapy to the mediastinum, cardiac surgery, and sequelae of a purulent or tuberculous infection of the pericardium.

Pathogenesis: Constrictive pericarditis is not an active inflammatory condition. It occurs as an exuberant healing after acute pericardial injury. The visceral and parietal layers of the pericardium become fused by a dense, rigid mass of fibrous tissue. This leads to the obliteration of the pericardial space. The scarred pericardium may be thickened (up to 3 cm) in such a way that it narrows the orifices of the venae cavae. The fibrous tissue may show calcified areas. Because of the dense fibrous scar neither cardiac hypertrophy nor dilation can occur.

MORPHOLOGY

The heart is small and the pericardium is thickened due to dense fibrosis. The fibrous scar can be up to a centimeter in thickness and obliterates the pericardial cavity/space. Sometimes calcification may be observed and in extreme cases, it can resemble a plaster mold *(concretio cordis)*.

Clinical features: Constrictive pericarditis may mimic right heart failure. Patients have small, quiet hearts and venous inflow is restricted. The rigid pericardium limits the diastolic volume of the heart. Thus, its clinical features are due to a combination of right-sided venous distention and low cardiac output (similar to the clinical features in restrictive cardiomyopathy). Cardiac output may be reduced at rest and the heart is not capable of increasing its output in response to increased systemic demands. Signs of constrictive pericarditis include distant or muffled heart sounds, raised jugular venous pressure (JVP), small pulse pressure, low cardiac output, and fluid retention with ascites and peripheral edema. There may or may not be a previous history of pericarditis.

Treatment consists of surgical resection of the shell of constricting fibrous tissue (total pericardiectomy).

Chronic or Healed Pericarditis

In some cases of chronic pericarditis, the organization produces either plaque-like fibrous thickenings of the serosal membranes ("soldier's plaque") or thin, delicate adhesions. They do not produce any impairment of cardiac function. **Adhesive pericarditis:** It is a milder form of healing of an inflamed pericardium. It is usually found as an incidental finding at autopsy. It is the outcome of many different types of pericarditis. The pericarditis after healing produces fibrosis in the form of mesh-like stringy adhesions between the visceral and parietal surfaces. This may completely obliterate the pericardial sac; but does not affect cardiac function.

Adhesive Mediastinopericarditis

Etiology: It may follow infectious pericarditis, previous cardiac surgery, or mediastinal irradiation.

Pathophysiology: In this type of pericarditis, the pericardial sac is obliterated, and the external aspect of the parietal layer of the pericardium is adherent to surrounding structures. This produces strains on the cardiac function. During each systolic contraction, the heart pulls both the parietal pericardium and the attached surrounding structures.

Clinical features: These include, systolic retraction of the rib cage and diaphragm, pulsus paradoxus, etc. The increased workload may occasionally lead to severe cardiac hypertrophy and dilation.

Pericardial Effusion and Hemopericardium

Normally, the pericardial sac contains less than 50 mL of pericardial fluid. It is thin, clear, straw-colored.

Definition: Pericardial effusions are defined as accumulations of excess fluid within the pericardial cavity.

The fluid accumulated may be either a transudate or an exudate. If the accumulated fluid is serous fluid it is termed pericardial effusion, if pus is termed purulent pericarditis, and if blood is accumulated it is termed hemopericardium. Pericardial effusion can occur in all forms of pericarditis.

Pericardial Effusions

Etiology: Various types and causes of pericardial effusions are presented in **Table 16.10**.

Rate of accumulation of fluid: If the pericardium is slowly distended (long-standing) with fluid, the pericardium has time to dilate. This allows chronic pericardial effusions to accommodate even up to 2 L of fluid without any significant hemodynamic consequences or interference with cardiac function. Clinically, chronic effusions of less than 500 mL may produce only a characteristic globular enlargement of the heart shadow on the chest radiograph. However, if the fluid accumulation is rapid, even 150–200 mL of fluid or blood [e.g., due to hemopericardium caused by a ruptured myocardial infarction (MI) or aortic dissection] may significantly increase intrapericardial pressure. This restricts diastolic filling, especially of the right atrium and ventricle. This can lead to fatal cardiac tamponade.

Cardiac Tamponade

Definition: It is a syndrome caused due to rapid accumulation of pericardial fluid, that restricts the filling of the heart. Tamponade refers to external compression of the heart chambers such that filling is impaired.

Pathophysiology: Rapid accumulation of fluid in the pericardial cavity raises the pericardial pressure. When the pressure increase exceeds central venous pressure, the return of blood to the heart is limited. This, in turn, reduces cardiac output and blood pressure and leads to **pulsus**

TABLE 16.10 Various types of pericardial effusion and their causes.

Type of pericardial effusion	*Causes*
Serous effusion (low protein content and few cells)	Congestive heart failure, hypoalbuminemia of any cause (e.g., nephrotic syndrome)
Serosanguineous (mixture of serous fluid and blood)	Blunt chest trauma (either accidentally or after cardiopulmonary resuscitation), malignancy, ruptured MI, or aortic dissection
Chylous effusion (fluid containing chylomicrons)	Communication of the thoracic duct with the pericardial space due to mediastinal lymphatic obstruction by tumor or infection
Hemopericardium (bleeding directly into the pericardial cavity)	Ventricular free wall rupture in myocardial infarct, penetrating cardiac trauma, rupture of a dissecting hematoma of the aorta, infiltration of a vessel by tumor, a bleeding diathesis

paradoxus (an abnormal decrease in systolic pressure with inspiration).

Consequences: Hemodynamic consequences can range from minimal symptoms to sudden cardiovascular collapse and death.

Beck's triad: It consists of three classic findings in cardiac tamponade—namely (i) hypotension, (ii) distended neck veins, and (iii) muffled heart sounds.

Acute cardiac tamponade is almost always fatal unless the pericardial pressure is relieved by aspirating/removing offending pericardial fluid, via needle pericardiocentesis or surgery.

Diagnosis of Pericardial Effusion

- Chest radiograph shows a "water bottle" configuration
- ECHO is useful for the detection of pericardial effusion and for determining the amount of fluid
- ECG may be useful
- Pericardial fluid analysis is similar to other body fluids (*refer* page 463-5).

CONGENITAL HEART DISEASE

Definition: Abnormalities of the heart or great vessels that are **present from birth** are termed congenital heart diseases. Congenital means "born with."

Incidence: Congenital heart diseases are the **most important and common type of heart disease in children.** They constitute about 20% to 30% of all birth defects.

Manifestations: Congenital heart diseases range from severe anomalies to lesions with few or no symptoms. **Severe** congenital heart diseases are incompatible with intrauterine (result in **intrauterine death)** or perinatal survival. Some produce clinical manifestations soon after birth, but some may not be evident until adulthood (e.g., ASD).

Etiology and Pathogenesis

In embryogenesis, major cardiovascular structures form and begin to function during 3–8 weeks of gestation. Hence, most congenital heart disease (CHD) arises from defective embryogenesis during this period. The cause of CHD is not known in about 90% of cases. Risk factors for CHD are:

- **Prematurity**
- **Family history**
- **Maternal conditions:** These include diabetes, hypertension, obesity, phenylketonuria, thyroid disorders, and systemic connective tissue disorders; exposure to teratogens including therapeutic drugs taken during pregnancy (e.g., phenytoin, retinoic acid), smoking and alcohol ingestion.
- **Assisted reproductive technology**: For example, in vitro fertilization.
- **Genetic disorders:** The congenital heart disease can be due to sporadic genetic abnormalities. These may be single gene mutations, small chromosomal deletions, and additions or deletions of whole chromosomes (trisomies and monosomies). The **most common genetic cause of congenital heart disease is trisomy 21 (Down syndrome).** Others include trisomy 18,13, and Turner syndrome.
- **In utero infections**: These include rubella, cytomegalovirus, coxsackie virus, human herpesvirus 6, parvovirus B19, herpes simplex, and toxoplasmosis.
- **Nutritional factors: During pregnancy**, consumption of multivitamins containing **folate may reduce the risk,** whereas heavy consumption of **alcohol increases the risk** of congenital heart defects.

Classification (Box 16.17)

Based on the hemodynamic and clinical consequences, the structural anomalies in congenital heart disease may be divided into three major categories: **Malformations causing (1) a left-to-right shunt, (2) a right-to-left shunt (cyanotic congenital heart diseases), and (3) an obstruction.**

Shunt: It is an abnormal communication between chambers of the heart or blood vessels. Depending on pressure, shunts allow the flow of blood from the left to the right side (high-pressure to the low-pressure side) of the heart or vice versa.

General Features

Left-to-right shunt: These are characterized by the flow of blood from the left (systemic) side to the right (pulmonary) side of the circulation. Its consequences are:

- **Pulmonary hypertension:** Left-to-right shunt causes **increased pulmonary blood flow** and does not produce cyanosis at least initially. Increased pulmonary blood flow **increases the volumes and pressures in**

BOX 16.17: Classification of congenital heart diseases.

Type of congenital heart disease

1. **Left-to-right shunt**
   - Ventricular septal defect
   - Atrial septal defect
   - Patent ductus arteriosus
2. **Right-to-left shunt**
   - Tetralogy of Fallot
   - Transposition of the great arteries
   - Persistent truncus arteriosus
   - Tricuspid atresia
   - Total anomalous pulmonary venous connection
3. **Obstructive congenital heart disease**
   - Coarctation of the aorta
   - Aortic stenosis
   - Pulmonary stenosis

the pulmonary circulation. It causes **pulmonary hypertension.**

- Pulmonary hypertension **leads to right ventricular hypertrophy and right-sided failure.**
- **Shunt reversal if not corrected**: Later, when the **pressure in the right ventricle reaches systemic levels**, the shunt changes to a new **right-to-left (shunt reversal).** It diverts the unoxygenated blood into the systemic circulation and results in **late-onset cyanosis.** Hence this CHD is known as **late cyanotic congenital heart disease, or Eisenmenger syndrome**.
- When pulmonary hypertension becomes irreversible, the structural defects of congenital heart disease become irreparable.

Right-to-left shunt: If the pressure on the right side rises more than that on the left, the blood flows from the right to the left side (right-to-left shunt) resulting in hypoxemia and **cyanosis** (blue discoloration of the skin and mucous membranes) due to the mixing of poorly oxygenated venous blood with systemic arterial blood (called **cyanotic congenital heart disease**). Its consequences are:

- **Paradoxical embolism:** It is a condition in which emboli from the peripheral veins can bypass the lungs and enter directly into the systemic circulation (*refer* page 156). It may result in infarction and abscess in the brain.
- **Clubbing and polycythemia:** Severe, long-standing cyanosis causes clubbing of the tips of the fingers and toes (called **hypertrophic osteoarthropathy**) and **polycythemia**.

Obstructive congenital heart disease: These are characterized by abnormal narrowing of chambers, valves, or blood vessels. If the obstruction is complete, it is called an atresia.

In some CHD, there may be coexistence of (e.g., tetralogy of Fallot) both obstruction (pulmonary stenosis) and a shunt (right-to-left through a VSD).

Malposition of the heart are very rare type of congenital heart disease.

Left-to-Right Shunts

Left-to-right shunts are the most common type of congenital cardiac heart disease. The common left-to-right shunt includes **atrial septal defects (ASDs)**, **ventricular septal defects (VSDs),** and **patent ductus arteriosus (PDA)**.

Atrial Septal Defect

Q. Write a short note on atrial septal defect.

An atrial septal defect (ASD) is an abnormal, fixed opening in the atrial septum. It is due to the incomplete formation of tissue in the atrial septum. It allows the **unrestricted flow of blood between the left and right atria.**

MORPHOLOGY

Classification: It is classified into three major types according to their location: Secundum, primum, and sinus venosus.

- **Ostium secundum ASDs** (90% of ASD): These result from a deficient or fenestrated oval fossa near the center of the atrial septum. The size varies and may be single or multiple, or be fenestrated.
- **Ostium primum ASDs** (5%) occur at the lowest part of the atrial septum near the AV valves.
- **Sinus venosus ASDs** (5%) are seen high in the atrial septum near the entrance of the superior vena cava.

Clinical features: ASDs are **usually asymptomatic till adulthood** (before 30 years of age). Initially, ASDs cause a left-to-right shunt and result in increased pulmonary blood flow by about two to four times normal. A murmur may be heard due to increased blood flow through the pulmonary valve.

Complications: (1) heart failure, (2) paradoxical embolization, and (3) irreversible pulmonary vascular disease.

Prognosis: Mortality is low.

Ventricular Septal Defect

Q. Write a short note on ventricular septal defect.

Incomplete closure of the ventricular septum is known as ventricular septal defect (VSD). It is the **most common form of congenital cardiac anomaly** diagnosed at birth. Most (70–80%) VSDs are associated with other congenital cardiac anomalies (e.g., tetralogy of Fallot). VSD causes free blood flow from the left-to-right ventricles.

Classification: Ventricular septal defects are classified according to their size and location.

- **Membranous VSD (90%):** They involve the membranous (basal) region of the interventricular septum.
- **Infundibular VSD (10%):** They lie below the pulmonary valve or within the muscular part of the interventricular septum.

Clinical features: The clinical features depend on the size of the defect.

- **Large ventricular septal defect:**
  - Usually **membranous or infundibular type** and manifest from birth.
  - Cause **left-to-right shunt** leading to right ventricular hypertrophy and pulmonary hypertension.
  - Irreversible pulmonary vascular disease develops later, in all patients resulting in **reversal of shunt, cyanosis, and death.**
- **Small ventricular septal defect:**
  - May not be recognized until adult life.
  - About 50% of small muscular VSDs may close spontaneously.

Patent Ductus Arteriosus

Q. Write a short note on patent ductus arteriosus.

Normal function of ductus arteriosus: In the fetus, it is an essential structure that carries the blood from the left pulmonary artery to the aorta just distal to the origin of the left subclavian artery. Thus, it bypasses the flow of blood to the unoxygenated lungs (like the patent foramen ovale). Within 1–2 days of birth in healthy term infants, it spontaneously closes and the blood from the pulmonary artery flows to the lung. It leaves behind only a strand of residual fibrous tissue known as the *ligamentum arteriosum.*

Patent (persistent) ductus arteriosus: It is a congenital anomaly in which the **ductus arteriosus remains open after birth (Fig. 16.36)**. PDAs may occur as an **isolated anomaly** (about 90%), **or associated with VSD, coarctation of the aorta, or pulmonary or aortic valve stenosis.** PDA produces a **characteristic continuous harsh murmur known as "machinery-like"**.

Clinical features: Depends on the diameter of the PDA and the cardiovascular status of the patient. PDA is **usually asymptomatic at birth.** A narrow PDA may not affect the child's growth and development. **First, the shunt is from left to right** and there is no cyanosis. However, additional volume and pressure overload produce obstructive changes in small pulmonary arteries, leading to a reversal of flow and its associated consequences. Thus, it leads to Eisenmenger syndrome with cyanosis and congestive heart failure.

Preservation of ductal patency (by administering prostaglandin E) is essential for the survival of infants with congenital malformations that obstruct the pulmonary or systemic blood flow tracts. Example: In aortic valve atresia, preserved PDA supplies the major blood into the systemic circulation. Consequences of patent ductus arteriosus are presented in **Figure 16.37.**

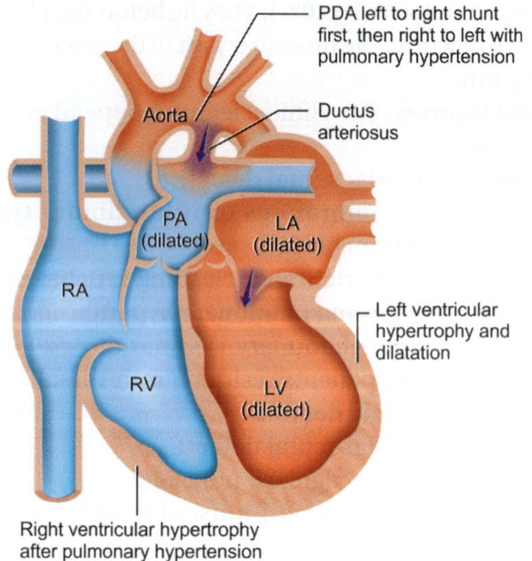

Fig. 16.37: Patent ductus arteriosus (PDA).

(LA: left atrium; RA: right atrium; LV: left ventricle; RV: right ventricle; PA: pulmonary artery).

Patent Foramen Ovale

The normal function of foramen ovale: In **the fetus, there is an essential small hole in the atrial septum at the oval fossa** that produces a right-to-left shunt, through which the oxygen-rich blood from the placenta directly travels from the right-to-left atrium without passing through the non-inflated lungs. The **foramen ovale closes at birth** due to increased blood pressure on the left side of the heart.

Consequences of a patent foramen ovale: Sustained pulmonary hypertension or transient increase in right-sided pressures (as occurs during a bowel movement, coughing, or sneezing), can produce transient right-to-left shunting, and paradoxical embolism.

Right-to-Left Shunts

Right-to-left shunts congenital diseases cause **cyanosis early in postnatal life** (cyanotic congenital heart disease). Cyanosis occurs because poorly oxygenated blood from the right side of the heart flows directly into the arterial circulation. Two important cyanotic congenital heart diseases are tetralogy of Fallot and transposition of the great vessels and others include transposition of the great arteries, persistent truncus arteriosus, tricuspid atresia, and total anomalous pulmonary venous connection.

Tetralogy of Fallot

Q. Write a short note on the tetralogy of Fallot's features and complications.

It is the most common cause of cyanotic congenital heart disease.

Components (Fig. 16.38): The **four characteristic features** of the tetralogy of Fallot (TOF) are:

1. **Ventricular septal defect:** Usually large and lies near the membranous portion of the interventricular septum.
2. **Subpulmonic stenosis (pulmonary valvular stenosis):** It obstructs the right ventricular outflow tract.
3. **Aorta overriding the VSD:** The aortic valve lies immediately over the VSD (**overriding aorta—**opening from both ventricular chambers). It is the major site of outflow of blood flow from both ventricles.
4. **Right ventricular hypertrophy:** It is due to the obstruction to right ventricular outflow most commonly due to narrowing of the infundibulum **(subpulmonic stenosis).**

MORPHOLOGY

Enlarged boot-shaped heart: The heart is enlarged and may be **"boot-shaped"** due to **marked right ventricular hypertrophy**, particularly of the apical region. The proximal aorta is dilated, and the pulmonary trunk is hypoplastic.

Left-sided cardiac chambers: They are normal in size.

Marked right ventricular hypertrophy: The thickness of the hypertrophied right ventricle, sometimes may be more than the thickness of the left ventricle.

Clinical features: The **consequences of tetralogy of Fallot are right-to-left shunting, reduced pulmonary blood**

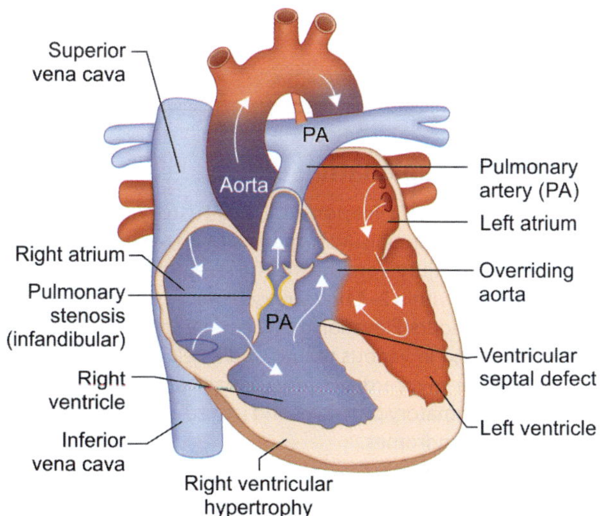

Fig. 16.38: Diagrammatic representation of tetralogy of Fallot. Four components are (1) Ventricular septal defect; (2) Subpulmonic stenosis/pulmonary valvular stenosis; (3) Aorta overriding the VSD; (4) Right ventricular hypertrophy.

(RA: right atrium; LA: left atrium; RV: right ventricle; LV: left ventricle).

flow, and increased blood volume flow through the aorta. The clinical features mainly depend on the severity of the subpulmonary stenosis because this decides the direction of blood flow.

- **Mild subpulmonary stenosis:** It clinically resembles an isolated VSD, and the shunt may be from left to right, **without cyanosis** (so-called pink tetralogy).
- **Moderate subpulmonary stenosis:** It produces increased resistance to right ventricular outflow. When the right-sided pressures approach or exceed that of left-sided pressures a right-to-left shunt develops. This **produces cyanosis** (classic TOF). **The majority of infants with TOF have cyanosis from birth or soon thereafter.**
- **Severe subpulmonary stenosis**: Pulmonary arteries become progressively hypoplastic with small and thin walls. The aorta becomes progressively larger in diameter. As the child grows, the size of the heart increases, but the pulmonary orifice does not expand proportionally. This results in progressive worsening of the obstruction.

Cardiac Abnormalities with Transposition of the Great Arteries are presented online along with **Figures 16.39A and B.**

CARDIAC MYXOMA

Q. Write a short note on cardiac myxoma.

Primary cardiac tumors are uncommon. Cardiac myxomas are the **most common primary cardiac tumor** of the adult heart. They are **benign tumors** arising from primitive multipotent mesenchymal cells.

MORPHOLOGY

Gross

Site: About 90% of myxomas arise in the atria, **more common in the left atrium** in the region of the fossa ovalis in the atrial septum.

Number: Usually single, but can rarely be multiple.

Size: Range from **small (<1 cm) to large (≥10 cm).**

Sessile or pedunculated (Fig. 16.40A): Vary from globular hard masses with hemorrhage to soft, translucent, papillary, or villous lesions having a gelatinous appearance. The pedunculated type may be mobile during systole into the atrioventricular valve producing intermittent obstruction or producing a "wrecking ball" effect that damages the valve leaflets.

Microscopy (Fig. 16.40B)

Composed of stellate or globular myxoma cells embedded within an abundant acid mucopolysaccharides ground substance. It frequently contains multinucleate cells typically with hyperchromatic nuclei. Vessel-like and glandlike structures are characteristically observed.

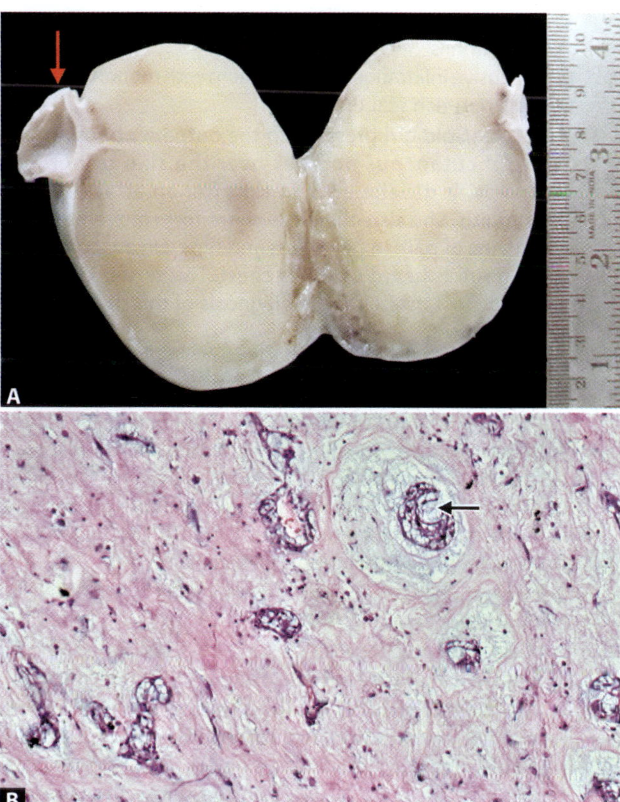

Figs. 16.40A and B: Cardiac myxoma: (A) Cut section of bisected cardiac myxoma. It shows a pedunculated solid tumor with a stalk (arrow). The cut section shows a pearly white appearance; (B) Microscopically shows cytologically bland myxoma cells surrounded by capillaries (arrow) and embedded in an abundant myxoid stroma.

Clinical features: Mainly due to **valvular "ball-valve" obstruction, embolization**, or constitutional symptoms, such as fever and malaise. Treatment is by surgical removal.

SCENARIO-BASED MCQs

1. **A 52-year-old man complains of crushing substernal chest pain. The pain persists for the next 4 hours and begins to radiate to his left arm. He becomes diaphoretic and breathless. He for another 8 hours and then comes to the hospital. The most useful serum laboratory tests that will be most useful for the diagnosis on admission to the hospital is:**
   A. ALT
   B. AST
   C. Troponins I
   D. C-reactive protein
2. **A 52-year-old man presents to the casualty with 1 hour of acute chest pain. Laboratory studies show an increased leukocyte count and increased serum levels of troponin I and CK-MB fraction. ECG confirms a diagnosis of massive transmural myocardial infarction of the left ventricle. The patient dies after 2 days. Autopsy shows atherosclerosis of the epicardial region of coronary arteries. Microscopic examination of the infarcted region is likely to show:**
   A. No obvious changes by light microscopy
   B. Coagulative necrosis of cardiac myocytes and infiltrates of neutrophils
   C. Extensive infiltration of myocardium with mononuclear cells
   D. Collagen-rich scar tissue
3. **An 11-year-old girl presents to the outpatient department with subcutaneous nodules over the skin of her arms and torso. It developed 3 weeks after an attack of acute pharyngitis. She also manifests choreiform movements and complains of pain in her knees and hips. On auscultation, a friction rub is heard over her chest. The serum laboratory findings most useful for the diagnosis of this disease is:**
   A. Creatinine level
   B. Troponin I level
   C. Antinuclear antibody titer
   D. Antistreptolysin O antibody titer
4. **A 24-year-old previously healthy man undergoes a tooth extraction. After 4 days, he develops a fever. He is a known case of congenital heart disease. A probable diagnosis of sub-acute infective endocarditis is made. The lesion likely to be seen in the heart of this patient is:**
   A. Vegetations
   B. MacCallum patch
   C. Calcified aortic stenosis
   D. Verrucae along the line of closure
5. **A 19-year-old man complains of a low-grade fever for 3 weeks. On examination, the spleen is tender and slightly palpable. Splinter hemorrhage under the fingernails and tender hemorrhagic nodules on the palms and soles are also detected. A heart murmur is heard on auscultation. The infectious agents that are most likely to be causing the condition is:**
   A. Coxsackievirus B
   B. *Streptococcus viridans*
   C. *Mycobacterium tuberculosis*
   D. *Pseudomonas aeruginosa*

Answers and Explanation

1. **The answer is C: Troponins T & I.** History suggests acute myocardial infarction (MI Troponins T & I) is a specific marker for myocardial injury from the MI. The levels of this enzyme begin to increase within 2–4 hours of ischemic myocardial injury and peak at 48 hours. Elevation of ALT is more specific for liver injury. AST is found in various tissues and its elevated levels are not specific for myocardial injury. C-reactive protein is elevated with inflammatory processes and is used as a predictor of acute coronary syndromes.
2. **The answer is B: Coagulative necrosis of cardiac myocytes and infiltrates of neutrophils.** The diagnosis in this case is acute myocardial infarction. Two days after myocardial infarction, the affected heart muscle will show coagulative necrosis of myofiber, edema, and focal hemorrhage. Polymorphonuclear leukocytes infiltrate at the border of the zone of infarction and the necrotic tissue. Lack of changes by light microscopy (choice A) is during the first 24 hours but not at 2 days. The other changes (choices C, and D) occur after longer periods.
3. **The answer is D: Antistreptolysin O antibody titer.** The girl is suffering from acute rheumatic fever. Acute rheumatic fever follows group A β-hemolytic streptococcal infections. It shows the elevation of anti-hyaluronidase, anti-DNase, and anti-streptolysin O (ASO) titers. Creatinine levels are elevated in renal diseases including post-streptococcal glomerulonephritis. Cardiac troponins are markers for ischemic myocardial injury. The ANA level is elevated in systemic lupus erythematosus, which can cause serious pericarditis.
4. **The answer is A: Vegetation.** Infective endocarditis is present in this man with a known cardiovascular congenital anomaly. The dental procedures may be preceded by prophylactic antibiotic therapy. Vegetations are characteristic lesions of infective endocarditis. MacCallum patch is observed in the posterior wall of the left atrium and verrucae develop along the line of closure in rheumatic fever. Calcified aortic stenosis occurs at an older age.
5. **The answer is D: *Streptococcus viridans*.** Prolonged fever, heart murmur, mild splenomegaly, and splinter hemorrhage are suggestive of infective endocarditis. The time course of 3 weeks suggests subacute bacterial endocarditis due to infection with a less virulent organism, such as *Streptococcus viridans*. Coxsackievirus B causes myocarditis. Tuberculosis involving the heart usually produces pericarditis. *Pseudomonas aeruginosa* is more likely to cause acute bacterial endocarditis that worsens over days, not weeks.

CHAPTER 17

Respiratory Disorders

CHAPTER OUTLINE

- Pneumonia
- Lung Abscess
- Obstructive Lung Diseases
- Tuberculosis
- Sarcoidosis
- Pneumoconioses
- Lung Tumors
- Metastatic Tumors
- Miscellaneous
- Pleural Tumor

PNEUMONIA

PA 26.1 (CC): Define and describe the etiology, types, pathogenesis, stages, morphology, and complications of pneumonia.

Introduction: Respiratory tract infections are the most frequent infections. In pulmonary infections, the causative agents may enter the lung parenchyma by following routes and mechanisms:

- **Through the respiratory tract:**
  - **Aspiration of oropharyngeal contents:** Most frequent.
  - **Inhalation of aerosolized droplets:** Second most frequent.
- **Hematogenous spread**: Bloodstream infection is less common.
- **Local spread.**

Definition: Pneumonia is defined as an **infection of the lung parenchyma.** It causes the alveoli to be filled with inflammatory exudates and **usually results in consolidation** (solidification) of the lung.

Classification of Pneumonia (Box 17.1)

Q. Classify pneumonia.

Community-Acquired Acute Pneumonia

Definition: Community-acquired pneumonia is **lung infection in healthy individuals** and infection is **acquired from the normal environment.**

Etiology and Pathogenesis of Pneumonia

Q. Etiology and pathogenesis of pneumonia.

The lung parenchyma is normally sterile because of several immune and nonimmune defense mechanisms. These mechanisms are observed throughout the respiratory system from the nasopharynx to the alveolar air spaces. Despite these, the lung is susceptible to infection because (1) many microbes are airborne and inhaled into the lungs; (2) even in healthy individuals, nasopharyngeal flora is subjected to regular aspiration during sleep; and (3) lung diseases usually lower local immune defenses.

Causative microorganisms (Box 17.1): These may be bacteria or viruses. Bacterial infection of the lung parenchyma **causes the alveoli to be filled with an inflammatory exudate, producing consolidation** (solidification) of the pulmonary parenchyma.

Factors favoring the development of pneumonia: These are as follows:

- **Lowered systemic resistance of the host:** It may be due to:
  - **Chronic diseases**
  - **Inherited or acquired immunological defects**: These may be in (a) innate immunity (including neutrophil and complement defects), (b) humoral (adaptive) immunity, and (c) cell-mediated immunity.
  - **Treatment with immunosuppressive agents.**
  - **Leukopenia.**
- **Impaired local defense mechanisms:**
  - **Loss or suppression of the cough reflex:** It is observed in conditions such as **coma, anesthesia, drugs, chest pain**, or neuromuscular disorders. It may lead to aspiration of gastric contents into the lung.
  - **Damage or injury to the mucociliary apparatus:** It may be due to **cigarette smoke** (also impairs the function of pulmonary macrophages)**, viral diseases, inhalation of hot or corrosive gases,** or genetic defects of ciliary function (e.g., the immotile cilia syndrome).

BOX 17.1: Classification of pneumonia based on the clinical setting and examples of causative pathogens.

Community-acquired bacterial pneumonia
- *Streptococcus pneumoniae or pneumococcus* (most common cause)
- *Haemophilus influenzae* (the most common bacterial cause of COPD)
- *Moraxella catarrhalis (in elderly)*
- *Staphylococcus aureus* (secondary bacterial pneumonia following viral respiratory illnesses)
- *Legionella pneumophila* (organ transplant recipients)
- *Enterobacteriaceae (Klebsiella pneumoniae* in debilitated and malnourished people) and *Pseudomonas* spp (common in patients with neutropenia)
- *Mycoplasma pneumoniae*

Community-acquired viral pneumonia
- COVID-19 (SARS-CoV-2), respiratory syncytial virus, human metapneumovirus, parainfluenza virus (children); influenza A and B (adults); adenovirus

Healthcare-associated pneumonia
- *Staphylococcus aureus,* methicillin-sensitive or methicillin-resistant
- *Pseudomonas aeruginosa*
- *Streptococcus pneumoniae*

Hospital-acquired (nosocomial) pneumonia
- Gram-negative rods belonging to Enterobacteriaceae (*Klebsiella* spp., *Serratia marcescens, Escherichia coli)* and *Pseudomonas* spp.
- *Staphylococcus aureus* (usually methicillin-resistant): commonest cause

Aspiration pneumonia
- Anaerobic oral flora *(Bacteroides, Prevotella, Fusobacterium, Peptostreptococcus)*, along with aerobic bacteria (*S. pneumoniae, S. aureus, H. influenzae,* and *Pseudomonas aeruginosa)*

Chronic pneumonia
- Nocardia
- Actinomyces
- Granulomatous: *Mycobacterium tuberculosis* and atypical mycobacteria, *Histoplasma capsulatum, Coccidioides immitis, Blastomyces dermatitidis*

Necrotizing pneumonia and lung abscess
- Anaerobic bacteria (extremely common) with or without admixed aerobic infection
- *S. aureus, K. pneumoniae, Streptococcus pyogenes,* and type 3 pneumococcus (uncommon)

Pneumonia in immunocompromised host
- Cytomegalovirus
- *Pneumocystis jirovecii*
- *Mycobacterium avium* complex (MAC)
- Invasive aspergillosis
- Invasive candidiasis
- "Usual" bacterial, viral, and fungal organisms (mentioned above)

Classification based on the anatomic distribution
- Lobar pneumonia
- Bronchopneumonia
- Interstitial pneumonia

(COPD: chronic obstructive pulmonary disease)

- **Accumulation of secretions:** Cystic fibrosis and bronchial obstruction.
- **Interference with the phagocytic or bactericidal action of alveolar macrophages**: It may be due to **alcohol intoxication, tobacco smoke, anoxia, or oxygen intoxication.**
- **Pulmonary congestion and edema.**

❖ **Other predisposing conditions**: These include the following:
- **Extremes of age infants and old age.**
- **Chronic diseases,** e.g., congestive heart failure, COPD, and diabetes.
- **Decreased or absent splenic function,** e.g., sickle cell disease or post-splenectomy (risk for infection with encapsulated bacteria).

Classification of bacterial pneumonia based on the anatomic distribution: Depending on the patterns of anatomic distribution, bacterial pneumonia can be divided into lobar pneumonia and lobular pneumonia (bronchopneumonia). In pneumonias, the term "consolidation" is used frequently for the "solidification" of the lung due to the replacement of the air by an exudate in the alveoli.

❖ **Lobar pneumonia:** It is defined as fibrinosuppurative **consolidation of a large portion of a lobe or an entire lung lobe (Fig. 17.1A).**

❖ **Bronchopneumonia:** It is characterized by **patchy** (scattered solid foci) **area consolidation in the same or several lobes** of the lung **(Fig. 17.1B).**

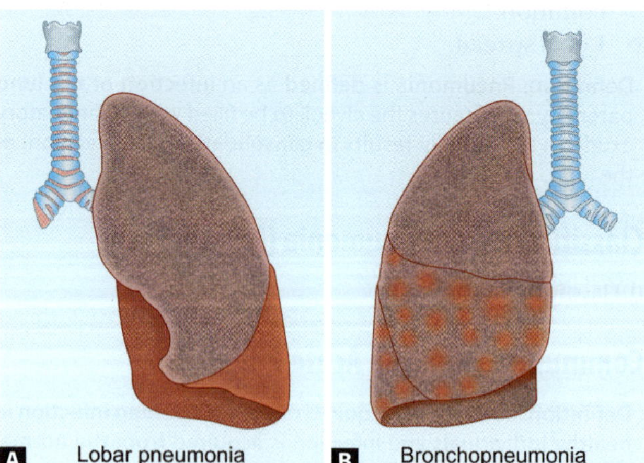

Figs. 17.1A and B: (A) Lobar pneumonia, anatomically involves whole or part of a lobe; (B) Bronchopneumonia, anatomically shows patchy area of consolidation.

These two anatomic patterns may overlap in the same lung. The same organisms may produce either pattern, which depends on the susceptibility of the patient. Identifying the causative agent and the extent of the disease is important.

MORPHOLOGY

Lobar Pneumonia

Q. Write a short note on the lung's morphology (stages, gross and microscopic features) in lobar pneumonia.

Lobar pneumonia is characterized by **diffuse inflammation** affecting the **part or entire lobe, usually the lower lobes (Fig. 17.1A).**

Morphological Stages

The inflammatory response is classically divided into four stages: **(i) Congestion, (ii) red hepatization, (iii) gray hepatization, and (iv) resolution (Box 17.2).**

Congestion

It is the first stage that lasts for less than 24 hours.

Gross: The involved lobe of the lung is **heavy, boggy, wet, and red. A blood-stained frothy fluid oozes from the cut surface.**

Microscopy: It is characterized by:

- **Dilatation and congestion of capillaries** in the alveolar walls.
- The air spaces in the **alveoli are filled with pale eosinophilic fluid with few neutrophils, red cells, and numerous bacteria.**

Red Hepatization

It is the next stage and lasts for 2–3 days.

Gross: The lobe appears distinctly red, firm, and airless. The firm consistency of the affected lobe of the lung resembles that of the liver. The cut section shows a red and granular appearance. Thus, this stage has been termed red hepatization (red in color and consistency like the liver). **The pleura may show serofibrinous pleurisy.**

Microscopy (Figs. 17.2A and B):

- **Alveoli** show **exudate** and interlacing strands of fibrin (formed from clotted fibrinogen present in fluid exudate)
- **Numerous neutrophils** and **red cells** are found in the fibrin meshwork.

Gray Hepatization

It is the third stage and is seen in 5–7 days

Gross (Fig. 17.3A): The affected lobe gradually loses its red color and appears grayish brown. In this stage also the involved region **is firm in consistency and resembles that of the liver. The cut surface shows a gray, dry, and granular appearance.** Hence has been termed gray hepatization (gray in color and consistency like the liver).

Microscopy (Figs. 17.3B and C):

- **Progressive disintegration of red cells.**
- **Fibrinosuppurative exudate in the alveoli** in which **neutrophils are replaced by macrophages.**
- There is a **clear space between the alveolar wall and the exudate** due to the contraction of the fibrin thread (formed from fibrinogen in the exudate) present in the exudate.

Resolution

It occurs by 8–9 days of infection. Resolution occurs by **liquefaction** of the previously **solid, fibrinous constituents of the exudate in the air spaces.** The fibrinous exudate within the air spaces undergoes progressive digestion to produce granular and semifluid debris. The liquefaction is due to fibrinolytic enzymes liberated from neutrophils. The liquefied material is **removed, partly by expectoration,** but mainly **ingested by macrophages** and drained through lymphatics. **If not removed, it may become organized** by ingrowth of capillaries and fibroblasts into the exudate.

Gross: The **affected lobe becomes more crepitant** as the air spaces reopen. The cut section appears frothy.

Microscopy: The alveolar space shows granular material and semifluid debris.

BOX 17.2: Four stages of lobar pneumonia.

1. Congestion
2. Red hepatization
3. Gray hepatization
4. Resolution

MORPHOLOGY

Bronchopneumonia

Q. Write a short note on bronchopneumonia.

It affects extremes of age (infants or old).

Gross (Fig. 17.1B)

- Bronchopneumonia is characterized by **widespread** focal/**patchy areas** of **acute suppurative inflammation.**
- The consolidation **may be restricted to one lobe** but is **more commonly multilobar and frequently bilateral. They are larger and more numerous in the lower lobes (basal).** This is because of the tendency of secretions to gravitate to the lower lobes.
- They are **centered on bronchioles and bronchi** with subsequent spread to surrounding alveoli. The involved alveoli show **consolidation.**
- **Cut section**: It appears slightly **raised above the surface of the surrounding lung** and measures several millimeters in diameter. They are **dry, solid, granular, gray-red to yellow, and poorly delimited at their margins.**

Microscopy

The bronchi, bronchioles, and adjacent alveolar spaces are filled with exudate rich in neutrophils **(Fig. 17.4).**

Complications of Pneumonia (Box 17.3)

Q. Write a short note on complications of pneumonia.

1. **Lung abscess:** Pneumonia may undergo extensive tissue destruction and necrosis resulting in lung abscess.
2. **Organization:** Delayed and incomplete resolution can cause **ingrowth of granulation tissue into the alveolar**

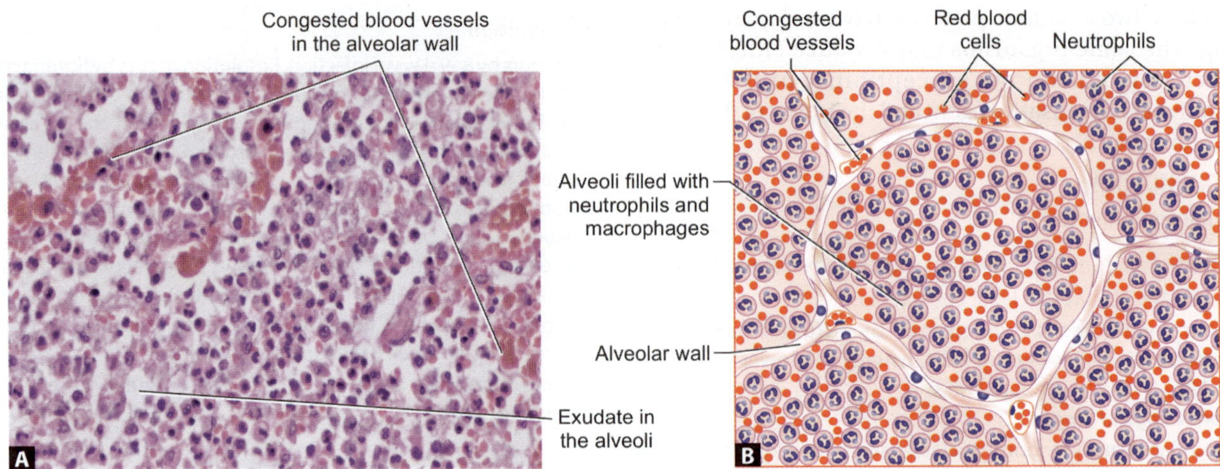

Figs. 17.2A and B: (A) Red hepatization in lobar pneumonia (H and E); (B) Diagrammatic.

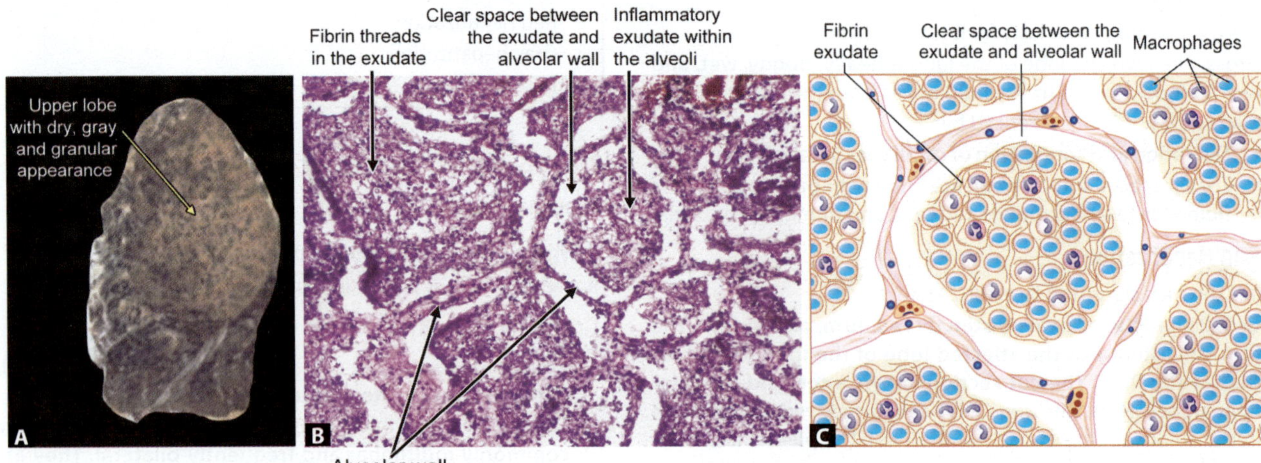

Figs. 17.3A to C: Gray hepatization of lung: (A) Gross appearance; (B) (H&E); (C) Microscopic appearance (diagrammatic).

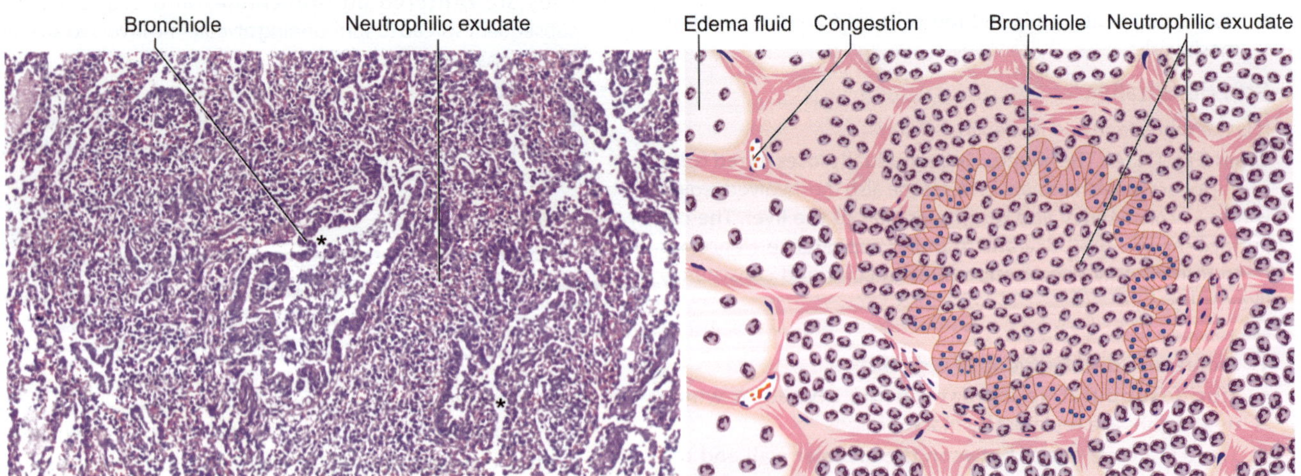

Fig. 17.4: Bronchopneumonia characterized by infiltration of bronchi, bronchioles, and adjacent alveoli by acute inflammatory exudate.

BOX 17.3: Complications of pneumonia.

- Lung abscess
- Organization
- Spread of infection to the pleural cavity
- Bacteremic dissemination (bacteremia)

exudate. The intra-alveolar plugs of granulation tissue are known as organizing pneumonia. Gradually, **increased alveolar fibrosis leads to a shrunken and firm lobe, and is called carnification.**

3. **Spread of infection to the pleural cavity**: It may result in:
   - **Pleuritis** (inflammation of the pleura) due to extension of inflammation from the lung. It may resolve or more often undergoes organization, and fibrous thickening or permanent adhesions.
   - **Pleural effusion** (fluid in the pleural space) is common and usually resolves.
   - **Pyothorax (pus in the pleural space):** It results from an infection of a pleural effusion and may heal with extensive fibrosis.
   - **Empyema:** It is a loculated collection of pus (intra-pleural fibrinosuppurative reaction) with fibrous walls and may result from the persistence of pyothorax.
4. **Bacteremic dissemination (bacteremia):** It can cause:
   - **Endocarditis (heart valves).**
   - **Pericarditis (pericardium).**
   - **Meningitis (meninges).**
   - **Metastatic abscesses in kidneys or spleen.**
   - **Suppurative arthritis (joint).**

Clinical Features

The major symptoms of typical community-acquired acute bacterial pneumonia are as follows:

- **Sudden onset of high fever, chills, and cough** with **mucopurulent (or rusty) sputum.**
- If fibrinosuppurative pleuritis is present, it causes pleuritic pain and accompanied by pleural friction rub.
- **Radiography:** It is the **gold standard** for diagnosing pneumonia. The **involved lobe appears radiopaque in lobar pneumonia and focal opacities in bronchopneumonia.**
- Positive Gram stain on sputum is more useful than culture.

Differences between lobar pneumonia and bronchopneumonia are depicted in **Table 17.1**.

Q. Differences between lobar pneumonia and bronchopneumonia.

SCENARIO-BASED ESSAY QUESTION

Q. A 63-year-old male complained of fever with chills and rigors, fatigue, increasingly severe productive cough, with rusty sputum for the last 5 days. On examination, crepitations and rhonchi were heard on the lower lobe of the left lung. He was treated in the hospital and was completely recovered.

a. What is the probable diagnosis? (Ans: Lobar pneumonia)
b. Which is the most common causative bacteria? *(refer Box 17.1)*.

TABLE 17.1 Differences between lobar pneumonia and bronchopneumonia.

Feature	*Lobar pneumonia*	*Bronchopneumonia*
Definition	Diffuse inflammation affecting the part or the entire lobe/s (usually lower lobes)	Widespread focal/patchy area of acute suppurative infection of terminal bronchioles extending into adjoining alveoli
Age group affected	More common in adults	Commonly develops at extremes of age (infants and old age)
Predisposing factors	Usually develops in healthy individuals	Usually accompany pre-existing diseases (e.g., chronic debility influenza)
Common causative organisms	Pneumococci, *Klebsiella pneumoniae* staphylococci, streptococci	Staphylococci, streptococci, *Pseudomonas*, *Haemophilus influenzae*
Pathologic features	Usually passes through four stages, namely (i) congestion, (ii) red hepatization, (iii) gray hepatization, and (iv) resolution	Patchy consolidation. Bronchi, bronchioles, and adjacent alveolar spaces are filled with exudate rich in neutrophils
Blood findings	Neutrophilic leukocytosis and positive blood culture	Neutrophilic leukocytosis, positive blood culture
X-ray	Shows consolidation	Shows mottled focal opacities
Complications	Less common and include pleural effusion, empyema, lung abscess	Bronchiectasis and complications similar to lobar pneumonia
Response to treatment	Better	Variable
Prognosis	Good	Poor

c. **Describe the gross and microscopic features of the lung in various stages of this condition** *(refer page 543).*
d. **What are the likely complications?** *(refer pages 543-5).*

Community-acquired Viral Pneumonia

Q. Write a short note on community-acquired pneumonia.

Etiology (*refer* Box 17.1): Before the COVID-19 pandemic, the most common causes of community-acquired viral pneumonia were influenza virus types A and B, the respiratory syncytial viruses, human metapneumovirus, adenovirus, rhinoviruses, rubeola, and varicella viruses. During the year 2020, SARS-CoV-2 (the agent of COVID-19), became the leading cause of community-acquired viral pneumonia.

Predisposing factors for the extension of the infection into the lower respiratory tract include **extremes of age, malnutrition, alcoholism, and underlying debilitating illnesses.**

Pathogenesis

- **Damage to respiratory lining cells:** The viruses causing community-acquired pneumonia have an affinity to attach and enter respiratory lining cells. Viral replication leads to cytopathic changes, leading to the death of cells and secondary inflammation. Then the process extends to the alveoli and causes interstitial inflammation.
- **Secondary bacterial infection:** The damage produced by the virus impairs the local pulmonary defensive forces (e.g., mucociliary clearance) and predisposes to superinfection by bacteria. Thus, secondary bacterial infection usually becomes more serious than the viral infection itself.

MORPHOLOGY

Gross

The lung may show either patchy or involvement of entire lobes bilaterally or unilaterally. The affected region appears red-blue and congested. Pleuritis or pleural effusions are infrequent.

Microscopy

Depends on the severity of the disease.

- **Interstitial inflammatory reaction:** Involvement of the alveolar walls by inflammatory cells is the **predominant feature.** The alveolar septa show widening, edema and mononuclear inflammatory infiltrate composed of lymphocytes, macrophages, and occasionally plasma cells. In acute cases, neutrophils may also be seen.
- The alveoli may show intra-alveolar proteinaceous material and a cellular exudate. If a patient develops ARDS, pink hyaline membranes may form lining the alveolar walls.
- Eradication of the viral infection results in resolution and return of the normal lung architecture.
- If there is superimposed bacterial infection, ulcerative bronchitis, bronchiolitis, and bacterial pneumonia may develop.

Clinical Course

Extremely varied. Many present as severe upper respiratory tract infections with fever, headache, muscle aches, and pains in the legs. Cough may be absent. Usually, viral infections are mild and resolve spontaneously without any sequelae. However, interstitial viral pneumonia may assume epidemic proportions and can lead to morbidity and mortality.

Hospital-acquired Pneumonia

Definition: Hospital-acquired (nosocomial) pneumonia are pulmonary infection acquired in the course of a hospital stay.

Predisposing factors: Severe underlying disease, immunosuppression, prolonged antibiotic therapy, patients on mechanical ventilation, or invasive access devices, such as intravascular catheters. The hospital-acquired pneumonia is serious and may be life-threatening.

The common causative organisms causing hospital-acquired pneumonia are listed in **Box 17.1.**

Pneumonia in the Immunocompromised Host

Pneumocystis Pneumoniae

Q. Write a short answer on *Pneumocystis pneumoniae*.

- Pneumocystis pneumonia is an opportunistic fungal infection of the lungs by inhalation of ***Pneumocystis jirovecii.***
- It usually **infects neonates and immunosuppressed individuals** (HIV/AIDS, immunosuppression by chemotherapy for organ transplants and tumors, malnutrition, agammaglobulinemia, etc.). In HIV, *Pneumocystis pneumoniae* usually develops when the CD4+ count is <200 cells/mm^3.

MORPHOLOGY

Gross

The affected parts of the lung are consolidated, dry, and gray.

Microscopy

- Interstitial pneumonitis with thickening and mononuclear infiltration of the alveolar walls.
- Alveoli contain **pink frothy fluid** with the organisms. On staining by **Grocott's methenamine-silver (GMS) stain,** they appear as oval or crescentic cysts, about 5 µm in diameter, and **surrounded by numerous tiny black dotlike organisms.** *P. jirovecii* is demonstrable in the frothy fluid.
- No significant inflammatory reaction in the air spaces.

Clinical Course

- Rapid onset of dyspnea, tachycardia, cyanosis, and nonproductive cough. Chest X-ray shows diffuse alveolar and interstitial infiltrate.
- If untreated, death occurs in one or two weeks.

LUNG ABSCESS

PA 26.2 (CC): Describe the etiology, gross and microscopic appearance, and complications of lung access.

Q. Write a short note on lung abscess.

Definition: Lung (pulmonary) abscess is a **local suppurative process within the lung parenchyma with the destruction of lung tissue.** It is characterized by the **formation of one or more large cavities containing pus.**

Etiology and Pathogenesis

Causative organisms: Any pathogen can produce lung abscesses. It is usually due to aerobic and anaerobic organisms normally found in the oral cavity (gram-negative organisms). Mixed infections occur when lung abscess develops due to inhalation of foreign material. Various agents causing lung abscess are:

- **Common: Anaerobic bacteria** (extremely common), with or without mixed aerobic infection. The most frequent anaerobes are commensals normally found in the oral cavity. They include *Prevotella, Fusobacterium, Bacteroides, Peptostreptococcus,* and microaerophilic streptococci.
- **Uncommon:** *Staphylococcus aureus, Klebsiella pneumoniae, Streptococcus pyogenes,* and type 3 *Pneumococcus.*

Pathogenesis

A lung abscess may be **primary or secondary**.

Secondary Lung Abscess

It develops as a complication of several conditions. Various **mechanisms** by which causative organisms may be introduced into the lung are as follows:

- **Aspiration of infective material: The infective material may be** from **infected nasal sinuses or tonsils,** periodontitis, or gingivitis. These may be aspirated into the lung during oral surgery, general anesthesia, coma, head injury, or neurological disease causing loss of consciousness, alcoholic intoxication, or in debilitated patients with depressed cough reflexes.
- **Aspiration of gastric contents:** It usually occurs along with infectious organisms from the oropharynx.
- **As a complication of necrotizing pneumonia:** The microbes usually associated are as follows: *S. aureus, Streptococcus pyogenes, K. pneumoniae,* and *Pseudomonas* spp.
- **Bronchial obstruction**: It may be by a **bronchial neoplasm** (primary or secondary) or foreign body (post-obstructive pneumonia). Impaired drainage, distal atelectasis, and aspiration of blood and tumor fragments can lead to the development of abscesses. An abscess also may form within a necrotic region within a tumor. Bronchiectasis may also be complicated by an abscess.
- **Septic embolism**: The source of embolus may be from thrombophlebitis in any part of the systemic venous circulation or from the vegetation of infective bacterial endocarditis on the right side of the heart. The embolus may be trapped in the lung causing multiple pyemic abscesses.
- **Hematogenous spread of bacteria:** Disseminated pyogenic infection (e.g., staphylococcal bacteremia) may produce lung abscess and often results in multiple lung abscesses.
- **Miscellaneous:** These include direct penetrating trauma to the lungs, and the spread of infections from neighboring organs (e.g., suppuration in the esophagus, spine, subphrenic space, or pleural cavity).

Primary Cryptogenic Lung Abscesses

These types of lung abscesses have no apparent cause for the abscess formation. These are termed *primary cryptogenic lung abscesses.*

MORPHOLOGY

Gross (Fig. 17.5)

- **Location and number:** Lung abscess may develop in **any part of the lung** and may be **single or multiple.** The location and number of abscesses depend on the mode of development of the abscess.
  - Abscess due to **aspiration** are more common on the **right** (because of the more vertical right main bronchus) and are most often **single.** They usually occur in the posterior segment of the right upper lobe and the apical segments of the right lower lobe. These locations are the sites of aspirated material in a recumbent individual.
  - Abscesses that complicate **pneumonia or bronchiectasis** are usually **multiple, basal, and diffusely scattered.**
  - **Septic emboli** and pyemic abscesses are **multiple** and may affect **any region** of the lungs.
- **Size: Vary from a few millimeters to large cavities measuring** 5–6 cm.
- **Content:** Abscess cavity may contain **suppurative debris.**
  - If **communication** with an air passage, the abscess may be partially drained to produce an **air-containing cavity.**
  - **Continued infection** may result in **gangrene of the lung.**

Microscopy

- **Cardinal feature: It is characterized by suppurative destruction of the lung parenchyma within the central area of cavitation.**
- Abscess shows **numerous polymorphonuclear leukocytes** and variable numbers of **macrophages.** The abscess is **surrounded by a fibrous wall infiltrated by inflammatory cells (lymphocytes, plasma cells).**

Clinical Course

- Like bronchiectasis, it is characterized by a **prominent cough**, **fever**, and **large amounts of foul-smelling purulent or sanguineous sputum**.

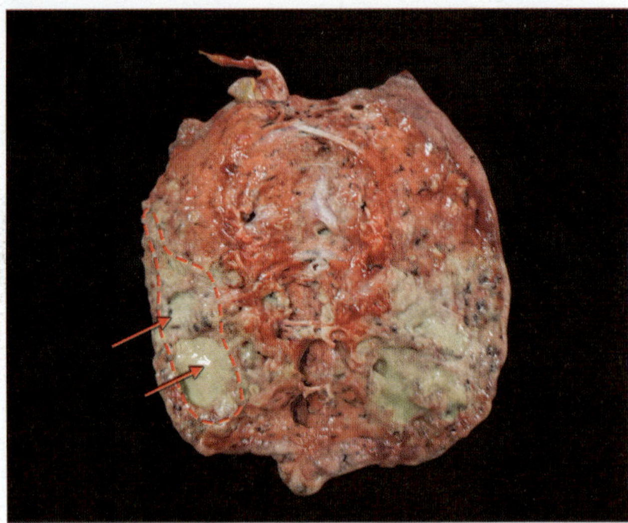

Fig. 17.5: Lung with suppurative abscess (arrows).

- **Fever, chest pain, and weight loss** are common.
- **Clubbing of the fingers and toes** may appear. Lung abscess in older individuals may be associated with carcinoma.

Complications

- **Extension of the infection into the pleural cavity** leading to **empyema/pneumothorax/bronchopleural fistula.**
- **Hemorrhage into the abscess cavity.**
- **Septic emboli** may cause **brain abscesses or meningitis.**
- **Secondary amyloidosis** (type AA).

OBSTRUCTIVE LUNG DISEASES

PA 26.3 (CC): Define and describe the etiology, types, pathogenesis, stages, morphology, complications, and evaluation of obstructive airway disease (OAD).

Introduction: Diffuse pulmonary diseases are classified into two categories:

1. **Obstructive (airway) disease:** It is characterized by an **increase in resistance to airflow.** It is caused by **partial or complete obstruction** at any level in the respiratory tract.
2. **Restrictive disease:** It is characterized by **reduced expansion of lung parenchyma, and decreased total lung capacity.**

Q. Define and enumerate chronic obstructive pulmonary diseases.

Definition: Chronic obstructive pulmonary/lung disease (COPD) is defined as a disease state characterized by airflow limitation that is not fully reversible. It is also called obstructive lung (airway) disease.

Obstructive lung (airway) diseases (OAD): The four major diffuse obstructive disorders are **(i) emphysema, (ii) chronic bronchitis, (iii) asthma, and (iv) bronchiectasis.** The expiratory flow rate in the lung is measured by forced expiratory volume at 1 second (FEV_1). In these patients, the forced expiratory volume at 1 second (FEV_1), is markedly decreased. But forced vital capacity (FVC) is either normal or slightly decreased. Thus, the ratio of FEV_1 to FVC (FEV_1/FVC) is decreased. Usually, an FEV_1/FVC ratio of less than 0.7 indicates obstructive disease. Expiratory obstruction due to airway narrowing occurs in asthma or from loss of elastic recoil in emphysema. Two diseases namely (i) emphysema and (ii) chronic bronchitis are grouped under **chronic obstructive pulmonary disease (COPD).**

World Health Organization (WHO) definition of chronic obstructive pulmonary disease (COPD): COPD is a common, preventable, and treatable disease that is characterized by persistent respiratory symptoms and airflow limitation that is due to airway and/or alveolar abnormalities caused by exposure to noxious particles or gases.

Emphysema

Q. Define emphysema. Write the types of emphysema and describe its pathogenesis.

Emphysema is defined based on morphological and radiological features. Different parts of the airway are presented in **Figures 17.6A and B.** In the lung, acinus is the structure distal to terminal bronchioles, and a cluster of three to five acini is termed a *lobule*.

Definition: Emphysema is a **chronic lung disease** characterized by **abnormal irreversible (permanent) enlargement (dilatation) of the airspaces distal to the terminal bronchioles.** This is **associated with the destruction of their walls but without obvious fibrosis.** Recent evidence shows that small airway fibrosis contributes to airflow obstruction.

Q. Classify/mention the types of emphysema.

Types (classification) of emphysema (Figs. 17.6B to F and Box 17.4): Emphysema is **classified according to its anatomic distribution** (location of the lesions) within the lobule into **four major types:** (i) centriacinar, (ii) panacinar, (iii) distal acinar (paraseptal), and (iv) irregular.

1. **Centriacinar (centrilobular) emphysema:** Enlargement (dilatation) **involves the central or proximal parts of the acini** (formed by respiratory bronchioles), whereas distal alveoli are not involved. Thus, **both emphysematous and normal airspaces are present within the same acinus and lobule.**
   - **Location:** It is more common and severe in the **upper lobes,** especially in the **apical segments.**
   - **Association:** Occurs in **heavy smokers** and in association with **chronic bronchitis** and **coal-worker's pneumoconiosis.** The walls of the emphysema often show **black pigment. Inflammation around the bronchi and bronchioles** is common.
2. **Panacinar (panlobular) emphysema: All the airspaces beyond the terminal bronchiole** (from the level of the respiratory bronchiole to the terminal blind alveoli) are more or less **uniformly/equally dilated.**

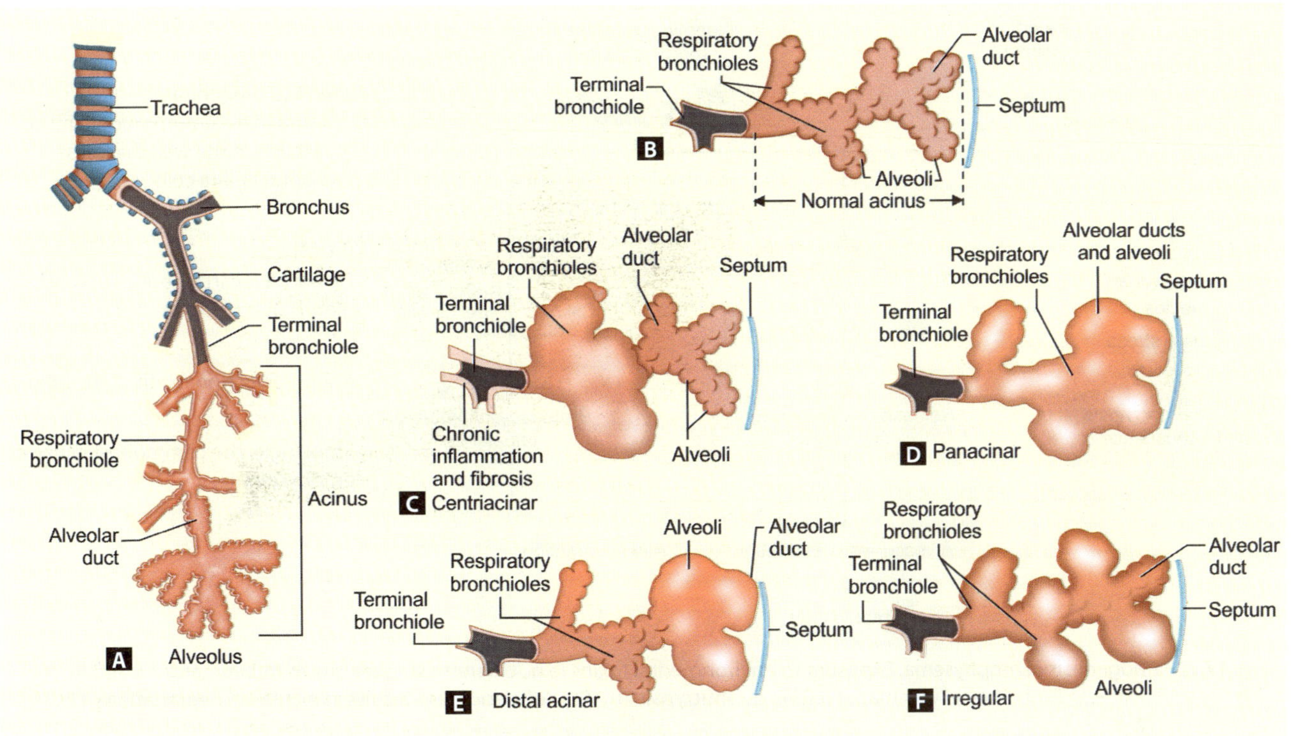

Figs. 17.6A to F: Four major types of emphysema: (A and B) Normal; (C) Centriacinar; (D) Panacinar; (E) Distal acinar; (F) Irregular emphysema

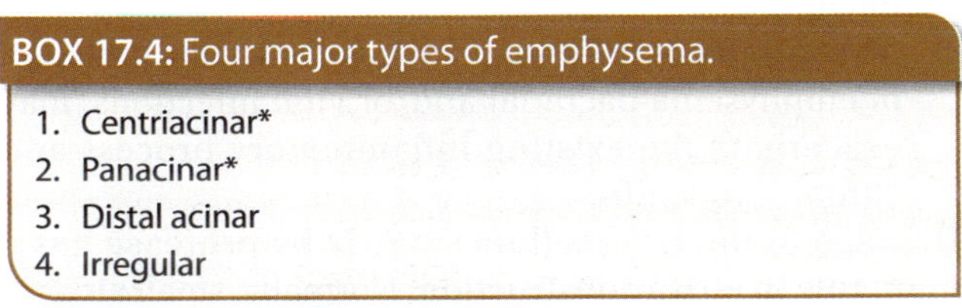
BOX 17.4: Four major types of emphysema.

1. Centriacinar*
2. Panacinar*
3. Distal acinar
4. Irregular

*Only these are associated with COPD (chronic obstructive pulmonary disease)

- **Location:** In contrast to centriacinar emphysema, it is more common in the **lower lobes**, and is usually **most severe at the bases.**
- **Association:** It is associated with **α_1-antitrypsin (α_1-AT) deficiency.**

3. **Distal acinar (paraseptal) emphysema:** Dilatation affects the **distal airspace** at the periphery of the lobule and the proximal portion is normal.
   - **Location:** More commonly **adjacent to septa, pleura,** along the lobular connective tissue septa, and at the **margins of the lobules. More severe in the upper half of the lungs.**
   - **Association:** It results from forces pulling on the septa and occurs **adjacent to fibrosis, scarring, or atelectasis areas.**
   - **Dimension**: It forms multiple, enlarged airspaces ranging **from less than 0.5 to more than 2.0 cm in diameter. Dilated spaces of more than 1 cm in size** are known as **bullae** (*refer* **Fig.17.8B**) which may rupture and cause spontaneous pneumothorax.
4. **Irregular (scar or cicatricial) emphysema:** Acinus is **irregularly involved** and may be asymptomatic.
   - **Most common form** of emphysema.
   - **Association: Occurs near the scar** and is commonly found **around old healed inflammatory processes like tuberculous scars.**

Etiology and Pathogenesis (Fig. 17.7)

Q. Write a short note on the etiopathogenesis of emphysema.

A clear-cut association between heavy cigarette smoking and the development of emphysema is observed. Inhaled **cigarette smoke and other toxic substances** produce **damage to the lung and produce inflammation**, particularly in patients with a **genetic predisposition.** This leads to the destruction of the lung parenchyma (emphysema) and disease of the airway (bronchiolitis and chronic bronchitis). The major event in emphysema is the destruction of the alveolar wall. Factors involved in the pathogenesis of emphysema are as follows:

1. **Inflammatory cells and mediators:**
   - **Inflammatory mediators:** Many inflammatory mediators are released in the lung [e.g., leukotriene B4, the chemokine IL-8, the cytokine tumor necrosis factor (TNF), and others]. The sources of these mediators are resident epithelial cells and macrophages.

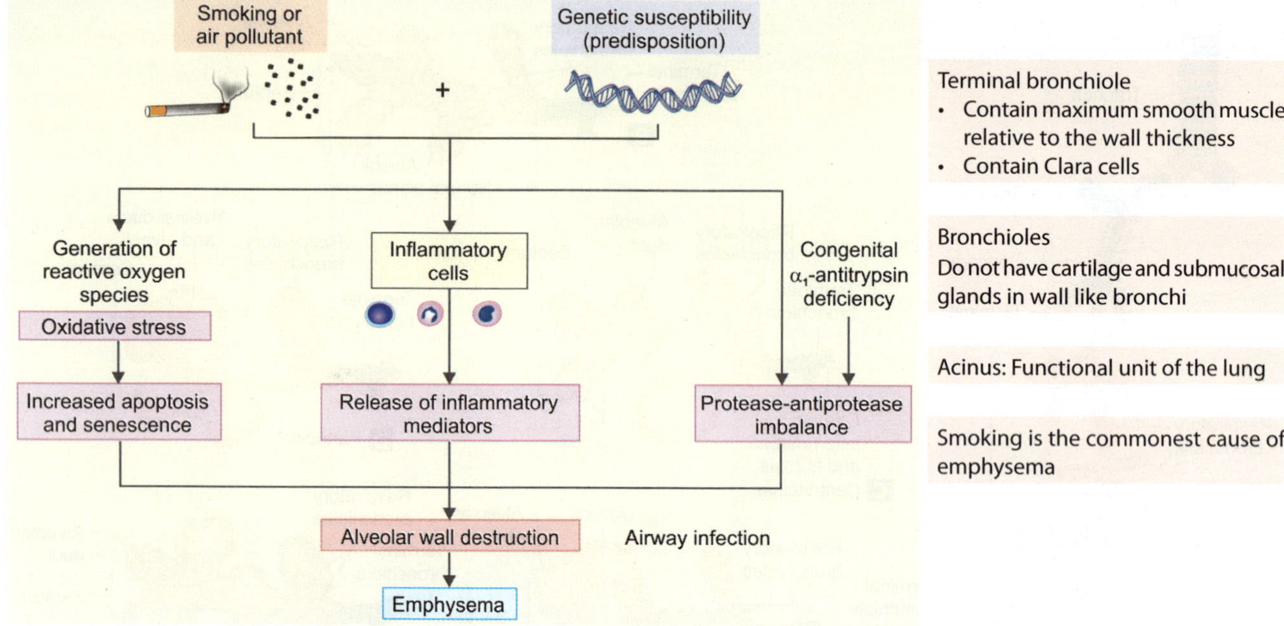

Terminal bronchiole
- Contain maximum smooth muscle relative to the wall thickness
- Contain Clara cells

Bronchioles
Do not have cartilage and submucosal glands in wall like bronchi

Acinus: Functional unit of the lung

Smoking is the commonest cause of emphysema

Fig. 17.7: Pathogenesis of emphysema. Exposure to environmental toxins (e.g., cigarette smoke) causes inflammatory reactions, cell death, and proteolysis of extracellular matrix (ECM). α_1-antitrypsin (α_1-AT) deficiency also results in increased degradation of ECM.

- **Attraction of inflammatory cells:** Chemotactic factors (e.g., leukotriene) attract inflammatory cells from the circulation and proinflammatory cytokines exaggerate the inflammatory process. They produce structural changes. The inflammatory cells include neutrophils, macrophages, and CD4+ and CD8+ T cells.

2. **Protease-antiprotease imbalance:** Injury (e.g., by smoking or other toxic substances) activates and favors the accumulation of inflammatory cells (e.g., neutrophils) and damages the epithelial cells. This leads to the **local release of proteases by inflammatory cells and damaged epithelial cells**. The proteases can damage the connective tissue. Normally, the damage by proteases is prevented by antiprotease (e.g., α_1-antitrypsin is a major inhibitor of proteases). About 1% of patients with emphysema have a deficiency of protective antiproteases.
   - **Genetic deficiency of α_1-antitrypsin:** α_1-antitrypsin is normally present in serum, tissue fluids, and macrophages. A balance is maintained between protease and antiproteases. α_1-antitrypsin is encoded by a gene in the proteinase inhibitor (*Pi*) locus on chromosome 14. The *Pi* locus is polymorphic, and individuals homozygous for the Z allele, have markedly decreased serum levels of α_1-antitrypsin. This deficiency is inherited as an autosomal recessive disorder. In these patients with the absence of α_1-antitrypsin activity, there is excessive digestion of elastic tissues which produces emphysema. The damage is aggravated by smoking.
3. **Oxidative stress:** Reactive oxygen species and other substances in cigarette smoke, stimulate the release of additional reactive oxygen species from inflammatory cells such as macrophages and neutrophils. These cause damage to the alveoli (apoptosis) and aggravate inflammation.
4. **Airway infection:** Though not involved in the initiation of emphysema bacterial and/or viral infections, may exacerbate the existing inflammatory process and chronic bronchitis.

Damage to the extracellular matrix by protease has a main role in airway obstruction. Normally, small airways are held open by the elastic recoil of the lung parenchyma. **Small airway obstruction in emphysema** is due to the loss of elastic tissue in the walls of the alveoli that surround respiratory bronchioles. Small airway inflammation may narrow the bronchiolar lumen.

MORPHOLOGY

The diagnosis and classification of emphysema is mainly by the macroscopic appearance of the lung. Emphysema can easily be seen on the cut surface of formalin-inflated fixed lung.

Gross (Figs. 17.8A to C)

- Usually, **the upper two-thirds of the lungs** are more severely involved than the lower lungs.
- **Bullae** are found in irregular and distal acinar emphysema.
- Advanced and panacinar emphysema produces **voluminous lungs.**

Microscopy (Figs. 17.9A and B)

- Lung shows **abnormally large alveoli** separated by thin septa without fibrosis. There is the **destruction of alveolar walls** and loss of attachments of the alveoli to the outer wall of small airways. **The pores of Kohn** (interalveolar connections or alveolar pores are discrete holes in walls of adjacent alveoli) **are enlarged.**

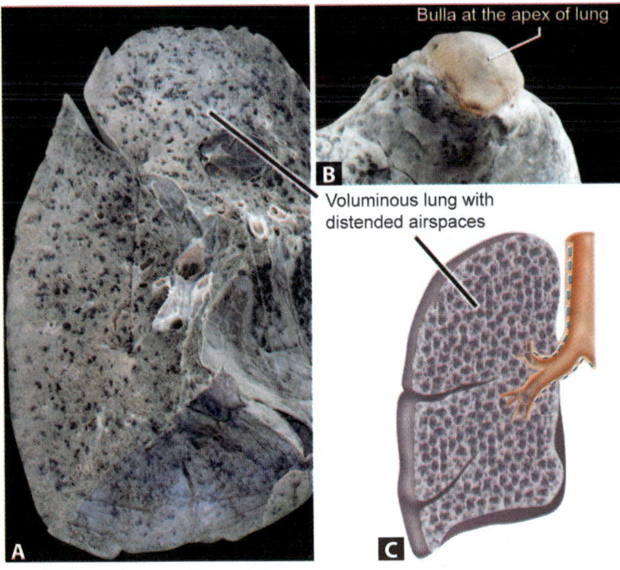

Figs. 17.8A to C: Voluminous lung in emphysema; (A) Cut section shows voluminous lung; (B) Part of lung bulla on the apex of lung; (C) Cut section (diagrammatic).

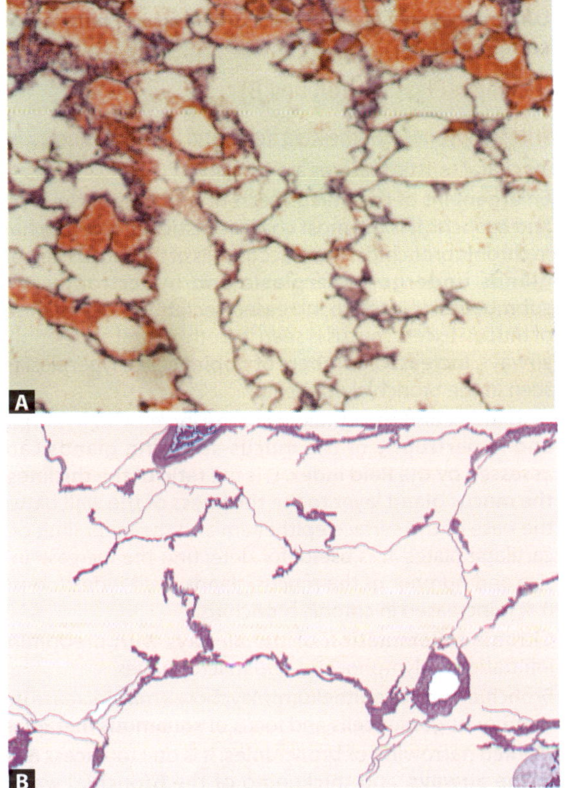

Figs. 17.9A and B: Microscopy of emphysema with destruction of alveolar walls forming large alveoli. (A) H & E; (B) Diagrammatic.

- In advanced disease, **bullae may be seen.**
- There may be inflammatory changes in small airways and submucosal fibrosis in advanced lesions.

Clinical Course

Manifestations appear late until at least one-third of the functioning pulmonary parenchyma is damaged.

- **Dyspnea** begins insidiously and steadily progresses.
- **Cough and expectoration.**
- **Weight loss** is common.

Clinical examination: Barrel-shaped chest, dyspnea with prolonged expiration, and breathes through pursed lips. The expiratory airflow limitation is helpful in diagnosis. The patient sits forward in a hunched-over position.

Complications: (i) **Cor pulmonale,** (ii) **congestive heart failure** due to secondary pulmonary hypertension and (iii) pneumothorax.

Cause of death: (i) Respiratory acidosis and coma, (ii) right-sided heart failure, and (iii) massive collapse of the lungs secondary to pneumothorax.

Other Forms of Emphysema

- **Compensatory hyperinflation: It is characterized by dilation of alveoli without destruction of septal walls.** It develops as a compensatory response to loss of lung substance elsewhere (e.g., removal of a diseased lung or lobe).
- **Bullous emphysema (Fig. 17.8B):** The air**spaces >1 cm in diameter** in the distended state are known as blebs or bullae. They can occur in any type of emphysema. They **may rupture and produce pneumothorax.**
- **Interstitial emphysema:** It is characterized by the **entry of air into the connective tissue stroma** of the lung, mediastinum, or subcutaneous tissue. It may result from alveolar tears in pulmonary emphysema, which occurs during coughing.

Chronic Bronchitis

It is defined on a clinical basis in contrast to emphysema which is defined based on morphologic and radiologic features.

Definition: Chronic bronchitis is defined clinically as **persistent cough with sputum** production (chronic productive cough) **for at least 3 consecutive months in at least 2 consecutive years**, in the absence of any other identifiable cause.

Etiology

- **Cigarette smoking:** It is the most important risk factor and **about 90%** of **chronic bronchitis patients are smokers.**
- **Air pollutants:** Chronic bronchitis is more common in individuals in regions with **significant air pollution** [e.g., sulfur dioxide (SO_2) and nitrogen dioxide].
- **Toxic industrial inhalants:** Occupational dust exposure.
- **Respiratory tract infection:** It may initiate and promote chronic bronchitis.

Pathogenesis (Flowchart 17.1)

Q. Discuss the pathogenesis of chronic bronchitis.

- **Irritation by inhaled air pollutants:** The initiating factor is irritation of large airway mucosa by inhaled air pollutants, such as **tobacco smoke** (90% of patients are smokers), **dust, cotton, sulfur dioxide, nitrogen dioxide,** and **silica.** Irritants cause **inflammation and infiltration by CD8+ T lymphocytes, macrophages, and neutrophils.**
- **Hypersecretion of mucus: It begins in the large airways and is the distinctive feature of chronic bronchitis.** The environmental irritants produce the following changes:
  - **Hyperplasia/hypertrophy of the submucosal glands** in **large airways (trachea and bronchi):** Develops in response to inhaled **environmental irritants** and **proteases released from neutrophils** (e.g., elastase, cathepsin histamine, and IL-13). This leads to **hypersecretion of mucus.**
  - **Marked increase of mucin-secreting goblet cells in small airways (small bronchi and bronchioles): They produce excessive mucus secretion and mucus plugging of the bronchial lumen.** This induces inflammation and fibrosis of the bronchial wall **leading to airway obstruction.**

Both the submucosal gland hypertrophy and the increase in goblet cells are thought to be protective metaplastic responses against air pollutants (e.g., tobacco smoke, sulfur dioxide, and nitrogen dioxide).

Flowchart 17.1: Pathogenesis of chronic bronchitis.

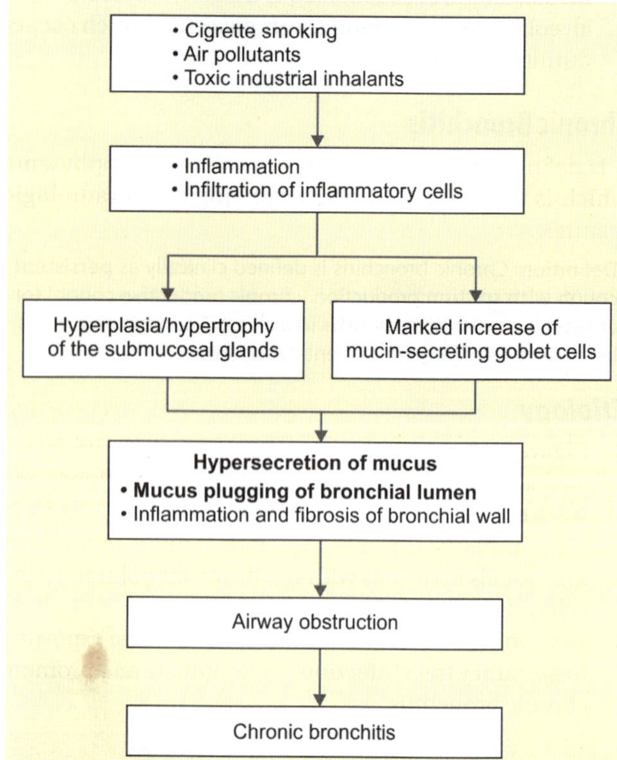

Role of Inflammation

Inhalants producing chronic bronchitis cause damage to cells and cause acute as well as chronic inflammation (neutrophils, lymphocytes, and macrophages). Chronic inflammation and accompanying fibrosis involving small airways can produce chronic airway obstruction.

Role of Infection

- Cigarette smoke predisposes to infection in several ways.
- **Infection may be secondary** rather than primary and probably important in maintaining and producing acute exacerbations.
- **Infection may cause direct damage to airway epithelium** and interfere with ciliary action of the respiratory epithelium and **defective clearance of bacteria** by leukocytes.

MORPHOLOGY

Gross

Airways (large and small) changes include:

- **Mucous membrane:** It shows **hyperemia, swelling, and edema.** It appears dusky red.
- **Lumen:** They are **filled with excessive mucus or mucopurulent secretion.**

Microscopy (Figs. 17.10A and B)

Q. Write a short note on the Reid index and its importance.

Major characteristic features are as follows:

- **Enlargement of the mucus-secreting glands of the trachea and bronchi:** It is the **most characteristic pathologic change in chronic bronchitis.** The mucous cells of the **mucus-secreting glands undergo hyperplasia and hypertrophy in the submucosa.** It leads to increased secretion (hypersecretion) of mucus. Excess mucus is seen in both central and peripheral airways. **Increased numbers of goblet** cells (hyperplasia) are seen in the bronchial epithelium.
- **Reid index and its significance:** The increase in **hyperplasia and hypertrophy of the mucus-secreting glands** can be **assessed by the Reid index.** It is the **ratio of the thickness of the mucus gland layer to** the **thickness of the wall** between the base of the surface epithelium and the inner limit of the cartilage plates. It is useful for detecting the increase in the size and number of the mucus glands. Reid index (normally 0.4) is increased in chronic bronchitis.
- **Chronic inflammation of the airways** with predominant infiltration by lymphocytes and macrophages.
- **Bronchial surface epithelium:** May show a **mild increase in the number of goblet cells** and focus of **squamous metaplasia.**
- **Marked narrowing of bronchioles:** It is due to: **excess mucus in the airways,** and **thickening of the bronchial wall** due to hyperplasia of mucus glands, edema, inflammation, and fibrosis. In severe cases, there may be obliteration of the lumen due to fibrosis **(bronchiolitis obliterans).**

Clinical Features

Usually affects **middle-aged** men who are **heavy smokers. Early symptoms: Persistent productive cough** (sputum) for many years.

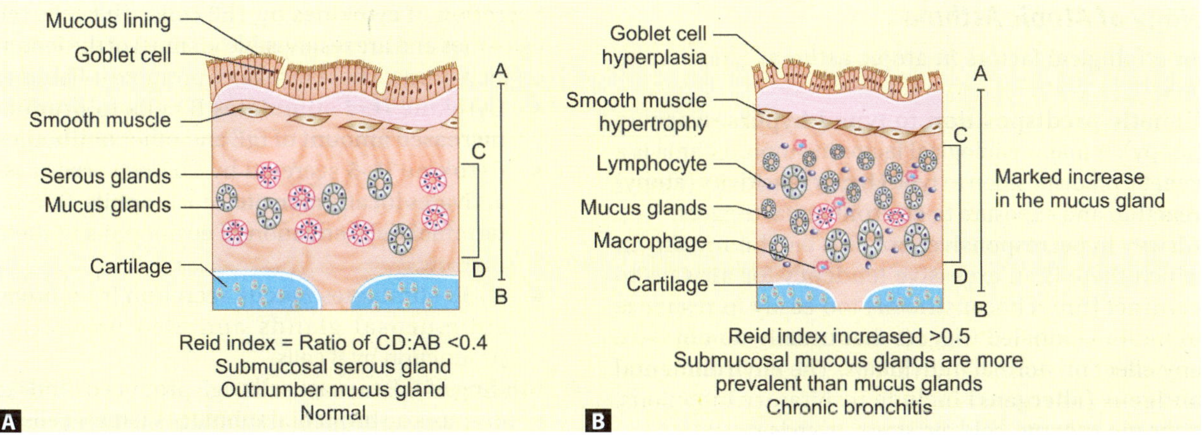

Figs. 17.10A and B: (A) Normal bronchial wall. Normally, airway submucosal serous glands outnumber mucous glands, and the epithelium consists of ciliated cells; (B) Microscopic features of chronic bronchitis. The bronchial submucosa is markedly expanded by hyperplasia of submucosal glands and constitutes more than 50% of the thickness of the bronchial wall. The Reid index is the ratio of the mucus gland layer's thickness to the wall's thickness between the base of the surface epithelium and the inner limit of the cartilage plates. Thus, the Reid index equals the maximum thickness of the bronchial mucus glands internal to the cartilage (C to D) divided by the bronchial wall thickness (A to B).

Later stage: Dyspnea on exertion and less prominent than in "pure" emphysema.

Blue bloaters: Patients develop **hypercapnia, hypoxemia, and mild cyanosis**. Such patients are called 'blue bloaters'.

Pink puffers: These patients have more emphysema than bronchial obstruction. Therefore, they **hyperventilate to produce** a relatively **normal blood gas profile**.

Complications

- Progression to **chronic obstructive pulmonary disease** (COPD).
- Long-standing cases lead to **cor pulmonale** with cardiac failure.
- May develop squamous **metaplasia and dysplasia** of the respiratory epithelium and acts as a rich soil for cancerous transformation.

Asthma

Definition: Asthma is a **heterogeneous, chronic inflammatory disorder** of the bronchial tree (airways) **that causes recurrent episodes of bronchospasm** (reversible bronchoconstriction). It is **clinically characterized by wheezing, breathlessness, tightness of the chest, and cough.**

Asthma is common but is a relatively rare cause of death. It usually develops at night and/or in the early morning. Characteristics features of asthma are listed in **Box 17.5**.

BOX 17.5: Characteristics features of asthma.

- Intermittent (episodes of) reversible airway obstruction (bronchoconstriction). Obstruction of airways may occur either spontaneously or after treatment
- Chronic inflammation of the bronchial wall with eosinophils
- Hypertrophy and hyperreactivity of bronchial smooth muscle cell
- Increased mucus secretion

Classification (Box 17.6)

Q. Classify bronchial asthma.

BOX 17.6: Classification of asthma.

According to the type of antigen:
- **Atopic** (allergic or extrinsic)
- **Non-atopic or intrinsic** (without evidence of allergen sensitization)

According to the agents or events that trigger broncho-constriction:
- Atopic (allergic or extrinsic), also known as seasonal
- Drug-induced (e.g., aspirin)
- Exercise-induced
- Occupational asthma
- Infectious asthma
- Asthmatic bronchitis in smokers

Atopic Asthma

- **It is the most common type** of asthma that usually begins in **childhood.** Atopy is the tendency to produce an exaggerated IGE immune response to an otherwise harmless environmental substance.
- **A family history of asthma or allergic diseases** (e.g., eczema, urticaria, or hay fever) is common.
- It is a classic example of a **type I IgE-mediated hypersensitivity reaction**. IgE antibodies against specific allergens can be recognized.
- **Exogenous substances (allergens)** causing asthma **can be recognized.** Asthmatic attacks are usually preceded by allergic rhinitis, urticaria, or eczema.
- **Triggering environmental allergens**: These include **dust, pollens**, animal dander, foods, or infections.
- **Skin test** with the causative allergen **results in an immediate wheal-and-flare reaction.**

Etiology of Atopic Asthma

Major etiological factors in atopic asthma: These are as follows:

- **Genetic predisposition** to **type I hypersensitivity** (atopy): A major etiological factor in atopic asthma is a genetic predisposition to **type I hypersensitivity (atopy) reaction** and exposure to environmental triggers.
- **Airway hyperresponsiveness**: It is an abnormality in which there is an **excessive tendency for airways to contract** (bronchoconstrictor) too easily in response to multiple inhaled triggers that usually do not have any effect on normal individuals. The **environmental antigens (allergens)** include respiratory infections, airborne irritants, cold air, stress, exercise
- Acute and chronic **airway inflammation. Inflammation** involves many cell types and inflammatory mediators.

Environmental risk factors: Several stimuli trigger asthmatic attacks. These include inhaled allergens, upper respiratory tract viral infections, air pollution, passive smoking, and drugs (e.g., β-adrenergic blockers and aspirin).

Hygiene Hypothesis

It proposes that individuals with a **lack of infections in early childhood** are more prone to asthma than children brought up on farms who are exposed to a high level of endotoxin. Intestinal parasite infection may also be associated with a decreased risk of asthma.

Pathogenesis of Atopic Asthma (Figs. 17.11A to C)

Q. Discuss the pathogenesis of atopic bronchial asthma.

Genetic predisposition: Atopic asthma is the **most common type of disease.** It **develops in genetically predisposed individuals** and is **caused by a Th2-mediated IgE response to environmental allergens.** It is a **classic example of a type I IgE-mediated hypersensitivity reaction.**

- **Gender: More common in boys** than girls and, after puberty, women slightly more commonly than men.
- **Age:** Most cases **begin before the age of 25 years.**

Th2 Responses, IgE, and Inflammation

Exaggerated type 2 helper T (Th2) cell response: The **main abnormality in asthma is a magnified Th2 response to normally harmless environmental antigens or various stimuli**. The various steps in the pathogenesis of atopic asthma are as follows:

Sensitization

- **Sensitization against antigen:** Genetically predisposed individuals are sensitized against many environmental antigens (allergens).
- **Allergen is taken up by dendritic cells:** Inhaled allergen (antigen) is taken by antigen-presenting cells (dendritic cell/macrophage) and **elicits a Th2-dominated response**. This favors the **production of IgE by B cells.**
- **Secretion of cytokines by Th2 cells:** Th2 cells secrete cytokines and are responsible for most of the features of atopic asthma. These cytokines promote inflammation.
  - **Cytokine IL-4 stimulates B cells to produce an increased amount of IgE** and other **antibodies.**
  - **Cytokine IL-5** secreted by Th2 cells **recruits and activates locally recruited eosinophils.** IL-5 causes terminal differentiation of eosinophils in the bone marrow.
  - **IL-13 stimulates mucus secretion** from bronchial submucosal glands and also promotes IgE production by B cells.
- **Binding of IgE to mast cells:** IgE produced binds to the Fc receptors on **bronchial submucosal mast cells**. Thus, mast cells are sensitized to allergens.

On re-exposure

Binding of allergen to IgE antibodies bound to mast cells: When a sensitized individual is **re-exposed to the same allergen** (antigen), the **inhaled allergen binds to the IgE antibody bound to the surface of bronchial submucosal mast cells.**

Release of mediators from mast cell granules during repeat exposure to the allergen: The allergen triggers the mast cells to release its granule contents. This consists of cytokines and other mediators. These mediators lead to two waves of reaction, an early (immediate hypersensitivity) phase and a late phase.

Early phase (immediate hypersensitivity) reaction: Mast cell mediators lead to the following results:

1. **Prominent bronchoconstriction:** This is by mediators released from mast cells, including **histamine, prostaglandin D_2, leukotrienes (LTC4, LTD4, and LTE4**), and also by reflex neural pathways.
2. Increased mucus production
3. **Vasodilation**
4. **Increased vascular permeability:** It produces edema.

Late-phase reaction: It is inflammatory in nature and characterized by the following:

- **Recruitment of leukocytes and release of additional inflammatory mediators:** During the late-phase reaction, there is the recruitment of leukocytes, **mainly eosinophils, basophils, monocytes, neutrophils, and more T cells**. Leukocytes recruited to the site of the reaction (neutrophils, eosinophils, and lymphocytes) release additional inflammatory mediators. These inflammatory mediators stimulate epithelial cells to produce various cytokines. Examples include:
  - **Eotaxin:** It is a powerful chemoattractant and activates eosinophils. Several factors released from eosinophils (e.g., major basic protein, eosinophil cationic protein) also damage the epithelium of airways.
  - **Chemokines**: They also promote the recruitment of Th2 cells, eosinophils, and other leukocytes. Thus, they exaggerate the inflammatory reaction.
- **Airway remodeling** (*refer* page 555): Repeated attacks of inflammation produce structural changes in the

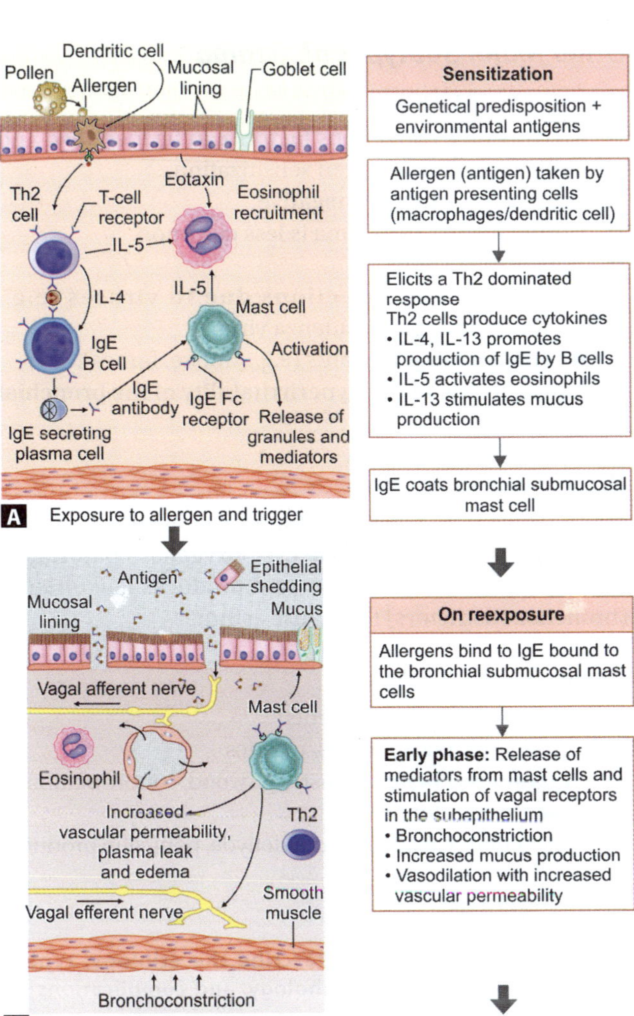

Figs. 17.11A to C: Pathogenesis of asthma. (A) Sensitization: Inhaled allergens (antigen) are taken up by antigen-presenting cells (macrophage/dendritic cells) and elicit a Th2-dominated response. This causes the production of IgE and the recruitment of eosinophils. (B) On reexposure to antigen (allergen), the immediate (early) phase is triggered within minutes. During this, antigens-induced cross-linking of IgE bound on Fc receptors present on mast cells. These mast cells release preformed mediators that directly and through neuronal reflexes produce bronchospasm, increased vascular permeability, mucus production, and recruitment of leukocytes. (C) Leukocytes accumulated at the site of the reaction (neutrophils, eosinophils, and basophils; lymphocytes and monocytes) release additional mediators. These mediators initiate the late-phase reaction. Many factors released from eosinophils (e.g., major basic protein, eosinophil cationic protein) also produce damage to the lining epithelium.

bronchial wall. These are together known as *airway remodeling*. These changes include (i) hypertrophy of bronchial smooth muscle and mucus glands and (ii) increased vascularity and deposition of subepithelial collagen.

MORPHOLOGY

Gross

- **Airways** (bronchi and bronchioles) are **occluded by sticky, thick mucous plugs.**
- In patients who die due to status asthmaticus, the lungs are markedly distended due to overinflation and show small areas of atelectasis (collapse).

Microscopy

Major processes which contribute to the narrowing of airways are as follows:

1. **Increased amount of mucus forms mucus plugs** and are seen in the bronchioles or bronchi. **The mucus plug contains desquamated epithelial cells and eosinophils and forms a spiral-shaped cast of the airways** and are called **Curschmann spirals.** These may be found in the sputum.
2. **Inflammation: Numerous eosinophils** are found in the walls of the bronchi and bronchioles. **Charcot–Leyden crystals,** which are **crystalloids derived from an eosinophil lysophospholipase** binding protein called galectin-10 are also found. There is also edema and congestion of the airways.
3. **Airway remodeling:** It is the **group of structural changes in the bronchial wall due to repeated bouts of inflammation** and consists of:
   - Thickening of the wall of the airways
   - Fibrosis below the basement membrane
   - Increased submucosal vascularity
   - An increase in size and number (hypertrophy/hyperplasia) of the submucosal glands and goblet cell metaplasia of the airway epithelium
   - Hypertrophy and/or hyperplasia of the bronchial wall smooth muscle.

- **Charcot-Leyden crystals as a pro-inflammatory factor:** Charcot-Leyden crystals are derived from a protein galectin-10 that is produced by eosinophils. This may be an important pro-inflammatory factor.
  Refer to type I hypersensitivity reactions on pages 170-3.

Clinical Course

- Acute asthmatic attack presents with severe dyspnea and wheezing due to bronchoconstriction and mucus plugging. It usually lasts **up to several hours.**
- Some patients may present with a **mild degree of chest tightness, dyspnea, wheezing, and cough** with or without sputum production.
- **Between the asthmatic attacks,** patients may be **asymptomatic.**
- **Status asthmaticus:** It is the **most severe form of asthma** in which the severe acute paroxysm persists for days and even weeks. The **bronchoconstriction does not respond to the drugs.** It may cause **severe airflow obstruction leading to severe cyanosis and even death.**

Diagnosis

- Demonstration of an increase in airflow obstruction (from baseline levels).
- Difficulty with exhalation (prolonged expiration, wheeze).
- **Elevated eosinophil count** in the peripheral blood.

Q. Add a note on sputum findings in bronchial asthma.

- **Sputum (Fig. 17.12):** It is sticky (viscous) and yellow and is **rich in eosinophils.** Microscopy shows:
  - **Charcot–Leyden crystals** are mainly seen in atopic asthma. They have the shape of a pair of **long, narrow, six-sided pyramids placed base-to-base.** They are crystalloids derived from an eosinophil lysophospholipase binding protein called galectin-10.
  - **Curschmann spirals** are **corkscrew-shaped twists of condensed mucus several centimeters long** that are usually **surrounded by an elongated mass of clear or opalescent material.** They form a spiral-shaped cast of the airways. The mucus plug contains desquamated epithelial cells and eosinophils.
  - **Creola bodies** are **compact clusters or strips of columnar epithelial cells** shed from the bronchus.

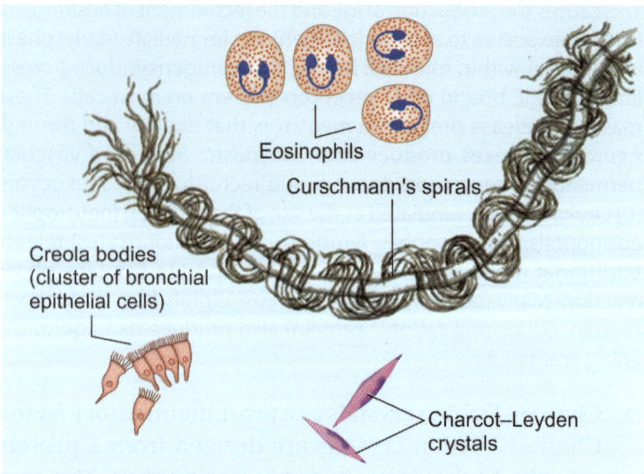

Fig. 17.12: Diagrammatic appearance of sputum in asthma showing Curschmann's spirals, Charcot–Leyden crystals, Creola bodies, and eosinophils.

Other Major Subtypes of Asthma

Non-atopic Asthma

- **No causative exogenous factors** can be identified and it does not show allergen sensitization.
- **Skin tests** are usually **negative.**
- **Family history** of asthma is **less common.**
- **Triggering events:**
  - **Respiratory infections due to viruses** (e.g., rhinovirus, parainfluenza virus).
  - **Inhaled air pollutants** (e.g., smoke, fumes).
- It may be **due to the hyperirritability of the bronchial tree.**

Drug-induced Asthma

Many drugs may trigger asthma (e.g., aspirin-sensitive asthma). Aspirin inhibits the cyclooxygenase pathway of arachidonic acid metabolism and produces leukotrienes (bronchoconstrictors) that cause asthma.

Occupational Asthma

Triggering occupational agents:

- **Fumes,** e.g., epoxy resins, plastics
- **Organic and chemical dust,** e.g., wood, cotton, platinum.
- **Gases,** e.g., toluene.
- **Other chemicals,** e.g., formaldehyde, penicillin products.

Bronchiectasis

PA 26.3 (CC): Define and describe the etiology, types, pathogenesis, stages, morphology, and complications of bronchiectasis.

Q. Define bronchiectasis.

Definition: Bronchiectasis is characterized by **irreversible** (permanent), **abnormal dilation of bronchi and bronchioles.** This **permanent dilation is due to the destruction of smooth muscle and elastic tissue of bronchi and bronchioles by inflammation that originated from persistent or severe infections.**

Etiology

Q. Discuss the etiopathogenesis of bronchiectasis.

The dilatation of bronchi and bronchioles is caused by the **destruction of the smooth muscle and supporting elastic tissue of the bronchial wall. It usually results from or is associated with chronic necrotizing infections.** It is not a primary disorder. It always develops secondary to persistent infection or obstruction caused by a various unrelated condition. Bronchiectasis may be either a focal (localized) or a diffuse (generalized) process. It may be divided into nonobstructive (postinflammatory) and obstructive.

Nonobstructive (Postinflammatory) Bronchiectasis

It is **usually of diffuse type** characterized by dilatation throughout the lung.

Postinfectious: It may be the result or associated with chronic necrotizing pneumonia.

- **Bacteria:** Bronchiectasis occurs as a complication of infection by virulent organisms such as *Staphylococcus aureus, Klebsiella* spp., *Haemophilus influenzae*, or *Pseudomonas*. Post-tuberculosis (*Mycobacterium tuberculosis)* bronchiectasis occurs in endemic areas.
- **Viruses:** Examples include adenovirus, influenza virus, [human immunodeficiency virus (HIV)]. Advanced bronchiectasis is also one of the complications after SARS-CoV-2 pneumonia.
- **Fungi** (*Aspergillus* species).

Focal nonobstructive bronchiectasis usually develops as a **complication of childhood infections, such as measles and pertussis.**

Genetic causes: These include the following:

Q. Write a short note on Kartagener's syndrome.

- **Kartagener or immotile cilia syndrome (primary ciliary dyskinesia):** It is an **autosomal recessive** syndrome with a **lack of ciliary function** (due to the absence of inner or outer dynein arms of cilia). This causes retention of secretions and recurrent infections. It comprises **sinusitis, bronchiectasis, dextrocardia** (with or without situs inversus), and **male infertility** (sperm dysmotility).
- **Young's syndrome**: Patients develop bronchiectasis, sinusitis, and obstructive azoospermia. The cause is not known.
- **Other dyskinetic ciliary syndromes:** These have deficient cilia throughout the body and include radial spoke deficiency (Sturgess syndrome) and absence of the central doublet of cilia.

Immunodeficiency: Patients with hypogammaglobulinemia, HIV infection, and bronchiolitis obliterans after lung transplantation have increased susceptibility to infections. This may lead to localized or diffuse bronchiectasis.

Autoimmune and immune-mediated diseases: These include autoimmune diseases such as rheumatoid arthritis, Sjögren's syndrome, systemic lupus erythematosus, and inflammatory bowel disease; and immune-mediated disease such as allergic bronchopulmonary aspergillosis.

Obstructive Bronchiectasis

It is **localized** to the obstructed segment of the lung.

Airway (bronchial) obstruction: Partial or total obstruction of the bronchial lumen may be caused by tumors, foreign body aspiration, and impacted mucus plugs. It may also develop as a complication of atopic asthma and chronic bronchitis.

Congenital or hereditary conditions: For example, major respiratory diseases in cystic fibrosis (CF) are sinusitis and bronchiectasis. Bronchiectasis occurs as a result of obstruction caused by abnormally viscid mucus and secondary infections.

Flowchart 17.2: Pathogenesis of bronchiectasis.

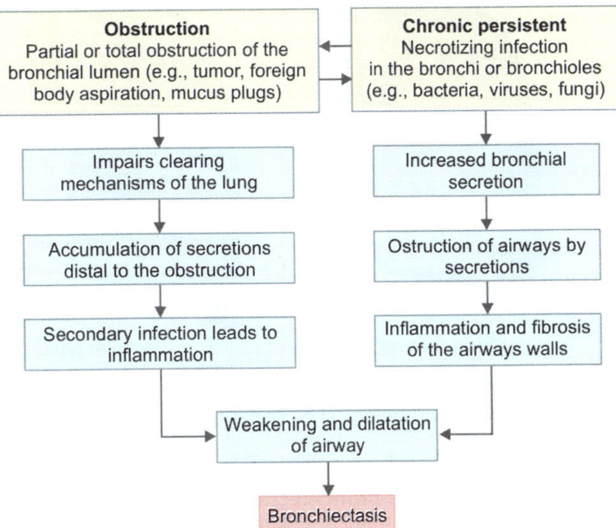

Pathogenesis (Flowchart 17.2)

Bronchiectasis is a **complex process.** Both **obstruction and chronic persistent infection** are the two major etiological conditions that seem to be necessary for the development of bronchiectasis.

1. **Obstruction:** It **impairs the clearing mechanisms** of the lung and results in the **accumulation of secretions** distal to the obstruction. This favors **secondary infection.** The accompanying inflammation weakens the bronchial wall. The accumulated exudate further distends the airways and leads to irreversible dilation of the airway.
2. **Chronic persistent necrotizing infection:** Chronic infection in the bronchi or bronchioles increases bronchial secretion. Poor clearance of secretion obstructs the airways. This produces inflammation and fibrosis of the airway walls leading to weakening and dilatation of airways.

Bronchiectasis associated with cystic fibrosis: It shows the **importance of both infection and obstruction.** In cystic fibrosis, there is a defect in the mucociliary action and there is an accumulation of thick viscid secretions. This leads to obstruction of the airways and favors microbial infections. With repeated infections, the walls of the airway are damaged and lead to dilatation of bronchi and bronchioles.

In patients with asthma and cystic fibrosis, hypersensitivity reactions to the fungus may cause allergic bronchopulmonary aspergillosis. This may predispose to proximal bronchiectasis.

MORPHOLOGY

Q. Write a short note on the gross and microscopic pathology of bronchiectasis.

Classification

A. **According to the shape of the bronchial dilation (Figs. 17.13A to D):**
   1. **Cylindrical (tubular) bronchiectasis:** It shows uniform and moderate dilation.

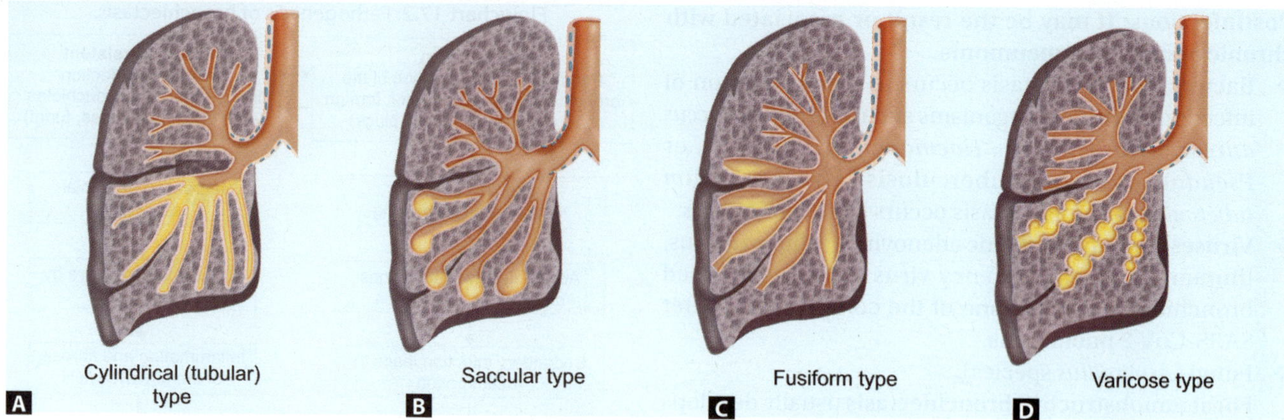

Figs. 17.13A to D: Morphological types of bronchiectasis: (A) Cylindrical (tubular) type; (B) Saccular type; (C) Fusiform type; (D) Varicose type.

2. **Saccular (cystic) bronchiectasis:** It is characterized by markedly dilated bronchi which end blindly in dilated sacs.
3. **Fusiform:** Characterized by fusiform dilatation.
4. **Varicose bronchiectasis:** It shows irregular dilations and constrictions. They resemble varicose veins when seen by radiologic bronchography.

B. According to the extent of involvement (Figs. 17.14A to D)

1. **Generalized:** It is **usually bilateral** and commonly affects the **lower lobes. The left lobe is more commonly involved than the right.** It is most severe in the more distal bronchi and bronchioles.
2. **Localized:** It is **restricted to a single segment of the lung** and usually occurs in association with obstruction (tumors or aspiration of foreign bodies).

Gross (Figs. 17.14A to D)

- **Dilatation of bronchi and bronchioles:** These **can be traced almost up to the pleural surfaces.** In the normal lung, the bronchioles cannot be followed by eye (or by ordinary gross dissection) beyond a point 2–3 cm from the pleural surfaces of the lung.
- **Extent of dilatation:** It may be up to four times the size of normal lumen.
- **Cut surface:** The **dilated bronchi and bronchioles** appear as saccular, cylindrical, or varicose (depending on the type). **The wall of the bronchi is thickened** by fibrosis. The **lumen is filled with thick, mucopurulent secretions** and the mucosal surface is congested.

Microscopy (Figs. 17.15A and B)

Varies with the activity and chronicity of the disease.

Bronchial Wall

- **Dilatation of bronchi and bronchioles** and destruction of their wall due to severe inflammation. If severe it may lead to lung abscess.
- **Dense infiltration of chronic inflammatory cells:** It mainly consists of **lymphocytes and plasma cells** within the **walls of the bronchi and bronchioles.** Sometimes, prominent lymphoid follicles may be seen.
- **Fibrosis of the bronchial and bronchiolar wall:** It occurs in chronic cases and may result in partial or complete obliteration of bronchiolar lumens.

Mucosal Changes

- **Desquamation of the lining epithelium** and areas of ulceration are seen.
- **Lining columnar cells** may show **pseudostratification** and squamous **metaplasia in the surrounding epithelium.**

Microbes: Culture of content from the involved bronchi **may show mixed microbes.** These include staphylococci, streptococci, pneumococci, enteric organisms, and (particularly in children) *Haemophilus influenzae* and *Pseudomonas aeruginosa.*

In allergic bronchopulmonary aspergillosis, fungal hyphae can be seen on special stains.

Clinical Course

- **Severe persistent productive cough:** It is the most common clinical feature.
- **Relation of cough to posture:** Paroxysms of cough occur, **especially when the patient rises in the morning.** This is because the changes in position lead to the drainage of collections of pus and secretions into the bronchi.
- **Copious foul-smelling sputum,** sometimes bloody. In severe cases, the patient presents with dyspnea and orthopnea.
- **Dyspnea, wheezing, orthopnea, and cyanosis:** These are variable and depend on the extent of the disease. These develop in severe cases of bronchiectasis Symptoms are precipitated by upper respiratory tract infections.
- Complications of bronchiectasis are presented in **Box 17.7.**

Q. Write a short note on complications of bronchiectasis.

BOX 17.7: Complications of bronchiectasis.

- Lung abscess
- Pneumonia
- Empyema
- Septicemia and brain abscesses
- Meningitis, osteomyelitis
- Metastatic abscesses (e.g., brain)
- Cor pulmonale
- Aspergilloma
- Hemoptysis
- Respiratory failure
- Pulmonary hypertension
- Generalized amyloidosis

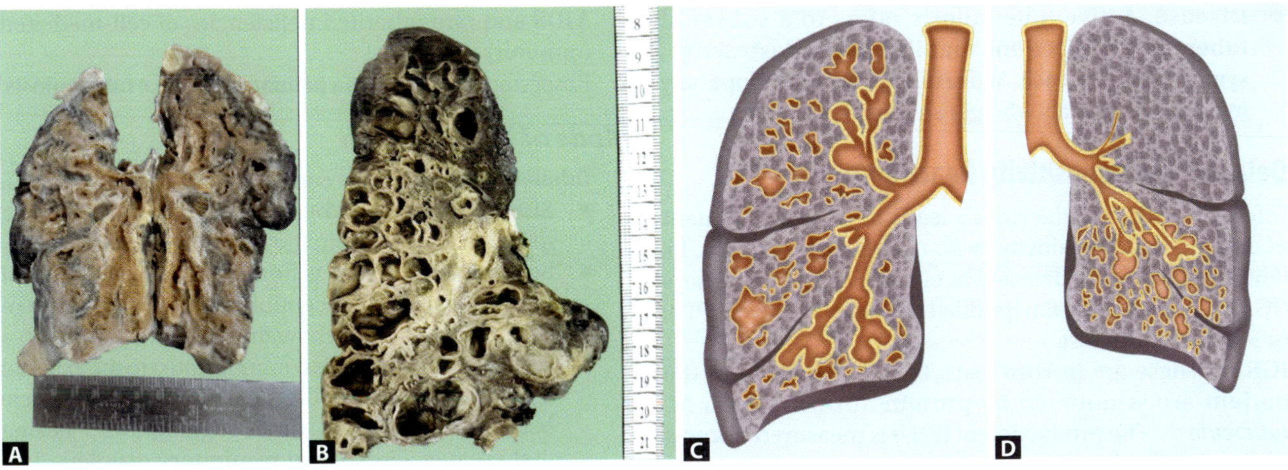

Figs. 17.14A to D: Gross appearance (cut section) of bronchiectasis with dilated bronchi and bronchioles: (A) Longitudinal section of dilated airways; (B) Markedly dilated bronchi and bronchioles, some forming cystic spaces; (C) Diffuse bronchiectasis (diagrammatic); (D) Localized bronchiectasis (diagrammatic).

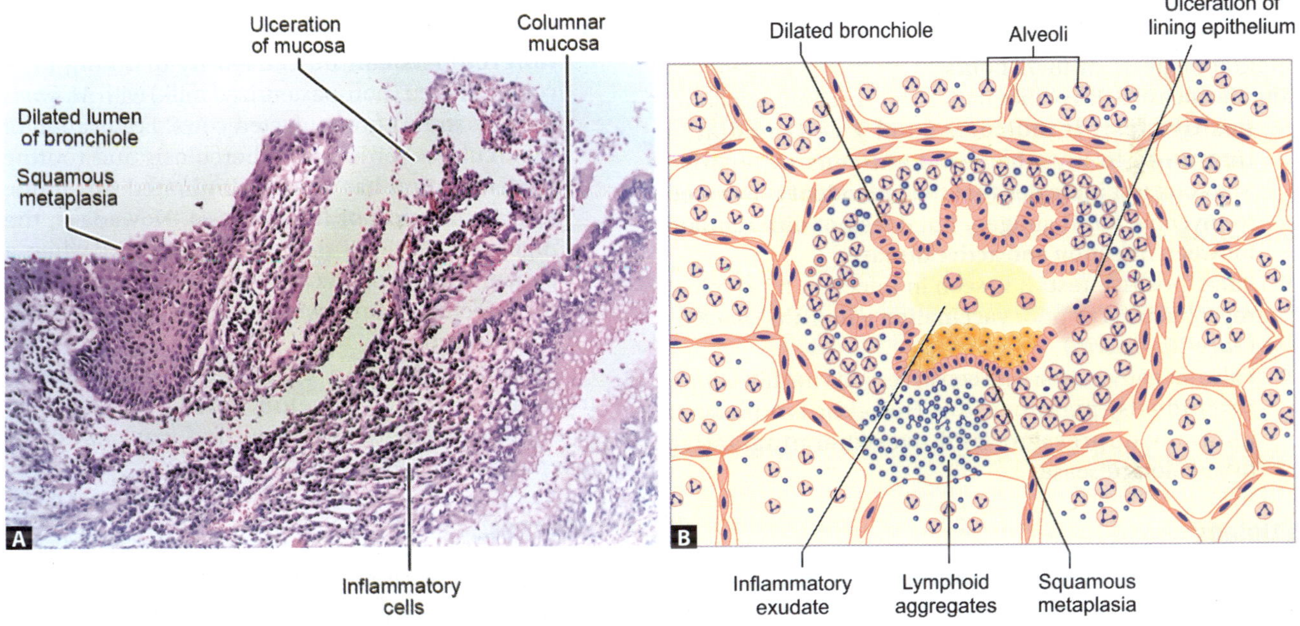

Figs. 17.15A and B: Microscopic features of bronchiectasis: (A) H&E; (B) Diagrammatic: (A) Shows wall of the bronchiole with infiltration by chronic inflammatory cells. There is also squamous metaplasia of the lining epithelium; (B) Shows bronchiole with dilated lumen and squamous metaplasia of the lining epithelium. The wall shows chronic inflammation.

A summary of disorders associated with airflow obstruction is presented (*refer* online Table 17.2).

TUBERCULOSIS

PA 26.4 (CC): Define and describe the etiology, types, pathogenesis, stages, morphology microscopic appearance, and complications of tuberculosis.

Definition: Tuberculosis (also called Koch's disease) is a **communicable, chronic granulomatous disease** caused by ***Mycobacterium tuberculosis***. Tuberculosis (TB) usually involves the lungs. But it can affect any organ or tissue in the body.

Epidemiology: Tuberculosis is common in India. The incidence of tuberculosis is high wherever there is **poverty, overcrowding, and chronic debilitating illness.**

- **Diseases that are associated with increased risk for tuberculosis**: Diabetes mellitus, Hodgkin lymphoma, malnutrition, immunosuppression, alcoholism, chronic lung disease (e.g., silicosis), and chronic renal failure. **HIV is the most important risk factor**.

Infection versus disease: Infection with *M. tuberculosis* is to be differentiated from disease.

- **Infection**: Tuberculous infection **indicates the presence of organisms in a person**, which **may or may not cause symptomatic disease**.

- **Disease**: Active tuberculosis refers to a subset of **tuberculous infections manifested by destructive, symptomatic disease.** Active tuberculosis develops only in a few individuals who get an infection.

Delayed Hypersensitivity Reaction

Infection with *M. tuberculosis* leads to the development of delayed hypersensitivity to *M. tuberculosis* antigens. Its development can be detected by either IFN-γ release assays (IGRAs) or the tuberculin [purified protein derivative (PPD), or Mantoux] skin test.

IGRAs: These are in vitro tests. In this, T cells from the patient are stimulated by protein antigens from *M. tuberculosis*. The production of IFN-γ is measured to know the level of T-cell immunity.

Tuberculin (Mantoux) test: It is performed by intracutaneous **injection of 0.1 mL of a purified protein derivative of *M. tuberculosis*.** In infected individuals, it produces a **visible and palpable induration of 10 mm diameter or more at the site of injection of PPD**. This induration peaks in 48–72 hours.

Significance of IGRA or tuberculin test: These are as follows:

- **Positive test: It indicates** good **T cell-mediated immunity** to mycobacterial antigens. A positive Mantoux test **indicates that the individual is exposed to mycobacterial antigen**. But **does not differentiate between infection and active disease.**
- **False-positive test:** It is seen in infection by **atypical mycobacteria** or prior **vaccination with BCG** (*Bacillus Calmette-Guerin*).
- **False-negative tests:** It is seen in certain viral infections, sarcoidosis, malnutrition, Hodgkin lymphoma, immunosuppression, and overwhelming active tuberculous disease.

Etiology

Characteristics of mycobacteria: It has the following features:

- It is an **aerobic, slender, rod-shaped bacteria** measuring 2–10 μm in length.
- **Acid-fast bacillus**: It has a high content of complex lipid coat which makes it difficult to stain. Once stained, this lipid binds tightly to the carbol fuchsin present in **Ziehl-Neelsen stain** and **resists decolorization** (not decolorized) **by acids and alcohol**. Hence, it is termed as acid-fast bacilli (AFB).
- Most cases of tuberculosis are caused by ***Mycobacterium tuberculosis hominins*** (human strain). The source of infection in patients with **active open cases of tuberculosis.**
- ***Mycobacterium bovis*** causes oropharyngeal and intestinal tuberculosis.
- *Mycobacterium avium complex* which is less virulent and nonpathogenic to normal individuals. However, they may cause disseminated infection **in patients with AIDS** and rare inherited deficiencies of cell-mediated immunity.
- Reservoir of infection is a patient with active tuberculosis.

Mode of Transmission

1. **Inhalation:** It is the **most common mode** of transmission.
   - **Site of infection:** When an individual inhales the droplets, they lodge in the lung and cause infection.
   - **Source of organisms** is from an **active open case of tuberculosis** to a susceptible host. An open case of tuberculosis is a patient with tuberculosis in which a cavitatory lung lesion is communicated to the external environment through the patient's airways. Tubercle bacilli will be expelled while coughing, and sneezing that creates aerosolized respiratory droplets. The source may also be from contaminated secretions.
2. **Ingestion:** It is not a common mode of infection.
   - **Site of infection:** *Mycobacterium bovis* causes oropharyngeal and intestinal tuberculosis.
   - **Source of organisms: Oropharyngeal and intestinal tuberculosis** can be caused by drinking milk contaminated (non-pasteurized milk) with ***M. bovis*** (bovine strain) from infected cows. Eradication of tuberculous herds with tuberculosis and routine **pasteurization** has almost **eliminated this mode of transmission** of tuberculosis. Nowadays, the ingestion mode of transmission occurs when a patient with an open case of tuberculosis swallows the infected sputum which results in tuberculosis of the intestine.
3. **Inoculation: It is an extremely rare mode** of transmission. May develop during postmortem examination, while cuts resulting from handling tuberculous infected organs.

Pathogenesis

Q. Write a short note on the pathogenesis of tuberculosis.

Cell-mediated immunity and hypersensitivity: Infection with tubercle bacillus results in two simultaneous immunological responses (i) cell-mediated immunity and (ii) Type IV hypersensitivity reaction. The effector cells for both cell-mediated immunity and hypersensitivity reaction are **Th1** cells.

- **Cell-mediated immunity:** Tuberculosis developing first time (newly exposed to tuberculosis) in an immunocompetent individual depends on the development of cell-mediated immunity. This immunity produces resistance to the mycobacteria and leads to the development of tissue hypersensitivity to tubercular antigens. Cell-mediated immunity is protective.
- **Type IV hypersensitivity reactions:** It develops against mycobacterial antigens and is **responsible for** typical pathologic features. This includes **tissue destruction, such as caseating granulomas and cavitation**. These are the result of the destructive tissue hypersensitivity

of the host immune response. **The effector cells in both protective immunity and damaging hypersensitivity are the same**. Hence, the appearance of type IV hypersensitivity reaction also indicates the development of protective immunity. In tuberculosis, immunity (resistance to infection) and hypersensitivity are two different manifestations of the same mechanism.

The Sequence of Events in Tuberculosis

Tuberculosis is a chronic granulomatous disease, caused by *M. tuberculosis*. The lung is commonly involved in tuberculosis; the pathogenesis is considered with respect to pulmonary tuberculosis.

Infection Before Activation of Cell-mediated Immunity (Fig. 17.16 and refer page 179-80 and Figs. 6.9 and 6.10)

Initial infection with *Mycobacterium tuberculosis* **in a nonsensitized individual** is called **primary tuberculosis.** The following sequence of events occurs:

Entry of mycobacteria into macrophages

The first time, when the **virulent tubercle bacilli** are inhaled, they are deposited in the alveoli of the lung. They primarily **infect** the alveolar **macrophages and undergo endocytosis**. They enter the macrophage endosomes by a process mediated **through several macrophage receptors.** These receptors include:

- **Mannose receptors** bind lipoarabinomannan (LAM), a glycolipid in the cell wall of tubercle bacilli.
- **Complement receptors** (C3b receptor) which bind mycobacteria opsonized by C3b.

The proliferation of mycobacteria within macrophages:

Prevention of the fusion of the lysosomes with the phagocytic vacuole: After internalization, the tubercle bacilli block the fusion of the lysosomes with the phagocytic vacuole. This inhibits normal microbicidal responses and allows the *Mycobacterium* to persist in the phagocytic vacuoles and proliferate.

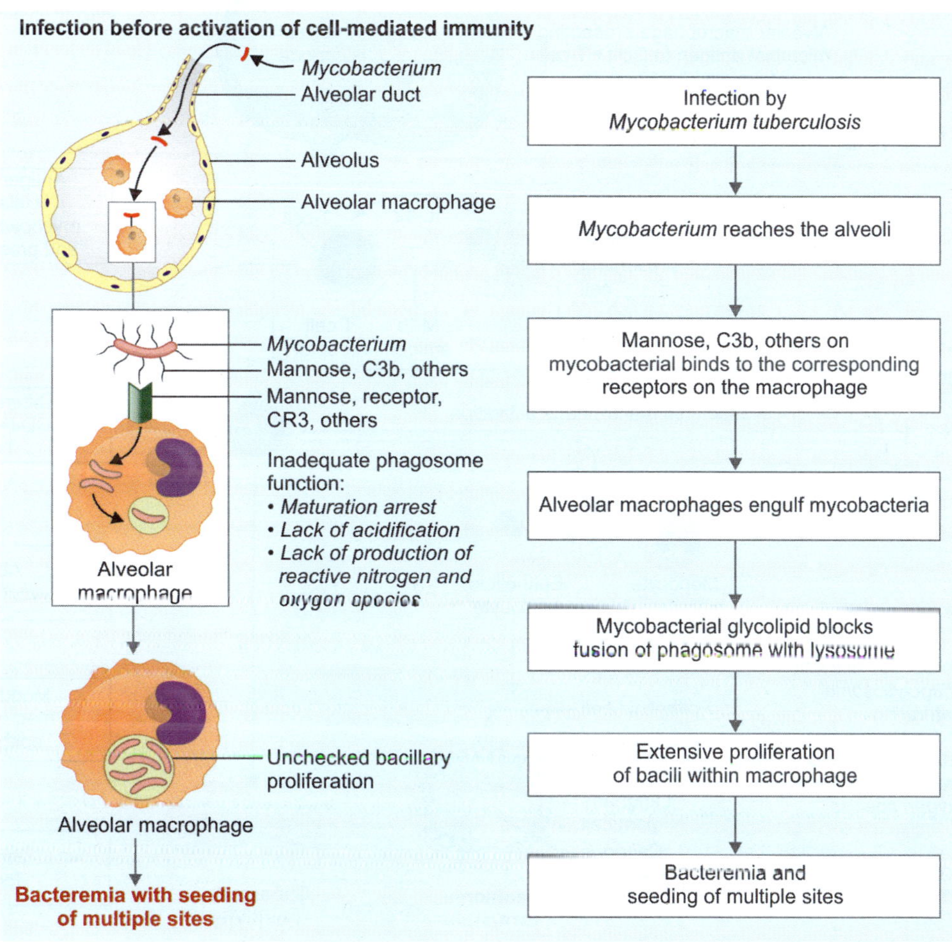

Fig. 17.16: Sequence of events in primary tuberculosis of the lung. Events occurring in the first weeks after exposure before activation of cell-mediated immunity.

(CR3: complement receptor 3).

Bacteremia with seeding at multiple sites: Mycobacteria proliferate freely within alveolar macrophages and air spaces. It results in bacteremia and seeding of tubercle bacilli at many sites. This bacteremia may be either asymptomatic or may have a mild flu-like illness.

Initiation and Consequences of Cell-mediated Immunity (Fig. 17.17)

Development of cell-mediated immunity

Cell-mediated immunity develops about 3 weeks after exposure to mycobacteria.

- **Presentation of antigen to CD4+ T-cells:** Mycobacterial antigens (MTb antigens) reach the draining lymph nodes. In the lymph nodes, these antigens are processed by antigen-presenting cells namely dendritic cells and macrophages, and presented to CD4+ T cells.
- **Differentiation of CD4+ T-cells into T-helper 1 (Th1) cell:** IL-12 secreted by macrophages cause differentiation of CD4+ T cells of the Th1 subset It is due to the action of IL-12 secreted by macrophages. Th1 cells secrete IFN-γ.

T cell-mediated macrophage activation and killing of bacteria

Activation of macrophages: IFN-γ released by the Th1 cells is important for the activation of macrophages.

Anti-mycobacterial effects by mediators and upregulated genes: Activated macrophages become bactericidal and release various mediators and upregulate the expression of genes having anti-mycobacterial effects. These include:

1. **TNF:** It recruits monocytes and activates them into the macrophages that characterize the granulomatous response.

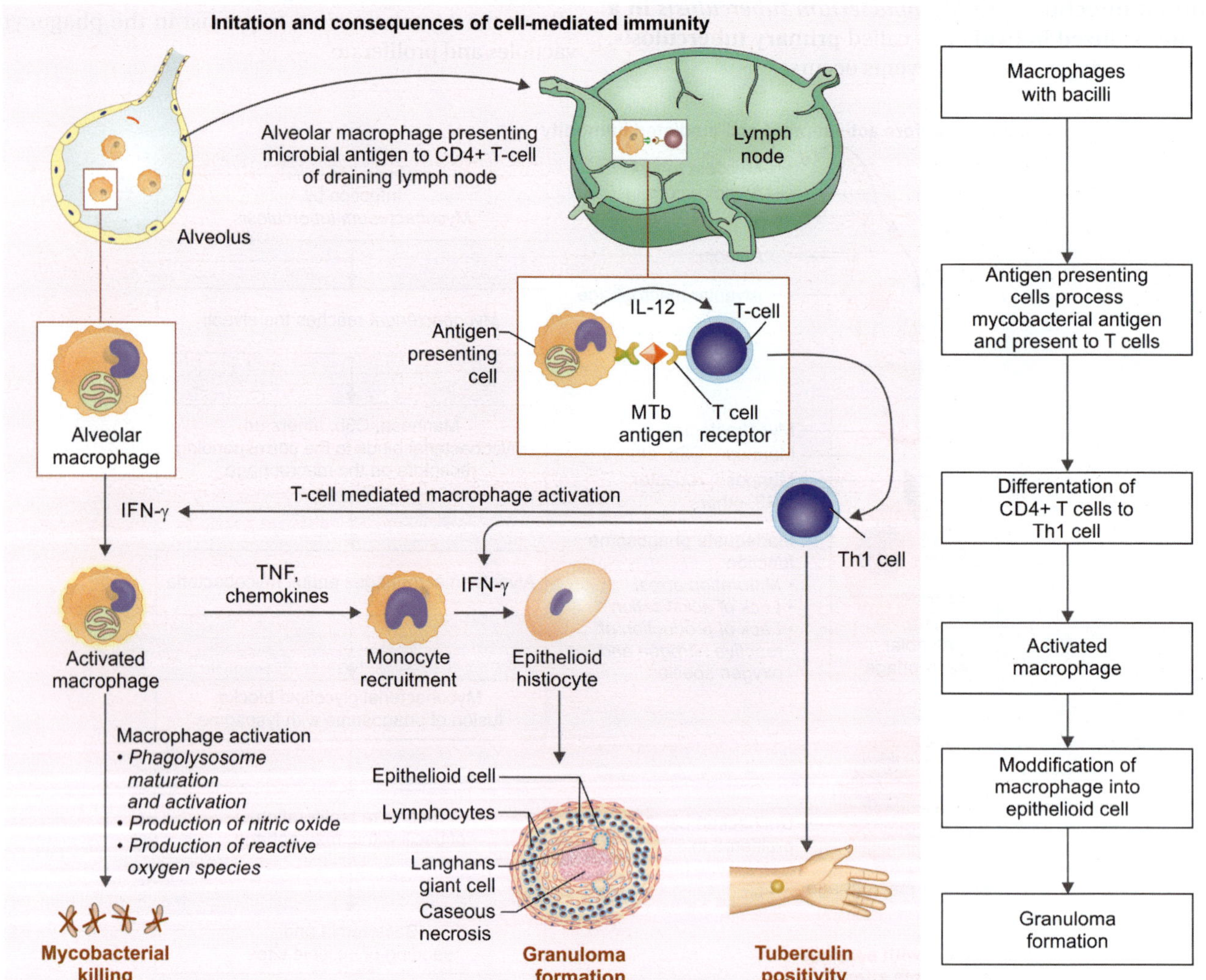

Fig. 17.17: Sequence of events in primary tuberculosis of lung: Events after 3 weeks of infection. The development of resistance to the *Mycobacterium* is accompanied by conversion to a positive result on tuberculin skin testing.

(IFN-γ: interferon γ; MTb: *Mycobacterium* tuberculosis; TNF: tumor necrosis factor).

2. **Stimulates inducible nitric oxide synthase (iNOS):** It raises levels of nitric oxide (NO) and produces reactive nitrogen intermediate. These are important in the killing of mycobacteria.
3. **Antimicrobial peptides (defensins):** These are toxic to mycobacteria.
4. **Phagolysosome maturation and activation** in infected macrophages. This exposes the bacteria to an acidic environment.
5. **Generation of reactive oxygen species** that are anti-bacterial.

Granulomatous inflammation and tissue damage

Apart from stimulating macrophages to kill mycobacteria, the Th1 response is involved in the formation of granulomas.

- **Differentiation of macrophages into epithelioid cells:** Macrophages activated by IFN-γ differentiate into the "epithelioid histiocytes" (epithelioid cells). Some of these "epithelioid cells" may fuse to form giant cells.
- **Granuloma formation**: A microscopic aggregate of epithelioid cells, surrounded by a rim of lymphocytes, is referred to as a granuloma and this pattern of inflammation, is known as **granulomatous inflammation**. Activated macrophages also secrete TNF and chemokines. They recruit more monocytes. **Hypersensitivity reaction results in tissue destruction leading to caseation and cavitation.**

The importance of TNF: Patients with rheumatoid arthritis and inflammatory bowel disease can be treated with TNF antagonists. These patients are at increased risk for TB reactivation.

Primary Tuberculosis

Q. Write a short note on primary tuberculosis.

Definition: Initial infection that occurs on first exposure to the organism **in an unsensitized** (previously unexposed) **immunocompetent individual** is known as primary tuberculosis.

In most, primary tuberculosis is asymptomatic. About 5% of newly infected people develop clinically significant disease. It develops when immune defenses are lowered, and the infection may produce potentially life-threatening disease.

- **The source** of the organism is always **exogenous.** Pulmonary tuberculosis is spread by droplet infection.

MORPHOLOGY

Sites of primary tuberculosis: Lung, intestine, tonsil, and skin (very rare).

Q. Write a short note on Ghon focus.

Lung

It is the **most common site** of primary tuberculosis.

Ghon lesion (Ghon focus): Following inhalation, tubercle bacilli get deposited in the distal airspaces.

- **Site of deposit:** Usually the bacilli lodge in the airspaces of the **lower part of the upper lobe or** the **upper part of the lower lobe. usually near the pleural surface** (subpleural).
- **Ghon focus (Figs. 17.18A and B):** About 2–4 weeks after the infection (during the development of sensitization), a circumscribed **gray-white area of consolidation** appears **in the lung** known as the Ghon focus. It measures about **1–1.5 cm.** In most cases, the **center of this Ghon focus undergoes caseous necrosis.** The term Ghon focus is restricted only to primary tuberculosis of the lung. In other organs, it is called primary focus.
- **Regional lymphadenitis:** Tubercle bacilli, either free or within phagocytes (macrophages) are carried along the lymphatics to the regional draining lymph nodes. These nodes also often show caseous necrosis.

Ghon complex: It is the combination of subpleural parenchymal lung lesion (**Ghon focus**) and **regional lymph node lesion.**

Q. Write a short note on the Ghon complex.

Fate of Ghon complex:

- **Healing:** In the **majority** (about 95%), cell-mediated immunity controls the infection and primary tuberculosis **heals.** The **hallmark of healing is fibrosis** and Ghon complex undergoes progressive fibrosis, followed by radiologically detectable **calcification** (detectable as a **Ranke complex**), and **very rarely ossification.** Thus, the majority of the healthy individuals who develop primary TB show a focus on pulmonary scarring.

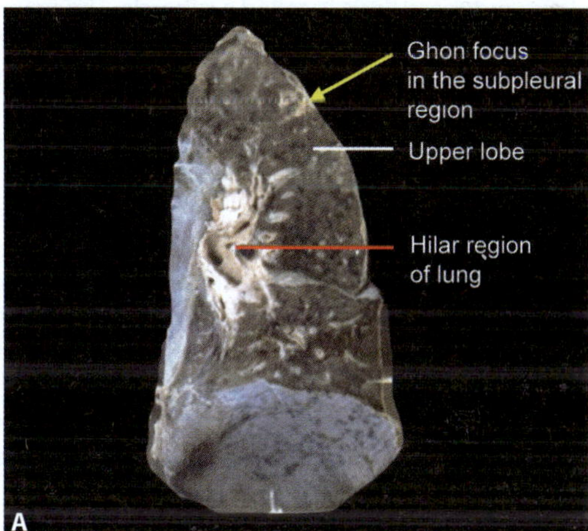

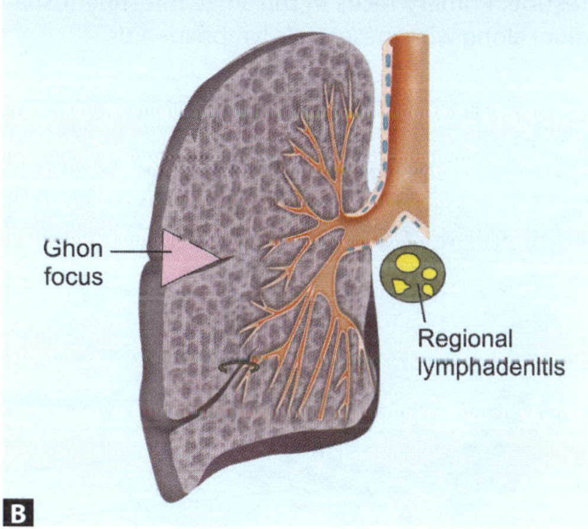

Figs. 17.18A and B: (A) Gross appearance of primary pulmonary tuberculosis; (B) Diagrammatic. Ghon complex consists of gray-white parenchymal focus under the pleura and enlarged hilar lymph nodes with caseation.

- **Spread:** During the first few weeks, lymphatic **and hematogenous dissemination** occurs to other organs or parts of the body.
  - **No lesions:** Despite dissemination and deposition of bacilli in other organs, no lesions develop.
  - **Progressive primary tuberculosis:** Uncommonly, individuals **who do not produce an effective immune response** against the initial infection lead to *progressive primary tuberculosis*. This complication occurs in patients who are immunocompromised or have minor defects in host defenses (e.g., severe acute malnutrition). The incidence of progressive primary TB is high in HIV-positive patients with significant immunosuppression (i.e., CD4+ T cell counts below 200 cells/μL). Immunosuppression decreases the ability to elicit a CD4+ T cell-mediated response. As a result, the lesions in such patients usually **do not form characteristic granulomas of tuberculosis.** Instead, the lesions **show sheets of macrophages containing numerous bacilli.**

Microscopy (Figs. 17.19A and B)

The sites of infection that are involved in infection show a characteristic inflammatory reaction. This is characterized by the presence of granuloma.

Granuloma in tuberculosis is called a tubercle. The granuloma may be **caseating** (show the central area of caseous necrosis/soft tubercle) **or noncaseating granulomas** (without caseation/hard tubercle). Individual tubercles are identified only by microscopic examination. When multiple granulomas coalesce, they may be grossly identified. **Caseating granuloma** consists of:

- **Central area of caseous necrosis**
- **Surrounded by epithelioid macrophages** (modified macrophages), some of which may fuse to form **multinucleate giant cells.** The **giant cells may be Langhans type** (nuclei arranged in horse- shoe pattern) **or foreign body type** (nuclei in the center).
- The epithelioid cells are **surrounded by a rim of lymphocytes.**
- These granulomas are usually **enclosed within fibroblasts.**

Other Sites of Primary Complex

- **Intestine:** Primary focus in the small intestine (usually ileal region) along with mesenteric lymphadenitis.
- **Tonsils:** Primary focus in the pharynx and tonsils with cervical lymph node enlargement.
- **Skin:** Primary focus on the skin along with regional lymph node involvement.

Secondary Tuberculosis

Q. Describe the morphological types of secondary tuberculosis.

(Synonyms: Reactivation tuberculosis or post-primary tuberculosis).

Definition: A pattern of tuberculosis that arises in a previously sensitized individual is known as secondary tuberculosis.

Source of infection:

- **Reactivation of a latent infection:** Secondary tuberculosis may appear shortly after primary TB. But more commonly arises many years after initial primary tuberculosis, usually when host resistance decreases. The most common source is the reactivation of a latent infection. Only a few patients (<5%) with primary tuberculosis develop secondary TB.
- **Reinfection:** Rarely, it may result from exogenous reinfection. It may occur either because the protection by the primary disease has disappeared or because of exposure to a large dose of virulent tubercle bacilli.

MORPHOLOGY

Q. Morphology of secondary tuberculosis.

Gross (Figs. 17.20A to C)

- **Location:** Any location may be involved in secondary tuberculosis, but the lungs are by far the most common site. In the lungs, secondary tuberculosis usually involves the **apex of the upper lobes** of one or both lungs, **within 1–2 cm of the apical pleura.** This may be because of high oxygen tension in the apices that helps in their multiplication.
- **Appearance**
  - **Focus of consolidation: The initial lesion shows a small focus (less than 2 cm in diameter) of consolidation.** It is sharply **circumscribed, firm,** and **gray-white to yellow** in color.

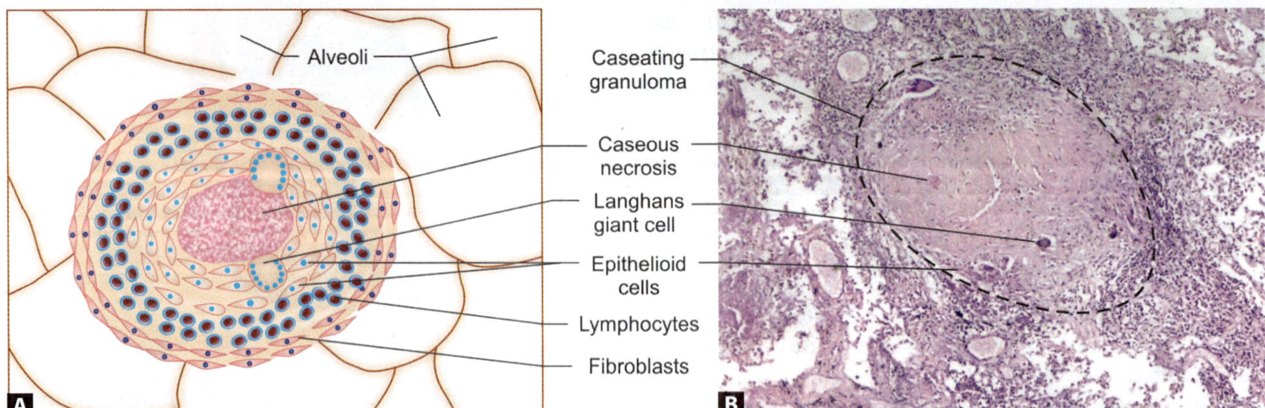

Figs. 17.19A and B: Microscopic appearance of tuberculous lung: (A) Diagrammatic; (B) Photomicrograph. The central area of caseation is surrounded by epithelioid and multinucleated giant cells.

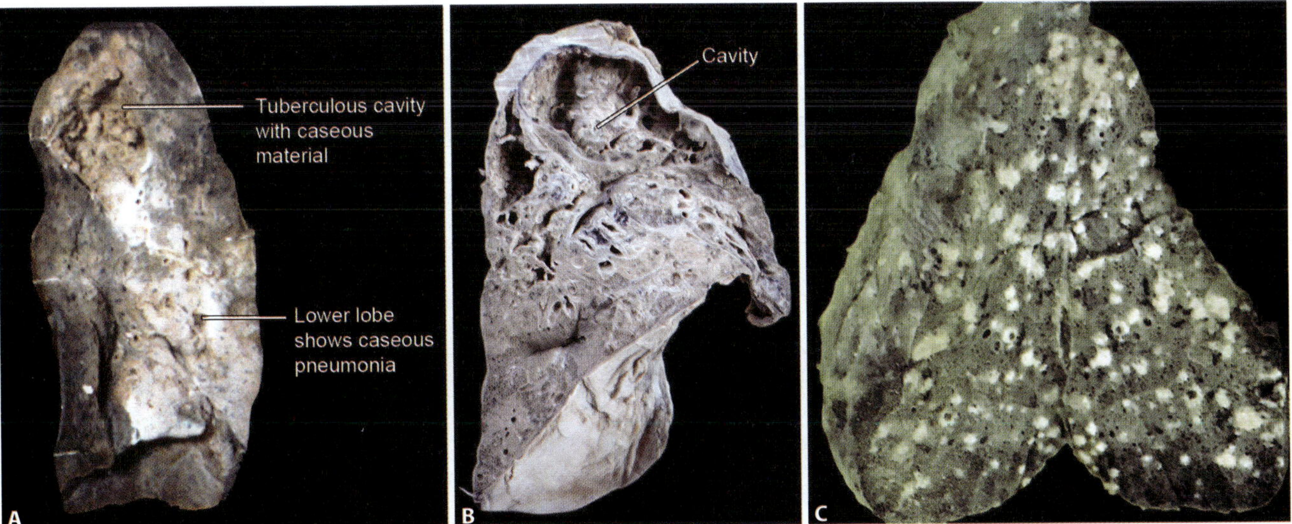

Figs. 17.20A to C: Secondary pulmonary tuberculosis: (A) Early; (B) Advanced. The lung shows gray-white areas of caseation with a cavity in the upper lobe; (C) Miliary tuberculosis of the lung. The cut surface shows numerous gray-white granulomas.

It shows variable amounts of central caseation and peripheral fibrosis.

- **Cavitation**: The infected region and associated inflammation usually undergo cavitation and erode into the airways. Such changes act as an important source of infectivity because these patients produce sputum containing the bacilli (open case of tuberculosis).

- **Regional lymph node involvement is less prominent** than in primary tuberculosis. Because, patients with secondary tuberculosis have preexistent hypersensitivity, and the bacilli elicit a prompt tissue response and try to wall off the focus. Thus, regional lymph nodes are less prominently involved than in primary TB.

Microscopy

Active lesions show **caseating granulomas** (*refer* **Figs. 17.19A and B**) and **acid-fast stain** often shows **tubercle bacilli**. Bacilli are not seen in late, fibrocalcific stages.

Fate of Secondary Tuberculosis (Fig. 17.21)

Healing

In immunocompetent individuals, localized, apical, secondary tuberculous focus may **heal with fibrosis and calcification,** rarely ossification. Heal may occur either spontaneously or after therapy.

Progress

Secondary tuberculosis of the lung may progress along several different pathways (**Box 17.8**).

Progressive pulmonary tuberculosis

It occurs mainly in the elderly and immunosuppressed. The apical lesion and caseous area may expand into the surrounding lung. It may erode into bronchi and vessels.

- **Erosion into bronchi:** It releases the central area of caseous necrosis into the bronchi. It creates a **ragged, irregular apical cavity (Figs. 17.20A and B). This cavity is lined by caseous material** and surrounded by fibrous tissue. This produces an **important source of infection**, because when the patient coughs, sputum may contain tuberculous bacilli.
- **Erosion of blood vessels:** This may result in hemoptysis. With prompt treatment, it may undergo healing by fibrosis.

Spread of infection

If the treatment is inadequate or if host defenses are impaired, the secondary tuberculous infection may spread locally and/or via (i) airways, (ii) lymphatics, or (iii) blood vessels.

1. **Local/direct spread:** Tuberculosis can directly spread to the surrounding tissue. In the lung, local spread to the pleura leads to serous **pleural effusions, tuberculous empyema**, or **obliterative fibrous pleuritis.**
2. **Spread through bronchi/airways:** It may produce tuberculous pneumonia. It can spread to other parts of the same lung as well as the opposite lung.
   - **Intestinal tuberculosis** (*refer* **Fig. 18.25**)**:** In the past, intestinal tuberculosis resulted from the drinking of contaminated milk and unpasteurized milk, now it is rare. Nowadays caused by the **swallowing of coughed-up infective material in patients with open cases of advanced pulmonary tuberculosis. Mainly develops in the ileum.**
3. **Spread along mucosal lining:** Spread through lymphatic channels or along the mucosal lining from mycobacteria present in the expectorated infectious material may lead to **endobronchial, endotracheal,** and **laryngeal tuberculosis.**
4. **Lymphatic spread:** Spread through lymphatic channels mainly reaches regional lymph nodes. It may also cause disseminated disease.
   - **Miliary pulmonary disease:** It is the disseminated form of tuberculosis. When the dissemination occurs only to the lungs, it is called miliary pulmonary disease (**Fig. 17.20C**).
     - **Mechanism of development**: Tubercle bacilli draining through lymphatics enter the venous blood. Then to the right venous side of the heart and through the pulmonary artery to the lung.

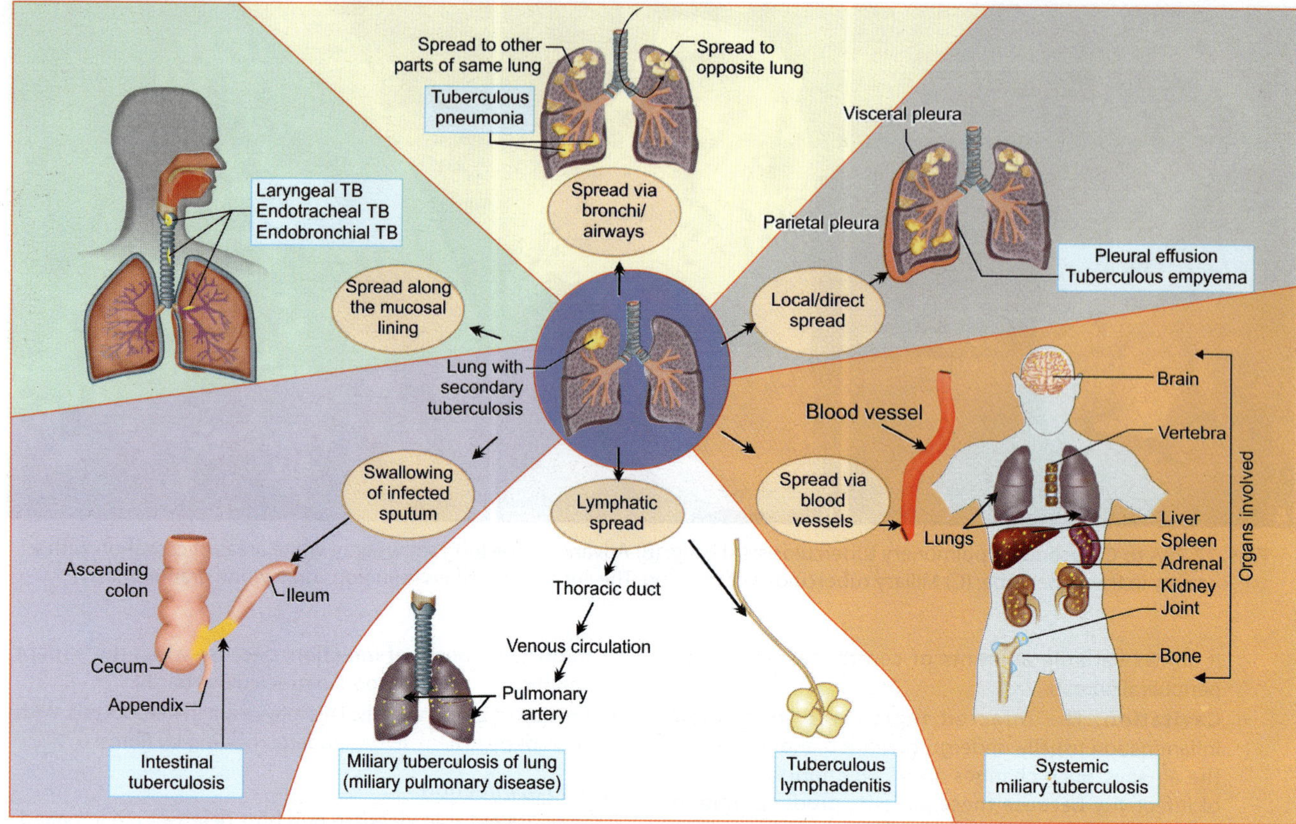

Fig. 17.21: Progress and complications of secondary tuberculosis of the lung.

- **Lesions:** It produces **multiple, small, yellow, nodular** lesions in the parenchyma of both lungs. Each lesion is either microscopic or small, visible (2 mm) foci of **yellow-white consolidation**. These lesions **resemble millet seeds, hence named "miliary"**.

– **Lymphadenitis**: It is the most frequent presentation of extrapulmonary tuberculosis, and usually occurs in the cervical region (scrofula).
- HIV-negative individuals: Unifocal and localized.
- HIV-positive individuals: Multifocal and systemic disease.

5. **Spread via blood vessels**

– **Systemic miliary tuberculosis** occurs when tubercle bacilli disseminate through the systemic arterial system. Miliary tuberculosis most commonly involves the liver, bone marrow, spleen, adrenals, meninges, kidneys, fallopian tubes, and epididymis. But no organ is exempt and can involve any organ.

– **Isolated-organ tuberculosis:** Dissemination of tubercle bacilli through blood may seed any organ or tissue resulting in isolated organ tuberculosis. Commonly involved organs are as follows:
- Meninges (tuberculous meningitis).
- Kidneys (renal tuberculosis).
- Adrenals.
- Bones (osteomyelitis): When it involves the vertebrae, the disease is referred to as **Pott disease**. Paraspinal "cold" abscesses may track along tissue planes and present as an abdominal or pelvic mass.
- Fallopian tubes (salpingitis), epididymis (epididymitis).

BOX 17.8: Various ways of the spread of tuberculosis.

- Local spread
- Along airways
- Along the mucosal lining
- Lymphatic spread
- Blood spread (hematogenous)

Clinical Features

- Localized secondary tuberculosis may remain asymptomatic. When it manifests, the symptoms usually are insidious in onset. It gradually develops both systemic and localizing symptoms and signs.
- **Systemic symptoms of secondary pulmonary tuberculosis**: Systemic symptoms are probably due to cytokines released by activated macrophages (e.g., TNF and IL-1). Various symptoms are as follows:
  - **Nonspecific**: Malaise, anorexia, weight loss and fever.
  - **Low-grade fever:** It is usually low grade and **remittent** (appearing late each afternoon and

then subsiding-commonly known as **evening rise of temperature**). It is accompanied by drenching **night sweats**.

- **Sputum:** With progressive involvement of the lung, increasing amounts of sputum are produced. At first, it is mucoid and later becomes purulent. When cavitation develops, the sputum contains tubercle bacilli. AFB stain for the sputum sample is used for its diagnosis.
- **Hemoptysis:** Some degree of hemoptysis is present in 50% of cases of pulmonary tuberculosis.
- **Pleuritic pain:** It may develop due to the extension of infection to the pleural surfaces.

❖ **Extrapulmonary manifestations** depend on the organ/system involved. For example, infertility (tuberculous salpingitis), headache and neurologic deficits (tuberculous meningitis), and back pain and paraplegia [spine involvement (Pott disease)]. Patients with HIV infection have an increased risk of tuberculosis.

Diagnosis of Pulmonary Disease

Q. Write a short note on the diagnosis of tuberculosis.

❖ Based on the **history, physical and radiographic** findings (consolidation or cavitation in the apices of the lungs).

❖ **Sputum for AFB**: Detection of **acid-fast tubercle bacilli in the sputum** is the most common method for diagnosis of active mycobacterial infection. Zeihl–Neelsen stain is an acid-fast bacilli (AFB) stain for demonstration of mycobacteria.

❖ Acid fastness of the *Mycobacterium* is due to mycolic acid. Staining with fluorescent auramine rhodamine also can be used.

❖ **Culture of the sputum:** Conventional cultures require up to 10 weeks. But liquid media-based radiometric assays can detect mycobacterial metabolism and provide the result within 2 weeks. Culture is the gold standard because it can identify the occasional PCR-negative case and is also useful for testing drug susceptibility. Multidrug resistance (MDR) is defined as resistance of mycobacteria to two or more of the primary drugs used for the treatment of TB. It is a common problem encountered in recent times. The most common cause of drug-resistant tuberculosis is previous antituberculous treatment (ATT).

❖ **PCR amplification** of *M. tuberculosis:* DNA is the rapid method of diagnosis. PCR can detect as few as 10 organisms in clinical specimens.

❖ **Cartridge-based nucleic acid amplification test (CB-NAAT)** is an automated cartridge-based molecular technique that not only detects *Mycobacterium tuberculosis* but also rifampicin resistance within two hours. This has been endorsed by WHO as an initial diagnostic test for tuberculosis.

TABLE 17.3 Main difference between primary and secondary tuberculosis of the lung.

Characteristics	*Primary TB*	*Secondary TB*
Type of infection	Initial infection in an unsensitized individual	Infection in a previously sensitized individual
Source of infection	Exogenous	Usually, endogenous activation of latent infection
The site of the lung involved	The lower part of the upper lobe or upper part of the lower lobe and subpleural	Apex and posterior segments of the upper lobe and superior segments of the lower lobe
Regional lymph node involvement	Significant and prominent	Not prominent
Sputum for AFB	Rarely positive	Commonly positive
Cavity formation	Rare	Common
Healing	Mainly by calcification	By fibrosis
Extrapulmonary complications	Very common	Lesions are usually localized to the lung

Complications of Secondary Tuberculosis

❖ **Hemoptysis** due to erosion into small pulmonary arteries adjacent to the tuberculous cavity.

❖ **Bronchopleural fistula:** It may develop when a tuberculous cavity in the subpleural region ruptures into the pleural space. It may lead to tuberculous empyema and pneumothorax.

❖ **Aspergilloma:** It is a fungal mass produced due to superinfection of a persistent open cavity with *Aspergillus*. It may fill the entire cavity and form a fungal ball.

❖ **Secondary amyloidosis** can also develop.

Prognosis: The prognosis depends on the extent of the infection (localized versus widespread), the immune status of the host, and the antibiotic sensitivity of the mycobacteria. Generally, the prognosis is good if infections are localized to the lungs. All stages of HIV infection are associated with an increased risk of tuberculosis.

The main differences between primary and secondary tuberculosis of the lung are presented in **Table 17.3**.

Assman focus: Infraclavicular lesion of tuberculosis.
Primary complex: Lesion of the primary tuberculosis in parenchymal tissue and the regional lymphadenitis.
Rich focus: Tuberculous granuloma occurring on the cortex of the brain that ruptures into the subarachnoid space.

Simon focuses: Healed calcified caseous nodules of tuberculosis at the apex of the lung.
Simmond focus: Healed foci of TB in the liver.
Weigart (Wigard) focus: Healed foci of TB in the intima of blood vessels.

Puhl's lesion: Isolated lesion in lung apex and supraclavicular without lymph node involvement.
Miliary tuberculosis: Disseminated form of tuberculosis.
Reactivated/secondary TB is most commonly located near the apex.
Ranke complex: Healed primary complex consisting of calcified peripheral and calcified hilar nodes, detected radiographically.
Rasmussen aneurysm: Aneurysm of a pulmonary artery within the tuberculous cavity. May rupture and cause hemoptysis.

SCENARIO-BASED ESSAY QUESTION

Q. A 56-year-old male has a 4-month history of evening rise of temperature (fever), night sweats, weight loss, and chronic productive cough with hemoptysis on and off. The sputum examined for the causative agent was positive. His X-ray chest showed right upper lobe cavitation. He was treated and completely recovered from his illness within 6 months.

a. **What is the probable diagnosis? (Ans: Secondary tuberculosis with cavitation)**
b. **What is the morphological appearance of the right lung in this case? *(refer pages 564-5).***
c. **What are the methods of spread of this lesion? *(refer pages 565-6).***
d. **What are the investigations that would aid in reaching a diagnosis? *(refer page 567).***

SARCOIDOSIS

Definition: Sarcoidosis is a **multisystem disease of unknown cause** characterized by the presence of **noncaseating granulomas** in **many tissues and organs.**

- **Organs involved:** Sarcoidosis can affect every organ of the body. **It most commonly** affects the **lung** and the **lymph nodes** in the **mediastinum and hilar regions**. Other organs commonly affected are the liver, skin, and eye.
- **Age and gender:** Most patients are **young (from 20 to 40 years of age)** and **more common in women** than in men. A higher prevalence is seen among nonsmokers.

Etiopathogenesis

The exact cause of sarcoidosis is **not known**. Factors that play a role in its pathogenesis are as follows: (i) environmental, (ii) genetic, and (iii) immunological.

- **Environmental factors:** Environmental agents (infectious and noninfectious) have been suggested as possible causes. Infectious inciting agents include Mycobacteria (both *Mycobacterium tuberculosis* and nontuberculous mycobacteria), *Propionibacterium acnes, Borrelia burgdorferi,* viruses, fungi, spirochetes, and *Rickettsia.*
- **Genetic factors:** Certain specific HLA genotypes (e.g., HLA-A1 and HLA-B8) are associated with an increased risk of developing sarcoidosis.
- **Immunological factors:** The granuloma is the pathologic hallmark of sarcoidosis. A characteristic feature of sarcoidosis is the local accumulation of inflammatory cells. Immunological factors are important in pathogenesis. The most likely etiology is an environmental agent (infectious or noninfectious) that triggers a **cell-mediated immune response to an unidentified antigen in a genetically susceptible host.**

  The sequences of events in the development of sarcoid granuloma are as follows:

- An unknown antigen is taken up by antigen-presenting cells (APCs).
- APC presents the unknown antigen to the CD4+ helper T cells. This results in antigen-driven proliferation of CD4+ helper T cells and accumulation of activated monocytes.
- CD4+ helper T cells release several cytokines, such as:
  - Interleukin (IL)-2 results in T-cell expansion.
  - Interferon-γ (IFN-γ) causes macrophage activation.
- Local increase of several cytokines (IL-8, TNF, macrophage inflammatory protein 1α) favors recruitment of additional T cells and monocytes. They contribute to the formation of granulomas.

Systemic immunological abnormalities: Patients with sarcoidosis may also show:

- **Anergy to common skin test antigens,** such as tuberculosis purified protein derivative (PPD) or *Candida.*
- **Polyclonal hypergammaglobulinemia** (another manifestation of helper T-cell dysregulation).

MORPHOLOGY

Noncaseating Granulomas (Figs. 17.22A and B)

- The involved tissues show the classical well-formed **noncaseating granulomas.** This is the cardinal histopathologic feature of sarcoidosis.
- These granulomas are composed of an **aggregate of epithelioid macrophages surrounded by CD4+ T cells.** Epithelioid macrophages characteristically have abundant eosinophilic cytoplasm and vesicular nuclei.
- Langhans or foreign body-type multinucleate giant cells formed by fusion of macrophages may also be seen.
- A thin layer of laminated fibroblasts is seen peripheral to the granuloma. Later, these fibroblasts proliferate and produce down collagen and may replace the entire granuloma with a hyalinized scar.

Other findings: Two other microscopic findings of sarcoidosis include:

- **Schaumann bodies:** These are laminated concretions of calcium and proteins.
- **Asteroid bodies:** These are stellate inclusions within giant cells found in about 60% of the granulomas.
- They are not pathognomonic because they can be seen in other conditions.
- Rarely, foci of central necrosis may be seen in sarcoid granulomas, especially in the nodular form.

Diagnosis

- **Involvement of two or more organs is necessary.** Kveim test was used for the diagnosis of sarcoidosis.
- **Histologic diagnosis** is made **after the exclusion** of organisms that are known to be associated with granuloma formation. Noncaseating (hard) granuloma is

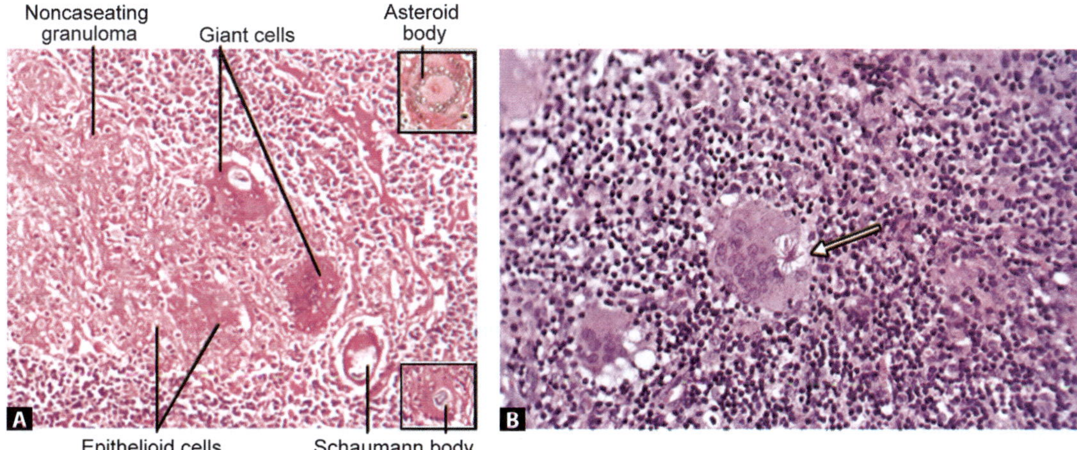

Figs. 17.22A and B: Microscopic appearance of sarcoidosis of the lymph node: (A) A noncaseating granuloma is composed of epithelioid cells surrounded by lymphocytes and giant cells. The inset shows a giant cell with an asteroid body (upper right) and a Schaumann body (lower right); (B) High-power appearance showing one giant cell in the center with an asteroid body (arrow).

not specific for sarcoidosis and may be seen in (i) mycobacterial infections, (ii) fungal infections, (iii) malignancy, and (iv) environmental agents (e.g., beryllium).

Clinical Features

- Variable clinical manifestations.
- Insidious onset of respiratory symptoms (shortness of breath, cough, chest pain, hemoptysis) or of constitutional signs and symptoms (fever, fatigue, weight loss, anorexia, night sweats).
- May be detected on **routine chest films as bilateral hilar lymphadenopathy** or may present with peripheral lymphadenopathy, skin lesions, eye involvement, splenomegaly, or hepatomegaly. It is associated with increased ACE and (2) hypercalcemia due to hypervitaminosis D.

Prognosis: Variable and is good for the majority of patients. Recovery with resolution of the disease: Occurs either spontaneously or induced by steroid therapy in about 65–70% of patients. Chronic or progressive course may lead to permanent loss of some lung function or some permanent visual impairment in about 25% of patients. Less than 3% of patients may die due to cardiac or pulmonary involvement.

PNEUMOCONIOSES

PA 26.5 (CC): Define and describe the etiology, types, exposure, environmental influence, pathogenesis, stages, morphology, microscopic appearance, and complications of occupational lung disease.

Q. Define and classify pneumoconiosis.

Occupational lung diseases: They constitute a broad group of diseases caused by the inhalation of dust, chemicals, or proteins. Among these occupational lung diseases, "Pneumoconiosis" (pneumo means air and Konis means dust) is the main and discussed in this session.

TABLE 17.4 Most common lung diseases caused by mineral dust.

Causative agent	*Disease*	*Occupation/ exposure*
Coal dust	Simple coal worker's pneumoconiosis (macules and nodules)	Coal mining
	Complicated coal worker's pneumoconiosis: Progressive massive fibrosis (PMF)	
Silica	Silicosis	Sandblasting, stone cuttings
Asbestos	Asbestosis	Mining, fabrication, and installation and removal of insulation
	Pleural plaques	
	Mesothelioma	
	Carcinoma of the lung, larynx, stomach, colon	

Definition: Pneumoconioses are defined as **chronic fibrosing lung diseases produced by exposure to organic and inorganic particulates. Some include those induced by chemical fumes and vapors.**

Originally, the term pneumoconiosis (or dust diseases of the lung) was used for non-neoplastic lung reactions to inhalation of mineral dust. A few disease caused by mineral dust is shown in **Table 17.4**. The coexistence of rheumatoid arthritis with pneumoconiosis is termed Caplan syndrome.

Pathogenesis

Only a small percentage of exposed individuals develop pneumoconiosis. This indicates a genetic predisposition. The development of pneumoconiosis depends on:

- **Amount of dust retained in the lungs and airways:** It depends on the concentration of dust in the air, the duration of exposure, and the efficiency of host clearance mechanisms.

- **Size, shape, and floating capacity of the particles:** Particles smaller than 0.5 µm reach in and out of alveoli. Particles that **range in size from 1–5 µm in diameter** tend to lodge at the bifurcation of the distal airways. They may reach the terminal small airways and air sacs and settle in their linings which are likely to be dangerous. The particles more than 5–10 µm in size usually do not reach distal airways.
- **Solubility and physiochemical reactivity of the particles:** It is influenced by their size.
  - **Smaller particles** that are soluble in pulmonary fluids can reach toxic levels rapidly and **produce acute lung injury.**
  - **Larger particles** that are not soluble persist within the lung parenchyma for years and produce pneumoconioses (e.g., silicosis).
- **Additional effects of other irritants,** e.g., accompanying **tobacco smoking worsen the effects of all inhaled mineral dusts.**

Alveolar macrophage: It is a key cell involved in the initiation and prolongation of inflammation, lung injury, and fibrosis. The dust particles are phagocytosed by pulmonary alveolar macrophages. Many particles activate inflammasome and release inflammatory mediators and fibrogenic cytokines (e.g., pro-inflammatory cytokine IL-1). They initiate an inflammatory response. This leads to fibroblast proliferation and collagen deposition.

Coal Workers' Pneumoconiosis

Definition: Coal workers' pneumoconiosis (CWP) is the **parenchymal lung disease caused by inhalation of carbon particles** (coal mine dust).

Pathogenesis

The pathogenesis of CWP is not completely known. In most cases, carbon dust itself is the major culprit. However, carbon mine dust contains various trace metals, inorganic minerals, and crystalline silica.

MORPHOLOGY

Spectrum of lung lesions in coal workers: A group of lung diseases caused by coal mine dust is commonly referred to as black lung. Lung lesions due to the progressive accumulation of carbon particles range from asymptomatic anthracosis, and simple CWP to complicated CWP, or progressive massive fibrosis (PMF).

1. Pulmonary Anthracosis

- It is a harmless, asymptomatic, coal-induced lesion in the lungs of coal miners. It is also seen in persons residing in urban areas and tobacco smokers.
- Inhaled carbon pigment is engulfed by macrophages present in the alveoli or interstitium of the lung. These carbon-laden macrophages accumulate in the connective tissue and are also carried by the lymphatics to the regional lymph nodes.

2. Simple CWP

It is a coal-induced lesion with little/no pulmonary dysfunction.

Gross

- **Coal macule:** It appears as a characteristic **nonpalpable lesion** that measures **1–2 mm in diameter.**
- **Coal nodule:** It is **larger than coal macule, but less than 2 cm.** It is a **palpable, round or irregular, and firm lesion.**

Both are mainly seen in the **upper lobes and upper zones of the lower lobes**, adjacent to respiratory bronchioles. As the lesion progresses, dilation of adjacent alveoli may produce **centrilobular emphysema.**

Microscopy

- **Coal macule:** It consists of **focal collections of** many **carbon-laden macrophages** surrounding respiratory bronchioles. It also shows small amounts of delicate network of collagen fibers.
- **Coal nodule:** It consists of carbon-laden macrophages and **small amounts of collagen and reticulin fibers.**

3. Complicated CWP

Complicated CWP (progressive massive fibrosis/PMF) develops in individuals with simple CWP and may have impaired respiratory function. It is formed by the fusion of coal nodules and usually develops over many years.

Gross (Fig. 17.23)

Lung shows **multiple, dark black scars larger than 2 cm.** Sometimes, they may be up to 10 cm in greatest diameter.

Microscopy

Shows **carbon pigment**, carbon-laden macrophages, **dense collagen,** and **disrupted lung architecture.** Dust cells are alveolar macrophages with anthracotic (carbon) pigment.

Clinical Course

CWP is usually a benign disease and is associated with minimal loss of lung function. However, in less than 10%, PMF develops leading to pulmonary dysfunction, pulmonary hypertension, and cor pulmonale.

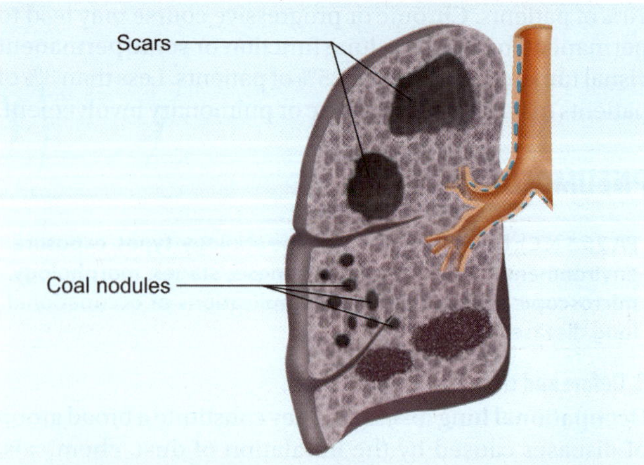

Fig. 17.23: Complicated coal worker's pneumoconiosis showing two large black scars in the upper part of the lung.

Silicosis

Q. Write a note on silicosis.

Definition: Silicosis is a **common parenchymal lung disease** associated with **inhalation of proinflammatory crystalline silicon dioxide** (silica).

- **Most prevalent slowly progressive pneumoconiosis** and usually present many years after exposure.
- Crystalline silicon dioxide is abundant and found in the earth's crust and is used in a variety of industrial applications.
- **Susceptible individuals**: Sandblasters, stone cutting, polishing and sharpening of metals, ceramic manufacturing, foundry work, tunneling through hard-rock with high quartz content, and the cleaning of boilers.
- **Forms of silica:** It occurs in both **crystalline** and **amorphous** forms. The crystalline forms including **quartz**, cristobalite, and tridymite are much more toxic and fibrogenic.

Pathogenesis (Fig. 17.24)

- **Inhalation**: Of all the crystalline forms, **quartz is the most common cause of silicosis.** These particles reach the lungs by inhalation.
- **Interaction with alveolar macrophages**: Silica is cytotoxic to alveolar macrophages. After inhalation, the particles reach the alveoli. They are ingested by alveolar macrophages.
- **Release of inflammatory mediators**: Silica particles activate macrophages and produce damage to lysosomes. They activate the inflammasome and **release inflammatory mediators** (IL-1, TNF, lipid mediators, oxygen-derived free radicals, and fibrogenic cytokines). These mediators **stimulate fibroblast proliferation and collagen formation.**

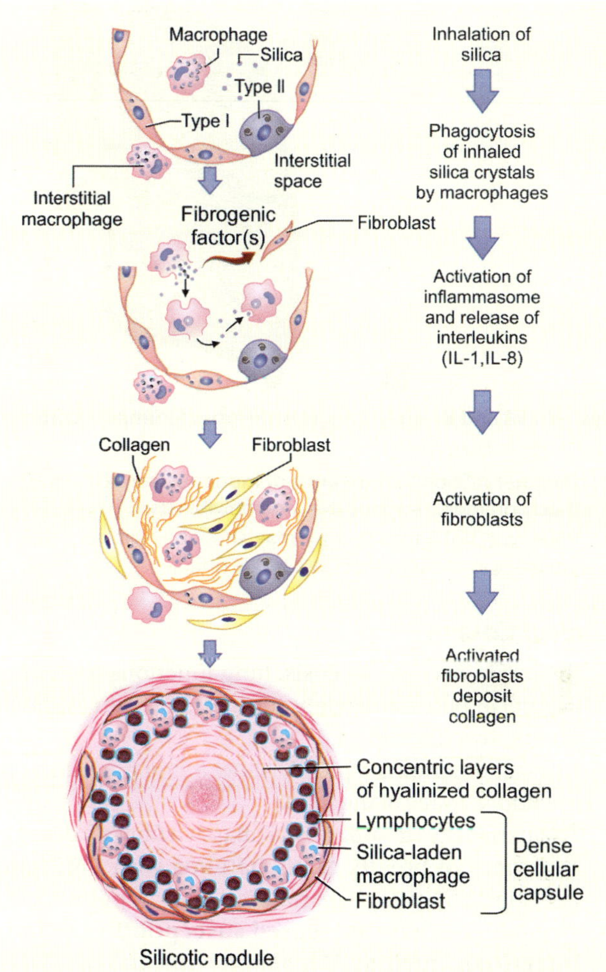

Fig. 17.24: Pathogenesis of silicosis. Silica particles (especially crystalline form) are toxic to macrophages. Silica damages macrophages and releases a fibrogenic factor. The dead macrophages release the silica, which is again phagocytosed by other macrophages. The fibrogenic factors activate fibroblasts which deposit collagen and form a characteristic dense fibrotic nodule termed a silicotic nodule. The silicotic nodule comprises concentric whorls of dense, sparsely cellular collagen. The edge of the nodule shows silica-laden macrophages and lymphocytes.

MORPHOLOGY

Chronic silicosis occurs in **two forms**, namely, **simple** form and **progressive massive fibrosis.** Simple silicosis is not associated with significant respiratory dysfunction.

Gross

Simple Nodular Silicosis (Fig. 17.25A)

Represents the early stage.

- **Silicotic nodules in lung parenchyma:** The upper zones of the lungs show **tiny, barely palpable, discrete** pale to blackened (if coal dust is also present) **silicotic nodules** (usually 2–4 mm).
- **Hilar lymph nodes with eggshell calcification:** They may become enlarged. The periphery of the lymph node may show a thin rim of calcification and are seen radiographically as **eggshell calcification** (i.e., calcium deposition surrounding a zone lacking calcification).

Progressive Massive Fibrosis (Fig. 17.25B)

As the disease progresses, the expansion and coalescence of lesions may produce progressive massive fibrosis.

- **Progressive massive fibrosis** is defined radiologically as nodular masses of more than 2 cm diameter in a background of simple silicosis.
- **Coalesce of silicotic nodules:** The smaller silicotic nodules coalesce to form large lesions, which range from 5 to 10 cm in size. These lesions are hard and some of them may undergo central softening and cavitation. These changes may be due to superimposed tuberculosis or ischemia.
- **Honeycomb pattern:** The intervening lung parenchyma between silicotic nodules may be compressed or over-expanded. This produces a honeycomb appearance.
- **Fibrotic lesions** may also develop in **the hilar lymph nodes and pleura**.

Microscopy

Silicotic nodule (Fig. 17.24): It has a characteristic **whorled appearance**.

- **Center:** It consists of **concentric layers of hyalinized acellular collagen** surrounded by a **dense cellular capsule** of more condensed collagen.

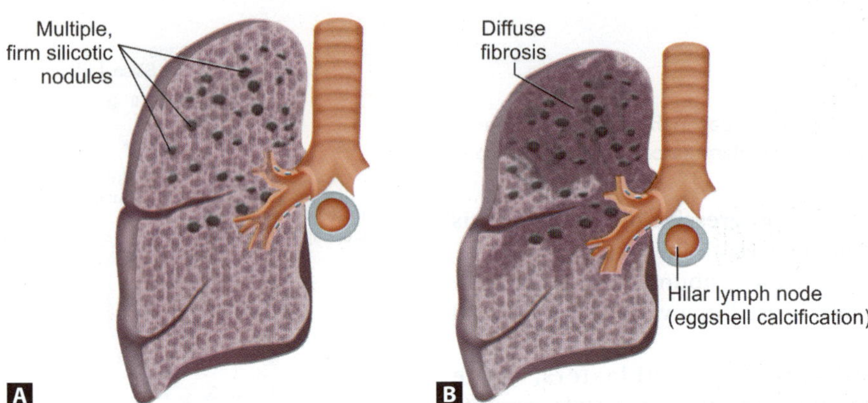

Figs. 17.25A and B: Gross changes in silicosis: (A) Simple nodular silicosis; (B) Progressive massive fibrosis shows scarring at the upper lobe.

- **Periphery:** Shows **aggregates of mononuclear cells,** mostly **macrophages, lymphocytes, and fibroblasts.**
- **Polarized light microscopy** may show **birefringent silica particles** in the center of the silicotic nodule.

Clinical Course

- In simple nodular silicosis, lung functions are either normal or only moderately affected. Silicosis is a slowly progressive disease.
- Chest radiographs typically show a fine nodularity in the upper zones of the lung.
- The patients with progressive massive fibrosis develop shortness of breath. Many patients with PMF may develop pulmonary hypertension and cor pulmonale.
- The patients have **increased susceptibility to lung infections, such as *Mycobacterium tuberculosis*, atypical mycobacteria, and fungi.**
- The crystalline silica is also carcinogenic.

Asbestosis and Asbestos-related Diseases

Q. Write a note on asbestosis.

Definition: Asbestosis is defined as **interstitial fibrosis of the lung caused by exposure to asbestos dust.** It does not include asbestos-induced pleural diseases and carcinoma of the lung that are found in asbestos-exposed workers.

Asbestos Use and Exposure

Q. Write a note on asbestos-related diseases.

- Asbestos is a family of crystalline hydrated silicates that form fibers.
- They have unique physical-chemical properties that make them effective for insulation, reinforcing materials, and friction products.
- Asbestos is used for fireproofing, in heat and sound insulations, and for strengthening plastics and cement.
- **Asbestos-related occupational lung diseases:** Occupational exposure to asbestos can cause different lung diseases. They are listed in **Box 17.9.**

BOX 17.9: Asbestos-related occupational lung diseases.

1. Parenchymal interstitial fibrosis (asbestosis
2. Localized fibrous plaques (rarely, diffuse fibrosis in the pleura)
3. Pleural effusions
4. Carcinoma of the lung
5. Malignant pleural and peritoneal mesotheliomas
6. Laryngeal carcinomas

Asbestos Types

Asbestos is a generic term used for naturally occurring fibrous silicates. Two major forms are **Serpentine and amphibole.**

Serpentine form: Chrysotile (white asbestos) is the most important serpentine form of asbestos are used in industry. Chrysotile consists of **long, curly, flexible structures that are likely to become impacted in the upper respiratory passages** and removed by the mucociliary action. They are less readily carried to the lungs and even if trapped in the lungs, they fragment into short particles and are easily ingested by macrophages. They are also more soluble than amphiboles.

Amphibole form: The **main amphibole forms are crocidolite (blue asbestos) and amosite (brown asbestos).** Amphibole form **consists of straight, rigid, brittle fibers** that may align themselves in the airstream and remain stable in the lung. They neither fragment nor are soluble and thus reach deeper into the lungs, where they can penetrate epithelial cells and reach the interstitium. Though they are not commonly used, they are **more pathogenic than chrysotiles,** particularly with respect to the induction of malignant pleural tumors (mesotheliomas).

Pathogenesis (Fig. 17.26)

Q. Discuss the pathology and complications of asbestosis.

Asbestos has both fibrogenic and oncogenic effects.

Fibrogenic effects: Inhaled asbestos fibers reach the air spaces. The macrophages (alveolar and interstitial) phagocytose the asbestos fibers. They **activate the inflammasome and phagolysosomal membranes.**

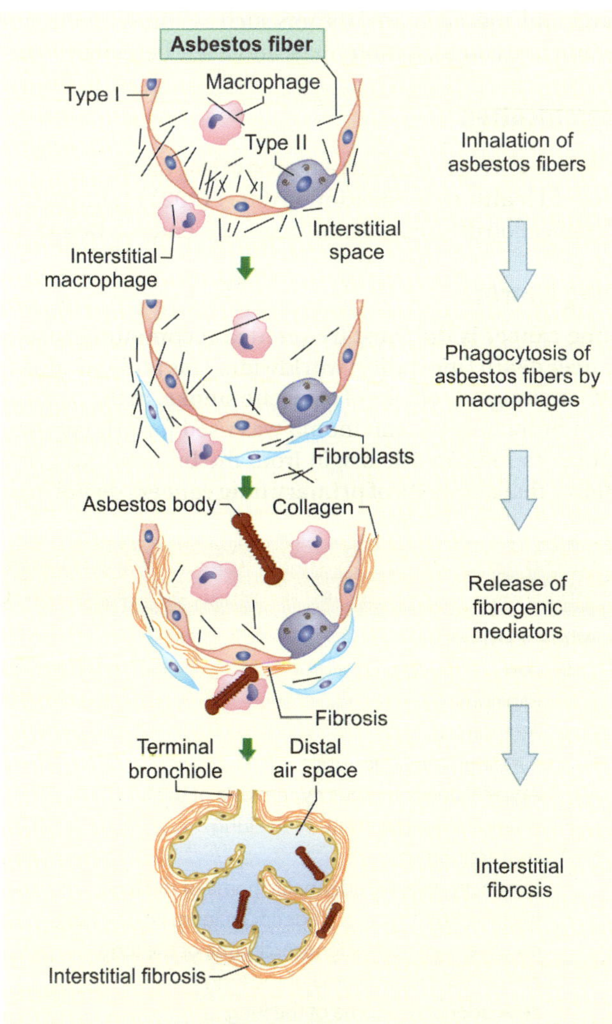

Fig. 17.26: Pathogenesis of asbestosis. Asbestosis is characterized by significant interstitial fibrosis and asbestos bodies.

They stimulate the release of pro-inflammatory factors and fibrogenic mediators. Both amphibole and serpentine forms are fibrogenic. The initial injury occurs at bifurcations of small airways and ducts, where the asbestos fibers land and penetrate. Chronic exposure and deposition of asbestos fibers lead to the persistent release of fibrogenic mediators. **The end result is generalized interstitial pulmonary inflammation and interstitial fibrosis.**

Oncogenic effects: Asbestos can act both as a tumor **initiator and as a promoter.** Some of the oncogenic effects of asbestos on the mesothelium are mediated by **free radicals** generated by asbestos fibers. They preferably localize in the distal lung close to the mesothelial layer. Inhaled **potentially toxic chemicals** are adsorbed onto the asbestos fibers and may be oncogenic. For example, the adsorption of carcinogens present in **tobacco smoke** onto asbestos fibers **increases the risk of lung carcinoma in asbestos workers.**

MORPHOLOGY

Lung

Gross (Fig. 17.27A)

Locations: Lesions **begin** in the **lower lobes and subpleura. This is in contrast with CWP and silicosis.** As the fibrosis progresses, the lesion spreads to the middle and upper lobes of the lungs.

Early stages

- **Mineral dust-induced small airway disease:** Interstitial fibrosis may not be apparent on gross examination. Begins as interstitial **fibrosis around respiratory bronchioles and alveolar ducts** and extends to involve adjacent alveolar sacs and alveoli. The lesions are **termed mineral dust-induced small airway disease.**

Later stages

- **Diffuse pulmonary interstitial fibrosis:** The **interstitial fibrosis becomes more extensive and may involve the entire lung.**
- **Honeycombed appearance**: The fibrosis may **destroy the normal architecture of the lung** to produce **dilated airspaces (cystic spaces) surrounded by** thick **fibrous walls.** This produces a **honeycomb** appearance to the involved regions. The lungs become small.

Microscopy

Asbestos Bodies (Fig. 17.27B)

- The asbestos fibers after reaching the finer bronchioles and alveoli may form asbestos bodies.
- The asbestos bodies are formed when macrophages attempt to phagocytose asbestos fibers. Asbestos bodies **consist of a translucent center of asbestos fibers coated with a film of proteins rich in iron.** The iron is derived from ferritin. The process of asbestos body formation occurs in the lysosome, which is normally the site of the degradation of ferritin.
- Asbestos bodies appear as **golden brown, fusiform, or beaded rods.**
- The coating is thickest at the ends of the fibers, giving a **dumbbell appearance.**

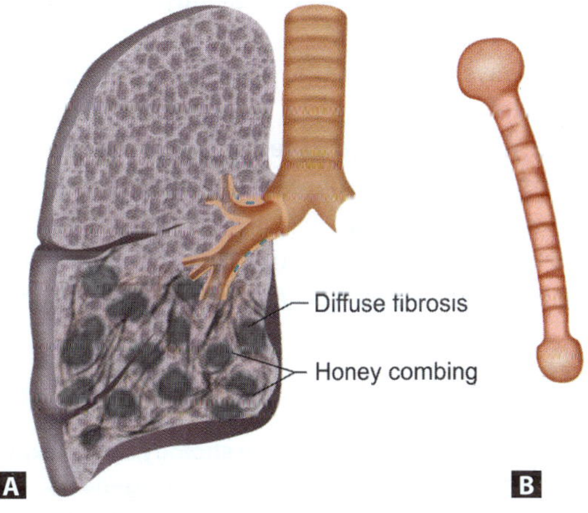

Figs. 17.27A and B: (A) Asbestosis of lung showing honeycomb appearance in the lower lobe; (B) Asbestos body is a ferruginous body, golden brown, beaded, and having dumb-bell shape.

- They form when macrophages attempt to phagocytose asbestos fibers; the iron is probably derived from phagocyte ferritin.

Ferruginous Bodies

Other inorganic particulates/fibers such as talc, mica, and glass (not asbestos) may also become coated with similar iron-protein complexes and are called **ferruginous bodies.**

Fibrosis of the Lung

Lung shows **diffuse pulmonary interstitial fibrosis** with multiple **asbestos bodies.**

Complications: The fibrous scarring may trap and narrow pulmonary arteries and arterioles. This may lead to pulmonary hypertension and cor pulmonale.

Pleural Plaques

They are the most **common manifestation of asbestos exposure.**

Gross

Pleural plaques appear as **pearly white; well-circumscribed plaques** (may be over 10 cm in diameter). **Usually bilateral** and most frequent on the **anterior and posterolateral aspects of the parietal pleura** and **over the domes of the diaphragm.**

Microscopy

It consists of **acellular, dense, hyalinized fibrous tissue**, with many **slit-like spaces** arranged in a parallel fashion (**basket-weave pattern**). They may contain calcium. It may show calcification. They **neither show asbestos bodies nor** do they **progress to mesotheliomas.**

Lung cancer and mesothelioma: The workers exposed to asbestos may develop lung carcinomas and mesotheliomas (pleural and peritoneal). Concomitant cigarette smoking markedly increases the risk of lung carcinoma but not that of mesothelioma.

Clinical Features of Asbestosis

- Initially patients present with **dyspnea on exertion**, but **later** it is present **even at rest**. Usually, it is accompanied by a productive cough.
- Chest X-rays show irregular linear densities, particularly in both lower lobes.
- As **the disease progresses, a honeycomb pattern** develops and may progress to respiratory failure, cor pulmonale, and death.
- Pleural plaques are usually asymptomatic and are visualized on radiographs as circumscribed densities.

LUNG TUMORS

PA 26.6 (CC): Define and describe the etiology, types, exposure, genetics, environmental influence, pathogenesis, stages, morphology, microscopic appearance, metastases, and complications of tumors of the lung and pleura.

About 95% of primary lung tumors are carcinomas. The remaining 5% include miscellaneous groups (e.g., carcinoid, mesenchymal tumors such as fibrosarcoma, and leiomyosarcoma), lymphomas, and a few benign lesions.

Classification

Q. Write a short note on the classification of lung cancer.

World Health Organization (WHO) (2021) (simplified) classification of tumors of the lung is presented in **Box 17.10.**

Lung Cancer

Lung cancer is the most frequent and common cause of cancer death (mortality) worldwide. This is mainly due to the carcinogenic effects of **cigarette smoke**. In the past, the term bronchogenic carcinoma was used for primary lung cancer to indicate the origin from the bronchi. Now, it is known that **about 5% of primary lung cancers do not arise**

BOX 17.10: World Health Organization (WHO) (2021) (simplified) classification of tumors of the lung.

Epithelial tumors:
- Benign
  - Papillomas
  - Adenomas
- Precursor glandular lesions
  - Atypical adenomatous hyperplasia of the lung
  - Adenocarcinoma in situ of the lung
- Adenocarcinomas
  - Minimally invasive adenocarcinoma of the lung
  - Invasive non-mucinous adenocarcinoma of the lung
  - Invasive mucinous adenocarcinoma of the lung
  - Colloid adenocarcinoma of the lung
  - Fetal adenocarcinoma of the lung
  - Enteric-type adenocarcinoma of the lung
- Squamous precursor lesions
  - Squamous dysplasia and carcinoma in situ of the lung
- Squamous cell carcinomas
  - Squamous cell carcinoma of the lung
  - Lymphoepithelial carcinoma of the lung
- Large cell carcinomas of the lung
- Adenosquamous carcinoma of the lung
- Salivary gland-type tumors

Lung neuroendocrine neoplasms:
- Precursor lesion
  - Diffuse idiopathic pulmonary neuroendocrine cell hyperplasia
- Neuroendocrine tumors
  - Carcinoid/neuroendocrine tumor of the lung
- Neuroendocrine carcinomas
  - Small cell lung carcinoma
  - Large cell neuroendocrine carcinoma of the lung

Tumors of ectopic tissues

Mesenchymal tumors specific to the lung

Hematolymphoid tumors

Metastasis in the lung

from the bronchus. Hence, the term lung cancer (cancer of the lung) is used.

Age and gender: Lung cancer is generally a disease of older adults. It occurs most often between ages **50 and 80 years**, and the peak incidence is between 60 and 70 years. More common in males, but there is a recent increase in females due to increased smoking among females.

Etiology and Pathogenesis

Q. Discuss etiopathogenesis of carcinoma of the lung.

Tobacco smoking is a well-known carcinogen. Most (but not all) lung cancers are associated with cigarette smoke. Apart from smoking, other genetic and environmental factors are also involved in the development of lung cancer.

Tobacco Smoking

About 80% of lung cancers occur in active smokers or in those **individuals who stopped smoking recently**. Thus, **carcinoma of the lung is strongly associated with tobacco smoking.**

Smoking habit: There is almost a linear correlation between the frequency of lung cancer and smoking habits. Smoking habit includes the **amount of daily smoking (packs per day), the tendency to inhale, and the duration (years) of the smoking**. In habitual heavy smokers (who smoke two packs a day for 20 years), the risk of lung cancer is 60 times higher than nonsmokers. It is observed that women are more susceptible to carcinogens present in tobacco than men. **Cessation of smoking reduces the risk of lung cancer over time**. But, in these individuals, the risk may never return to baseline levels. There is also a moderate risk of lung cancer in pipe and cigar smokers, but the risk is less than that of cigarette smoking. The long-term effects of electronic cigarette aerosols are not yet established because "vaping" is a relatively recent phenomenon. Vaping is the practice of **inhaling** and **exhaling** vapor containing nicotine and flavorings produced by a device. The **strongest association** of smoking is with **squamous cell and small cell carcinoma**. Adenocarcinoma is also associated with smoking. **Cigarette smoking is also associated with carcinoma of the mouth, pharynx, larynx, esophagus, pancreas, uterine cervix, kidney, and urinary bladder.**

Second-hand smoke or environmental tobacco smoke: It contains several carcinogens, and nonsmoking adults may develop lung cancer due to breathing second-hand smoke. Smoking also multiplies the risk of other carcinogenic influences, such as asbestos and uranium.

Major carcinogens in tobacco smoke: These include both initiators and promoters (such as phenol derivatives). These include **polycyclic aromatic hydrocarbons** [e.g., benzo(*a*) pyrene, dibenzanthracene] and. **radioactive elements and other contaminants** (e.g., arsenic, nickel, cadmium, molds, and vinyl chloride).

Lung cancer develops in only 10–15% of smokers. It suggests that probably **other factors that interact with smoking predispose individuals to lung cancer**. The mutagenic effect of carcinogens in cigarette smoke is modified by genetic variants.

Industrial Hazards

Certain industrial exposures increase the risk of developing lung cancer. These include asbestos, arsenic, chromium, uranium, nickel, vinyl chloride, mustard gas, polyaromatic hydrocarbons, chloromethyl ethers, cadmium, formaldehyde, and dioxin.

Ionizing radiation: A high dose of ionizing radiation is carcinogenic. Increased incidence of lung cancer was reported among survivors of the Hiroshima and Nagasaki atomic bomb blasts. **Radon** is a radioactive gas, and indoor air pollution by radon is associated with **increased lung cancer in miners exposed to high concentrations.**

Uranium: It is weakly radioactive. Uranium miners (both nonsmokers and smokers) have a four times higher risk of lung cancer than the general population. Uranium miners who are smoking have about 10 times higher risk. Lung cancer may develop after a latent period of 10–30 years.

Asbestos: Lung cancer is the most frequent malignancy in individuals exposed to asbestos. This risk increases further when associated with smoking.

Air Pollution

It is not clear whether air pollution, by itself, increases the risk of carcinoma of the lung. Major air pollutants include polycyclic hydrocarbons from fossil fuels and motor vehicle exhaust, especially diesel smoke. Probably air pollution adds to the risk for smokers or those exposed to second-hand smoke.

Radon: It is a ubiquitous radioactive gas that may contribute to air pollution. Epidemiologically, an increased risk of lung cancer was found in uranium miners due to exposure to radon gas. Others who have an increased risk for radon exposure are underground miners and workers in locations below ground. These include subways, tunnels, and basements. Low-level exposure (e.g., in well-insulated homes in regions with high levels of radon in soil) may also increase the incidence of lung cancer.

Acquired Mutations In Lung Cancer (Refer Online Table 17.5)

Smoking-related lung cancers occur by a **stepwise accumulation of oncogenic "driver" mutations** in the **pulmonary epithelial cells**. Large areas of the respiratory mucosa undergo genetic mutations due to exposure to carcinogens in tobacco smoke. This is called the **"field effect."** On this fertile soil, some cells acquire all the hallmarks of cancer and progress to carcinomas. **Tumor cells contain many genetic abnormalities and only certain abnormalities are required for tumor cell survival,** which are **called driver mutations.** Inactivation of one or more tumor suppressor genes located on the short arm of chromosome

3 (3p) is a very common early event in lung cancer. Mutations in the *TP53* tumor suppressor gene and the *KRAS* (rare in neuroendocrine carcinoma) oncogene occur relatively late. Certain genetic alterations, such as loss of chromosomal material on 3p, are observed even in benign bronchial epithelium of smokers without lung cancer. Each major histologic subtype of lung cancer has distinctive molecular features.

Adenocarcinoma

It is one of the histologic types of lung cancer that is **less associated with tobacco smoking** than other histologic subtypes. Adenocarcinoma is the most **common subtype in never-smokers**. For the last two decades, the incidence of adenocarcinoma has significantly increased.

Alterations in driver genes (oncogene) (growth signaling pathway)

Gain-of-function mutations in genes involved in tyrosine kinase signaling: About one-third of adenocarcinomas reveal **oncogenic gain-of-function mutations** involving components of **growth factor receptor signaling pathways**. Examples include ***EGFR* (higher in nonsmoking women), *ALK, MET,* and *RET***. Other tumors that have **gain-of-function mutations** include ***BRAF* and *PI3K* or the *KRAS* gene**. All these genes encode signaling molecules that lie downstream of receptor tyrosine kinases in growth factor signaling pathways.

- **Mutations in epidermal growth factor receptor (EGFR): EGFR is a** receptor tyrosine kinase that stimulates downstream pro-growth pathways involving RAS, PI3K, and other signaling molecules. **EGFR mutations are more common in adenocarcinomas in nonsmoker** women. These tumors are sensitive to drugs that inhibit EGFR signaling.
- **Mutations in KRAS:** KRAS is involved in the receptor tyrosine kinase/RAS/RAF pathways. Mutations in this oncogene, occur in adenocarcinomas (5–25%), large cell carcinomas, and squamous carcinomas (5%), but it is rare in small cell carcinomas [small cell lung carcinoma (SCLC)]. These mutations correlate with cigarette smoking, and patients with adenocarcinoma with these mutations have a **poor prognosis**. Presently, no effective targeted molecular therapy is available for *KRAS* mutations.
- **Activating rearrangements of *ALK* gene:** Fusion between echinoderm microtubule-associated protein-like 4 (*EML4*) and *ALK* is seen in 3–7% of adenocarcinomas. It is also most frequent in **nonsmokers**. Adenocarcinomas with *EML4-ALK* translocation are responsive to targeted therapy.
- **Mutations in *BRAF* gene:** These may be found in 2–20% of lung carcinoma.
- **Other gene alterations:** These include **somatic activating *ERBB2* mutations and alterations in** *ROS1, RET, NTRK1,* and *NRG1*.

Growth inhibitory pathway (p53/RB1/p14/STK11)

- Mutations of the tumor suppressor gene *TP53* occur in approximately 45% of lung adenocarcinoma.
- Like the adenoma–carcinoma sequence in the colon, it is possible that some invasive adenocarcinomas of the lung also arise through atypical adenomatous hyperplasia–adenocarcinoma in situ–invasive adenocarcinoma sequence. Lung injury models in experimental mice have identified a population of multipotent cells in the lung periphery at the bronchioloalveolar duct junction. These are termed *bronchioalveolar stem cells (BASCs)*. After lung injury, multipotent BASCs proliferate and restore the normal cell types (bronchiolar Clara cells and alveolar cells) in this location, thereby replacing the epithelial cells. regeneration. Possibly, these BASCs undergo the first mutation that initiates the changes that eventually develop into a full-blown malignancy.

Squamous Cell Carcinoma

Inactivation of tumor suppressor gene

Loss-of-function mutations: This histologic type is **highly associated with exposure to tobacco smoke**. It shows **diverse genetic aberrations**. Many of these aberrations are **chromosome deletions involving tumor suppressor loci**. These chromosomal losses are due to deletions, especially those involving **3p, 9p (site of the CDKN2A gene), and 17p (site of the *TP53* gene)**. They occur during the early stages of tumor evolution. They are frequently detected in the histologically normal respiratory mucosal cells of smokers.

- ***TP53* mutations:** Most SCCs have mutations in *TP53*. It is **found in 10–50% of squamous dysplasia and 60–90% of SCC in situ**.
- ***CDKN2A* mutations:** *CDKN2A* is a tumor suppressor gene and encodes the cyclin-dependent kinase inhibitor p16. It is mutated in **65% of SCC**.

Activation of oncogenes

Amplification of fibroblast growth factor receptor 1 (*FGFR1*): Many SCCs (15–25%) also have amplification of *FGFR1*. The *FGFR1* gene encodes the fibroblast growth factor receptor tyrosine kinase. **Amplification of the *EGFR* gene** can also occur.

Neuroendocrine Tumors (Small Cell Carcinoma)

It is a neuroendocrine carcinoma **almost always smoking-related carcinoma**. Small cell carcinoma has the **highest mutational burden** among all lung cancers.

Inactivation of tumor suppressor gene

Mutations in tumor suppressor gene *TP53* and *RB*: Small cell carcinoma is distinct from other forms of lung carcinoma, in that these tumors almost always have loss of function mutations in both important tumor suppressor genes *TP53* and *RB*. Thus, inactivation of both *TP53* and *RB* is observed in more than 90% of small cell carcinoma.

- **Mutations in *RB*:** An unusual transformation of non-small cell carcinoma to small cell carcinoma is usually associated with acquiring *RB* loss-of-function mutations. This indicates the importance of *RB* inactivation in small cell carcinoma of the lung. Loss of chromosome 3p also occurs in almost all of these tumors, which can even be found in histologically normal lung epithelium. This suggests that this also is an early critical event.
- **Mutations of TP53 are identified in 30–40% of adenocarcinoma and 50–80% of SCC.**

Activation of oncogenes

Activation of oncogenes-overexpression *MYC*: Small-cell carcinoma is also commonly associated with the amplification of genes of the *MYC* family. *MYC* is an oncogene and is overexpression in **20–30% of small cell carcinomas.** However, it is rare in other types of lung cancer. **Mutations in *KRAS*** can also occur.

In small cell carcinoma, precursor lesions have not been clearly described except diffuse idiopathic pulmonary neuroendocrine cell hyperplasia. Small cell carcinoma has high growth rates and is associated with early development of widespread metastases.

Precursor (Preinvasive) Lesions

Morphologic precursor (preinvasive) epithelial lesions exist in the lung **(Box 17.11)**. The precursor lesions need not always progress to cancer. It is not possible to distinguish between precursor lesions that progress to cancer and those that remain localized or regressed.

MORPHOLOGY

Precursor Glandular Lesions

Atypical Adenomatous Hyperplasia (AAH)

Gross: It is a precursor lesion that is **small in size (≤5 mm)** with mild fibrosis. It may be **single or multiple** and can be seen in the lung adjacent to an invasive tumor or away from it. It occurs in the peripheral lung, **often close to the pleura.**

Microscopy: It shows alveolar walls lined by dysplastic pneumocytes. They are cuboidal to low-columnar cells showing nuclear hyperchromasia, pleomorphism, and prominent nucleoli. It may progress in a stepwise fashion to adenocarcinoma in situ, minimally invasive adenocarcinoma, and invasive adenocarcinoma.

BOX 17.11: Morphologic precursor epithelial lesions in the lung.

Precursor glandular lesions
- Atypical adenomatous hyperplasia
- Adenocarcinoma in situ

Squamous precursor lesions
- Squamous dysplasia and carcinoma in situ

Precursor neuroendocrine lesion
- Diffuse idiopathic pulmonary neuroendocrine cell hyperplasia

Adenocarcinoma in situ (AIS)

It was formerly called bronchioloalveolar carcinoma (BAC and is obsolete). It has distinct gross, microscopic, and clinical features. It is a preinvasive form of adenocarcinoma.

Gross: It occurs in the **periphery of the lung** and is often close to the pleura. It is a **poorly defined single nodule** (coin lesion) measuring **up to 3 cm in diameter.**

Microscopy (Figs. 17.28A and B): It is entirely composed of **dysplastic cells that grow along preexisting alveolar septa (walls) without destruction of alveolar architecture.** This growth pattern is known as **lepidic**, where the neoplastic cells resemble butterflies sitting on a fence. **There is no evidence of stromal, vascular, or pleural invasion.** The lining cells show more dysplasia than observed in AAH. They may be subdivided into nonmucinous and mucinous variants.

- **Nonmucinous:** Most of them are nonmucinous types and consist of columnar, peg-shaped, or cuboidal cells.
- **Mucinous:** It consists of distinctive, tall, columnar cells with intracellular mucin growing along the alveolar septa.

Squamous Precursor Lesions

Squamous dysplasia and carcinoma in situ: Precursor lesions that give rise to invasive SCC may occur in the bronchial epithelium and are well characterized. In response to injury such as cigarette smoking, the bronchial epithelium undergoes regeneration from the pluripotent basal squamous cell layer with stem cell-like properties. The intensity of exposure to cigarette smoke and the appearance of progressive severe epithelial changes have a linear correlation. The epithelial changes begin with **benign-appearing basal cell hyperplasia and squamous metaplasia.** This later progresses to **squamous dysplasia and carcinoma in situ.** Finally, this progresses to **invasive cancer (Figs. 17.29A to F).** This phase may last for years. During this phase, atypical cells may be found in cytologic smears prepared from sputum or bronchial lavage fluids or bronchial brushings. However, this lesion is asymptomatic and cannot be detected by radiography. Finally, they develop into an invasive SCC.

Precursor Neuroendocrine Lesion

Diffuse idiopathic pulmonary neuroendocrine cell hyperplasia: Diffuse idiopathic pulmonary neuroendocrine cell hyperplasia (DIPNECH) is a generalized proliferation of pulmonary neuroendocrine cells (PNCs). This may be restricted to the mucosa of airways and may or may not protrude into the lumen.

Epithelial Tumors

Q. Write a short note on the morphology of lung cancer.

MORPHOLOGY

Gross

Location of Lung Cancer (Figs. 17.30A to C)

Lung carcinomas may arise in the lung's peripheral or central/hilar region.

- **Central (hilar):** Lung cancers arising **in and around the hilus of the lung** are the most common. About 75% arise from first, second, and third-order bronchi. More often, they are SCC.
- **Peripheral:** Lung cancers may also arise in the periphery of the lung from the alveolar septal cells or terminal bronchioles. They are **usually adenocarcinomas, including adenocarcinoma in situ.**

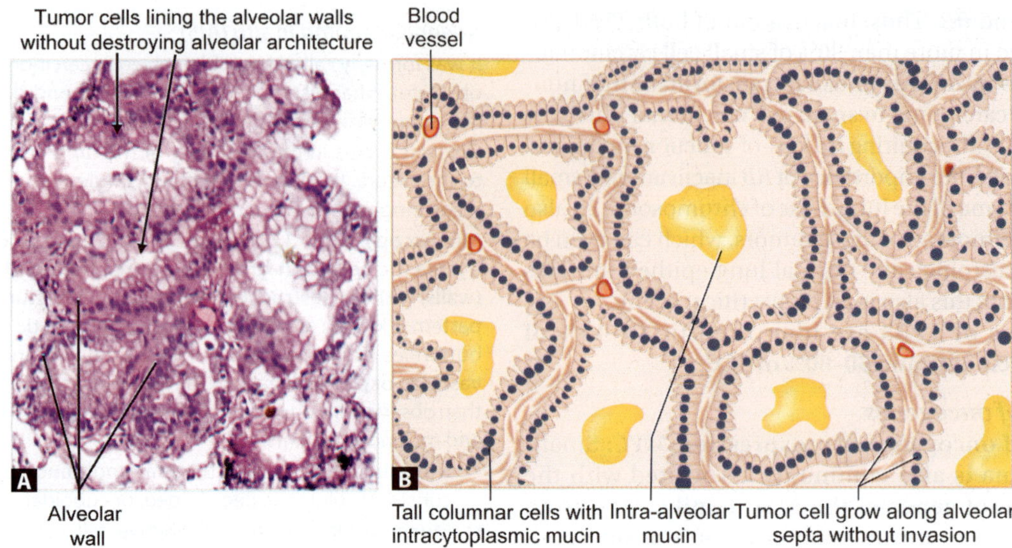

Figs. 17.28A and B: Adenocarcinoma in situ: (A) Photomicrograph; (B) Diagrammatic.

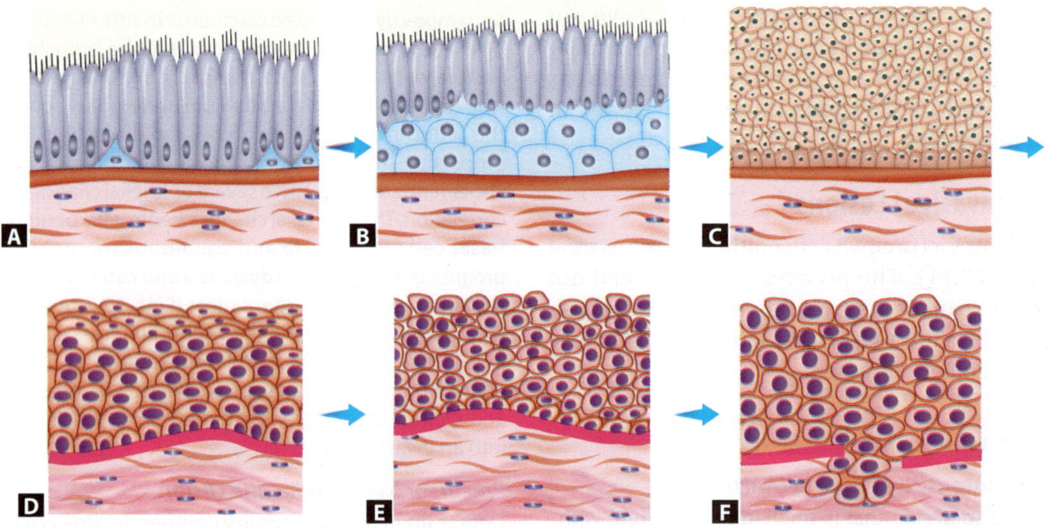

Figs. 17.29A to F: Sequential changes during the pathogenesis of lung cancer: (A) Normal epithelium; (B) Basal cell (or reserve cell) hyperplasia; (C) Squamous metaplasia; (D) Dysplasia (characterized by the presence of disordered squamous epithelium, with loss of nuclear polarity, nuclear hyperchromasia, and pleomorphism) may progress through the stages of mild, moderate and severe dysplasia; (E) Carcinoma-in-situ (CIS); (F) Invasive squamous carcinoma.

Adenocarcinoma

Q. Discuss the pathology of adenocarcinoma of the lung.

Minimally Invasive Adenocarcinoma

Minimally invasive adenocarcinoma (MIA) is defined as a lepidic—predominant adenocarcinoma tumor as in AIS but with foci of invasion less than or equal to 5 mm in maximal dimension and without any pleural or lymphovascular invasion and necrosis. These tumors are single and discrete and usually non-mucinous.

Invasive Adenocarcinoma

Adenocarcinoma is an invasive malignant epithelial tumor in which tumor cells show glandular differentiation or mucin production. It is the most **common type of carcinoma in women and nonsmokers.**

MORPHOLOGY

Gross (Figs. 17.31A and 17.30B)

- **Location:** Usually more **peripherally located** (in contrast to squamous cell carcinoma), and **tend to be smaller.**
- **Appearance**: They appear as **irregular masses** ranging from **2 to 5 cm in diameter**. They are often associated with pleural fibrosis and subpleural scars which represent a desmoplastic response to the tumor.
- **Cut section**: Nonmucinous tumors appear **grayish-white** and mucinous tumors may appear glistening or gelatinous (depending on the amount of mucus).

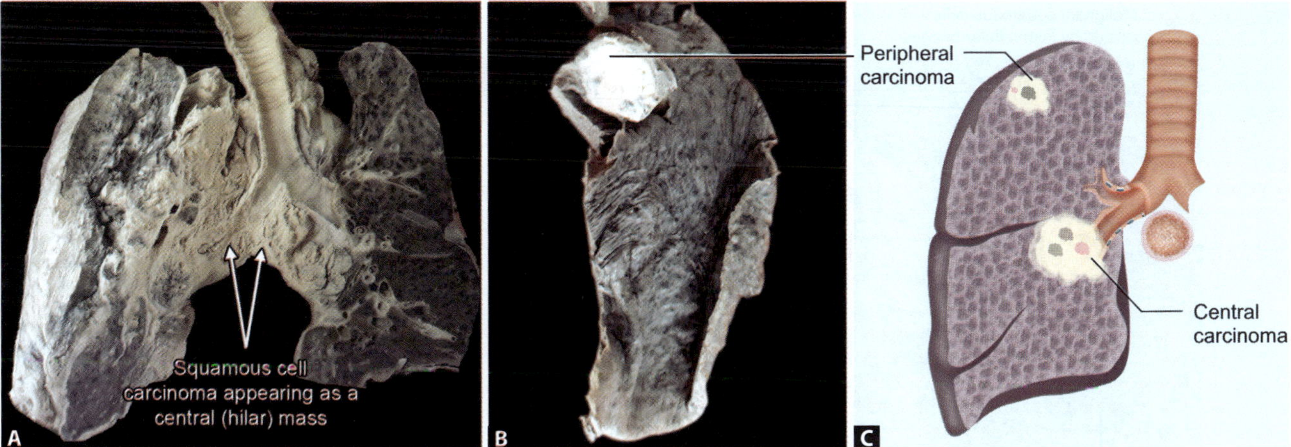

Figs. 17.30A to C: Gross types of carcinoma lung namely, central and peripheral: (A) Squamous cell carcinoma appearing as a central (hilar) mass which has invaded the contiguous lung parenchyma; (B) Peripheral carcinoma of the lung; (C) Diagrammatic.

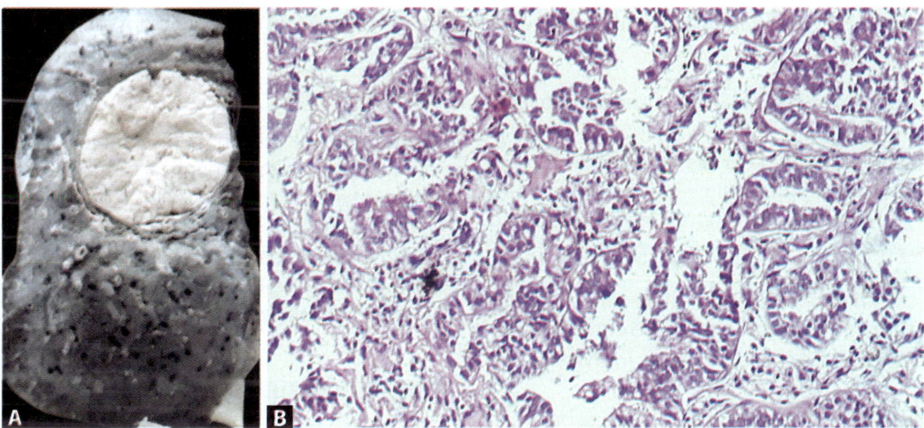

Figs. 17.31A and B: Adenocarcinoma of the lung: (A) Gross; (B) Microscopy: Tumor cells are arranged in a glandlike (acinar) pattern.

Microscopy (Fig. 17.31B)

Growth patterns: Adenocarcinoma are classified based on the predominant growth pattern namely: lepidic, acinar, papillary, solid, and micropapillary.

Most adenocarcinomas show mixtures of the above patterns: (i) **lepidic**—predominant tumors show prominent lepidic growth patterns (**cells grow along the surface of alveolar cells**), (ii) **acinar—predominant** tumor patterns, consists of regular glands lined by cuboidal or columnar cells, (iii) **papillary** adenocarcinomas show a single cell layer covering a fibrovascular connective tissue core, (iv) **micropapillary** carcinomas consist of small papillary tufts of tumor cells without fibrovascular core, and (v) **solid** adenocarcinomas with mucus formation are poorly differentiated tumors.

Immunohistochemistry: The majority of tumors are **positive for thyroid transcription factor-1 (TTF-1).**

Spread: They **grow more slowly than squamous cell carcinomas but metastasize widely and earlier.**

Squamous Cell Carcinomas

Squamous cell carcinoma is **most common** in **men** and is most **strongly related to cigarette smoking.** They are likely to arise from basal squamous cells. It spreads first to local hilar nodes and spreads outside the thorax occurs later than with other histologic types of lung cancer. Its precursor lesions are discussed on page 577.

MORPHOLOGY

Q. Discuss the morphology of squamous cell carcinoma of the lung.

Gross (Fig. 17.30A)

- **Location and pattern of growth:** Most tumors arise in the **central portion of the lung from the major bronchi** (main to segmental bronchus).
  - **Peribronchial growth:** In which the tumor appears as ulcerated lesions in the bronchi that penetrate the wall of the involved bronchus and infiltrate along the peribronchial tissue into the adjacent carina or mediastinum.
  - **Intraprenchymal growth:** In this pattern, the tumor grows like a cauliflower-like intraparenchymal mass which pushes the surrounding lung substance.
  - **Exophytic growth:** It starts as an endobronchial tumor projecting into the lumen of the bronchi producing an intraluminal mass. As it enlarges, it obstructs the involved bronchus leading to atelectasis and infection distal to the obstruction.

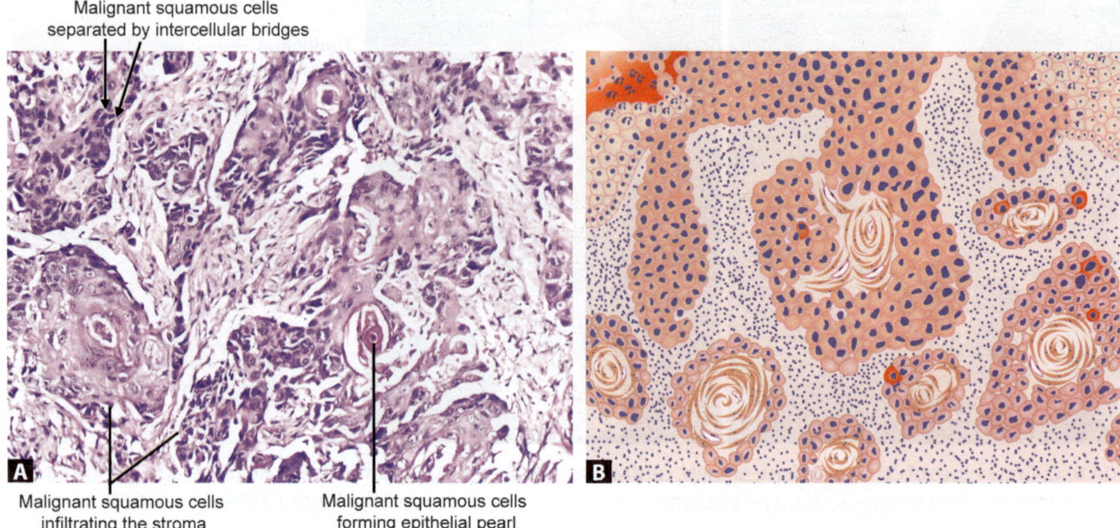

Figs. 17.32A and B: Well-differentiated squamous cell carcinoma of the lung: (A) Photomicrograph; (B) Diagrammatic.

- **Color and consistency**: **Gray-white** in color and **firm to hard** in consistency.
- **Cut section:** It may show focal **areas of hemorrhage or necrosis**. It may produce red or yellow-white mottling and softening. Large tumors may show central necrotic foci and may form a cavity.

Microscopy (Figs. 17.32A and B)

The characteristic features of squamous cell differentiation are:

- **Keratinization**: **Epithelial keratin pearls** or **individual cell keratinization.**
- **Intercellular bridges**: They are seen as slender gaps between adjacent cells.

Grades: Based on the amount of keratinization, SCCs are graded as:

1. **Well-differentiated**: These tumors show keratinization in the form of **keratin/squamous pearls.** They **appear as small round nests of brightly eosinophilic aggregates of keratin surrounded by concentric (onion skin) layers of squamous cells.**
2. **Moderately differentiated**: These tumors show **individual cell keratinization.** This appears as cells with intensely eosinophilic, glassy, and dense cytoplasm.
3. **Poorly differentiated**: These tumors may show only intercellular bridges without any foci of keratinization. **Mitotic activity is higher** in these tumors.

Large Cell Carcinoma

- Large cell carcinoma is an **undifferentiated malignant epithelial tumor** of the lung.
- **Diagnosis is by exclusion**: The tumor cells do not have the characteristics of neuroendocrine carcinoma and without any evidence of glandular, or squamous cell differentiation. Its diagnosis is by exclusion and they constitute about 10% of lung cancer.

MORPHOLOGY

Gross: Large cell carcinoma arises more frequently in the **periphery of the lung.** It forms a spherical tumor with well-defined borders. The cut section shows a bulging, fleshy, homogeneous, rather sarcomatous appearance.

Microscopy (Fig. 17.33): Tumor **cells are large with a moderate amount of cytoplasm, large nuclei, prominent nucleoli, and vesicular chromatin.**

Neuroendocrine Neoplasms

Neuroendocrine neoplasms of the lung include: (i) neuroendocrine tumors (carcinoid/neuroendocrine tumors of the lung); and (ii) neuroendocrine carcinoma.

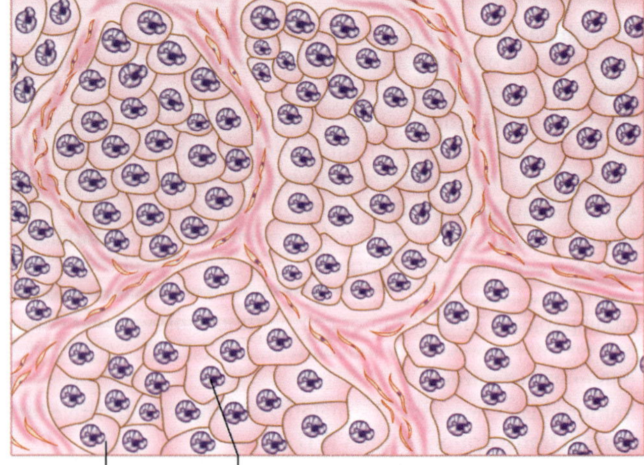

Fig. 17.33: Large cell carcinoma of the lung consisting of large tumor cells with a moderate amount of cytoplasm, large nuclei with vesicular chromatin, and prominent nucleoli.

Neuroendocrine carcinomas may be highly aggressive small-cell carcinoma or large-cell neuroendocrine carcinoma of the lung.

Carcinoid/Neuroendocrine Tumor of the Lung

Q. Write a short note on bronchial carcinoid.

- Carcinoid tumors are malignant neoplasms **composed of cells containing dense-core neurosecretory granules in their cytoplasm. They occasionally secrete hormonally active polypeptides.** They may occur as part of the multiple endocrine neoplasia (MEN) syndrome.
- These are considered **low-grade neuroendocrine carcinoma** and are subclassified as **typical or atypical**. They are usually resectable and curable.
- **Age and gender**: Most common below 40 years of age and both males and females are equally affected. There is no relation to cigarette smoking and about 20–40% of patients are nonsmokers.

MORPHOLOGY

Gross

Location: Carcinoids may arise centrally or may be peripheral.

- **Central tumors:** They are well-circumscribed, **round to ovoid, and sessile or pedunculated** (finger-like or spherical polypoid masses) in the mainstem bronchi covered by an intact mucosa. They are **predominantly endobronchial** neoplasms that project into the lumen of the bronchus. Size rarely exceeds 3–4 cm in diameter. Some may show limited penetration into the bronchial wall to fan out in the surrounding peribronchial tissue. This may produce a so-called **collar-button lesion.**
- **Peripheral tumors:** They are solid and nodular.

Microscopy

Microscopically, carcinoid tumors are well-circumscribed with limited invasion.

Growth pattern: Tumor cells are arranged in various patterns. These include organoid, trabecular, compact nests, ribbons, and palisading.

Stroma: The tumor cells are separated by a delicate fibrovascular stroma. Vascularity is pronounced.

Subcategories: They have more prominent nucleoli. Depending on the microscopic appearance they are subclassified into:

1. **Typical carcinoids:** The tumor cells are similar to the carcinoid tumors of the gastrointestinal tract. The individual tumor cells are quite regular, uniform, intermediate size in size, and have a polygonal shape. The tumor cells have central uniform round nuclei with finely granular "salt-and-pepper" chromatin. They show a moderate amount of eosinophilic and finely granular cytoplasm. These tumors have less than two mitoses per 10 high-power fields and lack necrosis.
2. **Atypical carcinoids:** They differ from typical carcinoids by (i) increased mitoses (2–10 mitoses per 10 high-power fields), (ii) foci of necrosis, (iii) increased pleomorphism, (iv) increased cellularity, and (v) tendency to grow in a disorganized fashion and invade lymphatics. They have more prominent nucleoli. Unlike typical carcinoids, these tumors have *TP53* mutations in 20–40% of cases.

Electron microscopy: Tumor cells contain dense-core granules.

Immunohistochemistry: Shows positivity for serotonin, neuron-specific enolase, chromogranin A and B, synaptophysin, bombesin, calcitonin, or other peptides.

Clinical Features

Carcinoid tumors grow slowly and about 50% of patients are asymptomatic at presentation. They are often discovered incidentally. If a patient is symptomatic, symptoms are due to:

- **Intraluminal growth:** It may manifest with a persistent cough, hemoptysis, secondary infections, dyspnea, bronchiectasis, emphysema, and atelectasis.
- **Metastasis and secretion of vasoactive amines:** The majority neither metastasize nor have secretory activity and follow a relatively benign course. In about 10% of cases, they may produce classic carcinoid syndrome, characterized by intermittent attacks of diarrhea, flushing, and cyanosis.

Prognosis: The 5-year survival rate is about 95% for typical carcinoids, and70% for atypical carcinoids.

Small Cell Lung Carcinoma

Q. Write a short note on small cell carcinoma of the lung.

It was previously known as oat cell carcinoma.

- **Highly malignant, most aggressive lung tumor with neuroendocrine features** and is **strongly associated with cigarette smoking**. They **widely metastasize** and are **almost always fatal**. SCLC has no known preinvasive phase. The male-to-female ratio is 2:1.
- **Molecular genetics:** At the molecular genetic level, SCLC shows a deletion in chromosome 3 (p14–p23) in almost 100% of cases, mutation of *TP53* in >80%, inactivating mutations of the *RB* gene in >50%, and amplification of *MYC, SOX2,* and *FGFR1* in few cases. Mutations in *KRAS* and *EGFR* are rare.

MORPHOLOGY

Q. Discuss the morphology of neuroendocrine tumors (small cell carcinoma).

Gross

Location: Usually, SCLC appears as a **large perihilar mass** in the **major bronchi**. Subsequently, it produces peribronchial compression and obstruction and involvement of nodes. In about 5% of cases, it presents as a solitary peripheral nodule.

Cut section: It is **soft, friable, and white,** and shows **extensive hemorrhage and necrosis.**

Light Microscopy (Figs. 17.34A and B)

Characteristics of tumor cells are as follows:

- **Size and shape:** Small cell carcinoma comprises relatively small cells. These cells are **round, oval, or spindle-shaped (fusiform cells)**. The small cell is termed an **oat cell**. There is no absolute size for the tumor cells to call it a small cell.

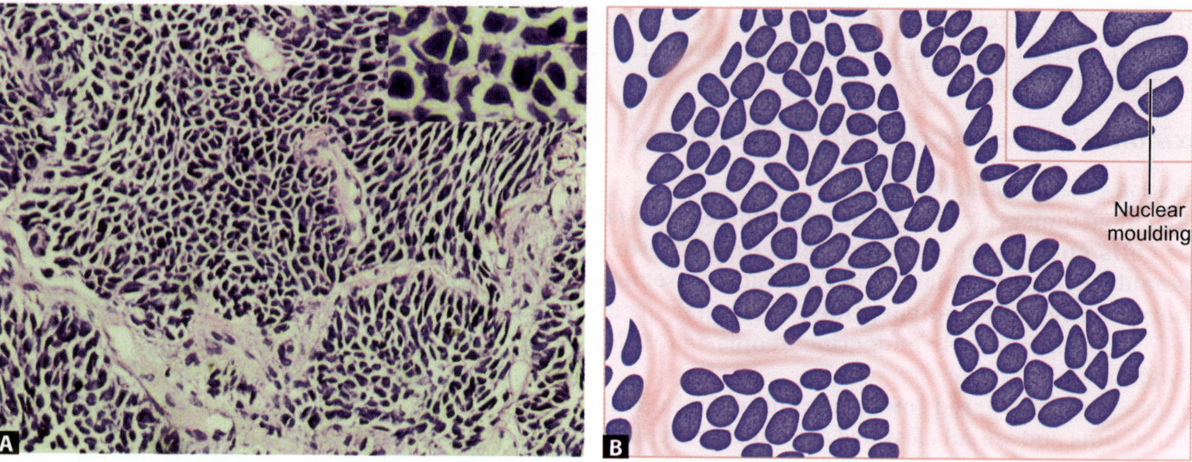

Figs. 17.34A and B: Microscopic appearance of small cell carcinoma. The inset shows nuclear molding. (A) Photomicrograph; (B) Diagrammatic.

But generally, **their diameter or size is less than three times the diameter of a small resting lymphocyte** (a size of about 25 microns). **Cells are fragile and show fragmentation and crush artifacts,** particularly prominent in small biopsy specimens.

- **Cytoplasm:** These cells have **scanty, faintly stained cytoplasm and have ill-defined cell borders.**
- **Nucleus:** It is round, ovoid, or spindle-shaped. It is **hyperchromatic with finely granular chromatin** (**salt and pepper pattern**) and **nuclear molding (better seen in cytology specimens)** is prominent. Nuclear molding **(distortion of the shape of adjacent cell nuclei to one another)** is a consequence of scant cytoplasm relatively free of intermediate filaments.
- **Nucleolus:** Absent or **inconspicuous.**
- **Mitotic count: High** with an average of 60–70 mitosis per 10 high-power fields.
- **Necrosis: Common and extensive.** The **blood vessel wall may stain blue due to the deposition of DNA** from necrotic tumor cells (**Azzopardi effect**).
- **Growth pattern:** The tumor cells grow in **sheets or clusters.** The stroma is delicate, vascular, and scanty.

Immunohistochemistry

Tumor cells express neuroendocrine markers such as **chromogranin, synaptophysin, and CD56.**

Electron Microscopy

The tumor cell shows **membrane-bound neurosecretory granules** similar to the neuroendocrine cells.

- **Origin of tumor:** Small cell carcinoma **arises from neuroendocrine progenitor cells present in the lining bronchial epithelium.** The evidence for this includes (i) the presence of neurosecretory granules, (ii) expression of neuroendocrine markers (e.g., chromogranin, synaptophysin, and CD56), and (iii) secretion of hormones (e.g., parathormone-related protein which produces paraneoplastic hypercalcemia) by some tumors.
- **Paraneoplastic syndrome: Small cell carcinoma is one of the most common lung cancers associated with ectopic hormone production and paraneoplastic syndromes.**
- **Behavior:** All small cell carcinomas are **high-grade** and are the most aggressive lung tumors. They **widely metastasize** and are **incurable by surgery** but are **markedly sensitive to chemotherapy.**

Secondary Pathology

Carcinoma of the lung produces local effects and may cause **pathologic changes in the lung distal to the point of bronchial involvement.**

- **Obstruction** of the **lumen of a major bronchus.**
  - **Partial** obstruction of the bronchus may cause **focal emphysema.**
  - **Total** obstruction may lead to **atelectasis** (collapse of the lung) distal to obstruction.
- **Suppuration:** It occurs **due to impaired drainage** of the airways. It may produce **severe suppurative or ulcerative bronchitis or bronchiectasis.** Sometimes it may produce **pulmonary abscesses.**
- **Compression or invasion of the superior vena cava:** It produces marked dilation of the veins of the head, neck, and arms, and cyanosis results in a characteristic clinical complex known as **superior vena cava syndrome.**

Spread of Tumor (Fig. 17.35)

Q. Write a short note on the mode of spread of lung cancer.

Local Spread (Table 17.6)

- Extension to the **pleural surface**, pleural cavity **(pleuritis),** or into the pericardium (pericarditis) associated with **effusions.**

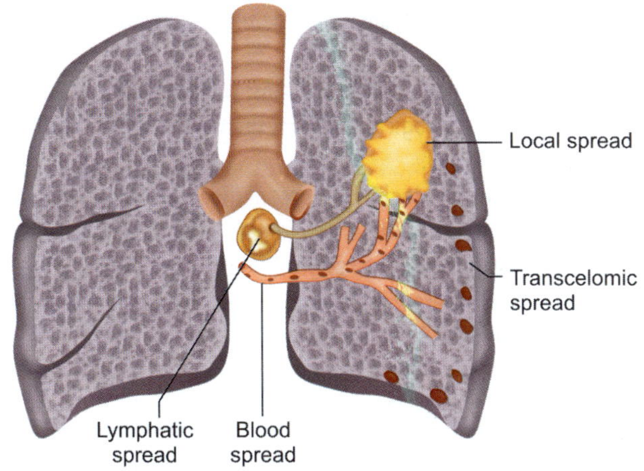

Fig. 17.35: Various routes of spread of lung cancer.

TABLE 17.6 Local effects of lung cancer.	
Pathological basis	***Local effects***
Obstruction of the airway by tumor	Pneumonia, abscess, atelectasis, focal emphysema
Local spread into pleura	Pleuritis and effusion
Local spread to pericardium	Pericarditis, effusion, tamponade
Compression of superior vena cava (SVC) by tumor	Superior vena cava syndrome
Structures invaded	**Effects**
Recurrent laryngeal nerve	Hoarseness
Phrenic nerve	Diaphragm paralysis
Sympathetic ganglia	Horner syndrome
Esophagus	Dysphagia
Chest wall	Destruction of rib

- **A tumor at the apex of the lung** may invade the **neural structures around the trachea** and the **cervical sympathetic plexus**. They may produce **severe pain in the distribution of the ulnar nerve** and **Horner syndrome** (ipsilateral enophthalmos, ptosis, miosis, and anhidrosis) on the same side as the tumor. **Such tumors are** also called **Pancoast tumors**.

Lymphatic Spread

The tumor may spread into the **tracheal, bronchial, hilar, and mediastinal** nodes. It may also spread to lymph nodes in the neck (scalene node) and clavicular region. Involvement of the supraclavicular node (**Virchow node**) may call attention to the primary.

Hematogenous Spread

Common sites of metastases are **adrenals (in more than 50%), liver, brain, and bone.**

Staging: The TNM system is used for staging cancer.

Clinical Course

Lung cancer is insidious in onset and aggressive in nature. It is usually discovered in the fifth decade. The symptoms are often of several months in duration.

Major clinical manifestations: The most common symptoms, in decreasing order of frequency, are **cough** (50–75%) due to involvement of central airways; **hemoptysis** (25–50%) due to hemorrhage from the tumor in the airway; **weight loss** (40%); **chest pain** (40%) due to the extension of tumor into the mediastinum, pleura, or chest wall; increased sputum production; and dyspnea (20%). Some of the more local manifestations of lung cancer are listed in **Table 17.7**. The tumor may also present with symptoms due to metastasis.

TABLE 17.7 Paraneoplastic syndromes—systemic effects and their most commonly related histologic type of lung carcinoma.	
Effects (elaborated hormones or hormone-like factors)	***Tumor type***
Cushing syndrome [adrenocorticotropic hormone (ACTH)]	Small cell carcinoma, carcinoid tumor
Carcinoid syndrome (serotonin and bradykinin)	Carcinoid tumor, small cell carcinoma
Hyponatremia [inappropriate secretion of antidiuretic hormone (ADH)]	Small cell carcinoma
Hypercalcemia (parathormone, parathyroid hormone-related peptide)	Squamous cell carcinoma
Gynecomastia (gonadotropins)	All tumor types
Clubbing of fingers and hypertrophic pulmonary osteoarthropathy (peculiar abnormality of connective tissue)	Unrelated to tumor type; mainly dependent on proximity to the pleural surface
Sensory neuropathy	Small cell carcinoma
Myopathic–myasthenia syndrome (Lambert–Eaton syndrome*)	Small cell carcinoma
Coagulation abnormalities: migratory thrombophlebitis (Trousseau syndrome), nonbacterial endocarditis, and disseminated intravascular coagulation Leukemoid reactions	Adenocarcinoma
Acanthosis nigricans (immunologic; secretion of epidermal growth factor)	May be seen with any type of lung cancer. Common with gastric carcinoma

*It is characterized by muscle weakness due to auto-antibodies directed against the neuronal calcium channel.

Investigations

- **Radiologic examination** of the chest.
- **Cytologic examination of sputum, bronchial washings or brushings or fine needle aspiration, or bronchoscopy biopsy** for demonstration of malignancy. **Transbronchial needle aspiration (TBNA)** is a procedure used to obtain cellular material

Prognosis: Poor for most patients with lung carcinoma. In general, the adenocarcinoma and squamous cell carcinomas remain localized and have a slightly better prognosis than small cell carcinoma.

Paraneoplastic Syndromes

Q. Write a short note on paraneoplastic syndromes associated with lung cancer (hormones elaborated).

Q. Write a short note on paraneoplastic syndromes produced by squamous cell carcinoma or oat cell carcinoma of the lung.

Lung carcinoma is sometimes associated with several extrapulmonary manifestations **(Table 17.7)** remote from the sites of primary or metastatic tumors. These are known as paraneoplastic syndromes. Any histologic types of tumors may produce any one of the hormones. **Usually, ACTH and ADH are produced by small cell carcinomas, whereas hypercalcemia is mostly observed in squamous cell carcinomas.**

Clinical Subgroups of Lung Cancer

Until recently, lung carcinoma was divided into two clinical subgroups based on the likelihood of metastases and response to therapies.

- **Small cell lung carcinomas (SCLC) (highly metastatic, high response to chemotherapy).**
- **Non-small cell lung carcinomas (NSCLC) (less metastatic, less responsive).** This group includes adenocarcinoma, squamous and large cell carcinoma, and large cell neuroendocrine carcinomas. However, **presently therapies are available that target specific oncoproteins found in a subset of NSCLC** (adenocarcinomas and squamous cell carcinomas).

Differences between small-cell lung carcinoma and common form of non-small-cell lung carcinoma (adenocarcinoma and squamous cell carcinoma) are summarized (*refer* **online Table 17.8).**

SCENARIO-BASED ESSAY QUESTION

Q. A 55-year-old male complains of a persistent productive cough of 1-year duration. He had episodes of intermittent blood in the sputum for the last 2 months. He also complains of progressive loss of weight and appetite for 1 month and occasional right-sided chest pain. He was a chronic smoker, smoking about 20 cigarettes/day for the last 25 years. On examination he was pale and there was clubbing of fingers. On inspection, the right half of the chest is not moving equally with respiration. On auscultation, breath sounds are absent on the right side. He was transferred to the oncology ward for further management.

a. What is the probable diagnosis? (Ans: Lung cancer)
b. What are the etiological factors responsible for this condition? *(refer pages 575-7).*
c. Discuss the morphological features of the lesion in the lung. And: The strongest ssociation of smoking is with squamous cell and small cell carcinoma. *(refer pages 579-82).*
d. What are the different methods of investigation that are helpful for the diagnosis? *(refer page 584).*

METASTATIC TUMORS

Q. Write a short note on metastatic tumors of the lung.

- The lung is the most common site for metastasis. Both carcinomas and sarcomas from any site may spread to the lungs via the blood or lymphatics or by direct invasion.
- Local spread into the lungs occurs in carcinoma of the esophagus, carcinomas, and mediastinal lymphomas.

Sources of Metastases to Lung

- **Common:** Carcinoma of the gastrointestinal tract, breast, thyroid, kidney, pancreas, and liver.
- **Other tumors**: Osteogenic sarcoma, neuroblastoma, Wilms tumor, melanoma, lymphomas, and leukemias.
- The microscopic appearance of metastases usually resembles that of the primary tumor.

MORPHOLOGY

The pattern of metastatic growth is variable.

- **Multiple nodules (Fig. 17.36):** Usually they appear as multiple **discrete nodules, distributed throughout all lobes**, more being at the periphery. Radiologically, when large nodules are seen in the lungs, they are known as **cannonball metastases.**
- **Other patterns:** They may also present as solitary nodule, endobronchial, pleural, pneumonic consolidation, or mixtures of any of these patterns.

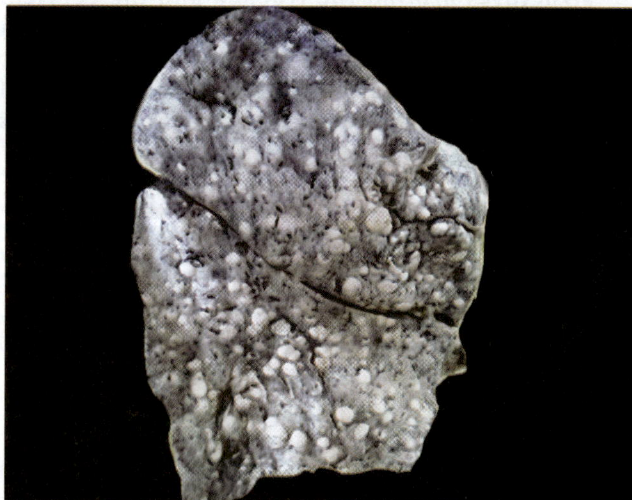

Fig. 17.36: Lung with multiple secondaries.

MISCELLANEOUS

Atelectasis (Collapse)

Q. Write a short note on atelectasis.

Atelectasis is the term used for either **incomplete expansion of the lungs** (neonatal atelectasis) or the **collapse of a previously expanded (inflated) lung** (acquired atelectasis). It produces relatively airless areas in the lung parenchyma.

Main Types of Acquired Atelectasis

- **Resorption atelectasis:** Develops due to complete obstruction of an airway. Causes include obstruction due to excessive secretions (e.g., mucus plugs) or exudates within smaller bronchi (e.g., bronchial asthma, chronic bronchitis, bronchiectasis, and postoperative states), aspiration of foreign bodies, and fragments of bronchial tumors (rare). Air in the dependent alveoli distal to obstruction gets resorbed and causes collapse of alveoli. There is reduced lung volume which shifts the mediastinum toward the atelectatic lung.
- **Compression atelectasis:** Develop due to **compression of the lung from the external aspect.** Causes include **accumulation of significant volumes of fluid** (transudate, exudate, or blood) or **air** (pneumothorax) **in the pleural cavity** and compression by tumor. In this type of atelectasis, the mediastinum is shifted away from the affected lung.
- **Contraction atelectasis** develops when **focal or generalized pulmonary or pleural fibrosis prevents full expansion of the lung.**

Significance

- Significant atelectasis **reduces oxygenation** and **predisposes to infection.**
- In long-standing atelectasis, the collapsed area of the lung becomes fibrotic and bronchi dilate, in part owing to infection distal to the obstruction—**bronchiectasis.**
- It is usually a reversible disorder except for contraction atelectasis.

Acute Lung Injury and Acute Respiratory Distress Syndrome (Diffuse Alveolar Damage)

Q. Write a short essay/note on acute lung injury/ARDS/diffuse alveolar damage.

Definition: Acute lung injury (ALI) is also termed as noncardiogenic pulmonary edema characterized by: **(1) abrupt onset of significant hypoxemia and (2) bilateral pulmonary infiltrates in the absence of cardiac failure.**

Acute respiratory distress syndrome (ARDS) is a severe form of ALI. ARDS as well as ALI has an inflammation-associated increase in pulmonary vascular permeability, edema, and death of epithelial cells. Histologically they show ***diffuse alveolar damage*** **(DAD).**

Etiology

ALI is triggered by diverse conditions **(Box 17.12).**

Pathogenesis

ALI/ARDS starts when there is an injury to pneumocytes and pulmonary endothelium and creates a vicious cycle of inflammation and pulmonary damage.

- **Endothelial cell injury/activation:** It is an important early event.
- **Adhesion and extravasation of neutrophils:** Neutrophils adhere to the activated endothelium and migrate into the interstitium and the alveoli. In the alveoli, neutrophils release inflammatory mediators, proteases, reactive oxygen species, and cytokines. This further recruits leukocytes, causing further damage to the endothelium. This cycle of inflammation and endothelial damage is the basic mechanism of ALI/ARDS.
- **Formation of hyaline membrane:** Endothelial activation and injury causes leakage of fluid from pulmonary capillaries into the interstitial tissue of the lung. Loss of type I pneumocytes permits fluid to enter the alveolar spaces. Injury to type II alveolar pneumocytes produces surfactant abnormalities which compromises the

BOX 17.12: Etiological factors of acute respiratory distress syndrome.

Infection
- Sepsis* (gram-negative septicemia, other bacterial infections, viral infections)
- Diffuse pulmonary infections* (e.g., pneumonia)
- Viral, *Mycoplasma*, and *Pneumocystis* pneumonia; miliary tuberculosis
- Aspiration of gastric contents*

Physical injury
- Severe trauma* (e.g., head injury, burns, multiple bone fractures with fat embolism, severe mechanical trauma to the chest wall)
- Pulmonary contusions
- Near-drowning (aspiration)
- Shock due to any cause
- Ionizing radiation

Inhalation of toxic gases and chemicals
- **Chemical injury**
  - Overdose of heroin, methadone, barbiturate
  - Acetylsalicylic acid
  - Cytotoxic drugs
- **Hematological conditions**
  - Transfusion-associated lung injury (TRALI)
  - Disseminated intravascular coagulation (DIC)
- **Pancreatitis**
- **Uremia**
- **Hypersensitivity reactions**

*Major conditions associated with ARDS.

alveolar gas exchange. The protein-rich (derived from leaked plasma) edema fluid and debris from dead alveolar epithelial cells form hyaline membranes which are characteristic of ALI/ARDS.

- **Resolution of injury:** If the patient survives the acute phase, macrophages remove intra-alveolar debris and release fibrogenic cytokines [e.g., transforming growth factor β (TGF-β) and platelet-derived growth factor (PDGF)]. These cytokines stimulate fibroblast growth and collagen deposition in the alveolar walls resulting in fibrosis of alveolar walls. Bronchiolar stem cells replace pneumocytes and uninjured capillary endothelium replace the endothelial cells.

MORPHOLOGY

Gross

Lungs are heavy, firm, red, and boggy.

Microscopy

Exudative Stage

- Congestion, interstitial and intra-alveolar edema, accumulation of inflammatory cells, fibrin deposition, and **diffuse alveolar damage.** Interstitial and intra-alveolar edema is prominent by the first day.
- **Hyaline membranes:** The alveolar walls become lined with waxy hyaline membranes which appear by the second day and are the **most conspicuous morphologic feature.** Alveolar hyaline membranes are eosinophilic and glassy. They consist of precipitated fibrin-rich plasma proteins in the edema fluid mixed with the cytoplasmic, nuclear, and lipid debris from sloughed necrotic epithelial cells.

Organizing Stage

In this stage, type II pneumocytes proliferate, and granulation tissue grows in the alveolar walls and into the alveolar spaces. In the majority, the granulation tissue resolves with only minimal functional impairment.

Clinical Course

Patients who develop ALI are usually admitted to the hospital for their predisposing conditions. Presenting features include severe dyspnea and tachypnea, increasing cyanosis and hypoxemia, respiratory failure, and the appearance of diffuse bilateral infiltrates on chest X-ray.

PLEURAL TUMOR

The pleura may be affected by primary or secondary tumors. Secondary metastatic tumors are more frequent than the primary tumors. The most common primary neoplasms metastasizing to the pleura are from the lung and breast. These metastatic tumors usually produce a serous or serosanguineous effusion containing neoplastic cells. Hence, careful cytologic examination of the sediment prepared from pleural effusion (*refer* pages 463-4) is of diagnostic value.

Solitary fibrous tumor characteristics are presented online.

Malignant Mesothelioma

PA 26.7 (CC): Define and describe the etiology, types, exposure, genetics, environmental influence, pathogenesis, morphology, microscopic appearance, and complications of mesothelioma.

Q. Write a short note on malignant mesothelioma.

Mesothelial tumors are classified into benign or preinvasive tumors and mesotheliomas. **Malignant mesothelioma** is called mesothelioma. **It is a rare malignant tumor of mesothelial cells.**

Sites: Mesotheliomas can arise in the **pleura** (most common), **peritoneum, pericardium,** tunica vaginalis of the testis, and genital tract (benign adenomatoid tumor). **Thoracic mesothelioma** arises from either the visceral or the parietal pleura.

Etiology

Q. Write a short note on the etiology of malignant mesothelioma.

- **Exposure to asbestos**: Mesothelioma is more prevalent in individuals heavily exposed to asbestos. There is a long latent period of 25–45 years for developing asbestos-related mesothelioma.
- Several cytogenetic abnormalities have been identified in mesothelioma. The most common is the homozygous **deletion of the tumor suppressor gene *CDKN2A/INK4a*** involving chromosome *9p* (in about 80% of mesotheliomas).

MORPHOLOGY

Gross (refer online Fig. 17.37A)

- Malignant pleural mesothelioma is a **diffuse lesion** that arises either from the visceral or parietal pleura. It usually **spreads widely in the pleural space** and is associated with extensive pleural effusion and direct invasion of thoracic structures.
- It appears as a **thick layer of soft, gelatinous, grayish-pink tumor tissue** that often encases and compresses the affected lung. It may also extend into fissures and interlobar septa, a distribution often termed as a "pleural rind" (rind = the tough outer skin of certain fruit, especially citrus fruit).

Microscopy

Q. Write a short note on microscopy of malignant mesothelioma.

Types

1. **Epithelioid type (60%):** Consists of, **or flattened cells** forming **tubular, glandular, or papillary** structures resembling adenocarcinoma. Immunohistochemistry is essential for differentiating mesothelioma from adenocarcinoma of the lung. Most mesotheliomas are strongly positive for keratin proteins, calretinin, Wilms tumor 1 (WT-1), cytokeratin 5/6, and D2-40.
2. **Mesenchymal (sarcomatoid) type (20%):** Consists of **spindle cells** similar in appearance to a fibrosarcoma. They have lower expression of many of the markers described under the epithelioid type mentioned above.
3. **Mixed (biphasic) type (20%):** Consists of both epithelioid and sarcomatoid patterns (*refer* **online Fig. 17.37B**).

Clinical Course

- Average age is 60 years.
- Chest pain, dyspnea, recurrent pleural effusions, and nonspecific symptoms, such as weight loss and malaise.

Spread

- Direct local invasion of the lung.
- Lymphatic spread to the hilar lymph nodes.
- Hematogenous spread to the liver, bones, peritoneum and adrenals.

The prognosis is poor and 50% die within 12 months of diagnosis.

SCENARIO-BASED MCQs

1. **A 58 -year-old man presents with fever, chills, shortness of breath, and pleuritic chest pain. Examination shows dullness on percussion over the lung fields. On auscultation, crackles are heard, and breath sounds over both lung fields are decreased. The patient also has tachypnea, with flaring of the nares. The sputum is rusty-yellow and shows numerous neutrophils and RBCs. The most common pathogens that are likely to cause a patient's lung infection are:**
   A. *Staphylococcus aureus*
   B. *Streptococcus pneumoniae*
   C. *Pseudomonas aeruginosa*
   D. *Mycoplasma pneumoniae*
2. **A 48-year-old alcoholic man is brought to the hospital having severe respiratory distress. He coughs constantly and expectorates rusty sputum. He is febrile. Physical examination shows bilateral crackles, dullness to percussion over both lung fields, and use of accessory muscles. A chest X-ray shows bilateral diffuse pulmonary consolidation. The patient subsequently dies due to bacterial sepsis. At autopsy, his left lung is red, with a liver-like consistency of the lower lobe. Probable diagnosis is:**
   A. Lobar pneumonia B. Bronchopneumonia
   C. Atypical pneumonia D. Pulmonary abscess
3. **A 52-year-old man complains of fever, night sweats, and a 3-kg weight loss over the past 3 months. Last month, he had episodes of hemoptysis. On physical examination, rales are heard over the upper lobe. The chest radiograph shows a prominent cavitatory lesion in the upper lobe. He is most likely to have an infection with the following organisms:**
   A. Influenza A
   B. *Mycoplasma pneumoniae*
   C. *Mycobacterium tuberculosis*
   D. *Legionella pneumophila*
4. **A 48-year-old man complains of gradually increased dyspnea and a 5-kg weight loss for the past 2 years. He has an occasional cough with minimal sputum production. He has smoked two packs of cigarettes per day for 20 years, but not for the past 1 year. The patient's face is puffy and red, and he has pitting edema of the legs. On physical examination, the anteroposterior diameter of the chest is increased and the lungs are hyperresonant. On auscultation of the chest, the breath sounds are decreased. A chest radiograph shows bilateral hyperlucent lungs and the lucency is more prominent in the upper lobes. Pulmonary function tests show markedly decreased FEV1, but FVC is normal, and the FEV1/FVC ratio is decreased. The mechanism that contributes to the pathogenesis of this condition is:**
   A. Release of elastase from neutrophils
   B. Impaired release of α1-antitrypsin from liver
   C. Abnormal epithelial cell chloride ion transport
   D. Decreased ciliary motility with irregular dynein arms
5. **A 14-year-old girl has a 6-year history of cough, wheezing, and repeated attacks of difficulty breathing. The attacks are common in the spring. During an episode of wheezing, a physical examination shows that she is afebrile. On percussion, her lungs are hyperresonant. A chest radiograph shows increased lucency of all lung fields. She has a history of allergies to cats and wool. Laboratory tests show raised levels of serum IgE and eosinophilia. Microscopic examination of sputum shows increased numbers of eosinophils. The histologic features that are most likely to be characteristic of her condition are:**
   A. Inflammatory destruction of bronchial walls
   B. Remodeling of airways with smooth muscle hyperplasia
   C. Dilation of respiratory bronchioles with loss of elastic fibers
   D. Patchy areas of consolidation with leukocytic exudates in alveoli.
6. **A 38-year-old woman has had multiple attacks of severe necrotizing pneumonia since childhood. Now, she has a productive cough with large amounts of purulent sputum. On physical examination, dullness is present on percussion with decreased breath sounds over the right mid to lower lung fields. A chest radiograph shows areas of consolidation in the right lower lobe. A bronchogram shows marked dilation of the right lower lobe bronchi. The mechanisms that are the most likely cause of her disease are:**
   A. Diffuse infiltration by adenocarcinoma in situ of lung
   B. Congenital malformation of the bronchial walls
   C. Recurrent inflammation with bronchial wall destruction
   D. Unopposed action of neutrophil-derived elastase on bronchi
7. **A 28-year-old man with AIDS complains of persistent cough, night sweats, low-grade fever, loss of weight, and malaise. A chest X-ray shows an area of consolidation in the periphery of the left upper lobe and hilar lymphadenopathy. Sputum examination and cultures show acid-fast bacilli. The most likely diagnosis is:**
   A. Lung abscess B. Tuberculosis
   C. Bronchiectasis D. Bronchopneumonia
8. **A 65-year-old man with small cell carcinoma of the left mainstem bronchus begins chemotherapy. During the treatment, he develops a fever and a productive cough. A CBC shows leukocytosis (WBC = 16,800/cu mm). The patient's cough worsens, and he expectorates large amounts of foul-smelling sputum. A chest X-ray shows a distinct cavity with an air/fluid level distal to the tumor area. The likely cause of these findings in a cancer patient is:**
   A. Atelectasis B. Lung abscess
   C. Bronchiectasis D. Lobar pneumonia
9. **A 68-year-old man, who is a chain-smoker, complains of a cough and a 5 kg weight loss over the past 4 months. Physical examination shows clubbing of the fingers. He is afebrile. A chest radiograph shows cavitation within a 3 cm lesion near the right hilum of the lung. Laboratory studies show**

a serum calcium of 12.3 mg/dL and phosphorus of 2.4 mg/dL. Bronchoscopy shows a lesion occluding the right main bronchus. The most likely neoplasms in this patient is:

A. Squamous cell carcinoma
B. Adenocarcinoma in situ
C. Large cell anaplastic carcinoma
D. Small cell carcinoma

Answers and Explanation

1. **The answer is B: *Streptococcus pneumoniae*.** All of the four choices can cause pneumonia. But, the most common cause of pneumonia is *Streptococcus pneumoniae (Pneumococcus)*. Pneumococcal pneumonia is acute in onset of is acute and presents with fever, chills, and shortness of breath. The pleuritic chest pain is due to the involvement of pleura-causing pleuritis.
2. **The answer is A: Lobar pneumonia.** Lobar pneumonia presents with a diffuse consolidation of one or more pulmonary lobes. Bronchopneumonia (choice B) is characterized by scattered, multiple, solid foci in the same or several lobes. Atypical pneumonia (choice C) is usually caused by mycoplasma pneumonia. Pulmonary abscess (choice D) may be a complication of lobar pneumonia or bronchopneumonia.
3. **The answer is C: *Mycobacterium tuberculosis*.** History of fever, night sweats, and a 3-kg weight, episodes of hemoptysis, and radiographic findings of prominent upper lobe cavitation are typical of reactivation-reinfection tuberculosis in adults. Influenza viral infections mainly show interstitial mononuclear inflammation and are usually of short duration. Bacterial organisms such as *Legionella* are more likely to produce widespread bronchopneumonia with alveolar neutrophilic exudates. Mycoplasma infection produces mainly interstitial mononuclear inflammation.
4. **The answer is A: Release of elastase from neutrophils.** The findings in this patient are predominantly those of emphysema, with a centrilobular pattern of predominantly upper lobe involvement. Smoking is a major etiologic agent of this disease. The subtle but long-term inflammation accompanying smoking leads to increased neutrophil and macrophage secretion of elastase. This is not sufficiently inhibited by the antiprotease action of $\alpha_1$antitrypsin. This leads to a loss of lung tissue over decades. α1-antitrypsin deficiency is uncommon and causes panlobular emphysema. Abnormal chloride ion transport is a feature of cystic fibrosis, and this causes widespread bronchiectasis. Decreased ciliary motility with irregular dynein arms occurs in Kartagener syndrome, which leads to bronchiectasis.
5. **The answer is B: Remodeling of airways with smooth muscle hyperplasia.** The girl has atopic asthma which is a type I hypersensitivity reaction. In this condition, presensitized, IgE-coated mast cells are present in the mucosal surfaces and submucosa of airways. Re-exposure to an allergen results in degranulation of the mast cells. It immediately releases (minutes) mediators such as histamine and causes bronchoconstriction. The delayed release (an hour or more) of leukotrienes and prostaglandins via the arachidonic acid pathway; attracts leukocytes, particularly eosinophils, and promotes bronchoconstriction. The characteristic microscopic changes in the bronchi consist of remodeling of airways and smooth muscle hyperplasia. Inflammatory destruction of bronchial walls with bronchial dilation is a feature of bronchiectasis Dilation of the respiratory bronchiole is a feature of centrilobular emphysema. Neutrophilic exudates with patchy consolidation are seen in pneumonia, typically from bacterial infections.
6. **The answer is C: Recurrent inflammation with bronchial wall destruction.** Bronchiectasis is a chronic obstructive airway disease characterized by irreversible dilation of bronchi. It results from inflammation and destruction of bronchial walls after prolonged infections or obstruction. Pneumonia can predispose to bronchiectasis. Adenocarcinoma in situ of the lung may mimic infiltrative pneumonia because of its lepidic pattern of spread. But it mainly produces a mass effect, and it does not begin in childhood. Congenital malformation of the bronchial wall weakening is rare. The unopposed action of neutrophil-derived elastases damages the elastic tissue of the alveoli. This leads to emphysema.
7. **The answer is B: Tuberculosis.** Tuberculosis is caused by Mycobacterium tuberculosis. The Ghon complex includes the area of parenchymal consolidation and enlargement of ipsilateral hilar lymph nodes. The sputum contains *M. tuberculosis*, which is acid-fast in smears stained by the Ziehl-Neelsen method. None of the other choices feature acid-fast organisms.
8. **The answer is B: Lung abscess.** A lung abscess is a localized collection of pus accompanied by the destruction of lung parenchyma. The most common cause of lung abscess is aspiration. It is also a common complication of lung cancer. Abscess cavities are usually partially filled with pus and air. This produces an "air/fluid level" on X-ray. Foul-smelling sputum may be expectorated if an abscess is communicating to a bronchus. Other choices do not present as cavitary lesions.
9. **The answer is A: Squamous cell carcinoma** of the lung is strongly associated with smoking and is most likely to produce paraneoplastic hypercalcemia. They can undergo central necrosis and form a cavity. Adenocarcinomas and large-cell carcinomas usually produce peripheral masses and are less likely to be associated with paraneoplastic syndromes. Small cell carcinomas often produce various paraneoplastic syndromes but are less likely hypercalcemia.

CHAPTER 18

Oral Cavity and Gastrointestinal Tract

Chapter Outline

- Oral Cavity
- Salivary Gland Neoplasms
- Odontogenic Tumors

Gastrointestinal Tract

- Esophagus
- Stomach
- Intestine
- Polyps of Colon
- Genetic Tumor Syndromes
- Colorectal Adenocarcinoma
- Acute Appendicitis

ORAL CAVITY

Oral cavity diseases can be divided into those affecting oral mucosa; salivary glands; teeth, and their support structures; and the jaw. Only more common conditions affecting these sites are described below.

Precancerous Lesions of the Oral Cavity

Q. Write a short note on premalignant lesions of the oral cavity.

Premalignant (precancerous) lesions of the upper oropharynx include two squamous lesions: (1) leukoplakia (white lesion), and (2) erythroplakia (red lesion):

Age and gender: Both leukoplakia and erythroplakia may be found in adults of any age, but they are usually seen between **40 and 70 years**. Male to female ratio is 2:1.

Etiology: Both have **multifactorial** origins and are associated with the use of **tobacco** (e.g., cigarettes, pipes, cigars), including smokeless tobacco (e.g., chewing tobacco).

Leukoplakia

Q. Write a short note on the definition and morphology of leukoplakia.

The term leukoplakia is derived from *the Greek* leukos, "white," and plax, "plaque." It is an asymptomatic white lesion seen on the surface of a mucous membrane. If any white patches in the oral cavity can be given a specific diagnosis, it is not a leukoplakia.

WHO defines: It as "a white patch or plaque that cannot be scraped off and cannot be characterized clinically or pathologically as any other disease."

MORPHOLOGY

Gross

Locations: These may be seen **anywhere in the oral cavity.** The most common sites are the buccal mucosa, the floor of the mouth, the ventral surface of the tongue, the palate, and the gingiva.

Number: It may be **single or multiple.**

Appearance: They appear as **white patches or plaques** having **sharply defined borders**. The surface may be smooth or wrinkled.

Microscopy

Changes in surface stratified squamous epithelium: It shows a spectrum ranging from **hyperkeratosis and acanthosis** to lesions with variable degrees of dysplastic changes (including carcinoma in situ). Until proven otherwise by microscopic examination, leukoplakia is considered precancerous.

Subepithelial inflammatory infiltrate: The subepithelial region shows **inflammatory infiltration of lymphocytes and macrophages**, the intensity of which is proportional to the degree of dysplasia.

Erythroplakia

It is a **less common** lesion related to leukoplakia. It is associated with a much higher risk for malignant transformation than leukoplakia.

MORPHOLOGY

Gross

It appears as a **red, velvety area within the oral cavity.** It remains at a level with or slightly depressed in relation to the surrounding mucosa.

Microscopy

The **epithelium is atypical** and has an **increased risk of malignant transformation** than leukoplakia.

Erythroplakia

- **Epithelium shows erosions with dysplasia, carcinoma in situ, or frank carcinoma.**
- **The subepithelial region** shows **intense inflammatory reaction** and **vascular dilatation, responsible for the reddish clinical appearance.**

Intermediate forms, which have the characteristics of both leukoplakia and erythroplakia, are termed speckled leukoerythroplakia.

Hairy Leukoplakia

Hairy leukoplakia is a **distinctive oral lesion caused by Epstein-Barr virus (EBV) and usually occurs in immunocompromised patients.** It may also occur in patients who are immunocompromised for other reasons (e.g., cancer therapy, transplant-associated immunosuppression, and advanced age).

MORPHOLOGY

Gross

Site: Located mostly on the **lateral edges/border of the tongue.**
Appearance: They appear as **white, confluent patches of fluffy ("hairy") thickenings,** which cannot be scraped off.

Microscopy

It shows **shaggy hyperparakeratosis, parakeratosis, and acanthosis** with **"balloon cells"** in the **upper spinous layer** of the epithelium. The **"balloon cells"** have dense central eosinophilic inclusions and vacuolated or ground-glass cytoplasm. Superimposed candidal infection may add to the "hairiness" of the lesion.

Squamous Cell Carcinoma

PA 24.1 (NC): Describe the etiology, pathogenesis, pathology, and clinical features of oral cancers.

In India, oral cavity cancer is the most common malignant tumor (buccal mucosa > anterior tongue > lower alveolus). The majority are squamous cell carcinomas.

Etiology

Q. Write a short note on the etiology of squamous cell carcinoma of the oral cavity.

Squamous cell carcinoma (SCC) of the oral cavity is a **multifactorial disease** usually seen in middle-aged men.

Risk Factors

1. **Tobacco products and smoking:** Any irritating smoked product increases the risk for tumors of the oral cavity. Nicotine in tobacco and other tobacco leaf components causes cancer. **Carcinogens in tobacco can act as initiators, as well as promoters.** Risk increases with the amount and duration of tobacco use. Tobacco may be used either for **smoking** or as **smokeless tobacco.**
   - **Smoking:** It may be in the form of cigarette, beedi, cigar, or pipe smoking, or reverse smoking (smoking a cheroot with the burning end inside the mouth is practiced in certain regions of India). Regular marijuana use has also been associated with oropharyngeal cancer.
   - **Smokeless tobacco:** It is in the form of a **betel quid**/pan that contains several ingredients such as areca nut, slaked lime, and tobacco, which are wrapped in a betel leaf. It is commonly used in India and Southeast Asia and is associated with a marked increase in oral cancer. **Betel quid appears to be the major carcinogen.** However, it may also be related to slaked lime and the areca nut. Other methods of tobacco consumption include snuff dipping and tobacco chewing.

   Oral cancers are found on the **buccal and gingival** surfaces in the sites **where tobacco products** are held in **contact** with the mucosa for long periods.
2. **Alcohol consumption:** It is another important etiologic factor and acts synergistically with tobacco as either a cocarcinogen (increasing the risk) or a promoter (decreasing the lag time). The risk of oral SCC is magnified in individuals who smoke as well as consume alcohol.
3. **Other risk factors:**
   - Radiation exposure and solar actinic radiation (sunlight).
   - Welding, metal refining, diesel exhaust, wood stove, and asbestos exposure.
   - Chronic irritation of the mucosa: It may be due to ill-fitting dentures, jagged teeth, or chronic infections.
   - Vitamin A deficiency and immunosuppression.
   - Poor nutrition.

Role of oncogenic HPV virus infection: High-risk HPV types 16 and 18 and, less commonly low-risk HPV types 6 and 11 have been found in oral carcinomas.

Inherited genomic instability: A family history of head and neck cancer is a risk factor and is thought to be due to inherited genomic instability.

Pathogenesis

The development of squamous cell carcinoma is a **multi-step process.** It involves sequential activation of oncogenes and inactivation of tumor suppressor genes in a clonal population of cells.

- **Inactivation of the *p16* gene** (about 80% of the cases): It causes stratified squamous epithelium to undergo hyperplasia/hyperkeratosis.
- **Mutation of the *p53* tumor suppressor gene:** It is associated with the progression of hyperplasia/hyperkeratosis to dysplasia.
- **Amplification and overexpression of the cyclin D1** gene constitutively activates cell cycle progression.

MORPHOLOGY

Location: Anywhere in the oral cavity. Common sites are the **lower lip, the ventral surface of the tongue, the floor of the mouth,** the buccal mucosa, the soft palate, and the gingiva.

Gross

Early stages: It appears either as raised, firm, pearly plaques or as irregular, roughened, or verrucous areas of mucosal thickening. May be superimposed on a leukoplakia or erythroplakia.

Later: It may appear as **ulcerated and protruding gray-white** masses with **irregular and indurated** (rolled) **borders.**

Microscopy

Squamous cell carcinomas **(Figs. 18.1A and B)** range from well-differentiated keratinizing neoplasms to poorly differentiated/anaplastic tumors. However, the histological grading does not correlate with behavior (*refer* page 951 for a general microscopic description of squamous cell carcinoma).

Spread

- **Local:** The tissue involved depends on the primary site.
- **Lymph node:** The involved site of the lymph node depends on the location of the primary tumor. The more anterior the tumor, the more is spread to the cervical nodes. Carcinomas of the base of the tongue and oropharynx metastasize to the deep retropharyngeal lymph nodes.
- **Blood spread:** It spreads to the lungs, liver, and bones.

Verrucous Carcinoma

Verrucous carcinoma (Ackerman tumor) is **a variant of well-differentiated squamous cell carcinoma**.

Site: Most common in the buccal mucosa and lower gingiva.

Age and gender: Most are elderly males.

Etiology: Tobacco, especially chewing or snuff dipping, and HPV infection.

MORPHOLOGY

Gross: It appears as a large, fungating, soft papillary growth (warty appearance).

Microscopy (Fig. 18.1C): The surface epithelium shows hyperkeratosis, acanthosis, and benign-appearing papillomatosis. Rete pegs are swollen and voluminous and extend into the deeper tissues (pushing infiltrative margins).

Spread: May infiltrate the soft tissues of the cheek, mandible, or maxilla, and invade perineural spaces. **Regional lymph node metastases are exceedingly rare,** and **distant metastases have not been reported**.

SALIVARY GLAND NEOPLASMS

Salivary gland neoplasms are relatively uncommon and constitute less than 2% of tumors.

Incidence: The parotid gland is the most common site for tumors of the salivary gland. **About 65–80% occur in the parotid gland and approximately 15–30% of parotid tumors are malignant.** Approximately 40% of the submandibular gland, 50% of the minor salivary gland, and 70–90% of sublingual tumors are malignant. Malignancy in the salivary gland is inversely proportional to the size of the gland.

Classification of salivary gland tumors is presented in **Table 18.1.**

Q. Classify salivary gland tumors.

Clinical presentation: Parotid gland neoplasms produce swellings in front of and below the ear. Both benign and malignant tumors range in size from 4–6 cm in diameter. Most tumors are mobile except advanced malignant tumors.

- **Age:** Benign tumors occur in the fifth to seventh decades of life. The malignant tumors appear later.
- **Sex: Slight female predominance**, except for **Warthin tumor, which occurs more often in males than in females**.

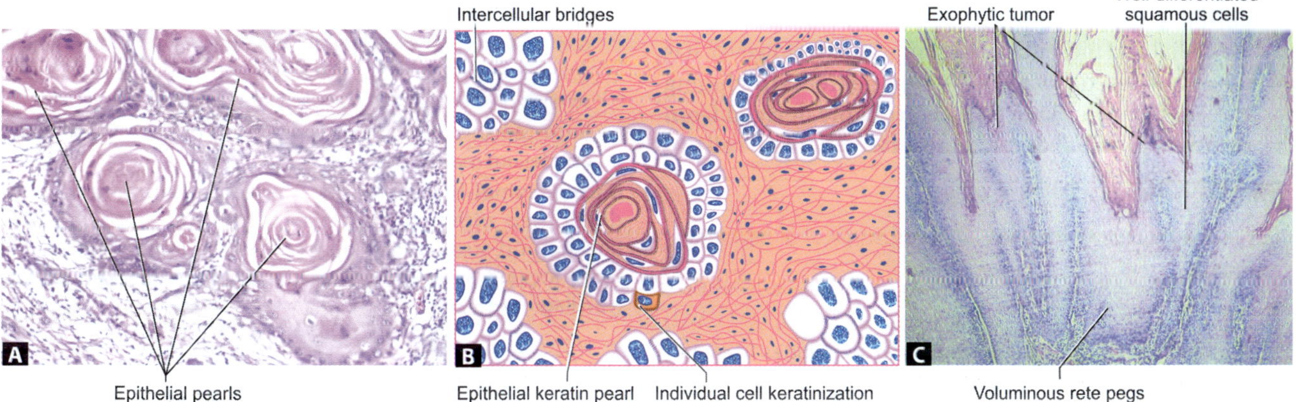

Figs. 18.1A to C: Well-differentiated squamous cell carcinoma microscopic appearance: (A) H&E; (B) Diagrammatic; (C) Verrucous carcinoma showing exophytic growth, swollen and voluminous rete pegs extending into the deeper tissues.

TABLE 18.1 Classification of common tumors of the salivary glands.

Benign	*Malignant*
Pleomorphic adenoma (mixed tumor) (50%)	Mucoepidermoid carcinoma (15%)
Warthin tumor (5%)	Acinic cell carcinoma (6%)
Oncocytoma (2%)	Adenocarcinoma (6%)
Basal cell adenoma (2%)	Adenoid cystic carcinoma (4%)
Cystadenoma	Malignant mixed tumor

Pleomorphic Adenoma

Q. Write a short note on pleomorphic adenoma.

Pleomorphic adenoma is the **most common benign tumor of the salivary glands.** It consists of a **mixture of ductal (epithelial) and myoepithelial cells. They usually show differentiation towards both epithelial and myoepithelial elements.** It is also called a **mixed tumor**. In pathology, the term "pleomorphic" is used to indicate nuclear variation (size and shape of nuclei) in neoplasm. However, **the term pleomorphic adenoma is used because of the variable cell type seen in this lesion.**

Age and gender: It occurs usually during the **third to fifth decade** of life (middle age). It is most frequent in **females.**

Location: It depends on the type of salivary gland.

- **Major salivary gland:** It is the common site and constitutes about **60% of tumors in the parotid.** Usually arises in the **superficial lobe of the parotid.** Less common in the submandibular glands and very rare in the sublingual gland.
- **Minor salivary gland:** It can also occur in various minor salivary gland sites. The most common minor salivary gland sites are the palate, cheek, tongue, and floor of the mouth.

Etiology and histogenesis: The origin of PAs is **not known.** Exposure to radiation increases the risk.

- **Cell of origin:** Histogenesis is also uncertain. It **was called a mixed tumor**, because of the mixture of epithelial and mesenchymal components. However, it is now considered that **all the tumor elements** (including mesenchymal and ductal) are **probably derived from the myoepithelial or ductal reserve cell** (stem cell).

MORPHOLOGY

Q. Write a short note on gross and microscopy of pleomorphic adenoma.

Gross

- **Size and shape:** It is usually **round** and size ranges from **2.5 to 6 cm in diameter.**
- **Consistency:** It depends on the relative number of epithelial cells and stroma. **Usually rubbery, resilient (tough) mass** with a **bosselated surface.**

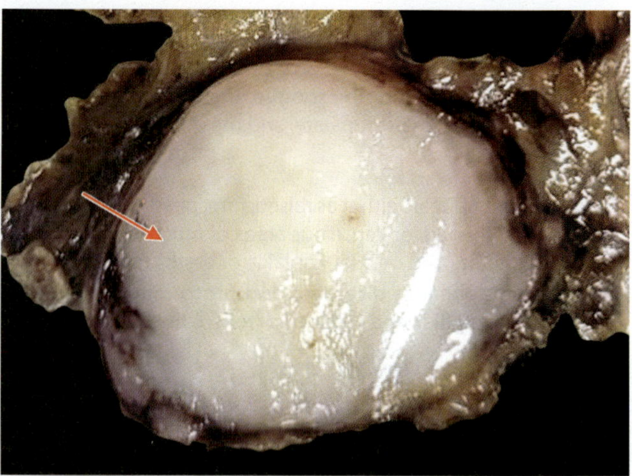

Fig. 18.2: Pleomorphic adenoma of the salivary gland. The cut section shows a well-circumscribed gray-white tumor with a blue-glistening area (arrow).

- **Capsulated or well-circumscribed:** It is well-demarcated and usually capsulated. In some locations (e.g., palate), the capsule is not fully developed, and small extensions can be seen protruding into the surrounding salivary gland. This makes the enucleation of the tumor difficult.
- **Cut surface (Fig. 18.2):** It shows **gray-white** with **myxoid and blue glistening, translucent chondroid** (cartilage-like) **areas.**

Microscopy (Figs. 18.3A and B)

A characteristic feature is the **pleomorphic** (heterogeneity/varied) **appearance.** Neoplastic cells show varying **mixtures of epithelial tissue components intermingled with cells showing mesenchymal differentiation.**

Epithelial element: This component consists of **ductal cells and myoepithelial cells.** The epithelial elements may predominate in some tumors and in others, they are present only in widely dispersed foci.

- **Epithelial elements resemble ductal or myoepithelial cells.** These are **arranged in the form of ducts, acini, irregular tubules, strands, or sheets.**
- **Myoepithelial cells:** The **ducts are lined by epithelial** (cuboidal to columnar) **cells** and **surrounded by myoepithelial components** (a layer of deeply chromatic, small myoepithelial cells). In some tumors, the myoepithelial cells may form **strands or sheets** with a plasmacytoid or spindled appearance.
- **Rare feature:** Islands of well-differentiated squamous epithelium may also be seen.

Mesenchymal-like elements: The epithelial elements are distributed within a varying amount of mesenchyme-like background stroma. This may contain variable mixtures of **loose myxoid (mucoid) tissue, islands of hyaline, chondroid (cartilaginous),** and rarely bone (osseous) tissue.

Clinical Features

- **Presentation:** Pleomorphic adenoma presents as a **painless, slow-growing, mobile, discrete** tumor in the **parotid or submandibular** areas or the buccal cavity.

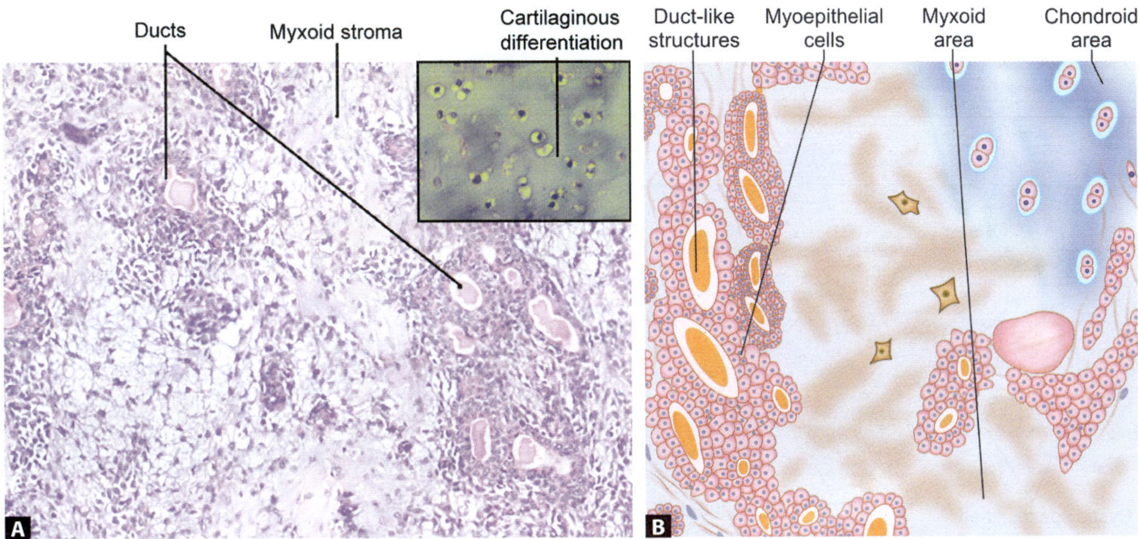

Figs. 18.3A and B: Mixed tumor (pleomorphic adenoma) of the parotid, gland: (A) H&E; (B) Diagrammatic shows epithelial cells forming ducts surrounded by myxoid stroma and cartilaginous differentiation (inset A).

- **Recurrence:** The tumors tend to protrude focally from the main tumor into adjacent tissues. Failure to recognize these minute protrusions at surgery is responsible for the recurrence of these tumors.

Carcinoma ex pleomorphic adenoma: Rarely, a carcinoma may arise in pleomorphic adenomas. This is called a **carcinoma ex pleomorphic adenoma or a malignant mixed tumor**. The incidence of carcinoma increases with the duration of the tumor. Microscopically, these tumors show poorly differentiated adenocarcinoma or undifferentiated carcinoma in an otherwise benign pleomorphic adenoma.

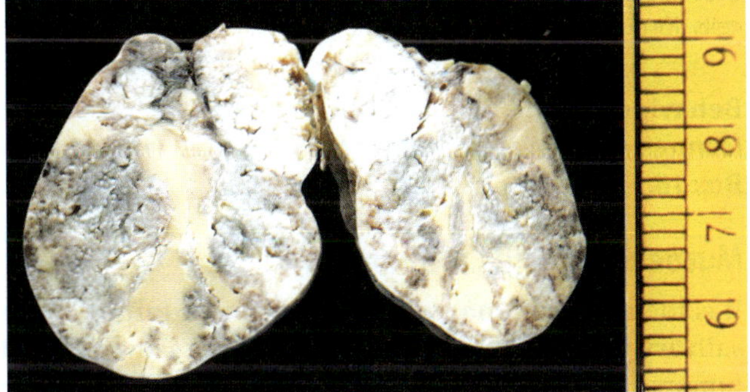

Fig. 18.4: Gross appearance of Warthin's tumor. Cut section showing a circumscribed, lobulated, solid yellow-to-brown colored mass with multiple, tiny cystic spaces.

Warthin Tumor

Q. Write a short note on Warthin tumor.

Warthin tumor (**papillary cystadenoma lymphomatosum, adenolymphoma**) is a **benign** and the **second most common salivary gland neoplasm.**

Age and gender: These tumors commonly occur during the **fifth to seventh decade of life.** Warthin's tumor is the **only salivary gland tumor that is more common in males than in females.**

Etiology: Warthin's tumors may be associated with **radiation exposure** and have a near-universal relationship with cigarette **smoking** (eightfold increased risk).

Histogenesis: Warthin tumor may represent an **aberrant incorporation of lymphoid tissue in the parotids.**

MORPHOLOGY

Gross

Location: It almost **exclusively** arises in the **parotid gland.** Usually arises in the **superficial parotid gland** and is readily palpable. About 10% are multifocal and 10% are bilateral.

Size and shape: It ranges from **2 to 5 cm** in diameter. It appears as a round to oval, **encapsulated** (or well-circumscribed) **mass.**

Cut section (Fig. 18.4): It is a soft, **pale gray** tumor **with few narrow cystic or cleft-like spaces.** These spaces may be filled with a mucinous or serous secretion or even resemble used (dark) motor oil.

Microscopy (Figs. 18.5A and B)

Tumors consist of cystic glandular spaces embedded in dense lymphoid stromal tissue.

1. **Cystic spaces:** Cystic glandular spaces show **papillary or polypoid projections.** Cystic spaces are **lined by a distinctive double layer of neoplastic epithelial cells** consisting of:
   - **Surface superficial layer of columnar cells** with **abundant, finely granular, eosinophilic cytoplasm** (oncocytes). Oncocytes have **abundant mitochondria** and are responsible for the **granular appearance** of the cytoplasm.
   - **Second (outer) layer** below the superficial layer consisting of **cuboidal to polygonal cells.**
2. **Lymphoid stromal tissue:** Cystic spaces are embedded in a dense lymphoid stroma that **closely resembles a normal lymph node.** The lymphoid tissue is prominent with germinal centers and is composed of B and a few T cells.

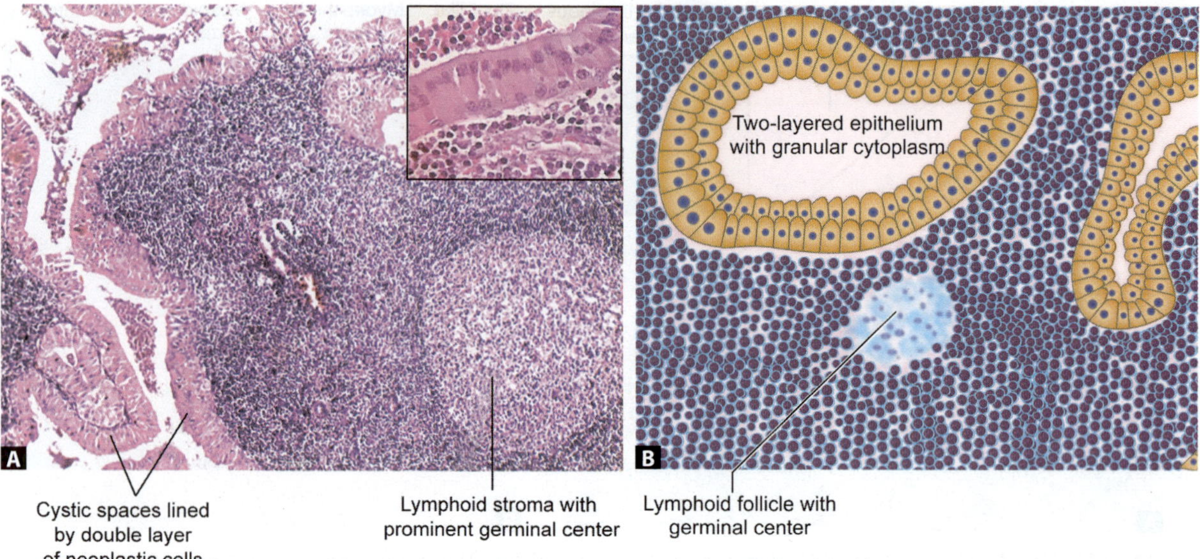

Figs. 18.5A and B: Microscopic appearance of Warthin tumor: (A) H&E; (B) Diagrammatic. Shows epithelial and lymphoid elements. Note the follicular germinal center in the center of lymphoid aggregates. The cystic spaces are lined by a double layer of eosinophilic epithelial cells (inset A) separated by reactive lymphoid stroma.

Behavior: It is **benign**, and about 2% may recur. Salient features of the Warthin tumor are presented (*refer* **online Box 18.1**).

Mucoepidermoid Carcinoma

It is the **most common primary malignant tumor of the salivary glands**. Constitute about 15% of all salivary gland tumors. Occur mainly (60–70%) in the parotids. Account for a major fraction of the minor salivary gland tumors.

MORPHOLOGY

Gross

- **Size:** It can grow as large as 8 cm in diameter.
- **Appear circumscribed**, but do not show well-defined capsules and are often infiltrative at the margins.
- **Cut section:** It is **pale gray to white** and frequently contains **small, mucin-containing cysts.**

Microscopy (Fig. 18.6)

Composed of variable mixtures of **(1) squamous cells, (2) mucus-secreting cells, and (3) intermediate cells**. These tumor cells are arranged in cords, sheets, or cystic structures. The intermediate cells have squamous features, with small to large mucus-filled vacuoles. The mucus stains are positive with mucin stains. The tumor cells may appear regular and benign or highly anaplastic and malignant.

Grading: These tumors are graded as low, intermediate, or high grade. Clinical features and prognosis depend on the grade of the neoplasm.

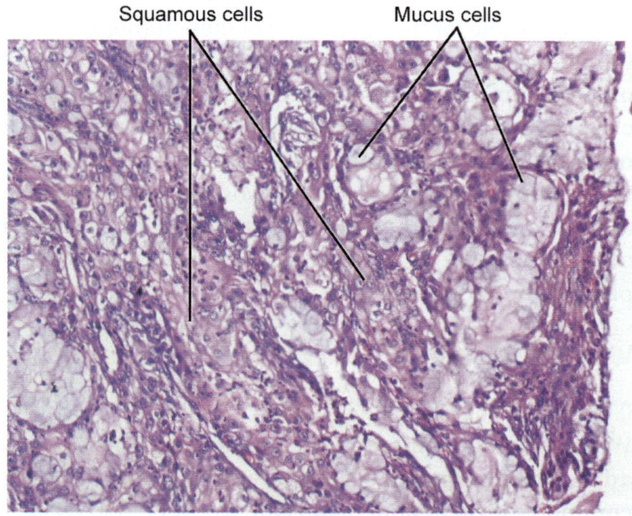

Fig. 18.6: Mucoepidermoid carcinoma composed of squamous cells as well as clear vacuolated cells containing mucin.

ODONTOGENIC TUMORS

Odontogenic tumors are a group of lesions with diverse microscopic appearances and clinical behavior. Some are true neoplasms (both benign and malignant) and others are hamartomas. Odontogenic tumors are derived from odontogenic epithelium, odontogenic mesenchyme, or both.

Ameloblastoma

Ameloblastoma is the **most common clinically significant odontogenic tumor**. It is a benign **intraosseous progressively, slow-growing, locally invasive neoplasm epithelial odontogenic neoplasm.** It is characterized by expansion and a tendency or local recurrence if not adequately removed.

Cell of origin: Ameloblastoma **arises from dental lamina.**
Sites: About 80% of all ameloblastomas occur in the mandible. Other may occur in the maxilla.

MORPHOLOGY

Gross

Ameloblastomas may range from **entirely solid to variably cystic.**

Microscopy (Figs. 18.7A and B)

It has **many subtypes or patterns.** Two predominant patterns are follicular and plexiform.

1. **Follicular type:** It is the **most common subtype.** In this type, there is an attempt to mimic the dental organ epithelium. It comprises **nests of epithelium that resemble the inner dental epithelial component of the enamel organ of the developing teeth.** These cells are dispersed in a mature fibrous connective tissue (fibrous) stroma. The peripheral (outermost) cells are tall columnar to cuboidal and resemble those of the developing tooth follicle (i.e., the ameloblastic layer). These **ameloblast-like cells have hyperchromatic nuclei and are arranged in a palisading pattern with reverse polarity** (nuclei of these cells are placed away from the basement membrane). The **central core of the nests is reminiscent of the stellate reticulum and is composed of loosely arranged angular cells** that resemble the stellate reticulum of the enamel organ. They often show cystic change. Cyst formation is common.
2. **Plexiform type:** It is the second most common type. It comprises irregular masses and anastomosing strands (interdigitating cords) of ameloblastomatous epithelium. The central portion of the epithelial island is composed of an inconspicuous loose network of cells resembling the stellate reticulum. It may show cyst-like stromal degeneration.

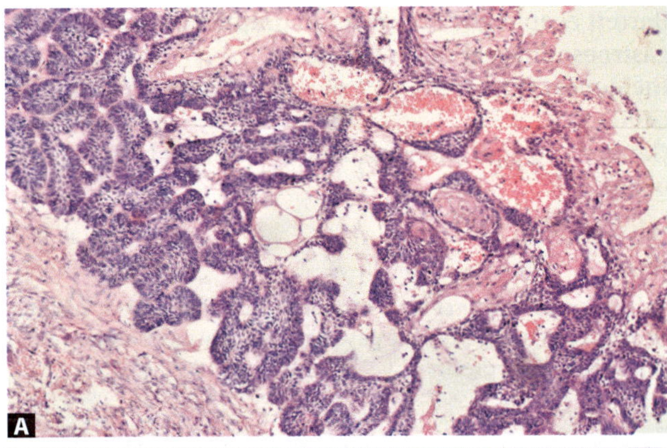

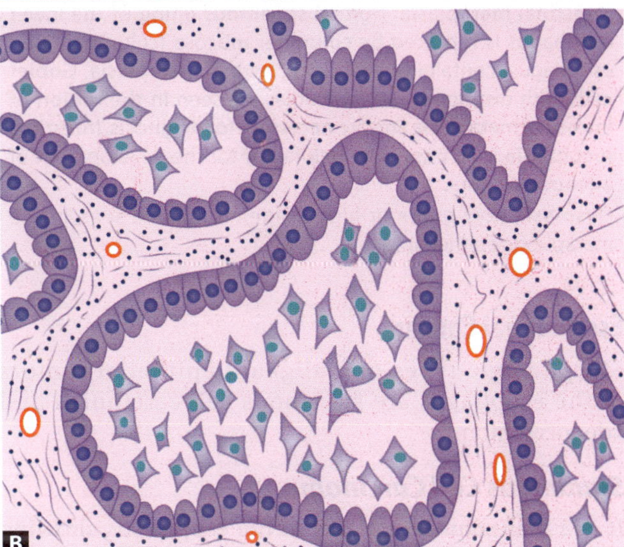

Figs. 18.7A and B: Ameloblastoma: (A) H&E; (B) Diagrammatic. It is composed of nests of epithelium that resemble the inner dental epithelial component of the enamel organ of the developing teeth. These cells are dispersed in a mature fibrous connective tissue (fibrous) stroma. The central portion of the epithelial island is formed of an inconspicuous *loose* network of cells resembling the stellate reticulum.

Clinical features: Ameloblastoma develops over a wide age range without gender predilection. It is rare in children and most commonly occurs in the **third to the seventh decades** of life. It **manifests as a slow, painless expansile lesion** of the jaw. Radiographically, it produces a corticated multilocular **radiolucent lesion**, so-called soap-bubble or honeycomb radiolucency.
Prognosis: Ameloblastoma has **invasive properties and a high tendency to recur unless it is removed in its entirety.** They are treated by complete surgical resection with a tumor-free margin.

GASTROINTESTINAL TRACT

ESOPHAGUS

Lacerations: Mallory–Weiss Tears

Q. Write a short note on Mallory-Weiss syndrome.

Mallory–Weiss tears are **nontransmural longitudinal tears** in the esophagus at the **gastroesophageal region.**
Etiology: Associated with **severe/vigorous retching** or **vomiting** secondary to acute alcohol intoxication or vigorous coughing.

MORPHOLOGY

Site of tears: Usually at the **gastroesophageal junction** but may also be located in the proximal gastric mucosa.
The appearance of tear: Superficial, **longitudinally oriented lacerations of variable length.**

Clinical features: They present with hematemesis. Usually, they do not require surgical intervention. It heals rapidly and completely.

Barrett Esophagus

Q. Write a short note on Barrett esophagus.

Barrett esophagus is defined as the **replacement of esophageal squamous mucosa by metaplastic columnar epithelium with goblet cells** (intestinal metaplasia).

Barrett esophagus occurs as a **complication of chronic gastroesophageal reflux** (GERD).
Incidence: Occurs in ~10% of patients with symptomatic GERD.
Gender and age: Males, usually between **40 and 60 years of age**.

MORPHOLOGY

Gross

It appears as **one or several tongues or patches of red, velvety mucosa** extending **from the gastroesophageal junction upwards into the esophagus**.

Microscopy (Fig. 18.8)

Intestinal metaplasia: Normal **squamous lining** of the lower esophagus **is replaced by columnar mucosa** (columnar lined esophagus) containing **areas of intestinal metaplasia. Goblet cells** with distinct mucous vacuoles are seen **in the region of intestinal metaplasia and are necessary for diagnosis. Intestinal metaplasia** is an important **risk factor** for the development of **adenocarcinoma.**
Dysplasia (low grade or high grade): It may be seen in the metaplastic epithelium.

Esophageal Cancer

Morphologic types of malignant epithelial tumors of the esophagus are squamous cell carcinoma and adenocarcinoma.

Squamous Cell Carcinoma

It is a malignant neoplasm of the esophagus showing squamous differentiation. Squamous cell carcinoma of the esophagus is **more frequent in males** (four times more frequent than in females) over 50 years of age. The most common type of esophageal cancer in India is squamous cell carcinoma. Investigation of choice in esophageal cancer is endoscopy and biopsy.

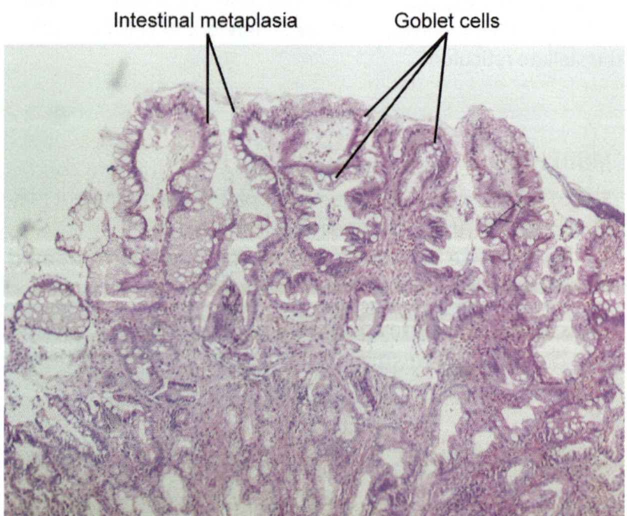

Fig. 18.8: Barrett esophagus with intestinal metaplasia containing goblet cells.

Etiology

Q. Write a short note on the etiology of esophageal cancer.

Risk factors
High alcohol intake and tobacco smoking: These are the two important and well-known environmental risk factors.
Nutrition: Poverty, **diet deficient in vitamins** and certain trace elements, **polycyclic hydrocarbons, nitrosamines**, fungal toxins in pickled vegetable foods, etc.
Hot beverages: Frequent consumption of burning-hot beverages causes thermal injury and may be a risk factor.
Other risk factors: Caustic esophageal injury, **Plummer-Vinson syndrome** (iron deficiency anemia, esophageal webs, and glossitis), **achalasia cardia**, celiac disease, and **previous radiotherapy** to the mediastinum. **Human papillomavirus (HPV)** infection is an etiologic agent in high-risk areas but not in low-risk regions.

MORPHOLOGY

Gross (Figs. 18.9A to C)

Localization: Esophageal SCC is most common in the **middle-third of the esophagus (~50%).**
Patterns of growth: They may be endophytic or exophytic.
1. **Fungating or exophytic:** Tumors protrude into and obstruct the lumen.
2. **Ulcerative:** Growth with elevated ulcer edges.
3. **Infiltrating, or stenotic:** Least common, predominantly intramural.

Mixed gross growth patterns also occur.

Microscopy (Fig. 18.10)

Malignant squamous cells with varying degrees of differentiation (well to poorly differentiated type) (*refer* page 868 for a general microscopic description of squamous cell carcinoma).

Spread

- **Local spread:** Into a respiratory tree, aorta, mediastinum, and pericardium.
- **Lymphatic spread:** Through lymphatics, the tumor spreads to regional lymph nodes.
    - Cancers in the upper third spread to cervical lymph nodes
    - Middle third to mediastinal, paratracheal, and tracheobronchial nodes
    - Lower third to gastric and celiac nodes.
- **Hematogenous spread**: Occurs late; to the liver, lungs, adrenals, kidneys, and bones.

Clinical features: Insidious in onset. Dysphagia, odynophagia (pain on swallowing) and obstruction. Barium swallow in esophageal cancer produces a rat tail appearance.

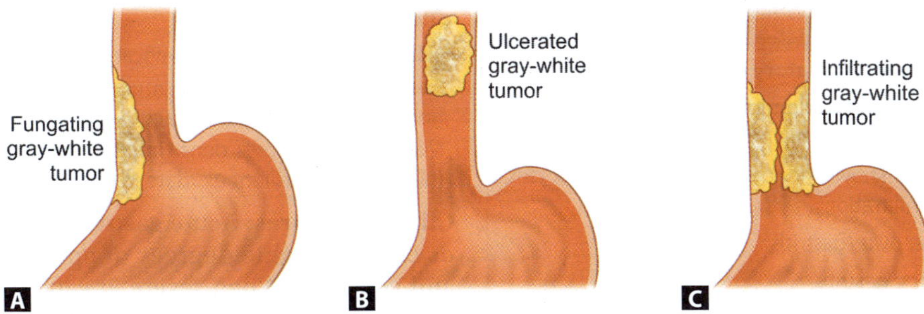

Figs. 18.9A to C: Gross types of carcinoma esophagus: (A) Fungating or exophytic type; (B) Ulcerative type; (C) Infiltrative/stenotic type.

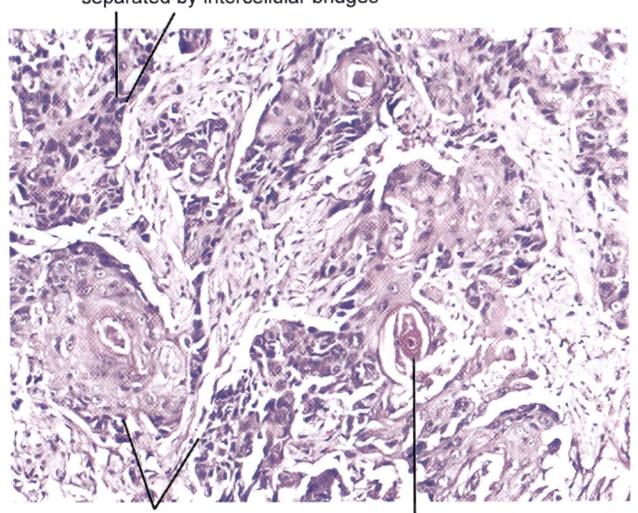

Fig. 18.10: Microscopic appearance of well-differentiated squamous cell carcinoma.

Adenocarcinoma

Q. Write a short note on the adenocarcinoma of the esophagus.

Carcinoma displays glandular differentiation and usually arises in a background of Barrett esophagus and long-standing gastroesophageal reflux diseases (GERD).

Etiology

Risk factors include dysplasia, tobacco use, GERD leading to Barrett esophagus, obesity, scleroderma, prior radiation therapy, and a diet rich in animal fat and cholesterol. Risk is reduced by diets rich in fresh fruits and vegetables.

Pathogenesis

Progression of Barrett esophagus to adenocarcinoma develops in a stepwise pattern with genetic and epigenetic changes.

- **Genetic changes** include chromosomal abnormalities and mutation or overexpression of *TP53*, amplification of *ERBB-2*, cyclin D1, cyclin E genes, etc.
- **Epigenetic changes** include silencing by hypermethylation of p16/INK4a.

MORPHOLOGY

Gross

Site: Usually in the distal third of the esophagus.

Appearance: Early lesions—flat or raised patches later **infiltrate diffusely or ulcerate.**

Microscopy

It consists of a malignant tumor with an **intestinal-type morphology of cells forming glands.** Tumors most commonly produce mucin. Barrett esophagus may be present adjacent to the tumor.

Clinical features: Pain or difficulty in swallowing, chest pain, progressive weight loss, hematemesis, or vomiting.

STOMACH

Various cells in the mucosa of the stomach and their secretions are presented (*refer* **online Table 18.2**).

Definitions

- **Erosion:** Loss of the superficial epithelium which produces a small defect in the mucosa that is **limited to the lamina propria** (do not penetrate the muscularis mucosae).
- **Ulcer:** Break in the mucosal surface **more than 5 mm in size, with depth up to the submucosa** (i.e., they penetrate the muscularis mucosae). It leads to a local defect or excavation due to active inflammation. **Gastric ulcers (GUs) and duodenal ulcers** (DUs) may be acute or chronic.
  - **Stress ulcers** occur with **shock, sepsis, or severe trauma.**
  - **Curling ulcers** develop in the proximal duodenum with **severe burns or trauma** (head injury/intracranial disease).
  - **Cushing ulcers** develop in the stomach, duodenum, and esophagus in patients with **intracranial disease.** Highly prone to perforation.
- **Gastritis: Inflammation of the gastric mucosa** and is **usually a histological diagnosis.** The term gastropathy is used when inflammatory cells are rare or absent (hypertrophic gastropathy).
- **Gastropathy:** This term is used when cell injury and regeneration are present but inflammatory cells are rare or absent.

BOX 18.2: Various ways of classifying gastritis.

A. **Depending on the inflammatory cells and duration**
   - Acute gastritis shows predominately acute inflammatory cells
   - Chronic gastritis shows mononuclear cell (lymphocytes, plasma cells) infiltration
     - *Helicobacter pylori* gastritis
     - Autoimmune gastritis
     - Others

B. **Depending on the segment of the involved stomach**
   - Antral-predominant gastritis
   - Corpus-predominant gastritis
   - Pangastritis

C. **Depending on the absence or presence of premalignant stages**
   - Nonatrophic
   - Atrophic gastritis may progress to carcinoma

Gastritis

Gastritis is inflammation of the gastric mucosa and is usually diagnosed by a histological examination.
Classification of gastritis is presented in **Box 18.2**.

Acute Gastritis

Q. Discuss the etiology, pathogenesis, and complications of acute gastritis.

Definition: Acute gastritis is a transient inflammation of gastric mucosa.

Etiology

- **Drugs:** Aspirin, nonsteroidal anti-inflammatory drugs (NSAIDs), and other drugs (e.g., iron preparations). NSAIDs interfere with protection provided by prostaglandins or reduce bicarbonate secretion.
- *H. pylori* and uremia **inhibit gastric bicarbonate transporters.**
- Alcohol causes direct cellular injury
- Bile reflux (e.g., following gastric surgery)
- Accidental or suicidal ingestion of chemicals (particularly acids or bases) **directly injure mucosal epithelium.**
- Severe physiological stress (e.g., burns)
- Radiation therapy, and chemotherapy (causes insufficient epithelial regeneration)
- Viral infections (e.g., cytomegalovirus—CMV).
- **Reduced synthesis of mucin and bicarbonate secretion (e.g., during old age)**

Pathogenesis of acute gastritis, chronic gastritis, and peptic ulcer disease is discussed together on pages 600-2.

MORPHOLOGY

Mild acute gastritis: No significant changes.
Severe gastritis: Severe mucosal damage, erosions, and hemorrhage and is termed **acute erosive hemorrhagic gastritis.**
Microscopy: It shows, dense infiltration by neutrophils within the mucosa and purulent exudate in the lumen.

Clinical features: Acute gastritis may be asymptomatic or cause variable degrees of epigastric pain, nausea, and vomiting. When severe, it causes mucosal erosion, ulceration, hemorrhage, hematemesis, and melena.

Chronic Gastritis

Chronic gastritis is a chronic inflammation of the stomach associated with mucosal injury. Microscopically, there is an increase in inflammatory cells (**mainly lymphocyte and plasma cell infiltrate) in the lamina propria of the gastric mucosa.**
Causes: A common cause of chronic gastritis is due to **infection by *Helicobacter pylori*.** Other causes include **autoimmune gastritis** (the most common cause in patients without *H. pylori* infection)**, and chronic NSAID use.** Less common are **radiation injury, chronic bile reflux, and mechanical injury (e.g., an indwelling nasogastric tube).**

Helicobacter pylori Gastritis

Q. Write a short essay/note on *Helicobacter pylori* gastritis.

Q. Write a short note on the role of *Helicobacter pylori* in the pathogenic mechanism of peptic/gastric ulcer.

Helicobacter pylori (H. pylori): These are **short, spiral-shaped, or curved (Figs. 18.11A to C) gram-negative bacilli** with multiple **flagella** at one end. They are noninvasive and **reside on the mucin of the surface and neck regions of the foveolar cells.** In gastric biopsies examined, they are found in all patients with duodenal ulcers and the majority with gastric ulcers or chronic gastritis.

- **Acute *H. pylori* infection**: It usually does not produce noticeable symptoms.
- **Chronic *H. pylori* infection:** It produces symptoms. *H. pylori* can be demonstrated in about 90% of patients with chronic gastritis of the pyloric antrum.
- ***Predisposing factors* for *H. pylori* infection**: These include poverty, overcrowding, and limited education. Humans are the primary carriers of infection and transmission is mainly through the fecal-oral route.
- **Mode of spread: Oro-oral or fecal-oral route** by either kissing or ingestion of contaminated vomitus.
- **Source of *H. pylori*:** Humans are the only known host for *H. pylori.*

Pathogenesis

Helicobacter pylori may cause **acute gastritis, mainly involving the antrum, or atrophic gastritis, involving the body and fundus.**

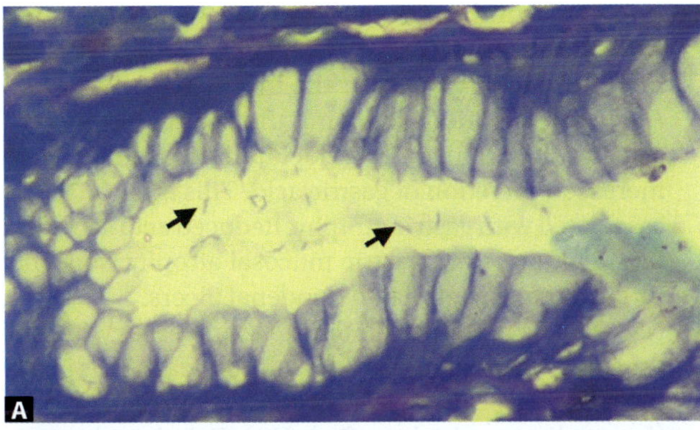

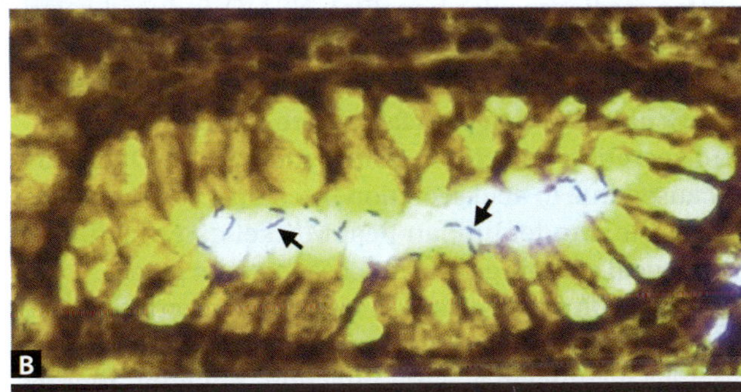

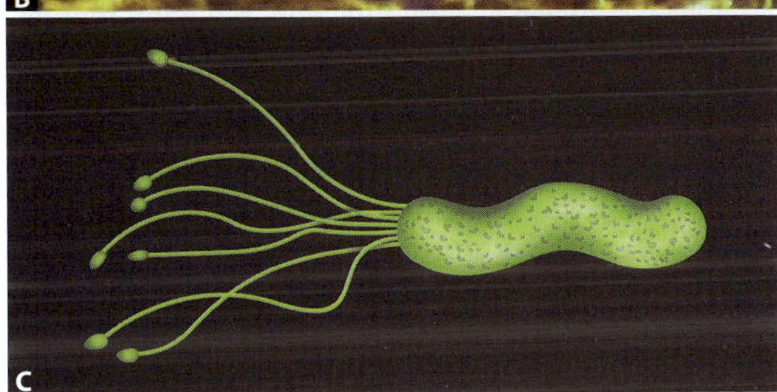

Figs. 18.11A to C: Photomicrograph shows *H. pylori* (arrows) in the lumen of gastric glands: (A) Giemsa stain; (B) Warthin–Starry stain; (C) Diagrammatic.

1. **Antral gastritis:** *Helicobacter* gastritis is **predominantly localized** and **mostly affects the antrum** causing **antral gastritis.** There may be **normal or increased acid production.** If inflammation is limited to the antrum, there may be an increase in parietal cell mass within the gastric body with increased production of acid. This is likely to cause a duodenal peptic ulcer. Local production of gastrin may be increased without increased serum gastrin (hypergastrinemia).
2. **Multifocal (patchy) atrophic gastritis:** With advancing time, antral gastritis may progress to involve the more proximal stomach (i.e., body and fundus) producing multifocal atrophic gastritis. This is characterized by **patchy mucosal atrophy, reduced parietal cell mass and acid secretion, intestinal metaplasia,** and an **increased risk of developing adenocarcinoma of the stomach.** Thus, there is an inverse relationship between duodenal ulcers and gastric adenocarcinoma. *H. pylori* do not invade and they are not found in the absence of foveolar cells or in association with intestinal-type epithelium. Thus, wherever there is intestinal metaplasia, *H. pylori* is not found.

Mechanism of action of H. pylori

- **Flagella:** It makes them motile, and allows them to move in viscous mucus. They burrow and live beneath the mucus layer above the epithelial surface.
- **Urease:** Produced by *H. pylori* releases ammonia (strong alkali) from endogenous urea. This ammonia raises the local gastric pH around the organisms. This in turn protects these bacteria form the acid pH of the stomach, and enhances bacterial survival. Raised local gastric pH acts on the antral G cells and releases gastrin leading to hypergastrinemia and resulting in **hypersecretion of gastric acid.**
- **Adhesins:** They help *H. pylori* to bind to the surface of the foveolar cells of gastric epithelium.
- **Cytotoxins:** Products of genes, namely—**cytotoxin-associated gene A (*cagA*), *CagE*, and vacuolating agent (*vacA*) gene** involved in the progression of the disease and cause gastritis, peptic ulceration, and cancer. These toxins stimulate the release of cytokines such as IL-8, a potent chemotactic factor for neutrophils. They initiate and sustain innate and adaptive immune responses and damage the mucosa.

Host factors: Play a role in the outcome of *H. pylori* infection.

- **Increased expression of proinflammatory cytokines:** Normally, *H. pylori* does not invade the cells/tissues. It causes increased production of proinflammatory cytokines [e.g., interleukin-1β (IL-1β) and tumor necrosis factor (TNF)] by the mucosal epithelial cells.
- **Decreased expression of the anti-inflammatory cytokines:** For example, interleukin-10 (IL-10).

The above mechanism activates neutrophils and macrophages (inflammatory response in the gastric mucosa) and impairs mucosal defense leading to pangastritis, atrophy, and gastric cancer. Thus, the development and course of *H. pylori* gastritis depend on the interplay between gastroduodenal mucosal defenses, inflammatory responses, and bacterial virulence factors.

MORPHOLOGY

Gross: *H. pylori* most commonly infects the antral mucosa. Hence, the antrum is the preferred biopsy site for the evaluation of *H. pylori* gastritis. The **involved mucosa is usually erythematous** and has a coarse or even nodular appearance on endoscopic examination.

Microscopy

- Initially, *H. pylori* gastritis is limited to the gastric antrum (the most common site of colonization) and later may extend to involve the body and fundus. *H. pylori* are **concentrated within the superficial mucus covering the epithelial cells in the surface and neck regions.** *H. pylori* have an affinity for gastric epithelium and are generally not found in association with intestinal metaplasia or duodenal epithelium. Biopsy of the antral region is preferred for evaluation of *H. pylori* gastritis.

- The presence of **intraepithelial neutrophils** and **subepithelial (superficial lamina propria) plasma cells** are **characteristics of *H. pylori* gastritis.** Neutrophils may accumulate in the lumen of gastric pits to produce **pit abscesses.**
- In **long-standing cases, gastritis may extend proximally to involve the body and fundus. Then the mucosa** can become **atrophic with loss of parietal and chief cells. Microscopically, it is accompanied by lymphoid aggregates,** some with germinal centers. These lymphoid aggregates represent an induced form of **mucosa-associated lymphoid tissue** or MALT, which **can transform into lymphoma.**
- **Special stains for demonstration of *H. pylori* (*Figs. 18.11A to C*):** Organisms can be easily demonstrated with special stains.
  - **Modified Giemsa stain and Diff–Quik stain** are popular, quick, cheap, and easy to perform.
  - **Silver stains: Warthin–Starry, Genta stain.**
  - **Immunohistochemistry for *Helicobacter*.**

Diagnostic tests for *H. pylori* are listed (*refer* **online Box 18.3**).

Significance of H. pylori infections

- **Peptic ulcer disease (PUD):** Chronic *Helicobacter* gastritis most commonly leads to PUD.
- **Gastric cancer and lymphoma:** *H. pylori* infection involving the body of the stomach increases the risk for gastric cancer. It is also associated with the risk of gastric lymphoma.

Complications of chronic gastritis: Important complications of chronic gastritis are **peptic ulcer disease, mucosal atrophy, intestinal metaplasia, and dysplasia.**

Peptic Ulcer Disease

PA 24.2 (CC): Describe the etiology, pathogenesis, pathology, microbiology, clinical and microscopic features of peptic ulcer disease.

Q. Define peptic ulcer disease.

Definition: A peptic ulcer disease (PUD) is defined as a chronic focal mucosal ulceration/defect measuring **at least 5 mm in diameter that penetrates the muscularis mucosae. It usually affects the duodenum (duodenal ulcer) or stomach (gastric ulcer).**

Q. Discuss the pathogenesis of peptic ulcer.

Etiology

The imbalances between mucosal defenses and damaging forces cause chronic gastritis. Peptic ulcer disease (PUD) is **one of the complications of chronic gastritis.**

***H. pylori* infection and NSAIDs:** PUD is often associated with *H. pylori* infection or NSAIDs. These factors compromise mucosal defense mechanisms and predispose patients to peptic ulcers.

- ***H. pylori* infection (*refer* pages 598-9): The most common form of PUD occurs within the antrum of the stomach or duodenum** because of chronic *H. pylori*-induced antral gastritis. This gastritis is associated with increased gastric acid secretion and decreased bicarbonate secretion in the duodenum. However, *H. pylori* infection involving the fundus or body of the stomach is usually associated with moderately increased secretion of gastric acid. This is because it is associated with gastric atrophy. Reduced acid secretion in individuals with gastric mucosal atrophy is usually protected from antral and duodenal ulcers.
- **NSAID:** The risk of developing PUD increases with age, especially in individuals older than 60 years. This is due to the increased use of NSAIDs such as low-dose aspirin (for cardiovascular benefits). NSAID-induced gastric injury can be further increased by *H. pylori* infection. *H. pylori* and NSAIDs work synergistically to increase the risk of PUD when both factors are present.

Acid secretion by ectopic gastric mucosa: PUD may also be caused due to acid secretion by ectopic gastric mucosa within the duodenum, an ileal Meckel diverticulum, or esophageal ectopic gastric mucosa (an inlet patch).

Less common causes: These include **hypersecretory states** [e.g., Zollinger–Ellison syndrome (ZES)], Crohn disease, vascular insufficiency, viral infection, radiation therapy, and cancer therapy.

Other factors: These may be involved in the development of PUD. PUD is also associated with **cigarette smoking and cardiovascular disease due to reduced mucosal blood flow**, oxygenation, and healing. Cigarette smoking impairs ulcer healing and increases the risk of recurrence. Other factors that play a relatively minor role include psychological stress, personality type, alcohol consumption, occupation, and diet.

Diseases associated with PUD: Certain chronic diseases are positively correlated with PUD. These include **chronic obstructive pulmonary disease, systemic mastocytosis, alcoholic cirrhosis, chronic renal failure (uremia), alpha 1-antitrypsin deficiency, and nephrolithiasis.**

Normal Process in the Stomach

Several mechanisms protect the gastric mucosa.

Two opposing sets of forces keep the stomach in a normal state: Damaging forces and defensive forces (**Fig. 18.12**).

Damaging Forces

These forces can induce mucosal injury. They consist of two gastric secretory products: (1) Gastric acidity due to hydrochloric acid (HCl) and (2) peptic enzymes produced from pepsinogen.

Gastric acidity: Gastric juice mainly comprises hydrochloric acid (HCl). The gastric lumen pH is about 1 which is several times more than the pH of blood. HCl plays the **main role in digestion,** but it also **can damage the gastric mucosa.**

- Enzyme H^+/K^+ ATPase is a proton pump responsible for producing a large concentration of H^+. Acid is secreted by the parietal cell located in the oxyntic gland.

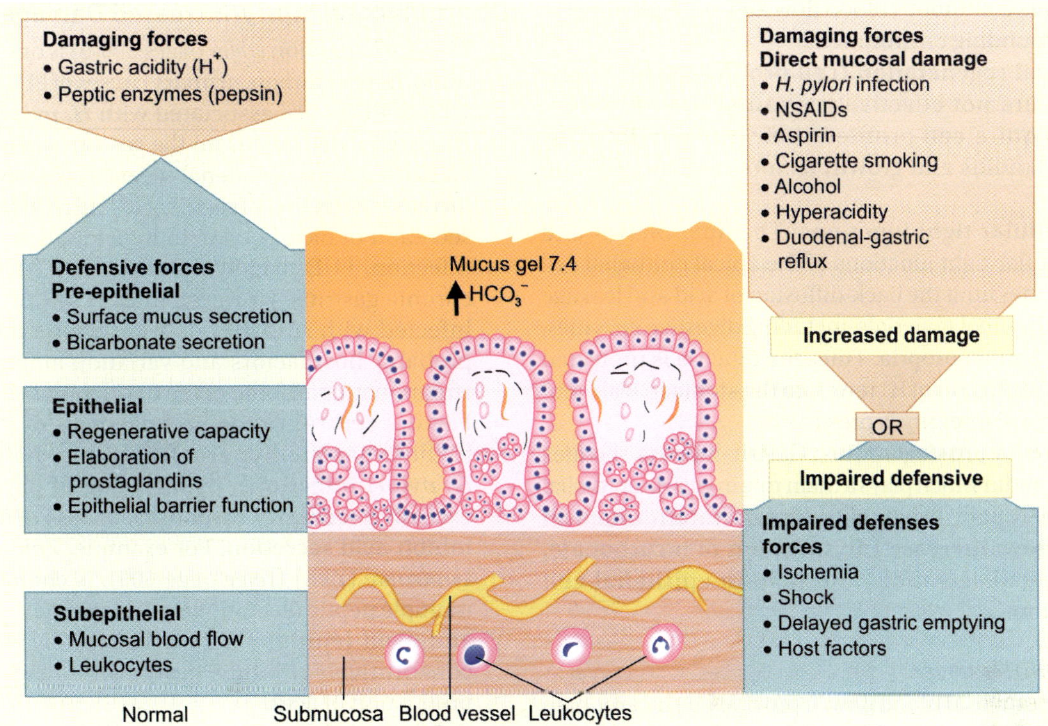

Fig. 18.12: Components involved in mucosal defense and repair in normal (left side) and in acute or chronic gastritis (right side). The gastric mucus barrier consists of viscid mucus (which forms an unstirred layer between the epithelium and the gastric lumen) and bicarbonates (HCO_3^-).

- Parietal cell expresses receptors for many stimulants of acid secretion, including histamine (H2), gastrin (cholecystokinin B/gastrin receptor), and acetylcholine (muscarinic receptor, M3).

Peptic enzymes: They can also damage the gastric mucosa.

- Pepsinogen, which is an inactive precursor of pepsin, is synthesized and secreted by the chief cell, found mainly in the gastric fundus.
- The acid environment within the stomach leads to the conversion of pepsinogen to pepsin and provides the low pH (<2.0) required for the activity of pepsin. Pepsin helps in digestion by breaking down proteins into peptides and amino acids. They are also capable of damaging the gastric mucosa.
- Pepsin activity decreases as the pH increases; it is markedly decreased at a pH of 4 and inactivated at a pH of 7 and above. Many of the substances, that stimulate acid secretion, also stimulate pepsinogen release.

Defensive Forces

These are a three-level barrier composed of (1) pre-epithelial, (2) epithelial, and (3) subepithelial elements.

Pre-epithelial barrier

It is a mucus-bicarbonate layer of the stomach. It is formed by several factors produced by surface epithelial cells, such as: (a) production of mucus, (b) bicarbonate secretion, (c) epithelial cell ionic transporters that maintain intracellular pH, and (d) intracellular tight junctions.

- **Surface mucus secretion:** Mucin is secreted by surface foveolar cells. Actions of mucus are:
  - **Prevents the direct contact of large food particles to the epithelium.**
  - Thick, alkaline, aqueous mucus-rich fluid **lubricates the mucosa and neutralizes acid at the epithelial level.**
  - The mucus layer **promotes the formation of an "unstirred" protective layer** of fluid on the mucosa.
  - Impedes the diffusion of ions and molecules such as pepsin.
- **Bicarbonate secretion:** Surface epithelial cells secrete bicarbonate into the mucus. The bicarbonate diffuses into the unstirred mucus and buffers the hydrogen ions entering from the luminal aspect. It results in a pH gradient, ranging from 1 or 2 at the gastric luminal surface, and reaching to a neutrality of 6 to 7 along the epithelial cell surface.

Epithelial barrier

It consists of surface epithelial cells that act through the following mechanisms:

- **Restitution of damaged gastric epithelial cells:** It is the process of restoration of a damaged region by migration of gastric epithelial cells bordering a site of injury.

It requires continuous blood flow and an alkaline pH in the surrounding environment.

- **Epithelial regeneration (cell proliferation):** Larger defects are not effectively repaired by restitution. They require cell proliferation. It is regulated by prostaglandins and growth factors such as EGF and TGF-α.
- **Intracellular tight junctions:** The lipid bilayer and intracellular tight junctions of the apical epithelial cell membranes limit the back-diffusion of acid and leakage of other luminal materials, including digestive enzymes, into the lamina propria. Thus, the mucosa is protected from the diffusion of H^+ ions into the stomach wall, and the mucosal integrity is preserved.
- **Secretion of prostaglandins:** Gastric mucosa secretes prostaglandin which plays a main role in gastric epithelial defense/repair. **Prostaglandins maintain mucosal blood flow, increase** the secretion of bicarbonate, inhibit acid secretion, **and help in epithelial cell restitution.**

Subepithelial barrier

Rich gastric mucosal blood flow: It provides (1) bicarbonate (HCO^-), which neutralizes the acid generated by parietal cells, (2) an adequate supply of nutrients and oxygen, and (3) removes toxic metabolic by-products. The rich blood supply of the gastric mucosa also buffers any protons that diffuse back into the lamina propria.

Pathogenesis of PUD/Acute or Chronic Gastritis

Q. Discuss the role of *H. pylori* in gastric ulcers (*refer* pages 598-9).

Components of the normal process involved in the maintenance of the balance of two opposite forces of the gastric mucosa are discussed above. The imbalances between mucosal defenses and damaging forces cause chronic gastritis and PUD. **Thus, PUD can occur due to direct mucosal injury or disruption of any of the protective mechanisms.** Risk factors for peptic ulcer disease are listed in **Box 18.4**.

BOX 18.4: Risk factors for peptic ulcer disease.

- *Helicobacter pylori* infection
- Cigarette smoking (synergizes with *H. pylori* for gastric PUD)
- NSAIDs (potentiated by corticosteroids)
- Chronic obstructive pulmonary disease (COPD)
- Alcoholic cirrhosis (primarily duodenal PUD)
- Psychological stress (increased gastric acid secretion)
- Zollinger-Ellison syndrome (PUD of stomach, duodenum, and jejunum)
- Viral infection: CMV, herpes simplex virus

(CMV: cytomegalovirus; NSAIDs: nonsteroidal anti-inflammatory drugs; PUD: peptic ulcer disease).

Direct Mucosal Injury/Increased Damage

- ***H. pylori* infection** (*refer* pages 598-9) is one of the **most important, common, primary causes** of PUD. **More than 70% of PUDs are associated with *H. pylori* infection.** *H. pylori* is detected from the gastric antrum in almost all patients with duodenal ulcers. It is associated with increased secretion of gastric acid and reduced duodenal secretion of bicarbonate. In individuals with *H. pylori* infection, PUD usually develops on a background of chronic gastritis. However, only 5–10% of individuals infected with *H. pylori* develop peptic ulcers. Thus, probably host factors and variation among *H. pylori* strains may contribute to the development of PUD.
- **Factors central to the pathogenesis of PUD:** These include **gastric hyperacidity (may be caused by *H. pylori* infection), hyperplasia of parietal cells, excessive secretory responses, or loss of signals that inhibit acid secretion.** For example, *Zollinger-Ellison syndrome* (ZES) (*refer* page 605), is characterized by multiple peptic ulcerations in the stomach, duodenum, and even jejunum. ZES is caused by tumors that constitutively produce gastrin and lead to massive production of acid.
- **Cofactors in peptic ulcerogenesis**: These include the following:
  - **Chronic use of nonsteroidal anti-inflammatory drugs (NSAIDs) and aspirin:** They cause (1) **direct chemical irritation of mucosa,** (2) **suppresses mucosal prostaglandin synthesis** and (3) **reduces the bicarbonate secretion**. NSAIDs inhibit cyclooxygenase (COX)-dependent synthesis of prostaglandins E_2 and I_2. These prostaglandins protect the gastric lining by stimulating mucus and bicarbonate secretion, mucosal blood flow, and epithelial restitution.
  - **Cigarette smoking: It decreases the blood flow to the mucosa** and healing of mucosal damage.
  - **High-dose corticosteroids:** They suppress the synthesis of prostaglandin and impair healing.
  - **Others:** Peptic ulcers are more frequent in patients with **alcohol-related cirrhosis, chronic obstructive pulmonary disease**, psychologic stress, alpha 1-antitrypsin deficiency, and nephrolithiasis. Hypercalcemia **in chronic renal failure, and hyperparathyroidism**, stimulate gastrin production and increase secretion of gastric acid.

Impaired Defense

It may be due to:

- **Ischemia**: Decreased oxygen delivery (e.g., at high altitudes and shock)
- **Shock**
- **Delayed gastric emptying**
- **Host factors:** Reduced mucin synthesis in the elderly leads to increased susceptibility to gastritis.

MORPHOLOGY

Q. Write a short note on the morphology of peptic ulcers.

Gross (Fig. 18.13)

Locations (sites) of peptic ulcer disease (Box 18.5): They can develop in any portion of the gastrointestinal tract exposed to acidic gastric juices. Size and location cannot differentiate benign peptic and malignant ulcers (ulcerating carcinoma).

- **Duodenum: Four times more common in the first portion of the duodenum than in the stomach**). They occur within a **few centimeters of the pyloric valve** and **involve the anterior wall.** Kissing ulcers are peptic ulcers occurring at both the posterior and anterior walls of the duodenum.
- **Stomach:** Gastric peptic ulcers predominantly occur on the **lesser curvature** near the junction (transitional zone) of the body and antrum:
  - **Proximal ulcers:** Located in the body of the stomach.
  - **Distal ulcers:** Located in the **antrum and angulus of the stomach.**
- **Gastroesophageal junction of the esophagus:** Peptic (acid-induced) injury may occur in the esophagus because of acid reflux (GERD) or acid secretion by ectopic gastric mucosa.
- **Anastomotic site:** It can develop at the anastomotic site in patients who have undergone a distal gastric resection. Occur at margins of the gastroduodenal anastomosis/ gastrojejunostomy (anastomotic ulcer). These are rare nowadays because of the present efficient acid—suppressing therapies available for peptic ulcers.
- **Multiple ulcers:** In the duodenum, stomach, and/or jejunum in Zollinger-Ellison syndrome.

BOX 18.5: Sites of peptic ulcer disease.

- Duodenum
- Stomach
- Esophagus
- Jejunum
- Gastric mucosa in Meckel diverticulum

- **At metaplastic or heterotopic gastric mucosa:** For example, Meckel diverticulum within ileum having ectopic gastric mucosa.

Number: Solitary in more than 80% of patients, **but may be more than one.**

Size: Lesions less than 0.3 cm in diameter are shallow and those larger than 0.6 cm are likely to be deeper ulcers.

Shape: Round to oval, sharply punched-out defect (Figs. 18.13A to C).

Margin: Usually **in level with the surrounding mucosa**. The gastric mucosal folds can be traced up to the margins of the ulcer and the radiating folds of mucosa from the ulcer **(Figs. 18.13A to C)** appear like a spoke wheel. In contrast, **heaped-up margins are more characteristic of gastric cancers.**

Depth: The depth of ulcers varies and correlates with the diameter and deep extension. It may be limited by the thick gastric muscularis propria, adherent pancreas, omental fat, or the liver.

Base: It is **smooth and clean** because of the peptic digestion of exudate.

PA 24.3 (CC): Describe and identify the microscopic features of peptic ulcer.

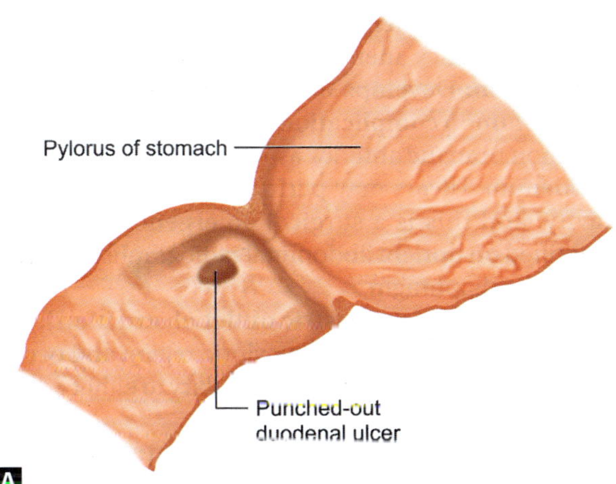

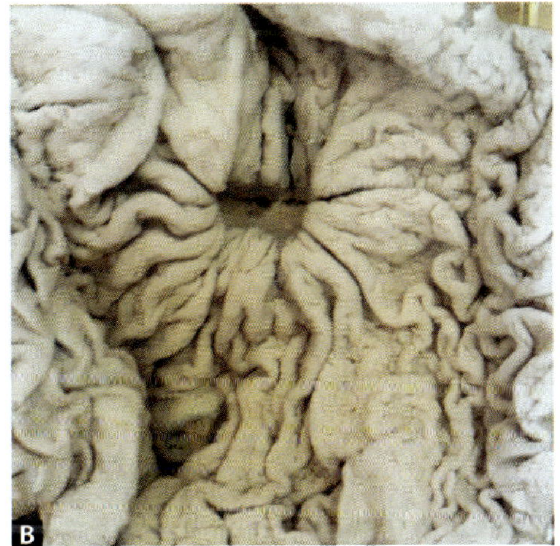

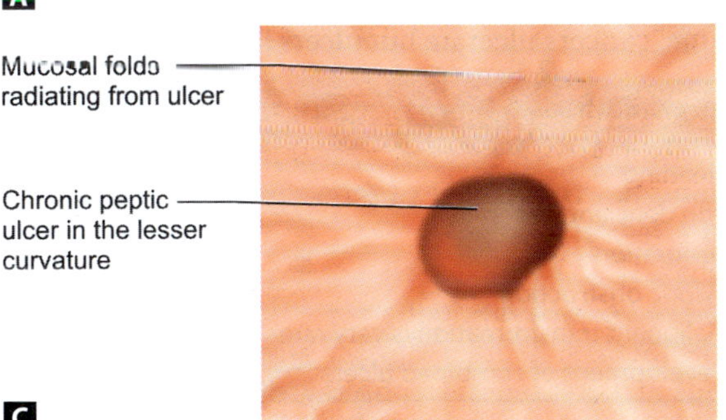

Figs. 18.13A to C: Gross appearance of peptic ulcer: (A) Duodenal ulcer In the first part of duodenum showing characteristic sharp demarcation from the surrounding mucosa (diagrammatic); peptic ulcer of the stomach; (B) specimen; (C) Diagrammatic showing characteristic sharp demarcation from the surrounding mucosa. Note the gastric mucosal folds can be traced up to the margins of the ulcer and the radiating folds of mucosa from the ulcer appear like a spoke wheel.

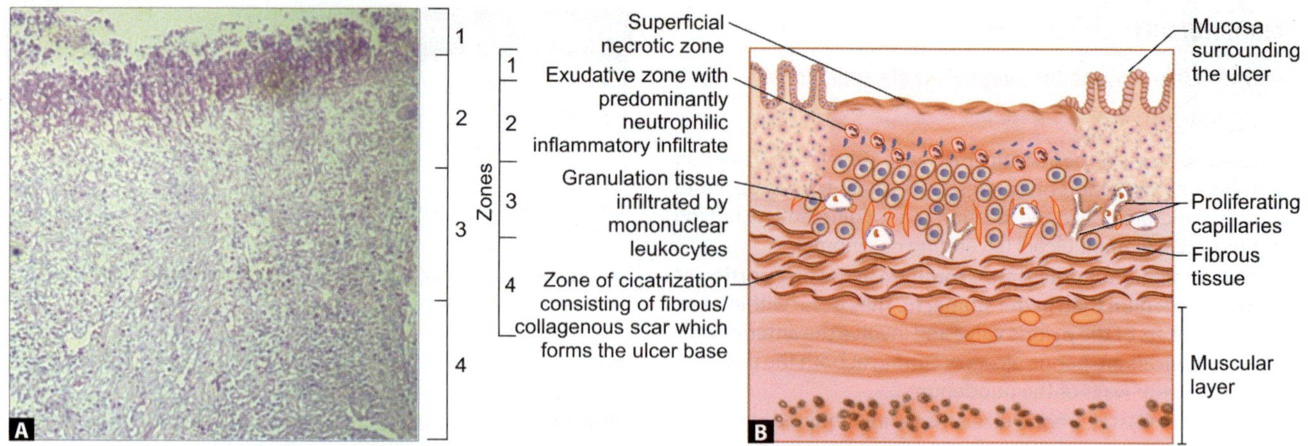

Figs. 18.14A and B: Microscopic features of a peptic ulcer: (A) Photomicrograph; and (B) diagrammatic, showing four layers of chronic gastric ulcer.

Microscopy (Figs. 18.14A and B)

Gastric and duodenal ulcers are microscopically similar. From the lumen outward **four layers** can be identified and are known as **Askanazy zones.**

1. **Necrotic zone:** It is the most superficial zone and consists of a surface coat of purulent exudate, bacteria, and necrotic debris.
2. **Superficial exudative zone:** It consists of **fibrinopurulent exudates with predominantly neutrophilic inflammatory infiltrate.**
3. **Granulation tissue zone:** It consists of granulation tissue infiltrated with mononuclear leukocytes.
4. **Zone of cicatrization:** It consists of **fibrous tissue or collagenous scar** which forms the base of the ulcer and may show chronic inflammatory cells.

   At the edges, the muscularis mucosae are seen to fuse with the muscularis externa. The mucosa surrounding the ulcer is of pyloric type.

Clinical Features

Peptic ulcers are **chronic, recurring lesions with more morbidity than mortality.**

- **Age:** Peptic ulcers occur most commonly in middle-aged to older adults without any obvious precipitating conditions other than chronic gastritis.
- **Pain:** Most patients with peptic ulcers present with epigastric burning or aching pain. Pain usually occurs 1–3 hours after meals during the day, and is worse at night between 11 pm and 2 am. It is relieved by alkali or food.
- **Periodicity:** After a period of weeks to months of active disease, healing may occur with or without treatment. There is a tendency to develop additional ulcers.
- **Other symptoms:** These include nausea, vomiting, bloating, belching, and significant weight loss.

PUD causes more morbidity than mortality. Current treatments consist of the eradication of *H. pylori* with antibiotics and the neutralization of gastric acid by ton pump inhibitors. Surgical management is reserved mainly for the treatment of ulcers that produce uncontrollable bleeding or perforation.

Complications of Peptic Ulcer Disease (Box 18.6)

Q. Write a short note on complications of gastric ulcer.

- **Bleeding:** A most common complication of peptic ulcer. Severe bleeding may cause "coffee ground" vomitus or melena and may be life-threatening. The gastroduodenal artery is the source of bleeding in duodenal ulcers. The left gastric artery is the source of bleeding in gastric ulcers.
- **Iron deficiency anemia:** Chronic blood loss may lead to iron deficiency anemia.
- **Perforation:** Develops in ~5% of patients and is the **most common complication of gastric ulcer**. It is most common from the anterior aspect of the first part of the duodenum. Ulcers may perforate into the peritoneal cavity, and this is a surgical emergency. It may be identified on upright abdominal radiographs as free air under the diaphragm.
- **Pyloric obstruction (gastric outlet obstruction):** It is associated with ulcers in the pyloric region and occurs in ~10% of ulcer patients. It is secondary to either edema or scarring.
- **Rarely malignant transformation:** Malignant transformation of peptic ulcers is very rare. The dictum is that 'cancers ulcerate but ulcers rarely cancerate.'

BOX 18.6: Complications of peptic ulcer disease.

- Bleeding
- Iron deficiency anemia
- Perforation
- Pyloric obstruction
- Malignant transformation is very rare
- Development of combined ulcers

TABLE 18.3 Differences between gastric and duodenal peptic ulcer.

Features	*Gastric ulcer*	*Duodenal ulcer*
Most common site	Along the lesser curvature	The first part of the duodenum
Incidence	Less common	More common
Age	Beyond 6th decade, M > F	Between 25 and 50 years, M > F
Association with *H. pylori* infection	Less common	Strong association
Acid level	Usually, normal	High
Clinical features		
Relationship of pain to antacids	Relief of pain not consistent	Prompt relief of pain
Relationship of pain to food	Aggravates the pain	Relieves the pain
Night pain	Not observed	Common
Heartburn	Not common	Common
Hematemesis/melena	Hematemesis more common	Melena more common
Vomiting	Common	No vomiting
Weight loss	Present	Absent
Complication	Rarely undergo malignant change	No malignant change

- **Development of combined ulcers**: In the stomach and duodenum of the same patient.

Differences between gastric and duodenal peptic ulcers are given in **Table 18.3**.

SCENARIO-BASED ESSAY QUESTION

Q. A 38-year-old male executive working in a public sector company complains of a long history of heartburn (dull pain in the midepigastric region) and dyspepsia for the last 1 year. The pain used to occur 2–3 hours after a meal and is relieved if he takes antacids or eats more food. There is no weight loss. On enquiry, he has been consuming analgesics (about 1–2 tablets per week) for headaches and consumes alcohol regularly. He underwent an upper GI endoscopy and was found to have a lesion in the anterior wall of the first part of the duodenum. He recovered from this illness after a few days of treatment with drugs and a modified lifestyle. He felt better and discontinued treatment. Three weeks later, the epigastric pain recurs.

a. **What is the probable diagnosis? (Ans: Peptic ulcer disease)**
b. **Describe the etiopathogenesis. What bacterial infection can be an etiological factor?** *(refer pages 600-2)*.
c. **Describe the gross and microscopy of the duodenum in this disease** *(refer pages 603-4)*.
d. **Mention the complications** *(refer pages 604-5)*.

Zollinger–Ellison Syndrome (ZES)

Q. Write a short note on Zollinger–Ellison syndrome.

Zollinger–Ellison syndrome consists of a triad: (1) hypergastrinemia caused by gastrin-secreting tumors (gastrinomas), (2) increased acid production, and (3) severe peptic ulcer disease.

- **Gastrinomas with hypergastrinemia: Gastrinomas** (gastrin-secreting tumors) are commonly seen in the small intestine or pancreas. It causes increased gastrin secretion and leads to the massive secretion of **acid and pepsin.** Fasting serum gastrin level greater than 1,000 pg/mL is diagnostic.
- **Increased acid (HCl) secretion:** Its inactivation of pancreatic enzymes and bile salts leading to malabsorption and diarrhea. The stomach shows an **increase in the number of parietal cells.**
- **Multiple, severe, and recurrent peptic ulcers** in the duodenum, stomach, and/or jejunum.

Gastric Adenocarcinoma

PA 24.4 (CC): Describe and etiology and pathogenesis and pathologic features of carcinoma of the stomach.

Gastric adenocarcinoma is a **malignant epithelial neoplasm of the gastric mucosa with glandular differentiation**. It is the **most common malignant tumor of the stomach** and constitutes >90% of all gastric cancers.

Epidemiology

More common in Japan and in males. Overall **decrease in the incidence** of gastric cancer is noted and may be due to:

- **Reduced prevalence of *H. pylori* infection.**
- **Dietary factors:**
  - **Decreased consumption of dietary carcinogens,** such as (1) N-nitroso compounds and benzo[a] pyrene, (2) reduced use of salt and smoking food, (3) decreased use of preservatives due to easy availability of food refrigeration.
  - **Intake of green, leafy vegetables and citrus fruits** that contain antioxidants such as vitamin C, vitamin E, and beta-carotene.

Though overall there is a reduction of cancer of the stomach, the cancer of the cardia region is on the rise. This may be due to the esophagus, increased incidence of chronic GERD, and obesity.

Etiology and Pathogenesis

Q. Discuss the etiology and pathogenesis of gastric carcinoma.

Gastric cancer is a multifactorial disease. About 90% are sporadic; the remaining 10% develop in a familial/ hereditary setting.

Q. Write a short note on risk factors for carcinoma of the stomach.

Risk Factors (Box 18.7)

Environmental factors: These include the following:

- ***Helicobacter pylori* infection:** It **increases the risk by five- to six-fold.** However, most individuals infected with *H. pylori* do not develop cancer.

BOX 18.7: Risk factors of gastric carcinoma.

A. Environmental factors
1. *H. pylori* infection (intestinal-type carcinoma and Epstein–Barr virus infection)
2. Dietary/nutritional: Nitrites derived from nitrates (water, preserved food), smoked foods (due to benzpyrene) and excess of salt (salted pickled vegetables, chili peppers), and deficiency of fresh fruit, vegetables, vitamins A and C, refrigeration
3. Low socioeconomic status: Low fat or protein consumption, high complex carbohydrate consumption
4. Rubber and coal workers

B. Host factors/predisposing conditions (precancerous conditions)
1. Chronic gastritis (especially atrophic gastritis), pernicious anemia, hypochlorhydria favors colonization with *H. pylori*. Intestinal metaplasia is a precursor lesion.
2. Partial gastrectomy (postmastectomy, post-vagotomy, postgastrojejunostomy): Favors bile reflux, alkaline intestinal fluid
3. Gastric dysplasia, gastric polyps, and adenomas more than 2 cm
4. Ménétrier's disease (hypertrophic gastropathy)
5. Barrett esophagus

C. Genetic factors
Blood group A, family history of gastric cancer, hereditary nonpolyposis colon cancer (HNPCC) syndrome, familial gastric carcinoma syndrome [germ line mutation in E-cadherin gene *(CDH1)*], Li–Fraumeni syndrome.

- **Epstein–Barr virus (EBV):** It is **associated with about 10% of gastric adenocarcinomas**. The exact role of EBV in the development of gastric adenocarcinomas is not known. Probably EBV infection preceded neoplastic transformation. *TP53* mutations are uncommon in EBV-positive gastric tumors, suggesting that the molecular pathogenesis of these cancers is distinct from that of other gastric adenocarcinomas. EBV-positive tumors tend to develop in the proximal stomach and most commonly are of diffuse type with a marked lymphocytic infiltrate.
- **Nitrites: High concentrations of nitrates are found in dried, smoked, and salted foods.** The long-term ingestion of nitrates appears to be associated with a higher risk of gastric cancer. The nitrates present in the diet can be converted to carcinogenic nitrites by bacteria (*refer* **online Box 18.8**). The source of these bacteria may be exogenous such as ingestion of partially decayed foods (consumed especially by the lower socioeconomic classes) or infection by bacteria such as *Helicobacter pylori*. *H. pylori* causes chronic inflammatory atrophic gastritis, and loss of gastric acidity, and favors the growth of bacteria that convert nitrate into carcinogenic nitrite. Though the risk for gastric carcinoma is 6 times higher in individuals infected with *H. pylori*, it is not known whether eradication of the bacteria in an individual already infected with *H. pylori* reduces the risk of gastric cancer.

Host factors/predisposing conditions: Gastric cancer is more common in **lower socioeconomic groups** and in patients with **multifocal mucosal atrophy and intestinal metaplasia**. Peptic ulcer disease does not increase the risk of gastric cancer, but patients who underwent partial gastrectomies for peptic ulcer disease have a slightly higher risk for gastric cancer in the residual gastric stump. This is mainly due to hypochlorhydria, bile reflux, and chronic gastritis.

Pathogenesis

H. pylori Infection

It is responsible for most gastric carcinomas. The possible mechanism of the development of carcinoma stomach by *H. pylori* infection is presented in **Flowchart 18.1**. It is observed that eradication of *H. pylori* reduces the risk of gastric carcinomas. Chronic *H. pylori* infection may cause DNA mutations and epigenetic changes in epithelial cells of the stomach (field cancerization).

Genetic Factors

Most gastric cancers have no hereditary basis and they are genetically heterogeneous. However, certain molecular alterations are frequently observed.

Familial gastric cancer: Mutations detected in familial gastric cancer have helped in understanding the mechanisms of carcinogenesis in sporadic cases.

Flowchart 18.1: Possible mechanism of development of carcinoma stomach by *H. pylori* infection.

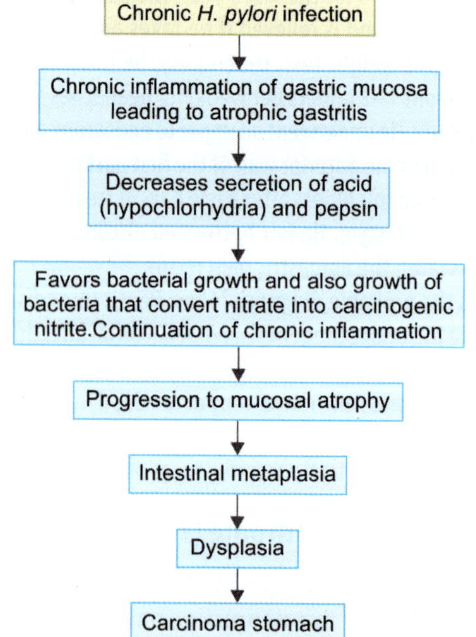

- **Germline mutations** in *CDH1* **gene: germline loss-of-function mutations** in the tumor suppressor gene *CDH1* are strongly associated with familial gastric cancer (usually diffuse type). Gene *CDH1* encodes E-cadherin. This is an epithelial intercellular adhesion protein.

Sporadic diffuse gastric cancers: Loss of E-cadherin is the key step in the development of diffuse gastric cancer. This may be by the following mechanisms:

- **Somatic mutations in *CDH1* gene**: These are observed in about 50% of sporadic diffuse gastric tumors.
- **Markedly decreased expression of E-cadherin**: It in found in 50% of sporadic diffuse gastric tumors. Their reduced expression is usually **by methylation and silencing of the *CDH1* promoter.**

CDH1 mutations are also commonly observed in sporadic and familial lobular carcinoma of the breast. These breast tumors are similar to diffuse GC, and tumor cells infiltrate as single cells.

Sporadic intestinal-type gastric cancers: These may show the following genetic abnormalities.

- **Mutations causing increased signaling via the WNT pathway (*refer* Fig. 18.47):** Unlike diffuse gastric cancers, sporadic intestinal-type gastric cancers are strongly associated with mutations that lead to increased signaling via the WNT pathway. This may be due to:
  - **Loss-of-function mutations in the adenomatous polyposis coli (*APC*) tumor suppressor gene.** FAP patients with germline *APC* mutations have an increased risk of developing intestinal-type gastric cancer, particularly in those who reside in high-risk areas such as Japan.
  - **Gain-of-function mutations in the gene encoding β-catenin.**
- **Mutation of *TP53*** in most sporadic gastric cancers of both diffuse and intestinal types.
- **Loss-of-function mutations or silencing in other genes:** These include other tumor suppressor genes, genes involved in the regulation of apoptosis (*BAX*), those involved in TGF-β signaling (TGFβRII), and cell cycle control (*CDKN2A*).
- ***HER2* gene amplification:** A subset of tumors (5–15% of all GCs of intestinal type) show strong membrane immunostaining for HER2. This is due to the amplification of the *HER2* gene. Usually, gastric cancers with overexpression of HER2 are associated with a poor prognosis.

MORPHOLOGY

Q. Write a short note on the morphology of gastric carcinoma.

Localization: The location of gastric carcinoma varies geographically according to the incidence of gastric cancer. **Pylorus and antrum (50–60%),** cardia (25%), body and fundus (15–25%). **Lesser curvature** is involved more often (in ~40%) than the greater curvature (~12%). The most favored site is the lesser curvature of the **antropyloric region.**

BOX 18.9: Various classifications of gastric carcinoma.

Based on depth of invasion
- Early gastric carcinoma (**Fig. 18.15**)
- Advanced gastric carcinoma (Bormann classification)

Lauren classification depending on the histologic subtype
- Intestinal type
- Diffuse or infiltrating gastric adenocarcinoma
- Mixed type

WHO classification (**Box 18.10**)

Classification of Gastric Carcinoma (Box 18.9)

Q. Classify gastric carcinoma.

There are several classifications of carcinoma of the stomach. Classification is done according to depth of invasion, location, and gross and histological subtype (microscopic appearance).

A. Based on Depth of Invasion

Q. Write a short note on early gastric carcinoma.

The important morphological feature that decides the clinical outcome of gastric cancer is the depth of invasion. According to this, gastric cancer can be divided into early gastric cancer and advanced gastric cancer.

1. **Early gastric carcinoma:** It is defined as an invasive **cancer that is limited to the mucosa and submucosa, with or without** perigastric **lymph node metastases.** It is not synonymous with carcinoma in situ (which is confined to the surface epithelial layer). Early gastric cancer is a **pathologic diagnosis** based on the depth of invasion and is associated with a better prognosis. Macroscopically, early gastric carcinomas (type 0) may be subclassified into three main types: 0-I, 0-II, and 0-III **(Fig. 18.15).** Early gastric carcinoma does not refer to the duration of the disease, its size, the presence of symptoms, and the absence of metastases or curability.
2. **Advanced gastric carcinoma**: It is a neoplasm that has **extended below the submucosa into the muscular wall.** All cancers may begin as "early" lesions, which develop into 'advanced' lesions. It is associated with poor prognosis. **Bormann classification** of growth patterns of advanced gastric carcinoma is presented in **Figures 18.16 and 18.17.**

B. Lauren Classification Depending on the Histologic Subtype

According to Lauren classification, gastric adenocarcinomas may be subdivided into **three pathologically defined categories: (1) Intestinal type, (2) diffuse type, and (3) mixed type.** The *diffuse type* is characterized by the absence of cell cohesion so that individual cells infiltrate and thicken the stomach wall without forming a discrete mass.

1. **Intestinal type:** Its gross and microscopic features are as follows:
   - **Gross:** It forms a **polypoid (exophytic) bulky tumor** or may be **ulcerated.** More commonly, they appear in the antrum and have lesser curvature of the stomach. They are often preceded by a prolonged precancerous process, often initiated by *H. pylori* infection.

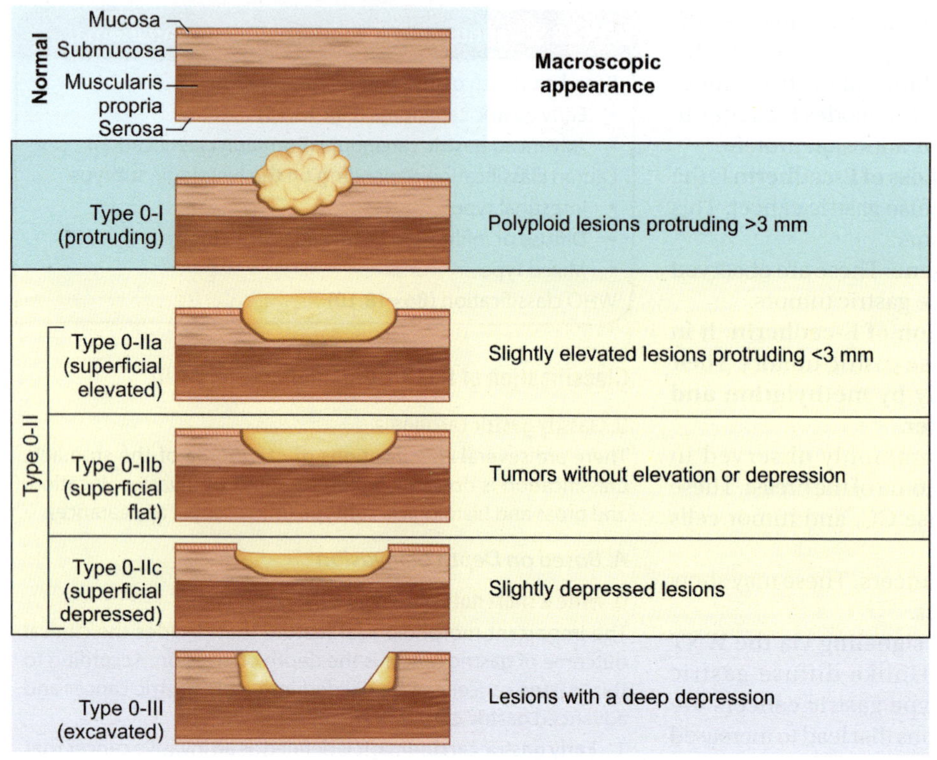

Fig. 18.15: Subclassification of early gastric carcinoma (type 0).

H. pylori
- Humans are the only known hosts
- Histology is the gold standard for its detection
- The special stains include non-silver stains (e.g., Giemsa, Diff Quick, Gimenez, Acridine orange) and silver stains (e.g., Warthin-Starry, Steiner)

Normal
Mucosa
Submucosa
Muscularis propria
Serosa
Type 1 Mass
Type 2 Ulcerative
Type 3 Infiltrative ulcerative
Type 4 Diffuse infiltrative

Gastric carcinoma
- Most important risk factor in intestinal metaplasia
- Antrum is the most common location

Linitis plastica or "leather bottle" appearance of the stomach seen in diffuse or infiltrating gastric adenocarcinoma.

Fig. 18.16: Macroscopic subtypes of advanced gastric cancer. Type 1 (mass): Localized tumor growth with polypoid appearance. It is sharply demarcated from the surrounding mucosa. Type 2 (ulcerative): Localized ulcerated tumor with raised margins. The surrounding wall of the stomach is thickened with clear margins. Type 3 (infiltrative ulcerative): Ulcerated tumors with raised margins. It is surrounded by a thickened gastric wall but without clear margins. Type 4 (diffuse infiltrative): Tumors do not show marked ulceration or raised margins. The gastric wall is thickened and indurated, and the margin is unclear.

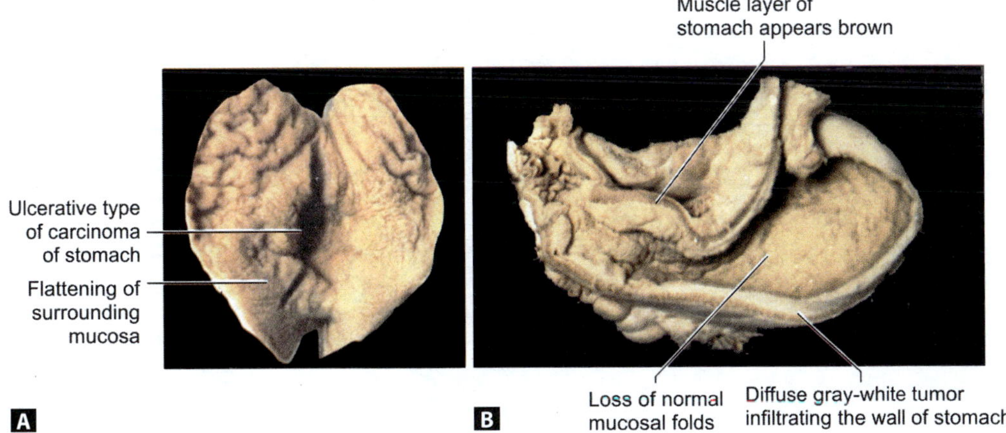

Figs. 18.17A and B: Gastrectomy specimen showing: (A) Infiltrative ulcerative type of carcinoma (Borrmann type 3); (B) Diffuse infiltrative type of carcinoma stomach with leather bottle appearance (Borrmann type 4); (C) Diagrammatic representation of the diffuse infiltrative type of carcinoma stomach.

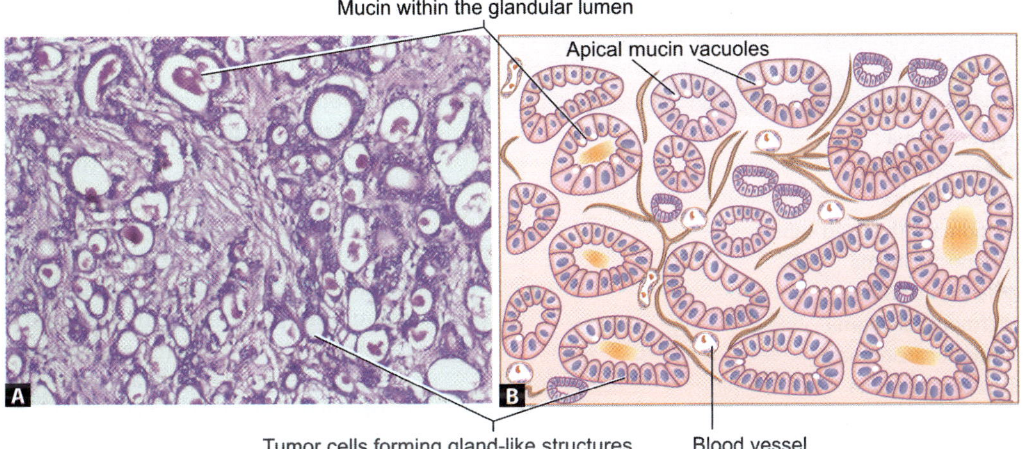

Figs. 18.18A and B: Microscopic appearance of an intestinal type of gastric carcinoma: (A) Photomicrograph; (B) Diagrammatic.

- **Microscopy (Figs. 18.18A and B):** The **term "intestinal" mainly describes the architecture rather than the cell type.** It consists of cohesive tumor cells that **form gland-like tubular structures,** resembling adenocarcinoma of the colon. It probably **arises in areas of intestinal metaplasia.** The tumor cells show **apical mucin vacuoles,** and mucin may be present in the lumen of the glands.

Q. Write a short note on linitis plastica.

2. **Diffuse or infiltrating gastric adenocarcinoma**: They occur more often in younger patients and carry a poorer prognosis. They are **not associated with *H. pylori*.**
   - **Gross:** Diffuse gastric cancer **infiltrates deeply into the stomach without forming obvious mass** lesions. It involves a broad region or entire stomach (throughout the stomach including the cardia) with local rigidity of the wall. They elicit a **desmoplastic reaction that** produces diffuse **flattening of rugal folds** in the mucosa and rigid, widespread **thickening of the wall.** If the entire stomach is involved, it may become nondistensible (loss of distensibility of the stomach wall) and the lumen is narrowed producing a **leather bottle appearance** termed **linitis plastica (Fig. 18.17B).** Currently, it is designated as signet ring (adeno)carcinoma.

Q. Write a short note on the signet ring cell.

Microscopy: It is composed of **discohesive** (cohesion is absent because of loss of E-cadherin) **tumor cells** that **do not form glands.** The tumor cells infiltrate and thicken the stomach wall without forming a discrete mass.

- **Signet-ring cells:** The **tumor cells contain abundant mucin** which expands the cytoplasm and pushes the nucleus to the periphery creating a **signet-ring appearance to the malignant cells (Figs. 18.19A and B).**
- **Signet-ring cell carcinoma:** If the signet-ring cells constitute **more than 50%** of the tumor, it is classified as **signet-ring cell carcinoma.**

C. WHO Classification of Gastric Tumors

It is **based on the histological features** and is presented in **Box 18.10.**

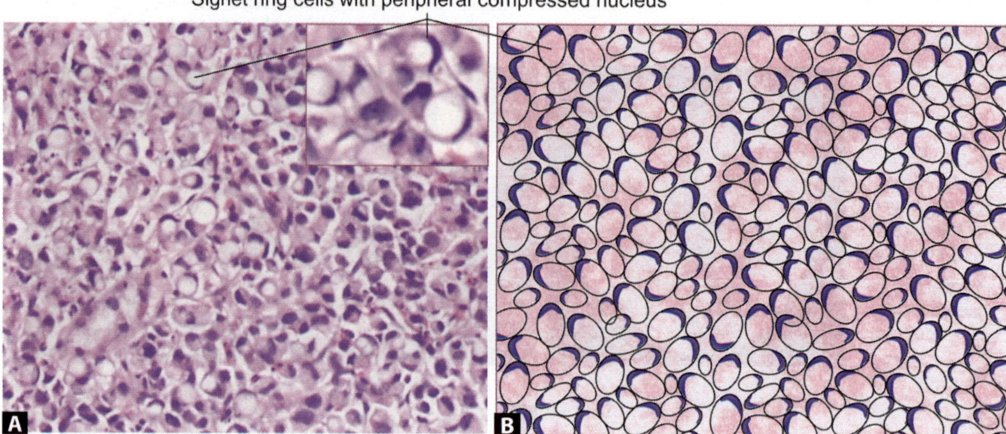

Figs. 18.19A and B: (A) Microscopic appearance of a diffuse type of gastric carcinoma predominantly consisting of signet ring cells (signet ring carcinoma). Inset shows signet ring cells (upper right); (B) Diagrammatic appearance of signet ring carcinoma.

BOX 18.10: World Health Organization (WHO) classification (2019) of malignant epithelial tumors of the stomach.

Gastric adenocarcinoma
- Tubular adenocarcinoma
- Parietal cell carcinoma
- Adenocarcinoma with mixed subtypes
- Papillary adenocarcinoma
- Micropapillary carcinoma
- Mucoepidermoid carcinoma
- Mucinous adenocarcinoma
- Signet-ring cell carcinoma
- Poorly cohesive carcinoma
- Medullary carcinoma with lymphoid stroma
- Hepatoid adenocarcinoma
- Paneth cell carcinoma

Gastric squamous cell carcinoma
Gastric adenosquamous carcinoma
Gastric undifferentiated carcinoma
Gastroblastoma
Gastric neuroendocrine neoplasms

Spread of Carcinoma Stomach

Q. Write a short note on modes of spread of gastric cancer (carcinoma stomach).

- **Local/direct spread:** It spreads into the muscularis and serosa of the stomach. It can invade the duodenum, pancreas, liver, colon, and retroperitoneum.
- **Lymphatic spread:** It spreads via the submucosal and subserosal lymphatics to both regional and distant lymph nodes. The pattern of lymph node involvement depends on the site of the tumor (*refer* **online Table 18.4**).
  - Frequently metastasizes to the **supraclavicular sentinel (Virchow) node** and **may be the first clinical manifestation of an occult neoplasm (Troisier's sign).**
    - Left axillary lymph node—Irish node
  - Metastasize to the **periumbilical lymph nodes**: This forms a subcutaneous nodule called **Sister Mary Joseph nodule** (after the nurse who noted this lesion as a marker of metastatic carcinoma) **(Fig. 18.20).** This nodule represents metastasis from GI tract malignancies (in about 50% of cases) and includes carcinoma of the stomach (most common), colon, and pancreas. Other primary sites include carcinoma of the ovary and uterus. Sister Mary Joseph nodule/node is associated with multiple peritoneal metastases and a prognosis poor.
  - Krukenberg tumor: Metastasis of signet-ring carcinoma to both ovaries. Primary may be in the stomach, breast, pancreas, and gallbladder.
  - Metastasis to the pouch of Douglas (Blumer shelf).
- **Blood spread:** It can spread via the portal vein into the **liver**. Other sites are **lungs** and **bones**.
- **Transperitoneal spread:** Via the transperitoneal route, the tumor may involve any intra-abdominal site (particularly the pelvis). The ovary is the favored site.

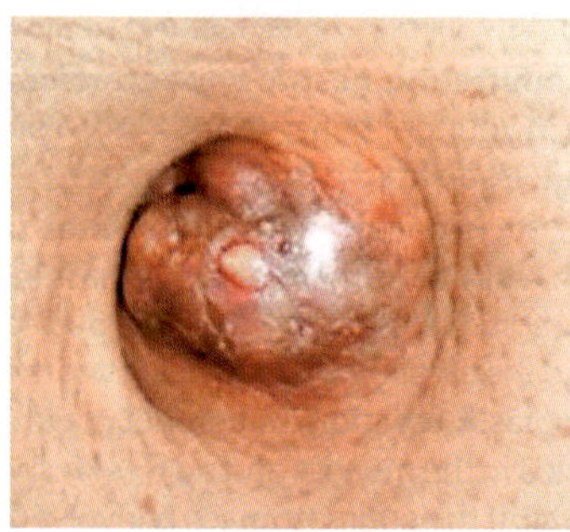

Fig. 18.20: Sister Mary Joseph nodule which represents metastasis to periumbilical lymph node from GI tract cancers.

- **Krukenberg tumor:** It is metastasis of a signet-ring carcinoma to both ovaries and in most cases, the primary tumor originates in the stomach. Other primary sites include the breast, pancreas, and gallbladder. If carcinoma of the stomach penetrates the serosa, peritoneal implants generally flourish. Bilateral massive involvement of the ovary (Krukenberg tumor) in carcinoma of the stomach can result from **either transperitoneal or hematogenous spread.**

Clinical Features

Age and gender: Most patients are usually over 50 years of age (the mean age of presentation is 55 years of age). However, rare cases can occur in younger individuals and even children. The male-to-female ratio is 2:1.

- **Intestinal-type gastric cancer: In high-risk areas, intestinal-type gastric cancer may arise from precursor lesions (e.g., flat dysplasia and adenomas).**
- **Advanced cancer:** It presents with **early satiety, bloating, distension, and vomiting. The tumor frequently bleeds causing iron-deficiency anemia.** Tumor in the pyloric region may present with **gastric outlet obstruction**.
- **Troisier's sign:** Metastatic lymph nodes may be palpable in the left supraclavicular fossa (Virchow's node, Troisier's sign).
- **Trousseau's sign:** Non-metastatic effects may be in the form of **migrating thrombophlebitis** (Trousseau's sign) and **deep venous thrombosis**. These are due to the effects of the tumor on thrombotic and hemostatic mechanisms.

Tumor markers include: (1) carcinoembryonic antigen (CEA), (2) CA-19.9, (3) CA-125, (4) CA72-4, and (5) beta-hCG.

Prognosis: It depends on the **depth of invasion, and the extent of nodal and distant metastasis.**

Q. List the differences between benign and malignant ulcers of the stomach.

Differences between benign and malignant ulcers of the stomach are listed in **Table 18.5**

TABLE 18.5 Differences between benign and malignant ulcers of the stomach.

Characteristics	*Benign ulcer*	*Malignant ulcer*
Age	Usually in younger age	Older age
Duration of symptoms	Weeks to years	Weeks to months
Location/usual site	Lesser curvature of pylorus and antrum	Greater curvature of pylorus and antrum
Gross		
1. Size	Small	Large
2. Shape	Regular	Irregular
3. Surrounding mucosa	Mucosal rugae projects outwards (radiates) from the margins of the ulcer	Mucosal rugae stop far from the ulcer and show flattening
4. Floor of the ulcer	Clean	Necrotic
5. Margins	Overhanging like spokes of a wheel	Heaped up and everted
Acidity	Normal to low	May show achlorhydria

SCENARIO-BASED ESSAY QUESTION

Q. A 55-year-old male laborer presents with early satiety, bloating, distension nausea, vomiting, and midepigastric pain for the last five months. He was treated by a local doctor for peptic ulcer disease without any relief. He has lost significant weight for the last 2 months. On examination, an epigastric mass was found and there was also an enlargement of the left supraclavicular lymph node. An abdominal CT scan showed gastric outlet obstruction. He underwent an upper gastrointestinal endoscopy and was found to have an ulcerated 2 × 4 cm bulky mass in the lesser curvature of the antrum at the pylorus. A biopsy taken from the stomach confirmed the clinical diagnosis. He died within 3 years of diagnosis.

a. **What is the probable diagnosis? (Ans: Carcinoma of the stomach)**
b. **Describe the gross and microscopy of the stomach in this disease** *(refer pages 607-10)*.
c. **How does this disease spread?** *(refer pages 610-1)*.

Q. A 65-year-old female complains of 9 kg weight loss with severe nausea, vomiting, and early satiety over the past 4 months. Upper gastrointestinal endoscopy reveals that the entire gastric mucosa is eroded and has an erythematous and leather bottle appearance. She underwent a total gastrectomy.

a. **What is your diagnosis? (Ans: Diffuse or infiltrating gastric adenocarcinoma). Give reasons for your diagnosis (Ans: clinical features and leather bottle appearance)**
b. **What are the risk factors involved in the disease?** *(refer pages 605-7)*
c. **Describe the gross appearances and microscopy of this lesion** *(refer page 609)*.
d. **Enumerate the classification of tumors of this organ** *(refer pages 607-9)*.
e. **What is Krukenberg tumor?** *(refer pages 611 and 833)*

Gastrointestinal Stromal Tumor

Gastrointestinal stromal tumor (GIST) is the **most common mesenchymal tumor of the abdomen. The most common location** of GIST is the **stomach.**

The cell of origin: The term stromal is a misnomer. This is because GISTs arise from the **interstitial cells of Cajal**, which are located in the muscularis propria. These cells serve as **pacemaker cells** of the gastrointestinal muscularis propria **and involved in gut peristalsis.**

- **Carney triad:** It of (1) gastric GIST, (2) paraganglioma, and (3) pulmonary chondroma.
- **Increased incidence** of GIST in patients with **neurofibromatosis type 1**.

Pathogenesis

Gastrointestinal Stromal Tumors with Mutated *KIT* or *PDGFRA*

- **Gain-of-function mutation in the gene encoding the receptor tyrosine kinase KIT**(C-kit/c-KIT)**: Tyrosine kinase KIT** is a receptor for stem cell factor. **About 80%** of all GISTs have this oncogenic, gain-of-function **mutations of the gene encoding this receptor.**
- **Other mutations:** About 8% of GISTs have mutations that activate a related tyrosine kinase, platelet-derived growth factor receptor A (PDGFRA).

KIT and *PDGFRA* gene mutations cause **constitutive activation** of **KIT or PDGFRA receptor tyrosine kinases.** They produce intracellular signals that activate the same downstream signaling (RAS and PI3K/AKT) pathways and **promote tumor cell proliferation and survival.**

Gastrointestinal Stromal Tumors without Mutated *KIT* or *PDGFRA*

- **Mutations in genes encoding components of the mitochondrial succinate dehydrogenase (SDH):** These mutations are observed rarely in GISTs without *KIT* or *PDGFRA* mutations.
- **DOG1 (Discovered on GIST-1):** More recently, DOG1 is described as an immunohistochemical marker for GIST. It has both high sensitivity and specificity for GIST.

MORPHOLOGY

Gross (Fig. 18.21A)

Size varies and may be quite large (up to 30 cm in diameter). Usually solitary, well-circumscribed, fleshy mass covered by intact or ulcerated mucosa, but can also project outward toward the serosa.

Microscopy (Fig. 18.21B)

Consists of thin elongated **spindle cells or** epithelial-appearing **(epithelioid)** cells **or mixtures** of these two types of cells.

Diagnostic markers: GISTs and Cajal cells express **KIT** (also known as **CD117**) and CD34. The most **useful diagnostic marker is KIT (Fig. 18.21C)**, and immunohistochemically detected in 95% of gastric GISTs.

Clinical Features

- **Age and gender**: The peak age for GIST in the stomach is about 60 years. It is slightly more common in males. Nonhereditary syndrome is seen in young females.
- Symptoms may be due to mass effects. Mucosal ulceration can cause blood loss.
- **Investigations**: Best diagnosed with CT scan and PET scan.

Prognosis: It correlates with:

- **Tumor size**: Recurrence or metastasis is rare when size **is less than 5 cm.**
- **Mitotic index: Mitotically active** tumors **larger than 10 cm commonly metastasize or recur.**
- **Location**: **Gastric** GISTs are **less aggressive** than those of the small intestine.

INTESTINE

Meckel Diverticulum

Q. Write a short note on Meckel diverticulum.

Meckel diverticulum is the most common type of true diverticula of the GI tract and occurs in the ileum.

Rule of 2s: It is used to remember characteristics of Meckel diverticulae.

- Occur in about **2%** of the **population.**
- Generally present within **2 feet (60 cm)** of the **ileocecal valve.**
- Approximately **2 inches long** (varies from 2 to 15 cm).

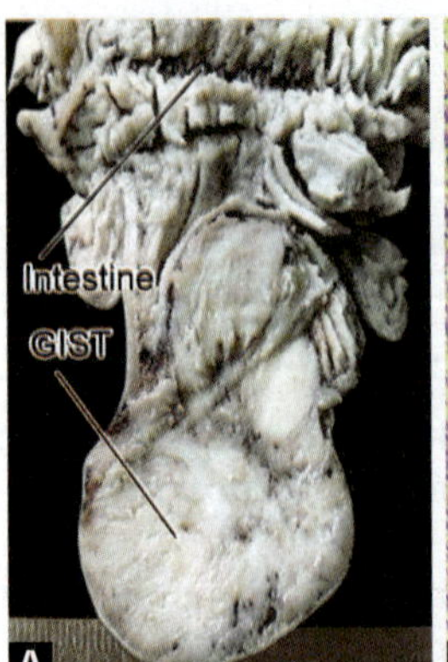

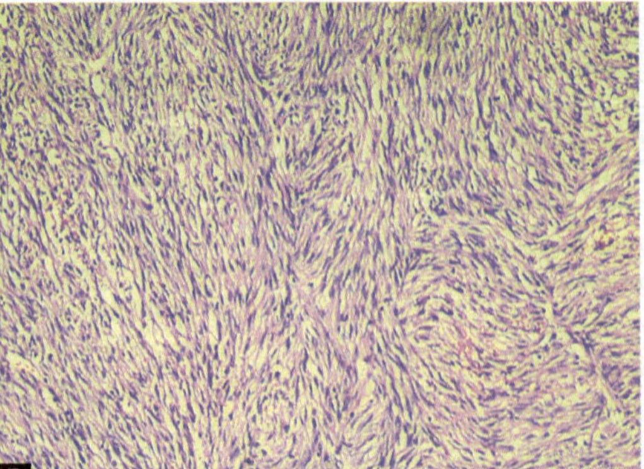

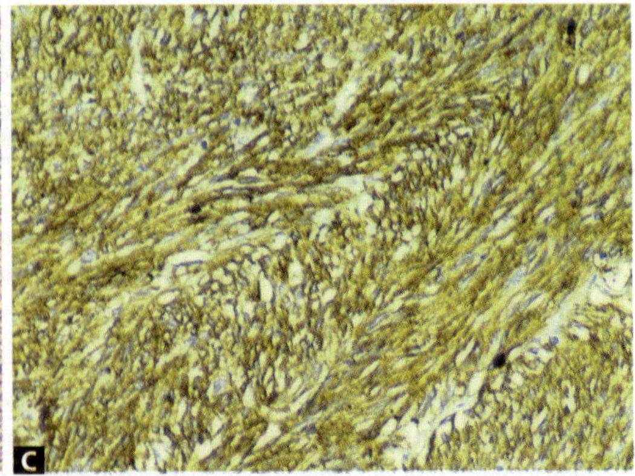

Figs. 18.21A to C: Gastrointestinal stromal tumor: (A) Intestine with GIST; (B) GIST showing bundles and fascicles of spindle-shaped tumor cells; (C) Tumor cells showing KIT (CD117) positivity.

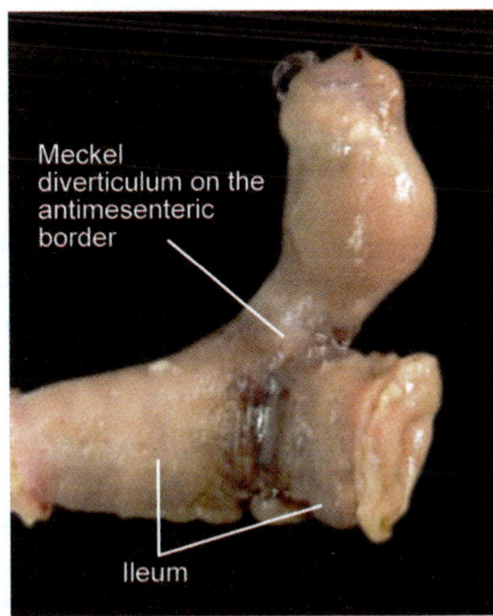

Fig. 18.22: Meckel diverticulum on the antimesenteric border.

- **Two times more common in males** than in females.
- Most often **symptomatic** by age **2**.

MORPHOLOGY

Single and always lies on the **antimesenteric** side of the bowel (**Fig. 18.22**). It is a true diverticulum and its wall consists of mucosa, submucosa, and muscularis propria and has its own blood supply. **Mucosal lining of Meckel diverticula:** The lining of **epithelium resembles** that of **normal small intestine**, but **ectopic pancreatic or gastric tissue is common. Heterotopic gastric mucosa** may lead to **peptic ulceration** of adjacent small intestinal mucosa and present with **bleeding, or perforation.**

Clinical features: Most Meckel diverticula are asymptomatic. Its symptoms may mimic acute appendicitis. The complications are as follows:

- **Severe hemorrhage:** Bleeding is the most common complication. It develops if the diverticulum contains acid-secreting gastric epithelium with peptic ulceration and presents with maroon-colored painless bleeding per rectum.
- **Meckel's diverticulitis:** Develops secondary to peptic ulcerations or obstruction of the orifice of the diverticula and symptoms appear similar to acute appendicitis.
- **Intestinal obstruction:** Results from intussusception, volvulus, adhesions, or the presence of a tumor or ectopic tissue or enteroliths.

Typhoid Fever

Q. Enumerate the different ulcerative lesions of the intestine.

Ulcerative lesions of small intestine: These include (1) tuberculosis, (2) typhoid, (3) Crohn disease, and (4) peptic ulcer.

Typhoid fever (enteric) is an **acute systemic disease** caused by infection with *Salmonella typhi*. Paratyphoid fever is a clinically similar but milder disease caused by *Salmonella paratyphi*. **Enteric fever** is the general term, which includes **both typhoid and para-typhoid** fever.

Etiology

Causative agent: Enteric fevers are caused by ***Salmonella typhi* and *Salmonella paratyphi*.** *Salmonella* are gram-negative, motile bacilli (rods). Boiling or chlorination of water and pasteurization of milk destroys the bacilli.

Source of infection: Humans are the only natural reservoir and include:

- **Patients suffering from disease:** Infected urine, feces, or other secretions from patients.
- **Chronic carriers of typhoid fever:** *S. typhi* or *S. paratyphi* **colonizes in the gallbladder** or biliary tree and may be associated with gallstones and the chronic carrier state.

Mode of transmission: From **person-to-person contact.**

- **Ingestion** of **contaminated food** (especially dairy products) and shellfish or **contaminated water**.
- **Direct spread:** Rare by **finger-to-mouth contact** with feces, urine, or other secretions.

Incubation period: Usually 7–14 days.

Pathogenesis (Fig. 18.23)

Q. Write a short note on the pathogenesis of typhoid fever.

- The typhoid bacilli (*Salmonella*) are **ingested through contaminated food or water**. They can **survive in gastric acid of the stomach** and reach the mucosa of the small intestine.
- **Events during the incubation period**:
  - During the initial asymptomatic period (about 2 weeks), the *Salmonella* **attach to the microvilli.** They penetrate the **ileal mucosa** of the small intestine and reach lamina propria and submucosa.
  - *Salmonella* is **phagocytosed by the macrophages** (mononuclear phagocytes) present in the lymphoid tissue and **Peyer's patches** in the submucosa of the small intestine.
  - *Salmonella* **multiply within the macrophages** and are **carried to the mesenteric lymph node** via lymphatics. They multiply in the lymph nodes and **via the thoracic duct** enter the **bloodstream** causing **transient bacteremia.**
- **During bacteremia**, the bacilli are **seeded in many organs.** They colonize reticuloendothelial tissues (**liver, gallbladder, spleen, bone marrow**), where bacilli multiply further causing **massive bacteremia** (occurs towards the end of the incubation period) and disease clinically manifests.
- **Bile is a good culture medium for the typhoid bacillus**, and bacilli **multiply in the gallbladder** bacilli are continuously shed through the bile into the intestine.

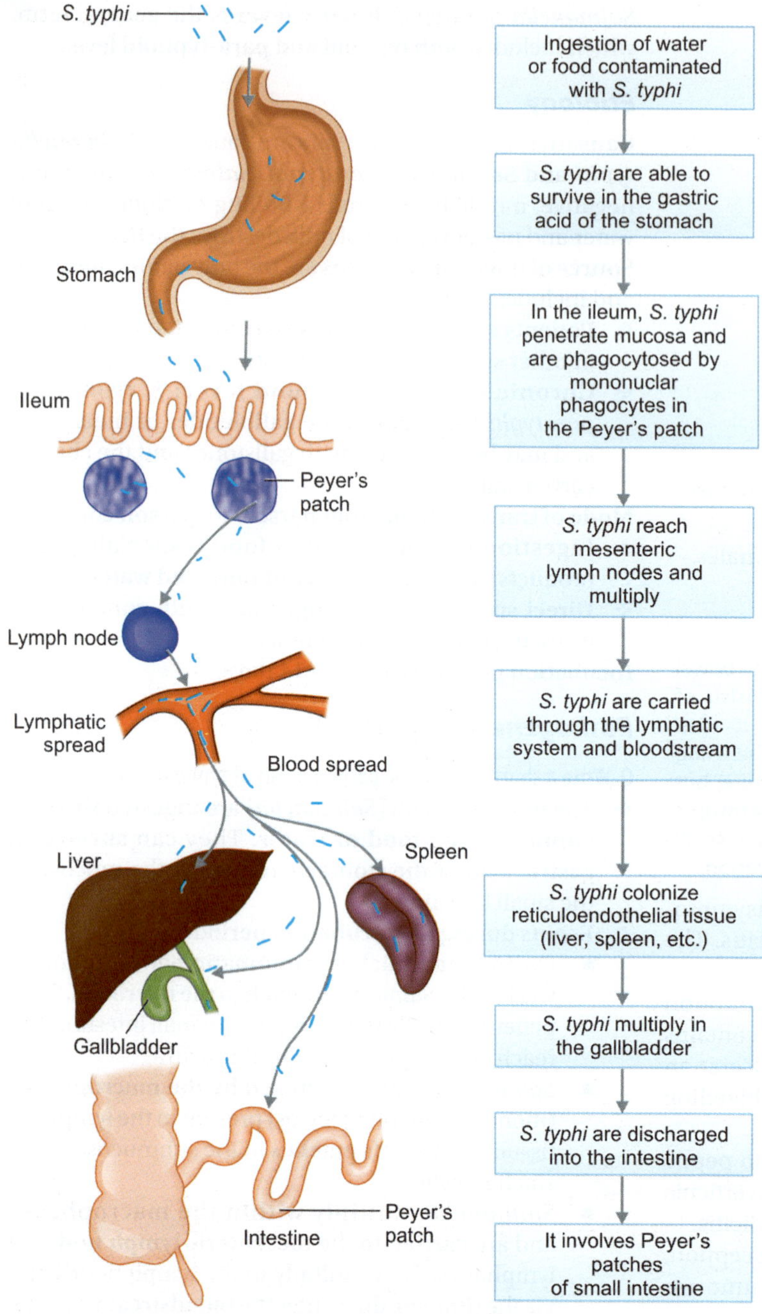

Fig. 18.23: Pathogenesis of typhoid fever.

- In the intestine, the bacilli are localized to the **Peyer's patches and lymphoid follicles** of the terminal ileum. They cause inflammation, plateau-like elevations of Peyer's patches, and necrosis, which results in characteristic **oval typhoid ulcers.**

MORPHOLOGY

Q. Morphology of intestine in typhoid fever.

Lesions may be (1) intestinal and (2) extraintestinal.

Intestinal Lesions

Gross (Fig. 18.24)

Q. Write a short note on the pathology of ileum in typhoid fever.

- **Location:** Most commonly, lesions occur in the **terminal ileum**, but may be seen in the jejunum and colon.
- **Appearance**: Peyer's patches in the terminal ileum enlarge into sharply delineated, plateau-like elevations. Ulceration and necrosis of mucosa over Peyer's patches mucosa produce typhoid ulcers.
- **Characteristics of typhoid ulcer:**
  - **Number: Varies.**
  - **Orientation: The ulcers are oval and oriented along** (parallel to) **the long axis of the bowel** (tuberculous ulcers of the small intestine are transverse).
  - **Base of the ulcer:** It is **black** due to sloughed mucosa.
  - **Margins: Slightly raised** due to inflammatory edema and cellular proliferation.
  - **No fibrosis:** Hence, narrowing of the intestinal lumen seldom occurs in healed typhoid lesions.

Microscopy

- **Mucosa: Oval ulcers** over the Peyer's patches.
- **Lamina propria:**
  - **Macrophages** containing bacteria, red blood cells (erythrophagocytosis is a characteristic feature of typhoid) and nuclear debris
  - **Lymphocytes and plasma cells**
  - **Neutrophils** within the superficial lamina propria.

Extraintestinal Lesions

- **Typhoid nodules:** Systemic dissemination of the bacilli leads to the **formation of focal granulomas** termed **typhoid nodules.** These nodules are composed of **aggregates of macrophages** (typhoid cells) containing ingested bacilli, red blood cells, and lymphocytes. They are **common in the lymph node, liver, bone marrow, and spleen.**
- **Mesenteric lymph nodes**: They are enlarged due to the accumulation of macrophages, which contains typhoid bacilli.
- **Liver:** It shows small, scattered foci of hepatocyte necrosis replaced by **typhoid nodules.**
- **Spleen:** It is enlarged and soft.
- **Abdominal muscles**: Zenker's degeneration (severe glassy or waxy hyaline degeneration or necrosis of skeletal muscles).
- **Gallbladder: Typhoid cholecystitis.** Gallbladder colonization with *S. typhi* or *S. paratyphi* may be associated with chronic carrier state.

Clinical Features

- Onset is gradual and patients present with anorexia, abdominal pain, bloating, nausea, vomiting, and diarrhea.

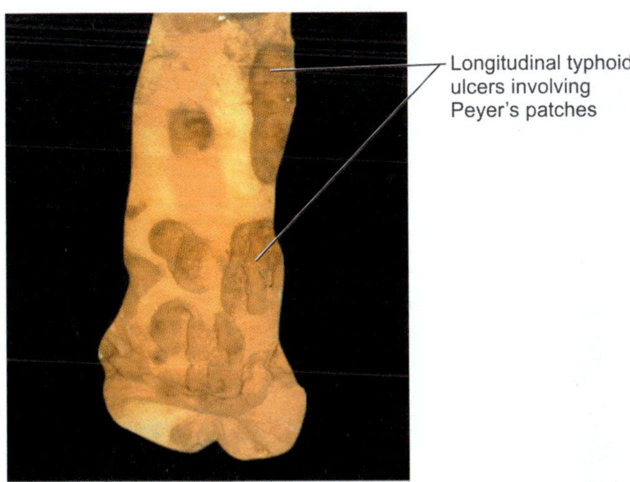

Fig. 18.24: Gross appearance of typhoid ulcers in the ileum of small intestine.

- **Fever: Continuous temperature rise** (step-ladder fever).
- **Rose spots:** These are small erythematous maculo-papular lesions on the skin that fade on pressure, appear on the chest and abdomen, and occur during the second or third week.
- **Spleen:** It is soft and palpable and may be accompanied by hepatomegaly.

Complications

1. **Intestinal complications:** It can be fatal. They can occur during the third week.
   - **Perforations of ulcer:** Typhoid fever is the most common cause of ileal perforation in tropical countries, e.g., India.
   - **Hemorrhage from the ulcer.**
2. **Extraintestinal complications**: **Encephalopathy, meningitis, seizures, endocarditis, myocarditis, pneumonia, and cholecystitis. Sickle cell disease** patients are **susceptible to *Salmonella* osteomyelitis**
3. **Carrier state:** Persistence of bacilli in the **gallbladder or urinary tract** may result in the passage of bacilli in the feces or urine causes a **'carrier state'** and is a source of infection to others.

Laboratory Diagnosis

Investigations in enteric fever: (1) blood culture; (2) stool culture; (3) urine culture; (4) widal test, and (5) total WBC count.

Isolation of bacilli

- **Blood culture:** It is positive in the **first week** of fever in 90% of patients and remains positive in the second week till the fever subsides. Blood culture rapidly becomes negative on treatment with antibiotics.
- **Stool cultures:** It is almost as valuable as blood culture and becomes positive in the **second and third** weeks.
- **Urine culture**: It reveals the organism in approximately 25% of patients by the **third week**.

Other tests

- **Widal reaction:** Classic Widal test **measures antibodies against O and H antigens** of *S. typhi*, but **lacks sensitivity and specificity**. The widal test (immunological reactions) becomes positive from the end of the first week till the fourth week. There are many false-positive and occasional false-negative Widal reactions.
- **Other serologic tests**: They are available for the rapid diagnosis of typhoid fever with a higher sensitivity.
- **Total leukocyte count**: It shows **leukopenia with relative lymphocytosis**. Eosinophils are usually absent. Absolute lymphocytosis is NOT seen in enteric fever.

Intestinal Tuberculosis

PA 24.5 (NC): Describe and etiology and pathogenesis and pathologic features of tuberculosis of the intestine.

Q. Write a short note on intestinal tuberculosis.

Forms of intestinal tuberculosis: There are three main forms, namely: Primary, secondary, and hyperplastic cecal tuberculosis.

Primary Intestinal Tuberculosis

It is uncommon in developed countries, but **common in developing countries** including India.

Mode of infection: In the pre-pasteurization era, ingestion of cow's unpasteurized milk infected with ***Mycobacterium bovis.*** Nowadays due to the eradication of tuberculosis in cattle and pasteurization of milk, all intestinal tuberculosis is caused by ***Mycobacterium hominis.***

MORPHOLOGY

Predominant changes are in the **regional mesenteric lymph nodes without any significant intestinal lesions.**

Gross: Lymph nodes are enlarged, matted, and caseous (tabes mesenteric). They may heal by fibrosis and calcification.

Microscopy: The primary complex shows a focus on the intestinal mucosa and mesenteric lymph nodes show typical **tuberculous granuloma** with caseation necrosis **(Fig. 18.25C).**

Secondary Intestinal Tuberculosis

Mode of infection: Swallowing of sputum in patients with active pulmonary tuberculosis. The lesions are most **common in the terminal ileum.**

MORPHOLOGY

Gross (Figs. 18.25A and B)

- **Lesions of the intestine are more prominent than** those of **regional lymph nodes.**

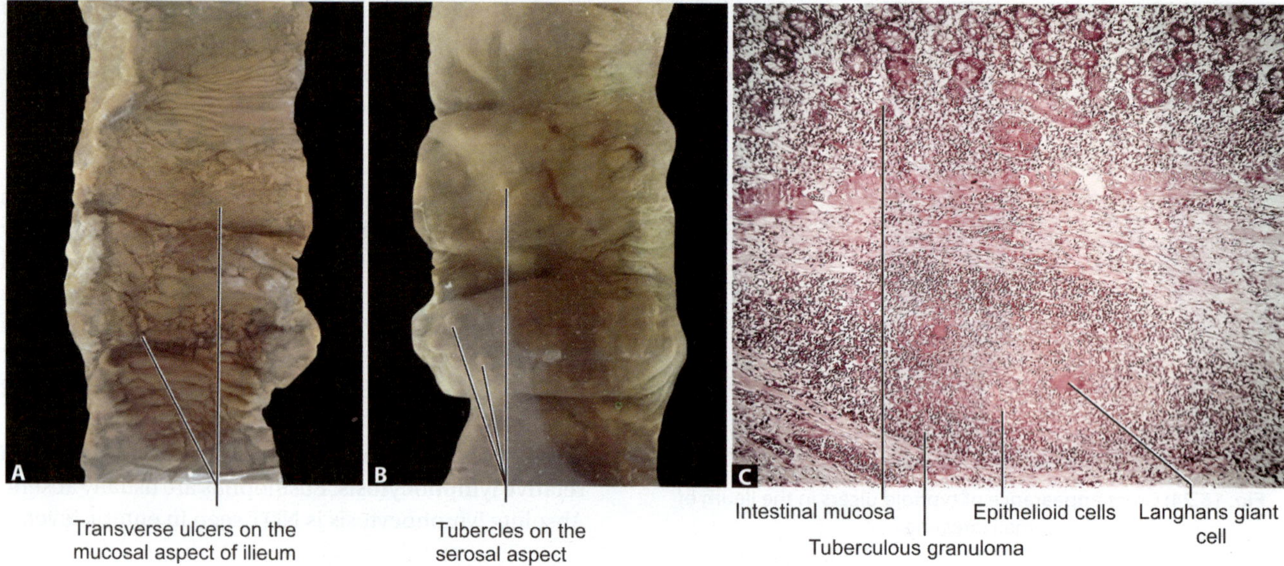

Figs. 18.25A to C: Ileum with a tuberculous ulcer on the mucosal aspect: (A) Specimen; (B) Serosal aspect shows tubercles; (C) Microscopy of tuberculosis of intestine.

- **Large ulcers** that are **transverse to the long axis of the bowel.** The surface of ulcers may be coated with caseous material. **The serosal surface may show visible tubercles (Fig. 18.25B).**
- **Healed lesions** may show transverse **fibrous strictures** and intestinal obstruction.

Microscopy

Mucosa and submucosa show ulceration and typical granulomas of tuberculosis (Fig. 18.25C). The muscularis propria may show a variable degree of fibrosis.

Hyperplastic Cecal Tuberculosis

It is a variant of secondary tuberculosis.

MORPHOLOGY

Gross: Lesions are seen mainly in the **cecum and/or ascending colon.** It produces **thickening of the wall and mucosal ulceration. Clinically**, the lesion presents as a palpable mass and may be **mistaken for carcinoma.**

Microscopy (Fig. 18.25C): It shows **caseating tubercles** and should be **distinguished from Crohn disease in which granulomas are non-caseating.**

Differences between typhoid and tuberculous ulcers are listed in **Table 18.6**.

Q. List the differences between tuberculous and typhoid ulcers of the intestine.

Shigellosis-Bacillary Dysentery

Q. Enumerate the different ulcerative lesions of the large intestine.

Ulcerative lesions of the large intestine: These are bacillary ulcers, amebic ulcers, ulcerative colitis, and Crohn disease Bacillary dysentery is **a necrotizing infection** of the **distal small bowel and colon** caused by ***Shigella.***

Etiology

- *Shigella* causes bacillary dysentery and is one of the **most common causes of bloody diarrhea.**
- *Shigella* is an unencapsulated, nonmotile, facultative anaerobic gram-negative bacilli. They belong to the Enterobacteriaceae and are closely related to *enteroinvasive E. coli.*
- *Shigella* species that cause colitis are classified into four major subgroups, namely, *S. dysenteriae* (most virulent), *S. flexneri*, *S. boydii*, and *S. sonnei.*

Source of infection: Humans are the only natural reservoir.

Mode of transmission: By **ingestion** through fecal–oral route or via fecally contaminated water and food. It can be acquired by oral contact with any contaminated surface (e.g., clothing, towels, or skin surfaces).

Incubation period: It ranges from **1 to 3 days.**

Pathogenesis

- *Shigella* is the **most virulent** enteropathogen that produces a toxin that has cytotoxic, neurotoxic, and enterotoxic effects. Ingestion of a few (10–100 organisms) produces disease.
- After ingestion, *Shigella* reaches the stomach. They are **resistant to the action of acid in the stomach**. Small intestinal infections do not occur unless the patient has a disturbance in the motility of the intestine.
- **In the colon**, the bacteria penetrate the intestinal mucous epithelium and are **taken up by M or microfold epithelial cells.** They proliferate inside the cytoplasm of these epithelial cells. These bacteria then penetrate the lamina propria and are phagocytosed by macrophages. *Shigella* induces apoptosis of macrophages and causes

TABLE 18.6 Differences between typhoid and tuberculous ulcers.

Characteristics	*Typhoid ulcer*	*Tuberculous ulcer*
Site	The small intestine involves Peyer's patches	Anywhere in the intestine but common is in the terminal ileum and ileocecal region. The involved segment becomes thickened and serosal aspects show tubercles
Orientation	**Longitudinal** to the long axis, because it involves Peyer's patch	**Transverse** to the long axis, because it spreads through lymphatics, which are arranged circumferentially
Microscopy	Macrophages and lymphocytes and plasma cells	Granulomas are composed of a central area of caseous necrosis, surrounded by epithelioid cells, Langhans giant cells, and lymphocytes
Differential count	Neutropenia	Lymphocytosis
Intestinal complications		
Perforation	Common as it is an acute process associated with thinning of the bowel wall	Not seen, because chronic inflammation results in healing by fibrosis
Hemorrhage	Common	Does not occur
Obstruction	Not seen	Stricture formation leads to obstruction
Extraintestinal	May develop carrier state	May develop tuberculous peritonitis

inflammatory reactions. This loosens the intercellular barriers and damages surface epithelium leading to superficial ulcers. This allows entry of *Shigella* in the intestinal lumen to the colonocyte basolateral membrane.

- *Shigella* **produces a toxin** that has cytotoxic, neurotoxic, and enterotoxic effects. When inflammation is severe, ileus, toxic megacolon, gross hemorrhage, and perforation may develop.

MORPHOLOGY

Gross (Fig. 18.26)

- **Site of lesions:** Most prominent in the **left colon** mainly in the **rectosigmoid area.** Mostly, the **lesions are continuous and diffuse.**
- **Characteristics of ulcer:** Mucosa shows **edema, and ulceration** and appears **friable granular, and hemorrhagic.** In severe infections, a gray mucopurulent exudate covers the mucosa. **Ulcers** appear first on the edges of mucosal folds, **perpendicular to the long axis of the colon.**

Microscopy

Changes are predominant in the **mucosa.**

- **Early-stage:** It shows erosions and **small aphthous ulcers** (microulcers), with **infiltration by neutrophils** below the microulcers.
- **Advanced stage**
  - **Necrosis of epithelial cells** and the damaged **mucosa is covered by purulent exudate** (composed of detached epithelial cells, neutrophils, and red blood cells).
  - **Ulcers:** They are **superficial, or may extend down to the muscularis mucosae.** May show superficial crypt abscess, edema, and mild plasma cell infiltrates.

Clinical features: It presents as diarrhea, fever, and abdominal pain. The initial watery diarrhea progresses to a dysenteric phase. Bacillary dysentery is the most common cause of bloody diarrhea. A stool culture is required for confirmation of *Shigella* infection.

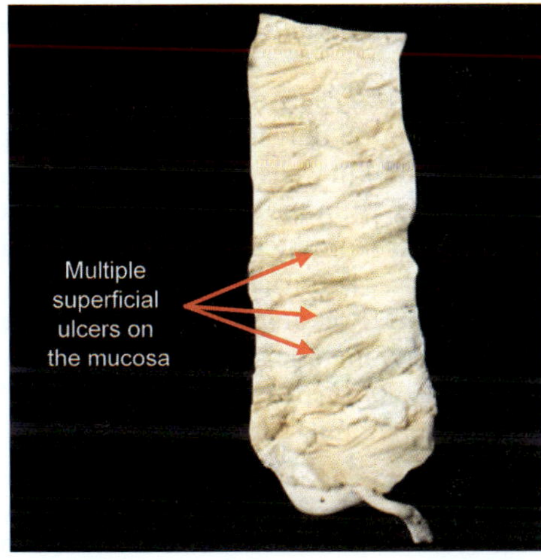

Fig. 18.26: Bacillary dysentery. Specimen of cecum and ascending colon (with appendix). The mucosa shows multiple superficial ulcerations with intervening normal mucosa.

Complications: They are **uncommon.** These are as follows:

- **Reiter syndrome:** A triad of **sterile arthritis, urethritis, and conjunctivitis.**
- **Hemolytic-uremic syndrome (HUS):** It is **due to toxins** secreted by *Shigella* organisms.

Amebiasis

Q. Write a short note on the amebic ulcer of the intestine.

Amebiasis is an **infection caused by the protozoan *Entamoeba histolytica*** (named so because of its lytic actions on involved tissue).

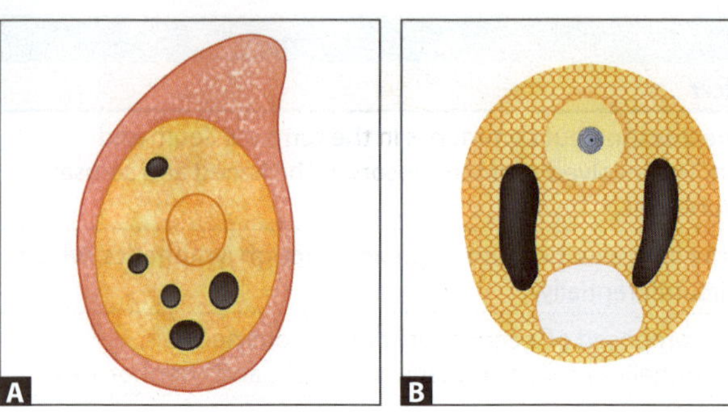

Figs. 18.27A and B: (A) Trophozoite; (B) Cyst of *E. histolytica*.

Etiology

E. histolytica has three distinct stages:

1. **Trophozoite stage (Fig. 18.27A):** Amebic trophozoites are spherical or oval. They are seen in the stools of patients with acute symptoms. The cytoplasm of the trophozoites stain positively by PAS.
2. **Precyst stage**: In the colon, the trophozoite develops into a cyst through an intermediate form termed the precyst.
3. **Cyst stage (Fig. 18.27B): Amebic cysts are the infecting stage** and are found only in stools. They are spherical and have thick chitin walls and usually four nuclei.

Source of infection: Humans are the only known reservoir for *E. histolytica*. It is reproduced in the colon of an infected individual and passes in the feces.

Mode of infection: It is **acquired by fecal-oral route** through ingestion of materials contaminated with human feces containing *E. histolytica*.

Incubation period: About 8–10 days.

Pathogenesis

The amebic cysts are passed in the stool and the **cysts can contaminate water, food, or fingers.**

- On ingestion, *E. histolytica* cysts traverse the stomach. They are **resistant to the action of gastric acid** and they pass to the colon.
- **Amebic cysts then colonize the epithelial surface of the colon and release trophozoites**. Each cyst containing four nuclei divides to form four small, immature trophozoites which then mature to full size. In the colon, they feed on bacteria and human cells. They may colonize any part of the large intestine, but **most frequently in the cecum and ascending colon causing amebic colitis**. These patients pass both cysts and trophozoites in the stool.
- **Trophozoite attaches the colonic epithelial cell** and **invades crypts, and burrows laterally into the lamina propria**. The trophozoite kills the intestinal cell by producing a lytic protein that damages the cell membrane and creates a superficial ulcer. Recruitment of neutrophils causes tissue damage and creates a **flask-shaped ulcer** with a narrow neck and broad base.
- **Trophozoite may penetrate blood vessels and reach the liver** to produce **abscesses** in about 40% of patients with amebic dysentery.

MORPHOLOGY

Q. Write a short note on gross and microscopy of amebic ulcer intestine.

E. histolytica can produce intestinal or extraintestinal disease.

- **Intestinal disease:** It mainly involves the **colon** (mainly cecum and ascending colon) and ranges from **asymptomatic colonization to severe invasive infections** causing bloody dysentery.
- **Extraintestinal disease:** It can produce **amebic liver abscesses.**

Colon

- Amebic lesions start as small **foci of necrosis,** which progress to **ulcers.** The ulcer floor is **gray and necrotic.** Chronic **amebic ulcers** are described as **flask-shaped ulcers** with a narrow/ bottle neck and broad base resembling a **flask (Figs. 18.28A and B).** Trophozoite invades crypts and burrows laterally in the lamina propria to produce a flask-shaped ulcer.
- Trophozoites can be detected on the surface of the ulcer and in the exudate. The ulcers show infiltration by acute and chronic inflammatory cells. PAS stain shows trophozoites of ameba in the exudate **(Fig. 18.28C).**
- **Ameboma:** It is a **rare complication** of amebiasis. The intestinal wall shows thickening due to inflammation (napkin-ring constriction) and may **resemble colon cancer.** Microscopically, **it consists of granulation tissue, inflammatory cells, fibrosis, and clusters of trophozoites.**

Clinical features of intestinal amebiasis: It may be asymptomatic or produce dysentery of varying severity. The incubation period for acute amebic colitis is about 8–10 days. Amebic dysentery may present with **abdominal pain, bloody diarrhea, or weight loss.** Liquid stools (up to 25 a day) contain blood and mucus.

An Amebic Liver Abscess (Fig. 18.29 and refer page 682 and Fig. 19.30)

Q. Write a short note on complications of amebic ulcer of the intestine.

It is a **major complication of intestinal amebiasis.**

- *E. histolytica* trophozoites **from the colon** may reach the liver **through the portal circulation.**
- **Trophozoites kill hepatocytes** and produce **abscess.**
- Abscess cavity is filled with a dark brown, odorless, semisolid necrotic material, which resembles **anchovy paste (sauce) in color and consistency.** The size of an amebic liver abscess may vary and can exceed 10 cm in diameter.
- **Spread of amebic liver abscess:**
  - **Local spread**: It may expand and rupture through the capsule of the liver and may directly **spread into the peritoneum, diaphragm, pleural cavity, lungs, or pericardium.**
  - **Hematogenous spread**: Rare and may spread to the **brain** and kidneys to produce necrotic lesions.

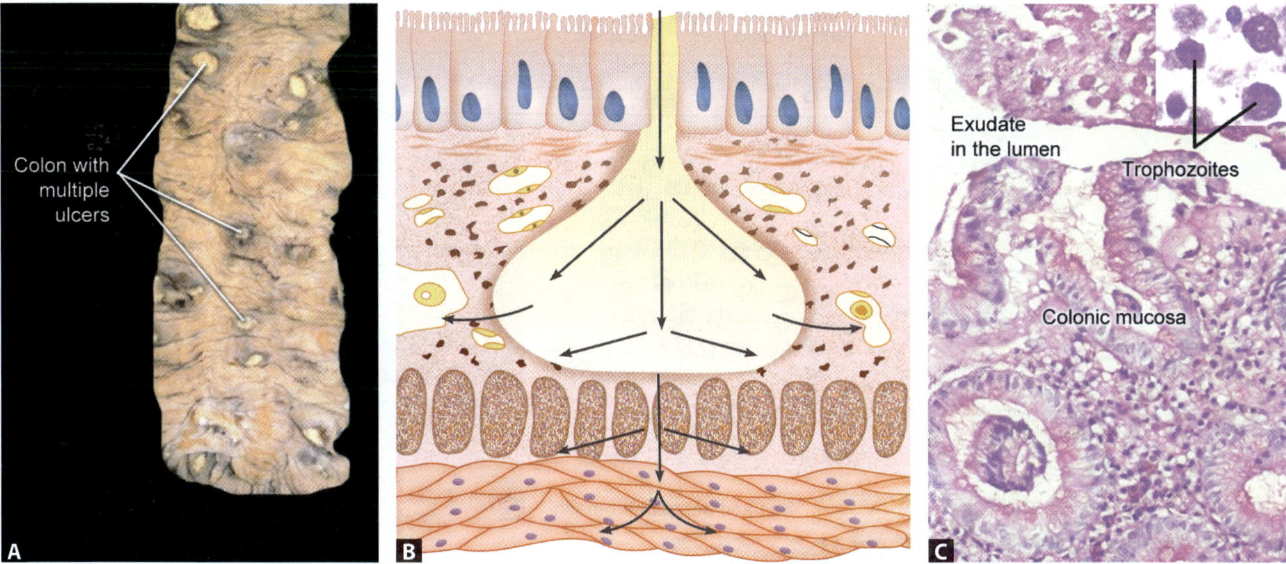

Figs. 18.28A to C: (A) Gross appearance of multiple amebic ulcers in the colon; (B) Microscopically appear as flask-shaped amebic ulcer (diagrammatic); (C) Microscopic appearance of amebic ulcer (PAS stain) shows PAS-stained trophozoites of ameba in the exudate (inset).

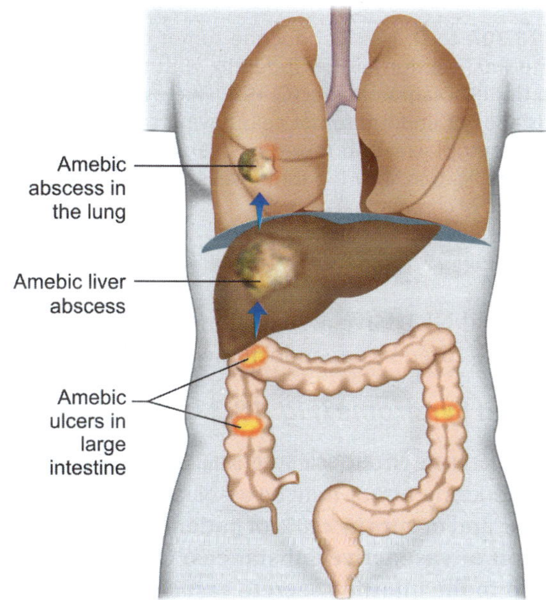

Fig. 18.29: Complications of amebiasis (diagrammatic).

Clinical features of amebic liver abscess: It may present with severe right upper quadrant pain, low-grade fever, and weight loss. The diagnosis is usually made by radiologic or ultrasound demonstration of the abscess, in conjunction with serologic testing for antibodies to *E. histolytica*.

Neuroendocrine (Carcinoid) Tumor

Q. Write a short note on neuroendocrine (carcinoid) tumor.

Neuroendocrine tumors (NET) were originally termed carcinoid, or "carcinoma-like," because these tumors are slowly growing and thought to be more indolent clinical course than GI carcinomas. Current WHO classification refers these tumors as low- or intermediate-grade neuroendocrine tumors. High-grade neuroendocrine tumors are termed as *neuroendocrine carcinoma*. They resemble small cell carcinoma of the lung.

Origin: Carcinoid tumors **arise from neuroendocrine cells. These cells are located in many organs** (e.g., endocrine pancreas and the GIT).

Common sites of neuroendocrine tumors: These include:

- Gastrointestinal (**GI**) **tract**: It is the major site.
  - **Small intestine** (more than 40%) mostly in the appendix.
  - **Stomach**: Gastric carcinoids may be associated with endocrine cell hyperplasia, chronic atrophic gastritis, and Zollinger-Ellison syndrome.
  - **Colon-rectum** (preferential site)
- **Tracheobronchial tree and lungs** (*refer* page 581): They are the next most involved sites.

MORPHOLOGY (FIGS. 18.30A TO D)

Gross

- Neuroendocrine tumors are **intramural or submucosal masses.** They usually present as a small polypoid lesion. Mucosa covering the tumor may be intact or ulcerated
- **Yellow or tan color**
- **Very firm in consistency** due to intense desmoplastic reaction
- May invade the wall deeply to involve the mesentery.

Microscopy

Patterns: It may classically show **solid islet (islands) structure** (composed of islets and nests), **trabecular structure** (composed of anastomosing trabeculae and ribbons) **glandular structure**

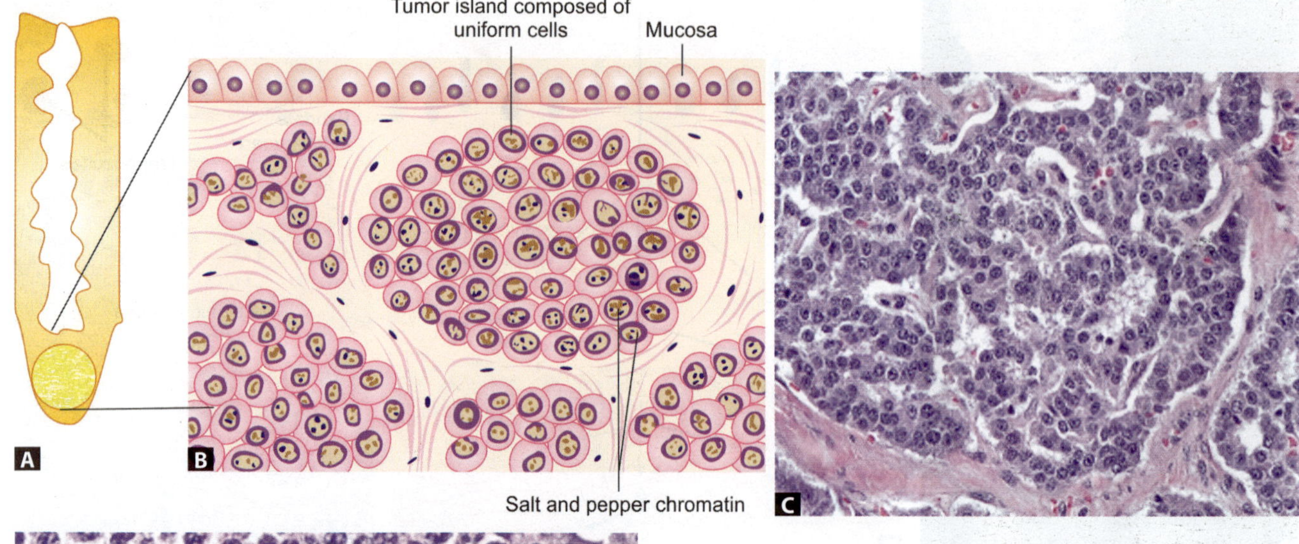

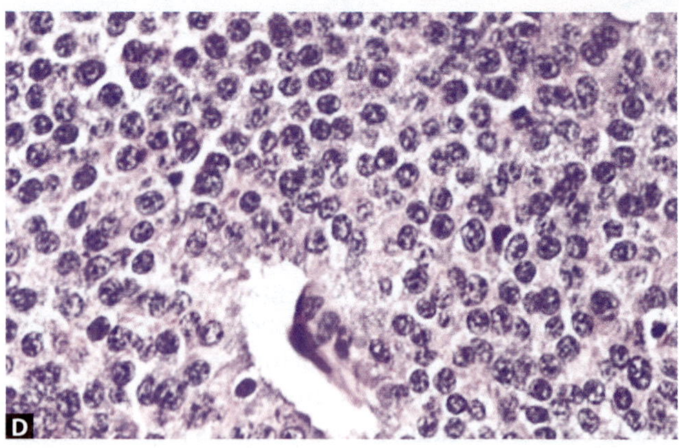

Figs. 18.30A to D: Neuroendocrine tumor of appendix: (A) Longitudinal section of the appendix with carcinoid tumor at the tip; (B) Diagrammatic; (C) H&E: Microscopically shows solid islands of uniform tumor cells having scant, pink, finely granular cytoplasm, and round to oval stippled nuclei; (D) High magnification showing tumor cells with salt and pepper appearance of chromatin.

(consisting of tubules, acini, and rosette-like structures), **strands or sheets** of tumor cells.

Tumor cells: The cellular characteristics are as follows:

- **Uniform cells of medium size:** NET is composed of **uniform (monomorphic), polygonal shaped cells of medium size.** Most tumors show **minimal pleomorphism but rarely may show anaplasia.**
- **Scant and pink granular cytoplasm:** The tumor cells have **abundant eosinophilic, sometimes granular cytoplasm.**
- **Round regular nuclei with salt and pepper chromatin:** The nuclei are round, regular with dispersed, granular, "salt and pepper" chromatin. They usually have inconspicuous nucleoli.

Other features: It is **uncommon to see mitoses** and when found indicate higher grade NET. Necrosis is usually absent. There may be minor mucin production.

Immunohistochemical stains: Tumor cells are positive for endocrine granule markers, such as **synaptophysin** and **chromogranin A.**

Clinical features: Peak incidence in the **sixth decade**, but can occur at any age. Symptoms depend on the hormones produced.

Prognosis: Location is the most **important prognostic factor** for GI carcinoid tumors. Most patients with appendiceal NET have an excellent prognosis and the majority are cured by appendectomy.

Carcinoid Syndrome (Fig. 18.31)

Q. Write a short note on carcinoid syndrome. List its symptoms.

Neuroendocrine tumor may be associated with *carcinoid syndrome* and **occurs in <10% of patients.**

Secretion of vasoactive substances: Carcinoid tumors confined to the intestine **secrete vasoactive substances.** These are **metabolized to inactive forms by the liver.**

Carcinoid syndrome: It develops when tumors secrete hormones into a non-portal venous circulation. Therefore, it is **strongly associated with metastatic disease.** These metastatic deposits produce a large amount of tumor products to bypass the portal circulation and liver. In such a situation, vasoactive secretion enters the systemic circulation (nonportal venous circulation).

Substances secreted: The carcinoid syndrome is due to **serotonin** secreted by the tumor cells and easily detectable in the urine in the form of its catabolite 5 hydroxyindoleacetic acid. Other substances such as **tachykinins, prostaglandins, and histamine**, may also be

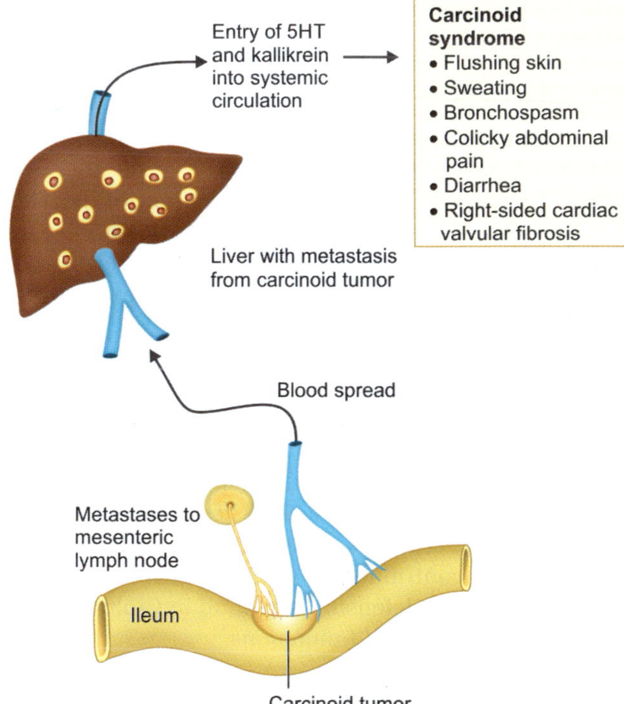

Fig. 18.31: Mechanism of development of carcinoid syndrome and its clinical features.

responsible for the syndrome. The tumor cells also secrete some substance that elicits the deposition of extracellular connective tissue around the tumor and sometimes at a distance. This is responsible for extensive fibrosclerosis, usually found in the tumor itself, and fibrosclerosis of the right sided cardiac valves that produce so called **carcinoid heart disease**.

Clinical features: Carcinoid syndrome is characterized by **flushing of the skin, sweating, facial edema, lacrimation, headache, bronchospasm (bronchoconstriction), colicky abdominal pain, diarrhea**, cyanosis of the face and anterior part of the chest, intermittent hypertension, palpitation, and frequent watery stools. It can produce **right-sided cardiac valvular fibrosis.**

Inflammatory Bowel Disease

PA 24.6 (CC): Describe and etiology and pathogenesis and pathologic and distinguishing features of inflammatory bowel disease.

Q. What are inflammatory bowel diseases?

Definition: Inflammatory bowel disease (IBD) is an **immune-mediated chronic intestinal inflammatory condition**. It is **triggered by the host immune response to intestinal microbes in genetically predisposed individuals.** These individuals have an inappropriate mucosal immune activation.

Major types of IBD: It consists of two entities: **(1) Ulcerative colitis (UC)** and (2) **Crohn disease (CD)**. They are distinguished mainly based on the distribution of affected sites and the morphologic expression of disease at those sites (*refer* **Table 18.8**).

Epidemiology

- **Age of onset:** Both UC and CD occur between **15 and 30 years** of age. A second peak is between the ages of **60 and 80 years**.
- **Cigarette smoking:** It may prevent ulcerative colitis, whereas smoking may cause Crohn disease.
- **Oral contraceptive use** increases the risk of Crohn disease.
- The prevalence of IBD is **higher in urban than rural areas** and **higher prevalence in high socioeconomic classes** than in lower socioeconomic classes.
- **Appendectomy: It is protective against UC** but is associated with **a higher risk of CD.**

Etiology and Pathogenesis

Q. Describe the etiopathogenesis of inflammatory bowel disease.

Normally, homeostasis exists between the three major host compartments namely—(i) commensal (intestinal) microbiota, (ii) epithelial cells lining the intestines [intestinal epithelial cells (IECs)], and (iii) immune cells within the tissues that produce mucosal immune responses. These three (microbiota, IECs, and immune cells) function together. They may be affected by environmental and genetic factors in a susceptible host and produce inflammatory bowel disease (IBD). The exact causes of IBD are not yet defined. Currently, IBD is due to an inappropriate host immune response to the endogenous (intestinal) commensal microbiota within the intestines, with or without some autoimmunity. Major factors involved in the pathogenesis of inflammatory bowel disease **(Box 18.11)** are discussed below.

Genetic Factors

Genetic **predisposition/susceptibility** contributes to IBD. **Affected familial member**: The risk for IBD is increased when there is an affected family member. IBD is **more common among relatives of patients with IBD** than in the general population. However, in ~85–90% of cases, IBD develops as a sporadic disease.

BOX 18.11: Major factors involved in the pathogenesis of inflammatory bowel disease.

1. Genetic factors, e.g., mutated *NOD2* (nucleotide oligomerization binding domain 2) gene
2. Abnormal mucosal immune responses: CD4+ T cells and its differentiation into Th1, Th2, and Th17 types
3. Epithelial defects: Defects in intestinal epithelial tight junction barrier function, and abnormal intestinal defensins
4. Changes in the microbiota in the intestinal lumen

- **Crohn disease:** Genetic factors **play a prominent role.** The concordance rate for monozygotic twins is about 50%.
- **Ulcerative colitis:** Genetic factors are **less prominent than in Crohn disease.** The concordance of monozygotic twins is approximately 16%. Concordance for dizygotic twins for both Crohn disease and ulcerative colitis is less than 10%.

Susceptibility genes

Molecular linkage analyzes of affected families have identified susceptibility genes in Crohn disease. These include **genes associated with innate immunity and autophagy such as *NOD2/CARD15, ATG16L1,* and *IRGM*.** They respond to infection and clear the infective agents such as bacteria, mycobacteria, and viruses.

- ***NOD2* (nucleotide oligomerization binding domain 2) gene:** It is the first Crohn disease susceptibility gene identified. The ***NOD2* gene** (on chromosome 16q, also known as IDB-1 locus) **codes for a NOD2 protein, which is required for normal recognition and response against microbes in the intestinal lumen.** NOD2 protein binds to intracellular bacterial peptidoglycans and subsequently activates NF-κB. The actions of *NOD2* protein are:
    - **Prevents the entry of microbes** into the wall of the intestine
    - **Regulates innate immune responses**
    - **Prevents excessive immune response** against luminal microbes.
- **Disease-associated form of *NOD2*:** It is produced due to **mutations.** This defective *NOD2* leads to the following:
    - Mutant forms are **ineffective at protecting against intestinal bacteria.**
    - Allows the **entry of luminal microbes into the lamina propria of the intestinal wall and stimulates inflammatory reactions.**
- **Two other genes**, namely—***ATG16L1*** (autophagy-related 16-like) and ***IRGM*** (immunity-related GTPase M) are involved in the recognition and response to intracellular pathogens.

Abnormal Mucosal Immune Responses

The normal regulatory immune response of gut mucosa: A normal uninflamed intestine contains many immune cells in a unique state of activation, thereby the **gut is prevented from producing a full immunologic/inflammatory response against the commensal microbiota and dietary antigens** in the intestinal lumen.

Defective immune regulation (Fig. 18.32): The immunosuppressive and immunomodulatory agents are useful therapeutic agents in IBD. This supports that inappropriately sustained immune responses are involved in the pathogenesis of IBD. The defective immune regulation probably contributes to the chronic inflammation in IBD. The role of autoimmunity is unclear.

Epithelial Defects

A **variety of epithelial defects** can develop in Crohn disease, ulcerative colitis, or both IBD.

Defects in intestinal epithelial tight junction barrier function: These are observed in patients with Crohn disease and a few of their healthy first-degree relatives. It **can activate innate and adaptive mucosal immunity and sensitize individuals to disease.**

Abnormal intestinal defensins: Paneth cell granules contain **antimicrobial peptides termed defensins** and affect the composition of luminal microbiota. These antimicrobial peptides normally protect the mucosa against adherent and invading bacteria. These defensins are abnormal in some patients with Crohn disease. These findings suggest that a defective "crosstalk" between the epithelium and the microbiota contributes to the pathogenesis of Crohn disease. **Abnormal defensins** are found in Crohn disease patients carrying *ATG16L1* mutations.

Changes in the Microbiota

The **gut lumen** contains **abundant commensal bacteria.** This endogenous commensal microbiota in the intestines plays a main role in the pathogenesis of IBD. Humans are born sterile and the commensal microbiota are acquired initially from the mother during passage through the birth canal and subsequently from environmental sources. Each individual possesses a unique combination of species and a stable species of bacteria is achieved by 3 years of age. This composition within individuals is likely to persist into adult life and remain stable for several years.

Control of microbiota: The composition and function of the commensal intestinal microbiota are under the control of **host** (e.g., immune, and epithelial responses), **environmental** (e.g., diet and antibiotics), and likely **genetic** (e.g., *NOD2*) factors.

Influence on epithelial and immune function of the host: The microbiota has major influences on the epithelial and immune function of the host through its structural components and metabolic activity. Many of the changes in the commensal microbiota occur as a result of inflammation.

Modification (alteration) of intestinal microflora/ microbiota:

- **It can be modified by diet and disease. IBD is associated with an alteration in the bacterial flora.**
- **Improved food storage conditions and decreased food contamination:** It has **reduced the frequency of enteric infections** with a 'clean' environment in the intestinal lumen. The **immune system may not be exposed to microorganisms** (pathogenic or non-pathogenic) and **inadequate development of regulatory processes** limits mucosal immune responses.

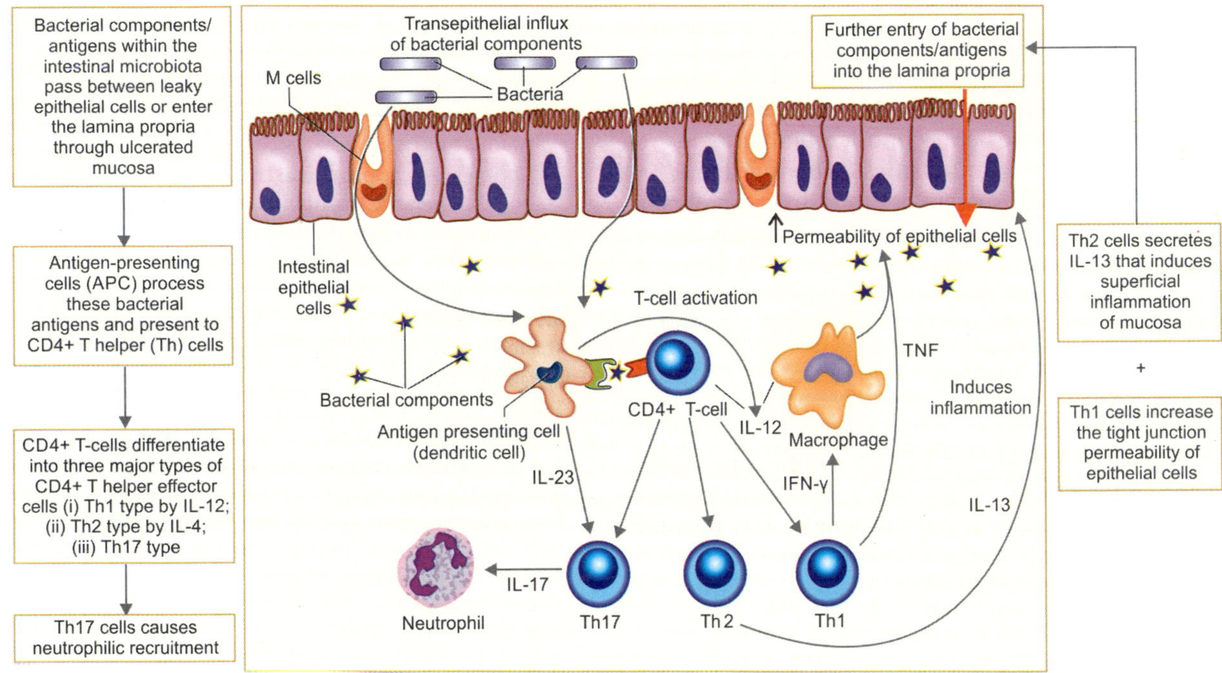

Fig. 18.32: Hypothesis for pathogenesis of inflammatory bowel disease (IBD). (IFN-γ: interferon-gamma; IL: interleukin; TNF: tumor necrosis factor)

Environmental Factors

It includes enteropathogens, antibiotics, diet, hygiene, psychological factors, and smoking.

Psychosocial factors: It can contribute to worsening of symptoms in IBD. Major life events (e.g., illness or death in the family, divorce, or separation) are associated with an increase in symptoms such as pain, bowel dysfunction, and bleeding.

Smoking: CD patients are more likely to be smokers and smoking exacerbates CD. In contrast, an increased risk of UC is observed in non- or ex-smokers.

Hypothesis for Pathogenesis of IBD

The IBD is characterized by **abnormal mucosal immunological response** and shows lymphocytes, macrophages, and other cells of the immune system infiltrating the lamina propria. However, the antigens that trigger the immune response are not yet identified. Whatever the antigenic trigger, **activated T-cells in the lamina propria are involved** in the pathogenesis of IBD.

Hypothesis (Fig. 18.32): One hypothesis signifies the role of intestinal microbiota, epithelial function, and mucosal immunity in the pathogenesis of IBD. The various events are:

- **Transepithelial influx of luminal bacterial components** (antigens) within the intestinal microbiota pass. The bacterial components pass between leaky epithelial cells or enter the lamina propria through ulcerated mucosa. It activates both innate and adaptive immune responses.
- **Presentation of microbial antigens to CD4+ helper T cells: Antigens** from the lumen of the bowel are **transported by M (microfold) and dendritic cells.** Probably, this is the initial trigger.
- **Processing of bacterial antigens: Antigen-presenting cells** (APC) in the lamina propria **process** these **bacterial antigens** and **present them to CD4+ T cells.**
- **Differentiation of CD4+ T cells into Th1 and Th17 cells:** Cytokines secreted by APCs cause differentiation of the CD4+ T cells into Th1 (by IL-12), Th2 (by IL-4), and Th17 (by IL-23) cells.
  - **Th1 cells:** They secrete interferon-gamma (IFNγ), which is the most powerful cytokine that activates macrophages; and, proinflammatory cytokines such as tumor necrosis factor (TNF). In a **genetically susceptible individual**, the release of TNF and other immune-mediated signals **increases the tight junction permeability of epithelial cells.** This causes a further **increase in the entry of bacterial components** into the lamina propria. These events may result in a **self-amplifying cycle** which may be sufficient to initiate IBD. They continue the inflammatory process with the activation of non-immune cells and the release of other important cytokines.
  - **Th2 cells:** They secrete IL-13 that **induces superficial inflammation of the mucosa.**

- **Th17 cells:** They secrete IL-17 and recruit neutrophils. **IL-23** secreted by APCs is essential for the **development and maintenance of Th17 cells.**

Defect in epithelial barrier function and uncontrolled inflammation: It causes entry of microbial antigens to the lamina propria and intensifies inflammation. The development of ulcerative colitis or Crohn disease probably depends upon differences in the cytokine milieu that is produced in response to microbial products. The mucosa shows increased production of the Th2-derived cytokine IL-13 in ulcerative colitis, and, to a lesser extent in Crohn disease.

Crohn Disease

Crohn disease (regional enteritis) is a **chronic multifocal relapsing and remitting, progressive inflammatory bowel disease** of unknown cause that **can involve any portion of the gastrointestinal tract**. Crohn disease has also been referred to as regional enteritis because it frequently involves the ileal region.

MORPHOLOGY

Q. Write a short note on morphological (gross and microscopic) features of Crohn disease.

Gross

- **Sites (Fig. 18.33A):** It can involve any area of the GI tract **from mouth to anus. Most commonly** in the **terminal ileum, ileocecal valve,** and **cecum (Fig. 18.33B)** Small intestine alone in ~40%; small intestine and colon in ~30%, and only the colon in ~30%.
- **Number of lesions:** Usually **multiple** and each lesion is **sharply demarcated** from intervening normal bowel giving rise to **characteristic skip lesions.** It **helps in differentiating it from ulcerative colitis.**
- **Mucosal lesions (Fig. 18.34A)**
- **Aphthous ulcer:** It is the **earliest lesion. Multiple lesions may coalesce** longitudinally to form elongated, linear, or **serpentine** (snake-like)/train track/rake **ulcers oriented along the axis of the bowel.**
  - **Fissures and fistula: Later** the ulcer becomes deeper and forms linear clefts or **fissures** that may extend deeply **to become fistula tracts or sites of perforation.**
  - **Mucosal edema**: Mucosa shows edema and loss of the normal mucosal fold.
  - **Cobblestone appearance:** Ulcers may fuse longitudinally and transversely. The **islands of normal mucosa between the ulcers** show edema and produce a **cobblestone** appearance **(Fig. 18.34B).**
- **Fibrotic thickening of the intestinal wall (Fig. 18.33B):** In the **involved region, it** shows **fibrotic thickening** and is **rubbery.** The **lumen is narrowed** and strictures are common. It appears **like a hosepipe** produces a characteristic radiological **'string sign.'**
- **External surface/serosa with serositis and creeping fat**: It appears red, opaque, hyperemic, and covered with serosal exudate-producing **serositis.** When the disease shows extensive transmural involvement, the mesenteric fat is often firm and contracted over areas of involvement. It becomes adherent to the serosal surface and may encircle around the antimesenteric serosal surface producing a pattern known as **creeping fat (Fig. 18.34C).**
- **Adhesion:** Involved loops of bowel may adhere to each other.
- **Strictures:** These can occur commonly in Crohn disease. The presence of strictures may also help differentiate Crohn disease from ulcerative colitis.

Microscopy (Figs. 18.35A and B)

Crohn disease is a **chronic inflammatory process.**

- **Abundant infiltration of neutrophils and crypt abscesses:** The presence of numerous/**clusters of neutrophils within a crypt** is termed a **crypt abscess.** These neutrophils may infiltrate and damage crypt epithelium and are often associated with crypt destruction.
- **Mucosal aphthous ulcers and inflammation:** They appear as small, superficial ulcers called **aphthous ulcers.** During early phases, the inflammation may be limited to the mucosa and submucosa. There may be a sudden transition between ulcerated and normal mucosa.

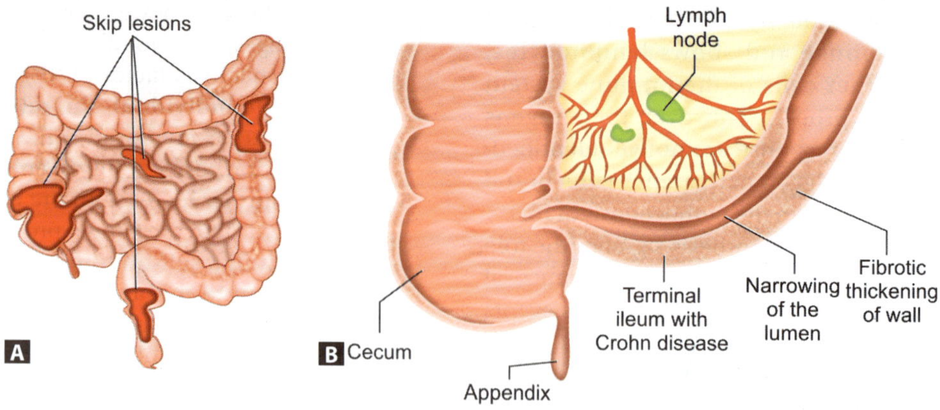

Figs. 18.33A and B: Diagrammatic appearances of Crohn disease: (A) Distribution of lesions; (B) Gross features.

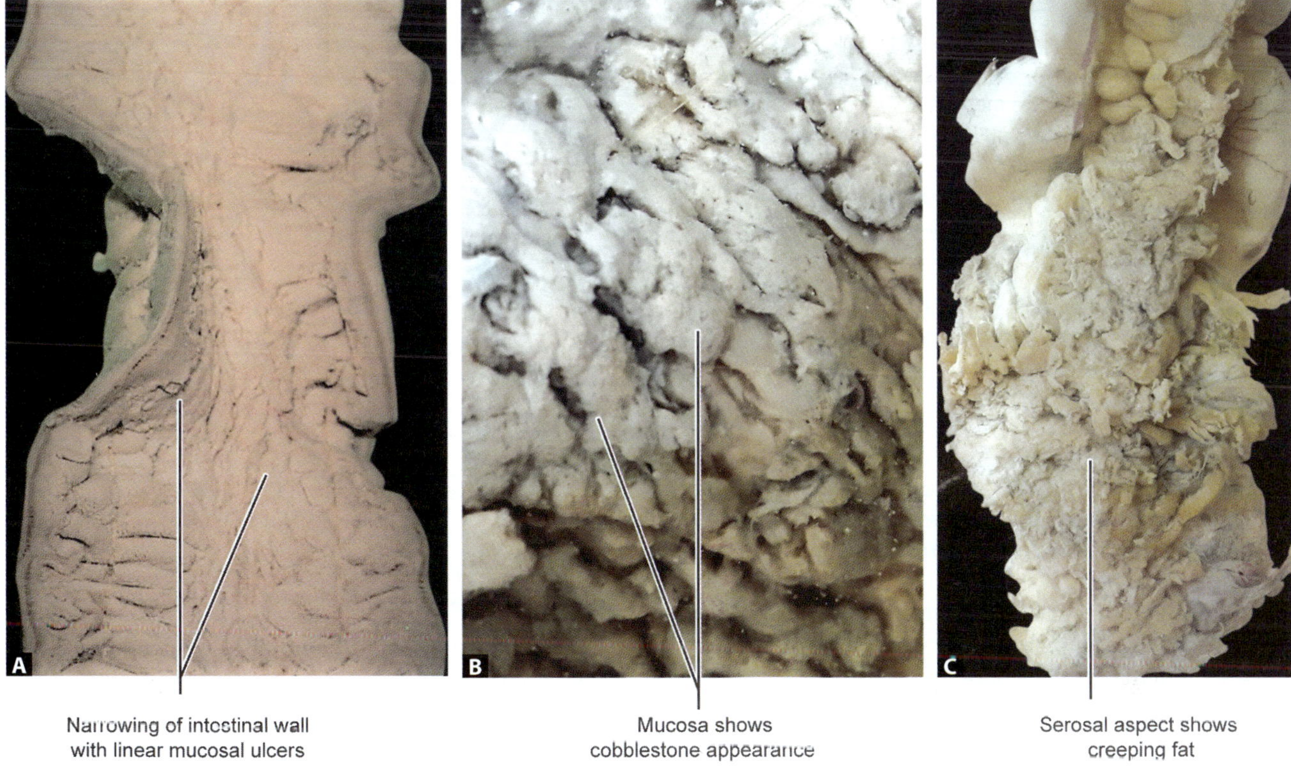

Figs. 18.34A to C: (A) Small-intestinal stricture with linear mucosal ulcers and thickened intestinal wall; (B) Mucosa showing cobblestone appearance; (C) Creeping fat pattern on the serosal aspect of the small intestine.

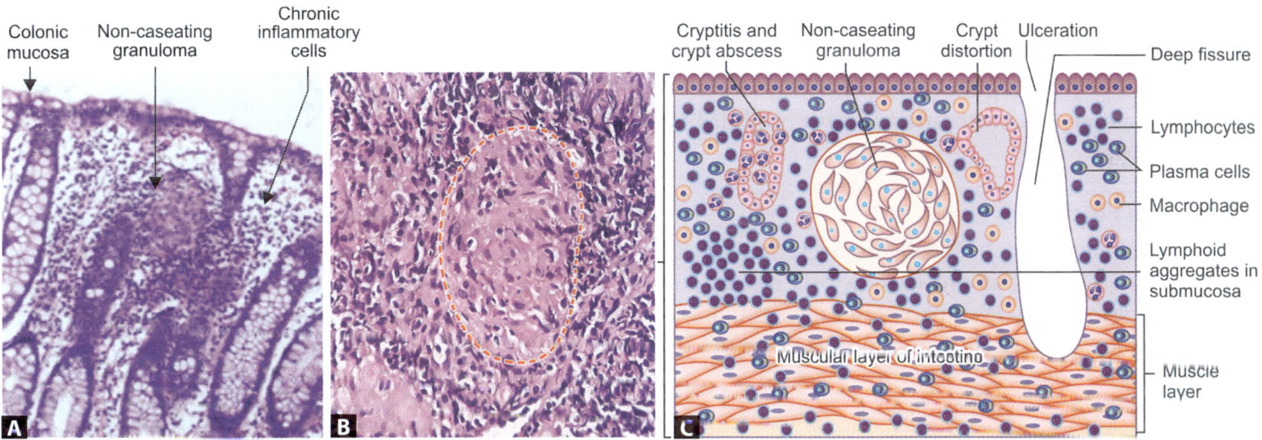

Figs. 18.35A to C: (A) Photomicrograph of Crohn disease showing one non-caseating granuloma; (B) High power of granuloma (dotted outline); (C) Microscopic features of Crohn disease (diagrammatic).

- **Distortion of mucosal crypt architecture:** Normally, crypts are straight and parallel to each other. Repeated cycles of crypt destruction and regeneration lead to **bizarre branching shapes and unusual orientations to one another** referred to as distortion of the mucosal crypt.
- **Epithelial metaplasia:** It develops because of chronic injury.
  - **Pseudopyloric metaplasia:** It is characterized by the occurrence of **glands, which appear like** those in the **gastric antrum and** may be seen in the involved segment of the intestine.
  - **Paneth cell metaplasia:** Paneth cells are normally absent in the left colon. Paneth cell metaplasia may appear in the left colon.
- **Noncaseating granulomas (Figs. 18.35A to C):** It is a **hallmark of Crohn disease.** They are **mostly seen in the submucosa** (but may be located at any level of the bowel wall) and are found in ~35% of cases. These granulomas when present, are typically poorly formed and consist of focal aggregates of epithelioid cells, surrounded by a thin rim of lymphocytes. Multinucleated giant cells may also be present. They may occur in areas

of active disease or uninvolved regions in any layer of the intestinal wall. Granulomas also may be found in mesenteric lymph nodes. Granulomas in the skin may form nodules and are called (misleading) as metastatic Crohn disease.

- **Transmural inflammation (Fig. 18.34C):** It is characterized by **chronic inflammation involving all layers of the intestinal wall** and may show **lymphoid aggregates** in the submucosa or subserosa.
- **Mucosal atrophy, with loss of crypts:** It may be seen after years of disease.

A summary of morphologic features of Crohn disease is presented (*refer* **online Box 18.12 and Fig. 18.33C).**

Clinical Features

Intestinal Manifestations

The clinical manifestations of Crohn disease are variable. The most common symptoms are as follows:

- Intermittent attacks of **mild diarrhea, fever,** and **abdominal pain.**
- About 20% present with **acute right lower quadrant pain, fever, and bloody diarrhea.** It may mimic acute appendicitis or bowel perforation.
- **Remission and exacerbations**: Periods of active disease are usually interrupted by asymptomatic periods that last for weeks to many months. The disease may be re-activated by external triggers, such as physical or emotional stress, NSAID, specific diets, and cigarette smoking.

Extraintestinal Manifestations

These include **uveitis, migratory polyarthritis, sacroiliitis, ankylosing spondylitis, erythema nodosum, and clubbing of the fingertips.**

Laboratory Findings

ESR and CRP are raised. In severe diseases, there may be hypoalbuminemia, anemia, and leukocytosis. Barium study may show a string sign. Histopathological examination of endoscopic biopsy will show microscopic features of Crohn disease.

Complications

Q. Write a short note on complications of Crohn disease.

- **Iron-deficiency anemia**: It may develop in patients with colonic disease due to loss of blood.
- **Malabsorption:** Extensive involvement of the small intestine may result in loss of protein, hypoalbuminemia, generalized nutrient malabsorption, or vitamin B12 deficiency.
- **Fibrosing stricture formation:** It may occur in the terminal ileum.
- **Fistula formation:** It may form between loops of the intestine and surrounding structures such as the urinary bladder uterus, vagina, and abdominal or perianal skin.

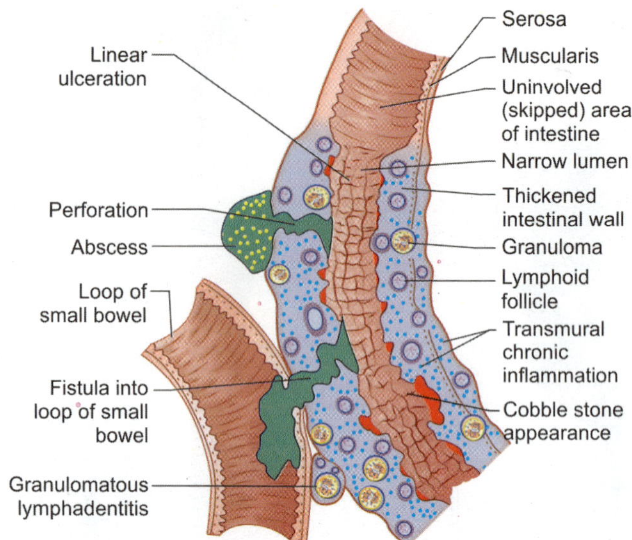

Fig. 18.36: Diagrammatic representation of major features of Crohn disease involving the small intestine.

Lesions in the distal rectum and anus may produce perianal fistulas. Perforations and peritoneal abscesses are common.

- **Acute complications:** Perforation and hemorrhage.
- **Development of carcinoma:** It is rare and the risk of carcinoma colon is increased in patients with long-standing colonic disease.
- **Systemic amyloidosis:** It is rare.

A diagrammatic representation of major features of Crohn disease involving the small intestine is presented in **Figure 18.36.**

Ulcerative Colitis

Ulcerative colitis (UC) is a **severe, chronic crypt destructive, ulcerating inflammatory** bowel disease of unknown cause. It is **limited to the colon and rectum** and inflammation **involves** only the **mucosa and submucosa** of the intestinal wall. It is clinically associated with exacerbations and remissions of bloody diarrhea.

MORPHOLOGY

Q. Write a short note on the morphology of ulcerative colitis.

Gross (Figs. 18.37A and B)

Site: Ulcerative colitis is a **diffuse disease limited to the colon and rectum.** Usually involves the rectum and extends proximally for a variable distance (continuous lesion) to involve part or the entire colon. **Skip lesions are not seen** in UC. The terminology used depends on the region involved as shown in **Table 18.7. No skip lesions.**

- **Mucosa in early colitis appear red and fine granular:** Involved colonic mucosa may appear **slightly red** and **fine granular (resembles sandpaper).** There may be an abrupt transition between diseased and uninvolved segments of the colon. Mucosa is **frequently covered with a yellowish exudate** and bleeds easily.

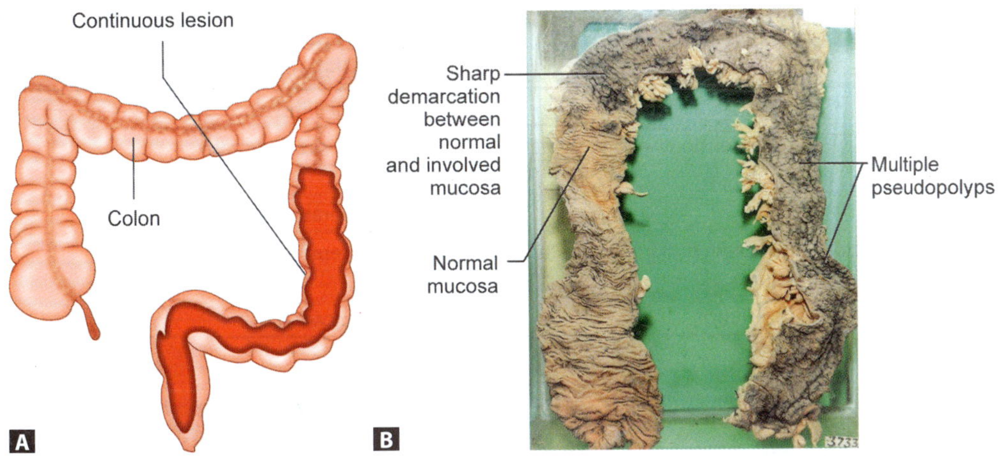

Figs. 18.37A and B: Gross features of ulcerative colitis: (A) Diagrammatic; (B) Transverse and descending colon showing numerous pseudopolyps.

- **Progressive colitis shows erosions or broad-based ulcers:** Later, **small, superficial erosions or broad-based ulcers** may develop. **Ulcers are aligned along the colon's long axis but do not form serpentine ulcers of Crohn.** Tissue repair accompanies tissue destruction. Granulation tissue develops in denuded areas of mucosa. Chronic ulcerative colitis may lead to mucosal atrophy with a smooth mucosal surface without normal folds.
- **Pseudopolyps (inflammatory polyps):** They develop in long-standing disease. **Isolated islands of regenerating mucosa** may **project into the lumen** of the bowel to produce small elevations termed **pseudopolyps (Fig. 18.37B)**.
- **Inflammation affects only mucosa and submucosa: The inflammatory process** is **diffuse** (without skip lesion) and **limited to the mucosa** and **superficial submucosa**.
- **Bowel wall is not thickened, the serosa is normal, and strictures do not develop**.
- **In severe cases**, inflammation, and inflammatory mediators may damage the muscularis propria and disturb neuromuscular function. This may lead to **colonic dilation** and **toxic megacolon** which can undergo perforation.
- **Mucosal atrophy in longstanding disease**: Chronic disease may lead to **mucosal atrophy.** This atrophied mucosa appears flat, with a smooth surface lacking normal folds.
- In contrast to Crohn disease, **no mural thickening, no strictures, and the serosal surface is normal.**

Microscopy [Figs. 18.38A and B (refer online Fig. 18.38C)]

Microscopic features of ulcerative colitis are like colonic Crohn disease. These include inflammatory infiltrates, crypt abscesses, crypt distortion, and pseudopyloric epithelial metaplasia. However, **the inflammatory process is diffuse and usually seen in the mucosa, and superficial submucosa and granulomas are not found.**

- **Inflammation limited to the mucosa and submucosa: Mucosal shows** the inflammation limited to the mucosa and submucosa. Both mucosa and submucosa show edema and an increase in the number of lymphocytes, plasma cells, and macrophages.
- **Changes in the crypt**
  - **Cryptitis: Neutrophils** are the **hallmark of acute disease.** They are in the epithelium of crypts and damage the crypt epithelium giving rise to **cryptitis. Neutrophils within crypt epithelium are termed cryptitis.**
  - **Crypt abscess:** Clusters of neutrophils are seen within a dilated crypt and are known as **crypt abscesses (Figs. 18.38A and B)** and are **usually associated with the destruction of crypts.** The term chronic active colitis is used when acute activity is superimposed on a background of chronic changes.
- **Histological hallmarks of chronicity: The regenerating epithelium is immature and as such does not contain mucin (mucin depletion).**
  - **Distortion of crypt architecture:** It is **due to repeated destruction and regeneration of the crypt**. The crypts may **appear shortened, tortuous with bizarre branching** (bifid), and **decreased** in number. Often a gap is seen between the crypt bases and the muscularis mucosae.
  - **Chronic inflammatory infiltrate:** A chronic inflammatory infiltrate of **lymphocytes, plasma cells,** and **macrophages** is seen **in the mucosa and superficial submucosa. Distortion of crypt architecture and increased mucosal chronic inflammation** are the two characteristic microscopic findings of UC.
  - **Basal plasmacytosis and multiple basal lymphoid aggregates**. Plasma cells extend into the muscularis mucosae.
- **Mucosal atrophy:** It occurs in **late stages.** The mucosa surface appears smooth, and flat without any normal folds.
- **Paneth cell metaplasia:** It is common, and may occur in the left colon (where Paneth cells are normally not found).
- **Loss of goblet cells and mucin depletion:** The regenerating epithelium is immature and does not contain mucin, and is called mucin depletion (typical mature goblet cells contain mucin).
- **Dysplastic changes in epithelium may appear and progress to carcinoma.**

A summary of morphologic features of Ulcerative colitis is presented (*refer* **online Box 18.13**).

TABLE 18.7 Terminology used for ulcerative colitis depending on the region involved.

Region involved	*Terminology*
Entire colon	Pancolitis
Only the left side of the colon (without extension beyond the transverse colon)	Left-sided disease
Limited to the rectum	Ulcerative proctitis
The disease process extends from the rectum proximally toward the splenic flexure	Ulcerative proctosigmoiditis
Mild mucosal inflammation of the distal ileum	Backwash ileitis

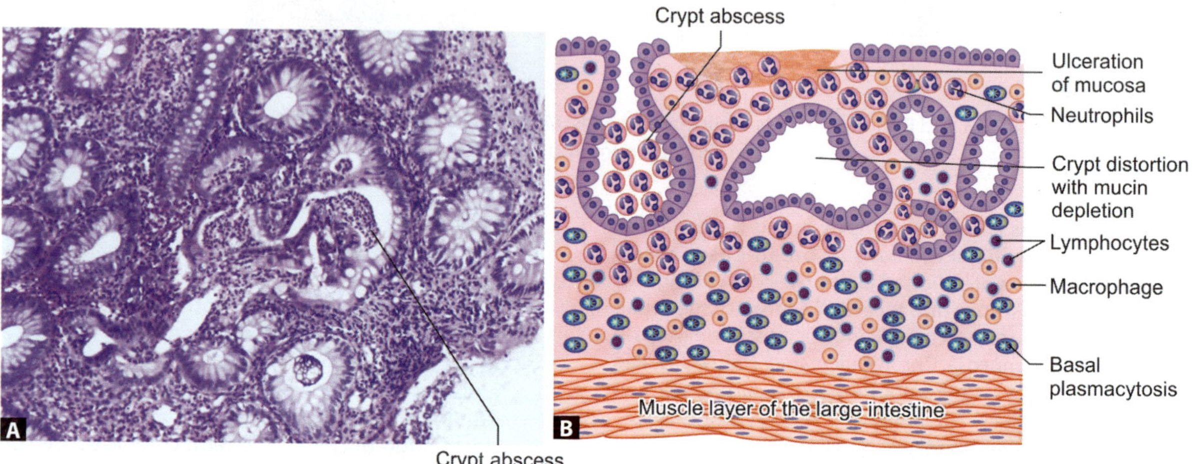

Figs. 18.38A and B: Ulcerative colitis: (A) Photomicrograph showing crypt abscess (arrow) and dense inflammatory infiltrate surrounding crypts; (B) Diagrammatic shows microscopic features of ulcerative colitis.

Clinical Features

Occurs mainly in young adults. UC is a relapsing disorder with **exacerbations and remissions.**

Triggering event: Infectious enteritis and psychological stress.

Intestinal manifestations: It presents with **attacks of bloody diarrhea** with mucoid material, **lower abdominal pain,** and cramps.

Extraintestinal manifestations: These include the following:

- **Migratory polyarthritis, sacroiliitis, ankylosing spondylitis.**
- **Eye:** Inflammation of the eye (mostly **uveitis**).
- **Skin:** Erythema nodosum and pyoderma gangrenosum.
- **Liver:** Primary sclerosing cholangitis and pericholangitis.
- **Thromboembolic phenomena:** Deep vein thrombosis of the lower extremities.

Complications

Q. Write a short note on complications of ulcerative colitis.

Complications of ulcerative colitis: (1) toxic megacolon, (2) development of colorectal carcinoma, (3) intestinal hemorrhage, and (4) electrolyte imbalances.

- **Toxic megacolon:** In fulminant cases, the inflammation and inflammatory mediators can damage the muscularis propria and disturb neuromuscular function. This may lead to colonic dilation, toxic megacolon, and perforation.

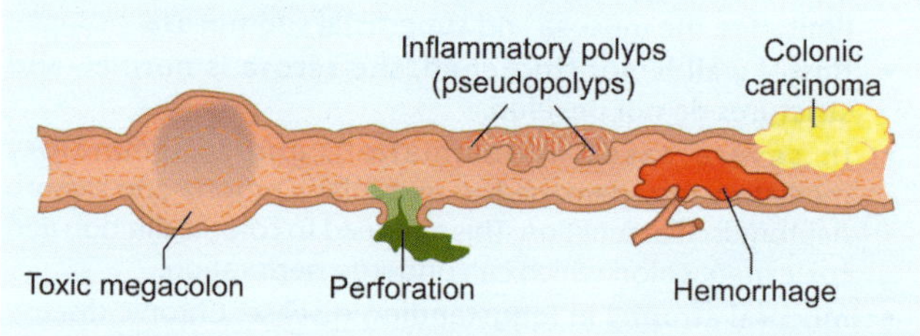

Fig. 18.39: Diagrammatic representation of salient features and complications of ulcerative colitis.

- **Colorectal cancer:** It may develop in long-standing UC.
- **Hemorrhage** from intestinal lesions and blood loss.
- **Electrolyte disturbances** due to diarrhea.

Salient features and complications of ulcerative colitis are presented in **Figure 18.39.**

Prognosis: It depends on the severity of active disease and disease duration.

Differences between ulcerative colitis and Crohn disease are listed in **Table 18.8.**

Q. Mention the differences between ulcerative colitis and Crohn disease.

TABLE 18.8 Differences between Crohn disease and ulcerative colitis.

Characteristics	*Crohn disease*	*Ulcerative colitis (UC)*
Macroscopic		
Bowel region involved	• Any area of the gastrointestinal tract (ileum ± colon) • Rectum is usually spared	• Colon and rectum (rectum almost always involved) • Rectal involvement (proctitis) is the hallmark of UC
Pattern of involvement (distribution)	Focal (skip), segmental lesions	Diffuse (continuous), no skip lesions
Luminal narrowing/stricture	Typical	Rare
Involved bowel wall	Thickened or normal	Thin
Depth of involvement	Transmural	Mucosa and submucosa
Mucosal appearance	Cobblestone appearance	Irregular ulcers, friable, atrophy
Creeping mesenteric fat	Common	Absent
Microscopic		
Inflammation	Transmural	Limited to mucosa and submucosa
Pseudopolyps	Few	Many
Ulcers	Deep, fissures (knife-like)	Superficial, broad-based
Lymphoid reaction	Marked	Moderate
Fibrosis	Marked	Minimal to none
Serosal inflammation (serositis)	Marked	Absent
Granulomas	Seen in ~35%	Absent
Fistulae/sinuses/fissures	Seen	Absent
Crypt abscess	Uncommon	Usual
Pyloric gland metaplasia	Common	Uncommon
Clinical		
Fissure, fistula and stricture	May be observed with colonic involvement (e.g., perianal fistula)	Usually, absent
Fat/vitamin malabsorption	Seen	Absent
Development of malignancy	In colonic involvement	Yes
Recurrence after surgery	Common	Not observed
Toxic megacolon	No	Yes
Rectal bleeding	Uncommon	Common
Smoking	Worsens course	Protective

Note: All features may not be seen in a single case.

Intussusception

Q. Write a short note on intussusception.

Intussusception is an **invagination (telescoping) of one segment of intestine into another** immediately **adjacent distal segment**. The highest incidence is between 4 and 10 months of age.

Causes

- **Infants and children**: Usually, there is **no underlying anatomic defect**.
- **Older children and adults**: A **mass or tumor in the wall of the bowel** disturbs normal peristaltic contractions forcing the lesion and a segment of the proximal bowel into a distal segment of the intestine. The lesion acts as the point of traction and causes intussusception. These lesions **include polyps, ingested foreign bodies**, Meckel diverticulum, etc.

MORPHOLOGY

Sites: In children, the most common site is **ileocolic** and **in adults** it is **colocolic.**

Gross (Figs. 18.40A and B): An intussusception consists of **three parts:**

1. Entering/inner tube (intussusceptum)
2. Returning or middle tube
3. Sheath or outer tube (intussuscipiens)

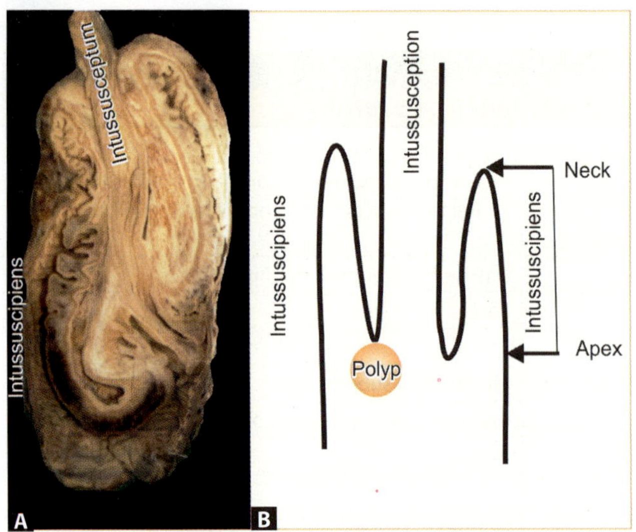

Figs. 18.40A and B: Intussusception: (A) Ileoileal intussusception; (B) Mechanism and nomenclature of intussusception.

Effect: Untreated intussusception may lead to intestinal obstruction, compression of vessels, and infarction of the bowel.

Hirschsprung Disease

Q. Write a short note on Hirschsprung disease.

Hirschsprung disease is a **congenital abnormality** that is also known as a **congenital aganglionic megacolon.** It may occur as isolated or in combination with other developmental abnormalities. About 10% of all cases are found in children with Down syndrome and serious neurologic abnormalities are present in another 5%. It is **more common in males.** When occurs in females, is usually severe and ends to involve longer aganglionic segments.

Pathogenesis

The neural crest cells migrate into the intestinal wall during embryogenesis. The enteric neuronal plexus develops from these neural crest cells.

- **Premature arrest of migration of neural crest cells:** Hirschsprung disease results **from a congenital defect in colonic innervation.** When **the normal migration of neural crest cells from the cecum to the rectum is arrested prematurely or when the ganglion cells undergo premature death**. This produces a **distal intestinal segment without** both **Meissner's submucosal** and the **Auerbach myenteric plexus** ("aganglionosis"). The defect usually begins at the rectum but extends proximally for variable lengths.
- **Consequences**: The above abnormality leads to the **absence of coordinated peristaltic contractions and functional obstruction.** This leads to **dilation proximal to the affected segment.**

Mechanisms: The cause of defective neural crest cell migration is not known. A genetic component may be present. Heterozygous loss of function **mutations in the receptor tyrosine kinase RET is responsible for the majority of familial cases** and about 15% of sporadic cases. Mutations in other genes encoding proteins involved in enteric neurodevelopment, including disease-modifying genes, as well as environmental factors are also involved.

MORPHOLOGY

The segment involved: Hirschsprung disease always affects the rectum and, in most cases, it is limited to the **rectum and sigmoid colon.** But it may additionally involve the variable length of the colon and in severe cases, it can involve the entire colon.

Appearance (Fig. 18.41): The **affected aganglionic region may be grossly normal or contracted.** Normally innervated **proximal colon may undergo progressive dilation** because of functional distal obstruction.

Diagnosis: By demonstrating the absence of ganglion cells in the affected segment.

Clinical Features

Present in neonates as **failure to pass meconium** in the immediate **postnatal period.** This is followed by obstructive constipation often with visible, ineffective peristalsis. It may progress to abdominal distension and bilious vomiting.

Complications: These include enterocolitis, fluid and electrolyte disturbances, perforation, and peritonitis.

Treatment: Surgical resection of the aganglionic segment with anastomosis of the normal proximal colon to the rectum.

POLYPS OF COLON

Definition: Polyp is a clinical term or gross description used for any circumscribed tumor or growth that projects above the surrounding mucosa. A gastrointestinal polyp is a **mass that protrudes into the lumen of the gut.**

Polyps are most common in the colon but may occur in the esophagus, stomach, or small intestine. They are of

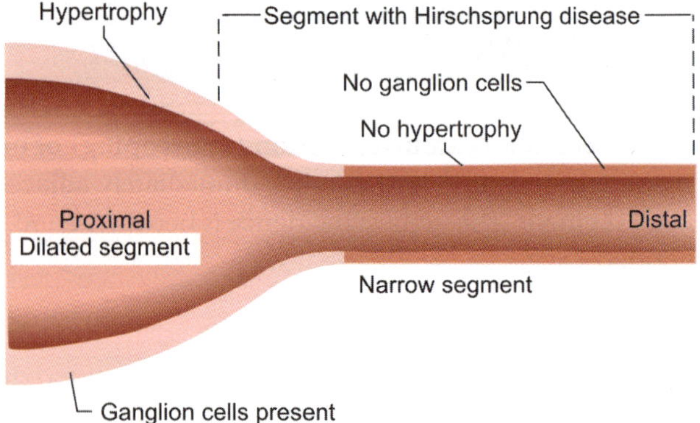

Fig. 18.41: Diagrammatic representation of the segment involved by Hirschsprung disease and the dilated proximal segment.

clinical importance because they tend to undergo malignant transformation.

Classification of Polyps (Box 18.14)

Q. Classify colorectal polyps.

Non-neoplastic Polyps

Inflammatory Polyps

These are raised nodules of inflamed, regenerating epithelium. They are associated with the solitary rectal ulcer syndrome. They present with the triad of rectal bleeding, mucus discharge, and an inflammatory polyp on the anterior rectal wall. These lesions are not precancerous. **Microscopy:** It is composed of inflamed and reactive mucosal tissue.

Hamartomatous Polyps

These are **rare tumor-like growths**. Hamartomatous polyps are composed of **mature tissues that are normally present at the site's anatomic location) where they develop**. Generally, they have both stromal and epithelial elements. Hamartomatous polyps may occur sporadically or as components of genetically determined or acquired syndromes. These syndromes are listed (*refer* **online Box 18.15**). They may be associated with **intestinal and extraintestinal manifestations**.

Juvenile Polyps

Q. Write a short note on juvenile polyposis colon.

These are the most common types of hamartomatous polyps. They are **focal hamartomatous malformations of the mucosal epithelium and lamina propria**.

Sporadic or syndromic: Juvenile polyps may be sporadic or occur as a component of the syndrome.

- **Sporadic juvenile polyps**: They are usually solitary. The majority occurs in **children** less than 5 years of age. They are located in the **rectum** and commonly present with rectal bleeding.
- **Juvenile polyposis syndrome:** It is an autosomal dominant syndrome. It is diagnosed if there are: any number of juvenile polyps plus a positive family history of juvenile polyposis, polyposis involving the entire GIT, or three or more juvenile polyps in the colorectum. It may be associated with dozens of polyps. It is associated with an **increased risk of colonic adenocarcinoma and carcinoma in other sites.**

BOX 18.14: Classification of gastrointestinal polyps.

According to gross appearance
- Sessile: Polyps do not have a stalk
- Pedunculated: Polyps have a well-defined stalk

According to histopathological appearance
- Non-neoplastic
  - Inflammatory
  - Hamartomatous: Juvenile polyp, Peutz–Jeghers polyp
  - Hyperplastic
- Neoplastic
  - Benign: Adenoma (tubular, tubulovillous and villous)
  - Malignant: Adenocarcinoma, lymphomas

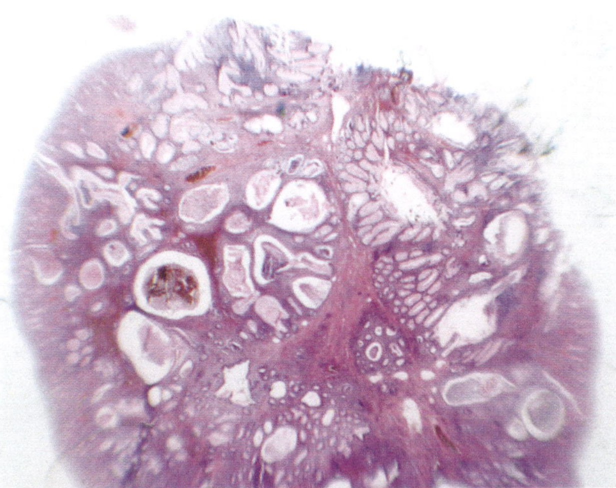

Fig. 18.42: Whole-mount view of a juvenile polyp showing cystically dilated glands.

MORPHOLOGY

The appearance of sporadic and syndromic juvenile polyps is similar.

Gross: They are **pedunculated, spherical, smooth-surfaced,** and **red in color.** Most are **less than 3 cm** in diameter. The cut section shows **cystic spaces**.

Microscopy (Fig. 18.42): They are composed of **cystically dilated glands** filled with mucin and inflammatory debris. **Lamina propria** is expanded due to **mixed inflammatory infiltrates.**

Peutz–Jeghers (PJ) Syndrome (Figs. 18.40A and B)

Q. Write a short note on Peutz–Jeghers syndrome and its components.

- It is a rare **autosomal dominant** syndrome.
- **Characteristic features:** Presence of (i) **multiple gastrointestinal (GI) hamartomatous polyps (Figs. 18.43A and C)**, (ii) **mucocutaneous** (mouth, buccal mucosa, and genitalia region) **hyperpigmentation (Fig. 18.43B), and (iii) an increased risk for the development of several malignancies.** These malignancies include cancers of the colon, pancreas, breast, lung, ovaries, uterus, and testes.
- **Median age** of presentation **is 11 years.**
- **Germline loss-of-function mutations in the** ***LKB1/ STK11*** **gene**: The *LKB1/STK11* gene is on chromosome 19. It encodes a tumor-suppressive protein kinase that regulates cellular metabolism. Its mutations are present in approximately half of the patients with the familial form of Peutz-Jeghers syndrome.

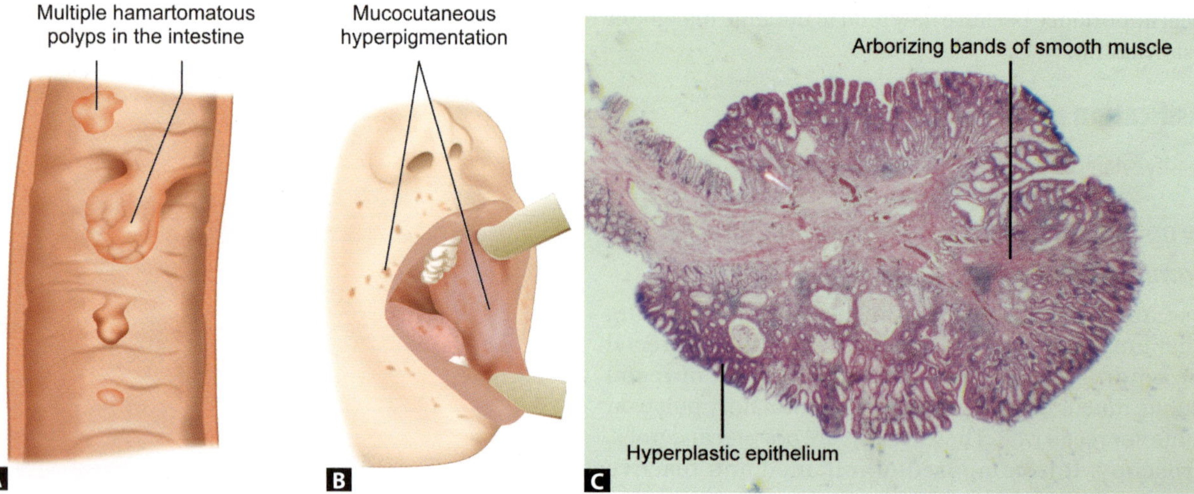

Figs. 18.43A to C: (A) Multiple hamartomatous polyps in the intestine; (B) Mucocutaneous hyperpigmentation; (C) Whole-mount view of PJ polyp showing arborizing bands of mature smooth muscle lined by hyperplastic epithelium.

MORPHOLOGY

Q. Write a short note on the microscopic appearance of Peutz-Jeghers (PJ) polyps.

Gross

Site: Most common in the **small intestine.**

Number: Intestinal polyps are usually present in **dozens.**

Size: Varies from a few millimeters to several centimeters in diameter.

Appearance: Large and pedunculated with a lobulated contour.

Microscopy

Consists of **hyperplastic mature epithelium** appropriate to the anatomic site (where it develops) and is **divided by broad bands of mature smooth muscle.**

Small intestinal PJ polyps consist of crypts and villi of varying lengths divided by **characteristic arborizing bands of smooth muscle fibers (commonly fan out from the center of the polyp and have tree-like appearance) intermixed with lamina propria (Fig. 18.43C).** They are **likened to trees in which the trunk and branches are smooth muscle fibers.**

Hyperplastic Polyps

- Most common non-neoplastic polyps of the colon and are frequently seen in the rectum. No malignant potential. Their pathogenesis is not completely known.
- **Age:** Sixth and seventh decades of life.

MORPHOLOGY

Gross

Location: Most common in the left colon.

Size: Usually less than 5 mm in diameter.

Number: They may be single but more commonly multiple, particularly in the sigmoid colon and rectum.

Appearance: They are smooth, nodular protrusions of the mucosa.

Microscopy

They are composed of an expanded population of mature goblet and absorptive cells. The crowding of these cells produces a serrated surface and is the characteristic morphologic feature.

Neoplastic Polyps

Q. Write a short note on neoplastic polyps of the intestine.

- The most **common and important** neoplastic polyps are **colonic adenomas** (benign neoplasms of intestinal epithelium). These are the precursor lesions of **colorectal adenocarcinomas.**
- Polyps can occur singly, synchronously in few numbers, or as part of a familial polyposis syndrome.

Classification: Colorectal adenomatous polyps are classified depending on the following:

1. **Growth pattern:** (a) Pedunculated, (b) sessile, or (c) flat or depressed. Pedunculated adenomas have thin fibromuscular stalks containing prominent blood vessels derived from the submucosa.
2. **Architecture:** Adenomas can be classified as **tubular, tubulovillous,** or **villous.**

MORPHOLOGY

General Features

- **Size and appearance:** Adenomas range from 0.3 to 10 cm in diameter. They may be sessile or pedunculated. They have a velvety texture and bumpy surface.
- **Site: Almost 50% of** all adenomatous polyps of the colon are located **in the rectosigmoid region.** The remaining 50% is evenly distributed throughout the rest of the colon.

Microscopy

- **All colorectal adenomas are low-grade dysplastic lesions** characterized by the presence of epithelial dysplasia.
- **Epithelial dysplasia:** It is characterized by nuclear hyperchromasia, elongation, and stratification. It may be classified as mild, moderate, and severe dysplasia.
- **Pedunculated adenomas:** They have thin fibromuscular stalks with prominent blood vessels derived from the submucosa. The stalk is covered by nonneoplastic epithelium.

Classification: Based on the architecture, adenomas can be classified as **tubular, tubulovillous,** or **villous.**

Tubular Adenomas (Adenomatous Polyps)

They constitute two-thirds of the adenomas of the large intestine.

- **Gross:** Appear as **small, smooth-surfaced, pedunculated polyps.** They are usually **less than 2 cm** in diameter **(Fig. 18.44A)**. Tubular adenomas over 2 cm have a higher risk of invasive carcinoma. It is like a raspberry on a stalk.
- **Microscopy:** It consists of **closely packed** small **rounded or tubular glands (Fig. 18.44B)** embedded in a **stroma** (increase in the number of glands and cells per unit area compared to the normal mucosa). The cells lining the glands are crowded and contain enlarged hyperchromatic nuclei. May **show variable degrees of epithelial dysplasia (Fig. 18.44C)**.

Villous Adenomas (Villous Papilloma)

Q. Write a short note on villous adenoma.

They constitute one-tenth of colonic adenomas and are **predominantly** found **in the rectosigmoid region**.

- **Gross: Large, broad-based, sessile**, elevated lesions with **cauliflower-like surface (Fig. 18.45A). Most are over 2 cm** but may be as large as 10–15 cm in diameter.
- **Microscopy:** Composed of **thin, long, finger-like projections,** (papillary, crown-like growth) which superficially **resemble the villi of the small intestine (Fig. 18.45B).** The lining epithelium shows dysplasia similar to tubular adenomas. However, **villous adenomas** (larger than 2 cm) likely **contain foci of carcinoma more commonly than tubular adenomas.**

Q. List the differences between villous adenoma and tubulovillous adenoma.

Tubulovillous Adenomas

They show a **mixture of both tubular and villous elements. Polyps with more than 25% and less than 75% villous component** are called tubulovillous.

Sessile Serrated Adenomas

They are more common in the right colon and histologically overlap with hyperplastic polyps. They have malignant potential but do not show dysplasia.

Microscopy

They consist of serrated architecture throughout the full length of the glands, including the base of the crypt, dilatation of the crypt, and lateral growth.

Risk for malignancy

Size of the polyp: It is the most **important feature that correlates with risk for malignancy**. For example, cancer is very rare in adenomas less than 1 cm in diameter. Almost 40% of lesions larger than 4 cm in diameter may contain foci of invasive cancer.

High-grade dysplasia: It is a second risk factor for the presence of cancer in a polyp.

Intramucosal Carcinoma

It is a term used when dysplastic epithelial cells break the basement membrane and invade the lamina propria or muscularis mucosae. Since there are no functional lymphatic channels in the colonic mucosa, intramucosal carcinomas do not have metastatic potential and complete polypectomy is usually curative.

GENETIC TUMOR SYNDROMES

Many syndromes are associated with polyps in colon and are associated with increased rates of colon cancer. These may be sporadic or genetic tumor syndrome (*refer* **online Table 18.9**). The most common familial colorectal syndromes include familial adenomatous polyposis and hereditary nonpolyposis colorectal cancer syndrome (Lynch syndrome).

Familial Adenomatous Polyposis

Q. Write a short note on familial adenomatous polyposis.

Definition: Familial adenomatous polyposis (FAP) is an **autosomal dominant** inherited syndrome characterized by **hundreds to thousands of adenomas** throughout the colorectum **(Fig. 18.46)** as well as numerous **extracolonic manifestations.**

FAP is **also known as polyposis coli**. Patients develop few adenomas by the age of 21 (*refer* page 636).

Genetic features: It is caused by **germ-line** inactivation (5q) **mutations** of the ***adenomatous polyposis coli (APC)* gene.** *APC* is a tumor suppressor gene and its products modulate a specific signaling cascade (WNT signaling) that regulates cell proliferation (*refer* **Fig. 18.47**). Every cell of FAP patient has one inactive APC allele and the inactivation of the second allele initiates the early phase of neoplastic change.

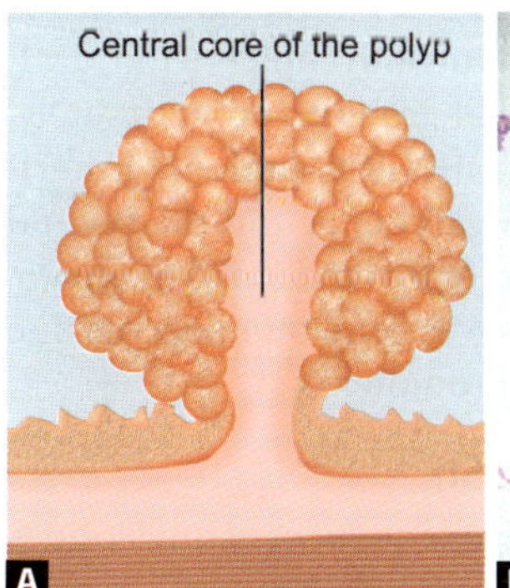

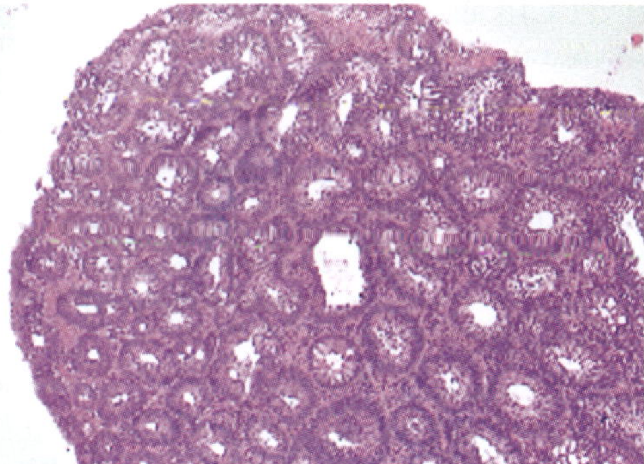

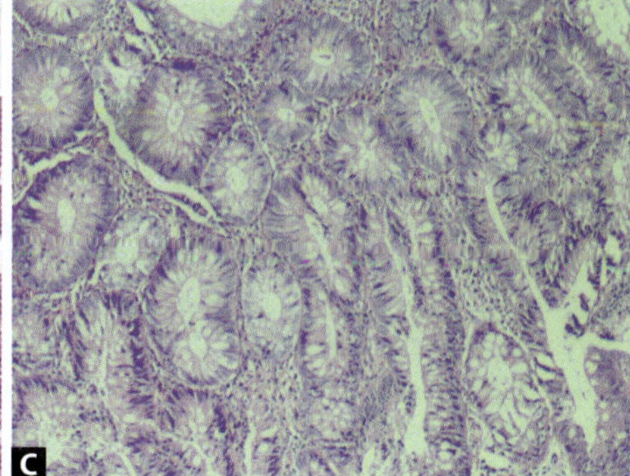

Figs. 18.44A to C: Tubular adenoma: (A) A pedunculated tubular adenomatous polyp cut section, which shows a central core (diagrammatic); (B) Photomicrograph shows closely packed tubular glands; (C) Tubular adenoma with low-grade dysplasia of lining epithelium.

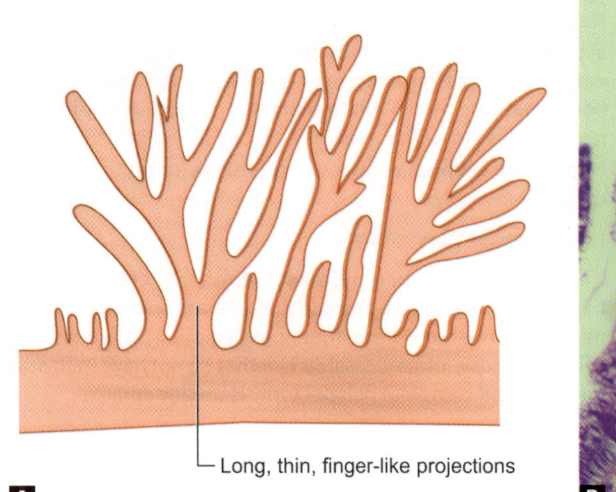

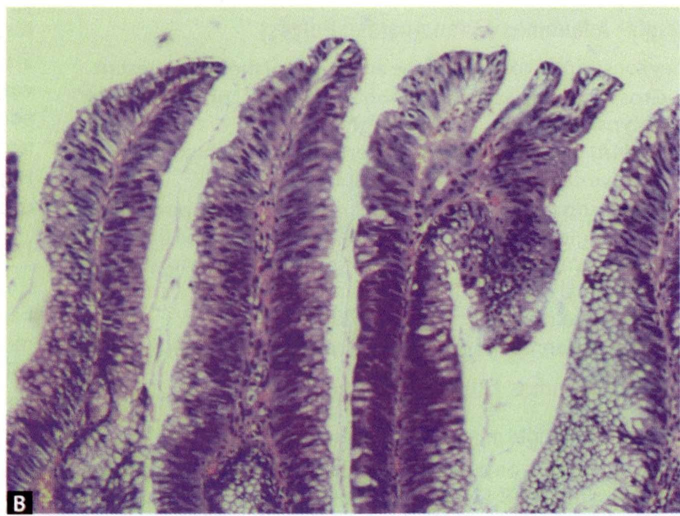

Figs. 18.45A and B: Villous adenoma: (A) Diagrammatic; (B) Thin, long, finger-like projections covered by dysplastic epithelium.

Number of polyps: A minimum of **100 polyps are necessary for a diagnosis** of FAP.

Sites of polyp: Adenomas occur throughout the colorectum.

Nature of polyp: FAP-associated polyps are morphologically indistinguishable from sporadic adenomas.

Progression to colonic adenocarcinoma: All untreated FAP patients **develop colorectal adenocarcinoma**, often before age 30. Prophylactic colectomy prevents colorectal cancer.

Variants of FAP

- **Gardner syndrome**: When the **extraintestinal manifestations of FAP are prominent**, the condition is known as Gardner syndrome. The extraintestinal lesions include **osteomas of the mandible, skull, and long bones, epidermal cysts, desmoid tumors in the abdominal wall, thyroid tumors, etc.**
- **Turcot syndrome:** It is a rare syndrome characterized by **colonic adenomas** with **tumors of the central nervous system** (particularly medulloblastomas).

Hereditary Nonpolyposis Colorectal Cancer

Hereditary nonpolyposis colorectal cancer (HNPCC) is also known as *Lynch syndrome* is transmitted as an **autosomal dominant** condition. "Nonpolyposis" means that colorectal cancer can occur when only a small number (not in large numbers) of polyps are present (or polyps are not present at all). **Despite the name hereditary nonpolyposis** colorectal cancer, **adenomas do develop** (though not in large numbers) in HNPCC patients.

Increased risk of cancers in HNPCC syndrome: Hereditary nonpolyposis colorectal cancer is associated with an increased risk of colorectal cancer as well as an increased risk of other epithelial cancers at several sites.

- **Colorectal cancer (***refer* **page 636):** HNPCC patients develop colonic cancer at **younger ages** than sporadic type and are often found in the **right proximal colon**. HNPCC-associated carcinoma is relatively nonaggressive, despite being poorly differentiated and mucinous type.
- **Extra-colonic cancers:** These include **cancers of the endometrium, ovary, stomach and small intestines, and urinary bladder.**

Genetics and Molecular Pathogenesis of HNPCC

Germline Mutations in DNA Mismatch Repair (MMR) Genes

HNPCC is caused by **germline (inherited) mutations** in one of the **DNA mismatch repair (MMR) genes.**

- **Mismatch repair (MMR) genes:** There are about six MMR genes. These are designated as *hMSH2, hMSH6, hMLH1, hMLH3, hPMS1, and hPMS2,* but the majority of HNPCC cases involve two genes namely—***MSH2 and MLH1.***
- **Normal function of MMR:** The MMR genes **encode proteins involved in the detection, excision, and repair of errors that occur during the replication of DNA.**
- **Mutation of *MMR* gene:** Mismatch repair genes **act as tumor suppressors.** The loss of both copies of the MMR genes results in uncontrolled growth and, ultimately, neoplastic transformation. HNPCC patients inherit one defective copy of an MMR gene, and the second copy of the MMR gene is lost or inactivated as a somatic event. Loss of the second MMR gene often occurs due to methylation of the gene promoter.

Microsatellite Instability (MSI)

Microsatellites: Simple repetitive sequences of nucleotides are termed microsatellites.

Microsatellite instability: The **appearance of abnormally long** (due to an increase in the number of nucleotide repeats) **or short** (due to a decrease in the number of nucleotide repeats) **microsatellites in a DNA** (in normal tissue versus tumor) is referred to as **microsatellite instability** (MSI). **One result of defective DNA MMR** gene is **microsatellite instability (MSI)** and MSI occurs in about 90% of cancers in HNPCC.

- **Groups of MSI**: It is divided into three groups depending on the alterations in microsatellite length: MSI-High (MSI-H), MSI-Low (MSI-L), and MS-Stable (MS-S).

COLORECTAL ADENOCARCINOMA

PA 24.7 (CC): Describe the etiology, pathogenesis, pathology, and distinguishing features of carcinoma of the colon.

Adenocarcinoma of the colon (colorectal carcinoma) is the **most common malignant tumor of the GI tract**. Colon cancer is the third most common cause of death due to cancer. The small intestine is an uncommon site for benign and malignant tumors. World Health Organization (WHO) (2019) (abridged) classification of epithelial tumors of the colon and rectum is presented in **Box 18.16**.

Q. Classify tumors of the large intestine.

BOX 18.16: World Health Organization (WHO) (2019) (abridged) classification of epithelial tumors of the colon and rectum.

Benign epithelial tumors and precursors
- Colorectal serrated lesions and polyps
  - Hyperplastic polyp
  - Sessile serrated lesion
  - Sessile serrated lesion with dysplasia
  - Traditional serrated adenoma
- Conventional colorectal adenoma
  - Tubular adenoma, low grade
  - Tubular adenoma, high grade
  - Villous adenoma, low-grade
  - Villous adenoma, high-grade
  - Tubulovillous adenoma, low grade
  - Tubulovillous adenoma, high grade
  - Advanced adenoma
- Inflammatory bowel disease-associated dysplasia of the colorectum

Malignant epithelial tumors
- Colorectal adenocarcinoma
  - Serrated adenocarcinoma
  - Adenoma-like adenocarcinoma
  - Micropapillary adenocarcinoma
  - Mucinous adenocarcinoma
  - Signet-ring cell carcinoma
  - Adenosquamous carcinoma
- Colorectal neuroendocrine neoplasms

Etiology and Risk Factors (Box 18.17)

Q. Write a short note on the etiopathogenesis (including molecular changes) of carcinoma of the colon.

The rate of colorectal cancer has increased significantly, probably because of changes in lifestyle and diet.

Dietary Factors

Dietary Factors that Increase the Risk

The etiology of most cases of colorectal cancer appears to be related to environmental factors. Dietary factors are closely associated with increased colorectal cancer rates.

- **Low intake of dietary fiber (unabsorbable vegetable fiber):** It is associated with decreased stool bulk that leads to **slower transit of fecal contents** through the colon and altered composition of the intestinal microbiota. These changes may **increase the synthesis of toxic oxidative** by-products of bacterial metabolism, which **remains in contact with the colonic mucosa for longer periods**. The dietary fiber may bind to potential mutagens and dilute their concentration by increasing stool bulk. However, studies have *failed* to show any value for dietary fiber in preventing the recurrence of colorectal adenomas or the development of colorectal cancer.
- **High intake of refined carbohydrates and fat:** High level of animal fat (found in red meats and processed meat) in the diet is associated with an **increased incidence of colorectal cancer.** High-fat intake increases the hepatic synthesis and secretion of bile into the intestine. The contents present in the bile such as cholesterol and bile acids can be converted into carcinogens by intestinal

BOX 18.17: Risk factors for colorectal cancer.

Dietary factors
- Factors that increase the risk
  - Fiber
  - Animal fat
  - Insulin resistance
  - Deficiencies of vitamins A, C and E
- Factors that reduce the risk
  - Diets rich in cruciferous vegetables (e.g., cauliflower, Brussels sprouts, and cabbage) and vitamin A
  - Protective effect of aspirin or other NSAIDs

Hereditary factors and syndromes
- Familial adenomatous polyposis (polyposis coli)
- MYH-associated polyposis
- Nonpolyposis syndrome (Lynch syndrome)

Inflammatory bowel disease: Ulcerative colitis and Crohn disease

Others
- *Streptococcus bovis* bacteremia
- Increasing age
- Family history of colonic cancer in a first-degree relative.
- Prior colorectal cancer

Flowchart 18.2: Sequence of events due to ingestion of animal fat involved in the risk of colorectal cancer.

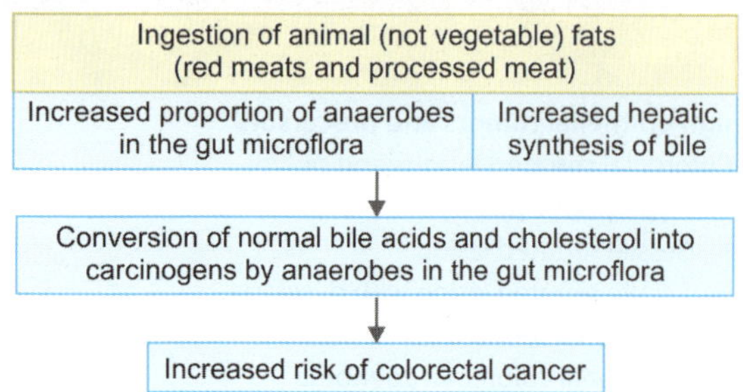

bacteria. The sequence of events due to the ingestion of animal fat involved in the risk of colorectal cancer is presented in **Flowchart 18.2**.

- **Insulin resistance:** Increased calorie intake along with physical inactivity is associated with a higher prevalence of obesity. Obese individuals develop insulin resistance and increased circulating levels of insulin. This leads to higher circulating concentrations of insulin-like growth factor type I (IGF-I). IGF-I may stimulate the proliferation of the intestinal mucosa.

Dietary Factors that Reduce the Risk

- **Diets rich in cruciferous vegetables** (e.g., cauliflower, Brussels sprouts, and cabbage) and **vitamin A** may be associated with a lower incidence of colorectal cancer. Deficiencies of vitamins A, C, and E, which act as antioxidants (free-radical scavengers) may increase the damage caused by oxidants.
- **Protective effect of aspirin or other NSAIDs**: Pharmacologic chemoprevention by ingestion of therapeutic agents, such as aspirin or other nonsteroidal anti-inflammatory drugs (NSAIDs) may reduce the risk of colorectal cancer. It may be due to these agents causing inhibition of the enzyme cyclooxygenase-2 (COX-2), which is highly expressed in 90% of colorectal carcinomas and 40–90% of adenomas. COX-2 is required to produce prostaglandin E_2, which promotes epithelial cell proliferation, particularly after injury.

Hereditary Factors and Syndromes (Refer Online Table 18.10)

A family history of colorectal cancer is found in up to 25% of patients which suggests the possibility of a hereditary predisposition. Inherited colorectal cancers can be divided into two main groups: (i) uncommon polyposis syndromes and (ii) the more common nonpolyposis syndromes.

1. **Familial adenomatous polyposis (polyposis coli/ familial polyposis of the colon)**: Familial adenomatous polyposis (FAP) is a rare **autosomal dominant** inherited syndrome characterized by the appearance of thousands of adenomatous polyps (adenomas) throughout the colorectum (**Fig. 18.46**) as well as numerous **extracolonic manifestations.** It is caused by **germ-line** inactivation (5q) **mutations** of the ***adenomatous polyposis coli (APC)*** **gene**. Colectomy should be performed as the primary therapy/prevention. **If the polyposis is not treated surgically, colorectal cancer will develop in almost all patients** aged <40. It is discussed on page 633-4.

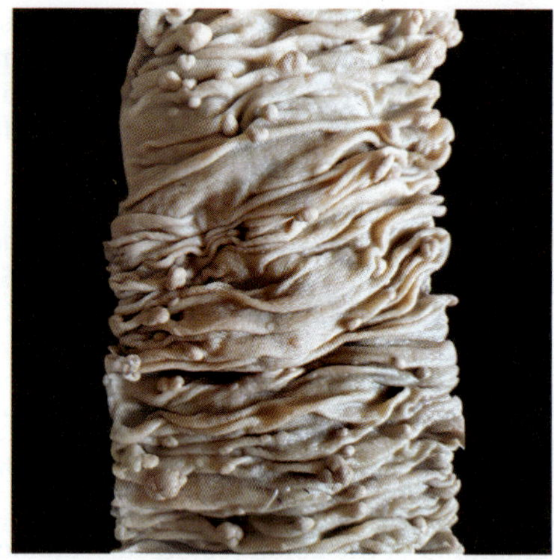

Fig. 18.46: Familial adenomatous polyposis with numerous polyps in the colon.

2. ***MYH*-associated polyposis (MAP):** It is a rare autosomal recessive condition caused by to **mutation in the *MUTYH* gene**. This condition may be one of the risk factors for colorectal cancer occurring in younger individuals.
3. **Hereditary nonpolyposis colorectal cancer (HNPCC):** HNPCC is also known as *Lynch syndrome* and is transmitted as an autosomal dominant condition. **Despite the name** hereditary **nonpolyposis** colorectal cancer, **adenomas do develop** (though not in large numbers) in HNPCC patients. **Colon cancers** in HNPCC patients **develop at younger ages** than sporadic colon cancers and are often found in the **right colon** (*refer* page 634).

The colonic adenocarcinoma may evolve from the pre-existing adenomas, referred to as the adenoma-carcinoma sequence discussed below (*refer* pages 637-8) under pathogenesis.

Inflammatory Bowel Disease

Patients with long-standing inflammatory bowel disease (IBD) have an increased risk of colorectal cancer. Cancers develop more commonly in patients with ulcerative colitis than in those with Crohn disease. In the case of ulcerative colitis, the risk is higher in younger patients with pancolitis.

Other Factors

- ***Streptococcus bovis*** **bacteremia:** Patients who develop endocarditis or septicemia from this fecal bacterium have been found to have a high incidence of occult colorectal tumors. The reason is unknown.

BOX 18.18: Precancerous lesions of the colon (large intestine).

- Hereditary cancer syndromes
- Familial adenomatous polyposis (FAP)
- Gardner syndrome, hereditary nonpolyposis colorectal cancer (HNPCC) (Lynch syndrome)
- Inflammatory bowel disease, especially chronic extensive ulcerative colitis
- Sporadic adenomatous polyps, especially villous and tubulovillous polyps

- **Increasing age:** It is the most important risk factor. Risk is low before age 40 and it increases steadily to age 50, after which it doubles with each decade.
- **Family history of colonic cancer** in a first-degree relative.
- **Prior colorectal cancer:** It increases the risk for a subsequent tumor.
- **Tobacco smoking:** Cigarette smoking is linked to the development of colorectal adenomas, particularly after >35 years of tobacco use. No biological explanation for this association has yet been proposed.
- **Alcohol consumption and obesity.**

Precancerous lesions of the colon (large intestine) are listed in **Box 18.18**.

Q. List the precancerous conditions of carcinoma colon.

Pathogenesis

Most colorectal cancers develop from the **combination of multiple molecular alterations**. They can be mainly divided into: (1) **genetic abnormalities** (that **activate oncogenes** or **inactivate tumor suppressor genes**) and (2) **epigenetic abnormalities**.

Genetic Pathways

Two distinct genetic pathways have been described: (i) the APC/β-catenin pathway (classic adenoma-carcinoma sequence), and (ii) the microsatellite instability pathway. Both pathways are characterized by the **stepwise accumulation of multiple mutations**. However, the genes involved and the mechanisms of the mutations are different.

APC/β-catenin Pathway (Adenoma-carcinoma Sequence)

Q. Write a short note on adenoma-carcinoma sequences in colonic carcinoma.

Most colorectal cancers (regardless of etiology) arise from adenomatous polyps. The classic adenoma-carcinoma sequence is seen in **about 80% of sporadic colonic cancers. According to this pathway, the morphologic progression in a specific step-wise sequence from normal mucosa to adenoma to invasive cancer** is accompanied by a **series of multiple molecular alterations** (at least 8–10 mutational events). Invasive cancers develop more frequently in sessile, serrated (i.e., "flat") polyps and villous adenomas.

1. **Inactivation of *APC* tumor suppressor gene (Figs. 18.47A to C)**
   - **Normal function of APC:** The adenomatous polyposis coli (*APC*) gene is a **member of the class of tumor suppressor genes** present on the short arm of chromosome 5 (*APC* locus 5q21), and it produces APC protein. **APC** is an important **negative regulator of β-catenin,** a component **of the WNT signaling pathway.** Normally, the product of the *APC* gene (APC protein) binds to and causes degradation of β-catenin and prevents the proliferation of cells.

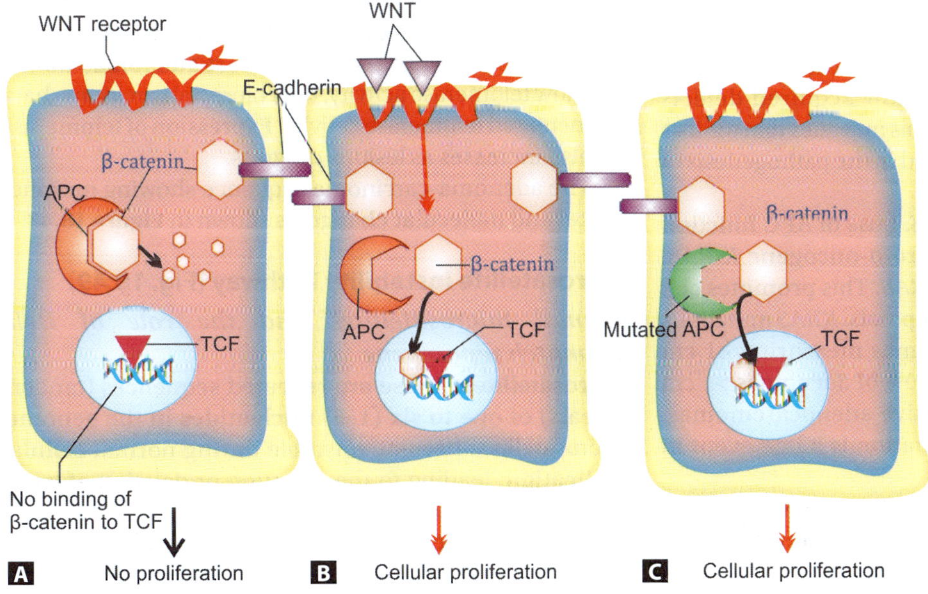

Figs. 18.47A to C: Role of APC in regulating the β-catenin. APC and β-catenin are components of the WNT signaling pathway. (A) In resting cells, β-catenin forms a complex with APC protein. This complex destroys β-catenin; (B) When cells are stimulated by WNT molecules, the β-catenin is not destroyed and its cytoplasmic levels increase. β-catenin translocate to the nucleus, where it binds to TCF, a transcription factor that activates cell cycle progression; (C) When *APC* is mutated or absent, the β-catenin cannot be destroyed and the cell enters the cell cycle.

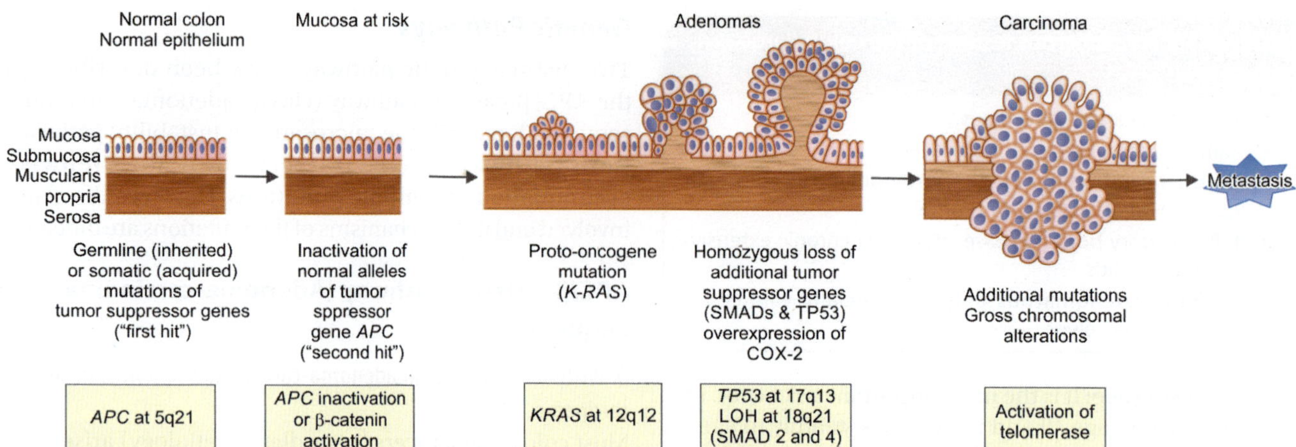

Fig. 18.48: Adenoma-carcinoma sequence showing morphological and molecular changes. Loss of one normal copy of the tumor suppressor gene *APC* occurs early. Individuals with familial adenomatous polyposis are born with one mutant allele of the *APC* gene. These individuals are extremely prone to the development of colon cancer. This mutation is followed by mutations of *K-RAS, SMAD2,* and *SMAD4*, and the tumor suppressor gene *TP53*. Later in the sequence, activation of telomerase leads to the formation of cancer.

(APC: adenomatous polyposis coli; COX-2: cyclooxygenase-2; LOH: loss of heterozygosity).

- **Inactivation of both copies of the *APC* gene:** For the development of adenoma, both copies of the *APC* gene must be functionally inactivated. This inactivation may be either by mutation or epigenetic silencing (by methylation). This causes the absence of production of APC protein. Lack of APC protein (which normally binds to β-catenin) leads to the **accumulation of β-catenin**. The accumulated β-catenin translocate to the nucleus and forms a complex with TCF. This **activates the transcription of genes, such as those encoding MYC and cyclin D1, that promote proliferation.** Thus, with the loss of APC function, cells behave as if they are being continuously stimulated by WNT. One of the syndromes associated with APC inactivation is familial adenomatous polyposis (*refer* pages 633 and 636). Apart from hereditary forms of colon cancer, 70–80% of nonfamilial colorectal carcinomas and sporadic adenomas also show acquired defects involving both *APC* genes. This indicates that the loss of function of APC is involved in the pathogenesis of colonic tumors.

2. **Activating mutations in *K-RAS*: Loss of APC function is followed by mutations in proto-oncogene *K-RAS*, which results in oncogene *K-RAS*.** This **promotes cell proliferation and prevents apoptosis.** *KRAS* mutations occur in about 10% of adenomas measuring <1 cm in diameter but are found in 50% of adenomas >1 cm in diameter and 50% of invasive adenocarcinomas. This indicates that ***K-RAS* mutation is a late event** in neoplastic progression.
3. **Mutations in other tumor suppressor genes:** Following tumor suppressor genes may be inactivated by **chromosomal deletions.**
   - ***SMAD2* and *SMAD4* mutations: *SMAD2* and *SMAD4*** are **tumor suppressor genes.** Mutations in these genes may develop as the neoplasm progresses. These genes encode effectors of TGF-β signaling. Normally, TGF-β signaling is a potent inhibitor of cell proliferation. The loss of these tumor suppressor genes may lead to uncontrolled cell proliferation.
   - **Mutation of *TP53*: *TP53* is a tumor-suppressor gene. It is mutated in 70–80% of colon cancers,** but its mutation is uncommon in adenomas. This suggests that *TP53* mutations also occur at late stages of tumor progression.
4. **Activation of telomerase:** Telomere plays a role in stabilizing the chromosome. It shortens with each cell division until cell senescence develops (*refer* pages 247-8). Telomerase is required to maintain telomere stability and hence cell immortality. Most adenomas do not show telomerase activity, but colorectal carcinoma have increased telomerase activity. **Expression of telomerase** also increases as lesions progress.

The adenoma-carcinoma sequence showing morphological and molecular changes is shown in **Figure 18.48.**

Microsatellite Instability Pathway (Fig. 18.49)

Normal microsatellites and the role of DNA mismatch repair gene

Microsatellites: These are repeated sequences (tandem repeats) of **one to six (1–6) nucleotides in the genome.** Microsatellites become **unstable during normal cellular replication,** leading to the insertion or deletion of bases within these regions.

DNA mismatch repair (MMR) genes: They **rapidly correct the errors that occur in microsatellites and maintain**

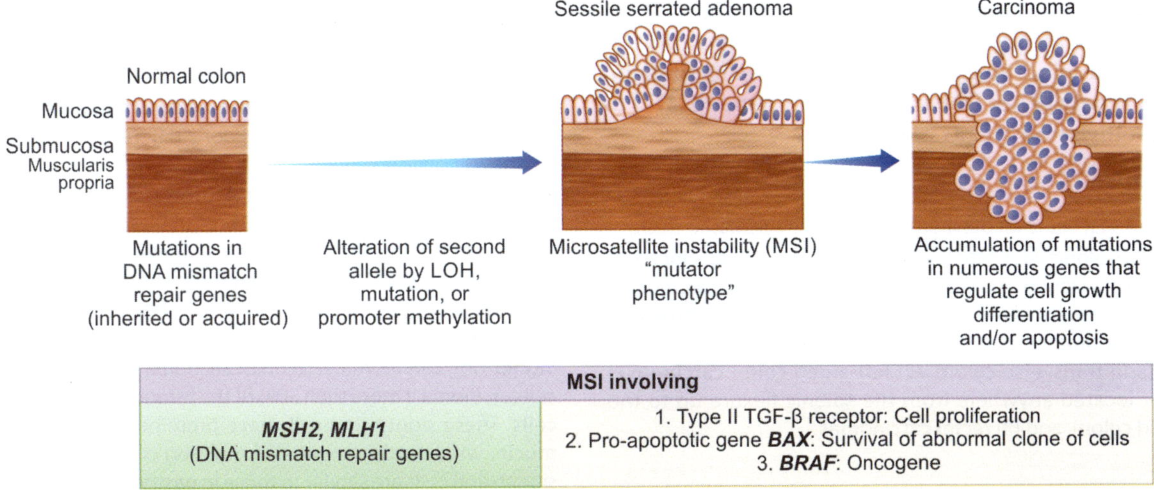

Fig. 18.49: Morphological and molecular changes in the microsatellite instability pathway of colon carcinogenesis. Defects in mismatch repair genes result in microsatellite instability. This leads to the accumulation of mutations in numerous genes involved in cell survival and proliferation.

(LOH: loss of heterozygosity; TGF-β: transforming growth factor beta).

microsatellite length. About six **mismatch repair (MMR) genes** have been identified, which are designated as *hMSH2, hMSH6, hMLH1, hMLH3, hPMS1,* and *hPMS2* (*refer* HNPCC in pages 634 and 636).

Microsatellite instability (MSI)

Microsatellite instability: The **appearance of abnormally long** (due to an increase in the number of nucleotide repeats) **or short** (due to a decrease in the number of nucleotide repeats) **microsatellites in a DNA** (in normal tissue versus tumor) is referred to as **microsatellite instability** (MSI). Molecular alterations of MSI are common in sessile serrated lesions and cancers that arise from them.

Cause of microsatellite instability (MSI): MSI may be due to mutations in DNA mismatch repair genes or hypermethylation of the promoter region of the mismatch repair genes such as MLH*1*.

1. **Loss of DNA mismatch repair genes: One result of defective DNA MMR gene is microsatellite instability (MSI).** In patients with DNA mismatch repair deficiency due to loss of mismatch repair genes, mutations accumulate in microsatellite repeats. This **mutation accumulations in microsatellite repeats are referred to as microsatellite instability** (MSI).
   - **Consequences of microsatellite instability:** Microsatellites are typically located in noncoding regions. However, some microsatellite sequences are in the coding or promoter region of genes involved in the regulation of cell growth. **Mutations in microsatellite sequences located in noncoding regions are generally silent**. However, **mutations of microsatellite sequences located in the coding or promoter regions of genes can produce cancer.** For example, **microsatellite instability** involving:
     - **Type II TGF-β receptor:** Normally, **TGF-β** inhibits colonic epithelial cell proliferation, and type II TGF-β receptor mutation can lead to uncontrolled cell growth.
     - **Pro-apoptotic gene *BAX*:** Its mutation can lead to loss of *BAX*, which may increase the survival of genetically abnormal clones of cells.
2. **CpG island hypermethylation phenotype (CIMP):** This is a subset of colon cancers with microsatellite instability in which there are **no mutations in DNA mismatch repair enzymes**. In these tumors, there is **hypermethylation of the *MLH1* promoter region.** This reduces MLH1 expression and repair function. These features constitute the CpG island hypermethylation phenotype (CIMP). These tumors commonly have **activating mutations in the *BRAF* oncogene**. *KRAS* and *TP53* are not usually mutated. **CpG sites or CG sites** are regions of DNA where a cytosine (C) nucleotide is followed by a guanine(G) nucleotide in the linear sequence of bases along its 5′ to 3′ direction (In the DNA segment, the 5′ to 3′ directions indicate down the left strand and up the right strand).

Thus, a combination of microsatellite instability, *BRAF* mutation, and methylation of specific targets, such as *MLH1*, are seen in this pathway of carcinogenesis.

Epigenetic Abnormalities

Epigenetics is a **reversible, heritable alteration in gene expression that occurs without mutation**. It is unrelated to the gene nucleotide sequence. Epigenetic changes involve histone modification and DNA methylation, both of which affect gene expression. The most common is methylation-induced gene silencing which may enhance progression along both the genetic pathways (i.e., *APC/β-catenin pathway and microsatellite instability pathway).* Another example of epigenetic mechanisms is the **silencing of DNA repair genes** (mismatch-repair gene MLH1) **by hypermethylation** of CpG island.

MORPHOLOGY

Q. Write a short note on the morphology of the carcinoma colon.

Location: Colonic adenocarcinomas can be found in **any location** of the colon. Depending on the location, colorectal carcinomas can be divided into three groups: (1) **Right-sided or proximal colon carcinomas** (includes those arising in the cecum, ascending colon, and transverse colon), (2) **left-sided colon carcinomas** (cancer located anywhere from the splenic flexure up to the sigmoid colon), and (3) **rectal carcinomas.**

Gross

Types: Gross appearances of colonic carcinomas are variable. Grossly colonic carcinomas can be categorized into three general types:

1. **Exophytic polypoid mass in the right side of the colon (Fig. 18.50A):** Tumors in the proximal colon usually grow into the lumen as bulky, **exophytic (cauliflower-like), polypoid masses.** They extend along one wall of the cecum and ascending colon. They rarely cause intestinal obstruction. They have a sharp dividing line with the normal bowel.
2. **Annular and constricting tumors in the left-side of the colon (Fig. 18.50C):** Carcinomas in the distal colon are annular lesions that produce the characteristic **"napkin-ring"** or **"apple core" constrictions** and luminal narrowing. It **may be associated with intestinal obstruction** and dilatation with attenuation and flattening of the mucosal folds of the colon proximal to the tumor. The tumors are firm due to associated desmoplasia.
3. **Infiltrative and ulcerating tumors (Fig. 18.50B):** These cancers are **usually raised, have irregular edges,** and have a **central, excavated ulcerated area** that often infiltrates the deep layers of the bowel wall. The ulcerated tumors show rolled edges extending around the circumference of the colon.

Cross-section: On the cross-section, the gray–white tumor tissue may be seen replacing the bowel wall. The edges of the tumor may be well demarcated or may show finger-like projections extending from the main tumor mass. Highly mucinous tumors produce a gelatinous, glaring appearance, and layers of mucus may be seen separating the layers of the bowel wall.

Microscopy (Figs. 18.51A and B)

Adenocarcinoma NOS (not otherwise specified): The majority (90%) of colonic cancers are **adenocarcinomas** and are similar on microscopic examination. Most cases are diagnosed as adenocarcinoma not otherwise specified (NOS).

- **Differentiation:** Adenocarcinoma may be **well-differentiated (grade I), moderately (grade II), or poorly differentiated (grade III).**
- **Microscopic features:** Most of the tumors show **glands of variable size and configuration** separated by a moderate amount of stroma. The glands are composed of tall columnar cells that resemble dysplastic epithelium found in adenomas.
- The **lumen** of the glands is usually **filled with inspissated eosinophilic mucus** and **nuclear and cellular debris ("dirty" necrosis). Mitotic figures are usually abundant.** The **invasive component of these tumors may show stromal desmoplasia and cause firm consistency.** Poorly differentiated carcinoma shows only a few glands.

Mucinous adenocarcinomas: A tumor is called mucinous adenocarcinoma if more than 50% of the lesion is composed of abundant pools of extracellular mucin. These mucins are secreted by tumor cells that accumulate within the intestinal wall and are associated with poor prognosis. This is because mucin aids in tumor extension.

Signet-ring carcinoma: A colonic carcinoma is called a signet-ring cell carcinoma if more than 50% of the tumor cells are **signet-ring cells.** These signet-ring cells have prominent intracytoplasmic mucin, with displacement and molding of the nucleus. These signet-ring cells are similar to those in gastric cancer. Carcinomas with signet-ring cells in less than 50% of the tumor are called adenocarcinomas with a signet-ring cell component.

Clinical Features

Q. Differences between the carcinoma of the colon on the right and left side.

Colorectal cancers develop slowly and may therefore not be detected for long periods.

- **Cancers in the cecum and other right-sided colon:** These cancers may grow large without causing obstruction, especially in the cecum, where the lumen is large and fecal contents are liquid. They usually present with **fatigue and weakness** due to **iron deficiency anemia**. Thus, iron deficiency anemia in an older man or postmenopausal woman must **be considered due to GI cancer until otherwise proven**.
- **Left-sided colorectal cancers:** These tumors may produce narrowing of the lumen, and feces are more solid, often constrict the lumen, and produce **obstructive symptoms.** These include changes in bowel habits (**altered bowel habits**), cramping left lower quadrant discomfort, and abdominal pain. They may cause **occult bleeding** (occult blood and **bright red blood** in the feces may occur if carcinoma is in the distal colorectum). Colorectal cancers may **perforate** early, leading to peritonitis.

Methods of investigation of colon cancer: These include the following:

1. **Occult blood loss in the stool by Guaiac test.** A positive test for fecal occult blood suggests the presence of cancer or an adenoma in 50% of cases.
2. **Tumor markers: Elevated levels of carcinoembryonic antigen (CEA) and CA 19-9.**
3. **Flexible sigmoidoscopy**

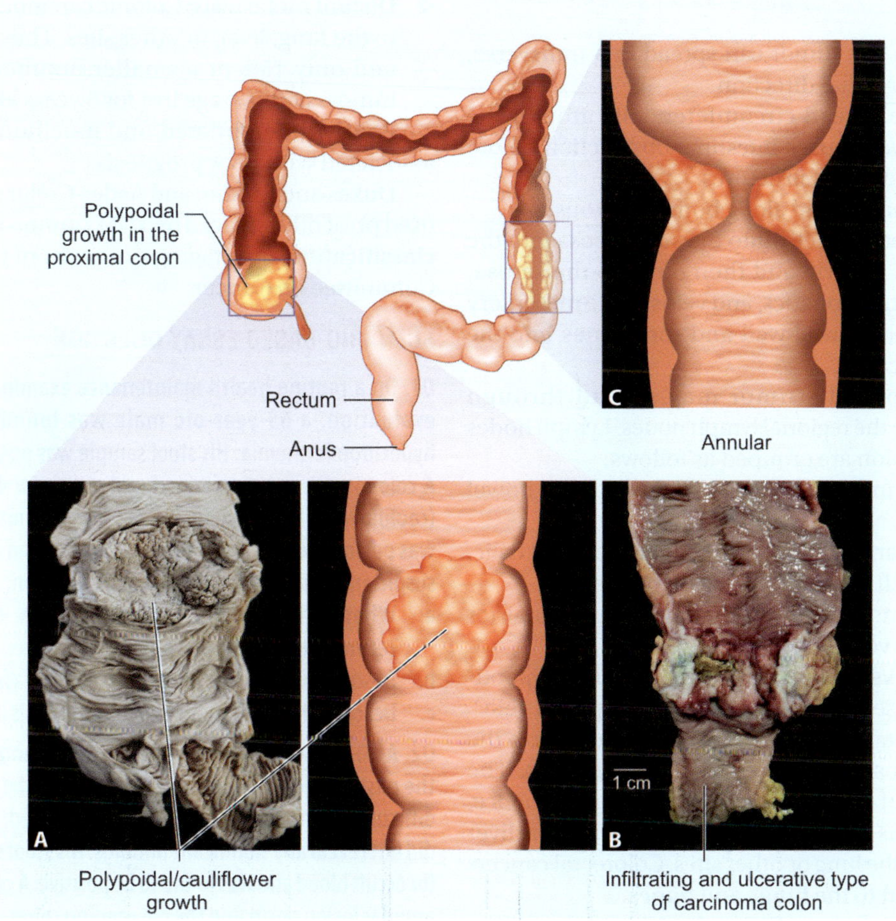

Figs. 18.50A to C: Common macroscopic varieties of carcinoma of the colon: (A) Exophytic/cauliflower/polypoidal in the right colon (specimen and diagrammatic representation of the same). Carcinoma of the proximal colon is usually polypoidal and exophytic. (B) Infiltrating and ulcerative (gross specimen), and (C) annular (diagrammatic). Carcinoma of the distal colon is usually annular.

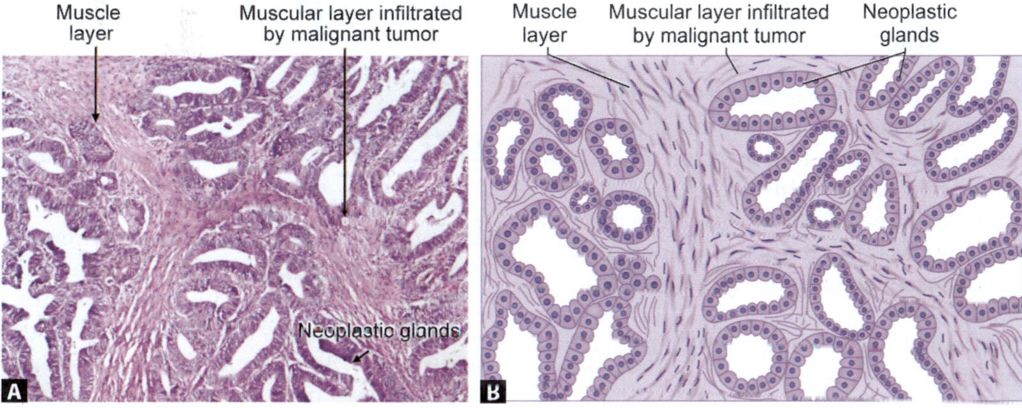

Figs. 18.51A and B: Adenocarcinoma of the colon composed of tumor cells arranged in glandular pattern: (A) H & E photomicrograph; (B) Diagrammatic.

4. **Fiberoptic colonoscopy** helps in direct visualization of cancer and may be used to take a biopsy. It is the investigation of choice.
5. **Radiology:**
   - **Double-contrast barium enema:** It is the radiological investigation of choice when colonoscopy is contraindicated. It characteristically shows an **"apple core" appearance.**
   - **Ultrasonography:** Used as a screening investigation for liver metastases.
   - **Spiral CT:** In elderly patients when contrast enemas or colonoscopy are not diagnostic or are contraindicated.

Spread

- **Direct spread:** The tumor can spread in a transverse, longitudinal, or radial direction.
  - **Transverse spread** circumferentially around the intestinal wall causes intestinal obstruction before it invades adjacent structures.
  - **Longitudinal spread** along both directions.
  - **Radial spread** directly into the submucosa into the muscularis propria and then out into the serosa, pericolic fat, lymphatics, and veins in the mesentery alongside the bowel wall and sometimes into the peritoneal cavity.
- **Lymphatic spread:** Tumor may spread through lymphatics into the regional lymph nodes. Lymph nodes draining the colon are grouped as follows:
  - N1: Nodes in the immediate vicinity of the bowel wall.
  - N2: Nodes arranged along the ileocolic, right colic, midcolic, left colic and sigmoid arteries.
  - N3: Apical nodes around the superior and inferior mesenteric vessels.
- **Blood spread: Venous invasion** may give rise to blood-borne metastases in the **liver** (through a portal vein). Because of portal drainage of the colon, the liver is the most common site of distant metastatic lesions. The rectum does not drain via the portal circulation; hence, anal carcinomas that metastasize often bypass the liver and deposit in the lung or other sites. Colorectal cancers may also spread to the **lungs and bones.**
- **Transcoelomic spread:** Rarely, it can spread by dislodging tumor cells from the serosa of the bowel or via the subperitoneal lymphatics to other structures within the peritoneal cavity.

Staging and Prognosis

Q. Write a short note on the staging of carcinoma of the colon.

Important prognostic factors: The two most important prognostic factors are: (i) depth of invasion and (ii) the presence or absence of lymph node metastases.

- **Depth of invasion**. Five-year survival rates for carcinoma limited to the mucosa (i.e., those that do not cross the muscularis mucosae) are approaching 100%, whereas the tumors that have invaded into the submucosa or muscularis propria it is 95% and 70–90%, respectively (for tumors limited to the primary site). Survival is further reduced for tumors that have invaded through the visceral serosal surface or into adjacent organs and tissues.
- **The presence of lymph node metastases:** It also reduces survival rate. Therefore, most patients with lymph node metastases are given radiation or chemotherapy. In some patients, these treatments are given before the resection of the primary tumor. This process is termed neoadjuvant therapy.
- **Distant metastasis**: Colonic carcinoma can metastasize to the lung, liver, or other sites. They limit the survival, and only 15% or a smaller number of patients with tumors at this stage live for 5 years after diagnosis.

Poorly differentiated and mucinous carcinomas are associated with poor prognosis.

Dukes and Kirklin, and Astler-Coller staging were being used presently replaced by **TNM (tumor-nodes-metastasis) classification** and staging system from the American Joint Committee on Cancer.

SCENARIO-BASED ESSAY QUESTION

Q1. On a routine health maintenance examination and laboratory evaluation, a 65-year-old male was found to have microcytic hypochromic anemia. His stool sample was positive for occult blood. A colonoscopy was performed and showed a 4 cm bulky, exophytic (cauliflower-like), polypoid lesion projecting into the cecum. A biopsy was performed and a microscopic examination confirmed the clinical suspicion. It was followed by colonic resection.

a. What is the probable diagnosis? (Ans: Carcinoma of colon/cecum—exophytic polypoid type).
b. Describe the etiopathogenesis of the disease *(refer pages 635-40)*.
c. Describe the morphological features of this lesion *(refer page 640)*.

Q2. A 70-year-old man complained of a change in bowel habits for the past one year. He also complained that the defecation was more difficult and the caliber of stools has decreased. Physical examination did not reveal any significant findings. His stool sample was examined for occult blood and was found to be positive. A colonoscopy showed an annular lesion encircling the descending colon. A biopsy examination confirmed the diagnosis and was followed by colonic resection.

a. What is the probable diagnosis? (Ans: Carcinoma of descending colon—annular type).
b. Describe the morphological features of this lesion *(refer page 640)*.
c. Mention the various methods of investigation of this condition *(refer pages 640-1)*.

ACUTE APPENDICITIS

Q. Write a short note on acute appendicitis.

The appendix is prone to acute and chronic inflammation. Acute appendicitis is an acute inflammatory process involving the appendix. **Acute appendicitis can occur in any age group but is most common in adolescents and young adults.** Acute appendicitis is a common abdominal surgical emergency.

Pathogenesis

The etiology of appendicitis is multifactorial and may involve obstruction, ischemia, infections, and hereditary factors.

- **Initiating event is a progressive increase in intraluminal pressure**: Acute appendicitis is thought to begin with luminal obstruction due to the factors, which progressively increase the intraluminal pressure.

The obstruction is usually caused by the small stone-like mass of stool, or *fecalith*, or less commonly, a gallstone, tumor, or mass of worms *(Oxyuriasis vermicularis)*.

- **Ischemic injury and stasis favor bacterial proliferation:** Increased intraluminal pressure compromises venous outflow. Ischemic injury and stasis of luminal contents favor bacterial proliferation and trigger an inflammatory response.
- **Inflammatory response**: Inflammation produces edema and neutrophilic infiltration of the lumen, muscular wall, and periappendiceal soft tissues. The pressure produced by inflammation and edema predisposes to the development of gangrene, perforation, and peritonitis.

MORPHOLOGY

Gross

The appendix may be **swollen and erythematous.**

The **serosa** initially appears dull and gray due to inflammatory reaction. Later, it may be **covered by a purulent exudate.**

Microscopy (Figs. 18.52A to C)

Mucosal neutrophils, erosion, and focal superficial ulceration: The early lesions may have these findings. But they are not specific.

Inflammation of lamina propria: Later, the inflammation extends into the lamina propria, and collections of neutrophils may also be seen in the lumen of the appendix.

Inflammation of muscularis propria is diagnostic: Diagnosis of acute appendicitis should be made when **muscularis propria shows infiltration by neutrophils.**

Congested subserosal vessels and neutrophilic infiltrate within all layers of the wall.

Complications

Acute suppurative appendicitis: In severe cases, neutrophilic exudate produces a fibrinopurulent reaction in the serosa. When focal abscesses develop within the wall, it is termed **acute suppurative appendicitis.**

Acute gangrenous appendicitis: When the appendix shows large areas of hemorrhagic ulceration and gangrenous necrosis that extend to the serosa, it is known as **acute gangrenous appendicitis.** Perforation secondary to gangrene can follow and form an abscess. This may rupture can also lead to suppurative peritonitis.

Clinical Features

Acute appendicitis presents with **pain in the periumbilical region**, which **ultimately moves to the right lower quadrant.** This is followed by **nausea, vomiting, low-grade fever, and mild leukocytosis.**

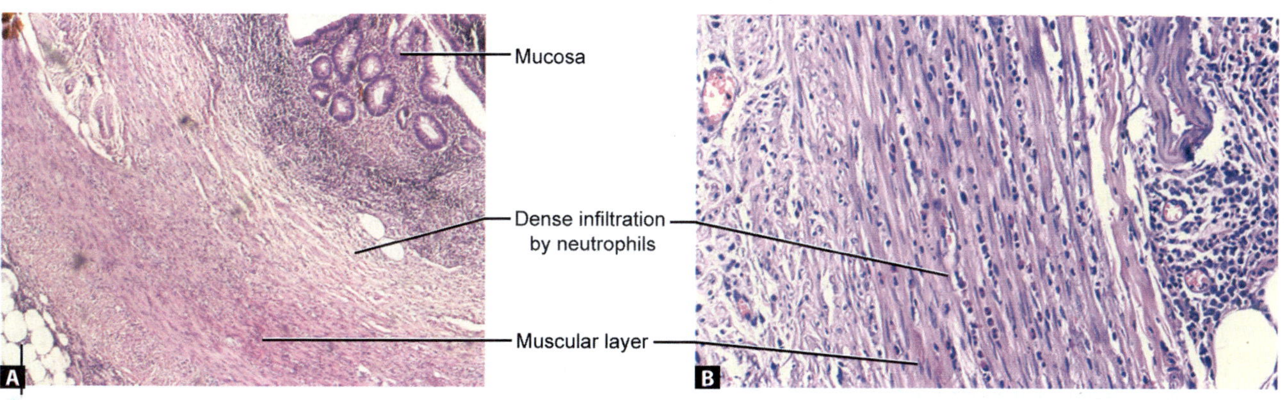

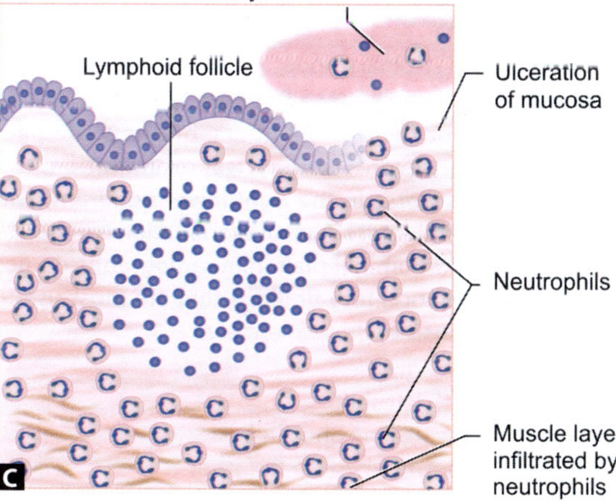

Acute appendicitis
Inflammation of muscularis propria is diagnostic.

Figs. 18.52A to C: (A) Photomicrograph (low power) of acute appendicitis showing inflammation of the mucosa, submucosa, and muscular layer; (B) (High power view) shows numerous neutrophils in the muscular layer; (C) Diagrammatic appearance of acute appendicitis.

McBurney's sign: A classic physical finding is a **deep tenderness located two-thirds of the distance from the umbilicus to the right anterior superior iliac spine** (McBurney's point).

Imaging studies: CT scanning helps narrow the differential diagnosis.

Complications: Gangrenous appendicitis, perforation, pyelophlebitis, portal venous thrombosis, liver abscess, and bacteremia. Worldwide, perforated appendicitis is the leading general surgical cause of death.

Laboratory findings in acute appendicitis: Raised WBC count, microscopic hematuria is common. Gross hematuria may indicate kidney stones.

SCENARIO-BASED MCQs

1. **A 42-year-old woman complains of sudden onset of severe mid-epigastric abdominal pain. She had a long history of heartburn and dyspepsia. On physical examination, the abdomen shows guarding and reduced bowel sounds. An abdominal plain film radiograph shows free air under the left diaphragm. She is immediately taken to operation theaters, and a perforated duodenal ulcer is repaired. The organisms that most likely produced these findings are:**

   A. *Giardia lamblia* B. *Helicobacter pylori*
   C. *Salmonella typhi* D. *Shigella flexneri*

2. **A 32-year-old man complains of epigastric pain for more than 1 year. The pain tends to occur 2–3 hours after a meal and is relieved by taking antacids or eating more food. The result of a urea breath test is positive, and a gastric biopsy specimen contains urease. The likely diagnosis is:**

   A. Peptic ulcer disease B. Carcinoid tumor
   C. Carcinoma stomach D. Autoimmune gastritis

3. **A 56-year-old woman complains of nausea, vomiting, and midepigastric pain for 6 months. The pain does not respond to antacids or H2-receptor antagonists. Physical examination does not reveal any significant findings. Laboratory studies show iron-deficiency anemia. An abdominal CT scan shows gastric outlet obstruction. An upper gastrointestinal endoscopy was performed. It shows an ulcerated 2 × 3 cm bulky mass in the antrum at the pylorus. A urease test is positive. A biopsy was performed on the mass. Most likely it shows microscopic features of:**

   A. Squamous cell carcinoma
   B. Adenocarcinoma
   C. Neuroendocrine carcinoma
   D. Non-Hodgkin lymphoma

4. **A 62-year-old woman complains of severe nausea, vomiting, early satiety, and a 7 kg weight loss over the past 5 months. On physical examination, she is pale and has muscle wasting. Laboratory studies show a microcytic, hypochromic anemia. On upper gastrointestinal endoscopy, the entire gastric mucosa is eroded with loss of rugosity. An abdominal CT scan shows a small and shrunken stomach. Microscopic examination of the gastric biopsy specimen is likely to show:**

   A. Chronic atrophic gastritis
   B. Primary gastric lymphoma
   C. Gastrointestinal stromal tumor
   D. Signet ring cell adenocarcinoma

5. **A 42-year-old woman complains of abdominal cramps and diarrhea with six stools per day for the past 1 month. She gives a history of similar episodes of self-limited pain and diarrhea, which have occurred multiple times during the past 12 years. Each episode used to last for about 2 weeks and resolves without treatment. Her stool sample is positive for occult blood. Laboratory studies do not show any ova or parasites in the stool. Colonoscopy shows diffuse, uninterrupted, bleeding, friable colonic mucosa, and superficial ulceration. It extends from the rectum to the ascending colon. Colonic biopsy from the affected area shows a diffuse, predominantly mononuclear infiltrate in the lamina propria along with a crypt abscess. She is at greatest risk for developing the following complications:**

   A. Adenocarcinoma B. Fat malabsorption
   C. Primary biliary cirrhosis D. Perirectal fistula formation

6. **A 26-year-old man complains of intermittent cramping abdominal pain and low-volume diarrhea for 3 weeks. On physical examination, mild lower abdominal tenderness was noticed without any mass, and bowel sounds were present. The stool was positive for occult blood. The symptoms subside within 1 week. Six months later, the abdominal pain recurs with perianal pain. On physical examination, there a perirectal fistula is detected. Colonoscopy shows many areas of mucosal edema and ulceration and some areas appear normal. Microscopically, a biopsy specimen from an ulcerated area shows a patchy acute and chronic inflammatory infiltrate, crypt abscesses, and noncaseating granulomas. The most likely underlying disease processes responsible for this presentation are:**

   A. Shigellosis B. Amebiasis
   C. Crohn disease D. Ulcerative colitis

7. **A 62-year-old man complains of progressive weakness and stools tinged with blood. His family members have noticed that he has become pale, and lost weight. On abdominal palpation, a fullness was observed in the right lower abdominal quadrant. Laboratory studies show iron-deficiency anemia and a hemoglobin value of 7.4 g/dL. The stool examination is positive for occult blood. A colonoscopy shows an elevated and centrally ulcerated lesion of the sigmoid colon. The most likely microscopic diagnosis of the lesion is:**

   A. Lymphoma
   B. Carcinoid tumor
   C. Adenocarcinoma
   D. Gastrointestinal stromal tumor

8. **An 18-year-old girl complains of nausea and vague lower abdominal pain for the past 24 hours, but now the pain has become more severe. On physical examination, the abdominal pain is worse in the right lower quadrant, and there is rebound tenderness. A stool examination is negative for occult blood. Abdominal plain film radiographs do not show free air. The laboratory findings that are most useful to aid in the diagnosis of this patient are:**

   A. Increased serum amylase
   B. Neutrophilia with left shift
   C. Increased serum alkaline phosphatase
   D. Entamoeba histolytica cysts in the stool

Answers and Explanation

1. **The answer is B: *Helicobacter pylori*.** These are not found in the duodenum, but they alter the microenvironment of the stomach, causing the stomach and duodenum to be susceptible to peptic ulcer disease. Almost all peptic ulcers in the duodenal are associated with *H. pylori infection*. In the present case, peptic ulcers have undergone perforation. The other organisms listed are not involved in the pathogenesis of peptic ulcer disease. They produce infectious diarrheal illnesses. *Salmonella typhi* may produce typhoid fever. It produces more systemic symptoms and the marked ulceration of Peyer patches may lead to perforation.
2. **The answer is A: Peptic ulcer disease.** The clinical symptoms suggest peptic ulcer disease and most of them are associated with *Helicobacter pylori infection*. These bacteria secrete urease, which can be detected by urea breath test. In the biopsy urease test is positive. Carcinoid tumors can rarely occur in the stomach, but they are not related to peptic ulcer disease. Peptic ulcers rarely progress to gastric carcinoma. Features, in this case, do not favor autoimmune gastritis
3. **Answer is C: Adenocarcinoma.** The most likely cause of a large mass in the stomach is gastric carcinoma which accounts for more than 95% of all malignant gastric tumors. Microscopically, it is an adenocarcinoma, likely to be the intestinal type found in the antral region. Adenocarcinoma is related to *Helicobacter pylori infection*. Squamous cell carcinomas usually occur in the esophagus. Neuroendocrine carcinomas are rare in the stomach. Non-Hodgkin lymphomas are less common and usually form bulky masses in the fundus.
4. **Answer is D: Signet ring cell adenocarcinoma.** The endoscopic and radiologic findings are in favor of the linitis plastica ("leather bottle") appearance of diffuse gastric carcinoma. In linitis plastica, no true tumor mass is seen macroscopically. Microscopically, these carcinomas are composed of tumor cells with a signet ring appearance. In these cells, the cytoplasmic mucin pushes the nucleus to one side. The invading tumor cells induce extensive fibrosis in the submucosa and muscularis of the stomach wall. In chronic atrophic gastritis, the rugal folds are lost, but there is no significant scarring or shrinkage of the stomach. Primary gastric lymphomas are less common than adenocarcinoma and they do not involve the stomach in a diffuse pattern. Gastrointestinal stromal tumors tend to produce bulky lesions.
5. **The answer is A: Adenocarcinoma.** Ulcerative colitis can cause relapsing and remitting episodes of low-volume diarrhea containing blood and mucus. It shows diffuse inflammation and ulceration of the rectal and colonic mucosa. One of the complications of ulcerative colitis is the development of colonic adenocarcinoma. Fat malabsorption usually does not occur in ulcerative colitis because the ileum is not involved. Ulcerative colitis is associated with several extraintestinal manifestations. These include sclerosing cholangitis but have no relationship to primary biliary cirrhosis. Perirectal fistula formation is usually seen in Crohn disease.
6. **The answer is C: Crohn disease.** The clinical and histologic features are suggestive of Crohn disease. Crohn disease is characterized by segmental bowel involvement and transmural inflammation that leads to strictures, adhesions, and fistula. Noncaseating granulomas are more typical of Crohn disease. Amebiasis and shigellosis are infectious processes that can cause mucosal ulceration, but they do not produce granulomas or fissures. Ulcerative colitis involves mucosa and in contrast to Crohn disease, the mucosal involvement is diffuse and does not show "skip areas." Fissures and fistulas are not frequent in ulcerative colitis.
7. **The answer is C: Adenocarcinoma.** Adenocarcinoma of the rectum or sigmoid colon usually presents as a circumferential mass that narrows the lumen of the intestine. Bleeding typically causes iron deficiency anemia. The microscopic appearance of the colorectal cancer is adenocarcinoma. In either case, Choices A, B, and D are mainly lesions involving the wall of the intestine.
8. **The answer is B: Neutrophilia with left shift.** This girl has acute appendicitis. This can be accompanied by a raised WBC count with neutrophilia and left shift. Increased serum amylase occurs in acute pancreatitis. The alkaline phosphatase level may be increased in conditions with obstruction of the biliary tract. Amebiasis is usually associated with a history of diarrhea, with blood in the stool.

Plummer vinson syndrome:
1. Iron deficiency anemia
2. Esophageal webs
4. Glossitis

Barrett's esophagus: Most important risk factor to the development of esophageal adenocarcinoma.

Histology: Gold standard for detection of *H. pylori*

Special stains for *H. pylori*:
- Non-silver stains (Giemsa, Diff Quick, Gimenez, Acridine orange)
- Silver stains (Warthin-Starry, Steiner, etc.)

Linitis plastica or leather bottle stomach: Diffuse involvement of the stomach in cancer.

Guaiac test: Used for occult blood loss in the stool

Krukenberg tumor:
- Metastasis of a signet ring carcinoma to both ovaries.
- In most cases, the primary tumor is in the stomach.

Inflammatory bowel disease:
- Crohn disease
- Ulcerative colitis

Pathogenesis of colonic cancer:
- APC/β-catenin pathway (classic adenoma carcinoma sequence)
- Microsatellite instability pathway.

CHAPTER 19

Hepatobiliary and Pancreatic Disorders

Chapter Outline

Liver
- Bilirubin Metabolism
- Jaundice
- Hepatic (Liver) Failure
- Viral Hepatitis
- Alcohol-related Liver Disease
- Nonalcoholic Fatty Liver Disease
- Cirrhosis
- Portal Hypertension
- Inherited Metabolic Liver Diseases
- Autoimmune Cholangiopathies
- Liver Abscesses
- Malignant Neoplasms of Liver
- Metastatic Tumors

Gallbladder
- Cholelithiasis (Gallstones)
- Cholecystitis
- Carcinoma of the Gallbladder

Pancreas
- Pancreatitis
- Pancreatic Carcinoma
- Interpretation of Liver Function and Viral Hepatitis Serology Panel

LIVER

BILIRUBIN METABOLISM (FIG. 19.1)

PA 25.1 (CC): Describe bilirubin metabolism, enumerate the etiology and pathogenesis of jaundice, and distinguish between direct and indirect hyperbilirubinemia.

Q. Write a short note on bilirubin metabolism.

Bilirubin Production

Sources of bilirubin: Bilirubin is the end product of heme degradation. Its sources are as follows:

- **Major** (85% = 0.2–0.3 g): It is derived from the **catabolism of hemoglobin** during the breakdown of senescent red cells by macrophages in the spleen, liver, and bone marrow.
- **Minor** (15–20%): It is derived from the turnover of hepatic heme or hemoproteins (e.g., the P-450 cytochromes) and from premature destruction of hemoglobin in developing red cell precursors in the bone marrow.

Bilirubin formation: Heme liberated from the above sources is oxidized to **biliverdin** by intracellular heme oxygenase. **Biliverdin** is immediately **reduced to bilirubin** by the enzyme biliverdin reductase. The bilirubin formed is known as **unconjugated bilirubin**.

Transport of Bilirubin (Bilirubin Binding)

Unconjugated bilirubin formed in the periphery is liberated into the circulation. This **unconjugated bilirubin** reversibly **binds to serum albumin** (albumin–bilirubin complex). Unconjugated bilirubin is **insoluble in aqueous solutions** at physiologic pH and is also highly toxic to tissues. The albumin carries unconjugated bilirubin and is transported to **the liver**.

Hepatic Processing of Bilirubin

Excretion of bilirubin from the body is one of the major functions of the liver. Metabolism of bilirubin in the liver consists of four separate but interrelated events:

- **Hepatic uptake from the circulation**: On reaching the sinusoidal plasma membrane of the hepatocyte, the unconjugated bilirubin (albumin–bilirubin complex) is dissociated and enters the hepatocytes.
- **Binding:** Within the hepatocyte, bilirubin binds to several proteins in the cytosol known collectively as **glutathione-S-transferases** (also termed ligandin).
- **Conjugation with glucuronic acid**: **Unconjugated bilirubin** (not water-soluble) combines with one or two molecules of glucuronic acid in the presence of uridine diphosphate (UDP)–glucuronyltransferase (UGT1A1) in the endoplasmic reticulum. It forms **water-soluble bilirubin diglucuronide (conjugated bilirubin).**

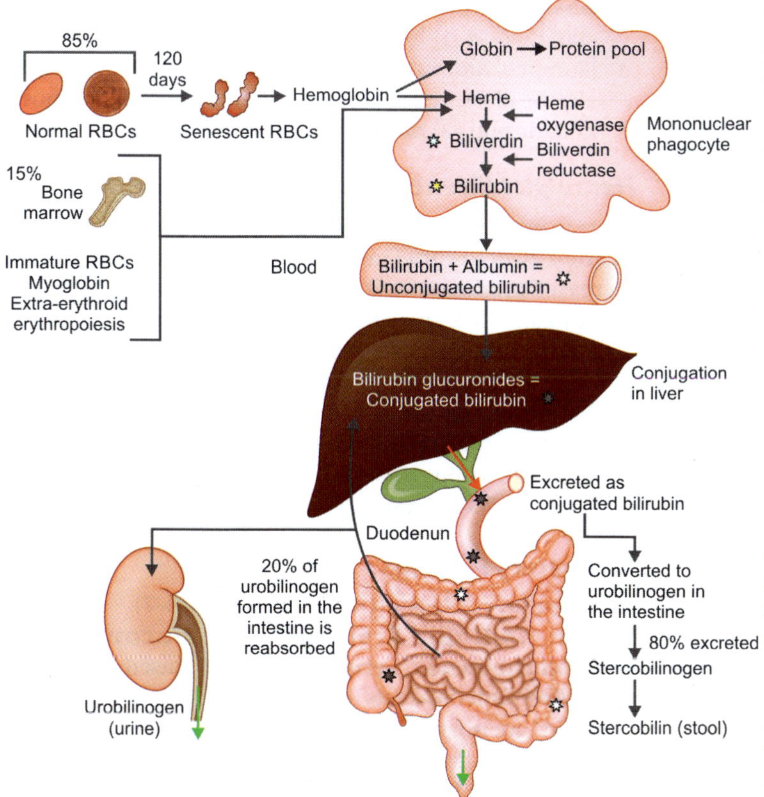

Lobule
- The function unit of the liver
- Hexagonal shape
- Have hepatic vein at its center and portal tract (composed of hepatic artery, portal vein and bile duct) at its periphery

Bilirubin has affinity for elastin
Hence, jaundice is observed in skin and sclera

Inherited causes of unconjugated hyperbilirubinemia:
- Gibert syndrome
- Crigler-Najjar syndrome.

Fig. 19.1: Bilirubin metabolism. Major bilirubin is derived from the breakdown of senescent circulating RBCs. The bilirubin binds to serum albumin and is delivered to the liver. In the liver, bilirubin forms conjugated water-soluble bilirubin and excreted into bile. In the gut, bacteria deconjugate the bilirubin and degrade it to colorless urobilinogen. About 80% of urobilinogen is excreted in the stool, and about 20% is reabsorbed. A minor fraction of reabsorbed is excreted into urine as urobilinogen.

- **Biliary excretion/secretion:** Conjugated bilirubin (water-soluble, nontoxic bilirubin glucuronides) is excreted into bile and reaches the small intestine.

Intestinal Phase of Bilirubin Metabolism

In the intestine, conjugated bilirubin has two fates:

1. **Deconjugation of bilirubin glucuronides in the gut: Most of the conjugated bilirubin deconjugated** (in the lumen of the distal small intestine and colon) by bacterial β-glucuronidases. It is degraded **to a colorless urobilinogen**. The urobilinogen has two fates:
   i. **Excretion of urobilinogen: Most (80%)** of the urobilinogen is **excreted in the feces as** stercobilinogen (is responsible for the normal color of the stool).
   ii. **Reabsorption of urobilinogen**: About 20% of urobilinogen formed are reabsorbed in the terminal ileum and colon into the portal circulation. It is returned to the liver and re-excreted into the bile.
      - A small amount of reabsorbed urobilinogen is excreted in the urine as urobilinogen.

      Note: (1) In obstructive jaundice, urine does not contain urobilinogen. (2) In hepatocellular and hemolytic jaundice, urinary urobilinogen is markedly increased (more than 4 mg/day).
2. **Part of the conjugated bilirubin is excreted in the stool** as such (bilirubin glucuronide).

Renal excretion of bilirubin: Unconjugated bilirubin is tightly bound to albumin; cannot be filtered by the glomeruli and is not excreted in the urine. **Conjugated bilirubin is filtered by the glomeruli** and appears in the urine (bilirubinuria).

JAUNDICE

Q. Write a short note on hyperbilirubinemia.

Definition: Jaundice is defined as **yellowish pigmentation** of **skin, mucous membranes, and sclera** due to **increased levels of bilirubin** in the blood. The scleral involvement is because it is rich in elastic tissue that has a special affinity for bilirubin.

Normal serum bilirubin level: In the normal adult range from 0.3 to 1.2 mg/dL. The rate of bilirubin production is equal to the rate of hepatic uptake, conjugation, and its biliary excretion. **Hyperbilirubinemia** means **increased blood levels of bilirubin** (>1.0 mg/dL).

- **Jaundice:** Clinically detected when the serum bilirubin level is above 2.0–2.5 mg/dL. With severe disease, the levels may be as high as 30–40 mg/dL. The **term jaundice may be used for yellow discoloration of the skin and icterus for yellowish coloration of the sclera.** Jaundice becomes clinically evident when there is an imbalance between production and excretion of bilirubin. This causes elevation of serum bilirubin levels above 2–2.5 mg/dL. In severe jaundice, it may be as high as 30–40 mg/dL.

Mechanism of jaundice: Normal bilirubin level is maintained by a balance between the rate of bilirubin production and the rate of biliary excretion Jaundice occurs whenever there is a disturbance in the equilibrium between bilirubin production and clearance. This may be due to (i) **increased bilirubin production (e.g., extravascular red cell hemolysis), (ii) hepatocyte dysfunction (e.g., hepatitis), or (iii) obstruction of the bile flow (e.g., obstruction by gallstone).** Various mechanisms can produce jaundice (**Box 19.1**). Generally, one of these mechanisms predominates. However, more than one mechanism may be responsible for jaundice.

Classification of Jaundice

Q. Write a short note on the classification of jaundice.

Q. Enumerate the etiology and pathogenesis of jaundice

1. **Based on the underlying cause (Box 19.1):** Depending on the underlying etiology, the elevation can predominantly involve unconjugated (indirect) or conjugated (direct) bilirubin.
   - Predominantly unconjugated
   - Predominantly conjugated

BOX 19.1: Classification of jaundice based on the underlying cause.

Predominantly Unconjugated Hyperbilirubinemia

- **Increased production of bilirubin:**
  - Hemolytic anemias
  - Resorption of blood from internal hemorrhage (e.g., bleeding in the gastrointestinal tract, large hematomas)
  - Ineffective erythropoiesis (e.g., pernicious anemia, thalassemia)
- **Reduced hepatic uptake of bilirubin:** Drugs that interfere with membrane carrier systems
- **Impaired bilirubin conjugation in the liver:**
  - Physiologic jaundice of the newborn (decreased UGT1A1 activity, decreased excretion)
  - *Diffuse hepatocellular disease,* e.g., viral or drug-induced hepatitis, cirrhosis

Predominantly Conjugated Hyperbilirubinemia

- Decreased hepatocellular excretion
  - *Hepatocellular damage or toxicity,* e.g., viral or drug-induced hepatitis, total parenteral nutrition, systemic infection
- **Impaired intrahepatic or extrahepatic bile flow:**
  - Inflammatory destruction of intrahepatic bile ducts (e.g., primary biliary cholangitis, graft-versus-host disease, liver transplantation)
  - Gallstones
  - External compression, e.g., Carcinoma of the pancreas

(UGT1A1: uridine diphosphate-glucuronyltransferase family, peptide A1)

2. **Based on pathological mechanism:** Jaundice is classified as (i) hemolytic jaundice, (ii) hepatocellular jaundice, and (iii) obstructive jaundice. Jaundice may also be classified as: (1) prehepatic, hepatic, and post-hepatic and (2) medical and surgical.

Hemolytic (Prehepatic) Jaundice

Increased destruction of red blood cells (hemolysis) **or their precursors** (ineffective erythropoiesis) causes increased production of bilirubin. **Unconjugated bilirubin** accumulates in the plasma and results in jaundice. **Jaundice is usually mild** because the normal liver can easily handle the increased bilirubin production. In **hemolytic disease of the newborn** (erythroblastosis fetalis), excessive unconjugated bilirubin crosses the blood-brain barrier to reach the brain. It leads to severe neurologic damage referred to as **kernicterus**.

Laboratory Findings

Show features of hemolysis (*refer* pages 344-7).

Serum findings: Predominantly unconjugated hyperbilirubinemia. Serum bilirubin is raised (<6 mg%). **Other liver function tests** (e.g., serum ALP, transferases, and albumin) are **normal**, however, **LDH is increased.**

Urine findings: No bilirubin in urine, because the unconjugated bilirubin is not water-soluble and cannot pass into the urine; hence the term **'acholuric jaundice.' Urinary urobilinogen is increased** (>4 mg/24 hours).

Hepatocellular (Hepatic) Jaundice

Dysfunction of any of the hepatic steps in bilirubin metabolism may cause jaundice. Hepatocellular jaundice occurs as a **consequence of parenchymal liver disease** which leads to an inability of the liver to transport bilirubin across the hepatocyte into the bile. Defects in bilirubin transport across the hepatocyte may occur at any point between the uptake of unconjugated bilirubin into the hepatocyte and the transport of conjugated bilirubin into biliary canaliculi.

Laboratory Findings

Serum findings: Raised transaminases (AST, ALT). Acute jaundice with AST >1,000 U/L is highly suggestive of an **infectious cause** (e.g., hepatitis A, B), **drugs** (e.g., paracetamol), or **hepatic ischemia. Both unconjugated and conjugated bilirubin level rises** in the blood.

Urine findings: Bilirubin and urobilinogen are present.

Cholestatic (Obstructive/Surgical/Posthepatic) Jaundice

Cholestasis means failure of bile flow: Its cause may be anywhere between hepatocyte and duodenum **(Fig. 19.2)**. Cholestatic jaundice is usually a **'surgical jaundice'** meaning a cause that requires surgical intervention. Cholestasis can be intrahepatic or extrahepatic.

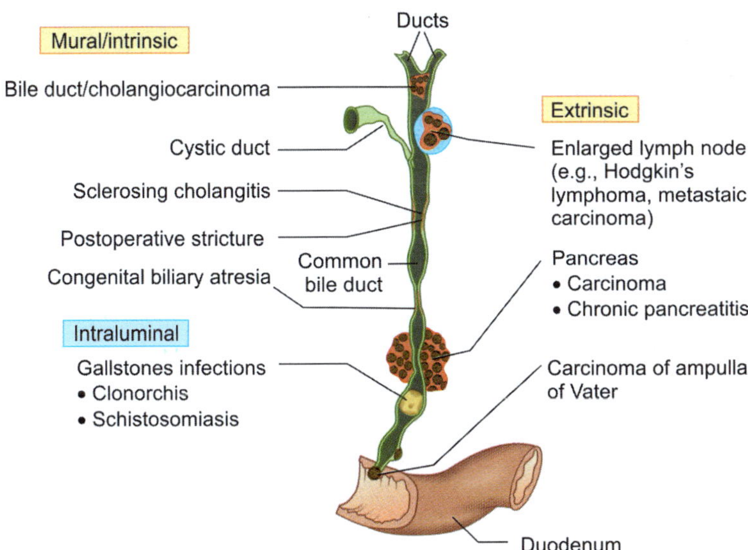

Fig. 19.2: Causes of obstructive jaundice.

Blood supply to the liver:
- About 60% supplied by portal vein
- About 40% is supplied by the hepatic artery.

Kupffer cells are found in the liver-derived from the macrophage–monocyte system

Hepatic stellate cells (Ito cell)
- Found in space of Disse
- High in lipid content
- Store vitamin A
- Synthesize extracellular collagen

Enterohepatic circulation: Process of excretion of bile by the liver into the intestine and return to the liver. Helps to maintain a large endogenous pool of bile acids for digestive and excretory purposes.

Consequences of cholestasis: Retention of bile acids and bilirubin in the liver and blood and **deficiency of bile acids in the intestine.**

Laboratory Findings

Serum findings

- **Serum bilirubin markedly raised** and is predominantly conjugated (representing >50% of the total bilirubin) hyperbilirubinemia.
- **Serum alkaline phosphatase (ALP) markedly raised** (3–4 times that of normal).
- Minimal biochemical changes of liver parenchymal damage.
- Increase in serum GGT/γ-GT (gamma-glutamyl transpeptidase), and 5'nucleotidase.
- Antimitochondrial antibody (in primary biliary cholangitis).

Urine findings

- **Bilirubin (bilirubinuria ++) present** (conjugated bilirubin is soluble in urine). Urine is yellow because of conjugated bilirubin.
- **Urobilinogen absent:** This is because conjugated bilirubin in bile does not enter the bowel. Therefore, the intestinal bacteria cannot convert conjugated bilirubin into urobilinogen. There is less reabsorption of urobilinogen (enterohepatic circulation), and less is excreted in the urine.

  Liver function tests are discussed in detail on pages 472-6.

Distinguishing Obstructive from Nonobstructive Jaundice Based on Liver Function Tests

Nonobstructive jaundice includes prehepatic and hepatic jaundice, whereas obstructive jaundice is usually posthepatic obstruction **(Fig. 19.2)**.

Serum transaminases: A **significant elevation of serum transaminases** out of proportion to the other liver enzymes indicates a **primarily hepatocellular disorder** (i.e., hepatitis). Alcoholic and other toxic hepatitis almost always are associated with marked elevation of the aspartate aminotransferase (AST) level compared to the alanine aminotransferase (ALT), whereas in viral hepatitis the reverse is usually true.

Serum alkaline phosphatase: Predominant elevation of alkaline phosphatase (ALP) level indicates intrahepatic cholestasis and is usually due to an infiltrative process (e.g., metastatic carcinoma) or drug reaction. **Serum ALP markedly raised in obstructive (posthepatic) jaundice.**

Serum bilirubin: Raised bilirubin level can result from either direct (conjugated) or indirect (unconjugated) causes. Although many liver disorders can produce elevations of both, as a practical matter unconjugated hyperbilirubinemia is due to significant hemolysis. A predominant elevation in conjugated bilirubin favors extrahepatic cholestasis from biliary obstruction.

Laboratory Investigations in Jaundice (Refer Online Table 19.1)

Q. Write a short note on laboratory investigations in jaundice.

PA 25.6 (CC): Interpret liver function and viral hepatitis serology panel. Distinguish obstructive from nonobstructive jaundice based on clinical features and liver function tests. The procedure requires certification.

Q. Distinguish between direct and indirect hyperbilirubinemia.

Differences between unconjugated and conjugated bilirubin: Both unconjugated (indirect) bilirubin and conjugated (direct) bilirubin may accumulate in systemic circulation. Distinguishing features between direct and indirect hyperbilirubinemia are presented in **Table 19.2.**

TABLE 19.2 Distinguishing features between direct and indirect hyperbilirubinemia.

Feature	*Unconjugated bilirubin*	*Conjugated bilirubin*
Definition	It is the bilirubin that is not conjugated in the liver	It is bilirubin diglucuronide formed by conjugation of unconjugated bilirubin with glucuronic acid in the liver
Normal serum level	More	Less (less than 0.25 mg/dL)
Water solubility	Not soluble in water and is present in the circulation forming tight complexes with serum albumin	Soluble in water, nontoxic, and only loosely bound to albumin in the plasma
Solubility in lipids and alcohol	Soluble in fat and alcohol	Insoluble in fat and alcohol
Serum albumin binding	High	Low
Presence in bile	Not present in bile	Present in bile
Presence in urine (renal excretion)	Cannot be excreted in the urine even when its levels are high in the blood	Not present in urine, but appear when they're in a high plasma level
van den Bergh reaction	Indirect (total minus direct)	Direct positive
Toxicity	Toxic to the tissues. It can cause brain damage leading to kernicterus (neurologic damage) in infants	Not toxic to the tissues

Van den Bergh Reaction

It was a colorimetric method of estimation of serum bilirubin level and was done to know the nature/type of jaundice. Presently, this method is not used.

Principle: It was a chemical reaction in which the serum of the patient is mixed with a diazo reagent (which contains diazotized sulfanilic acid). Bilirubin reacts with diazotized sulfanilic acid in the diazo reagent to produce purple-colored azobilirubin.

Interpretation

- **Direct positive:** If the serum contains conjugated bilirubin, a red color develops immediately and it is called direct positive.
- In an **indirect positive** test, the patient's serum is first treated with alcohol and later mixed with diazo reagent. The development of red color indicates the presence of unconjugated bilirubin in the serum.
- **Biphasic reaction:** If both conjugated and unconjugated bilirubin are present the reaction is termed biphasic reaction.

Clinical features and laboratory findings useful in differentiating different types of jaundice are presented in **Table 19.3**.

Hereditary Hyperbilirubinemias (Table 19.4)

Hereditary hyperbilirubinemia occurs due to genetic mutations. These genetic mutations can cause a defect in the uptake, conjugation, or secretion of bilirubin.

Crigler–Najjar Syndrome

Q. Write a short note on Criggler–Najar syndrome.

Crigler–Najjar Syndrome Type 1

Crigler–Najjar syndrome type 1 is a rare, **autosomal recessive** disorder due to the **complete absence of hepatic UGT1A1**. It is invariably fatal around birth.

- Characterized by **chronic, severe, unconjugated hyperbilirubinemia and** produces severe jaundice, icterus, and **death** secondary to kernicterus **within 18 months** of birth. Bile does contain conjugated bilirubin; hence, it is **colorless.** Treatment with **phenobarbital** (which induces microsomal enzymes including UGT), has **no effect.**
- **Liver** is **morphologically normal** by light and electron microscopy.

Crigler–Najjar Syndrome Type 2

Crigler–Najjar syndrome type 2 is a **less severe, nonfatal** disorder due to *partial deficiency of the UGT1A1 enzyme.* It is inherited as an **autosomal dominant** disorder with variable penetrance. Phenobarbital treatment can improve bilirubin glucuronidation by inducing hypertrophy of the hepatocellular endoplasmic reticulum.

Gilbert Syndrome

Relatively **common, harmless,** inherited disorder with no clinical consequences. It is transmitted as an **autosomal recessive** mode of inheritance. Caused **mutations in the promoter of the UGT1 gene.** This leads to inadequate synthesis of the UGT1A1 enzyme (activity is about 30% of normal), a less severe reduction than in Crigler–Najjar syndromes. Usually, asymptomatic. **Mild, chronic unconjugated fluctuating hyperbilirubinemia** not associated with functional derangements.

TABLE 19.3 Clinical features useful in differentiating different types of jaundice.

Feature	*Hemolytic (prehepatic)*	*Hepatocellular (intrahepatic)*	*Obstructive (posthepatic)*
Clinical features			
Jaundice: Color (depth)	Lemon yellow (mild)	Orange yellow (variable)	Greenish yellow (deep)
Pruritus	Absent	Variable	Present
Bleeding tendency	Absent	Present	Present (late)
Anemia	Present	Absent	Absent
Splenomegaly	Present	Variable	Absent (may develop later when cirrhosis develops)
Palpable gallbladder	Absent	Absent	May be present
Features of hepatocellular failure	Absent	Present (early)	Present (late)
Laboratory findings			
Conjugated bilirubin	Absent	Raised	Raised
AST or ALT	Normal	Increased	Normal
ALP	Normal	Normal	Raised
Urine bilirubin	Absent	Present	Present
Urine urobilinogen	Present	Present	Absent*

(AST: aspartate aminotransferase; ALT: alanine aminotransferase; ALP: alkaline phosphatase)
*The presence of urobilinogen in urine rules out obstructive jaundice.

TABLE 19.4 Hereditary hyperbilirubinemias.

Hereditary disorder	*Mode of inheritance*	*Defects in bilirubin metabolism*	*Characteristics*
Unconjugated hyperbilirubinemia			
Crigler–Najjar syndrome type 1	Autosomal recessive	Absent UGT1A1 activity	Fatal
Crigler–Najjar syndrome type 2	Autosomal dominant with variable penetrance	Decreased UGT1A1 activity	Usually, mild
Gilbert syndrome	Autosomal recessive	Decreased UGT1A1 activity	Harmless
Conjugated hyperbilirubinemia			
Dubin–Johnson syndrome	Autosomal recessive	Impaired biliary excretion of bilirubin glucuronides	Liver with pigmented granules in cytoplasm, harmless
Rotor syndrome	Autosomal recessive	Decreased hepatic uptake and decreased biliary excretion	Harmless

(UGT: uridine diphosphate–glucuronyl transferase; UGT1A1: UDP Glucuronosyltransferase Family 1 Member A1).

Dubin–Johnson Syndrome

Q. Write a short note on Dubin–Johnson syndrome.

It is a benign autosomal recessive disorder due to the **complete absence of multidrug resistance protein 2 (MRP2)**. It is characterized by a defect in the hepatocellular excretion of bilirubin glucuronides across the biliary canalicular membrane.

MORPHOLOGY

The liver is **darkly pigmented** because of **coarse melanin-like pigmented granules** within the enlarged lysosomes present in the cytoplasm of hepatocytes. **The pigment is composed of polymers of epinephrine metabolites and not bilirubin.**

Clinical features: It causes chronic or recurrent conjugated hyperbilirubinemia. Most patients are asymptomatic and have a normal life expectancy.

Rotor Syndrome

A rare form of asymptomatic **conjugated hyperbilirubinemia.** It may be due to many defects, such as hepatocellular uptake, intracellular binding, and excretion of bilirubin pigments. Inherited as an **autosomal recessive** trait. **The liver is morphologically normal.**

HEPATIC (LIVER) FAILURE

PA 25.2 (CC): Describe the pathophysiology and pathologic changes seen in hepatic failure and their clinical manifestations, complications, and consequences.

Hepatic failure is a clinical syndrome that is the most severe clinical consequence of liver disease. It occurs when the liver cannot sustain its vital activities and about 80–90% of hepatic functional capacity must be lost to produce hepatic failure.

Types of liver failure: It may develop as acute, chronic, and acute-on-chronic liver failure.

Acute Liver Failure

Definition: Acute liver failure is defined as an acute liver disease that produces encephalopathy (and coagulopathy) within 6 months (26 weeks) of the initial liver injury in the absence of pre-existing liver disease.

Acute liver failure is the result of sudden and massive hepatic destruction. Acute liver failure is termed fulminant **liver failure** when the encephalopathy develops within 2 weeks of the onset of jaundice, and **subfulminant liver failure** when the encephalopathy develops within 3 months.

Causes (refer online Box 19.2): Massive hepatic necrosis in acute liver failure is most commonly produced by:

- **Acute viral hepatitis:** Hepatitis A, B, and E infections.
- **Drugs or toxins:** Accidental or deliberate ingestion of acetaminophen (paracetamol).
- **Autoimmune hepatitis**

Mechanism of hepatocellular necrosis: It may be due to direct toxic damage (e.g., acetaminophen) to hepatocytes, but more often due to a combination of toxicity and immune-mediated hepatocyte destruction (e.g., hepatitis virus infection).

MORPHOLOGY

Acute liver failure shows **massive hepatic necrosis.**

Gross

Initially, the liver is enlarged due to swelling and edema produced by inflammation. This is followed by a dramatic decrease in the size (becomes small and shrunken) due to the destruction/loss of parenchyma.

Microscopy

It shows broad/large regions/zones of parenchymal loss/destruction surrounded by occasional islands of regenerating hepatocytes. Since it is an acute process scar is not seen.

Clinical Features

Acute liver failure presents first with nausea, vomiting, worsening jaundice, and fatigue. They are followed by the onset of life-threatening encephalopathy, coagulation defects, and portal hypertension associated with ascites. The end result is the development of multiorgan failure and death. Other manifestations of acute liver failure are as follows:

- **Jaundice** (yellow discoloration of the skin) and **icterus** (yellow discoloration of the sclera) due to retention of bilirubin. Jaundice (hyperbilirubinemia) in hepatic failure is mostly conjugated, although unconjugated bilirubin levels may also be increased. Cholestasis increases the risk of life-threatening bacterial infection.
- **Hepatic encephalopathy:** It is due to a disorder of neurotransmission in the central nervous system and neuromuscular system. It consists of a spectrum of disturbances in consciousness. They range from mild behavioral abnormalities to marked confusion and stupor, to deep coma and death. The progression of encephalopathy following acute injury may occur over days, weeks, or months. Impaired neuronal function and brain edema are correlated to raised levels of ammonia in blood. Associated fluctuating, neurologic signs include rigidity, hyperreflexia, and asterixis.
    - **Asterixis**: Asterixis is a characteristic sign characterized by the nonrhythmic rapid extension-flexion movement of the head and extremities. This is best seen as the "flapping" of the hands when the arms are held in extension with dorsiflexed wrists.
- **Coagulopathy**: The liver produces vitamin K-dependent and vitamin K-independent clotting factors. The production of these coagulation factors is massively decreased in acute liver failure because of impaired synthesis by damaged hepatocytes. This is responsible for coagulopathy. It presents as easy bruising and can lead to life-threatening or fatal intracranial bleeding. The liver also helps in removing activated coagulation factors from the circulation. The damaged liver cannot remove the activated coagulation factors, which may sometimes paradoxically produce disseminated intravascular coagulation, further exacerbating the bleeding tendency.
- **Portal hypertension**: It occurs when there is reduced blood flow through the portal venous system. This may be due to prehepatic, intrahepatic, or posthepatic obstruction. Though it can manifest in acute liver failure, portal hypertension is more common in chronic liver failure (*refer* page 653). In chronic liver disease, portal hypertension develops over months to years. If portal hypertension develops in acute liver failure within days to weeks, the site of obstruction is usually intrahepatic. Its major clinical consequences are ascites and hepatic encephalopathy.
- **Hepatorenal syndrome**: It is a type of renal failure developing in patients with liver failure. There will be neither intrinsic morphologic nor functional cause for this renal failure. The main renal functional abnormalities include sodium retention, impaired free-water excretion, and decreased renal perfusion and glomerular filtration rate. It presents with a decrease in urine output and rising blood urea nitrogen and creatinine levels.

Laboratory findings: Initially, the serum transaminase levels are markedly raised into the thousands. As hepatocytes are lost, serum transaminase levels decrease rapidly because of the disappearance of their source, namely—hepatocytes.

Chronic Liver Failure and Cirrhosis

Chronic liver failure follows years or decades of insidious, progressive liver injury.

Causes: These include **chronic hepatitis B, chronic hepatitis C, nonalcoholic fatty liver disease** (NAFLD), **and alcoholic liver disease. Liver failure in chronic liver disease is usually associated with cirrhosis.**

Cirrhosis is discussed in detail on pages 673-9. It must be noted that not all cirrhosis leads to chronic liver failure and not all end-stage chronic liver disease is associated with cirrhosis of the liver.

Child–Pugh classification (Child–Pugh score) is a system for assessing the prognosis of chronic liver disease primarily cirrhosis. Child–Pugh classification of cirrhosis distinguishes between class A (well compensated), B (partially decompensated), and C (decompensated). It correlates with different histological features histologically.

MORPHOLOGY

Liver failure in chronic liver disease is most commonly associated with cirrhosis (*refer* pages 673-9), the cause of which varies.

- **Fibrosis**: In cirrhosis with thin fibrous septa separated by large islands of intact hepatic parenchyma are less likely to develop portal hypertension. In cirrhosis with broad bands of dense scar, dilated lymphatic spaces, and with less intervening parenchyma are likely to develop portal hypertension and to end-stage disease.
- **Ductular reactions**: In chronic liver disease, as the disease progresses, there is an increase in ductular reactions which is usually most prominent in those with cirrhosis. These ductular reactions are derived from the activation and differentiation of stem cells. Ductular reactions may stimulate some amount of the scarring in chronic liver disease and may cause further progression of the liver disease.
- **Regression of fibrosis**: Although uncommon, regression of fibrosis may rarely occur even in a fully established cirrhosis. This is characterized by thinning, compactness, and eventual fragmentation of scars. As fibrous septa break apart, adjacent nodules of regenerating parenchyma may coalesce to form larger islands of parenchyma. All livers with cirrhosis show evidence of both progression and regression and their balance depends on the severity and persistence of the underlying disease.

Clinical Features

In about 40% of patients with cirrhosis, there may not be symptoms until the most advanced stages of the disease. Even at late stages when symptoms occur, the initial symptoms may be nonspecific as anorexia, weight loss, and weakness. Later patient may develop signs and symptoms of acute liver failure namely jaundice, encephalopathy, and coagulopathy (discussed under acute liver failure above on page 652). Apart from these symptoms, chronic liver failure may show the following additional features. Portal hypertension is more frequent and more complex in chronic liver failure than in acute liver failure. Portal hypertension and its consequences are discussed on pages 675-8.

Chronic liver diseases are one of the risk factors for the development of hepatocellular carcinoma (HCC) (*refer* page 683).

Acute-on-Chronic Liver Failure

It is the **sudden development of signs of acute liver failure in patients suffering from years of stable, well-compensated, and advanced chronic liver disease.**

Cause: These patients, usually suffer from well-established cirrhosis with extensive vascular shunting. There are large volumes of functioning liver parenchyma with a borderline vascular supply. Such liver is vulnerable to superimposed, potentially lethal insults. The short-term mortality in these patients is about 50%. The cause of sudden decompensation in patients with chronic liver disease is:

- Hepatitis D superinfection in patients with chronic hepatitis B
- Resistance to medical therapy in patients with medically suppressed viral hepatitis B in whom viral mutants arise.
- Ascending bacterial cholangitis in patients with primary sclerosing cholangitis
- Replacement of liver parenchyma by primary or metastatic carcinoma.
- **Systemic disorder,** e.g., sepsis and its attendant hypotension, acute cardiac failure, or a superimposed toxic injury in a patient with well-compensated cirrhosis.

VIRAL HEPATITIS

PA 25.3 (CC): Describe the etiology and pathogenesis of viral and toxic hepatitis: distinguish the causes of hepatitis based on the clinical and laboratory features. Describe the pathology, complications, and consequences of hepatitis.

Definition: Viral hepatitis may be defined as a viral **infection of hepatocytes** that produces necrosis and inflammation of the liver.

Q. Classify viral hepatitis. List the different causative viruses of hepatitis.

Causes of viral hepatitis (Box 19.3): Most cases of hepatitis are caused by a group of **five separate, unrelated viruses** that have a particular affinity for the liver known as **hepatotropic viruses** (hepatitis viruses A, B, C, D, and E). **All except HBV are RNA viruses.**

- Hepatitis **A and E** are transmitted mainly by the fecal-oral route or ingestion of contaminated water.
- Hepatitis **B, C, and D** are transmitted mainly by parenteral routes and less commonly by intimate or

BOX 19.3: Causes of viral hepatitis.

- Hepatitis A virus (HAV)
- Hepatitis B virus (HBV)
- Hepatitis C virus (HCV)
- Hepatitis D virus (HDV)
- Hepatitis E virus (HEV)

sexual exposure. They can produce chronic hepatitis, which may progress to cirrhosis and hepatocellular carcinoma.

- **In few cases** of acute viral hepatitis-like syndrome, the **known hepatitis virus cannot be identified** as an etiological agent. They are termed hepatitis of unknown cause.

Hepatitis A Virus

- **Hepatitis A virus (HAV):** It is a **nonenveloped, 27 nm, RNA virus.** The virus replicates mainly in the liver. It has outer capsid protein (HAVAg).
- **Source of infection**: The only source of infection is an **acutely infected person.** The virus is excreted through the bile into the **stool/feces of infected persons** for about 2–3 weeks before the onset of symptoms and then for a further 1 week after the onset of jaundice. The disease is **maximally infectious just before the onset of jaundice.**
- **Mode of transmission: Fecal-oral route** by ingestion of contaminated water and foods. HAV viremia is transient. Hence, blood-borne transmission does not occur.
- **Incubation period**: 2–6 weeks (mean ~4 weeks).
- **Outcome of HAV infection:** HAV causes mild, **benign, self-limited acute hepatitis.** HAV **does not produce chronic hepatitis or a carrier state b** cleared by the host immune response. Fulminant hepatitis develops only rarely.

Laboratory and Serological Findings for HAV Hepatitis

Q. Serological markers of hepatitis A with graphic form.

Prodromal Stage

- **Serum: Serum bilirubin** is **usually normal. Raised serum AST or ALT** precedes the jaundice.
- **Urine**: **Bilirubinuria** and **increased urinary excretion of urobilinogen.**
- **HAV in blood:** The period of viremia is short and occurs early in the disease.
- **Fecal shedding of HAV** follows its appearance in the liver by about a week and is present only for a brief period. It is demonstrated by electron microscopy.

Icteric Stage

- **Serum**: Serum **bilirubin is raised.** Serum **AST is raised** and maximum levels are reached within 1–2 days after the appearance of jaundice and may rise above 500 IU/L. **Serum ALP** is usually **less than 300 IU/L.**
- **IgM anti-HAV** is the first detectable immune response to HAV. Serum IgM anti-HAV in a patient with acute hepatitis confirms HAV as the cause. It is a **reliable marker of acute infection.** It appears in the blood at the onset of symptoms during the acute illness. It reaches peak levels in 2–3 weeks. IgM titers begin to decline within a few weeks and are undetectable by 3–6 months.

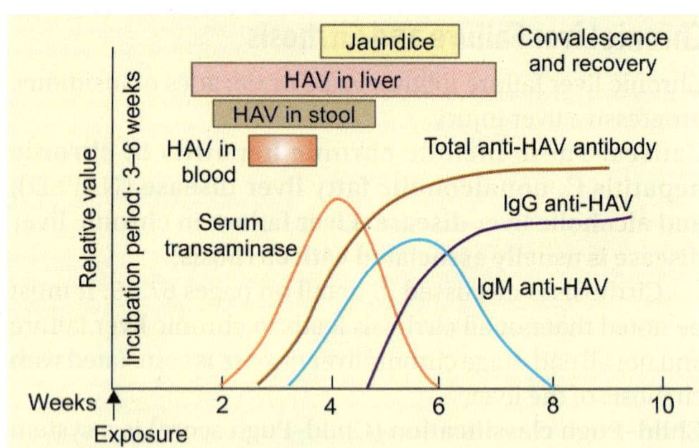

Fig. 19.3: Laboratory and serologic course markers in acute hepatitis A.

(IgG: immunoglobulin G; IgM: immunoglobulin M ALT: alanine aminotransferase; HAV: hepatitis A virus)

Recovery Stage

IgM anti-HAV is followed by the appearance of IgG anti-HAV. IgG anti-HAV appears as patients recover. It persists for years and **provides lifelong immunity** against reinfection by HAV.

Diagnosis (Fig. 19.3): It is done by demonstrating the virus in feces and detection of antibody in the serum. These are IgM anti-HAV during acute hepatitis and IgG anti-HAV during a recovery phase.

Prophylaxis: Improved sanitary practices and **prevention of fecal contamination of food and water**. The **HAV vaccine** is effective in preventing HAV infection.

Hepatitis B Virus

Q. Describe the structure of the hepatitis B virus.

Structure of HBV

Hepatitis B virus (HBV) is a **hepatotropic DNA virus** belonging to the family Hepadnaviridae. HBV **virion** is spherical and **double-layered.**

Genome and associated proteins of HBV: The genome of HBV consists of **partially double-stranded circular DNA** and has four genes **(Fig. 19.4)**. The **viral particle is a 42-nm sphere** and is termed a **Dane particle.** HBV genome encodes the following proteins:

- **Envelope glycoproteins (HBsAg, hepatitis B surface antigen):** HBsAg consists of three-related viral envelope glycoproteins, large, middle, and small HBsAg. Large HBsAg is usually associated with complete virions and is **immunogenic. Infected liver cells also synthesize and secrete large amounts of noninfective viral envelope proteins (mainly small HBsAg)** and these are free of viral core elements.

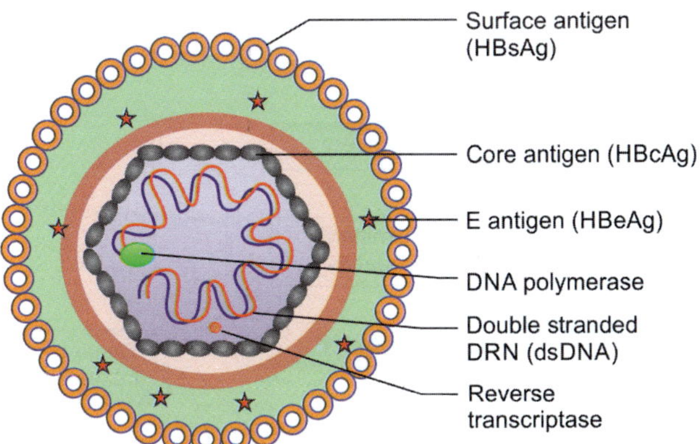

Fig. 19.4: Diagrammatic representation of hepatitis B virus (HBV) and its various genes.

- **Nucleocapsid "core" protein (HBcAg, hepatitis B core antigen)** and **hepatitis B e antigen** (HBeAg): **Hepatitis B core antigen** (HBcAg):
  - **HBeAg**: It is secreted into serum and is a surrogate (substitute) marker for high levels of viral replication. It is essential for the establishment of persistent infection.
  - **HBcAg**: It remains intracellular within the hepatocytes and participates in the assembly of virions. It does not circulate in the serum. Hence, not detectable in the serum of patients.
- **A polymerase (Pol):** It has both DNA polymerase activity and reverse transcriptase activity. It is required for the **virus replication** to occur. The genomic replication of HBV occurs in a unique DNA → RNA → DNA cycle via an intermediate RNA template. This polymerase is the target of drugs used in the treatment of hepatitis B infection.
- **HBx protein: HBx protein** is **necessary for virus** replication. It may act as a transcriptional transactivator for viral genes and various host genes. **HBx** protein has been **implicated in the pathogenesis of liver cancer in HBV infection.**

Source of infection: A human suffering from hepatitis B or a carrier of HBV is the only source of infection. HBV is 100 times as infectious as the human immunodeficiency virus (HIV) and 10 times as infectious as the hepatitis C virus (HCV).

Mode of transmission: The virus may be vertically or horizontally transmitted.

- **Vertical (congenital) transmission**: From the mother [who is a carrier for HBV (90% HbeAg+, 30% HbeAg–)] to a child may **occur in utero, during parturition, or soon after birth.**
- **Horizontal transmission**: **The parenteral mode of transmission is the dominant mode of transmission** of HBV. It may occur by the following routes:
  - **Unprotected sexual contact (or close personal contact):** HBV may be transmitted through unprotected heterosexual or homosexual intercourse. The virus can be found in semen and saliva. Anal sexual contact is an important mode of transmission.
  - **Percutaneous and mucous membrane:** Exposure to infectious body fluids, through minor cuts/abrasions in the skin or mucous membranes. HBV can survive for long periods on household articles, e.g., toys, and toothbrushes, and may transmit the infection. Most cases of hepatitis B are now transmitted by intimate or close bodily contact. Such contact transmission largely involves the direct transfer of the virus through breaks in the skin or mucous membranes
  - **Intravenous route:** HBV may also be transmitted through transfusion of unscreened infected blood or blood products. This mode of spread is rare now, because of routine screening of all blood donors for HBV and HBC. Other modes include intravenous drug abuse with the sharing of needles and syringes, tattooists, or acupuncturists.
  - **In children, horizontal transmission** can occur through minor breaks in the skin or mucous membranes following physical contact with infected individuals.

Incubation period: It has a long incubation period that ranges from **2 to 26 weeks**.

Pathogenesis

Hepatitis B virus attaches to host hepatocytes and then enters the hepatocyte. Inside the cytoplasm of hepatocytes, the virus uncoats. The viral genome then enters the nucleus of the hepatocyte. In the nucleus, the plus strand is synthesized and converted into a covalently closed circular DNA (cccDNA). This acts as the template for the transcription of viral messenger RNA (mRNA). HBV replication occurs through reverse transcription via an RNA intermediate. The persistence of cccDNA prevents clearance of HBV from the host, even with the use of potent antiviral pharmacotherapy.

Immune response: HBV is not directly cytopathic. The **main determinant of the outcome of the HBV infection is the host's immune response to the virus.** Asymptomatic chronic HBV carriers have a large load of infectious virus in their liver for years without any functional or biochemical evidence of liver cell injury.

High-level viral replication and high production of viral proteins in infected hepatocytes can produce cytopathic changes. Target viral antigens are expressed on the surface of infected hepatocytes. These viral antigens on infected cells are recognized by CD8+ CTLs. The CTLs cause hepatocyte injury by destroying hepatocytes and are also responsible for clinical liver disease. A strong host immune response by virus-specific CD4+ and CD8+ interferon-gamma (IFN-γ) producing cells is associated with the resolution of acute HBV infection.

The clinical course and sequelae (outcome) of HBV infection are presented in **Flowchart 19.1** and **Box 19.4**.

Flowchart 19.1: Potential outcomes of hepatitis B infection.

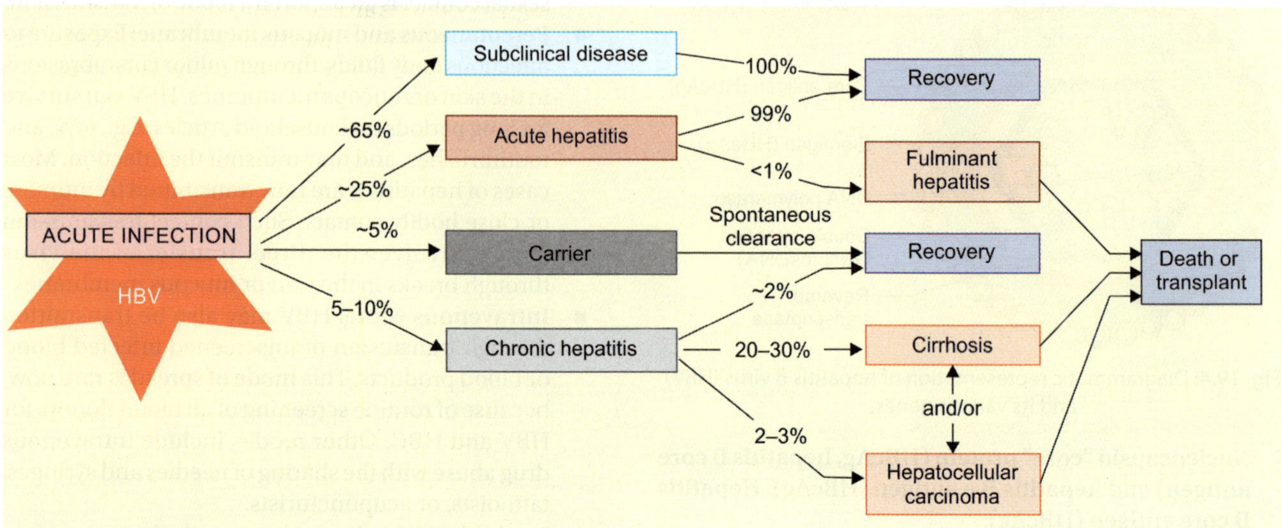

BOX 19.4: Clinical course and sequelae of hepatitis B virus (HBV) infection.

Clinical course
- Acute hepatitis with recovery and clearance of the virus
- Fulminant hepatitis with massive liver necrosis
- Chronic hepatitis

Sequelae
- Progressive chronic disease ending in cirrhosis
- Asymptomatic carrier state
- Hepatocellular carcinoma

Q. Write a short note on sequelae course/outcome of hepatitis B virus infection.

The Sequence of Serological Markers for HBV Hepatitis

Q. Discuss the laboratory diagnosis (serological markers) of hepatitis B virus infection.

Q. Mention the antibodies of hepatitis B infection.

The natural course of the HBV infection can be followed clinically by measuring viral antigens and monitoring serologic markers in the blood **(Figs. 19.5A and B).**

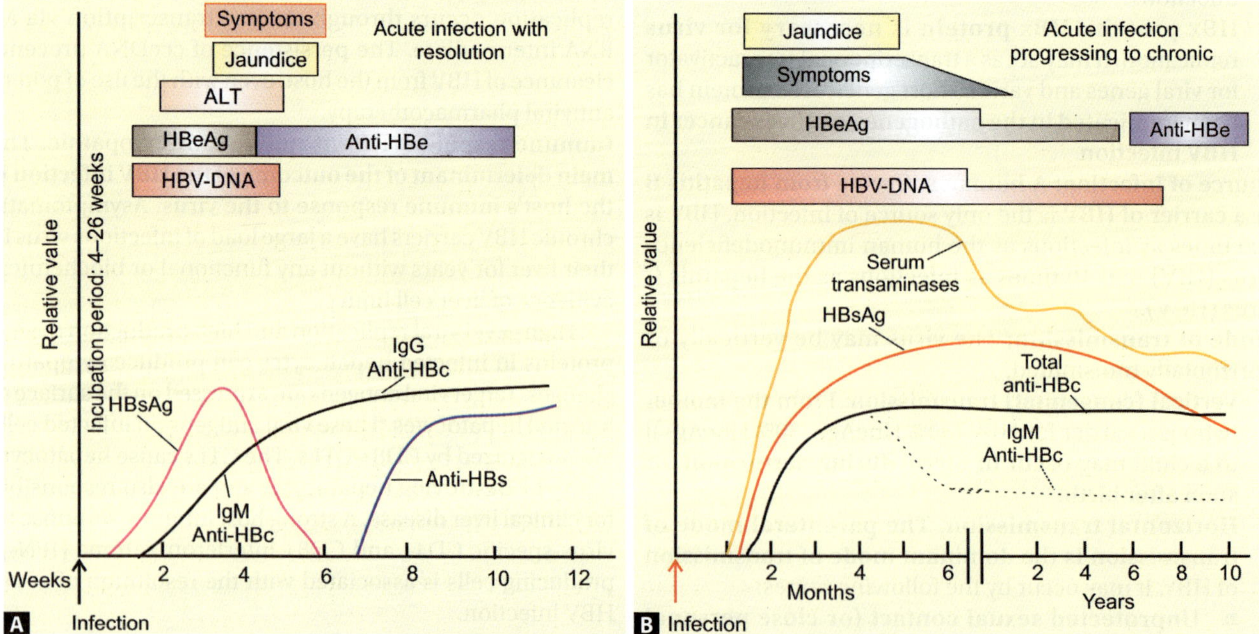

Figs. 19.5A and B: Sequence of serologic markers: (A) Acute hepatitis with resolution; (B) Chronic hepatitis caused by HBV. (ALT: alanine aminotransferase; DNA: deoxyribonucleic acid; HBc: hepatitis B core; HBeAg: hepatitis B e antigen; HBsAg: hepatitis B surface antigen; IgG: immunoglobulin G; IgM: immunoglobulin M)

HBsAg: It is the **first virologic marker.**

- **Significance:** It **appears in serum before the onset of symptoms.** It peaks during the symptomatic disease. It becomes undetectable within 12 weeks in individuals who clear the infection. **The persistence of HBsAg in the serum indicates progression to chronicity.**

Anti-HBs antibody: It is an antibody to HBsAg.

- **Significance**: It **appears in the serum after the acute disease is over**. It is usually not detected until a few weeks to several months after the disappearance of HBsAg. Anti-HBs is a **protective antibodies** and **may persist for life. This is the basis for current HBsAg-containing (noninfectious HBsAg) vaccination**. Anti-HBs antibodies are not produced in patients who progress to chronic liver disease.

HBeAg, HBV-DNA, and DNA polymerase: They appear in serum soon after HBsAg.

- **Significance: They** signify active viral replication. They are usually not helpful in the diagnosis of hepatitis B but may be **valuable in assessing prognosis**.
  - **HBeAg:** Their persistence 6 weeks after the onset of symptoms indicates infectivity and probably develops chronic hepatitis B. Their absence is a favorable serologic finding and if associated with the appearance of anti-HBe antibodies indicates low infectivity.
  - **Anti-HBe:** The presence of anti-HBe antibodies implies that an acute infection has peaked and is waning. It is present in the serum during the recovery phase.
  - HBV DNA by PCR helps confirm the diagnosis

Anti-HBc: HBcAg is not found in the serum. But its antibody, IgM anti-HBc appears in serum a week or two after the appearance of HBsAg. After about 6 months, the IgM anti-HBc antibody is replaced by IgG anti-HBc.

- **Significance**:
  - **IgM anti-HBc:** It is the **earliest antibody marker** seen in the serum, long before anti-HBe or anti-HBs. **IgM anti-HBc indicates a recent infection.** This antibody is detectable in serum shortly before the onset of symptoms along with the onset of raised serum aminotransferase levels (indicates destruction of hepatocyte).
  - **IgG anti-HBc:** Over a period of months, the IgM anti-HBc antibody is replaced by IgG anti-HBc. This antibody **indicates remote infection** (beyond 6 months). IgG anti-HBc remains lifelong in the serum and its presence **indicates previous infection with HBV** even when all the other viral markers are not detectable.

Prevention: Hepatitis B can be prevented by **vaccination** and by the **screening of donor blood, organs, and tissues.** The **vaccine is purified HbsAg** and induces a protective anti-HBs antibody response.

Treatment of chronic hepatitis B: It is treated with HBV polymerase inhibitors and IFN-α. These drugs can slow the progression of disease, reduce damage to the liver, and prevent liver cirrhosis or hepatocellular carcinoma. But they do not eliminate the HBV infection.

Hepatitis C Virus

HCV is a **small, enveloped (containing specific proteins), single-stranded RNA virus.** It is a member of the Flaviviridae family. It is the major cause of liver disease.

Mode of spread: It mainly spreads by the **parenteral route** as a blood-borne infection. It may also spread by **sexual contact**. The major route of infection in children is vertical perinatal transmission from the mother. The risk factors for HCV infection are intravenous substance use, needlestick injury, and perinatal transmission at the time of birth.

Incubation period: 4–26 weeks (mean 9 weeks).

Genome and associated proteins of HCV: The genome of HCV encodes a single polyprotein that is processed by several proteases into 10 functional proteins. These proteins include the following:

- **Protease:** It is required for complete processing of the polyprotein.
- **NS5A:** It is necessary for the assembly of HCV into mature virions.
- **RNA polymerase:** It is needed for replication of the viral genome.

Development of new genetic variants: Host immune response is not able to eliminate HCV. The HCV RNA polymerase has a low fidelity (accuracy/exactness). These two features make the viral genome inherently unstable and HCV can rapidly develop new genetic variants. The **emergence of an endogenous, newly mutated strain, its genomic instability, and antigenic variability make it difficult to produce an effective HCV vaccine.**

Life cycle of HCV (Fig. 19.6): The proteins in the viral envelope of HCV attaches to the receptor on the surface of the liver cell. The virus enters the liver cell through receptor-mediated endocytosis. They release their RNA genome into the cytoplasm of liver cells (hepatocytes). The genome of the virus encodes a single polyprotein that is processed by several proteases into 10 functional proteins. The most important of these viral proteins are: (i) viral protease (needed for complete processing of the polyprotein); (ii) NS5A (a protein that is required for assembly of HCV into mature virions); and (iii) a viral RNA polymerase (required for replication of the viral genome).

Targeted therapy for HCV: Like HIV, knowledge about the life cycle of HCV (viral replication and assembly) has helped in the development of highly effective anti-HCV drugs for the treatment of HCV infection. **These drugs specifically target the viral protease, RNA polymerase, and NS5A protein, all of which are required to produce the virus (Figs. 19.7A and B).** Combination therapy with these drugs (a strategy similar to triple-drug therapy for HIV) has

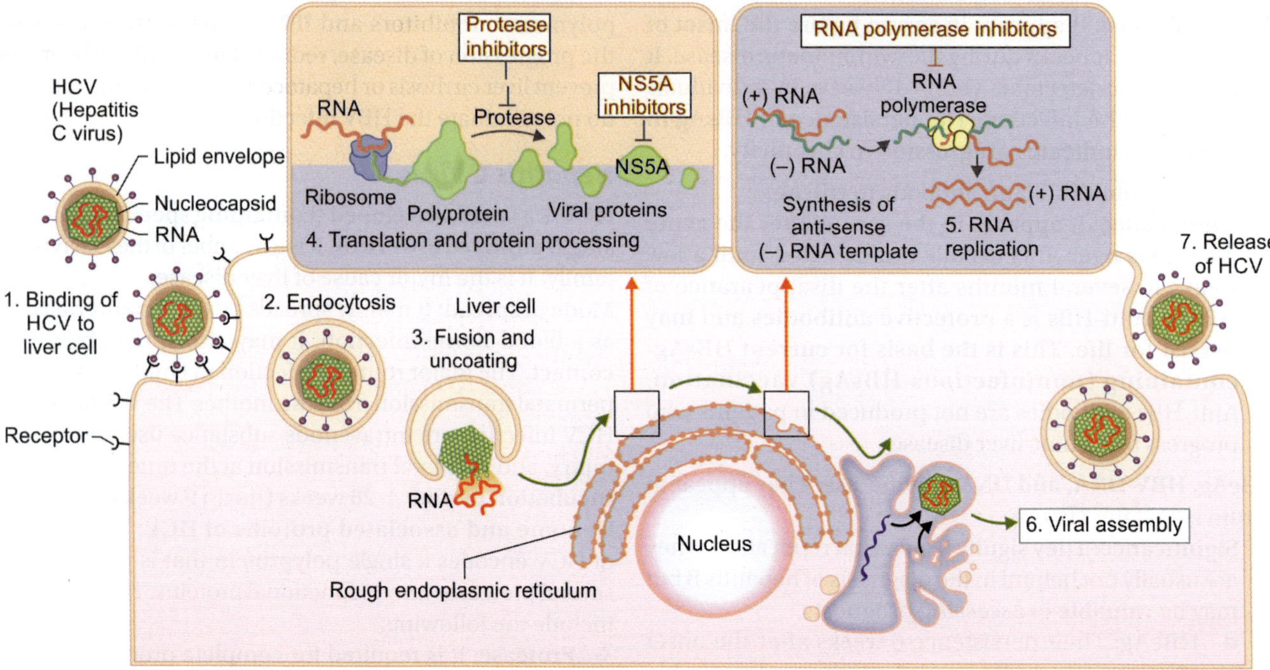

Fig. 19.6: Life cycle of hepatitis C. Various steps are shown along with steps that can be effectively targeted with antiviral drugs. Various steps in the life cycle include (1) Binding of HCV to liver cells, (2) Endocytosis of HCV, (3) Fusion and uncoating of viral RNA, (4) Translation and protein processing (5) RNA replication, (6) Viral assembly, and (7) Replication of HCV.

(NS5A: nonstructural protein 5A; RNA, ribonucleic acid).

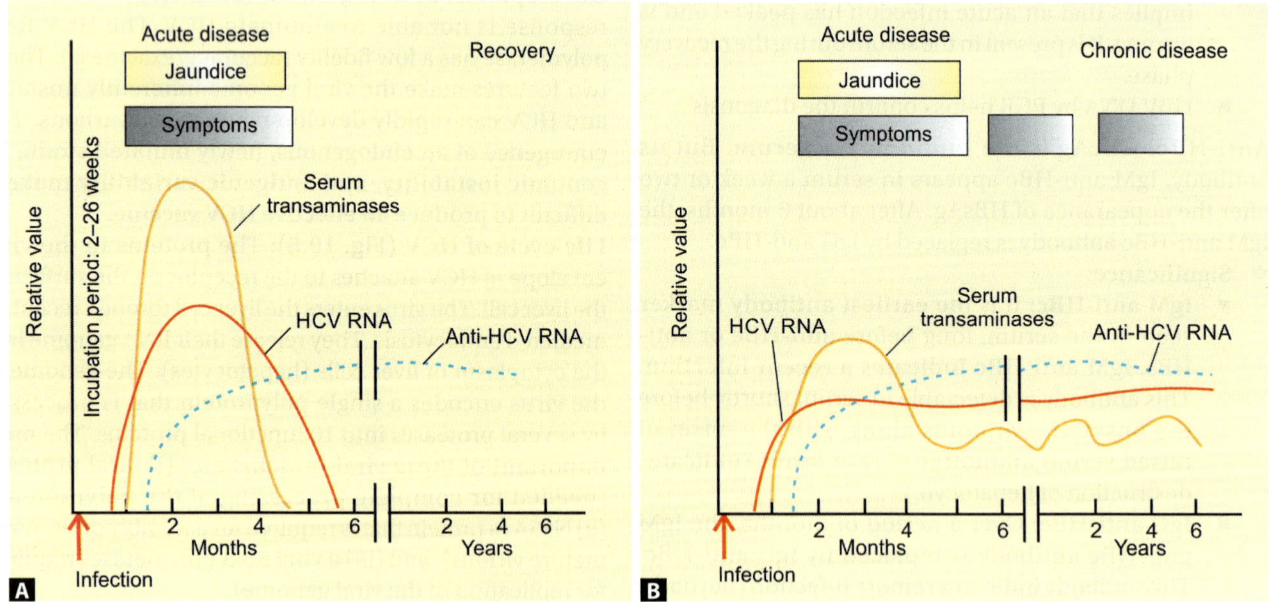

Figs. 19.7A and B: (A) Sequence of serologic markers for acute hepatitis caused by HCV; (B) Sequence of serologic markers for chronic hepatitis caused by HCV.

(HCV: hepatitis C virus; RNA: ribonucleic acid)

proven to be very effective. The goal of current therapy is to eradicate HCV RNA, which is defined by the absence of detectable HCV RNA in the blood 6 months after treatment is stopped. This is associated with a high probability of cure. **Presently, more than 95% of HCV infections are curable**, and this can be expected to improve further as new antiviral drugs become available. The major disadvantage is that these drugs are very expensive.

BOX 19.5: Sequelae of hepatitis C virus infection.

- Acute hepatitis
- **Chronic hepatitis:** It occurs in many individuals (80–90%) infected by HCV. Screening procedures can prevent it
- Fulminant hepatic failure is rare
- **Cirrhosis:** It develops over 5–20 years in approximately 20% of patients.
- **Hepatocellular carcinoma:** Patients with cirrhosis due to HCV have a risk for the development of hepatocellular carcinoma.

Sequelae of hepatitis C virus infection are presented in **Box 19.5**.

Q. Sequelae of hepatitis C virus infection.

Serum markers HCV hepatitis (Figs. 19.7A and B): The elevated titers of **IgG anti-HCV** after an active infection **do not confer effective immunity**. Diagnosis is confirmed by PCR for HCV DNA.

Hepatitis D Virus

Hepatitis D virus (HDV) also called **delta agent** is a **defective RNA virus.** It requires and depends on HBV for its replication and expression. HDV is found only in HBV carriers. The duration of HDV infection is determined by the duration of HBV infection.

Mode of spread: Parenteral route and sexual contact.

Patterns of HDV hepatitis and outcome: HDV causes hepatitis with two clinical settings:

1. **Acute coinfection**: It develops when an individual is **exposed simultaneously** to serum containing **both HDV and HBV**. The HBV infection first becomes established and the HBsAg is necessary for the development of complete HDV virions.
   - **Acute hepatitis B + D**: It is usually transient and self-limited and clinically similar to acute hepatitis B. It usually clears both viruses (HBV and HDV).
   - **Acute hepatic failure**: It may occur in intravenous drug users.
   - **Increased risk for cirrhosis and hepatocellular cancer** (HCC).
2. **Superinfection**: It occurs when an **individual already a chronic carrier of HBV** is exposed to a **new dose of HDV**. It produces disease 30–50 days after superinfection.
   - **Severe acute hepatitis**: It may occur in an asymptomatic HBV carrier, or as an exacerbation of chronic hepatitis B infection.
   - **Chronic hepatitis**: Chronic HDV infection occurs in more than 80% of superinfections. It may present with two phases:
     1. **Acute phase**: It is characterized by active HDV replication and suppression of HBV. It is associated with high levels of serum transaminase.
     2. **Chronic phase**: During this phase, replication of HDV decreases, and HBV replication increases. The levels of serum transaminase fluctuate.

Serological Markers of HDV

Q. Write a short note on serological markers of hepatitis D viral hepatitis.

- **HDV RNA:** It is detectable in the blood and liver **before and in the early days of acute disease.**
- **Anti-HDV: IgM anti-HDV-most reliable indicator of recent HDV exposure.**

Acute coinfection by HDV and HBV: It is associated with IgM against HDAg and HBcAg (indicating infection with hepatitis B).

Chronic hepatitis due to HDV superinfection: It shows HBsAg in serum, and anti-HDV antibodies (IgG and IgM) persist for months or longer.

Prevention: HDV infection depends on HBV. Hence, HDV infection is prevented by vaccination against HBV.

Hepatitis E Virus

Hepatitis E virus (HEV) is an **unenveloped, RNA virus** in the Hepevirus genus. Viral particles are 32–34 nm in diameter HEV infection is responsible for **more than 30–60% of cases of sporadic acute hepatitis in India**. Hepatitis E occurs primarily in young to middle-aged adults.

Source of infection: HEV is a **zoonotic disease with animal reservoirs**, such as monkeys, cats, pigs, and dogs. Virions are shed in stool during the acute illness.

Mode of transmission: It is an **enterically transmitted, water-borne** infection.

Incubation period: ~6 weeks.

The outcome of HEV infection: It causes self-limiting acute hepatitis. It *does not cause chronic liver disease.* However, it has a **high mortality rate (about 20%) among pregnant women.**

Diagnosis of HEV: It is by following investigations:

- **Before the onset of clinical illness: HEV RNA and HEV virions can be detected in stool and serum.**
- **After the onset of clinical illness: Raised levels of serum aminotransferases** and elevated IgM anti-HEV titers also occur simultaneously.
- **After recovery**: The IgM is replaced with a **persistent IgG anti-HEV** titer PCR for HEV RNA.

The salient features of hepatitis viruses are presented in **Table 19.5**.

Clinical Features of Viral Hepatitis

Infection with hepatitis viruses can produce a range of outcomes **(Box 19.6)**. Diagnosing and distinguishing viral hepatitis is based on the various types of serologic and molecular studies.

TABLE 19.5 Summary of features of hepatitis viruses.

Type	*Type of virus*	*Route of transmission*	*Mean incubation period*	*Frequency of chronic liver disease*	*Diagnosis*
A	ssRNA	Fecal-oral (contaminated food or water)	2–6 weeks	Never	IgM anti-HAV
B	Partially dsDNA	Parenteral, sexual contact, perinatal	2–26 weeks (mean 8 weeks)	5–10%	HBsAg or antibody to HBcAg, PCR for HBV DNA
C	ssRNA	Parenteral	4–26 weeks (mean 9 weeks)	More than 80%	ELISA for anti-HCV, PCR for HCV RNA
D	Circular defective ssRNA	Parenteral	Same as HBV	10% (coinfection); 90–100% (superinfection)	Anti-HDV, HDV RNA in serum, or HDAg in liver biopsy. Coinfection: IgM anti-HBc and anti-HDV Superinfection: IgG anti-HBc and anti-HDV
E	ssRNA	Fecal-oral	4–5 weeks	In immunocompromised hosts only	Serum IgM/IgG anti-HEV; PCR for HEV RNA

(SS: single-stranded; DS: double-stranded DNA; HBcAg: hepatitis B core antigen; HBsAg: hepatitis B surface antigen; HBV: hepatitis B virus; HCV: hepatitis C virus; HDAg: hepatitis D antigen; HDV: hepatitis D virus; HEV: hepatitis E virus)

BOX 19.6: Clinical course of viral hepatitis.

- Acute hepatitis (all hepatotropic viruses)
  - Asymptomatic acute infection with recovery (serologic evidence only)
  - Symptomatic acute hepatitis (anicteric or icteric) with recovery
- Acute liver failure with massive to submassive hepatic necrosis: HAV, HBV, or HDV. In pregnant women HEV infection
- Chronic hepatitis (without or with progression to cirrhosis): HCV and HBV. HAV and HEV do not cause chronic hepatitis.
- Chronic carrier state

Acute Hepatitis

Acute hepatitis may be caused by any hepatotropic viruses. Acute infections by all the hepatotropic viruses may be asymptomatic or symptomatic. In pregnant women, HEV can cause acute liver failure.

Asymptomatic acute infection with recovery (serologic evidence only): It is usually incidentally discovered because of mild elevation of serum transaminases or the presence of antiviral antibodies after recovery. Infections by HAV and HBV, particularly in childhood, are usually subclinical. Acute asymptomatic infection with recovery.

Symptomatic acute infection with recovery: It can be caused by any one of four hepatotropic viruses (HAV, HBV, HCV, and HEV) and follows a similar course. Their course can be divided into four phases:

1. **Incubation period** (varies depending on the type of virus).
2. **Symptomatic preicteric phase:** It presents with non-specific symptoms, such as malaise, nausea, poor appetite, and vague abdominal pain.
3. **Symptomatic icteric phase:** Jaundice and yellow sclera, dark-colored urine (conjugated hyperbilirubinemia), and pruritis (bile salt retention).
4. **Convalescence:** Peak infectivity is during the last asymptomatic period of the incubation period and the early days of acute symptoms.

Laboratory Findings in Acute Viral Hepatitis

Biochemical (liver function) tests: These include the following:

- **Serum aminotransferases (AST, ALT): Raised** and maximum levels are observed during the prodromal phase (400–4,000 IU/L). They progressively decline during the icteric and recovery phases. Serum ALT is more specific for necrosis of liver cells than serum AST. Serum ALT is the last liver enzyme to return to normal.
- **Serum bilirubin:** When jaundice appears, the serum bilirubin usually rises to levels ranging from 5–20 mg/dL. It may continue to rise despite falling serum aminotransferase levels. Both conjugated and unconjugated bilirubin levels are equally **raised.** Bilirubin levels >20 mg/dL extending and persisting late into the course of viral hepatitis are likely to be associated with severe disease.
- **Serum alkaline phosphatase:** It may be normal or only mildly elevated (less than two times the normal).
- **Serum protein: Normal**

Urine: Bilirubinuria (in early stages), and **increased urinary urobilinogen.**

Hematological tests: These include the following:

- **Neutropenia and lymphopenia** are transient. These are followed by a **relative lymphocytosis.**

- **Prothrombin time** (PT) measurement is important in acute viral hepatitis. This is because it is **prolonged in severe cases** which signifies extensive hepatocellular necrosis damage and indicates a worse prognosis.
- **Erythrocyte sedimentation rate (ESR) is raised.**

Serological findings: They are discussed under each type of hepatitis.

Liver biopsy: It is not necessary, except when the diagnosis is questionable or when clinical evidence suggests chronic hepatitis.

MORPHOLOGY

Q. Morphology of liver in viral hepatitis.

General morphological features: The majority of microscopic changes caused by hepatotropic viruses (A, B, C, D, and E) are generally similar.

Gross

- Liver may be **normal or may be swollen** in acute hepatitis. **Involvement** may be **diffuse or patchy.** The liver is shrunken in massive liver necrosis due to acute liver failure.
- Cut section muddy-red, mushy with yellow or green discoloration due to jaundice.

Microscopy (Fig. 19.8)

Q. Write a short note on microscopy of acute viral hepatitis.

Q. Write a short answer on the Councilman body.

1. **Hepatocyte injury: Ballooning degeneration** is seen with mild injury. It is characterized by **swelling of hepatocytes**, empty and pale-stained cytoplasm, with clumping of cytoplasm around the nucleus. The **hallmark of acute viral hepatitis** is the death of liver cells. The type of cell death varies:
   - **Dropout necrosis**: Rupture of the cell membrane of ballooned hepatocytes leads to cell death and focal loss of hepatocytes. These necrotic cell dropout are associated with **the** collapse of the sinusoidal collagen reticulin framework. **Aggregates of macrophage** surround these necrotic hepatocyte.
   - **Acidophilic or apoptotic or Councilman body:** It is caused by antiviral cytotoxic (effector) T cells. Apoptotic hepatocytes shrink and become **intensely eosinophilic.** They have densely staining **pyknotic or fragmented nuclei**. They may be surrounded by effector T cells. The remnants of apoptotic hepatocytes may be extruded into the sinusoids and appear as **acidophilic or Councilman bodies.** Acidophilic bodies are **characteristic of viral hepatitis** but **may also be seen in many other liver diseases.**
   - **Confluent necrosis:** In most common forms of acute viral hepatitis, liver cell necrosis is random and patchy. In severe cases of acute viral hepatitis, **necrosis of groups of hepatocytes** may be seen. It is **termed confluent necrosis.** It is characterized by the death of many hepatocytes in a geographical distribution.
   - **Bridging necrosis (Fig. 19.9):** It is a **confluent band (uniting band/zone) of necrosis of hepatocytes** and is observed in severe acute hepatitis**.** This **band/zone of necrosis** may extend from **portal tract to portal tract, central vein to central vein, or portal-to-central regions of adjacent lobules.**
2. **Portal and lobular inflammation:** Inflammation involves **all areas** of the lobule and portal region. It is a **characteristic and prominent feature** of acute hepatitis.
   - **Mononuclear inflammatory cells:** The inflammatory cells in acute hepatitis mainly consist of **lymphocytes and macrophages.** It may show a variable number of plasma cells and eosinophils.
   - **Lobular hepatitis:** It is **inflammation** involving **liver parenchyma away from the portal tract.** Unlike chronic hepatitis, the inflammatory infiltrate is usually not concentrated in portal tracts but is seen scattered throughout the lobule. It is termed "spotty necrosis" or lobular hepatitis.
   - **Interface hepatitis:** It can **occur in acute and chronic hepatitis** (*refer* page 663).
3. **Hypertrophy and hyperplasia of Kupffer cells:** These show **hypertrophy and hyperplasia** and contain lipofuscin pigment as a result of phagocytosis of hepatocellular debris.
4. **Lobular disarray**: Loss of normal regular liver cell pattern is called lobular disarray and is a diagnostically helpful feature. It is due to a combination of necrosis of hepatocytes, accompanying regeneration, and mononuclear inflammatory infiltrate. This disrupts the normal orderly architecture of the liver cell plates.

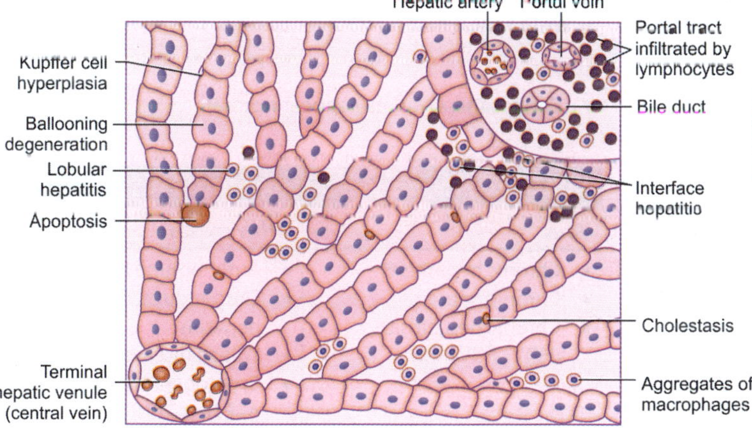

Interface hepatitis: Spill over of inflammatory from the portal tract into the adjacent parenchyma at the limiting plate.

Fig. 19.8: Chronic HBV carrier showing few liver cells with diffuse granular cytoplasm giving rise to ground-glass hepatocytes due to abundant HBsAg in the smooth endoplasmic reticulum. The inset shows hepatocyte nuclei with a sanded appearance due to the accumulation of HBcAg.

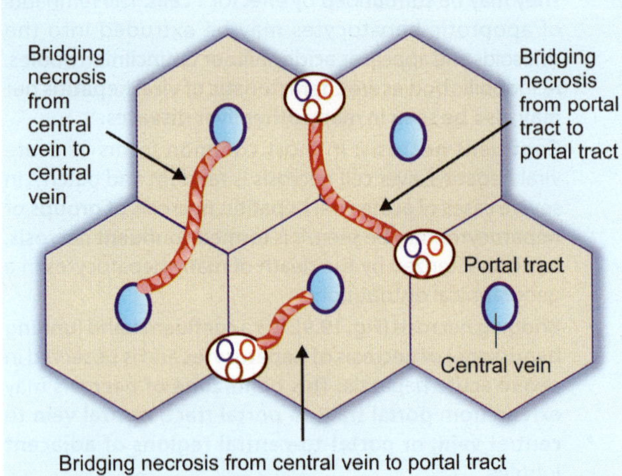

Fig. 19.9: Patterns of bridging necrosis (schematic) in severe hepatitis.

BOX 19.7: Salient microscopic features of acute viral hepatitis.

- Hepatocyte injury
  - Ballooning degeneration
  - Hepatic necrosis
    - Drop-out necrosis
    - Acidophilic or apoptotic or councilman body
    - Confluent necrosis
    - Bridging necrosis
- Portal and lobular inflammation: Mononuclear inflammatory cells (lymphocytes, macrophages), lobular hepatitis
- Hypertrophy and hyperplasia of Kupffer cells
- Lobular disarray
- Cholestasis (rare)

5. **Cholestasis:** Rarely cholestasis may be found, characterized by the bile plugs in canaliculi and brown pigmentation of hepatocytes.

The above changes are gradually reversed during recovery, and the normal architecture of the liver is completely restored. It is usually not possible to microscopically diagnose with certainty the etiology of acute viral hepatitis. Diagnosis requires serologic and/or molecular testing. Salient microscopic features of acute viral hepatitis are presented in **Box 19.7**.

Acute Liver Failure with Massive to Submassive Hepatic Necrosis

It is rare and may occur with HAV, HBV, or HDV infections. Viral hepatitis is responsible for about 10% of cases of acute hepatic failure. Liver failure can develop with massive hepatic necrosis. Acute liver failure is unusual and is seen mainly with HAV and HBV infection, depending on the region. HEV can cause acute liver failure in pregnant women. It may also be caused by acetaminophen toxicity.

MORPHOLOGY

Morphological features are almost similar irrespective of the causative agent. It can be subdivided into submassive and massive necrosis.

Gross

- Distribution of liver destruction varies. May involve **the entire liver or only random areas.**
- **Massive necrosis: Liver may shrink to 500–700 g.** It appears **shrunken, red covered by a wrinkled, too-large capsule. Cut section,** the **necrotic areas appear muddy red, and mushy** with areas of hemorrhage.

Microscopy

- **Massive necrosis** of **hepatocytes** in contiguous lobules and the reticulin framework is collapsed in these regions.
- **Minimal inflammatory reaction.**
- If the patient survives for several days, there may be inflammatory cells that phagocytose the necrotic cells.
- If the parenchymal framework is preserved, regeneration can completely restore the liver architecture.

Prognosis: The mortality is ~80% without liver transplantation and ~35% with transplantation.

Chronic Hepatitis

Definition: Chronic hepatitis is defined as **symptomatic, biochemical, or serologic evidence of** continuing or relapsing **hepatic disease present** for **more than 6 months.** Microscopically, there should be inflammation and necrosis in the liver.

Causes: Chronic hepatitis (without or with progression to cirrhosis) may be caused by viruses. **HCV** is the most common cause of chronic viral hepatitis and is mostly asymptomatic. Only 5–10% of adults infected with HBV develop chronic hepatitis. Chances of chronic hepatitis are high if the HBV **infection occurs at a younger age and with maternal-to-infant transmission.** HAV and HEV do not cause chronic hepatitis. Apart from viruses' chronic hepatitis may be caused by other etiologic agents **(Table 19.6).**

MORPHOLOGY

Q. Write a short note on chronic hepatitis.

Gross

- **Early stage:** Liver may appear **normal.**

TABLE 19.6 Major causes of chronic hepatitis.

Virus	*Other causes*
• Chronic hepatitis B • Chronic hepatitis C • Chronic hepatitis D (HDV+HBV)	• Autoimmune hepatitis • Drug-induced chronic hepatitis • Wilson disease • Cryptogenic hepatitis (non-A–E hepatitis)

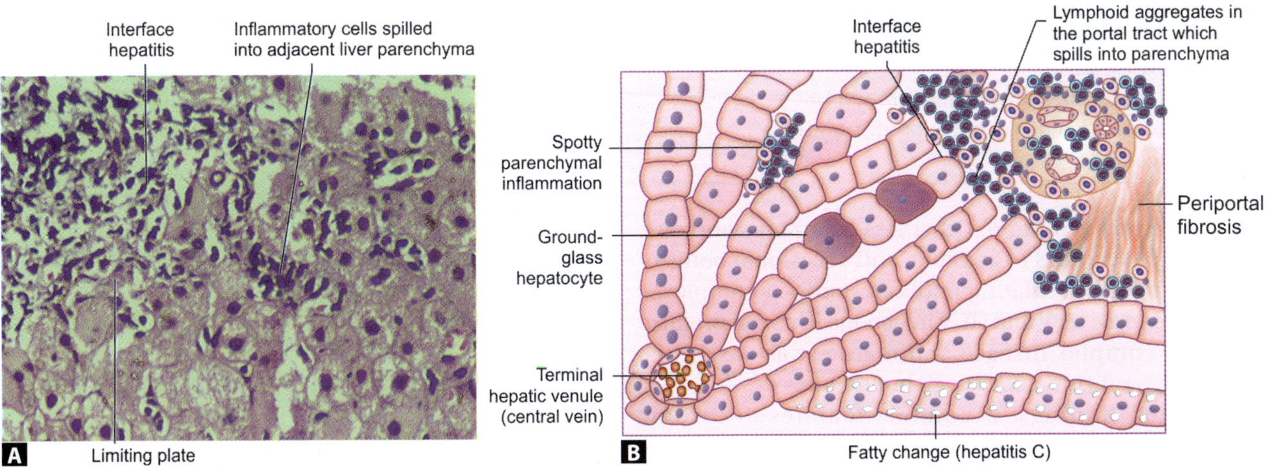

Figs. 19.10A and B: Microscopic features of chronic hepatitis: (A) Photomicrograph; (B) Diagrammatic.

- **Later stage:** Liver feels **firm** because of increased fibrosis and may progress to macronodular cirrhosis.

Microscopy (Figs. 19.10A and B)

A liver biopsy is usually done to confirm the diagnosis of chronic hepatitis and to assess inflammatory activity and fibrosis. Microscopic changes range from mild to severe hepatitis. Regardless of etiology, it is characterized by a combination of (1) portal inflammation, (2) interface hepatitis, (3) parenchymal inflammation and necrosis, and (4) fibrosis.

1. **Portal inflammation:** In **mild hepatitis,** inflammation is **limited to portal tracts** and predominantly consists of **lymphocytes, macrophages, and occasional plasma cells.**
2. **Interface hepatitis (periportal necrosis and formerly called piecemeal necrosis):** It is an **important feature** characterized by the **spillover (crossing) of inflammatory cells** (lymphocytes and plasma cells) **from the portal tract into the adjacent parenchyma** at the limiting plate. It is called interface activity or interface hepatitis. It is associated with degenerating and apoptosis of periportal hepatocytes.
3. **Parenchymal inflammation and necrosis:** It is variable in severity but usually spotty. Mononuclear inflammatory cells surround the damaged hepatocytes. **Bridging necrosis** between portal tracts and portal tracts-to-terminal hepatic veins **may be seen.**
4. **Fibrosis:** It is the **hallmark of chronic liver damage:** Continued inflammation and associated necrosis lead to progressive fibrosis at the limiting plate and enlargement of the portal tract.
   - **Initially:** Fibrosis is seen only in the portal tracts or periportal region.
   - **Later:** Periportal fibrosis is followed by bridging/linking of fibrous septa (bridging fibrosis) between adjacent fibrotic portal tracts (i.e., portal to portal) or portal-central. It eventually leads to cirrhosis.

Specific features: Some morphologic features are characteristic of the specific subtypes of chronic viral hepatitis.

- **Chronic hepatitis B (Fig. 19.11):** It shows **"ground-glass" hepatocytes** and **"sanded nuclei."** The ground-glass hepatocytes are liver cells with a pale, homogeneous, more finely granular appearance in part or all of their cytoplasm. These cells have endoplasmic reticulum swollen by HBsAg. These cells **stain orange with Orcein stain.** The presence of viral antigens in these hepatocytes can be demonstrated by immunohistochemistry. Sanded nuclear appearance is due to HBcAg.
- **Chronic hepatitis C:** It usually shows **large lymphoid aggregates** and is associated with a **fatty change** in scattered hepatocytes. It may also show bile duct damage.

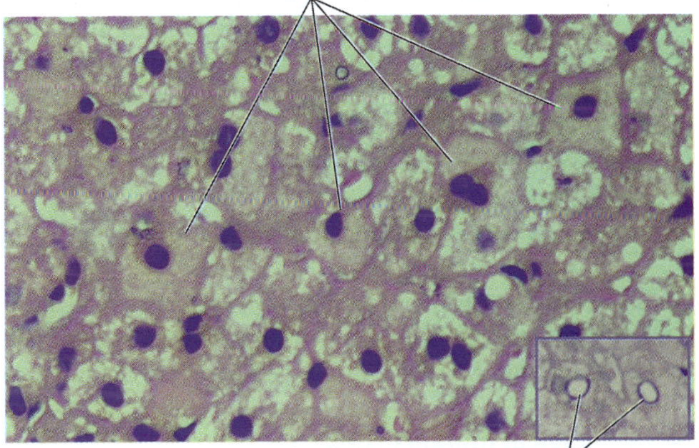

Fig. 19.11: Chronic hepatitis B showing ground-glass hepatocytes. The liver cells show cytoplasmic inclusions that stain light pink and finely granular appearance on hematoxylin and eosin staining and give rise to ground-glass hepatocytes. It is due to the accumulation of hepatitis B surface antigen (HBsAg) in the smooth endoplasmic reticulum. The inset shows hepatocyte nuclei with a sanded appearance due to the accumulation of hepatitis B core antigen (HBcAg).

Clinical features of chronic hepatitis: These are highly variable. In some individuals, persistently raised levels of serum transaminases may be the only clinical evidence of chronic hepatitis. In symptomatic patients, **fatigue is the**

BOX 19.8: Serological markers of chronic hepatitis B.

- Positive HBsAg
- Positive IgG anti-HBc, negative IgM anti-HBc
- Positive HBe antigen or rarely, positive anti-HBe
- Positive HBV-DNA

most common symptom. Other less common symptoms include malaise, loss of appetite, and occasional bouts of mild jaundice. Circulating antibody–antigen complexes occur in chronic HBV and HCV infections. This can produce immune complex disease and manifest as vasculitis, glomerulonephritis, and cryoglobulinemia.

Laboratory findings: Laboratory features of chronic hepatitis B cannot adequately distinguish mild from severe hepatitis.

- **Biochemical investigations:** These include the following:
  - **Serum aminotransferase: Mild** to moderate **elevation** and may fluctuate in the range of 100–1,000 units/dL. ALT (SGPT) tends to be more raised than compared to AST (SGOT). Once cirrhosis develops AST levels exceed ALT.
  - **Serum alkaline phosphatase:** Normal or only marginally elevated.
  - **Serum bilirubin:** May be normal or raised in the range of 3–10 mg/dL.
  - **Serum proteins: Hypoalbuminemia** in severe cases and hyperglobulinemia in severe or end-stage cases
  - **Prothrombin time:** Prolonged in severe or end-stage cases.
- **Serological markers** (**Box 19.8** and *refer* pages 656-7, and 659 for different hepatotropic viral hepatitis).
- **Urine** shows increased bilirubin and urobilinogen.

Consequences: Continued loss of hepatocytes and fibrosis results in **cirrhosis.** Cirrhosis is characterized by irregularly sized nodules separated by broad fibrous scars and is referred to as **postnecrotic cirrhosis.** It is usually **macronodular or mixed micro- and macronodular** type. The term postnecrotic is not specific and is applied to any cirrhosis in which the liver shows large, irregular-sized nodules with broad scars.

Carrier State

Definition: A "carrier" is an individual **who harbors** and **can transmit an organism (HBV)**, but **does not manifest symptoms.**

Types of carriers: The carrier state constitutes reservoirs for infection. For hepatotropic viruses, carrier states are of two separate types:

1. **Inactive carriers (healthy carriers)**: These individuals carry one of the hepatotropic viruses but have no liver disease. For healthy carriers in HBV have **normal or** only **mildly raised serum aminotransferase** values. They also **have HBsAg and anti-HBe** but **without HBeAg** but **show anti-HBe.** The majority do not progress to liver disease.

   In HCV, there is no state equivalent to the HBV "healthy carrier."
2. **Active carriers**: They harbor the viruses and have non-progressive liver damage. They are usually asymptomatic but show intermittent or persistent **elevation of serum aminotransferase levels.**

Factors determining carrier state: These include the following:

- **Age at infection:** If infection occurs **in children perinatally**, there is likely a high rate of developing carrier state. The carrier rate is lowest when adults are infected.
- **Impaired immunity** may be associated with the carrier state.

The general morphologic changes of viral hepatitis are diagrammatically shown in **Figures 19.12A and B.** Mnemonics of hepatotropic viruses are presented (*refer* **online Box 19.9**).

ALCOHOL-RELATED LIVER DISEASE

PA 25.4 (CC): Describe the pathophysiology, pathology, and progression of alcoholic liver disease including cirrhosis.

Chronic and excessive alcohol (ethanol, ethyl alcohol) consumption is **one of the major causes of liver disease.** The most important adverse effects of chronic alcohol consumption are alcohol-related fatty liver disease. This alcohol-related liver disease (also called alcoholic liver disease/ALD) constitutes a **spectrum of disorders** consisting of **three major, distinctive, but overlapping lesions (Fig. 19.13):** (1) Hepatic steatosis (fatty liver), (2) steatohepatitis (formerly termed alcoholic hepatitis), and (3) fibrosis and alcohol-related cirrhosis.

Interrelation between alcohol-related liver disease: Approximately 90% to 100% of individuals who chronically consume excess alcohol develop fatty liver (i.e., hepatic steatosis). Of these, 10% to 35% develop steatohepatitis, and 8–20% of these individuals develop cirrhosis. Steatosis, steatohepatitis, and fibrosis may develop sequentially or independently. They need not represent a sequential continuation of changes. Hepatocellular carcinoma may occur in 10–20% of patients with cirrhosis due to excessive alcohol use.

Metabolism of Ethanol (Fig. 19.14)

The liver is the main organ involved in the ethanol (alcohol) metabolism.

Formation of acetaldehyde: Ethanol is metabolized to acetaldehyde by three enzyme systems present in the liver, namely—(1) Alcohol dehydrogenases (ADHs), (2) cytochrome P-450 2E1 (CYP2E1), and (3) catalase (least important).

1. **Alcohol dehydrogenase (ADH):** It is present in the cytoplasm of the liver and is the **main enzyme system involved in alcohol metabolism at low concentrations.**

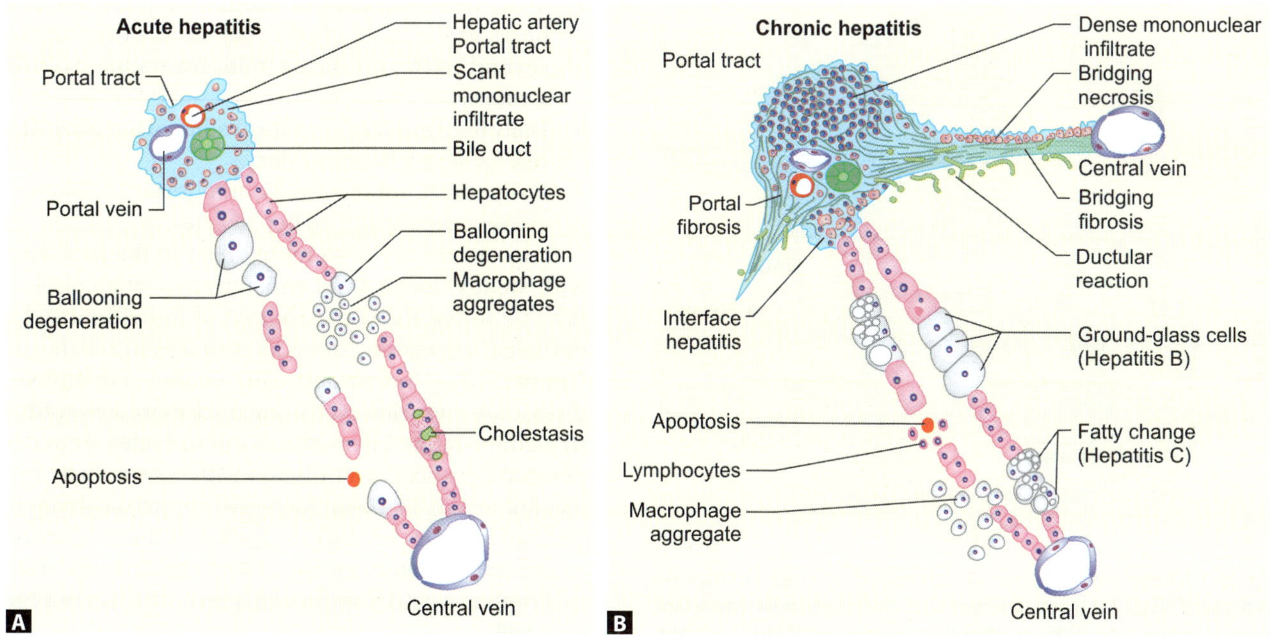

Figs. 19.12A and B: Diagrammatic representation of the general morphologic changes in acute and chronic hepatitis: (A) Acute hepatitis is characterized by lobular inflammation, minimal mononuclear infiltration in the portal tract, and hepatocellular injury; (B) Chronic hepatitis shows dense inflammation in the portal region. Bridging necrosis occurs in chronic hepatitis, but can also occur in severe acute hepatitis. In chronic hepatitis, fibrosis, and ductular reaction are usually present in areas of fibrosis.

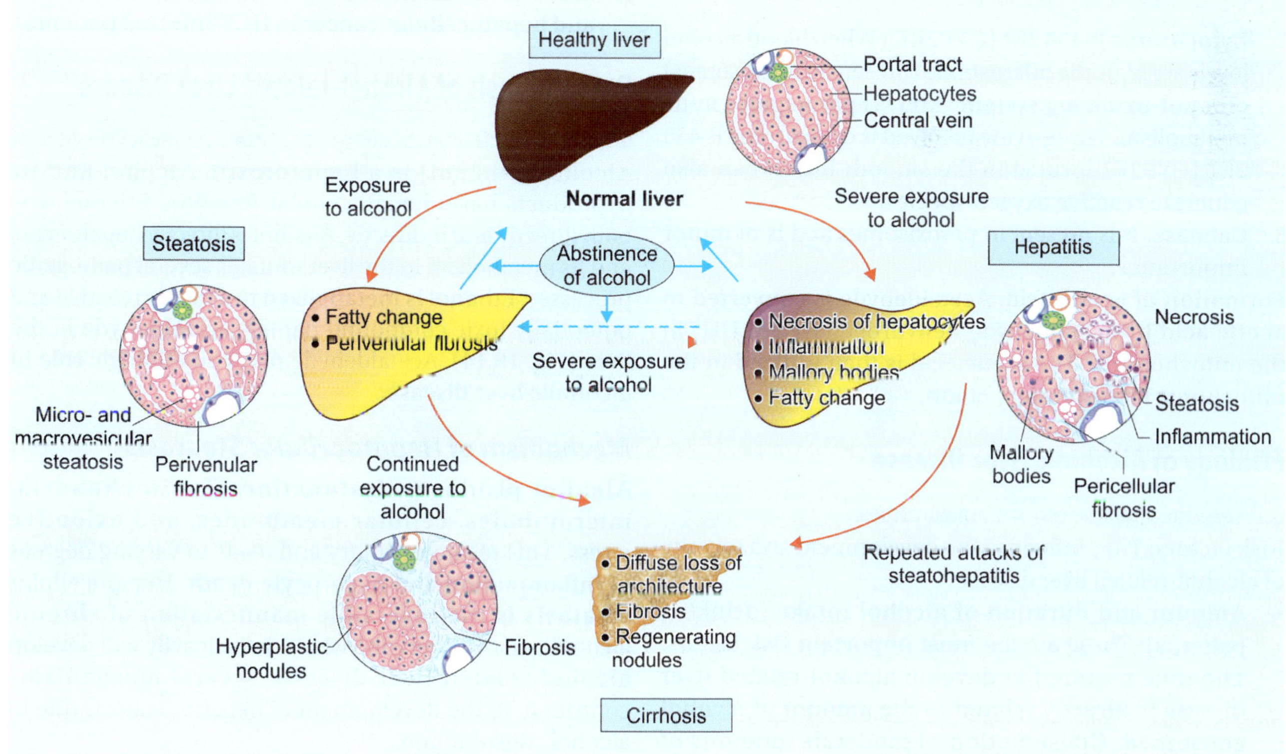

Fig. 19.13: Alcohol-related liver disease. Interrelationships among steatosis, steatohepatitis, and alcohol-related cirrhosis.

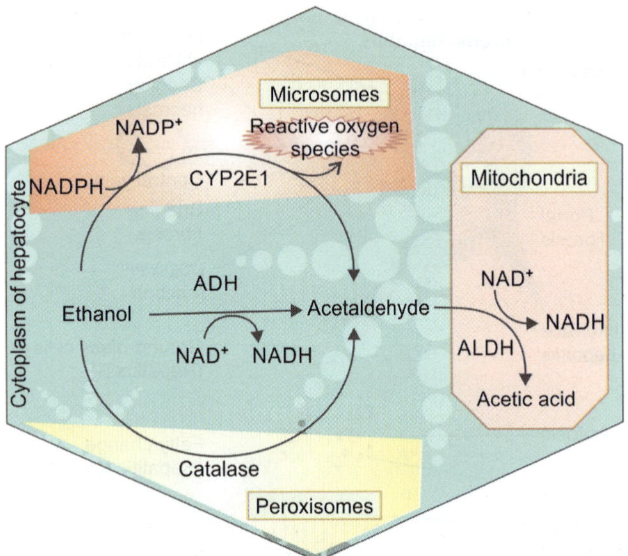

Fig. 19.14: Ethanol metabolism in hepatocytes. Ethanol is converted to acetaldehyde by three different routes: (1) the most important route is in the cytosol by alcohol dehydrogenase (ADH) (2) in the microsomes (by CYP2E1), and (3) in the peroxisomes (by catalase). Acetaldehyde is oxidized by aldehyde dehydrogenase (ALDH) to acetic acid in mitochondria. Oxidation through CYPs in the microsomes may also generate reactive oxygen species.

($NADP^+$: Nicotinamide-adenine dinucleotide phosphate; NADPH: reduced form of nicotinamide-adenine dinucleotide phosphate; NAD^+: nicotinamide adenine dinucleotide; NADH: reduced form of nicotinamide adenine dinucleotide)

2. **Cytochrome P-450 2E1 (CYP2E1):** When blood alcohol levels are high, the **microsomal** (present in microsomes) **ethanol-oxidizing system** (MEOS) participates in its metabolism. The enzyme involved is cytochrome P-450 2E1 (CYP2E1 located in the smooth ER). It **can also generate reactive oxygen species**.
3. **Catalase**: It is present in peroxisomes and is of **minor importance**.

Formation of acetic acid: Acetaldehyde **is converted to acetic acid** by acetaldehyde dehydrogenase (ALDH) in the mitochondria. The acetic acid is then **utilized in the mitochondrial respiratory chain.**

Etiology of Alcoholic Liver Disease

Q. Discuss the pathogenesis of alcoholic cirrhosis.

Risk factors: They influence the development and severity of alcohol-related liver disease.

- **Amount and duration of alcohol intake** (drinking patterns): These are the **most important risk** factors. The time required to develop alcohol-related liver disease **is directly related to the amount of alcohol consumed**. Consumption of moderate amounts of alcohol is usually not injurious, but excessive amounts cause damage.
  - Short-term ingestion of about 80 g of alcohol (six beers or 8 ounces of 80-proof liquor) over one to several days ° produces mild, reversible hepatic steatosis.
  - Daily intake of 80 g or more of ethanol increases the risk for severe hepatic injury.
  - Daily consumption of 160 g or more for 10–20 years causes severe injury to hepatocytes.

  Binge drinking causes more injury to the liver than with steady, lower-level consumption of alcohol. It is to be noted that only 10–15% of individuals who chronically consume excess alcohol develop cirrhosis.
- **Gender:** Most individuals with alcohol-related liver disease are men. However, **women are more susceptible** to alcohol-related liver disease than males. Females develop advanced liver disease with substantially less alcohol intake. Estrogen increases gut permeability to endotoxins (gut-derived) and increases the production of pro-inflammatory cytokines and chemokines (from macrophages and Kupffer cells) resulting in injury to liver cells.
- **Genetic factors:** Genetic predisposition is likely and **polymorphisms in detoxifying enzymes** (aldehyde-dehydrogenase-ALDH) have been identified.
- **Associated conditions: Iron overload** and **chronic infections with HCV and HBV** can **increase the severity** of ALD and **hasten the progression** of alcohol-related liver disease to cirrhosis in chronic alcoholics. Even **moderate alcohol intake increases the risk of cirrhosis and hepatocellular cancer in HCV-infected patients.**

Pathogenesis of Alcohol-related Liver Disease

Q. Write a short note on the etiopathogenesis of alcoholic liver disease.

Alcohol (ethanol) is a **hepatotoxin**. Alcohol and its byproducts harm hepatocellular function. Ethanol acts both directly and indirectly. Alcohol is directly hepatotoxic, and its metabolism in the liver initiates several pathogenic processes. **Ethanol is metabolized** to a highly reactive and potentially toxic compound namely **acetaldehyde** in the liver **(Fig. 19.14)**. Acetaldehyde **plays an etiologic role in alcoholic liver disease**.

Mechanism of Hepatocellular Steatosis

Alcohol produces dysfunction of mitochondria, microtubules, cellular membranes, and oxidative stress. This results in injury and leads to varying degrees of **inflammation and hepatocyte death**. Hepatocellular **steatosis is** the **reversible** manifestation of chronic alcoholism. Not everyone who drinks heavily will develop alcohol-related liver disease. Several mechanisms contribute to the development of hepatic steatosis due to alcohol consumption.

Increased redox (NADH: NAD^+) ratio due to increased generation of NADH: Metabolism of alcohol-by-alcohol dehydrogenase (ADH) and acetaldehyde dehydrogenase (ALDH) produces large amounts of nicotinamide-adenine dinucleotide (NADH). This causes decreased nicotinamide adenine dinucleotide (NAD^+) in both the cytoplasm as well as the mitochondria of hepatocytes. The **acetaldehyde** formed from ethanol **is converted to acetic acid in mitochondria**. This reaction also increases, causes NADH/NAD^+ ratio in the mitochondria, and generates reactive oxygen species (superoxide ions). Normally, antioxidant glutathione is transported from the cytoplasm into the mitochondria and can neutralize oxidants. This transport of glutathione is impaired in alcoholic liver disease. Due to the **depletion of glutathione,** the generated reactive oxygen species produce **mitochondrial dysfunction.** Increased NADH and reduced NAD have several effects that favor lipogenesis (***refer*** **Fig. 2.28**).

1. **Shunts fatty acid precursors away from catabolism and toward lipid biosynthesis:** Decreased NAD^+ in the cytoplasm **suppresses the oxidation of fatty acid** and increases the expression of enzymes that favor the synthesis of fatty acid in the liver. The increased fat/lipid generated accumulates in the cytoplasm of hepatocytes.
2. **Ethanol impairs the assembly and secretion of lipoproteins:** Ethanol may impair lipoprotein assembly and secretion and may lead to further accumulation of lipids.
3. **Alcohol also increases the catabolism of fat in peripheral tissues** (lipolysis) and increases the delivery of free fatty acids to the liver. Most of the fat deposited in the liver is derived from the diet.
4. **Increases fatty acid synthesis from acetate:** Acetaldehyde formed from ethanol is oxidized into acetate via ALDH. Ethanol increases fatty acid synthesis from acetate.
5. Decreases the oxidation of fatty acids by mitochondria.
6. Increases the production of triglycerides.

Mechanism of Steatohepatitis and Cirrhosis (Fig. 19.15)

The exact pathogenesis of *steatohepatitis* secondary to alcohol is not known. It may be produced due to one or more of the following toxic byproducts of ethanol and its metabolites:

Acetaldehyde: It is a major metabolite of ethanol. It causes lipid peroxidation and forms **chemical adducts with cellular proteins** (acetaldehyde-protein adduct) in hepatocytes. These adducts may disrupt cytoskeleton and membrane function.

Mitochondrial damage: *Alcohol* can directly affect mitochondrial function and membrane fluidity.

Reactive oxygen species (oxidative stress): Oxidation of alcohol in the liver by the microsomal ethanol oxidizing

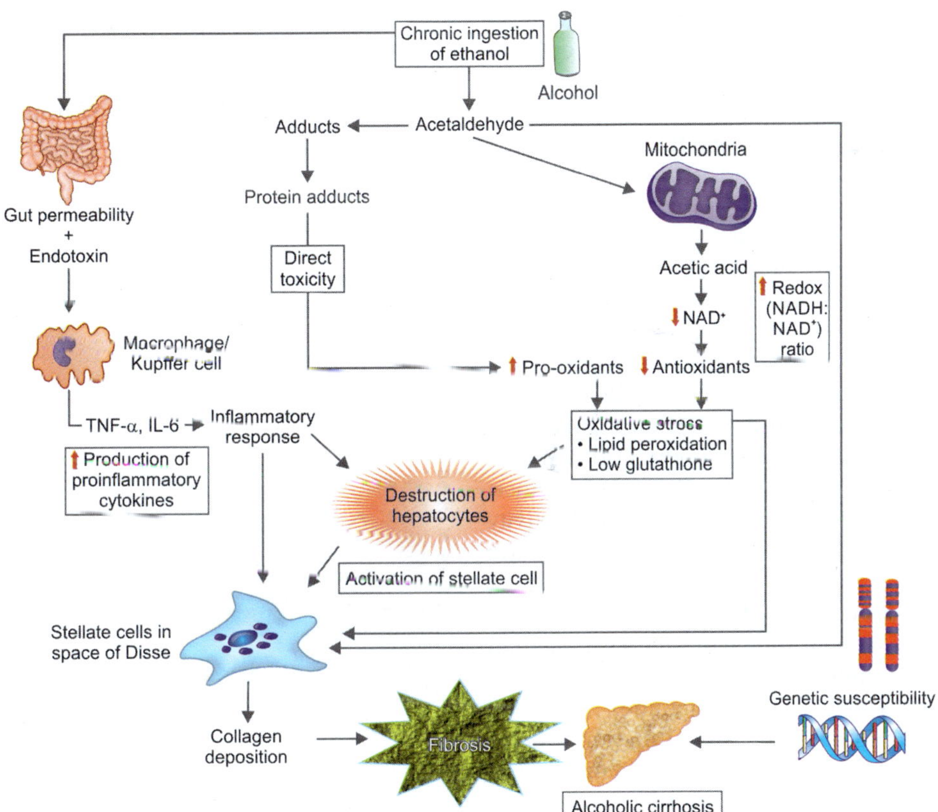

Fig. 19.15: Pathogenesis of alcoholic-related liver disease.

system produces **reactive oxygen species** (such as hydrogen peroxide and superoxide ions). They react with and damage membranes (by **lipid peroxidation**) and proteins. Reactive oxygen species are also generated by neutrophils, which infiltrate in the region of hepatocyte necrosis.

The production of acetaldehyde and free radicals is maximum in the centrilobular region. Therefore, the centrilobular region is most susceptible to alcohol-induced injury. Pericellular and sinusoidal fibrosis also occurs first in this region of the hepatic lobule. Concurrent viral hepatitis, particularly hepatitis C, increases alcohol-related liver disease.

Increased production of proinflammatory cytokines: It may occur in two ways:

1. **Lipopolysaccharide (endotoxin) from gram-negative bacteria**: In the intestinal flora, alcohol increases the uptake of bacterial endotoxin (lipopolysaccharide-LPS) from gram-negative bacteria present in the gut. **LPS enters** the **portal circulation and stimulates the production** of **TNF-α** and other **cytokines** [interleukin (IL)-6 and transforming growth factor (TGF)-α] from macrophages and Kupffer cells. They produce inflammatory responses and **injure the liver cells.**
2. **Impaired proteasome function:** The normal function of the ubiquitin-proteasome pathway is to remove irregular and damaged proteins. In alcohol-related liver disease, the function of the proteasome is impaired. This **causes inefficient degradation of ubiquitin and accumulation of large amounts of ubiquitin** in the hepatocytes **in the form of Mallory bodies.** Impaired proteasome function also causes the death of hepatocytes and releases cytokines, such as IL-8 and IL-18. IL-8 attracts neutrophils, and IL-18 sustains inflammation and causes damage to liver cells.

Other factors: These are as follows:

- **Hypoxic damage:** The centrilobular area of the hepatic lobule has the lowest oxygen tension and high susceptibility to hypoxia-induced damage. Chronic alcohol consumption increases oxygen demand by the liver resulting in hypoxia of the centrilobular region.
- **Reduced levels of ADH and ALDH isozymes:** The efficiency of alcohol metabolism in the liver depends on the expression levels of ADH and ALDH isozymes. Persons having genetic variants with low ALDH activity cannot oxidize acetaldehyde and cannot tolerate alcohol.
- **Malnutrition and deficiencies of vitamins:** When alcohol becomes a major source of calories in the diet of an alcoholic, the individual may develop malnutrition and vitamin deficiencies (such as thiamine). Additional factors, such as impaired digestive function (due to chronic gastric and intestinal mucosal damage and pancreatitis), may further contribute to these defects.

Damage caused by the factors mentioned above leads to inflammation. When it becomes chronic, fibrosis and deranged vascular perfusion occur in the liver. Alcohol-related liver disease can be considered a maladaptive state in which hepatocytes respond in an increasingly pathologic manner to a stimulus (alcohol) that originally was only marginally harmful.

Mechanisms of Fibrosis/Cirrhosis (Fig. 19.16)

Stellate cells (Ito cells or perisinusoidal cells) are present in the space of Disse between hepatocytes and sinusoidal endothelial cells. Normally, the stellate cells are quiescent and store vitamin A.

Activation of stellate cells: One of the characteristic features of cirrhosis is fibrosis. Alcohol activates hepatic stellate cells **transformed into highly fibrogenic cells with myofibroblast-like contractile properties.** They produce collagen (fibrosis) and lose their stored vitamin A. Myofibroblasts are also capable of constricting sinusoidal vascular channels thereby increasing vascular resistance within the liver. The causes of **stellate cell activation are as follows:**

- **Cytokine and chemokine:** It is produced by Kupffer cells, endothelial cells, hepatocytes, and bile duct epithelial cells. For example, transforming growth factor β (TGF-β).
- **Inflammatory cytokines:** These are produced by chronic inflammation and include: Tumor necrosis factor (TNF), lymphotoxin, interleukin 1β (IL-1β), and lipid peroxidation products.
- **Oxidative stress.**

Cirrhosis develops after 10–15 years in only a small percentage of individuals who chronically drink excess alcohol. The reason is unknown. With complete abstinence,

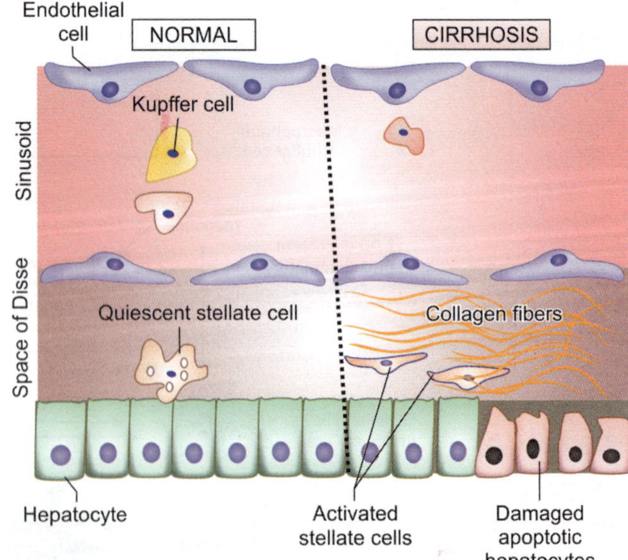

Fig. 19.16: Pathogenesis of fibrosis in cirrhosis of the liver. Activation of the stellate cell is followed by the proliferation of fibroblasts and the deposition of collagen in the space of Disse.

partial regression of scarring occurs, and rarely, there is complete regression of cirrhosis.

MORPHOLOGY

Q. Write a short note on the morphology of alcoholic (alcohol-related) liver disease.

Hepatocellular Steatosis (Fatty Change)

Gross: The **liver** with widespread steatosis **is enlarged** (can cause massive enlargement of the liver and may weigh about 4–6 kg or more), **soft, yellow, and greasy** (*refer* Fig. 2.29).

Microscopy (Figs. 19.17 and *refer* Fig. 2.30)

Accumulation of fat usually begins in centrilobular hepatocytes. The lipid droplets in hepatocytes range from small (microvesicular) to large (macrovesicular).

1. **Microvesicular steatosis (Fig. 19.17A):** It is the **accumulation of small, clear vacuoles of lipids within the cytoplasm of hepatocytes.** It is the initial and most common histologic response. It affects **acinar zone 3 (perivenular/centrilobular region of lobule)** where alcohol dehydrogenase (the major enzyme responsible for alcohol metabolism) is located and hence, affected first. The **nuclei of affected hepatocytes are centrally located and the cytoplasm looks foamy.**
2. **Macrovesicular steatosis (Fig. 19.17B):** It **develops with continuing alcohol ingestion.** This creates **clear large, lipid vacuole/s** (single or multiple), which **compress and displace the hepatocyte nucleus to the periphery** of the cell. With more extensive steatosis, the lipid accumulation in hepatocytes spreads outward from the central vein to hepatocytes in the mid-lobule and then the periportal regions. However, with the abstention from further intake of alcohol, fatty changes are **completely reversible,** and the liver returns to normal.
3. **Absence of inflammation or fibrosis:** There is usually neither inflammation nor fibrosis, but continued alcohol intake leads to **fibrosis around the terminal hepatic veins (perivenular)** and adjacent to sinusoids.

Steatohepatitis (Alcoholic Hepatitis)

Q. Write a short note on the morphology of alcoholic hepatitis.

Steatohepatitis can be caused by alcohol as well as NAFLD (nonalcoholic fatty liver disease). It is usually more prominent with alcohol use than in NAFLD. Alcoholic steatohepatitis **may be a precursor** to the development of **cirrhosis.**

MORPHOLOGY

Gross

The liver may be **enlarged; yellow** due to steatosis and **firm** due to increased fibrosis.

Q. Write a short note on Mallory body, its microscopic appearance, and conditions associated with Mallory body.

Microscopy (Figs. 19.18A and B)

Alcoholic steatohepatitis has the following characteristic features **(Box 19.10)** and the lesions are predominantly centrilobular.

1. **Hepatocyte ballooning:** It is characterized by single or scattered foci of **swollen liver cells** (hepatocytes) having pale-stained, finely granular, or clumped cytoplasm. This is **due to the accumulation** of **fat, water, and proteins.** Like steatosis, it is predominant in the centrilobular region (zone 3 of acinus). Severe ballooning degeneration may lead to hepatocyte necrosis.
2. **Mallory hyaline bodies (Mallory–Denk bodies/Mallory hyaline):** They consist of **tangled skeins (mesh/coil) of cytokeratin intermediate filaments** (**such as cytokeratin 8 and 18).** They appear as **dense, eosinophilic ropey cytoplasmic inclusions/clumps,** usually situated in a **perinuclear** location, in the degenerating hepatocytes **(Figs. 19.18** and *refer* **Fig. 2.33A).** Mallory bodies are a **characteristic but not a specific** feature of alcoholic liver disease.
3. **Neutrophilic infiltration:** They are commonly seen **around ballooned hepatocytes,** particularly those containing Mallory bodies. The **portal tracts or parenchyma** may be infiltrated by **lymphocytes and macrophages** but this is not a prominent feature.

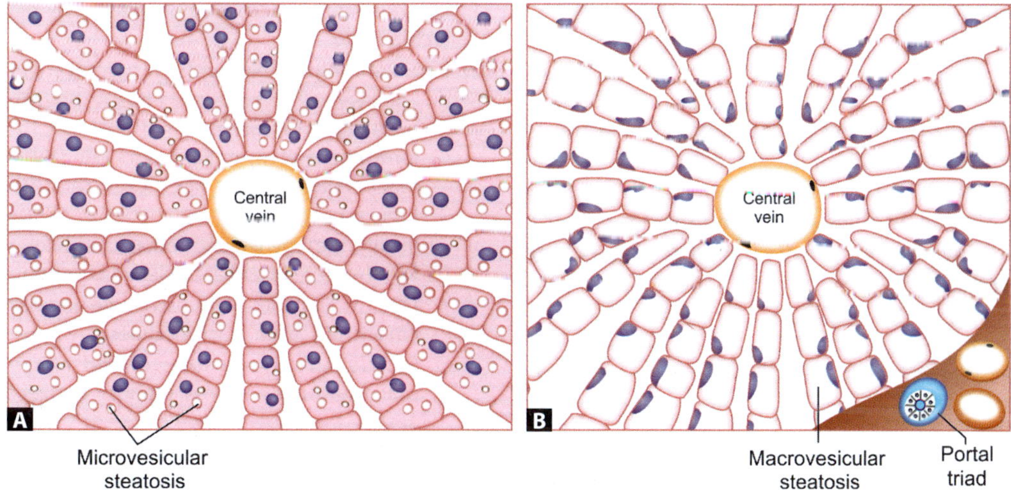

Figs. 19.17A and B: Hepatic steatosis: (A) Diagrammatic appearance of microvesicular steatosis; (B) Macrovesicular steatosis.

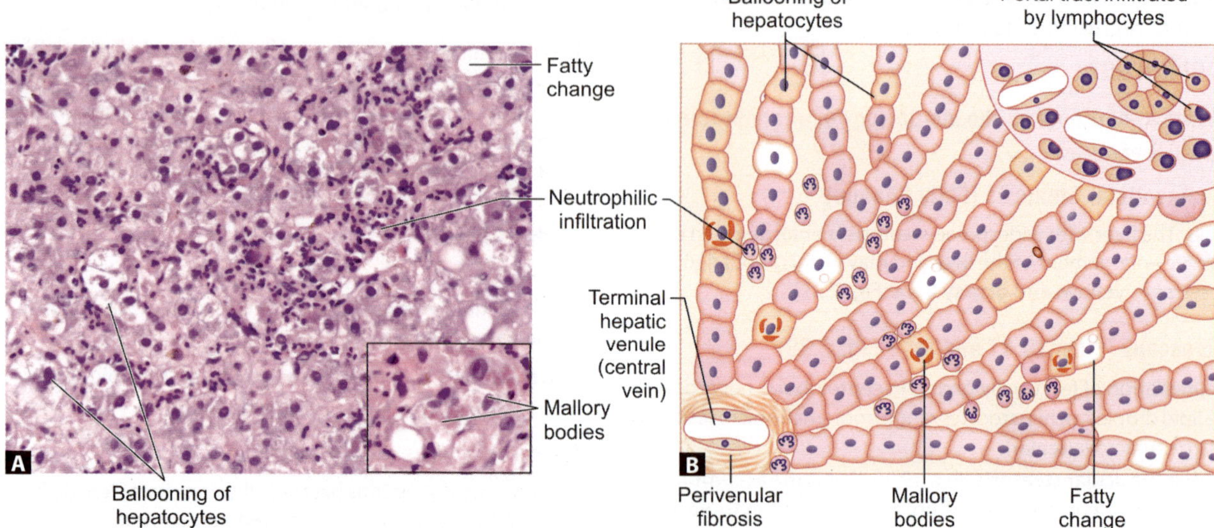

Figs. 19.18A and B: Alcoholic hepatitis showing ballooning degeneration of hepatocytes, fatty change, Mallory bodies, and neutrophilic infiltration: (A) Photomicrograph and inset shows Mallory bodies; (B) Diagrammatic.

BOX 19.10: Microscopic features of steatohepatitis.

- Hepatocyte ballooning
- Mallory bodies
- Neutrophilic infiltration
- Steatofibrosis
- Variable degree of steatosis

4. **Alcoholic steatofibrosis:** Alcoholic hepatitis may activate sinusoidal stellate cells and portal fibroblasts. This produces fibrosis which **initially starts in the centrilobular region as central vein sclerosis.** This is followed by perisinusoidal fibrosis in the space of Disse of the centrilobular region. Then fibrosis spreads further outward to the periphery of the lobule, enclosing **single or small groups of hepatocytes in a chicken wire fence pattern.** In late stages, fibrosis may link fibrous tissue from the **central vein to portal tracts.** Eventually, nodularity may develop leading to cirrhosis.
5. **Variable degree of steatosis:** Described earlier under steatosis.

Alcoholic Cirrhosis

Cirrhosis is **chronic, irreversible,** and **end-stage** of alcoholic liver disease. It is characterized by diffuse loss of architecture with fibrosis and parenchymal nodular regeneration. Usually evolves slowly and insidiously. It is also known as **Laennec cirrhosis, portal cirrhosis, and nutritional cirrhosis**.

MORPHOLOGY

Q. Write a short note on the morphology (pathology) of alcoholic cirrhosis.

Gross

Early stage: Liver appears **yellow-tan, fatty, and enlarged,** usually weighs above 2 kg.

Late stage (Figs. 19.19A and B): Liver appears brown, nonfatty (loses fat), **diffusely nodular,** and **firm.** The **size** of the liver progressively becomes **smaller** than normal **(shrunken).** The weight may be sometimes less than 1 kg.

- **Micronodular cirrhosis: The capsular surface** of the liver is **nodular** or may have a pig-skin texture. As it advances, the nodularity becomes more prominent and nodules are less than 3 mm (**micronodular**) and have a **"hobnail"** appearance on the surface of the liver.
- **Mixed micronodular and macronodular pattern:** With time, the nodules may coalesce to form larger nodules and form a **mixed micronodular and macronodular pattern.**
- End-stage alcoholic cirrhosis resembles cirrhosis due to other causes and the underlying etiology cannot be determined by both gross and microscopic examination.

Microscopy (Figs. 19.20A to C)

1. **Diffuse loss of architecture:** The hepatocyte injury and consequent fibrosis involve the entire liver diffuse loss of the architecture.
2. **Regenerating nodules without normal architecture:**
   - The liver cell damage and fibrosis stimulate the surviving hepatocytes to regenerate and proliferate. These hepatocytes form regenerating nodules surrounded by fibrous septa. The regeneration nodules lack the normal structure of the liver lobules or acini.
   - Initially, the regenerating nodules are uniform with diameters less than 0.3 cm and are called **micronodules.**
   - Later wider bands of fibrosis create nodules larger than 0.3 cm and are called **macronodules.**
   - Finally, the liver shows **mixed micronodular and macronodular patterns. Mallory bodies** are usually **not seen** at this stage.
3. **Fibrosis:** It is initially delicate and extends through sinusoids from **central-to-portal regions as well as from portal tract to portal tract.** Later, there are **broad bands of fibrosis.**

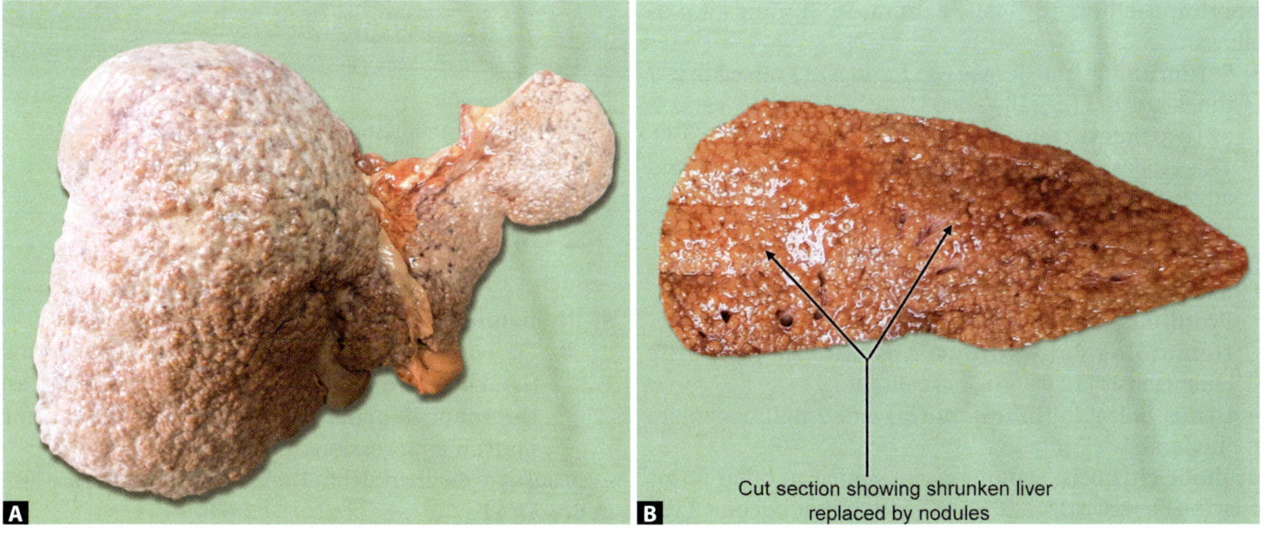

Figs. 19.19A and B: Gross appearance of alcoholic cirrhosis showing diffuse replacement of parenchyma by micronodules: (A) Outer aspect; (B) Cut section.

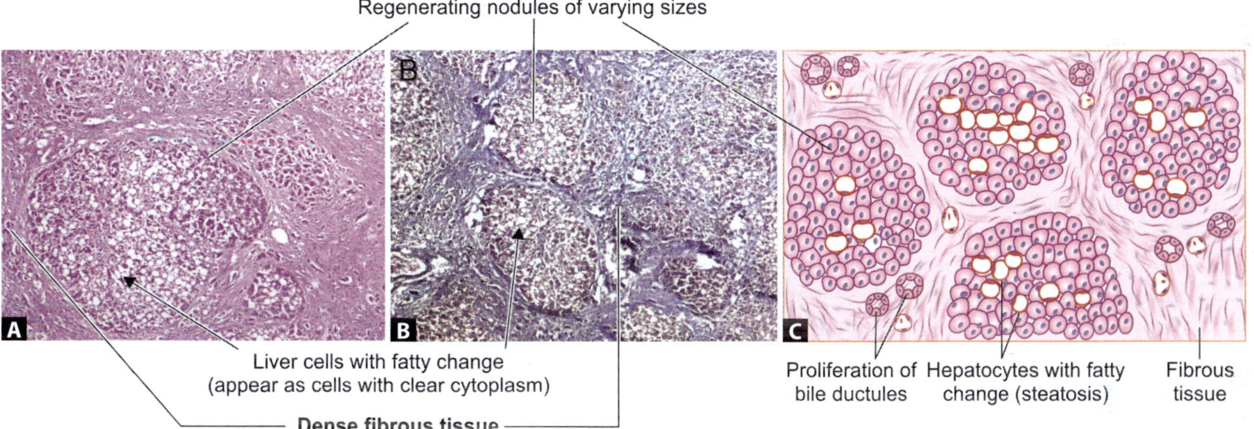

Figs. 19.20A to C: Microscopic appearance of alcoholic cirrhosis: (A) Photomicrograph; (B) Masson trichrome; (C) Diagrammatic showing abnormal regenerating nodules of varying sizes separated by fibrous tissue. In B, fibrous tissue appears blue (Masson trichrome).

4. **Vascular reorganization:** The parenchymal damage and fibrosis disrupt the vascular architecture of the liver. New vascular channels will be formed in the fibrotic septa, which connect the vessels in the portal region (hepatic arteries and portal veins) to terminal hepatic veins, shunting blood from the parenchyma.

Clinical Features

Steatosis (fatty liver): It may produce hepatomegaly and there may be mild elevation of serum bilirubin, alkaline phosphatase, and γ-glutamyl transpeptidase (GGTP). Alcohol cessation and with the provision of an adequate diet, the liver can return to normal. Laboratory findings are as follows:

- Moderately **raised ALT and aspartate aminotransferase (AST) with AST: ALT >1.**
- **γ-GT (gamma-glutamyl transpeptidase)** level is a sensitive test to determine whether the individual is taking alcohol. There is increased synthesis of this due to the induction of the smooth endoplasmic reticulum by alcohol.
- **Liver biopsy:** It shows the accumulation of fat in perivenular hepatocytes and later in the entire hepatic lobule.

Steatohepatitis: It can develop after just weeks or months of heavy alcohol use. It appears acutely, usually following a bout of heavy drinking. Symptoms may be nonspecific, such as malaise, anorexia, weight loss, upper abdominal discomfort, fever, and tender hepatomegaly. The outlook is unpredictable. Each attack of alcohol-related hepatitis carries a 10–20% risk of death. Repeated bouts of alcohol-related hepatitis may lead to cirrhosis in about one-third of patients within a few years. Steatohepatitis may be superimposed on cirrhosis. Laboratory findings are as follows:

- **Serum aminotransferase (AST and ALT) raised** to 2–7 times normal (usually <500 U/mL). **AST: ALT ratio is >2** (two times greater increase in serum AST than ALT). This is because AST is located in the mitochondria, and alcohol damages the mitochondria in hepatocytes.
- **Serum bilirubin**: Raised
- **Serum alkaline phosphatase**: Mildly elevated
- **Serum albumin**: Decreased
- **Prothrombin time**: Prolonged
- **Hematological findings**: Absolute neutrophilic leukocytosis (12,000–14,000 cells/μL).
- **Urine:** Bilirubin (**bilirubinuria**) and urobilinogen are moderately elevated.

Alcoholic cirrhosis: Symptoms are similar to other forms of cirrhosis (*refer* page 675). When ethanol becomes the major source of calories in the diet, it causes malnutrition and vitamin deficiencies (e.g., thiamine, and folate). It may also produce chronic gastric and intestinal mucosal damage and pancreatitis. Investigations help assess the severity and type of liver disease.

- **Hyperbilirubinemia**: Due to the rise in both conjugated and unconjugated bilirubin. Not very common with cirrhosis. Could suggest superadded hepatitis, hepatocellular carcinoma, congestive or obstructive etiology.
- **Serum proteins:** Show **reversal of the A: G ratio.**
  - **Serum albumin is decreased** (hypoalbuminemia) and is due to reduced synthesis by the liver.
  - **Serum globulin is increased** (hyperglobulinemia) due to stimulation of the reticuloendothelial system.
- **Serum transaminases:**
  - **AST (SGOT) is raised**
  - **ALT (SGPT) is raised** and usually less than 300 units/dL.
  - **AST: ALT ratio: More than 2 in alcoholic cirrhosis** and **less than 2 in cirrhosis complicating viral hepatitis**.
- **Alkaline phosphatase:** It may be slightly elevated.
- **Prothrombin time: Prolonged** due to reduced synthesis of clotting (especially vitamin K-dependent) factors.
- **Serological markers:** For hepatitis B and C.
- **Blood ammonia** estimation: It is a reliable investigation when hepatic encephalopathy is suspected. Raised blood ammonia is due to:
  - Decreased clearance by liver
  - Shunting of portal venous blood to the systemic circulation.
- **Serum electrolytes**: Low sodium (hyponatremia) indicates severe liver disease and is due to either a defect in free water clearance or to excess diuretic therapy. Other findings include hypokalemia, hypomagnesemia, and hypophosphatemia.

BOX 19.11: Causes of death in alcohol-related liver disease.

- Hepatic coma
- Massive gastrointestinal hemorrhage
- Intercurrent infection
- Hepatorenal syndrome
- Hepatocellular carcinoma

- **Hematological tests:**
  - *Peripheral blood picture:* **Anemia and acanthocytosis** (spur-like projections on RBC), **leukopenia, and thrombocytopenia** due to hypersplenism and bone marrow suppression by alcohol).

Causes of death in alcohol-related liver disease are listed in **Box 19.11**.

NONALCOHOLIC FATTY LIVER DISEASE

- **Nonalcoholic fatty liver disease (NAFLD) is a common disease in which fatty liver develops in association with insulin resistance and metabolic syndrome. It occurs in individuals who do not drink alcohol.** The liver can show any of the three types of changes that occur in alcohol-related liver disease. These include steatosis, steatohepatitis (usually inflammation is less prominent than in alcohol-related liver disease), and cirrhosis.
- **Nonalcoholic steatohepatitis (NASH):** The term is used when there are clinical features of liver injury (e.g., elevated serum transaminases), and the histological features of hepatitis.

Systemic metabolic dysfunction is involved in NAFLD. Hence, the term **metabolic dysfunction-associated steatohepatitis (MASH)** replaces NASH and nonalcoholic fatty liver disease (NAFLD) is replaced **by metabolic (dysfunction)-associated fatty liver disease** (MAFLD).

Characteristic features associated with NAFLD are presented in **Box 19.12**.

Q. List four abnormalities associated with nonalcoholic fatty liver disease (NAFLD).

BOX 19.12: Characteristic features associated with NAFLD.

1. Association with insulin resistance
2. Metabolic syndrome
3. Type 2 diabetes (or family history of diabetes)
4. Obesity, primarily central obesity
5. Dyslipidemia (hypertriglyceridemia, low high-density lipoprotein cholesterol, high low-density lipoprotein cholesterol)
6. Hypertension

Pathogenesis (Refer Online Figs. 19.21A and B)

Increased release of free fatty acids from adipocytes: The main initiating events in NAFLD are **(i) the development of obesity and (ii) insulin resistance** (within both adipose tissue and the liver). Insulin resistance increases the mobilization of free fatty acids from adipose tissue due to overactivity of lipoprotein lipase.

Increased free fatty acid uptake by hepatocytes: Mobilization of free fatty acids from adipose tissue is associated with decreased production of the hormone adiponectin from adipocytes. It **decreases oxidation of free fatty acids by skeletal muscle** and increases free fatty acid uptake into hepatocytes. In the liver, the fatty acids are stored as triglycerides.

Inflammasome activation and release of the proinflammatory cytokine in the liver: Hepatocytes in patients with NASH show inflammasome activation. This may be due to the direct or indirect effects of lipids. This leads to the local release of the proinflammatory cytokine IL-1.

Other products of lipid metabolism: These may be directly toxic to hepatocytes. These products include increased production of reactive oxygen species, induction of ER stress, and disruption of mitochondrial function.

Alterations in the gut microbiome and increased production of gut-derived endotoxin: They may induce inflammation and injury to liver cells.

Hepatic fibrosis: Hepatocyte injury due to various mechanisms causes activation of stellate cells in the space of Disse, deposition of collagen, and hepatic fibrosis. This leads to the development of NASH.

Clinical Features

Incidental elevation of serum transaminases: NAFLD is the most common cause of **incidental elevation of serum transaminases.**

The AST to ALT ratio is less than one: In alcohol-related fatty liver disease, this ratio is more than two.

May be asymptomatic: Most of the patients with hepatic steatosis are asymptomatic and those with active steatohepatitis or fibrosis may also be asymptomatic.

Symptoms of chronic liver disease: Some patients may complain of fatigue, malaise, right upper quadrant discomfort, or symptoms of chronic liver disease.

Liver biopsy: It is needed to detect NASH and distinguish it from uncomplicated NAFLD. NAFLD is a significant contributor to the pathogenesis of "cryptogenic" cirrhosis.

Current therapy: It is directed toward the reduction of weight and reversal of insulin resistance. Lifestyle modifications to reduce weight (diet and exercise) are the most effective form of treatment.

Pediatric NAFLD: It is becoming more common due to increased problems of obesity and metabolic syndrome.

CIRRHOSIS

Q. Define cirrhosis.

Definition: Cirrhosis is a **diffuse process** (the entire liver is involved) characterized by the **transformation of the liver into abnormal regenerative parenchymal nodules surrounded by fibrous bands.**

Cirrhosis is the morphologic change associated with chronic liver disease. It is the leading causes of chronic liver failure that include chronic hepatitis B, chronic hepatitis C, nonalcoholic fatty liver disease (NAFLD), and alcohol-related liver disease. Cirrhosis is a common feature of many chronic liver diseases and is not a specific entity.

Morphological Characteristics

Cirrhosis involves the entire liver and is characterized by the formation of abnormal regenerative parenchymal nodules surrounded by fibrous bands. The three main morphologic characteristics of cirrhosis (**Figs. 19.22A and B**) are as follows:

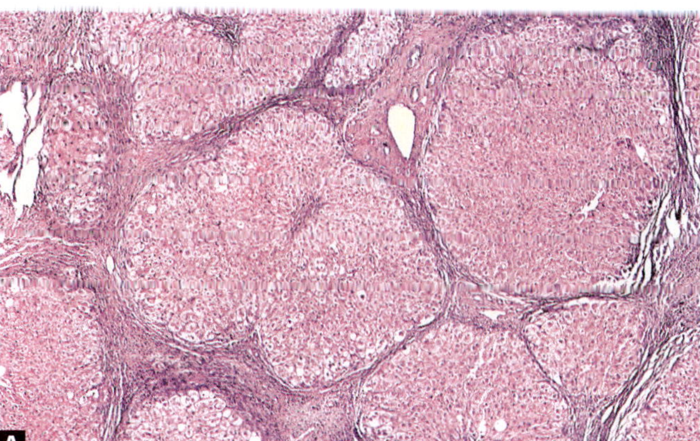

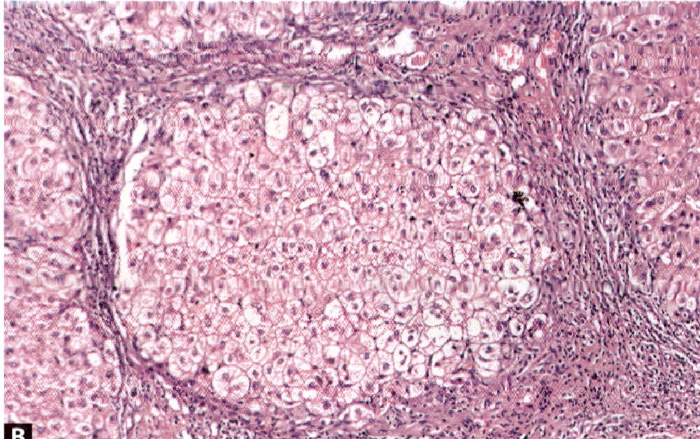

Figs. 19.22A and B: Microscopic characteristic features of cirrhosis: (A) The liver shows a loss of architecture and is replaced by numerous regenerating nodules of varying sizes. These regenerating nodules are separated by fibrosis; (B) Shows regenerating nodule surrounded by fibrosis. The regenerating nodule does not have normal architecture.

1. **Fibrosis**: It is the characteristic feature of progressive liver damage. The fibrous tissue forms delicate bands or broad scars and links portal tracts with one another and portal tracts with terminal hepatic veins.
   - **Regression of fibrosis:** Fibrosis in cirrhosis was considered as irreversible. However, it was discovered that fibrosis can regress and even in a fully established cirrhosis, the disease may undergo remission or cure. The fibrous scars may become thinner, more densely compacted, and may fragment. As fibrous septa break apart, adjacent nodules of regenerating parenchyma may coalesce and form larger islands.
2. **Regenerating nodules**: Liver cell damage is compensated by the regeneration of hepatocytes. These regenerating hepatocytes form nodules and are surrounded by fibrosis. Nodularity results from cycles of hepatocyte regeneration and scarring. The regenerating liver cells do not maintain the normal architecture. The size of nodules varies from very small (<0.3 cm, micronodules) to large (several centimeters, macronodules). The pattern of scarring may be scars either linking portal tracts to each other or linking portal tracts to central veins.
3. **Loss of architecture**: The hepatocyte injury and consequent fibrosis are diffuse processes, which occur in the entire liver. This disrupts the architecture of the **entire liver**.

Classification (Box 19.13)

Q. Classify cirrhosis.

Morphological Classification (Fig. 19.23)

Depending on the size of the regeneration nodules cirrhosis is classified as (i) micronodular, (ii) macronodular, and (iii) mixed.

1. **Micronodular cirrhosis**: It is characterized by **regular** and **small nodules** measuring **less than 3 mm in diameter**. The **fibrous tissue septa** are **usually thin** and fibrous septa bridge portal tracts and central veins (portal-portal and/or portal-central) resulting in a small nodule without central structures (e.g., alcoholic cirrhosis).

BOX 19.13: Classification of cirrhosis.

Morphologic classification
- Micronodular
- Macronodular
- Mixed

Etiological classification (depending on the etiology)
- Alcohol is one of the most common causes
- Chronic viral hepatitis (HBV and HCV)
- Nonalcoholic steatohepatitis (NASH)
- Autoimmune hepatitis
- Biliary cirrhosis, e.g., primary biliary cholangitis
- Inherited metabolic disorders:
  - Hemochromatosis
  - Wilson disease
  - α1-antitrypsin deficiency
- Cystic fibrosis
- Cryptogenic (hidden cause) or idiopathic
- Indian childhood cirrhosis
- Cardiac cirrhosis

(HBV: hepatitis B virus; HCV: hepatitis C virus)

2. **Macronodular cirrhosis:** It is characterized by the presence of nodules of variable size, more **irregular** than in micronodular cirrhosis, and usually **larger than 3 mm in diameter**. The **fibrous tissue septa are broad** and the nodules are more variable in composition and are often composed of multiple acini. Micronodular cirrhosis can be converted into a macronodular form by continued regeneration and expansion of existing nodules. For example, cirrhosis is associated with chronic hepatitis. The macronodular cirrhosis has an **increased risk** of developing **carcinoma** of the liver.
3. **Mixed cirrhosis:** It consists of both micronodules and some macronodules.

Depending on the activity, each of these forms may subclassified as an active and inactive form.

- **Active form:** It is characterized by evidence of continuing liver cell necrosis and inflammatory reaction.
- **Inactive form:** It shows neither liver cell necrosis nor inflammation.

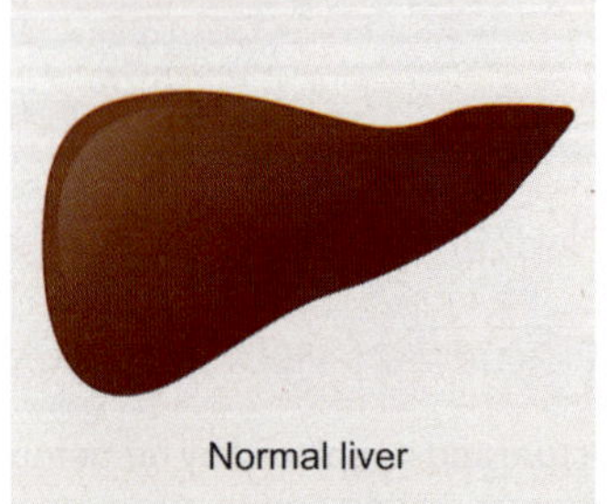

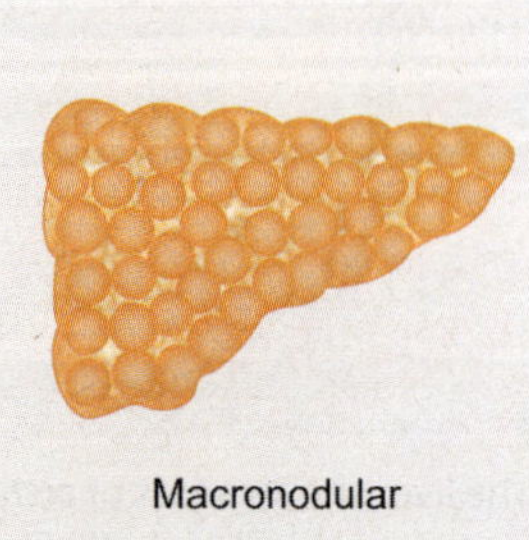

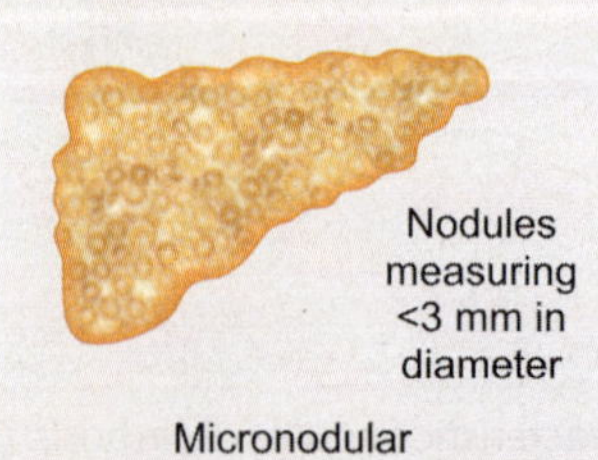

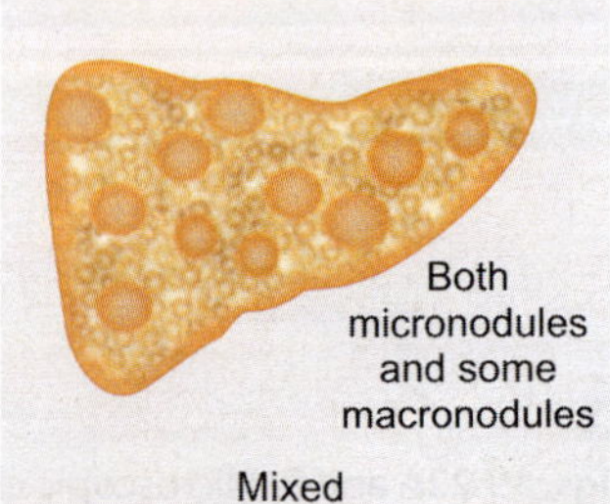

Fig. 19.23: Morphological classification of cirrhosis.

Etiological Classification

This classification takes into consideration clinical, biochemical, immunological, or biopsy features. The main causes of cirrhosis are shown in **Box 19.13**.

Pathogenesis

Four important processes are involved:

1. **Death of liver cells with loss of architecture**: The pathogenesis of hepatocyte injury varies depending on the etiological agent. The mechanism by which alcohol causes hepatocyte injury is discussed on pages 616-18.
2. **Fibrosis (Fig. 19.16):** It is mainly due to the **activation of hepatic stellate cells,** which are transformed into highly fibrogenic cells called myofibroblasts. It is discussed in detail on page 668.
3. **Regenerating nodules:** The liver cell damage and fibrosis stimulate the surviving hepatocytes to regenerate and proliferate to form regenerating nodules (*refer* page 670).
4. **Vascular reorganization:** The parenchymal damage and fibrosis disrupt the vascular architecture of the liver (*refer* page 670).

The net outcome is the formation of a fibrotic and nodular liver. The blood supply to hepatocytes is severely compromised, as well as the ability of liver cells to secrete substances into the blood.

Clinical Features

The clinical features of cirrhosis range widely:

- **Initial phase:** It is termed as "**compensated**" cirrhosis, the patient may be asymptomatic.
- **Later phase:** It is termed as "**decompensated**" cirrhosis, and presents with complications of portal hypertension or liver dysfunction (or both).

Nonspecific clinical manifestations: Anorexia, weight loss, weakness, and in advanced disease, symptoms and signs of hepatic failure may develop. Hepatic failure is usually precipitated by systemic infection or gastrointestinal hemorrhage.

PORTAL HYPERTENSION

PA 25.5 (CC): Describe the etiology, pathogenesis, and complications of portal hypertension.

Q. Write a short note on portal hypertension.

Definition: Portal hypertension is defined as the **elevation of the hepatic venous pressure** above 7 mm Hg. It leads to increased resistance to portal blood flow.

Causes of Portal Hypertension

The causes of portal hypertension can be divided into three categories:

1. **Prehepatic causes:** Obstructive thrombosis of the portal vein before it ramifies within the liver or massive splenomegaly with increased splenic vein blood flow.
2. **Posthepatic causes:** Severe right-sided heart failure, constrictive pericarditis, and hepatic vein outflow obstruction.
3. **Intrahepatic causes:** Cirrhosis (main cause), schistosomiasis, massive fatty change, and diffuse fibrosing granulomatous disease (e.g., sarcoidosis).

Pathogenesis of Portal Hypertension in Cirrhosis

It is produced by a combination of two simultaneously occurring processes:

1. **Increased intrahepatic resistance to blood flow through the liver:**
   - **Active vasoconstriction: Contraction of vascular smooth muscle cells and myofibroblasts** (functional component) also **increases the sinusoidal vascular resistance**. Intrahepatic vasoconstriction is jointly due to a deficiency in intrahepatic nitric oxide (NO) by sinusoidal endothelial cells as well as increased production of the vasoconstrictor ET-1. Intrahepatic vasoconstriction increases resistance to portal blood flow into the liver.
   - **Deposition of fibrous tissue** (scarring): Fibrosis and compression by regenerative nodules (fixed component) **increases the sinusoidal vascular resistance. In the fibrous septa, anastomosis develops between the arterial and portal system.** These impose arterial pressures on the low-pressure portal venous system and contribute to portal hypertension.
   - **Formation of regenerating parenchymal nodules:** Regenerative nodules in the cirrhotic liver impinge on the hepatic veins. This produces obstruction of blood flow beyond the hepatic lobules.
2. **Increase in portal venous inflow (flow): It results from the hyperdynamic circulation/consequences of portal hypertension**.

Major Consequences of Portal Hypertension

Q. What are the complications of cirrhosis?

Q. Write a short note on complications of portal hypertension.

Portal hypertension affects many organ systems. The consequences of portal hypertension (**Fig. 19.24**) are listed in **Box 19.14**.

Ascites

Q. Write a short note on the pathogenesis of ascites due to alcoholic cirrhosis.

Ascites is defined as the **accumulation of excess fluid** in the **peritoneal cavity**. The **most common** (85% of cases) **cause** of ascites is **portal hypertension caused by cirrhosis**.

Pathogenesis of Ascites in Cirrhosis (Fig. 19.25)

The pathogenesis of ascites is a complex process and involves the following mechanisms:

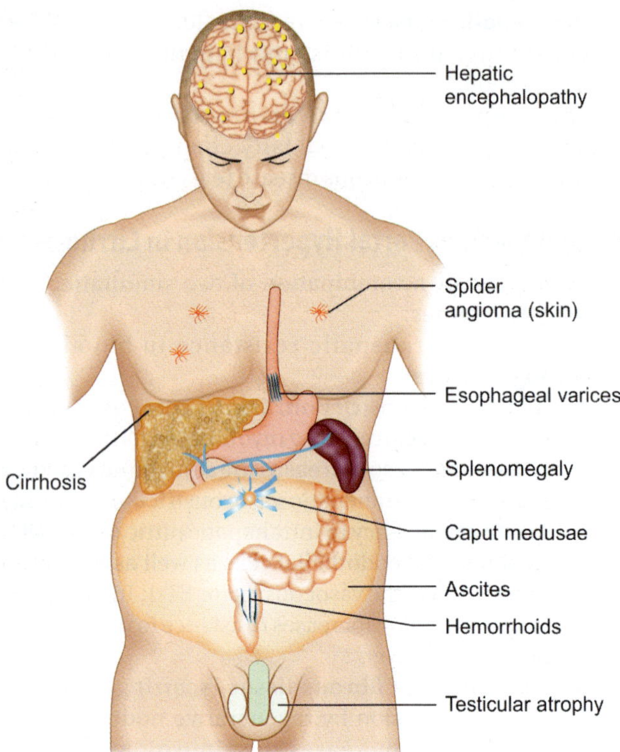

Fig. 19.24: Major clinical consequences of portal hypertension in cirrhosis.

BOX 19.14: Major consequences of portal hypertension.

- Ascites
- Formation of portosystemic venous shunts
- Congestive splenomegaly and hypersplenism
- Hepatic encephalopathy
- Endocrine complications

1. **Portal hypertension (sinusoidal hypertension):** It increases the hydrostatic pressure in the portal vein and increases the hydrostatic pressure in the portal vein and causes sinusoidal hypertension.
2. **Hypoalbuminemia:** It is due to decreased synthetic function in a cirrhotic liver that reduces the plasma oncotic pressure.
3. **Increased hepatic lymph flow:** In cirrhosis, hepatic lymphatic flow exceeds thoracic duct capacity. The excess lymph may percolate (pass through the liver) into the peritoneal cavity and cause ascites.
4. **Splanchnic vasodilation and hyperdynamic circulation**. It reduces systemic arterial blood pressure and activates the **renin-angiotensin-aldosterone system.** The development of hyperaldosteronism leads to **sodium retention,** fluid accumulation and expansion of the extracellular fluid volume.

The combination of portal hypertension, splanchnic arterial vasodilation, and sodium and water retention increases the hydrostatic pressure as well as the permeability of interstitial capillaries. It causes extravasation of fluid into the peritoneal cavity.

Portosystemic Shunts

It is one of the complications of portal hypertension due to cirrhosis. In portal hypertension, increased portal vascular resistance leads to an increase in the portal system pressure the blood flow is reversed from portal to systemic circulation by dilation of collateral vessels and the development of new vessels. Portosystemic shunting/bypasses occur at the sites where the systemic and portal circulation share common capillary beds.

Main Sites of Portosystemic Shunting/Bypasses

Portosystemic shunting/bypasses appear at the sites where the systemic and portal circulation share common capillary beds. They arise when collateral portal–systemic vascular channels open to relieve pressure in the portal circuit. The main sites are as follows **(Fig. 19.25)**:

1. **Esophagogastric junction:** These collaterals produce gastroesophageal varices (in about 40% of patients). They can cause massive, frequently fatal hematemesis (especially when there is associated coagulopathy).
2. **Veins around and within the rectum:** It results in rectal varices (manifest as hemorrhoids).
3. **Retroperitoneum:** Collaterals may form in the retroperitoneum, especially in females, and communicate between the ovarian vessels and iliac veins.
4. **Umbilicus:** Produce prominent collaterals around the umbilicus. They appear as dilated subcutaneous veins extending from the umbilicus toward the rib margins (**caput medusae**).

Splenomegaly and Hypersplenism

Portal hypertension is associated with long-standing congestion and may cause **congestive splenomegaly**. The spleen is enlarged and varies in size. Massive splenomegaly may give rise to the syndrome of **hypersplenism**. Hypersplenism is characterized by a decrease in the lifespan of all of the formed elements of the blood (pancytopenia). **Pancytopenia** of hypersplenism is due to the prolonged transit time of blood through the hyperplastic spleen.

MORPHOLOGY

Gross

The **spleen is firm and enlarged**; up to 1,000 g. The cut surface is uniformly deep red (**Fig. 19.26**).

Microscopy

The spleen shows dilated sinusoids with thickening of the wall due to fibrous tissue (*refer* **Fig. 5.11**). Focal areas of hemorrhages may lead to the formation of **fibrotic, iron-laden nodules.** These are known as **Gamna–Gandy bodies** (*refer* **Fig. 5.11C**).

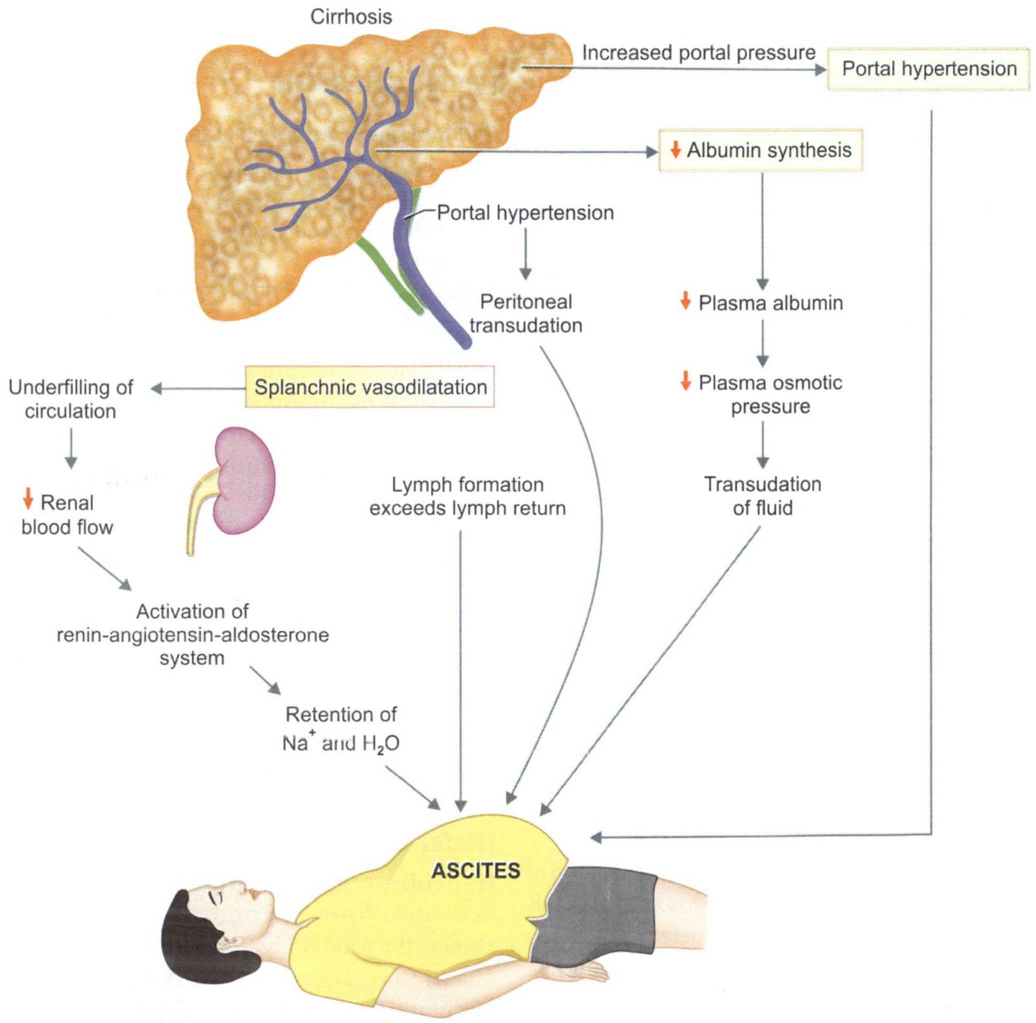

Cirrhosis
Increased portal pressure
Portal hypertension
↓ Albumin synthesis
Portal hypertension
Peritoneal transudation
↓ Plasma albumin
↓ Plasma osmotic pressure
Underfilling of circulation
Splanchnic vasodilatation
↓ Renal blood flow
Lymph formation exceeds lymph return
Transudation of fluid
Activation of renin-angiotensin-aldosterone system
Retention of Na^+ and H_2O
ASCITES

Fig. 19.25: Pathogenesis of ascites in cirrhosis.

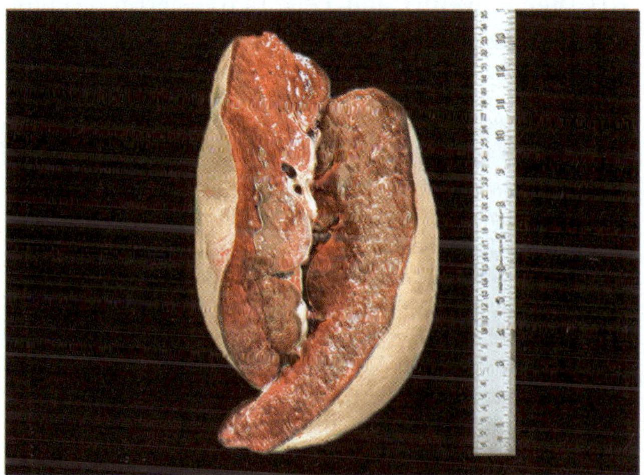

Fig. 19.26: Congestive splenomegaly: The cut section of the enlarged spleen appears deep red.

Endocrine Complications Associated with Cirrhosis

It may be either due to the direct effects of alcohol abuse or hepatic dysfunction.

In Men

Hyperestrogenism: Chronic liver failure is associated with **reduced hepatic catabolism of estrogens**, and weak **androgens are converted to estrogenic compounds in peripheral tissues**. This leads to hyperestrogenism and leads to **feminization**. The portosystemic shunts secondary to portal hypertension in cirrhosis allow these hormones to bypass the liver. Feminization is characterized by **gynecomastia, a female body habitus, and a female distribution of pubic hair**. Hyperestrogenism also causes **vascular manifestations, which include spider angiomas** (commonly seen on the face, neck, or upper chest) and **palmar erythema** (due to local vasodilatation).

Hypogonadism: Chronic alcoholics also develop hypogonadism, manifested as testicular atrophy, impotence, and loss of libido. These are due to the direct toxic action of alcohol.

In Women

They may show features of **gonadal failure**, presenting as oligomenorrhea, amenorrhea, infertility, ovarian atrophy, and loss of secondary sex characteristics. These effects are **due to the direct toxic action of alcohol on gonads.**

Others

Pruritus: Chronic severe jaundice can cause pruritus (itching). Its intensity may be very severe and the skin scratch may be too deep to produce raw areas in the skin. These are prone to repeated potentially life-threatening infection. In some patients, severe pruritus can be relieved by and is a primary indication for liver transplantation. Pruritus may also develop in other disorders associated with cholestasis and may be due to the increased bile salts in the body.

Cause of death: Hepatic encephalopathy, bleeding from esophageal varices and bacterial infections (resulting from damage to the mucosa in the GIT and Kupffer cell dysfunction), and **development of hepatocellular carcinoma.**

SCENARIO-BASED ESSAY QUESTIONS

Q. A 62-year-old male with a history of alcohol abuse, complained of gradual weakness, anorexia, and weight loss. He has been a chronic alcoholic for the last 22 years. On examination, there was jaundice, spider angiomas on the skin, and gynecomastia. Abdominal palpation revealed ascites and splenomegaly.

a. What is your probable diagnosis? (Ans: Alcoholic cirrhosis with portal hypertension).
b. Discuss the etiopathogenesis of this condition *(refer pages 666-9)*.
c. List the different forms of liver diseases associated with alcohol intake *(refer page 664)*.
d. Describe the morphological changes in the target organ involved *(refer pages 670-1)*.
e. What are the clinical manifestations of portal hypertension? *(refer pages 675-8)*.

Q. A 65-year-old male with a history of alcohol abuse was brought to casualty with a history of hematemesis 2 hours back. Physical examination revealed mild jaundice, spider angiomas, mild pedal edema, and gynecomastia. There was distension of the abdomen due to ascites. The liver was firm nodular liver and spleen was just palpable. Upper GI endoscopy revealed dilated bleeding blood vessels in the esophagus. Sclerotherapy was done and bleeding was controlled.

a. What is your probable diagnosis? (Ans: Alcoholic cirrhosis with bleeding from esophageal varices).
b. Describe the morphological changes in the liver *(refer pages 670-1)*.
c. What is the cause of hematemesis? *(refer page 676)*.
d. List the complications *(refer pages 675-8)*.

INHERITED METABOLIC LIVER DISEASES

Hemochromatosis

Q. Write a short note on hemochromatosis.

Definition: Hemochromatosis is defined as a **group of genetic diseases that predispose to iron overload, potentially leading to fibrosis and organ failure.**

Classification of Iron Overload

Hemochromatosis is an **iron-storage disorder caused by to excessive absorption of iron. This excess iron is usually deposited in organs such as the liver and pancreas. It may be also deposited in the heart, joints, and endocrine organs.** Hemochromatosis may be a primary (hereditary hemochromatosis) or secondary to other acquired or genetic disorders **(Box 19.15)**. It is most commonly due to an inherited disorder, hereditary hemochromatosis.

Primary (hereditary) hemochromatosis (hemochromatosis): It is a homozygous-recessive inherited disorder due to excessive absorption of iron.

Secondary (acquired) **hemochromatosis (hemosiderosis):** Accumulation of iron in tissues may occur secondary to other disorders.

Pathogenesis of Hereditary Hemochromatosis (Refer Online Fig. 19.27)

Hepcidin regulates intestinal iron absorption: Iron excretion from the body is not a regulated process. Hence, the total body iron is tightly regulated by intestinal absorption. This intestinal iron uptake is controlled by **circulating negative regulator peptide hormone termed hepcidin. It is encoded by the *HAMP* gene.**

The iron sensor in the liver: ***HFE*** [for *Hereditary Fe* (iron)], ***HJV*** **(hemojuvelin)**, and ***TFR2*** (a transferrin receptor) are the three main membrane proteins expressed on hepatocytes. They function together as a sensor for iron.

BOX 19.15: Classification of iron overload.

1. **Hereditary hemochromatosis**
   - Mutations of genes encoding HFE, transferrin receptor 2 (TfR2), or hepcidin
   - Mutations of genes encoding HJV (hemojuvelin: Juvenile hemochromatosis)
2. **Hemosiderosis (secondary hemochromatosis)**
   - Parenteral iron overload: Transfusions, long-term hemodialysis, aplastic anemia, sickle cell disease
   - Ineffective erythropoiesis with increased erythroid activity: β-thalassemia, sideroblastic anemia
   - Increased oral intake of iron
   - Chronic liver disease: Chronic alcoholic liver disease
   - Miscellaneous: Increased oral intake of iron as in African iron overload (Bantu siderosis)

When body iron is sufficient, signals are transmitted from these sensors. They stimulate the expression of *HAMP* transcripts and hepcidin is secreted. This in turn reduces the intestinal absorption of iron.

Loss of function mutations in hereditary hemochromatosis: In hereditary hemochromatosis, there may be **mutations in *HFE, HJV,*** and ***TfR2*** which leads to the absence of hepcidin. This causes absorption of iron even when there is substantial elevation of body iron stores. The excess iron accumulates mainly in the liver. Symptoms develop usually when the stored iron exceeds 20 g.

Mechanism of Tissue Damage

Excessive iron is directly toxic to host tissues. Mechanisms of liver injury due to excessive iron include the following:

1. **Lipid peroxidation:** Free radicals formed damage the tissue by lipid peroxidation.
2. **Stimulates collagen formation**: It is by **activation of hepatic stellate cells.**
3. **DNA damage by reactive oxygen species:** Interaction of reactive oxygen species and iron with DNA, leads to lethal cell injury or predisposes to hepatocellular carcinoma.

Organs (tissues) affected: Hemosiderin gets deposited in the following organs (in decreasing order of severity): **The liver, pancreas, myocardium,** pituitary gland, adrenal gland, thyroid, and parathyroid glands, joints, and skin. Mainly it presents with **cirrhosis** and **pancreatic fibrosis.**

MORPHOLOGY

Liver

Gross: In the early stages, the liver may appear grossly normal or slightly darker in color. With the progressive accumulation of iron, the liver (other organs, such as the pancreas) becomes **chocolate-brown in color. Cirrhosis** due to hemochromatosis is **initially micronodular** and **later** becomes **macronodular** cirrhosis.

Microscopy: Iron deposits first appear as a **finely granular golden-yellow hemosiderin pigment in the cytoplasm** of periportal hepatocytes. **Hemosiderin is easily recognized** with **Prussian blue stain** (histochemical stain, *refer to* **Fig. 2.31**), which stains them blue. As iron continues to accumulate, iron accumulates in hepatocytes throughout the lobule, within the bile duct epithelium and Kupffer cells. Fibrosis develops slowly. Initially, fibrosis develops at the periportal region, later forms portal-portal bridging fibrosis and leads to **micronodular cirrhosis.**

Clinical Features

- Excessive iron accumulation is a **slow and progressive process** and symptoms usually develop during the fifth to sixth decades of life. Males are more affected than females (5 to 7:1). This is because in females menstrual bleeding limits the accumulation of iron until menopause.
- Classic triad is characterized by:
  a. **Micronodular cirrhosis** in all patients
  b. **Diabetes mellitus** (75–80%) termed bronze diabetes
  c. **Skin pigmentation** (75–80%) particularly in sun-exposed areas.
- **Laboratory findings in hemochromatosis**: It can be diagnosed long before irreversible tissue damage occurs. Laboratory findings include raised serum iron, raised percent saturation of transferrin, raised serum ferritin, and reduced total iron binding capacity (TIBC).

The actions of iron on cells are reversible and if damage is not severe, removal of excess iron with therapy promotes recovery of tissue function. Regular phlebotomy results in the removal of excess tissue iron. Death may result from cirrhosis, cardiac disease, or hepatocellular carcinoma.

Wilson Disease

Q. Write a short note on Wilson disease.

Wilson disease (hepatolenticular degeneration) is an **autosomal recessive disorder of copper metabolism.** It is a **disorder of copper** (one of the trace elements) **transport.**

Etiology

Wilson disease is due to **impaired excretion of copper into bile and a failure to incorporate copper into ceruloplasmin. Ceruloplasmin is a protein synthesized in the liver** and carried to various parts of the body. Ceruloplasmin constitutes 90–95% of plasma copper.

- **Major method of elimination of copper from the body**: It is by **excretion of copper in the bile** and is regulated by the Wilson disease gene, ***ATP7B.***
- **Loss-of-function mutations of the *ATP7B* gene in Wilson disease (*refer* online Fig. 19.28):** This mutation causes deficiency in the ATP7B protein. It results in impaired **excretion of copper into bile and impaired incorporation of copper into ceruloplasmin.** This inhibits the secretion of ceruloplasmin into the blood. These defects lead to (1) a decrease in circulating levels of ceruloplasmin and (2) the **accumulation of copper within the liver.** Accumulated copper causes toxic **liver injury through the ROS** produced by the **Fenton reaction.**

MORPHOLOGY

Organs affected: Wilson disease is characterized by the progressive accumulation of toxic levels of copper in various tissues. **Copper** (one of the trace elements) **causes tissue toxicity** and end-organ damage. It mainly involves the **liver.** The extrahepatic sites include the central nervous system (**brain**), **eye**, kidneys, endocrine organs, heart, and musculoskeletal system.

Liver

It is the main organ involved.

Gross: In the early stages, the liver may be grossly normal or show a mild degree of steatosis. In later stages, progressive fibrosis leads to **macronodular cirrhosis.**

Microscopy: In early Wilson disease, the changes may be mild. The changes may be as follows:

- **Fatty change (steatosis):** Mild to moderate steatosis is common and may be microvesicular or macrovesicular.
- **Acute liver failure can mimic acute viral hepatitis,** except for accompanying fatty change.
- **Chronic hepatitis:** It is common. It usually shows moderate-to-severe portal inflammation and hepatocyte necrosis, admixed with fatty change and features of steatohepatitis (i.e., ballooned hepatocytes, prominent Mallory hyaline, and perisinusoidal fibrosis).
- **Cirrhosis:** As the **disease progresses, periportal fibrosis** may develop. This may progress to bridging fibrosis and **cirrhosis.** Cirrhosis may develop rapidly, even in childhood.
- **Massive liver necrosis:** It is rare and is similar to that caused by viruses or drugs.

Brain: Affects the **basal ganglia**, particularly the **putamen,** and shows **atrophy.**

Q. Write a short note on Kayser–Fleischer ring.

Eye lesions: Kayser–Fleischer rings are formed **due to green-to-brown deposits of copper in Desçemet's membrane** (in the limbus) of the cornea.

Clinical Features

- **Age at onset:** It ranges between 6 and 40 years of age.
- **Liver involvement:** It can produce **acute or chronic liver disease.**
- **Neuropsychiatric manifestations:** These include: Mild behavioral changes, frank psychosis, or **Parkinson disease–like syndrome** (such as tremor).

Biochemical Findings

- **Decreased serum ceruloplasmin.**
- **Increased copper content in the liver** (the most sensitive and accurate test).
- **Increased urinary excretion of copper** (the most specific screening test).
- **Serum copper levels:** It is **not useful for diagnosis,** since they may be low, normal, or elevated, depending on the stage of the disease.

AUTOIMMUNE CHOLANGIOPATHIES

Autoimmune cholangiopathies consist of two distinct immunologically mediated disorders that involve intrahepatic bile ducts. These are (i) primary biliary cholangitis and (ii) primary sclerosing cholangitis.

Primary Biliary Cholangitis

Definition: Primary biliary cholangitis (PBC) is an autoimmune liver disease. It is mainly characterized by **nonsuppurative, inflammatory destruction of small- and medium-sized intrahepatic bile ducts** (cholangitis).

PBC **does not involve large intrahepatic ducts and the extrahepatic biliary tree.** Previously, PBC **was known as primary biliary cirrhosis.** Since, most patients do not progress to cirrhosis, the term primary biliary cholangitis is preferred.

Gender and age: It usually affects **middle-aged women,** with a female-to-male ratio of more than 6:1. It may occur between 20 and 80 years of age, with peak incidence between **40 and 50 years of age.**

Etiology and Pathogenesis

- **Autoimmune disorder:** It is thought to be **an autoimmune disorder, the** triggers that initiate PBC are not known. **Genetic and environmental factors play a role** in the pathogenesis of the PBC. Family members of PBC patients have an increased risk.
- **Mechanism of intrahepatic bile destruction: PBC results from the destruction of small interlobular bile ducts by autoreactive T lymphocytes.** The bile duct injury causes retention of bile salts and leads to secondary hepatocellular injury. It can produce **fibrosis** and progress to cirrhosis. Cirrhosis develops several years after the onset of the disease and most patients are diagnosed at a precirrhotic stage. Hence, the older term primary biliary cirrhosis is somewhat misleading.
- **Antimitochondrial antibodies (AMA): They are detected in 90–95% of patients.** Though they are characteristic **autoantibodies** of PBC, their role in the pathogenesis is not clear. There is no correlation between the antibody titers with disease severity or disease progression, or response to therapy.

MORPHOLOGY

Gross

- **Early-stage,** PBC may have **few gross findings,** weight may be normal or mildly increased (because of inflammation).
- In **late-stage** PBC, the liver shows uniform and bile stasis stains the **liver green.**

Microscopy

The morphologic hallmark of PBC is lymphocytic infiltration and epithelial injury involving the small interlobular bile ducts. The classic staging systems for PBC consist of four stages.

Stage 1: Florid duct lesion:

- **Chronic cholangitis:** This stage is characterized by **inflammation and injury to interlobular bile duct epithelial cells.** The bile ducts are **actively destroyed** and surrounded by a dense collection of **lymphocytes, macrophages, and plasma cells.** Lymphocytes may form **lymphoid follicles and a few with germinal centers.**
- **Florid duct lesion:** The pathognomonic feature is a florid **duct lesion** consisting of granulomatous (**noncaseating epithelioid granulomas)** or lymphocytic infiltration of duct epithelium. The lesion is quite patchy in distribution.

Stage 2: Periportal stage

- **Destruction of small intrahepatic bile ducts:** As the disease progresses, the **inflammatory process destroys small bile ducts.** This leads to the loss of small intrahepatic bile ducts, which are reduced in number ("ductopenia"). This is accompanied by a **proliferation of bile ductules** at the periphery of the portal triad and **obstruction to intrahepatic bile flow.**
- **Feathery degeneration:** Stasis of bile salts (cholestasis) leads to swelling of periportal hepatocytes. These hepatocytes have clear cytoplasm with granular strands **(feathery degeneration)** and may develop Mallory hyaline.

Stage 3: Septal stage: Destructive inflammation in stages 1 and 2 leads to the disappearance of small bile ducts. It is common to find scarring of medium-sized bile ducts. Collagenous septa from the portal tracts extend into the lobular parenchyma. They begin to encircle some liver lobules.

Stage 4: Cirrhosis: The end stage of PBC is cirrhosis. The liver consists of dark green bile-stained nodules. Like other biliary diseases, cirrhotic nodules in PBC are elongated ("garland-shaped") in contrast to the round nodules in hepatic diseases. Microscopically, it shows mainly portal-to-portal bridging fibrous septa. This fibrosis gives a **"jigsaw puzzle" appearance** to the cirrhotic nodules. Small bile ducts are very few, and medium-sized ducts are conspicuously fewer in number. There is little inflammation within either the fibrous septa or the parenchymal nodule.

Clinical Features

Insidious in onset. Commonly present with **pruritus (itching), fatigue**, and **abdominal discomfort. Other features** include skin pigmentation (due to melanin deposition), eyelid xanthelasmas (cholesterol-rich macrophages), steatorrhea, osteomalacia, and/or osteoporosis (due to malabsorption of vitamin D).

- **Cirrhotic stage:** Jaundice, hepatic decompensation, portal hypertension, and variceal bleeding develop.

Laboratory Findings

Most patients are diagnosed in the early stages of disease by laboratory findings.

- **Raised levels of serum alkaline phosphatase** (markers of cholestasis), **γ-glutamyltransferase, and cholesterol (hypercholesterolemia).** Hyperbilirubinemia occurs in the late stages.
- **Antimitochondrial antibodies** are **characteristic and are essential for the diagnosis** of PBC. They are found in 90–95% of patients.
- **Liver biopsy:** PBC is confirmed by liver biopsy and the lesion is considered diagnostic if a florid duct lesion is present.

Prognosis: PBC is associated **with an increased risk of hepatocellular carcinomas.**

Cause of death: Liver failure, massive hemorrhage from esophageal varices, and intercurrent infection.

Treatment: Early treatment with oral ursodeoxycholic acid results in dramatically improved outcomes by slowing the progression of the disease. Liver transplantation is the best treatment for advanced liver disease.

Primary Sclerosing Cholangitis

Definition: Primary sclerosing cholangitis (PSC) is characterized by inflammation and obliterative fibrosis of intrahepatic and extrahepatic bile ducts.

Age and gender: PSC usually occurs in the third to fifth decades of life and has a 2:1 male predominance.

Beading appearance in MRI: Irregular biliary strictures in PSC **lead to dilation of preserved segments of the liver.** This produces characteristic **"beading" of the intrahepatic and extrahepatic biliary tree in MRI.**

Coexistence with inflammatory bowel disease: Most commonly ulcerative colitis, coexists in about 70% of patients with PSC.

Pathogenesis: PSC is probably due to an **immunologically mediated injury to bile ducts**. Features that suggest immunologically mediated injury to bile ducts are as follows:

- **Presence of T cells in the periductal stroma.**
- **Presence of autoantibodies:** About 75% of patients with PSC have antismooth muscle antibodies and antinuclear antibodies. Antibodies directed against cytoplasmic and nuclear antigens of neutrophils (ANCA) are observed in up to 80% of patients.
- **Coexistence with ulcerative colitis.**
- **Genetic factors**: First-degree relatives of patients with PSC are at increased risk for developing the disease. This may be due to genetic factors. Several autoantibodies are present in PSC.

MORPHOLOGY

Morphologic changes seen in large ducts (intrahepatic and extra-hepatic) are different from those seen in smaller intrahepatic ducts.

- **Large duct inflammation:** It is **similar to that of ulcerative colitis.** It consists of **neutrophils infiltrating** into the epithelium in the **background of a chronic inflammatory infiltrate.** Inflamed areas progress to strictures as scarring narrows the lumen.
- **Smaller ducts with onion skin fibrosis:** They usually show a striking **circumferential, "onion skin" fibrosis** around an atrophic duct lumen which may eventually obliterate the lumen, leaving a "tombstone" scar. Inflammation is minimal.
- **Cirrhosis:** As the disease progresses, the liver becomes markedly cholestatic, leading to cirrhosis.
- **Risk of cholangiocarcinoma:** Biliary intraepithelial neoplasia and cholangiocarcinoma may develop in up to 7% of patients.

Clinical features: Patients may be asymptomatic and may show **persistent elevation of serum alkaline phosphatase.** Some may present with progressive fatigue and pruritus. Liver transplantation is the only definitive treatment.

LIVER ABSCESSES

Q. Write a short note on liver abscesses.

Definition: A localized collection of pus inside the liver parenchyma is known as a liver abscess. Liver abscesses are common in developing countries.

Etiology

- *Entamoeba histolytica:* Amebic liver abscess is caused by ***Entamoeba histolytica***.
- **Liver abscess by other protozoa and helminthic organisms:** Secondary infection of hydatid cyst caused by echinococci and less commonly other organisms.
- **Pyogenic abscess:** Bacterial infections in the liver may manifest as pyogenic abscess. Such abscesses usually represent a complication of bacterial infection elsewhere.
- **Fungal abscess:** *Candida*.

Mode of infection: The causative agent may reach the liver by any one of the following routes:

- **Portal vein:** The majority of hepatic abscesses used to result from portal spread of intra-abdominal infections (e.g., appendicitis, diverticulitis, colitis).
- **Artery:** Through hepatic artery, e.g., during septicemia.
- **Ascending infection** in the biliary tract (ascending cholangitis).
- **Direct invasion of the liver** from a nearby source or a penetrating injury.

MORPHOLOGY

Gross and microscopic appearances are similar to abscesses in other sites and are usually filled with purulent debris. Bacteria may be demonstrated with special stains.

Gross (Fig. 19.29)

- Liver abscesses may be **multiple or solitary**. Bacteremic spread through the arterial or portal system produces multiple small abscesses, whereas direct extension and trauma usually cause solitary large abscesses.
- More common in the right lobe.
- Size is variable, ranging up to 10 cm.

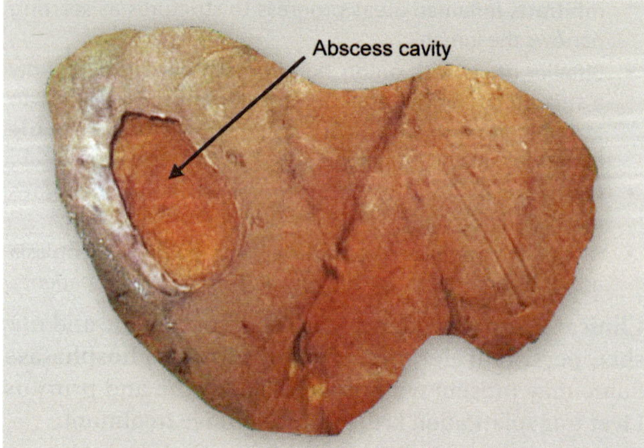

Fig. 19.29: Liver with an abscess cavity in the right lobe.

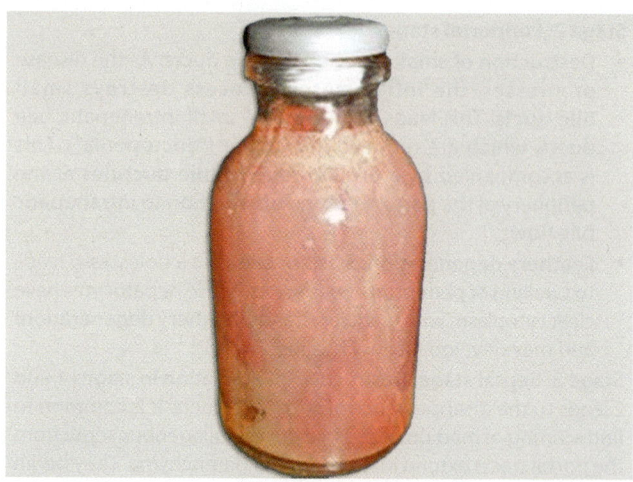

Fig. 19.30: Anchovy sauce appearance of amebic liver abscess.

Clinical features: They present with **fever, right upper quadrant pain,** and **tender hepatomegaly.** Jaundice may develop when there is extrahepatic biliary obstruction.

Amebic Liver Abscess

Q. Write a short note on amebic liver abscess.

Most common extraintestinal complication of amebic dysentery (*refer* pages 617-9 and **Figs. 18.28 and 18.29**).

Q. Write a short note on morphology (gross and microscopy) of amebic liver abscess.

Gross

Amebic abscess ranges from 8–12 cm in diameter and appears well circumscribed. **Amebic abscesses are usually located in the subdiaphragmatic region.** The **abscess cavity contains** thick, dark material that has been likened to **anchovy paste (sauce) (Fig. 19.30) or chocolate.**

Microscopy

The trophozoites can be demonstrated in the periphery of the necrotic debris.

Clinical features: The symptoms are similar to pyogenic abscesses. Surgical drainage of large abscesses is important.

Complications: If an amebic abscess continues to grow, it may rupture into the **(1) thoracic cavity to produce empyema or a lung abscess, (2)** may rupture into the **peritoneal cavity**, where it produces **peritonitis**, a complication associated with a mortality rate as high as 40%. The amebae may also invade the blood, in which case **abscesses of the brain and lungs** may ensue.

MALIGNANT NEOPLASMS OF LIVER

Malignant tumors of the liver can be primary or metastatic. Most primary cancers of the liver arise from hepatocytes and are termed **hepatocellular carcinoma** (HCC). Less common are cancers that arise from bile ducts known as cholangiocarcinomas. Two rare primary liver cancers are hepatoblastomas and angiosarcomas.

Hepatoblastoma

Q. Write a short note on hepatoblastoma.

Hepatoblastoma is a rare **malignant primary hepatic blastomatous tumor** that **recapitulates hepatic ontogenesis** (development features from the earliest stage to maturity). It consists of variable **combinations of epithelial and mesenchymal elements.** It is the most common liver tumor arising in young childhood. It is a **malignant tumor** and is usually fatal.

MORPHOLOGY

Gross

Appears as a **solitary, well-circumscribed, large mass** in the **right lobe.**

Microscopy

Two variants

1. **Epithelial type:** It consists of small **polygonal fetal cells or smaller embryonal cells.** These tumor cells form **acini, tubules, or papillary** structures.
2. **Mixed epithelial and mesenchymal type:** It is characterized by areas of **both epithelial and mesenchymal differentiation.** The mesenchymal component may be **primitive, mesenchyme** (with spindle or stellate cells with little cytoplasm), or show differentiation towards osteoid, cartilage, or striated muscle.

Clinical features: Hepatoblastoma may present as abdominal enlargement (swelling) in an asymptomatic infant or child.

Hepatocellular Carcinoma

Definition: Hepatocellular carcinoma (HCC) is a primary malignant tumor of the liver **composed of epithelial cells showing hepatocellular differentiation.** It is **derived from hepatocytes or their precursors.** HCC was inappropriately known as *hepatoma.*

Age and gender: Most HCCs are seen in patients older than 40 years, with a peak at 70 years of age. **Predominantly occurs in males** with an M: F ratio of 2.4:1.

Etiology and Pathogenesis

Q. Write a short note on the etiopathogenesis of HCC.

Predisposing and associated factors (Box 19.16): In about 90% of the patients, HCC can be related to a defined cause, either **chronic liver disease or exogenous exposure.** Only in a minority of cases, HCC develops in a normal or near-normal liver. **Most HCCs occur in chronic liver disease with cirrhosis.** Male gender, age, and duration of cirrhosis are the major risk factors for HCC in patients with cirrhosis.

Chronic Liver Diseases

Chronic liver diseases are the most common condition associated with the development of HCC. Probably chronic inflammation, with associated growth factors and cytokines, promotes the proliferation of normal cells and predisposes to the acquisition of mutations.

BOX 19.16: Predisposing and associated factors for hepatocellular carcinoma.

Chronic liver diseases: Various causes include:
- Chronic hepatitis: HBV/HCV
- Alcoholic steatohepatitis
- Metabolic syndrome and its attendant obesity, diabetes mellitus, and NAFLD
- Inherited diseases: Hereditary hemochromatosis, glycogen storage disease, a_1-antitrypsin deficiency, hereditary tyrosinemia, Wilson disease

Exogenous substances
- Aflatoxin B_1

Precursor lesions
- Hepatocellular adenoma
- Cellular dysplasias: Large-cell change and small-cell change
- Dysplastic nodules: Low-grade and high-grade

Others
- Oral contraceptives
- Cigarette smoking

(HBV: hepatitis B virus; HCV: hepatitis C virus; NAFLD: nonalcoholic fatty liver disease)

Hepatotropic viruses, namely **HBV and HCV:** These are the most common disease-causing chronic liver diseases (chronic viral hepatitis B and C).

- **HBV infection:** Chronic HBV infection is strongly associated with HCC, especially **vertical transmission** from infected mothers to their children.
  - **Repeated cycles of liver cell necrosis and regeneration** in chronic hepatitis B are the soil for HCC. HBV-associated cirrhosis is another major risk factor.
  - The **genome of HBV is integrated** into the **host DNA of liver cells** and may **activate protooncogenes into an oncogene**, which causes tumors.
  - **X gene of HBV encodes HBV X-protein**, which is a transcriptional activator of many genes. **It can inactivate tumor suppressor genes** and **cause cell transformation.**
- **HCV infection**: Most patients with HCV who develop HCC have underlying cirrhosis. **HCV core protein may interact with many cellular proteins** to cause HCC.

Steatohepatitis due to chronic alcohol abuse: Heavy alcohol intake is a well-established risk factor for the development of HCC. There is a synergistic effect of heavy alcohol use and HBV or HCV infection.

Inherited disorders: Particularly hereditary hemochromatosis and α_1AT deficiency, and, to a lesser degree, Wilson disease are the risk factors for HCC. The majority of the risk factors for HCC result in cirrhosis. Over 80% of patients with HCC have cirrhosis.

Metabolic syndrome and its attendant obesity, diabetes mellitus, and **nonalcoholic fatty liver disease** (NAFLD) also increase the risk of HCC, even without cirrhosis.

Exogenous Substances

Many exogenous substances have hepatocarcinogenic effects.

Aflatoxin B_1: Dietary exposure to aflatoxin B_1 is an important risk factor for HCC. **Aflatoxin B_1 (chemical carcinogen)** is a toxin produced by the fungus ***Aspergillus flavus***. This fungus **contaminates improperly stored peanuts and grains**. The incidence of liver cancer correlates roughly with the dietary content of aflatoxin. The presence of aflatoxin B_1 metabolites in urine is associated with a threefold increased risk of HCC. **Aflatoxin** can **bind covalently with the cellular DNA of hepatocytes** and cause a specific **mutation of the *TP53* tumor suppressor gene**. Aflatoxin B_1 acts synergistically with alcohol and hepatitis B in the pathogenesis of HCC.

Precursor Lesions of HCC

Q. Write a short note on precursor lesions of HCC.

Hepatocellular adenoma: In the noncirrhotic liver, HCC can arise in hepatocellular adenoma, particularly those with β-catenin-activating mutations.

Cellular dysplasias in chronic liver disease: This may be seen in chronic liver disease, before or after the development of cirrhosis. There are two types of liver cell dysplasia, namely large-cell change and small-cell change.

1. **Large-cell change:** These cells are larger than normal liver cells having large, multiple, moderately pleomorphic nuclei with a normal nuclear–cytoplasmic ratio. It is a marker of increased risk of HCC in the liver and hepatitis B. They may also be directly premalignant.
2. **Small-cell change:** It is probably premalignant. There are two types of liver cell dysplasia, namely large-cell change and small-cell change. These liver cells have a high nuclear–cytoplasmic ratio and mild nuclear hyperchromasia and/or pleomorphism.

Dysplastic nodules: These are nodules having a different appearance than cirrhotic nodules, that are usually detected radiologically or in resected specimens of cirrhosis. Some HCCs arise in dysplastic *nodules*.

- **Low-grade dysplastic nodules:** They may or may not transform into higher-grade lesions. However, they have a higher risk for the development of HCC. They do not have cytological or architectural atypia.
- **High-grade dysplastic nodules:** They are the most important precursor of HCC in viral hepatitis and alcohol-related liver disease. The cells of these nodules have cytological (e.g., small-cell change) or architectural features suggestive of, but not sufficient for diagnosis of frank HCC.

Mechanisms of Carcinogenesis

Hepatocarcinogenic mechanisms have been suggested for the various causes of HCC. In most cases, HCC follows an evolution starting from chronic liver disease and final progression to HCC. HCC can develop by acquired mutations in oncogenes and tumor suppressor genes. No single sequence of molecular or genetic alterations leads to the development of HCC. The mechanism of carcinogenesis can be divided into etiology-specific and nonspecific mechanisms.

- **Nonspecific mechanisms:** The changes caused by chronic liver disease may act in sequence. The sequences are chronic injury, inflammation, hepatocellular death, regeneration, acquisition of mutations, oncogenic factors derived from the inflammatory milieu, and effects due to fibrosis and vascular rearrangement. These contribute to the acquisition of driver mutations that lead to the development of HCC.
- **Specific oncogenic mechanisms:** HCC in developing hepatitis B transactivates viral factors and viral integration with constant cis- and trans-activation of oncogenic factors. Aflatoxin has direct genotoxic effects (e.g., mutation of *TP53*), leading to HCC. The proposed mechanism for hepatitis C is the oncogenic effects of core antigen and NS5A.

Mutations: As with other cancers, HCC is associated with complementary **sets of driver mutations.** This leads to the acquisition of cancer hallmarks.

- **Activating mutations involving the β-catenin gene:** It is the most common mutation that is found in about 40% of tumors.
- **Mutations in the *TERT* (telomerase transcriptase) gene promoter:** It occurs in 50–60% of tumors and it upregulates telomerase activity. Cells may become immortal, through activation of the cellular telomerase enzyme.
- **Inactivating mutations in *TP53*** (up to 60% of tumors): It is strongly associated with exposure to aflatoxin. In many cases, aflatoxin is responsible for the *TP53* mutations.
- **Fusion gene:** One unusual subtype of hepatocellular carcinoma is **fibrolamellar HCC**. It often occurs in adolescents and young adults without preexisting liver disease. It is **strongly associated with a fusion gene that leads to aberrant activity of protein kinase A**. This is an enzyme that participates in a signaling pathway regulated by cyclic adenosine monophosphate (cAMP).

MORPHOLOGY

Gross

Q. Write a short note on the morphology of HCC.

Four main macroscopic patterns. All patterns may **cause enlargement of the liver. Areas of necrosis and hemorrhage** are common in all patterns.

1. **Single distinct nodule (unifocal):** The tumor appears as a **large circumscribed single mass** in a portion of the liver **(Figs. 19.31A and 19.32A).**
2. **Large dominant nodule of HCC with multiple smaller satellite nodules (multifocal):** The satellite nodules are usually present within 2 cm of the dominant nodule **(Figs. 19.31B and 19.32B).**
3. **Many small nodules of HCC (dozens to hundreds) (diffusely infiltrative):** They are approximately the same size and shape as cirrhotic nodules. This growth pattern is called diffuse or cirrhotomimetic **(diffusely infiltrative).** This type is characterized by a **large part of the liver or sometimes the entire liver infiltrated by homogeneous indistinct tumor nodules.** The tumor may diffusely infiltrate the liver and blend into a cirrhotic liver background. It may be difficult to differentiate from the regenerating nodules of cirrhosis **(Fig. 19.31C).**
4. **Multiple distinct nodules of HCC:** They represent independent primaries. Tumors are clearly separate from each other and do not fit a dominant tumor/satellite tumor pattern or a diffuse pattern. **Multiple** discrete masses of variable sizes are widely distributed **(Fig. 19.31D).**

Color: HCCs are usually **light brown, yellowish-white, or gray** in color. **Production of bile** by tumor cells may cause **greenish-brown discoloration** of the tumor.

Size: Due to recent progress in radiographic procedures, an increased number of small (<2.0 cm) HCCs are detected. Tumors measuring >2 cm are more likely associated with vascular invasion and intrahepatic metastases.

Microscopy (Figs. 19.33A to C)

Hepatocyte differentiation: The tumor cells in HCC show hepatocytic differentiation by morphology and/or immunohistochemistry. The tumor shows a loss of normal hepatic architecture.

Histologic growth pattern: HCCs show mainly four histological growth patterns, namely: (1) **Trabecular**, (2) **solid**, (3) **pseudoglandular**, and (4) **macrotrabecular**. About 50% of tumors show mixed patterns.

- **Trabecular pattern:** It shows malignant hepatocytes arranged in trabeculae **(several layers of malignant cells)** or **irregular anastomosing plates**. The tumor **cells are polygonal** and have **abundant, slightly granular cytoplasm.** The **nuclei** are **large** and **hyperchromatic** and show **prominent nucleoli.** Endothelium-lined sinusoids separate the liver plates.
- **Solid variety:** The tumor cells usually are small and may show considerable variation in shape. Bile production is rare.
- **Pseudoglandular pattern** (pseudo-acinar adenoid): In this pattern, malignant hepatocytes are arranged around **a lumen and resemble glands.** The lumen may contain bile. The acini formed by the tumor cells are not true glands, hence the name pseudoglandular.

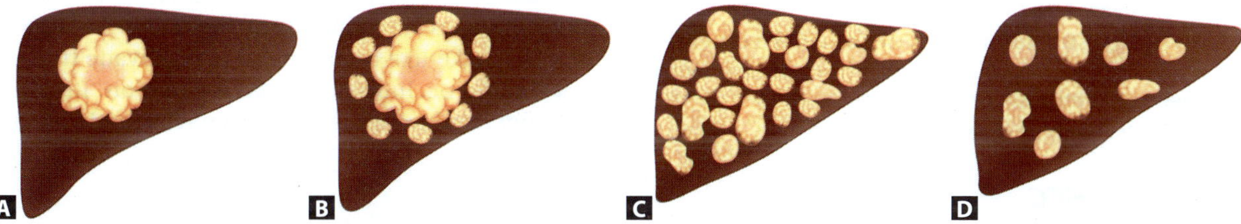

Figs. 19.31A to D: Gross patterns of hepatocellular carcinoma (HCC): (A) Single distinct nodule (unifocal); (B) Large dominant nodule of HCC with multiple smaller satellite nodules (multifocal); (C) Many small nodules of HCC (diffuse infiltrative); (D) Multiple distinct nodules.

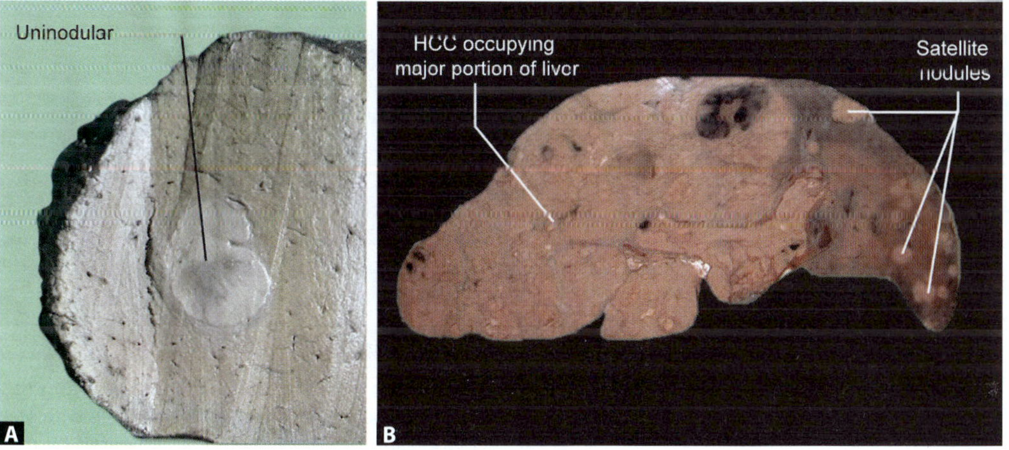

Figs. 19.32A and B: Hepatocellular carcinoma: (A) Uninodular; (B) Liver with a large gray-white tumor occupying the major portion of the liver along with satellite nodules.

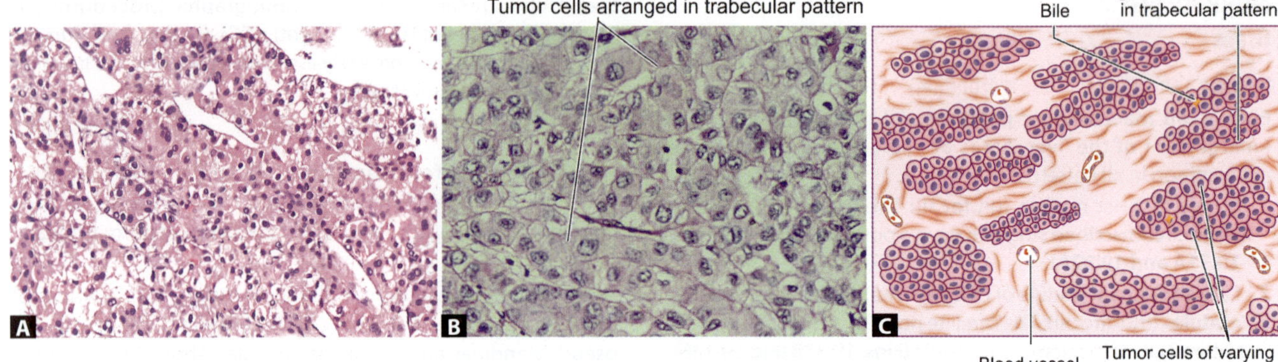

Figs. 19.33A to C: Hepatocellular carcinoma: (A) Low magnification, and (B) higher magnification shows a tumor composed of malignant hepatocytes arranged in a trabecular pattern. (C) Diagrammatic.

Histological Grading

Hepatocellular carcinoma is graded as well-differentiated, moderately differentiated, and poorly differentiated.

1. **Well-differentiated HCC: Tumor cells can be recognizable as hepatocytic in origin** and resemble normal hepatocytes. **Bile production by tumor cells** is the **hallmark** of hepatocellular carcinoma. Tumor cells are arranged in trabecular and acinar (pseudoglandular) patterns. The pseudoglandular pattern recapitulates poorly formed, ectatic bile canaliculi.
2. **Moderately differentiated HCC:** This grade may show a solid, scirrhous, and clear-cell pattern.
3. **Poorly or undifferentiated** HCC: It consists of **pleomorphic cells with great variation in size and shape.** The nuclei also are extremely variable in size and shape. Many bizarre-looking anaplastic giant cells can be seen.

Globular hyaline structures: It may be seen in the cytoplasm of all types of hepatocellular carcinoma. They represent **alpha-fetoprotein, α_1-antitrypsin,** or other proteins.

Mallory's hyaline may be occasionally seen.

Fibrolamellar HCC

Q. Write a short note on fibrolamellar HCC.

- It is a **distinctive uncommon variant** of **HCC** and constitutes about 5% of HCCs.
- **Age and sex**: It occurs in **young patients without cirrhosis.**
- **Etiology:** Unknown.

MORPHOLOGY

Gross

Single large, hard "scirrhous" well-circumscribed tumor with a central stellate fibrous scar.

Microscopy

It shows a characteristic triad of features: (1) **large, eosinophilic** (oncocytic), **polygonal cells with granular cytoplasm** due to abundant mitochondria (tumor cells are arranged **in nests or cords**); (2) **vesicular nuclei with prominent nucleoli**; and (3) **parallel lamellae of abundant, dense collagen bundles (Fig. 19.34).** Tumor marker for fibrolamellar HCC is neurotensin.

- **Prognosis:** It grows slowly and is **better** than the conventional HCC.

Spread of Hepatocellular Carcinoma

- **Local spread:** HCC may first spread within the liver itself and develop satellite nodules. **Intrahepatic metastases (by vascular invasion/direct extension) are** more likely to occur when the size of tumors reaches 3 cm. Local invasion of the diaphragm is common.
- **Lymphatic spread: HCC may spread** to portal lymph nodes, perihilar, peripancreatic, and para-aortic nodes.
- **Blood spread: All patterns of HCCs have a strong tendency for invasion of vessels**. This may result in extensive intrahepatic metastases. The portal vein and its branches are infiltrated by the tumor. Occasionally, long, snake-like tumor masses may **invade the portal vein** and occlude the portal circulation. Rarely, the tumor may invade the inferior vena cava and extend into

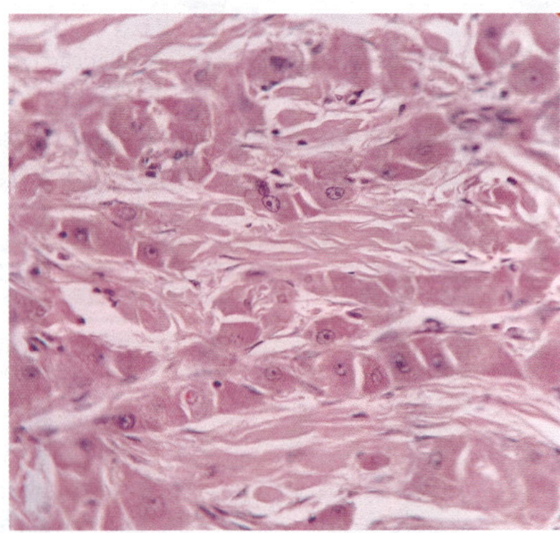

Fig. 19.34: Fibrolamellar carcinoma showing nests and cords of large polygonal malignant-appearing cells with granular (oncocytic) cytoplasm. The tumor cells are separated by parallel lamellae of dense collagen bundles.

the right side of the heart through the hepatic veins. It may metastasize to the **lungs**.

Clinical Features

Most patients present with **ill-defined upper abdominal pain, malaise, fatigue, weight loss,** and hepatomegaly. On examination, the liver appears enlarged, irregular, or nodular.

Paraneoplastic syndromes: HCC may cause paraneoplastic syndromes due to ectopic hormone production by the tumor. Associated paraneoplastic syndromes include **polycythemia [parathyroid hormone (PTH)-related protein], hypoglycemia (insulin-like factor), hypercalcemia, and erythrocytosis [erythropoietin (EPO)].**

Laboratory findings and serum markers: These include:

- **Alpha-fetoprotein (AFP):** Elevated serum levels of AFP are frequent in advanced HCC. However, it is not a sensitive screening test for early tumors and is not found with the fibrolamellar variant of HCC. It may also be elevated in other benign and malignant liver diseases and some extrahepatic disorders. **Lectin fraction-3 of AFP** is highly specific to HCC, an indicator of poorly-differentiated HCC, and unfavorable prognosis.
- **α-L-fucosidase:** It is raised in HCC and also in cirrhosis.
- **Serum des-gamma-carboxy prothrombin:** It is raised in most HCCs.
- **Hep-par 1 (hepatocyte paraffin 1):** Specific for hepatocyte mitochondria and is considered the most specific and sensitive marker of normal and neoplastic hepatocytes. It is used in diagnosing hepatocellular carcinoma.

The TNM staging system is widely used but is limited as it does not take into account important clinical factors.

Causes of death: These include cachexia, gastrointestinal or esophageal variceal bleeding, liver failure with hepatic coma, and rupture of the tumor with fatal hemorrhage (rare).

Cholangiocarcinoma (CCA)

It is the **second most common hepatic malignant tumor of the liver.**

Subtypes: It may **arise anywhere in the biliary tree** from intrahepatic and extrahepatic bile ducts. Cholangiocarcinoma is classified according to its location.

- **Intrahepatic** (about 10%).
- **Extrahepatic forms** (about 80–90%): **Perihilar tumors** (50–60% of all CCAs) are known as **Klatskin tumors** and are located at the **junction of the right and left hepatic ducts** forming the common hepatic duct. **Distal bile duct (bile duct carcinomas) tumors** (20–30%): They arise **near the ampulla of Vater**. They **also include periampullary carcinomas,** which consist of adenocarcinoma of the duodenal mucosa and pancreatic carcinoma.

Risk factors: These include the following conditions:

- **Primary sclerosing cholangitis** (PSC).
- **Congenital fibropolycystic diseases of the biliary system,** such as Caroli disease and choledochal cysts.
- **HCV infection.**
- Previous **exposure to thorotrast** (formerly used in radiography of the biliary tract).
- **Chronic infection** of the biliary tract by the liver fluke **opisthorchis sinensis.**
- **Premalignant lesions:** Biliary intraepithelial neoplasias (low to high grade, BilIN-1, -2, or -3).

MORPHOLOGY

Gross

- **Extrahepatic CCAs: These** are **usually small lesions** and appear as **firm, gray nodules within the bile duct wall.**
- **Intrahepatic CCAs**: They develop in the intrahepatic portal tract **(refer online Figs. 19.35A to C).**

Microscopy

- **Adenocarcinomas**: Well-differentiated adenocarcinomas consist of well-defined **glandular and tubular structures lined by cuboidal to low columnar epithelial cells.**
- **Marked desmoplasia:** It is characterized by dense collagenous stroma separating the glandular structures.

METASTATIC TUMORS

Q. List four common primary sites of metastatic tumors.

- Metastasis to the liver is **more common than primary tumors of the liver**. Apart from the liver, the lungs are also most often involved in the metastatic spread of cancers.
- **Most common sites of primary tumor-producing hepatic metastases** are the (i) **gastrointestinal tract (colon), (ii) breast, (iii) lung, and (iv) pancreas.** However, any cancer in any site of the body may spread to the liver, including leukemias, melanomas, and lymphomas.

MORPHOLOGY

Gross (Fig 19.36)

- The liver is **enlarged** and may weigh several kilograms.
- The liver may show only **one nodule or** may be completely replaced by **multiple nodules of metastatic deposits.**
- On the surface of the liver, the metastatic **nodules appear as umbilicated masses.**
- **Central umbilication is due to** necrosis (outgrow blood supply) and hemorrhage in the central area of the nodule.

Microscopy

The metastatic deposits usually appear **similar to the primary tumor.** Occasionally, they may be so undifferentiated that the primary site cannot be determined.

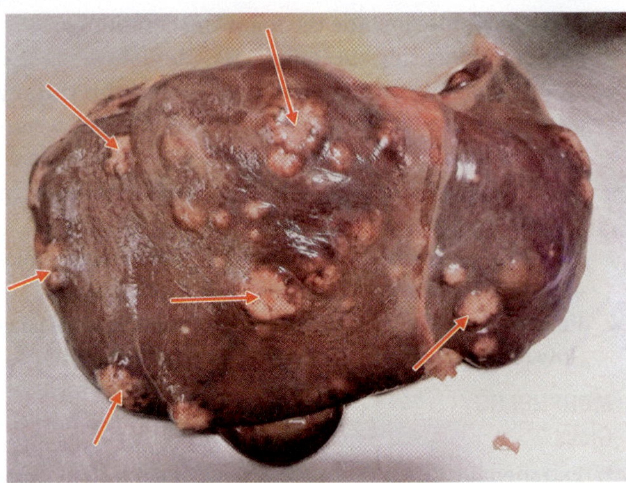

Fig. 19.36: Metastasis to liver showing multiple nodules (arrows) with umbilication.

Clinical Features

- **Weight loss:** It is a common early finding.
- **Portal hypertension with splenomegaly, ascites**, and **gastrointestinal bleeding** may occur.
- **Jaundice**: It may be either due to obstruction of the bile ducts or replacement of most of the liver parenchyma.
- Hepatic failure may develop.

Laboratory findings: May show an **increase** in the **serum alkaline phosphatase** level.

Prognosis: Most patients die within a year.

GALLBLADDER

CHOLELITHIASIS (GALLSTONES)

Q. Discuss the etiopathogenesis of cholelithiasis. Describe the morphology of different kinds/types of gallstones. List the complications.

Cholelithiasis means stones in the lumen of the gallbladder or the extrahepatic biliary tree. Cholelithiasis is a **common disorder** and found in ~10 to 20% of adult populations in developed countries and constitutes >95% of biliary tract disease. **The majority (>80%) of them are "silent"**.

Classification of Gallstones

Q. Classify gallstones/cholelithiasis.

Depending on the Chemical Composition (Box 19.17)

Basic chemical constituents of gallstones: These include **cholesterol, calcium bilirubin, and other calcium salts (carbonate, phosphate, and palmitate).** Almost all gallstones contain a variable amount of cholesterol.

BOX 19.17: Classification of gallstones.

Cholesterol stones
- Pure cholesterol stones
- Mixed cholesterol stones

Pigment stones
- Black pigment stones
- Brown pigment stones

The most widely used classification is based on the amount of cholesterol in the stones. There are two main types of gallstones, namely (1) cholesterol stones (75–85%) and (2) pigment stones (15–25%).

Cholesterol stones: They contain **>50% of crystalline cholesterol monohydrate**. They may be subclassified as pure or mixed cholesterol stones.

- **Pure cholesterol stones (about 10% of cholesterol stones):** Stones containing **>90% of** crystalline **cholesterol monohydrate** are termed **pure cholesterol stones.** The **remaining chemical component** of pure cholesterol stones is **calcium bilirubinate and calcium carbonate**. These cholesterol stones being mainly composed of cholesterol are **radiolucent**.
- **Mixed cholesterol gallstones (70–90% of cholesterol stones):** Stones with a lower cholesterol content (less than that in pure cholesterol stones, i.e., <90% cholesterol) are called mixed cholesterol stones. They contain a **mixture of cholesterol (60–89%), calcium bilirubinate, calcium carbonate, and mucin glycoprotein**.

More than 80% of cholesterol stones **lack calcium carbonate** and are **radiolucent**, and about 20% are radiodense (containing calcium).

Pigment gallstones: They are **predominantly composed of bilirubin calcium (calcium bilirubinate) salts**. Apart from calcium bilirubinate (calcium salts of unconjugated bilirubin), they also contain **calcium carbonate** and **<20% of cholesterol**. They develop when there is increased unconjugated bilirubin. Pigment stones are subclassified as black and brown pigment stones. They **constitute 15–25% of gallstones.**

- **Black pigment stones:** They are **common in India** (40%). Generally, they occur in patients with older age, cirrhosis, and **chronic hemolytic states (increased unconjugated bilirubin)**. They **contain 10–90% calcium bilirubinate (calcium salts of unconjugated bilirubin), other calcium salts** (50–75%—such as **phosphate and carbonate**), and mucin glycoprotein. They have very low cholesterol concentrations. **About 50–75% are radiopaque** because of calcium salts.
- **Brown pigment stones:** These are more common in Asia. They form in the bile duct and are associated with bile stasis and infections in the gallbladder and biliary tree. They are rare in the gallbladder. They **comprise calcium bilirubinate, calcium palmitate (calcium salts**

of free fatty acids), mucin glycoprotein, fatty acids, and less than 20% cholesterol. Calcium phosphate and calcium carbonate are usually not present (in contrast, they are present in black pigment stones). They are **usually radiolucent.**

Depending on the Location

- **Intrahepatic stones:** They are predominantly **brown pigment stones.**
- **Gallbladder stones:** These are **mainly cholesterol stones** and a **few are black pigment stones.**
- **Choledocholithiasis** (bile duct stones): Composed mostly of **mixed cholesterol stones.**

Risk Factors for Cholesterol Stones (Box 19.18)

Q. Write a short note on risk factors for cholesterol stones.

Cholesterol gallstones are uncommon in developing countries. They are formed probably due to a combination of genetic susceptibility and environmental factors.

1. **Advancing age:** It is one of the **major risk factors.** The prevalence of cholesterol gallstones increases with age until, 60 years. They are seen in individuals of **middle to older age.** As age advances increase in gallstones is associated with metabolic syndrome and obesity as well as hypersecretion of biliary estrogen.

BOX 19.18: Risk factors for gallstones.

Cholesterol Stones

1. Advancing age
2. **Female sex hormones:** Female, pregnancy, parity and oral contraceptives
3. **Hereditary factors:** Familial predisposition, inborn disorders of bile acid metabolism
4. **Environmental factors:** Drugs (octreotide, ceftriaxone, clofibrate therapy), obesity and metabolic syndrome, rapid weight reduction, diet high in calories and cholesterol
5. **Acquired disorders:** Gallbladder stasis or hypomotility, rapid weight reduction
6. Genetic predisposition
7. **Metabolic abnormalities:** Diabetes, obesity, insulin resistance, genetic hyperlipoproteinemias and primary biliary cholangitis (PBC)

Pigment Stones

1. **Chronic hemolysis** (e.g., sickle cell anemia, hereditary spherocytosis)
2. **Demography:** More common in Asians and in rural regions than in urban
3. Chronic biliary tract infections
4. **Gastrointestinal diseases:** Ileal disease (e.g., crohn disease), ileal resection or bypass, cystic fibrosis with pancreatic insufficiency
5. Alcoholic cirrhosis
6. Pernicious anemia
7. Advancing age

2. **Female sex hormones: Five Fs of cholesterol stone** are Fat, Fertile, Forty, Female, and Familial.
   - **Female gender:** Gallstone is **two times more** common in females than in males and higher prevalence is observed in premenopausal women and both may be due to the effect of estrogen. **Estrogen** increases the secretion of cholesterol and decreases the secretion of bile acids by the liver. This favors lithogenic bile secretion by the liver.
   - **Pregnancy:** In the last trimester of pregnancy, the **gallbladder empties more slowly** and causes **stasis,** and increases the **precipitation of cholesterol crystals.** Progesterone, which is the predominant hormone during pregnancy inhibits the discharge of bile from the gallbladder.
   - **Oral contraceptives:** They **increase** both the **uptake and synthesis of cholesterol.**
3. **Hereditary factors: Familial predisposition** is observed in cholesterol stones and is twice as common in first-degree relatives of patients with gallstones. ***ABCG5* and *ABG2* genes** participate in biliary cholesterol secretion and their **variants increase the risk** for the development of cholesterol gallstones.
4. **Environmental factors:**
   - **Drugs: Clofibrate,** used to lower blood cholesterol results in **excessive secretion of cholesterol in the bile.** Drugs, such as octreotide and ceftriaxone also predispose to gallstones.
   - **Obesity and rapid weight loss:** These are strongly associated with **increased biliary cholesterol secretion.** Obesity enhances cholesterol absorption, synthesis, and secretion. There is probably a linear relation between body weight and the risk of gallstones.
   - **Diet high in calories and cholesterol:** They are associated with increased risk.
5. **Acquired disorders: Gallbladder stasis** (neurogenic or hormonal) or hypomotility (occurs in pregnancy, rapid weight loss, and spinal cord injury) promotes cholesterol and pigment gallstones.
6. **Genetic predisposition:** The prevalence of cholesterol stones is highest in North American Indians and Chilean Indians.
7. **Metabolic abnormalities:** These are associated with high blood cholesterol levels (e.g., diabetes, some genetic hyperlipoproteinemias, and PBC).

Pathogenesis of Gallstones

Pathogenesis of the two main forms (cholesterol and pigment) of gallstones differs and is briefly discussed separately.

Pathogenesis of Cholesterol Stones (Fig. 19.37)

Q. Write a short note on the pathogenesis of cholesterol stones.

The cholesterol stone formation is a **complex multifactorial process.** Cholesterol gallstone formation involves four

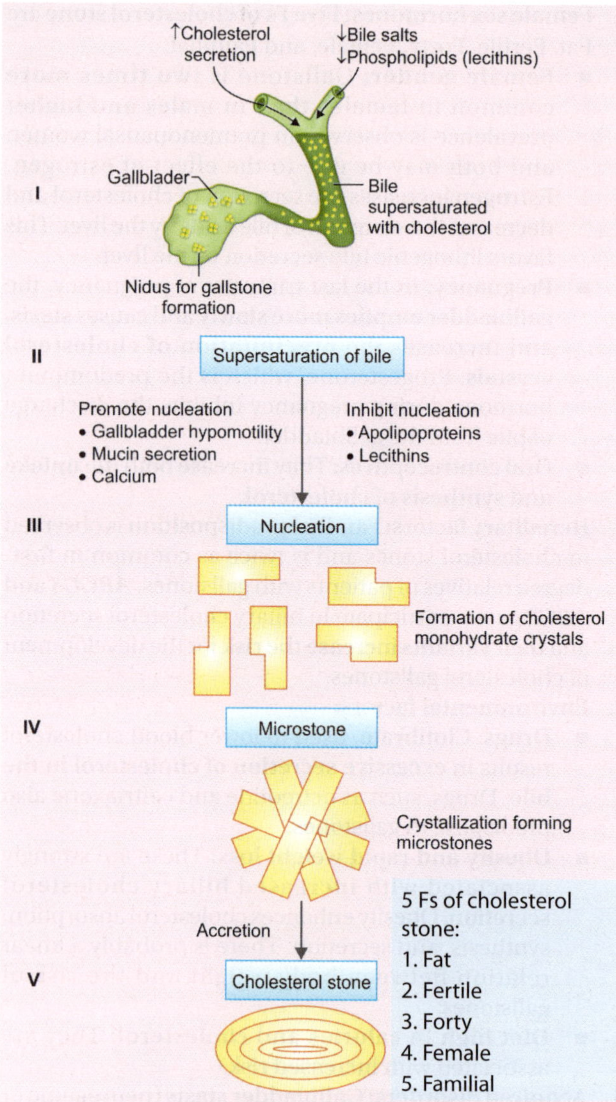

Fig. 19.37: Pathogenesis of cholesterol stones.

simultaneous processes namely, (1) supersaturation of bile with cholesterol (cholesterol supersaturation), (2) gallbladder hypomotility, (3) accelerated cholesterol crystal nucleation (nucleation and crystallization of cholesterol), and (4) hypersecretion of mucus in the gallbladder.

Supersaturation of Bile with Cholesterol

Excretion of excess cholesterol: Significant excretion of excess cholesterol from the body is by the formation of bile formation. This may be excreted either as free cholesterol or as bile salts (water-soluble products of cholesterol metabolism). **Cholesterol is secreted by the hepatocytes as vesicles** (unilamellar or multilamellar) **or micelles.**

- **Vesicles**: They are spherical structures **consisting of cholesterol surrounded by one or more layers of phospholipid bilayers but do not contain bile salts.** Unilamellar vesicle consists of cholesterol surrounded by one phospholipid bilayer. Multilamellar vesicle consists of cholesterol surrounded by more than one phospholipid bilayer.
- **Micellation**: Bile acids are water-soluble sterols and are the major catabolic products of cholesterol. They act as detergents and solubilize water-insoluble lipids (secreted by hepatocytes) in the bile and dietary lipids in the lumen of the gut. Micellation is the **process of conversion of vesicles into complex aggregates of water-soluble molecules** known as mixed **micelles** by **the detergent-like action of bile acids and lecithins.** Mixed micelles consist of a combination of bile acids, phospholipids, and cholesterol. In mixed micelles, the lipophilic (fat-soluble) portions of the three molecules aggregate in the center of the structure while the hydrophilic (water-soluble) portions are oriented at the periphery, thus allowing solubility in bile.

Supersaturation: It is a condition in which **cholesterol concentrations of bile exceed** the **solubilizing** (achieved by phospholipids and bile acids) **capacity of bile**. It is one of the important mechanisms in the formation of lithogenic (stone-forming) bile. With supersaturation, cholesterol can no longer remain dispersed in bile. Cholesterol nucleates into solid cholesterol monohydrate crystals. **Cholesterol supersaturation** may be due to **increased biliary cholesterol secretion** (the most important cause), **decreased bile acid synthesis, or both**. It may be due to decreased biliary lecithin.

- **Increased biliary cholesterol secretion**: It is observed in obesity, high-calorie diets, cholesterol-rich diets, certain drugs (e.g., clofibrate), pregnancy, oral contraceptives, rapid weight loss, and increased activity of hMG-CoA reductase (the rate-limiting enzyme of hepatic cholesterol synthesis).
- **Decreased bile salts: Primary biliary cholangitis** (PBC), mutation of *CYP7A1* gene, oral contraceptive pills, and impaired enterohepatic circulation (e.g., Crohn's disease, ileal resection) are associated with decreased bile salts.
- **Decreased biliary lecithin:** For example, *MDR3* gene mutation. The solubility of cholesterol in bile depends on the concentration of phospholipids (lecithins) and bile acids.

Gallbladder Hypomotility

- Normal motility of the gallbladder empties and completely excretes its bile along with all supersaturated bile or crystals. Thus, motility does not allow stones to grow.
- Abnormalities in gallbladder emptying (decreased motility/hypomotility) **cause gallbladder stasis.** Causes of gallbladder hypomotility/stasis include total parental nutrition (TPN), prolonged fasting, pregnancy,

massive burns, oral contraceptive pills, and the drug octreotide. Hypomotility **promotes cholesterol crystals' aggregation and biliary sludge formation** (also known as **microlithiasis**).

Accelerated Cholesterol Crystal Nucleation (Nucleation and Crystallization of Cholesterol)

Nucleation: With supersaturation, cholesterol can no longer remain soluble. Excess of cholesterol is carried as unilamellar cholesterol-rich vesicles, which fuse into large multilamellar vesicles. They nucleate to form solid microscopic cholesterol monohydrate crystals. The **nucleation** is the first and crucial step in gallstone formation and is **accelerated in lithogenic bile.** Accelerated nucleation may be due to either an excess of pronucleating factors or a deficiency of antinucleating factors.

- **Pronucleating factors: Mucin** and **certain nonmucin glycoproteins** and **biliary calcium** are important pronucleating factors.
  - **Hypersecretion of mucus** (discussed below).
  - **Calcium salts:** Calcium carbonate, calcium bilirubinate, and calcium phosphate in the bile can **serve as a nidus for cholesterol crystallization.**
- **Antinucleating factors:** These include apolipoproteins A-1 and A-2, other glycoproteins and lecithins.

Growth to stone-sized aggregates: It involves different steps.

- **Biliary sludge:** It is defined as a **suspension of precipitates of cholesterol monohydrate crystals or calcium bilirubinate granules in bile.** Before the appearance of stones, there is always the formation of a 'biliary sludge'. It implies supersaturation of bile with either cholesterol or calcium bilirubinate. Biliary sludge can resolve, persist, or progress. When it progresses to stones its crystals grow to form plates, in part because of impairment in gallbladder contractility.
- **Microlithiasis: After nucleation, crystallization** occurs, and **cholesterol monohydrate crystals grow into microstones** (microlithiasis/crystals in bile). Microlithiasis is identified by the presence of sludge by ultrasonography (US) or the presence of birefringent cholesterol crystals in bile.
- **Gallstone:** The **microstones increase** in size by the gradual addition of more cholesterol and other constituents to **form macroscopic gallstones.**

Hypersecretion of Mucus in the Gallbladder

Mucin glycoproteins usually are secreted continuously from the gallbladder. Hypersecretion of mucin **accelerates the growth and precipitation of cholesterol monohydrate crystals.** Mucus traps the nucleated crystals and favors their aggregation into stones. It leads to more cholesterol accretion and the formation of macroscopic gallstones.

Pathogenesis of Pigment Stones

Q. Write a short note on the risk factors/pathogenesis of pigment stones.

Pigment stones are subclassified as **black and brown pigment** stones. Risk factors for pigment stones are listed in **Box 19.18. Pigment stones mainly develop in the setting of bacterial infections or parasitic infestations of the biliary tree**, as well as in individuals with diseases that lead to **chronic hemolysis.**

Black Pigment Stones

Increased production of unconjugated bilirubin: Unconjugated bilirubin is usually a minor component of bile and is **insoluble in bile**. Under **normal physiologic conditions, it is not secreted into bile** and constitutes less than 1% of total bile pigment. **Increased production of unconjugated bilirubin** may **precipitate as calcium bilirubinate** probably **around a nidus of mucinous glycoproteins to form black pigment stones.**

- **Causes of increased unconjugated bilirubin in bile:** These include **chronic hemolysis** (e.g., β-thalassemia, hereditary spherocytosis, sickle cell disease), cirrhosis, severe ileal dysfunction (or bypass), and pancreatitis. In most patients, the predisposing cause is not known.

Brown Pigment Stones (Refer Online Flowchart 19.2)

It can be **found in the gallbladder or within the biliary tree**. Brown pigment stones develop **secondary to stasis and infection.**

Stasis: It **favors the bacterial infection** as well as the accumulation of mucus.

Biliary infections

These include bacterial infections and parasitic infections.

Bacterial infections of the biliary tract: Unconjugated bilirubin in bile increases biliary tract infection. Bacterial infections of the biliary tract by enteric bacteria (predominantly *Escherichia coli*) with ascending cholangitis favor pigment stone formation.

- **Actions of bacterial enzymes on bile constituents:** In bile, bacterial enzymes have different actions on bile constituents.
  - **Bacterial enzyme β-glucuronidases** from microbia **hydrolyze bilirubin glucuronides** (conjugated bilirubin) in the bile to **unconjugated**, insoluble bilirubin.
  - **Bacterial phospholipases hydrolyze phospholipids** and **liberate free fatty acids** (such as palmitic acid and stearic acid).
  - **Bacterial enzymes hydrolyze bile salts** (glycine or taurine-conjugated) into **free (unconjugated) bile acids.**

- **Products formed from the bacterial actions**: These include (1) unconjugated insoluble bilirubin, (2) free fatty acids, and (3) unconjugated bile acids. They **combine with calcium** to produce a **water-insoluble calcium bilirubinate** and form a brown stone.

Parasitic infestations: Brown stones may be found in association with **infestation by *Ascaris lumbricoides* or *Clonorchis sinensis***, and other helminths, which may invade the biliary tract.

Dead bacteria and parasites may act as nuclei and accelerate the precipitation of calcium bilirubinate.

MORPHOLOGY

Cholesterol Stones

- **Sites:** They occur only in the **gallbladder.**
- **Chemical composition and appearance:** They consist of 50% to 100% cholesterol. Their **appearance varies depending on the cholesterol content;** either purely cholesterol (100%—rare) or have cholesterol as the major chemical component.

Pure Cholesterol Stones

They account for 10% of gallstones. They are **radiolucent.**

Appearance (Fig. 19.38A): They are **typically single, pale yellow, round to ovoid (spheroidal), and coarsely nodular.** They have **finely granular** and **hard external surfaces.** They are **large** and measure **2–4 cm** in diameter.

Cut surface: They have a **glistening bluish-white color** with a **crystalline or laminated** cut surface. They show **long, thin, radiating cholesterol monohydrate crystals.**

Mixed Cholesterol Gallstones

Stones with **lower cholesterol content than pure cholesterol stones** are designated mixed. They are composed of **60–89% cholesterol and proportions of calcium carbonate, phosphates, and bilirubin.** They are **slightly more common than pure cholesterol stones.**

Appearance (Figs. 19.38B and C): They are often **multiple and gray-white to black.** They are **smaller than pure cholesterol stones** and range from **0.2 to 3.0** cm in diameter. **Surfaces may be rounded or faceted** because of tight apposition.

Cut surface: They have **a laminated cut surface** with a dark core.

Stones composed mainly of cholesterol without calcium carbonate are radiolucent, but those with sufficient calcium carbonate are radiopaque (10–20%).

Pigment Gallstones

By definition, pigment stones contain <25–30% cholesterol. They are composed of calcium bilirubinate, phosphate, and carbonate. Black pigment stones are **formed in sterile gallbladder bile,** and **brown stones are formed in infected intrahepatic or extrahepatic ducts.**

Sites: They may arise anywhere in the biliary tree.

Black Pigment Stones (Fig. 19.38D)

Black stones contain **calcium salts of unconjugated bilirubin (calcium bilirubinate),** small amounts of calcium carbonate, calcium phosphate, mucin glycoprotein, and some cholesterol monohydrate crystals. In general, black pigment stones are found in sterile gallbladder bile.

Appearance: They are **multiple** with **an inverse relationship between size and number.**

- They have a shiny, **black, or deep brown** color.
- **Usually,** they are **irregular, spiculated** ("jack-like"), **molded,** and may crumble on touch (quite friable).
- They are **relatively small** and range from **0.2 to 1.5** cm **in diameter.** They **arise in sterile gallbladder bile.**
- Because they contain enough calcium carbonates and phosphates, **approximately 50–75% are radiopaque.**

Brown Pigment Stones (Fig. 19.38E)

They are composed of **calcium salts of unconjugated bilirubin, palmitate, and stearate,** with **varying amounts of cholesterol** (higher cholesterol concentration than in black stones) **and protein.** Brown stones tend to be single or few in number.

- **Appearance:** They are **multiple, dull brown, laminated, and soft** (much softer than black stones). They may have a **soap-like or greasy consistency** (due to the presence of fatty acid salts released from biliary lecithins by bacterial phospholipases). These stones are **easy to crush endoscopically.** They range from **0.2 to 1.5** cm **in diameter.**
- **Usually, radiolucent.**
- Usually **associated with infection of the biliary tract** (*E. coli* and biliary flukes), and they are generally found in **infected large bile ducts (intrahepatic or extrahepatic ducts).**

Clinical Features

Asymptomatic: The majority of patients with gallstones remain **asymptomatic** throughout their lives.

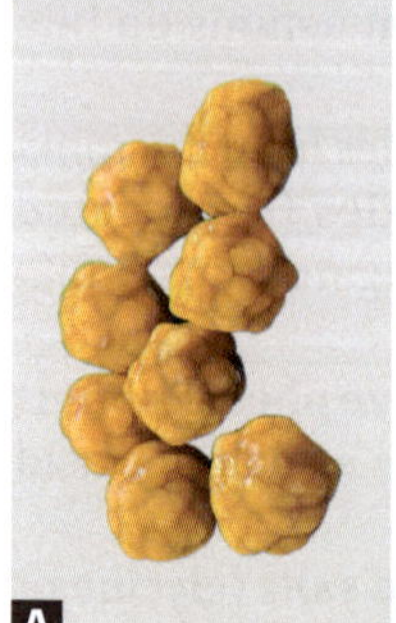

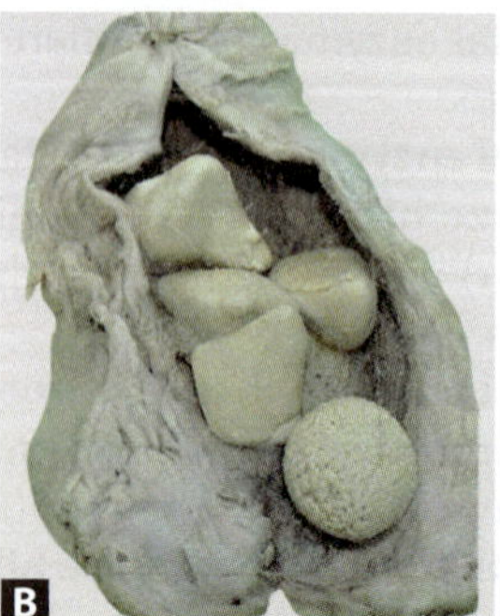

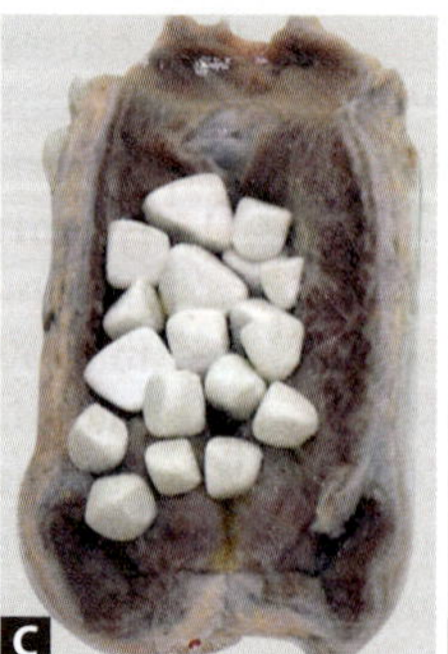

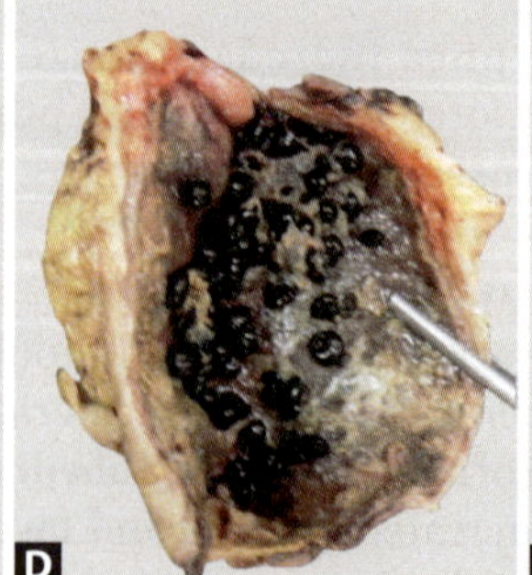

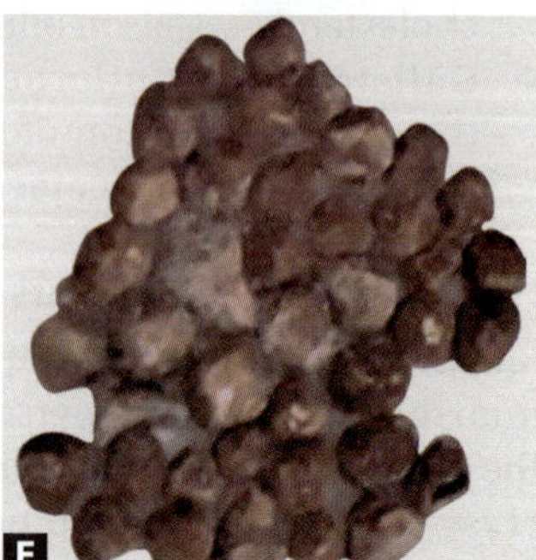

Figs. 19.38A to E: Types of gallstones: (A) Pure cholesterol stones; (B and C) Gallbladder with mixed cholesterol stones; (D) Gallbladder with multiple black pigment stones; (E) Brown stones.

Symptoms: Gallstones usually produce symptoms by causing inflammation or obstruction when they pass into the cystic duct or CBD. In a minority of patients, it presents with right upper quadrant or epigastric pain, often severe. The characteristic symptom is **biliary colic** which is a constant and often long-lasting pain. Large gallstones usually cannot enter the cystic or common ducts to produce obstruction. Pain usually develops after a fatty meal that produces contraction of the gallbladder, and presses a stone against the gallbladder outlet, leading to increased pressure and pain.

Complications

Q. Write a short note on complications of gallstones.

In the Gallbladder

- **Cholecystitis**: It can cause both **acute and chronic cholecystitis.** Rarely it may cause gangrenous or emphysematous cholecystitis.
- **Empyema of the gallbladder**: It is characterized by distention of the gallbladder with pus.
- **Hydrops of the gallbladder**: Gallbladder distended with clear watery fluid.
- **Mucocele:** Gallbladder distended by cloudy, mucoid material.
- **Perforation of gallbladder**.
- **Carcinoma:** Gallstones may **increase the risk of carcinoma** of the gallbladder.

In the Bile Ducts

- **Biliary obstruction** (obstructive cholestasis).
- **Acute cholangitis** (inflammation of the biliary tree).
- **Acute pancreatitis.**

In the Intestine

- **Biliary fistulas:** Fistula may develop **between the biliary system and bowel or gallbladder and skin.**
- **Gallstone ileus** or **Bouveret's syndrome**: Rarely, a large gallstone may erode directly into an adjacent loop of the small intestine and produce intestinal obstruction (**"gallstone ileus" or Bouveret's syndrome**)

CHOLECYSTITIS

Inflammation of the gallbladder is cholecystitis. It may be acute, chronic, or acute superimposed on chronic. Almost always, cholecystitis occurs in association with gallstones.

Acute Cholecystitis

Definition: Acute cholecystitis is an acute **diffuse inflammation** of the gallbladder.

Q. Write a short note on cholecystitis.

Types: Acute cholecystitis may be acute calculous or acalculous type.

- **Acalculous cholecystitis:** It is not associated with gallstones and may occur in severely ill patients.

Acute Acalculous Cholecystitis

Acute calculous cholecystitis is associated **with gallstones in the gallbladder.** It is the most common serious complication of gallstones.

Pathogenesis

Acute inflammation of the gallbladder develops in **about 90% of cases as a complication due to obstruction of the neck or cystic duct by gallstones**. Acute calculous cholecystitis is particularly common in diabetic patients who have symptomatic gallstones. The inflammation of the gallbladder may be brought out by **three factors**, namely (1) chemical inflammation, (2) mechanical inflammation, and (3) bacterial inflammation.

1. **Chemical inflammation:** Acute calculous cholecystitis results from chemical irritation and inflammation of a gallbladder obstructed by gallstones.
   - **Production of lysolecithin:** As a consequence of the obstruction, the enzyme phospholipase is released from the mucosal epithelium of the gallbladder. This enzyme may act on lecithin present in bile and **release toxic lysolecithin**. It is a membrane-active toxin and can cause chemical inflammation.
   - **Decreased glycoprotein: Normally, a glycoprotein** produced by gallbladder mucosa has a **protective role**. Its **decreased production** leads to exposure of the mucosal epithelium to the **direct detergent action of concentrated bile salts. Supersaturation of bile with cholesterol** may cause **toxic damage** to the epithelium.
   - **Prostaglandins:** These are **released within the wall of the distended gallbladder** and contribute to **inflammation of the mucosa and the wall of the gallbladder.**
2. **Mechanical inflammation: Obstruction of the cystic duct** increases intraluminal pressure and distention of the gallbladder. It leads to **mucosal and mural inflammation**. It also disturbs the motility (dysmotility) of the gallbladder. Increased intraluminal pressure also compromises blood flow to the mucosa. It obstructs the venous flow and ischemia of the gallbladder mucosa and wall. These events initially occur even in the absence of bacterial infection.
3. **Bacterial inflammation:** It may play a role in acute cholecystitis, but **a bacterial invasion is usually a secondary event exacerbating the inflammatory process**. The most frequent organisms include *E. coli*, *Klebsiella* species, *Streptococcus* species, and *Clostridium* species.

Acute Acalculous Cholecystitis

Gallstones are not seen in 5–10% of patients with acute cholecystitis. **Ischemic injury** is probably the **main pathogenic event** in acute acalculous cholecystitis. The cystic artery is an end artery without collateral circulation. Ischemia may occur due to obstruction of blood flow.

Contributing factors include inflammation and edema of the wall-compromising blood flow, dehydration, gallbladder stasis due to the accumulation of microcrystals of cholesterol (biliary sludge), viscous bile, and mucus, causing cystic duct obstruction in the absence of stones. It usually develops in acutely ill patients who are hospitalized for unrelated conditions.

Risk factors for acute acalculous cholecystitis: These are severe debilitating conditions and are as follows:

- Nonbiliary major surgical operations
- Major trauma and burns
- Severe burns
- Sepsis with hypotension and multisystem organ failure
- Immunosuppression
- Diabetes mellitus
- Vasculitides
- Systemic infections (tuberculosis, syphilis, hemolytic streptococcal septicemia, actinomycosis, etc.)
- End-stage renal disease

MORPHOLOGY

Both **acute acalculous** and **calculous cholecystitis** are **morphologically similar**, except that stones are not seen in the acalculous form.

Gross

- **Size:** Gallbladder is usually **enlarged, tense,** and **edematous.**
- **Serosa:** It is covered by **fibrinous exudate** and the serosa may appear bright red due to subserosal hemorrhage. In severe cases, serosa may be covered by suppurative exudate.
- **Wall:** It is **thickened** (up to 2 cm) due to edema and hemorrhage.
- **Mucosa:** It is **red or purple** and may show **ulcerations.**
- **Lumen:** In **calculous cholecystitis,** the lumen may contain one or more **stones.** The lumen is filled with turbid fluid.

Q. Write a short note on microscopy of acute cholecystitis.

Microscopy (Figs. 19.39A and B)

- Mucosa shows focal **ulcerations.**
- **The wall of the gallbladder** shows **edema, hemorrhage,** and **acute inflammatory cells.** Secondary bacterial infection may lead to suppuration in the gallbladder wall.
- **Widespread necrosis** is found in **gangrenous cholecystitis.**

Clinical Features

Acute cholecystitis presents with **progressive right upper quadrant** or epigastric pain. It is frequently associated with **mild fever, anorexia, nausea**, and **vomiting**. Acute calculous cholecystitis may also **appear suddenly** as an **acute surgical emergency. Acute acalculous cholecystitis** tends to be **more insidious in onset**.

Laboratory findings: Mild to moderate leukocytosis and mild elevations in serum alkaline phosphatase values may be seen.

Complications

Q. Write a short note on complications of acute cholecystitis.

- **Empyema of the gallbladder:** The gallbladder with an obstructed cystic duct may be distended with pus (purulent exudate).
- **Gangrenous cholecystitis:** Gallbladder transformed into a green-black necrotic organ **(Fig. 19.39C)**.
- **Acute gaseous or emphysematous cholecystitis**: It is due to invasion of gas-forming organisms (such as clostridia and coliforms).
- **Perforation of the gallbladder:** It is due to secondary bacterial infection.
- **Bile peritonitis:** It may result from the discharge of bile from the distended gallbladder into the peritoneal cavity.
- **Pericholecystic abscess, abscesses in the liver or abdominal cavity**.
- **Fistula into the intestine or duodenum**: Perforations may lead to fistula formation with neighboring

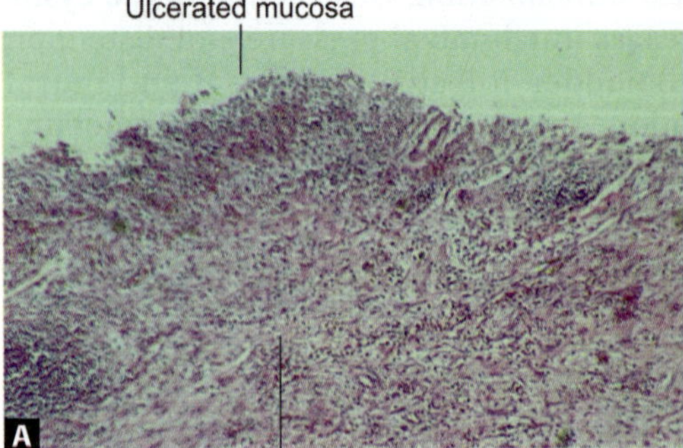

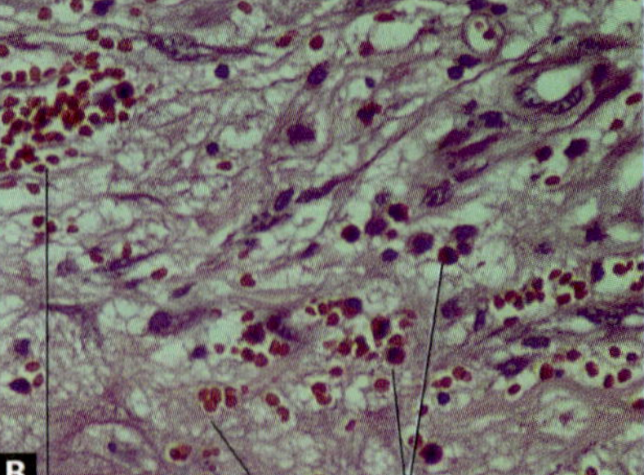

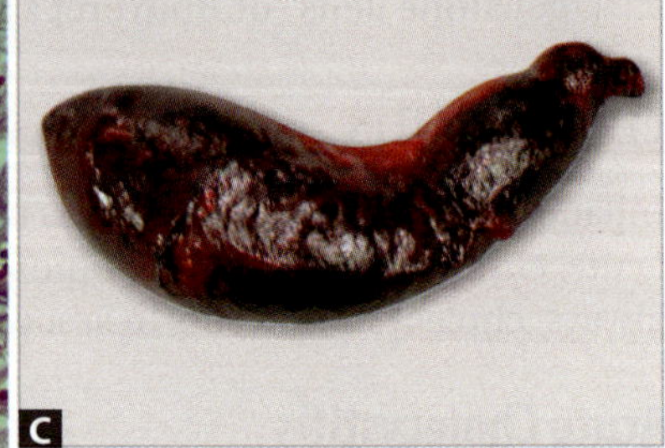

Gangrenous cholecystitis in which the gallbladder is transformed into a green-black necrotic organ

Figs. 19.39A to C: (A) Microscopy of acute cholecystitis showing ulceration of mucosa; (B) High-power view showing edema, hemorrhage, and acute inflammatory infiltrate; (C) Gangrenous cholecystitis.

organs, such as the small or large intestine creating a **cholecystenteric fistula.**

- **Gallstone ileus: Through the fistula,** a large gallstone can **pass into the bowel** → resulting in gallstone ileus or intestinal obstruction.

Chronic Cholecystitis

Chronic cholecystitis is characterized by persistent chronic inflammation of the gallbladder. It is the **most common disease of the gallbladder.** Associated with **gallstones in ~90%** of the cases. It may also develop following recurrent attacks of acute cholecystitis.

MORPHOLOGY

Extremely variable and depends on the severity and the duration of the disease.

Gross (Fig. 19.40)

- **Size:** Gallbladder may be **normal** or may be **shrunken** in severe cases.
- **Serosa:** It is usually **smooth and glistening**, but may be dull due to fibrosis.
- **Cut section:** The **wall is thickened, opaque, and gray-white.**
- **Lumen:** It usually shows **stones.**

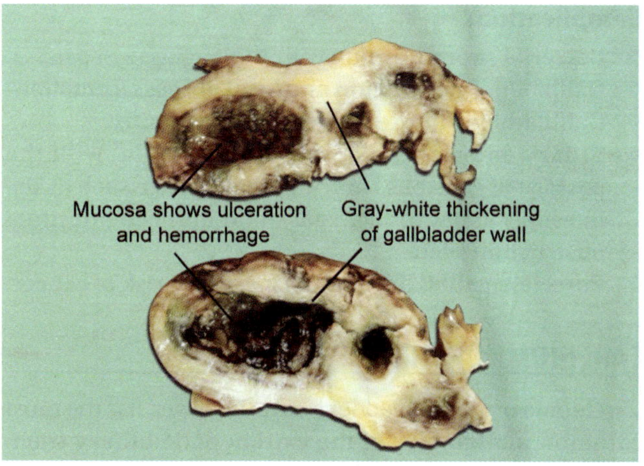

Fig. 19.40: Gross appearance of chronic cholecystitis.

Microscopy (Figs. 19.41A and B)

Q. Write a short note on microscopy of chronic cholecystitis.

Mild cases: The inflammation is **scanty** and shows **lymphocytes, plasma cells, and macrophages** in the **mucosa and the subserosal fibrous tissue.**

Advanced cases: It shows **marked subepithelial and subserosal fibrosis,** associated with **mononuclear cell infiltration.**

- **Mucosal epithelium:** It may be **normal or atrophic** or show focal ulceration.
- **Rokitansky–Aschoff sinuses:** These are **irregularly shaped, tubular structures** formed due to **invagination of mucosal epithelium deep into the wall** of the gallbladder. They represent herniations or diverticula resulting from increased intraluminal pressure.

Morphological Variants

- **Cholecystitis glandularis:** In this variant, **mucosal folds fuse** and form crypts of epithelium buried in the gallbladder wall.
- **Porcelain gallbladder:** It is characterized by **extensive dystrophic calcification** within the gallbladder wall (predominantly in the muscle and lamina propria).
- **Acute on chronic cholecystitis:** Superimposition of acute inflammation on chronic inflammation indicates acute on chronic cholecystitis.
- **Xanthogranulomatous cholecystitis:** It is characterized by **marked thickening of the wall** and **diffuse or nodular collections of macrophages containing neutral fat and lipofuscin** (ceroid) pigment.

Clinical Features

- Usually present as **recurrent attacks** of either **steady or colicky epigastric or right upper quadrant pain.**
- Other features **include nausea**, vomiting, and **intolerance for fatty foods.**

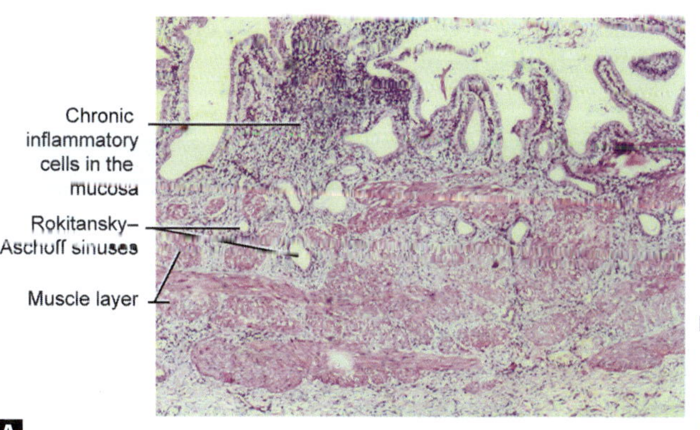

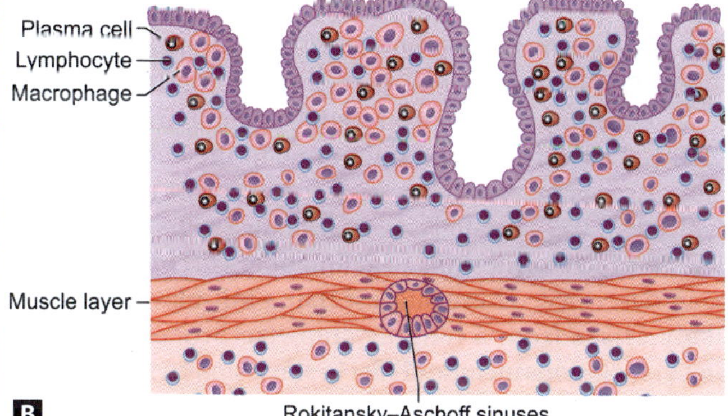

Figs. 19.41A and B: Microscopic appearance of chronic cholecystitis. Outpouching of the mucosa through the wall forms the Rokitansky–Aschoff sinus. Mucosa is infiltrated by inflammatory cells: (A) Photomicrograph; (B) Diagrammatic.

Complications

- **Bacterial superinfection** with cholangitis or sepsis.
- **Gallbladder perforation and local abscess** formation.
- **Gallbladder rupture with diffuse peritonitis.**
- **Biliary enteric (cholecystenteric) fistula**, with the passage of gallstones into adjacent organs, such as the intestine. It may result in **gallstone-induced intestinal obstruction (ileus).**
- **Porcelain gallbladder has an increased risk of cancer.**

CARCINOMA OF THE GALLBLADDER

Carcinoma of the gallbladder is **rare**; however, it is the **most common malignancy of the extrahepatic biliary tract**. It is slightly **more common in females** and occurs most frequently during the seventh decade of life. It is common in parts of northern India.

Etiology

Risk Factor

- **Gallstones**: They predispose to **carcinoma by causing chronic irritation, chronic inflammation, and epithelial damage**.
- **Genetic factors:** Prevalence of the gallbladder cancer in American Indians, Hispanic Americans, and parts of north India probably reflects the role of genetic factors.
- **Carcinogen: Present in the bile acids** are believed to play a role.
- **Primary sclerosing cholangitis:** It may predispose to gallbladder cancer.
- **Calcification of the gallbladder**.
- **Gastrointestinal disorders:** Ulcerative colitis and polyposis syndromes also have an association with gallbladder adenocarcinoma.

Molecular Genetics

Carcinoma of the gallbladder develops through the accumulation of **multiple genetic alterations**. Relatively common driver mutations include gain-of-function aberrations affecting members of the epidermal growth factor (EGF) receptor gene family (including *HER2*) and genes encoding downstream signaling components such as RAS. Loss-of-function mutations in the *TP53* tumor suppressor gene are also present in up to 50% of tumors. Typically, *TP53*-mutated cancers exhibit aneuploidy.

Several **precursor lesions of gallbladder carcinoma** have been described. These suggest that a full-blown cancer likely arises from a lengthy stepwise process. These precursor lesions include (1) flat in situ lesions with varying degrees of dysplasia, (2) mass-forming adenoma-like lesions termed intracholecystic papillary tubular neoplasm, and (3) intestinal metaplasia.

MORPHOLOGY

Gross

- **Sites: Most arise in** the **fundus and neck** (60%), followed by the body (30%).
- **Usually shows calculi** and marked fibrosis of the wall.

Two patterns of growth.

- **Diffusely infiltrating (70%):** It usually appears as a **poorly defined area of diffuse thickening of the gallbladder wall** (due to **prominent desmoplasia**) and is similar to linitis plastica of the stomach. These tumors are **scirrhous, gray-white,** and have a very firm consistency. Deep ulceration can cause fistula formation in adjacent viscera.
- **Exophytic/polypoid (30%):** It grows into the lumen as an **irregular, cauliflower mass** and also invades the underlying wall of the gallbladder. The luminal portion of the tumor mass may show areas of necrosis, hemorrhage, and ulceration.

Microscopy

- Most gallbladder cancers are **adenocarcinomas** showing varying degrees of differentiation.
- The well-differentiated carcinomas consist of well-formed glands lined by a layer of cuboidal cells and often embedded in a desmoplastic stroma.
- Other tumors may be infiltrative and poorly differentiated to undifferentiated.

Spread

- **Direct spread**: The tumor may spread to the liver, peritoneal surfaces, cystic duct, and adjacent bile ducts. Biliary-enteric fistulas may develop when the tumor penetrates the intestine.
- **Lymphatic spread**: It may spread to perihilar lymphatics and portal-hepatic lymph nodes and in later stages, mediastinal and supraclavicular lymph nodes.
- **Blood spread**: **Liver** (both local spread and hematogenous spread) and **lungs**.

Clinical Features

- **Right upper quadrant abdominal pain, anorexia and nausea, and vomiting.**
- Laboratory investigation shows **elevated alkaline phosphatase level.**

PANCREAS

PANCREATITIS

Inflammatory disorders of the pancreas are termed pancreatitis. It may be divided into acute (acute pancreatitis) and chronic types (chronic pancreatitis). In *acute pancreatitis,* the function of the pancreas can return to normal if the cause of inflammation is removed. In *chronic pancreatitis,* there is an irreversible destruction of the exocrine pancreas.

Acute Pancreatitis

Definition: Acute pancreatitis is a reversible, **acute inflammation of the exocrine pancreas** due to injury to the parenchyma of the pancreas.

Acute pancreatitis is relatively common. **It is a reversible inflammatory condition and its severity varies from focal edema and fat necrosis to widespread hemorrhagic necrosis.**

Etiology

Q. Discuss the etiology and pathogenesis of acute pancreatitis.

Various causes of acute pancreatitis are presented in **Box 19.19. Alcoholism and gallstones account for** about **80% of the cases.**

- **Alcohol:** It causes acute pancreatitis usually in individuals who consume large quantities of alcohol. **A polymorphism in the detoxifying enzyme uridine 5-diphosphate (UDP) glucuronyl transferase increases the risk for alcoholic-induced pancreatitis.** The male-to-female ratio is 6:1.
- **Gallstones within the common bile duct:** It is responsible for acute pancreatitis **in about 30–60% of cases.** The frequency of acute pancreatitis is inversely proportional to the size of gallstones. The male-to-female ratio is 1:3. The gallstone slows the flow of pancreatic enzymes through the ampulla of Vater ("gallstone pancreatitis").
- **Nongallstone-related obstruction of the pancreatic ducts:** It may be due to pancreatic cancer or other periampullary neoplasms, biliary sludge, parasites (e.g., *Ascaris lumbricoides* and *Clonorchis sinensis*).
- **Genetic factors:** No cause is identified in about 10–20% of patients and are termed idiopathic. Some of these may have a genetic basis. Three susceptibility genes have been identified:
  1. **Mutation in cationic trypsinogen (*PRSS1*) gene:** It is the **most common genetic defect,** which results in resistance to trypsin hydrolysis.
  2. **Mutation in the pancreatic trypsin inhibitor gene** (serine protease inhibitor, Kazal type 1; *SPINK1*): *SPINK1* gene is essential for the inactivation of trypsin and for the prevention of the autodigestion of the pancreas by activated trypsin. Mutation of this gene **causes inappropriate activation of trypsin,** which in turn can **activate other digestive proenzymes** resulting in pancreatitis.
  3. **Mutations in the cystic fibrosis transmembrane regulator (*CFTR*)** gene.
- **Metabolic disorders:** These include hypertriglyceridemia (above 1,000 mg/dL), hyperparathyroidism, and other hypercalcemic states.
- **Medications:** These include anticonvulsants, cancer chemotherapeutic agents, thiazide diuretics, estrogens, and many others. They cause pancreatitis **either by a hypersensitivity reaction** or by the generation of **toxic metabolites.**
- **Infections with mumps virus or coxsackievirus:** They may directly infect pancreatic exocrine cells.
- **Idiopathic pancreatitis:** No identifiable cause.

BOX 19.19: Causes of acute pancreatitis.

Metabolic
- **Alcoholism**
- Hyperlipoproteinemia (hypertriglyceridemia)
- Hypercalcemia (e.g., hyperparathyroidism)
- Obesity, type 3 diabetes mellitus, smoking
- Drugs (e.g., azathioprine, ACE inhibitors, statins, GLP-1 agonists, DPP-4 inhibitors, 6-mercaptopurine, estrogens, tetracycline, valproic acid, 5-ASA, thiazide diuretics)

Genetic
- Mutation in cationic trypsinogen (*PRSS1*) and trypsin inhibitor (*SPINK1*) gene

Mechanical
- **Gallstones**
- Traumatic acinar injury
  - Blunt abdominal trauma
  - Iatrogenic injury
    - During operative surgery
    - Endoscopic procedures with dye injection (e.g., ERCP)
    - Fine needle aspiration biopsy of the pancreas
- Periampullary neoplasms (e.g., pancreatic cancer)
- Parasites (*Ascaris lumbricoides* and *Clonorchis sinensis* organisms)

Medications and toxins
- Drugs: Furosemide, azathioprine
- Toxins: Insecticides, methanol, organophosphates

Vascular
- Shock
- Atheroembolism, thrombosis, and embolism
- Polyarteritis nodosa

Infectious
- Viral infections: Mumps, coxsackie virus

Idiopathic (~10–20%)

(ACE: angiotensin-converting enzyme; DPP-4: dipeptidyl peptidase-4; ERCP: endoscopic retrograde cholangiopancreatography; GLP-1: glucagon-like peptide-1; 5-ASA: 5-aminosalicylic acid)

Pathogenesis (Fig. 19.42)

Q. Write a short essay on the pathogenesis of acute pancreatitis.

The exact mechanisms by which the above causes trigger inflammation of the pancreas are not completely known.

Inappropriate release and activation of pancreatic enzymes: Pancreatic enzymes are synthesized in an inactive proenzyme form (e.g., trypsinogen, chymotrypsinogen, proelastase, and lipolytic enzymes, such as phospholipase A_2) and become active when converted into an enzyme form. **Acute pancreatitis results from inappropriate**

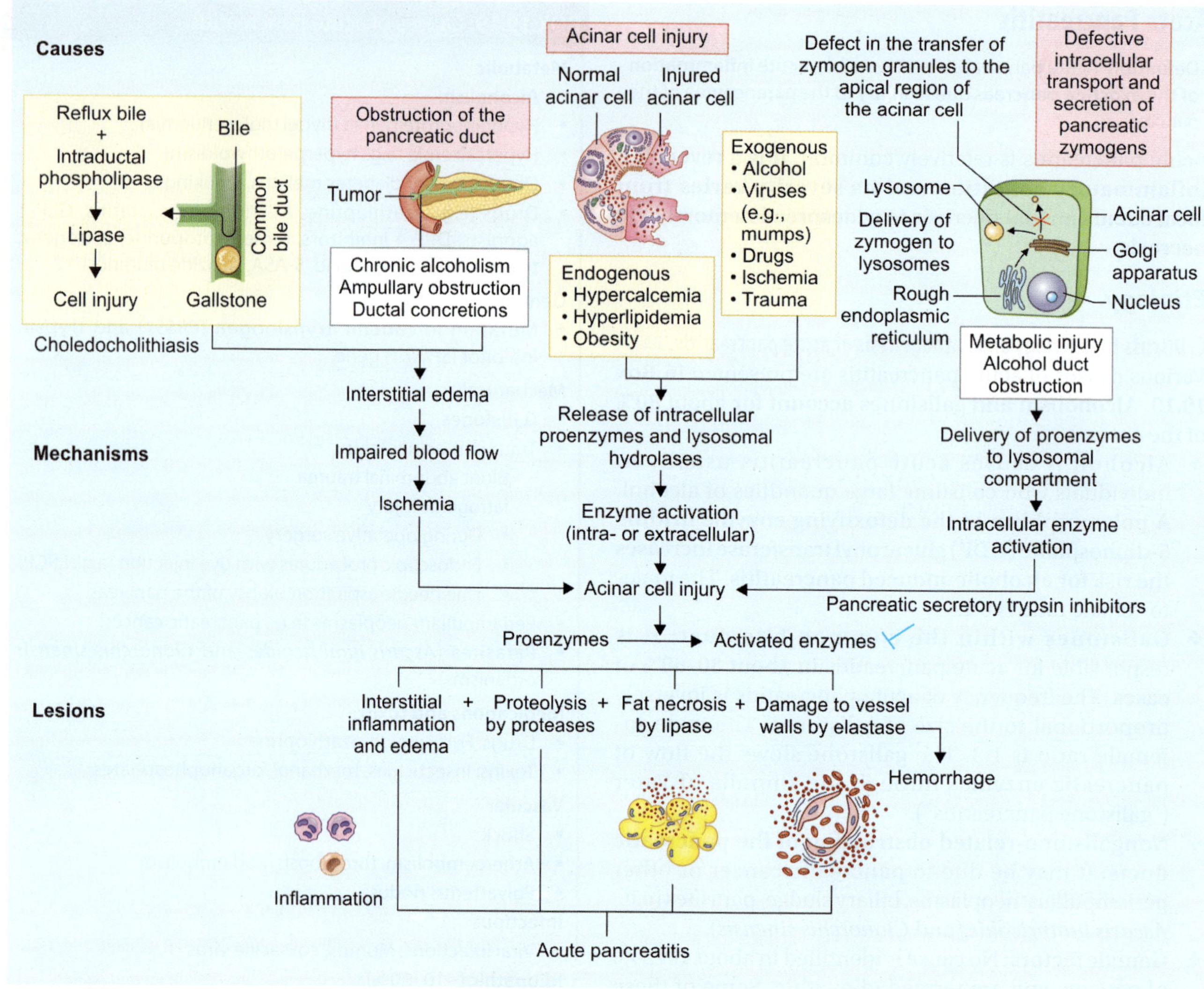

Fig. 19.42: Pathogenesis of acute pancreatitis.

release and activation (premature activation means activation before their secretion from the acinar cells) **of pancreatic enzymes. These enzymes destroy pancreatic tissue and bring out an acute inflammatory reaction.**

- **Inappropriate activation of trypsin:** One of the pancreatic **proenzyme trypsinogen is prematurely activated to trypsin.** It is an **important triggering event** in the pathogenesis of **acute pancreatitis.**
- **Actions of trypsin:** Inappropriate activation of trypsin within the pancreas can activate other proenzymes. Trypsin can **convert many proenzymes into active forms** [e.g., proelastase to elastase (damages the elastic fibers of blood vessels) and prophospholipase A2 to phospholipase (degrades fat cells)]. So, **trypsin is central to the pathogenesis of acute pancreatitis.** Examples of **factors that activate trypsin** include endotoxins, exotoxins, viral infections, ischemia, and anoxia. Trypsin also can be spontaneously activated.

Activation of coagulation, complement, kinin, and fibrinolytic system: Once tissue damage starts, trypsin can also directly or indirectly activate factors found in the blood. These include the activation of components of the coagulation, complement, kallikrein, and fibrinolytic pathways. They produce inflammation and small-vessel thrombosis. They produce further damage to acinar cells and amplify intrapancreatic enzyme activation.

Major Initiating Events that Trigger Intrapancreatic Enzyme Activation in Sporadic Acute Pancreatitis

The exact mechanisms of activation of pancreatic enzymes are not well-understood. However, there is evidence that at least three major initiating events trigger intrapancreatic enzyme activation in sporadic acute pancreatitis:

1. **Pancreatic duct obstruction:** It is most commonly caused by **gallstones and biliary sludge.** But it may also be due to periampullary neoplasms (e.g., pancreatic cancer), choledochoceles (congenital cystic dilation

of the common bile duct), parasites (particularly *A. lumbricoides* and *C. sinensis*), and probably a congenital anomaly, namely pancreas divisum.

- **Rupture of ductules and acini: Pancreatic duct obstruction can raise upstream intrapancreatic ductal pressure,** exacerbate back diffusion across the ducts, and lead to the **rupture of ductules and acini.**
- **Accumulation of enzyme-rich fluid within the interstitium of the pancreas**: The **rupture of ductules and acini** leads to the accumulation of enzyme-rich fluid within the interstitium of the pancreas. **Inappropriate activation of digestive proenzymes** causes injury to initiate local inflammation and interstitial edema. Edema may decrease the local blood flow and cause vascular insufficiency and ischemic injury to acinar cells.

2. **Primary acinar cell injury:** Any injury to the acinar cell leads to the release of digestive enzymes, inflammation, and tissue autodigestion. A variety of endogenous, exogenous, and iatrogenic insults can damage acinar cells. Direct acinar cell injury may be caused by certain **viruses (e.g., mumps), drugs, alcohol,** hypertriglyceridemia, **and direct trauma** to the pancreas. Injury may also follow ischemia or shock. Many of these factors that damage acinar cells result in oxidative stress and the production of intracellular free radicals. Cellular injury **initiates the inflammatory process** and leads to pancreatic edema, hemorrhage, and necrosis.

   Increased calcium flux: It is another essential trigger that can cause inappropriate activation of the pancreatic enzyme. Calcium plays a crucial role in trypsin regulation. When calcium levels are low, trypsin tends to cleave and inactivate itself, called autoinhibition. But when calcium levels are increased, this autoinhibition is lost, and trypsin gets autoactivated. Any factor that increases calcium within acinar cells may lead to excessive trypsin activation. Examples include inherited abnormalities that affect calcium levels. Mechanisms by which hypercalcemia can cause acute pancreatitis include excessive activation of trypsin, secretory block, intracellular zymogen accumulation, and activation of proteases.
3. **Defective intracellular transport of proenzymes within acinar cells:** The pancreatic acinar cell is highly compartmentalized to produce and process pancreatic enzymes. In normal pancreatic acinar cells, digestive enzymes and lysosomal hydrolases are transported through separate pathways. However, pancreatic proenzymes and lysosomal hydrolases become packaged together in some animal models of metabolic injury. This activates proenzyme and leads to the rupture of lysosomes (by the action of phospholipases). Thus, activated enzymes are locally released. Probably similar events may occur in human acute pancreatitis.

Mechanism of Alcohol-induced Pancreatitis

Several mechanisms contribute to alcohol-induced pancreatitis.

- **Transient increase of pancreatic exocrine secretion with obstruction of small pancreatic ductules and ducts**: Alcohol is a pancreatic secretagogue (promotes secretion) and increases pancreatic exocrine secretion. Chronic ingestion of alcohol results in the hypersecretion of protein-rich pancreatic fluid by acinar cells without increased fluid. This abnormal secretion can precipitate to form **inspissated "protein plugs"** in small pancreatic ducts. These deposits obstruct small pancreatic ductules and ducts. They lead to acute pancreatitis similar to duct obstruction described above.
- **Abnormal spasm of the sphincter of Oddi:** Alcohol consumption transiently increases and causes **contraction of the sphincter of Oddi** (the muscle at the ampulla of Vater that regulates the flow of pancreatic secretions through the papilla of Vater) and may cause pancreatitis.
- **Direct toxic effects on acinar cells:** Alcohol-induced oxidative stress may produce free radicals within acinar cells. This causes lipid oxidation of the acinar cell membrane and also activation of the proinflammatory transcription factors. The transcription factors induce the expression of chemokines that attract mononuclear cells.
- **Delivery of proenzymes to a lysosomal compartment with intracellular activation of trypsin and other digestive enzymes**: Oxidative stress may also promote the fusion of lysosomes and zymogen granules. This, in turn, increases intracellular calcium levels, probably by damaging the mitochondria. Raised intracellular calcium promotes the intracellular activation of trypsin and other digestive enzymes.
- **Increased amounts of proteases in pancreatic secretions** are found in alcoholic patients. However, most alcoholics never develop pancreatitis. In alcoholics, pancreatitis usually develops after many years of alcohol abuse. Thus, the main pathophysiology of alcohol-induced pancreatitis is not known.

MORPHOLOGY

Q. Write a short note on the morphology of acute pancreatitis.

The changes in the pancreas in acute pancreatitis depend on the duration and severity of the process.

Basic changes in acute pancreatitis: These include the following:

1. Microvascular leak and edema
2. Fat necrosis (by lipases)
3. Acute inflammatory reaction (neutrophils)

4. **Proteolytic destruction of pancreatic parenchyma (proteases) and blood vessels (elastases) leading to interstitial hemorrhage.**

The extent of each of these changes depends on the duration and severity of acute pancreatitis.

Morphologic classification of acute pancreatitis: It is classified into 3 types, namely—**(i) interstitial/edematous, (ii) necrotizing, and (iii) hemorrhagic.**

Acute Interstitial or Edematous Pancreatitis

A more limited form of acute interstitial pancreatitis is a **mild and reversible** process. The pancreas is swollen and edematous. The blood supply to the pancreas is maintained.

Microscopy: It shows **interstitial edema** and **mild infiltration** by **polymorphonuclear leukocytes. Necrosis or hemorrhage is not seen**). Enzymatic destruction of fat cells by lipase produces fat necrosis. The released fatty acids combine with calcium to form insoluble salts.

Acute Necrotizing Pancreatitis

Gross

Pancreas

- It is **enlarged** and **swollen** and shows red-black **areas of hemorrhage** with foci of yellow-white, chalky **fat necrosis** (*refer* page 20 and **Fig. 2.9**). Fat necrosis is due to the action of lipase on triglycerides, which release fatty acids from the fat cells.
- The **fatty acids combine with calcium to form insoluble salts** (calcium soaps). This process of soap formation is known as **saponification.** The calcification **may reduce the level of blood calcium**, sometimes to such an extent as causing neuromuscular irritability.

Extrapancreatic lesions

- **Foci of fat necrosis** (*refer* **Fig. 2.9**): It may also be seen in **extrapancreatic fat** (omentum and the mesentery of the bowel) and outside the abdominal cavity (subcutaneous fat).
- **Fluid:** The **peripancreatic tissue or peritoneal cavity** may contain a **serous, slightly turbid, brown-tinged fluid.**
- This fluid may show necrotic fat globules, which are produced by the action of enzymes on adipose tissue. The necrotic tissue appears **"putty-like,"** and is similar to **"canned dog food"**.

Microscopy (Fig. 19.43A and B)

The damage in acute necrotizing pancreatitis also involves acinar and ductal cells, the islets of Langerhans, and blood vessels. Microscopic findings are as follows:

- Edema of interstitial tissue: It is due to leakage of fluid from the microvasculature.
- **Acute inflammation:** Seen in the interstitial tissue.
- **Enzymatic fat necrosis** (*refer* **Fig. 2.9**): It appears as **granular blue with ghost outlines of the necrotic cells.**
- **Destruction of the parenchyma of the pancreas:** Acinar and ductal tissues as well as the islets of Langerhans are necrotic **due to proteolytic digestion.**
- **Destruction of blood vessels:** The **activated elastase** destroys blood vessels and **leads to interstitial hemorrhage.**

Acute Hemorrhagic Pancreatitis

Q. Write a short note on acute hemorrhagic pancreatitis.

It usually develops in **middle age** (peak incidence at 60 years) and is associated with **high morbidity and mortality.**

Gross (Fig. 19.44A): It shows extensive necrosis, hemorrhage, and fat necrosis within the **pancreatic parenchyma.** In severe cases, marked hemorrhage may convert the pancreas into a large retroperitoneal hematoma.

Microscopy (Fig. 19.44B): It shows extensive necrosis of pancreatic parenchyma, accompanied by **intraparenchymal hemorrhage** due to vascular injury. Necrosis is usually patchy and rarely involves the entire gland. The pancreatic necrotic foci can undergo secondary infection, termed **infected pancreatic necrosis. Fat necrosis** appears as chalky white plaques and nodules. It is observed within the **pancreatic parenchyma.** The pancreas appears red–black colored with interspersed foci of yellow–white, chalky fat necrosis. In severe cases, marked hemorrhage may convert the pancreas into a large retroperitoneal hematoma with barely recognizable pancreatic tissue.

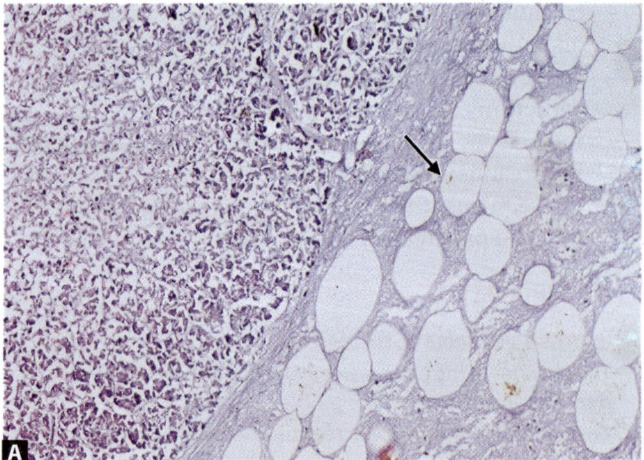

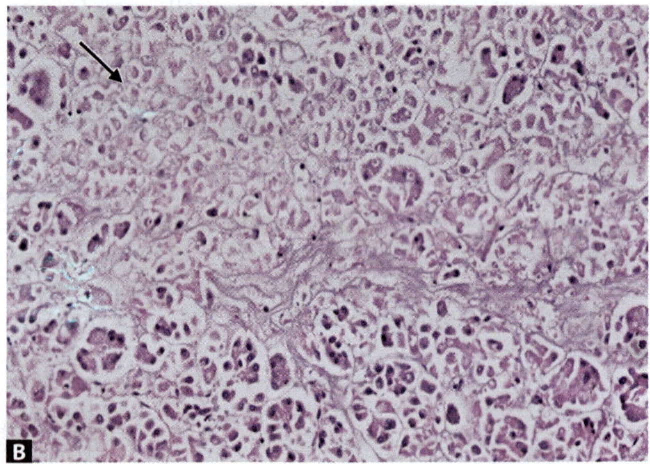

Figs. 19.43A and B: Acute necrotizing pancreatitis: (A) The pancreas shows acinar necrosis and enzymatic fat necrosis in the right half. Fat necrosis appears granular blue with ghost outlines of the necrotic cells (arrow); (B) Pancreas showing foci of necrosis (arrow) and pancreatic acini.

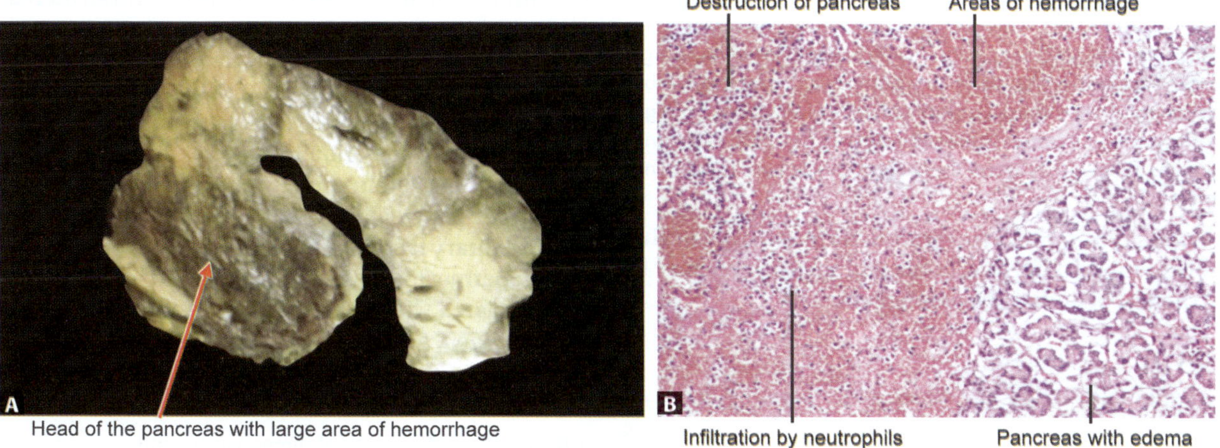

Figs. 19.44A and B: Acute hemorrhagic pancreatitis: (A) The longitudinal section of the pancreas shows dark areas of hemorrhage in the head of the pancreas (left); (B) Microscopic appearance of acute hemorrhagic pancreatitis. Histology shows numerous neutrophils, hemorrhage, and destruction of parenchyma (left side) and pancreas with edema (right side).

Clinical Features

Abdominal pain: Patients present with severe abdominal pain, which is the cardinal manifestation of acute pancreatitis. Characteristically, the pain is constant and intense in the **epigastric region**. It is referred to as the **upper or mid back** and, occasionally, the left shoulder. The severity ranges from mild discomfort to incapacitating severe pain. Severe acute pancreatitis is an acute abdominal medical emergency. Patients usually present with acute abdomen and systemic findings.

Other symptoms: These include anorexia, nausea, and vomiting.

Laboratory Findings

- **Leukocytosis:** It is usually found in moderate to severe acute pancreatitis.
- **Serum amylase:** It is markedly elevated during the **first 24 hours**. Amylase can be elevated in other conditions (e.g., peptic ulcer disease, mesenteric ischemia, salpingitis).
- **Serum lipase:** It is raised **within 72–96 hours** and follows elevated amylase. A three-fold or higher elevation of amylase and lipase levels confirms the diagnosis. Lipase is a more specific/diagnostic marker and lasts longer (**remain elevated for 8–14 days**).
- **C-reactive protein level >130 mg/mL** indicates severe pancreatitis.
- **Glycosuria:** It occurs in 10% of cases.
- **Hypocalcemia:** It is **due to precipitation** of calcium soaps in necrotic fat. Persistent hypocalcemia is a poor prognostic sign.

Direct visualization of the pancreas: By radiography. **Computed tomography (CT) scanning or** magnetic resonance imaging (MRI): Enlarged, inflamed pancreas can be directly visualized. It is helpful in the diagnosis of pancreatitis.

Complications of Acute Pancreatitis (Table 19.7)

Q. Write a short note on complications of acute pancreatitis.

TABLE 19.7 Complications of acute pancreatitis.

Local complications	*Systemic complications*
• Pancreatic and peripancreatic necrosis (sterile or infected), sterile pancreatic abscess • Pancreatic pseudocyst (occurs after 3–5 weeks) • Infection by gram-negative organisms from the alimentary tract • Splenic and portal vein thrombosis	• Systemic inflammatory response syndrome (SIRS) due to increased vascular permeability from a cytokine, platelet aggregating factor, and kinin release • Shock with acute renal tubular necrosis during the first week • Acute respiratory distress syndrome • Acute renal failure • Hemolysis • Disseminated intravascular coagulation (DIC) • Diffuse fat necrosis • Hypocalcemia due to the sequestration of calcium in fat necrosis, fall in ionized calcium

Chronic Pancreatitis

Definition: Chronic pancreatitis is a **chronic (long-standing) fibroinflammatory state of the pancreas** characterized by **permanent and progressive morphologic or functional damage to the pancreas.** It causes **irreversible destruction of the exocrine pancreas, followed by loss of the islets of Langerhans (endocrine pancreas).**

The pancreas shows **irreversible damage of exocrine parenchyma and fibrosis.** In the **late stages**, there may be **destruction of endocrine parenchyma**.

Etiology

Most etiologic factors that cause acute pancreatitis (*refer* **Box 19.19**) also cause chronic pancreatitis. This may evolve from repeated episodes of acute pancreatitis with scarring. However, in about 50% of patients, there is no history of acute pancreatitis.

Chronic excessive alcohol consumption: It is the **most common (about 70%) cause** and usually develops in middle-aged males.

Less common causes: These include the following:

- **Long-standing obstruction of the pancreatic duct:** By pseudocysts, calculi, trauma, or carcinoma.
- **Autoimmune injury to the pancreas**: Causes autoimmune pancreatitis (AIP). Autoimmune pancreatitis is one feature of IgG4-related disease that may involve multiple tissues.
- **Chronic injury to acinar cells:** For example, **hemochromatosis is associated with pancreatic fibrosis and atrophy.**
- **Chronic renal failure:** It is associated with an **increased incidence of acute and chronic pancreatitis.**
- ***CFTR* gene mutations: Cystic fibrosis** is caused by inherited mutations in the cystic fibrosis transmembrane conductance regulator (*CFTR*) gene. This **decreases bicarbonate secretion by pancreatic ductal cells** and **promotes protein plugging** and the development of chronic pancreatitis.
- **Hereditary factors**
- **Idiopathic:** It constitutes about 20% of cases. It may be associated with germline mutations in *CFTR*, *PRRS1*, and *SPINK1* genes.

Pathogenesis (Fig. 19.45)

Q. Discuss the pathogenesis of chronic pancreatitis.

The pathogenesis of chronic pancreatitis is not clear. **Repeated attacks of acute pancreatitis may lead to chronic pancreatitis. Different theories** have been suggested and it is unlikely that all cases of chronic pancreatitis can be explained by a single theory.

Oxidative stress: The pancreas is exposed to "oxidative stress" through systemic circulation or the reflux of bile into the pancreatic duct. Oxidative stress generates **free radicals** in acinar cells with the following consequences:

- Leads to membrane lipid oxidation and acinar cell necrosis
- Recurrent inflammation, tissue damage and fibrosis, and the fusion of lysosomes and proenzymes
- **Alcohol abuse** is one of the etiological factors that induces oxidative stress.

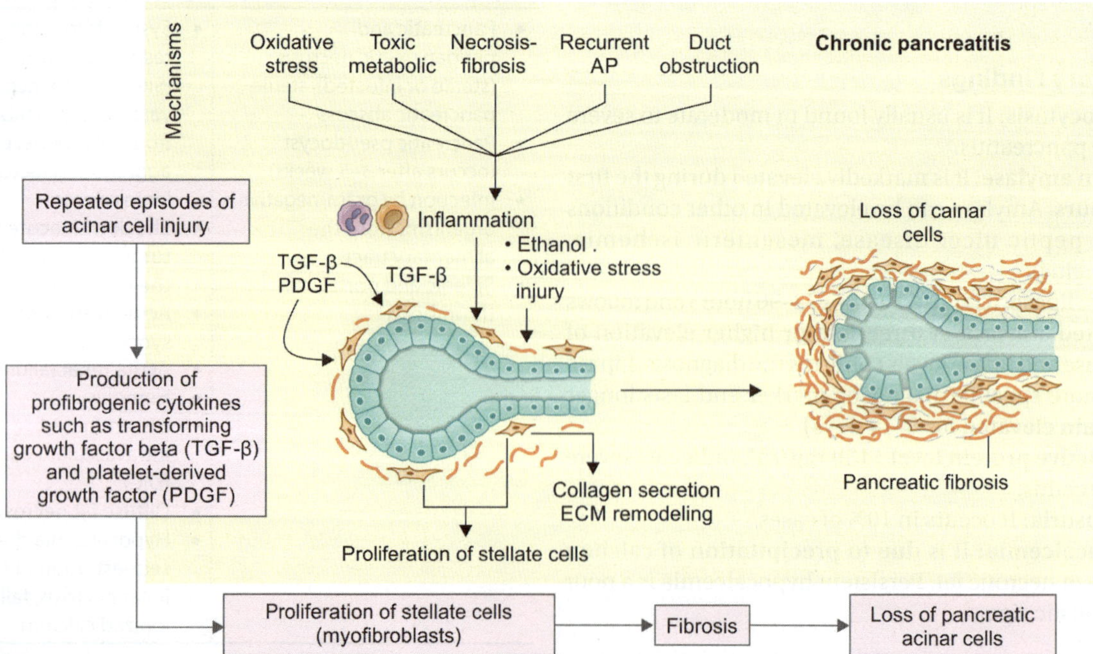

Fig. 19.45: Pathogenesis of chronic pancreatitis. In chronic pancreatitis, repeated episodes of acinar cell injury produce profibrogenic cytokines such as transforming growth factor beta (TGF-β) and platelet-derived growth factor (PDGF). This causes the proliferation of stellate cells (myofibroblasts) and produces fibrosis. It is followed by the loss of pancreatic acinar cells.

Toxic–metabolic: Toxins such as alcohol and its metabolites can cause direct toxic damage to acinar cells. This **produces necrosis of cells and, eventually, fibrosis.**

Necrosis–fibrosis: The inflammation and scarring may result from **bouts of acute pancreatitis.** This causes **obstruction and stasis within the ducts and forms stones in the duct.**

Recurrent acute pancreatitis: Chronic pancreatitis may develop following repeated attacks of acute pancreatitis. In acute pancreatitis, acinar injury releases digestive enzymes. This leads to a cascade of events. These events include activation of the clotting cascade, acute and chronic inflammation, vascular injury, and edema. In most patients with acute pancreatitis, there is complete resolution of the acute injury to the pancreas. This restores acinar cell mass **(Fig. 19.45).** Probably recurrent attacks of acute pancreatitis initiate a sequence of perilobular fibrosis, duct distortion, and altered secretions. Recurrent injury due to recurrent pancreatitis may lead to loss of exocrine parenchyma and fibrosis.

Duct obstruction: Some etiological agents cause **increased protein concentrations** and protein precipitation. This forms **ductal plugs** and calcification of ductal plugs to form calculi. This further **obstructs the pancreatic ducts.** Obstruction may develop in **alcoholic-induced chronic pancreatitis.**

Chronic injury to the pancreas due to any cause is associated with the **local production of inflammatory mediators.** These mediators **promote fibrosis and cause loss of acinar cells.** There is some overlap between the cytokines released during acute and chronic pancreatitis. However, in chronic pancreatitis, repeated episodes of acinar cell injury produce more profibrogenic cytokines than in acute pancreatitis. These **fibrogenic cytokines mainly include transforming growth factor beta (TGF-β) and platelet-derived growth factor (PDGF).** Fibrogenic factors activate and cause the **proliferation of pancreatic stellate cells** (periacinar myofibroblasts). This causes collagen synthesis, deposition, and extracellular matrix (ECM) remodeling, **leading to fibrosis (Fig. 19.45).** Repeated injury to the pancreas leads to irreversible loss of acinar cell mass, fibrosis, and (exocrine) pancreatic insufficiency.

MORPHOLOGY

Gross

Chronic pancreatitis can be subdivided into two major forms:

Nonobstructive Chronic Pancreatitis

It is by far the **most common form of chronic pancreatitis** (~95%) and about 80% of the patients are alcoholics.

- Pancreas is **nodular, hard,** and may be either enlarged or atrophic.
- **Cut section** may show **dilated ducts** and **calcified concretions.**
- **When the calcification is extensive,** it is termed **chronic calcifying pancreatitis.**

Obstructive Chronic Pancreatitis

It is the result of narrowing or occlusion of the pancreatic ducts. It is most **commonly due to carcinoma and stones** in the ductal system.

Microscopy

Chronic pancreatitis is characterized by:

- **Parenchymal fibrosis:** The pancreas shows large irregular areas of fibrosis (periductal, intralobular, and interlobular). It is a major feature.
- **Reduced number and size of acini:** Acinar loss is seen. The islets of Langerhans are relatively resistant to chronic pancreatitis in comparison with the pancreatic acini. However, as the disease progresses, they may be reduced or disappear.
- **Variable dilation of the pancreatic ducts:** The **interlobular and intralobular pancreatic ducts are frequently dilated** and their **lumen shows protein plugs.**
- **Alterations in the duct epithelium:** It shows **atrophy/hyperplasia/squamous metaplasia.**
- **Chronic inflammatory infiltrate:** Fibrotic areas show infiltration by **lymphocytes, plasma cells, and macrophages.**

Autoimmune pancreatitis

Microscopy: Infiltration of the pancreas by lymphocytes and plasma cells, many of which are positive for IgG4. It also shows a "swirling" fibrosis and venulitis **(lymphoplasmacytic sclerosing pancreatitis).**

Clinical Features

- **Repeated attacks of abdominal pain** or persistent abdominal and back pain.
- **Silent until severe functional damage** develops:
  - **Pancreatic exocrine insufficiency:** Characterized by **weight loss** and **hypoalbuminemic edema** due to chronic malabsorption.
  - **Pancreatic endocrine insufficiency: Diabetes mellitus** may develop.

Complications of chronic pancreatitis are listed in **Box 19.20.**

Prognosis: Long-term outlook is poor.

Pseudocyst of Pancreas (Figs. 19.46A and B)

Q. Write a short note on pancreatic pseudocyst.

- Pseudocysts constitute about 75% of cysts in the pancreas.
- Pseudocyst is **not a true cyst** and **does not have any epithelial lining.** It is intimately associated with the pancreatic tissues.
- **Causes:** Complication of **acute and chronic pancreatitis,** and **traumatic injury to the pancreas.**

BOX 19.20: Complications of chronic pancreatitis.

- Chronic abdominal pain
- Exocrine pancreatic insufficiency: Malabsorption, steatorrhea
- Secondary diabetes mellitus
- Pseudocyst
- Pancreatic cancer
- Biliary stricture and/or biliary cirrhosis
- Pancreatic duct stricture
- Splanchnic venous thrombosis
- Metabolic bone disease (osteoporosis)

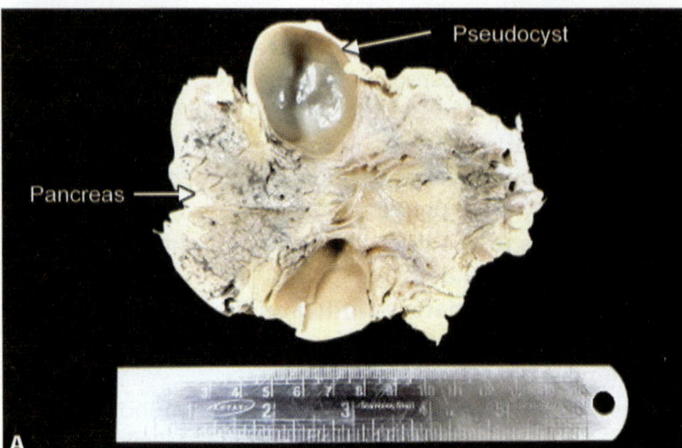

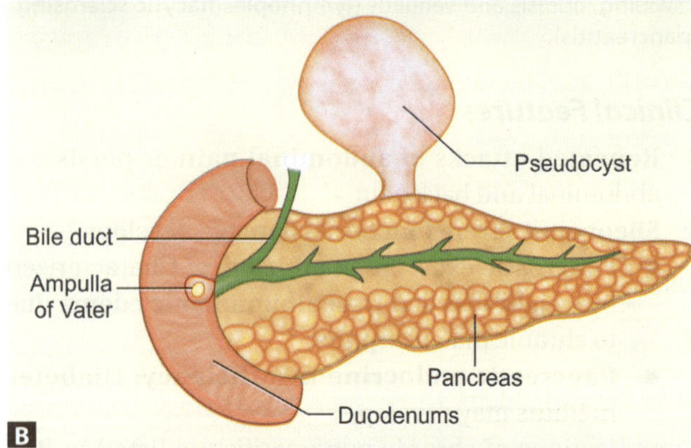

Figs. 19.46A and B: Pseudocyst of the pancreas.

MORPHOLOGY

Gross

- Number: It is usually **single**.
- Size: It ranges from 2 to 30 cm in diameter.
- Sites **(Figs. 19.46A and B)**: May be seen **within the substance of the pancreas**, or **more commonly in the lesser omental sac or the retroperitoneum** between the stomach and transverse colon or between the stomach and liver.
- Lumen: It contains **necrotic-hemorrhagic material rich in pancreatic enzymes** (amylase).

Microscopy

The wall of the pseudocysts shows nonepithelial-lined fibrous connective tissue and necrotic pancreatic debris.

Complications: The majority of pseudocysts resolve spontaneously.

- Pseudocyst may **enlarge and compress** or obstruct the duodenum or even perforate into **adjacent structures**.
- May be **secondarily infected and** form an **abscess**.
- Rarely **may rupture resulting in chemical or septic peritonitis** or both.

PANCREATIC CARCINOMA

PA 32.6 (NC): Describe the etiology, pathogenesis, manifestations, laboratory, morphologic features, complications, and metastases of pancreatic cancer.

Carcinoma of the pancreas may be **duct adenocarcinoma or acinar cell carcinoma. More than 85%** of pancreatic malignancies are **duct adenocarcinomas** (ductal adenocarcinoma).

Pancreatic Ductal Adenocarcinoma

The infiltrating duct adenocarcinoma of the pancreas is more commonly known as "**pancreatic cancer**." It is an invasive pancreatic epithelial neoplasm. It **shows glandular (ductal) differentiation** and usually demonstrates **luminal and/or intracellular mucin production**. It is one of the leading causes of cancer deaths. The 5-year survival rate is about 10%.

Age: It is usually found in **elderly patients** and about 80% of cases occur between the ages of **60 and 80 years**.

Etiology

Risk factors for pancreatic carcinoma are listed in **Box 19.21**.

Pathogenesis (Fig. 19.47)

Precursors to pancreatic cancer (pancreatic intraepithelial neoplasias): Pancreatic cancer develops as a result of inherited and acquired mutations in cancer-associated genes. Similar to the multistep progression of colon cancer, there is a progressive accumulation of genetic changes. It shows progression in the pancreas from non-neoplastic epithelium to well-defined noninvasive lesions in small ducts and ductules to invasive carcinoma. The precursor lesions are called "pancreatic intraepithelial neoplasias"

BOX 19.21: Risk factors for pancreatic carcinoma.

- Cigarette smoking and alcohol use
- Consumption of a diet rich in fats
- Chronic pancreatitis
- Diabetes mellitus
- Inherited genetic defects:
  - *BRCA2* mutations
  - Mutations in *CDKN2A (p16)*
  - Mutation in the *PALLD* gene.

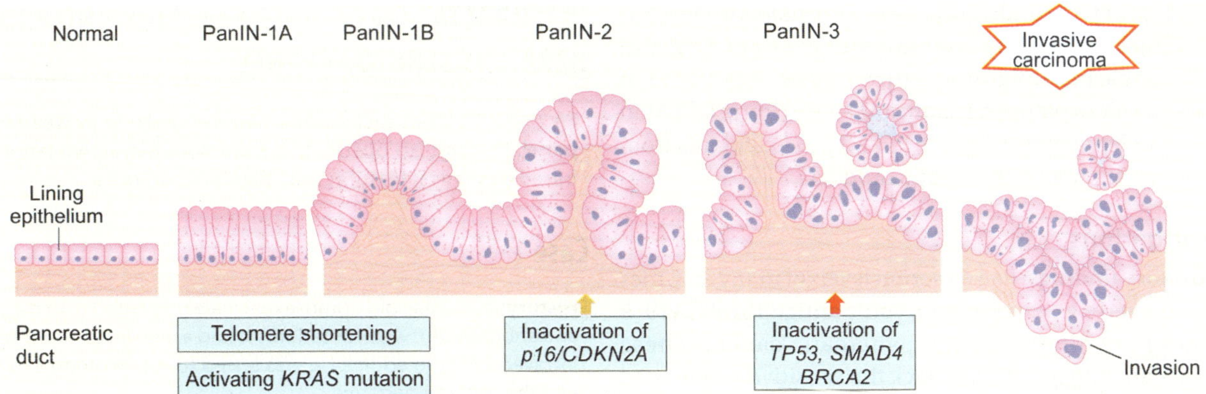

Fig. 19.47: Genetic progression of pancreatic carcinogenesis. The progression from normal epithelium to low-grade pancreatic intraepithelial neoplasia (PanIN) (PanIN1 and PanIN2), to high-grade PanIN3, to invasive carcinoma (left to right) is associated with the accumulation of specific genetic alterations. Telomere shortening and mutations of the oncogene *KRAS* occur at early stages. It is followed by the inactivation of the p16 (tumor suppressor gene) at intermediate stages, and the inactivation of the *TP53, SMAD4 (DPC4)*, and *BRCA2* tumor suppressor genes occur at late stages.

(PanINs). However, the majority of PanINs do not progress to frank malignancy. The epithelial cells in PanINs show **critical shortening of telomere length.** It predisposes these lesions to accumulate progressive chromosomal abnormalities and to develop invasive carcinoma.

Genetic Factors

Pancreatic cancer is a genetic disease. It is caused by inherited (germline) and somatic mutations along with epigenetic alterations. These mutations alter the expression of oncogenes and tumor suppressor genes. The four most common recurrent abnormalities in the pancreatic cancer genome are (1) oncogenic mutations of ***KRAS***, (2) ***CDKN2A/p16***, (3) ***SMAD4 (DPC4)***, and (4) loss-of-function mutations and/or deletions of tumor suppressor genes ***TP53.***

Activation of oncogene

Oncogenic mutations of *KRAS*: *KRAS* mutations are one of the earliest genetic alterations in the multistep progression of pancreatic cancer. Oncogenic activating point mutations of *KRAS* are most frequent in pancreatic cancer and are observed in >90% of pancreatic cancers. It results in constitutive **activation of the RAS signaling pathway** that increases autonomous cell growth and survival.

Inactivation of tumor suppressor gene

Inactivation of *CDKN2A*: *CDKN2A* is a tumor suppressor gene. This is inactivated **in 30–40% of pancreatic cancers.** *CDKN2A* complex locus encodes two tumor suppressor proteins: p16/INK4a and ARF. The p16/INK4 is a cyclin-dependent kinase inhibitor that antagonizes cell cycle progression. ARF is a protein that augments the function of the p53 tumor suppressor protein.

Inactivation of *SMAD4 (DPC4)*: *SMAD4* is inactivated in 55% of pancreatic cancers. *SMAD4* encodes a tumor suppressor. It plays an important role in signal transduction from the TGFb family of cell surface receptors. SMAD4 is only rarely inactivated in other cancer types

Inactivation of *TP53*: The *TP53* gene is inactivated in 70–75% of pancreatic cancers by the loss of one allele coupled with an intragenic mutation in the second allele. *TP53* gene encodes the tumor suppressor p53. It is a nuclear DNA-binding protein. p53 can respond to DNA damage by arresting cell growth, inducing cell death (apoptosis), or causing cellular senescence. ***BRCA2*** is also mutated late in a few pancreatic cancers.

MORPHOLOGY

Location: About **60% in the head, 15% in the body,** and 5% in the tail; in about 20% of cancers diffusely involve the entire pancreas.

Gross: Pancreatic carcinomas usually appear as **hard, stellate, gray-white, poorly delineated, and firm masses.**

Microscopy (refer online Figs. 19.48A and B): Pancreatic ductal adenocarcinoma is graded microscopically into **well-differentiated, moderately differentiated, and poorly differentiated. The tumor cells form abortive tubular structures (Fig. 19.45) or cell clusters and show infiltration**. The malignant glands are poorly formed and are usually lined by pleomorphic cuboidal-to-columnar epithelial cells. **Dense stromal fibrosis (desmoplasia) accompanies tumor invasion.**

Clinical Features

Pancreatic cancers usually remain silent until they infiltrate into adjacent structures.

- **Pain:** It is usually the first and the **outstanding symptom.**
- **Obstructive jaundice:** It is associated **with carcinoma of the head** of the pancreas.
- **Advanced stage:** Symptoms include: Weight loss, anorexia, and generalized malaise and weakness.
- **Carcinomas of the body and tail of the pancreas: They remain silent in the initial period.**

- **Migratory thrombophlebitis (Trousseau sign):** It is **characterized by spontaneously appearing and disappearing (migratory) thrombosis**. It is found in about 10% of patients. It is attributable to the production of platelet-aggregating factors and procoagulants from the carcinoma or its necrotic products.

Investigations

Laboratory findings: Raised serum levels of many enzymes and antigens (e.g., **carcinoembryonic antigen and CA19–9 antigen**) are often found in pancreatic cancer. These markers are nonspecific and lack the sensitivity. However, they are useful in follow-up of a patient's response to treatment.

Imaging techniques: Many imaging techniques, such as endoscopic ultrasonography and computed tomography, are useful for the diagnosis, but are not useful as screening tests.

Spread

- **Local spread:** Pancreatic cancers usually show **perineural invasion**. They grow along nerves and invade into the retroperitoneum. They can directly spread into peripancreatic soft tissues, spleen, adrenals, vertebral column, transverse colon, and stomach. The most common carcinoma that may show perineural invasions is listed in **Box 19.22**.
- **Lymphatic spread:** Through lymphatics, it spreads to peripancreatic, gastric, mesenteric, omental, and portohepatic lymph nodes.
- **Blood spread:** It may spread to the liver, lungs, adrenal, and bones.

Prognosis: The **course is brief and progressive**.

BOX 19.22: Most common carcinoma that may show perineural invasions.

Perineural invasion:

1. Pancreatic cancer
2. Prostatic cancer
3. Adenoid cystic carcinoma
4. Carcinoma of gallbladder
5. Cholangiocarcinoma

Trousseau's syndrome/migrating thrombophlebitis: Spontaneously appearing and disappearing (migratory) thrombosis.

Associated malignancies are:

1. The most common is carcinoma of the pancreas
2. Carcinoma of the lung
3. GI tract malignancies
4. Prostatic cancer
5. Ovarian cancer
6. Lymphoma

INTERPRETATION OF LIVER FUNCTION AND VIRAL HEPATITIS SEROLOGY PANEL

PA 25.6 (CC): Interpret liver function and viral hepatitis serology panel. Distinguish obstructive from nonobstructive jaundice based on clinical features and liver function tests.

Case 1

History: A 28-year-old homosexual male presented with malaise and anorexia of 1-week duration. He had a mild fever. He is not an intravenous drug addict. He was tested for HIV 6 months earlier and the test was negative.

Examination: He has a mild temperature (38.6°C) and with mild jaundice.

Investigations:

Liver function tests

Test	*Results*	*Normal range*
Serum aspartate aminotransferase	250 IU/L	12–38 U/L
Serum alanine aminotransferase	300 IU/L	7–41 U/L
Total bilirubin	6 mg/dL	0.3–1.3 mg/dL
Direct (conjugated)	4.5 mg/dL	0.1–0.4 mg/dL
Indirect (unconjugated)	1.5 mg/dL	0.2–0.9 mg/dL
Alkaline phosphatase	106 IU/L	33–96 U/L
Proteins—total	7.0 g/dL	6.7–8.6 g/dL
Albumin	5.0/g/dL	3.5–5.5 g/dL
Globulins	2.0 g/dL	2.0–3.5 g/dL
Albumin/globulin ratio	2.5:1	1.5-3: 1
Prothrombin time (PT) (Quick's one stage method)	17 seconds	11–16 seconds

Other tests

Urine	
Bile pigments	++
Bile salts	+
Urobilinogen	+ (traces)
Feces	Normal colored

HIV test: Negative

Total WBC count: 11,500/μL (4,000–11,000/μL)

Questions

1. What is the probable diagnosis?
2. Interpret the liver function test.
3. What further investigations will help in arriving at the diagnosis?

Answers

1. The probable diagnosis is **hepatocellular jaundice** due to **acute viral hepatitis.**
2. The liver function test is abnormal with a marked rise in the alanine aminotransaminases (high AST/ALT indicates hepatocyte damage) and moderately elevated bilirubin. A normal or mild increase of serum alkaline phosphatase indicates that there is no biliary obstruction. This indicates a hepatocellular jaundice rather than an obstructive jaundice. The raised total WBC count suggests acute viral hepatitis. Acute viral hepatitis may be caused by A, B, or C. Since, this patient is a homosexual (a risk factor) probably it may be either hepatitis B or C.
3. Serological tests can be used to know whether there are immunoglobulin M (IgM) antibodies indicating acute infection with hepatitis B or hepatitis C viruses, to confirm the diagnosis. This patient has an acute hepatitis B infection. Other serological markers to be performed.

Case 2

History: A 55-year-old woman complained of intermittent dull central epigastric pain of 2-month duration. The pain was not radiating and there was no relationship of pain to eating. Her appetite was normal and there was no history of nausea, vomiting, or loss of weight. Her bowel habits were normal. Investigations showed normal blood count, urea, creatinine and electrolytes, and liver function tests. An H2 antagonist was prescribed and follow-up was advised.

She was slightly relieved of pain at first, but after 1 month, the pain became more frequent and severe. This time, the patient noticed that the pain was relieved by sitting forward and began to radiate through to the back. The patient's husband noticed that her eyes had become slightly yellow. A few days later, she noticed that her urine had become dark and her stools pale. She also complains of itching.

Examination: Her sclerae was yellow with a slight yellow tinge to the skin. There were scratch marks on the skin and there were no other significant findings.

Investigations: Routine hematological investigations were normal.

Liver function tests

Test	Results	Normal range
Serum aspartate aminotransferase	80 IU/L	12–38 U/L
Serum alanine aminotransferase	90 IU/L	7–41 U/L
Total bilirubin	12 mg/dL	0.3–1.3 mg/dL
Direct (conjugated)	10.0 mg/dL	0.1–0.4 mg/dL
Indirect (unconjugated)	2.0 mg/dL	0.2–0.9 mg/dL
Alkaline phosphatase	162 IU/L	33–96 U/L
Proteins—total	6.6 g/dL	6.7–8.6 g/dL
• Albumin	4.4/g/dL	3.5–5.5 g/dL
• Globulins	2.2 g/dL	2.0–3.5 g/dL
Albumin/globulin ratio	2:1	1.5–3: 1
Prothrombin time (PT) (Quick's one stage method)	25 seconds	11–16 seconds
• After parenteral Vitamin K administration	18 seconds	

Other Tests

Urine	
• Bile pigments	Present
• Bile salts	++
Feces	Clay-colored

Questions

1. What is the probable diagnosis?
2. What are other causes that can produce this type of change in liver function tests?
3. What further investigations should be performed?

Answers

1. Points favor a probable diagnosis of **obstructive jaundice**. Features that point to obstructive jaundice are markedly raised serum alkaline phosphatase (suggestive of biliary obstruction) and serum bilirubin, presence of dark urine (indicates a conjugated hyperbilirubinemia arising from biliary obstruction), and pale stools (because conjugated bilirubin is not entering the bowel because of obstruction). The conjugated bilirubin is water soluble and excreted in the urine. Prolonged prothrombin time is reduced after parenteral vitamin K indicates failure of absorption of vitamin K due to bile salt deficiency (bile salts are needed for the absorption of the fat-soluble vitamins A, D, E, and K) due to biliary obstruction. Retention of bile salts is responsible for itching. The objective is to define the site of obstruction and its cause. Carcinoma of the pancreas in its early stages can present with nonspecific symptoms. The pain has two characteristic features of carcinoma of the pancreas: relief by sitting forward and radiation to the back. Pancreatic **carcinoma** is an important cause of obstructive jaundice. An alternative diagnosis could be gallstones, but the pain is not typical.
2. Other causes of obstructive jaundice (*refer* **Fig. 19.2**).
3. Further investigations: These include an abdominal ultrasound, computed tomography (CT) scan, and magnetic resonance cholangiopancreatography (MRCP).

Case 3

History: A 62-year-old male is brought to the emergency department at 2 am for vomiting fresh red blood. He is continuing to vomit large amounts of blood. He has no associated abdominal pain. His stools have been dark black for the last 2 days. **On enquiry, he was a chronic alcoholic for the last 20 years.**

Examination: He is anemic and mildly jaundiced. There are spider nevi on his upper trunk and **gynecomastia**. **Abdominal palpation shows ascites** and the spleen is palpable at 4 cm below the costal margin (**splenomegaly**). His pulse rate is 72/min and the blood pressure is 90/60 mm Hg lying down, dropping to 76/48 on standing.

Liver function tests

Test	*Results*	*Normal range*
Serum aspartate aminotransferase	40 IU/L	12–38 U/L
Serum alanine aminotransferase	80 IU/L	7–41 U/L
Total bilirubin	2.1 mg/dL	0.3–1.3 mg/dL
Direct (conjugated)	0.9 mg/dL	0.1–0.4 mg/dL
Indirect (unconjugated)	1.2 mg/dL	0.2–0.9 mg/dL
Alkaline phosphatase	344 IU/L	33–96 U/L
Proteins—total	5.6 g/dL	6.7–8.6 g/dL
Albumin	1.6/g/dL	3.5–5.5 g/dL
Globulins	4.0 g/dL	2.0–3.5 g/dL
Albumin/globulin ratio	1:2.5	1.5–3: 1
Prothrombin time (PT) (Quick's one stage method)	22 seconds	11–16 seconds
Gamma-glutamyl transpeptidase	467 IU/L	9–58 IU/L

Questions

1. What is the likely diagnosis?
2. Give reasons.
3. What are the complications of this condition?

Answers

1. The most likely diagnosis is a variceal bleed due to underlying chronic liver disease secondary to alcohol.
2. The patient has signs of chronic liver disease and his liver function tests are consistent with this. The synthetic function of the liver is markedly reduced. This is reflected in the reduction of serum proteins, reversal of albumin globulin ratio (1:2.5), and prolonged prothrombin time. Raised gamma-glutamyl transpeptidase is a good guide to alcohol intake of more than 60 g alcohol/day.
3. Complications of cirrhosis [**Ans:** These include portal hypertension or liver dysfunction (or both). They are discussed on pages 675-8].

Case 4

A 24-year-old woman presents with a history of fever, malaise, and brown-colored urine of a 2-week duration. Physical examination shows jaundice, mild hepatomegaly, and tenderness in the right upper quadrant. The serum bilirubin is 8.2 mg/dL, with 60% in the conjugated form. AST and ALT levels in the serum are markedly elevated (380 and 378 U/L, respectively). Serum albumin level is normal. Serum IgM antihepatitis A virus (anti-HAV) is positive and also IgG antihepatitis B surface antigen (anti-HBsAg) antibodies are positive. Antihepatitis C virus antibodies are negative. The most likely diagnosis is:

A. Acute viral hepatitis A
B. Acute viral hepatitis B
C. Chronic viral hepatitis B
D. Acute viral hepatitis C

The answer is A: Acute viral hepatitis A. HAV is transmitted by the fecal-oral route. Hepatitis A does not progress to chronic hepatitis and does not have a carrier state. IgM anti-HAV indicates an acute infection by HAV. The presence of serum IgG anti-HBsAg indicates prior exposure to the hepatitis B virus but does not favor active disease (choice B). Individuals with chronic hepatitis B (choice C) do not have detectable anti-HBsAg in their serum. Acute viral hepatitis C (choice C) is ruled out because of the negative serology.

Case 5

A 30-year-old man presents with a history of fatigue and recurrent fever for the last 9-month. He noticed yellow skin and sclerae, and dark urine. Physical examination reveals jaundice, abdominal tenderness, and mild hepatomegaly. Laboratory studies reveal elevated serum bilirubin (3.4 mg/dL), decreased serum albumin (2.5 g/dL), and prolonged prothrombin time (17 seconds). Serologic tests show positive HBsAg and HBeAg; and antibodies to hepatitis B core antigen (IgG anti HBcAg). Serum anti-HCV negative. The most likely diagnosis is:

A. Acute hepatitis B
B. Chronic hepatitis B
C. Acute hepatitis C
D. Acute hepatitis E

The answer is B: Chronic hepatitis B. Chronic hepatitis B is an infection with the hepatitis B virus (HBV) and shows necrosis and inflammation in the liver for more than 6 months. Most patients with HBV infection recover completely from acute infection, but some develop chronic infection. Surface antigen (HBsAg) is present in the serum of patients with chronic hepatitis B. The presence of HBeAg is usually associated with the progression of the disease. Duration of disease for 9 months is against acute hepatitis B (choice A), C (choice C), and hepatitis E (choice D).

SCENARIO-BASED MCQ

1. **A 43-year-old obese woman complains of severe abdominal pain that radiates to the back. She is neither an alcoholic nor a drug addict. The blood pressure is 88/46 mm Hg, and the pulse is 100 per minute. Physical examination reveals abdominal tenderness, guarding, and rigidity. Laboratory examination shows elevated serum amylase (850 U/L) and lipase (675 U/L), and hypocalcemia (7.8 mg/dL). The most likely diagnosis is:**
   A. Acute cholecystitis
   B. Acute pancreatitis
   C. Alcoholic hepatitis
   D. Chronic calcifying pancreatitis

Answer and Explanation

1. **The answer is B: Acute pancreatitis.** The sudden onset of pain abdomen, accompanied by signs of shock (hypotension, and tachycardia) favors acute condition. The release of amylase and lipase from the injured pancreas into the serum provides a sensitive marker for the diagnosis of acute pancreatitis. Other choices do not feature increases in serum amylase and lipase.

Stellate cells (Ito cells):
- Store vitamin A
- Get transformed into collagen producing myofibroblasts during hepatic inflammation.

HBV: Microscopically, HBsAg is responsible for "ground glass" hepatocytes and HBcAg gives "sanded nuclei" appearance.

Most useful indicator of prior infection with HBV: Anti-HBcAg.

Amebic liver abscess: Anchovy paste (sauce) or chocolate colored pus.

Alcoholic-related liver disease:
1. Hepatic steatosis (fatty liver)
2. Steatohepatitis (formerly termed alcoholic hepatitis)
3. Fibrosis and alcohol-related cirrhosis

Most common cause of portal hypertension in adults: Cirrhosis

Microscopic features of cirrhosis:
1. Fibrosis
2. Regenerating nodules
3. Loss of architecture

Mallory bodies are tangled skeins of cytokeratin intermediate filaments (such as cytokeratin 8 and 18). Seen in:
- Alcoholic hepatitis
- Nonalcoholic fatty liver disease (NAFLD)
- Primary biliary cirrhosis (PBC)
- Wilson disease
- Chronic cholestatic syndromes
- Hepatocellular tumors

Tumors of liver:
- Most common benign tumor of the liver: Hemangioma.
- Most common primary malignant tumor of the liver: HCC
- Most common primary hepatic tumor of childhood.

Hepatoblastoma:
- Angiosarcoma of the liver is highly aggressive neoplasms, associated with exposure to vinyl chloride (plastic pipes), arsenic, or thorotrast
- Hepatocellular carcinoma: Most common symptom—abdominal pain > weight loss

- HCC: Tumor cells recapitulate varying degrees of normal liver architecture. Bile production by neoplastic cells is the hallmark.
- Strong tendency for invasion of vessels.

Four main macroscopic patterns of HCC:
1. Single distinct nodule (unifocal)
2. Large dominant nodule of HCC with multiple smaller satellite nodules (multifocal)
3. Many small nodules of HCC (dozens to hundreds) (diffusely infiltrative)
4. Multiple distinct nodules of HCC

Fibrolamellar type of HCC:
- Best prognosis
- Not associated with HBV/cirrhosis
- Normal AFP levels

AFP: Marker of choice for differentiating between hepatocellular cancer and its fibrolamellar variant.

Metastasis to the liver: Most common malignant tumors of the liver. Common primary include the GI tract, breast, lung, and pancreas.

Acute pancreatitis: An important triggering event is the premature activation of pancreatic proenzyme trypsinogen to trypsin.

Acute pancreatitis:
- Gallstones most common cause
- Alcohol abuse 2nd most common cause

Kidney and Urinary Tract Disorders

Chapter Outline

- Histology of the Kidney
- Glomerular Diseases
- Nephritic Syndrome
- Nephrotic Syndrome
- Glomerular Lesions Associated with Systemic Diseases
- Diseases Affecting Tubules and Interstitium
- Acute Kidney Injury
- Acute Tubular Injury
- Chronic Kidney Disease
- Vascular Diseases of the Kidney
- Horseshoe Kidneys
- Cystic Diseases of the Kidney
- Urolithiasis (Renal Calculi, Stones)
- Urinary Tract Obstruction (Obstructive Uropathy)
- Malignant Tumors of the Kidney
- Nephroblastoma (Wilms Tumor)
- Urothelial Tumors
- Common Urinary Abnormalities in a Clinical Specimen

HISTOLOGY OF THE KIDNEY

PA 28.1 (CC): Describe the normal histology of the kidney.

Nephron

The nephron is the microscopic structural unit of the kidney (Fig. 20.1). The nephron is a **tubular structure with five major subunits.** These **subunits include** (i) glomerulus, (ii) proximal convoluted tubule (PCT), (iii) loop of Henle, (iv) distal convoluted tubule (DCT), and (v) collecting ducts. The renal artery supplies each kidney with blood.

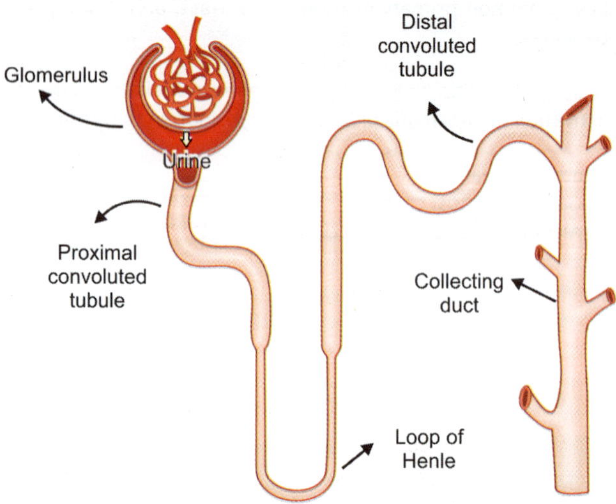

Fig. 20.1: Different components of nephron.

Main structural components of the kidney: The four main structural components of the kidney are (i) glomerulus, (ii) tubules, (iii) interstitium, and (iv) blood vessels.

Glomerulus

The glomerulus [**Figs. 20.2 and 20.3 (*refer* online Figs. 20.2A and 20.4)**] is a vascular structure and is the **basic filtering unit** of the kidney. It consists of a **tuft of an anastomosing network of capillaries** formed by branching of the afferent arteriole. **Each lobule of the glomerulus consists of a cluster of capillaries supported by the mesangium.**

Bowman capsule: The Bowman capsule is a **double-membrane chamber and is the enlarged portion of the proximal convoluted tubule** (PCT) of the kidney. **Bowman capsule has two layers of epithelial cells,** namely **an inner**

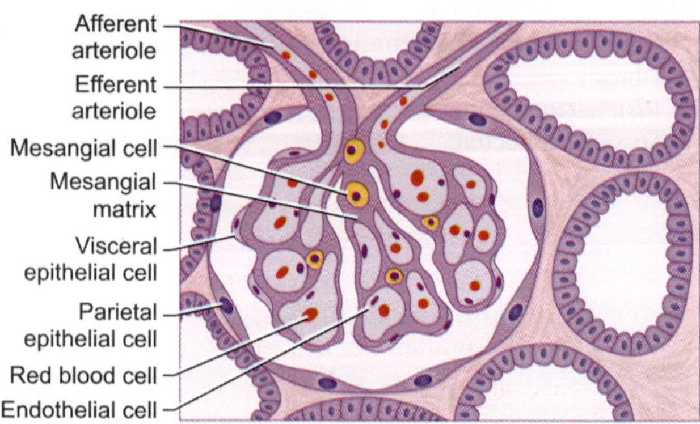

Fig. 20.2B: Diagrammatic. Light microscopic appearance of the glomerulus.

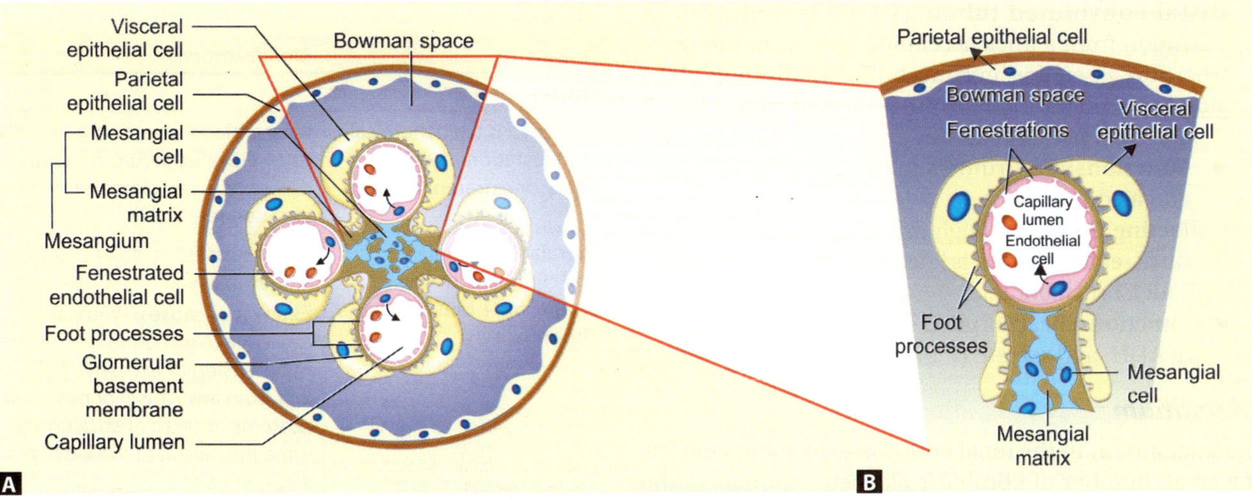

Figs. 20.3A and B: Diagrammatic representation of electron microscopic view of normal renal glomerulus: (A) Four glomeruli with a core of mesangium; (B) The relationship of the different cell types to the glomerular basement membrane and a mesangial matrix is illustrated using a single glomerular loop.

visceral layer and an outer parietal layer. Bowman space is the cavity **(space) between these two layers is called Bowman space.**

- **Visceral epithelium:** It is a specialized cell called podocytes. They have interdigitating foot processes embedded in the outer layer of the GBM. Adjacent foot processes are separated by 20- to 30-nm-wide gaps. These are bridged by a thin *slit diaphragm.* The visceral cells surround the tuft of capillaries of the glomerulus. It constitutes part of the capillary wall and covers the entire **outer surface of GBM.** The visceral epithelial cells line the glomerular side of Bowman space. These visceral epithelial cells are separated from the endothelial cells of capillaries by a basement membrane.
- **Parietal epithelium:** It surrounds Bowman space (urinary space) in which the plasma filtrate collects. The parietal epithelium is continuous with tubular epithelium.

Glomerular capillaries: The wall of the glomerular capillary is the filtering membrane. It consists of the following structures.

- **Fenestrated glomerular endothelial cells:** The capillaries are lined by **fenestrated (window-like openings) endothelium** lying on a **glomerular basement membrane** (GBM). The outer portions of the fenestrated endothelial cell are in contact with the inner surface of the GBM, whereas the central part is in contact with the mesangial cell and mesangial matrix.
- **Glomerular basement membrane (GBM):** It is the **main component of the filtration barrier**. It separates endothelial cells from the podocytes (visceral epithelial cells of the Bowman capsule) in the peripheral capillary walls, and it also separates podocytes from the mesangium. GBM has three ultrastructurally definable layers. The **central thick electron-dense layer is termed the lamina densa.** It is **bordered by two thinner** (narrow) **electron-lucent peripheral layers, namely the *lamina rara interna*** (inner electron-lucent zone) **and *lamina rara externa*** (outer electron-lucent zone). GBM consists of collagen (mostly type IV), laminin, polyanionic proteoglycans, fibronectin, and several other glycoproteins.

Mesangium: It **supports the entire glomerular tuft.** This mesangium **lies between the capillaries.** It consists of **mesangial cells** and a basement membrane-like **mesangial matrix.**

Tubules

The tubules constitute the greatest amount of the renal parenchyma. The structure of renal tubular epithelium varies in different parts of the nephron and is correlated with the functional capacity of that part of the tubule.

- **Proximal convoluted tubule (PCT):** It is the first part arising from the glomerulus. It is lined by cuboidal cells with a brush border composed of microvilli.
  - **Functions: Active reabsorption** of filtered sodium, potassium, glucose, amino acids, proteins, vitamins, bicarbonate, phosphate, calcium, and uric acid. **Passive reabsorption** of 80% of filtered water.
- **Loop of Henle:** The PCT drains into the straight part of the loop of Henle. It consists of thin descending, and thin and thick ascending limbs. The descending limb is a continuation of PCT and the ascending limb continues further into the distal convoluted tubule (DCT). The descending segment of the loop of Henle is lined by simple epithelium whereas the ascending limb is lined by columnar cells.
  - **Functions: Active reabsorption** of sodium, potassium, and chloride, and **passive diffusion** of water resulting in concentrated filtrate of urine.

- **Distal convoluted tubule (DCT):** It represents a transition from a thick ascending limb from the point where the ascending limb meets the vascular pole of the glomerulus of its origin, to the early collecting ducts. It is lined by cuboidal cells.
  - **Functions:** Contributes to urinary concentration and acidification.
- **Collecting ducts:** Through these ducts urine reaches the tip of renal papilla. It is lined by cuboidal epithelium without a brush border.
  - **Functions:** Reabsorption of water under the control of ADH, and secrete H^+ and K^+ ions.

Interstitium

The interstitium in the renal cortex is scanty and consists of a small number of fibroblast-like cells whereas in the medulla, it is more and contains stellate interstitial cells.

Blood Supply

Blood is supplied to each kidney by a main **renal artery** which arises from the aorta at the level of the 2nd lumbar vertebra. It usually divides into anterior and posterior divisions at the hilum. The anterior and posterior divisions divide into segmental branches from which interlobar arteries arise which course between the lobes.

Diseases of the kidney can be divided into four major groups depending on the basic morphologic components affected namely: glomerular diseases, tubules diseases, interstitial diseases, and diseases of blood vessels. Clinical manifestations of renal diseases are presented in **Table 20.1**.

Q. Write a short note on azotemia and uremia.

TABLE 20.1 Clinical manifestation of renal diseases.

Disease	*Manifestations*
Glomerular syndromes	
1. Nephritic syndrome (glomerular disease)	**Hematuria** (red blood cells in urine), diminished GFR, **mild to moderate proteinuria (with or without edema), azotemia**, renal failure, and **hypertension**
2. Rapidly progressive glomerulonephritis	Nephritic syndrome with a rapid decline in GFR (within hours to days)
3. Nephrotic syndrome (glomerular disease)	Heavy/massive proteinuria (more than 3.5 g/day), hypoalbuminemia, severe edema, hyperlipidemia, and lipiduria (lipid in the urine)
4. Chronic kidney disease (previously termed chronic renal failure)	Progressive renal failure (uremia)
5. Asymptomatic hematuria or proteinuria, or both	Usually due to mild glomerular abnormalities
Others	
Azotemia is a biochemical manifestation of kidney injury or extrarenal causes	Raised blood urea nitrogen (BUN) or an elevated serum creatinine due to reduced glomerular filtration rate (GFR)
Uremia is azotemia and clinical signs and symptoms + biochemical abnormalities	**Renal causes:** Acute or chronic kidney injury **Extrarenal causes:** Prerenal azotemia (e.g., due to hypotension or excessive fluid loss from any cause) or postrenal azotemia (due to obstruction to urine flow distal to the kidney)
Acute kidney injury	Abrupt onset of renal failure, oliguria/anuria. It may be due to glomerular, interstitial, vascular, or acute tubular injury
Urinary tract obstruction and renal tumors	Features depend on anatomic location and nature of the lesion
Urinary tract infection. It may affect the kidney (pyelonephritis) or the bladder (cystitis)	Bacteriuria and pyuria (bacteria and leukocytes in the urine) Infection may be symptomatic or asymptomatic
Nephrolithiasis (renal stones)	Spasms of severe pain (renal colic) and hematuria

GLOMERULAR DISEASES

PA 28.5 (CC): Define and classify glomerular diseases. Enumerate and describe the etiology, pathogenesis, mechanisms of glomerular injury, pathology, distinguishing features, and clinical manifestations of glomerulonephritis.

Q. Classify glomerulonephritis.

Glomerular diseases may be broadly divided into primary and secondary. The most common forms of glomerulonephritis are listed in **Box 20.1**.

- **Primary glomerulonephritis or glomerulopathy:** The kidney is the only or predominant organ involved.
- **Secondary glomerular diseases:** In these disorders, glomeruli are involved secondary to a systemic disease.

Clinical manifestations are grouped into the **five major glomerular syndromes (Table 20.1)**.

Pathologic Responses of Glomerulus to Injury

Various types of glomerular diseases are either **glomerulopathies (noninflammatory) or glomerulonephritis (inflammatory)**. These are characterized by one or more basic tissue reactions namely: (1) hypercellularity (increased cellularity), (2) basement membrane thickening, and (3) hyalinization or sclerosis.

Hypercellularity (increased cellularity): It is characterized by an **increase in the number of cells in the glomerular tufts.**

BOX 20.1: Common glomerular diseases.

PRIMARY GLOMERULONEPHRITIS/GLOMERULOPATHIES
- Acute proliferative glomerulonephritis: Postinfectious, others
- Rapidly progressive (crescentic) glomerulonephritis (RPGN)
- Minimal-change disease (MCD)
- Focal segmental glomerulosclerosis (FSGS)
- Membranous glomerulonephritis (MGN)
- Membranoproliferative glomerulonephritis (MPGN)
- C3 glomerulopathy
- Dense deposit disease
- C3 glomerulonephritis
- Immunoglobulin A (IgA) nephropathy
- Chronic glomerulonephritis

SYSTEMIC DISEASES WITH GLOMERULAR INVOLVEMENT
- Systemic immunological diseases (e.g., systemic lupus erythematosus)
- Metabolic diseases (e.g., diabetes mellitus)
- Vasculitis: Microscopic polyarteritis/polyangiitis, Wegener granulomatosis, Henoch–Schönlein purpura
- Amyloidosis
- Goodpasture syndrome
- Bacterial endocarditis

HEREDITARY DISORDERS
- Alport syndrome
- Thin basement membrane disease
- Fabry disease

Such a **lesion is called proliferative glomerulonephritis.** Hypercellularity may result from one or more of the following:
- **Proliferation of cells:** It may involve any of the cells of glomeruli (mesangial, endothelial, or epithelial cells).
- **Infiltration of leukocytes:** These include neutrophils, monocytes, and lymphocytes.
- **Crescent formation:** These are formed due to the **proliferation of parietal epithelial cells and infiltration by leukocytes** (*refer* **Fig. 20.10**). This develops **as a response to fibrin** that **leaks into the urinary space through ruptured basement membranes.**

Basement membrane thickening: It may be due to:
- **Deposition of amorphous electron-dense** (immune complexes) **material**: The deposits may be on the **endothelial or epithelial side of the** GBM **or within the GBM** itself.
- **Thickening of the basement membrane** (e.g., in **diabetic glomerulosclerosis**).

Hyalinosis and sclerosis: Its features are as follows:
- **Hyalinosis:** It is the **accumulation of homogeneous and eosinophilic material in the glomeruli** and **consists of plasma proteins** that have leaked from the circulation into glomerular structures. It is usually due to endothelial or capillary wall injury.

BOX 20.2: Terms used in glomerulopathies/glomerulonephritis.

- **Diffuse or generalized:** A lesion affecting/involving all of the glomeruli in the kidney
- **Global:** Involving the whole/entire individual glomeruli
- **Focal:** A lesion involving only a some/proportion of the glomeruli in the kidney but leaving others unaffected
- **Segmental:** Affecting a part/segment of each glomerulus
- **Capillary loop or mesangial:** Affecting predominantly capillary or mesangial regions.

- **Sclerosis:** It is characterized by **deposition of the extracellular collagenous matrix**, either in the **mesangium** (e.g., diabetic glomerulosclerosis) **or in the capillary loops, or both.**

The cause of the majority of the primary glomerulopathies is not known and they are classified by their microscopic features. Nomenclature of glomerular injury is used to describe the distribution/pattern of injury in glomeruli (**Box 20.2**).

Mechanism of Glomerular Injury and Disease (Fig. 20.5)

Q. Write a short essay on the pathogenesis of glomerulonephritis.

Various mechanisms involved in glomerular injury are presented in **Box 20.3. Immune mechanisms** are responsible for **most of the primary** glomerulopathy and **many of the secondary** glomerular disorders.

Antibody-Mediated Injury

Antibodies bind to the GBM by different mechanisms. Antibody-associated glomerular injury is of two forms:
1. Deposition of circulating antigen-antibody complexes:
2. **Glomerular injury by antibodies reacting in situ within the glomerulus:** The antibodies may bind **either to:**
   - **Insoluble fixed (intrinsic) glomerular antigens** or
   - **Extrinsic molecules (antigens) planted within the glomerulus**
3. Deposition of anti-glomerular basement membrane antibody

Consequences: The deposition of immune complexes or antibodies causes complement and/or Fc receptor-mediated inflammation and leukocyte activation. This results in injury to the glomerulus which is characteristic of nephritis (nephritic syndrome). In some cases, the antibodies or immune complexes impair the glomerular permeability to cause the nephrotic syndrome, even without overt inflammation.

Deposition of Circulating Immune Complexes

Q. Write a short essay on circulating immune complex glomerulonephritis.

A major cause of glomerulonephritis is the result of the deposition of preformed immune complexes.

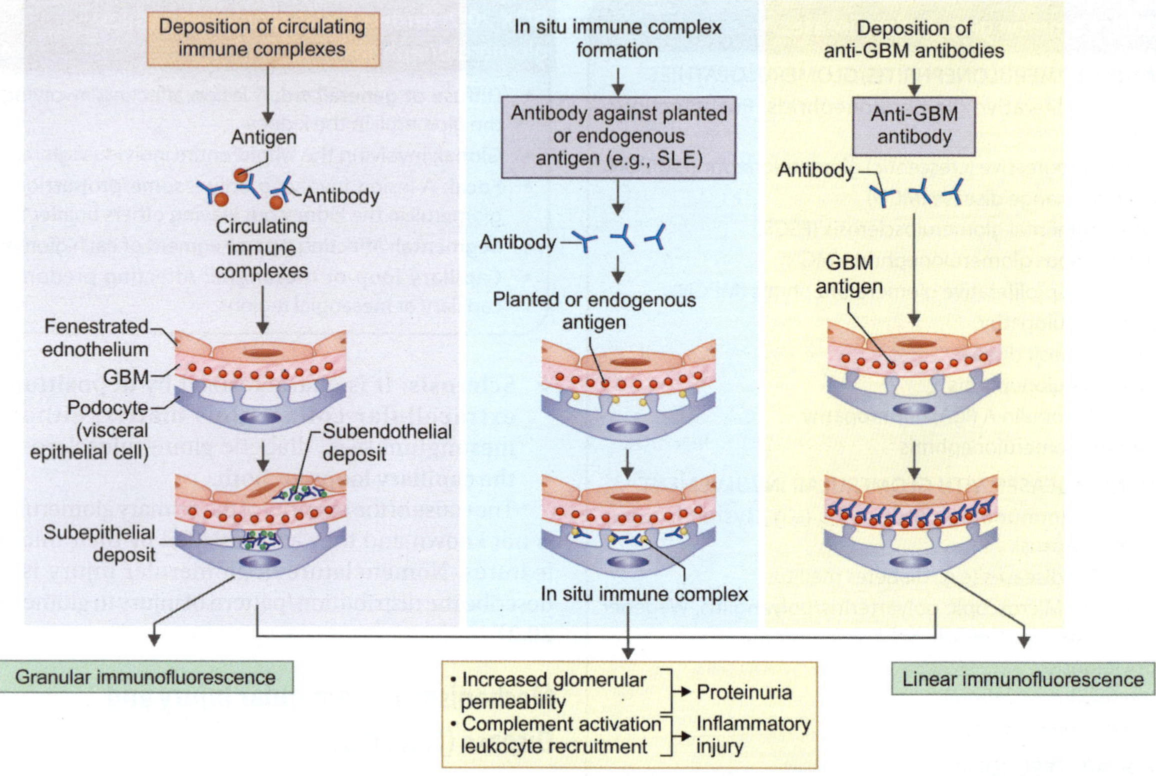

Fig. 20.5: Various immunological mechanisms of antibody-mediated glomerulonephritis. Glomerular injury can be either due to the deposition of circulating immune complexes or from antibody-binding to glomerular components followed by the formation of complexes in situ. Deposition of circulating immune complexes produces a granular immunofluorescence pattern. Anti-glomerular basement membrane (anti-GBM) antibody glomerulonephritis produces a linear immunofluorescence pattern and it is not accompanied by an immune deposit.

(GBM: glomerular basement membrane; SLE: systemic lupus erythematosus).

BOX 20.3: Various mechanisms involved in glomerular injury.

IMMUNE MECHANISM

1. **Antibody-mediated injury**

   Circulating immune complex deposition
   - Endogenous antigens (e.g., DNA, tumor antigens)
   - Exogenous antigens (e.g., infectious products.

   Formation of immune complex in situ
   - Intrinsic (endogenous) glomerular antigens (e.g., membranous glomerulopathy)
   - Planted antigens
     - Exogenous (e.g., infectious agents, drugs)
     - Endogenous (e.g., DNA, nuclear proteins)

   Deposition of anti-glomerular basement membrane antibody (e.g., anti-GBM nephritis)
2. **Cell-mediated immune injury**

NONIMMUNE GLOMERULAR INJURY

1. **Activation of the alternative complement pathway**
2. Direct injury

(GBM: glomerular basement membrane).

Origin of antigens*:* The source of the antigens that trigger the formation of circulating immune complexes may be endogenous or exogenous.

- **Endogenous origin,** e.g., glomerulonephritis associated with autoimmune diseases [e.g., systemic lupus erythematosus (SLE)] and IgA nephropathy. Some tumor antigens may cause immune complex-mediated nephritis.
- **Exogenous origin,** e.g., glomerulonephritis that follows certain infections. Exogenous microbial antigens include **bacterial products** (streptococcal proteins), **the surface antigen of the hepatitis B virus, hepatitis C virus antigens**, and antigens of *Treponema pallidum*, *Plasmodium falciparum*, and many viruses.
- **Unknown:** The inciting antigen is unknown in many cases.

Mechanisms of glomerular injury following immune complex formation: Antibodies are produced against the antigens. They form **antigen–antibody complexes** in the **circulation** which get **trapped in the glomeruli** and **produce injury**. The damage is through **type III hypersensitivity**. The injury is by local activation of toll-like receptors on glomerular cells, deposition of immune complexes, or activation of complement cascade.

Sites of immune complex deposits in glomeruli: Fluid from the blood passes through the GBM at high pressure (to produce urine). Since the GBM is a continuous barrier, it is a common site of deposition of circulating immune complexes. These circulating **antigen-antibody complexes are deposited** either on the **subendothelial or subepithelial side of GBM**. Subendothelial deposits are usually associated with more inflammation, possibly because of easier access to complement proteins and leukocytes from the blood. The subepithelial complexes usually produce proteinuria with little or no inflammation, probably because they interfere with the function of the slit diaphragm or epithelial cells.

Factors affecting the localization of antigens, antibodies, or immune complexes: Many factors are involved and the most important are the (i) molecular charge and (ii) size of these reactants.

- **Molecular charge**:
  - **Highly cationic antigens:** They can cross the GBM and the immune complexes get **localized in a subepithelial location.**
  - **Highly anionic macromolecules:** They cannot cross the GBM and are **trapped subendothelial** or are not nephritogenic at all.
  - **Molecules of neutral charge:** Immune complexes and molecules with neutral charge tend to **accumulate in the mesangium.**
- **Molecular size: Large circulating immune complexes are usually not nephritogenic**. This is because they are often cleared by the mononuclear phagocyte system. Thus, they do not enter the GBM in significant quantities. **Immune complexes** of **medium size** and with **slight antigen excess** are the **most pathogenic**.

Electron microscopy: It shows **electron-dense deposits**, presumably containing immune complexes. The immune complexes appear as electron-dense deposits of immunoglobulins and complement. They may lie in three different locations in the glomeruli **(Fig. 20.6)**. These include.

- **Subendothelial deposits** between the endothelial cells and the GBM.
- **Subepithelial deposits** between the outer surface of the GBM and the podocytes.
- **Mesangium** (mesangial deposits).

Deposits may be present in more than one site in a given case.

Immunofluorescence microscopy: The immune complexes appear as **granular deposits** (deposits of immunoglobulins and complement) along the basement membrane **(Fig. 20.5)**, in the mesangium, or in both locations. The deposits are described as "lumpy-bumpy" deposits by pathologists.

The fate of immune deposits: Immune complexes deposits in the glomerulus may eventually be degraded. This degradation may be brought out mostly by infiltrating neutrophils and monocytes/macrophages, mesangial cells, and endogenous proteases. After the degradation of immune complexes, the inflammatory reaction may subside.

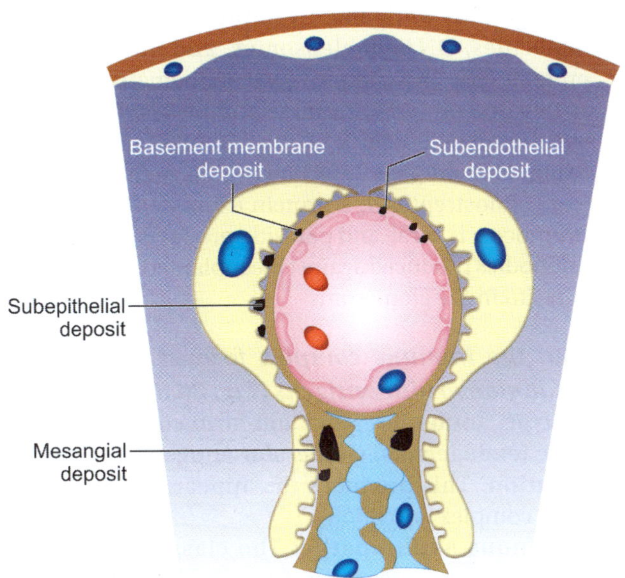

Fig. 20.6: Various locations of immune complex deposition in the glomerulus include: subepithelial, subendothelial, basement membrane, and mesangial.

- **Short-lived exposure to antigens:** Degradation of immune complexes and eventual recovery occurs when the exposure to the inciting, (provoking) antigen is short-lived and limited (e.g., in most cases of post-streptococcal glomerulonephritis).
- **Repeated and prolonged exposure to antigens:** If there are repeated and prolonged periods of deposition of immune complexes, many cycles of glomerular injury may occur. This leads to a more chronic membranous or membranoproliferative type of glomerulonephritis (e.g., glomerulonephritis occurring in SLE or viral hepatitis).

Formation of Immune Complexes In Situ

This form of glomerular injury is the result of the formation of immune complexes locally (in situ immune complexes) in the glomerulus. The **antibodies react either with (1) extrinsic antigens (molecules) "planted" in the glomerulus from the circulation or (2) intrinsic glomerular antigens** in a patchy distribution. They produce the appearance of in situ immune complex formation.

In situ immune complexes formed against planted antigens (Fig. 20.5)

Planted antigens: Some antigens may not be normally present in the glomerulus but are "planted" (nonglomerular antigens) in the glomerulus. Such planted antigens may interact with various intrinsic components of the glomerulus. These antigens may be endogenous or exogenous.

- **Endogenous antigens**: Examples include cationic molecules, DNA, nucleosomes, and other nuclear proteins (e.g., in systemic lupus erythematosus), large aggregated proteins, immune complexes themselves, and immunoglobulin A.
- **Exogenous antigens:** Infectious agents such as bacterial (e.g., endostreptosin, a protein expressed by group A streptococci), viral, and parasitic products; and drugs.

Antibodies produced against these planted antigens can react in situ in the glomerulus.

In situ, the immune complex formed against the intrinsic glomerular antigens (Fig. 20.5)

In this type, **antibodies react and form complexes with intrinsic (endogenous) glomerular antigens in a patchy distribution**. This produces the appearance of in situ immune complex formation.

Membranous nephropathy: The classic example of glomerular disease resulting from the local formation of immune complexes containing antibodies reactive with endogenous (intrinsic) antigens is membranous nephropathy (MGN). In MGN, immune complexes are formed in the subepithelial portion of the GBM. It causes a severe increase in the permeability of the glomerulus, resulting in nephrotic syndrome, with little or no inflammation. It is discussed on pages 721-3.

Immunofluorescence (IF) microscopy: In both types of in situ immune complexes, bound antibodies appear granular by immunofluorescence microscopy, similar to the circulating immune complex nephritis.

Deposition of Anti-glomerular Basement Membrane Antibody

Antibody-mediated GN is caused due to the glomerular deposition of autoantibodies directed against protein components of the GBM. A classic example is an anti-GBM antibody–mediated GN, also known as *Goodpasture disease.*

Goodpasture syndrome: It results from the formation of **autoantibodies against** intrinsic (fixed) GBM antigens. It is characterized by conformational changes in the α_3 chains of type IV collagen of GBM. This fixed altered GBM antigen (Goodpasture antigen) can trigger the formation of **anti-GBM antibodies.** This GN is an example of type II hypersensitivity. These antibodies may sometimes cross-react with not only renal GBM but also with the basement membrane of lung alveoli, resulting in simultaneous production of lung and kidney lesions and this is known as Goodpasture syndrome (*refer* pages 720-1).

Immunofluorescence (IF) microscopy: In anti-GBM antibody-induced glomerulonephritis, antibodies bind to intrinsic antigens. These **antigens are continuously,** (homogeneously) **distributed along the entire length of the GBM.** Under IF, it produces produce a **diffuse linear pattern of immunofluorescence**. This is in contrast to the granular lumpy pattern of immunofluorescent staining seen in circulating immune complexes (described below).

Cell-mediated Immunity in Glomerulonephritis

Antibody-mediated immune complex-mediated injury may initiate most forms of glomerulonephritis. However, cell-mediated immunity may also be involved in its pathogenesis. Cell-mediated immunity is a delayed hypersensitivity (type IV hypersensitivity) reaction and can damage the glomerulus.

Nonimmune Glomerular Injury

Apart from immune mechanisms, nonimmune mechanisms also can cause glomerular injury. It may be due to ischemia, metabolic disorders (e.g., diabetes mellitus), toxin exposure, drugs, vascular disorders (e.g., vasculitis), and infection with direct injury to glomerular cells. Different causes of glomerular injury may produce more than one type of glomerular lesion. Thus, a particular form of glomerular lesion need not be specific to a disease.

Activation of Alternative Complement Pathway

An alternative complement pathway is activated by a nonimmunological mechanism in the absence of an antibody. Activation of alternative complement pathways occurs in the clinicopathologic entity called dense-deposit disease and in C3 glomerulopathies. Dense deposit disease was earlier known as MPGN type II. Alternative complement pathway activation is discussed on page 730 (*refer* **Fig. 3.12 and Flowchart 20.3**).

NEPHRITIC SYNDROME

Definition: Nephritic syndrome is **characterized by hematuria** (gross or microscopic), dysmorphic red cells, red cell casts in the **urine, azotemia,** and **oliguria** (due to decreased glomerular filtration rate), and **mild to moderate hypertension.** Proteinuria and edema are common, but they are not as severe as in the nephrotic syndrome.

The main features of the nephritic syndrome are presented in **Box 20.4**.

One of the causes of the nephritic syndrome is acute proliferative glomerulonephritis.

BOX 20.4: Main features of nephritic syndrome.

- **Hematuria:** Either gross hematuria (red blood cells in urine) or microscopic hematuria with dysmorphic red cells and red cell casts in the urine
- **Proteinuria:** Mild-to-moderate proteinuria, usually in the subnephrotic range. It is associated with or without edema.
- **Azotemia:** Biochemical abnormality with elevated blood urea nitrogen (BUN) and creatinine levels resulting from reduced glomerular filtration rate (GFR)
- **Hypertension**
- **Diminished glomerular filtration rate (GFR) and oliguria**

Acute Proliferative Glomerulonephritis

It is a group of diseases characterized histologically by the **diffuse proliferation of glomerular cells accompanied by infiltration (exudation) of glomerulus by leukocytes.**

Immune complex diseases: Acute proliferative GNs are usually immune complex-mediated diseases. The triggering antigen may be exogenous or endogenous.

- **Exogenous** (e.g., postinfectious glomerulonephritis, which commonly follows streptococcal infection).
- **Endogenous** [e.g., systemic lupus erythematosus (SLE)].

Poststreptococcal (Postinfectious) Glomerulonephritis

Poststreptococcal glomerulonephritis is a common disorder in developing countries.

Age group: It is most frequent in **children between 6 and 10 years of age**, but may develop in adults of any age.

Etiology and Pathogenesis (Flowchart 20.1)

Q. Discuss the etiopathogenesis of acute poststreptococcal glomerulonephritis.

Follows streptococcal infection: Poststreptococcal GN is caused by immune complexes: These immune complexes **contain streptococcal antigens and specific antibodies.** It **follows streptococcal infection** (hence poststreptococcal) rather than direct primary infection of the kidney by streptococci.

Primary streptococcal infection of the pharynx or skin: It usually involves the **pharynx** (pharyngitis) **or the skin** (impetigo/pyoderma). Skin infections are usually associated with overcrowding and poor hygiene.

Nephritogenic strains of group A β-hemolytic streptococci: Only **certain strains** of **group A β-hemolytic streptococci are nephritogenic**. More than 90% are due to **types 12, 4, and 1**. These can be identified by typing of M protein of the streptococcal cell wall.

Immune complex nephritis: It is an **immunologically mediated** disease. Both have an affinity for glomerular proteins and plasmin.

Flowchart 20.1: Pathogenesis of poststreptococcal glomerulonephritis

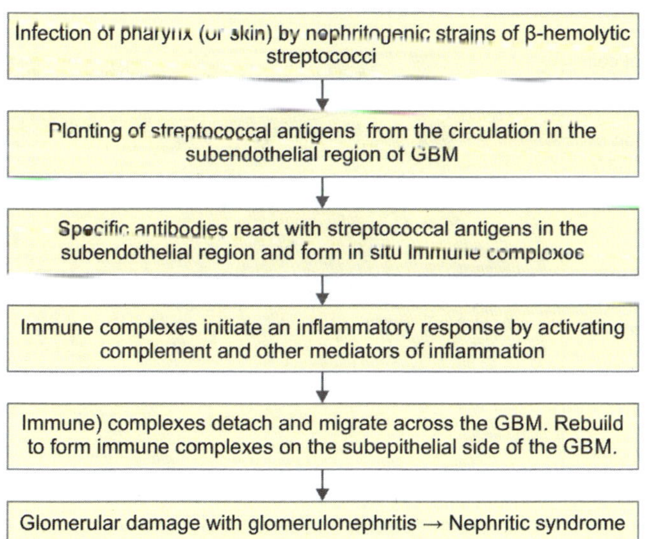

Evidence to support immunological basis

- **Latent period:** It **usually develops** after a **latent period of 1–4 weeks after a primary streptococcal infection of the pharynx** (pharyngitis) **or skin** (impetigo/pyoderma). This period is compatible with the **time required for the production of antibodies and the immune complex formation.**
- **Antibodies against streptococcal antigens:** Raised titers of antibodies against one or more streptococcal antigens are present in the majority of patients with GN. These antibodies include the following:
  - Anti-streptolysin O (ASO)
  - Anti-deoxyribonuclease B (anti-DNase B)
  - Anti-streptokinase
  - Anti-hyaluronidase
  - Anti-nicotinyl adenine dinucleotidase.
- **Hypocomplementemia:** In **more than 90% of patients,** serum complement levels are low. This indicates the activation and utilization of complement components by immune complexes.
- **Immune-complex deposits:**
  - **Electron microscopy shows** glomeruli with **electron-dense deposits** of immune complexes.
  - **Immunofluorescence shows granular fluorescence** to the immune deposits (IgG and complement).
- **Streptococcal antigens in the glomeruli:** Many cationic antigens unique to nephritogenic strains of streptococci, can be demonstrated in the glomeruli. The antigenic component is responsible for immune reaction in post-streptococcal glomerulonephritis. Examples:
  - **Streptococcal pyogenic exotoxin B (SpeB)** (main antigenic determinant responsible for immune reaction in most cases of poststreptococcal glomerulonephritis) and its zymogen precursor **(zSpeB).**
  - **Nephritis-associated streptococcal plasmin receptor (NAPlR).**
  - **Streptococcal glyceraldehyde-3-phosphate dehydrogenase (GAPDH)** in most but not all cases.

Mechanism of glomerular damage

Initially, the triggering **exogenous antigens** (e.g., streptococcal antigens) **are planted** from the circulation in the **subendothelial region in glomerular capillary walls**. The antibodies react with these antigens in the subendothelial region of the glomerular basement membrane (GBM) and **form in situ immune complexes.** The immune complexes **initiate an inflammatory response** by activating complement and other humoral and cellular mediators of inflammation and produce glomerular damage. Subsequently, through an unknown mechanism, the **antigen-antibody (immune) complexes detach and migrate across the GBM**. They **rebuild to form immune complexes on the subepithelial side of the GBM**. Besides forming in situ immune complexes, circulating immune complexes may also be deposited in the glomerulus. They may also contribute to the lesions. Granular immunofluorescent deposits and subepithelial humps are characteristic of immune-complex nephritis.

MORPHOLOGY

Q. Describe the morphology (light microscopy, electron microscopy, and immunofluorescence findings) of the kidney in acute diffuse proliferative glomerulonephritis.

Gross

The kidneys are enlarged and show a pale capsular surface and cortex.

Q. Write a short answer on microscopy of the kidney in acute post-streptococcal glomerulonephritis.

Light Microscopy (Figs. 20.7A and B)

The classic histologic features of poststreptococcal GN are as follows.

Glomeruli: They are **enlarged and hypercellular (increased cellularity)**. It is the classical diagnostic feature. The **hypercellularity is due to:**

- **Infiltration by leukocytes:** It includes both **neutrophils and monocytes.**
- **Proliferation and swelling of endothelial and mesangial cells. This along with leukocyte infiltration obliterates the glomerular capillary lumens.**
- **Crescent formation in severe cases:** Rarely, the **proliferation of parietal cells lining the Bowman capsule** leads to the formation of epithelial crescents. The presence of crescents is a **poor prognostic feature.**

The proliferation of cells (endothelial and mesangial) and leukocyte (neutrophils and monocytes) infiltration is generally **global and diffuse (involves nearly all glomeruli)**. Thus, they involve all lobules of all glomeruli.

Tubules: They may contain **red cell casts** in the lumen and the tubular epithelial cells may show degenerative changes.

Interstitium: It may show edema and inflammatory cell infiltrate.

Blood vessels: Unremarkable.

Immunofluorescence Microscopy (Fig. 20.8)

Granular deposits of immunoglobulin G (IgG) and C3, and sometimes IgM, are seen **in the mesangium and along the GBM**. It produces **granular fluorescence**. Immune complex deposits are almost present in all cases. But they are usually focal and sparse

Electron Microscopic Findings (Fig. 20.9)

- **Subepithelial deposits:** The characteristic feature is the presence of **discrete, amorphous, electron-dense deposits on the epithelial side of the GBM**. These deposits appear as dome-shaped "humps," often termed **"humps" or "lumpy" deposits.** They correspond to the granular IgG and C3 demonstrated by the immunofluorescence. These deposits are usually cleared by about 2 months after the resolution of the infection.
- **Subendothelial deposits:** They are also commonly seen during the early phase of the disease. Intramembranous and mesangial deposits may also be observed.

Refer online **Box 20.5** for the main morphologic features of poststreptococcal glomerulonephritis.

Clinical Features

The clinical presentation varies from asymptomatic to acute nephritic syndrome.

- Affected **child abruptly develops malaise, fever, nausea, oliguria, and hematuria (smoky or cola-colored urine) 1–2 weeks** after recovery from a **sore throat.**
- **Periorbital edema**, and **mild to moderate hypertension** are usually observed.
- In adults, clinical features are atypical.

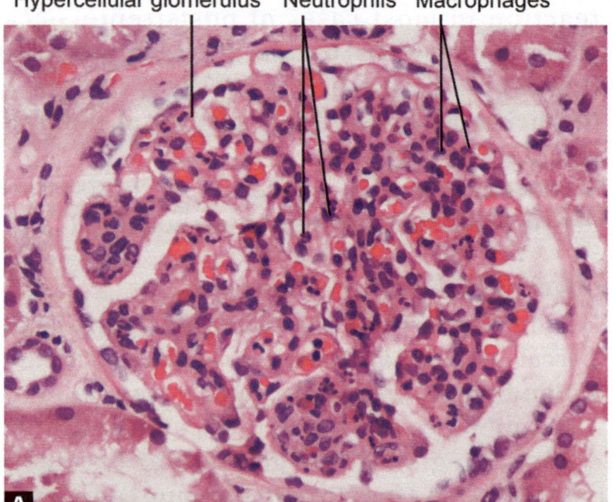

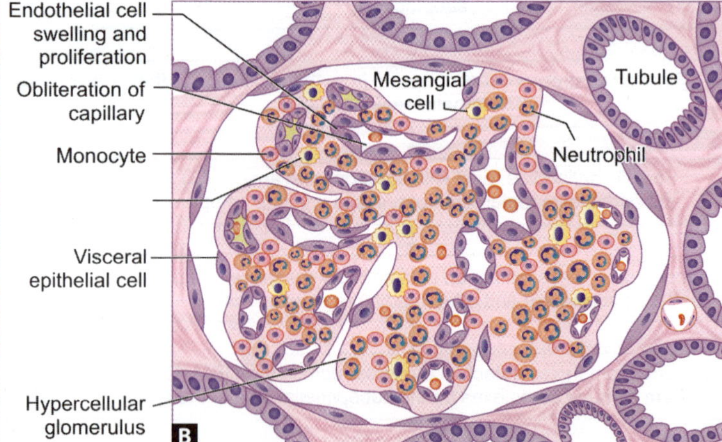

Figs. 20.7A and B: Light microscopic appearance of acute poststreptococcal glomerulonephritis: (A) (Hematoxylin and eosin stain); (B) (diagrammatic). The glomerulus is hypercellular due to the proliferation of intrinsic glomerular cells and infiltration by leukocytes.

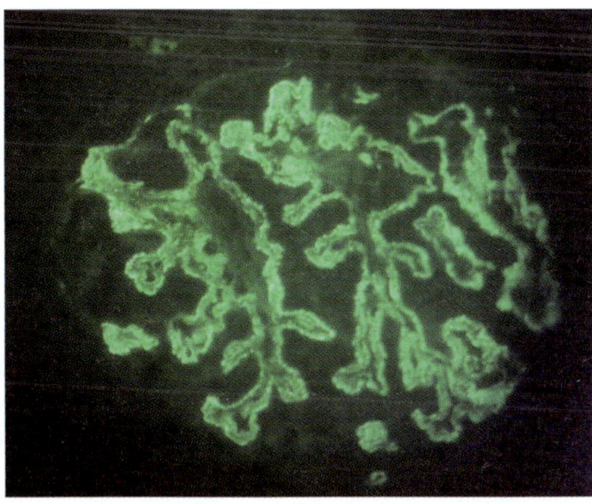

Fig. 20.8: Granular immunofluorescence characteristic of circulating or in situ immune complex nephritis.

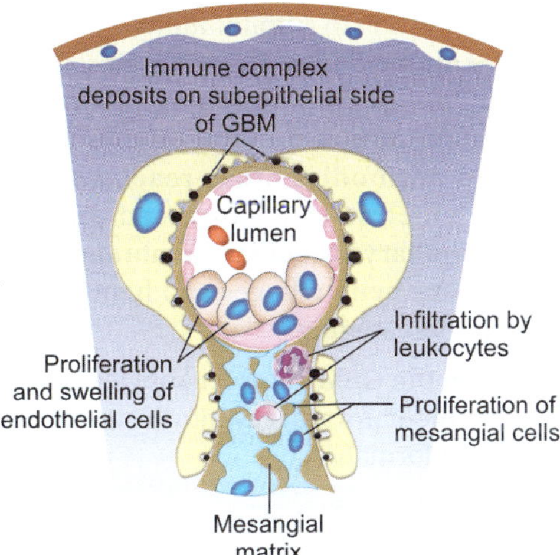

Fig. 20.9: Diagrammatic electron microscopic appearance of post-streptococcal glomerulonephritis. Subepithelial immune complexes appear as characteristic hump-like structures. Other features are endothelial and mesangial cell proliferation with narrowing of the lumen.

(GBM: glomerular basement membrane)

Laboratory Findings

Q. Laboratory findings in nephritic syndrome.

Blood findings

- **Raised antistreptococcal antibody titers** [e.g., anti-streptolysin O (ASO) titer], but the level may be low in GN that follows streptococcal skin infection.
- **Hypocomplementemia:** Significant **reduction in serum** concentration of **complement (C3)** components.
- **Raised blood urea and serum creatinine** indicate renal impairment.

Urinary findings

Q. Write a short answer on urinary findings in acute nephritis.

- **Oliguria**
- **Mild** (variable degree) **proteinuria** (usually <1 g/day).
- **Hematuria (smoky or cola-colored urine):** RBCs in urine.
- **Microscopy: Red cell casts or dysmorphic red cells (red cells with cellular protrusions or fragmentation).**

Prognosis

- **Children:** Prognosis is **good** in children and more than 95% totally recover.
- **Adults:** In adults, it is **less benign**. They may recover promptly or develop rapidly progressive glomerulonephritis or progress to chronic glomerulonephritis.

SCENARIO-BASED ESSAY QUESTION

Q. A 10-year-old boy was brought by the mother to pediatric outpatient with chief complaints of puffiness of the face, particularly more marked in the morning, mild pitting edema on both legs, malaise with nausea, and a slight fever for about one month. The mother also complained that he passed dark brown (red or cola) colored (smoky) urine and the urine output was reduced (oliguria). On enquiry, the mother informed that about 2 weeks back the child had a severe sore throat (upper respiratory tract infection). On examination, the blood pressure was 160/100 mm Hg (moderate hypertension). Urine examination revealed mild (or moderate) albuminuria/proteinuria and microscopy showed RBC ++ and RBC cast +. Laboratory investigation showed a raised serum antistreptolysin O titer and a low serum complement level.

a. What is the most probable diagnosis? (Ans: This is a case of nephritic syndrome in the setting of acute poststreptococcal glomerulonephritis)
b. Discuss the etiopathogenesis of these lesions *(refer pages 717-8)*.
c. Describe the light microscopy, immunofluorescence, and electron microscopic findings *(refer page 718)*.
d. List the investigations. What is the prognosis of this disease? *(refer page 719)*.

Nonstreptococcal Acute Glomerulonephritis (Postinfectious Glomerulonephritis)

Acute proliferative glomerulonephritis may also occur in association with other infections:

- **Bacteria:** Examples, staphylococcal endocarditis, pneumococcal pneumonia, and meningococcemia.
- **Virus:** Examples, hepatitis (B and C), mumps, HIV infection, varicella, and infectious mononucleosis.
- **Parasite** (e.g., malaria, toxoplasmosis).

The morphological changes are similar to post-streptococcal glomerulonephritis.

Rapidly Progressive (Crescentic) Glomerulonephritis

Q. Write a short note on rapidly progressive glomerulonephritis.

Definition: Rapidly progressive glomerulonephritis (RPGN) is a clinical syndrome, characterized by **acute renal failure (rapid and progressive loss of renal function), features of the nephritic syndrome, and often severe oliguria.** If not treated, death occurs due to renal failure within weeks to months.

RPGN does not represent a specific etiologic type of glomerulonephritis. The most common microscopic feature in many cases is the presence of glomerular (epithelial) crescents in most of the glomeruli. Hence also termed crescentic glomerulonephritis.

Pathogenesis

The RPGN is a syndrome caused by **primary glomerular diseases as well as systemic diseases**. Pathogenetic mechanism varies but most are immunologically mediated and it indicates severe glomerular damage.

Q. Write a short essay on classification.

Classification: In most cases of RPGN, the glomerular injury is immunologically mediated. RPGN is classified into three types based on immunological findings **(Box 20.6)**. Each type may be idiopathic or associated with a known disorder.

Q. Write a short note on the etiology and pathogenesis of rapidly progressive glomerulonephritis.

Type I RPGN: It is an uncommon, aggressive type **caused by an anti-GBM antibody**. One of the examples is Goodpasture syndrome.

Type II RPGN: It is due to **immune complex deposition** and may complicate any of the immune complex nephritides (e.g., postinfectious glomerulonephritis, systemic lupus erythematosus, IgA nephropathy, and Henoch-Schönlein purpura). **Immunofluorescence** shows **granular fluorescence** characteristic of immune complex nephritis.

Type III RPGN: It is also known as the pauci-immune type. It **neither shows anti-GBM antibodies nor immune complexes** by immunofluorescence and electron microscopy. Majorities are **idiopathic** and have circulating **antineutrophil cytoplasmic antibodies (ANCAs)**. Some may be a component of systemic vasculitis, such as Granulomatosis with polyangiitis (formerly Wegener's granulomatosis).

BOX 20.6: Classification of rapidly progressive glomerulonephritis.

Type I (Anti-GBM antibody)
- Limited to kidney
- Goodpasture syndrome with involvement of lung

Type II (Immune complex)
- Idiopathic
- Known disorder
  - Postinfectious glomerulonephritis
  - Lupus nephritis
  - Henoch–Schönlein purpura
  - IgA nephropathy
  - Others

Type III (Pauci-immune)
- ANCA-associated
  - Idiopathic
- Vasculitis associated
  - Granulomatosis with polyangiitis (formerly Wegener's granulomatosis)
  - Microscopic polyangiitis

(ANCA: antineutrophil cytoplasmic antibodies; GBM: glomerular basement membrane; IgA: Immunoglobulin A).

Goodpasture Syndrome

Q. Write a short essay on Goodpasture syndrome.

In Goodpasture syndrome, **anti-GBM antibodies cross-react with pulmonary alveolar basement membranes** causing pulmonary hemorrhage associated with acute renal failure.

Pathogenesis

Genetic predisposition: The high prevalence of certain HLA subtypes (e.g., **HLA-DRB1**) in these patients points toward genetic predisposition to autoimmunity.

- **Anti-GBM antibodies** are formed **against Goodpasture antigen**. This antigen results from conformational changes in the α3 chains of type IV collagen of GBM.
- **Anti-GBM antibodies cross-react** with the **target antigen,** which is also expressed on pulmonary **alveolar-capillary basement membranes.** This results in **pulmonary hemorrhages** and **hemoptysis**, which may be life-threatening.

Ruptures in the GBM allow **leukocytes, proteins**, and **inflammatory mediators to leak** into the urinary space and initiate crescent formation.

MORPHOLOGY OF RPGN

Gross

Kidneys are enlarged and pale (large white kidney). They may show **petechial hemorrhages on the cortical surfaces (flea-bitten kidney).**

Microscopy (Figs. 20.10A to C)

Q. Write a short note on epithelial crescent.

Microscopic features depend on the underlying cause.

Glomeruli: Its characteristic feature is **crescents** in most of the glomeruli. Hence, the term crescentic glomerulonephritis.

- **Crescents:** These are formed by the (i) **proliferation of the parietal epithelial cells** lining the Bowman capsule and (ii) infiltration of **monocytes and macrophages** into the urinary space.
  - **Stimulus: Fibrin** leaked into the Bowman space is the stimulus and is found between the cellular layers. Fibrin is derived from fibrinogen, which escaped through the **ruptured GBM** into Bowman space.
  - **Significance:** It indicates **severe glomerular injury** and does not represent any specific etiological factor.

Tubules: The tubular lumen may show casts and red cells.

Interstitium: It shows edema with few inflammatory cells.

Blood vessels: Normal.

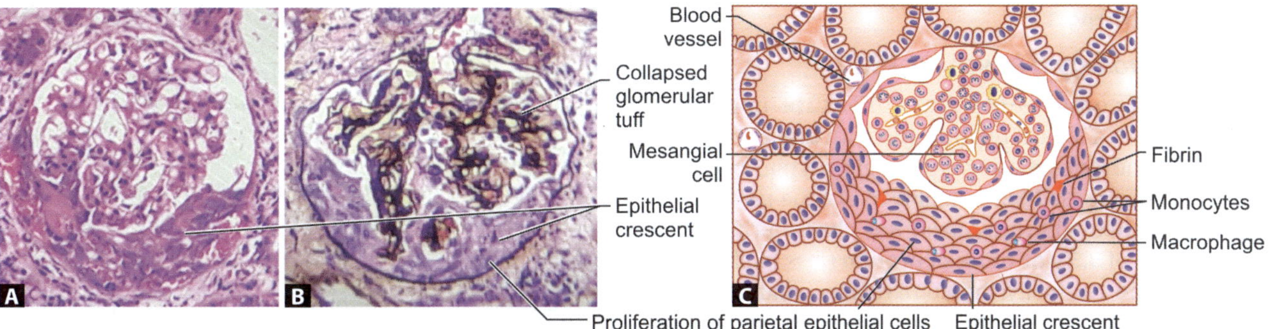

Figs. 20.10A to C: Crescentic glomerulonephritis showing a crescent-shaped mass of proliferating parietal epithelial cells and leukocytes internal to Bowman capsule: (A) Hematoxylin and eosin stain (H & E stain); (B) Silver methenamine stain; (C) Diagrammatic representation.

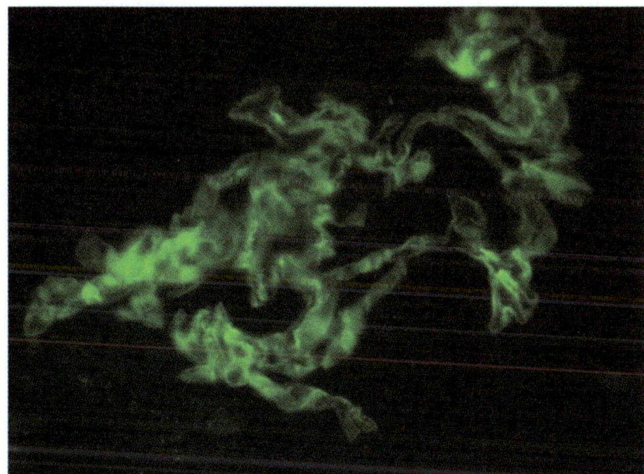

Fig. 20.11: Linear immunofluorescence for immunoglobulin G is seen along the GBM in Goodpasture syndrome.

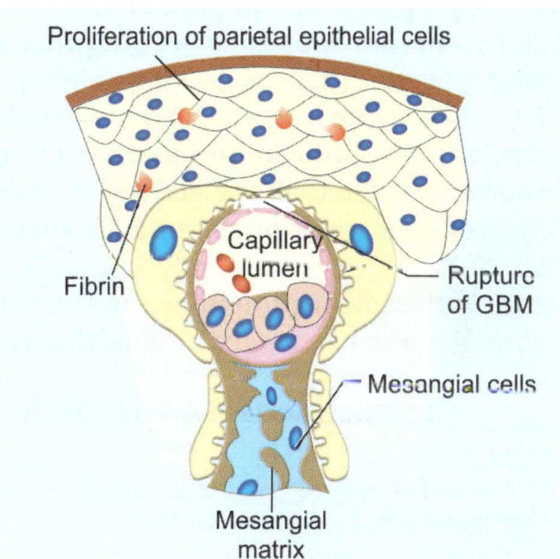

Fig. 20.12: Diagrammatic electron microscopic appearance of crescentic (rapidly progressive) glomerulonephritis. Shows disruption of GBM and proliferation of parietal epithelial cells to form a crescent.

Immunofluorescence Microscopy

Goodpasture syndrome: It shows **linear GBM fluorescence (Fig. 20.11)** for IgG and C3 complement.

Immune complex-mediated RPGN: It shows granular immune deposits.

Pauci-immune RPGN: It has **little or no deposition** of immune reactants.

Electron Microscopy

Break or ruptures in the GBM (Fig. 20.12).

Type II (immune complex) RPGN shows immune complex deposits.

Clinical Features

All forms of crescentic GN present with hematuria, RBC casts in the urine, moderate proteinuria (occasionally massive in the nephrotic range), and variable degrees of hypertension and edema.

Goodpasture syndrome: It may present with **recurrent hemoptysis or life-threatening pulmonary hemorrhage.**

Laboratory diagnosis: The diagnosis of specific subtypes depends on the detection of anti-GBM antibodies, antinuclear antibodies, and ANCAs.

- **Urine findings** include (1) hematuria, (2) RBC casts and dysmorphic RBCs, and (3) moderate proteinuria.

Prognosis: Milder forms may recover, but the renal involvement usually progresses within weeks and causes severe oliguria. The prognosis depends upon several crescents as it correlates with oliguria. Uremia is the cause of death in Goodpasture syndrome.

NEPHROTIC SYNDROME

Q. Define nephrotic syndrome. List the causes of nephrotic syndrome. Add a note on its pathophysiology. What are the causes of nephrotic syndrome in the pediatric age group?

Definition: Nephrotic syndrome is a clinical disorder **caused by a derangement in glomerular capillary walls that leads to increased permeability to plasma proteins.** The various components of the nephrotic syndrome are as follows:

1. **Massive/heavy proteinuria (>3.5 g of protein/24 hours).** This is less in children.
2. **Hypoalbuminemia** with plasma levels of albumin <3 g/dL
3. Generalized edema
4. Hyperlipidemia and lipiduria

General Features

Pathophysiology (Flowchart 20.2)

The various components that constitute nephrotic syndrome have a logical relationship with one another. In nephrotic syndrome, damage to the glomerular capillary walls causes increased permeability to plasma proteins.

1. **Massive (heavy) proteinuria:** It is characterized by a **daily loss of 3.5 g or more** of **protein** (less in children) in the **urine.** Normally, the glomerular capillary wall acts as a size and charge-dependent barrier for the plasma filtrate.
   - Proteinuria is **due to the increased permeability of the glomerular capillary wall to plasma proteins.**
   - The major proportion of protein lost in the urine is **albumin (low-molecular-weight proteins)**, and rarely globulins (high-molecular-weight proteins). The ratio between low- and high-molecular-weight proteins in the urine in various cases of nephrotic syndrome is due to the selectivity of proteinuria. Types of glomerular proteinuria are presented in **Box 20.7**.

   Albumin is the major protein lost in the urine, but globulins may also be excreted in some diseases.

BOX 20.7: Types of glomerular proteinuria.

- **Highly selective proteinuria:** In this type, only low-molecular-weight/intermediate-sized (<100 kDa) proteins (such as albumin 70 kD, transferrin 76 kD molecular weight) leak through the glomerulus, e.g., minimal-change disease
- **Nonselective (poorly-selective) proteinuria:** It is characterized by leakage of a range of different proteins (proteins of any size) including larger/higher molecular-weight serum proteins (e.g., immunoglobulins) in addition to albumin through the glomerulus, e.g., membranous nephropathy

2. **Hypoalbuminemia: Plasma albumin levels less than 3 g/dL.** Massive proteinuria **decreases serum albumin** levels (hypoalbuminemia) at a rate beyond the compensatory synthetic capacity of the liver. Hypoalbuminemia **decreases the colloid osmotic pressure** of the blood.
3. **Generalized edema:** It is soft and pitting. Edema is most marked in the **periorbital regions (Fig. 20.13)** and **dependent portions of the body.** When edema is **massive and generalized, it is called anasarca**, and it

Flowchart 20.2: Various characteristic features of nephrotic syndrome and its mechanism.

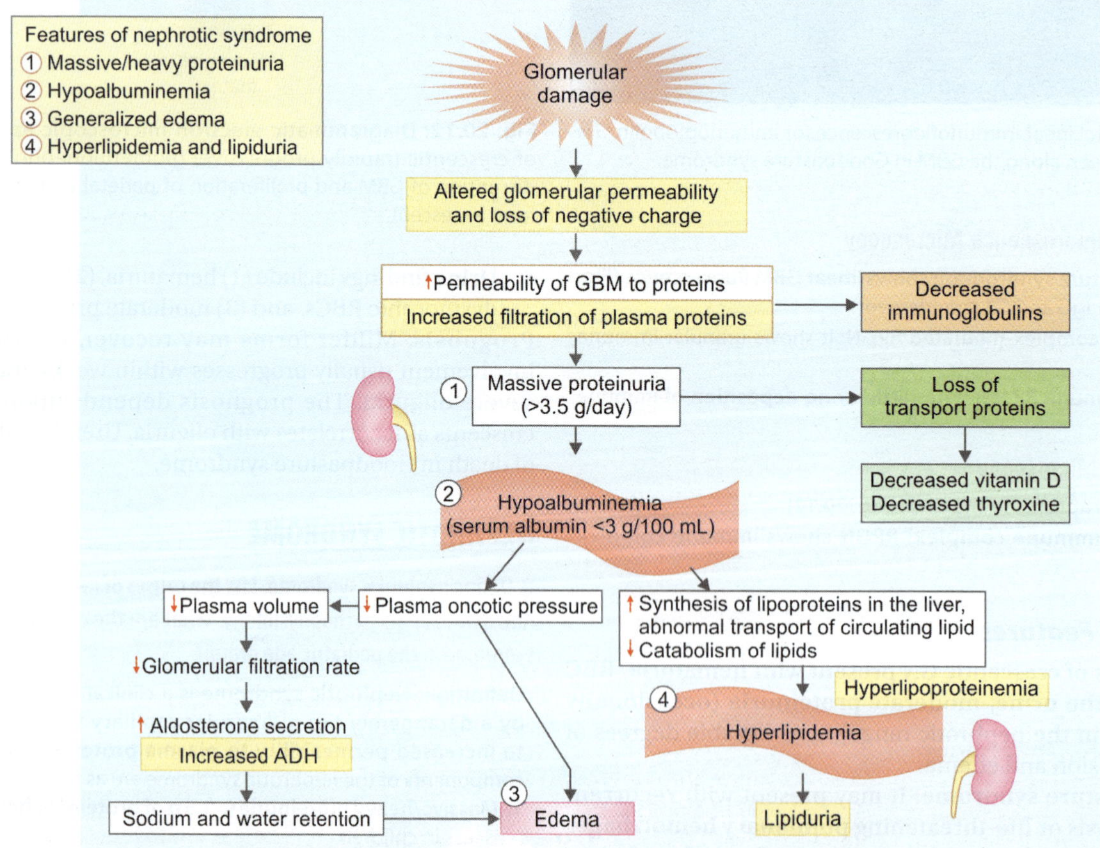

(GBM: glomerular basement membrane).

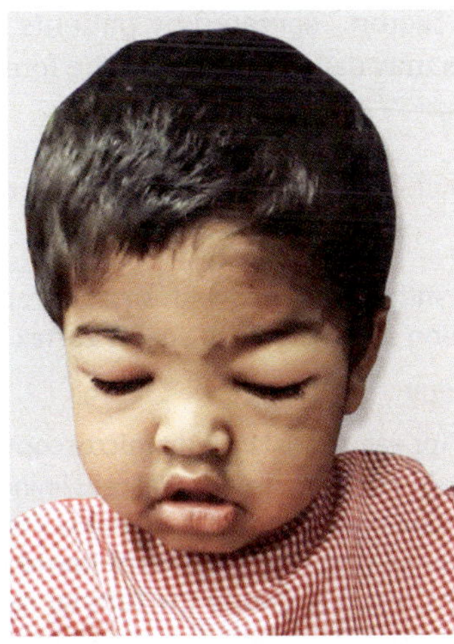

Fig. 20.13: Facial and periorbital puffiness in nephrotic syndrome.

may be associated with pleural effusions and ascites. **The causes of generalized edema are as follows:**

- **Decreased colloid osmotic pressure of the blood:** It leads to the accumulation of fluid in the interstitial tissues and produces generalized edema.
- **Sodium and water retention:** In nephrotic syndrome, there is also retention of sodium and water, and this aggravates the edema. Several factors are responsible for the retention of sodium and water. These include (1) hypovolemia which increases the secretion of renin which in turn leads to the **compensatory secretion of aldosterone**, (2) stimulation of the sympathetic system, and (3) reduction of the secretion of natriuretic factors such as atrial peptides.

4. **Hyperlipidemia and lipiduria**
   - **Hyperlipidemia:** Most patients with nephrotic syndrome have raised blood levels of cholesterol, triglyceride, very-low-density lipoprotein, low-density lipoprotein, Lp(a) lipoprotein, and apoprotein. Hyperlipidemia is due to (i) increased synthesis of lipoproteins in the liver, (ii) abnormal transport of circulating lipids, and (iii) decreased catabolism of lipids.
   - **Lipiduria:** Hyperlipidemia is followed by leakage of lipoproteins across the glomerular capillary wall. The leaked lipoproteins are reabsorbed by tubular epithelial cells and then shed along with the injured tubular cells that have detached from the basement membrane. These **lipids appear in urine either as free fat or as fat oval bodies.**

Q. Write a short note on selective and nonselective proteinuria.

Major complications of nephrotic syndrome are as follows:

- **Coronary atherosclerosis:** Hyperlipidemia predisposes to atherosclerosis of the coronary artery.
- **Infections:** Nephrotic patients are susceptible **to infection**, especially staphylococci and pneumococci. It may be **due to loss of immunoglobulins in the urine.**
- **Thrombotic and thromboembolic complications:** This may be due to the loss of endogenous anticoagulants (e.g., antithrombin III) and antiplasmins in the urine.

Causes of Nephrotic Syndrome (Table 20.2)

Q. Write a short note on the causes of nephrotic syndrome.

- The most common systemic causes of nephrotic syndrome are **diabetes, amyloidosis, and systemic lupus erythematosus (SLE).**
- The most important primary glomerular lesions causing nephrotic syndrome are **minimal-change disease, membranous glomerulopathy**, and **focal segmental glomerulosclerosis (FSGS).**

Minimal Change Disease

Minimal change disease (MCD) is a relatively benign disorder and is the most frequent cause of nephrotic syndrome in children. It is less common in adults. **It is characterized by glomeruli that appear normal appearance (changes are minimal or absent) by light microscopy.** Hence, is named minimal change disease (sometimes known as *nil lesion*). However, under electron microscopy, it shows **diffuse effacement (loss) of foot processes of visceral epithelial cells** (podocytes).

Age: It may develop at any age but most commonly occurs between 2 and 6 years of age.

TABLE 20.2 Causes of nephrotic syndrome.

Primary glomerular diseases	*Systemic diseases*
Minimal-change disease (~75% in children)	Diabetes mellitus
Focal segmental glomerulosclerosis (~35% in adults)	Amyloidosis
Membranous glomerulopathy (~30% in adults)	Infections (malaria, syphilis, hepatitis B and C, HIV)
Membranoproliferative glomerulonephritis and dense deposit disease	Systemic lupus erythematosus
Other proliferative glomerulonephritis (focal, pure mesangial, IgA nephropathy)	Drugs (penicillamine, "street heroin")
	Malignancy (carcinoma, melanoma)
	Others (bee-sting allergy, hereditary nephritis)

Pathogenesis

Q. Write a short note on the etiology and pathogenesis of minimal-change disease.

Probably has an immunologic basis: The pathogenesis of MCD remains unknown. The electron microscopic changes indicate that the **primary injury is to the visceral epithelial cells.** There are no immune deposits in the glomerulus. This may probably exclude the possibility of immune complex-mediated injury. However, **several features of the MCD favor an immunologic basis.** These are as follows:

- MCD **may follow a respiratory infection and routine prophylactic immunization.**
- It **dramatically responds to corticosteroids** and/or **other immunosuppressive therapy**.
- It may **develop in association with other atopic disorders.** For example, eczema and rhinitis.
- There is an **increased prevalence of MCD in certain human leukocyte antigen** (HLA) haplotypes in patients with atopy. This suggests a genetic predisposition.
- There is an **increased incidence of MCD in adult patients with Hodgkin lymphoma** (associated with T-cell dysfunction), **thymoma, leukemias, and T-cell lymphoma.**

Secondary MCD may develop following nonsteroidal anti-inflammatory drug (NSAID) therapy. It is usually associated with acute interstitial nephritis.

Mechanism of proteinuria: According to the leading hypothesis circulating molecules injure podocytes. The proteinuria occurs secondary to foot process effacement. However, effacement of the foot process is commonly seen in many causes of nephrotic syndrome. Therefore, it is not entirely known whether effacement of the foot process is the primary lesion or is secondary to proteinuria. Probably "permeability factors" secreted by patients' lymphocytes and other cells may cause damage to the foot process.

MORPHOLOGY

Q. Write a short note on the morphology of minimal-change disease.

Gross

- Kidneys are **mildly enlarged** with smooth capsular surface. The cut section shows a **pale to yellow cortex.**

Light Microscopy

- **Glomeruli:** Appear **normal by light microscopy (Fig. 20.14A).**
- **Tubules:** The **cytoplasm of epithelial cells** lining the **proximal tubules contain lipid vacuoles and glassy (hyaline) protein droplets (hence,** the **historical term lipoid nephrosis** for this disease). These are **due to the tubular reabsorption of lipoproteins** passing through damaged glomeruli.
- **Interstitium:** May show mild edema.
- **Blood vessels:** Appear normal.

Electron Microscopy [Fig. 20.14C (refer online 20.14B)]

- **GBM appears normal** without any electron-dense deposit.
- **Changes in the visceral epithelial cells:** The most **characteristic feature is uniform and diffuse effacement of foot processes in the visceral epithelial cells.** This change is wrongly called as "fusion" of foot processes. The cytoplasm shows vacuolization and swelling.

Immunofluorescence

Does not show immunoglobulin or complement deposits.

Clinical Features

- Classically, it presents as **nephrotic syndrome**. The onset of nephrotic syndrome may be **preceded by upper respiratory tract infection or immunization.** Despite massive proteinuria, renal function remains good.

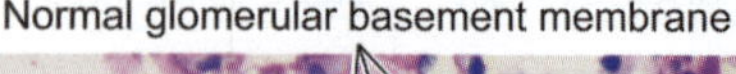

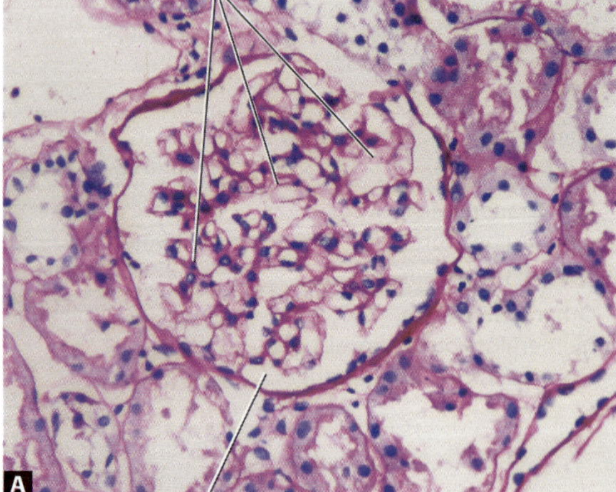

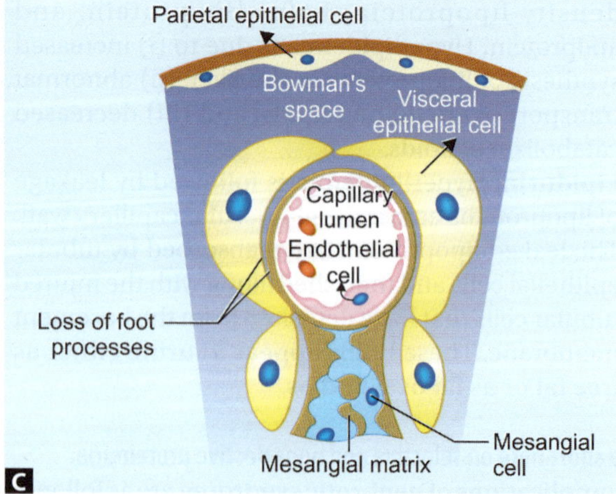

Figs. 20.14A and C: Minimal change disease: (A) Light microscopy. Periodic acid–Schiff (PAS) stain shows normal GBM without any cellular proliferation; (C) Diagrammatic electron microscopic appearance. It shows effacement of the foot processes of visceral epithelial cells. All other glomerular structures appear normal (*refer* **online Fig. 26.14B**).

- **Other features: Generalized edema, hypoalbuminemia, and hyperlipidemia.**

Urine findings: Proteinuria, oval fat bodies, and fatty casts are urinary findings. The **proteinuria is usually highly selective (selective proteinuria, albumin more than globulins) and mostly albumin with minimal amounts of higher-molecular-weight proteins.**

Prognosis: Excellent.

SCENARIO-BASED ESSAY QUESTION

Q. A 6-year-old boy child is brought to the hospital with a complaint that he has become less active over the past 10 days. On physical examination, the boy had facial puffiness which is more prominent around his eyes, swelling of the abdomen, and swelling of both ankles. There was neither a history of fever nor hypertension. An X-ray film of the chest showed bilateral pleural effusions, without evidence of lung disease. Urinalysis showed 4+ proteinuria and there were no blood, glucose, or ketone bodies. Microscopic examination of urine showed fat globules and there were no cells, casts, or crystals. The protein in a 24-hour urine sample revealed 4.8 g of protein. The serum creatinine and blood urea levels were normal. He responded well to corticosteroid therapy.

a. What is the most probable diagnosis? (Ans: Steroid-responsive proteinuria in a child is a feature nephrotic syndrome due to minimal change disease)
b. Discuss the etiopathogenesis of this disease *(refer page 724)*.
c. Describe the light microscopic, electron microscopic, and immunofluorescence findings in this condition *(refer page 724)*

Focal Segmental Glomerulosclerosis

Q. Write a short answer on focal segmental glomerulosclerosis.

Focal segmental glomerulosclerosis (FSGS) shows **sclerosis of some (but not all) glomeruli (focal) that involve only a part of each affected glomerulus (segmental, part of the capillary tuft).**

Classification (Refer Online Box 20.8)

FSGS is not a specific disease. It represents a pattern of injury that is usually seen in adults and children with nephrotic syndrome. There are several forms of FSGS.

Primary FSGS: Primary FSGS has no identifiable predisposing cause. It may produce nephrotic syndrome. This can progress to end-stage renal disease.

Secondary: FSGS may follow various insults. Examples are as follows:

- **Maladaptive response to nephron loss**: Any type of chronic kidney disease causes loss of functional renal mass and may develop FSGS. It can also occur in severely obese patients who develop proteinuria. In these situations, there is increased filtration pressure in residual glomeruli. This may result in FSGS.
- **Infections**: FSGS occurs in 5–10% of patients infected with HIV.
- **Drugs**: Specifically, it may develop with heroin use.

Genetic: The inherited forms usually occur as an autosomal recessive disease. Genetic disorders affect the genes that encode proteins involved in podocyte function (e.g., nephrin, podocin, cytoskeletal proteins).

Pathogenesis

Injury to podocytes: Probably, the initiating event in primary FSGS is an unknown injury to podocytes. This injury produces a fusion of the foot process and is associated with increased glomerular permeability. This may progress to loss of podocytes and slit diaphragms.

Permeability-inducing factors produced by lymphocytes: In FSGS, the deposition of hyaline in the glomeruli is due to the entrapment of plasma proteins and lipids in the foci of injury where sclerosis develops. The recurrence of proteinuria in patients undergoing renal transplantation for FSGS, sometimes within 24 hours of transplantation, suggests the possibility of a circulating mediator which leads to podocyte damage in some cases.

MORPHOLOGY

Light Microscopy

Glomerular involvement: Primary FSGS **initially involves only the juxtamedullary glomeruli** and with the progression of the disease, it affects all levels of the cortex. The **lesions occur in only some tufts within a glomerulus while other tufts appear normal on light microscopy.**

Microscopic Features (Figs. 20.15A and B)

The affected glomeruli show: **(i) increased mesangial matrix, (ii) obliterated capillary lumina, (iii) deposition of hyaline (hyalinosis)** which is characterized by extracellular accumulation of **homogeneous and eosinophilic material** in the glomeruli. It represents **leaked plasma proteins** due to endothelial or capillary wall injury] and **(iv) foamy (lipid-laden) macrophages.**

Advanced stages: As the FSGS progresses, the **sclerosis of the glomeruli involves other glomeruli** (global sclerosis), and there will be pronounced **atrophy of the tubules, and fibrosis of the interstitium.** At this stage, it is difficult to differentiate it from other forms of chronic glomerular disease.

Collapsing glomerulopathy: It is a morphologic variant of FSGS characterized by collapse of the glomerular tuft and epithelial cell hyperplasia. This severe form of FSGS may be idiopathic or may be seen with HIV infection, drug-induced toxicities, and some microvascular injuries. It has a poor prognosis.

Electron Microscopy

Both sclerotic and nonsclerotic areas show **diffuse effacement of foot processes** of podocytes of visceral epithelial cells of glomeruli as in minimal-change disease.

Immunofluorescence Microscopy

It usually shows **nonspecific trapping of immunoglobulins**, usually IgM, and complement in the areas of hyalinosis.

Clinical Course

It is necessary to **distinguish FSGS from minimal-change disease**, because of markedly different clinical courses

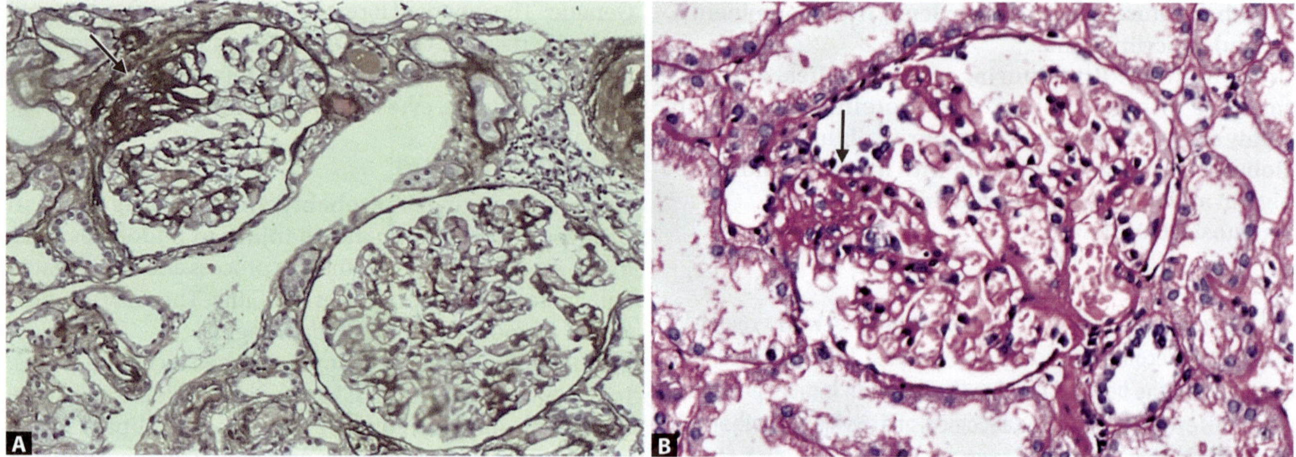

Figs. 20.15A and B: Focal segmental glomerulosclerosis: (A) Silver stain (Jones) shows two glomeruli. One glomerulus on the left shows sclerosis of the capillary loops (arrow). Other right glomeruli are essentially normal; (B) Periodic acid–Schiff (PAS) stain showing one glomerulus with focal segmental glomerulosclerosis (arrow).

Courtesy: Part B Dr Alok Sharma, Director, Renal Pathology and Electron Microscopy, National Reference Laboratory, Dr Lal PathLabs Ltd, New Delhi, India.

and responses to therapy. Both present with nephrotic syndrome, but hematuria and hypertension are more frequent in FSGS. In contrast to minimal change disease, **FSGS-associated proteinuria is nonselective, and it shows poor response to corticosteroid therapy**. About 50% of FSGS patients progress to end-stage renal disease within 10 years of diagnosis.

Urine findings: Proteinuria, microscopic hematuria, oval fat bodies and, fatty casts.

Prognosis: Children have a better prognosis than adults.

Membranous Nephropathy

Q. Write a short note of membranous glomerulopathy.

Membranous nephropathy (membranous glomerulopathy) is characterized by **uniform diffuse thickening of the glomerular capillary wall**. This is **due to the accumulation of electron-dense deposits of antigen-antibody complexes along the subepithelial side of the glomerular basement membrane**.

Age: It usually presents in adults between 30 and 60 years of age. Membranous nephropathy is the **common cause (~30%) of nephrotic syndrome in adults**.

Causes (Box 20.9): About 80% of membranous nephropathy is caused due to primary glomerular diseases. Primary **membranous nephropathy is caused by autoantibodies against podocyte antigens.** The remaining 20% develop in association with other systemic diseases. In these systemic diseases, there is an identifiable etiologic agent. Hence, they are called secondary membranous nephropathy.

Q. Write a short essay on the etiology and pathology of membranous glomerulopathy.

BOX 20.9: Causes of membranous glomerulopathy.

Primary membranous glomerulopathy
- Anti-phospholipase A_2 receptor (PLA_2R) autoantibodies

Secondary membranous glomerulopathy
- **Infections:** For example, chronic hepatitis B, hepatitis C, syphilis, schistosomiasis, malaria
- **Malignant tumors:** For example, carcinomas of the lung, colon, breast, stomach, kidney, esophagus; B cell tumors such as chronic lymphocytic leukemia
- **Autoimmune diseases:** Membranous glomerulopathy constitutes about 10–15% of glomerulonephritis in systemic lupus erythematosus (SLE), rheumatoid arthritis
- **Exposure to inorganic salts:** For example, gold, mercury
- **Drugs:** For example, penicillamine, captopril, nonsteroidal anti-inflammatory drugs (NSAIDs)
- **Other systemic diseases:** Fanconi's syndrome, sickle cell anemia, diabetes

Pathogenesis

Primary membranous nephropathy: It was **formerly called idiopathic**. Now it is identified as an **autoimmune disease caused in most cases by antibodies** reacting **in situ usually to an endogenous glomerular antigen (autoantigen).**

Autoantibodies against phospholipase A_2 receptor (PLA_2R): Autoimmune reactions by autoantibodies are most often directed against phospholipase A2 receptor antigen (PLA2R) on the podocyte (autoantibodies against podocyte antigen). It results **in the situ formation of the immune complex**. These autoantibodies are observed in 70–80% of cases. In the rest of the primary cases, antibodies are against several other glomerular antigens.

Mechanism of Glomerular Injury

- **No inflammatory cells: Glomeruli do not show** any **inflammatory cells** (like neutrophils, monocytes), or platelets.
- **Membrane attack complex (MAC)**: Membranous nephropathy shows subepithelial immune deposits that activate the complement system on the surface of podocytes and generate **C5b-C9** (membrane attack complex/MAC). MAC **has an important role in damage to the glomerulus.** They activate podocytes of glomerular epithelial cells and mesangial cells and liberate proteases and oxidants. They cause capillary wall injury and leakage of protein.

MORPHOLOGY

Light Microscopy (Figs. 20.16A to C)

1. **Glomeruli:** They show the following features:
   - **Uniform, diffuse thickening of the glomerular capillary wall.**
   - **Normocellular glomeruli:** There is **neither proliferation nor inflammation.**
   - **Special stains: Silver stains (black color) (Fig. 20.16C) or periodic acid-Schiff stains (pink color)** show **characteristic spikes** in all glomeruli, **between the deposits of the immune complex on the epithelial side of the GBM in all glomeruli.**
   - As the disease progresses glomeruli may become totally sclerosed.
2. **Tubules:** The **epithelial cells of the proximal tubules** show **droplets of reabsorbed protein**. Later tubules undergo atrophy.
3. **Interstitium:** It shows mononuclear cell inflammatory cells and interstitial fibrosis in late stages.
4. **Blood vessels**: Early stages vessels appear normal.

Electron Microscopy (Figs. 20.17A and B)

Thickening of the glomerular capillary wall: This is **due to irregular electron-dense deposits of immune complexes** between the basement membrane and the overlying visceral epithelial cells (**subepithelial**). The **visceral epithelial cells show effaced foot processes.**

Spike and dome pattern: In **between the immune deposits, the basement membrane material is laid down**, which appear as **irregular spikes protruding from the GBM. This is termed a spike and dome pattern.** Changes due to subepithelial immune complexes are divided into stages:

- **Stage I: Capillary walls are normal or show mild thickening** and subepithelial dense deposits.
- **Stage II: Projections of GBM material around dense deposits,** that **appear as spikes** on the epithelial surface of the basement membrane, which stain with silver.
- **Stage III:** As the disease progresses, the **basement membrane encircles the deposits** and is laid over the immune deposits. This will bury (incorporate) them within a markedly thickened, irregular membrane. In silver stain, they appear as dome-like protrusions.
- **Stage IV:** Later in the disease, the incorporated immune deposits undergo **degradation and lysis** leaving cavities within the GBM.

If the deposition of the basement membrane matrix continues, it causes progressive thickening of basement membranes. This may result in sclerosis of the glomeruli.

Immunofluorescence Microscopy

It shows **granular deposits** of both **immunoglobulins (IgG) and complement (C3)** in the **subepithelial** (between the visceral epithelial cell and the GBM) region. There is also intense staining for the membrane attack complex.

Clinical Features

- Present as sudden onset **nephrotic syndrome.**
- **Nonselective proteinuria** (which is selective in minimal-change disease).
- **Does not respond to corticosteroid** therapy.
- **Serologic findings of anti-PLA2R:** It is helpful in the diagnosis and the titer is useful in monitoring response to therapy.

Course: Variable but generally follows an indolent and slowly progressive course.

SCENARIO-BASED ESSAY QUESTION

Q. A 45-year-old man complained of swelling in the extremities for 2 months and face especially eyelids (facial puffiness) for the past 3 months. Protein estimation of a 24-hour urine sample revealed 4.1 g of

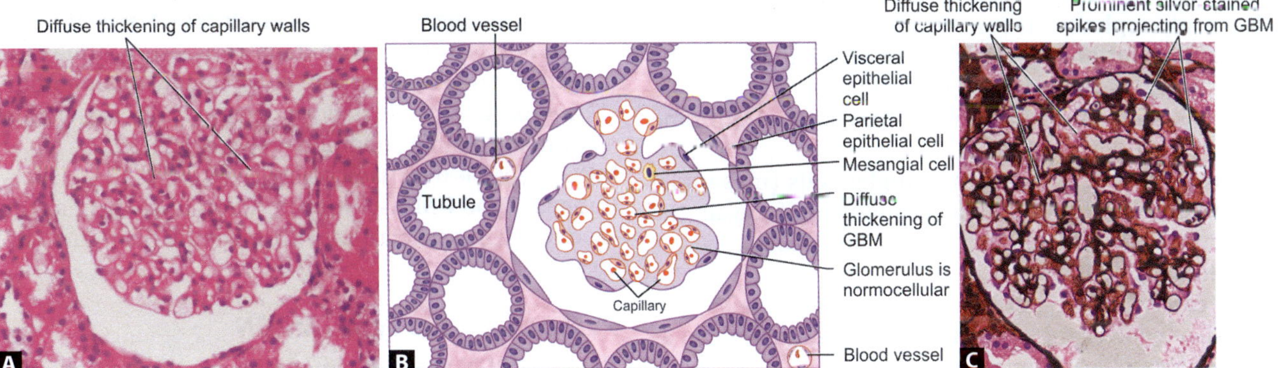

Figs. 20.16A to C: Light microscopy of membranous nephropathy: (A) Hematoxylin and eosin stain (H & E); (B) Diagrammatic of membranous nephropathy showing marked diffuse thickening of the GBM without an increase in the number of cells; (C) Silver methenamine stain showing marked thickening of capillary walls and prominent silver-stained spikes projecting from GBM.

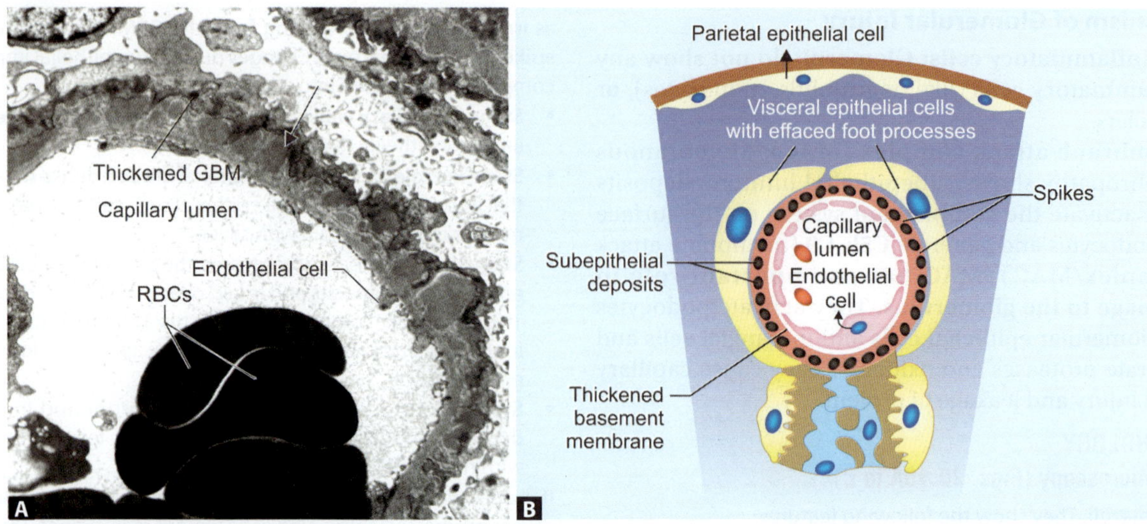

Figs. 20.17A and B: Electron microscopic appearance of membranous nephropathy: (A) Electron micrograph showing electron-dense deposits *(arrow)* along the epithelial side of the glomerular basement membrane (GBM); (B) Diagrammatic representation of electron microscopy of membranous glomerulopathy. Electron-dense deposits are seen along the epithelial side of the basement membrane. The visceral epithelial cells show effacement of foot processes overlying deposits.

Courtesy: Fig. A Dr Alok Sharma, Director, Renal Pathology and Electron Microscopy, National Reference Laboratory, Dr Lal PathLabs Ltd, New Delhi, India.

protein (albumin and globulins). His serum albumin level was 2.0 g/dL. Urine microscopy showed fat globules. A course of corticosteroid therapy was given and there was no response. A renal biopsy was performed and microscopic examination showed diffuse thickening of the glomerular basement membrane. Immunofluorescence staining with antibody to the C3 component of complement was positive in a granular pattern in the glomerular capillary loops.

a. **What is the probable diagnosis? (Ans: One of the most common causes of nephrotic syndrome in adults is membranous nephropathy).**
b. **Discuss the etiopathogenesis of this disease *(refer pages 726-7).***
c. **Describe the light microscopic, electron microscopic, and immunofluorescence findings in this condition *(refer page 727).***

Membranoproliferative Glomerulonephritis

Membranoproliferative glomerulonephritis **is a pattern of glomerular injury rather than a specific type of glomerulonephritis.** It **constitutes 5–10% of idiopathic nephrotic syndrome in children and young adults**. MPGN is histologically characterized by the following:

- **Thickening** of the **glomerular basement membrane (GBM).**
- **Proliferation** of mainly **mesangial cells (mesangial hypercellularity)** and accumulation of mesangial matrix. Also, proliferation of endothelial cells.
- **Leukocyte infiltration.**

Because the proliferation is mainly mesangial cells and also involves the capillary loops, it is also known as **mesangiocapillary glomerulonephritis**.

Former subclassification of MPGN: In the past, MPGN was subclassified based on distinct pathologic findings into two types (I and II). **Now, these two are recognized to be distinct entities.**

- **MPGN type I**: It shows the presence of immune complexes. It is more common and forms about 80% of cases.
- **Dense deposit disease (formerly MPGN type II)**: Type II is now termed a dense-deposit disease. It is due to the activation of the complement system without immune complexes. Dense deposit disease is discussed along with the related condition on pages 729-30.

MPGN type I is discussed below.

Causes: Type I MPGN may be idiopathic (primary) or secondary in association with systemic disorders (**Box 20.10**).

BOX 20.10: Causes of type I membranoproliferative glomerulonephritis (MPGN).

Idiopathic MPGN (Minority of Cases)

Secondary MPGN

- Chronic immune complex disorders: Autoimmune diseases (e.g., systemic lupus erythematosus), hepatitis B infection, hepatitis C infection
- Neoplasms: Cancer of the lung, breast; lymphoid tumors such as chronic lymphocytic leukemia; monoclonal gammopathy
- Human immunodeficiency virus (HIV) infection, schistosomiasis

Pathogenesis of Type I MPGN

Type I MPGN may be caused by the deposition of (i) circulating immune complexes or (ii) by the formation of an **in situ immune complex against a planted antigen.**

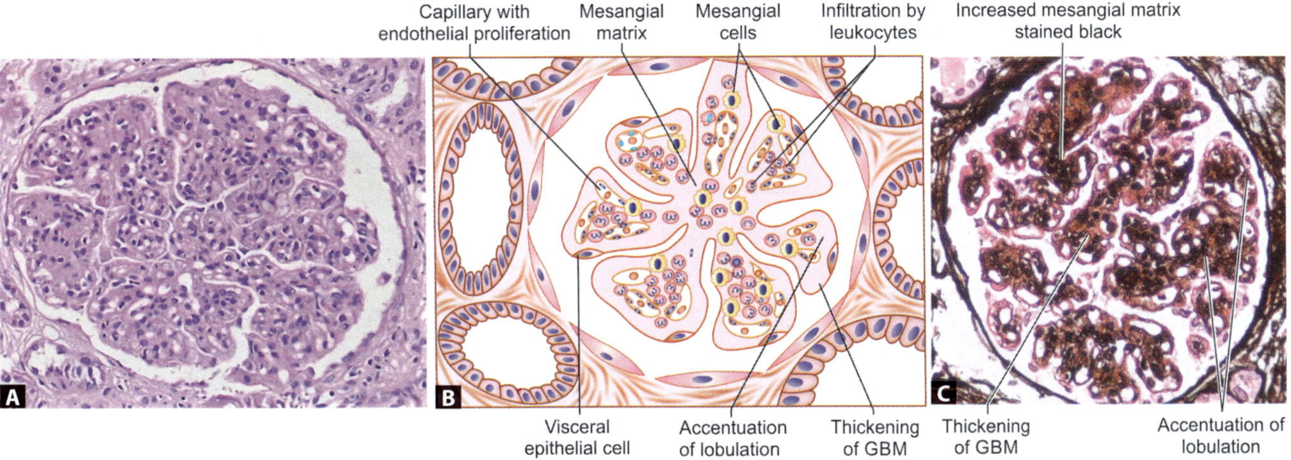

Figs. 20.18A to C: Type 1 membranoproliferative glomerulonephritis: (A) Hematoxylin and eosin (H & E); (B) Diagrammatic; (C) Silver methenamine stain. The glomerulus shows mesangial cell proliferation, increased mesangial matrix, thickening of GBM, accentuation of lobular architecture, and infiltration by leukocytes.

Courtesy: Fig. A Dr Alok Sharma, Director, Renal Pathology and Electron Microscopy, National Reference Laboratory, Dr Lal PathLabs Ltd, New Delhi, India.

They activate both classical and alternative complement pathways. In the majority of cases, it is secondary to an underlying disorder (*refer* **Box 20.10**). It is idiopathic in a minority of cases.

MORPHOLOGY

Light Microscopy

Glomeruli (Figs. 20.18A to C): The glomerular changes are as follows:

- **Large and hypercellular glomeruli:** It is due to:
  - Proliferation of (mesangial and endothelial) cells
  - Infiltration of **leukocytes**
  - **Epithelial crescents** are seen **in many cases.**
- **Accentuation of lobular architecture (lobular distortion or hypersegmentation):** It is due to the proliferating mesangial cells as well as an increased mesangial matrix.
- **Thickening of GBM:** It may be segmental and most prominent in the peripheral capillary loops.
- **Subendothelial immune complex deposits** stimulate the synthesis of new basement membrane producing **"duplication" of the basement membrane** (commonly called splitting). It produces a **"double-contour" or "tram-track"** appearance. This is better appreciated with **special stains such as silver or PAS**. The "splitting" of the GBM is due to: (i) the extension of mesangial processes and inflammatory cells into the peripheral capillary loops, (ii) the deposition of mesangial matrix, and (iii) subepithelial immune complexes.

Tubules: Epithelial cells of tubules may show vacuolation and droplets of hyaline.

Interstitium: It may show mild focal chronic inflammatory cells.

Blood vessels: During early stages appear normal but later may show changes due to hypertension.

Electron Microscopy

Shows discrete **subendothelial electron-dense deposits [Fig. 20.19B (*refer* online 20.19A)].**

Immunofluorescence

Deposits of **IgG and C3 produce a granular fluorescence pattern.** Early complement components (C1q and C4) are also usually found. These findings **suggest immune complex pathogenesis and activation of the classic complement pathway.**

Clinical Features

Age: Mostly found in adolescents or young adults.

Presentation: It presents with **nephrotic syndrome**, some only with hematuria or proteinuria in the non-nephrotic range, but many have a combined **nephrotic-nephritic picture.**

Urine findings: Proteinuria, oval fat bodies and, fatty casts.

The course of disease: Few remissions may occur spontaneously. The disease **usually follows a slowly progressive but unremitting course.** About 50% develop chronic renal failure. Some may develop crescents and develop RPGN.

C3 Glomerulopathy

The C3 glomerulopathy is a recent disease classification.

Sole or dominant staining for C3: C3 glomerulopathy is defined as the **glomerular accumulation of C3 with little or no Ig.** Kidneys with C3 glomerulopathy show sole or dominant staining for C3.

Classification of C3 glomerulopathy (Box 20.11): It consists of two conditions: (i) **dense deposit disease** (formerly called MPGN, type 2) and (ii) **C3 glomerulonephritis (C3 GN).** Both are relatively rare and **share certain clinical, morphologic, and pathogenic features.** However, **they differ in the electron microscopic appearance.**

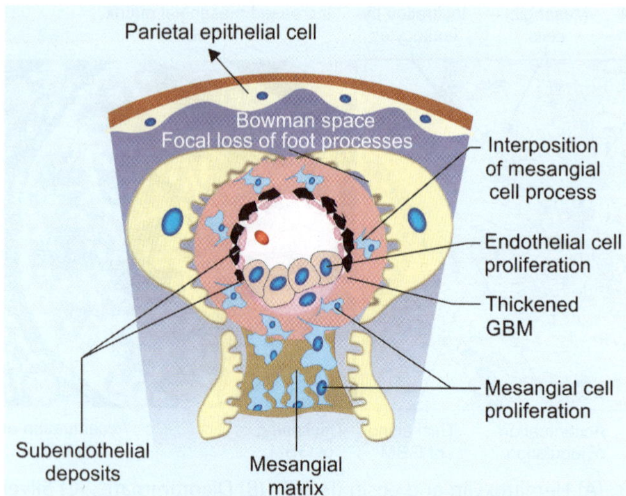

Fig. 20.19B: Type 1 membranoproliferative glomerulonephritis (MPGN): Diagrammatic electron microscopic appearance of MPGN characterized by hypercellular glomeruli (proliferation of endothelial and mesangial cells), thickened glomerular basement membrane (GBM), and narrowing of the capillary lumen (asterisk). Type I MPGN shows large subendothelial deposits of immune complexes, which extend along the inner border of the basement membrane.

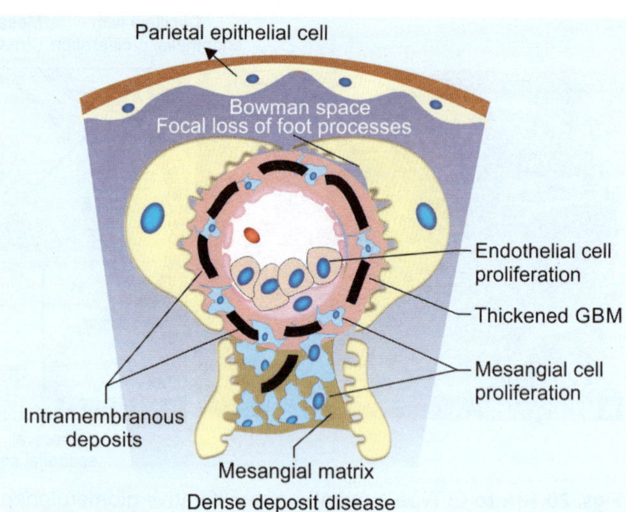

Fig. 20.20B: Dense deposit disease: Diagrammatic electron microscopic appearance of dense deposit disease [formerly called type II membranoproliferative glomerulonephritis (MPGN)] intramembranous deposits.

(GBM: glomerular basement membrane)

BOX 20.11: Classification of C3 glomerulopathy (C3 dominant, nonimmunoglobulin mediated).

Dense deposit disease (C3 dominant)
- Idiopathic
- Specific genetic mutations and/or autoantibodies to factors involved in the alternate complement pathway or regulatory factors of the alternate complement pathway

C3 glomerulonephritis

Specific genetic mutations and/or autoantibodies to factors involved in alternate complement pathway or regulatory factors of alternate complement pathway

Pathogenesis

Both dense deposit disease and C3 GN are **caused by complement dysregulation.** This may **either be due to acquired or hereditary abnormalities of the alternative pathway of complement activation [Fig. 20.20B (*refer* online Fig. 20.20A)]**. The supporting evidence for this is:

- **Consistently decreased serum C3 but normal C1 and C4**. The early components of complement (C1 and C4) are used only in the activation of the classical complement pathway.
- **Decreased serum levels** of **factor B and properdin**, which are the **components of the alternative complement pathway.**
- **Glomeruli with deposits of C3 and properdin but not IgG:** In the alternative complement pathway, C3 is directly cleaved to C3b. The glomeruli show deposits of C3 and properdin but not IgG.

The sequence of events of complement dysregulation **(Flowchart 20.3):**

- **Cleavage of C3 to C3b by alternate pathway:** Substances like **bacterial polysaccharides, endotoxin, and aggregates of IgA cleave C3 to C3b.**
- **Formation of alternative pathway C3 convertase: C3b in the presence of factors B and D generates C3bBb** (alternative pathway C3 convertase).
- **Degradation or stabilization of C3 convertase: C3bBb is labile** and **degraded by factors I** and **H** but **stabilized by properdin.**
- **C3 nephritic factor (C3NeF):** Some patients with C3 glomerulopathy have an activating autoantibody against C3 convertase in the serum. This is known as **C3 nephritic factor (C3NeF). C3NeF** acts at the same step as properdin and **stabilizes C3bBb and prevents its degradation.**
- **Uncontrolled and prolonged cleavage of C3:** C3NeF causes uncontrolled and prolonged cleavage of C3 by the alternative complement pathway.

In other patients, the cause of unregulated activation of the alternative pathway of complement may be due to mutations in various complement regulatory proteins. These include mutations in Factor H, Factor I, and membrane cofactor protein (MCP). It may also be due to autoantibodies to Factor H.

MORPHOLOGY

Light Microscopy

Dense deposit disease and C3 GN show a wide spectrum of microscopic changes. The classic light microscopic appearance is similar to that of the MPGN type I described earlier on page 729.

Flowchart 20.3: The alternative complement pathway in C3 glomerulopathy. Patients show C3NeF antibody in the serum, which acts at the same step as properdin and stabilizes the alternative pathway C3 convertase. This enhances C3 activation and consumption, resulting in hypocomplementemia.

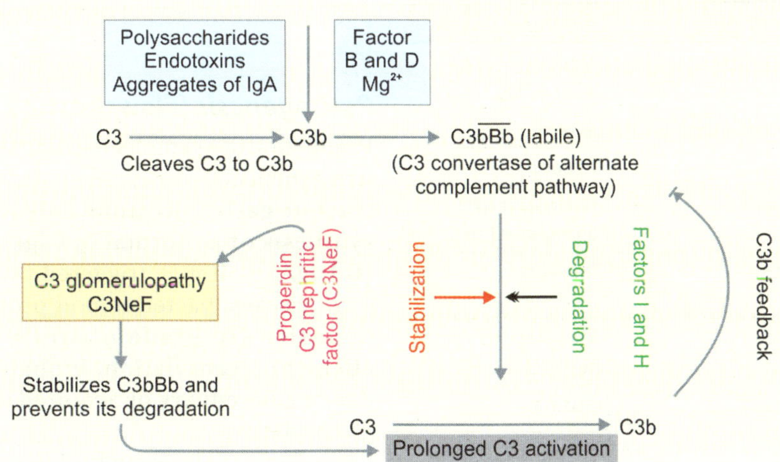

Glomeruli

- **Hypercellular glomeruli:** The glomeruli are hypercellular.
- **Duplication of the basement membranes of capillary walls.**
- **Mesangial proliferation**: The majority of cases show a mesangial proliferative pattern of injury, with an increase in the mesangial matrix or they may show **membranoproliferative patterns** (hypercellular with capillary walls showing duplicated **basement** membranes).
- **Inflammation and focal crescents**: It may be seen in some cases and others may show dense deposits of cellular material in the glomerular basement membranes.

Election Microscopy

The **defining feature of dense deposit disease and C3 GN by electron microscopy. Both differ in electron microscopic appearance.**

Dense deposit disease (Fig. 20.21): It shows **dense deposits** forming ribbons in the GBM. The lamina densa central zone of GBM is transformed into an **irregular, ribbon-like, homogeneous, extremely electron-dense** material structure resulting from the **deposition of C3-containing material.**

- **C3 glomerulonephritis:** It shows **mesangial and subendothelial electron dense "waxy" deposits.** Similar deposits also may be seen along the basement membranes of renal tubules.

Immunofluorescence

Its appearance suggests the activation of an alternate complement pathway.

- **Bright C3 staining is seen in the mesangial** (forms characteristic **circular aggregates termed mesangial rings) and glomerular capillary wall** in both dense deposit disease and C3 GN. In dense deposit disease, C3 staining also may be seen along the tubular basement membranes.
- **IgG and early complement components (C1q and C4) are absent in both conditions.** This indicates that there is no activation of the classical pathway of the complement system.

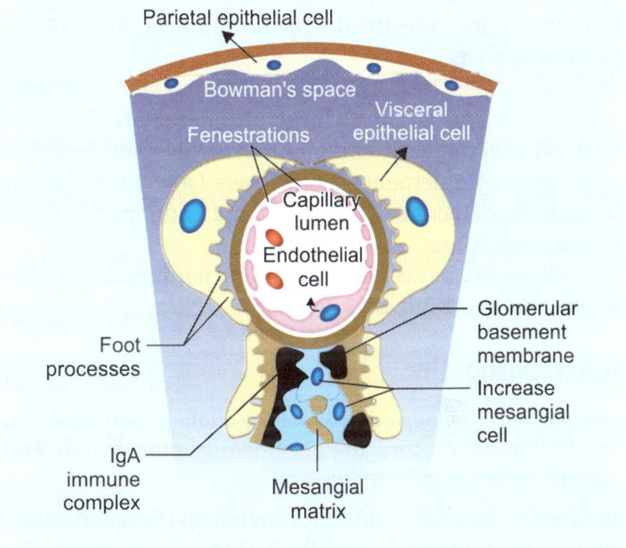

Fig. 20.21: Diagrammatic appearance of electron microscopic findings in immunoglobulin A (IgA) nephropathy. It shows the significant accumulation of IgA in the mesangium, most commonly between the mesangial cells and the glomerular basement membrane.

Clinical Features

Dense deposit disease (DDD): It mainly affects **children and young adults**. It manifests as a **nephritic syndrome with hematuria and/or nephrotic syndrome with proteinuria**. Clinical features overlap with those of MPGN. It is more likely to have **low serum C3 levels than patients with C3 GN**. The **prognosis is poor,** and >50% of cases progress to end-stage renal disease (ESRD). DDD recurs in 90% of transplant recipients.

C3 glomerulonephritis: They are reported in an **older age group** (mean age 30 years). They are clinically less

TABLE 20.3 Differences between nephritic and nephrotic syndrome.

Features	*Nephritic syndrome*	*Nephrotic syndrome*
Proteinuria	1–2 g/day	Massive; >3.5 g/day
Hematuria	Present	Absent
Hypertension	Present	Absent
Hypoalbuminemia	Absent	Present; serum albumin <3 g/dL
Hyperlipidemia and lipiduria	Not seen	Present
Edema	Mild	Moderate to severe
Azotemia and oliguria	Present	Absent
Microscopy of urine	RBC and RBC casts	Fatty casts

well-defined. About two-thirds of patients present with hematuria and one-third with proteinuria. They have a **poor prognosis.**

Investigations: These include **renal biopsy and serological and genetic evaluation. C3 levels are characteristically low with normal C4** (early complement involved in the classic pathway of complement system) levels. Other investigations include the detection of C3NeF, factor H, and specific CFHR genetic mutations.

Differences between nephritic and nephrotic syndrome is presented in **Table 20.3**.

IgA Nephropathy

PA 28.6 (CC): Define and describe the etiology, pathogenesis, pathology, laboratory, urinary findings, progression, and complications of IgA nephropathy.

Berger first described glomerulonephritis (Berger disease), now termed **immunoglobulin A (IgA) nephropathy**. IgA nephropathy is one of the **most common types of** primary **glomerulonephritis** revealed by renal biopsy **worldwide.**

Hallmark: IgA nephropathy is **characterized by prominent deposition of IgA-anti-IgA immune complexes in the mesangium. Clinically,** it manifests with **recurrent** episodic **hematuria (microscopic or gross)**.

Etiology

Immune complexes of poorly glycosylated IgA and autoantibodies: IgA is the main immunoglobulin (Ig) present in mucosal secretions. In plasma, it is present at low concentrations. IgA nephropathy is **caused by immune complexes consisting of an abnormally glycosylated IgA1 [i.e., galactose-deficient IgA1 (Gd-IgA1)] immunoglobulin and autoantibodies against this IgA.**

Genetic susceptibility: IgA nephropathy is **predominantly a sporadic disease**. However, genetic susceptibility may be uncommonly observed. Familial forms of IgA nephropathy can occur in families and in HLA identical siblings. More than 25% of blood relatives of IgA nephropathy patients have increased serum levels of poorly glycosylated IgA.

Pathogenesis (Flowchart 20.4)

Production of IgA molecules with abnormal glycosylation: In a genetically susceptible individual, **upper respiratory tract or gastrointestinal infections cause increased synthesis of abnormal IgA]galactose-deficient IgA1 (Gd-IgA1)]**. It may triggered by environmental agents (e.g., viruses, bacteria, food proteins). The **glomerular deposits are predominantly IgA molecules with aberrant glycosylation.** Probably, IgA nephropathy is due to a **hereditary or acquired defect causing aberrant glycosylation.**

Deposition of abnormally glycosylated IgA molecules in the mesangium or elicit the formation of autoantibody formation: Abnormal aberrantly glycosylated IgA1 is either (i) **directly deposited by itself in the mesangium** of glomeruli **or** (ii) **generates an autoimmune response** to produce IgG autoantibodies.

Formation of immune complexes: Immune complexes of IgA may be of two types:

- **Abnormal IgA1 directly deposited in the mesangium:** The abnormal IgA1 deposited in the mesangium is recognized by IgG and **forms in situ immune complexes.**
- **Autoimmune response:** Autoantibodies may be formed against abnormal IgA1. They form immune complexes in the circulation. These immune complexes get deposited in the mesangium of the glomerulus. This unusual location in mesangium may be due to the physicochemical characteristics of IgA and may be facilitated by an IgA1 receptor (CD71) on mesangial cells.

Activation of mesangial cells and recruitment of leukocytes: The mesangial immune deposits activate mesangial cells. These mesangial cells proliferate, produce excessive amounts of ECM, and secrete several cytokines and growth factors. The mediators further activate mesangial cells and may also recruit inflammatory cells into the glomeruli. The leukocytes injure the glomerulus and also stimulate a reparative response (includes opsonization and removal of the immune complexes).

Activation of alternate complement pathway: The deposited IgA cannot activate the classical complement pathway. The IgA-deposited and IgA-containing immune complexes activate the alternative and lectin complement pathway. It shows C3 in the mesangium and there is the absence of early components of complement, namely C1q and C4 points (involved in the classical pathway). This suggests the activation of the alternative complement pathway in its pathogenesis.

Flowchart 20.4: Various steps involved in the pathogenesis of immunoglobulin A (IgA) nephropathy.

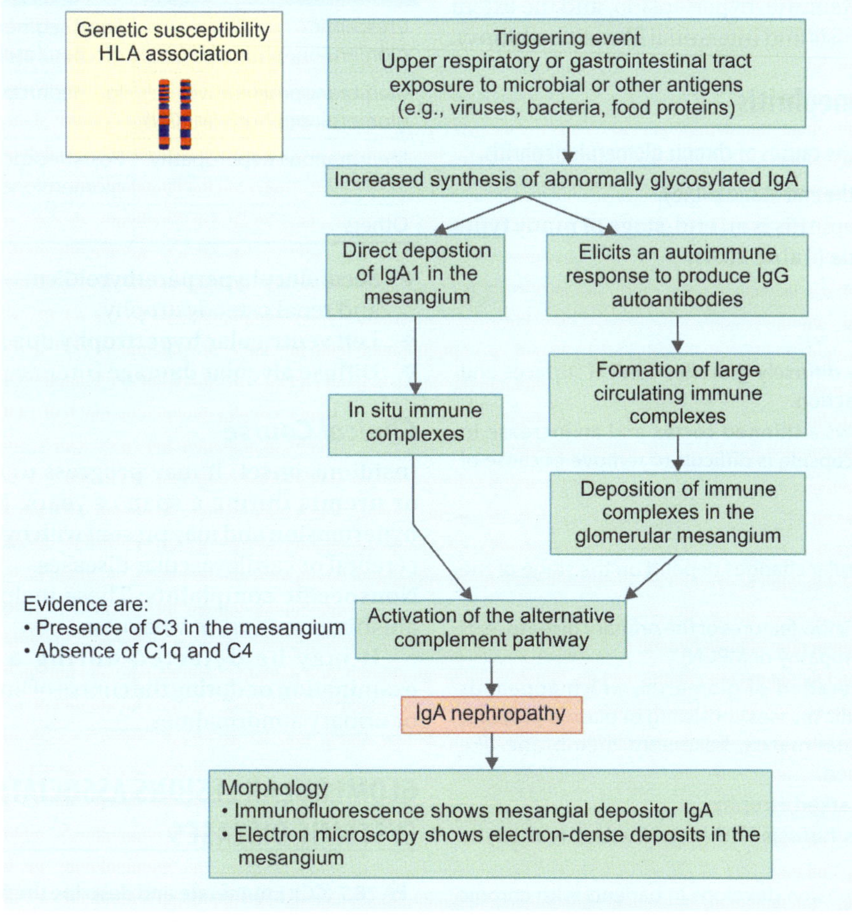

(HLA: human leukocyte antigen; IgG: immunoglobulin G)

The above concept is supported by the fact that increased frequency of IgA nephropathy occurs in individuals with celiac disease (there is a defect in intestinal mucosa), and in liver disease (where there is defective hepatobiliary clearance of IgA complexes).

MORPHOLOGY

Light Microscopy

The lesions are variable.

Glomeruli

- **Mesangial widening and hypercellularity**: Glomeruli may appear normal or **may show mesangial widening, and hypercellularity.**
- **Segmental inflammation**: Inflammation may be restricted to some glomeruli (focal proliferative GN)
- **Diffuse mesangial proliferation (mesangioproliferative** GN); or (rarely) **frank crescentic GN.**

Immunofluorescence: It is essential for the diagnosis of IgA nephropathy. It shows a **mesangial deposit of IgA**, usually with C3 and properdin and smaller amounts of IgG or IgM. Early components of the classical complement pathway are usually not seen.

Electron microscopy (Fig. 20.21): Shows **electron-dense deposits in the mesangium.**

Clinical Features

- Occurs in **children and young males.**
- Presents with **asymptomatic/painless microscopic hematuria or recurrent macroscopic hematuria** generally within 1–2 days after a nonspecific upper respiratory or gastrointestinal viral infection. The hematuria usually lasts for several days and initially subsides. Then hematuria periodically recurs usually in association with a viral infection.
- Proteinuria occurs and in 5% it can be in the nephrotic range.
- Occasionally, it may present as acute renal failure (ARF) or nephritic syndrome.

Diagnosis by renal biopsy: Immunofluorescence microscopy shows prominent **IgA deposits** in the mesangial regions.

Course and prognosis: Course is highly variable.

- **Prognosis is usually good** and many patients maintain normal renal function for decades.
- **Risk of development of** slowly progressing **end-stage renal failure** in about 25% of patients over a period of 20 years.

- **Poorer prognostic indicators** are onset at old age, male gender, heavy proteinuria, hypertension, and the extent of glomerulosclerosis and interstitial fibrosis on biopsy.

Chronic Glomerulonephritis

Q. Write a short note on the causes of chronic glomerulonephritis.

Q. Write a short note on the end-stage kidney.

Chronic glomerulonephritis is an **end-stage of many types of glomerulonephritis (Table 20.4).**

MORPHOLOGY

Gross (Figs. 20.22A to C)

- **Both kidneys** show **diffusely granular** cortical surfaces and **symmetrical contraction.**
- **Cut section:** It shows a **thinned cortex** and an **increase in peripelvic fat.** The **capsule is difficult to remove** because of adhesions.

Microscopy

Glomeruli: The glomerular changes depend on the stage of the disease:

- **Early stages:** It may show features of the **primary disease** (e.g., membranous nephropathy or MPGN).
- **Late stages: Obliteration of glomeruli,** which appear as **acellular eosinophilic masses** consisting of plasma proteins, increased mesangial matrix, basement membrane-like material, and collagen.

Tubules: They show **marked atrophy.**

Interstitium: It shows fibrosis and mononuclear leukocytic infiltration.

Blood vessels: Hypertension develops in patients with chronic glomerulonephritis and the **vascular changes of hypertension** such as **arterial and arteriolar sclerosis** may be seen (*refer* page 494).

Uremic complications: Patients with chronic renal failure may show complications due to uremia (for features of uremia, *refer* **Table 20.1**). These include:

- Uremic **pericarditis**
- Uremic **gastroenteritis**

TABLE 20.4 Causes of chronic glomerulonephritis.

Crescentic glomerulonephritis (RPGN)	Focal segmental glomerulosclerosis (FSGS)
Membranoproliferative glomerulonephritis (MPGN)	IgA nephropathy
Membranous nephropathy	Poststreptococcal glomerulonephritis—rare
Others	

- **Secondary hyperparathyroidism** with nephrocalcinosis and renal osteodystrophy
- **Left ventricular hypertrophy** due to hypertension
- **Diffuse alveolar damage** (uremic pneumonitis).

Clinical Course

Insidious onset: It may **progress to renal insufficiency or uremia** during a span of years. Most patients have **hypertension** and may present with hypertension-induced cerebral or cardiovascular diseases.

Nonspecific complaints: These include loss of appetite, anemia, vomiting, or weakness.

It **may be detected during a routine medical examination or** during the course of investigation of edema or urinary abnormalities.

GLOMERULAR LESIONS ASSOCIATED WITH SYSTEMIC DISEASES

PA 28.7 (CC): Enumerate and describe the findings in glomerular manifestations of systemic disease.

Lupus Nephritis

Q. Write a short note on lupus nephritis.

- **SLE is an autoimmune disease**: Systemic lupus erythematosus (SLE) is an autoimmune disease. In this, autoantibodies are produced against their own nuclear proteins and other self-antigens. **Renal (kidney)**

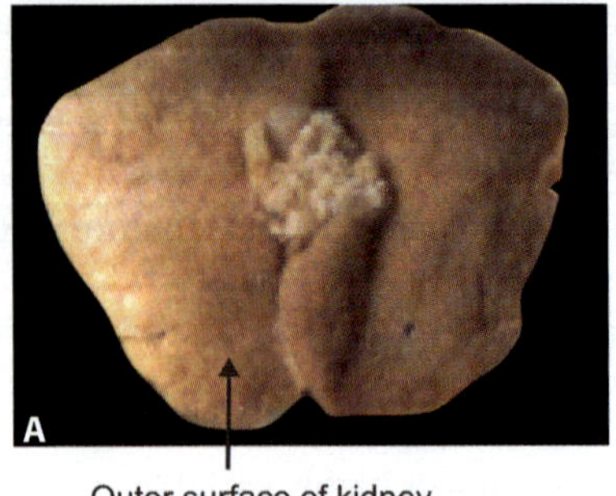

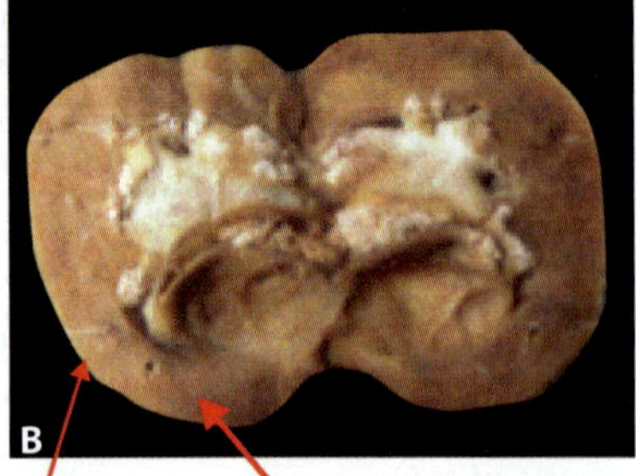

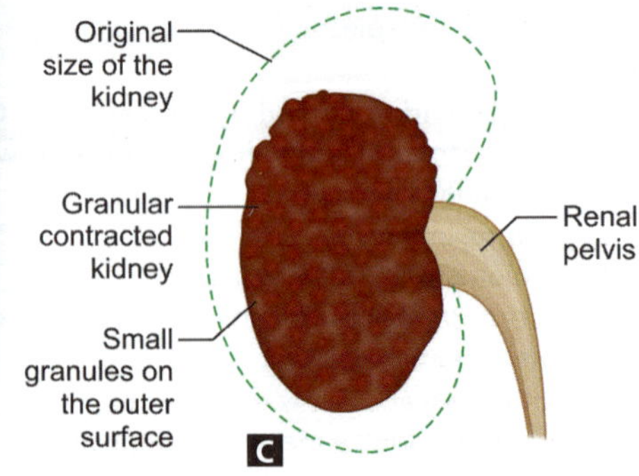

Figs. 20.22A to C: Gross features of chronic glomerulonephritis: (A) Outer aspect shows contracted kidney with diffusely granular surface; (B) Cut section shows thinned cortex and loss of demarcation between cortex and medulla; (C) Diagrammatic appearance of chronic GN.

changes in systemic lupus erythematosus (SLE) are known as lupus nephritis and are seen in up to 50% of SLE patients.

- It is an **immune complex-mediated** (type III hypersensitivity reaction) disease. The main mechanism of renal injury is by immune complex, which consists of **DNA and anti-DNA antibodies.** Morphological features are presented on page 207.

Diabetic Nephropathy

Diabetic nephropathy is the term used for **collective lesions that often occur together in the diabetic kidney**. Diabetic nephropathy can develop in both insulin-dependent type 1 diabetes and type 2 diabetes.

Pathogenesis

Diabetic glomerulosclerosis represents a part of the generalized diabetic microangiopathy that involves small vessels throughout the body (*refer* page 892).

In diabetes, **insulin deficiency, hyperglycemia (or glucose intolerance), and metabolic defects** cause **biochemical alterations.**

- **Nonenzymatic glycosylation and formation of advanced glycation end-products:** In diabetics, glucose binds to protein nonenzymatically to form advanced glycation end-products (AGEs). These AGEs produce their effects either by binding to their specific receptors (RAGE) or by direct action and include: **increased synthesis of extracellular matrix, increased production of reactive oxygen species, and direct cross-linking with extracellular matrix proteins.**
  - **Consequences: Cross-linking with collagen type IV** in glomerular basement membrane (GBM) results in increased collagen type IV and fibronectin and decreased heparin sulfate proteoglycans. This results in the **thickening of GBM and increased mesangial matrix.**
- **Hemodynamic changes:** They cause **glomerular hypertrophy** and may also be responsible for the initiation and progression of diabetic glomerulosclerosis. Both **advanced glycosylated end-products and hemodynamic changes** contribute to the **loss of podocytes.** This may occur due to apoptosis of podocytes in response to metabolic abnormalities and exposure to reactive oxygen species.
- **Disturbances in polyol pathways: This increases** the glomerular cells' **susceptibility** to oxidative stress.

Renal Changes in Diabetes

Q. Write a short note on renal changes in diabetes mellitus (diabetic nephropathy).

The **kidneys** are the **main targets** of diabetes. **Renal failure** is second only to myocardial infarction as a **cause of death** in diabetes.

MORPHOLOGY

Renal lesions in diabetes can involve any component. Four varieties of lesions are encountered namely:

- Glomerular lesions
- Renal vascular lesions (mainly arteriolosclerosis)
- Pyelonephritis (including necrotizing papillitis)
- Tubular lesions.

Glomerular Lesions (Figs. 20.23 and 20.24)

They are the most **important and common renal lesions.** These include: (a) thickening of capillary basement membrane (GBM), (b) diffuse mesangial sclerosis, and (c) nodular glomerulosclerosis (Kimmelstiel–Wilson nodules).

Diffuse widespread thickening glomerular capillary basement membrane (Figs. 20.23A to C): It occurs in almost all cases of diabetic nephropathy. It represents part and parcel of diabetic microangiopathy. This can be observed under electron microscopy within a few years of the onset of diabetes.

Diffuse mesangial sclerosis: It is characterized by a **diffuse increase in the PAS-positive mesangial matrix associated with the proliferation of mesangial cells and thickening of GBM.** As the disease progresses, the mesangial areas can expand to assume a nodular appearance. It is seen in most diabetics of more than 10 years' duration. It is more common in older

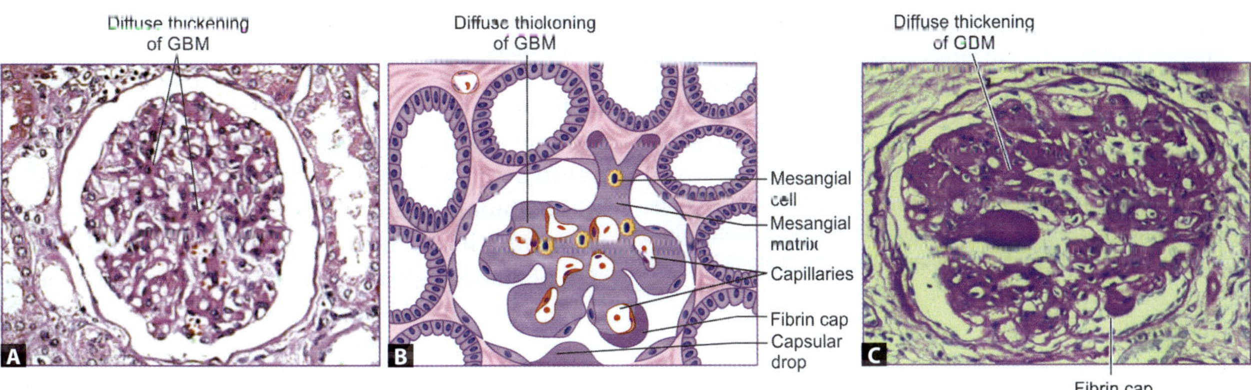

Figs. 20.23A to C: (A) Hematoxylin and eosin (H & E stain); (B) Diagrammatic; (C) PAS stain. Diabetic nephropathy glomeruli with diffuse widespread thickening glomerular capillary basement membrane and insulative lesions (fibrin cap and capsular drop).

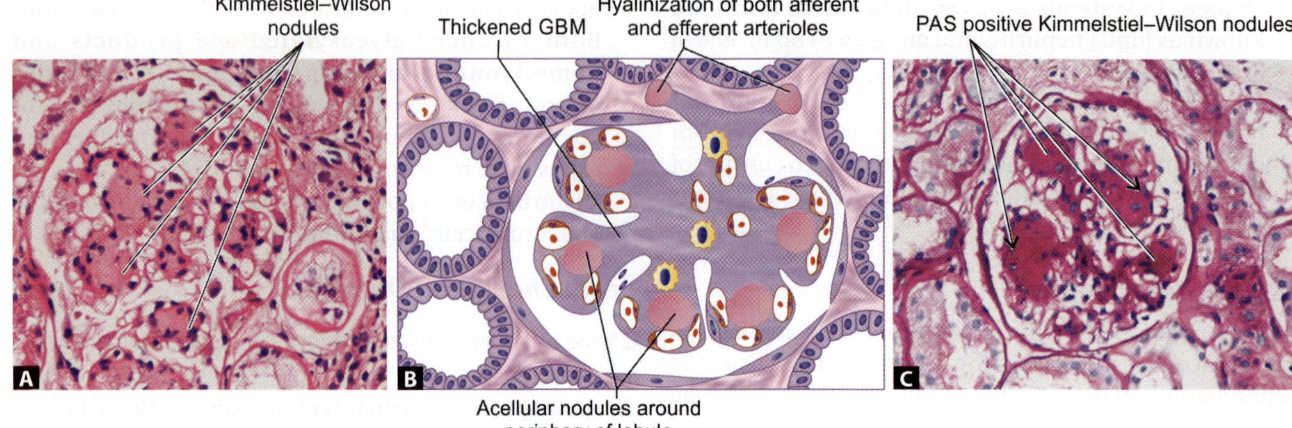

Figs. 20.24A to C: Diabetic nephropathy: (A) Hematoxylin and eosin (H & E stain); (B) Diagrammatic; (C) PAS stain. Nodular glomerulosclerosis shows oval nodules of the mesangial matrix at the periphery of the glomerulus, (C) Nodules are PAS positive.

patients and those with hypertension. Severe glomerulosclerosis leads to the development of nephrotic syndrome (proteinuria, hypoalbuminemia, and edema).

Nodular glomerulosclerosis (Figs. 20.24A to C): It is also called **intercapillary glomerulosclerosis or Kimmelstiel–Wilson disease** and **is pathognomonic of diabetic nephropathy.**

Q. Write a short note on Kimmelstiel–Wilson (KW) lesion.

- Glomerular lesion consists of **ovoid or spherical**, often laminated, **nodules of mesangial matrix** seen within the mesangial core and **situated in the periphery of the glomerulus.** These nodules can be surrounded by peripheral capillary loops with patent or dilated lumen. The nodules are **PAS-positive (Fig. 20.24C).** As the disease advances, the individual nodules increase in size and compress the surrounding capillaries.
- **Develops in about 15–30%** of long-term diabetes and is **mostly associated with renal failure.**

Insudative lesions: These include fibrin cap and capsular drop.

- **Fibrin caps:** These are **prominent subendothelial** accumulations of **hyaline material** in/along capillary loops.
- **Capsular drops:** They consist of **round nodules adherent to Bowman's capsules** and are **seen between Bowman's capsule and the parietal epithelium.**

Renal Vascular Lesions

- **Hyaline arteriosclerosis** (hyalinosis): It involves **both the afferent and the efferent arteriole** at the hilum of glomeruli. **Arteriolosclerosis of efferent arteriole is rare in nondiabetics.**
- **Renal atherosclerosis:** It constitutes part of the macrovascular disease in diabetics. It involves arteries and arterioles and is similar to those found in other parts of the body.

Glomerular and arteriolar lesions together produce **renal ischemia** leading to atrophy of tubules, interstitial fibrosis, and contraction of the kidney. It manifested as a kidney with finely granular cortical surface (nephrosclerosis).

Pyelonephritis

It is a tubulointerstitial inflammation of the kidneys.

- Both **acute and chronic pyelonephritis** occur in nondiabetics as well as in diabetics. It is **more common** and tends to be **more severe** in diabetics than in the general population.
- **Necrotizing papillitis** (or papillary necrosis): It is one **special pattern of acute pyelonephritis** and is much more frequent in diabetics compared to nondiabetics. **Hyaline arteriolosclerosis** narrows blood vessels and **reduces the blood supply** to the renal medulla. The ischemia causes **necrosis of the tips of papillae** (papillary necrosis).

Tubular Lesions

The basement membrane of the tubules shows thickening. In patients with high blood sugar levels, the **epithelial cells of the proximal convoluted tubules show extensive deposits of vacuoles of glycogen.** These are known as **Armanni–Ebstein lesions.**

Renal changes in diabetes mellitus (diabetic nephropathy) are summarized in **Box 20.12.**

Electron Microscopy (Fig. 20.25)

- **Thickening of the lamina densa** of the glomerular basement membrane.
- **Increase in the mesangial matrix**, particularly in nodular lesions.
- **Insudative lesions** appear as electron-dense masses.

Immunofluorescence Microscopy

It reveals IgG, albumin, fibrinogen, and other **plasma** proteins in the GBM.

Clinical features: Glomerular lesions in diabetic nephropathy may present with **non-nephrotic proteinuria, nephrotic syndrome, and chronic renal failure. Microalbuminuria** is urinary excretion of 30–300 mg of albumin/24 hours. Microalbuminuria is the **first laboratory sign of diabetic glomerulopathy.** Liver-fatty acid binding protein (L-FABP) is a biomarker of diabetic nephropathy and chronic kidney disease.

Amyloidosis: The kidney is the most common and the most serious form of organ involvement in amyloidosis (renal amyloidosis—*refer* page 210).

BOX 20.12: Renal changes in diabetes mellitus (diabetic nephropathy).

1. Glomerular lesions:
   - Diffuse thickening of glomerular capillary basement membrane
   - Diffuse mesangial sclerosis
   - Nodular glomerulosclerosis (pathognomonic)
   - Insudative lesions: Fibrin cap and capsular drop
2. Renal vascular lesions:
   - Hyalinization of afferent and efferent glomerular hilar arterioles
   - Arteriolosclerosis of renal arteries and arterioles
3. Pyelonephritis:
   - Acute and chronic pyelonephritis
   - Necrotizing papillitis
4. Tubular lesions:
   - Armanni–Ebstein lesions

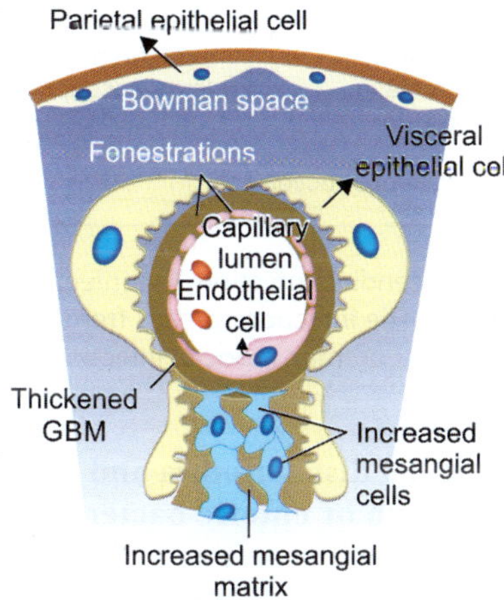

Fig. 20.25: Diagrammatic electron microscopic appearance of diabetic glomerulosclerosis showing thickened glomerular basement membrane, increased mesangial cells, and mesangial matrix.

Causes of necrotizing papillitis:

- Diabetes mellitus
- Analgesic nephropathy
- Sickle cell anemia
- Obstructive uropathy

DISEASES AFFECTING TUBULES AND INTERSTITIUM

PA 28.8 (CC): Enumerate and classify diseases affecting the tubular interstitium.

Most types of tubular injury also affect the interstitium of the kidney. Therefore, they are considered together as tubulointerstitial diseases **(Box 20.13)**.

Major categories: Three major categories of tubulointerstitial diseases are: (1) infection of the kidney and urinary tract *(pyelonephritis)*, (2) noninfectious inflammation affecting the tubules and interstitium *(tubulointerstitial nephritis)*, and (3) ischemic or toxic tubular injury, leading to *acute tubular injury* and the clinical syndrome of *acute kidney injury.*

BOX 20.13: Classification of tubular and interstitial diseases.

- Acute kidney injury
- Tubulointerstitial diseases
- Pyelonephritis and urinary tract infections
- Tubulointerstitial nephritis
- Other tubulointerstitial diseases
  - Urate nephropathy
  - Hypercalcemia and nephrocalcinosis

Urinary tract infection (UTI) can be classified as:

- **Lower urinary tract infections:** These include **cystitis** (bladder) and **urethritis**. Bacterial infection of the lower urinary tract may be completely asymptomatic (asymptomatic bacteriuria). In most cases, it remains localized to the bladder. However, lower urinary tract infection always carries the risk of spread to the kidney.
- **Upper urinary tract infections (pyelonephritis):** It involves **kidneys and their collecting systems.** Or
- **Both upper and lower UTI.**

Pyelonephritis

Q. Write a short essay on pyelonephritis.

Definition: Pyelonephritis is an **inflammatory disease** of the kidney **affecting the tubules, interstitium, and renal pelvis.**

Pyelonephritis is one of the most common diseases of the kidney.

Classification of pyelonephritis: Pyelonephritis may be acute or chronic.

- **Acute pyelonephritis:** It is caused by bacterial infection and is associated with urinary tract infection.
- **Chronic pyelonephritis:** It is a more complex disorder. However, bacterial infection plays a major role, but other factors (vesicoureteral reflux, obstruction) are also involved in its pathogenesis.

Acute Pyelonephritis

PA 28.10a (CC): Describe the etiology, pathogenesis, pathology, laboratory findings, and complications of acute pyelonephritis.

Acute pyelonephritis is an **acute suppurative inflammation of the kidney** (affecting the tubules, and interstitium), **and renal pelvis caused by bacterial infections.**

Etiology and Pathogenesis (Figs. 20.26A and B)

Q. Write a short note on the etiopathogenesis of acute pyelonephritis.

Causative organisms: The majority (~85%) of urinary tract infections are caused by gram-negative bacilli, which are normal inhabitants of the intestinal tract (enteric origin). Sometimes, it may be caused by viral (e.g., polyomavirus) infection.

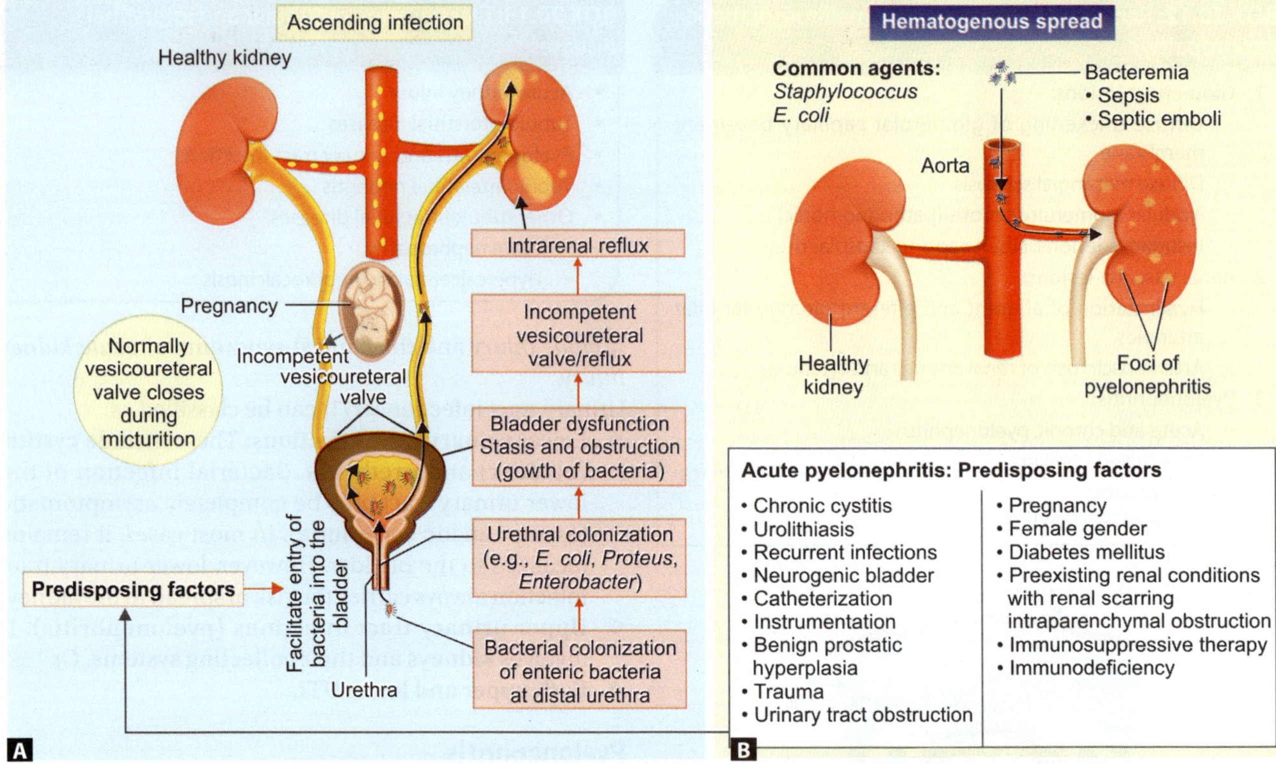

Figs. 20.26A and B: Pathogenesis of acute pyelonephritis: (A) A more common mode is ascending infection. This infection develops due to a combination of urinary bladder infection, vesicoureteral reflux, and intrarenal reflux. The infection spreads from renal calyces into the renal cortex; (B) Hematogenous infection results from the bacteremic spread. It is a less common mode of infection and leads to foci of pyelonephritis that may form abscesses.

- **Common pathogens:** ***Escherichia coli*** (most common), ***Proteus, Klebsiella, and Enterobacter***, and *Pseudomonas*.
- **Less common:** *Streptococcus faecalis*, staphylococci, and fungi.
- **In immunocompromised patients: Viruses** (polyomavirus, cytomegalovirus, and adenovirus).

Recurrent infections may develop in patients who undergo urinary tract manipulations or have congenital or acquired anomalies of the lower urinary tract.

Source and Route of Infection

Bacteria can reach the kidney by two routes namely (1) by ascending infection (from the lower urinary tract) or (2) through hematogenous infection (through the bloodstream).

Ascending infection (Fig. 20.26A)

It is the **most common route** of infection of pyelonephritis. It is a form of endogenous infection, where the source of infecting organisms is the **patient's own fecal flora**. The infection ascends from the lower urinary tract into the renal parenchyma. **Different steps** in the pathogenesis of pyelonephritis are:

Colonization of the distal urethra and introitus (in the female) **by coliform or enteric bacteria**: By enteric or coliform bacteria from the perineum due to poor hygiene and hormonal effects. It produces cystitis (inflammation of the urinary bladder).

Entry from the urethra to the urinary bladder: Bladder infections (cystitis) usually precede the development of acute pyelonephritis. Organisms may enter the bladder with instrumentation or without instrumentation.

- **With instrumentation:** Instrumentation includes urethral catheterization or other instrumentation through which organisms can enter from the urethra to the bladder. Notably, long-term catheterization carries a risk of infection.
- **Without instrumentation**: In the absence of instrumentation, urinary infections **more commonly occur in females. Reasons include** any combination of the following factors:
  - Shorter urethra and its closeness to the rectum in the females. Prostatic fluid has antibacterial properties, and it is absent in females.
  - Hormonal changes in women can affect the adherence of bacteria to the mucosa.
  - Trauma to the urethra during sexual intercourse facilitates the migration of bacteria.

Ascent of microbes from the bladder to the ureters: Normally, the urinary bladder empties all but 2–3 mL of residual urine. If organisms enter the bladder, adding sterile urine from the kidneys dilutes the organism. The organism is cleared by continual voiding of urine and by antibacterial mechanisms. However, if the volume of the residual urine is increased, sterile urine from the kidneys may be insufficient to dilute residual bladder urine to prevent the accumulation of organisms. Similar to an obstruction, the residual urine in the urinary bladder favors bacterial growth. Conditions that predispose to the ascent of infection include **obstruction to the outflow of urine in the urinary tract or bladder dysfunction.** It causes **incomplete emptying** and **increased residual volume of urine.**

- **Lower urinary tract obstruction:** Urinary tract infection is frequent in patients with lower urinary tract obstruction. Examples of obstructions include **benign prostatic hypertrophy, tumors, or calculi.**
- **Neurogenic bladder dysfunction:** For example, diabetic neuropathy or spinal cord injury such as paraplegia. Diabetic glycosuria also favors a rich bacterial growth medium.
- **Stasis: Organisms** introduced into the bladder **can multiply** when there is stasis.

Vesicoureteral reflux: The organism in bladder urine usually does not ascend into the ureter. The normal vesicoureteral valve acts as a one-way valve. During micturition, the intravesicular pressure rises and occludes the lumen of distal ureters and prevents retrograde flow of urine from the bladder to the ureter. Obstruction is an important predisposing factor in ascending infection. An **incompetent vesicoureteral orifice/valve results in vesicoureteral reflux (VUR). This VUR allows the infected bladder urine into the ureters and is an important cause of ascending infection.** Then it **propels into the renal pelvis.** Incompetent vesicoureteral orifice/valve may be congenital or acquired.

- **Congenital vesicoureteral reflux** (e.g., congenital absence or shortening of the intravesical portion of the ureter). This reflux can force the urine into the renal pelvis and calyces.
- **Acquired vesicoureteral reflux:** Vesicoureteral reflux may be acquired by infection of the bladder. In adults, acquired vesicoureteral reflux may be observed due to persistent bladder atony caused by spinal cord injury.

Infections usually remain localized in the urinary bladder in individuals without vesicoureteral reflux. Thus, most of individuals with repeated or persistent bacterial colonization of the urinary tract develop cystitis and urethritis (lower urinary tract infection) without pyelonephritis.

Intrarenal reflux: Even if vesicoureteral reflux pressure delivers bacteria to the calyces, the renal parenchyma need not be contaminated. Intrarenal reflux allows easier passage of infecting organisms through open ducts at the tips of papillae deep into the renal parenchyma through to the collecting system. **Intrarenal reflux is most common at both the poles of the kidney**, namely the upper and lower poles.

Hematogenous route (Fig. 20.26B)

Bacteria and other pathogens can produce pyelonephritis through the bloodstream, causing hematogenous pyelonephritis. It is a less common route of infection of pyelonephritis. Because of the rich blood supply, bacteria can seed the kidneys **during septicemia** or localized infections such as **infective endocarditis** through the bloodstream. It occurs with **nonenteric organisms** (e.g., gram-positive organisms such as staphylococci), fungi (*Candida* and *Aspergillus*), and viruses. Hematogenous infections occur in the presence of ureteral obstruction, debilitated patients, and patients receiving immunosuppressive therapy (e.g., fungi, such as *Aspergillus*). Hematogenous infections preferentially affect the cortex, whereas ascending infection affects the renal medulla.

MORPHOLOGY

Gross

- Acute pyelonephritis may be **unilateral or bilateral.** The involved kidney may be normal in size or enlarged.
- **Focal, discrete, yellowish raised abscesses (Fig. 20.27A):** These may be seen on the **subcapsular surface** that appears small and **white.** In pyelonephritis associated with reflux, they are **most common in the lower and upper poles.**
- **Pelvic and calyces:** They may be **hyperemic and covered by purulent exudate.**

Microscopy

The pathognomonic features of acute pyelonephritis are: (1) **patchy suppurative inflammation of interstitium, (2) intratubular aggregates of neutrophils, (3) neutrophilic tubulitis, and (4) injury to tubules**

- **Interstitium: It shows patchy interstitial neutrophilic infiltration,** which may later become extensive.
- **Tubules: Intratubular aggregates of neutrophils (Fig. 20.27 B)** form abscess with the destruction of the involved tubules and **necrosis of tubular epithelial cells.**
- **Glomeruli:** They appear normal because they are relatively resistant to the infection.

Complications

Q. Write a short note on complications of acute pyelonephritis.

1. **Papillary necrosis:** It is the **necrosis of the tips of the renal papillae.**
   - Seen mainly in **diabetics,** with **urinary tract obstruction,** and sickle cell anemia.
   - **Usually bilateral** but may be unilateral. One or all of the pyramids of the affected kidney may be involved.
   - **Cut section**: The **tips or distal two-thirds of the renal pyramids** show areas of gray-white to yellow **necrosis.**

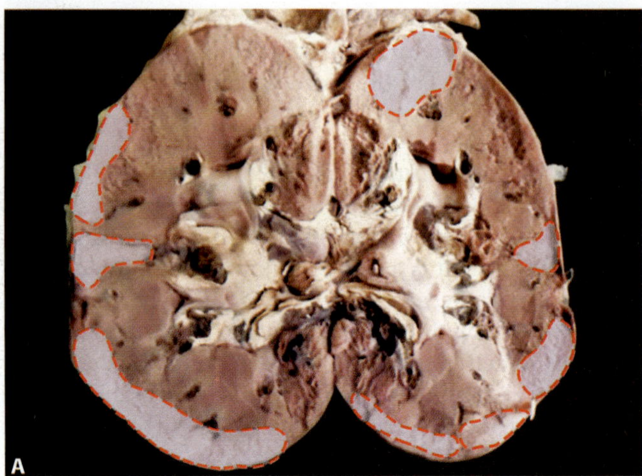
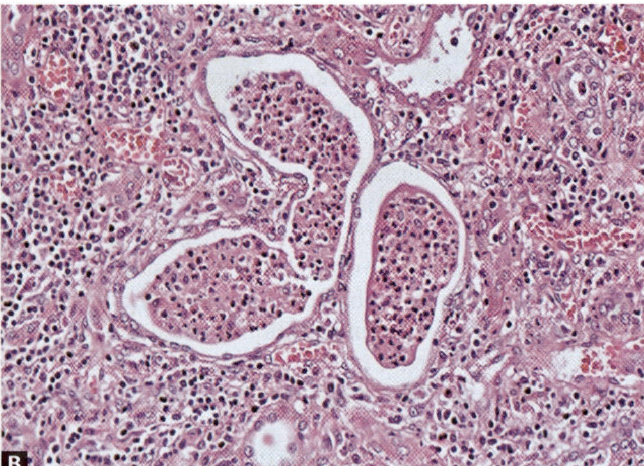

Figs. 20.27A and B: (A) Gross appearance of acute pyelonephritis showing focal abscesses (dotted outlines) in the cortical region; (B) A case of acute on chronic pyelonephritis showing neutrophilic exudates within two tubules. The interstitium shows mainly chronic inflammatory cells.

- **Microscopy**: The necrotic area shows **coagulative necrosis**, with preservation of tubular outline.

2. **Pyonephrosis:** It is characterized by the accumulation of **pus** (suppurative exudates) **within the renal pelvis, calyces, and ureter.** The kidney becomes distended with pus and the pus does not drain. This complication develops when there is a total or complete obstruction to the urinary drainage high in the urinary tract near the kidney.
3. **Perinephric abscess**: It develops when the **suppurative infection breaks the renal capsule** and spreads into the perinephric tissue.

Clinical Features

These include a **sudden onset of pain at the costovertebral angle** and systemic evidence of infection. These include **fever, chills, sweats, and malaise**. Usually, there are features indicative of bladder and urethral irritation. These symptoms are **dysuria, frequency, and urgency**.

Urinary Findings

Microscopy

- **Pus cells:** Urine shows many leukocytes (**pyuria**), but it does not differentiate upper from lower urinary tract infection.
- **WBC casts:** Casts are formed only in tubules and the finding of leukocyte casts, which are rich in neutrophils (pus cells), **indicates renal involvement** (i.e., pyelonephritis).

Culture and sensitivity: It can **establish the causative organism**.

Course of the disease: Usually, follows a benign course.

Chronic Pyelonephritis and Reflux Nephropathy

PA 28.10b (CC): Describe the etiology, pathogenesis, pathology, laboratory findings, distinguishing features progression, and complications of chronic pyelonephritis and reflux nephropathy.

Q. Discuss the etiopathogenesis, gross, and microscopy of chronic pyelonephritis.

Definition: Chronic pyelonephritis is a **clinicopathologic entity characterized by interstitial inflammation associated with grossly seen scarring of the kidneys and deformity of the pelvicalyceal system (renal calyces, and pelvis) in patients with a history of UTI.**

The pelvicalyceal damage is an important diagnostic clue for the diagnosis of chronic pyelonephritis.

Types and pathogenesis: Chronic pyelonephritis is an **important cause of end-stage renal disease (ESRD)**. Chronic pyelonephritis may be of two types:

- **Chronic reflux-associated pyelonephritis (reflux nephropathy) (Fig. 20.28A):** It is the most common cause of chronic pyelonephritis.
    - **Reflux with superadded infection:** This type **develops** due to the **superimposition of urinary infection on congenital vesicoureteral reflux and intrarenal reflux**.
    - **Unilateral or bilateral:** Reflux **may be unilateral or bilateral** and accordingly causes scarring of one or both kidneys, leading to chronic renal insufficiency.
- **Chronic obstructive pyelonephritis (Fig. 20.28B):** It develops due to **recurrent and persistent bacterial infections superimposed on obstructive lesions**, which lead to renal inflammation parenchymal atrophy, and scarring.
    - **Unilateral or bilateral obstruction**: An example of bilateral obstruction is congenital anomalies of

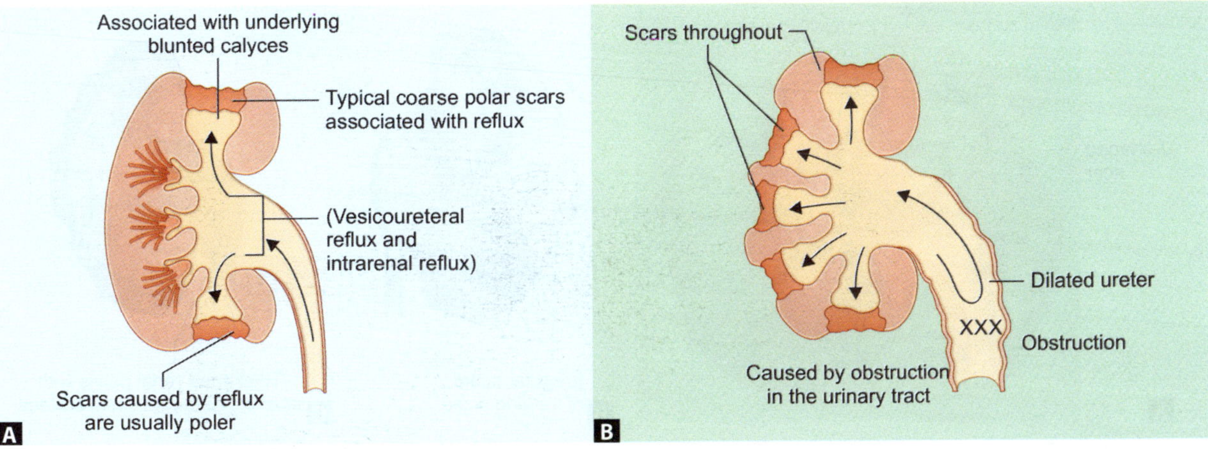

Figs. 20.28A and B: Two major types of chronic pyelonephritis: (A) Reflux (vesicoureteral and intrarenal reflux associated) causes infection, and scars are seen in the poles of the kidney; (B). Obstruction of the urinary tract produces high-pressure backflow of urine. This causes infection of all papillae leading to diffuse scarring of the kidney and thinning of the cortex.

the urethra (e.g., posterior urethral valves). More common is unilateral obstruction, secondary to calculi or unilateral obstructive lesions of the ureter.

MORPHOLOGY

Q. Describe the gross and microscopy of chronic pyelonephritis.

Gross (Figs. 20.29A to C)

Chronic pyelonephritis produces characteristic gross changes. They show **broad, irregular depressed areas of cortical fibrosis and atrophy overlying a dilated calyx (caliectasis).**

- May be **unilateral or bilateral.** When bilateral, the involvement is **asymmetric**. In contrast, both kidneys are diffusely and symmetrically scarred in chronic glomerulonephritis.
- **Size:** Kidney is **reduced** in size due to **irregular scars**.
- **Nature of scars:** May affect one or both kidneys. The scars vary from one to several in number.
  - Most are seen in the **upper and lower poles in reflux-associated chronic pyelonephritis.**
  - Scars are **coarse, well-defined,** and can vary from one to several in number.
- **Calyces and renal pelvis:** It may appear **thickened and irregular** with **scarring of the mucosal surface. Calyces below the scars are dilated, blunted, or deformed. Papillae are flattened.**

In obstructive uropathy, all the calyces and the renal pelvis are dilated. The renal parenchyma is uniformly thinned. In chronic pyelonephritis associated with vesicoureteral reflux, the calyces are preferentially expanded at the poles of the kidney. They are associated with overlying discrete, coarse scars. They produce indentation of the surface of the kidney.

Microscopy (Figs. 20.30A to C)

Q. Write a short note on microscopic features of chronic pyelonephritis.

Changes are predominant in the interstitium and tubules.

Interstitium: It shows dense **chronic inflammatory infiltrate** of **lymphocytes and macrophages and fibrosis**. Few neutrophils may be found with active infection.

Tubules: It may show **atrophy** in some places and hypertrophy or dilation in others.

- **Thyroidization:** The characteristic (but not specific) tubular change is thyroidization. The **dilated tubules** with flattened epithelium may be **filled with pink to blue, glassy-appearing, casts. These are PAS-positive and resemble the colloid inside the thyroid follicles.** They are known as colloid casts.

Blood vessels: They may show **endarteritis obliterans** and in the presence of hypertension may show **hyaline arteriosclerosis.**

Glomeruli: It may appear normal except for **periglomerular fibrosis or sclerosis.**

Calyces: Shows calyceal epithelium surrounded by **fibrosis** and infiltrated by **dense chronic inflammatory infiltrate.**

Q. Write a note on xanthogranulomatous pyelonephritis.

Xanthogranulomatous pyelonephritis: It is an **unusual and rare form of chronic pyelonephritis** associated with ***Proteus*** infections.

MORPHOLOGY

Gross

The cut surface shows large, yellowish-orange nodules, which may be **confused with renal cell carcinoma.**

Microscopy

Interstitium shows foamy **macrophages, plasma cells, and lymphocytes** (*refer* **online Fig. 20.31**).

Clinical Features

Chronic pyelonephritis associated with reflux **may be silent** onset. The usual symptoms are **back pain, fever, pyuria, and bacteriuria.**

Reflux-associated pyelonephritis: It is usually diagnosed early while investigating the cause of hypertension in children. Due to the loss of tubular function, especially the concentrating ability, it presents with polyuria and nocturia.

Chronic obstructive pyelonephritis: It may be silent

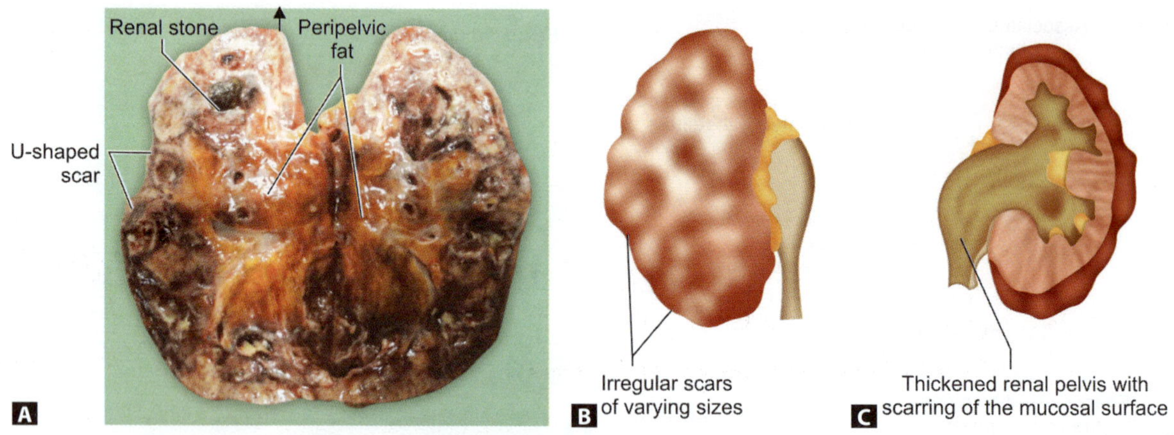

Figs. 20.29A to C: Gross appearance of chronic pyelonephritis: (A) Cut section of kidney showing scars and a renal stone in the calyces; (B) Outer aspect (diagrammatic); (C) Cut section (diagrammatic).

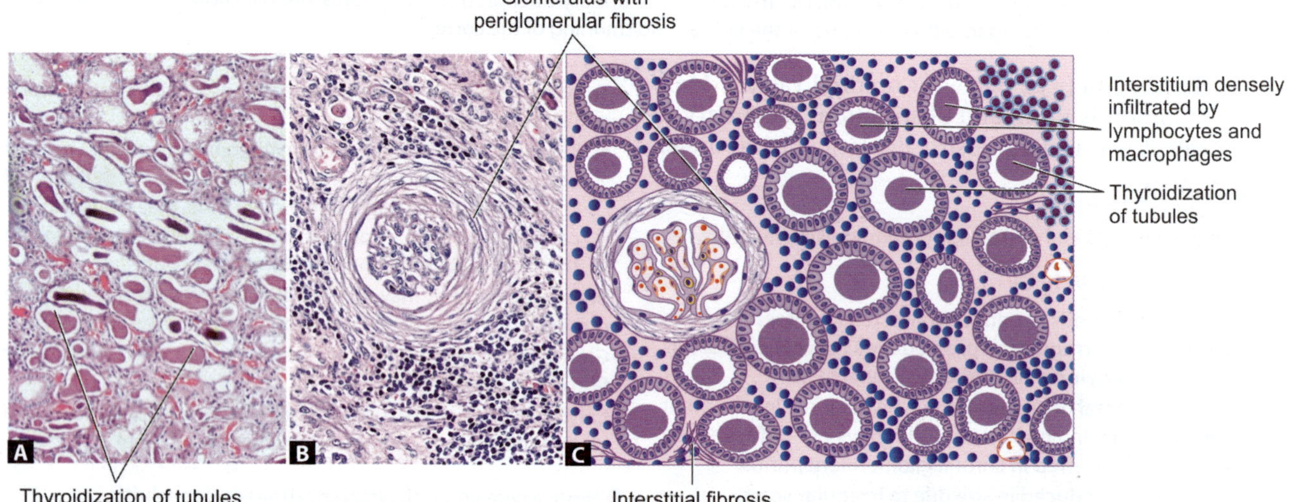

Figs. 20.30A to C: Microscopic appearance of chronic pyelonephritis: (A) Tubules containing hyaline material resembling the colloid of thyroid follicles (thyroidization); (B) Glomerulus with periglomerular fibrosis and interstitium with chronic inflammatory cell infiltrate; (C) Diagrammatic.

in onset or present with features of acute recurrent pyelonephritis. These symptoms include **back pain, fever, pyuria, and bacteriuria**. Patients with silent onset are diagnosed relatively late because of the gradual onset of renal insufficiency and hypertension.

Urinalysis

It shows **leukocytes (WBCs) and leukocyte casts**. Significant bacteriuria may be present, but it is often absent in the late stages. **Proteinuria:** It is **usually mild**.

ACUTE KIDNEY INJURY

PA 28.2 (CC): Define and describe the etiology, precipitating factors, pathogenesis, pathology, laboratory urinary findings, progression, and complications of acute renal failure.

Acute kidney injury (AKI) was previously known as acute renal failure. The term AKI is now preferred because the severity of damage varies and is not always associated with renal failure.

Definition: Acute kidney injury (AKI) is a **clinicopathologic entity, characterized clinically by rapid** (abrupt, over days to few weeks) **reduction of renal function** [decreased glomerular filtration rate (GFR)] **and excretory function.**

The deterioration in renal function in AKI is sufficiently severe to result in the retention of nitrogenous wastes in the body (uremia) and other waste products normally cleared by the kidneys (elevation of serum creatinine). AKI is a clinical diagnosis and not a structural one. It is **usually** but not invariably accompanied by **oliguria**.

Acute kidney injury is a clinical diagnosis and not a structural one. AKI may be with or without injury to the kidney parenchyma. Its severity can range from asymptomatic to rapidly fatal conditions.

Common diagnostic features of AKI: AKI is not a single disease. It consists of a heterogeneous group of conditions that have the following common diagnostic features:

1. **Acute rise in serum creatinine and blood urea nitrogen (BUN) concentration.**
2. **Often associated with a reduced volume of urine.**

Etiology and Pathophysiology

Classification of causes of AKI (*refer* online Flowchart 20.5): AKI may be secondary to intrinsic diseases of the kidney or extrarenal causes. AKI may be secondary to intrinsic diseases of the kidney or extrarenal (prerenal or postrenal) causes. Thus, the causes of AKI are traditionally divided into three broad categories: (i) prerenal azotemia (prerenal causes), (ii) intrinsic disease of the kidney (intrarenal/renal causes), and (iii) postrenal obstruction (postrenal causes). The most **common causes of AKI are acute tubular necrosis (ATN) and acute tubular injury (ATI), followed by prerenal causes**. ATI may produce oliguria (defined as urine output of <400 mL/day).

Prerenal Causes (Prerenal Azotemia)

Prerenal azotemia (the term azotemia is derived from "azo", meaning nitrogen, and "-emia", meaning in the blood) is the **most common form of AKI**.

- **Reduced fluid volume and reduced GFR**: Prerenal causes are associated with reduced fluid volume and therefore reduced glomerular perfusion.
- **Raised serum creatinine and BUN**: Prerenal azotemia is characterized by a **rise in serum creatinine or blood urea nitrogen (BUN) concentration**. These are elevated due to inadequate (reduced) blood flow to the kidneys and reduced intraglomerular hydrostatic pressure to support normal glomerular filtration.
- **Oliguria**: Inadequate perfusion and markedly reduced GFR produce oliguria (urine output <400 mL/day).
- **No damage to renal parenchyma**: Prerenal azotemia **does not produce damage to renal parenchyma** and is rapidly reversible once parenchymal blood flow and intraglomerular hemodynamics are restored. However, prolonged periods of prerenal azotemia may lead to ischemic injury, often termed acute tubular necrosis (ATN).

Various causes are as follows:

- **Systemic causes:** The most common precipitating clinical event is **renal hypoperfusion** due to a **reduction in the volume of extracellular fluid** [e.g., hypovolemia due to massive hemorrhage, severe dehydration, severe burns, prolonged diarrhea) or **impaired cardiac function** (e.g., congestive heart failure, acute myocardial infarction, massive pulmonary embolism).
- **Local causes:** Prerenal azotemia may also occur with medications that interfere with renal autoregulatory responses. These include nonsteroidal anti-inflammatory drugs (NSAIDs) and inhibitors of angiotensin II.

Renal Causes (Intrinsic AKI)

Intrinsic diseases of the kidney causing AKI (intrarenal causes) are classified according to the primary histologic site of injury: **tubules, interstitium, vasculature, or glomerulus.**

- **Renal tubular epithelial cell injury:** It is commonly known as **acute tubular injury (ATI)**. It occurs more commonly due to **ischemia** of any cause. Other causes include **sepsis and nephrotoxins** (specific renal toxins). Nephrotoxins may be endogenous or exogenous. ATN results in ischemia and necrosis of the tubular epithelial cells. However, when the causative factors are removed the tubular cells can regenerate.
- **Interstitium:** Acute tubulointerstitial nephritis (ATIN) such as in hypersensitivity reaction to drugs can cause AKI.
- **Vascular causes:** These include **vasculitis**, such as in microscopic polyangiitis, microangiopathies [e.g., hemolytic uremic syndrome (HUS) or thrombotic thrombocytopenic purpura (TTP)] or **malignant hypertension.**
- **Glomerular causes:** These include acute glomerulonephritis (GN), rapidly progressive GN (RPGN), and lupus nephritis.

Postrenal Causes (Postrenal AKI)

Normally, urine flow is unidirectional from the kidneys to the tip of the urethra. Postrenal AKI occurs when this downward flow is acutely blocked, either partially or totally. The blockage leads to increased retrograde hydrostatic pressure, interfering with glomerular filtration.

Causes of Obstruction

Obstruction of the urinary tract may be functional or structural and may be extrarenal or intrarenal. Obstruction may occur at any point in its course, from the renal pelvis to the tip of the urethra. It may be intraluminal or extraluminal.

- **Extraluminal obstruction:** Examples of obstructions include benign nodular hyperplasia of the prostate, cancer of the prostate, ureteral obstruction (e.g., by ureteral stones, invasive cervical cancer, bladder cancer), and neurogenic bladder.
- **Intraluminal obstruction**: Ureteric obstruction can be an intraluminal obstruction [e.g., ureteral stones (calculi), urethral strictures, blood clots, sloughed renal papillae], infiltration of the wall of the ureter (e.g., neoplasia), or compression from the outside (e.g., retroperitoneal fibrosis, neoplasia, abscess, or damage by the surgical procedure).

Urinary findings in different types of acute kidney injury are presented (*refer* **online Table 20.5**).

Complications of AKI are presented in **Box 20.14**.

BOX 20.14: Complications of acute kidney injury.

- **Metabolic:** Hyperkalemia, hypocalcemia, hyperphosphatemia, hypermagnesemia, hyperuricemia, metabolic acidosis (increased anion gap)
- **Cardiovascular:** Cardiac arrhythmias, pulmonary edema, pericarditis/pericardial effusion
- **Gastrointestinal:** Gastrointestinal hemorrhage
- **Neurologic:** Encephalopathy, neuropathy, seizures
- **Hematologic:** Anemia, bleeding—platelet dysfunction
- **Miscellaneous:** Infections (pneumonia, urinary tract infection, septicemia)

ACUTE TUBULAR INJURY

PA 28.9 (CC): Define and describe the etiology, pathogenesis, pathology, laboratory, urinary findings, progression, and complications of acute tubular necrosis.

Definition: Acute tubular injury (ATI) is characterized by damage to renal tubular epithelial cells and an acute decline in renal function. Urine usually shows granular casts and tubular cells.

Terminology: Frank necrosis is rarely observed in a kidney biopsy in patients with *acute tubular injury*. Hence, the older term ***acute tubular necrosis*** **is not used.**

Findings in acute kidney injury: It clinically manifests as **decreased GFR with elevation of serum creatinine. ATI is the most common cause of acute kidney injury** (AKI described above) **and may produce oliguria** (urine output of <400 mL/day).

Etiology and Pathogenesis

Forms of ATI

It is of two types that differ in the underlying causes. But they have similar outcomes.

Ischemic ATI

- **Prerenal causes of inadequate blood flow to the kidney:** Ischemic ATI usually develops when there is inadequate blood flow to the kidney. This may occur when there is severe hypotension and shock (*refer* **online Flowchart 20.5**). Events that initiate ischemic ATI include severe trauma, blood loss, acute pancreatitis, and septicemia.
- **Vascular causes:** Ischemia to tubules may also occur due to reduced intrarenal blood flow. It may be due to vascular causes such as small vessel vasculitis (e.g., microscopic polyangiitis), malignant hypertension, and thrombotic microangiopathies.
- **Other causes:** These include mismatched blood transfusions, other hemolytic crises, and myoglobinuria.

Nephrotoxic ATI

It is caused by various poisons or toxins. The toxin may be endogenous and exogenous. Exogenous toxins include many poisons, including heavy metals (e.g., mercury); organic chemicals (e.g., ethylene glycol, carbon tetrachloride); many drugs (e.g., gentamicin and other antibiotics), and radiographic contrast agents.

Pathogenesis (Refer Online Flowchart 20.6)

Two important features occur in both ischemic and nephrotoxic ATI. These are **(1) injury to tubular cells and (2) persistent and severe disturbances in blood flow.**

Injury to the Tubular Epithelial Cells

Proximal tubular epithelial cells **are highly susceptible to ischemia and toxic injury.** Factors that predispose the epithelial cells of renal tubules to injury in AKI are:

- Raised intracellular concentrations of various molecules that are resorbed in the proximal tubule.
- Exposure to high concentrations of solutes in the lumen. These solutes are concentrated because of the resorption of water from the glomerular filtrate.
- High rate of oxygen consumption, which is needed for the production of the ATP required for transport and reabsorption functions.

Structural alterations in epithelial cells due to ischemia: These include **loss of cell polarity in the tubular epithelial cells, decreased GFR, recruitment of leukocytes, tubular obstruction by cellular debris, and interstitial edema.**

Disturbances in Blood Flow

Ischemic renal injury produces hemodynamic alterations and reduces GFR. One of the important alterations is intrarenal vasoconstriction. This leads to reduced glomerular blood flow as well as reduced oxygen supply to the functionally important tubules in the outer medulla.

Decreased sodium reabsorption: Damage of the plasma membrane of proximal tubular epithelial cells by ischemia and toxins results in decreased sodium reabsorption and increased delivery of sodium to distal tubules.

- **Triggering of tubuloglomerular feedback**: Increased sodium in distal tubules triggers a tubuloglomerular feedback mechanism involving the renin-angiotensin pathway.
- **Afferent arteriolar vasoconstriction**: The renin-angiotensin pathway causes *intrarenal vasoconstriction*. This decreases glomerular blood flow and oxygen delivery to the tubules in the outer medulla (thick ascending limb and straight segment of the proximal tubule).
- **Further ischemic injury to tubules**: The reduced GFR further reduces the blood flow and causes more ischemic injury to tubules.

Luminal obstruction by casts: Injury to the tubular epithelial cells causes **necrosis and detachment of the damaged cells from the basement membranes**. They are shed into the urine. When there is sufficient build-up of tubular debris, it can block the outflow of urine (obstruction by forming casts) in the tubules. **Obstruction results in**

(1) **increased intratubular pressure,** (2) further **decrease in GFR,** and (3) **decreased urine outflow.**

Fluid leak from the lumen into the interstitium: Fluid from the damaged tubules may leak back into the interstitium. This **increases the interstitial pressure** and **causes collapse of the tubules.** This results in decreased urine output.

Recovery: The tubular necrosis is patchy and there is maintenance of the integrity of the basement membrane along many segments. This allows repair of the injured foci of tubular epithelial cells and recovery of function if the precipitating cause is removed.

MORPHOLOGY

A characteristic morphological feature of ATI is a **tubular epithelial injury at multiple focal points** along the nephron. There are **large normal skip areas** between these involved segments of the nephron. Often, the involved segments of nephrons show **rupture of basement membranes** (tubulorrhexis) **and occlusion of tubular lumens by casts.** Tubular injury in ischemic and toxic ATI shows distinct patterns.

Ischemic ATI

Gross

Both kidneys are **swollen** and show a **pale cortex** and a **congested medulla.**

Microscopy

Glomeruli: Appear normal.

Tubules: It shows the following changes:

- **Areas of tubules involved (Fig. 20.32A):** Tubules show **focal and multiple areas of damage** along the nephron, **with large skip areas** in between. The lesions are **most marked in the straight portions of the proximal tubules** and the **ascending thick limbs of the loop of Henle** in the **outer medulla.**
- Tubular epithelial alterations:
  - **Epithelial simplification** It is characterized by **focal flattening** and **loss of proximal tubule brush borders.** The cytoplasm of cells shows vacuolization.
  - **Blebbing and sloughing of the brush borders (apical cytoplasm)** of non-necrotic tubular cells into the lumen of the tubules.
  - **Formation of proteinaceous casts:** Sloughed apical cytoplasm, non-necrotic and necrotic cells form **hyaline casts and brown pigmented granular casts.** The casts are seen in the **lumen of distal tubules,** collecting ducts, and in the urine. These casts are **composed of Tamm–Horsfall protein** (a urinary glycoprotein normally secreted by the cells of ascending thick limb and distal tubules) **and other plasma proteins.**
  - **Occlusion of tubular lumens:** The casts occlude the lumen and result in **dilation of the lumen.**
  - Necrosis of tubular epithelial cells **[Fig. 20.33A** (*refer* **online Fig. 20.33B)].**
  - **Rupture of basement membranes** (tubulorrhexis): It can occur in later stages.
  - **Epithelial regeneration:** If the precipitating cause is removed, the tubular epithelium can regenerate and tubules may return to normal without any residual evidence of damage.

Interstitium: It shows edema and a mild inflammatory infiltrate consisting of neutrophils, lymphocytes, and plasma cells.

Blood vessels: Normal.

Nephrotoxic ATI

Microscopy

- Areas involved **(Fig. 20.32B):** The most **common site of toxic injury** is seen in the **proximal convoluted tubules.** The **necrosis** of tubular epithelium is **more extensive** in toxic ATN than seen in ischemic ATN.
- Tubular necrosis is limited to certain segments of tubules that are most sensitive to the particular toxin.
- **ATN due to hemoglobin or myoglobin** shows many **red-brown colored** (due to heme pigments) **tubular casts.**

Q. Write a short answer on Tamm–Horsfall protein.

Urinary casts in urine sediment provide important clues for differentiating renal diseases. Casts are formed in the tubule of the nephron. The cast is composed of a protein meshwork with entrapped cells or cell fragments. Cells in the ascending thick limb of Henle and distal tubules produce and secrete small amounts of a glycoprotein called *Tamm–Horsfall* protein into the tubular lumen. Tamm–Horsfall protein forms the meshwork that entraps cells in the tubule to form casts and is found in normal urine. Normal protein casts that do not have cells in them are called *agranular casts.*

Changes in tubular epithelial cells induced by a few poisons and organic solvents are presented (*refer* **online Table 20.6**).

Clinical Features

The clinical course of ATI may be divided into three stages namely: (1) initiation, (2) maintenance, and (3) recovery phases.

Initiation phase: Clinical features depend on the initiating cause of ATI. There is a mild reduction of urine output, with an increase in BUN, and serum creatinine. This phase lasts for about 36 hours.

Maintenance phase: During this phase, there is a **sustained decrease in urine output** in the range of 40–400 mL/day (oliguria), **salt and water overload, rising BUN levels, hyperkalemia, metabolic acidosis,** and other features of uremia. This oliguric crisis can be overcome with appropriate management.

Recovery phases: During this phase, there is a **steady increase in urine volume,** which may reach up to 3 L/day. There is a **loss of large amounts of water, sodium, and potassium** (leading to hypokalemia) in the urine (because the tubular epithelium has not fully recovered). Once the renal tubular function returns to normal, BUN and creatinine levels also return to normal.

Prognosis: ATN is a **potentially reversible condition** and with modern therapy (supportive treatment or dialysis), most patients recover.

Refer **online Table 20.7** for common causes of acute renal failure and associated urinary findings.

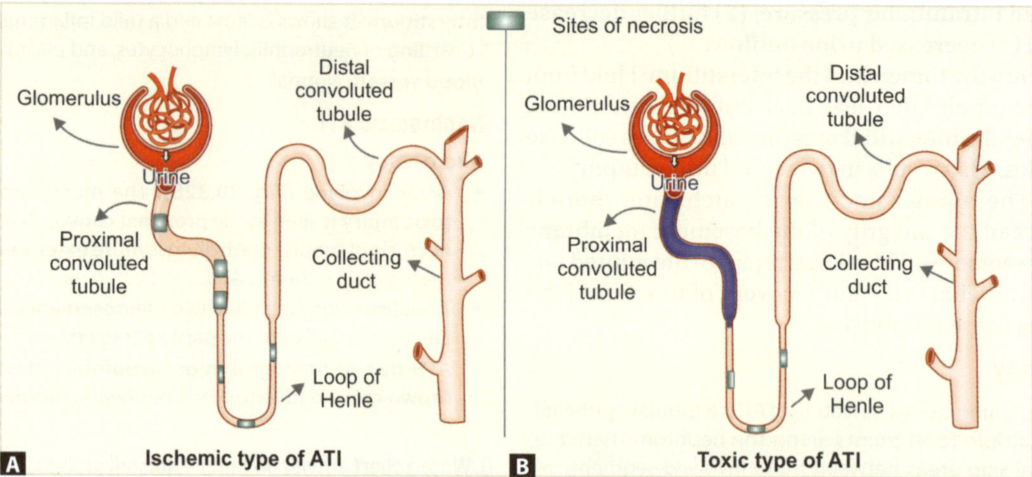

Figs. 20.32A and B: Patterns of tubular damage in ischemic and toxic acute tubular injury: (A) In ischemic type, tubular necrosis is patchy, relatively short lengths of tubules are affected, and most marked in the straight segments of proximal tubules and ascending limbs of the loop of Henle; (B) In toxic acute tubular injury, extensive necrosis involves the proximal convoluted tubule segments.

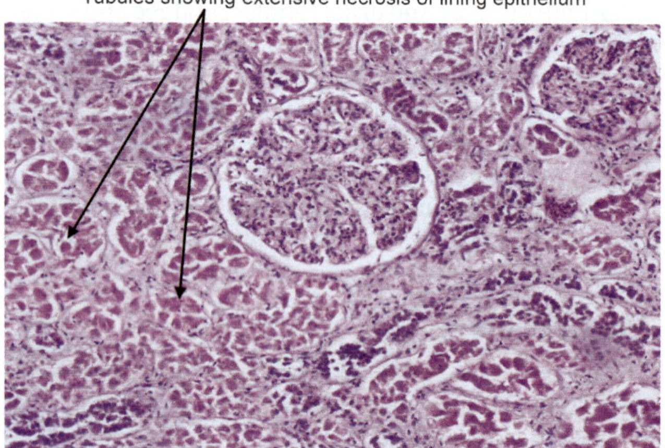

Fig. 20.33A: Microscopic appearance of acute tubular injury: Low magnification.

CHRONIC KIDNEY DISEASE

PA 28.4 (CC): Define and describe the etiology, precipitating factors, pathogenesis, pathology, laboratory urinary findings, progression, and complications of chronic renal failure.

Chronic kidney disease (CKD) was previously termed chronic renal failure or chronic renal insufficiency.

Definition: Chronic kidney disease (CKD) is a broad term used to describe the final common pathway of progressive nephron loss resulting from any type of severe kidney disease.

Chronic kidney disease refers to a spectrum of **longstanding** (>3 months), usually **progressive** processes associated with **irreversible worsening of renal function** and decline in glomerular filtration rate (GFR). **CKD spectrum ranges from abnormalities detectable only by laboratory testing to uremia.** Unless CKD is treated with dialysis or transplantation, death occurs due to uremia, electrolyte disturbances, or other complications.

Important causes of chronic kidney disease are listed in **Box 20.15.**

BOX 20.15: Important causes of chronic kidney disease.

- **Glomerulopathies***
  - *Proliferative GN*
  - *Crescentic GN*
  - *Membranoproliferative GN*
  - *Immunoglobulin A (IgA) nephropathy*
- **Systemic and metabolic diseases**
  - *Diabetes**
  - *Systemic lupus erythematosus (SLE)*
  - *Polyarteritis nodosa (PAN)*
  - *Amyloidosis*
  - *Gout*
- **Interstitial**
  - *Chronic interstitial nephritis**
  - *Chronic pyelonephritis**
  - *Analgesic*
  - *Tuberculosis*
  - *Nephrocalcinosis*
- **Obstructive***
  - *Calculus*
  - *Tumors*
  - *Retroperitoneal fibrosis*
  - *Prostatic enlargement*
- **Renovascular diseases**
  - *Essential hypertension (accelerated)**
  - *Renovascular vasculitis (SLE, PAN, scleroderma)*
- **Congenital**
  - *Autosomal dominant polycystic kidney disease **
  - *Medullary cystic disease*
  - *Alport's syndrome*
- **Unknown**

* Common causes of chronic renal failure.

Pathogenesis

In chronic kidney disease (CKD), there is progressive renal damage. It destroys more and more nephrons as the disease progresses. Two broad mechanisms of damage are involved in CKD. These are (1) initiating mechanisms and (2) adaptive mechanisms.

Initiating mechanism: The initiating mechanism depends on the underlying etiology. For example, it may be abnormalities in the development or integrity of the kidney, immune complex deposition followed by inflammation in glomerulonephritis, exposure to toxins in certain diseases of the renal tubules and interstitium, or metabolic defects as in diabetes mellitus.

Adaptive mechanisms: Till there is a critical loss of nephrons, the following adaptive mechanisms are initiated. They try to maintain homeostasis until the late stages of chronic kidney disease.

- **Glomerular hyperfiltration:** It tends to compensate for decreased glomerular filtration rate.
- **Increase in the rate of excretion of solutes per nephron:** It may be through the following mechanism (i) increased plasma concentrations for creatinine, (ii) decreased tubular reabsorption for sodium, phosphate, and calcium, or (iii) increased tubular secretion for potassium and hydrogen ions.

Progressive deterioration of renal function: Renal function usually deteriorates progressively even when the original cause is controlled. Uncontrolled hypertension (regardless of the etiology) in chronic kidney disease produces a more rapid decline in renal function.

MORPHOLOGY

Q. Write a short note on the granular contracted kidney.

Causes of the granular contracted kidney: These include (i) **chronic GN, (ii) nephrosclerosis, and (iii) chronic pyelonephritis.** Differentiating features of granular contracted kidneys are presented in **Table 20.8.**

Gross

Chronic GN and nephrosclerosis: Chronic GN is a glomerular disorder and nephrosclerosis is a vascular disorder of the kidney. In both conditions, kidneys are **symmetrically contracted. Their outer surface is red-brown and diffusely granular.** Their granules are small, regular, and fine.

Chronic pyelonephritis: In this, the kidneys are usually **unevenly (asymmetrically) involved** and have **deep, irregular, coarse, and large scars.**

Microscopy

The feature is common to all cases of chronic kidney disease irrespective of the underlying cause.

Scarring of the glomeruli: Common to all is the advanced scarring of the glomeruli. The **obliteration** (sometimes complete obliteration) **of the glomeruli** is the end-point of many diseases, and it is not possible to determine the nature of the initial lesion.

Atrophy and dropout of tubules: It is found in many of the tubules in the cortex.

Interstitial fibrosis and inflammation: It may be marked. Lymphocytic (and, rarely, plasma cell) infiltrates are seen in the fibrotic interstitial tissue.

Thickening of the wall with narrowing of the lumina of blood vessels: These occur in small- and medium-sized arteries, secondary to hypertension.

As damage progresses, it may become difficult to identify whether the primary lesion was glomerular, vascular, tubular, or interstitial. Such markedly damaged kidneys are termed **end-stage kidneys.**

Clinical Features

Chronic kidney disease may develop insidiously. Initially, most patients with slowly progressive disease are often asymptomatic and manifest only as a biochemical abnormality. It is frequently suspected when proteinuria, hypertension, or azotemia is detected during a routine medical examination. Azotemia is a biochemical abnormality characterized by the **elevation of BUN and creatinine levels**. It is mainly due to a decreased GFR. Some degree of proteinuria is present in almost all cases, and hypertension is very common. Microscopic hematuria is usually present. BUN and creatinine are commonly used to measure the excretory capacity of the kidneys.

Laboratory Urinary Findings

Physical examination: Fixed specific gravity around 1.010 (isosthenuria) is seen in CRF.

Chemical examination: Hematuria may indicate glomerulonephritis. Proteinuria, if heavy, is strongly suggestive of glomerular disease. Glycosuria with normal blood glucose level is common in CRF.

TABLE 20.8 Differentiating features of granular contracted kidney.

Features	*Chronic glomerulonephritis*	*Nephrosclerosis*	*Chronic pyelonephritis*
Size of the kidney	Reduced	Reduced	Reduced
Involvement	Bilateral	Bilateral	Unilateral or bilateral
Nature of involvement	Diffuse, and symmetrical involvement	Diffuse, and asymmetrical atrophy	Asymmetrical involvement when bilateral
Appearance of scars	Fine, uniform, and small granular scars	Fine, uniform, and small granular scars	Large, irregular, coarse, and discrete
Shape of scars	–	V-shaped	U-shaped

Urine Microscopy

Cells

- **White cells** in the urine usually indicate **bacterial urinary infection**, sterile pyuria suggests papillary necrosis or renal tuberculosis.
- **Eosinophils** indicate **allergic tubulointerstitial nephritis** or cholesterol embolization.
- **Red cell** source may be from anywhere in the urinary tract between the glomerulus and the urethral meatus.

Casts

Red-cell casts are suggestive of **glomerulonephritis**. **Granular casts** indicate **active renal disease**. **Broad casts** are seen in CRF.

A urine culture should be performed. Early-morning urine samples should be cultured for tuberculosis.

Prognosis of chronic kidney disease: Without treatment, the prognosis is poor. They progress to uremia and death.

Complications of Chronic Kidney Disease

- **Anemia of chronic disease**
- **Metabolic bone disease (renal osteodystrophy):** It includes (1) hyperparathyroid bone disease (osteitis fibrosa cystica), (2) osteomalacia, and (3) osteoporosis.
- **Gastrointestinal complications:** (1) reduced gastric emptying and increased risk of reflux esophagitis, (2) increased risk of peptic ulceration and acute pancreatitis, (3) constipation, and (4) gastrointestinal bleeding.
- **Metabolic abnormalities:**
  - **Gout:** Urate retention is common.
  - **Insulin requirement and resistance:** Insulin is catabolized by and to some extent excreted via the kidneys. Thus, insulin requirements in diabetic patients reduce as renal failure progresses. By contrast, end-organ resistance to insulin is observed in advanced renal impairment.
  - **Lipid metabolism abnormalities:** Include (1) impaired clearance of triglyceride-rich particles and (2) hypercholesterolemia.
- **Endocrine abnormalities:** Include (1) hyperprolactinemia, (2) increased luteinizing hormone (LH) levels in both sexes, (3) decreased serum testosterone levels, (4) absence of normal cyclical changes in female sex hormones, resulting in oligomenorrhea or amenorrhea, (5) abnormalities of growth hormone secretion and action, and (6) abnormal thyroid hormone levels.
- **Proximal myopathy.**
- **Nervous system:** Median nerve compression in the carpal tunnel due to β2-microglobulin-related amyloidosis.
- **Cardiovascular disease: Increased incidence of cardiovascular disease,** particularly myocardial infarction, cardiac failure, sudden cardiac death and stroke, uremic pericarditis, or dialysis pericarditis. Hypertension develops in about 80% of patients with CRF.
- **Malignancy: Raised** incidence of malignancy. Malignant change can occur in polycystic kidney disease. Lymphomas, primary liver cancer, and thyroid cancers can also develop.

VASCULAR DISEASES OF THE KIDNEY

PA 28.11 (CC): Define classify and describe the etiology, pathogenesis, pathology, laboratory, urinary findings, distinguishing features progression, and complications of vascular disease of the kidney.

Almost all kidney diseases secondarily affect the renal blood vessels, as well as systemic vascular diseases (e.g., various vasculitis) can also involve renal blood vessels. The kidney is also involved in the pathogenesis of both essential and secondary hypertension and the kidney can both be a cause and consequence of increased blood pressure. Classification of vascular diseases of the kidney is presented in **Box 20.16**.

Hypertensive Renal Disease

Systemic hypertension produces pathologic and functional effects on the kidneys. Long-standing hypertension has been termed essential or benign, but the preferred term is *primary hypertension*. A small proportion of patients with primary hypertension develop a rapid rise in blood pressure that causes organ damage. This is called *malignant hypertension* and is a medical emergency. Both chronic primary hypertension and malignant hypertension produce similar renal manifestations but with some significant differences.

Pathogenesis

Primary (Benign) Hypertension

The arterial lesions in primary hypertension are mainly due to endothelial dysfunction and platelet activation.

BOX 20.16: Classification of vascular disease of the kidney.

- Hypertensive renal disease
  - Nephrosclerosis (previously known as benign nephrosclerosis)
  - Malignant nephrosclerosis
- Thrombotic microangiopathies
- Renal artery stenosis
- Other vascular disorders
  - Atherosclerotic ischemic renal disease
  - Atheroembolic renal disease
  - Sickle-cell nephropathy
  - Diffuse cortical necrosis.
  - Renal infarcts

- **Endothelial dysfunction:** Long-standing hypertension produces injury to endothelium. This **increases the permeability** of the vessels **to plasma proteins and platelet deposition**. Platelets and other cells produce growth factors that stimulate the proliferation of vascular smooth muscle cells and the synthesis of extracellular matrix proteins. This leads to thickening of the tunica media and intima. These changes may be worsened by the hemodynamic effects of high blood pressure and aging.
- **Platelet activation**: Platelets that are deposited on the injured endothelium are activated. They produce growth factors and may cause repeated attacks of thrombus formation.

Vascular changes

Hyaline arteriosclerosis: Two processes participate in the arterial lesions of **sclerosis of renal arterioles and small arteries.** These include (i) the leakage of plasma proteins through injured endothelium and (ii) increased deposition (production) of basement membrane matrix in the vessel wall (arterioles). These changes lead to the morphologic changes in the vessels that are termed as hyaline arteriosclerosis.

Renal changes

Nephrosclerosis: Hyaline arteriosclerosis with thickened walls narrows the lumen of the blood vessels. This causes ischemia of renal parenchyma with subsequent atrophy of tubules and fibrosis of the interstitium (scarring). This results in a reduction in functional renal mass. These changes in the gross appearance of the involved kidney are termed *nephrosclerosis*. Thus, nephrosclerosis is the **renal pathology associated with sclerosis of renal arterioles and small arteries**. It was previously termed benign nephrosclerosis. It is **strongly associated with hypertension**. However, nephrosclerosis may develop in any disease with chronic ischemia that causes atrophy and fibrosis in the kidney. A mild degree of nephrosclerosis is present in many individuals above 60 years of age in the absence of hypertension. The frequency and severity of these lesions increase with age and in patients with hypertension or diabetes. Many primary renal diseases cause hypertension. Hence, nephrosclerosis is usually superimposed on other primary diseases of the kidney.

Malignant Hypertension

Malignant hypertension (blood pressure usually >200/120 mm Hg) occurs in a small percentage of patients with primary hypertension. Malignant or accelerated phase of hypertension is relatively uncommon.

Vascular changes

Hyperplastic arteriosclerosis: In severe "malignant" hypertension, the **vascular smooth muscle cells proliferate** and produce a morphologic appearance known as *hyperplastic arteriosclerosis*. The **hyperplasia (proliferation) of intimal smooth muscle cells may be due to mitogenic factors from platelets** (e.g., PDGF), **plasma and other cells**

Fibrinoid necrosis of arterioles and small arteries: Apart from hyperplastic arteriosclerosis, the vascular injury may be severe enough to produce *fibrinoid necrosis* of arterioles and small arteries. It may be associated with intravascular thrombosis.

Renal changes

Raised plasma rennin: Severe **narrowing of renal afferent arterioles causes ischemia. These** vascular changes activate the **renin-angiotensin system and are associated with raised levels of plasma renin.** It increases vascular tone and systemic blood pressure. Thus, hypertension acts on the kidneys to cause more hypertension, thereby producing a vicious cycle.

MORPHOLOGY

Q. Write a short note on kidney changes in hypertension.

Primary Hypertension (Nephrosclerosis)

Gross: The changes in kidneys in long-standing hypertension are as follows:

- **Involvement**: Bilateral.
- **Size and weight:** Kidneys are either **normal or smaller** (atrophic). **Weight** is between 110 and 130 g (normal 150 g).
- **Outer surface:** It shows a diffuse, **fine, even granularity** resembling grain leather.
- **Cut section:** It shows a **thinned cortex with scarring**.

Microscopy

Blood vessel: Changes in the kidney depend on the size of the vessel.

- **Hyaline arteriosclerosis: Arterioles and small arteries** show **homogeneous, pink hyaline thickening of the walls** called **hyaline arteriolosclerosis** (*refer* **Figs. 16.11A and B**). These vessels show a loss of underlying cellular detail and narrow the lumen of the vessels.
- **Larger blood vessels (interlobar and arcuate arteries):** They show thickening of intima with replication of internal elastic lamina. The media shows fibrous thickening.

Tubules: They show diffuse atrophy due to ischemia.

Interstitium: Shows fibrosis with scant or no inflammatory infiltrates.

Glomeruli: Most of them appear normal and in advanced stages may show **sclerosis of glomeruli**.

Malignant Hypertension

Q. Write a short answer on kidney changes in malignant hypertension.

Q. Write a short answer on flea-bitten kidney and its causes.

Gross

- **Size**: The size of the kidney may be normal or shrunken. It depends on the duration and severity of the hypertension.
- **Flea-bitten kidney:** It is characterized by the presence of **small, pinpoint petechial hemorrhages on the cortical surface.** It is due to a **rupture of arterioles or glomerular capillaries.** The causes of the flea-bitten kidney are listed in **Box 20.17**.

BOX 20.17: Causes of the flea-bitten kidney.

- Malignant hypertension
- Subacute bacterial endocarditis
- Rapidly progressive glomerulonephritis
- Henoch–Schönlein purpura

MORPHOLOGY

Q. Write a short note on the granular contracted kidney.

Causes of the granular contracted kidney: These include (i) **chronic GN, (ii) nephrosclerosis, and (iii) chronic pyelonephritis.** Differentiating features of granular contracted kidneys are presented in **Table 20.8.**

Gross

Chronic GN and nephrosclerosis: Chronic GN is a glomerular disorder and nephrosclerosis is a vascular disorder of the kidney. In both conditions, kidneys are **symmetrically contracted. Their outer surface is red-brown** and **diffusely granular.** Their granules are small, regular, and fine.

Clinical Features

Primary hypertension: Uncomplicated nephrosclerosis may be asymptomatic. Long-standing hypertension shows some impairment of renal function, such as loss of urine concentrating ability or a diminished GFR. There may be mild proteinuria, but renal failure or uremia is rare.

- **Laboratory findings:** Mild proteinuria, hematuria (no RBC casts), increase in serum blood urea nitrogen (BUN), and creatinine (renal azotemia).

Malignant hypertension: Patients with severely elevated blood pressure or a second underlying disease (especially diabetes), have an increased risk of developing renal failure. The full-blown syndrome of malignant hypertension is characterized by papilledema, retinal hemorrhages, encephalopathy, cardiovascular abnormalities, and renal failure. Initial symptoms are due to raised intracranial pressure and include headaches, nausea, vomiting, and visual impairments. Later renal failure may develop.

- **Laboratory findings:** Urine examination may show marked proteinuria and hematuria with RBC casts without any significant alteration in renal function. Increase in serum BUN and creatinine.

Thrombotic Microangiopathies

PA 28.15 (NC): Describe the etiology, genetics, pathogenesis, pathology, presenting features, and progression of thrombotic angiopathies.

Thrombotic microangiopathy (TMA) is characterized by widespread microvascular thrombosis, microangiopathic hemolytic anemia, thrombocytopenia, and sometimes renal failure.

Classification

Primary forms: No underlying disease.

- **Shiga toxin-mediated hemolytic uremic syndrome (HUS):** Caused by Shiga toxin-producing *E. coli* or *Shigella dysenteriae.*
- **Complement-mediated TMA (previously termed atypical HUS):** Due to excessive complement activation, can be inherited or acquired.
- **Thrombotic thrombocytopenic purpura (TTP):** Can be inherited or acquired.
- **Drug-mediated TMA:** Caused by drugs like mitomycin, cisplatin, cyclosporine, tacrolimus, and anti-VEGF therapy.

Secondary forms: Associated with other diseases or conditions. Examples: Malignant hypertension, scleroderma, pregnancy, chemotherapy, anti-phospholipid antibodies, and transplant rejection.

Importance: Timely diagnosis is crucial to avoid sudden death.

Pathogenesis

Major Factors

- **Endothelial cell injury:** Can be caused by toxins, drugs, autoantibodies, or inherited mutations.
- **Platelet activation and aggregation:** Leads to thrombosis in small vessels, resulting in ischemic injury and organ dysfunction.

Classic Manifestations

- **Platelet-rich thrombi in small vessels.**
- **Thrombocytopenia:** Due to platelet consumption.
- **Microangiopathic hemolytic anemia:** Red cell fragmentation as they pass through narrowed vessels.

Secondary forms: Present with features of underlying disorders, e.g., severe hypertension, systemic sclerosis, pregnancy complications, chemotherapy effects, antiphospholipid antibodies, and transplant rejection.

Consequences of Thrombotic Microangiopathy (TMA)

1. **Thrombocytopenia:** Due to widespread platelet consumption.
2. **Intravascular thrombi:** Excessive formation in small vessels (capillaries and arterioles).
3. **Microangiopathic hemolytic anemia:** Caused by mechanical injury to red cells in narrowed vessels.
4. **Ischemic injury and organ damage:** Microvascular occlusions lead to tissue ischemia and organ damage, such as renal failure.

MORPHOLOGY

Thrombi: Found in glomerular capillaries, arterioles, and larger arteries in severe cases.

HUS-specific changes: Include endothelial injury, widening of the subendothelial space, splitting of the glomerular basement membrane (GBM), and mesangial cell lysis. Severe cases may show cortical necrosis.

Clinical Features

General symptoms: Fever, thrombocytopenia, hemolytic anemia, transient neurologic deficits, and renal failure.

Shiga toxin–associated HUS: Acute kidney injury, bleeding manifestations, severe oliguria, hematuria, microangiopathic hemolytic anemia, and sometimes neurologic changes. Typically follows a gastrointestinal or flu-like prodrome.

- **Prognosis:** Most recover with dialysis, but 25% may develop renal insufficiency over 15–25 years.

Complement-mediated TMA: Sudden onset without prodromal diarrhea. Managed with plasma exchange, liver transplantation, and antibody inhibitors of the membrane attack complex.

- **Prognosis:** Generally poorer than Shiga toxin-mediated HUS.

Thrombotic thrombocytopenic purpura (TTP) (*refer* **online Fig. 20.34**)**:** Sudden onset with central nervous system involvement and less renal involvement. Treated with plasma exchange to replace deficient ADAMTS13.

- **Prognosis:** Without treatment, it is rapidly fatal with a 10% survival rate. Plasma exchange improves prognosis and typically leaves no residual renal abnormalities.

HORSESHOE KIDNEYS

Q. Write a short note on the horseshoe kidney.

Horseshoe kidneys are a **common congenital anomaly** in which there is a fusion of the upper (10%) or lower poles (90%) of the kidneys. It gives a horseshoe appearance to kidneys (**Fig. 20.35**), which are continuous across the midline anterior to the great vessels. When the kidney is fused at the lower pole, the ureters cross over the junction between the two kidneys. It **increases the risk of urinary obstruction and renal infection** (pyelonephritis).

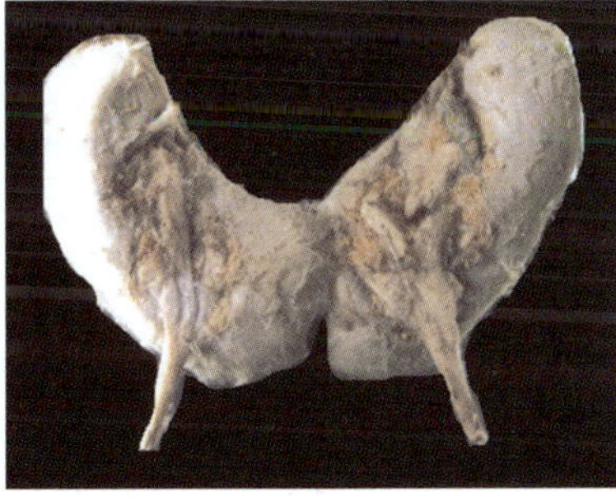

Fig. 20.35: Horseshoe kidney showing fusion of the lower poles.

CYSTIC DISEASES OF THE KIDNEY

PA 28.12 (CC): Define classify and describe the genetics, inheritance, etiology, pathogenesis, pathology, laboratory, urinary findings, distinguishing features, progression, and complications of cystic disease of the kidney.

Q. Write a short note on the cystic disease of the kidney.

Definition: Cystic diseases of the kidney represent a heterogeneous group of **hereditary, developmental, and acquired disorders** characterized by the **presence of cysts in one or both kidneys** (unilateral or bilateral).

Classification of renal cystic disease is presented in **Box 20.18**.

Autosomal Dominant (Adult) Polycystic Kidney Disease

Q. Write a short note on polycystic kidney disease.

Definition: Autosomal-dominant (adult) polycystic kidney disease (ADPKD) is a **hereditary disorder** characterized by **multiple cysts in both kidneys.** These cysts expand and destroy the intervening kidney parenchyma and lead to renal failure.

It is a common condition responsible for about 5–10% of cases of end-stage renal disease (ESRD) that need renal transplantation or dialysis.

Pathogenesis (Fig. 20.36)

ADPKD is a **genetically heterogeneous disorder** and is inherited as an autosomal dominant disorder. **It is associated with mutations in *PKD1* and *PKD2* gene.**

PKD* gene:** It is a tumor suppressor gene. ADPKD is caused by **mutations in one of the two *PKD1 (85% of cases) **and *PKD2* genes** (15%). ***PKD1* gene** encodes a cell membrane-associated protein called **polycystin-1** and the ***PKD2* genes** encodes **polycystin-2.**

- **Polycystin-1:** It is the protein product of the *PKD1* gene. It is localized to the primary cilium of tubular cells

BOX 20.18: Classification of renal cystic disease.

1. Polycystic kidney disease
   - Autosomal dominant (adult) polycystic disease
   - Autosomal recessive (childhood) polycystic disease
2. Medullary cystic disease
   - Medullary sponge kidney
   - Nephronophthisis
3. Multicystic renal dysplasia
4. Acquired (dialysis-associated) cystic disease
5. Localized (simple) renal cysts
6. Renal cysts in hereditary malformation syndromes (e.g., tuberous sclerosis)
7. Glomerulocystic disease
8. Extraparenchymal renal cysts (pelvicalyceal cysts, hilar lymphangitic cysts)

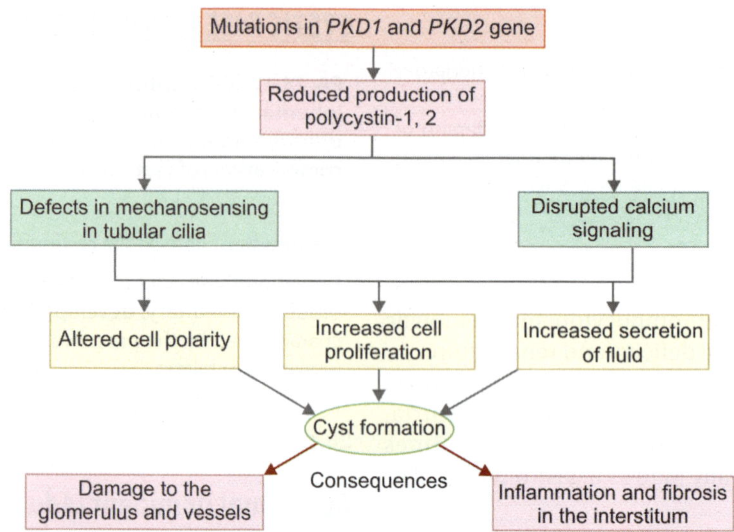

Fig. 20.36: Mechanisms of cyst formation in polycystic kidney disease.

(similar to nephrocystins linked to medullary cystic disease). Cilia are hairlike organelles that project into the lumina from the apical surface of tubular cells. They **act as mechanosensors of fluid flow in the lumen of the tubules.** They are also **involved in cell-cell or cell-matrix adhesion.**

PKD1 Gene Mutations

PKD1 gene encodes a cell membrane-associated protein called *polycystin-1. PKD1* gene mutations are responsible for 85% to 90% of cases.

Germline mutations in the *PKD1* gene: They are present in all renal tubular epithelial cells of affected individuals. Cysts develop only in some tubules. This may be because the *PKD* gene (tumor suppressor gene) also requires a second hit for the loss of the second allele of the gene to develop the disease. The loss of the second allele is by the sporadic somatic event.

Consequences of mutations of the *PKD1* gene: It causes **reduced production of polycystin-1.** When the reduction of polycystin-1 function reaches below a critical threshold, it causes **defects in mechanosensing** by tubular epithelial cells. It **disrupts calcium signaling** (calcium is essential for the maintenance of epithelial cell differentiation and normally inhibits renal tubule growth). This in turn leads **to altered cell polarity, increased cell proliferation, and increased secretion of fluid**. These changes favor the formation of cysts that progressively enlarge as time passes.

PKD2 Gene Mutations

It occurs in 10–15% of cases. Structurally, polycystins-2 is distinct from polycystin-1, but they act together. Thus, mutation in either gene gives rise to ADPKD, although patients with *PKD2* mutations have a slower rate of progression of disease than those with *PKD1* mutations.

MORPHOLOGY

Q. Write a short answer on gross features of adult polycystic kidney disease.

Gross (Figs. 20.37A and B)

- **Bilateral:** Involves both kidneys.
- **Size of the kidney: Markedly enlarged**; weight is increased and each may reach up to 4 kg.
- External surface: Bosselated.
- **Cut section:** The kidney is composed of **numerous cysts of varying sizes**, measuring up to 3–4 cm in diameter, with no intervening parenchyma.
- **Content of cysts:** The cysts are filled with fluid, which may be **clear, serous fluid, or more commonly** contain **turbid, red to brown**, sometimes hemorrhagic fluid.

Microscopy

Cysts

- **Number: Numerous cysts** with functioning nephrons between these cysts.
- **Origin:** Cysts can **arise at any level (or segments) of the nephron.** This includes proximal tubules, distal tubules, and collecting ducts, and therefore, they **show variable lining epithelia**. Occasionally, epithelial cells of Bowman capsules may be involved in cyst formation.
- **Lining: Cuboidal and columnar** epithelium.

Intervening renal parenchyma: The pressure of the expanding cysts causes ischemic atrophy of the intervening renal substance. The renal parenchyma may show foci of interstitial fibrosis and pyelonephritis.

Clinical Features

- **Majority** of patients remain **asymptomatic until the fourth decade** of life.
- It may present with **flank pain** (heaviness or dragging sensation), **bilateral abdominal masses, renal colic**

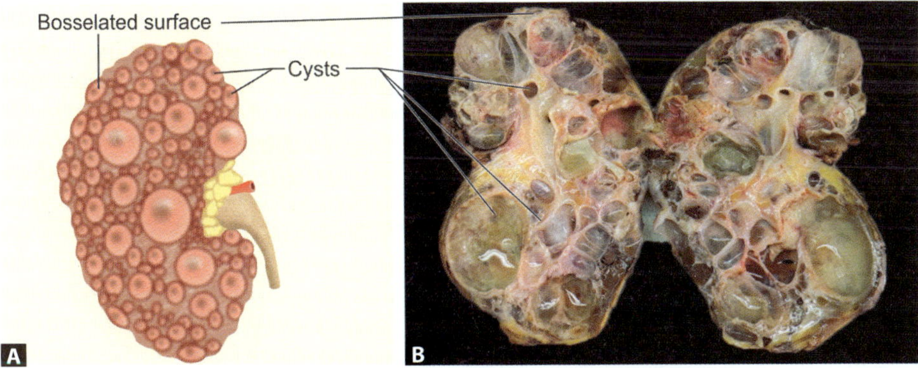

Figs. 20.37A and B: Autosomal-dominant adult polycystic kidney disease (ADPKD): (A) External surface (diagrammatic); (B) Cut section shows markedly enlarged kidneys with numerous dilated cysts of varying sizes that have replaced almost the entire renal parenchyma.

(due to passage of blood clots in the urine), and **hypertension**. When a sufficient quantity of nephrons is destroyed, the patient develops **renal failure**. Chronic renal failure develops between the ages of 40–60 years.

Extrarenal associated congenital anomalies: These include the following:

- Cysts in other organs such as the liver (**polycystic liver disease**).
- Intracranial **berry (saccular) aneurysms** in the **circle of Willis** which may rupture and cause subarachnoid hemorrhages.
- **Mitral valve prolapse** and other cardiac valvular anomalies.

Progress: Patients with **ADPKD progress to chronic kidney disease (CKD)**.

Autosomal Recessive (Childhood) Polycystic Kidney Disease

Autosomal recessive (childhood) polycystic kidney disease (ARPKD) is **genetically different from adult polycystic kidney disease** (ADPKD).

Subcategories: ARPKD can be categorized as **perinatal, neonatal, infantile, and juvenile**, depending on the time of presentation. The perinatal and neonatal categories are the most common and are usually fatal.

Pathogenesis

Mutation in PKHD1 Gene

In the **majority** of cases, ARPKD is caused by **mutations of the polycystic kidney hepatic disease (*PKHD1*) gene**. PKHD1 **encodes for a protein called fibrocystin [polyductin complex (FPC)]**. It is highly expressed in the epithelial cells of the collecting ducts and thick ascending loops of Henle.

Fibrocystin: It is localized to the primary cilia of epithelial cells of renal tubules (cortical and medullary collecting ducts) and cholangiocytes of bile ducts. Probably, it may be a cell surface receptor involved in collecting duct and biliary differentiation.

MORPHOLOGY

Gross

- **Both kidneys** are **markedly enlarged** and have a **smooth external appearance**. Thus, they retain their **reniform configuration**.
- **Cut section (Figs. 20.38A and B):**
  - **Medulla and cortex** are completely **replaced by numerous small cysts.**
  - The cysts tend to be **linear and radiate from the medulla to the outer cortex** (right angles to the cortical surface). It gives a **sponge-like appearance to the kidney.**

Microscopy

- **Shape: Cyst is cylindrical** and appears as a dilated tubular structure or, less commonly saccular.
- **Lining: All the cysts are lined** by **cuboidal epithelial cells,** reflecting their **origin from the collecting ducts.**

In almost all patients, the liver also shows cysts, portal fibrosis, and proliferation of portal bile ducts.

Clinical Features

ARPKD patients have **large, cystic kidneys at birth**. Patients who survive infancy (infantile and juvenile forms), may develop **congenital hepatic fibrosis.** It is characterized by bland periportal fibrosis and the proliferation of well-differentiated biliary ductules. Older children may develop portal hypertension with splenomegaly. Usually, death occurs in infancy or childhood.

Medullary Diseases with Cysts

Q. Write a short answer on the medullary sponge kidney.

Two major types of cystic disease affect the medulla: (1) nephronophthisis-medullary cystic disease complex and (2) medullary sponge kidney.

1. **Nephronophthisis-medullary cystic disease complex:** It usually begins in childhood. It is associated with renal dysfunction and progresses to chronic kidney disease. Depending on the time of onset, it is divided into (i) infantile, (ii) juvenile (most common), (iii) adolescent, and (iv) adult.

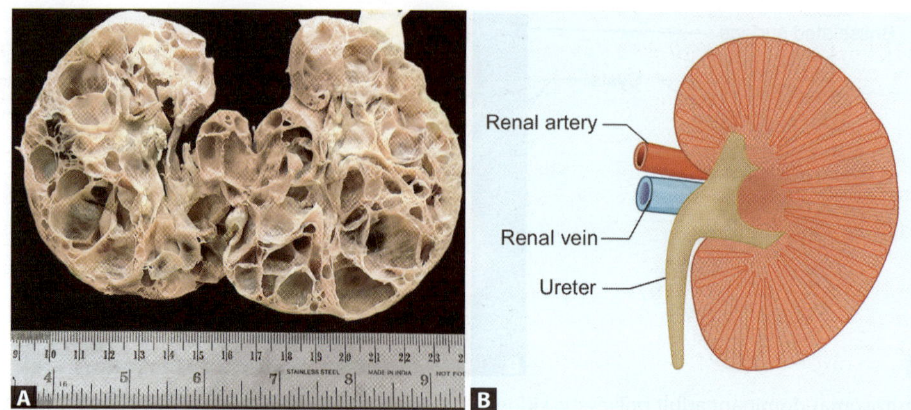

Figs. 20.38A and B: Gross appearance of a cut section of autosomal recessive polycystic kidney disease (ARPKD): (A) Showing smaller cysts and an outer smooth surface; (B) Diagrammatic representation showing dilated channels at right angles to the cortical surface.

2. **Medullary sponge kidney:** It is relatively common and usually harmless. It is characterized by dilation of terminal collecting ducts and medullary cysts of variable size. Symptomatic cases are often associated with renal stones (nephrolithiasis).

MORPHOLOGY

Gross

Kidneys are **small and contracted.** Numerous small cysts are seen at the corticomedullary junction.

Microscopy

These cysts are lined by flattened or cuboidal epithelium. Other nonspecific findings include chronic tubulointerstitial nephritis, tubular atrophy, thickening of the tubular basement membranes, and interstitial fibrosis.

Clinical Features

It usually manifests with polyuria and polydipsia due to reduced tubular function. Over a period of 5–10 years, it progresses to end-stage renal disease.

UROLITHIASIS (RENAL CALCULI, STONES)

PA 28.13 (CC) (a): Define classify and describe the etiology, pathogenesis, pathology, laboratory, urinary findings, distinguishing features progression, and complications of renal stone disease.

Q. Write a short note on renal stones.

Urolithiasis is the formation of calculus (stone) at any level in the urinary collecting system. Most commonly calculi arise in the kidney (renal pelvis and calyces). **Peak is between 20 and 30 years old.** They are more common in men than in women.

Terminology

- **Nephrolithiasis (renal stones):** Stones that occur **within the collecting system of the kidney**.
- **Urolithiasis (urinary calculi/stones):** Stones occurring **anywhere in the collecting system** of the urinary tract.
- **Primary stone:** It is the stone that **develops in sterile urine and often originates in the kidney**.
- **Secondary stone:** It is the stone that **occurs in the presence of infection, outflow obstruction, impaired bladder emptying, or a foreign body**.

Etiology

Q. Write a short note on the etiopathogenesis of renal stones.

The cause of stone formation in the kidney is usually unknown, particularly in calcium-containing stones.

Familial and hereditary predisposition: Stone formation has an association with family history. Hereditary diseases such as inborn errors of metabolism may predispose to stone formation. For example, in cystinuria and primary hyperoxaluria, there is excessive production and excretion of stone-forming substances.

Other risk factors: These include the following:

- Individual factors
- Geography
- **Diet:** A deficiency of vitamin A causes desquamation of epithelium and these cells may form a nidus on which a stone can be deposited.
- Dehydration
- **Infection:** It favors the formation of calculi. Stone formation is common when urine is infected with urea-splitting streptococci, staphylococci, and, especially *Proteus*.
- Metabolic alterations
- **Altered urinary solutes and colloids:** Dehydration increases the concentration of urinary solutes which are liable to precipitate.
- **Decreased urinary citrate:** Citrate in urine is present as citric acid and is under hormonal control. It tends to keep otherwise relatively insoluble calcium phosphate and citrate in solution. Urinary excretion of citrate is decreased during menstruation.

- Changes in urinary pH.
- **Urinary stasis:** It favors stone formation.

Q. Write a short note on types of renal stones.

Types of Renal Stones (Box 20.19)

These include (i) calcium stones, (ii) magnesium stones, (iii) uric acid, (iv) cystine stones, and (v) others.

Calcium Stones (Calcium Oxalate and/or Calcium Phosphate)

Most (80%) renal stones are **composed of calcium oxalate alone or mixed with calcium phosphate**. These stones are radiopaque. The etiological factors **(Box 20.19)** are as follows:

- **Hypercalciuria without hypercalcemia:** It is **observed in about 50% of patients with calcium stones.** Most of these patients absorb excessive amounts of calcium from the gut (absorptive hypercalciuria) and excrete it in the urine. Some have a primary renal defect in calcium reabsorption by renal tubules (renal hypercalciuria).
- **Hypercalcemia and hypercalciuria:** It is found in about 10% of patients and may be due to hyperparathyroidism, diffuse bone disease, or sarcoidosis.

Birefringent crystals in urine are seen in calcium oxalate stones.

Struvite Stones (Magnesium Stones)

Q. Write a short answer on struvite stones.

About 10% of stones are composed of magnesium ammonium phosphate (struvite) and are **known as struvite stones or triple phosphate stones**. They **develop** in individuals with persistently alkaline urine secondary to UTIs. **Infections of the urinary tract by urea-splitting bacteria** (e.g., ***Proteus vulgaris*** **and staphylococci**) convert urea to ammonia and produce alkaline pH. Slowing of urine flow causes precipitation of magnesium, ammonium, phosphate (struvite), and calcium phosphate (apatite). Bacteria may also serve as nidi for the formation of any type of stone. In vitamin A deficiency, desquamated cells from the metaplastic epithelium of the collecting system may act as nidi for stones.

BOX 20.19: Types and causes of renal stones.

1. **Calcium oxalate and/or calcium phosphate (80%)**
   - Idiopathic hypercalciuria without hypercalcemia (most common)
   - Hypercalciuria and hypercalcemia
   - Hyperoxaluria: Enteric or primary. It causes "nucleation" of calcium oxalate in the collecting ducts
   - Hyperuricosuria: Hereditary (primary oxaluria) or acquired
   - No known metabolic abnormality
2. **Struvite (magnesium, ammonium, phosphate) (~10%)**
   - Urinary tract infection
3. **Uric acid (~7%)**
   - Associated with hyperuricemia
   - Associated with hyperuricosuria
   - Idiopathic
4. **Cystine (~2%)**
5. **Others/Unknown (~1%)**

Uric Acid and Urate Stones

Uric acid stone is commonly found in patients **with hyperuricemia** and high urine uric acid levels (e.g., gout), treatment of **certain cancers involving rapid cell turnover**. (e.g., leukemias). However, more than 50% of patients have neither hyperuricemia nor increased urinary excretion of uric acid, but excrete a persistently acidic urine with a pH <5.5. **Uric acid is insoluble in acidic urine** and this low pH predisposes to uric acid stone formation.

Cystine Stones

Cystine stones are uncommon. It is almost always associated with cystinuria due to genetic defects in the renal transport of certain amino acids, including cystine. Stones form at low urinary pH (acidic urine).

Q. Write a short answer on the causes of renal stones (conditions in which it occurs).

Pathogenesis of Renal Stones

Q. Write a short note on the pathogenesis of renal stones.

There are two main steps involved in stone formation: Initiation and propagation of stones.

1. **Supersaturation:** Initiation starts with the supersaturation of urine.
   - **Increased urinary concentration of stone constituents:** It is the most important factor in stone formation and exceeds their solubility (supersaturation).
   - **Decreased urine volume:** It may also favor supersaturation.
2. **Precipitation of crystals:** Deficiency in inhibitors of crystal formation in urine enhances the precipitation of crystals. These inhibitors include pyrophosphates, citrates, glycosaminoglycans, osteopontin, and a glycoprotein called neprocalcin.

MORPHOLOGY

General Features of Renal Stones

- Stones are **unilateral** in **about 80%** of patients.
- **Number:** It may be **single or multiple**.
- **Common sites of formation:** Renal **calyces** and **pelvis** and in the **bladder**.
- **Size:** Calculi are usually small (average diameter, 2–3 mm)
- **Shape:** Stones may have **smooth contours (surface) or** may be **irregular, jagged masses of spicules**.

Calcium Oxalate and/or Calcium Phosphate (~80%)

Most (80%) renal stones are **composed of calcium oxalate alone or mixed with calcium phosphate.**

- **Calcium oxalate** stone **(Fig. 20.39A)**: It is irregular in shape, **hard,** and covered with **sharp projections. Hemorrhage** from the mucosa of the renal pelvis may be produced by its sharp edges and blood may cover the stone **making it appear black.** It is radiodense (radio-opaque). **Urine sediment** shows needle-shaped/square envelope-shaped oxalate.
- **Calcium phosphate** stone **(Fig. 20.39B)**: It is **soft and pale.**

Struvite Stones (Triple Stones/Magnesium, Ammonium, Phosphate Stones)

Q. Write a short answer on staghorn calculus.

- **Color: Yellow-white** and **solitary**
- **Consistency: Hard** to **soft** and **friable**
- **Size:** These are **the largest stones** because normally large amounts of urea are excreted. **Sometimes fill the pelvis and calyces** to **form a cast** of these spaces and is referred to as a **staghorn calculus (Figs. 20.39C and D).** Even a very large staghorn calculus may be clinically silent for years until it produces hematuria, urinary infection, or renal failure.
- Easily seen on radiographic films.
- **Urine sediment**: it shows coffin lid-shaped crystals

Uric Acid Stones

- Uric acid stones are **radiolucent;** this contrasts with radiopaque calcium stones.
- They are **smooth,** and **hard, and** vary from **yellow to reddish-brown.** Sometimes have a multifaceted appearance.
- They are usually **multiple** and are **less than 2 cm** in diameter.
- They show **lamination on the cut section.**
- **Urine sediment**: It shows diamond/barrel-shaped crystals.

Cystine Stones

- Cystine stones are **small, round, smooth,** and usually **multiple**
- **Yellow and waxy.**
- They are **very hard** and radiopaque because of their sulfur content.
- **Urine sediment:** It may show the characteristic **hexagonal cystine crystals** and crystal formation is favored in acidic urine (low pH).

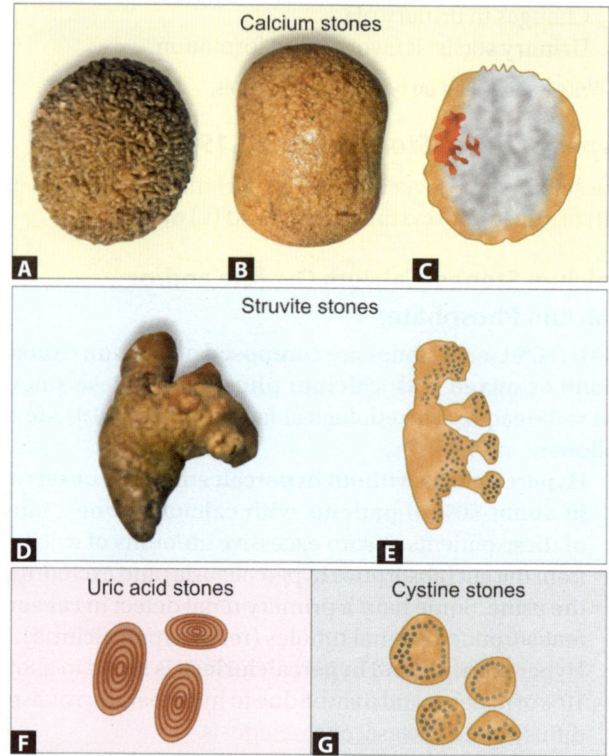

Figs. 20.39A to G: Calcium stones: (A) Calcium oxalate stone; (B) Calcium phosphate stone; (C) Diagrammatic calcium stone; (D) Staghorn calculus; (E) Staghorn calculus (diagrammatic); (F) Uric acid stone (diagrammatic); (G) Cystine stones (diagrammatic).

Clinical Features of Renal Stones

Age: The **peak age at onset is between 20 and 30 years.**

Sex: Renal stones are more common in men than in women.

Asymptomatic: Urolithiasis may be asymptomatic and incidentally discovered in an abdominal computed tomography (CT) or ultrasound examination for other purposes. Larger stones cannot enter the ureters and will likely **remain silent** within the renal pelvis.

Symptoms: The most common presenting symptoms are as follows:

- **Renal or ureteric colic:** Small stones **may pass into the ureters**, producing **severe colicky flank and/or abdominal pain** radiating to the anterior abdominal wall. This symptom complex is termed renal or ureteric colic. These symptoms are due to partial or complete obstruction of urinary flow produced by stones while passing through the ureter.
- **Hematuria (microscopic or gross):** Stone may produce **ulceration and bleeding**. Larger stones may present with **hematuria.**
- **Renal damage:** Obstruction may **lead to significant damage to the renal parenchyma**. Stones also **predispose to superimposed infection** both due to obstruction and trauma. This may also **cause significant renal damage.**

Laboratory tests: These include serum studies for renal function, electrolytes, calcium, magnesium, phosphate, and uric acid. If there is hypercalcemia, a parathyroid hormone (PTH) level should be obtained.

Complications of Renal Stones

1. **Hematuria**
2. **Hydronephrosis** due to obstruction
3. **Pyelonephritis and pyonephrosis**
4. **Carcinoma:** Stones can cause squamous metaplasia and later squamous cell carcinoma.

URINARY TRACT OBSTRUCTION (OBSTRUCTIVE UROPATHY)

PA 28.13b (CC): Define classify and describe the etiology, pathogenesis, pathology, laboratory, urinary findings, distinguishing features progression, and complications of obstructive uropathy.

Definition: Obstructive uropathy is a term used for **obstruction in the urinary passage** involving the urethra, bladder, ureters, or pelvicalyceal system.

Urinary tract obstruction is caused by **structural or functional abnormalities** and results in **obstruction of the flow of urine (Figs. 20.39A to G). Consequences of obstruction are** as follows**:**

- Unrelieved obstruction almost always leads to:
  - **Renal dysfunction (obstructive nephropathy)** and **permanent renal atrophy**.
  - **Dilation of the collecting system** (hydronephrosis).
- **Increased susceptibility to infection** and **renal stone formation**.

Hydronephrosis

Q. Write a short note on hydronephrosis.

Definition: Hydronephrosis is defined as an aseptic **dilation of the renal pelvis and calyces due to obstruction of urinary outflow,** associated with **progressive atrophy of the kidney**.

Q. Write a short note on the causes (etiology) and pathogenesis of hydronephrosis.

Causes of obstruction: Causes of urinary tract obstruction are presented in **Box 20.20 and Figure 20.40.** Obstruction may be due to a structural or functional disorder. Obstruction may be **complete or incomplete,** may be sudden or insidious, and may occur at any level of the urinary tract, from the urethra to the renal pelvis.

- **Bilateral hydronephrosis**: It occurs only when the obstruction is below the level of the ureters.
- **Unilateral hydronephrosis:** It occurs when the blockage is at the ureters or above.

BOX 20.20: Causes of urinary tract obstruction.

STRUCTURAL DISORDERS

Congenital Anomalies: These are as follows:

- **Urethra:** Atresia of the urethra, posterior urethral valves (in either the ureter or urethra) and urethral strictures, meatal stenosis
- **Bladder:** Bladder neck obstruction, severe vesicoureteral reflux
- **Ureter:** Obstructive megaureter, ectopic ureter, aberrant renal artery compressing the ureter, abnormal position of the kidney with torsion, or kinking of the ureter
- **Ureteropelvic junction:** Ureteropelvic junction narrowing or obstruction
- **Infundibular/pelvis:** Congenital narrowing

Acquired Conditions

- **Urinary calculi:** It may be at the ureter, ureteropelvic junction, or infundibular/pelvis.
- **Foreign bodies**, e.g., sloughed necrotic papillae
- **Proliferative lesions**
  - **Benign prostatic hypertrophy**
  - **Tumors:** These may be intrinsic or extrinsic. Examples are carcinoma of the prostate, bladder tumors (papilloma and carcinoma), contiguous malignant disease (retroperitoneal lymphoma, and carcinoma of the cervix or uterus)
- **Inflammatory lesions:** Prostatitis, urethritis, retroperitoneal fibrosis
- **Pregnancy, uterine prolapse and cystocele**

FUNCTIONAL DISORDERS

Neurogenic bladder (spinal cord damage or diabetic nephropathy).

Pathogenesis

Obstruction in the urinary tract (Fig. 20.40 and Box 20.12): It may be **complete or incomplete**. Obstruction in the urinary tract leads to the **accumulation of urine proximal to the obstruction**.

- **Initial stages show dilation of calyces and renal pelvis:** Even if there is complete urinary tract obstruction, glomerular filtration does not stop but continues for some time. This is because the filtrate in the nephrons subsequently diffuses back into the renal interstitium and perirenal spaces. This filtrate ultimately returns to the lymphatic and venous systems. Because of this continued glomerular filtration, the filtrate accumulates in the affected calyces and pelvis. This leads to the **dilation of the pelvis and calyces, often markedly due to back pressure.**
- **Later stages show renal atrophy and compression of renal vasculature:** Raised pressure in the renal pelvis and calyces is transmitted back through the collecting ducts into the renal parenchyma, and its consequences are:
  - **Renal atrophy**
  - **Compresses the renal vasculature of the medulla,** leading to reduced blood flow to the medulla. Initially, compression of vasculature in the medulla is reversible, but if it persists, it can lead to disturbances in medullary function.
  - **Functional disturbances:** The initial functional alterations caused due to urinary obstruction mainly involve tubular function. This manifests as impaired concentrating ability. Later, the **glomerular filtration rate (GFR)** will be **reduced.**
  - **Interstitial inflammation:** Obstruction also initiates an interstitial inflammatory reaction and leads to fibrosis of the interstitium.

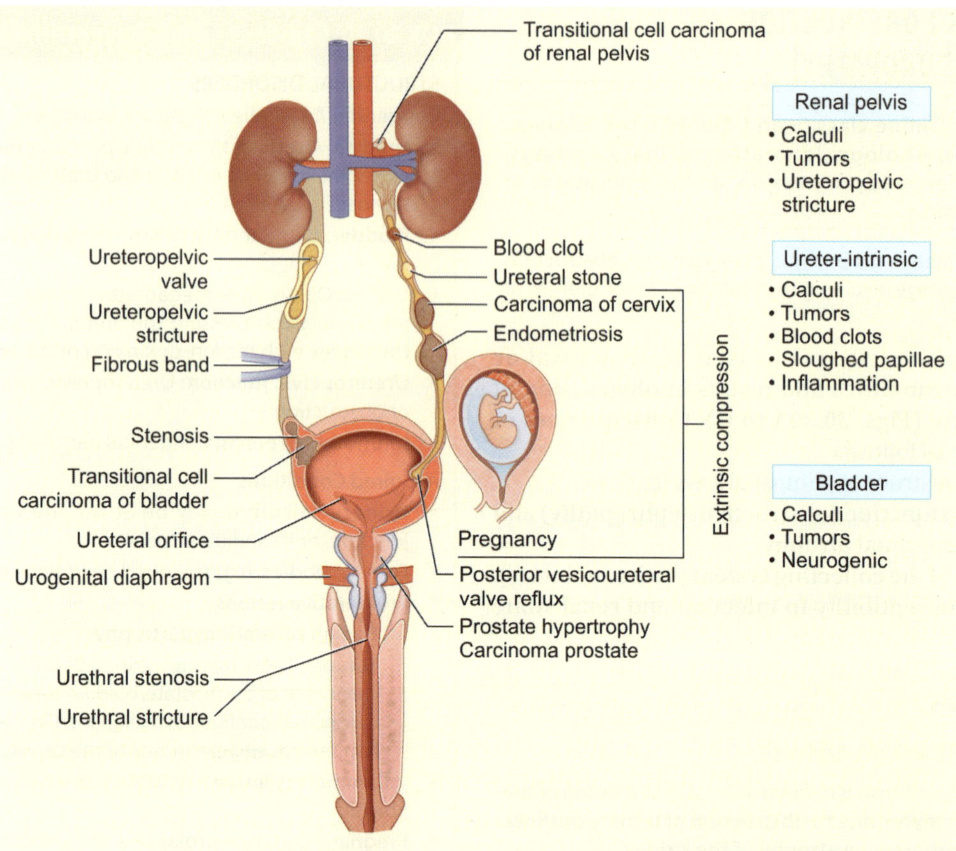

Fig. 20.40: Various common obstructive lesions of the urinary tract.

MORPHOLOGY

Q. Write a short answer on the morphology (gross and microscopy) of the kidney in hydronephrosis.

Type of Obstruction and its Consequence

- **Sudden and complete obstruction:** It reduces the glomerular filtration and leads to **mild dilation** of the pelvis and calyces.
- **Subtotal or intermittent obstruction:** It does not suppress glomerular filtration, and **produces progressive dilation.**

Level of Obstruction

Depending on the level of urinary obstruction, the dilation may first affect the bladder or ureter and then the kidney.

Gross

Depending on the level of obstruction, it may be **unilateral or bilateral** and **may be accompanied by dilatation of the ureter (hydroureter).**

Depending on the degree and the duration of the obstruction, the kidney may show **slight to massive enlargement.**

- **Early stage:** Simple **dilation of the pelvis and calyces** (pelvicalyceal system).
- **Late stage:** Progressive **blunting of the apices of the renal pyramids.**
- **Advanced stage: The kidney may appear** like a **thin-walled, cystic structure** having a diameter of up to 15–20 cm. **Renal parenchyma shows destruction due to severe pressure atrophy and thinning of the cortex.** A kidney destroyed by longstanding hydronephrosis appears as a thin-walled, lobulated, fluid-filled sac **(Fig. 20.41).**

Microscopy

- **Tubules:** The early lesions show dilation and atrophy of tubules.
- **Renal pelvis and calyces:** Progressive dilation of the renal pelvis and calyces leads to renal parenchymal atrophy.
- **Glomeruli:** They are usually spared and, in later stages, show partial or complete sclerosis followed by loss of the glomeruli.
- **Interstitium:** Marked chronic inflammatory infiltrate and fibrosis. Hydronephrotic kidneys are more prone to pyelonephritis. This further adds injury to renal parenchyma.

Clinical Features

Clinical features **depend on the cause of obstruction.** For example, calculi in the ureters may present with renal colic, and prostatic enlargements may present with bladder symptoms.

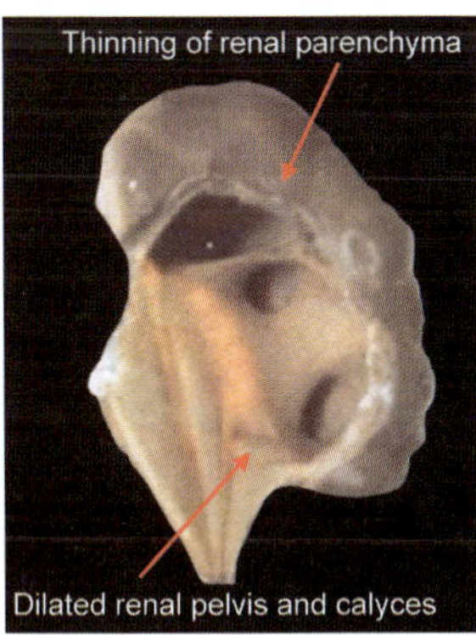

Hydronephrosis: The nature of obstruction may be:
- Congenital or acquired
- Sudden or insidious
- Partial or complete
- Unilateral or bilateral
- Intrinsic lesions or extrinsic lesions
- May occur at any level of the urinary tract from the urethra to the renal pelvis

Fig. 20.41: Marked hydronephrosis of the kidney showing marked dilation of the pelvis and calyces and thinning of the renal parenchyma.

Unilateral complete or partial hydronephrosis: It may be silent due to maintenance of adequate renal function by the unaffected kidney.
Bilateral partial obstruction: It may manifest as **polyuria and nocturia** due to the inability to concentrate the urine (tubular dysfunction).
Complete bilateral obstruction: It presents with **oliguria or anuria**.
Ultrasonography is **useful** in the diagnosis of obstructive uropathy.

MALIGNANT TUMORS OF THE KIDNEY

PA 28.14 (CC): Classify and describe the etiology, genetics, pathogenesis, pathology, presenting features, progression, and spread of renal tumors.

Q. Classify tumors of the kidney. Describe the etiopathogenesis and morphology of renal cell carcinoma.

Both benign and malignant tumors can occur in the kidney. The most common malignant tumors are renal cell carcinoma and nephroblastoma. WHO classification (2022) (abridged) of tumors of the kidney is presented in **Box 20.21.**

BOX 20.21: The World Health Organization (WHO) (2022) (abridged) classification of tumors of the kidney.

Renal cell tumors
- **Clear cell renal tumors**
  - Clear cell renal cell carcinoma
  - Multilocular cystic renal neoplasm of low malignant potential
- **Papillary renal tumors**
  - Renal papillary adenoma
  - Papillary renal cell carcinoma
- **Oncocytic and chromophobe renal tumors**
  - Oncocytoma of the kidney
  - Chromophobe renal cell carcinoma
  - Other oncocytic tumors of the kidney
- **Collecting duct tumors**
  - Collecting duct carcinoma
- **Other renal tumors**
  - Clear cell papillary renal cell tumor
  - Mucinous tubular and spindle cell carcinoma
  - Tubulocystic renal cell carcinoma
  - Acquired cystic disease-associated renal cell carcinoma
  - Eosinophilic solid and cystic renal cell carcinoma
  - Renal cell carcinoma NOS
- **Molecularly defined renal carcinomas**

Metanephric tumors
Mixed epithelial and stromal renal tumors

Renal mesenchymal tumors
- **Adult renal mesenchymal tumors**
- **Pediatric renal mesenchymal tumors**

Embryonal neoplasms of the kidney
- Nephroblastic tumors: Nephroblastoma

Miscellaneous renal tumors

Renal Cell Carcinoma

Q. Write a short note on renal cell carcinoma.

Renal cell carcinoma (RCC) is a **malignant tumor** of the kidney. Because of their **gross yellow color** and the **microscopic resemblance of the tumor cells to clear cells of the adrenal cortex**; these tumors were initially thought to arise from embryonic adrenal rests and **were called hypernephroma**. Outdated terminology used for RCC includes renal clear cell adenocarcinoma, Grawitz tumor, and hypernephroma.

- **Cell of origin:** The tumors arise from **renal tubular epithelium**. Hence, they are located predominantly in the cortex of the kidney.
- Renal cell carcinoma **represents 80–85% of all primary malignant neoplasms of the kidney**.
- **Age and gender:** RCC is most common from the **sixth to seventh decades** of life. **More common in males** with a male-to-female ratio of 2:1.

Risk factors for renal cell carcinoma are presented in **Box 20.22**.

BOX 20.22: Risk factors for renal cell carcinoma.

- Tobacco: Cigarette and pipe smoking
- Obesity (mainly in women)
- Hypertension
- Occupational exposure to cadmium. Exposure to asbestos, petroleum products, and heavy metals
- Unopposed estrogen therapy
- Chronic renal failure and acquired polycystic disease as a complication of chronic dialysis.
- Tuberous sclerosis.

Q. Write a short note on the classification of renal cell carcinoma.

Classification of renal cell carcinomas (Box 20.13): RCCs are classified based on morphology, growth patterns, and molecular origins. The three most common forms are clear cell carcinoma, papillary renal cell carcinoma, and chromophobe renal carcinoma.

Clear Cell Carcinoma

Clear cell carcinoma renal cell carcinoma is the most common type, and it accounts for 70–80% of renal cell carcinomas.

Definition: Clear cell RCC is a **morphologically heterogeneous group of malignant neoplasms** composed of **cells with clear or eosinophilic granular cytoplasm.** These neoplasms are nonpapillary and show typical vessel formation. These tumors have a characteristic molecular background, with **inactivation of VHL and upregulation of HIFs.**

Pathogenesis (Fig. 20.42)

Most cases (95%) of clear cell RCC are **sporadic**, but they can be **familial or occur in association with von Hippel-Lindau** (VHL) **disease.**

***VHL* gene:** von Hippel-Lindau (VHL) disease is an autosomal dominant disorder. It is caused by an inherited germline loss-of-function mutation of the *VHL* gene on chromosome 3p25. VHL disease is characterized by a predisposition to various neoplasms, especially hemangioblastomas of the cerebellum and retina. ***VHL* gene function is lost in familial clear cell RCC and the majority of sporadic clear cell carcinomas.**

***VHL* gene mutations:** The *VHL* gene is a tumor suppressor gene located in the short arm of chromosome 3. This gene is involved in sporadic and familial RCCs. The ***VHL* gene encodes a protein called VHL protein.** The VHL protein **forms a part of a ubiquitin ligase complex involved in the degradation of other proteins.** One of the important target proteins of the VHL protein is the **transcription factor HIF-1α. The molecular hallmark of clear cell carcinoma is the loss or inactivation of both copies of the *VHL* gene.** About 98% of clear cell carcinoma (familial, sporadic, or associated with VHL syndrome) show **loss of the short arm of chromosome 3 with loss of the *VHL* gene.** In up to 80% of clear cell cancers, a second allele of the *VHL* gene is inactivated (or lost) by somatic mutations or hypermethylation-induced inactivation.

Consequences of *VHL* gene mutations: When *VHL* is inactive, HIF-1α cannot be degraded, and it accumulates. High levels of HIF-1α cause inappropriate expression of many HIF target genes that are usually turned on by HIF. These include genes that **promote angiogenesis** (e.g., VEGF) and genes that **stimulate cell growth** [e.g., insulin-like growth factor-1 (IGF-1)]. Also, HIF collaborates in complex ways with the oncogenic factor MYC to "reprogram" cellular metabolism and promote cell growth.

Papillary Renal Cell Carcinoma

Papillary renal cell carcinoma is the **second most common subtype**, accounting for 10–15% of all renal cancers. It shows a characteristic papillary or tubulo-papillary growth pattern. These tumors are frequently multifocal and bilateral and present at early stages.

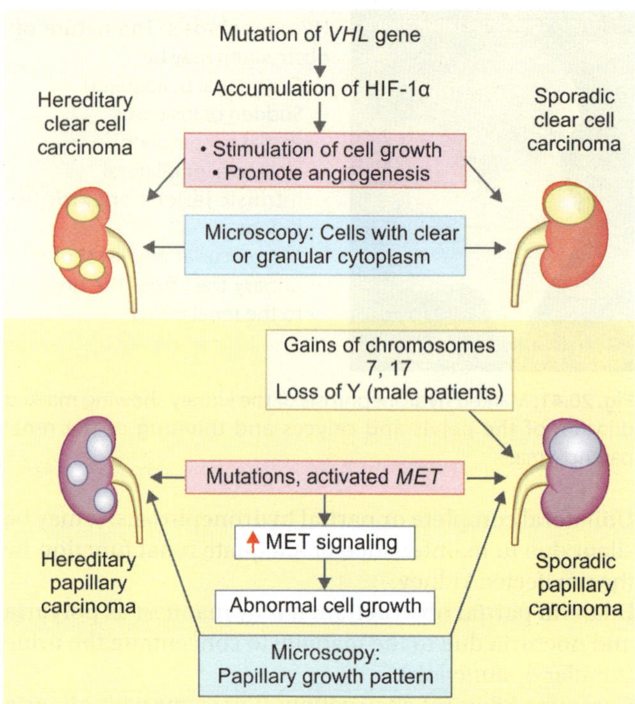

Fig. 20.42: Cytogenetics, genetics, and microscopic features of clear cell and papillary renal cell carcinoma.

Cell of origin: It arises from **distal convoluted tubule epithelial cells.**

Age: The age of presentation ranges from the pediatric age group to extreme old age. The mean age distribution among adults is 59–63 years.

Pathogenesis (Fig. 20.42)

Papillary renal cell carcinomas are molecularly heterogeneous. They also occur in familial and sporadic forms.

MET alterations

***MET* gene:** It is a proto-oncogene present on chromosome 7q. MET is a tyrosine kinase receptor encoded by the ***MET* gene.** The genetic abnormalities common in both forms are an **increase in the function of MET.** This increases MET signaling and causes abnormal growth of proximal tubular epithelial cells.

Sporadic tumors: Increased MET function in these tumors is usually due to increased *MET* copy number or from somatic activating mutations in *MET*.

Familial cases: They are usually caused by germline-activating *MET* mutations.

Others

Papillary renal cell carcinomas commonly have gains of chromosomes 7 and 17, and loss of the Y chromosome.

Chromophobe Renal Cell Carcinoma

Chromophobe renal cell carcinoma is the **least common type** of RCC. It constitutes about 5% of renal cell carcinomas.

Cell of origin: It arises from **intercalated cells of collecting ducts.**

Pathogenesis: Chromophobe renal cell carcinoma shows losses of chromosomes 1, 2, 6, 10, 13, 17, 21, and Y

Tumor cells: They have lightly eosinophilic tumor cells that appear pale (chromophobe). The cells do not appear clear as in clear cell carcinomas.

Prognosis: Chromophobe renal cell cancers have a favorable prognosis.

MORPHOLOGY

Q. Write a short note on the morphology of renal cell carcinoma.

Clear Cell Renal Cell Carcinoma

Gross

- **Site:** May arise in **any part** of the cortex of the kidney. More commonly affects the poles, **mostly the upper pole.**
- **Size varies from 3 to 15 cm in diameter.** High-resolution radiographic techniques may detect smaller tumors incidentally.
- **Outer surface:** It is usually **bosselated and** may distort the renal outline.
- Usually, they occur as **solitary** and **unilateral lesions**.

Cut Surface (Figs. 20.43A and B)

- Tumors may **appear as usually large, circumscribed, spherical masses with well-demarcated margins.** But may show some breach in the renal capsule and invasion into the perinephric fat.
- Tumor is **solid, bright yellow-gray-white,** and shows **areas of hemorrhage, necrosis,** and **cystic change**, which give a **variegated appearance.** The **yellow color** is due to **prominent lipids** in the tumor cells.

Venous Invasion

- **One of the characteristics of RCC** is its **tendency to invade the renal vein.** Sometimes, the tumor may grow as a continuous cord in the inferior vena cava and rarely may extend into the right atrium.

Microscopy (Figs. 20.44A and B)

Q. Write a short answer on microscopic variants of renal cell carcinoma.

Growth pattern: Varies from **solid to trabecular (cord-like), nests, or tubular** (resembling tubules or glands).

Tumor cells: Tumors are **composed of cells with clear or granular cytoplasm** and are **nonpapillary. Most tumors** are well-differentiated with **little cellular or nuclear pleomorphism.**

- **Cell shape:** The tumor cells are **round or polygonal** in shape with **distinct cell membranes.**
- **Cytoplasm: Abundant** either **clear or granular. Clear cells** have sharply outlined cell membranes ("vegetable cells"). The clear cytoplasm is due to **glycogen and lipids**; which are removed by the water and solvents (xylene) used during processing of tissue for histopathological examination. **Eosinophilic cytoplasm** may be seen in many tumors and is especially common in high-grade tumors.
  - **Special stains: Glycogen may be demonstrated with PAS and fat by oil red O stains.**
- **Nucleus:** It is **centrally located** and **small,** which falsely masks the malignant nature of this tumor.

Stroma: Consists of branching vasculature.

Papillary Renal Cell Carcinoma

Gross: Papillary renal cell carcinomas may be bilateral and multiple. They are usually well-circumscribed and often encapsulated. They may also show necrosis, hemorrhage, and cystic degeneration. They have less orange-yellow color on the cut section than clear cell carcinomas due to their lower lipid content.

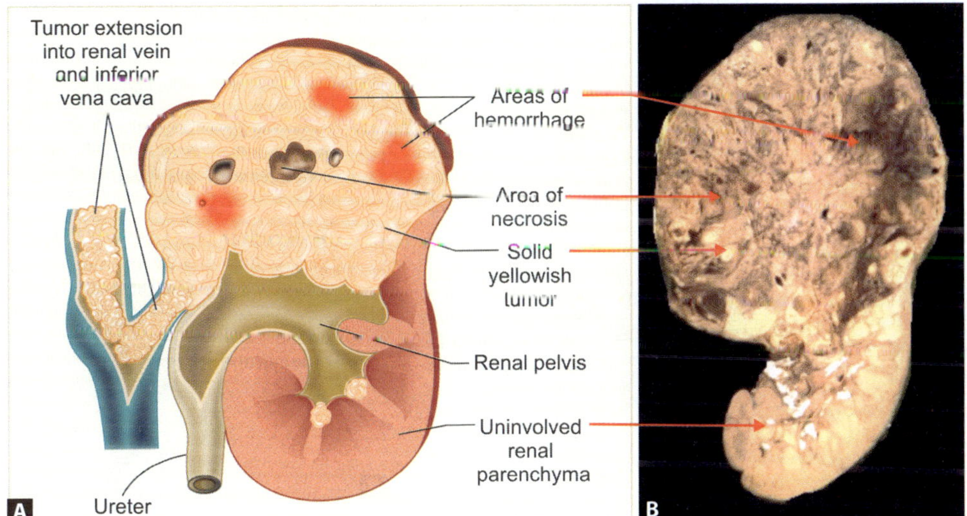

Figs. 20.43A and B: Cut surface of clear cell renal cell carcinoma showing a yellowish, spherical, circumscribed, variegated tumor at the upper pole of the kidney: (A) Diagrammatic; (B) Gross specimen.

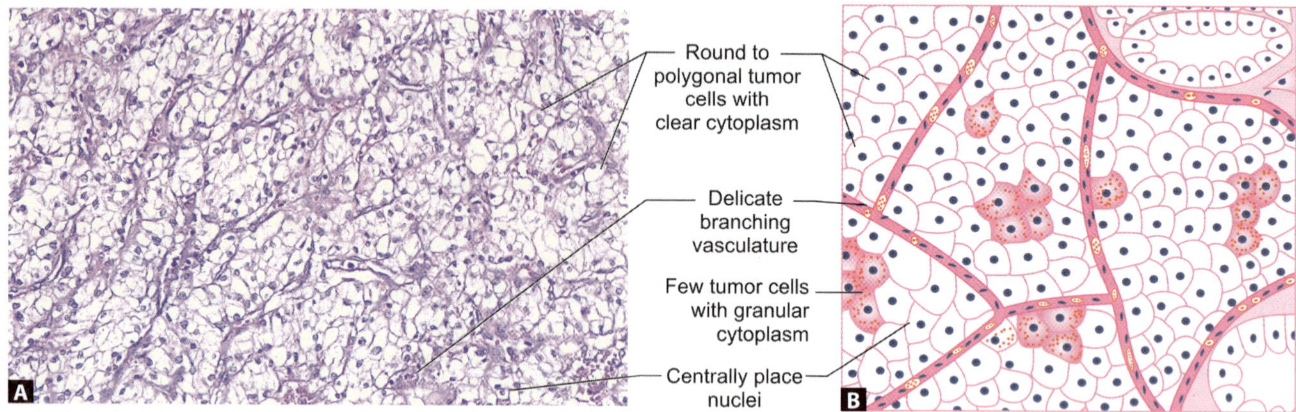

Figs. 20.44A and B: Clear cell renal cell carcinoma: (A) Photomicrograph; (B) Diagrammatic appearance of clear cell type showing solid alveolar arrangement of clear cells separated by vascular stroma.

Microscopy (Fig. 20.45A): It shows a **papillary growth pattern.**

- **Papillary configuration:** The tumor is composed of cuboidal or low columnar tumor cells arranged in complex papillary formations. The **fibrovascular core shows prominent infiltration by foamy macrophages** and may contain numerous psammoma bodies.
- **Cytoplasm** may be **eosinophilic or basophilic.**
- Stroma is usually scanty and highly vascularized.

Chromophobe Renal Cell Carcinoma

Gross: It is well circumscribed, unencapsulated, often large (average 7 cm in diameter), and solitary tumor. The cut surface is homogeneous gray to tan-brown and typically without hemorrhage or necrosis.

Microscopy: Tumor cells are characteristically arranged in a **broad "alveolar" pattern.** It is characterized by **tumor cells with prominent cell membranes, wrinkled nuclei with perinuclear halos,** and **pale to eosinophilic cytoplasm (Fig. 20.45B).**

Clinical Features

The signs and symptoms vary. Classical diagnostic triad (seen in only 10% of cases) of renal cell carcinoma are:

1. **Costovertebral or flank pain**
2. **Palpable abdominal mass**
3. **Hematuria (most reliable)** and occurs in more than 50% of patients.

Q. Write a short note on paraneoplastic syndromes produced by renal cell carcinoma.

Paraneoplastic syndromes (Box 20.23): RCC is one of the great mimics in medicine because it may produce diverse systemic symptoms unrelated to the kidney. Extrarenal manifestations include fever and polycythemia due to the production of erythropoietin by the neoplastic cells. RCCs produce rare systemic/paraneoplastic manifestations/ syndromes related to abnormal, ectopic production of hormones or other products.

These syndromes include polycythemia, hypercalcemia, hypertension, hepatic dysfunction, feminization or masculinization, Cushing's syndrome, systemic amyloidosis, polyneuromyopathy, gastrointestinal disturbances, and hepatosplenomegaly.

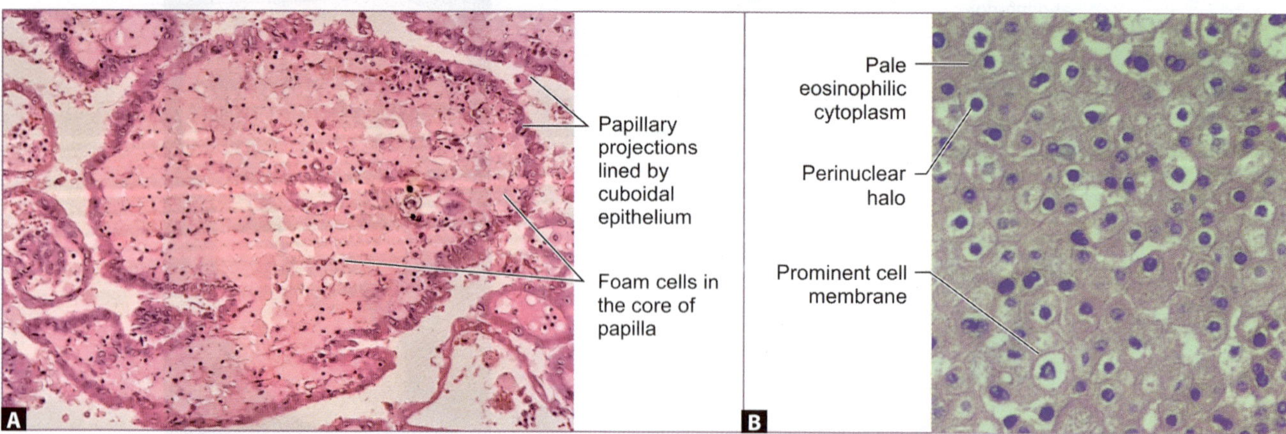

Figs. 20.45A and B: (A) Papillary carcinoma showing papillae lined by single-layer of cuboidal tumor cells and fibrovascular core with foam cell; (B) Chromophobe renal cell carcinoma showing tumor cells with prominent membrane, pale eosinophilic cytoplasm, and perinuclear halo.

BOX 20.23: Examples of paraneoplastic syndromes produced by renal cell carcinoma.

- Polycythemia (due to erythropoietin)
- Hypercalcemia (due to PTHrP)
- Hypertension (due to renin)
- Feminization or masculinization (due to sex hormones)
- Cushing's syndrome (due to ACTH)
- Eosinophilia, leukemoid reactions
- Nonmetastatic hepatic dysfunction (due to IL-6 leading to increased ALP, PT, and bilirubin)

(ALP: alkaline phosphatase; IL-6: interleukin 6; PT: prothrombin time; PTH-rp: parathyroid hormone-related protein)

Spread

Patients may **develop wide metastasis** before giving rise to any local symptoms or signs.

1. **Local spread:** It invades **perinephric fat and renal sinus**.
2. **Lymphatic spread:** Lymphatic metastases can involve the **hilar, aortic, and caval lymph nodes**. They can enter the thoracic duct or directly involve thoracic nodes.
3. **Hematogenous spread:** Most common route. The most common sites are the lungs (cannon ball deposits and pulsating secondaries), bones, liver, adrenal, and brain.

Prognosis: Prognosis is related to many clinicopathologic parameters including the extent of the tumor. The average 5-year survival rate for RCC is about 70% and may be 100% in the absence of distant metastases. With the invasion of the renal vein or extension into the perinephric fat, the 5-year survival rate is reduced to about 60%.

SCENARIO-BASED ESSAY QUESTION

Q. A 55-year-old man presents to the urology department with complaints of feeling fullness and pain in the right flank of his abdomen and gross painless hematuria. He also informed that he lost about 7 kg weight over the last 6 months.

On physical examination, a right-sided flank mass was palpable on bimanual examination. Urine examination showed 3+ hematuria, but no protein, glucose, or leukocytes. An abdominal CT scan showed a 9 cm mass in the upper pole of the right kidney. A right-sided nephrectomy was done.

a. What is the probable diagnosis? (Ans. Clear cell renal cell carcinoma).
b. How do you classify this disease of the kidney? *(refer Box 20.21)*.
c. Describe the gross and microscopic appearance of the kidney in this disease *(refer page 761)*.
d. List the paraneoplastic syndromes produced by this disease *(refer Box 20.23)*.

NEPHROBLASTOMA (WILMS TUMOR)

Q. Write a short note on Wilms tumor.

Definition: Nephroblastoma is a **highly malignant primary embryonal tumor** derived from nephrogenic blastemal cells that replicate the histology of developing kidneys and often show divergent patterns of differentiation. It is the **most common primary kidney tumor in childhood**.

Age group: Most common in children between **2 and 5 years of age**, and more than 95% occur below 10 years of age.

Pathogenesis and Genetics

In **most (90%)** cases, the nephroblastoma is **sporadic** (nonsyndromic) **and unilateral. About 5–10% are** syndromic, **bilateral** which involve either simultaneously (synchronous) or one after the other (metachronous).

Molecular Abnormalities in Syndromic and Congenital Anomalies

Mutations in *WT1* and *WT2*: Mutation in tumor suppressor genes is associated with nephroblastoma. These include **nephroblastoma-associated genes 1 (*WT1*) and *WT2*.** The *WT1* **gene is located on chromosome 11p13.** *WT1* is important for the normal development of kidneys and gonads. Constitutional inactivation of one copy of this gene results in genitourinary abnormalities.

Congenital Malformations Associated with an Increased Risk

In about 5% of cases, arises in three congenital syndromes at an early age and often bilaterally. These syndromes are:

1. **WAGR** (**W**ilms tumor, **a**niridia, **g**enital anomalies, and mental **r**etardation) **syndrome:** It has **germline deletions** of 11p13, a region where the **Wilms tumor gene *(WT1)*** is located.
2. **Denys–Drash syndrome (DDS)** (Wilms tumor, intersexual disorders, glomerulopathy)**: These individuals** have a dominant negative inactivating mutation in the *WT1* gene. This interferes with the function of normal WT1 protein encoded by the other *WT1* allele.
3. **Beckwith–Wiedemann syndrome (BWS):** It is associated with an increased risk for nephroblastoma. These patients have enlargement of individual body organs (e.g., tongue, kidneys, or liver) or entire body segments (hemihypertrophy). The genetic locus in BWS is on chromosome 11 distal to the *WT1* locus. This region contains several genes, including one that encodes insulin-like growth factor-2 (IGF2). Normally, the *IGF2* gene is expressed from the paternal allele (from the father), whereas the maternal allele (from the mother) is imprinted. Some nephroblastomas show loss of imprinting (i.e., re-expression of *IGF2* by the maternal allele). This leads to overexpression of the IGF-2 protein and is responsible for both organ enlargement and tumorigenesis. Patients with BWS also show an increased risk for the development of hepatoblastoma, adrenocortical tumors, rhabdomyosarcoma, and pancreatic tumors.

Molecular Abnormalities in Nonsyndromic (Sporadic) Nephroblastomas

These account for 90% of cases of nephroblastoma.

1. **Gain-of-function mutations of the β-*catenin* gene:** These occur in approximately 10% of sporadic cases of nephroblastomas.
2. **Recurrent mutations occur in genes encoding proteins involved in microRNA processing:** This occurs in 15–20% of cases. The genes involved in microRNA processing include *DROSHA*, *DGCR8*, and *DICER1*. These mutations lead to decreased levels of many mature microRNAs, particularly those involved in "mesenchymal to epithelial transformation" during renal morphogenesis. The absence of mesenchymal to epithelial transformation may lead to persistent blastemal "rests" in the kidney, which can progress into nephroblastoma. **Nephrogenic rests** (small foci of persistent primitive blastemal cells, which are precursor lesions of nephroblastomas) are seen in the renal parenchyma adjacent to bilateral nephroblastoma.
3. ***TP53* mutations:** These nephroblastomas have a poor prognosis and usually microscopically show anaplastic features.
4. Nephroblastoma was **also found in association with other malignancies** (e.g., osteosarcoma, retinoblastoma, hepatocellular carcinoma, and neuroblastoma).

MORPHOLOGY

Q. Write a short note on the morphology of Nephroblastoma.

Gross (Fig. 20.46)

- Nephroblastoma **usually appears as a large, single, round, well-circumscribed** mass. **Usually unilateral** but 10% is either bilateral or multicentric.
- **Cut section:** Tumor is **soft, bulging, homogeneous, and tan to gray.** Foci of hemorrhage, cyst formation, and necrosis may be seen.

Microscopy (Figs. 20.47A and B)

Microscopically, nephroblastomas show tumor cells that show recognizable attempts to recapitulate different stages of nephrogenesis. Tumor shows **three major components,** which resemble normal fetal tissue. The **three types of cells** are:

1. **Undifferentiated blastemal component:** It consists of **small, round to oval blue cells** with **scanty cytoplasm.** These cells are closely packed, and arranged in sheets, nests, and trabeculae.
2. **Immature stromal** (mesenchymal) **component:** It consists of **undifferentiated fibroblast-like spindle cells or myxoid tissue.** They **may show smooth muscle, skeletal muscle, or fibroblast differentiation.**
3. **Immature epithelial component: Epithelial cells show differentiation** in the form of **small abortive (embryonic) tubules or immature glomeruli.**

Classically, the tumor shows a **triphasic** (all three cell types) combination, although the percentage of each component varies. Occasionally, they contain only two elements (biphasic) or even only one (monophasic).

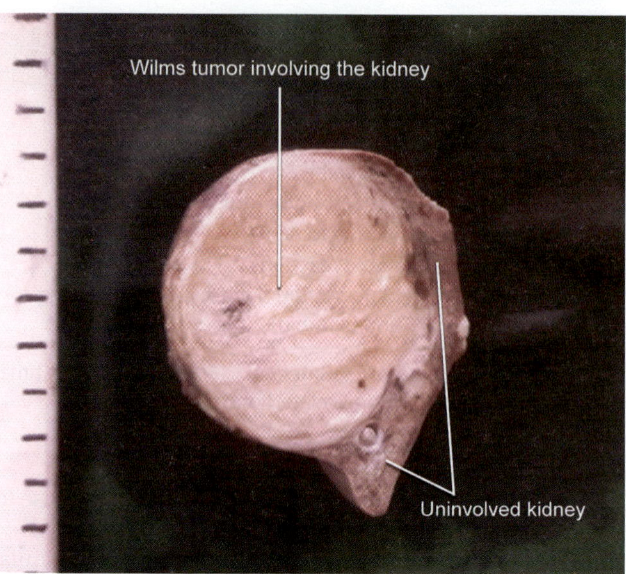

Fig. 20.46: Nephroblastoma of the kidney with well-circumscribed margins.

- **Anaplasia:** Approximately 5% of tumors show foci of **anaplasia.** It is defined as the **presence of cells with large, hyperchromatic, pleomorphic nuclei and atypical abnormal mitotic figures.** Anaplasia is **associated with acquired *TP53* mutations** and such tumors **do not respond to chemotherapy.**

Clinical Features

1. Most children present with a palpable **abdominal mass,** when large it may extend across the midline and down into the pelvis.
2. Others: **Hematuria,** fever, **pain in the abdomen,** intestinal obstruction, and pulmonary metastases are other patterns of presentation.

Spread

1. **Local spread:** It spreads to perirenal soft tissues.
2. **Lymphatics:** It spreads to regional lymph nodes.
3. **Hematogenous:** Lungs, liver and peritoneum.

Prognosis

1. **Clinical parameter:** Children **younger than 2 years** of age have a **better prognosis.**
2. **Histological parameter:**
   - **Invasion of the renal capsule** is associated with **poor prognosis.**
   - **Anaplasia** indicates a **poorer prognosis.**

UROTHELIAL TUMORS

PA 28.16 (NC): Describe the etiology, genetics, pathogenesis, pathology, presenting features, and progression of urothelial tumors.

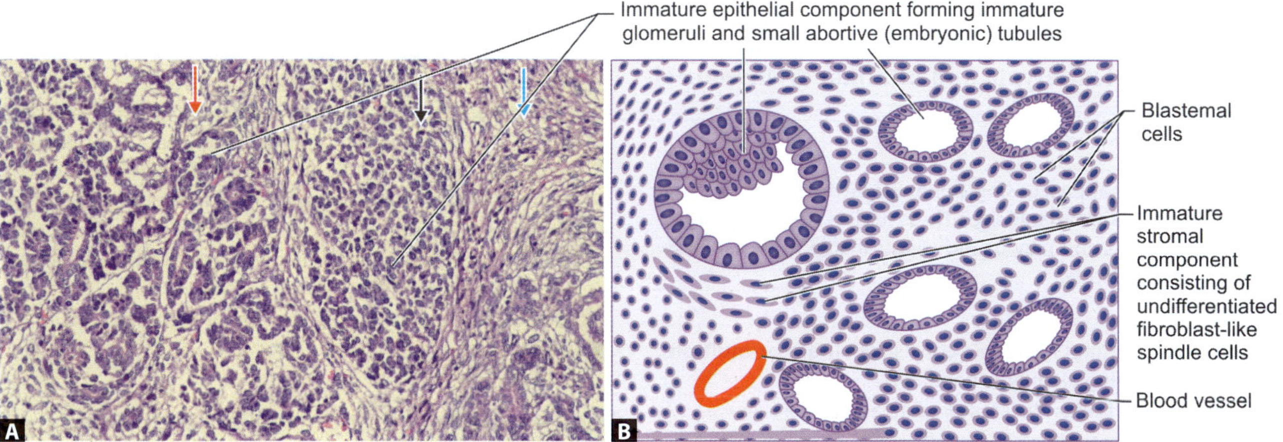

Figs. 20.47A and B: Nephroblastoma with triphasic growth pattern: (A) Hematoxylin and eosin (H & E); (B) Diagrammatic. Nephroblastoma shows highly cellular areas composed of tightly packed blue cells (undifferentiated blastema (black arrow in A) separated by loose stroma containing undifferentiated mesenchymal cells (blue arrow in A), and immature (primitive) tubules (red arrow in A).

Q. Write a short note on urothelial (transitional cell) carcinoma of the urinary bladder.

Urothelial neoplasms are most common and **constitute about 90% of all tumors of the urinary bladder**.

Localization: Urothelial neoplasms can occur in any part of the urinary tract lined by urothelium, from the renal pelvis to the distal urethra.

Behavior: Urothelial neoplasms **vary from small benign lesions that do not recur to aggressive cancers that are often fatal**. Many of these tumors are multifocal at the time of clinical presentation.

Appearance: The urothelial tumors vary in appearance from **purely papillary to nodular or flat.** Papillary lesions are red, elevated excrescences, and range in size from <1 cm in diameter to large lesions up to 5 cm in diameter. They may also occur as multiple discrete tumors.

The WHO (2022)/International Society of Urological Pathology Consensus classification of urothelial neoplasms is presented in **Box 20.24**.

BOX 20.24: The World Health Organization (WHO) (2022)/International Society of Urological Pathology (ISUP) consensus classification (abridged) of urothelial neoplasms

NONINVASIVE UROTHELIAL NEOPLASMS

Papillary Neoplasms
- Urothelial papilloma
- Inverted urothelial papilloma
- Papillary urothelial neoplasm of low malignant potential
- Noninvasive papillary urothelial carcinoma, low-grade
- Noninvasive papillary urothelial carcinoma, high-grade

Flat Lesions with Atypia
- Urothelial carcinoma in situ (CIS)

INVASIVE UROTHELIAL NEOPLASMS
- Invasive urothelial carcinoma

Noninvasive Urothelial Neoplasms

Papillary Neoplasms

Noninvasive papillary tumors are the most common precursor lesions of urothelial carcinoma. They may originate from papillary urothelial hyperplasia. These tumors show a range of atypical changes and are graded according to their biological behavior.

Urothelial Papilloma

Urothelial papilloma is a **solitary exophytic** (slender) **benign papillary urothelial neoplasm** having a delicate fibrovascular core. These **papillae are lined by urothelium of normal cytological features** and **thickness**. It has a benign clinical course and a very low recurrence rate.

MORPHOLOGY

Gross: Most papillomas are solitary and small (0.5–2 cm). They appear as delicate structures superficially attached to the mucosa by a stalk **(exophytic papillomas)**.

Microscopy

Papillae: They consist of a **simple, delicate, exophytic, branching papillary architecture.** The individual finger-like papillae have a **central fibrovascular core.**

Lining epithelial cells:
- **Normal urothelial lining:** The papillae are **covered by epithelium that is histologically identical to normal urothelium.**
- **Normal cellularity and normal cytologic features:** The thickening of the urothelial lining has **normal cellularity** (≤7 cell layers), and lining cells have **normal cytologic features.**

Papillary Urothelial Neoplasm of Low Malignant Potential

Papillary urothelial neoplasm of low malignant potential (PUNLMP) is a urothelial tumor with papillary fibrovascular structures. These papillae are lined by **thickened urothelium**

(commonly exceeds that of normal urothelium) or **increased cellularity**, with **mild cytological atypia (minimal nuclear atypia and minimal architectural abnormalities.**

MORPHOLOGY

Gross: PUNLMPs appear as **single or multiple** discrete **exophytic papillary lesions of variable sizes.** These tumors are usually **larger than papillomas** and may be indistinguishable from papillary cancers of the bladder.

Microscopy

Branching papillae: PUNLMPs consist of **single or multiple discrete branching exophytic papillae.**

Lining epithelial cells: Their features are as follows:

- **Thickened urothelium: The papillary structures** of PUNLMPs are **lined by thickened urothelium and/or more cellular than normal urothelium.**
- **Monotonous cells**: In contrast to normal urothelium, the tumor cells are almost identical to each other (**monotonous**).
- **No loss of polarity** (i.e., no loss of order).
- **Mitotic figures are rare.**

Noninvasive Papillary Urothelial Carcinoma, Low-grade

Low-grade, noninvasive papillary urothelial carcinoma is a **malignant urothelial neoplasm**. It is characterized by **papillary structures that are confined within the basement membrane** (i.e., not associated with invasion beyond the basement membrane). These papillae are lined by **urothelial cells with mild architectural disorder and nuclear atypia** that are visible at low-to-intermediate magnification.

MORPHOLOGY

Gross: It shows an **exophytic papillary tumor**. It may be **single or multiple and variable in size.**

Microscopy (Figs. 20.48A and B)

Papillae: Low-grade noninvasive papillary urothelial carcinoma has **delicate papillae. These papillae** may show **extensive branching or fusion of the papillary structures.**

Lining epithelial cells: Their features are as follows:

- **Variable thickness**: The **papillae** are **lined by neoplastic transitional epithelium** of variable thickness.
- **Variability in architecture or cytologic features:** The cells show an overall (relatively) **orderly appearance** but have **variability in architecture or cytologic features.** These cells are **cohesive and architecturally** show **some loss of polarity.**
- **Low-grade cytologic atypia:** The tumor cells show **low-grade cytologic atypia** with **mild nuclear variation in size, shape,** and **chromatin texture** (cytologic disorder).
- **Mitoses:** They **may or may not be present**, but there are usually no atypical mitoses.

Noninvasive Papillary Urothelial Carcinoma, High-grade

High-grade, noninvasive papillary urothelial carcinoma is a **malignant urothelial neoplasm**. It is characterized by **papillary structures lined by urothelial cells with marked architectural and cytological disorders**. The tumor cells are limited within the basement membrane.

MORPHOLOGY

Gross

These lesions appear **exophytic**. They may be either **single or multiple.**

Microscopy (Figs. 20.49A and B)

Complex papillae: High-grade, noninvasive papillary urothelial carcinoma is characterized by papillae that are **more complex than those in low-grade tumors.** There is **frequent branching and fusion of papillae.** The **thickness of the urothelium** lining papillae is **quite variable.**

Lining epithelial cells: The lining cells are characterized by a **disorderly appearance** because of **marked architectural and cytologic abnormalities.** The cytological features and not the architectural pattern determine the high-grade nature of the lesion.

- **Disorderly orientation with loss of polarity:** Tumor cells lining the papillae show disorderly orientation with loss of polarity.
- **Cellular pleomorphism:** Variation in size and shape ranges from **moderate to marked.**

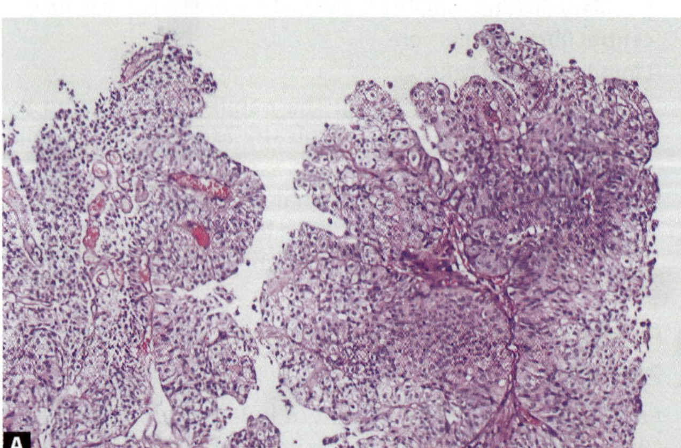

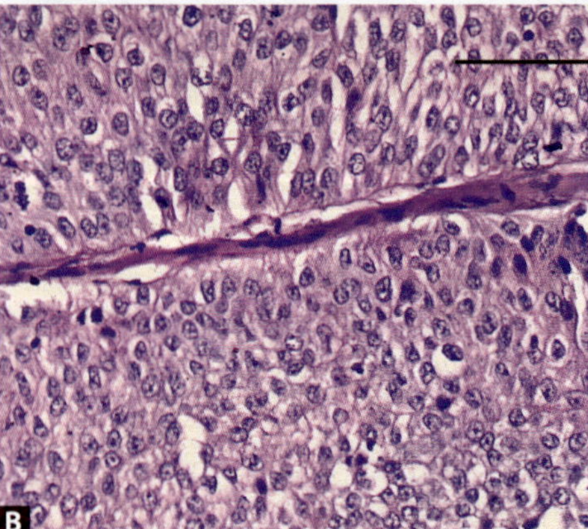

Figs. 20.48A and B: Low-grade, noninvasive papillary urothelial carcinoma: (A) Shows papillae lined by tumor cells with some loss of polarity; (B) High magnification shows some loss of polarity and low-grade cytologic atypia.

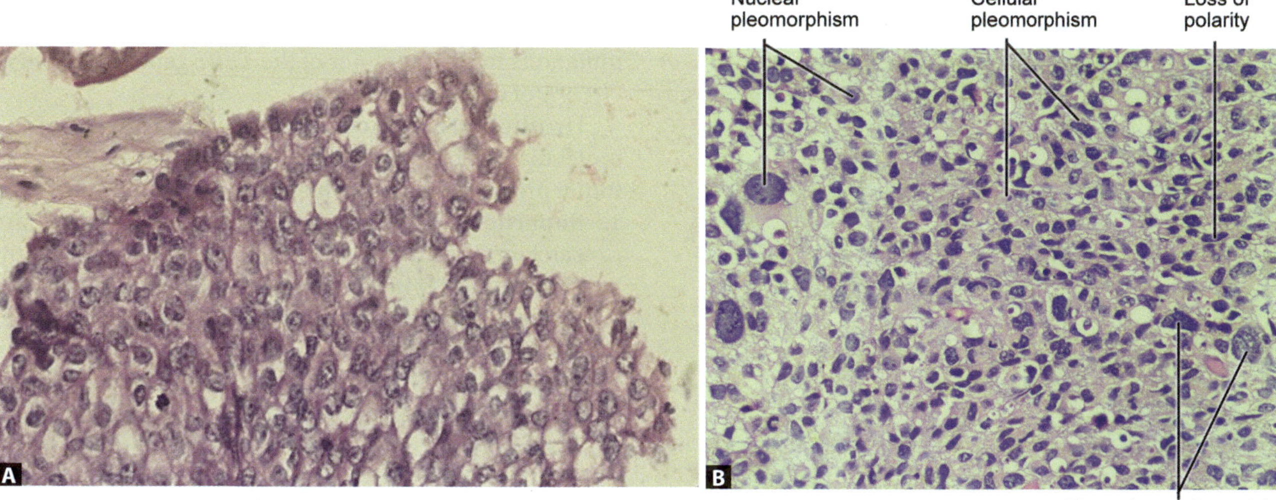

Figs. 20.49A and B: High-grade noninvasive papillary carcinoma: (A) Part of the papillae is lined by cells with much more pleomorphism and mitotic activity (left lower half); (B) Marked nuclear and cellular pleomorphism, hyperchromatic nuclei, and loss of polarity.

- **Irregular and pleomorphic nuclei:** The tumor cells show **variation in nuclear size and irregular, pleomorphic,** and **hyperchromatic nuclei.** They have **irregular nuclear contours** and **irregular prominent nucleoli.**
- **Numerous mitoses, including atypical forms,** are frequently seen **at all levels of the urothelium.**

Flat Lesions with Atypia namely Urothelial Carcinoma in situ is presented online.

Invasive Urothelial Carcinoma

Definition: Invasive urothelial carcinoma is the most common **malignant neoplasm, arising from the urothelial lining** of the urinary tract. The histologic diagnostic criteria are the **invasion beyond the basement membrane.** It was **formerly known as infiltrating transitional cell carcinoma (not recommended).**

Epidemiology: Bladder cancer may occur at any age. But most (about 80%) are between 50 and 80 years of age. Higher in males than in females (male-to-female ratio is 3:1). There is no genetic predisposition to bladder cancer, and no hereditary factors are identified in most cases.

Etiological Factors

Q. Write a short answer on the causes of urinary bladder (urothelial) tumors.

Several factors have been associated with the causation of urothelial carcinoma.

Environmental Factors

Environmental factors play an important role in the pathogenesis of urothelial carcinoma. These are as follows:

- **Cigarette smoking:** It is the **most important risk factor**. Multiple chemical agents, particularly aromatic amines (such as 2-naphthylamine and 4-aminobiphenyl), present in cigarette smoking are metabolized in the body. They trigger carcinogenesis.
- **Occupational exposure:** Exposure to **benzidine-based dyes** (or dyes that metabolize to benzidine), increases the risk of developing bladder cancer. Certain **organic chemicals such as arylamines** (aniline dye industry), particularly 2-naphthylamine and related compounds, are chemical carcinogens. The **aromatic amines (β-naphthylamine) and azo dyes** were widely used in the past **in the aniline dye and rubber industries.** Exposure to aromatic amines may occur among truck, taxi, and bus drivers (e.g., in diesel exhaust); painters (in paint products); and workers in some chemical industries. The metabolism of 2-naphthylamines has organ specificity. Arylamines are conjugated to glucuronic acid in the liver (**Flowchart 20.7**). These conjugates are excreted in the urine. In the bladder, β-glucuronidase hydrolyzes the glucuronic acid conjugate in acidic urine. This produces reactive aryl nitrenium ions. These ions act as mutagens and the cancers develop 15–40 years after the first exposure.
- **Radiation therapy:** Previous exposure of the bladder to irradiation (for other pelvic malignancies).
- **Immunosuppressive agent:** Heavy long-term exposure to an immunosuppressive agent such as **cyclophosphamide** causes hemorrhagic cystitis, and this increases the risk of bladder cancer.
- **Dietary and herbal medicine exposure:** Aristolochic acid is a carcinogenic and nephrotoxic nitrophenanthreneh carboxylic acid. It is produced by *Aristolochia* plants. Ingestion of *Aristolochia*-based herbal medicines or contaminated wheat grains may be associated with urothelial carcinoma.
- **Infection and chronic irritation:** Transitional epithelium of the bladder can undergo various forms

Flowchart 20.7: Mechanism of action of aromatic amines and azo dyes.

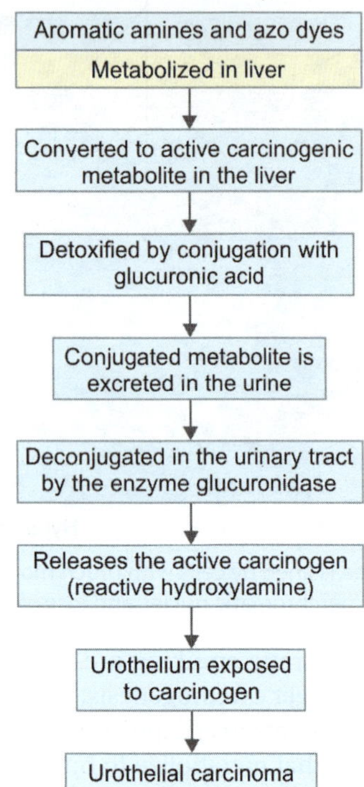

of metaplasia. For example, the urothelium can undergo squamous metaplasia as a response to injury, which is a precursor to dysplastic lesions and in situ and invasive squamous cell carcinoma. ***Schistosoma haematobium* infections** are a risk factor in endemic areas (Egypt, Sudan). More than three-fourths of the cancers are **squamous cell type** and the remaining urothelial type. Chronic inflammation associated with. ***S. haematobium* infections** predispose to neoplasia.

- **Analgesics:** Long-term use of **phenacetin** was strongly associated with upper urinary tract urothelial carcinoma. Phenacetin is presently being replaced by other analgesics.
- **Arsenic:** It is present in the drinking water and soil in certain parts of Bangladesh, India, China, and Hungary. It is an environmental risk factor.
- **Neurogenic bladder:** Patients with neurogenic bladder are at increased risk of bladder cancer.

A family history of bladder cancer is a known risk factor.

Precursor lesions (Figs. 20.50A to D): Two precursor lesions of invasive urothelial carcinoma are:

1. **Noninvasive papillary tumors:** They show a range of atypical changes in the urothelial cells, and are graded according to their biological behavior.
2. **Flat noninvasive urothelial carcinoma in situ (CIS):** It is characterized by cytologic changes of malignancy.

Molecular Pathways of Tumor Progression

Recurrent mutations in genes such as ***TP53, FGFR3, PIK3CA, RB1,* and *HRAS*** have been identified. The most common mutations are activating mutations in *FGFR3* and deactivating alterations of *TP53*, along with common mutations in the promoter of the *TERT* gene (observed in 70–79% of cases).

Urothelial carcinoma develops through unique molecular pathways. Two major molecular pathways of tumor progression parallel histopathological classification.

1. **Superficial papillary tumors:** Low-grade papillary carcinoma recurs frequently but progresses infrequently. ***FGFR3/RAF/RAS* signaling***:* This signaling pathway is activated **predominantly in low-grade, nonmuscle-invasive papillary tumors.** Activating **gain-of-function mutations in *FGFR3*** (fibroblast growth factor receptor gene) is found in as many as 77% of tumors. These alterations increase signaling through growth factor receptor pathways, such as amplifications of the FGFR3 tyrosine kinase receptor gene and activating mutations in the genes encoding *RAS* and *PI3-kinase catalytic subunit a (PIK3CA)*. The FGFR3/RAF/RAS pathway regulates many genes involved in the cell cycle through MAP kinases. These tumors frequently recur but muscle invasion only occurs in about 20% of cases in association with *TP53* mutations.
2. **Carcinoma in situ:** High-grade papillary carcinoma and carcinoma in situ (CIS) are associated with higher rates of progression. These are the precursor lesions for muscle-invasive bladder cancer. In this tumor progression, urothelial carcinoma develops from flat (i.e., not papillary) lesions with **mutations that disrupt the function of p53 and RB.**
   p53/RB: This pathway regulates cell cycle progression. ***TP53* gene is predominantly mutated or deleted in CIS and high-grade invasive tumors**. Inactivation of *RB* is also mainly seen in invasive bladder tumors. The majority of muscle-invasive bladder cancers develop by progression from "flat" CIS. Mutations that alter the function of p53 and RB occur in 93% of all muscle-invasive cancers.

Mutations in the promoter of the *TERT* gene: It is observed in 70–79% of cases. Telomerase activity is important for the initiation of bladder cancer. *TERT* gene encodes the catalytic subunit of telomerase, which is responsible for the elongation of telomeres at the ends of chromosomes. *TERT* mutations are one of the most common mutations in bladder cancer.

MORPHOLOGY

Gross (Fig. 20.51): Can be unifocal or multifocal. It can have a variety of gross appearances. These include **polypoid, sessile, nodular, papillary, or ulcerative morphology.**

Microscopy (Figs. 20.52A and B)

Infiltrating urothelial carcinoma shows a **remarkable diversity of morphological appearance.** Most of these tumors are **cytologically high-grade tumors.**

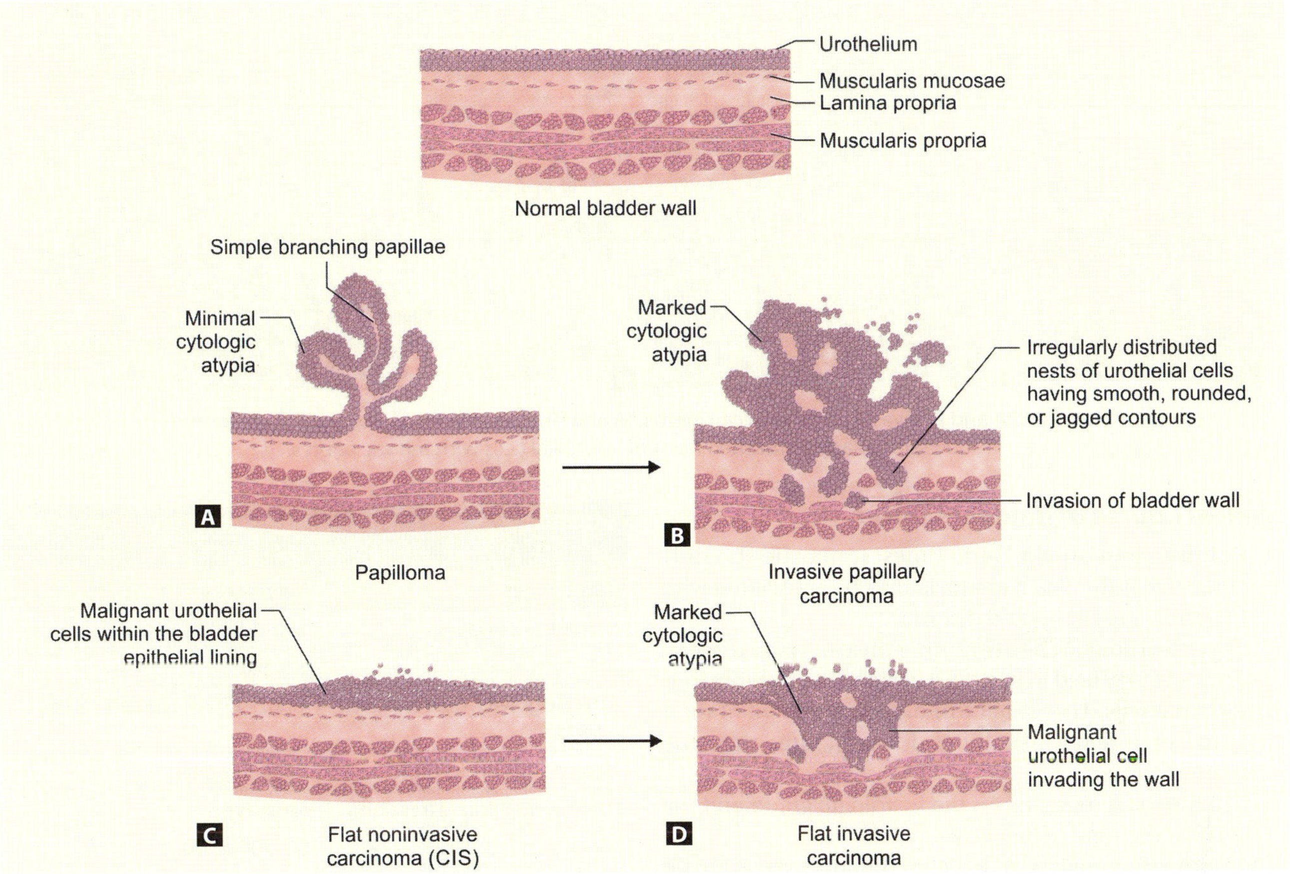

Figs. 20.50A to D: Diagrammatic representation of two distinct precursor lesions of invasive urothelial carcinoma, namely: (A) noninvasive papillary tumors that can progress to invasive papillary carcinoma; (B and C) flat noninvasive urothelial carcinoma in situ that can result in flat invasive carcinoma (D).

(CIS: carcinoma in situ)

Architecture: Urothelial carcinomas present as variably sized **nests, sheets, trabeculae, cords, and individual** cells. Most commonly, they show **irregularly distributed nests of urothelial cells** having either **smooth, rounded, or jagged contours.**

Cytological features: Invasive urothelial neoplastic cells show high-grade features.

- **Nuclei**: Characteristically, they show **striking nuclear pleomorphism** with variably sized and shaped **hyperchromatic nuclei.** Nuclei are irregular.
- **Cytoplasm**: Usually pale to eosinophilic and moderate to abundant. This can produce a squamoid appearance, which should be distinguished from true squamous differentiation.
- **Mitotic figures: Numerous** mitotic figures and **abnormal mitotic figures** are present.

Grade: Most invasive urothelial carcinomas are **high-grade.** Since significant **outcome differences have been found between low- and high-grade invasive tumors,** it is necessary to identify the grade of tumor.

The pattern of invasion: Irregular infiltration into the muscularis propria (muscle wall) is the single diagnostic feature of malignancy. The pattern of invasion has prognostic significance. Tumors with **more infiltrative cords and single-cell patterns have a worse prognosis.**

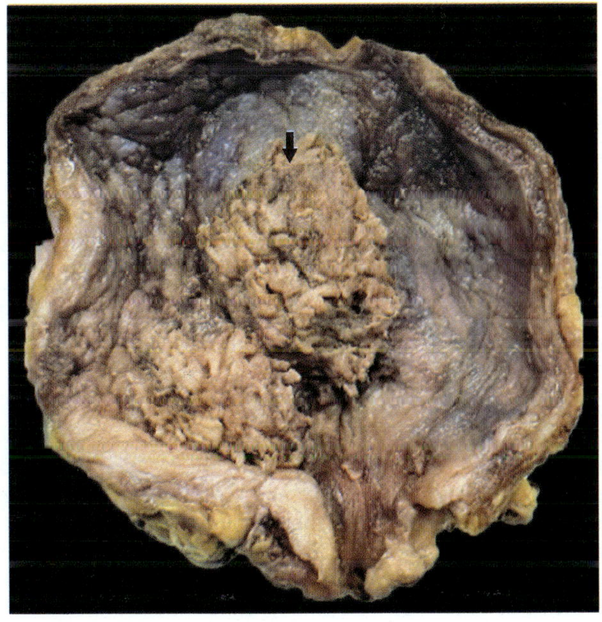

Fig. 20.51: Urothelial carcinoma of the urinary bladder. A large exophytic tumor is situated above the neck of the bladder (arrow).

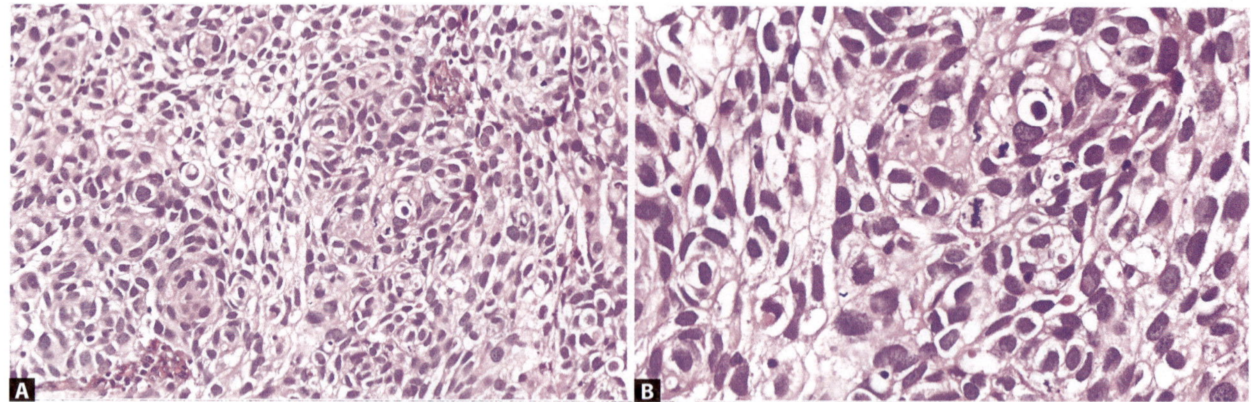

Figs. 20.52A and B: Invasive urothelial carcinoma: (A and B) Shows cytologically high-grade tumor. It shows irregularly distributed nests of urothelial cells with mitotic figures.

Clinical Course of Bladder Cancer

- **Painless hematuria**: Sometimes, it may be the only clinical feature. The hematuria may be associated with frequency, urgency, and dysuria.
- **Complications:** When the tumor obstructs the ureteral orifice, it may lead to pyelonephritis or hydronephrosis.
- **Recurrences:** Urothelial tumors, irrespective of their grade may recur, usually at different sites than the original tumor.
- **Prognosis:** It depends on the histologic grade and the stage at the time of diagnosis.

Laboratory diagnosis: Cytologic examinations of urine for malignant cells and biopsy of the tumor.

- **Newer markers:** Bladder tumor antigen (BTA) test, urinary nuclear matrix protein (NMP22) detects cancer-specific proteins in urine (BTA/NMP22).
- Hyaluronidase and Lewis-X antigen on exfoliated urothelial cells.
- Determination of telomerase activity in exfoliated cells.

TABLE 20.9 Various normal components of normal urine with their reference value.

Component	*Reference value*
Volume—24 hours	600–1,800 mL (variable)
pH	5.0–9.0
Specific gravity, quantitative (random)	1.002–1.028 (average 1.018)
Protein—24 hours urine	<150 mg/day
Protein, qualitative (random)	Negative
Glucose, quantitative—24 hours urine	50–300 mg/day
Glucose, qualitative (random)	Negative
Urobilinogen—24-hour urine	1.0–3.5 mg/day
Microalbuminuria (24 hours)	0–30 mg/24 hours (0–0.03 g/day) (0–30 µg/mg creatinine) (0–0.03 g/g creatinine)

COMMON URINARY ABNORMALITIES IN A CLINICAL SPECIMEN

PA 23.1 (SH): Describe abnormal urinary findings in disease states and identify and describe common urinary abnormalities in a clinical specimen.

Various normal components of normal urine with their reference value are presented in **Table 20.9**.

Case 1

History: An 8-year-old boy was brought by his mother to pediatric outpatient with chief complaints of puffiness of the face, particularly more marked in the morning, mild pitting edema on both legs, malaise with nausea, and a slight fever for about one month. The mother also complained that he passed dark brown (red or cola) colored (smoky) urine and the urine output was reduced (oliguria). On enquiry, the mother informed me that about 2 weeks back the child had an upper respiratory tract infection. On examination, the blood pressure was 140/100 mm Hg (moderate hypertension).

Urine Examination

Urine color	Brown (smoky)
Quantity	700 mL/day (reduced)
Proteinuria	+
Glucose	Nil
Microscopy	
RBC	++
RBC cast	+
WBC (leukocyte)	Occasional

Serological examination: Raised anti-streptolysin O titer and low serum complement level.

Questions

1. What is the most probable diagnosis?
2. Describe the light microscopy, immunofluorescence, and electron microscopic findings.
3. What is the prognosis of this disease?
4. What are the causes of hematuria?

Answers

1. Nephritic syndrome due to acute poststreptococcal glomerulonephritis. The points in favor of nephritic syndrome are hematuria (gross or microscopic), RBC casts in the urine, and oliguria (due to decreased glomerular filtration rate), and mild to moderate hypertension. Two weeks back the child had an upper respiratory tract infection, favoring poststreptococcal disease.
2. Describe the light microscopy, immunofluorescence, and electron microscopic findings (*refer* page 718)
3. What is the prognosis of this disease? (*refer* page 719)
4. Causes of hematuria (*refer* **Box 15.16** on page 458).

Case 2

History: A 6-year-old child was brought to the hospital for a complaint of increased puffiness around his eyes and he has become less active over the past 10 days.

Examination: On physical examination, the boy had facial puffiness which is more prominent around his eyes, and also had swelling of both ankles. There was neither a history of fever nor hypertension.

Urine Examination

Albuminuria/proteinuria	++++
Glucose	Nil
Microscopy	
RBC	–
RBC cast	–
Fat globules/oval fat bodies	+
Protein in a 24-hour urine sample	3.8 g of protein

Serological examination: Serum creatinine and blood urea levels were normal.

He responded well to corticosteroid therapy.

Questions

1. What is the most probable diagnosis?
2. Describe the light microscopic, electron microscopic, and immunofluorescence findings in this condition.
3. What are the causes of proteinuria?

Answers

1. Steroid-responsive proteinuria in a child features nephrotic syndrome due to minimal change disease and is the most common cause of nephrotic syndrome in children. Points favoring nephrotic syndrome are the presence of massive/heavy proteinuria (>3.5 g of protein/24 hours), generalized edema (due to hypoalbuminemia), and the presence of fat globules in urine (due to lipiduria). The leakage of large amounts of protein (>3.5 g per day) in urine results in hypoalbuminemia. The subsequent fall in plasma oncotic pressure leads to the redistribution of extracellular fluid to the interstitial compartment, producing edema. Treatment with steroids achieves a complete remission in the majority of children. *The nephrotic* syndrome should be distinguished from *nephritic* syndrome (characterized by hematuria, uremia, and a degree of renal failure).
2. In *minimal change disease, glomeruli* look normal under a light microscope. However, electron microscopy shows effacement of podocyte foot processes (fusion of podocyte foot processes) in the glomerulus and is the only pathologic finding found on electron microscopy.
3. Causes of proteinuria (*refer* **Box 15.10**).

Case 3

History: A 57-year-old female was admitted to the hospital with a history of increasing back pain and fevers for the last 3 days. She is a type 2 diabetic on oral hypoglycemic agents and has mild hypertension. There is no history of burning micturition or colicky abdominal pain or chronic ingestion of analgesics.

Examination: The patient is febrile (37.9°C) [Normal body temperature is about 37°C (98.6°F)]. On palpation, there is tenderness over the left loin without any tenderness on the anterior abdomen.

Investigations

Type of investigation	*Value (normal range)*
Serum creatinine	0.9 mg/dL (0.6–1.2 mg/dL)
Serum urea	26 mg/dL (20–40 mg/dL)
Urine analysis	
Protein	+
Sugar	++
Ketone bodies	–
Urine microscopy	
Leukocytes	Plenty
RBCs	Occasional
Leukocyte casts	+
Granular cast	+

Questions

1. What is the likely diagnosis in this patient?

2. What is the significance of casts on examination of the urinary sediment?
3. What other investigation will help confirm the diagnosis?

Answers

1. History and urine findings suggest that it is an episode of acute pyelonephritis. Diabetic and immunocompromised patients are predisposed to urinary tract infections. The symptoms of increasing back pain and fevers without burning micturition suggest an upper tract rather than a lower urinary tract infection.
2. The presence of casts indicates renal parenchymal disease. There are different types of cast and their significance is presented in **Figure 15.15** on page 462. The leukocytic casts are indicative of an infective renal parenchymal episode.
3. Urine for culture and sensitivity will help in identifying the causative organism and sensitivity of the organism to the antibiotics.

Case 4

History: A 29-year-old female complains of fever and burning sensation when passing urine for the last 3 days. She also complains that she voids urine more often than usual without any sense of urgency and suffers from severe lower back pain that started 1 day back. She has not noticed any blood in her urine. She has never had this problem in the past and she is not taking any regular medications. There is no history of vaginal discharge or urinary incontinence except for an episode of cystitis 3 months ago. She is sexually active and has two children and is currently not pregnant.

Examination: Her temperature is 39.4 °C [normal body temperature is about 37°C (98.6°F)]. Her pulse is 120 beats/min, and her blood pressure is 106/70 mm of Hg. Abdominal examination shows suprapubic tenderness and marked tenderness in both loins. There was no tenderness at the renal angle on either side. Examination of the cardiovascular and respiratory systems is unremarkable. Bowel sounds are normal.

Investigations

Type of investigation	*Value (normal range)*
Hemoglobin	13.5 g/dL (12.0–15.0 g/dL)
WBC count	22,000/μL (4,000–11,000/μL)
Platelets	334,000/μL (150,000–450,000/μL)
Serum creatinine	0.8 mg/dL (0.6–1.2 mg/dL)
Serum urea	24 mg/dL (20–40 mg/dL)
Urine analysis	
Protein	+
Sugar	–
Blood	+
Ketone bodies	–
Urine microscopy	Midstream urine was collected for microscopy, culture, and sensitivity
Leukocytes	Plenty
RBCs	Occasional
Leukocyte casts	+
Granular cast	+
Urine culture and sensitivity	
E. coli grew after one day	Sensitivity to nitrofurantoin, trimethoprim, gentamicin, and co-amoxiclav

Blood was sent for culture and sensitivity.

Questions

1. What is the probable diagnosis?
2. List the common organisms causing this disease.
3. What are the complications of this disease?
4. What is Tamm-Horsfall protein?

Answers

1. This patient is probably suffering from an uncomplicated urinary tract infection (UTI). UTIs are classified by anatomy into lower and upper UTIs. Upper UTIs refer to infection above the bladder and include the ureters and kidneys. Infection of the kidney and renal pelvis is known as pyelonephritis. Lower UTIs refer to infections at or below the level of the bladder and include cystitis, urethritis, prostatitis, and epididymitis. In this patient, the recent onset of fever and back pain suggest an upper UTI. Plenty of leukocytes and leukocyte in the urine favors acute pyelonephritis. Acute pyelonephritis is much more common in females than males and occurs due to ascending bacterial infection from the lower to upper urinary tract.
2. *Escherichia coli* causes 80–90% of UTI. Other causative organisms include other enteric gram-negative bacteria such as *Proteus, Klebsiella, Enterobacter, and Pseudomonas* species.
3. Complications of acute pyelonephritis (*refer* pages 739-40).
4. Tamm-Horsfall protein (*refer* page 745).

Case 5

History: A 65-year-old male complained of a vague history of generalized weakness anorexia, bony pains, and impotence for the past few months. He informs that he had hypertension for the past 20 years which was poorly controlled. He has not visited any medical professionals for the past 6 years. Irregularly he used to take diuretics for his blood pressure.

Examination: Physical examination reveals conjunctival pallor and his blood pressure is 180/100 mm of Hg.

Investigations

Type of investigation	Value (normal range)
Hemoglobin	10.2g/dL (13.0–17.0 g/dL
WBC count	8,000/μL (4,000–11,000/μL)
Platelets	210,000/μL (150,000–450,000/μL)
Mean cell volume	92 fL (82–100 fL)
Sodium	132(136–146 mEq/L)
Potassium	5.6 mEq/L (3.5–5.0 mEq/L
Urea	62 mg/dL (20–40 mg/dL)
Creatinine	37 mg/dL (0.6-1.2 mg/dL)
Urine analysis	
Urine specific gravity	1010 fixed specific gravity
Protein	+++
Urine microscopy	Granular casts and broad casts

Ultrasound shows both kidneys smaller than normal.

Questions

1. What is the likely diagnosis?
2. What are the common causes of this condition?
3. What are the likely complications of this condition?
4. What is the mechanism of fixed specific gravity of 1010?

Answers

1. The blood tests show high serum creatinine and urea. The renal ultrasound shows small kidneys bilaterally, which suggests that this condition is long-standing. The probable diagnosis is chronic kidney disease (CKD). It develops due to progressive impairment of renal function with a decrease in the number of functioning nephrons. Usually, the patients are asymptomatic until a late stage of CKD. In this patient, the blood pressure is 180/100 and there is associated pallor [normocytic anemia due to reduced erythropoietin (EPO) production by kidney in chronic kidney disease] most likely underlying cause of CKD is hypertension. The symptoms of generalized weakness anorexia, bony pains, and impotence are the consequences of complications of chronic kidney disease.
2. Common causes of CKD are (1) diabetes mellitus, (2) hypertension, and (3) glomerulonephritis (*refer* **Table 20.4**).
3. Complications of chronic kidney disease (*refer* page 748).
4. When the specific gravity of urine is low and fixed at 1.010, this is known as isosthenuria. In this condition, the urine whose specific gravity (concentration) is neither greater (more concentrated) nor less (more dilute) than that of protein-free plasma (1.008–1.012). It is indicative of severe renal damage (chronic kidney disease) with disturbance of both the concentrating and diluting abilities of the kidney. It reflects damage to the kidney's tubules or the renal medulla.

SCENARIO-BASED MCQ

1. **A 54-year-old woman with diabetes mellitus has frequent urinary tract infections. She complained of flank pain, fever with chills, and general malaise for the past 3 days. Peripheral blood shows neutrophilic leukocytosis (13,500/cu mm). Urine cultures show numerous bacterial colonies, composed predominantly of gram-negative microorganisms. Blood pressure is 160/100 mm Hg, BUN is 32 mg/dL, and creatinine is 2.0 mg/dL. Fasting serum glucose is 190 mg/dL. Urinalysis shows 2+ sugar and 1+ protein. Microscopic examination of the urine sediment shows numerous neutrophils and few WBC (leukocyte) casts. The most likely diagnosis is:**
   A. Diabetic nephropathy
   B. Acute pyelonephritis
   C. Acute tubular necrosis
   D. Postinfectious glomerulonephritis

Answer and Explanation

1. **The answer is B: Acute pyelonephritis.** Pyelonephritis is a bacterial infection of the renal parenchyma and pelvis. The most common cause of acute pyelonephritis is gram-negative bacteria namely *Escherichia coli*. The infection reaches the kidney by ascending through the urinary tract. Diabetic patients with glucosuria are at increased risk for developing acute pyelonephritis. Acute bacterial infection is not a feature of the other options.

Nephritic syndrome:
- Most common a use in children is post poststreptococcal GN
- Most common cause in adults is IgA nephropathy.

Epithelial crescent:
- Composed of parietal cells, leukocytes (macrophage) and fibrin
- Characteristic of RPGN
- Number of crescents decides the prognosis

WBC casts in urine: Suggestive of renal involvement because casts are formed only in tubules

Causes of necrotizing papillitis:
- Diabetes mellitus
- Analgesic nephropathy
- Sickle cell anemia
- Obstructive uropathy

Shape of different types of renal stones:
- Calcium oxalate: Needle shaped/square envelop shape
- Struvite (triple) stone: Coffin Lid shaped
- Uric acid: Diamond/barrel shape
- Crystine stone: Hexagonal

Most common causes of nephrotic syndrome:
- In children: Minimal change disease
- In adults : Focal segmental glomerulosclerosis
- In Elderly: Membranous glomerulopathy
- Most common systemic cause: Diabetes mellitus

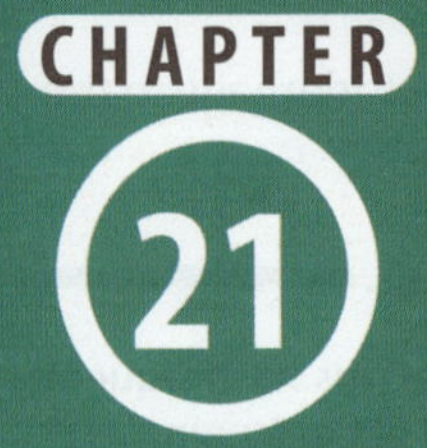

Male Genital Tract Disorders

Chapter Outline

Testis
- Cryptorchidism
- Testicular Tumors

Penis
- Tumors of the Penis

Prostate
- Prostatitis
- Benign Prostatic Hyperplasia
- Male Infertility

TESTIS

CRYPTORCHIDISM

Q. Write a short note on cryptorchidism.

Cryptorchidism is a congenital anomaly in which there is a complete or incomplete **failure of the intra-abdominal testes to descend into the scrotal sac.** It usually occurs as an isolated anomaly or may be with other malformations of the genitourinary tract (e.g., hypospadias in which the opening of the urethra is not located at the tip of the penis).

Normal descent of testis: Testicular descent occurs in two phases.

1. **Transabdominal phase:** In this first phase, the testis comes from the abdomen cavity to lie within the lower abdomen or brim of the pelvis. It occurs by the third month of gestation.
2. **Inguinoscrotal phase:** During this phase, the testes descend through the inguinal canal into the scrotal sac. It occurs during the last 2 months of intrauterine life.

Diagnosis of cryptorchidism: Testicular descent into the scrotum is not always complete at birth. Hence, cryptorchidism can be diagnosed with certainty after 1 year of age, particularly in premature infants.

Sites of arrest of testis: Testes may be arrested anywhere along their pathway of descent (**Fig. 21.1**). In most patients, the undescended testis is palpable in the inguinal canal. Cryptorchidism is asymptomatic, and it is found by the patient or the examining physician only when no testis is found while examining the scrotal sac.

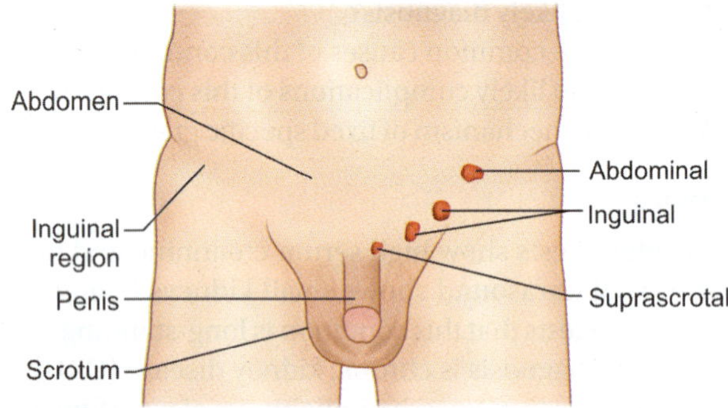

Fig. 21.1: Various sites of arrest of testicular descent resulting in cryptorchidism.

MORPHOLOGY

Gross

Cryptorchidism is unilateral in most of the cases, but it may be bilateral. The cryptorchid testis **appears small** and firm.

Microscopy

Atrophy of seminiferous tubules: It begins to appear by 5–6 years of age and is usually advanced by the time of puberty. These **atrophied tubules** arrest the development of germ cells.

Thickening of tubular basement membrane: It shows marked **hyalinization and thickening.**

Increase in interstitial stroma and prominent Leydig cells.

Germ cell neoplasia in situ: It may develop in cryptorchid testes and is a likely precursor of subsequent germ cell tumors. Hence, it is recommended for surgical repositioning (orchiopexy) at 6–12 months of age.

Complications

Q. Write a short note on complications of undescended testis.

- **Atrophy and infertility/sterility:** Undescended testes usually become atrophic. Hence, bilateral cryptorchidism leads to sterility. Even unilateral cryptorchidism may be associated with atrophy of the contralateral descended testis.
- **Susceptibility to trauma and crushing** against the ligaments and bones, may be accompanied by an **inguinal hernia**.
- **Increased risk of testicular cancer:** Cryptorchidism is associated **with testicular dysfunction.** It is associated with a **3–5-fold increased risk for testicular cancer** than the descended testis. Even unilateral cryptorchidism is also at increased risk for the development of cancer in the contralateral, normally descended testis. This suggests the possibility of some intrinsic abnormality, rather than a simple failure of descent, being responsible for the increased cancer risk. The risk of seminoma is higher for the abdominal than for the inguinal testis. Surgical placement of the undescended testis into the scrotum (orchiopexy) is recommended by 18 months of age to reduce the likelihood of testicular atrophy, infertility, and testicular cancer. The risk of testicular malignancy in undescended testes is **not reduced** by orchiopexy.

Causes of testicular atrophy: Cryptorchidism, chronic ischemia, trauma, irradiation, anticancer chemotherapy, and conditions associated with chronically elevated estrogen levels (e.g., cirrhosis).

TESTICULAR TUMORS

PA 29.1 (CC): Classify testicular tumors and describe the pathogenesis, pathology, presenting and distinguishing features, diagnostic tests, progression, and spread of testicular tumors.

Q. Classify testicular tumors.

Classification (Box 21.1)

The World Health Organization (WHO) (2022) classification of tumors of the testis is presented in **Box 21.1**. Testicular tumors form a spectrum of histologic types with numerous categories.

Two major categories: These constitute most tumors. These are as follows:

1. **Germ cell tumors** (GCTs): They arise from germ cells and **constitute about 95% of testicular tumors. Most of them are aggressive** and can rapidly disseminate, but with current therapy, most can be cured.
2. **Sex cord–stromal tumors:** These tumors are uncommon tumors derived from Sertoli or Leydig cells. They are generally benign.

BOX 21.1: WHO (2022) (abridged) classification of testicular tumors.

Germ cell tumors derived from germ cell neoplasia in situ (GCNIS)

- Noninvasive germ cell neoplasia
  - Germ cell neoplasia in situ
  - Specific forms of intratubular germ cell neoplasia (e.g., intratubular seminoma, intratubular embryonal carcinoma)
- The germinoma family of tumors
  - Seminoma
    - Seminoma with syncytiotrophoblast cells
- Nonseminomatous germ cell tumors
  - Embryonal carcinoma
  - Yolk sac tumor, postpubertal-type
  - Choriocarcinoma
  - Teratoma, postpubertal-type
  - Teratoma with somatic-type malignancy
- Mixed germ cell tumors of the testis
- Germ cell tumors of unknown type

Germ cell tumors unrelated to germ cell neoplasia in situ

- Spermatocytic tumor
- Teratoma, prepubertal-type
  - Dermoid cyst
  - Epidermoid cyst
- Yolk sac tumor, prepubertal-type
- Mixed teratoma and yolk sac tumor, prepubertal-type

Sex cord-stromal tumors of the testis

- Leydig cell tumor
- Sertoli cell tumors
- Granulosa cell tumors
- The fibroma thecoma family of tumors
- Mixed and other sex cord-stromal tumors

Metastatic tumors

Germ Cell Tumors

Age: Germ cell tumors predominantly affect males **between 15 and 45 years of age**. These are the most common malignant tumors in this age-group.

Subcategories: Testicular germ cell tumors are separated into two fundamentally different groups: **those derived from germ cell neoplasia in situ (GCNIS) and those unrelated to GCNIS.**

Etiology and Pathogenesis

The etiology of testicular tumors is not known. Both environmental factors and intrinsic (inherited and acquired genetic abnormalities) factors may predispose to the development of germ cell neoplasia.

Environmental factors: They may play a role in testicular germ cell tumors. The incidence of testicular tumors shows a geographic variation.

- **Cryptorchidism:** About 10% of testicular germ cell tumors are associated with **undescended testis** and are the **most important risk factor**. There is also an increased risk for cancer in the contralateral descended testis. The high incidence of testicular germ cell tumors may be due to its exposure to high temperatures in the abdomen or inguinal region compared to that in the scrotum.
- **Testicular dysgenesis:** Testicular germ cell tumors (TGCTs) have several well-defined positive associations. Five of these are— (1) **testicular dysgenesis syndrome**, (2) **a previous history** of **(prior testicular) germ tumor, (3) a familial history of TGCTs,** (4) **certain disorders of sex development** (intersex syndromes), and (5) **oligospermic infertility.** TGCTs are associated with testicular maldevelopment (disorders of gonadal development), the so-called "testicular dysgenesis syndrome." These conditions might be related to in utero exposures to pesticides and estrogens.

Genetic factors: Testicular germ cell tumors are partially heritable. There is a strong family or genetic predisposition with testicular germ cell tumors. Several genetic loci have been linked to familial GCT risk.

- **Oncogenic mutations in *KIT*:** It may be found in up to 25% of tumors.
- **Isochromosome 12 [i(12p)]:** Extra copies of the short arm of chromosome 12 usually due to the presence of an isochromosome 12 [i(12p)], are observed in almost all germ cell tumors.
- **Klinefelter syndrome:** It is **associated with a 50 times greater risk** (than normal) **for the development of mediastinal germ cell tumors**, but they **do not develop testicular tumors.**
- **Time of malignant transformation:** It may occur **during fetal development or** in the **peripubertal period.**

Molecular Pathogenesis

The interplay of environmental and genetic factors appears to lead to the stepwise development of GCTs **(Fig. 21.2)**.

Steps in the development of germ cell tumors

Acquired defect in primordial germ cell differentiation: The cell of origin of GCTs is a primordial germ cell with an acquired defect in differentiation (suboptimally differentiated germ cells). These primordial germ cells show a similar gene expression profile to malignant germ cells and are morphologically similar to seminoma cells.

Activation of growth factor receptor signaling: The next step in transformation consists of activation of growth factor receptor signaling. This is often by activating mutations in the KIT receptor tyrosine kinase, which **stimulate the proliferation** of suboptimally differentiated germ cells.

Germ cell neoplasia in situ: The proliferation of these germ cells is involved in the genesis of a precursor lesion termed germ cell neoplasia in situ (GCNIS). GCNIS consists of undifferentiated malignant germ cells confined to seminiferous tubules. This in situ precursor lesion is seen in about 90% of testes involved in germ cell neoplasms. GCNIS is also frequently detected in testes at high risk for developing GCTs (e.g., in 2–4% of patients with cryptorchid testes). GCNIS is believed to arise in utero and remain dormant until puberty. Like invasive GCTs, GCNIS is also associated with i(12p). GCNIS may also evolve into intermediate precursor lesions before the invasive disease is established. These intermediate precursors are intratubular forms of seminoma or embryonal carcinoma (EC).

Germ cell neoplasia in situ is found in association with all types of GCTs in the testis except spermatocytic tumors (spermatocytic seminoma), teratomas of prepubertal testes, or yolk sac tumors (YSTs) of infancy. Probably, these neoplasms develop directly from altered germ cells without an in situ phase.

Progression to invasive germ cell tumor: During puberty, hormonal influences may stimulate the growth of germ cells. The lesional cells retain the expression of the transcription factors OCT3/4 and NANOG. These transcription factors are essential in the maintenance of pluripotent stem cells. About 70% of individuals with GCNIS (e.g., in cryptorchid testes) very likely (if not inevitably) progress to develop invasive

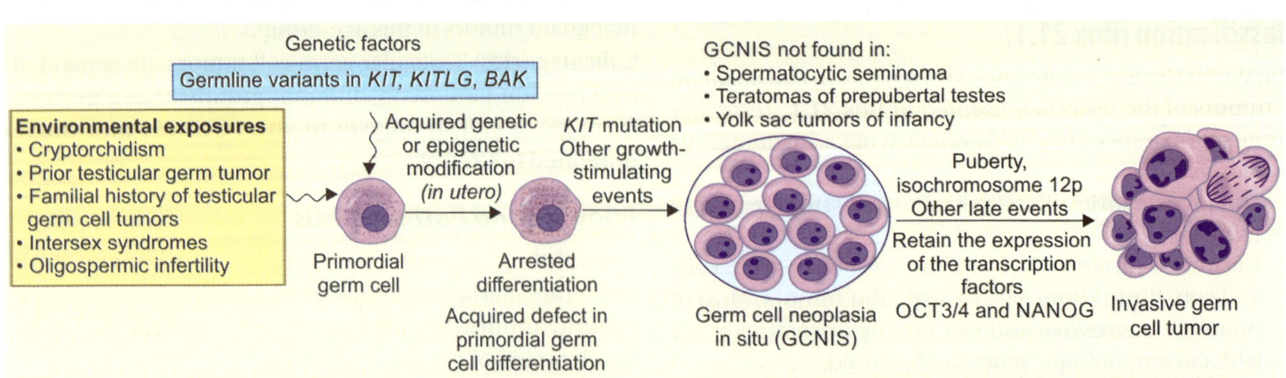

Fig. 21.2: Various steps in the development of germ cell tumors. Environmental and genetic risk factors and acquired genetic and epigenetic alterations lead to the development and progression of germ cell tumors.

GCTs within 7 years of the diagnosis. Seminoma and embryonal carcinoma (EC) contain primitive pluripotent stem cells. These stem cells can differentiate into somatic or extraembryonic tissue, forming mixed GCTs, teratomas, YSTs, or choriocarcinomas. Embryonic carcinoma cells also share significant similarities with human embryonic stem cells.

In most postpubertal testicular germ cell tumors, progression to full-blown GCTs is strongly associated with full or partial gains in the short arm of chromosome 12 (12p).

Major groups of invasive testicular germ cell tumors: They are divided into two major groups.

1. **The germinoma family of tumors:** It consists of seminoma. They are composed of cells that resemble primordial germ cells or early gonocytes.
2. **Nonseminomatous tumors:** These tumors may be composed of undifferentiated cells that resemble embryonic stem cells, as in the case of embryonal carcinoma (EC), but the malignant cells may also differentiate along other lineages. This may produce YSTs, choriocarcinomas, and teratomas.

Germ cell tumors may be composed of a single cell type or mixtures of seminomatous and/or nonseminomatous components.

Germ Cell Tumors Derived from GCNIS

Noninvasive Germ Cell Neoplasia

Noninvasive germ cell neoplasia includes germ cell neoplasia in situ, and specific forms of intratubular germ cell neoplasia **(Box 21.1)**.

Germ Cell Neoplasia In Situ (GCNIS)

Q. Write a short essay on GCNIS of the testis (in situ carcinoma of testis).

Germ cell neoplasia in situ is a preinvasive form (precursor) of invasive germ cell tumors (GCTs).

Sites of germ cell tumors: It usually occurs in the testis and ovary. But germ cell tumors can also occur in extragonadal site **(Box 21.2)**.

BOX 21.2: Extragonadal site of germ cell tumors.

1. Mediastinum (most common)
2. Retroperitoneum
3. Pineal gland

Definition: Germ cell neoplasia in situ **consists of gonocyte-like germ cells with abundant clear cytoplasm and large (10–11 µm) angulated nuclei with coarse chromatin clumps.** These cells are located along the base of the seminiferous tubules.

MORPHOLOGY

Germ cell neoplasia in situ is **grossly not recognizable.**

Microscopy

Patchy distribution: In adults, GCNIS occurs in a patchy distribution throughout the testis. It usually affects <10–30% of seminiferous tubules.

Tumor cells inside the seminiferous tubules: GCNIS cells are localized inside the seminiferous tubule of the testis. Usually, it is one layer thick and broadly attached to the basal lamina. Later, the GCNIS tumor cells **form several layers** and appear in the tubular lumen. Seminiferous tubules with GCNIS have **thick basement membranes** and replace normal germ cells. Hence, they **do not contain sperm** (normal spermatogenesis is absent).

Tumor cells of GCNIS: They resemble spermatogonia or fetal germ cells, but these are much larger.

- **Cytoplasm:** The tumor cells have **abundant, clear cytoplasm** and their clear appearance is due to the presence of considerable **glycogen.**
- **Nuclei:** The nuclei are **central, polyploid, with finely dispersed chromatin** and **prominent nucleoli.**

Immunohistochemistry: Like fetal germ cells, these cells are **placental alkaline phosphatase** (PLAP) **positive** on the plasma membrane. Other markers include OCT3/4 (also called POU5F 1) and NANOG.

Specific Forms of Intratubular Germ Cell Neoplasia

- **Intratubular seminoma:** In this, there is complete filling of seminiferous tubules by neoplastic cells that are morphologically identical to those of GCNIS and seminoma. Intratubular seminoma is found adjacent to about 30% of seminomas and 15% of nonseminomas.
- **Intratubular nonseminoma:** Intratubular nonseminoma consists almost exclusively of pure embryonal carcinoma. Probably they result from reprogramming of a GCNIS cell. They usually show distortion and enlargement of the seminiferous tubules. There may be necrosis and calcification. The tumor cells are more pleomorphic than GCNIS cells. intratubular nonseminoma is only seen adjacent to tumors with nonseminomas.

The Germinoma Family of Tumors

Seminoma

Q. Write a short note on seminoma.

Most common type of germ cell tumor: Seminomas are the most common type of germ cell tumor (40–50% of germ cell tumors).

Definition: Seminoma is a **malignant germ cell tumor** (GCT) **composed of monomorphous cells** that are considered as the neoplastic counterparts of the primordial germ cells/gonocytes present during early embryonic development. They are composed of cells that **resemble spermatogonia**. It was previously known as classical seminoma.

- **Age-group:** Peak incidence is during the **fourth decade (between 30 and 40 years)**. They do not occur before prepuberty and never occur in infants.

- **Identical tumors in other sites:** An identical tumor arises in the ovary (called **dysgerminoma of the ovary**), and in the central nervous system (CNS), usually in midline structures such as the pineal gland (referred to as germinoma).

MORPHOLOGY

Q. Write a short note on the morphology of seminoma.

Gross (Figs. 21.3A and B)

Seminomas are **bulky, solid, rubbery-firm,** and **bosselated tumors.**

Size: It varies from **2 to 6 cm** and the **testis is enlarged**, sometimes up to 10 times the normal testis.

Cut Surface

- Tumor is **homogeneous, gray-white (cream colored)** or **grayish-yellow,** and **lobulated.** Their cut surface bulges above the surrounding parenchyma.
- Tumor is **sharply demarcated from normal testis,** which may be compressed, and atrophic.
- Usually, the **tunica albuginea** is **not penetrated.**
- **Areas of necrosis or hemorrhage** are **usually not seen.**

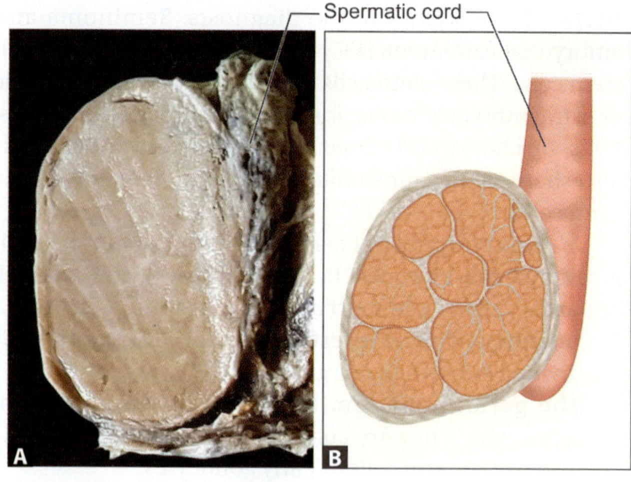

Figs. 21.3A and B: Gross appearance of seminoma of the testis: (A) Cut section of testis shows replacement of testis by a circumscribed, pale, fleshy, homogeneous tumor; (B) (Diagrammatic) shows a lobulated tumor.

Microscopy (Figs. 21.4A and B)

Seminoma appears **microscopically similar to dysgerminoma** of the ovary.

Pattern: The tumor is composed of **solid, diffuse sheets or separated into nests, clusters, or cords of a uniform population of seminoma cells.** The tumor cells form **poorly demarcated lobules.**

Seminoma (tumor) cells: They have the following features:

- **Uniform single population of large cells:** They **resemble spermatogonia. Cells** are **large, round to polyhedral, and have a distinct cell membrane.**
- **Cytoplasm:** Tumor cells have **abundant cytoplasm.** It may appear **pale and eosinophilic or clear** (watery). It contains **varying amounts of glycogen** (stain positive with PAS stain) and **some lipids.** An abundant amount of cytoplasm causes the nuclei to be well-spaced and nonoverlapping.
- **Nucleus:** The nuclei are **polygonal, large with finely granular chromatin with one or two large, centrally located prominent nucleoli.**
- **Mitoses:** They vary in number.
- **GCNIS** can be found in the residual seminiferous tubules in about 85–90% of cases.

Stroma: The seminoma cells are divided into poorly demarcated lobules by delicate fibrous septa. **Fibrous septa are infiltrated with a moderate amount of lymphocytes and plasma cells.**

Rare features:

- Syncytiotrophoblasts (~15%) with minimally elevated serum hCG (in about 10% of cases).
- Ill-defined granulomas with giant cells in the stroma.

Immunohistochemistry: Seminoma cells are diffusely positive for (i) cytoplasmic/plasma membrane including KIT and placental alkaline phosphatase (PLAP) and (ii) nuclear including OCT3/4 and SALL4.

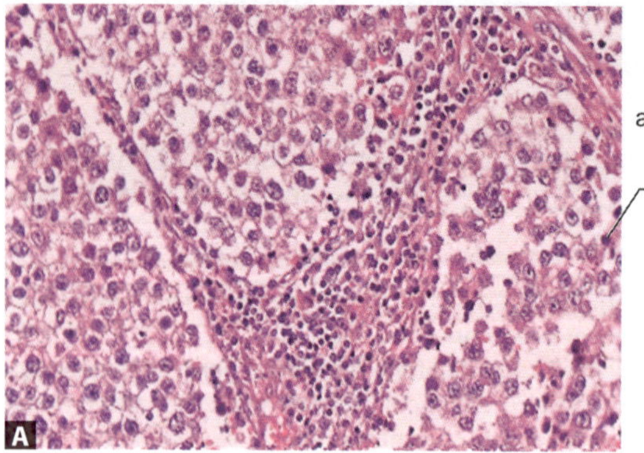

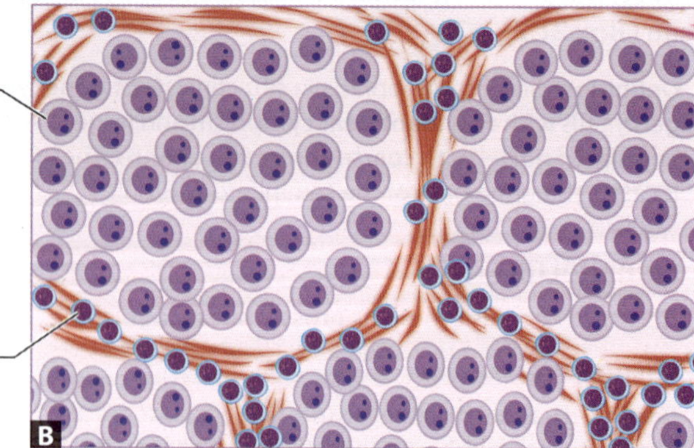

Figs. 21.4A and B: Microscopy of seminoma: (A) H&E and (B) diagrammatic. It shows seminoma cells divided into lobules separated by delicate septa with lymphocytic infiltrate. Seminoma cells are large and have pale to clear abundant cytoplasm with well-defined cytoplasmic membranes. The nuclei are polygonal, vesicular, much larger than the small round nuclei of the lymphocytes, pale, and often have flattened edges. Nucleoli are prominent.

Clinical features: Seminoma usually presents as a **progressively growing scrotal mass.** It is generally diagnosed while still curable by orchiectomy, with or without abdominal lymph node dissection. **Alpha-fetoprotein (AFP) is never elevated** in seminoma. Seminomas are highly radiosensitive and **melt like ice with radiotherapy**. Radiotherapy is important for treating seminomas that are not cured by surgery alone. In advanced stages, chemotherapy can be curative. Currently, the cure rate for all histologic subtypes of seminoma is >90%.

Spread

- **Local spread:** Seminoma remains localized to the testis for a long time. Locally it may spread as follows:
  - Invasion of the testicular parenchyma
  - Spread into rete testis
  - Invasion of the epididymis occurs later in the disease.
- **Lymphatic spread:** To abdominal lymph nodes
- **Hematogenous spread:** It occurs **late in the disease**.

Prognosis of seminoma

- The overall prognosis is excellent. It is extremely **radio-sensitive. Remains localized** to the testis for a long time.

SCENARIO-BASED ESSAY QUESTION

Q. A 26-year-old male complains of a vague feeling of painless heaviness in the right scrotum for the last 3 months. There is no history of antecedent trauma. Physical examination shows that the right testis was enlarged and measured 5 cm in size, firm, and nontender. The swelling is negative for transillumination. Ultrasound scan reveals a solid, circumscribed mass in the right testis. Regional lymph nodes were not palpable. Right orchiectomy was done.

a. What is the probable diagnosis? (Ans: Seminoma of right testis).
b. Discuss the morphological features of this condition. *(refer page 778)*.
c. How does this lesion spread and what is its prognosis? *(refer page 779)*.

Nonseminomatous Germ Cell Tumors

Q. Write a short essay on nonseminomatous germ cell tumors of the testis.

Nonseminomatous germ cell tumors of the testis may be derived from GCNIS, embryonal cells, or seminoma. These include several entities (*refer* **Box 21.1**), and they can be tumors of a single histologic type or >1 histologic type. Out of these tumors, two form most of the cases: (1) pure EC [nonseminomatous tumors of one of the tumors (NSTs) of a single histologic type] and (2) mixed GCT (NSTs of more than one histologic type). In mixed GCTs, it may show any combination of >1 GCT type. Therefore, any combination of seminoma, teratoma, EC, YST, and choriocarcinoma may be seen.

Embryonal Carcinoma

Definition: Embryonal carcinoma (EC) is a **malignant germ cell tumor (GCT)** composed of **tumor cells resembling embryonic stem cells.** It is composed of **primitive epithelial cells.**

- **More aggressive than seminomas.**
- **Age-group:** The peak incidence is seen in the **20–30 years of age-group.**

MORPHOLOGY

Gross

Size: Small or quite often enlarge the testis. The average diameter of 2–3 cm.

Cut surface (*refer* **online Fig. 21.5A**):

- It has a **variegated appearance. Areas of hemorrhage or necrosis** are common.
- **Poorly demarcated** at the margins. **The tumor extends into tunica albuginea, epididymis, or spermatic cord.**

Microscopy (*refer* online Fig. 21.5B)

Pattern: The tumor cells may be arranged in **broad, solid sheets, cords, gland-like tubules, and acini** (alveolar pattern), and sometimes even line papillary structures. But they lack well-formed glands with basally situated nuclei and apical cytoplasm. Combinations of two or more patterns are common.

Tumor cells:

- It consists of **undifferentiated cells** that have an **epithelial appearance.** These cells are **large and anaplastic cells.** They show considerable **variation in cell and nuclear size and shape.**
- **Cytoplasm**: It is dense amphophilic with poorly defined cytoplasmic membranes. **Cell borders** are usually **indistinct.**
- **Nuclei:** They are **large, pleomorphic,** and vesicular with **prominent single or multiple macronucleoli.** Nuclear crowding, overlapping, and marked pleomorphism are helpful features to distinguish it from other GCT types.
- **Mitotic figures** and **tumor giant cells** are **frequent.**

Immunohistochemistry: Positive for cytokeratin and CD30, and **negative for KIT** (CD117).

Clinical features. Most patients present with a testicular mass. It can be painful due to rapid growth and may be mistaken for testicular torsion. About 10% of patients present with manifestations of metastatic disease.

Teratoma

Q. Write a short note on the teratoma of the testis.

Definition: Teratoma is a germ cell tumor **composed of various cellular or organoid components representing derivatives of more than one germinal layer. These germ layers include endoderm, mesoderm, and ectoderm.**

Tissue components: Teratoma is a tumor which may contain **variable proportions of different tissues derived from three germ cell layers** (ectoderm, mesoderm, and endoderm) **(Table 21.1)**. The **neoplastic germ cells form somatic tissue elements of adult (mature) or fetal**

TABLE 21.1	Type of germ cells and their common tissue derivatives.
Type of germ cell	***Tissue derivatives from differentiation of germ cells***
Ectoderm	Skin, central nervous system, retinal pigment cells, and other related tissues
Mesoderm	Smooth and striated muscle, cartilage, and bone
Endoderm	Intestinal tissue, bronchial epithelium, salivary glands, etc.

(immature) development and are frequently encountered together.

Age: Teratomas may occur at any age, from infancy to adulthood. **Teratomas that occur early in life differ biologically and clinically from those that occur in adults.** Hence, it may be **broadly divided into postpubertal and prepubertal** types. Classification of testicular teratoma is presented in **Box 21.3**.

- **Prepubertal type**: Pure teratoma is generally common in **infants and children** and is referred to as the "prepubertal type."
- **Postpubertal type:** In **adults**, pure teratomas are rare (2–3% of germ cell tumors). More commonly teratomas are mixed with other tumor types such as embryonal carcinoma or yolk sac tumor.

Postpubertal type teratoma

It is thought to arise from the differentiation of other types of germ cell tumors (GCTs), particularly GCNIS, or seminoma. Only a minor fraction of teratomas occurring in adults share these features of prepubertal teratoma. Postpubertal adult teratomas are **generally considered malignant**, and metastasis occurs in 22–37% of cases.

Pure teratomas: These are **rare in adults** and constitute 2–3% of GCTs. In postpubertal patients, diagnosis of pure teratoma should be made only when teratomas show no cytologic atypia, not associated GCNIS, and no evidence of regressive or atrophic changes in the background parenchyma. It also lacks isochromosome 12p.

Mixed germ cell tumor (GCT): In adult patients, **postpubertal-type teratoma usually occurs as one component of a mixed GCTs.**

BOX 21.3: Classification of testicular teratomas.

Germ cell tumors derived from germ cell neoplasia in situ (GCNIS)
- Nonseminomatous germ cell tumors
  - Teratoma, postpubertal type
  - Teratoma with somatic-type malignancy

Germ cell tumors unrelated to GCNIS
- Teratoma, prepubertal type

- **Component of mixed GCT:** Teratomatous component is seen in >50% of all mixed GCTs. It may be composed exclusively of **well-differentiated, mature tissues or have immature, embryonic-type tissues.** Teratoma may contain syncytiotrophoblastic giant cells.

Clinical presentation: Postpubertal teratomas generally occur in **young patients**, present with a **testicular mass,** but may have symptoms due to metastasis and may have elevated serum markers (depending on the nature of the associated components).

MORPHOLOGY

Q. Write a short note on the morphology of the teratoma of the testis.

Gross

Appearance and size: Postpubertal-type teratomas in adult males are usually **large, firm, and often multinodular.** The size ranges from **5 to 10 cm in diameter.**

Cut surface: The presence of various tissues gives a **heterogeneous appearance.** The cut section shows **solid and cystic areas (Fig. 21.6A).** The cysts may be filled with clear or mucoid fluid or keratinous material. Solid areas may show nodules of translucent, white cartilaginous areas (*refer* **online Fig. 21.6B**), as well as bone. Areas of immature tissue may have a fleshy, and encephaloid character. Hair is not seen in postpubertal-type teratomas.

Hemorrhage and necrosis suggest mixed GCT: The presence of hemorrhage and necrosis usually points toward the mixed tumors such as embryonal carcinoma, choriocarcinoma, or both.

Microscopy (Figs. 21.7A and B)

In the World Health Organization (WHO) classification, the earlier characterization of testicular teratomas as "mature" or "immature" was removed. This is because **immaturity in the epithelial or stromal components has no prognostic significance.**

Types of tissue: Virtually **any epithelial or mesenchymal tissue type** including neural tissue. The tissues may be mature and/or fetal or embryonic-type derived from more than one germ cell. These **heterogeneous mature and immature tissues** are **arranged in a helter-skelter (haphazard) pattern. Tissue derivatives of three germ cell layers include:**

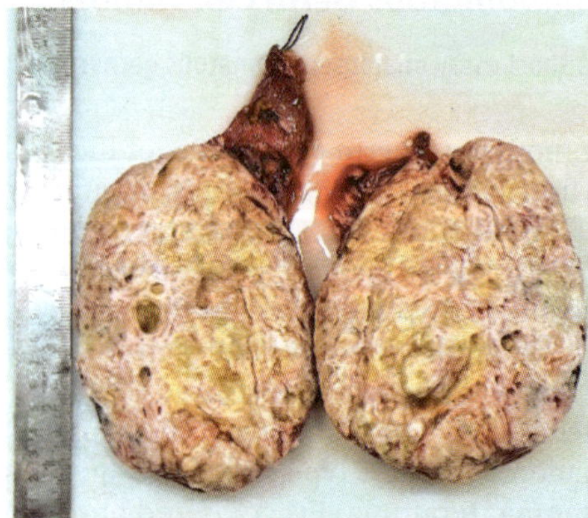

Fig. 21.6A: Cut section of postpubertal teratoma. (A) Multiple cysts and solid areas.

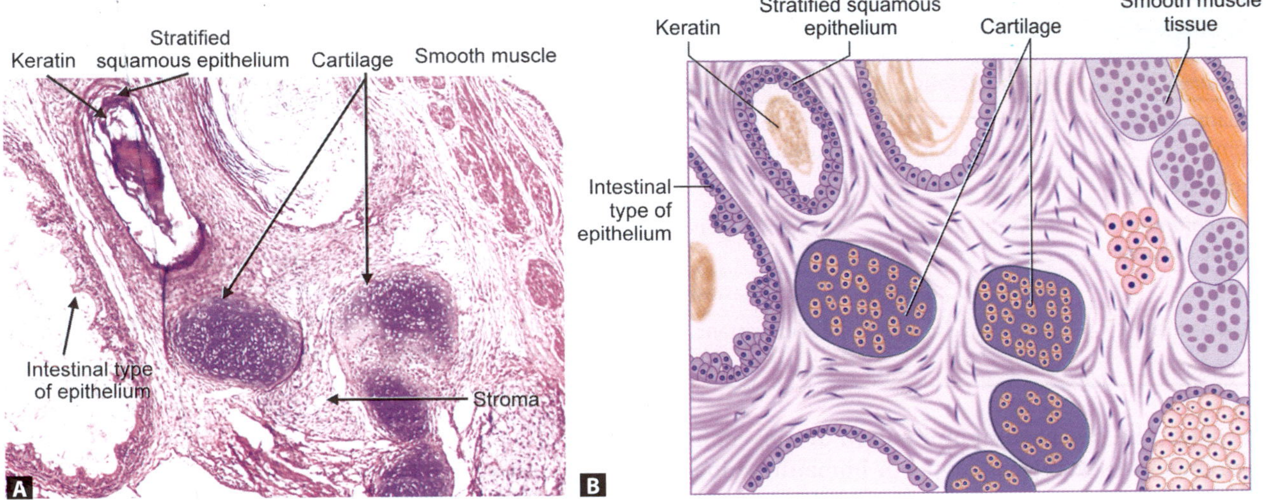

Figs. 21.7A and B: Microscopic features of postpubertal teratoma. (A) H&E and (B) diagrammatic appearance: (A) A disorganized collection of cysts lined by intestinal type of epithelium, keratin-filled cyst, foci of cartilage, and smooth muscle surrounded by stroma; (B) Immature tissue stroma with cytologic atypia and immature cartilage.

Type of tissue: Almost any epithelial or mesenchymal tissue type derived from more than one germ cell layer can be seen.

- **Mature elements (resembling somatic tissue):** They may show **well differentiated mature elements** or organoid structures (resembling various adult tissues) derived from one (monodermal) or all three germ layers (ectoderm, mesoderm, and endoderm).
  - **Ectodermal derivatives:** Structures or tissues derived from ectoderm include skin (clusters of squamous epithelia, sweat and sebaceous glands, and hair), tooth enamel, and brain substance (neural tissue, glia).
  - **Mesodermal derivatives**: These include smooth muscle bundles, islands of cartilage, bone, fat, blood vessels, and lymphatics.
  - **Endoderm elements**: These include respiratory tract (bronchial or bronchiolar epithelium), and gut (bits of the intestinal wall) structures.
- **Immature elements:** Tumor **may show immature tissue elements**. Immature tissues show histologic features of fetal or embryonic tissue. They can show islands of **immature neuroectoderm resembling embryonic neural tube or primitive tubules**, similar to those seen in nephroblastoma and often with accompanying renal blastema. Grading the degree of immaturity in the postpubertal teratoma is not needed, unlike in ovarian cases. This is because these immature elements are derived from invasive malignant GCTs.
- **Helter-skelter pattern**: The tissue elements are embedded in a fibrous or myxoid stroma. Pure teratomas are composed of tissues resembling somatic tissues.

Cytological atypia: Postpubertal teratoma frequently shows cytologic atypia. For example, mature glandular tissue may show features of high-grade dysplasia or in situ carcinoma, and cartilage may resemble chondrosarcoma. Cytologic atypia reflects their malignant potential and development from GCNIS. This is supported by the demonstration of aneuploidy.

Stroma: Commonly these tumors have primitive, mitotically active, cellular stroma cuffing glands.

Changes in the uninvolved region of the testis: In about 90% of cases, they show germ cell neoplasia in situ (GCNIS).

Mixed GCTs: In these tumors, teratoma is often found along with yolk sac tumor or embryonal carcinoma.

Immunohistochemistry: It gives the results depending on the specific elements examined. Examples include neural markers in neural tissues, CKs in epithelia, vimentin in stromal tissues, and desmin in muscle.

Invasion: Teratoma can invade paratesticular tissue and may invade intra- and extratesticular vessels.

Metastasis: These tumors, when they metastasize, follow the same routes of spread as other GCTs.

Teratoma with somatic-type malignancy

Definition: A teratoma with somatic-type malignancy is a **teratoma that develops a distinct secondary component that resembles a somatic (nongerm cell) type malignant neoplasm.** These somatic-type malignancies are similar to those in other organs and tissues (e.g., sarcomas and carcinomas).

Rarely, malignant nongerm cell (somatic) tumors may arise in postpubertal teratomas. This phenomenon is termed a teratoma with somatic-type malignant transformation. Transformation may develop if any of the somatic elements undergo malignant transformation. It was formerly termed a "teratoma with malignant transformation." This term is not recommended because it may lead to a misconception that teratomas without somatic-type malignancy are benign. Examples of somatic-type malignancy are **squamous cell carcinoma, mucin-secreting adenocarcinoma, sarcoma, or other cancers.**

Significance: When the non-germ cell malignancy spreads outside of the testis, it does not respond to chemotherapy.

Prognosis of postpubertal teratoma: All teratomas (both mature and immature) **are considered malignant** and **are capable of metastasis**. Metastases can develop in 22–37%

TABLE 21.2 Differences between seminomatous and nonseminomatous tumors of testis.

Features	*Seminomatous*	*Nonseminomatous*
Characteristic of tumor	Remain localized to testis for a long time	Some of them spread rapidly
Aggressiveness	Not very aggressive	Aggressive
The common mode of spread	By lymphatics	By hematogenous
Metastasis	Does not occur early	Early metastasis
Radiosensitivity	Highly radiosensitive	Radioresistant
Prognosis	Good	Poor

of cases. The presence of epithelium or mesenchymal elements with cytological atypia or immaturity does not affect prognosis.

Q. Differences between seminoma and nonseminomatous germ cell tumors.

Differences between seminomatous and nonseminomatous tumors of the testis are presented in **Table 21.2**.

Mixed Germ Cell Tumors of the Testis

Definition: Mixed GCTs are malignant tumors composed of more than one type of GCT component. All are clinically regarded as nonseminoma, regardless of the presence or absence of a seminoma component.

Various types of GCTs may occur as pure tumors. But it is much more common (except for seminoma) to see combinations of different neoplastic types. About 70–90% of nonseminomatous testicular tumors are mixed types.

- **Common mixed component**: The **most frequently encountered** mixed components are teratoma, embryonal carcinoma, and yolk sac tumor. Teratocarcinoma is an older term used to describe mixed GCTs characterized by a combination of EC and teratoma (mature and/or immature).
- **Prognosis:** Depends on the more aggressive component in the mixed tumor.

Germ Cell Tumors Unrelated to Germ Cell Neoplasia In Situ

Spermatocytic Tumor

Definition: A spermatocytic tumor is an **unusual, rare, distinctive germ cell tumor** (GCT) **derived from postpubertal-type germ cells**. The **tumor cells resemble** spermatogenic cells, most commonly **spermatogonia or early primary spermatocytes**.

- Spermatocytic tumor **formerly known as spermatocytic seminoma** (not recommended) is distinct from seminoma of testis clinically, morphologically, histochemically, and molecularly (its origin and pathogenesis).
- It is a **rare tumor** (~1–2% of all testicular germ cell tumors).
- **Origin:** Despite its original name, spermatocytic tumor is **unrelated to classical seminoma.** It originates **from germ cells undergoing spermatogenesis**. Represent more differentiated type of germ cell tumor. It is important to distinguish it from usual seminoma because treatment differs significantly.
- **Age:** The tumor occurs over **a wide patient age range** (19–92 years), with a peak incidence in the sixth decade of life (usually above 65 years of age). Most present with a painless testicular mass.

MORPHOLOGY

Gross

Size: Usually **3–5 cm**, but it may be larger.

Appearance: Spermatocytic tumors are **lobular to multinodular** (typical) tumors. These are **soft and pale gray**.

Cut surface: It varies from **gray-white to hemorrhagic** and from fleshy to myxoid. It may show mucoid cystic regions. It tends to be circumscribed.

Microscopy

Arrangement: The tumor cells are arranged in **diffuse to multinodular patterns**. These may be interrupted by edema-filled spaces. Cystic change is common.

Tumor cells: The most distinctive feature or hallmark is **cellular polymorphism**. It consists of a characteristic polymorphous population of tumor cells usually described as tripartite (composed of three intermixed types) **(Fig. 21.8)**. These three types are:

1. **Smaller lymphocyte-like cells:** These small cells (6–8 µm in diameter) have round, uniformly dense nuclei with smudged dense chromatin. They have a thin (narrow) rim of eosinophilic cytoplasm more than a true lymphocyte. They resemble secondary spermatocytes.
2. **Medium-sized (intermediate-sized) cells:** These are the **most numerous** and common cells seen in the tumor.

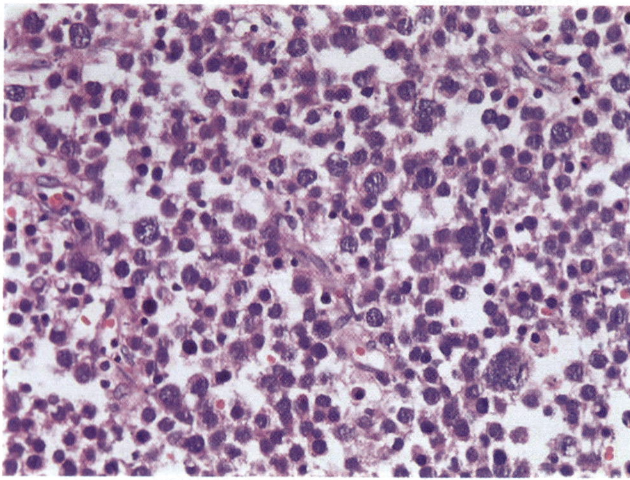

Fig. 21.8: Spermatocytic tumor composed of mixtures of small lymphocyte-like cells, medium-sized cells, and large cells.

The **nucleus is round, having finely granular to filamentous chromatin** and variably prominent nucleoli (occasional nucleoli). The chromatin in some tumor cells is distinctively filamentous in appearance, similar to the **"spireme" chromatin** seen in the meiotic phase of non-neoplastic primary spermatocytes. These cells show dense eosinophilic to amphophilic cytoplasm. The cytoplasmic membranes are often (but not always) poorly defined.

3. **Large (giant) cells:** Scattered giant cells are seen. Giant cells may have single (mononucleated) or multiple nuclei (multinucleated). They have nuclear features similar to that of intermediate-sized cells.

Mitotic rate: It is often high, including atypical forms, is usually frequent.

Stroma: It is usually scant, finely fibrous, and not typically conspicuous. The **regular fibrous septation of classic seminoma is not seen.**

Immunohistochemistry: The tumor cells do not express typical seminoma markers.

Differential diagnosis

Seminoma: In contrast to seminomas, the features in spermatocytic tumors are: (i) absent or scant interstitial lymphocytic infiltration; (ii) granulomatous inflammation is rare; (iii) not associated with germ cell neoplasia in situ; and (iv) rarely metastasize.

Clinical features: Most patients present with painless enlargement of the testis, which can be of several years' duration. Serum tumor markers are not elevated. Spermatocytic tumor only rarely metastasizes. Orchiectomy is curative for almost all patients.

Prognosis: Spermatocytic tumor is a slow-growing tumor. It rarely metastasizes. The prognosis is excellent.

Prepubertal-type Teratoma

Definition: Prepubertal-type teratoma is a germ cell tumor **that usually occurs in the prepubertal testis.** But it may also be found in postpubertal patients. It is **composed of elements resembling somatic tissue derived from one or more of the germ layers** (endoderm, mesoderm, and ectoderm).

In prepubertal patients, teratoma is **almost always pure neoplasms**. Among germ cell tumors, prepubertal teratomas (15% of testicular germ cell tumors) are second in frequency in infants and children, only to yolk sac tumors.

Age: Pure teratoma is common in the prepubertal testis of **infants and children**. The mean age at the time of diagnosis is 20 months, which is unusual beyond 4 years.

Features

No association with GCNIS: Prepubertal-type teratomas are **not associated with germ cell neoplasia in situ (GCNIS), dysgenetic parenchymal changes, scarring, or chromosome 12p amplification.**

Prepubertal-type versus postpubertal-type teratomas: Prepubertal teratomas are usually **distinct from postpubertal-type teratomas**. Both differ in terms of pathogenesis and clinical behavior.

- **More organized architecture:** In contrast to postpubertal testicular teratoma, prepubertal teratomas produce distinct elements arranged into structures **(more organized architecture)** that more closely resemble normal tissue. In an organoid pattern, the smooth muscle encircles the ciliated epithelium-lined cysts, sometimes splitting into distinct layers similar to muscularis mucosa and muscularis propria, with an intervening collection of connective tissue resembling submucosa. A lobular arrangement of glands resembling salivary or pancreatic acinar cells may be found.
- **Lack of significant cytologic atypia** in prepubertal teratomas.
- **Benign course**: Prepubertal teratomas **do not recur or metastasize.**
- **Mostly pure form**: Most prepubertal teratomas are pure. But rarely, they are admixed with prepubertal type yolk sac tumors.
- **Immature tissue has potential value:** Immaturity of tissue elements is not considered in the classification of postpubertal-type testicular teratomas. But it has **potential value in the prepubertal group**. This is mainly because they are closely related to teratomas of the ovary and sacrococcygeal region. The method for assessing the quantity of immature neuroectodermal tissue can be the same as that in ovarian and sacrococcygeal teratomas.

Specialized variants of prepubertal-type teratoma: Special types include dermoid cysts, epidermoid cyst, and well-differentiated neuroendocrine tumors (monodermal teratoma). Differences between prepubertal and post-pubertal type teratoma of testis are presented in **Table 21.3.**

Clinical Features of Testicular Germ Cell Tumors

Painless enlargement of testis: Germ cell tumors of the testis usually present as painless enlargement of the testis. **Nonseminomatous germ cell tumors** (NSGCTs): Most NSGCTs tend to **grow faster** than seminomas and **metastasize more readily and more widely**. In some NSGCTs, metastases may be the first clinical sign of the neoplasm.

Solid testicular mass: Any solid testicular mass **should be considered neoplastic until otherwise proved.**

Fine needle aspiration cytology (FNAC) contraindicated: FNAC is contraindicated in testicular tumors because it may result in inguinal lymph node metastasis.

For a biopsy of a testicular neoplasm: It is **necessary to excise the scrotal skin in addition to orchiectomy.** It is associated with a risk of tumor spillage. Hence, the standard management of a solid testicular mass is radical orchiectomy based on the presumptive diagnosis of malignancy. Occasionally, when there is suspicion of a benign lesion, it can be excised by partial orchiectomy. An intraoperative frozen section examination may be done to avoid an unnecessary radical orchiectomy.

TABLE 21.3 Differences between prepubertal and postpubertal type teratoma of testis.

Features	*Prepubertal teratoma*	*Postpubertal teratoma*
Manifestation	Majority in prepubertal testis of infants and children, rarely postpubertal (adults) patients	Postpubertal (adult) patients
GCNIS changes in the uninvolved region of the testis	No GCNIS	About 90% of cases show GCNIS
Association with dysgenetic parenchymal changes, scarring, or chromosome 12p abnormalities	No	Yes
Architecture of tumor	Organoid architecture	No organoid architecture
Cytologic atypia	Absent	May be present
Immature tissue elements	Potential value	Not considered in classification
As a component of mixed GCT	No	Usually occurs as one component of a mixed GCTs
Course	Benign	Malignant

(GCNIS: germ cell neoplasia in situ; GCT: germ cell tumor).

Mode of Spread of Testicular Tumors

Q. Write a short note on the spread of testicular tumors.

Testicular tumors have a characteristic mode of spread.

Lymphatic spread: It is **common to all forms of testicular tumors**. Usually, it **first spreads to retroperitoneal para-aortic nodes** and not inguinal lymph nodes. Subsequently, it spreads **to mediastinal and supraclavicular nodes**. Metastases from seminomas generally involve lymph nodes.

Hematogenous spread: Primarily, it spreads to the **lungs**, but the **liver, brain, and bones** may also be involved. Hematogenous spread occurs later in the course of seminoma. Nonseminomatous GCTs tend to metastasize through the hematogenous route earlier and more frequently. The microscopic appearance of metastases and distant recurrences may be different from that of the primary testicular tumor.

Tumor Markers (Table 21.4)

Q. Write a short note on serological markers/tumor markers of testicular tumors.

- Germ cell tumors of the testis may **secrete hormones and enzymes,** which can be detected in blood.

TABLE 21.4 Tumor markers of testicular germ cell tumors.

Type of tumor	*Tumor marker*
Seminoma	hCG, placental alkaline phosphatase
Teratomas and teratocarcinoma	AFP, hCG
Embryonal carcinoma	CEA
Yolk sac tumor	AFP
Choriocarcinoma	β-hCG

(AFP: α-fetoprotein; hCG: human chorionic gonadotropin; CEA: carcinoembryonic antigen).

- Tumor markers include **hCG**, **AFP**, and **lactate dehydrogenase**.
- They are **valuable in the diagnosis and management** of testicular neoplasms.
  1. **Lactate dehydrogenase:** The **level** of raised lactate dehydrogenase **correlates with the mass of tumor cells** and can be **used to assess tumor burden**.
  2. **AFP and hCG: Marked elevation** of these markers was found in more than 80% of individuals **with NSGCT**.
     - AFP: produced by yolk sac tumor.
     - hCG levels: Raised in tumor with choriocarcinoma elements. Seminomas with syncytiotrophoblastic giant cells may also cause mild elevation of hCG levels.
- **Importance of tumor markers:**
  - Evaluation of testicular masses
  - Staging of testicular germ cell tumors
  - Assessing tumor burden
  - Monitoring the response to therapy.

PENIS

TUMORS OF THE PENIS

Tumors of the penis are not common. The most frequent neoplasm is squamous cell carcinoma (SCC). WHO (2022) classification of tumors of the penis is presented in **Box 21.4**.

Q. Write a short essay on premalignant lesions of the penis.

Squamous Cell Carcinoma Precursors

Precursor squamous lesions may be squamous cell carcinoma precursors HPV-associated or HPV-independent. Squamous cell carcinoma precursors, HPV-associated are termed penile intraepithelial neoplasia (PeIN), HPV-associated.

Penile Intraepithelial Neoplasia

Q. Write a short note on premalignant lesions of the penis.

Penile intraepithelial neoplasia (PeIN) is a histological alteration of the penile squamous epithelium characterized

BOX 21.4: WHO (2022) classification (abridged) of tumors of the penis.

Precursor squamous lesions
- Squamous cell carcinoma precursors, HPV-associated
  - Penile intraepithelial neoplasia (PeIN), HPV-associated: Basaloid PeIN, Warty PeIN, and Warty-basaloid PeIN
- Squamous cell carcinoma precursors, HPV-independent
  - Differentiated penile intraepithelial neoplasia, HPV-independent

Invasive epithelial tumors of the penis
- Invasive squamous epithelial tumors
  - HPV-associated squamous cell carcinoma
    - Basaloid squamous cell carcinoma
    - Warty carcinoma
  - HPV-independent squamous cell carcinoma
    - Squamous cell carcinoma, usual type
    - Verrucous carcinoma
  - Squamous cell carcinoma NOS (not otherwise specified)
    - Other epithelial tumors

by **dysplastic changes throughout the epidermis without invasion** of the underlying stroma (basement membrane is **intact).**

PeIN is like that of carcinoma in situ (CIS) in other sites such as the uterine cervix. Morphologically, they can range from mild dysplasia to CIS. These lesions in the penis are termed under the umbrella term PeIN. PeIN is the precursor to the invasive SCC of the penis. The term **penile intraepithelial neoplasia (PeIN) is preferred over old terms** such as **squamous intraepithelial lesion** (SIL), **erythroplasia of Queyrat, and Bowen disease**. All are squamous lesions confined to the epidermis and show an intact basement membrane.

Penile Intraepithelial Neoplasia, HPV-associated

Human papillomavirus-associated PeIN is a rare HPV-driven precursor/premalignant lesion of penile squamous cell carcinoma (SCC). PeIN is histologically characterized by **dysplastic squamous epithelium with an intact basement membrane.**

Etiology and pathogenesis: HPV-associated **(HPV-related or undifferentiated)** PeIN is rare. It is most commonly associated with high-risk HPV types such as 16, and 18. The rate of its progression to cancer is low. But HPV-associated PeIN accounts for 70–89% of all PeIN. High-risk HPV produces two proteins namely E7 and E6 (*refer* page 258 and **Fig. 7.25**).

MORPHOLOGY

Gross

Lesions of HPV-associated PeIN may be **flat to slightly elevated macules, papules, or plaques.** They may be well-delineated with irregular outlines. Solitary lesions are more common.

Microscopy

HPV-associated PeIN shows more prominent morphologic changes and multiple patterns. Depending on the microscopic appearance, it can be subclassified into three types. Gross differentiation between the types and subtypes of PeIN is not easy.

1. **Basaloid** (undifferentiated) **PeIN:** The **epithelium** (usually the full-thickness epithelium) **is replaced** by a **monotonous population of small to medium-sized immature basaloid dysplastic squamous cells.** These cells have round to oval nuclei; inconspicuous nucleoli; and scant cytoplasm. They show a high nuclear to-cytoplasmic (N: C) ratio. Mitotic figures are prominent. They are positive for HPV16.
2. **Warty (Bowenoid) PeIN:** The involved epithelium has an **undulating/spiking surface** and shows **low papillary structures.** The **epithelium is replaced by striking pleomorphic cells with koilocytic atypia** (characterized by multinucleation, nuclei with irregular contours, and perinuclear halo). Mitoses tend to be numerous. They are usually positive for HPV, but unlike in basaloid PeIN, the genotypes are heterogeneous.
3. **Mixed (warty/basaloid) PeIN:** Frequently, lesions show combined features of both warty and basaloid. They have a spiking surface with koilocytic changes, whereas the lower half of the epithelium mainly consists of small basaloid cells. PeIN can be divided into **low-grade and high-grade lesions** depending on the thickness of epithelium involved by atypical cells. HPV is usually positive.

Clinical features: HPV-associated PeIN (previously known clinically as erythroplasia of Queyrat and Bowen disease) presents with one or more abnormal growths or sores (ulcers) on the penis.

Differentiated Penile Intraepithelial Neoplasia, HPV-independent

Differentiated penile intraepithelial neoplasia (PeIN) is an HPV-independent precursor/premalignant lesion of penile squamous cell carcinoma. It is characterized by **dysplastic squamous epithelium mainly in the basal and parabasal cells** within an otherwise well-differentiated epithelium with an intact basement membrane.

Etiology: It is associated with chronic inflammation and conditions producing chronic irritation/injury (e.g., phimosis, balanoposthitis, and lichen sclerosus) with chronic scarring.

MORPHOLOGY

Gross

Differentiated PeIN appears as a **single white or pink and plaque-like** in a circumcised specimen, with the atrophic appearing skin of lichen sclerosus.

Microscopy

Differentiated PeIN shows **thickened epithelium** (epithelial hyperplasia, hyperkeratosis, and parakeratosis), elongated and anastomosing (intercommunicating) rete ridges, **abnormal maturation** (enlarged keratinocytes with abundant eosinophilic cytoplasm). It creates a reticulated epithelial architecture. It also shows dyskeratosis (premature or abnormal differentiation of squamous cells), **keratin pearl** formation in deep rete ridges, and prominent intercellular bridges. **Atypical keratinocytes are restricted to the basal and parabasal layers of epithelium.** These atypical cells have abundant eosinophilic cytoplasm, enlarged hyperchromatic nuclei, and occasional prominent nucleoli. All cases of differentiated PeIN are considered high grade. It is usually negative for HPV.

Clinical features: Differentiated PeIN usually occurs in slightly older men than HPV-associated PeIN. Patients are usually uncircumcised and have a history of longstanding lichen sclerosus.

Bowen disease and erythroplasia of Queyrat: These are old terms used for penile intraepithelial neoplasia (PeIN). Carcinoma in situ involving the skin of the shaft and scrotum of older men was known as Bowen disease, and lesions in the glans were termed erythroplasia of Queyrat. These terms are not recommended and are replaced by the term PeIN.

Bowenoid papulosis

Bowenoid papulosis (HPV16/18-associated) is also an HPV-related proliferation that **occurs in sexually active men**. It is **usually caused by HPV serotypes 16, 18**, and/or 35. In contrast to penile intraepithelial neoplasia (PeIN), Bowenoid papulosis occurs **at a younger age and presents as multiple** (rather than solitary) reddish brown papular lesions. It is also related to HPV 16 and microscopically indistinguishable from penile intraepithelial neoplasia (PeIN). Bowenoid papulosis **never develops into invasive carcinoma** and **usually undergoes spontaneous regression.**

MORPHOLOGY

Gross

It affects the skin of the anogenital region of young adults. Bowenoid papulosis appears as **multiple, 2–10 mm, soft brownish or violaceous papules, or macules** that can coalesce to form plaques. They are usually multiple.

Microscopy

It shows features like PeIN, especially undifferentiated (warty/basaloid) PeIN. There is a **proliferation of atypical cells with a high nuclear-to-cytoplasmic ratio.** But Bowenoid papulosis is sharply demarcated from normal epidermis like HPV-induced warts.

These lesions are **benign, self-limited, and typically regress spontaneously.** They do not progress to invasive carcinoma.

Invasive Squamous Cell Carcinoma

PA 29.2 (CC): Describe the pathogenesis, pathology, presenting and distinguishing features, diagnostic tests, progression, and spread of carcinoma of the penis.

Squamous cell carcinoma (SCC) of the penis is not a common malignancy. It arises from the squamous mucosa of the glans and contiguous urethral meatus or the prepuce and skin covering the penile shaft.

Epidemiology: Carcinomas are commonly affecting middle-aged and older patients between **40 and 70 years of age**. Carcinoma of the penis is much more common in less developed countries than in developed countries. It is almost unknown in men circumcised at birth.

Types of invasive SCC: These include HPV-associated SCC, HPV-independent SCC, and SCC NOS (not otherwise specified) (*see* **Box 21.4**).

HPV-associated Squamous Cell Carcinoma

HPV-associated SCC is an invasive keratinizing carcinoma. It **arises from penile mucosal or cutaneous compartments** and is **associated with HPV infection.**

Etiology: High-risk HPVs are associated with about 33% of all penile cancers. The most frequent subtype is HPV16.

Pathogenesis: HPV-induced penile cancers develop from the noninvasive precursor lesion called PeIN. The transforming effects of high-risk HPV to develop penile carcinoma are identical to its role in cervical cancer. High-risk HPV encodes E6 and E7 proteins. E6 oncoprotein inhibits the p53 and E7 oncoprotein inhibits RB tumor-suppressor proteins. These lead to genomic instability and increased cell proliferation. E6 protein also stimulates increased expression of telomerase, leading to the immortalization of cells and ensuing autonomous cell proliferation (without G1 cell-cycle stops). E7 protein induces feedback loops that increase levels of the cyclin-dependent kinase inhibitor p16 (p16INK4a). These increased levels of p16 can be used as a surrogate for the presence of high-risk HPV in tumor cells.

MORPHOLOGY

There are 4 subtypes: Basaloid SCC, warty carcinoma, clear cell SCC, and lymphoepithelioma-like carcinoma

Basaloid SCC

Gross: It appears as a large, ulcerated, nonexophytic tumor mass. These tumors may be extensively papillary.

Microscopy: This subtype of tumor is composed of **solid nests of** relatively **small, monotonous (uniform) basaloid hyperchromatic cells.** It has a destructive pattern of invasion. It shows frequent vascular and perineural invasions are seen.

Warty Carcinoma

Gross: They typically appear as cauliflower-like, exophytic, white to grey tumors.

Microscopy: It is a verruciform neoplasm. Throughout the tumor (not only at the surface), it also shows a **parakeratotic papillomatous surface** with **conspicuous frankly atypical koilocytosis.**

HPV-independent Squamous Cell Carcinoma

HPV-independent SCC is an invasive keratinizing carcinoma. It arises from the mucosa of the penis or cutaneous compartments. It is not associated with HPV infection. Two major subtypes are squamous cell carcinoma, the usual type, and verrucous carcinoma.

Etiology: Various risk factors for HPV-independent SCC include phimosis, poor genital hygiene, chronic inflammation, lichen sclerosus smoking, ultraviolet (UV)

radiation, radiotherapy, condyloma, and lack of circumcision. These risk factors lead to chronic inflammation of the glans and prepuce. They promote the development of differentiated PeIN and non–non-HPV-associated penile cancer. Low-income status is also a salient risk factor.

- **Circumcision:** It has a **protective role**, and hence very rare among Jews and Muslims. Circumcision is associated with **better genital hygiene** and **reduces exposure to carcinogens** that may be concentrated **in smegma**. It also **decreases** the likelihood of **infection with** potentially **oncogenic types of HPV** (HPV type 16 and HPV 18).
- **Cigarette smoking:** It is also associated with a higher risk of carcinoma of the penis.
- **Other factors:** Poor hygiene and chronic inflammation probably contribute to cancers that are not HPV-related. Chronic inflammatory conditions such as *lichen sclerosus et atrophicus (BXO)* are also risk factors.

MORPHOLOGY

Squamous Cell Carcinoma, Usual Type

Gross (Figs. 21.9A and B)

Localization: It arises from the **mucosa of the glans penis or the** inner surface of the prepuce near the coronal sulcus.

Appearance: Squamous cell carcinoma may have a spectrum of clinical appearance. It may **vary from minute areas of induration, erythema, or exophytic growths to nodular and ulcerated lesions.** They have irregular margins.

Microscopy (Figs. 21.10A and B)

It is an invasive squamous cell carcinoma showing **varying degrees of differentiation.** It ranges from well- to poorly differentiated SCC. Penile SCCs are graded using the three-tiered WHO Classification of Tumors/International Society of Urological Pathology (WHO/ISUP) system.

- **Grade 1 (well-differentiated) carcinomas:** These are not common. These tumors show nests of squamous cells with extreme differentiation (keratin pearls).
- **Grade 2 (moderately differentiated) carcinomas:** This shows features between grade 1 and grade 3. The tumor cells show individual cell keratinization.
- **Grade 3 (poorly differentiated) carcinomas:** They consist of **small nests, cords, trabeculae, or isolated anaplastic cells.** Keratinization is rare, focal, or poorly developed in these tumors.

Verrucous Carcinoma

Gross

Verrucous carcinoma is a non-HPV-related variant of squamous cell carcinoma. It is an exophytic tumor showing papillomatous growth (papillary architecture) with a demarcation at the interface between the tumor and stroma.

Microscopy

Verrucous carcinoma is **a well-differentiated SCC** showing exophytic or endophytic papillary growth. The papillae do not have a prominent central fibrovascular core, and the tumor cells do not show any koilocytic atypia. The tumor shows a characteristically **broad-based pushing pattern of infiltration** (broad, rounded pushing deep border). The cross-section of the papillae shows a central keratin plug at the tip of the papilla and neoplastic cells at the periphery. There is no cytologic atypia.

Squamous cell carcinoma NOS (SCC-NOS): It is an invasive keratinizing carcinoma without any special histological features.

Clinical Features

- **Slowly growing and locally invasive tumor**: Invasive squamous cell carcinoma of the penis presents as a slowly growing and locally invasive lesion. They are often present for a year or more before it is brought to medical attention. They usually do not produce pain until they undergo ulceration and infection.
- They may metastasize to inguinal lymph nodes. Grade and stage are the most important prognostic factors for penile carcinoma.

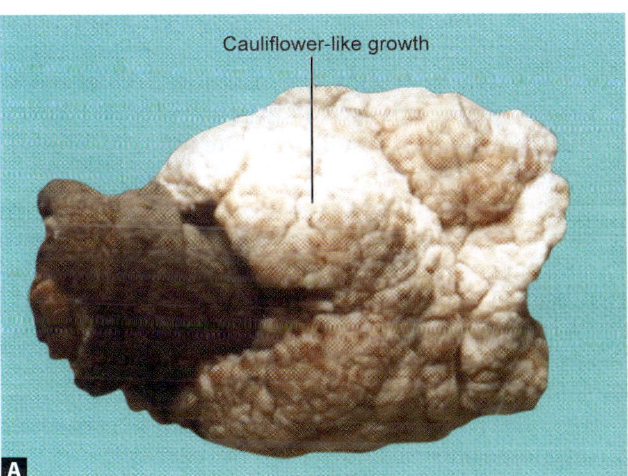

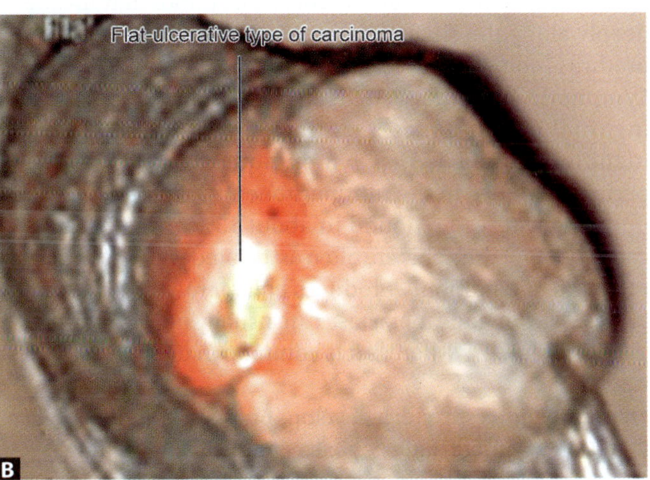

Figs. 21.9A and B: Carcinoma of the penis: (A) The exophytic fungating type shows a glans penis deformed by a cauliflower-like growth; (B) Ulcerative type of carcinoma.

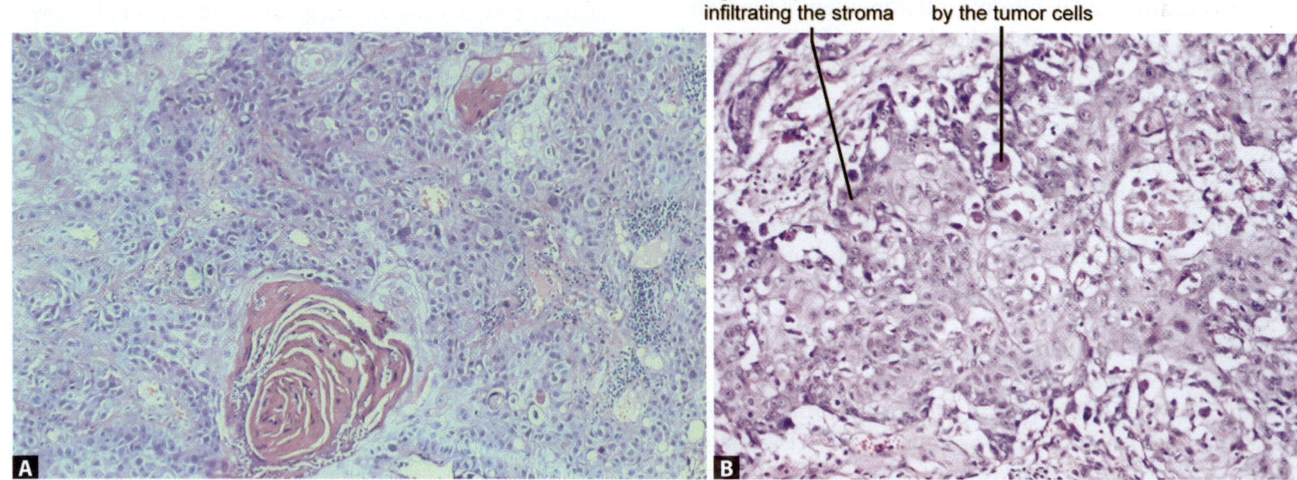

Figs. 21.10A and B: Microscopic appearance of squamous cell carcinoma of the penis: (A) Well-differentiated squamous cell carcinoma showing neoplastic squamous cells with epithelial pearls; (B) Moderately differentiated squamous cell carcinoma with pleomorphic malignant squamous cells.

SCC, usual type: It occurs most frequently in the sixth and seventh decades of life. It forms about 45–65% of penile SCCs. Prognosis depends on histological grade; anatomical level of infiltration (pathological stage); vascular, lymphatic, and perineural invasion; and inguinal lymph node metastasis.

Verrucous carcinoma: It is a rare tumor of the penis that accounts for 3–7% of all penile SCCs and 12–38% of all verruciform tumors. It occurs in older men. **Pure verrucous carcinoma is locally invasive and has no metastatic potential.**

Spread and Metastases

Local spread: It can occur from one epithelial compartment to the other and from superficial to deep anatomical levels. Spread may be horizontal or vertical. The tumor may invade deeply along the shaft of the penis. Local spread into the urethra is common.

Lymphatic spread: It usually first spreads to **superficial inguinal lymph nodes** ("sentinel node"), then to deep inguinal and pelvic iliac lymph nodes, and last to the periaortic nodes in the retroperitoneum. Inguinal lymph node metastases are found in about 15% of cases. Since carcinomas of the penis are often associated with secondary infection, it commonly produces enlargement of inguinal nodes. Lymph node metastases are usually not common in exophytic tumors whereas it is common in deeply invasive tumors.

Hematogenous spread: It develops only as a late event. The usual sites of metastatic deposits are the liver and lungs.

PROSTATE

PROSTATITIS

PA 29.5 (NC): Describe the etiology, pathogenesis, pathology, and progression of prostatitis.

Definition: Prostatitis is inflammation of the prostate.

Classification: Prostatitis may be divided into several categories, depending on the cause, patterns of tissue reaction, and clinical course. Often no etiology is found. Prostatitis can be generally classified into the following categories.

1. **Acute bacterial prostatitis:** It is caused by the organisms (coliform uropathogens such as *E. coli, Klebsiella, Proteus, Pseudomonas, Enterobacter,* gonococci, staphylococci, and streptococci) that produce acute urinary tract infections. It constitutes 2–5% of cases. **Usually, it develops as a complication of other urinary tract infections. It results from the reflux of infected urine into the prostate.**
2. **Chronic bacterial prostatitis**: It is also caused by common pathogens involved in urinary tract infections and they constitute 2–5% of cases. **It may or may not be preceded by an episode of acute prostatitis.**
3. **Chronic nonbacterial prostatitis: Sometimes in chronic prostatitis, no causative organism is identified.** Some of them may be due to *Chlamydia trachomatis, Mycoplasma,* or *Ureaplasma urealyticum.* It is usually diagnosed after excluding the other causes.

4. **Granulomatous prostatitis:** It is usually caused by the instillation of Bacille Calmette-Guérin (BCG) within the bladder for treatment of superficial bladder cancer. BCG is an attenuated tuberculosis strain that produces a granulomatous immune reaction. Microscopically it is indistinguishable from tuberculosis. Other causes of granulomatous prostatitis are tuberculosis *(M. tuberculosis)* and fungal (*Histoplasma capsulatum*) granulomatous prostatitis (in immunocompromised hosts).
   - **Nonspecific granulomatous prostatitis:** It may develop as a foreign-body reaction to fluids that leak into tissue from ruptured prostatic ducts and acini or following surgery (postsurgical prostatic granulomas).
5. **Chronic pelvic pain syndrome:** It forms the majority of prostatitis (90–95% of cases). It can be subdivided into (i) inflammatory (associated with leukocytes in prostatic secretions), and (ii) noninflammatory cases (no leukocytes in prostatic secretion). The etiology is not known and its diagnosis is by exclusion.

Diagnosis: It is usually not diagnosed based on biopsy because the microscopic findings are nonspecific and if biopsy is performed on an infected prostatitis, it can result in sepsis. However, in *granulomatous prostatitis,* which may cause induration of the prostate and biopsy should be done to rule out prostate cancer.

MORPHOLOGY

Microscopy

Acute prostatitis: Shows acute inflammatory infiltrate in the prostatic acini and stroma.

Chronic bacterial prostatitis: It shows infiltration by lymphocytes, plasma cells, and macrophages.

Clinical features of prostatitis: These are as follows:

- **Acute bacterial prostatitis:** It presents with sudden onset of fever, chills, dysuria (intense discomfort on urination), perineal pain, and bladder outlet obstruction. It may be complicated by sepsis. If acute prostatitis is suspected, the digital rectal examination should not be done because it can produce bacteremia. Most patients respond well to antibiotics.
- **Chronic bacterial prostatitis:** It usually presents with recurrent urinary tract infections interspaced by asymptomatic periods. Presenting features include low back pain, dysuria, perineal and suprapubic discomfort, and burning at the urethral meatus. The urine usually contains bacteria. Diagnosis is made by detection of more than 10–12 leukocytes/high power fields in expressed prostatic secretions, and by positive culture of urine specimen. It is treated also with antibiotics.
- **Chronic pelvic pain syndrome:** It is characterized by chronic pain localized to the perineum, suprapubic area, and penis. A prominent feature is pain during or after ejaculation. Therapy for chronic pelvic pain syndrome is empirical and depends on the nature of the symptoms.

BENIGN PROSTATIC HYPERPLASIA

PA 29.3 (CC): Describe the pathogenesis, pathology, hormonal dependency presenting and distinguishing features, urologic findings, and diagnostic tests of benign prostatic hyperplasia.

Stromal and glandular proliferation: Benign prostatic hyperplasia (BPH) or nodular hyperplasia is characterized by hyperplasia of both prostatic stromal and epithelial cells.

Nodules in the periurethral region: BPH forms large, fairly discrete (separate) nodules in the periurethral region of the prostate.

Partial or complete obstruction of urinary flow: BPH is an important cause of urinary obstruction. When the nodules of BPH become sufficiently large, they compress and narrow the urethral canal and cause partial or complete obstruction of the urethra and urinary outflow.

Occurs in men older than 50 years: BPH is a very common disorder in men older than 50 years of age. Its frequency progressively increases with age and reaches 90% by the eighth decade of life.

Etiology and Pathogenesis (Figs. 21.11A to C)

Q. Describe the etiology and pathogenesis of nodular hyperplasia/ benign hyperplasia of the prostate.

Increased number of epithelial cells and stromal cells: In BPH, there is an increased number of epithelial cells and stromal cells in the **periurethral area** of the prostate.

- **Increased number of epithelial cells:** The increased number of epithelial cells is **not due to increased epithelial cell proliferation but mainly due to the reduction of the rate of cell death.** It results in the **accumulation of senescent epithelial cells.**
- **Increased number of stromal cells:** It is due to the **proliferation of stromal cells.**

Role of Androgen

The cause and earliest pathogenic events in BPH are incompletely understood. However excessive androgen-dependent growth of stromal and glandular elements of the prostate plays a main role.

Androgens needed for the growth of the prostate: Androgen plays a key role in prostatic growth. It **increases cellular proliferation** and **inhibits cell death**. Testosterone is the most common androgen necessary for prostatic development and maintaining secretory function. The active androgen form of testosterone is dihydrotestosterone (DHT). It forms 90% of total prostatic androgens.

Dihydrotestosterone (DHT) is the active androgen: Dihydrotestosterone is the main androgen in the prostate. The main source of DHT in the prostate is testosterone, and DHT is 10 times more potent than testosterone.

Synthesis of dihydrotestosterone: DHT is synthesized in the prostate **from the conversion of testosterone** by the action of the enzyme type 2 5α-reductase, present mainly

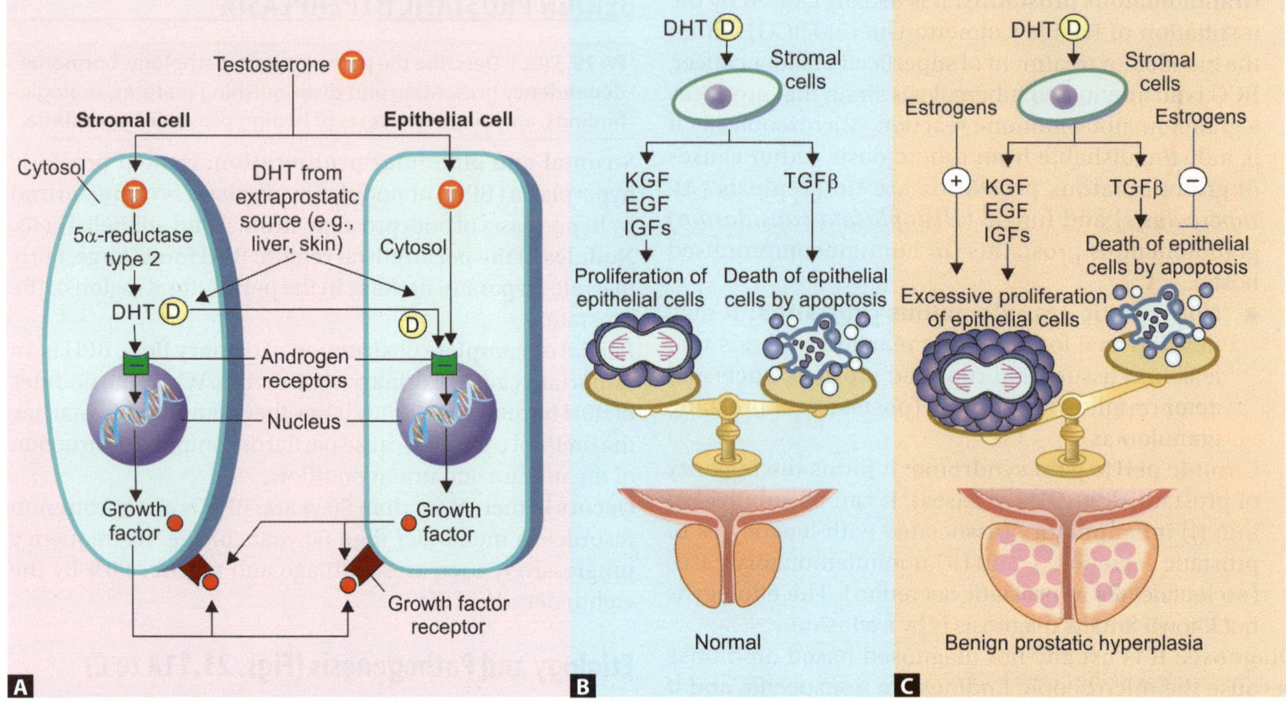

Figs. 21.11A to C: Pathogenesis of benign prostatic hyperplasia (BPH): (A) The stromal cells play a central role in the synthesis of dihydrotestosterone (DHT) from testosterone by type 2 5α-reductase. DHT may also be produced in the liver and skin by both mainly type 1 5α-reductase; (B) Role of DHT and estrogens in maintaining the normal balance between proliferation and death of epithelial cells; (C) Estrogens can shift the balance toward proliferation and reduce the death of epithelial cells. This may contribute to the pathogenesis of BPH. (AR: androgen receptor; EGF, Epidermal growth factor; IGFs, insulin-like growth factors; KGF, keratinocyte growth factor; TGFβ, transforming growth factor β).

in the stromal cells and a **few basal cells**. This **enzyme** (type 2 5α-reductase) is **not present in the epithelial cells** of the prostate. **Thus, stromal cells are responsible for the androgen-dependent growth of the prostate.**

- **Type 1 5α-reductase:** It is another enzyme that produces **DHT from testosterone in extraprostatic locations** (e.g., liver and skin). This is an additional source of DHT that reaches the prostate through the blood.

Actions of DHT: DHT binds to the nuclear androgen receptor (AR) present in **both epithelial and stromal cells** of the prostate. **DHT is more potent than testosterone** because (1) it has a **higher affinity for AR** and (2) **it forms a more stable complex with AR.** Nuclear androgen receptors also bind circulating testosterone.

Expression of genes involved in the growth and survival of prostatic epithelium and stromal cells: DHT binding to AR **activates the transcription of androgen-dependent genes,** which results in the **increased production of many growth factors and their receptors**. DHT-induced growth factors **increase the proliferation of stromal cells and decrease the death of epithelial cells.** The most important growth factor is the **fibroblast growth factor (FGF) family.**

- **FGF-7 (keratinocyte growth factor/KGF):** It is an important growth factor produced by stromal cells and mediates **prostatic growth by paracrine mechanism.**
- FGFs 1 and 2, and TGF-β cause fibroblast proliferation.

Role of Estrogens

With aging, estrogens act synergistically with DHT: Apart from androgens, estrogens also play a role in the pathogenesis of BPH. On prostate cells (both epithelial and stromal cells), two different forms of estrogen receptor (ER) are present. These are ERα and ERβ, and they have opposing proliferative and antiproliferative effects, respectively. With aging, testosterone levels decrease whereas estrogen levels remain unchanged. The unchanged levels of estrogens may be due to increased peripheral conversion of androgens to estrogens. Estrogens may act similarly to DHT and stimulate the growth of epithelial and stromal cells leading to proliferation.

MORPHOLOGY

Q. Describe the morphology of nodular hyperplasia of the prostate.

Gross (Figs. 21.12A to C)

- **Weight:** The normal weight of the prostate is about 20–30 g. In BPH, it usually weighs **2–4 times the normal weight** and ranges from 60 g to 100 g.
- **Sites of involvement:** Nodular hyperplasia begins in the **submucosa (the inner portions of the prostate) of the proximal urethra (laterally situated within the transition zone).** These nodules are seen in the periurethral region.

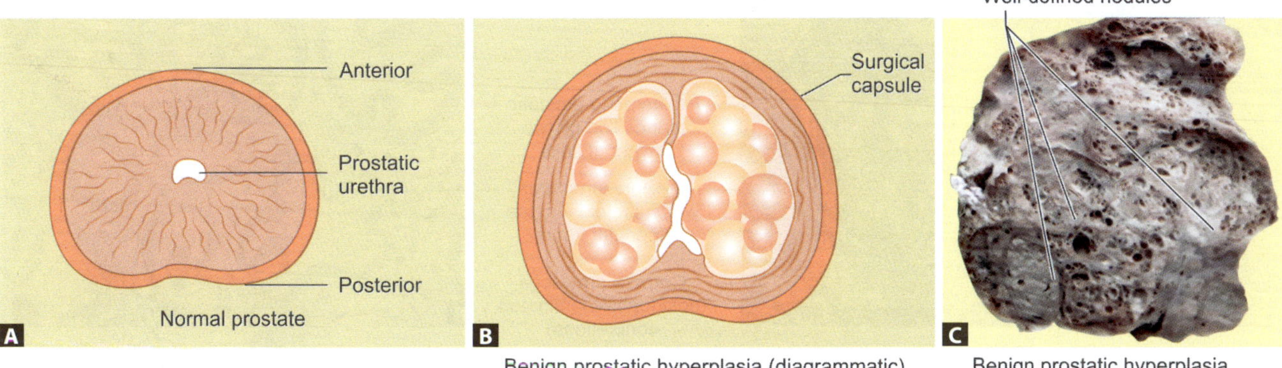

Figs. 21.12A to C: (A) Schematic representation of cut-section of normal prostate; (B) The diagrammatic appearance of benign prostatic hyperplasia. It shows numerous well-defined nodules, predominantly in the periurethral part of the gland. Hyperplastic nodules compress and distort the urethra into a slit-like lumen. Expansion of the central prostatic glands compresses the peripheral parts and the resulting fibrosis leads to the formation of a so-called surgical capsule; (C) Gross appearance of benign prostatic hyperplasia. Cut sections show many well-defined nodules.

- **Cut-section:** It shows **multiple circumscribed nodules** without any true capsules. These nodules compress the surrounding prostatic tissue, which creates a plane of cleavage between the nodule and the normal prostatic tissue. The **nodules may appear solid or contain cystic spaces** (representing dilated glands). **Nodules vary in color and consistency** depending on the predominant component.
  - **Nodule with predominant glands:** They appear **yellow-pink, honeycombed, and have a soft consistency**. Milky-white prostatic fluid oozes out from these areas.
  - **Nodule with predominant fibromuscular stroma:** They appear **pale gray, and are firm/tough in consistency**. These do not exude fluid.
  - **Median lobe hypertrophy:** Sometimes, hyperplastic **nodules may project up into the floor of the urethra** as a hemispheric mass directly beneath the mucosa of the urethra. This is called by the clinician's **median lobe hypertrophy** (**Figs. 21.14A** and *refer to* **Fig. 2.24B**). It does not correspond to the anatomical middle lobe.
- **Compression of the urethra:** As the hyperplastic **nodules enlarge**, they may **compress** the centrally located **urethra** to a slit-like orifice and also the more peripherally located normal prostate.

Microscopy (Figs. 21.13A and B)

Q. Write a short note on microscopy of benign hyperplasia of the prostate.

Nodularity: It is a **characteristic feature** of BPH.

Composition of the Nodules

Benign prostatic hyperplasia shows the proliferation of three types of cells in variable proportions.

1. **Epithelial cells (acini and ductules):** Their proliferation (adenomatous/glandular) of glandular epithelial cells leads to the formation of **small to large cystically dilated glands or acini.**
   - **Glands are lined by two layers of cells,** an inner tall columnar and an outer basal layer of cuboidal or flattened epithelium.
   - Characteristic features are **papillary structures,** which project into the glandular lumen and are lined by columnar epithelial cells.
   - **Corpora amylacea** (eosinophilic-laminated concretions) are commonly seen within the acini.
2. **Smooth muscle cells**
3. **Stromal fibroblasts.**

Types of Nodules

- Five types are recognized and depend on the proportion of the type of cells: **(1) stromal (fibrous), (2) fibromuscular, (3) muscular, (4) fibroadenomatous, and (5) fibromyoadenomatous (most common).**
- **Other findings:** (1) foci of lymphocyte infiltration, (2) areas of infarction, and (3) foci of squamous metaplasia at the edges of the infarcts.

Clinical Features

Clinical manifestations of prostatic hyperplasia occur in only about 10% of men with BPH. Nodular hyperplasia compresses the prostatic urethra and results in bladder outlet obstruction. Thus, the **main symptoms of BPH are due to urinary obstruction.**

- Increasing urinary frequency and nocturia.
- Difficulty in urination, difficulty in starting and stopping the stream of urine, overflow dribbling, and dysuria (painful micturition).
- Urine retention and increased risk of urinary infection by bacteria.

Complications (Figs. 21.14A and B and Box 21.5)

Q. Write a short note on complications (secondary effects) of nodular hyperplasia of the prostate.

- **Hypertrophy of bladder:** Obstruction to urinary outflow leads to hypertrophy and distension of the bladder accompanied by **retention of urine**.

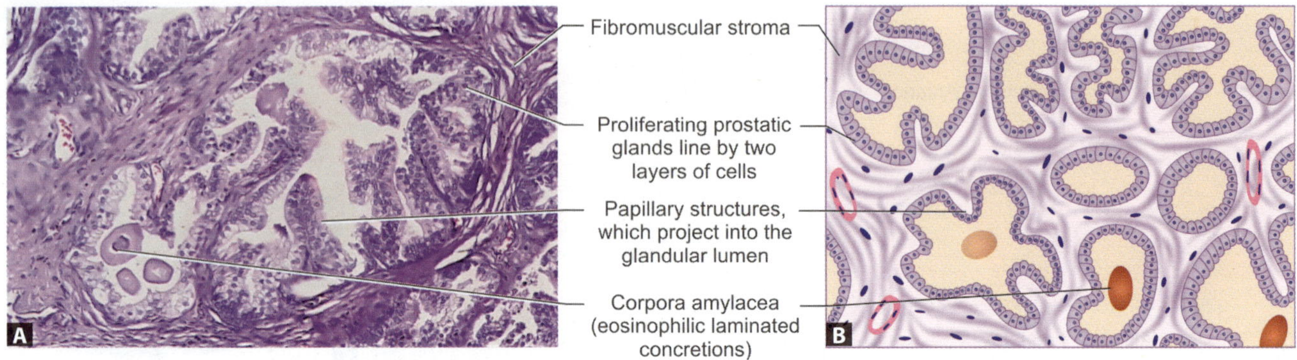

Figs. 21.13A and B: (A) Photomicrograph; (B) Diagrammatic appearance of benign prostatic hyperplasia showing proliferation of epithelial cells forming acini, few with papillary structures.

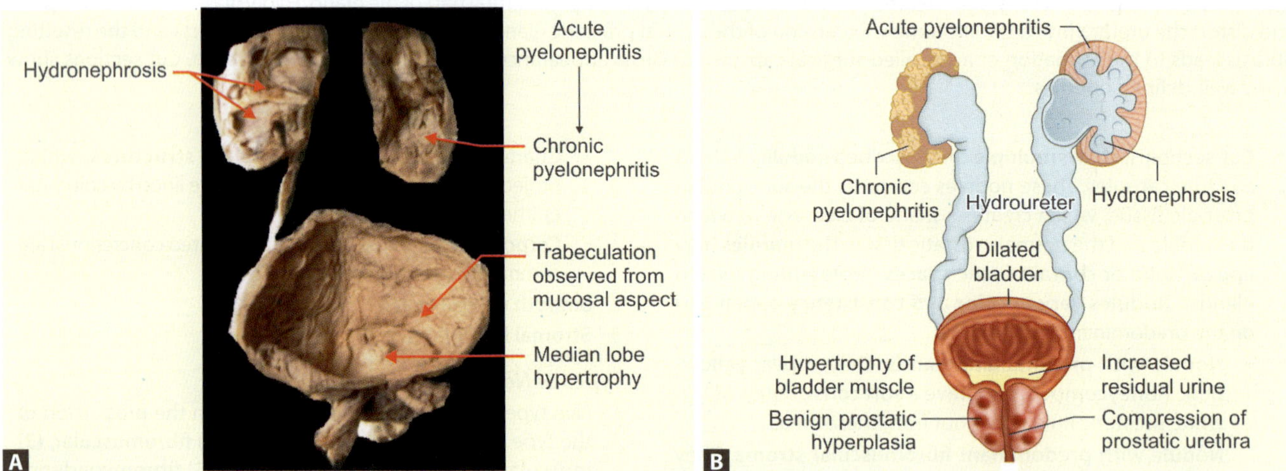

Figs. 21.14A and B: Complications of benign hyperplasia of the prostate (BPH): (A) Gross appearance of the hypertrophied bladder with a nodule projected up into the floor of the bladder. Both kidneys show hydronephrosis and chronic pyelonephritis; (B) Diagrammatic representation of various complications of BPH.

BOX 21.5: Complications of benign prostatic hyperplasia (BPH).

- Hypertrophy of the bladder
- Bladder diverticula
- Cystitis
- Pyelonephritis
- Hydroureter
- Hydronephrosis

- **Bladder diverticula:** Trabeculation of the bladder wall due to obstruction may develop. It can lead to diverticula.
- **Infection:** The inability to empty the bladder completely leads to residual urine in the bladder. The residual urine provides a culture medium for bacteria and is a common source of infection. This can cause bladder infection (**cystitis**) and consequent ascending infection may cause **pyelonephritis**.
- **Consequences of obstruction:** Prolonged severe obstruction with back pressure (in the absence of appropriate treatment) results in **hydroureter**, **hydronephrosis**, and ultimately death due to renal failure.

Treatment: Initial symptomatic BPH is managed medically with targeted therapeutic agents. These include α-adrenergic blockers which relax the prostatic smooth muscle by blocking α_1-1-adrenergic receptors, and 5α-reductase inhibitors which inhibit the formation of DHT from testosterone. Various surgical techniques include transurethral resection of the prostate, high-intensity focused ultrasound (HIFU), laser therapy, hyperthermia, transurethral electrovaporization, and radiofrequency ablation. These surgical treatments are reserved for severely symptomatic cases that do not respond to medical therapy.

Adenocarcinoma of Prostate

PA 29.4 (CC): Describe the pathogenesis, pathology, hormonal dependency presenting and distinguishing features, diagnostic tests, progression, and spread of carcinoma of the prostate.

The World Health Organization (WHO) (2022) (abridged) classification of prostate tumors is presented in **Box 21.6**.

BOX 21.6: World Health Organization (WHO) (2022) (abridged) classification tumors of the prostate.

Epithelial tumors of the prostate
- Glandular neoplasms of the prostate
  - High-grade prostatic intraepithelial neoplasia
  - Intraductal carcinoma of the prostate
  - Prostatic acinar adenocarcinoma
  - Prostatic ductal adenocarcinoma
- Squamous neoplasms of the prostate

Mesenchymal tumors unique to the prostate

Adenocarcinoma of the prostate (prostatic adenocarcinoma) is the **most common malignant tumor in men.** It is the second leading cause of cancer-related death in men, the first being lung cancer.

Age: Prostate cancer is mainly a disease of aging (of older men). The incidence of prostate cancer increases from 20% in men in their 50s to approximately 75% between **60 and 80 years of age**.

Histological types: Adenocarcinoma of the prostate is mainly two histological types namely acinar and ductal.

- **Acinar adenocarcinoma:** It is the **most common type.** Acinar adenocarcinoma is an invasive carcinoma consisting of neoplastic prostatic epithelial cells with secretory differentiation arranged in a variety of histomorphological patterns. These patterns include glands, cords, single cells, and sheets. Basal cells are typically absent.
- **Ductal adenocarcinoma**: It is a subtype of prostatic adenocarcinoma with **large glands lined by tall pseudostratified columnar cells**.

Etiology and Pathogenesis

Risk factors for adenocarcinoma: These include age, androgens, hereditary factors, environmental factors, and acquired somatic mutations. They are involved in the pathogenesis and progression of prostate cancer.

Androgens

Prostatic **cancer growth depends on androgens which are important in prostatic cancer.** Androgens bind to the androgen receptor (AR) and express **pro-growth and pro-survival genes.** Surgical or chemical castration (treatment with **antiandrogens) induces** disease **regression**. Most prostatic cancers eventually become resistant to androgen blockade. This is either by acquiring androgen receptor gene amplifications (which increase sensitivity to lower androgen levels) or mutations that permit ligand-independent androgen receptor activation. Other mutations or epigenetic changes can activate alternative signaling pathways and thus avoid the need for androgen receptor signaling.

Heredity

It also contributes to the pathogenesis of prostate cancer. Men with first-degree relatives affected by the carcinoma of the prostate have a 2-fold increased risk.

Germline variants: There are several germline variants associated with an increased risk of cancer. These include the following:

- **Activation of *MYC* oncogene:** MYC is a transcription factor encoded by the *MYC* gene. It promotes cell cycle progression. Relatively common variants that modestly increase risk are variants in **regulatory regions that influence the expression of MYC.** It is an important oncogene involved in prostate cancer.
- **Inactivation of DNA repair genes:** Other rare variants associated with a high risk of early onset; aggressive cancers have been identified. ***BRCA2*** is required for DNA repair by homologous recombination. Mutations that **interfere with proteins involved in homologous recombination** (e.g., loss-of-function mutations in **BRCA2**) and **DNA mismatch repair may be involved in prostate cancer.**

Environmental Factors

Exposure to carcinogens (such as dietary carcinogens), estrogens, and oxidants can damage prostatic epithelium. These damaged epithelial cells may acquire genetic and epigenetic changes that lead to the development of cancer.

Dietary factors: Increased consumption of charred **red meat and animal fat increases the risk** of prostate cancer. Diets that prevent or delay prostate cancer include lycopene (found in tomatoes), marine omega-3 fatty acids (in fish), soya products, and cruciferous vegetables (e.g., cauliflower, broccoli, Brussels sprouts), selenium, and vitamin D.

Infections: Sexually transmitted infections (e.g., trichomoniasis, chlamydia, and gonorrhea), and oxidative stress may initiate chronic inflammation of the prostate. Epithelial damage and accompanying inflammation are the common pathogenic link between environmental carcinogens and the development of prostate cancer.

Acquired Genetic and Epigenetic Abnormalities

Acquired genetic abnormalities are actual drivers of cellular transformation.

- ***TPRSS2-ETS* fusion gene:** It is the most common genetic change in a chromosomal rearrangement. In this rearrangement, the coding sequence of an ETS family transcription factor gene is placed next to the androgen-regulated promoter of the *TMPRSS2* gene. This leads to its overexpression of *TMPRSS2* in an androgen-dependent fashion. *TPRSS2-ETS* fusion gene is observed in 40–50% of prostate cancer and **occurs relatively early in tumorigenesis**.
- **Amplification of *MYC* and deletion of *PTEN*:** They increase cell growth and may contribute to resistance to antiandrogen therapy.

- **Loss of *TP53* (by deletion or mutation) and deletion of *RB,* amplifications of the androgen receptor gene:** These are common in late-stage prostate cancer.
- **Epigenetic events**: Epigenetic changes that modify gene expression are also common in prostate cancer.
  - **Epigenetic silencing of the *GSTP1* (glutathione-S transferase Pi 1) gene by DNA methylation:** GSTP1 is the product of this gene and is an antioxidant enzyme involved in the detoxification of xenobiotic compounds. Epigenetic silencing of the *GSTP1* gene by DNA methylation downregulates GSTP1 expression and probably enhances the genotoxic effects of environmental carcinogens.
  - **Epigenetic silencing of other genes:** Other genes are silenced by an epigenetic mechanism in a few prostate cancers. These include genes involved in cell cycle regulation (*RB, CDKN2A*), maintenance of genomic stability (*MLH1* and *MSH2*), and Wnt signaling (*APC*).

Precursor Lesions

Carcinoma prostate develops in a stepwise manner. It includes one of the presumed precursor lesions characterized by intraductal dysplastic epithelial proliferation termed PIN. PIN is a **proliferation of atypical epithelial cells in preexisting prostatic ducts and acini** (synonyms used in the past include atypical hyperplasia and dysplasia). It consists of architecturally benign prostatic acini or ducts lined by cytologically atypical luminal cells and a concomitant decrease in basal cells. Both PIN and prostate cancer usually predominate in the peripheral zone and are relatively uncommon in other zones of the prostate. PIN is graded as **low-grade PIN (LGPIN)** and **HGPIN**.

High-grade Prostatic Intraepithelial Neoplasia (HGPIN)

Q. Write a short answer on (high-grade) prostatic intraepithelial neoplasia.

High-grade PIN constitutes the preinvasive stage of the neoplastic proliferations of secretory cells lining the prostatic ducts and acini. HGPIN is a **precursor of invasive prostatic cancer**. HGPIN is mostly found in the peripheral zone of the prostate.

HGPIN consists of **benign prostatic acini** lined **by cytologically atypical cells with prominent nucleoli**. There is neoplastic proliferation of secretory cells within preexisting ducts and acini, with cytological changes resembling those seen in cancer, including enlargement of nuclei and numerous prominent nucleoli. The basal cell layer is often fragmented or lost.

The pathogenesis of prostate adenocarcinoma is complex. Multiple factors, including hereditary, environmental, hormonal, genetic, and epigenetic alterations, are involved in its pathogenesis. The salient genetic and epigenetic alterations during the development and progression of prostate cancer are illustrated (*refer* **online Fig. 21.15**).

MORPHOLOGY

Carcinomas detected clinically are usually not grossly visible. **More advanced cancers appear as firm, gray-white lesions with ill-defined margins that infiltrate the adjacent gland.**

Gross (Figs. 21.16A and B)

- **Localization:** Carcinoma of the prostate arises in the **peripheral zone of the gland** (70%), usually in a **posterior location**, (posterior/posterolateral peripheral zone). This makes it **palpable on rectal examination.** However, there is a relative increase in dominant anterior prostatic tumors (located in the anterior peripheral zone or transition zone).
- **Cut-section:** Tumor tissue is **gritty and firm.** When the tumor is embedded within the prostate, it may be more readily **appreciated on palpation than by visualization.**

Microscopy (Figs. 21.17A and B)

Most prostate cancers are **adenocarcinomas** and **consist of well-defined glandular patterns. Major criteria for the diagnosis of prostate cancer** are: **(i) architecture** (pattern of growth), **(ii) absence of basal cells**, and **(iii) nuclear atypia**. Perineural invasion is a specific finding, but in general, the diagnosis is made based on a combination of architectural, cytologic, and ancillary features.

Architectural Features

The finding of crowded small glands is suspicious but not diagnostic of carcinoma. A more specific feature is the presence of either a linear row of atypical glands or small atypical glands on both sides of a benign gland.

- **Neoplastic glands:** They are **usually smaller than benign glands— microacinar.** In contrast to benign glands, prostate cancer glands are **more crowded**, and **lack branching and papillary infolding.**
- **Single uniform layer of cuboidal or low columnar epithelial lining without the basal cell layer:** Glands are **lined by a single uniform layer of cuboidal or low columnar** cells. **The outer basal cell layer, which is seen in benign glands is absent** in cancer. This is **used as a criterion to distinguish benign and malignant prostate glands.**

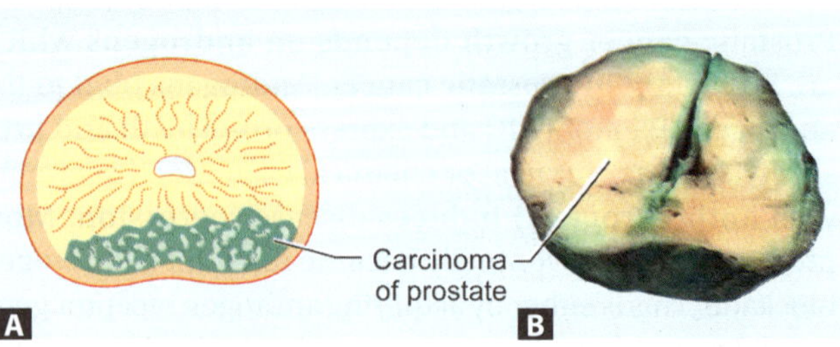

Figs. 21.16A and B: (A) Diagrammatic appearance of a cut section of prostate carcinoma shows a nodular, solid, irregular, gray-white tumor. (B) Cut section of the prostate with carcinoma. The green color is due to the dye used to paint the margins of the tumor.

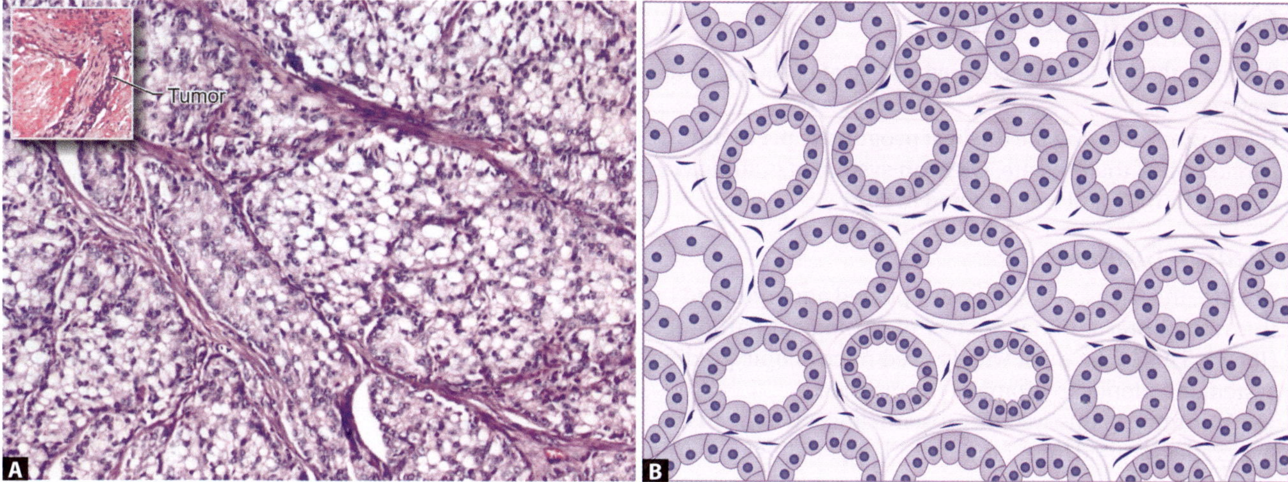

Figs. 21.17A and B: Microscopy of carcinoma of the prostate: (A) H& E and (B) diagrammatic. Prostate cancer consists of back-to-back uniform-sized malignant glands. Inset in A shows perineural invasion.

Tumor Cells

- **Cytoplasm** ranges from **pale-clear** (similar to benign glands) **to** a distinctive **amphophilic** (dark purple) **appearance** than the surrounding benign glands, which have pale to clear cytoplasm. An abundant cytoplasm with straight luminal borders in larger glands is also a helpful feature of carcinoma.
- **Nuclei** are **large** and **may contain** one or more large **nucleoli**. The presence of prominent nucleoli is an important cytological feature for the diagnosis of prostate adenocarcinoma. However, it should not be used as the sole criterion to establish the diagnosis. Mild variation in nuclear size and shape may be seen, but **pleomorphism is not marked**.

Intraluminal Contents

Prostatic crystalloids in the lumen are dense eosinophilic crystal-like structures and appear in various geometric shapes (such as rectangular, hexagonal, triangular, and rodlike structures) can also help in the diagnosis of prostatic adenocarcinoma. Crystalloids, although not diagnostic, are more common than in benign glands.

Mitotic figures are more common in high-grade prostate carcinoma.

As the grade increases, irregular or ragged glandular structures, cribriform glands, sheets of cells, or infiltrating individual cells are observed. In about 80% of cases, there are precursor lesions, called high-grade prostatic intraepithelial neoplasia (HGPIN) seen. Many of the molecular changes of invasive cancers are also found in HPIN.

Immunohistochemical Markers

The differentiation of benign from malignant prostate glands is that **benign glands have basal cells, whereas they are absent in glands in cancer.** This can be detected by using various immunohistochemical markers to label basal cells. One of the immunohistochemical markers namely, **α-methylacyl-coenzyme A-racemase (AMACR) is upregulated in prostate cancer.** Most of the prostate cancers are positive for AMACR.

Spread

Q. Write a short note on the spread of carcinoma of the prostate.

- **Local spread**: Various sites of local spread are as follows:
  - Invasion of prostatic **capsule.**
  - **Perineural tumor invasion** (*refer* **online Fig. 21.18**) both in the prostate and adjacent tissues.
  - Spreads into **periprostatic tissue (periprostatic fat), seminal vesicles, and** periurethral zones of the prostate. Locally advanced cancers may invade the adjacent soft tissues, the wall of the urinary bladder, or (less commonly) the rectum.
- **Lymphatic spread**: Three pathways of lymphatic spread are: (1) laterally to the iliac nodes, (2) inferiorly to the pudendal and iliac nodes, and (3) posteriorly to the presacral nodes.
  - First to the obturator nodes.
  - Later to the iliac and the para-aortic lymph nodes.
  - Metastases to the lung are due to lymphatic spread through the thoracic duct and through the prostatic venous plexus to the inferior vena cava.
- **Hematogenous spread**:
  - **Metastasis to axial skeleton:** Prostatic cancer mainly spreads to the **bones of the axial skeleton, but** is frequently late in the disease. The bony metastases are **osteoblastic** (bone-producing) in nature and strongly point towards prostatic cancer. It can be detected on *radionuclide bone scans.* Most other carcinoma bone metastases are osteolytic. The **bones involved, in descending order of frequency, are lumbar spine, proximal femur, pelvis, thoracic spine, and ribs.**
  - **Visceral metastasis**: Massive visceral dissemination is rare. Visceral metastasis most commonly to the lung, liver, and adrenal glands.

Grading of Prostatic Cancer

Q. Write a short note on grading and staging of carcinoma of the prostate.

Grading and staging are the **best prognostic predictors** of carcinoma of the prostate. **Gleason system** of grading was created in 1967 and was updated in 2014.

Gleason Grading

In 2014, the Gleason system was updated and modified by the WHO/International Society of Urological Pathology (ISUP). This is the most widely used microscopic grading system for adenocarcinoma of the prostate.

According to this system, prostate cancer is divided into five grades (graded from 1 to 5) based on glandular patterns of growth.

- **Gleason grade 1 and 2**: These are the most well-differentiated tumors and consist of uniform and round neoplastic glands that form well-circumscribed nodules. Gleason grades 1 and 2 are discontinued in the present new Gleason grade group system (see below).
- **Gleason grade 3:** It consists of single, separate, well-formed glands, small glands with pinpoint lumina, and medium-sized or large glands.
- **Gleason grade 4:** The main finding is the presence of coalescent or fused glands with >1 lumen and the absence of intervening stroma between adjacent glands. It consists of acinar structures and cribriform glands.
- **Gleason grade 5**: These tumors do not form glands and infiltrate the stroma in cords, sheets, and solid nests. It shows comedonecrosis.

More than one pattern in most tumors: Most tumors contain more than one pattern. In these tumors, a **primary grade** is assigned to the dominant pattern (predominant tumor pattern), and a **secondary grade** is assigned to the second-most frequent (prevalent) pattern. If a tumor has only one histological pattern, then, both the primary and secondary patterns are given the same grade.

Gleason Score or Sum

- In the biopsy, the **most common and highest-grade patterns on a given core are added.** The **combined Gleason grades** are called as Gleason score or sum. It is obtained by adding the two numbers of primary and secondary patterns. Gleason score in a pathology report as a mathematical equation (e.g., "Gleason score: 3 + 3 = 6").
- Many potentially treatable prostatic cancers are detected on needle biopsy because of screening and have Gleason scores of 6 or 7. Tumors with Gleason scores of 8 through 10 tend to be advanced cancers and are less likely to be cured.

New Gleason Grade Group System

In the new Gleason system, it was recommended to **discontinue Gleason grades 1 and 2 of prostate cancer and thereby Gleason score of 2–5 for prostate cancer in a needle biopsy.** This is because they do not predict better prostatectomy findings than grade 3 and these grades show marked interobserver variability. Presently, Gleason scores are combined into **five Grade Groups (Table 21.5).** Each has a different prognosis. Five Gleason score ranges from 6 (3 + 3) to 10 (5 + 5).

TABLE 21.5 The new Gleason grade group system with the histological definitions.

Gleason grade group	*Gleason score (Gleason pattern)*	*Histological definitions*
1	≤6 (≤3 + 3)	Cancers are composed only of individual discrete well-formed glands
2*	7 (3 + 4)	Cancers are composed predominantly of discrete and well-formed glands with lesser components of poorly formed/fused/cribriform glands
3*	7 (4 + 3)	Cancers with predominantly poorly formed/fused/cribriform glands with lesser components of well-formed glands
4	8 (4 + 4)	Cancers composed only of poorly formed/fused/glomeruloid/cribriform glands
	8 (3 + 5)	Tumors with discrete and well-formed glands and lesser components lacking glands (or with necrosis)
	8 (5 + 3)	Tumors predominantly lack glands (or with necrosis) and a lesser component of discrete, well-formed glands
5	9 –10 (4 + 5 or 5 + 4 or 5 + 5)	Cancers without gland/luminal formation or with necrosis, with or without poorly formed/fused/glomeruloid/cribriform glands

*Exact quantification of Gleason grade 4 tumor is necessary because of its independent prognostic implication (NCCN Guidelines Version 4.2022 Prostate Cancer). (GX, the grade cannot be assessed).

Significance: The Gleason score is a powerful predictor of the clinical behavior of prostate cancer.

WHO grading: A new grading system also based on glandular pattern was recently accepted by the World Health Organization (WHO). It was used initially in conjunction with the Gleason system. It ranges from 1 (excellent prognosis) to 5 (poor prognosis).

Staging of Prostatic Cancer

TNM system is used for staging. Staging is not only important for **predicting prognosis** but also important in the selection of the **appropriate form of therapy**.

Clinical Course

- **In the early stages**, it is **asymptomatic**. They are usually discovered during rectal examination or elevated serum PSA levels.
- **Advanced** prostatic cancer **may present** with **urinary symptoms**, like dysuria, frequency, or hematuria.
- **Vertebral metastases may present** as **back pain** and have fatal outcomes. **Detection of osteoblastic metastases by skeletal surveys or by radionuclide bone scanning is virtually diagnostic** of prostatic cancer.

Digital rectal examination, transrectal ultrasonography, and other imaging modalities (MRI) have both low sensitivity and specificity. MRI in patients with elevated PSA levels can help identify nonpalpable cancers.

Methods of tissue diagnosis: These include: fine-needle aspiration cytology (FNAC), needle core biopsy, transurethral resection, open (simple) prostatectomy/enucleation, and radical prostatectomy.

Tumor Markers

Prostate-specific antigen (PSA)

Q. Write a short note on prostate-specific antigen.

- PSA is the most **important tumor marker used for diagnosis and management**. Great value in assessing the response to therapy and detecting recurrence.
- **PSA is a serine protease produced by prostatic epithelium cells and normally secreted in the semen. Only minute amounts of PSA circulate in the serum** (a serum level of 4 ng/mL is the cutoff point between normal and abnormal). Serum PSA levels correlate strongly with the risk of prostate cancer.
- **Raised blood PSA levels: It occurs with localized as well as advanced prostatic cancer**. However, the PSA value may be normal or less. PSA measurement as a screening test for prostate cancer has suboptimal sensitivity and specificity. This is because PSA levels may be elevated in a variety of benign conditions **(Box 21.7)**.
- PSA is **organ-specific**, but **not cancer-specific**. PSA has limitations because it is commonly elevated in benign prostatic hyperplasia, prostatitis, and with mechanical manipulation of the prostate gland.
- **Useful for assessing the response to treatment and follow-up**: PSA assays are of **uncertain value as screening tests.** But, once prostate cancer is diagnosed, serial measurements of PSA are very useful in assessing the response to therapy. For example, an elevated PSA level after radical prostatectomy or radiotherapy for localized cancer indicates recurrence or dissemination of cancer.

BOX 21.7: Causes of raised PSA.

- Carcinoma prostate
- Benign hyperplasia of prostate
- Prostatitis
- Infarct of prostate
- Following instrumentation of the prostate
- Ejaculation

Prostate-specific Antigen Derivatives

- **PSA density**: It is the **ratio between the serum PSA value and the volume of the prostate gland.**
- **PSA velocity**: It is the **rate of change in PSA value with time**. A PSA velocity of 0.75 ng/mL/year best distinguishes between cancer and benign lesions of the prostate.
- **Age-specific reference ranges.**
- **Ratio of free and bound PSA in the serum.**

Prostatic Acid Phosphatase (PAP)

- It is secreted by prostatic epithelium. Its activity is 1,000-fold greater in the prostate than in any other tissue.
- It is elevated when the prostatic cancer has spread beyond the prostate or metastasized.
- Not prostate-specific and is increased in renal, liver, and bone malignancies.

Serum alkaline phosphatase levels: They are elevated in patients with osteoblastic bony metastases. This enzyme is released from osteoblasts forming new bone at a site of metastasis.

Urine Markers

PCA is a noncoding RNA that is overexpressed in 95% of prostate cancers. **Quantification of urine PCA3A** is also used as a diagnostic additional biomarker in patients suspected to have prostate cancer (because of raised PSA, but without cancer on prostate biopsy). The combination of urinary PCA3 with a screening of urine for TMPRSS2-ERG fusion DNA improves prostate cancer diagnosis.

Treatment: Prostate cancer can be treated with surgery or radiation, with or without hormonal therapy. With such therapy, more than 90% can live for 15 years. The growth and survival of prostate cancer cells depend on androgens. Therefore, androgen deprivation is a key therapeutic component in cancer of prostate. It is usually by administration of synthetic agonists of lutoinizing hormone-releasing hormone (LHRH). This regulates LH production, which is needed for the production of testosterone. Antiandrogen therapy induces remissions, but androgen-independent clones emerge and can lead to progression of disease and death.

Prognosis: Following radical prostatectomy, prognosis is based on the pathologic stage, margin status, and Gleason grade.

MALE INFERTILITY

Q. Write a short note on the causes of male infertility.

The causes of male infertility are listed in **Box 21.8**.

Investigations: These should be performed to determine the cause/precise nature. These include a testicular biopsy

BOX 21.8: Causes of male infertility.

- **Endocrine disorders:** Gonadotropin deficiency, estrogen excess (e.g., cirrhosis of the liver)
- **Testicular causes:** Cryptorchidism, Klinefelter's syndrome, maturation arrest of spermatogenesis (idiopathic), varicocele, irradiation, defective spermatozoa (e.g., immotile cilia)
- **Post-testicular causes:** Blockage of efferent ducts due to congenital cause or secondary to an inflammatory process, impotence (e.g., neurological disorders)

to assess the integrity of the seminiferous tubules and the degree of spermatogenesis, hormonal assessment, and other relevant investigations.

SCENARIO-BASED MCQs

1. **A 30-year-old man complains of a vague feeling of painless heaviness in the right scrotum for the past 5 months. On examination, the right testis is slightly larger than the left testis. A testicular mass is found and cannot be transilluminated. An ultrasound examination shows a solid, circumscribed, homogeneous, 1.4 cm mass in the body of the right testis. Serologic testing did not show any tumor markers. Cytogenetic analysis shows an additional fragment of chromosome 12 (isochromosome p12). An orchiectomy is performed. Microscopic examination of the mass shows uniform nests of cells with distinct cell borders, glycogen-rich cytoplasm, and round nuclei with prominent nucleoli. The stroma shows aggregates of lymphocytes. The most likely diagnosis is:**
   A. Seminoma B. Lymphoma
   C. Choriocarcinoma D. Embryonal carcinoma
2. **A 9-year-old boy is brought to the pediatric outpatient department because his parents noticed a mass on his left testicle. Physical examination shows a solid mass that cannot be transilluminated. A biopsy is performed and shows a haphazard arrangement of benign differentiated tissues. These include squamous epithelium, glandular epithelium, cartilage, smooth muscle cells, fat tissue, and neural tissue. This tissue shows the organoid arrangement. No cytologic atypia is noted. The testis surrounding the tumor did not show any germ cell neoplasia in situ (GCNIS). Following this, the left testicle was removed surgically, and the child is symptom-free 5 years later. The most probable diagnosis is:**
   A. Seminoma B. Yolk sac tumor
   C. Prepubertal teratoma D. Embryonal carcinoma
3. **A 62-year-old man presents with an irregular fungating mass on his penis that he has had for 5 months. Physical examination shows an irregular gray-white mass with indurated margins on the glans and foreskin. Biopsy of the lesion shows pleomorphic epithelial cells with hyperchromatic nuclei, connected by intercellular bridges, and invasion into the dermis. The probable histologic diagnosis for this patient's penile lesion is:**
   A. Melanoma B. Adenocarcinoma
   C. Urothelial cell carcinoma D. Squamous cell carcinoma
4. **A 72-year-old man presents dysuria, urinary frequency and hesitancy, and hematuria of 5 days duration. For the past few years, he has had repeated attacks of acute cystitis. Urine cultures are positive for *E. coli*. Ultrasound examination shows bladder diverticulum. The conditions most likely contributed to the formation of a bladder diverticulum in this patient, are:**
   A. Nephrolithiasis
   B. Diabetes mellitus
   C. Nodular prostatic hyperplasia
   D. Urothelial cell carcinoma of the bladder
5. **A 71-year-old, a previously healthy man, comes to the hospital for a routine health checkup. Rectal examination shows a nodule in his normal-sized prostate. Laboratory studies show a serum prostate-specific antigen (PSA) level of 17 ng/mL. No abnormalities were detected on routine urinalysis. The microscopic findings that are most likely to be seen in a subsequent biopsy specimen of his prostate are:**
   A. Adenocarcinoma B. Acute prostatitis
   C. Nodular hyperplasia D. Chronic abacterial prostatitis

Answers and Explanation

1. **The answer is A: Seminoma.** It is the most common testicular cancer and accounts for 40% of all germ cell tumors in that testis. The peak incidence is in men between 30 and 40 years of age. The age, non-transilluminated mass, detection of solid and homogeneous appearance on ultrasound examination, cytogenetic abnormality of an additional fragment of chromosome 12 (isochromosome p12), and the microscopic features favor seminoma. The other choices are less common than seminoma. Moreover, choriocarcinoma (choice A) releases tumor markers namely human chorionic gonadotropin (hCG) that can be identified in blood.
2. **The answer is C: Prepubertal teratoma.** Teratomas are the most common testicular tumor in the age-group between 4 and 12 years. The prepubertal age, tissue showing organoid arrangement without cytologic atypia, and surrounding testis without any germ cell neoplasia in situ (GCNIS) favor prepubertal teratoma. The mature somatic tissues represent the three embryonic germ layers (ectoderm, mesoderm, and endoderm). The other choices are malignant tumors. The clinical and histopathological findings along with symptom-free 5 years later are against these tumors.
3. **The answer is D: Squamous cell carcinoma.** The clinical finding of an irregular fungating mass with an indurated margin on the glans and foreskin in a 62-year-old male suggests a malignant tumor. Microscopic findings of pleomorphic epithelial cells with hyperchromatic nuclei, connected by intercellular bridges, and invasion into the dermis suggest penile squamous carcinomas. The other choices do not show either intracellular bridges or these characteristic physical signs.
4. **The answer is C: Nodular prostatic hyperplasia.** The age, and clinical features point towards nodular hyperplasia of the prostate. It is a common condition characterized by enlargement of the gland. The clinical symptoms result from compression of the prostatic urethra and the consequent obstruction to the flow of urine through the bladder outlet. Urinary obstruction leads to hypertrophy of the bladder wall. Diverticula which are solitary or multiple saclike outpouchings of the bladder wall may develop as a complication. Urine retained inside a diverticulum is often infected. The other choices do not produce structural changes in the bladder wall.
5. **The answer is A: Adenocarcinoma.** In this patient, the prostate-specific antigen (PSA) level is significantly elevated and most likely indicates prostatic adenocarcinoma. Many prostatic adenocarcinomas do not produce obstructive symptoms and may not be palpable on digital rectal examination. Inflammation (prostatitis) and nodular hyperplasias can increase the PSA level. However, the PSA levels are usually not very high.

CHAPTER 22

Female Genital Tract Disorders

CHAPTER OUTLINE

Cervix
- Normal Structure
- Inflammations of the Cervix
- Premalignant and Malignant Neoplasms of the Cervix

Uterus
- Menstrual Cycle
- Endometriosis
- Endometrial Hyperplasia
- Endometrial Carcinoma
- Uterine Leiomyomas
- Uterine Leiomyosarcoma

Ovaries
- Ovarian Tumors
- Epithelial Tumors
- Germ Cell Tumors
- Sex Cord-stromal Tumors
- Metastatic (Secondary) Tumors

Gestational Disorders
- Gestational Trophoblastic Disease

CERVIX

NORMAL STRUCTURE

The uterine cervix consists of the **ectocervix** which is the part exposed to the vagina and visible on vaginal examination. Ectocervix is lined by mature stratified squamous epithelium and is continuous with the squamous lining of the vaginal wall. In the center of the ectocervix, there is a small opening termed the **external os** that leads to the endocervical canal (or simply termed endocervix). The endocervix is lined by columnar, mucus-secreting epithelium. The endocervical mucosa has clefts and tunnels, commonly referred to as cervical glands and they secrete mucus. The junction of the ectocervix and endocervical canal is a point where the squamous epithelium of the ectocervix meets the columnar epithelium of the endocervix and is referred to as the **squamocolumnar junction.** In this region, there is a gradual transition between squamous and columnar epithelia. The position of this squamocolumnar junction is variable and changes with age and hormonal influence. Usually, this junction moves upwards into the endocervical canal with time. The columnar/glandular epithelium of the endocervix can be replaced by advancing squamous epithelium and this process is called **squamous metaplasia.** The area of the cervix where the columnar epithelium of the endocervix abuts the squamous epithelium of the ectocervix is termed the "*transformation zone*" and is significant both clinically and pathologically. It is highly susceptible to infections with human papillomavirus (HPV) which is one of the important etiological agents involved in cancer of the cervix. Immature squamous metaplastic epithelial cells in this transformation zone are most susceptible to infection by HPV and are the site where cervical precursor lesions and cancers can develop.

The most common lesions of the cervix are cervicitis, certain benign tumors, dysplasia, carcinoma in situ, and invasive carcinoma.

INFLAMMATIONS OF THE CERVIX

PA 30.6 (NC): Describe the etiology and morphologic features of cervicitis.

Inflammation of the cervix is termed as cervicitis and is an extremely common condition of the cervix. It is because of its constant exposure to bacterial flora in the vagina.

- **Glycogen in squamous cells favors the growth of organisms:** At the onset of menarche, the estrogens are secreted by the ovary. They stimulate maturation of the cervical and vaginal squamous mucosa and intracellular glycogen vacuoles are formed in the squamous cells. As these squamous cells are shed, the **glycogen** present *in* these **squamous cells provides a substrate for various endogenous vaginal aerobes and anaerobes**.
- **Lactobacilli produce acid pH and suppress the growth of organisms**: One of the **dominant microbial species**

in the normal vagina is **lactobacilli.** These lactobacilli produce lactic acid, which in turn, helps to maintain the vaginal pH below 4.5. This acidic/low pH suppresses the growth of other saprophytic and pathogenic organisms. Also, at this low pH, lactobacilli produce bacteriotoxic hydrogen peroxide (H_2O_2). If the pH becomes alkaline (e.g., due to bleeding, sexual intercourse, antibiotic therapy, or vaginal douching), there will be decreased production of H_2O_2 by lactobacilli. This, in turn, promotes the overgrowth of other microorganisms and can result in cervicitis or vaginitis.

- Some degree of inflammation is observed in the cervix of almost all multiparous women and some nulliparous women and is usually of little clinical significance. The normal intact ectocervical stratified epithelium is usually resistant to infection compared to the endocervical columnar epithelium.

Classification

Cervicitis can be subclassified in different ways.

- Infectious or noninfectious
- **Depending on the cause:** It may be a specific or nonspecific infection.
  - **Specific cervicitis**: These are caused by gonococci, *mycoplasmas, mycobacterium tuberculosis*, syphilis, granuloma inguinale, lymphogranuloma venereum, *chlamydia,* and chancroid.
  - **Nonspecific cervicitis**: It is more frequent and is generally divided into acute and chronic forms, the latter being quite common.
- **Depending on the onset:** It may be acute or chronic.
  - **Acute cervicitis** is usually associated with puerperal infection or gonococcal infection. Other causes include primary chancre and infection with herpes simplex.
  - **Chronic cervicitis**: Chronic nonspecific cervicitis is quite common and is the common cause of leukorrhea.
    - **Caused by organisms present in the vaginal flora**: Chronic nonspecific cervicitis is mostly caused by organisms present in the normal vaginal flora. These include streptococci, enterococci (e.g., *E. coli*), and staphylococci. Other organisms include gonococci, *Trichomonas vaginalis, Candida albicans,* and herpes simplex.
    - **Predisposing factors**: These include sexual intercourse, trauma of childbirth, instrumentation, and excess or deficiency of estrogen.
    - **Microscopy:** It shows a subepithelial inflammatory infiltrate composed of lymphocytes, plasma cells, large mononuclear cells, and a few neutrophils. In some, lymphoid follicles may be formed (*follicular cervicitis*). The surface epithelium may be either normal or may show squamous metaplasia.

PREMALIGNANT AND MALIGNANT NEOPLASMS OF THE CERVIX

PA 30.1 (CC): Describe the epidemiology, pathogenesis, etiology, pathology, screening, diagnosis, and progression of carcinoma of the cervix.

Carcinoma of the cervix is the fourth most common cancer in women. It can be detected in low stage and is a highly curable cancer. Remarkable benefits of effective screening, early diagnosis, and curative therapy are observed in carcinoma of the cervix. Most credit for these dramatic gains is because the cervix is accessible to Pap testing in detecting cervical precursor lesions and visual examination by colposcopy. Some of the precursor lesions (CIN or SIL) would have progressed to invasive carcinoma in the cervix if not treated. CIN usually slowly progresses to carcinoma, typically over decades. All these features and the introduction and widespread use of cytologic screening, detection, and preventive treatment have decreased the incidence of cervical carcinoma. The World Health Organization (WHO) (2020) (abridged) classification of the uterine cervix is presented in **Box 22.1**.

Etiology and Pathogenesis of Squamous Cell Tumors and Precursors

Q. Write a short essay on the etiology and pathogenesis of cervical cancer.

Epidemiologic, etiologic, and pathogenetic features of squamous intraepithelial lesion (SIL) and invasive cancer are similar and are discussed together.

Risk Factors

Common risk factors for SIL and carcinoma of the cervix include (1) human papillomavirus (HPV) and (2) environmental factors.

Human Papillomavirus Infection

Q. Discuss the role of HPV in carcinoma cervix.

HPV is **essentially a sexually transmitted DNA virus** belonging to the papovavirus family. The following features are associated with increased exposure to HPV and increased incidence of both SIL and cervical cancer. These features point out that HPV is a major risk factor. **Increased incidence of SIL and carcinoma cervix** is observed in women with:

- Multiple sexual partners
- Early age at first intercourse (coitus)
- High parity
- A male partner having multiple previous or current sexual partners
- Persistent infection with a high oncogenic risk HPV, e.g., HPV 16 or HPV 18

BOX 22.1: World Health Organization (WHO) (2020) (abridged) classification of the tumors of the uterine cervix.

Squamous epithelial tumors:
- Squamous cell tumors and precursors:
  - Squamous intraepithelial lesions of the uterine cervix
  - Squamous cell carcinoma, HPV-associated, of the uterine cervix
  - Squamous cell carcinoma, HPV-independent, of the uterine cervix
  - Squamous cell carcinoma NOS of the uterine cervix

Glandular tumors and precursors:
- Benign glandular lesions:
  - Endocervical polyp
  - Nabothian cyst
- Adenocarcinomas:
  - Adenocarcinoma in situ, HPV-associated, of the uterine cervix
  - Adenocarcinoma, HPV-associated, of the uterine cervix
  - Adenocarcinoma in situ, HPV-independent, of the uterine cervix
  - Adenocarcinoma, HPV-independent, gastric type, of the uterine cervix
  - Adenocarcinoma, HPV-independent, clear cell type, of the uterine cervix
  - Adenocarcinoma, HPV-independent, mesonephric type, of the uterine cervix
  - Other adenocarcinomas, of the uterine cervix

Other epithelial tumors:
- Carcinosarcoma of the uterine cervix

Mixed epithelial and mesenchymal tumors:
- Adenomyoma of the uterine cervix
- Adenosarcoma of the uterine cervix

Germ cell tumors of the uterine cervix

(HPV: human papillomavirus; NOS: not otherwise specified)

- **Inefficient immune response:** Most HPV infections are transient and are eliminated by the immune response, and immunosuppression may result in persistent HPV infection.

Classification of human papillomavirus

Based on the genotypes human papillomaviruses are classified into those of low and high oncogenic risk.

Low oncogenic risk: It causes sexually transmitted **condyloma acuminatum** in the vulva, perineal, and perianal regions. The **HPV genome is maintained in a nonintegrated free episomal** (extrachromosomal) **form. Virus freely replicates and causes the death of the host cell,** and it is known as a **productive infection.**

High oncogenic risk: Currently, 15 types of high oncogenic risk HPVs (high-risk HPVs) have been identified.

- **Most common HPV 16 and HPV 18:** Among 15 types, HPV 16 alone accounts for almost 60% of cases, and HPV 18 accounts for another 10% of cases of cervical cancer. Others include HPV 31 and 33.
- **Squamous cell carcinomas in other sites:** High oncogenic risk HPV can also cause squamous cell carcinoma at many other sites. These include the **vagina, vulva, penis, anus, tonsil, and oropharynx.**
- **Integration into the host DNA:** In cancers, the HPV genome (viral DNA) is integrated into the genome of the host cell, which is important for malignant transformation. **Integration causes overexpression of the oncoproteins E6 and E7 and genomic instability** in the host cell.

Environmental Factors

Only HPV infection is not sufficient for carcinogenesis, and it acts in association with environmental factors. The environmental factors include:

- **Presence of cocarcinogens:** A co-carcinogen is a chemical that promotes the effects of a carcinogen in the production of cancer. Cigarette smoke, which contains polycyclic hydrocarbons, acts as a cocarcinogen. Smoking increases the incidence of cancer of the cervix, but the exact mechanism is not known.
- **Coexisting microbial infections**
- **Dietary deficiencies**
- **Hormonal changes**
- **Use of oral contraceptives**

Pathogenesis

The **most important factor** in the development of cervical cancer is **high-risk HPV**. Most genital HPV infections are asymptomatic and do not produce any changes in tissue.

Features of Infection by Human Papillomavirus

Even though HPV is a causative factor for CIN and cancer of the cervix, only a few infected individuals will develop cancer. **Most HPV infections in women are transient**. These infections are cleared by immunological mechanisms.

Higher risk with longer duration of HPV infection: The longer the duration of infection (persistent) with high-risk HPVs, the higher the risk of cervical precursor lesions (SIL) and subsequent carcinoma. Infections with high oncogenic risk HPVs last longer, and take longer time to clear than infections with low oncogenic risk HPVs.

Cells and sites infected by human papillomavirus: Human papillomavirus **does not infect mature intact superficial squamous cells**. For productive and persistent HPV infection, the **virus should enter immature basal epithelial cells of the squamous epithelium.** Hence, surfaces covered with mature, intact squamous epithelium (e.g., ectocervix, vagina, vulva, penis, and oropharynx) are **generally resistant** to HPV infection. In areas of epithelial breaks or damage, the HPV can reach the immature cells in the basal layer of the epithelium.

Cells infected by HPV in the cervix: In the female genital tract, the sites susceptible to HPV infection include **areas of trauma and repair of squamous epithelium**. In such damaged sites, the virus may **reach basal cells**.

HPV-susceptible cell type is a **stem cell located in the region of the cervical transformation zone.** HPV may also infect the **immature metaplastic squamous cells present at the squamocolumnar junction** of the cervix. Thus, the cervix having relatively large areas of immature squamous metaplastic epithelium is particularly susceptible to HPV infection.

Replication of HPV *in* the maturing nonproliferating squamous cells: Human papillomavirus infects immature squamous cells. However, replication of HPV occurs in the maturing, nonproliferating squamous cells. Normally, these more **mature squamous cells are arrested in the G_1 phase of the cell cycle.** However, when these mature cells are infected with HPV, the infection prevents the growth arrest (arrest at the G1 phase) of these cells. These mature cells continue to actively progress through the cell cycle by using the host cell DNA synthesis machinery to replicate its own genome. This effect is necessary for the replication of the viral genome and the productive shedding of the virus.

Carcinogenicity of human papillomavirus

Integration of HPV genome into the host genome: Human papillomavirus infection induces SIL and cervical cancer. This requires the integration of the HPV genome (viral DNA) into the genome of the host cell. This is important for malignant transformation. Integration causes **overexpression of the oncoproteins E6 and E7.** The ability of high-risk HPV to act as a carcinogen depends on these **viral E6 and E7 proteins.** These proteins **are prooncogenic.** (*refer* page 258 and **Fig. 7.25**).

Actions of the E7 protein of HPV: Viral E7 protein **binds the hypophosphorylated (active) form of RB** and **promotes the degradation of RB. E7 also binds and inhibits two important cyclin-dependent kinase inhibitors** (p21, and p27). Removal of these controls not only increases the progression of the cell cycle but also impairs the capability of cells to repair DNA damage.

Actions of the E6 protein of HPV: Viral E6 protein **interferes with the activity of the tumor-suppressor protein p53. E6 binds p53 and promotes its degradation.** The DNA repair defect in infected cells caused by E7 is exacerbated by E6 proteins. **E6 also upregulates the expression of telomerase,** which leads to cellular immortalization.

The net effect of high-risk HPV infection is increased proliferation of cells **(Fig. 22.1).** These cells are prone to acquire additional mutations that may lead to the development of cancer. The physical state of the virus is another factor that contributes to malignant transformation by HPV.

Integration of viral DNA into host DNA: In most cancers (also HSIL), the viral DNA of HPV is integrated into the genome of the host cell. This integration has two main effects: (1) **increases the expression of two early (E) genes, namely E6 and E7 genes,** (2) may **also dysregulate oncogenes** (e.g., *MYC*) near the sites of viral insertion, and (3) integration is associated with increased genomic

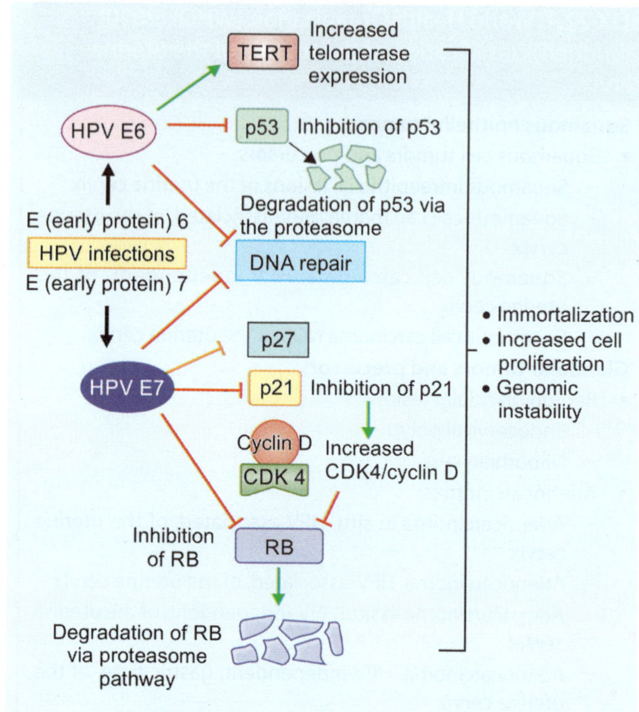

Fig. 22.1: Oncogenic effects of human papillomavirus *(HPV)* E6 and E7 proteins. E6 and E7 proteins of HPV immortalize cells and lead to increased cell proliferation.

(TERT: telomerase reverse transcriptase)

instability. This instability may lead to the acquisition of additional prooncogenic mutations.

Extrachromosomal (episomal) form of viral DNA: By contrast, it is observed that in precursor lesions associated with high-risk HPVs and condylomata associated with low-risk HPVs, the viral DNA is extrachromosomal (episomal). The consequences of HPV infection in the cervix are shown in **Figure 22.2.**

Low-risk HPVs: In infection by low-risk HPVs, their E7 proteins bind with lower affinity to RB, and E6 proteins fail to bind p53 altogether. In low-grade squamous intraepithelial lesion (LSIL) (*refer* below on page 803), HPV is an episomal form and replicates freely to cause cell death. Genital warts (condylomata acuminata) of the cervix often contain low-risk HPV types 6 or 11.

Other factors: Human papillomavirus is the major cause of cervical cancer. However, only a few women infected by HPV develop cancer. Thus, other factors such as exposure to cocarcinogens (e.g., cigarette smoking) and host immune status may be involved.

Squamous Intraepithelial Lesion (SIL) and Cervical Intraepithelial Neoplasia (CIN)

Q. Define and write a short note on cervical intraepithelial neoplasia (CIN)/squamous intraepithelial lesion.

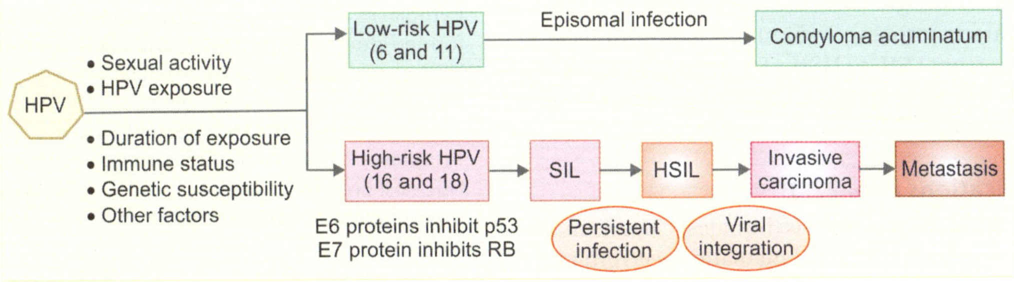

Fig. 22.2: Consequences of HPV infection in the cervix.
(LSIL: low-grade squamous intraepithelial lesion; HSIL: high-grade squamous intraepithelial lesion).

Definition: Squamous intraepithelial lesions (SILs) of the uterine cervix, **also known as cervical intraepithelial neoplasia (CIN),** are **proliferations of squamous cells driven by HPV infection.** These are **precancerous lesions** that show **maturation abnormalities and/or viral cytopathic change.** These abnormal changes **do not extend beyond the basement membrane.**

Squamous intraepithelial lesions may progress to cancer: HPV-related carcinogenesis begins with the precancerous epithelial change. These are termed as squamous intraepithelial lesions (**SILs).** These lesions **usually precede the development of an apparent cancer by many years, sometimes decades.** The peak incidence of SIL is at about 30 years of age, whereas invasive carcinoma peaks at about 45 years of age.

Classification of Cervical Precancer Lesions (Fig. 22.3)

Q. Write a short note on the classification of cervical intraepithelial neoplasia.

The categorization of cervical precursor lesions has undergone an evolution over time. Terminologies, namely CIN, dysplasia, carcinoma in situ (CIS), and squamous intraepithelial lesion (SIL) are commonly used interchangeably. The classification presently being used is **Bethesda system squamous intraepithelial lesion.**

Squamous Intraepithelial Lesion

The **Bethesda System** for Reporting Cervical/Vaginal Cytologic Diagnoses groups these cervical precursor lesions into a two-tier system: (1) **low-grade squamous intraepithelial lesions (LSIL), and (2) high-grade squamous intraepithelial lesions (HSIL).** Clinical management is based mainly on this two-tier system that reflects the biology of the disease.

Low-grade squamous intraepithelial lesion (LSIL): LSIL **corresponds to CIN I** (*refer* below) and is far **more common than HSIL.**

- **Most LSILs regress** spontaneously, but few may progress to HSIL.
- Associated with a **high level of viral replication.** It shows only mild alterations in the growth of the host cells.
- LSIL is **not considered a premalignant lesion.**

High-grade squamous intraepithelial lesion (HSIL): HSIL includes CIN II and III (see below).

- HSIL is associated with **increased proliferation, arrest of epithelial maturation, and lower levels of viral replication.**
- HSIL has a **high risk for progression to carcinoma** if not treated. Hence, it is a precancerous lesion. But, in most patients, it does not progress to cancer, and some cases even regress.

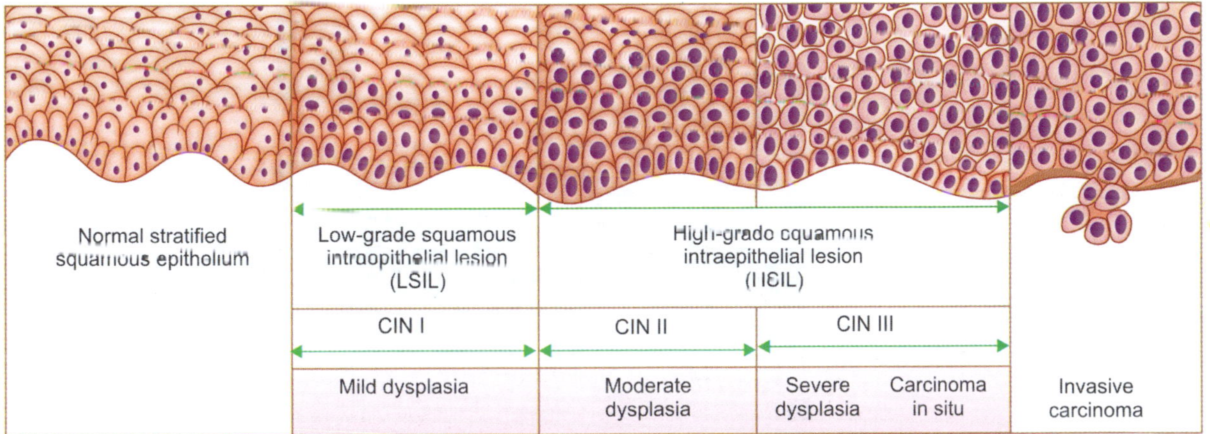

Fig. 22.3: Spectrum of cervical intraepithelial neoplasia with normal stratified squamous epithelium for comparison. LSIL (CIN I/mild dysplasia); HSIL (CIN II and CIN III/severe dysplasia and carcinoma in situ).

- **Risk factors for progression of HSIL to cancer**: These include cigarette smoking and immunocompromise.
- **Progression from LSIL to HSIL**: The majority of HSILs develop from LSILs. In about 20% of cases of HSIL develop de novo, without any pre-existing LSIL.

Other Classifications (Fig. 22.3)

Carcinoma in situ (CIS) system: It is the oldest classification in which **mild dysplasia** is on one end of the spectrum and severe **dysplasia/carcinoma in situ** on the other end.

Cervical intraepithelial neoplasia (CIN) classification: According to this, mild dysplasia is termed **CIN I**, moderate dysplasia **CIN II**, and severe dysplasia is termed **CIN III**.

MORPHOLOGY

Q. Write a short note on the morphology of squamous intraepithelial lesion (carcinoma in situ).

Squamous Intraepithelial Lesion (SIL)

The spectrum of morphologic changes in squamous intraepithelial lesions ranges from **normal, low-grade to high-grade** (*refer* **Fig. 22.3**).

Diagnosis of SIL: It is **based on the identification of atypical immature squamous cells** that have the following features:

Pleomorphism: It shows **variation in cell and nuclear size.**

Nuclear atypia: The characteristics of nuclear atypia are:
- **Nuclear enlargement.**
- **Pleomorphic nuclei: Variation of nuclear sizes and shapes.**
- **Hyperchromasia: Characterized by dark staining of nuclei.**
- **Heterogeneity of chromatin with coarse chromatin granules.**

Presence of mitoses, some atypical, **above the basal layer.**

Nuclear cytoplasmic ratio: Increased.

Loss of polarity.

Cytoplasmic change: The nuclear atypia mentioned above may be accompanied by a perinuclear cytoplasmic halo, which is termed **koilocytic atypia (Figs. 22.4A to C).** The **koilocyte** (from the Greek *koilos*, hollow) is **a superficial or intermediate mature squamous cell** characterized by:
- **Cytoplasm**: Sharply outlined **perinuclear halo (vacuolation)** formed **due to extensive cytoplasmic destruction** by an HPV-encoded protein E5 smallest transforming protein encoded by the human papillomaviruses that is localized to the membranes of the endoplasmic reticulum. **The peripheral cytoplasm** is **dense and shows irregular staining.**
- **Nucleus: Enlarged, wrinkled** with an **undulating** (raisin- or prune-like) **nuclear membrane** and **rope-like chromatin** pattern.

Koilocytes are absent in many cases of high-grade dysplasia and all invasive cancers.

Grading of SIL

The squamous intraepithelial lesion is graded as LSIL (low) and HSIL (high grade) based on the expansion of the immature cell layer from its normal basal location.
- **LSIL (Figs. 22.4A to C):** If the **atypical, immature squamous cells (dysplastic changes)** are **confined to the lower one-third of the epithelium**, the lesion is graded as LSIL. The **koilocytotic changes** are observed in **the superficial layers of the epithelium.**
- **HSIL [Fig. 22.5A** (*refer* **online Figs. 22.5B and C)]:** If the **atypical, immature squamous cells extend beyond the lower one-third of the epithelial thickness,** the lesion is graded as HSIL. **It may involve lower two-thirds to full-thickness of epithelium.** When the full thickness is involved, usually there is greater variation in cell and nuclear size, chromatin heterogeneity, disorderly orientation of the cells, and abnormal mitoses. Koilocytic change is usually absent.

These histologic features correlate with the cytologic appearances **[Figs. 22.6A and B** (*refer* **online Figs. 22.6C and D)].**

Markers of actively dividing cells are presented online.

Clinical Features

Squamous intraepithelial lesion (SIL is asymptomatic and usually detected through an abnormal Pap test result). SILs are followed up by colposcopy, in which acetic acid identifies lesions for biopsy. Colposcopic examination shows white epithelium and a mosaic pattern in the

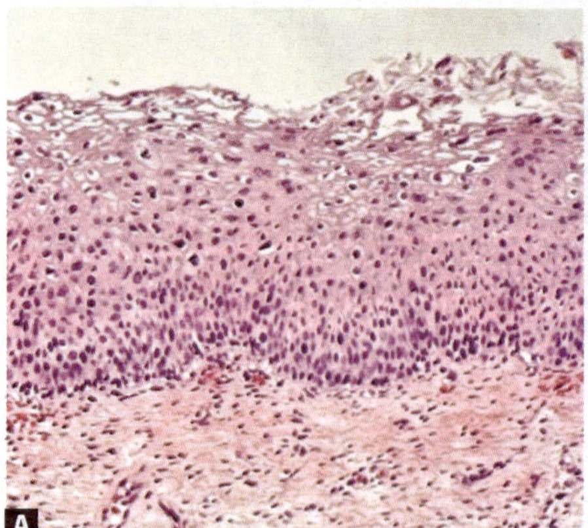

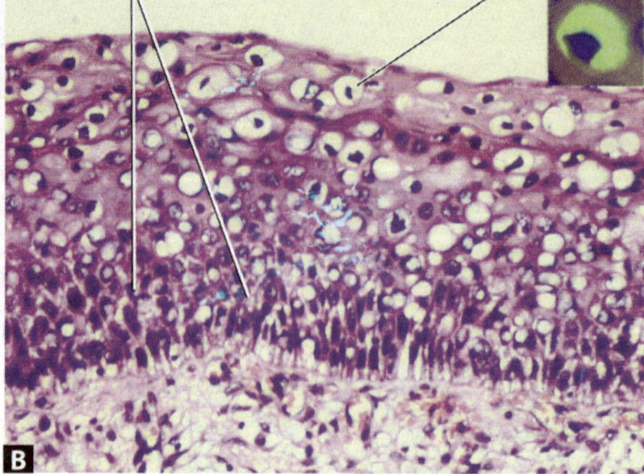

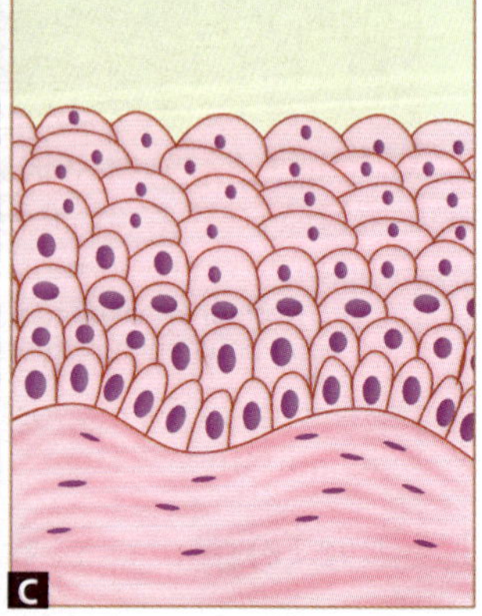

Figs. 22.4A to C: Low-grade squamous intraepithelial lesion (LSIL): (A) Low magnification; (B) High magnification with koilocyte. The koilocytotic changes are observed in the superficial layers of the epithelium; (C) The diagrammatic appearance of LSIL.

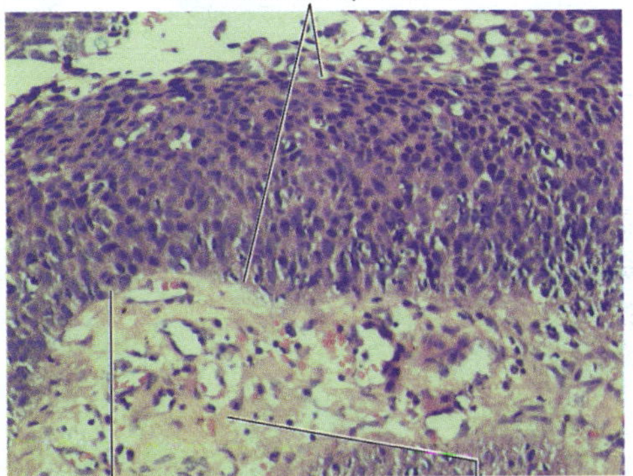

Fig. 22.5A: High-grade squamous intraepithelial lesion without koilocytic change: Low magnification.

Koilocyte with perinuclear cytoplasmic halo

Cells with pleomorphism and nuclear atypia

A B

Figs. 22.6A and B: Papanicolaou smears showing the cytology of squamous intraepithelial lesion (SIL). The cytoplasm of desquamated cells may be stained either red or blue. SIL shows a reduction in the cytoplasm and an increase in the nucleus-to-cytoplasm ratio. This increases as the grade of the lesion increases: (A) Cervical cytology of low-grade squamous intraepithelial lesion [LSIL; cervical intraepithelial neoplasia (CIN) I] with koilocytes; (B) LSIL shows nuclei greater than three times the size of an intermediate nucleus. Nuclear/cytoplasmic (N/C) ratios are relatively preserved despite the increased nuclear size. Nuclei are often hyperchromatic and may show irregular nuclear contours. Koilocytic halos are seen but not required.

transformation zone in LSIL. This mosaic (irregular surface resembling inlaid woodwork) pattern is characterized by a network of fine-caliber blood vessels that appear in close proximity to one another.

LSIL: Biopsy proved LSIL is managed conservatively with careful observation and follow-up.

HSILs and persistent LSIL: They are treated with surgical excision (cone biopsy), cryosurgery, and (rarely) hysterectomy. Follow ups are necessary in patients with HSIL, because of the risk for HPV-associated cervical, vulvar, and vaginal cancers.

Invasive Carcinoma of the Cervix

PA 30.1 (CC): Describe the epidemiology, pathogenesis, etiology, pathology, screening, diagnosis, and progression of carcinoma of the cervix.

Q. Describe the etiology, pathology, and spread of carcinoma of the cervix.

Squamous cell carcinoma is the most common histologic subtype of cervical cancer. It accounts for approximately 80% of carcinoma of the cervix. Other tumors of the cervix are adenocarcinoma, mixed adenosquamous carcinoma (15%), and small cell neuroendocrine carcinoma (<5%). All these tumors are caused by high-risk HPV. Squamous cell carcinoma of the cervix may be HPV-associated (>90–95%) or HPV-independent (5–10%). HPV-vaccinated women have reduced rates of HPV-associated precancers.

Age: Cervical cancer is usually found between **40 and 60 years** (mean age 54 years) with a peak at 45 years.

The etiology and pathogenesis of carcinoma of the cervix are discussed on pages 800-2.

MORPHOLOGY

Q. Write a short note on the morphology of carcinoma of the cervix.

Squamous Cell Carcinoma

Gross

Carcinoma of the cervix arises from the transformation zone. It ranges from microscopic foci of stromal invasion to grossly visible tumors. Three patterns of invasive cervical carcinoma are:

1. **Fungating (exophytic):** Forms a **nodular** and **exophytic cauliflower-like growth** protruding into the vagina (**Figs. 22.7A and B**).
2. **Endophytic (infiltrative) mass (Fig. 22.7C):** If the tumor is located **within the endocervical canal,** it may infiltrate the stroma and cause diffuse enlargement and hardening of the cervix.
3. **Ulcerative type:** It appears as an **ulcerated, granular, eroded lesion.**

Tumors encircling the cervix and penetrating the underlying stroma produce a **barrel-shaped cervix.** This can be identified by direct palpation.

Microscopy

The invasive tumors consist of tongues and nests of malignant squamous cells that produce a desmoplastic stromal response. The most common pattern of squamous cell carcinomas in HPV-associated carcinoma is nonkeratinizing. HPV-independent can show any histologic pattern. Grading of squamous cell carcinoma is based on the degree of squamous differentiation. It ranges from well-differentiated tumors with keratin pearls to poorly differentiated tumors. Depending on the cytological features, it can be divided into **keratinizing and nonkeratinizing carcinoma.** They **invade the underlying stroma** of the cervix

- **Keratinizing squamous cell carcinomas (Figs. 22.8A and B):** These are well-differentiated tumors composed of tumor **cells with abundant, dense, eosinophilic cytoplasm.** They show **keratin pearls** (concentric whorls of squamous cells) and nests of tumor cells with central keratin. The malignant cells are separated by intervening desmoplastic or inflammatory stroma. Nuclear pleomorphism and increased mitotic count are seen.
- **Nonkeratinizing carcinomas (Fig. 22.8C):** They **do not show keratin pearl** formation. But they **show individual cell keratinization or intercellular bridges.** They are typically moderately differentiated. Currently, the **distinction between**

Carcinoma cervix
Squamous cell carcinoma is the most common histological subtype.

Most common cancer in women in India: Carcinoma cervix

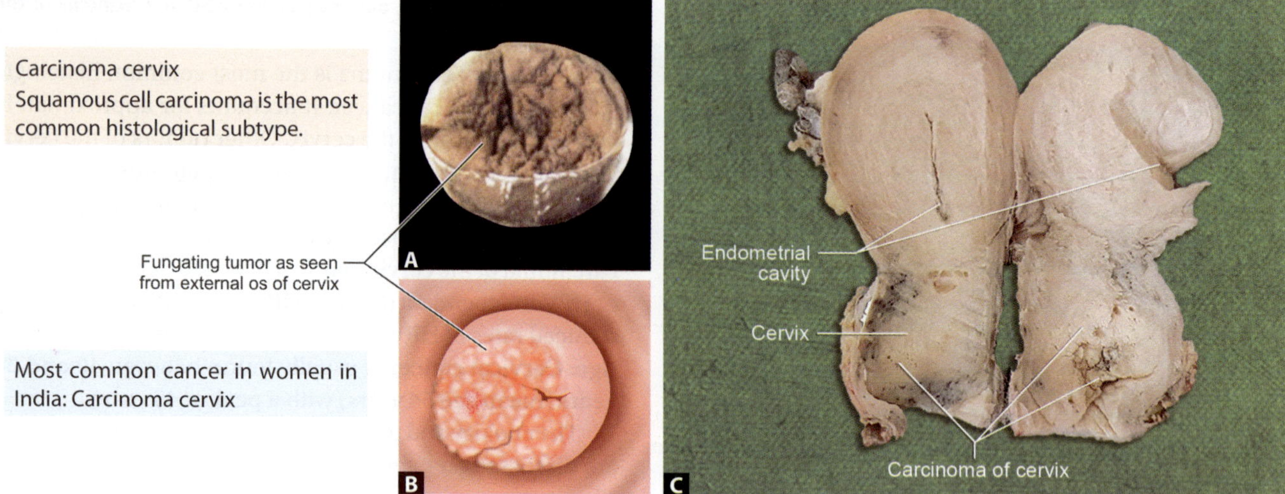

Figs. 22.7A to C: Invasive squamous cell carcinoma of the cervix: (A) Groos specimen and (B) Diagrammatic. Exophytic-carcinoma cervix presenting as a fungating growth projecting from the cervical os; (C) Hysterectomy specimen with endophytic cervical carcinoma involving the endocervix and extending into the lower uterine segment.

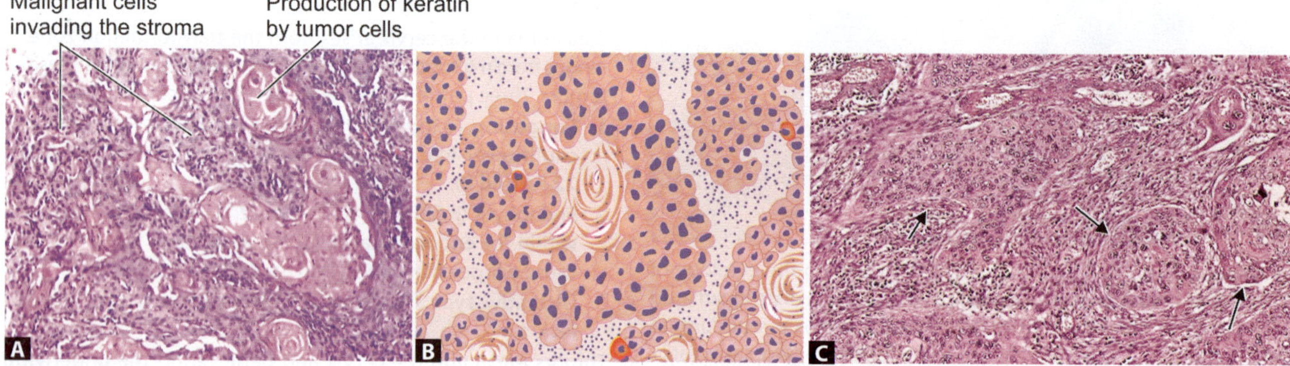

Figs. 22.8A to C: Invasive squamous cell carcinoma of the cervix: (A) H&E (B) Diagrammatic. Keratinizing squamous cell carcinoma shows infiltrating tumor cells with keratin pearls; (C) Nonkeratinizing squamous cell carcinoma consists of solid nests of large malignant squamous cells (arrows) without keratin pearls.

keratinizing and nonkeratinizing types has no clinical significance.

Adenocarcinoma

Second most common tumor type (~15%). It consists of **malignant endocervical cells forming a glandular pattern** (*refer* **online Figs. 22.9A and B**). Tumor cells have large, hyperchromatic nuclei with minimal mucin in the cytoplasm.

Spread of Carcinoma Cervix

Q. Write a short note on the spread of carcinoma of the cervix.

Overall, tumor growth and spread are relatively slow in cervical carcinoma.

Direct extension: Cervical cancer may spread into the surrounding tissues and organs.

- **Local extension into surrounding parametrial/ paracervical tissues.**
- **Urinary bladder and rectum:** Their involvement may lead to fistula formation.
- **Ureters:** Its involvement may lead to ureteral compression (obstruction) and cause clinical complications of hydroureter, hydronephrosis, pyelonephritis, and renal failure (uremia).
- Vagina

Lymphatics: Tumor may spread through lymphatic vessels to regional lymph nodes and leads to metastases in paracervical, hypogastric, and external iliac nodes.

Hematogenous spread: Only rarely cervical cancer spreads by the hematogenous route. It may spread to the liver, lungs, and bone marrow.

Clinical Features

- Early stages of cervical cancer: Patients most often present with **vaginal bleeding** after intercourse.
- Advanced cancer: Symptoms depend on the route and degree of spread.

The prognosis for invasive carcinomas depends largely on the stage of the carcinoma.

Cervical Cancer Screening

Q. Write a short note on the diagnosis of carcinoma of the cervix.

Cytologic Screening by Pap Smear Examination

Most cervical cancers are preceded by a precancerous lesion and **cytologic screening by Pap smear** is the **most reliable screening test for preventing and also detecting noninvasive stage of cervical cancer**.

Pap tests are **cytological preparations of exfoliated cells from the cervix** that are **stained with the Papanicolaou method** (*refer* pages 307-8). Using a spatula (*refer* **Fig. 10.1**) or brush, the transformation zone of the cervix is circumferentially scraped and the cells are smeared onto a slide. Following fixation and staining, the smears are screened **to identify cytologic abnormalities.** The cellular changes seen on the exfoliated cells obtained for the Pap test, illustrating the spectrum from LSIL to HSIL, are shown in **Figures 22.6A to D**. Papanicolaou smears showing the cytology of squamous cell carcinoma are shown (**Fig. 22.10C and *refer* online Figs. 22.10A and B**).

Testing for the presence of HPV DNA in cervical scrapes: It is a complementary molecular method of cervical cancer screening.

Histologic Diagnosis and Removal of Precancerous Lesions

Colposcopic examination: If **the Pap test shows abnormal cells**, a **colposcopic examination** of the cervix and vagina is performed to know the extent of the lesion, and the lesion is biopsied.

- Application of **acetic acid to the cervix highlights abnormal areas.**
- After confirmation by tissue biopsy, women with LSIL can be followed up with repeat smears.

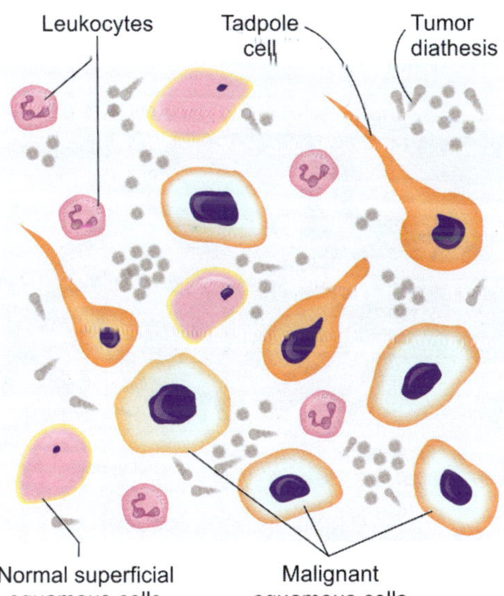

Fig. 22.10C: Papanicolaou smears showing the cytology of squamous cell carcinoma: Cytological appearance of squamous cell carcinoma of the cervix (diagrammatic).

Cervical conization of HSIL: HSILs are treated with cervical conization (excision) and follow-up smears and clinical examinations for life.

Treatment of cervical cancer: Superficially invasive squamous cell carcinomas may be treated by **cervical cone excision**. However, most **invasive localized cancers** are managed by **radical hysterectomy with lymph node dissection**, especially in younger women. Advanced cancers are treated with radiation and chemotherapy.

Cervical Cancer Prevention

Vaccination against high-risk HPV types: It is an important method and is recommended for boys and girls by 11–12 years of age and young men and women up to 26 years of age. Vaccination of males is important because of their role in the spread of HPV to women.

- **Nature of HPV vaccine:** Prophylactic quadrivalent HPV vaccine for HPV types 6, 11, 16, and 18 has been used to reduce the incidence of cervical cancer. The vaccine is prepared from noninfectious, DNA-free virus-like particles produced by recombinant technology. More recently a 9-valent vaccine is available and is very effective in preventing HPV infections. It produces high levels of serum antibodies in vaccinated individuals.

SCENARIO-BASED ESSAY QUESTION

Q. A-48-year-old woman complains of brownish, foul-smelling vaginal discharge for the last 6 months. She also gives a history of postcoital spotting. On per vaginal and per speculum examination, the cervix showed 3 cm ulceroproliferative growth which bleeds on touch to the cervix.

a. What is the probable diagnosis and give a reason? (Ans: Carcinoma cervix. Reasons: age, clinical features of foul-smelling vaginal discharge, history of postcoital spotting, and ulceroproliferative growth which bleeds on touch are features that favor carcinoma of the cervix).
b. Discuss the etiopathogenesis of the disease. *(refer pages 800-2)*
c. Describe the morphological features of this condition. *(refer pages 805-6)*
d. What screening methods/investigations will help in the diagnosis of this condition? *(refer page 807)*

UTERUS

MENSTRUAL CYCLE

The endometrium undergoes characteristic morphologic changes during the menstrual cycle due to sex hormones produced in the ovary. The normal menstrual cycle begins with the shedding of the upper half to two-thirds of the endometrium during menses. Different phases of the menstrual cycle are discussed below.

Proliferative Phase (Figs. 22.11A and B)

- **Endometrial glands:** During the proliferative phase, the endometrial glands are **straight, tubular, and**

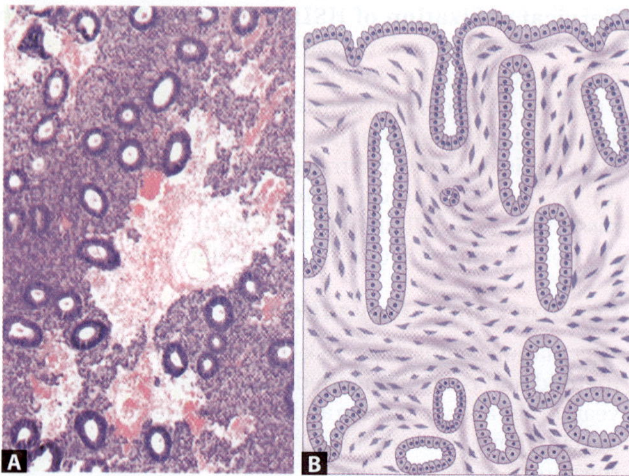

Figs. 22.11A and B: Proliferative phase composed of tubular endometrial glands lined by tall columnar cells (A, H&E; B, diagrammatic).

evenly distributed. Glands are **lined by regular, tall, pseudostratified columnar cells**. Mitotic figures are numerous.

- **Endometrial stroma:** Consists of **compactly arranged spindle cells** having scanty cytoplasm but abundant mitotic activity. Spiral arteries are narrow and mostly inconspicuous.

Secretory Phase

- **Endometrial glands: Enlarge, dilate**, and **become more coiled**. The lining cells develop abundant and prominent, glycogen-rich, **subnuclear vacuoles** (*refer* **online Fig. 22.12**). The **secretion increases** and the basal vacuoles progressively push past the nuclei. Later, the **secretions are discharged into the lumen** of the gland • the glands are dilated and tortuous, producing a serrated ("**saw-toothed**") appearance **(Figs. 22.13A and B)** when they are cut in their long axis.
- **Endometrial stroma:** The stromal cell enlarges (hypertrophy) and shows **large, round, vesicular nuclei and abundant eosinophilic cytoplasm** and the reappearance of stromal mitoses. These cells are the precursors of the decidual cells of pregnancy and are referred to as **predecidual change**.

Menstrual Phase

- In the absence of pregnancy, spiral arteries collapse, and the disintegration of the functionalis begins.
- The blood escapes into the stroma, marking the beginning of menstrual shedding. Menses commence on day 28, last 3–7 days.

ENDOMETRIOSIS

PA 30.7 (NC): Describe the etiology, hormonal dependence, features, and morphology of endometriosis.

Q. Write a short note on endometriosis.

Definition: Endometriosis is the **presence of "ectopic" benign endometrial glands and stroma** in a location **outside of the uterus.**

Age: Mainly occurs **during active reproductive life**, mostly in the **third and fourth decades**. It occurs in 5–10% of women and about 50% of them have infertility.

Localization: Endometriosis is frequently multifocal. Its various sites are listed in **Box 22. 2**.

Types of endometriosis: Three types of endometriosis are: (i) superficial peritoneal endometriosis, (ii) ovarian endometriosis, and (iii) deep infiltrating endometriosis. There is a risk of malignant transformation of deep infiltrating endometriosis.

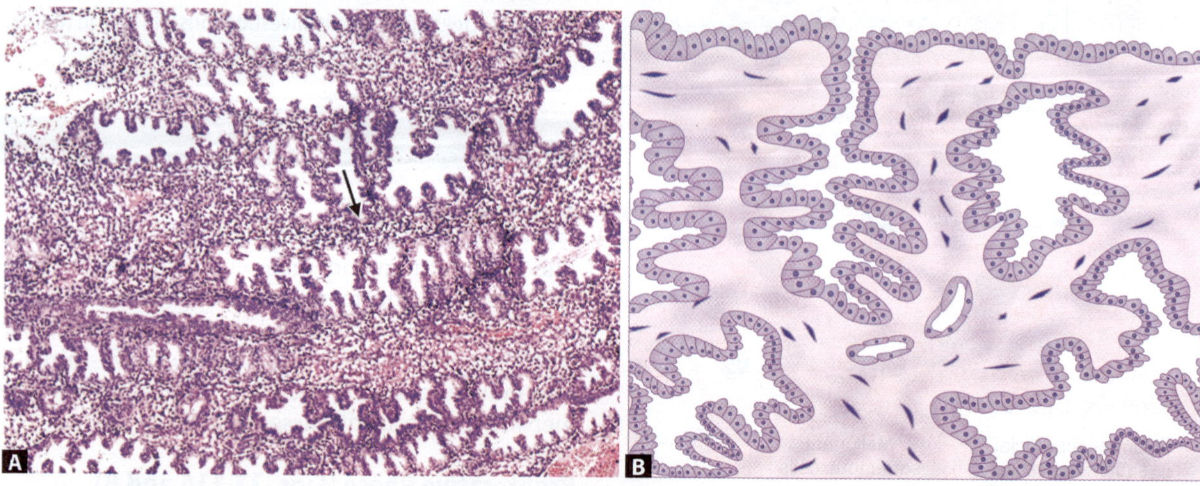

Figs. 22.13A and B: Late secretory endometrium saw-tooth appearance of the gland and predecidual changes in the stroma: (A) H&E; (B) Diagrammatic.

BOX 22.2: Various sites of endometriosis.

- Ovaries (more than 60%)
- Pouch of Douglas
- Uterine ligaments
- Fallopian tubes
- Rectovaginal septum
- Cul de sac
- Pelvic peritoneum and peritoneal cavity
- Large and small bowel and appendix
- Cervix, vagina
- Laparotomy, hysterectomy scars
- Periumbilical tissues

Pathogenesis

The pathogenesis of endometriosis is not completely known.

Proposed origin of endometriosis: The proposed origin of endometriosis may be from two main sources: (1) **from the uterine endometrium** and (2) from **outside the uterus from cells that can give rise to endometrial tissue.**

Main theories of endometriosis: These are as follows:

1. **Regurgitation theory:** According to this, the endometrial tissue by retrograde menstruation passes through the opening of the fallopian tubes and is implanted at an abnormal/ectopic site. It can explain the distribution of endometriosis within the peritoneal cavity. Retrograde menstruation occurs even in normal women.
2. **Benign metastases theory:** According to this, endometrial tissue can spread from the uterus to distant sites (e.g., bone, lung, and brain) through blood vessels and lymphatic channels.
3. **Metaplastic theory:** During embryonic development, Coelomic epithelium (mesothelium of pelvis or abdomen) gives rise to the Müllerian ducts and ultimately the endometrium. According to this theory, endometrium arises directly from the metaplasia of the coelomic epithelium. Also, mesonephric remnants may undergo endometrial differentiation and this may form ectopic endometrial tissue.
4. **Extrauterine stem/progenitor cell theory:** It is a recent theory according to which the endometrial tissue in an ectopic site represents the differentiation of stem/progenitor cells from the bone marrow.

Different characteristics of endometrial implants: The endometriotic tissue in endometriosis is not just misplaced but is also of **different characteristics than normally situated uterine endometrium.** They differ from normal in the following aspects:

- **Increased levels of proinflammatory and angiogenic factors:** For example, prostaglandin E_2 (PGE_2), vascular endothelial growth factor (VEGF), and matrix metalloproteinases (MMP). Some of these mediators are released by macrophages that are recruited to endometriotic implants by proinflammatory factors.
- **Secretion of aromatase by endometriotic stromal cells:** The stromal cells produce high levels of aromatase. These favor **increased local estrogen production from androgens.**

The above two factors increase the survival and persistence of the endometriotic tissue in a foreign location (important in the pathogenesis of endometriosis). This is supported by the fact that the use of COX-2 inhibitors (against PGE2) and aromatase inhibitors are found to be beneficial in the treatment of endometriosis. **An association between endometriosis and ovarian endometrioid and clear cell type carcinoma** is observed.

MORPHOLOGY

Gross

- **Endometriotic lesions bleed periodically:** Endometriotic lesions **respond to both extrinsic cyclic (ovarian) and intrinsic hormonal stimulation.** Hence, these lesions **bleed periodically**, similar to normal endometrial tissue. **Organization of hemorrhage** causing fibrosis and subsequent **fibrous adhesions** between neighboring structures (e.g., tubes, ovaries, and obliterates the pouch of Douglas).
- **Cystic nodules with a red-blue to yellow-brown appearance** (due to the breakdown of blood products) at the site of endometriosis.
- **Endometriosis of the ovary** is called a **chocolate cyst.**

Q. Write a short note on the endometriosis/chocolate cyst of the ovary.

- Ovaries may be distorted by numerous **cystic spaces** (1–5 cm in diameter) **filled with dark brown fluid** (due to previous hemorrhage).
- **Repeated hemorrhage** may form **large cysts** up to 15 cm in diameter, which **contain inspissated, chocolate-colored material and are** clinically known as **chocolate cysts** or endometriomas.

Microscopy

Commonly shows **both endometrial glands and stroma with or without** the presence of **hemosiderin-laden macrophages** at the ectopic site. Rarely, may show only endometrial stroma and/or hemosiderin-laden macrophages.

Scar Endometriosis

Q. Write a short answer on scar endometriosis.

Rarely, endometriosis can occur outside of the pelvis, and these are called extrapelvic endometriosis. Endometriosis occurring in scar tissue is rare and is called scar endometriosis. It occurs at the incision site, after obstetrical (especially after cesarean section) and gynecological surgeries. The term cesarean scar endometriosis (CSE) is an unusual manifestation of extrapelvic endometriosis. The patient may complain of the formation of a mass or lump (size varies) in the surgical scar. There is often pain in the abdominal wall at the incision site at the time of menstruation and is because of the bleeding in endometrial tissue. The bleeding is very irritating to the abdominal organs.

Clinical Features

Symptoms of endometriosis depend on the site of endometriosis. Symptoms include severe **dysmenorrhea** (painful menstruation), **dyspareunia** (pain with intercourse), **pelvic pain** (due to the intrapelvic bleeding and periuterine adhesions), pain on defecation (rectal wall involvement), dysuria (involvement of serosa of the bladder), intestinal disturbances (when the small intestine is affected), and menstrual irregularities.

Consequences: Infertility in ~30–40% of women and malignancy is uncommon.

Adenomyosis

PA 30.8 (NC): Describe the etiology and morphologic features of adenomyosis.

Q. Write a short note on adenomyosis of the uterus.

Definition: Adenomyosis is defined as the **presence of endometrial glands and stroma deep within the myometrium** (uterine wall).

Adenomyosis is seen in ~20% of uterine specimens.

Etiology and pathogenesis: The cause and pathogenesis of adenomyosis is **not known**. Adenomyosis is seen in continuation with the endometrium. So, it may develop due to downgrowth followed by proliferation of endometrial tissue into and between the smooth muscle fascicles of the underlying myometrium.

MORPHOLOGY

Gross

- **Enlarged uterus:** The uterus may show **mild to moderate enlargement.**
- **Cut section of the uterine wall:** It shows coarse **trabeculations with an ill-defined area of hemorrhage.**

Microscopy (Fig. 22.14)

- **Endometrial glands and stroma deep within the myometrium:** It shows irregular nests of benign endometrial glands and stroma deep within the myometrium.
- **Diagnostic criteria:** The minimum **distance between the basal endometrium and the endometrial tissue of adenomyosis should be one low-power microscopic field** (i.e., at least 2–3 mm).

Clinical Features

The clinical symptoms of adenomyosis may be similar to endometriosis. These include menometrorrhagia (irregular and heavy menses), colicky dysmenorrhea, dyspareunia, and pelvic pain, particularly during the premenstrual period. Many patients are asymptomatic.

ENDOMETRIAL HYPERPLASIA

PA 30.9 (NC): Describe the etiology, hormonal dependence, and morphology of endometrial hyperplasia.

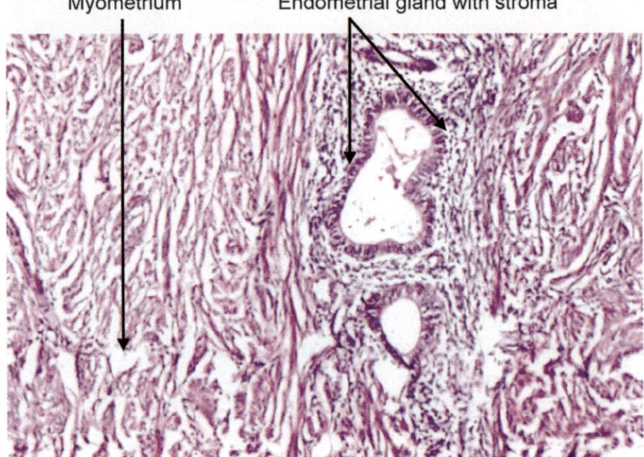

Fig. 22.14: Adenomyosis showing nests of endometrial glands and stroma deep within the myometrium.

Q. Write a short note on endometrial hyperplasia/causes/types of endometrial hyperplasia.

Definition: Endometrial hyperplasia is defined as an **abnormal proliferation of the endometrial glands relative to the stroma.** It results in an increased gland-to-stroma ratio when compared with normal proliferative endometrium and **increased thickness of the endometrium.**

- Endometrial hyperplasia is an **important cause of abnormal uterine bleeding**.
- **Precursor of endometrial carcinoma.**

Etiology

Prolonged or marked excess of estrogen relative to progestin: It can lead to ***excessive*** proliferation of endometrium (endometrial hyperplasia). Endometrial hyperplasia is an important **precursor of endometrial carcinoma**. Endometrial hyperplasia is a **soil for endometrial carcinoma** and both share specific acquired driver mutations in cancer genes. Causes of estrogen excess are listed in **Box 22.3**. Treatment with tamoxifen is associated with an increased risk of hyperplasia owing to its proestrogenic effects on the endometrium.

Mutation of PTEN: PTEN is a tumor-suppressor gene. It is mutated in both endometrial hyperplasias and carcinomas. Mutations in PTEN are seen in more than 20% of endometrial hyperplasias, both with and without atypia. It is observed in 30–80% of endometrial carcinomas. These findings suggest that alterations in PTEN occur at an early stage of endometrial tumorigenesis. Loss of PTEN function may activate cellular pathways normally activated by estrogen. Thus, inactivation of the PTEN and hyperestrogen may act in conjugation both in endometrial hyperplasia and endometrial carcinoma.

Classification of Endometrial Hyperplasia

According to the World Health Organization (WHO 2020), endometrial hyperplasia (*refer* **Box 22.4**) is classified into

BOX 22.3: Various conditions associated with increased estrogen that predispose to endometrial hyperplasia.

Endogenous source of estrogen:
- Obesity (increased peripheral conversion of steroid precursors into estrogens)
- Chronic anovulation
- Menopause
- Polycystic ovarian syndrome, e.g., Stein-Leventhal syndrome
- Functioning tumors of the ovary: Thecoma, granulosa cell tumor
- Excessive ovarian cortical function (cortical stromal hyperplasia)

Exogenous source of estrogen:
- Prolonged administration of estrogenic substances without counterbalancing progestin: For example, estrogen replacement therapy

two major categories: (1) **endometrial hyperplasia without atypia** and (2) **endometrial atypical hyperplasia** (also referred to as endometrial intraepithelial neoplasia). They differ in appearance and tendency to progress to carcinoma.

Endometrial Hyperplasia without Atypia

Definition: Endometrial hyperplasia without atypia (non-atypical endometrial hyperplasia) is defined as a **proliferation of endometrial glands of irregular size and shape without significant cytological atypia.**

Normally estrogenic stimulation of the endometrium is for the first 2 weeks of the menstrual cycle. If it is beyond the normal 2-week proliferative phase, it causes progressive changes in the endometrium. Endometrial hyperplasia without atypia is a functionally normal endometrium that responds to excess, abnormal stimulation by estrogen.

Pathogenesis: Hyperplasia without atypia develops due to prolonged estrogen exposure unopposed by progesterone or progestational agents acting on the entire endometrial tissue. It rarely progresses to adenocarcinoma (~1–3%).

MORPHOLOGY

Gross

The endometrium may have the uniform, tan appearance of the late proliferative phase. It appears highly thickened and sometimes polypoid or spongy with cysts.

Microscopy [Figs. 22.15A and 22.16 (*refer* online Fig. 22.15B)]

Endometrial hyperplasia without atypia **affects the entire endometrium.** It is characterized by **diffuse architectural and randomly distributed cytologic changes.** Three **diagnostic criteria are as follows:**

1. **Increased endometrial gland-to-stroma ratio:** It is the cardinal feature.
2. **Tubular, branching, and/or cystically dilated endometrial glands:** The **glands show variation in size and shape.** It shows **tubular glands admixed with branching and/or cystically dilated glands** resembling proliferative endometrium.

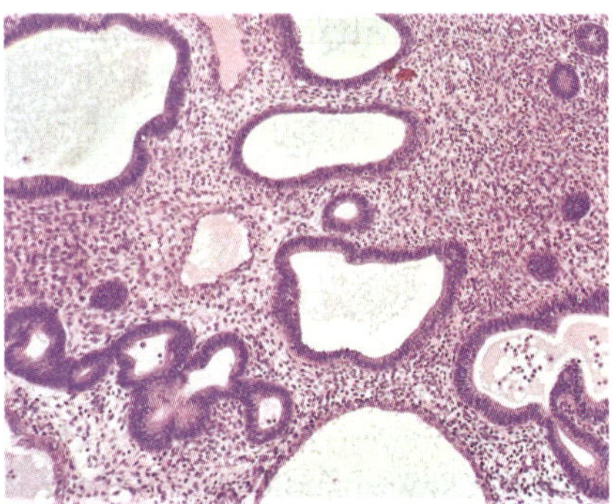

Fig. 22.15A: Endometrial hyperplasia without atypia: Shows cystic dilatation of glands.

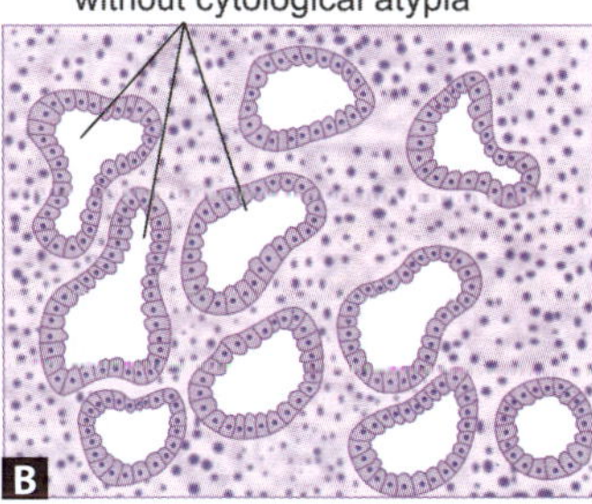

Figs. 22.16A and B: Endometrial hyperplasia without atypia (diagrammatic): (A) Shows cystic dilatation of glands; (B) Shows closely packed gland with increased gland-to-stroma ratio. The glands show mild variation in size.

   a. **Irregular distribution of glands:** The endometrial glands are often **irregularly distributed**, with variable ratios of glands to the stroma. The glands are crowded and are punctuated by cysts. Although **there may be a focal back-to-back arrangement of** glands, some intervening stroma is usually seen.
   b. **Glands lined by simple epithelium:** The glands are lined by simple epithelium, **without true stratification. No significant cytological atypia.**

3. **Uniform distribution of nuclear features: Higher levels of estrogen** drive mitoses, and nuclei appear **round,** whereas **decreased estrogen levels** produce mitotically quiescent **round or elongated nuclei.** They should have an inconspicuous nucleolus.

Most cases can be successfully managed with curettage or hormonal manipulation. When estrogen is withdrawn, hyperplasia may evolve into cystic atrophy.

Endometrial Atypical Hyperplasia (Endometrial Intraepithelial Neoplasia)

Definition: Endometrial atypical hyperplasia (endometrioid intraepithelial neoplasia) is defined as a **simultaneous change of epithelial cytology and an increased number of endometrial glands in comparison with the stroma** (crowded gland architecture). This is seen within a morphologically defined region in the endometrium, distinct from the surrounding endometrium or entrapped normal glands.

Endometrial atypical hyperplasia (endometrioid intraepithelial neoplasia) comprises genetically altered (mutated) precancerous cells that grow as a monoclonal neoplastic outgrowth of endometrial glands.

Pathogenesis: Endometrial atypical hyperplasia (endometrioid intraepithelial neoplasia) occurs as a clonal expansion of mutated glands. It **begins as a localized lesion** and may expand to occupy the entire endometrial compartment. It shows many of the genetic changes found in endometrioid endometrial carcinoma. These include microsatellite instability (including Lynch syndrome); *PAX2* inactivation; and *PTEN*, *KRAS*, and *CTNNB1* mutation.

MORPHOLOGY

Gross

Many of them have no distinguishing gross features. Others may appear as a **focal thickening resembling a polyp or within a diffusely thickened endometrium.**

Microscopy [Figs. 22.17B and C (*refer* online Fig. 22.17A)]

Endometrial atypical hyperplasia [endometrioid intraepithelial neoplasia (EIN)] is composed of complex patterns of proliferating glands that show **nuclear atypia.**

Crowded glandular architecture and altered epithelial cytology: It is composed of **crowded aggregates of cytologically altered tubular or slightly branching glands.** They **show both architectural and cytological alterations.** The glands often have complex outlines due to branching structures. They show back-to-back arrangements.

Background endometrium: These lesions **begin at a single point.** Then the lesion expands centripetally as proliferating neoplastic glands that displace and separate normal glands. The **normal glands may be adjacent to and/or admixed with the lesion.** The **endometrial changes endometrial atypical hyperplasia (endometrioid intraepithelial neoplasia) is distinct from the surrounding endometrium** and/or entrapped nonneoplastic glands.

Gland to stroma volume: The area of the glands exceeds the stroma. This leads to a reduction of the stromal volume. The glands **commonly show back-to-back arrangement.**

Lining epithelium: Individual cells lining the glands are rounded and lose the normal perpendicular orientation to the basement membrane. Cytoplasmic changes, such as various types of metaplasia, may be associated with nuclear atypia.

Nuclear atypia: Nuclear appearance is always distinct from that of the background from which the lesion has emerged. Cytologic changes in nuclei include **alterations in nuclear size, shape, and texture.** The nuclei have **open (vesicular) chromatin and conspicuous nucleoli.**

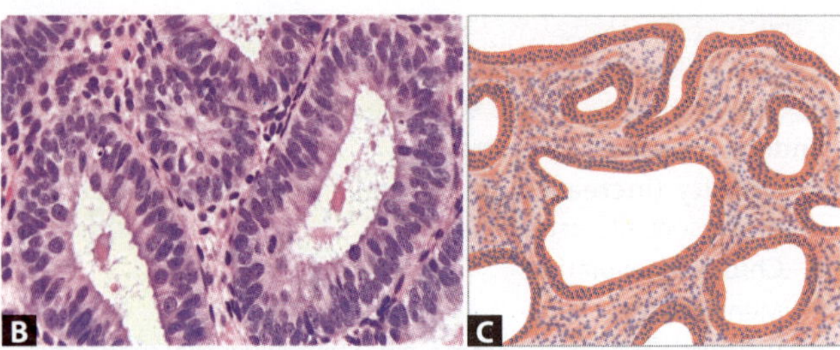

Figs. 22.17B and C: Endometrial atypical hyperplasia (endometrioid intraepithelial neoplasia): (B) higher magnification. It shows an altered gland-to-stroma ratio with predominant glands. The cells show nuclear enlargement and loss of polarity. (B) At higher magnification; (C) Diagrammatic appearance.

ENDOMETRIAL CARCINOMA

PA 30.2 (CC): Describe the pathogenesis, etiology, pathology, diagnosis, progression, and spread of carcinoma of the endometrium.

The WHO (2020) (abridged) classification of tumors of the uterine corpus is presented in **Box 22.4**.

BOX 22.4: World Health Organization (WHO) (2020) (abridged) classification of tumors of the uterine corpus.

Endometrial epithelial tumors and precursors
- Precursor lesions
  - Endometrial hyperplasia without atypia
  - Endometrial atypical hyperplasia/endometrioid intraepithelial neoplasia
- Endometrial carcinomas
  - Endometrioid carcinoma of the uterine corpus
  - Serous carcinoma of the uterine corpus

Tumor-like lesions
- Endometrial polyp
- Arias–Stella reaction of the uterine corpus

Mesenchymal tumors of the uterus
- Smooth muscle tumors
  - Uterine leiomyoma
  - Uterine leiomyosarcoma
- Endometrial stromal and related tumors
  - Low-grade endometrial stromal sarcoma
  - High-grade endometrial stromal sarcoma
- Miscellaneous mesenchymal tumors

Mixed epithelial and mesenchymal tumors
- Adenomyoma of the uterine corpus
- Adenosarcoma of the uterine corpus

Miscellaneous tumors

Q. Write a short note on the classification of tumors of the uterus.

- **Endometrial carcinoma is the most frequent gynecological cancer in higher-income countries.**
- **Age-group**: Carcinoma of the endometrium is uncommon before 40 years of age, and mainly occurs in postmenopausal **women** between **55 and 65 years**.
- **Postmenopausal bleeding:** Clinically endometrial carcinoma presents as abnormal (postmenopausal) bleeding.

Classification

Morphologic classification: Endometrial carcinoma is broadly classified into two morphologically distinct categories: (i) **endometrioid** (type I) and (ii) **serous**

carcinoma (type II). However, this classification is often either difficult to apply or poorly predictive of outcome. There is a substantial overlap between these tumors. Limitations of this approach are further highlighted by molecular data.

Endometrioid Endometrial Carcinoma

Definition: Endometrioid carcinoma is a malignant epithelial neoplasm that **shows varying proportions of glandular, papillary, and solid architecture.** These neoplastic **epithelial cells show endometrioid differentiation.**

Age: It occurs in **perimenopausal women.**
Most common type: Endometrioid endometrial carcinoma is the most common type (80–85%) of endometrial carcinoma.
Mostly well-differentiated: Most of these carcinomas are well-differentiated and mimic proliferative endometrial glands. Hence, the name endometrioid (**endometrial-like**).

Q. Risk factors for endometrial carcinoma.

Risk factors: Typically, endometrioid endometrial carcinoma arises in the setting **of endometrial hyperplasia with atypia.** Similar to endometrial hyperplasia, it is associated with **estrogen excess** [hyperestrogenic conditions such as obesity, estrogen-secreting ovarian tumors, exposure to exogenous estrogens (*refer* **Box 22.3**), early menarche, late menopause, and nulliparity] in which there is unopposed estrogenic stimulation of the endometrium. The most common associated condition **is obesity, hypertension**, and **type 2 diabetes mellitus.**
Pathogenesis (Fig. 22.18): Like in other cancers, endometrioid carcinoma develops from the stepwise acquisition of genetic alterations (mutations) in tumor-suppressor genes and oncogenes. The genetic alterations accumulate during the transition from normal to endometrioid intraepithelial neoplasia (atypical hyperplasia) to endometrioid carcinoma. These may occur over a period of years.

Early events in the stepwise development of endometrioid carcinoma are mutations in mismatch repair genes and the tumor-suppressor gene *PTEN*. In most cases, these mutations are acquired (somatic). It can occur in association with germline mutations of these genes. These include Cowden syndrome with germline mutations in *PTEN* and Lynch syndrome with germline mutations in DNA mismatch repair genes). *MLH1* gene encodes a component of the mismatch repair complex of proteins. Loss of function of *MLH1* results in microsatellite instability and is observed in about 20% of endometrioid carcinomas. *TP53* mutations also occur in endometrioid carcinomas but are relatively uncommon late events.

MORPHOLOGY

Gross (Figs. 22.19A to D)

Endometrioid endometrial carcinoma may be:

- **Diffuse tumor** involving the endometrial surface (infiltrative)
- **Localized polypoid growth or more discrete nodules (exophytic).**
  Large tumors usually **show areas of hemorrhage and necrosis.**

Microscopy

Most endometrial carcinomas (~85%) are **endometrioid adenocarcinomas [Figs. 22.20B and C (*refer* online Fig. 22.20A)]** and are **well differentiated.**

- **Glandular pattern:** Tumors consist of irregular, complex glandular, or villoglandular structures.
- **Tumor cells:** The glandular or villoglandular structures are lined by **columnar tumor cells with pseudostratified nuclei. Resembles normal endometrial epithelium.**
- Cytoplasm of the neoplastic cells—it is usually eosinophilic and granular.
- **Nuclei:** They are basophilic and range from oval **bland to markedly pleomorphic.** The nucleoli may be inconspicuous or may be prominent in high-grade carcinomas.
- **Mitotic figures:** The mitotic count is highly variable. It may be abundant and may be abnormal in less differentiated tumors.

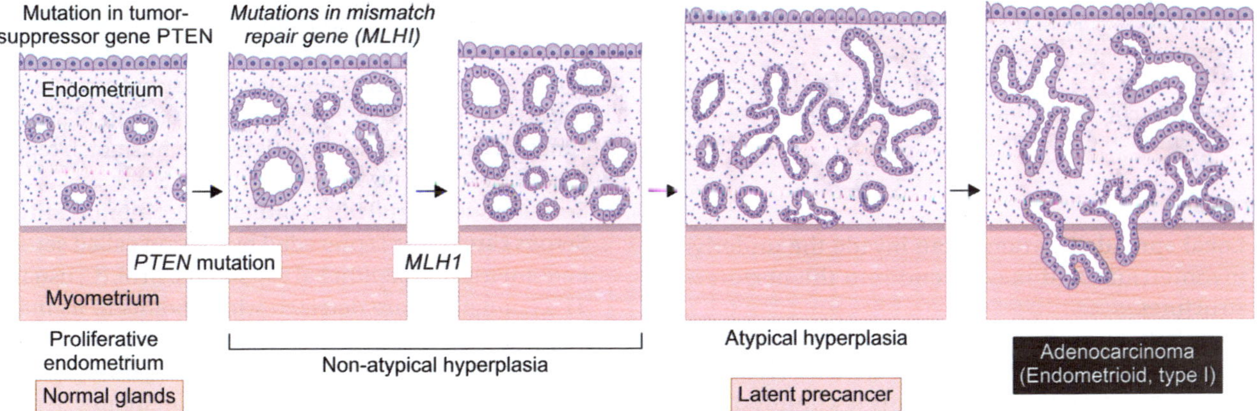

Fig. 22.18: Schematic diagram showing the development of endometrioid endometrial adenocarcinoma. The most common molecular genetic alterations that occur are mentioned. *MLH1* gene encodes a component of the mismatch repair complex of proteins. Loss of function of *MLH1* results in microsatellite instability and is observed in about 20% of endometrioid carcinomas.

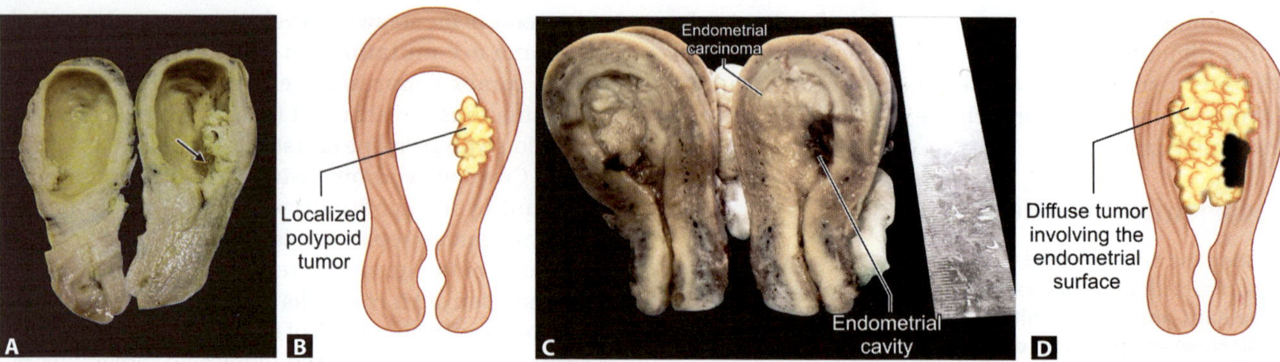

Figs. 22.19A to D: Endometrioid adenocarcinoma of the endometrium: (A) The bisected uterus shows a localized gray-white polypoid mass involving the body of the uterus (arrow). The uterine cavity is dilated due to the obstruction of the lower uterine segment caused by the tumor; (B) Diagrammatic appearance of localized polypoid tumor; (C) Carcinoma presents as a diffusely infiltrative and fungating gray-white tumor involving the entire endometrial surface of the uterine corpus projecting into the cavity; (D) The diagrammatic appearance of the diffuse infiltrative tumor.

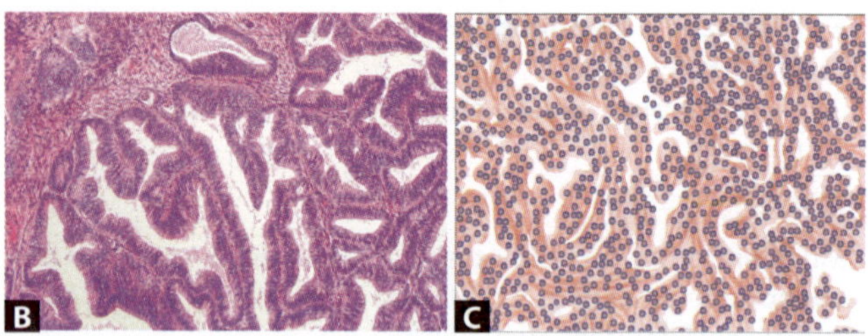

Figs. 22.20B and C: Well-differentiated endometrioid endometrial adenocarcinoma: (B) High magnification shows glandular and papillary formation with minimal stroma between the glands; (C) Diagrammatic appearance.

Grading: It is done according to the glandular differentiation alone.

- **Well-differentiated (grade 1/G1) adenocarcinoma:** It consists of tumor cells forming **easily recognizable glandular** patterns.
- **Moderately differentiated (grade 2/G2) adenocarcinoma:** It consists of a mixture of both **well-formed glands and solid sheets** of malignant cells.
- **Poorly differentiated (grade 3/G3) adenocarcinoma:** It consists of **solid sheets (more than 50%)** of cells **without recognizable glands.** They show a severe degree of nuclear atypia and numerous mitotic figures.

According to the binary grading system, endometrioid carcinoma can be divided into low-grade (includes grade 1 and grade 2) and high-grade (grade 3).

Spread

- **Local spread:** The tumor can invade the underlying myometrium and may extend into the periuterine structures.
- **Lymphatic spread:** To the regional lymph nodes. Serous carcinoma spreads to the extrauterine (lymphatic or transtubal) site, even when it is confined to the endometrium or its surface epithelium.
- **Hematogenous spread:** To the lungs, liver, bones, and other organs.

Serous Endometrial Carcinoma

Definition: Serous endometrial carcinoma is a carcinoma with **diffuse, marked nuclear pleomorphism**. It usually **shows papillary and/or glandular growth patterns.**

Age: Serous endometrial carcinoma usually occurs in **postmenopausal women** in their sixth and seventh decades of life. Usually, it occurs a **decade later than endometrioid carcinoma.**

No association with estrogen exposure: In contrast with endometrioid carcinoma, they usually arise **in the setting of endometrial atrophy** and are **not associated with estrogen exposure.**

High-grade and aggressive tumors: Serous tumors are considered as high-grade (grade 3) (poorly differentiated) aggressive tumors. Hence, their histologic grading is not clinically useful.

Less common: They are less common and account for up to 15% of cases of endometrial carcinoma. This subtype shows significant morphologic and biologic overlap with ovarian serous carcinoma.

Pathogenesis (Fig. 22.21): Most (more than 90% of cases) **serous endometrial carcinoma is associated with mutations in the *TP53* tumor-suppressor gene.** This mutation is an early event in the evolution of serous endometrial carcinoma. Mutations in DNA mismatch repair genes and *PTEN* are rare.

- **Serous endometrial intraepithelial carcinoma (SEIC):** Serous carcinoma is preceded by a lesion called serous endometrial intraepithelial carcinoma. In SEIC, usually *TP53* mutations are detected which points to its main role in the development of this form of endometrial carcinoma. It shows significant morphologic and biologic overlap with ovarian serous carcinoma. Serous carcinoma probably begins as a surface epithelial neoplasm that extends into adjacent gland structures and later invades endometrial stroma.

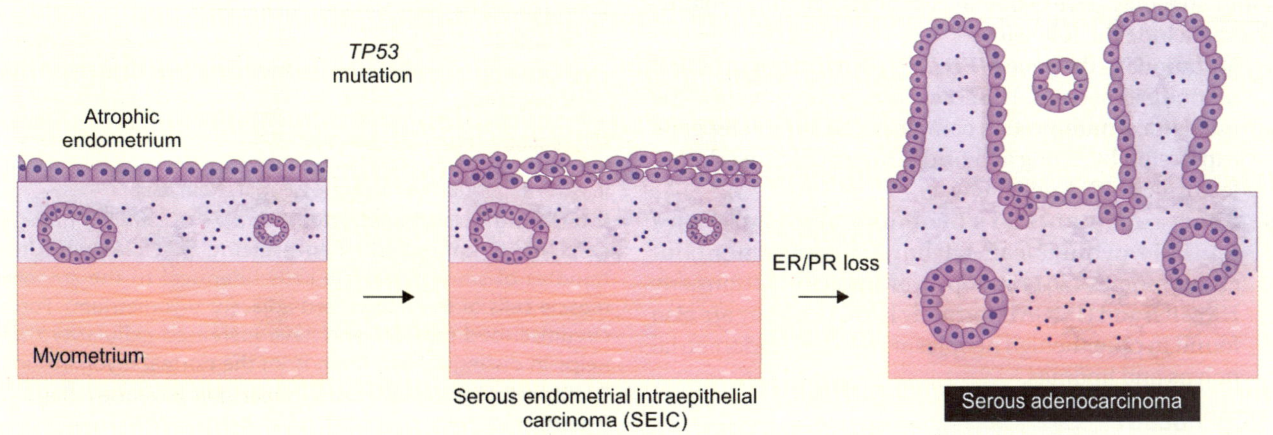

Fig. 22.21: Schematic diagram showing the development of serous endometrial carcinoma and alterations that are likely to occur during the progression of the disease.

MORPHOLOGY

Serous Endometrial Intraepithelial Carcinoma (SEIC)

It is the **precursor lesion that arises from a polyp or atrophic endometrium.** It is the noninvasive precursor lesion of serous endometrial carcinoma. It consists of malignant cells similar to those of serous carcinoma. These tumor cells are confined to the epithelial surface of the endometrium.

Serous Carcinomas

Gross: Serous carcinomas usually arise in small atrophic uteri. They form large bulky masses or deeply invade the myometrium.

Microscopy (refer online Figs. 22.22A and B)

Serous carcinoma histologically resembles and behaves like serous carcinoma of the ovary.

Growth pattern: These are invasive lesions and, in most cases, show **complex papillary and/or glandular architecture.** They may also show solid growth patterns.

Glands: The glands are typically **elongated and irregular, with slit-like luminal spaces.** When it shows a predominant glandular growth pattern resembling endometrioid carcinoma, they are distinguished because of the **marked cytologic atypia** in serous endometrial carcinoma. The cytologic atypia is characterized by a high nuclear-to-cytoplasmic ratio, atypical mitotic figures, hyperchromasia, and prominent nucleoli.

High grade: All the tumors are classified as grade 3, irrespective of the architectural pattern.

Spread: Serous carcinoma may show relatively superficial endometrial involvement. However, they may be associated with extensive peritoneal disease. This suggests that it spreads by routes other than direct invasion. They can shed malignant cells and metastasize to extrauterine sites by tubal regurgitation. It often shows transtubal spread to peritoneal surfaces.

Refer online **Table 22.1** for the differentiating features of endometrioid and serous endometrial carcinoma.

Clinical Features of Endometrial Carcinoma

- **Age:** Mostly seen in postmenopausal women between 55 and 65 years of age. Patients with serous carcinoma tend to be older and manifest between 65–70 years of age.
- **Irregular or postmenopausal vaginal bleeding** with excessive leukorrhea.
- **Diagnosis:** It is by histologic examination of **tissue obtained by biopsy or curettage.**

Prognosis: Stage determines survival in both types. Serous tumors more frequently produce extrauterine extension and have a worse prognosis than endometrioid carcinomas.

Malignant mixed Müllerian tumors (MMMTs): Also termed **carcinosarcomas** are **endometrial adenocarcinomas with a malignant mesenchymal component.** They resemble endometrial carcinoma genetically and have poor prognosis. Microscopically, they usually consist of adenocarcinoma (endometrioid, serous, or clear cell) along with the malignant mesenchymal (sarcomatous) component.

UTERINE LEIOMYOMAS

PA 30.3 (CC): Describe the pathogenesis, etiology, pathology, diagnosis, progression, and spread of leiomyomas and leiomyosarcomas.

Uterine leiomyomas (commonly called **fibroids or myomas**) are **benign smooth muscle neoplasms** and are the **most common tumors in women.**

Age: Leiomyomas predominantly occur in women during the reproductive period. They are rare before the age of 20 years. They occur in 75% of women over the age of 30 years. Most leiomyomas regress after menopause.

Pathogenesis: Estrogen and progesterone stimulate the growth of leiomyoma. Hence, these tumors shrink after menopause. Most leiomyomas have normal karyotypes, but about 40% may have a simple chromosomal abnormality. These include the following:

- **Mutations in the gene *MED12*:** It occurs in about 70% of uterine leiomyomas. *MED12* encodes a component of the mediator, a multiprotein complex. This stimulates gene expression by acting as a bridge between transcription factors and RNA polymerase.
- **Rearrangements of chromosomes 12q14 and 6p**: Leiomyomas can harbor rearrangements of chromosomes 12q14 and 6p involving *HMGA2* (formerly HMGIC) and HMGA1 (formerly HMGIY). They are also found in other benign neoplasms, such as endometrial polyps and lipomas.

MORPHOLOGY

Q. Write a short note on the morphology of leiomyoma (including its sites).

Sites (Figs. 22.23A and B)

- **Most common sites**: Uterine leiomyomas may be found in the following sites:
  - **Intramural: Within the myometrium** of the corpus.
  - **Submucosal**: Just **beneath the endometrium.** These may ulcerate and cause abnormal uterine bleeding.
  - **Subserosal: Beneath the serosa** or pedunculated. These tumors may extend out and may become attached to surrounding organs, from which they may get a blood supply (parasitic leiomyomas).
- **Rare sites:** Uterine ligaments, lower uterine segment, or cervix

Gross

- **Sharply circumscribed:** Leiomyomas are sharply (well) circumscribed (without encapsulation), **discrete, round, firm, gray-white** tumors.
- **Size varies:** They **vary** in size from small nodules to massive (vary from 1 mm to over 30 cm in diameter) tumors that fill the pelvis. They tend to enlarge during pregnancy since they have estrogen and progesterone receptors.
- **Number:** They may be single or multiple.
- **Whorled cut surface:** It has a characteristic **whorled pattern** of smooth muscle bundles and has a **raw (watered) silk appearance.**

Microscopy (Figs. 22.24A and B)

Q. Write a short answer on microscopy of leiomyoma.

Interlacing fascicles/whorled bundles of smooth muscle cells: It is composed of interlacing fascicles/whorled bundles of smooth muscle cells (identical to the smooth muscle cells of the uninvolved adjacent myometrium). Form circumscribed nodules and have increased cellularity that helps in distinguishing them from the normal myometrium.

Tumor cells: Individual muscle tumor cells have the following features:

- **Uniform in size and shape.** They are **uniform and spindle-shaped with indistinct borders.**
- **Moderate amount of eosinophilic cytoplasm:** They have abundant, eosinophilic cytoplasm with long, slender bipolar cytoplasmic processes.
- **Cigar-shaped nuclei:** The tumor cells have a characteristic **elongated oval nucleus with blunt ends.**

Mitotic figures: Usually not seen.

Secondary changes (Box 22.5): These include the following:

- **Hyaline change** (degeneration—refer **Fig. 2.34), mucoid or myxomatous degeneration, calcification, cystic changes, and fatty metamorphosis.**
- **Red degeneration:** It may be **observed in large tumors** and is characterized grossly by a bulging surface and a **homogeneous dark brown** (beefy-red/yellow-brown) **to red, softened appearance on the cut section.** It may be **associated with pregnancy or the use of contraceptive drugs.** It shows **extensive coagulative necrosis.**

Clinical Features

- **Age group:** Rare before age 20 and most regress after menopause.

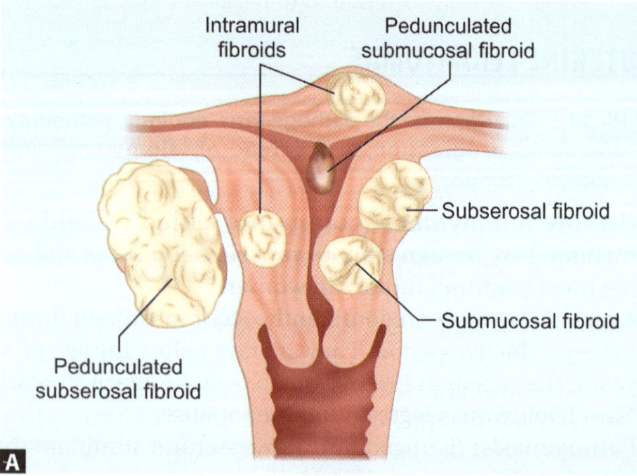

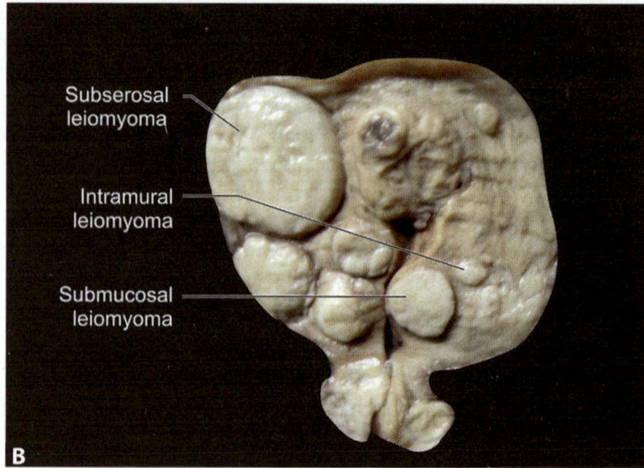

Figs. 22.23A and B: Leiomyomas of the uterine myometrium: (A) Diagrammatic appearance showing different sites of leiomyoma; (B) The gross specimen of cut-opened uterus displays multiple sharply circumscribed tumors in submucosal (bulging into the endometrial cavity), intramural, and subserosal locations. The cut section of these tumors has a firm, whorled, and homogeneous appearance.

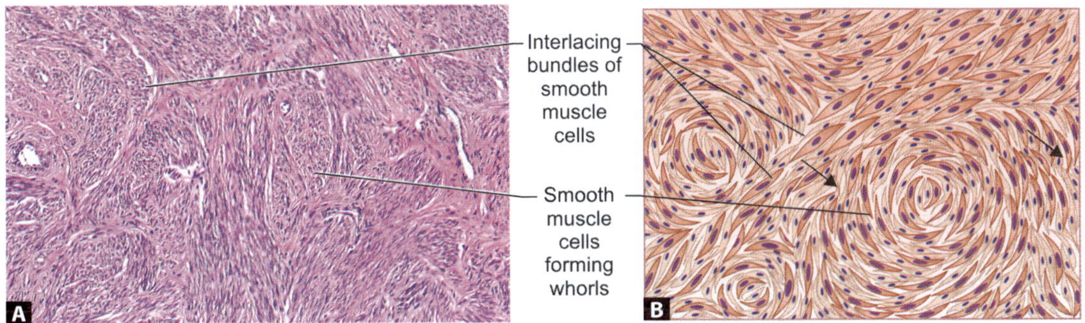

Figs. 22.24A and B: Microscopic appearance of leiomyoma showing well-differentiated, regular, spindle-shaped smooth muscle cells arranged in interlacing fascicles: (A) Hematoxylin and eosin (H and E); (B) Diagrammatic appearance.

BOX 22.5: Secondary changes in leiomyoma.

- Hyaline change
- Myxomatous change
- Calcification
- Cystic change
- Fatty metamorphosis
- Red degeneration

- Leiomyomas of the uterus **may be asymptomatic**. In symptomatic cases, common symptoms are **abnormal bleeding** (menorrhagia, with or without metrorrhagia), **urinary frequency** (compression of the bladder), and infertility. Malignant transformation (leiomyosarcoma) is extremely rare.

UTERINE LEIOMYOSARCOMA

Leiomyosarcoma of the uterus is an **uncommon malignant tumor**. These tumors probably **originate from the myometrium or endometrial stromal precursor cells.** They are **always solitary** and usually develop in **postmenopausal women**. This contrasts with its benign counterpart leiomyomas, which are frequently multiple and usually arise in premenopausal women. The genetics of leiomyosarcomas revealed that leiomyosarcoma **does not arise from leiomyomas.**

MORPHOLOGY

Gross

Leiomyosarcoma are **usually large** and measure about 10–15 cm in diameter. They are **soft and show areas of hemorrhage and necrosis.** They have irregular borders and invade the adjacent myometrium.

Microscopy

It varies widely from tumors that closely resemble leiomyoma to wildly anaplastic neoplasms. Well-differentiated tumors may show morphological features of leiomyoma in some areas along with leiomyosarcoma. The **diagnostic features include tumor necrosis, cytologic atypia, and mitotic activity.** More than 10 mitoses per 10 HPF with or without cellular atypia (if the tumor is more than 5 cm in diameter), or 5–10 mitoses per 10 HPF with cellular atypia and necrosis are considered for the diagnosis of leiomyosarcoma.

Prognosis: Recurrence is common and many tumors metastasize to the lungs.

OVARIES

OVARIAN TUMORS

PA 30.4 (CC): Classify and describe the etiology, pathogenesis, pathology, morphology, clinical course, spread, and complications of ovarian tumors.

Various types of tumors can occur in the ovary. **Ovarian cancer is the second most frequent gynecologic malignancy** after endometrial cancer. It is the eighth most common cancer death in women. It accounts for about 3% of all cancers in females. Ovarian cancer carries a higher mortality rate than all other female genital cancers combined. This is because by the time of diagnosis, in more than three-fourths of patients, ovarian cancers have spread beyond the ovary and fallopian tube into the pelvis or abdomen. They are rarely encountered during the early and curable stage.

Age group: About **two-thirds of ovarian tumors occur in women of reproductive age.** Less than 5% are seen in children. Approximately, 80% are benign, and they occur mostly in young women between 20 and 45 years of age. The single most common ovarian tumor is the mature cystic teratoma (dermoid cyst), and it mainly occurs in younger women. Within the epithelial group, borderline tumors (tumors of indeterminate malignancy) are often seen in women in their 30s and, occasionally, even in younger women, in whom epithelial carcinomas are relatively rare and are mostly of mucinous type. Almost 90% of malignant tumors are observed in women between 45 and 65 years of age. However malignant tumors may occur in younger women with a family history of the disease. Some ovarian neoplasms are largely restricted to certain age groups. For example, primitive germ cell tumors rarely occur in women >50 years of age.

Classification

Q. Classify ovarian tumors.

Q. Classify sex cord-stromal tumors of the ovary.
Q. Classify germ cell tumors of the ovary.

World Health Organization (WHO, 2020) histological classification of ovarian tumors is given in **Box 22.6**. Primary ovarian neoplasms are traditionally classified according to the most probable cell or tissue of origin **(Fig. 22.25)**. Most primary ovarian tumors arise from one of three major ovarian components.

1. **Multipotent surface/fallopian tube epithelium and endometriosis:** Most (~60%) are epithelial tumors that arise **directly or indirectly from Müllerian epithelium**. About 90% of ovarian malignancies are of epithelial origin, and the most common are high-grade serous carcinoma (HGSC). The term epithelial-stromal tumors is used to describe *epithelial tumors* with major stromal components.
2. **Pluripotent germ cells:** These cells migrate to the ovary from the yolk sac. They are pluripotent and the tumors arising from them form about 30% of ovarian tumors.
3. **Sex cord-stromal cells:** They constitute the endocrine apparatus of the postnatal ovary. These tumors form about 8% of ovarian tumors.

EPITHELIAL TUMORS

Most primary ovarian neoplasms arise from Müllerian epithelium. These epithelial tumors are **common primary** neoplasms and constitute >90% of ovarian cancers.

Classification of Epithelial Tumors

Q. Classify surface epithelial tumors of the ovary.

Epithelial tumors of the ovary are classified broadly based on both differentiation and the extent of epithelium cell proliferation.

Based on Differentiation of Epithelium

These may differentiate into any neoplastic Müllerian-type epithelium. These include the following:

- **Serous** (resembling epithelium of fallopian tube)
- **Mucinous** (resembling mucosa of the endocervix or that of the gastric pylorus)
- **Endometrioid** (resembling the glands of the endometrium)
- **Others:** These include **clear cells** (resembling glycogen-rich cells like endometrial glands in pregnancy), **Brenner** (resembling the mucosa of the bladder), or **mixed tumors**.

Based on the Extent of Proliferation of Epithelium

According to tumor cell proliferation, degree of nuclear atypia, and presence or absence of stromal invasion, these epithelial tumors are classified as **benign, borderline, and malignant** (i.e., carcinomas).

BOX 22.6: World Health Organization (2020) (abridged) histological classification of ovarian tumors.

Epithelial tumors
- **Serous tumors**
  - Benign serous tumors
    - Serous cystadenoma
    - Adenofibroma and cystadenofibroma
    - Surface papilloma of the ovary
  - Borderline serous tumors
  - Malignant serous tumors
    - Low-grade serous carcinoma of the ovary
    - High-grade serous carcinoma of the ovary
- **Mucinous tumors**
  - Benign mucinous tumors
    - Mucinous cystadenoma and adenofibroma
  - Borderline mucinous tumors
  - Malignant mucinous tumors
    - Mucinous carcinoma of the ovary
- **Endometrioid tumors**
  - Benign endometrioid tumors
    - Endometrioid cystadenoma and adenofibroma
  - Borderline endometrioid tumors
  - Malignant endometrioid tumors
    - Endometrioid carcinoma of the ovary
- **Clear cell tumors**
  - Benign clear cell tumors
    - Clear cell cystadenoma and adenofibroma
  - Borderline clear cell tumors
  - Malignant clear cell tumors
    - Clear cell carcinoma of the ovary
- **Seromucinous tumors**
  - Benign seromucinous tumors
    - Seromucinous cystadenoma and adenofibroma
  - Borderline seromucinous tumors
  - Malignant seromucinous tumors
    - Seromucinous carcinoma
- **Brenner tumors**
  - Benign Brenner tumors
  - Borderline Brenner tumors
  - Malignant Brenner tumors
- **Other carcinomas**

Mesenchymal tumors

Mixed epithelial and mesenchymal tumors

Sex cord-stromal tumors
- Pure stromal tumors
  - Ovarian fibroma
  - Thecoma
- Pure sex cord tumors
  - Adult granulosa cell tumor
  - Juvenile granulosa cell tumor
- Mixed-sex cord-stromal tumors
  - Sertoli–Leydig cell tumor
  - Sex cord-stromal tumor NOS
  - Gynandroblastoma

Contd...

Contd...

Germ cell tumors
- Mature teratoma of the ovary
- Immature teratoma of the ovary
- Dysgerminoma
- Yolk sac tumor
- Embryonal carcinoma
- Nongestational choriocarcinoma
- Mixed germ cell tumor of the ovary
- Monodermal teratomas and somatic-type tumors arising from a dermoid cyst
  - Struma ovarii
  - Ovarian carcinoid
- Germ cell-sex cord-stromal tumors
  - Gonadoblastoma
  - Mixed germ cell-sex cord-stromal tumor, unclassified

Miscellaneous tumors

Mesothelial tumors Tumor-like lesions

Metastases
- Metastases to the ovary

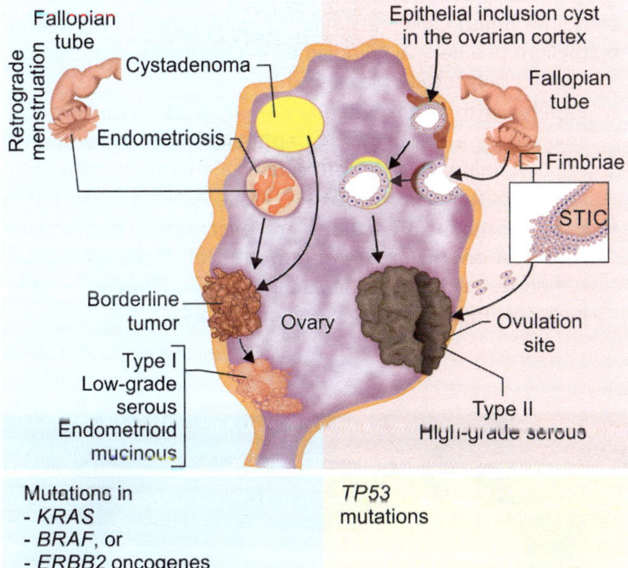

Fig. 22.25: Schematic of the proposed origin of various epithelial tumors of the ovary. Type I tumors progress from benign to borderline tumors and may progress to low-grade carcinoma. Retrograde menstruation leads to the development of endometriosis and borderline tumors. These can give rise to low-grade serous, endometrioid, and mucinous tumors. Type II tumors arise from ovarian surface epithelial inclusion cysts from the fimbrial epithelium of the fallopian tube. These epithelial cells from fimbria implant on the site of rupture on the ovary where ovulation occurred. These epithelial cells can invaginate and form a cortical inclusion cyst. Type II tumors also can arise via intraepithelial precursors (STIC = serous tubal intraepithelial carcinoma), which are often not identified. These tumors are high-grade and most commonly of serous type.

Benign tumors: About 80% of surface epithelial tumors of the ovary are benign. Mostly, they occur in young women between 20 and 45 years of age. These are usually further subclassified based on the components of the tumors.
- **Cystadenoma:** It is a tumor with **cystic areas.**
- **Cystadenofibroma:** It shows **both cystic and fibrous areas.**
- **Adenofibroma:** It consists of **predominantly fibrous areas.**

Cystadenoma and cystadenofibroma may contain mucinous, serous, endometrioid, or transitional (Brenner tumor) epithelium.

Borderline tumors: These tumors of indeterminate malignancy are characterized by the **proliferation of epithelial cells and nuclear atypia.** But it **does not show destructive stromal invasion.** They fall into an intermediate "gray zone" category. They occur at a slightly older age. The majority behave in a benign manner, some recur, and a few may progress to carcinoma.

Malignant tumors: They **can be solid or have a cystic component**. A malignant tumor with a cystic component is sometimes termed a **cystadenocarcinoma.** Carcinomas of the ovary are most common in women between 45 and 65 years of age and rare in women below the age of 35.
- **Based on light microscopy and molecular genetics:** Ovarian carcinomas are classified into five main subtypes. **They account for 98% of ovarian carcinomas.**
  1. **High-grade serous carcinoma** (HGSCs) (>70%)
  2. **Low-grade serous carcinomas** (LGSCs) (<5%)
  3. **Endometrioid carcinomas** (10%)
  4. **Mucinous carcinomas** (3–4%)
  5. **Clear cell carcinomas** (CCCs) (10%)
- **Based on the tumorigenic pathways and pathogenesis,** ovarian carcinomas can be further grouped into two types: types I and II **(Fig. 22.25).**
  - **Type I (low-grade) carcinoma**: These are **low-grade tumor** that usually **arise in association with borderline tumors or endometriosis**. These include **low-grade serous, endometrioid, and mucinous tumors.**
  - **Type II (high-grade) carcinoma**: These are most often **high-grade serous carcinoma** and they arise **from serous intraepithelial carcinoma.**

Risk factors for surface epithelial carcinomas: Important risk factors include:
- **Increasing age, early menarche/late menopause, and nulliparity**
- **Mutations in the *BRCA1* or *BRCA2* tumor-suppressor genes:** Family history, and germline mutations in certain tumor-suppressor genes such as *BRCA* increase the risk. About 5–10% of ovarian cancers are familial. Most of them have mutations in the *BRCA1* or *BRCA2* tumor-suppressor genes. These genes are also mutated in some hereditary breast cancers. These gene mutations are observed in only 8–10% of sporadic ovarian cancers.

- **Risk is reduced by prolonged use of oral contraceptives:** This may be due to suppression of ovulation.

Serous Tumors

Q. Write a short essay on serous tumors of the ovary.

Incidence: Serous tumors account for about **30% of all ovarian tumors** and about **over 50% of ovarian epithelial tumors**. Serous tumors are subclassified as benign, borderline, and malignant tumors. About **70% are benign or borderline**. About **30% are malignant**.

Age Group

- **Benign and borderline** tumors: Most common between **20 and 45 years.**
- **Serous carcinomas:** Usually occur **later** in life (except in familial cases).

Risk Factors

- **Risk factors** for **benign and borderline** tumors are **unknown.**
- **Risk factors for malignant** serous tumors (serous carcinomas):
  - **Parity: Nulliparous** and women with **low parity** have higher risk.
  - **Genetic factors:** Heritable mutations in tumor-suppressor genes ***BRCA1* and *BRCA2*** increase susceptibility to ovarian cancer.
  - **Family history** is a **risk factor.**

Oral contraceptives and sterilization during the reproductive period **reduce the risk.**

Grades of Serous Carcinoma (Fig. 22.25)

There are two types of serous carcinomas namely (i) low-grade and (ii) high-grade.

Low-grade: They **arise from benign or borderline** lesions. They **progress slowly to invasive carcinoma.**

- **Mutations in *KRAS, BRAF,* or *ERBB2* oncogenes:** These are observed in low-grade tumors arising in serous borderline tumors and they usually have wild-type (normal) *TP53* alleles.

High-grade: Many of these tumors **arise in the fimbriated end of the fallopian tube through a serous tubal intraepithelial carcinoma.** They develop rapidly.

- ***TP53* mutations:** These are present in more than 95% of cases of high-grade serous cancers. Ovarian carcinomas that develop in women with *BRCA1* or *BRCA2* mutations are high-grade serous carcinomas characterized by *TP53* mutations. Other frequently mutated genes include the tumor-suppressors NF1 and RB.

Morphological Features

The morphological features of benign, borderline, and malignant serous tumors are separately discussed below.

Q. Describe the morphological features of serous epithelial tumors of the ovary.

MORPHOLOGY

Benign Serous Tumors

Gross [Fig. 22.26A (refer online Fig. 22.26B)]

Benign serous cystadenoma

- **Size varies:** Tumor may measure from **1 to 10 cm in diameter.**
- **Cystic tumor:** Tumor contains **one (unilocular) or more thin-walled cysts.** The cyst **wall is smooth and glistening** without any epithelial thickening.
- **Content of cysts:** Lumen filled with **clear watery serous fluid.**
- **Cut section:** Shows **smooth outer and inner glistening surface** and **may show small papillae [Fig. 22.26A (*refer* online Fig. 22.26B)]** projecting into the cavity. Rarely papillae are seen projecting from the outer surface of the ovary (surface papilloma).
- **Bilaterality is common** and found in **about 20% of benign** serous cystadenomas.

Cystadenofibromas contain cysts surrounded by a variable amount of solid areas.

Microscopy

Benign serous tumors (Figs. 22.27A and B)

Cysts lined by nonstratified or stratified cuboidal to columnar cells. The lining cells are similar in appearance to the lining epithelium of a normal fallopian tube. Cilia are present though sometimes only focally. May also show:

- **Papillae with a fibrovascular core (Fig. 22. 27C):** They are covered by a single layer of epithelium similar to that of the cyst lining. Papillary projections are more prominent in malignant tumors.
- **Psammoma bodies:** They are dystrophic, concentric calcifications. They are common in all types of serous tumors but are not specific to these tumors. They are usually inconspicuous or absent in benign tumors.

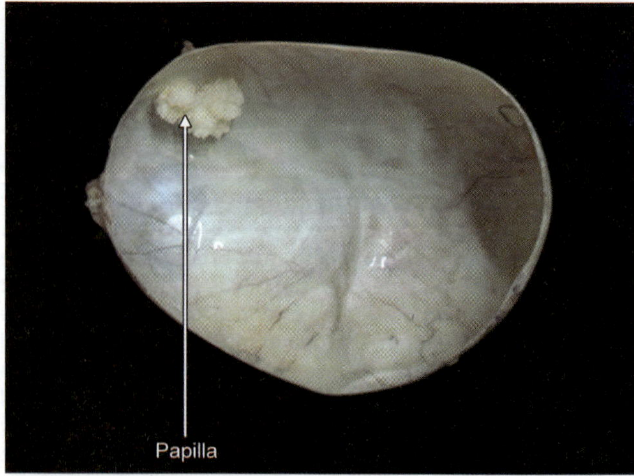

Fig. 22.26A: Serous cystadenoma of the ovary: The cut section shows an uniloculated cyst with a focus of the papilla.

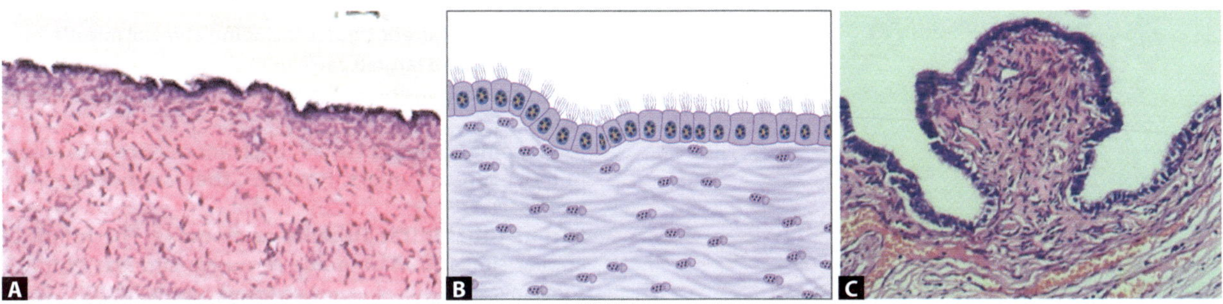

Figs. 22.27A to C: (A) H&E; (B) Diagrammatic. Microscopic appearance of serous cystadenoma showing cyst lined by a single layer of cuboidal epithelium; (C) Papillary serous cystadenofibroma shows broad, nonbranching, and simple stromal papillae embedded in the prominent fibromatous stroma. The cyst wall and papilla are lined by a single layer of cuboidal epithelium.

MORPHOLOGY

Borderline Serous Tumors

Gross

- **Vary in size, usually >5 cm and typically cystic.**
- Cut section shows **cystic cavities filled** by the increased number of **closely packed, papillary** projections. These papillae are extensive, fine, friable, confluent, soft, and form grape-like clusters in the cyst wall
- **Bilaterality:** Approximately **30%** are bilateral.

Microscopy (Figs. 22.28A and B)

They are noninvasive tumors with **greater epithelial proliferation and cytological atypia than benign but less than low-grade serous carcinoma.**

- **Complex branching papillae** with variable amounts of stroma in the cores.
- **Stratification of the epithelium (multilayering)** with the following features:
  - **Budding or cellular tufting:** These are tiny, irregular **tightly packed stroma-free clusters** of tumor cells that get detached **(detached buds of the epithelium)** and float into the lumen of the cyst.
  - **Mild-to-moderate cytological atypia** (nuclear atypia) **of the lining epithelial cells.** The neoplastic cells usually have scanty cytoplasm.
  - **Mildly increased mitotic activity**
  - **Psammoma bodies (Fig. 22.28C) frequently appear in about 25% of tumors.**
  - **Absence of stromal invasion:** But, tumors with exophytic growth may show implant on peritoneal surfaces in 30% of cases.
- **Papillary structures:** They resemble the papillary fronds seen in benign cystadenomas but show epithelial stratification, moderate nuclear atypia, and mitotic activity.
- **Micropapillary serous borderline tumors:** About 5–10% grow in a delicate papillary pattern and are called a micropapillary **(and/or a cribriform) pattern.**

MORPHOLOGY

Malignant Serous Tumors (Serous Carcinoma)

Serous ovarian carcinoma is classified into two major groups based on the degree of nuclear atypia. These are low-grade and high-grade serous carcinomas [*refer* **online Table 22.2** (50–60%)].

Low-grade Serous Carcinomas

Gross

They are **usually bilateral** and show **papillary growth.** They may be gritty due to calcification.

Microscopy [Fig. 22.29C (*refer* online Figs. 22.29A and B)]

Various architectural patterns: Low-grade serous carcinomas show a variety of architectural patterns. These include **single cells and small nests of irregular shape infiltrating the stroma,** and **micropapillae** (rarely macropapillae).

Tumor cells: They are **more uniform with mild to moderate nuclear atypia** and **limited nuclear pleomorphism.**

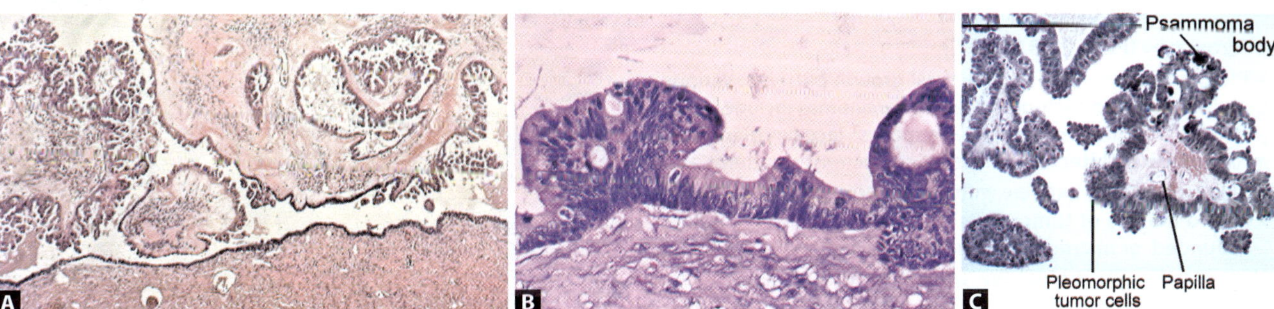

Figs. 22.28A to C: Serous borderline tumor of the ovary: (A) Branching papillae with variable amounts of stroma and detached buds of epithelium; (B) Epithelial stratification and the lining cells show mild-to-moderate cytologically atypical epithelium; (C) Papillae lined by multilayered columnar epithelium and one core of papilla with psammoma body.

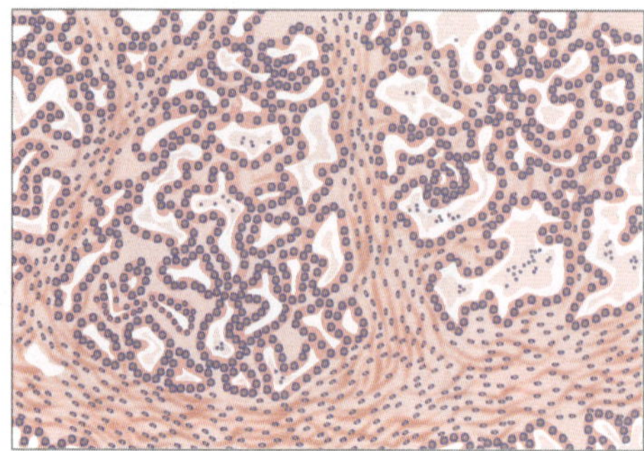

Fig. 22.29C: Low-grade serous carcinomas: Diagrammatic appearance.

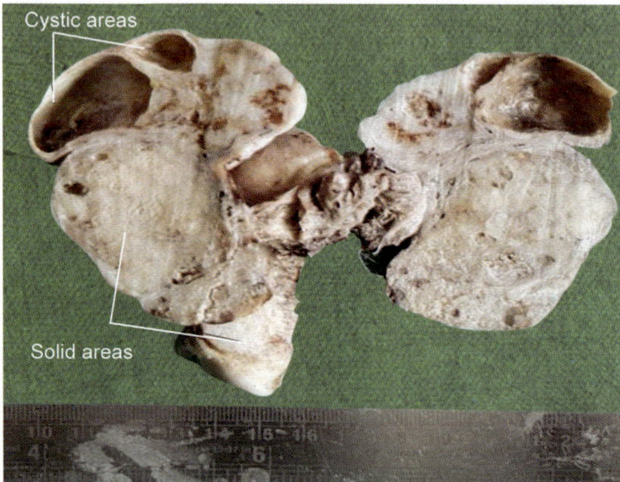

Fig. 22.30: High-grade serous carcinomas of the ovary. The tumors show both solid and cystic areas.

High-grade Serous Carcinomas

Gross (Fig. 22.30)

These tumors are **usually bilateral, large, and exophytic.** They show a **mixture of solid and cystic areas.**

Solid areas may show papillary growth. The **solid areas appear tan to white** and frequently show **areas of necrosis and hemorrhage.**

The **cysts may contain serous, turbid, or bloody fluid.** The tumor varies in size from microscopic to about 20 cm in the greatest dimension.

Bilateral: Approximately **66%** are bilateral.

Microscopy (Figs. 22.31A to C)

Wide range of complex architectural growth patterns: Various growth patterns in high-grade serous carcinomas include **solid, papillary, labyrinthine (with slit-like spaces), lacelike, glandular, or cribriform architecture.** The most characteristic patterns are:

- **Fine, disorderly papillae** with little or no stromal support
- **Solid masses of tumor cells with irregular, often slit-like, rounded, or microcystic glandular lumina.**

High-grade cytological features throughout tumor cells show marked cytologic atypia. The tumor cells may become undifferentiated and the serous features may not be evident on microscopic examination.

- **Nuclear features:** Tumor cells show **nuclear atypia, pleomorphism, and hyperchromatic nuclei.**
- **Numerous mitotic figures including atypical mitotic figures.**
- **Necrosis and large bizarre or multinucleated giant cells.**

Widespread invasion or frank effacement of the underlying stroma.

Psammoma bodies: These are concentric calcifications observed in most serous tumors. However, they are not specific for neoplasia.

Serous tubal intraepithelial carcinomas: The tumor cells appear similar to high-grade serous carcinomas but do not show invasion.

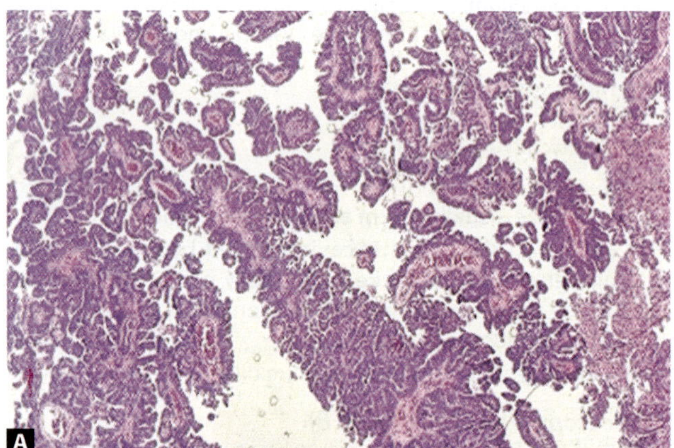

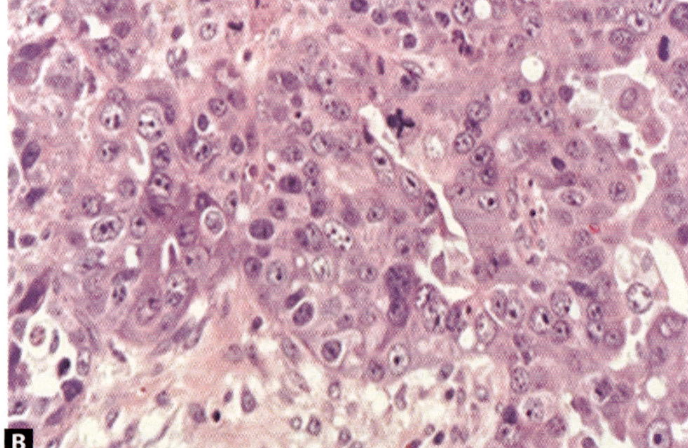

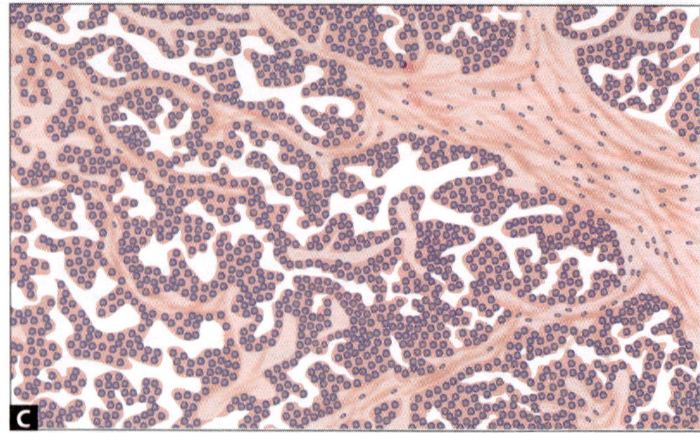

Figs. 22.31A to C: High-grade serous carcinomas: (A) Disorderly papillae with budding. The papillae are without stromal support; (B) Solid growth pattern with marked cytologic atypia and high mitotic activity; (C) Diagrammatic appearance.

Refer online **Table 22.2** for the molecular basis of the classification of serous carcinoma.

Spread of Ovarian Serous Carcinoma

Local spread: Both low- and high-grade carcinomas may spread to the peritoneal surfaces and omentum and are commonly associated with ascites. The extent of their spread outside the ovary determines the stage of the disease. It may spread to the following sites:

- **Umbilical metastasis ("sister Mary Joseph's nodule")** (*refer* page 610 and **Fig. 18.20**)
- Spread to **contralateral (opposite) ovary**
- Abdominal viscera (bowel, liver, spleen)

Lymphatic spread: It may spread to para-aortic and pelvic lymph nodes.

Hematogenous spread: To liver and lung

Prognosis: It depends on the histologic appearance of the tumor and the presence and extent of peritoneal disease.

Mucinous Tumors

Q. Describe the gross and microscopy of mucinous tumors of the ovary.

Primary ovarian mucinous tumors include benign mucinous cystadenomas, mucinous borderline tumors, and malignant mucinous carcinomas.

Incidence

- Mucinous tumors are **less common than serous tumors.** These are the second most common type of surface epithelial tumor and form about **20–25% of all ovarian neoplasms.**
- About **80% are benign, 10% borderline,** and about **10% are malignant**. Primary ovarian mucinous carcinomas are uncommon and account for less than 3% of all ovarian cancers.
- **Age group:** It is seen mainly during **middle adult life** and is rare before puberty and after menopause.

Main differences between mucinous and serous tumors of the ovary: These are as follows:

- The neoplastic epithelium is composed of mucin-secreting cells and the cyst contains mucinous material.
- Mucinous tumors are larger and multicystic (multiloculated). It shows hundreds to thousands of small cysts filled with sticky; gelatinous mucinous fluid rich in glycoproteins.
- Mucinous tumors are less likely to be malignant. The malignant component may be very focal.
- **Less bilateral:** Only 5% of mucinous cystadenomas and mucinous cystadenocarcinomas are bilateral.
- **Lack of ovarian surface involvement.**

Molecular Pathogenesis

- **Risk factor: Smoking.**
- ***KRAS* mutations:** *KRAS* is a proto-oncogene and may undergo mutation to form an oncogene. This **may occur early** and may be **observed in benign, borderline,** and **primary ovarian mucinous carcinomas.**

Morphological Features

The morphological features of benign, borderline, and malignant mucinous tumors are discussed below.

Q. Write a short note on the morphology of mucinous tumors of the ovary.

MORPHOLOGY

Benign Mucinous Cystadenoma (Figs. 22.32A and B)

Gross

- Usually **unilateral** (95%)
- **Large:** They measure from a few centimeters to >30 cm (even up to 50 cm and the mean size is 10 cm).
- **Multilocular**, thin-walled cysts with smooth outer surface.
- **Cyst content: Sticky semisolid mucinous** material.

Microscopy (Figs. 22.33A to C)

Many cysts and glands: The tumors are composed of many cysts and glands.

Type of lining epithelium: The epithelial lining may be gastric foveolar type/intestinal type or endocervical type.

- **Gastric foveolar-type, or intestinal epithelium (Fig. 22.33A):** Most tumors are lined by **simple nonstratified mucinous epithelium** resembling gastric foveolar type/intestinal type of epithelium. These cells have **bland, basally situated, small nuclei**. They do not show cytological atypia, and there are absent or minimal mitotic activity and apoptotic bodies. They contain goblet cells and sometimes neuroendocrine cells or Paneth cells.
- **Endocervical type (Fig. 22.33C):** These mucinous tumors are lined by a **single layer of simple, endocervical-type, nonstratified mucinous epithelium**. These cells **resemble** the Müllerian type of epithelium lining **endocervical mucosa**. These cells are columnar having **apical mucin and basally situated bland nuclei**.

Stroma: The stroma adjacent to cysts may be cellular.

Accompanying tumor: A component of a dermoid cyst or Brenner tumor may be found.

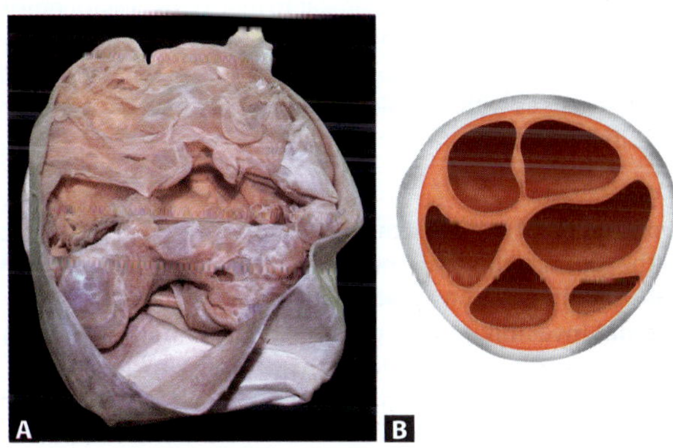

Figs. 22.32A and B: Cut section of mucinous cystadenoma of ovary: (A) Specimen; (B) Diagrammatic.

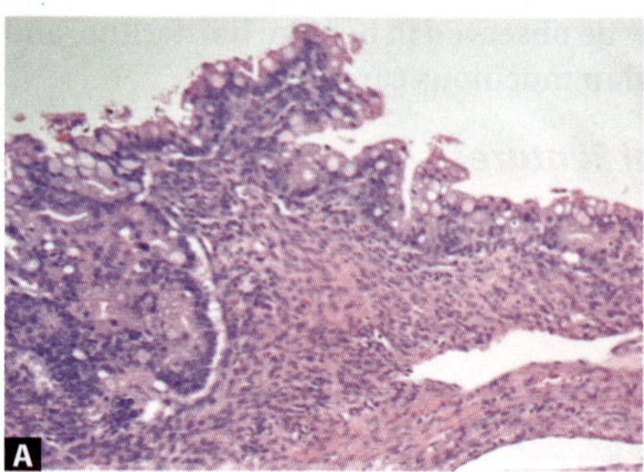

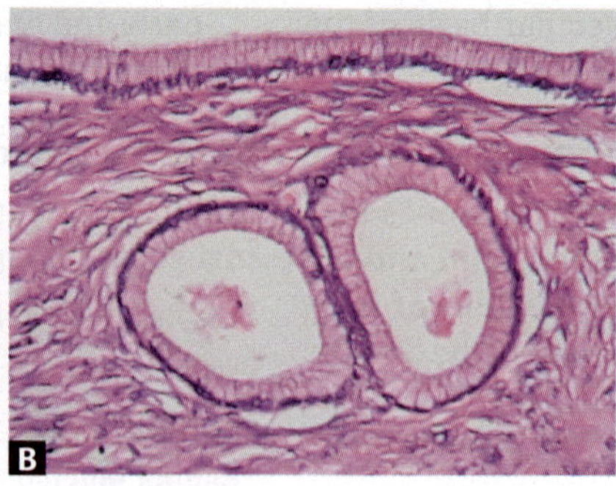

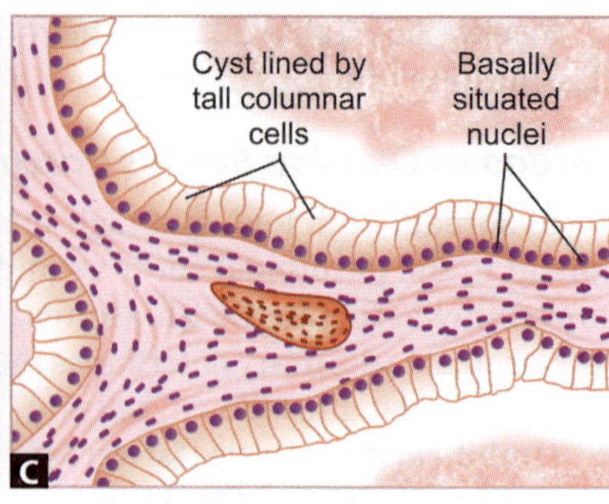

Figs. 22.33A to C: Microscopic appearance of mucinous cystadenoma of ovary: (A) Mucinous tumor lined by simple nonstratified mucinous epithelium resembling gastric foveolar type/intestinal type of epithelium. These cells have bland, basally situated, small nuclei. They also show goblet cells; (B) H& E; (C) Diagrammatic appearance of mucinous tumor with the endocervical type of epithelium. Simple cyst lined by uniform, nonstratified mucinous, columnar cells with small, bland, uniform basally situated nuclei and apical mucin.

Mucinous Borderline Tumors

Gross

Mucinous borderline tumors are unilateral (bilateral in only about 5% of cases), multiloculated tumors, and have thick cyst walls. Solid areas may be seen and should be preferentially sampled because these areas may show areas of invasion.

Microscopy (refer online Fig. 22.34)

The same criteria as borderline serous tumors are applied.

Stratification (multilayering) **of lining epithelium, budding, and tufting:** Mucinous borderline tumors contain multiple cysts and glands lined by atypical gastrointestinal-type mucinous epithelium. They are distinguished from cystadenomas by the presence of epithelium that shows variable degrees of stratification (generally to two or three layers) **and tufting** (clumping). It may show papillary intraglandular growth (appear similar to tubular adenomas or villous adenomas of the intestine).

Mild to moderate nuclear atypia: The mucinous epithelium usually shows mild-to-moderate (low-grade) nuclear atypia. Mitotic activity is typically predominantly present in crypt regions and is less prominent on the luminal surface.

Absence of stromal invasion.

Mucinous Carcinoma of the Ovary

Gross

Mucinous carcinomas are typically large, unilateral, and multiloculated cystic masses similar to mucinous cystadenomas. But they show additional **solid regions.** Solid areas may contain areas of **necrosis and hemorrhage.** The cut section shows solid and cystic areas with **mucoid contents.** They have an intact and smooth outer surface.

Microscopy

Stratification of epithelial cells and cytologic atypia: The atypical epithelium is more than four cells in thickness. Shows **loss of gland architecture and areas of necrosis.**

Stromal invasion: Mucinous carcinoma shows frank stromal invasion. There are **two different patterns of invasion:** (1) expansile (confluent) and (2) infiltrative (destructive). The expansile/confluent pattern is more common, and two patterns may coexist in the same tumor.

- **Expansile (confluent) invasive pattern** (*refer* **online Figs. 22.35A and B):** It is characterized by marked glandular crowding, with little or absent intervening stroma (confluent growth of back-to-back or almost back-to-back glands).
- **Infiltrative (destructive) pattern:** It is characterized by irregular infiltrating glands (often misshapen glands), nests, clusters, cords, and single cells with malignant cytological features, frequently with a desmoplastic stromal response.

Spread of Mucinous Carcinoma

Q. Write a short note on pseudomyxoma peritonei.

- **Peritoneal implant and local invasion**: Ruptured ovarian mucinous tumors may seed the peritoneum and invade into neighboring structures like bowel, abdominal wall, and bladder.
- **Pseudomyxoma peritonei:** It is characterized by:
  - **Extensive mucinous ascites**
  - **Stable implantation of mucinous tumor cells in the peritoneum.** The abdomen is filled with tenacious, semisolid mucin. Mostly it is caused by metastatic spread of tumors in the gastrointestinal tract, primarily the appendix.
  - **Peritoneal adhesions** can cause **intestinal obstruction.** It can also develop due to mucinous tumors of the appendix with secondary ovarian and peritoneal spread.
- **Metastases to distant organs are infrequent.**

Prognosis of mucinous carcinoma: It is a little better than that of its serous counterpart.

Endometrioid Ovarian Tumors

- Endometrioid tumors of the ovary include benign endometrioid tumors, borderline endometrioid and endometrioid cancers.
- **Benign** endometrioid tumors (endometrioid adenofibromas) and **borderline** endometrioid tumors **are rare.** The majority of endometrioid tumors of the ovary are **endometrioid carcinomas** and account for

approximately 20% of all ovarian cancers. Hence, only endometrioid carcinoma of the ovary is discussed below.

- These tumors may be solid or cystic.
- Microscopically, endometrioid tumors **show tubular glands resembling benign or malignant endometrium, within the lining of cystic spaces.**

Pathogenesis of Endometrioid Carcinoma

- About **15–20%** of cases, endometrioid **carcinoma develop in association with endometriosis.**
- About **15–20%** are **accompanied by carcinoma of the endometrium.**
- **Molecular changes in endometrioid carcinoma:** They are similar to endometrioid endometrial carcinoma and show frequent mutations in the PTEN tumor-suppressor gene and mismatch DNA repair genes. TP53 mutations are common in poorly differentiated tumors.

MORPHOLOGY

Endometrioid Carcinoma

Gross

- Size varies from 2–30 cm.
- **Most are solid** and exhibit necrotic areas, but some may show a combination of solid and cystic areas.
- **Usually unilateral** and bilateral in about 20% of cases

Microscopy

Show **glandular patterns resembling endometrial origin.** They are graded similarly to endometrial adenocarcinomas (*refer* page 813).

Brenner Tumor

Q. Write a short note on Brenner tumor of the ovary.

Brenner tumors contain neoplastic **epithelial cells resembling urothelium**. The epithelial cell type is characterized by a relatively uniform population of **stratified cells with ovoid nuclei showing nuclear grooves.** They may be benign, borderline, or malignant. **Nearly all are benign Brenner tumors.** Borderline and malignant forms are very uncommon.

Benign Brenner Tumor

It is a benign ovarian tumor composed of nests of bland **transitional/urothelial epithelium within a background of the dense fibromatous stroma.**

Age: It occurs at all ages, and 50% of cases are present in women over the age of 50.

MORPHOLOGY

Gross

- May be **predominantly solid or rarely may be cystic.**
- **Usually unilateral** (approximately 90%).
- **Vary in size** from small lesions >1 cm in diameter to massive tumors up to 20–30 cm.

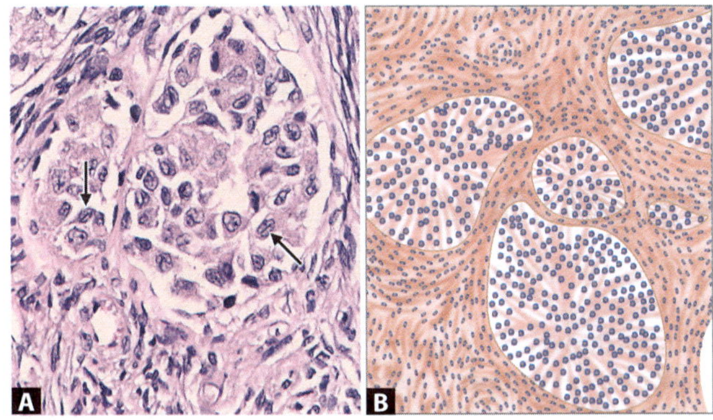

Figs. 22.36A and B: Brenner tumor: (A) H&E and (B) Diagrammatic. Microscopically showing nests of transitional-type cells separated by fibrous stroma. The tumor cells have nuclear grooves resembling coffee bean (arrow).

Microscopy (Figs. 22.36A and B)

- Brenner tumor shows nests of **bland epithelial cells resembling** the **epithelium of the urinary tract** (urothelium) **separated by fibrous stroma**, resembling that of the normal ovary.
- The **nuclei of epithelial cells show nuclear grooves** resembling **coffee-bean.**

Clinical Presentation of Surface Epithelial Tumors

Clinical manifestations of all ovarian carcinomas are similar. Ovarian tumors rarely produce symptoms until they become large and distend the abdomen. Benign tumors are most common and may be asymptomatic.

- May be unilateral or bilateral.
- Most tumors are nonfunctional and produce only mild symptoms. The most common symptoms are:
  - **Lower abdominal pain and distention/enlargement.**
  - **Due to compression produced by the tumor,** for example, urinary frequency, dysuria, and gastrointestinal tract symptoms
- Most **malignant ovarian tumors** are detected when they spread outside the ovary. Symptoms include:
  - **Progressive weakness, weight loss, and cachexia.**
  - **Massive ascites** due to cancer invasion are common and **ascitic fluid may show exfoliated tumor cells.**
  - **Metastasis:**
    - Regional nodes are often involved.
    - Hematogenous metastasis to the liver, lungs, gastrointestinal tract, and elsewhere.
    - Across the midline to the opposite ovary.

Biochemical Markers of Surface Epithelial Tumors

- **CA-125:** It is a high-molecular-weight glycoprotein **present in the serum of about 80% of patients with serous and endometrioid carcinomas.** It is **not a reliable marker** because it can be elevated with nonspecific irritation of the peritoneum (e.g., endometriosis, inflammation).

- **Osteopontin:** It is expressed at **higher levels** in ovarian cancer patients.

GERM CELL TUMORS

Q. Classify ovarian germ cell tumors. Describe germ cell tumors of the ovary.

Tumors derived from germ cells constitute about **25–30% of all ovarian tumors.** They are similar to germ cell tumors in the testis. Germ cell tumors include multiple subtypes (*refer* **online Flowchart 22.1**).

- **In adult women:** Most (95%) germ cell tumors are **benign** (mature cystic teratoma, dermoid cyst).
- **In children and young adults:** The most common is **malignant tumor.**

WHO (2020) Classification of germ cell tumors of the ovary is presented in **Box 22.7.**

Teratomas

Q. Write a short note on the teratoma of the ovary.

Teratoma is a tumor of germ cell origin. They contain **mature or immature cells or tissues representative of more than one germ cell layer** (at least two) and sometimes all three embryonic layers. These **cells or tissues are arranged in a helter-skelter fashion** (disorganized).

Origin of Teratoma

Primordial germ cell: Teratomas are believed to originate from the primordial germ cell. It is the primary undifferentiated stem cell type that will differentiate toward gametes: spermatozoa or oocytes.

Karyotype of 46,XX: The karyotype of almost all benign ovarian teratomas is 46,XX.

Arise from an ovum after the first meiotic division: Genetic analyses suggest that most teratomas arise from an ovum after the first meiotic division, whereas the remainder arises before the first division.

Mature teratomas develop by parthenogenesis: Parthenogenesis is a form of reproduction in which an egg can develop into an embryo without being fertilized by a sperm. Haploid (postmeiotic) germ cells duplicate to produce diploid genetically female tumor cells (46, XX).

Classification: According to WHO (2020), teratomas are divided into three categories **(Box 22.7).** More than 90% of teratomas are benign.

1. **Mature (benign) teratoma:** It consists of all **well-differentiated component** parts derived from two or three germ layers (ectoderm, mesoderm, and endoderm). Depending on the gross feature, they are further categorized as:
   - **Cystic** (mature cystic teratoma)
   - **Solid** (mature solid teratoma).
2. **Immature (malignant) teratoma:** It consists of **less well-differentiated or immature elements.**
3. **Monodermal teratoma and somatic-type tumors arising from a dermoid cyst."**

BOX 22.7: WHO (2020) Classification of germ cell tumors of the ovary.

Teratoma
- Mature teratoma of the ovary
- Immature teratoma of the ovary
- Monodermal teratomas and somatic-type tumors arising from a dermoid cyst
  - Struma ovarii, NOS
  - Struma ovarii, malignant
  - Ovarian carcinoid (strumal carcinoid)

Dysgerminoma
Yolk sac tumor
Embryonal carcinoma
Non-gestational choriocarcinoma
Mixed germ cell tumor of the ovary
Germ cell sex cord-stromal tumors

Mature (Benign) Teratomas

Q. Write a short note on dermoid cyst/benign cystic teratoma of the ovary.

A mature teratoma is a tumor **composed exclusively of mature somatic tissues derived from two or three germ layers** (ectoderm, mesoderm, and/or endoderm). Most contain mature tissues derived from at least two germ cell layers. These tumors **account for 20% of all ovarian neoplasms.**

- **Dermoid cyst: Most benign ovarian teratomas are cystic.** They are usually referred to as **dermoid cysts** (mature cystic teratoma) because they are almost always **lined by skin-like structures.**
- **Age group:** Usually detected in **young women** during the active reproductive years with a peak incidence in the **third decade.**
- Clinically they may be discovered incidentally. The karyotype of benign ovarian teratomas is 46,XX.

Q. Write a short answer on the morphology of benign cystic teratoma.

MORPHOLOGY

About 90% of benign teratomas are unilateral. They more commonly affect the right ovary. They may be solid or cystic.

Mature Cystic Teratoma (Dermoid Cyst)

Gross (Figs. 22.37A and B)

- Most mature teratomas are **usually 5–10 cm in diameter**
- **Appearance:** It is usually a **unilocular, thick-walled cystic tumor** with a smooth, shiny outer surface.

Cut section

- Unilocular cyst contains **yellow or gray, buttery, or cheesy sebaceous material** with a variable amount of **matted** (twisted) **hair.**

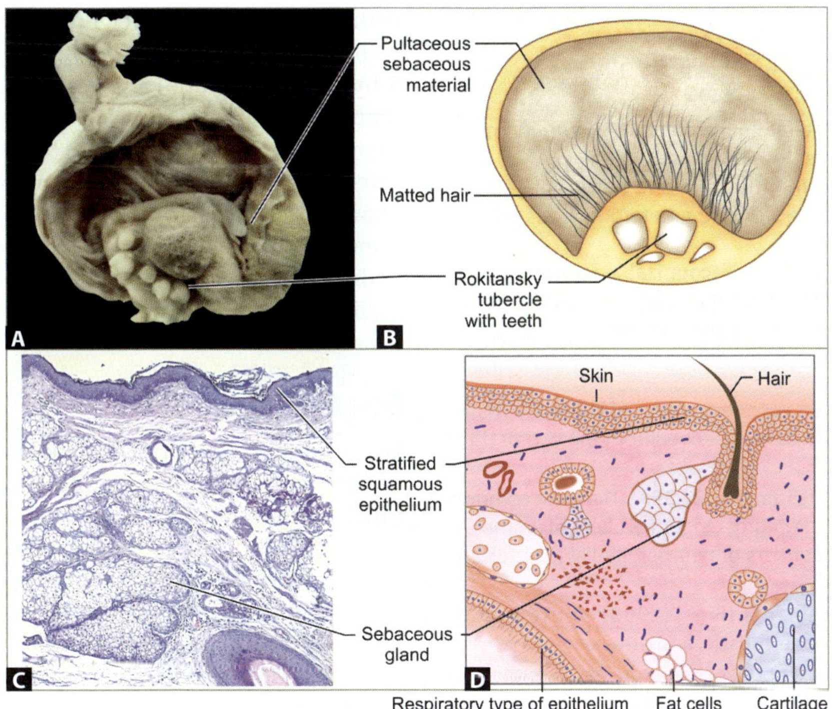

Figs. 22.37A to D: (A and B) Opened mature cystic teratoma (dermoid cyst) of the ovary; (C) Photomicrograph; (D) Diagrammatic appearance of dermoid cyst of the ovary.

- **Cyst is lined** by an opaque, gray-white, **wrinkled epidermis,** frequently with protruding hair shafts.
- **Tooth** and **areas of calcification** are common.
- **Rokitansky nodules/protuberance**: Sometimes, cystic teratomas show one or more **foci** of rounded **nodular** structure/s, **covered with hair protruding into the lumen** of the cyst. These are known as **Rokitansky nodules (protuberance),** mammillary body (**tubercle), or** dermoid **nipples.** Teeth tend to be located at this site and may protrude into the cystic cavity. It shows the greatest variety of tissue types from all three germ cell layers.

Microscopy (Figs. 22.37C and D)

- **Main differentiation along the ectodermal line:** These tumors mainly show differentiation along the ectodermal line. The **cyst wall consists of skin** (stratified squamous epithelium) **with skin appendages** (sebaceous glands, hair shafts, and other skin adnexal structures).
- **Structures from all three germ layers (*refer* Table 21.1):** In most cases, structures from all three germ layers can be identified, which include:
  - Ectoderm (e.g., skin, neural tissue, glia)
  - Mesoderm (e.g., smooth muscle, cartilage, bone, fat)
  - Endoderm (e.g., respiratory tract epithelium, gut, thyroid)

If Rokitansky protuberance is present, it usually contains tissue elements of all three germ cell layers. It is composed of adult-type tissue that represents all three germ layers.

Solid Teratoma

Rarely, mature (benign) teratoma can be solid with mature tissues derived from two or three germ layers. On gross examination, these tumors are difficult to differentiate from malignant, immature teratomas.

Complications of Benign Cystic Teratoma

Sometimes, teratomas may produce the following complications:

1. **Infertility**
2. **Torsion** in about 10–15% of cases: It constitutes an acute surgical emergency.
3. **Limbic encephalitis:** It may develop as a **rare paraneoplastic complication** with **teratomas containing mature neural tissue**. It usually resolves with the removal of the tumor. It is an autoimmune disorder and can also develop with certain other tumors, most commonly small cell carcinoma of the lung.

Malignant transformation: In about 1% of cases, malignant transformation, usually can occur. They tend to occur in older women and include **squamous cell carcinoma, thyroid carcinoma, melanoma,** basal cell carcinoma, and carcinoid tumor.

Immature (Malignant Teratomas)

Immature teratoma is a teratoma **containing immature and variable amounts of mature tissues derived from the three germ layers**. They differ from mature (benign) cystic teratomas in that the **component tissues resemble embryonal and immature fetal tissue.** Immature teratomas are rare tumors of the ovary. They are rapidly growing malignant tumors.

- **Age:** Mostly found in **prepubertal adolescents** and **young women**. The mean age is 18 years.

MORPHOLOGY

Gross (*refer* online Figs. 22.38A and B)

- **Usually, unilateral.**
- Immature (malignant) teratomas are **large, bulky,** round, ovoid tumors **with smooth external surfaces.**
- **Cut section: Predominantly solid** and has lobulated and **variegated appearance** showing a heterogeneous mixture of various tissues.
- Solid areas may show **grossly recognizable immature bone and cartilage, hair, sebaceous material, and calcification.**
- It shows **areas of hemorrhage and necrosis.**

Microscopy

Immature tissues: It shows varying amounts of immature tissues **mixed with some mature tissues** derived from the two or three germ layers.

- **Immature neuroepithelium (Fig. 22.39A):** The most common immature element is the neuroectodermal element (immature neuroepithelium). It consists of neuroepithelial rosettes and immature glia.
- **Other immature elements (Fig. 22.39B)**: These include immature cartilage, bone, muscle, and others.

Grading: It is based on the amount of immature neuroepithelium. The risk of metastasis depends on the proportion of the tumor that comprises immature neuroepithelium.

Monodermal Teratomas and Somatic-type Tumors Arising from a Dermoid Cyst

Q. Write short note on struma ovarii.

Monodermal (specialized teratomas) are rare tumors composed entirely of one tissue type. The most common among these are struma ovarii and carcinoid.

Struma ovarii: It is a cystic lesion composed entirely or predominantly of mature thyroid tissue (*refer* **online Figs. 22.40A and B**). These thyroidal neoplasms may hyperfunction and may lead to hyperthyroidism.

Ovarian carcinoid: It is a **well-differentiated neuroendocrine tumor** (NET) that resembles those occurring in the gastrointestinal tract. Probably arises from intestinal epithelium in a teratoma. They may be functional (producing 5-hydroxytryptamine) and result in carcinoid syndrome. Rarely, **strumal carcinoids** may occur in an ovary that shows a combination of struma ovarii (with thyroid follicles) and carcinoids in the same ovary. Most ovarian carcinoid is seen in postmenopausal (mean age: 53 years) women.

Somatic neoplasms arising from teratomas (teratoma with malignant transformation): They may be benign or malignant tumors arising from any of the elements within a teratoma.

Dysgerminoma

Dysgerminoma is a **primitive malignant germ cell tumor** of the ovary composed of **cells showing no specific differentiation**.

Dysgerminoma is the **ovarian counterpart of the seminoma of the testis**. It is the most common malignant germ cell tumor. It accounts for **about 2% of ovarian cancers** and roughly **50% of malignant ovarian germ cell tumors.**

- **Age group**: Dysgerminoma most commonly (75%) occurs in adolescents and young women in the second and third decades of life.
- **Predisposing factors**: These include **gonadal (ovarian) dysgenesis** (including pseudohermaphroditism), Turner syndrome, testicular feminization, and triple X syndrome.
- **Functional characteristics: Most do not show endocrine function.**

Pathogenesis: In 80% of dysgerminomas, chromosome 12 abnormalities are seen, typically, either an isochromosome 12p or 12p amplification (overexpression). In 30–50% of dysgerminomas, ***KIT*** **mutation** is present, and ***KIT*** **amplification** in 30% of patients. Like seminomas, dysgerminomas **express transcription factors, namely Oct3, Oct4, and Nanog**. These are responsible for pluripotency.

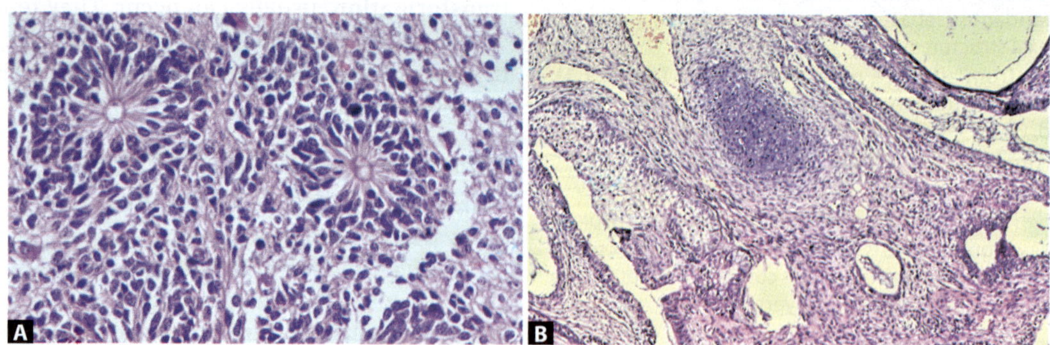

Figs. 22.39A and B: Immature teratoma of the ovary: (A) Immature neuroepithelium consisting of primitive neuroectodermal rosettes and masses. The rosettes are composed of mitotically active hyperchromatic cells with an increased nuclear–cytoplasmic (N:C) ratio; (B) Mesodermal elements, namely fetal-type cartilage, and fibrous tissue in the center. It also shows endodermal fetal-type epithelium elements such as respiratory and gastrointestinal epithelium.

MORPHOLOGY

Q. Write a short note on the morphology of dysgerminoma.

Gross

- Usually **unilateral** (80–90%)
- **Size: Varies** with a mean **diameter of 15 cm.**
- **Appearance:** These are **solid, firm, round to oval, encapsulated** tumors. **The external surface is smooth, nodular**, and **convoluted/bosselated.**
- **Cut section [Fig. 22.41B (*refer* online Fig. 22.41A)]: Soft, fleshy,** and uniformly **yellow-white to gray-pink (cream-colored).**

Microscopy (Figs. 22.42A to C)

Dysgerminoma is similar to testicular seminoma. It has a microscopic appearance identical to a seminoma.

Pattern: The tumor cells are arranged in **sheets, groups, cords, or nests** separated by **scant fibrous stroma.**

Tumor cells: They **resemble primordial germ cells** with the following characteristics:

- **Monotonous tumor cells**: Individual tumor cells are **monotonous (uniform).** They are **large, round to polygonal with well-defined cell membranes.**
- **Abundant cytoplasm:** These cells have **abundant clear to finely granular glycogen-filled** and sometimes fine droplets of fat.
- **Large nuclei:** They are **large, regular,** and **centrally placed nuclei** with **fine reticular chromatin.** It contains **one or more prominent nucleoli.**
- **Mitotic figures** are usually **common.**

Stroma: Similar to seminoma, the nests of tumor cells are separated by scant (thin) fibrous stroma, sometimes by broad bands of collagen. The **fibrous stroma is infiltrated by mature lymphocytes** (most are of T-cell type) (lymphocyte-rich fibrous stroma).

Spread

- **Local spread:** Dysgerminoma can spread into the peritoneal cavity and is associated with a decreased survival rate.
- **Lymphatic spread:** Through lymphatics, it spreads commonly to the contralateral ovary and retroperitoneal nodes.
- **Blood spread:** It can spread to the lungs.

Prognosis: All dysgerminomas are **malignant**. Dysgerminoma is treated surgically, and 5-year survival for patients with stage I is almost 100%. The tumor is **highly radiosensitive** and **responsive to chemotherapy**.

Yolk Sac Tumor

Yolk sac tumor is a **highly malignant primitive germ cell tumor** that is derived from undifferentiated and multipotential malignant germ cells. Commonly, it shows **endodermal extraembryonal differentiation** (secondary yolk sac and allantois) or, less commonly, endodermal somatic tissues (intestine, liver, and mesenchyme).

- Yolk sac tumor (also known as endodermal sinus tumor) is the **second most common malignant tumor of germ cell** tumor. Tumor is **rich** in **α-fetoprotein and α_1-antitrypsin**. They are **often a component of mixed germ cell tumors.**

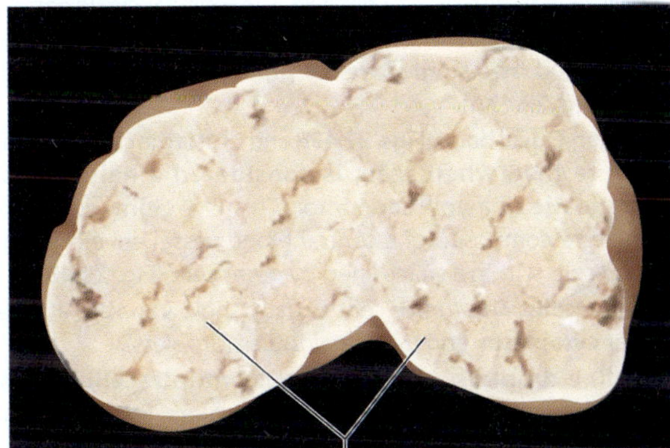

Fig. 22.41B: Dysgerminoma of the ovary: Diagrammatic appearance.

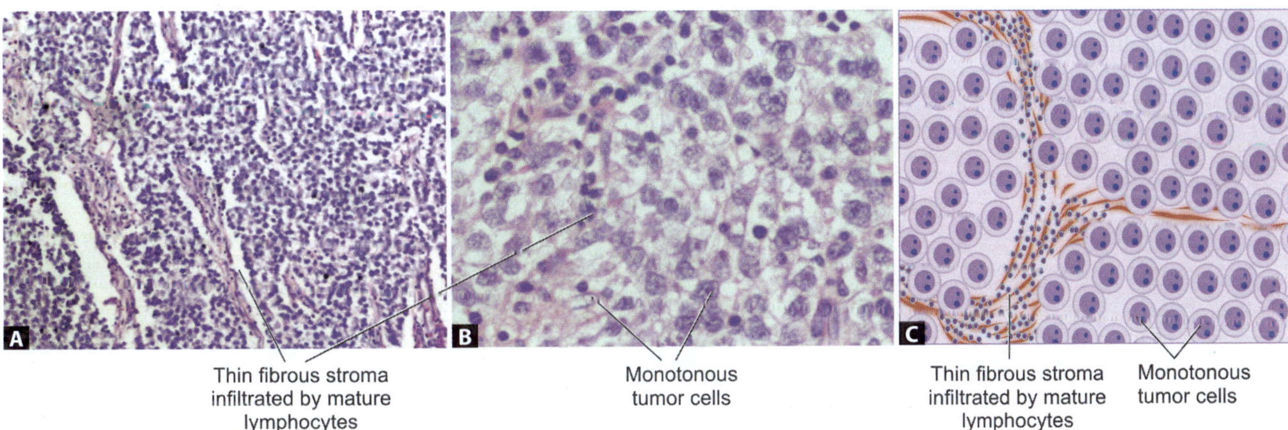

Figs. 22.42A to C: Dysgerminoma of ovary: (A) Low magnification; (B) High magnification—shows nests of polyhedral tumor cells with clear cytoplasm and centrally placed reticular nuclei. The adjacent thin, scanty fibrous stroma separating the tumor cells is infiltrated by lymphocytes; (C) Diagrammatic appearance.

❖ **Age:** It occurs in **children or young women** under the age of 30.

MORPHOLOGY

Sites: Yolk sac tumor, either **pure or combined** with other neoplastic germ cell elements, occurs in the **ovary and testis.** It may also arise in **extragonadal locations** where germ cell tumors are known to occur. These include the mediastinum, sacrococcygeal region, pineal gland, and vagina.

Gross

Usually **unilateral and solid** often contain cysts. It is typically **large, with an average size of 15 cm.** The external surface is usually smooth and glistening. It is round, ovoid, or globular and encapsulated.

Cut surface: It shows a **soft, friable, yellow-to-gray** tumor with **extensive areas of necrosis and hemorrhage.** It may be associated with other germ cell components (e.g., dermoid cyst, dysgerminoma). The presence of other neoplastic germ cell elements may alter the gross appearance of the tumor.

Microscopy

- **Patterns:** Yolk sac tumor usually shows **various** (multiple/wide ranges of) histologic **patterns.** The most **common pattern is the reticular/microcystic pattern.** The reticular cystic pattern consists of a **loose meshwork of anastomosing spaces and cysts lined by a single layer of primitive epithelial tumor cells (Fig. 22.43A).**
- **Schiller–Duval body (Figs. 22.43B and C):** It is the characteristic feature that, **when seen, is considered a hallmark or diagnostic** of a yolk sac tumor. This is a glomerulus-like structure composed of a central blood vessel enveloped by germ cells within a space lined by germ cells **(Fig. 22.43).**
- **Tumor cells:** The tumor cells usually show **variable atypia, clear cytoplasm,** and hyaline globules (droplets).
- **Hyaline droplets:** All show prominent **intracellular and extracellular PAS-positive hyaline droplets.** Some of these may stain for α-fetoprotein by immunoperoxidase techniques.

Tumor Marker

❖ **α-fetoprotein and α1-antitrypsin** in tumor cells by immunohistochemistry
❖ α-fetoprotein in the serum.

Prognosis: Yolk sac tumors grow rapidly and may spread outside the ovary. Once it was considered as uniformly fatal. However, with combination chemotherapy, the 5-year survival rate is more than 80%, independent of the disease stage.

Nongestational Choriocarcinoma of Ovary

Nongestational choriocarcinoma is a malignant tumor composed of cytotrophoblast and syncytiotrophoblast, which is not of gestational origin.

Choriocarcinoma in females may be:

- **Gestational:** More common of **placental origin.**
- **Nongestational:** Germ cell origin can be confirmed only in the prepubertal girl. This is because after puberty the origin of an ovarian, ectopic pregnancy cannot be ruled out.

Pure choriocarcinomas of the ovary are **extremely rare** and most **coexist with other germ-cell tumors.**

MORPHOLOGY

Gross: Solid with large areas of hemorrhage

Microscopy: Similar to gestational choriocarcinoma (*refer* page 838) and **consists of cytotrophoblast and syncytiotrophoblast without any villi.**

❖ **Behavior: Aggressive tumors** generally **metastasize through the bloodstream** to the **lungs, liver, bone,** and other viscera at the time of diagnosis.
❖ **Tumor marker:** These tumors **secrete high levels of chorionic gonadotropins (hCG)** which help in diagnosis or detecting recurrences.
❖ **Prognosis:** In contrast to gestational, these nongestational types generally do not respond to chemotherapy and are **fatal.**

Other Germ Cell Tumors

❖ **Embryonal carcinoma: Highly malignant** tumor of primitive embryonal elements, similar to that of testes.
❖ **Mixed germ cell tumors:** They show various combinations of dysgerminoma, teratoma, endodermal sinus tumor, and choriocarcinoma.

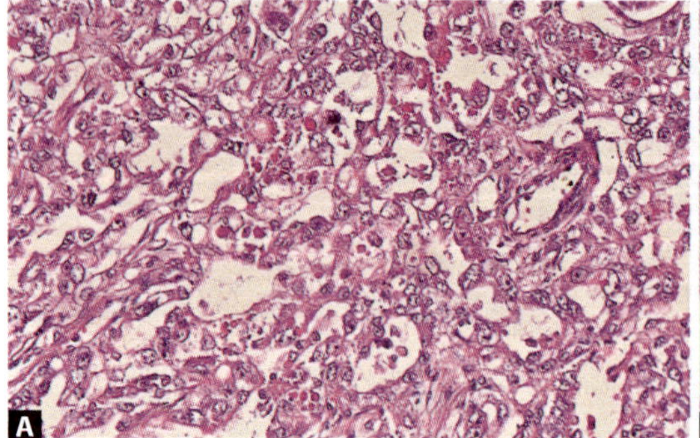

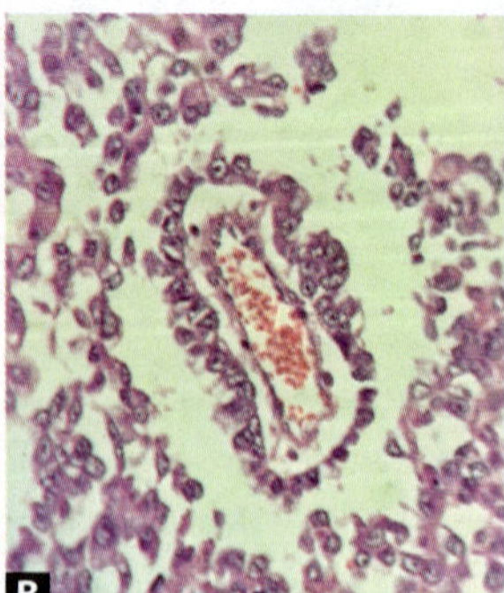

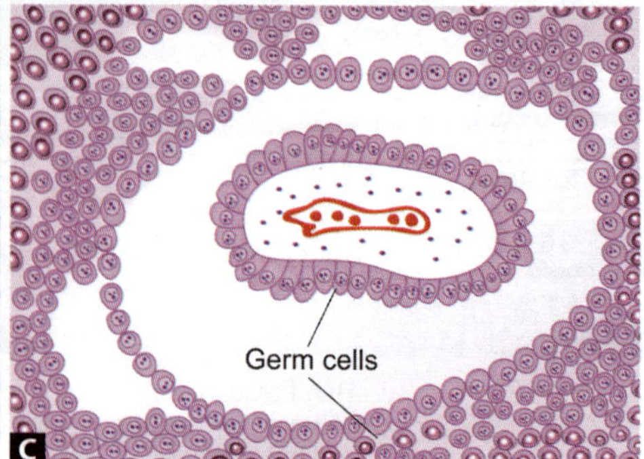

Figs. 22.43A to C: Yolk sac tumor: (A) Reticular cystic pattern composed of a loose meshwork of anastomosing spaces and cysts lined by a single layer of primitive epithelial tumor cells. There are few hyaline globules; (B) Yolk-sac tumor showing characteristic glomerulus-like structure known as Schiller–Duval body. This is composed of a central blood vessel enveloped by germ cells within a space lined by germ cells; (C) The diagrammatic appearance of Schiller–Duval body.

SEX CORD-STROMAL TUMORS

Sex cord-stromal tumors account for about 6–10% of all ovarian tumors.

Origin: Sex cord-stromal tumors originate from **either primitive sex cords** (which arise from the epithelium of the two gonadal ridges) **or from the mesenchymal stroma of developing gonads.** Thus, the term sex cord-stromal tumors **includes the neoplasms that contain elements of derivatives of either or both the sex cords and the stroma of the embryonic gonad.**

- **Sex cord derivatives:** The **undifferentiated gonadal mesenchyme** produces specific types of cells **in female (granulosa and theca) and male (Sertoli and Leydig) gonads.**
- **Stromal derivatives:** The components derived from the **stroma have the appearance of cellular gonadal stroma or** its specialized derivatives, namely the **theca and Leydig cells.**

Functioning tumors: Some of these cells of sex cord-stromal tumors normally secrete hormones (estrogens or androgens). Sex cord-stromal tumors are the **most common clinically functioning ovarian neoplasms.** They may be either feminizing or masculinizing.

- **Feminizing**, e.g., granulosa-theca cell tumors may secrete estrogens.
- **Masculinizing**, e.g., Leydig cell tumors may secrete androgens.

Classification: Sex cord-stromal tumors are mainly divided into (i) pure sex-cord tumors, (ii) pure stromal tumors, and (ii) mixed sex cord-stromal tumors.

Pure Sex Cord Tumors

These include all ovarian tumors composed of epithelial-type sex cord cells. These may differentiate along the female sex cord lineage (granulosa cell tumor) or along the male lineage (Sertoli and Sertoli–Leydig cell tumor).

Granulosa Cell Tumor

Q. Write a short note on the granulosa cell tumor of the ovary.

Granulosa cell tumor is a **low-grade malignant sex cord stromal tumor.** It is **composed of cells that resemble granulosa cells of a developing ovarian follicle.** It may contain a variable number of **fibroblasts and theca cells.**

- **Estrogen secretion:** It may be associated with estrogen secretion.
- **Incidence:** Account for about 1.5–5% of all ovarian tumors.
- **Subtypes:** Based mainly on the age of the patient, granulosa cell tumors are broadly divided into two morphologic types: (1) adult granulosa cell tumors and (2) juvenile granulosa cell tumors. About 95% of GCTs are of the adult type.
  - **Age group:** About two-thirds of adult granulosa cell tumors occur in **postmenopausal women.** Juvenile granulosa cell tumors occur in children and young adults.

Adult Granulosa Cell Tumor

An adult granulosa cell tumor is a tumor composed of granulosa cells admixed with a variable population of fibroblasts or theca cells. Mutations of the *FOXL2* gene are observed in 97% of adult granulosa cell tumors.

MORPHOLOGY

Gross (Figs. 22.44A and B)

- Usually, **unilateral.**
- **Size varies** from microscopic foci to large, solid, and cystic encapsulated masses.
- **Cut surface: Hormonally active tumors** have a **yellow color,** due to intracellular lipids (lipid-laden luteinized granulosa cells).

Microscopy

Adult granulosa cell tumors may be composed of only granulosa cells or, more often, an additional component of theca cells, fibroblasts, or both.

Granulosa Cell Component [Figs. 22.45B and C (refer online Fig. 22.45A)]

Tumor cells

- **Shape:** Tumor cells are **small, cuboidal to polygonal.**
- **Nuclear groove:** The nuclei of tumor cells are commonly **pale, round to oval** with an irregular nuclear membrane and **nuclear grooves (cleaved, elongated nucleus with coffee bean appearance—Fig. 22.45B inset).**
- **Cytoplasm:** They have scant cytoplasm, giving rise to a **densely cellular "blue" appearance.**

Stromal Component

- Granulosa cell tumors contain a **variable amount of fibromatous or thecomatous stroma.**
- **Reticulin stain:** It shows **reticulin fibers surrounding the nests of tumor cells,** except in stromal regions.

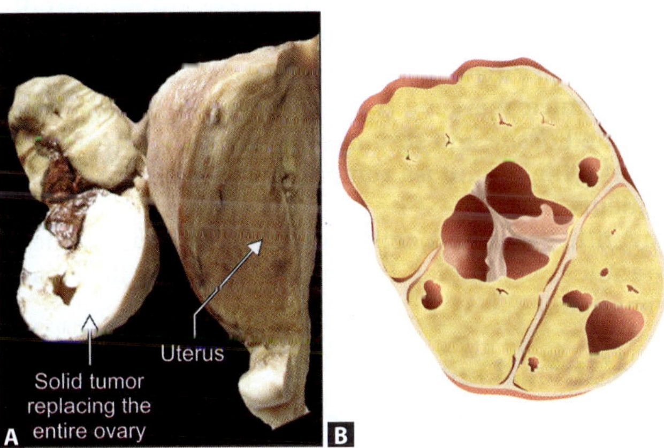

Figs. 22.44A and B: Granulosa cell tumor of the ovary: (A) The cut section shows a solid tumor in the ovary (left side) that appears soft and tan to yellow; (B) The diagrammatic appearance of granulosa cell tumor.

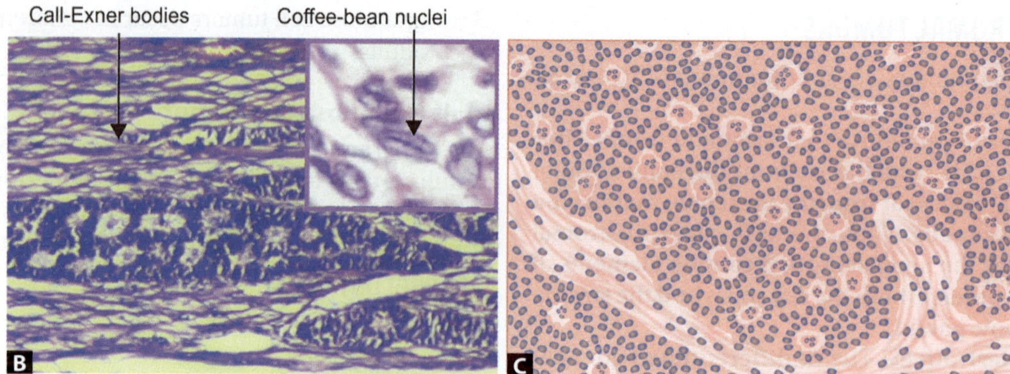

Figs. 22.45B and C: Adult granulosa cell tumor of the ovary: (B) H&E and (C) diagrammatic. Microfollicular pattern composed of tumor cells arranged in sheets punctuated by small follicle-like structures (Call–Exner bodies). The inset of Figure B shows the coffee-bean nucleus of tumor cells.

Growth Patterns

Tumors may show a variety of architectural (histologic) patterns. Common patterns are diffuse, corded to trabecular, insular (discrete islands), solid–tubular, or microfollicular.

- Diffuse (sarcomatoid) sheets are the most common pattern.
- Trabecular (anastomotic bands of granulosa cells) and insular (islands of cells in ribbons and nests) are the other common patterns.
- Microfollicular pattern: In this pattern, tumor cells surround small, distinctive, generally regular, gland-like spaces/structures (follicles/spaces) containing acidophilic material (fluid) with nuclear debris or hyalinized basement membrane-like material. They simulate the **Call–Exner bodies (Figs. 22.45B and C)** of the developing (immature) graafian follicle. **When** these well-known structures are **present, they are very useful for diagnosis.** They are **seen in a minority of tumors.**

Clinical Features

Adult granulosa cell tumors occur over a wide age range. The average age is 53 years. Typically, they present with **post-menopausal bleeding** in older women and **menorrhagia, metrorrhagia, or amenorrhea in younger patients.**

Behavior: All granulosa cell tumors are **potentially malignant** and are considered low-grade **malignant tumors** because they may spread locally as well as metastasize.

Biochemical markers: They secrete protein β-**inhibin** and **elevated tissue and serum** levels of which are useful for **identifying granulosa tumors and monitoring treated patients.**

Juvenile granulosa cell tumor is a distinctive type of granulosa cell tumor. It occurs mainly in children and young adults.

Pure Stromal Tumors

Fibromas and Thecomas

Q. Write a short note on Meigs syndrome.

Tumors arising in the ovarian stroma (pure stromal tumors) may be composed of either fibroblast **(fibromas)** or plump spindle cells with lipid droplets **(thecomas)**. They are **relatively common** and account for about 4% of all ovarian tumors. The majority of fibromas and thecomas are **benign.**

- **Fibroma:** Consists of **only fibroblasts** and are **hormonally inactive.**
- **Thecomas:** It is an ovarian stromal tumor composed predominantly of cells resembling theca cells (plump **spindle cells with lipid droplets)**. Pure thecomas are rare but **may be hormonally active.**
- **Fibrothecomas:** Many tumors contain a **mixture of fibroblasts and plump spindle cells with lipid droplets.** These are termed as fibrothecomas.

MORPHOLOGY

Fibroma

Gross

- **Unilateral** in about 90% of cases.
- Usually **solid, spherical, or slightly lobulated, encapsulated, hard, gray-white** masses covered by glistening, intact ovarian serosa (*refer* **online Fig. 22.46A**).

Microscopy

The tumor cells resemble the stroma of the normal ovarian cortex. It consists of **well-differentiated fibroblasts separated by scant collagenous connective tissue** (*refer* **online Fig. 22.46B**). The spindle cells are arranged in interlacing bundles and storiform patterns.

Thecoma

Gross

Thecomas are **unilateral solid** tumors. Cut surface is typically **solid, occasionally lobulated,** and **yellowish-tan** (owing to the many lipid-laden theca cells).

Microscopy

They are composed of theca cells in a fibromatous stroma. The theca cells appear uniform, large, and round to oval. They have **appreciable pale-gray cytoplasm** and indistinct (ill-defined) cell membranes (*refer* **online Fig. 22.46C). Oil Red O fat stains** (require fresh–frozen tissue) **highlight the intracellular lipid. The lipid appears red** (*refer* **online Fig. 22.46D).**

Clinical Features

Most fibromas come to attention as a **pelvic mass**, sometimes accompanied by pain. It may be associated with two decidedly curious syndromes: Meigs syndrome and basal cell nevus syndrome.

Meigs syndrome: It is the combination of **ovarian fibroma, hydrothorax, and ascites**. The mechanism is not known.

- **Ascites are** found in about 40% of cases when **tumors are larger than 6 cm** in diameter.
- **Uncommonly, hydrothorax** is seen usually only on the **right side**.

METASTATIC (SECONDARY) TUMORS

Ovarian metastases are malignant tumors metastasizing to the ovary from extraovarian primary sites. They constitute about 3% of ovarian tumors.

Source of Primary Tumor

- **From genital tumors:** Most common metastatic tumors are derived from tumors of the **uterus, fallopian tube**, and **contralateral (opposite) ovary**.
- **Extragenital tumors:** Most common extra-Müllerian tumors metastatic to the ovary are from **carcinomas of the breast and gastrointestinal tract** (including colon, stomach) biliary tract, and pancreas.

Routes of spread to the ovary: It depends on the primary tumor. Various routes by which a tumor can metastasize to the ovary are: (1) via direct invasion, (2) lymphovascular/hematogenous, (3) transcoelomic/transperitoneal, or (4) transtubal spread.

Gross features, which point to metastatic carcinoma: These include **bilateral ovarian involvement** and **multi-nodularity**.

Krukenberg Tumor

Q. Write a short note on the Krukenberg tumor.

Metastatic carcinoma to the ovary: Krukenberg tumors are metastatic carcinomas to the ovary **composed of signet ring cells** that comprise at least 10% of the tumor. First described by Krukenberg in 1896.

Age: Usually found between **30 and 60 years.**

Sources of primary: These are as follows:

- **Stomach** (*refer* page 611) is the most common primary site (in 75% of cases). It can spread from gastric carcinoma either by the transperitoneal or hematogenous route.
- **Large intestine, appendix**
- **Breast.**

MORPHOLOGY

Gross [Figs. 22.47A (*refer* online Fig. 22.47B)]

- Most (approximately 90%) are **bilateral.**
- **Appearance: Solid with a smooth or bosselated contour. The capsule** is **intact** and **smooth.**

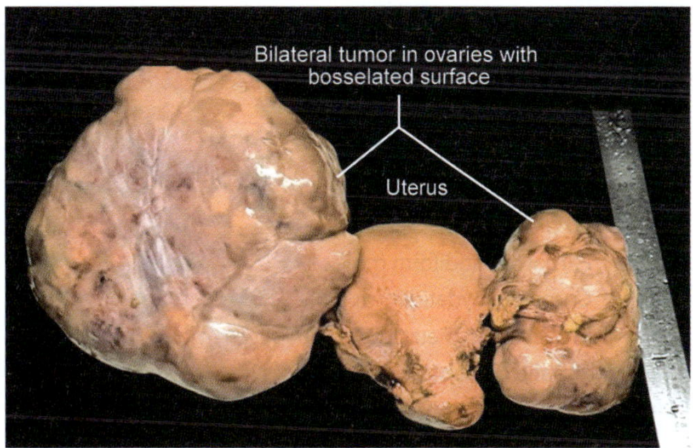

Fig. 22.47A: Krukenberg tumor: (A) Bilateral, solid ovarian tumor with a smooth or bosselated contour. The center shows the uterus.

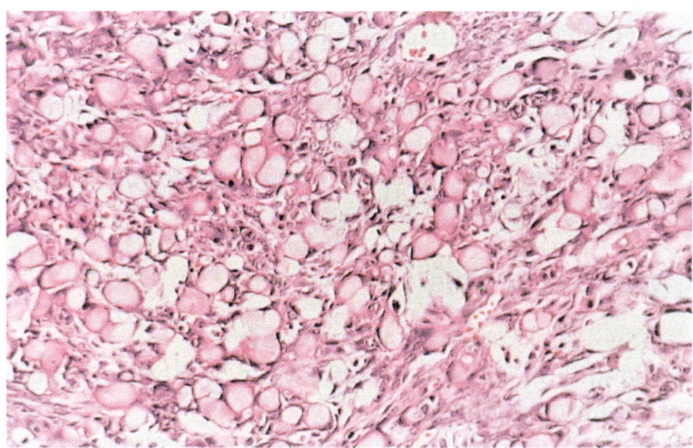

Fig. 22.48A: Krukenberg tumor: H&E showing nests of mucin-producing signet-ring cells within a cellular stroma.

- **Shape of the ovary is maintained.**
- **Cut surface:** Vary from **firm to soft and white to tan.**

Microscopy

It shows **nests of mucin-producing, signet-ring** cancer **cells surrounded by** a cellular **ovarian stroma [Figs. 22.48A** (*refer* **online Fig. 22.48B)].**

GESTATIONAL DISORDERS

GESTATIONAL TROPHOBLASTIC DISEASE

PA 30.5 (CC): Describe the etiology, pathogenesis, pathology, morphology, clinical course, spread, and complications of gestational trophoblastic neoplasms.

Q. Discuss the pathogenesis and morphology of trophoblastic disease.

Gestational trophoblastic disease (GTD) consists of a group of tumors and benign tumor-like lesions characterized by proliferation and maturation of placental tissue, either villous or trophoblastic.

BOX 22.8: WHO (2020) (abridged) classification of gestational trophoblastic disease (GTD).

Tumor-like lesions
- Non-neoplastic lesions
  - Exaggerated placental site reaction
- Molar pregnancies
  - Partial hydatidiform mole
  - Complete hydatidiform mole
  - Invasive and metastatic hydatidiform moles

Gestational trophoblastic neoplasms
- Placental site trophoblastic tumor
- Gestational choriocarcinoma

Classification

WHO (2020) classification of gestational trophoblastic disease is listed in **Box 22.8**. The major disorders include hydatidiform mole (complete and partial), invasive mole, choriocarcinoma, and placental site trophoblastic tumor (PSTT). They secret human chorionic gonadotropins (hCG) to varying degrees.

Hydatidiform Mole

Q. Write a short essay on the hydatidiform mole.

Hydatidiform moles are characterized by the **proliferation of villous trophoblasts**.

Significance: Hydatidiform mole is **important to recognize because it is associated with** an **increased risk of persistent trophoblastic disease (invasive mole) or choriocarcinoma.**

Age: It can develop at any age but is higher at the two ends of reproductive life (in **teenagers and between 40 and 50 years of age**).

Diagnosis: Usually diagnosed **during early pregnancy** (average 9 weeks) **by pelvic sonography.**

Subtypes: Depending on cytogenetic and histological features, there are two distinctive subtypes of hydatidiform moles: **complete and partial**. Invasive hydatidiform moles invade the uterine myometrium and/or uterine vasculature. Both subtypes of hydatidiform mole result from **fertilization with an excess of paternal genetic material.**

Complete Mole

Complete hydatidiform mole is an **abnormal gestation with diffuse trophoblastic proliferation** and **villous hydrops without the development of the embryo**. All cellular components show the **presence of paternal-only (androgenetic diploid) nuclear genome,** which is the fundamental etiology in most cases.

A complete hydatidiform mole is also known as a "classic" hydatidiform mole. It was traditionally described as a "hydatidiform mole" for the **grapelike structures observed at the time of evacuation**.

Q. Write a short answer on the etiopathogenesis of hydatidiform mole.

Etiology: The risk of hydatidiform mole **relates to maternal age** and shows two peaks. **Girls under 15 years** of age have a higher risk than women 20–35 years old. Risk **increases progressively for women over 40 years**. Most complete hydatidiform moles are sporadic (with a diploid paternal-only genome and maternal-only mitochondrial DNA), and familial biparental is rare.

Genetic (Molecular) Basis of Pathogenesis (Figs. 22.49A to C)

Complete mole results from **fertilization of an empty ovum** (an egg that has lost its female chromosomes and has no functional maternal DNA), **either by one or two sperm**. Thus, the **genetic material is completely paternally derived (from sperm)**, and there is a **complete absence of maternal chromosomes** (empty ovum). Complete moles are diploid (46,XX or 46,XY).

No fetal parts: Complete hydatidiform moles are not compatible with embryogenesis and do not contain fetal parts.

Diploid chorionic epithelial cells with 46,XX: All the chorionic villi are abnormal. The chorionic epithelial cells are diploid (46,XX or, uncommonly, 46,XY).

- **46,XX karyotype:** It is the **most common (~90%) karyotype, homozygous, and all 46,XX are derived from sperm.** This complete mole develops from the **fertilization of an empty egg**/ovum **by one sperm** (monospermy). The **genetic material (chromosomes) of one sperm (23,X, not 23,Y) undergoes duplication** (endoreduplication), and this phenomenon is called androgenesis. Thus, the complete mole formed has a **karyotype 46,XX** diploid pattern, all derived from sperm. It will **never have a karyotype of 46,YY.**
- **46,XX or 46,XY karyotype:** Less commonly (~10%), complete moles are **heterozygous**, formed by the **fertilization of an empty ovum** (egg) **by two sperm** (dispermy). Depending on the genetic material of the two sperms (23,X or 23,Y), the complete mole has **either karyotype 46,XX** (two sperms with 23,X) **or 46,XY** (one sperm with 23,X and other sperm with 23,Y).

In complete moles, **the embryo dies very early** in development. Hence, the **embryo is usually not identified.** These patients have a 2.5% **risk of** subsequent development of **choriocarcinoma** and a 15% risk of **persistent or invasive mole.**

MORPHOLOGY

Q. Write a short note on the morphology of hydatidiform/vesicular mole.

Localization: Commonly uterus and less commonly ectopic in the fallopian tube or ovary.

Gross

- **Larger uterus:** Classically, complete moles present as a larger uterus than expected for the gestational age.

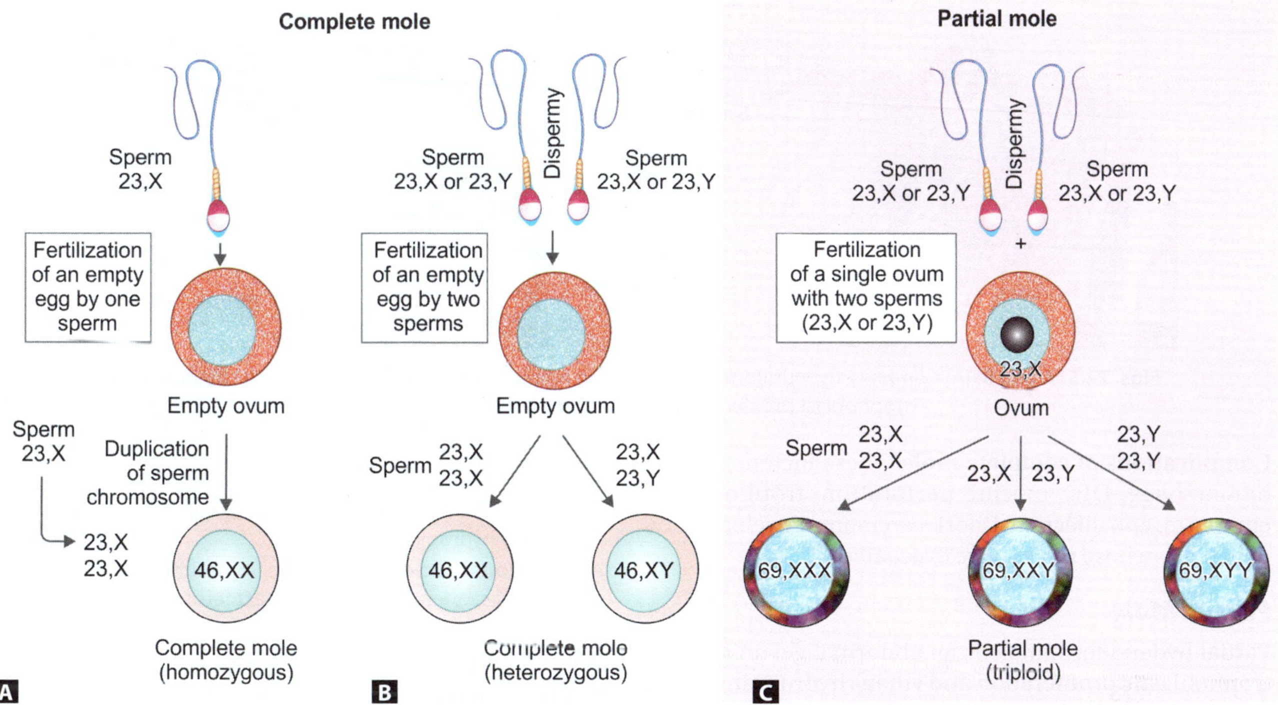

Figs. 22.49A to C: Schematic representation of the origin of complete and partial hydatidiform moles: (A) More commonly, complete moles develop from fertilization of an empty ovum by a single sperm (23,X) that undergoes duplication of its chromosomes (fertilization by single 23,Y is not compatible because its duplication results in 46,YY); (B) Less commonly, complete moles may arise from fertilization of an empty ovum by two sperms (dispermy); (C) Partial moles develop from fertilization of the single ovum by two sperms (possible combinations include: 23,X, 23,X; 23,X, 23,Y or 23,Y, 23,Y) and form partial mole with triploid karyotype.

- **"Hydatid" or grapelike appearance:** A complete hydatidiform mole represents a **placenta** with **grossly swollen, edematous (hydropic) chorionic villi. Hydropic chorionic villi appear delicate** and form **friable thin-walled, semitranslucent, cystic vesicles of variable sizes.** They resemble **bunches of grapes [Figs. 22.50A** (*refer* **online Fig. 22.50B)].**
- **Absence of fetal parts or normal placental structures**

Microscopy of Complete Mole (Figs. 22.51A and B)

1. **Diffuse villous hydrops and marked trophoblastic hyperplasia:** The villous hydropic changes **involve all chorionic villi.** These are the hallmarks of a well-developed complete mole.
2. **Hydropic, poorly vascularized, acellular, and enlarged villi:** Characteristics of villi are as follows:
   - **Significant increase in the size of villi.**
   - **Enlarged with irregular shape:** Individual chorionic villi are **round, oval, or irregular** (scalloped). They are **edematous, and enlarged.**
   - **Edematous acellular stroma of villi:** The **central areas** of the **villi** show loose, myxomatous, **extensively edematous stroma.** It frequently **forms cystic acellular, fluid-filled spaces** (central villous cavitation/cisterns/cisternae). The stroma is **acellular without cellular components** (lack mesenchymal cells). They occupy at least 50% of the villous stromal area
   - **Poorly vascularized chorionic villi.**

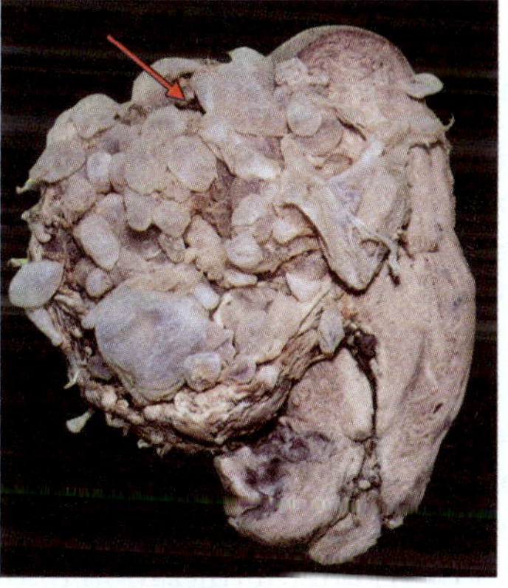

Fig. 22.50A: Specimen.

3. **Trophoblast proliferation**
   - **Irregular-to-diffuse, marked trophoblastic proliferation: The extensive trophoblast proliferation involves all or a significant portion of chorionic villi.** The trophoblastic hyperplasia is **nonpolar, multifocal, and frequently involves the entire circumference of the villi.**
   - Trophoblast consists of **intermediate trophoblast admixed with cytotrophoblast and syncytiotrophoblast.** They may show cellular atypia.
4. **Absence of fetal parts or nonvillous placental structures:** Embryos die before placental circulation has developed.

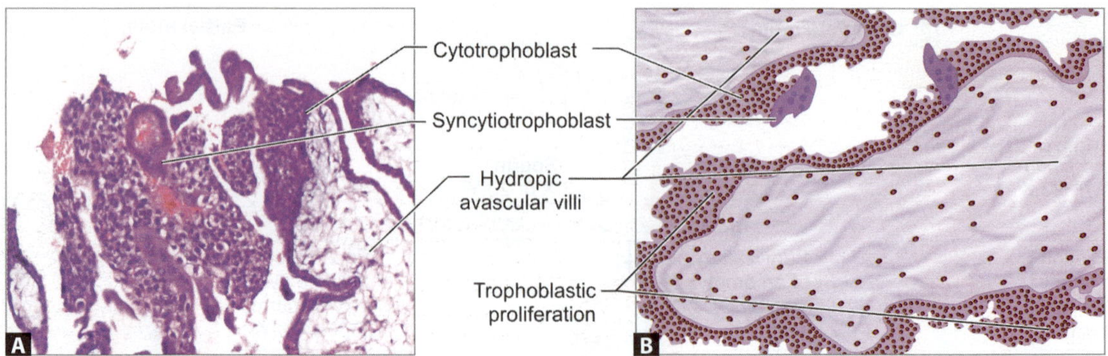

Figs. 22.51A and B: (A) Complete hydatidiform mole showing marked swollen chorionic villi and circumferential trophoblast proliferation; (B) Diagrammatic representation.

Complications of complete mole: These include uterine hemorrhage, DIC, uterine perforation, trophoblastic embolism, and infection. Choriocarcinoma develops in 2% of patients whose moles were evacuated.

Partial Mole

Partial hydatidiform mole is an abn**ormal gestation with trophoblastic proliferation and villous hydrops involving part of the chorionic villi.** It is **usually associated with fetal tissue or embryonic development.**

Etiology: The fundamental etiology in most cases of partial moles is **excess paternal chromosome complements**, resulting in a diandric monogynic triploid genome. Rarely, they may be tetraploid with three paternal haploid chromosome sets.

Genetic Basis of Pathogenesis (*refer* Fig. 22.49C)

Partial moles have **triploid genomes with 69 chromosomes** (triploidy)—**one haploid maternal set and two haploid paternal sets.**

- Most partial moles (>95%) result from **fertilization of a single, normal ovum with two sperms** (23,X or 23,Y) (dispermic/heterozygous).
- Remaining (<5%) partial moles result from **reduplication of the paternal chromosome** set (monospermic/homozygous) **due to failure of meiotic reduction** (meiosis I or II) after fertilization of one egg by one spermatozoon.

The karyotype in partial moles is triploid. These include 69,XXX [ova (23,X) + sperm (23,X + 23,X)], 69,XXY [ova (23,X) + sperm (23,X + 23,Y)], 69,XYY [ova (23,X) + sperm (23,Y + 23,Y)] or even occasionally tetraploid (92,XXXY). **Fetal tissues are usually present**. Even though partial moles have an increased risk of persistent molar disease, they are **not associated with evolution into choriocarcinoma.**

MORPHOLOGY

Localization: Uterus and less commonly ectopic in the fallopian tube.

Gross

Chorionic villi: Villous tissue may appear grossly normal or may show focal hydropic vesicles.

A gestational sac or fetal parts: Sometimes, it may show a gestational sac, fetal parts, or an intact fetus.

Microscopy (*refer* online Fig. 22.52)

- **Chorionic villi:** Partial moles are typically composed of an **admixture of two populations of chorionic villi:**
  - **Essentially normal or small fibrotic villi.**
  - **Enlarged, irregularly shaped, swollen claw-like villi** with scalloped contours. A variable degree of hydropic swelling (hydrops) is seen. The hydropic villi show central cavitation (at least focal) (*refer* **online Fig. 22.52**).
- **Trophoblastic hyperplasia:** Trophoblastic proliferation is **focal, moderate, and less marked** (pronounced) than in complete moles. Chorionic villi show fetal blood vessels **with fetal (nucleated) red blood cells.**
- **Fetal parts are frequently seen in partial moles.**

Clinical Features

Complete moles: Patients with complete moles commonly present at 11–25 weeks of pregnancy. They show excessive enlargement of the uterus (larger uterus than expected for the gestational age) and often have uterine bleeding. They often pass through tissue fragments resembling small, grapelike masses. On ultrasound examination, they have a so-called **snowstorm pattern without fetal parts**. High-resolution sonography usually reveals a complex intrauterine mass with many small cysts. This pattern, especially with a markedly elevated beta-hCG level, is clinically diagnostic of a hydatidiform mole.

Partial moles: Most patients with partial moles present with spontaneous miscarriages.

Comparative features of complete and partial hydatidiform mole are presented in **Table 22.3**.

Q. Write a short note on the differences between complete and partial mole.

TABLE 22.3 Comparative features of complete and partial hydatidiform mole.

Features	*Complete mole*	*Partial mole*
Karyotype	Diploid (46,XX or 46,XY)	Triploid (69,XXY or 69,XXX)
Parental origin of haploid genome sets	Both paternal	1 maternal, 2 paternal
Gross appearance		
Uterus	Large with voluminous specimen	Small, no gross abnormality
Embryo/fetal part	Absent	Present
Microscopy		
Chorionic villi	Enlarged with marked, generalized hydrops	Two populations: (1) enlarged villi with irregular, scalloped contours, and mild-to-moderate hydrops and (2) small fibrotic villi
Hydropic villi	All villi involved, frequently circumferential	Some
Hydropic swelling	Marked, cisterns present	• Less pronounced and focal • Cisterns' less prominent • Villous fibrosis
Trophoblastic proliferation (hyperplasia)	Diffuse, marked circumferential	Focal, mild-to-moderate
Fetal (villus) vessels	Absent	Often present
Other features		
hCG in tissue	4+	1+
Serum hCG	High	Less elevated
Risk of subsequent choriocarcinoma	2.5% after mole	No choriocarcinoma

(hCG: human chorionic gonadotropin)

Laboratory Diagnosis of Hydatidiform Mole

Q. Write a short answer on laboratory diagnosis of hydatidiform mole.

- **Human chorionic gonadotropin (β-hCG):**
  - **In complete moles, β-hCG levels are high** compared to normal pregnancy.
  - Serial hormone determination shows an increase in the β-hCG levels faster than for the pregnancy.
- **Monitoring serum concentrations of β-hCG is necessary** to determine the early development of invasive moles or gestational choriocarcinoma.

Treatment: Most moles are successfully removed by suction curettage of the uterus. Subsequently, serum hCG levels are monitored for 6 months to 1 year until the hCG levels decrease to nonpregnant levels. Continuous elevation of hCG levels may indicate persistent or invasive moles.

Invasive and Metastatic Hydatidiform Mole

An invasive hydatidiform mole is a **hydatidiform mole** (usually complete or less often partial) **that shows invasion** (penetration) or even perforates the **uterine wall** (invasion of the myometrium and/or uterine vessels by hydropic chorionic villi). In contrast to choriocarcinoma, it lacks the metastatic potential. Invasive mole is accompanied by a **proliferation of both cytotrophoblasts and syncytiotrophoblasts.**

The diagnosis of a metastatic mole is by identification of the molar chorionic villi at extrauterine sites (most commonly involving the vaginal wall or pelvis). Both invasive and metastatic hydatidiform moles are lesions included in the category of postmolar or persistent GTD or gestational trophoblastic neoplasia (GTN). Invasive mole is a sequela of molar pregnancy of either complete or partial hydatidiform mole.

MORPHOLOGY

Uterus

Gross: The villi of an invasive mole **extends into the myometrium.**

Microscopy: Most invasive hydatidiform moles are **complete hydatidiform moles.** They have villous with histological features of complete mole. The villus epithelium shows the proliferation of both trophoblastic and syncytiotrophoblast components. But it shows invasion into the myometrial and or vessels.

Ovary: Theca lutein cysts may occur with any form of tropho blastic disease. It is prominently observed with invasive moles. They are due to stimulation by hCG.

Spread

Local spread: Sometimes, the villi invade parametrial tissue and blood vessels beyond the uterine cavity, most commonly the vaginal wall/pelvis.

Metastasis: Invasive mole may even embolize to distant sites (e.g., lungs and brain), and about one-third spread to distant sites, mostly the lungs.

Clinical features: It manifests with **vaginal bleeding and irregular uterine enlargement.** It is associated with **persistently elevated serum hCG levels.**

Treatment: Invasive mole responds well to chemotherapy with a cure rate in more than 80% of cases.

Complication: The immediate complication is **severe hemorrhage**. Invasive moles may cause uterine perforation. It may cause uterine rupture, which is a major complication.

Choriocarcinoma

Q. Write a short note on choriocarcinoma.

Gestational choriocarcinoma is an uncommon, **highly aggressive, malignant tumor composed of neoplastic villous trophoblastic cells**. These include **anaplastic cuboidal cytotrophoblasts and syncytiotrophoblasts. It metastasizes widely and responds well to chemotherapy**

Types: Choriocarcinoma may be subdivided into gestational and nongestational.

- **Gestational:** It is preceded by:
  - **Complete hydatidiform moles**
  - **Previous abortions**
  - **Healthy (normal) pregnancies**
  - **Ectopic pregnancies.**
- **Nongestational:** It is **very rare** and **arises** from totipotential cells within the gonads **(ovaries/testis) or the mediastinum.**

MORPHOLOGY

Q. Describe the gross and microscopy of choriocarcinoma.

Localization: Most commonly, gestational choriocarcinoma occurs in the **uterus**. Rarely, it may arise in ectopic sites (fallopian tube, ovary, and cervix).

Gross

Uterine lesions of choriocarcinoma may be **single or multiple.**

Size: Choriocarcinoma in the uterus **ranges from microscopic foci to huge necrotic and hemorrhagic tumors.**

Appearance: Choriocarcinoma usually appears as a **hemorrhagic, dark-red soft, fleshy, necrotic uterine mass.** Viable tumors may be minimal.

Secondary changes: Tumor may show large pale areas of ischemic necrosis, extensive areas of hemorrhage, and foci of cystic softening.

Microscopy (Figs. 22.53A and B)

Q. Write a short answer on microscopy and laboratory diagnosis of choriocarcinoma.

- **Pattern:** The classic pattern of choriocarcinoma is **bilaminar, dimorphic, or biphasic**. These patterns are characterized by the distinctive alternating arrangement of mononuclear trophoblastic cells and syncytiotrophoblastic cells.
- **Trophoblastic cells:** They consist of **anaplastic cuboidal cytotrophoblasts and syncytiotrophoblasts.**
- **Absence of** chorionic **villi**
- **Mitosis: Abundant** and sometimes abnormal.
- **Secondary changes:** Due to rapid growth, it can undergo hemorrhage, ischemic necrosis, and secondary inflammation.
- **Invasion:** They can invade the underlying **myometrium, blood vessels, and lymphatics.**

Clinical Features

- Uterine choriocarcinoma usually manifests as **irregular vaginal spotting of a bloody, brown fluid.**
- May follow a normal pregnancy, after a miscarriage, or after curettage.
- By the time it is discovered, it might develop widespread vascular spread.

Laboratory findings: Serum and urine β-hCG is elevated more than that found in hydatidiform moles.

Spread

Widespread metastases through blood are characteristic of choriocarcinoma. **Frequent sites** include the **lungs, brain, bone marrow, liver (Fig. 22.53C)**, kidneys, **vagina,** and other organs. Lymphatic invasion is uncommon.

Treatment of gestational choriocarcinoma: It consists of evacuation of the contents of the uterus, surgery, and chemotherapy. Placental choriocarcinoma is very sensitive to chemotherapy. Nearly 100% of cure are observed even in patients with distant metastases. However, the response to chemotherapy in nongestational choriocarcinomas that arise in the gonads (ovary or testis) is relatively poor.

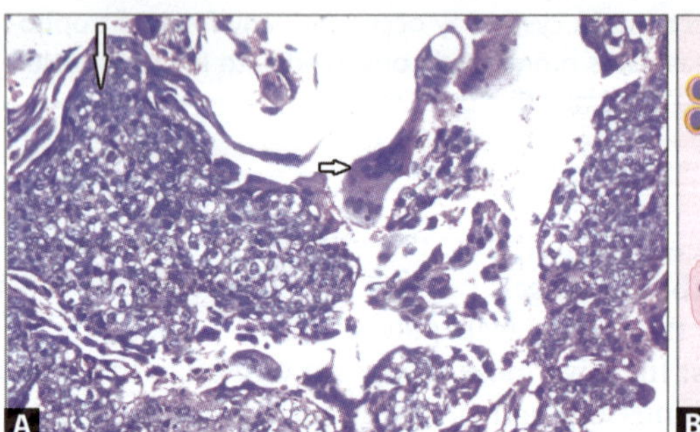

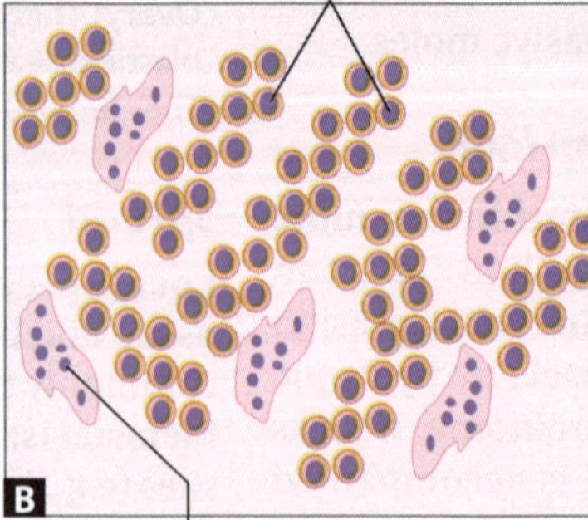

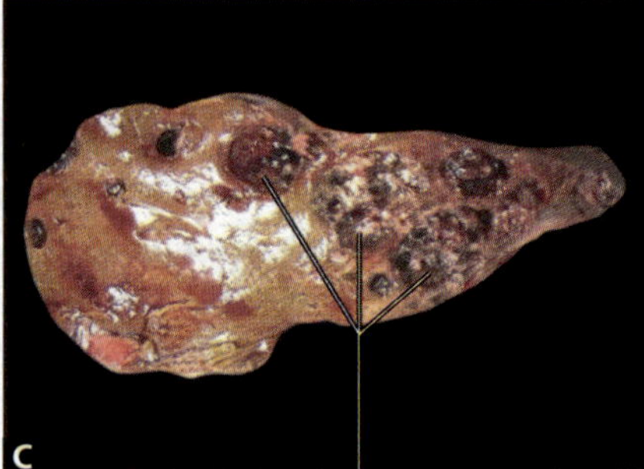

Figs. 22.53A to C: (A) H & E, and (B) Diagrammatic appearance of choriocarcinoma. Choriocarcinoma shows the dimorphic population of neoplastic cuboidal cytotrophoblast (long arrow in A) and syncytiotrophoblast (short arrow in A); (C) Liver showing multiple secondaries from choriocarcinoma.

Prognosis: It has an indolent clinical course, usually with a favorable outcome if the tumor is within the endomyometrium. These tumors are not as sensitive to chemotherapy when compared with other trophoblastic tumors. Hence, the prognosis is poor when it spreads beyond the uterus.

Placental site trophoblastic tumor (PSTT) is presented online.

Ectopic Pregnancy

Q. Write a short note on ectopic pregnancy.

Ectopic pregnancy (gestation) is the **implantation of a fertilized ovum** (developing blastocyst or fetus) **at a site other than the normal intrauterine endometrium** (of the fundus or lower uterine segment) of the uterus (extrauterine site).

Sites of Ectopic Pregnancy

Q. Write a short answer on sites of ectopic pregnancy.

- Within the **fallopian tubes [Fig. 22.54B (*refer* online Fig. 22.53A)]:** It is the most common site (~90%) mainly in the intrauterine portion of the fallopian tube (cornual pregnancy).
- **Other sites:** Ovary, and abdominal cavity. Ovarian pregnancies occur when the ovum is fertilized just as the Graafian follicle ruptures. Ectopic pregnancy within the abdominal cavity occurs when the fertilized egg drops out of the fimbriated end of the fallopian tube and gets implanted on the peritoneum.

Predisposing Conditions

- **Prior pelvic inflammatory disease** resulting in intraluminal fallopian tube scarring and narrowing/ obstruction (chronic salpingitis).
- **Other causes:** These include the following conditions:
  - Intrauterine tumors, endometriosis, and peritubal scarring and adhesions (due to appendicitis, previous surgery, etc.).
  - Intrauterine contraceptive devices also increase the risk of ectopic pregnancy.

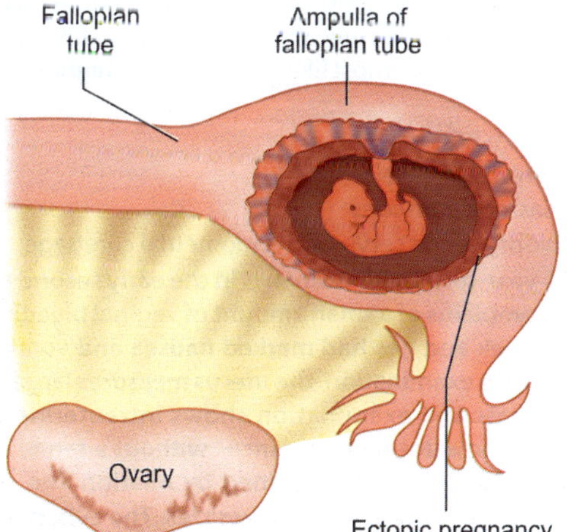

Fig. 22.54B: Tubal pregnancy: Diagrammatic appearance of tubal pregnancy.

Often, no anatomic cause is identified.

Pathogenesis of Fallopian Tube Pregnancy

- Initially the embryonal sac, surrounded by placental tissue gets **implanted in the lumen of the fallopian tube**.
- With time, trophoblastic cells and chorionic villi of the placenta **invade the fallopian tube** wall as they do in the uterus during normal pregnancy.
- The growth of the gestational sac **distends the fallopian tube** causing thinning and rupture.
- Fallopian tube **rupture usually results in massive intraperitoneal hemorrhage**.

MORPHOLOGY

Gross

Formation of placental tissue, the amniotic sac, and decidual changes: This occurs early in all sites of ectopic pregnancies.

Tubal pregnancy: In this site, the invading placenta burrows through the wall of the fallopian tube. This causes **intratubal hematoma (hematosalpinx**, blood-filled fallopian tube), **intraperitoneal hemorrhage,** or both. Tubal pregnancies are the most common **cause of hematosalpinx** and are usually distended by freshly clotted blood with bits of placental and fetal tissue.

Microscopy

It usually shows blood clots admixed with placental chorionic villi (*refer* **online Figs. 22.54C**) or, rarely the embryo.

Clinical Features

Tubal pregnancy: Its clinical presentation may be indistinguishable from a typical pregnancy characterized by cessation of menstruation and elevation of serum and urinary placental hormones. This may continue till a rupture occurs.

During rupture of tubal pregnancy: It most commonly develops about 6 weeks after a previous normal menstrual period. Rupture of an ectopic (tubal) pregnancy presents as **sudden onset of severe abdominal pain** due to rupture of the tube leading to pelvic hemorrhage. It causes signs of an acute abdomen and **constitutes a medical emergency**. The patient may rapidly develop **hemorrhagic shock**. Prompt surgical intervention is required to prevent death.

SCENARIO-BASED MCQs

1. **A 32-year-old woman comes for a routine gynecologic examination and a cervical Pap smear is taken. The cervical Pap smear shows numerous, loosely arranged cells with a high nuclear-to-cytoplasmic ratio. Few of these cells showed perinuclear vacuolation. Colposcopic examination shows white epithelium and a mosaic pattern in the transformation zone. The most likely diagnosis of this condition is:**

   A. Chronic cervicitis
   B. Herpes simplex virus infection
   C. Squamous intraepithelial lesion
   D. Adenocarcinoma of endocervix

2. A 31-year-old sexually active woman comes to the hospital for a routine gynecologic examination. She has been taking oral contraceptives for the past 8 years. Physical examination does not show any abnormal findings. A Pap smear shows a high-grade squamous epithelial lesion (HSIL). The most probable molecular pathogenesis for this HSIL is:
   A. Cell proliferation due to oral contraceptive
   B. Recurrent gonococcal cervicitis
   C. Inherited mutation *TP53* (tumor-suppressor gene)
   D. Inactivation of the *RB1* gene product by human papilloma viral protein
3. A 47-year-old woman comes with complaints of a mild amount of vaginal bleeding and a brownish, foul-smelling discharge for the past 1 month. On pelvic examination, a 3-cm ulcerative, exophytic lesion is seen on the ectocervix and projects into the vagina. Microscopic examination of the lesion showed sheets of anaplastic tumor cells with invasion of underlying tissue. The most likely diagnosis is:
   A. Chronic cervicitis
   B. Adenocarcinoma
   C. Squamous cell carcinoma
   D. High-grade squamous intraepithelial lesion
4. A 38-year-old woman comes with a history of menometrorrhagia for the past 2 months. She has no history of prior irregular menstrual bleeding. On physical examination, there is a right adnexal mass. But there are no lesions in the vagina or cervix, and the uterus appears normal in size. An abdominal ultrasound scan shows the presence of a 5 cm solid mass in the right ovary. Endometrial biopsy shows endometrial hyperplastic without atypia. The most likely lesion in the ovary that is responsible for her menstrual abnormalities is:
   A. Krukenberg tumor B. Serous cystadenoma
   C. Mature cystic teratoma D. Granulosa-theca cell tumor
5. A 60-year-old obese, nulliparous woman comes with a complaint of an episode of vaginal bleeding, which is about 5 mL of blood. On pelvic examination, the uterus is normal in size, and the cervix appears normal. A Pap smear shows cells with features of adenocarcinoma. The most likely pre-existing conditions that have contributed to the development of this adenocarcinoma are:
   A. Adenomyosis
   B. Chronic endometritis
   C. Endometrial hyperplasia
   D. Human papillomavirus infection
6. A healthy 42-year-old woman complains of pelvic heaviness for the past 11 months. There is no history of abnormal bleeding. A bimanual pelvic examination shows an enlarged uterus with multiple, irregular palpable masses. No abnormalities were seen in the Pap smear. A pelvic CT scan shows multiple solid uterine masses without any evidence of necrosis or hemorrhage. A total abdominal hysterectomy is performed. The uterus shows three circumscribed masses in the myometrium. The cut surface shows a whorled, watered silk appearance. The most likely diagnosis is:
   A. Endometrial polyp B. Leiomyomas
   C. Adenomyosis D. Endometriosis
7. A 38-year-old woman complains of increasing abdominal enlargement for the past 6 months. She feels that she is pregnant, but the urine for the pregnancy test is negative. On physical examination, shows abdominal distention with a fluid in the peritoneal cavity. A pelvic ultrasound scan shows bilateral ovarian masses, 10 cm on the right and 7 cm on the left. These masses are partly cystic with solid areas. The masses are surgically removed. On gross examination, the masses are partly solid and partly cystic. Microscopic examination shows that the cystic area shows papillae covered with atypical cuboidal cells that invade the underlying stroma. Psammoma bodies are present. The solid areas showed glandular structures lined by cells with cytologic atypia. The most probable diagnosis is:
   A. Dysgerminoma B. Endometrioid tumor
   C. Cystadenocarcinoma D. Mature cystic teratoma
8. A 32-year-old woman presents with a history of increasing abdominal girth and pelvic discomfort for the last 4 months. Ultrasound examination shows a mass replacing the left ovary. Surgical excision of the mass shows a multilocular tumor filled with thick, viscous fluid. Microscopically, glandular and cystic spaces are lined by mucinous, columnar epithelial cells. There is no evidence of cytologic atypia. Neither papillary structures nor stromal invasion is seen. The most probable diagnosis is:
   A. Mucinous cystadenoma
   B. Mucinous cystadenocarcinoma
   C. Serous cystadenocarcinoma
   D. Mature cystic teratoma
9. A 31-year-old woman has complained of dull, constant abdominal pain for the past 6 months. Physical examination shows a right adnexal mass. CT scan of the pelvis shows an 8 cm circumscribed cystic mass on the right ovary with an irregular area of calcifications. The right fallopian tube and ovary are surgically excised. A gross examination shows a cystic tumor. On opening the right ovary, it shows matted hairs and sebaceous material in the cystic cavity. Microscopic examination of this lesion is most likely to show:
   A. Mature squamous epithelium
   B. Papillary structures with psammoma bodies
   C. Primitive neuroepithelium
   D. Sheets of trophoblasts and syncytial cells
10. A 44-year-old woman complains of increasing abdominal girth for the last 6 months. Gynecologic examination shows large bilateral ovarian masses. The patient undergoes bilateral oophorectomy. The pathology report is "Krukenberg tumor," and microscopically it shows mucin-filled signet ring cells. The test that most likely provides the highest diagnostic yield is:
    A. Serum hCG level
    B. Serum AFP level
    C. Gastric endoscopy
    D. Biopsy of the cervix and endometrial curettage
11. A 24-year-old G2, P1 woman is in the early second trimester. She complains of a small amount of vaginal bleeding for the past week and has had marked nausea and vomiting for 3 weeks. On examination, the uterus measures large for dates. An ultrasound examination shows intrauterine contents with a "snowstorm appearance," without a fetus. The gross appearance of tissue obtained by dilation and curettage shows numerous grape-like vesicles. The substance that is most likely to be greatly increased in the serum of this patient is:

A. Estradiol
B. α-Fetoprotein
C. Human placental lactogen
D. Human chorionic gonadotropin

Answers and Explanation

1. **The answer is C: Squamous intraepithelial lesion (SIL).** It is characterized by intraepithelial abnormalities. The vacuolated cells in the cervical Pap smear are typical of HPV infection and are termed as koilocytes. SIL is often detected on colposcopic examination by epithelial mosaicism and vascular dots differentiated from the surrounding tissue surface by color and texture. The other choices do not show these gross morphologic features.
2. **The answer is D: Inactivation of the *RB1* gene product by human papillomavirus protein.** HSIL of the cervix should not be ignored because they naturally progress to invasive carcinomas. HSIL is strongly related to human papillomavirus (HPV) infections. Viral E6 and E7 proteins bind to Rb to up-regulate cyclin E. With HPV infection, the Pap smear may show changes in low-grade squamous intraepithelial lesions (LSIL). Oral contraceptives with low-dose estrogens and progestins do not increase the risk of squamous intraepithelial lesions. Cervicitis usually is due to bacterial or fungal organisms and is not a significant risk for squamous intraepithelial lesions or carcinoma. Though the *TP53* gene is involved, this is not due to inherited mutation.
3. **The answer is C: Squamous cell carcinoma.** The morphological features suggest the most likely diagnosis of an invasive squamous cell carcinoma that has infiltrated the subepithelial region. Chronic cervicitis produces erythematous lesions with forming masses. Adenocarcinoma is a glandular invasive lesion, which is much less common than squamous cell carcinoma of the cervix. Dysplastic changes restricted to the epithelium constitute squamous intraepithelial lesions and do not form mass lesions.
4. **The answer is D: Granulosa-theca cell tumor.** The mass in the right ovary is probably producing estrogen, which has led to endometrial hyperplasia. Estrogen-producing tumors of the ovary are mainly sex cord tumors, such as a granulosa-theca cell tumor and thecomas. Krukenberg tumor is a metastatic tumor of the ovary which is usually bilateral and serous cystadenoma is a surface epithelial tumor. They do not produce increased estrogen. Mature cystic teratomas can contain various histologic elements, but not estrogen-producing tissues.
5. **The answer is C: Endometrial hyperplasia.** Endometrial carcinomas can be associated with increased estrogen due to anovulatory cycles, nulliparity, obesity, and exogenous estrogen. These risk factors may initially produce endometrial hyperplasia. If the estrogenic stimulation continues, endometrial hyperplasia can progress to endometrial carcinoma. Adenomyosis increases the size of the uterus and does not progress to endometrial carcinoma. Chronic endometritis and human papillomavirus infection (associated with squamous intraepithelial lesion and squamous cell carcinoma) do not cause adenocarcinoma.
6. **The answer is B: Leiomyomas.** The well-circumscribed masses with whorled, watered silk appearance in the myometrium of the uterus suggest the presence of benign tumors namely uterine leiomyomas (fibroids). Leiomyomas are often asymptomatic, but submucosal leiomyomas may produce menometrorrhagia and chronic blood loss, leading to iron deficiency anemia. The endometrial polyp produces a lesion in the endometrial surface and projects into the endometrial cavity. Adenomyosis is the presence of endometrial glands and stroma in the myometrium. It does not form circumscribed nodules with a whorled appearance. Endometriosis is the presence of endometrial glands and stroma outside the uterus and does not produce myometrial lesions.
7. **The answer is C: Cystadenocarcinoma.** These are common ovarian tumors that are often bilateral. Serous carcinomas occur more frequently than mucinous carcinomas. Serous tumors may be benign, borderline, or malignant. Dysgerminoma is a solid tumor of germ-cell origin. Endometrioid tumors resemble endometrial carcinomas and may arise in the foci of endometriosis of the ovary. Mature cystic teratomas contain abundant hair and sebaceous fluid within the cystic cavity; surrounded by tissues derived from various germ layers.
8. **The answer is A: Mucinous cystadenoma.** Common benign epithelial tumors of the ovary are almost always serous or mucinous cystadenomas. The mucinous cystadenomas are multiloculated and may be massively enlarged. Benign epithelial tumors compared to malignant counterparts, tend to have thin walls and lack solid areas. The absence of stromal invasion and atypia in this case excludes mucinous cystadenocarcinoma (choice B). Serous cystadenocarcinoma shows invasion and cells do not show mucin. Mature cystic teratomas contain abundant hair and sebaceous fluid within the cystic cavity; surrounded by tissues derived from various germ layers.
9. **The answer is A: Mature squamous epithelium.** A cystic tumor with a mass of hair in the lumen is characteristic of a mature cystic teratoma. It is also known as a dermoid cyst because it is cystic and filled with hair and sebum derived from well-differentiated ectodermal structures. Teratomas with mature tissue elements are benign tumors of germ-cell origin. They can contain tissues derived from ectoderm, endoderm, and mesoderm. Papillary structures with psammoma bodies are seen in serous cystadenocarcinoma. Primitive neuroepithelium in a more solid and less cystic tumor of the ovary favors an immature teratoma. Sheets of trophoblasts and syncytial cells are observed in choriocarcinoma and are usually gestational in origin and have a hemorrhagic appearance.
10. **The answer is C: Gastric endoscopy.** Krukenberg tumors are ovarian metastases most commonly stomach is the primary site (gastric adenocarcinoma). Bilateral ovarian involvement and bosselated outer surface are important clues to the diagnosis of metastatic carcinoma. Microscopically, the tumor shows nests of mucin-filled "signet ring" cells within a cellular stroma derived from the ovary. Other options do not fit the findings in this case.
11. **The answer is D: Human chorionic gonadotropin.** A complete hydatidiform mole shows an enlarged uterus containing grapelike villi in the endometrial cavity. These trophoblastic tumor cells secrete large amounts of human chorionic gonadotropin (hCG). Molar pregnancies result from abnormal fertilization, with only paternal chromosomes present. Estrogens can be secreted by various ovarian stromal tumors, including granulosa cell tumors and thecomas. α-Fetoprotein is a marker for some germ cell tumors that contain yolk sac elements. A small amount of human placental lactogen is produced in the developing placenta, and its serum levels are usually not measured.

Breast Disorders

CHAPTER OUTLINE

- Female Breast
- Benign Epithelial Lesions
- Carcinoma of the Breast
- Types of Breast Carcinoma
- Invasive (Infiltrating) Carcinoma
- Paget Disease of the Nipple
- Fibroepithelial Tumors of Breast
- Male Breast

FEMALE BREAST

Normal Anatomy

Each breast consists of **15–25 lobes**, and each lobe has a branching structure like a flowering tree. **Each lobe** has two major components: (1) the **terminal duct–lobular unit (TDLU)** and (2) the **large duct system (Figs. 23.1A and B)**.

1. **TDLU:** It **consists of a lobule** (functional unit of the breast), together with **its terminal** (intralobular and extralobular) duct. Each **lobule consists of** a variable number of **terminal ductules/acini** embedded within the specialized intralobular stroma and is connected to the intralobular terminal duct.
2. **Large duct system:** The intralobular ducts emerge from the lobule as the extralobular duct and connect with the **subsegmental duct**, which in turn leads to a **segmental duct**. This leads to a **collecting (lactiferous or galactophorous) duct,** which opens onto the surface of the nipple. A fusiform dilation is seen beneath the nipple between the collecting and the segmental duct, known as the **lactiferous sinus**. The ducts carry the milk to the nipple.

Microscopy: It consists of the following:

- **Lining of ducts and lobules:** Entire ducts and lobules of the breast are lined by a specialized two-cell-type epithelial lining—the **inner epithelium** with secretory (produce milk during lactation) and absorptive functions (often simply called the epithelium), and the **outer** (basally located) **myoepithelial cells (Fig. 23. 1B)**. The myoepithelial cells have a contractile function that helps in ejection of milk and also support the basement membrane.
- **Breast stroma:** It consists of two types namely, **intralobular** and **extralobular**.

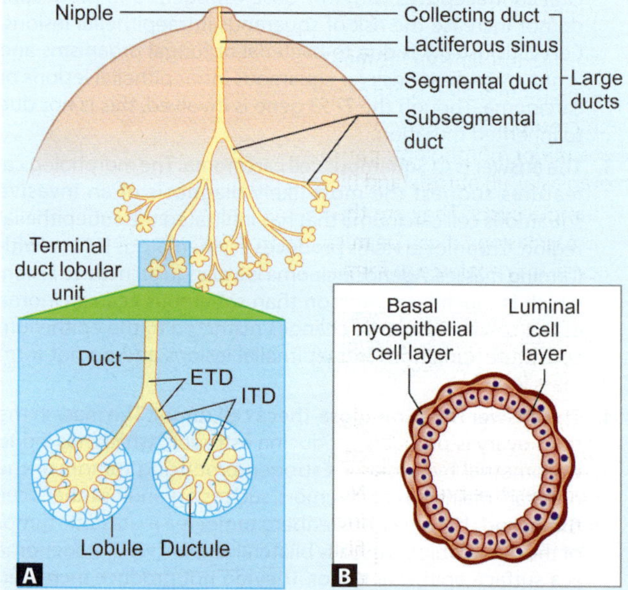

Figs. 23.1A and B: (A) Diagrammatic representation of the breast structure and terminal duct lobular unit (TDLU) structure; (B) Duct lined by a specialized two-cell-type—the inner epithelium, and the outer (basally located) myoepithelial cells.

(ETD: extralobular terminal duct; ITD: intralobular terminal duct)

Biopsy techniques for breast lesions: These include (i) fine needle aspiration cytology (FNAC), (ii) tru-cut (core-cut) biopsy, and excisional biopsy.

BENIGN EPITHELIAL LESIONS

PA 31.1 (CC): Classify and describe the types, etiology, pathogenesis, and hormonal dependency of breast pathology and benign breast disease.

Q. List benign epithelial lesions of the breast.

Classification: Based on the subsequent risk of developing breast carcinoma, the benign epithelial lesions of the breast can be divided into three groups **(Table 23.1)**.

Nonproliferative Breast Changes (Fibrocystic Changes)

Q. Write a short note on the fibrocystic disease of the breast (fibrocystic changes).

- **No proliferation of epithelium**: Termed "nonproliferative" because in these lesions only single layers of epithelial cells are seen, in contrast to the multilayered hyperplastic epithelium in proliferative lesions.
- It is a group that consists of many **common morphological changes observed in the breast** and is also termed as fibrocystic changes group.
- It is **not associated with an increased risk of carcinoma of the breast**.

MORPHOLOGY (FIGS. 23.2A TO D)

Q. Write a short note on the morphology of nonproliferative breast changes (fibrocystic disease of the breast).

Major morphologic patterns: Nonproliferative changes consist of **three major** morphologic **patterns:** (i) cysts (often with apocrine metaplasia), (ii) fibrosis, and (iii) adenosis.

1. **Simple cysts:** They are the most common nonproliferative breast lesions. It can be **microscopic or grossly visible**. Small cysts may coalesce to form larger cysts.
   - **Cysts contain turbid, cloudy yellow, and semitranslucent fluid.** Some of these cysts externally appear brown or blue in color (**'blue dome cysts' of Bloodgood**). Secretions within the cysts may calcify and be detected by mammography.
   - **Microscopically,** cysts are lined either by a **flattened atrophic epithelium** (especially the larger cysts) or by **metaplastic apocrine cells. Apocrine metaplasia** is a common change often seen in **dilated ducts and cystic structures.** Apocrine cells have an **abundant granular, eosinophilic**/acidophilic **cytoplasm** and **round nuclei with prominent nucleolus.** The apical portion of the cytoplasm shows the typical **'apocrine snout'**.
2. **Fibrosis: Cysts may rupture.** The **leakage of debris** may produce chronic inflammation and fibrosis. This **may produce a palpable nodularity** and firmness of the breast (so-called "fibrocystic changes" formerly known as fibrocystic disease).
3. **Adenosis:** It is defined as an increase in the number of acini (terminal ductules) per lobule. Adenosis is normal in pregnancy and may be seen focally in nonpregnant women.

Nonproliferative breast changes also include mild hyperplasia, duct ectasia, and fibroadenoma without complex features.

Proliferative Breast Disease without Atypia

These lesions include epithelial hyperplasia, sclerosing adenosis, complex sclerosing lesion, radial sclerosing lesion (radial scar), and papilloma. Each of these lesions shows varying degrees of epithelial cell proliferation. They are usually detected as mammographic densities, calcifications, or incidental findings in biopsies done for other reasons.

TABLE 23.1 Classification of benign epithelial lesions of the breast.

Group	*Risk of subsequent development of breast cancer*
Nonproliferative breast changes	Not associated with increased risk (e.g., fibrocystic change). The relative risk of about 1%
Proliferative breast lesions/disease (proliferative conditions without atypia)	Associated with a 1.5- to 2-fold increased risk of developing carcinoma over 5–15 years. The relative risk of about 1.5–2%
Proliferative disease with atypia (atypical hyperplasia): • Atypical ductal hyperplasia • Atypical lobular hyperplasia	Greater relative risk (three- to five-fold) of developing carcinoma. The relative risk of about 4–5%

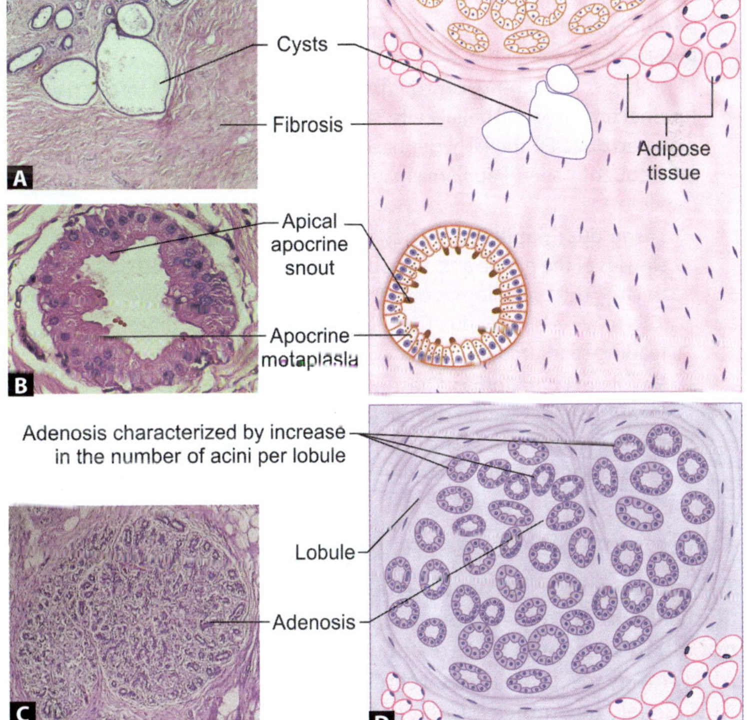

Figs. 23.2A to D: Microscopic features of nonproliferative breast change (fibrocystic changes): (A) Hematoxylin and eosin (H&E) showing cysts and fibrosis cysts; (B) (H&E) Showing cysts with apocrine metaplasia of the lining cells; (C) (H&E) Showing adenosis; (D) Diagrammatic appearance showing the above features.

MORPHOLOGY

1. **Epithelial hyperplasia:** Normal breast ducts and lobules are lined by two layers of cells: Inner (luminal) epithelial cells and outer myoepithelial cells.
   - **Epithelial hyperplasia** is defined as the **presence of more than two cell layers.** The additional cells consist of both luminal and myoepithelial cell types. These cells fill and distend ducts and lobules. **Irregular lumens can often be seen at the periphery of the cellular masses.**
   - **Degree of epithelial hyperplasia:** It may be mild (when made up of three or four epithelial cells in thickness), moderate, or severe (more pronounced).
2. **Sclerosing adenosis:** Sclerosing adenosis (SA) is a benign proliferative condition.
   - **Enlargement and an increase in the number of acini per lobule** (adenosis).
   - **Stromal proliferation:** The increased number of acini accompanied by stromal proliferation. It is **more cellular centrally than peripherally.** On occasion, stromal fibrosis may produce a microscopic **appearance mimicking invasive carcinoma.**
   - **Compression and distortion of acini at the center and dilatation at the periphery.**
3. **Complex sclerosing lesion:** It is known by a variety of terms and includes radial scar and radial sclerosing lesion. It is a benign lesion with fibroelastosis and entrapped glandular structures, with or without proliferative epithelial lesion. These microscopically complex lesions usually have sclerosis, adenosis, variable degrees of epithelial hyperplasia, and papilloma. These components are arranged in a radial or stellate configuration.
4. **Papillomas:** Papillomas are **localized, benign intraductal** lesions that grow within a dilated duct. They are composed of **multiple, branching, central fibrovascular cores lined by luminal and myoepithelial cells.** These **papillae grow within a dilated duct.** Epithelial hyperplasia and apocrine metaplasia are frequently seen. Papilloma may be large duct or small duct papilloma.
   - **Large duct papillomas:** They are seen in the lactiferous sinuses of the nipple and are **usually single.** More than 80% of large duct papillomas present with a **nipple discharge.** This may be bloody due to torsion of the stalk of papillae, leading to infarction.
   - **Small duct papillomas:** These are **commonly multiple** and located deeper within the ductal system. Most small duct papillomas present as small palpable masses or as densities or calcifications on mammography.

Proliferative Breast Disease with Atypia

This group includes **atypical ductal hyperplasia (ADH)** and **atypical lobular hyperplasia (ALH)**. They have **some, but not all, microscopic features of carcinoma in situ**. Thus, ADH closely resembles ductal carcinoma in situ (DCIS) and ALH closely resembles lobular carcinoma in situ (LCIS).

MORPHOLOGY

Atypical hyperplasia is a cellular proliferation, which **resembles carcinoma in situ.**

Atypical ductal hyperplasia

- It is an intraductal proliferation with cytological and architectural features similar to those of low-grade ductal carcinoma in situ (DCIS).
- **Cytological features of ADH:** These include **regularly (evenly) paced, relatively monomorphic** (monotonous) **cells with well-defined cell borders.** These cells have **round nuclei** with dense chromatin. Necrosis is unusual.
- **Architectural features: The ducts are only partially involved, and/or uniform involvement to a limited extent.** These features distinguish this from DCIS.

Atypical lobular hyperplasia

- It is a cellular proliferation identical to those of lobular carcinoma in situ (LCIS), but the **cells do not fill or distend more than 50% of the acini within a lobule.**
- **TDLUs are filled with a monotonous (monomorphic), low-grade, small, solid proliferation of dyscohesive epithelial cells.**

CARCINOMA OF THE BREAST

PA 31.2 (CC): Classify and describe the epidemiology, pathogenesis, classification, morphology, prognostic factors, hormonal dependency, staging, and spread of carcinoma of the breast.

Breast carcinoma is the most common malignant tumor in women. Its mortality in women is second only to lung cancer. Two important recent advancements are the availability of mammographic screening and more effective treatment modalities. **Almost all malignant tumors of the breast are adenocarcinomas.**

Classification of Breast Tumors

Q. Classify tumors of the breast.

World Health Organization (WHO) (2019)

WHO classification of epithelial tumors of the breast is presented in **Box 23.1**.

Molecular Classification

Breast carcinoma is divided into three major groups based on the expression of three proteins namely: (i) estrogen receptor (ER), (ii) progesterone receptor (PR), and (iii) HER2 (also known as ERBB2). They are grouped as follows:

1. **Luminal (50–65% of cancers):** They are **positive for ER and negative for HER2.** It constitutes **50–65% of cancers** and **is the most common molecular subtype of invasive breast cancer.** It is subdivided into two subgroups based on proliferation rates.

BOX 23.1: World Health Organization (WHO) (2019) (abridged) classification of epithelial tumors of the breast.

Epithelial tumors
- **Benign epithelial proliferations and precursors**
  - Atypical ductal hyperplasia
- **Adenosis and benign sclerosing lesions**
  - Sclerosing adenosis
  - Radial scar/complex sclerosing lesion
- **Adenomas**
  - Tubular adenoma
  - Lactating adenoma
  - Duct adenoma
- **Epithelial-myoepithelial tumors**
- **Papillary neoplasms**
  - Intraductal papilloma
  - Papillary ductal carcinoma in situ
  - Invasive papillary carcinoma
- **Noninvasive lobular neoplasia**
  - Atypical lobular hyperplasia
  - Lobular carcinoma in situ, NOS
- **DCIS (ductal carcinoma in situ)**
  - Intraductal carcinoma, noninfiltrating, NOS
    - DCIS of low nuclear grade
    - DCIS of intermediate nuclear grade
    - DCIS of high nuclear grade
- **Invasive breast carcinoma**
  - Invasive breast carcinoma of no special type (NST)
    - Medullary pattern invasive cancer
  - Invasive lobular carcinoma
  - Tubular carcinoma
  - Cribriform carcinoma, NOS
  - Mucinous adenocarcinoma
  - Metaplastic carcinoma, NOS
- **Rare and salivary gland-type tumors**
- **Neuroendocrine neoplasms**

Fibroepithelial tumors of the breast
- Fibroadenoma
- Phyllodes tumor

Tumors of the nipple
- Nipple adenoma
- Paget disease of the breast

(NOS: not otherwise specified)

a. **ER-positive/PR-positive tumors (40–55%):** Luminal cancers with high expression of ER usually also express high levels of PR. These tumors are **usually well differentiated and slow-growing with low proliferation. These tumors form the majority of cancers in older women and men.** Many of them are detected at an early stage. The local recurrence rate is very low and is usually cured by surgery.

b. **Low ER and absent PR (10%):** These luminal carcinomas tend to be at the other end of the spectrum. They are usually **poorly differentiated and have a high proliferative rate.**

2. ***HER2*-positive (10–20% of cancers):** These tumors are positive for HER2 and **positive or negative for ER.** It is the **second most common molecular subtype of invasive breast cancer.** They are more common in young women. They are identified by assays of *HER2* protein overexpression or *HER2* gene amplification. They can metastasize early (to the viscera and brain) and even when the tumor is small. About, one-third or more of these patients respond completely to antibodies that bind and block *HER2* activity and have an excellent prognosis.
3. **Triple-negative (10–20% of cancers):** These cancers are negative for ER, PR, and HER2. They are more common in young premenopausal women. This forms the majority of carcinomas in women with *BRCA1* mutations. They have high proliferation and rapid growth. Hence, they present as a palpable mass. These can metastasize when small in size, frequently to viscera and the brain.

These three groups show marked differences in patient characteristics, pathologic features, treatment response, metastatic patterns, time to relapse, and outcome **(Table 23.2).**

Etiology

Q. Discuss the etiopathogenesis of breast carcinoma.

Risk Factors

Many risk factors for breast cancer have been identified **(Fig. 23.3 and Box 23.2).**

Female gender: The **most important risk factor is gender** (99% of cancers are in females). Breast cancer cases occur in only 1% of males.

Age: Breast cancer is rare before the age of 25 years and is uncommon before the age of 30 years. Its incidence increases rapidly after the age of 30 years. Triple-negative and HER2-positive cancers constitute almost 50% of breast cancers in younger women and less than 20% of cancers in older women.

Prolonged exposure to estrogens: It **increases the risk of breast carcinoma.** It may be seen in the following conditions:

- **Endogenous hormone exposure** occurs with **long duration of reproductive life**:
  - **Early menarche** (<12 years) and **late menopause** (>55 years).
  - **Late age at first-term pregnancy (>35 years) and nulliparity.**
  - **Postmenopausal obese: Increased risk** due to the synthesis of estrogens in fat depots. However, obesity has no role among premenopausal women.
  - **Carcinoma of the contralateral breast or endometrium:** Both **produce prolonged estrogenic stimulation.**

TABLE 23.2 Summary of major biologic types of invasive breast carcinoma.

Feature	*ER positive/HER2 negative: "Luminal"*	*HER2 positive (ER positive or negative): "HER2"*	*Triple negative (ER, PR, and HER2 negative): "TNBC"*
Frequency	50–65%	20%	15%
Type of patient	Older women; men; detected by screening; germline *BRCA2* mutation	Young women; germline *TP53* mutation	Young women; germline *BRCA1* mutation carriers
Common somatic gene mutations	*PIK3CA* (29–45%), *TP53* (12–29%)	*TP53* (70–80%), *PIK3CA* (~39%)	*TP53* (70–80%), *PIK3CA* (9%)
Histological grade	Mainly grade 1 and 2	Mainly grade 2 and 3	Mainly grade 3
Pattern of metastasis (percentage)	Bone (70–80%), viscera (25–30%), brain (~10%)	Bone (70%), viscera (45%), brain (30%)	Bone (40%), viscera (35%), brain (25%)
A complete response to chemotherapy	~10%	• 15% (ER-positive) • 30–60% (ER-negative)	~30%
Recurrence	Low rate over many years; long survival possible with bone metastases	Bimodal with early and late (10 years) peaks	Early peak at <8 years, late recurrence rare, survival with metastases rare
Prognosis	Intermediate to excellent	Poor	Poor

(ER: estrogen receptor; PR: progesterone receptor; TNBC: triple-negative breast cancer)

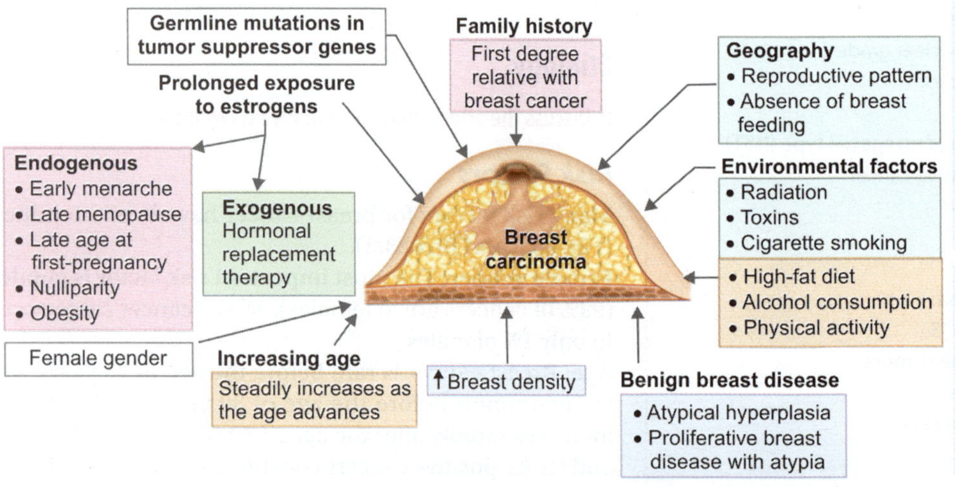

Breast cancer:
- Most common cancer in women in the world
- Most common cancer in urban women in India
- Second most common cause of cancer-related death in women
- The upper outer quadrant is the most common site for cancer

Factors that reduce the risk of breast carcinoma:
- Breastfeeding: Long duration of breastfeeding has a protective effect
- Exercise
- Healthy body weight

Fig. 23.3: Risk factors involved in the development of breast cancer.

- **Exogenous hormone exposure:** It may be due to **postmenopausal hormonal replacement therapy**. Estrogens stimulate the production of growth factors, which promote the development of carcinoma.

Germline mutations: About 5–10% of breast cancers develop in women with germline mutations in tumor-suppressor genes ***BRCA1*** and ***BRCA2*** (*refer* pathogenesis below on page 847).

Family history of first-degree relatives with breast cancer: First-degree relatives include mother, sister, or daughter. It is strongly associated with an increased risk for breast cancer. The risk is higher if the relative had breast cancer at a young age or developed bilateral breast cancer.

Geographic variations: They are observed and may be related to the following:

- **Reproductive patterns:** These include the number and timing of pregnancies.
- **Nursing habits/breastfeeding: The longer the women breastfeed**, the **greater the risk reduction**.
- **Physical activity (exercise)** may have a **protective role.**

Environmental risk factors: These include the following:

- **Radiation exposure:** Radiation to the chest due to cancer therapy, atomic bomb exposure, or nuclear accidents.
- **Environmental toxins:** Organochlorine pesticides have estrogenic effects.
- **Cigarette smoking:** Active smoking, particularly if started at an early age and continued for a prolonged period, increases the risk.

BOX 23.2: Risk factors for breast carcinoma.

Nonmodifiable
- Female gender
- Increasing age
- Prolonged exposure to estrogens
  - Early menarche (age <12 years)
  - Late menopause (age >55 years)
  - Late first pregnancy (age >35 years)
  - Nulliparity
- Germline mutations in tumor suppressor genes
- Family history
- Personal history of breast cancer
- High breast density, benign breast disease

Modifiable
- Absence of breastfeeding
- Exogenous hormone therapy
- Postmenopausal obesity
- **Environmental risk factors**
  - High-dose radiation to the chest at a young age
  - **Cigarette smoking**
  - High alcohol consumption
  - Physical inactivity (exercise)
  - High-fat diet

- **Type of diet: High total fat** may increase the risk, but it is likely to be small. It may modify levels of circulating estrogens. Consumption of **coffee (caffeine) may decrease the risk**.
- **Moderate or heavy alcohol consumption**: It may be associated with **relatively moderate increased risk.**
- **Physical activity:** Higher levels of physical activity **reduce breast cancer risk**, and there is a dose-response relationship.

Benign breast disease (Box 23.1): If previous breast biopsies had **atypical hyperplasia/proliferative breast disease with atypia/lobular carcinoma in situ**, they increase the risk.

Breast density: Women with very dense breasts (high density) on mammography have a four- to six-fold higher risk of (both ER positive and ER negative) breast cancer compared to women with the lowest density. High breast radiodensity indicates deficient involution of lobules at the end of each menstrual cycle.

Major factors that decrease the risk of breast cancer: These include **early pregnancy** (before 20 years of age) and **prolonged breastfeeding**.

Pathogenesis (Figs. 23.4A to C)

Breast cancer can be divided into three major subtypes depending on the differential expression of hormone receptors and HER2 (*refer* **Table 23.2**). These three major subtypes **arise through specific pathways that involve the stepwise acquisition of driver mutations in the epithelial cells of the duct/lobular system.** Driver mutations in cancer genes may be inherited and acquired and both are involved in breast carcinogenesis.

Contributing factors: The contributing factors involved in the development of breast cancer can be categorized as: (i) genetic and (ii) hormonal (estrogen).

Genetic Factors

The mutations in cancer genes that contribute to breast carcinogenesis can be divided into inherited (germline) and acquired mutations.

Familial breast cancer: The major germline mutations in breast cancer affect genes that regulate genomic stability or that are involved in pro-growth signaling pathways.

- ***BRCA1* and *BRCA2*:** These are tumor-suppressor genes and are normally expressed in many different cells and tissues. **Breast cancer develops only when both alleles are inactivated or defective.** *BRCA1* and *BRCA2* **encode proteins that are necessary for the repair of double-stranded DNA breaks.** Germline mutations in these genes **increase the risk of breast and serous ovarian cancer.**
- ***BRCA2* mutations:** These are **mainly associated with ER-positive tumors.**
- ***BRCA1* mutations:** These are strongly **associated with triple-negative cancers.**
- **Other mutated genes associated with familial breast cancer**: These include ***TP53*** ("guardian of the genome") and ***PTEN*** (an important negative regulator of the pro-growth PI3K-AKT pathway).

Sporadic breast cancers: The genes mutated in familial breast cancer are often disturbed in sporadic breast cancers.

- **Somatic mutations in *BRCA1* and *BRCA2***: These are **rare in sporadic cancers**. However, *BRCA1* is inactivated by methylation in up to 50% of triple-negative cancers.
- **Somatic mutations in *TP53*:** These are **common in breast cancer** (especially in triple-negative and HER2-positive tumors). Mutations that activate PI3K-AKT signaling are also found in sporadic ER-positive and HER2-positive breast cancers.

Amplification of the *HER2* gene. *HER2* is a receptor tyrosine kinase. It promotes the proliferation of cells and opposes apoptosis by stimulating the RAS- and PI3K-AKT signaling pathways. **A common driver mutation in breast cancer is an amplification of the *HER2* gene.** Cancers that overexpress *HER2* are **distinct tumors and highly proliferative.** In the past, they were considered to be having a poor prognosis. However, the availability of therapeutic agents that specifically target *HER2* receptors markedly improved the prognosis for these patients.

Role of Estrogen

The major risk factor for luminal breast cancer is exposure to estrogen. **Estrogens have an important role, particularly in breast cancer occurring after menopause.**

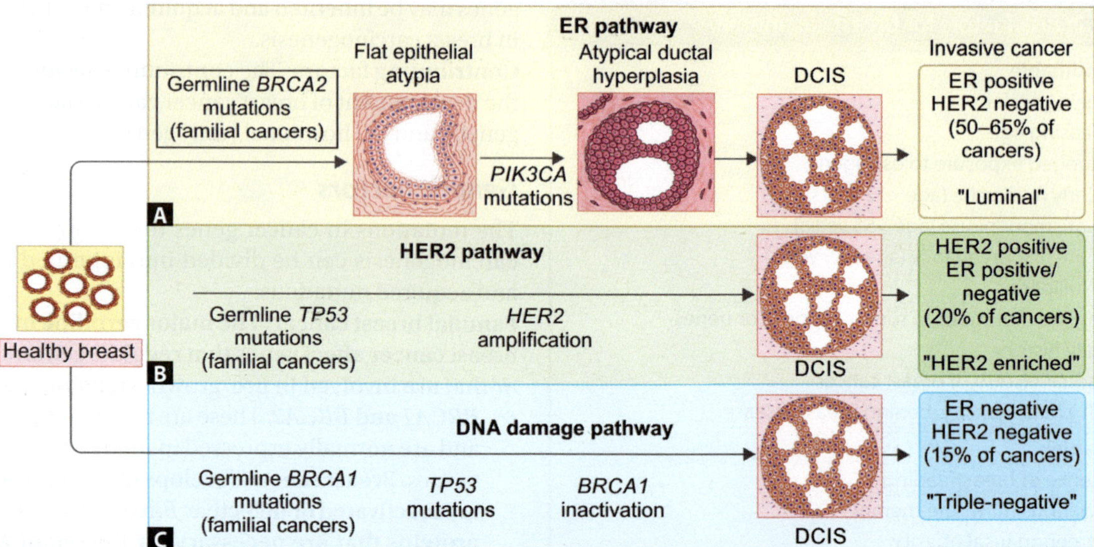

Figs. 23.4A to C: Major pathways involved in the development of ductal breast cancer: (A) The most common pathway leads to ER-positive cancers. The precursor lesions of this pathway include atypical ductal hyperplasia (ADH) and ductal carcinoma in situ (DCIS). Both these lesions have certain genomic events with invasive ER-positive carcinomas. These include mutations of *PIK3CA* (the gene encoding PI3K). These cancers are classified as "luminal" and they occur most commonly in individuals with germline *BRCA2* mutations; (B) Less common are cancers that overexpress HER2 because of gene amplification. These cancers may be positive or negative for ER. This type of cancer is most common in individuals with germline *TP53* mutations. (C) The least common but molecularly most characteristic type of breast cancer is negative for ER and HER2 ("triple negative"). In these carcinomas, there is a loss of BRCA1 and p53 function and they are genomically unstable. They are associated with germline *BRCA1* mutations.

(DCIS: ductal carcinoma in situ; ER: estrogen receptor).

The development of breast cancer can be promoted by estrogen through several mechanisms:

- **Proliferation of breast epithelial cells:** Physiologically, estrogen stimulates the proliferation of breast epithelial cells during puberty, menstrual cycles, and pregnancy. Estrogen binds to estrogen receptors (ER) and **stimulates the transcription of many target genes.** Thus, estrogens promote the proliferation and survival of breast epithelial cells.
- **Accumulation of mutations:** DNA replication during proliferation caused by excessive estrogenic stimulation may lead to the **accumulation of mutations.** The pause or interval in cell division that occurs during the latter part of the menstrual cycle may allow time for defective DNA repair to occur. Repetition of this process occurs during each menstrual cycle. The repeated process and a cumulative number of menstrual cycles occur more in women with early menarche and late menopause. This, in turn, increases the risk of developing luminal breast cancer
- **Benefits of estrogen antagonists:** Increased incidence of luminal cancers occurs in women treated with postmenopausal hormone therapy. Estrogen has a prooncogenic effect. The use of estrogen antagonists in therapy clearly observes the importance of estrogen. Estrogen antagonists reduce the development of luminal cancers in women at high risk.

Major Pathways of Breast Cancer (Figs. 23.4A to C)

1. **ER-positive, HER2-negative cancers (luminal): They constitute 50–65% of breast cancers.** The most common pathway leads to ER-positive cancers and these cancers are **classified as "luminal."** This type of cancer arises most commonly in individuals with germline *BRCA2* mutations. They show mutations of *PIK3CA* (the gene encoding PI3K).
2. **HER2-positive cancers (HER2 enriched): They arise through a pathway associated with amplifications of the *HER2* gene on chromosome 17q. They constitute about 20% (less common) of all breast cancers** and may be either ER-positive or ER-negative. They are usually associated with germline *TP53* mutations.
3. **ER-negative, HER2-negative cancers (Triple-negative): They arise via a distinct pathway that is independent of ER-mediated changes in gene expression and *HER2* gene amplifications.** They constitute ~15% (least common) of breast cancers but the molecularly most distinctive type of breast cancer is negative for ER and HER2 ("triple negative"). These cancers have a loss of *BRCA1* and *TP53* function and are genomically unstable. By gene expression profiling, the majority of triple-negative cancers are classified as "basal-like."

Role of stromal cells: Neoplastic epithelial cells are dependent on interactions with stromal cells in the local microenvironment. The stroma consists of fibroblasts, blood vessels, lymphatics, inflammatory cells, and extracellular matrix. The role of stroma is not yet completely known. However, it is observed that cancers develop in the areas with increased mammographic density (due to increased fibrous stroma) which suggests that stroma is both a marker of risk and biologically important for tumorigenesis. Focal changes in the stroma may create a microenvironment required for tumor development and growth. Angiogenesis and tumor-associated inflammation are commonly found with carcinoma even in the in situ stage.

TYPES OF BREAST CARCINOMA

The broad classification depends on a combination of histological patterns and cytological characteristics.

Carcinoma in situ (noninvasive carcinoma): It is characterized by the presence of **malignant epithelial cells within the ducts and lobules** and **has not penetrated the basement membrane.** It is a noninvasive cancer with no metastatic potential. **Carcinoma in situ** was originally classified as ductal (ductal carcinoma in situ/DCIS) or lobular (lobular carcinoma in situ/LCIS) based on the resemblance of the involved spaces to normal ducts or lobules (acini). Presently, these terms are based on differences in tumor cell biology; "lobular" refers to carcinomas of a specific type, and "ductal" is used more generally for adenocarcinomas that have no other designation. DCIS distorts the involved lobules into ductlike spaces. LCIS usually expands the involved lobules with bland, monomorphic cells.

Invasive carcinoma ("infiltrating" carcinoma): It is characterized by malignant cells that have **penetrated** through the **basement membrane** into the stroma. It may spread and kill the patient.

Ductal Carcinoma In Situ (DCIS; Intraductal Carcinoma)

Q. Write short note on ductal carcinoma in situ/intraductal carcinoma.

DCIS is a **noninvasive proliferation of cohesive neoplastic epithelial cells limited to the ducts** of the breast by the basement membrane. The myoepithelial cells are preserved.

- They usually **involve the small and medium-sized ducts**. DCIS can **spread throughout ducts and lobules**. Thus, it can produce extensive lesions involving an entire sector of a breast.
- DCIS does not produce a palpable mass. Most DCIS are detected by mammography due to calcifications forming on membrane fragments in secretions or in central necrosis ("comedonecrosis").

MORPHOLOGY

Ductal carcinoma in situ is characteristically a **unifocal disease and predominantly involves ducts. It shows the proliferation of cohesive (E-cadherin-positive) malignant epithelial cells within the ducts.**

Subtypes: It has the following subtypes: DCIS of low nuclear grade; intermediate nuclear grade; and of high nuclear grade.

Architectural patterns: It shows a range of architectural patterns and nuclear grades. According to architectural patterns, DCIS is categorized as **comedo, cribriform, micropapillary, papillary, or solid types. The majority of DCIS shows a mixture of these patterns.**

1. **Comedo DCIS:** Two features of comedo DCIS are **(1) tumor cells with pleomorphic, high-grade nuclei and (2) areas of central necrosis. Necrosis in the center of ducts** is called comedo-type necrosis.
   - **Gross:** Comedonecrosis appears grossly as distended ducts containing white necrotic material resembling comedos (a small defect on the skin usually containing a plug of sebum), hence the term comedonecrosis.
   - **Microscopy (Fig. 23.5A):** Ducts contain solid sheets of very **large, pleomorphic epithelial cells** having **pleomorphic, irregular hyperchromatic nuclei.** The **central areas** show **necrosis. The central necrotic area** commonly undergoes **dystrophic calcification.**
2. **Cribriform DCIS (Fig. 23.5B):** It is composed of cribriform ("cribriform" meaning "sieve-like" or "perforated") **spaces between the intraductal tumor**. These spaces **are round, evenly distributed, and regular in shape** (cookie cutter-like). These spaces tend to be crisp, rigid, and "punched-out," extracellular lumens (spaces are not always uniform). The neoplastic cells polarize around the spaces. These spaces are usually filled with calcified secretory material.
3. **Micropapillary DCIS (Fig. 23.5C):** It shows **bulbous protrusions without a fibrovascular core.**
4. **Papillary DCIS (Fig. 23.5D):** It shows **papillae with fibrovascular cores** and without the normal myoepithelial cell layer.
5. **Solid DCIS (Fig. 23.5E):** It shows **tumor cells completely filling the involved spaces.** The ducts contain a **monomorphic population of tumor cells** with **nuclear grades ranging from low to high. Necrosis is minimal or absent.**

Prognosis of DCIS: If untreated, women with small, low-grade DCIS may develop invasive cancer. **Mastectomy for DCIS is curative for over 95% of patients.**

Lobular Carcinoma In Situ (LCIS)

Arises in TDLU: LCIS is a noninvasive neoplastic proliferation of small, loosely cohesive, uniform cells that originate in TDLUs (terminal duct lobular units)**. These neoplastic cells have** homogeneous chromatin and inconspicuous nucleoli**. The proliferating cells fill (and often distend) >50% of the lobules in the involved TDLUs**

Lack of E-cadherin: E-cadherin is a transmembrane adhesion protein involved in the cohesion of normal epithelial cells in the breast and other glandular tissues. E-cadherin may be lost in neoplastic proliferation through different mechanisms. One mechanism is by mutation of the E-cadherin gene *(CDH1)*. The cells of atypical lobular hyperplasia, LCIS, and invasive lobular carcinoma (ILC) are identical and show loss of E-cadherin with **mutations of the E-cadherin gene**. Lack of E-cadherin in LCIS results in

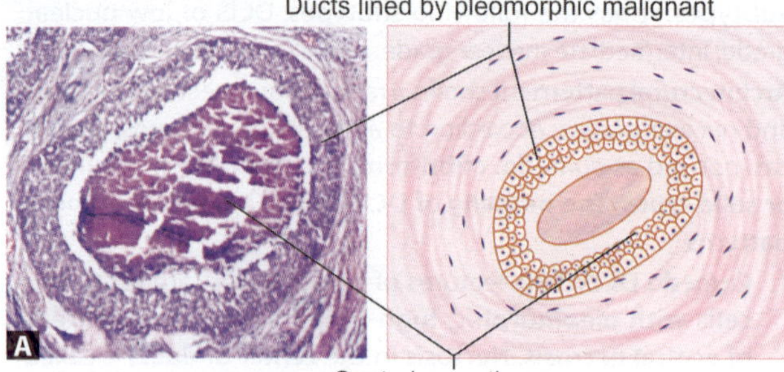

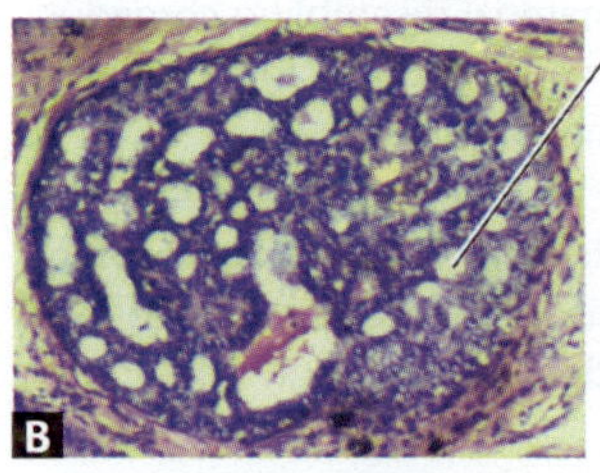

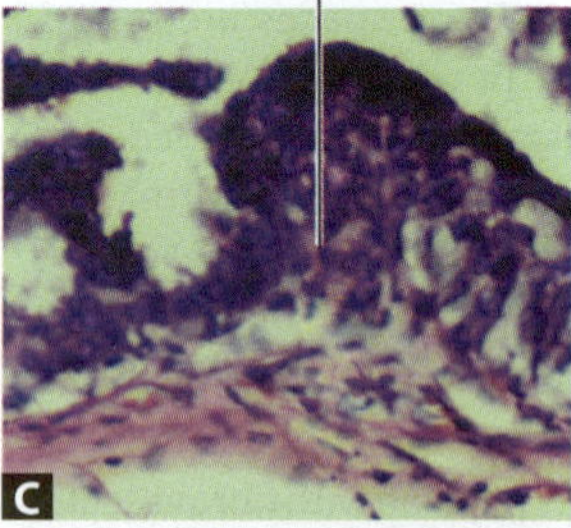

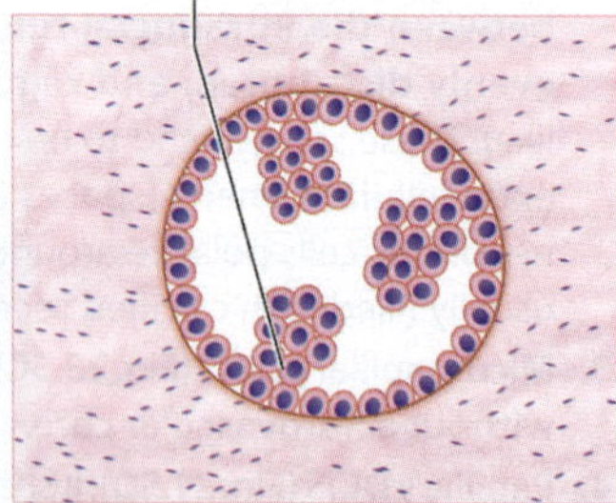

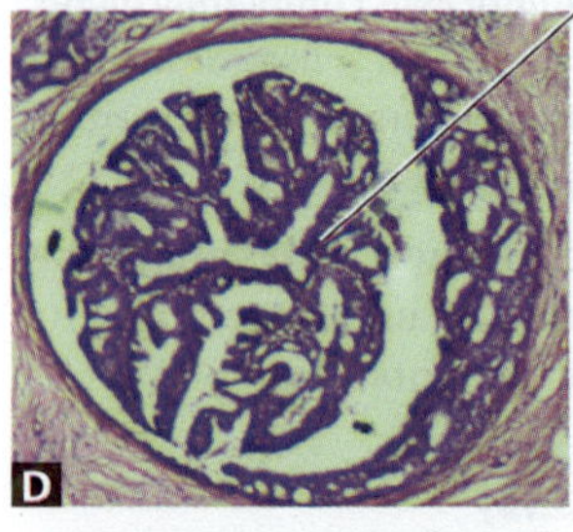

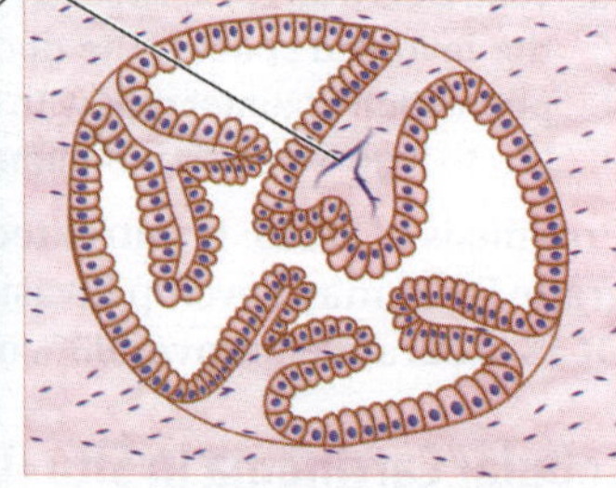

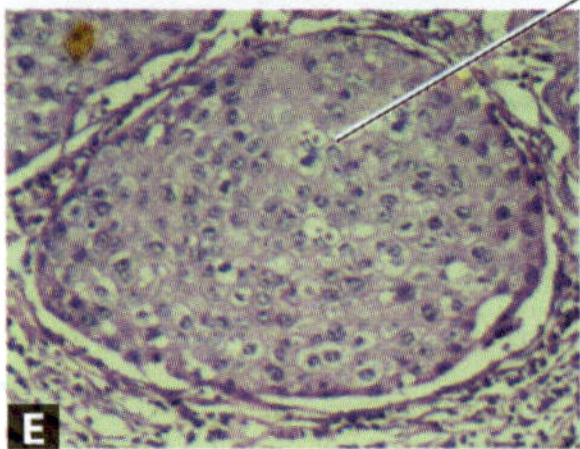

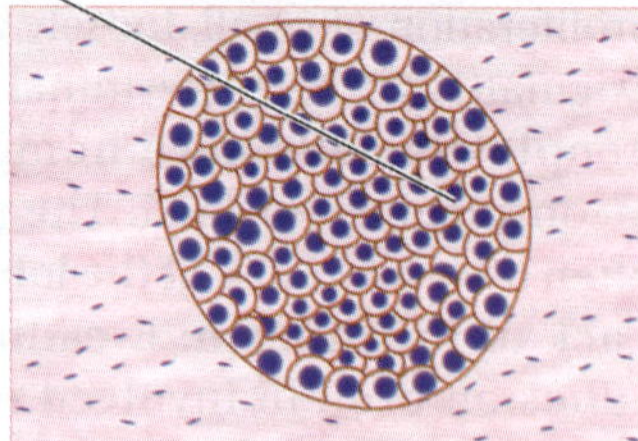

Figs. 23.5A to E: Photomicrographic (left of each) and diagrammatic (right of each) appearances of ductal carcinoma in situ (DCIS): (A) DCIS-comedo subtype showing ducts containing large, pleomorphic epithelial cells and central area of the duct with necrosis; (B) Cribriform; (C) Micropapillary; (D) Papillary; (E) Solid type.

rounded tumor cells due to loss of attachment to adjacent cells. Lack of E-cadherin expression confirms the lobular nature of neoplastic cells.

Tends to be bilateral in 20–40% of cases.

MORPHOLOGY

Gross

LCIS **does not usually produce grossly recognizable abnormalities.**

Microscopy (*refer* online Figs. 23.6A and B)

Retained lobular architecture: The overall lobular architecture is retained. However, **individual acini are enlarged and distended, and their lumina are obliterated.**

Tumor cells:

- **Monotonous cells:** The tumor consists of **a loose, noncohesive** (dyscohesive), **uniform population** of **cells.** Tumor cells are **smaller** and **more monotonous** than in DCIS.
- **Oval or round, regular nuclei with small nucleoli.**
- **Mucin-positive signet-ring cells** are commonly present.

No necrosis or calcification.

Immunohistochemistry: Lack of **E-cadherin,** almost always **expresses ER and PR, and does not overexpress HER2/neu.**

INVASIVE (INFILTRATING) CARCINOMA

Invasive breast carcinoma (IBC) is a **heterogeneous group of malignant epithelial neoplasms of the glandular elements** of the breast. Invasive ductal carcinoma is the **most common histological type** of breast carcinoma.

Common features of invasive carcinoma: They are as follows:

- **Invasion:** It is characterized by the presence of tumor cells outside of the duct-lobular units and into the surrounding breast stroma.
- **Desmoplasia:** It is characterized by marked stromal fibrosis.

Morphological classification: Invasive breast carcinoma can be broadly classified as (i) invasive breast carcinoma of no special type, and (ii) special histologic types of invasive carcinoma.

Invasive Breast Carcinoma of No Special Type (NST)

Q. Discuss the pathology of infiltrating duct (invasive breast) carcinoma.

Definition: Invasive breast carcinoma (IBC) of no special type (NST) is a **large and heterogeneous group of IBCs that cannot be classified morphologically as any of the special histological types.**

Invasive breast carcinomas (IBC) of no special type **constitute** about **70–80% of carcinomas** and the remaining can be classified into special histologic types.

PA 31.3 (CC): Describe and identify the morphologic and microscopic features of carcinoma of the breast.

MORPHOLOGY

Q. Write a short note on the morphology of invasive/infiltrating duct carcinoma of the breast.

Localization: Most (~90%) of breast cancers are unifocal. They can occur in any quadrant of the breast. **About 50% are located in the upper outer quadrant**, 10% in each of the remaining quadrants, and about 20% occur in the central or subareolar region.

Gross (Figs. 23.7A and B)

The appearance varies widely depending on the stromal reaction to the tumor.

- **Hard and irregular:** Most commonly, these cancers are **firm to hard in consistency.** They have an **irregular outline or border.**
- **Cut section:** They are **nodular or stellate on cut sections.** The cut surface appears **tan-white to gray, firm to hard, with a gritty surface (Figs. 23.7A and B).** When cut or scraped, they typically produce a characteristic **grating sound** (like cutting a water chestnut or unripened pear). This is due to small, central pinpoint foci or streaks of chalky-white desmoplastic stroma (dense fibrous stroma), and occasional foci of calcification.
- **Nipple retraction:** When the carcinoma involves the central portion of the breast, it **may produce retraction of the nipple.** Tumors may **retract below the surface.**

Microscopy (Figs. 23.8A and B)

Carcinoma of the breast is termed as no special type (NST), essentially through a process of exclusion of recognized special types.

Architecture

The growth pattern varies. The tumor cells may be **arranged in cords, sheets, nests, clusters, solids, trabeculae, and glands** (tubules).

Tumor Cells

Carcinoma cells have a variable appearance. They may have **abundant and eosinophilic cytoplasm. Nuclei may be regular, uniform, or highly pleomorphic with prominent, often multiple, nucleoli.** Mitotic counts vary and range from virtually absent to frequent. In up to 80% of cases, **foci of associated ductal carcinoma in situ (DCIS)** may be present. Their nuclear grade is the same as that of the invasive component.

Stroma

The stromal component surrounding the tumor cells is extremely variable. It can range from a highly cellular fibroblastic proliferation forming a **desmoplastic stroma to a scanty element of connective tissue** or marked hyalinization (collagenous).

Nottingham Histologic Score

The Nottingham grading system (Nottingham Histologic Score) is used for grading invasive breast cancers. Carcinomas are scored depending on (1) tubule formation, (2) nuclear pleomorphism, and (3) mitotic rate. The points are added and carcinomas are graded into grades I, II, and III.

- **Grade I (well-differentiated carcinomas):** They show tumor cells forming **prominent tubules.** The tumor cells have small round nuclei, and mitotic figures are rare.
- **Grade II (moderately differentiated carcinomas):** Tumor cells may form **tubules**, but they also show **solid clusters or single infiltrating cells.** The tumor cells show a greater degree of nuclear pleomorphism and also have mitotic figures.
- **Grade III (poorly differentiated carcinomas):** They consist of **nests or solid sheets of cells.** The tumor cells also show enlarged irregular nuclei, numerous mitotic figures, and areas of tumor necrosis.

Immunohistochemistry: About 70–80% are ER-positive, and 15% are HER2-positive.

Prognosis: Overall, 35–50% of patients survive 10 years. It varies according to tumor and lymph node stage, tumor grade, and the presence or absence of lymphovascular invasion (LVI).

Special morphologic patterns of invasive ductal carcinoma: Several special morphologic patterns of invasive carcinoma NST fall short of the criteria to classify them as separate special subtypes in the WHO (2019) breast tumor classification. The three most common patterns include: (1) *medullary pattern invasive cancer,* (2) *invasive carcinoma with neuroendocrine differentiation*, and (3) *carcinoma with osteoclast-like stromal giant cells.*

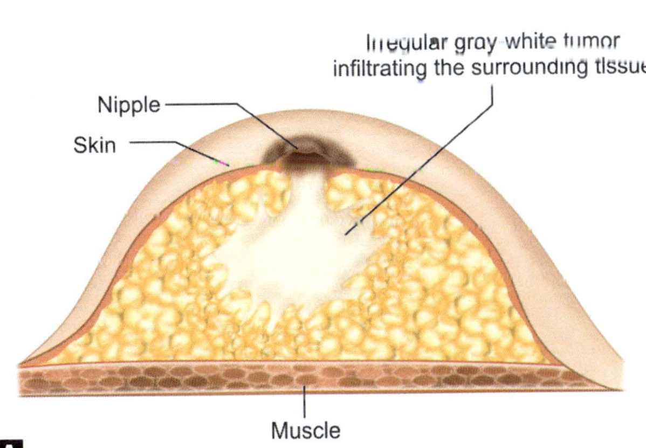

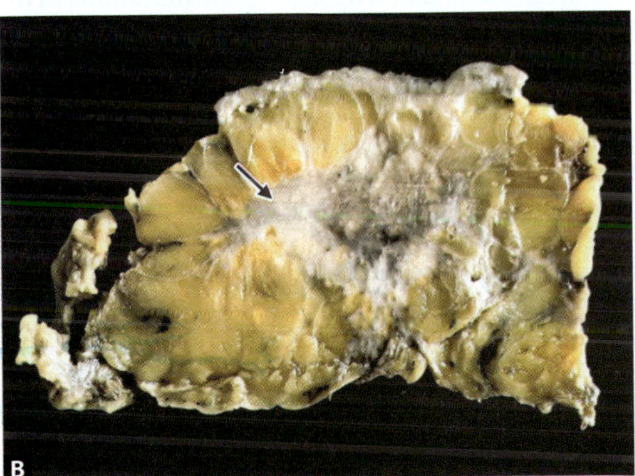

Figs. 23.7A and B: Gross appearance of invasive carcinoma of the breast: (A) Diagrammatic; (B) Mastectomy specimen with irregular, gray-white tumor.

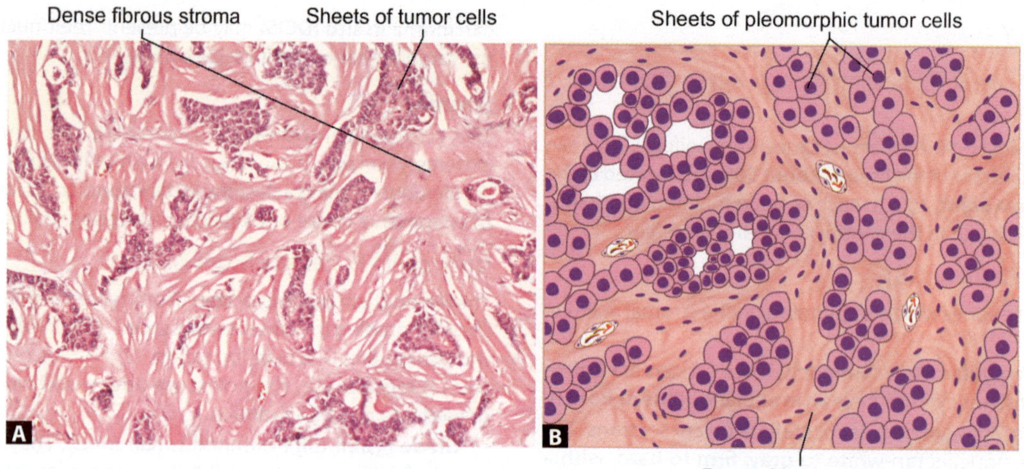

Figs. 23.8A and B: (A) Hematoxylin and eosin (H & E); (B) Diagrammatic. Microscopy of invasive carcinoma of breast showing irregular sheets of malignant cells separated by dense fibrous stroma (desmoplasia).

Medullary Pattern Invasive Cancer

Q. Write a short essay on the medullary pattern of invasive breast cancer.

Cancers **historically described as medullary carcinoma, atypical medullary carcinoma, or carcinoma with medullary features** were previously considered as a specific special type of breast cancer. The characteristic features of these tumors are presented in **Box 23.3.** It forms about 5% of all breast cancers. It has no resemblance to medullary carcinoma of the thyroid.

Tumor-infiltrating lymphocytes (TILs): The presence of unusually large numbers of tumor-infiltrating lymphocytes (TILs) in high-grade breast cancers is associated **with a better prognosis** for these cancers than other poorly differentiated carcinomas. These TILs are related to a host immune response to tumor antigens. ***For clinical purposes, these cancers are now categorized diagnostically as IDC with medullary patterns.***

***BRCA1*: More than 50% of *BRCA1*-associated carcinomas have this appearance.** Most carcinomas with the medullary pattern are not **associated with germline mutations in the *BRCA1* gene.** However, hypermethylation of the *BRCA1* promoter leading to downregulation of *BRCA1* expression is found in 67% of these tumors. Lymph node metastases are infrequent.

- **Age-group:** Most common in the **sixth decade.**
- **Clinical presentation:** Presents as a **well-circumscribed mass** and mimics a benign lesion. It may present as a rapidly growing mass.

BOX 23.3: Characteristic features of medullary pattern invasive carcinoma.

- Well-circumscribed cancers
- High histological grade with regions of necrosis
- Pushing margins
- Syncytial architecture with no glandular structures
- Prominent tumor-infiltrating lymphocyte (TIL) infiltrate
- Better clinical outcome than other stage-matched high-grade cancers
- Most often triple-negative [negative for hormone receptors (ER and PR) and HER2]

(ER: estrogen receptor; PR: progesterone receptor)

MORPHOLOGY

Q. Write a short note on the morphology of medullary carcinoma of the breast (medullary pattern invasive cancer).

Gross (Fig. 23.9)

Well-circumscribed soft tumor: Carcinoma with medullary (*medulla* is Latin for "marrow") pattern is a **well-circumscribed, fleshy, and soft** (softer than other carcinomas due to minimal desmoplasia).

Cut surface: On the cut section, shows a **bulging cut surface.** It is a **tan-brown to pale-gray mass.** Hemorrhage, necrosis, or cystic change may be seen.

No desmoplasia: It usually **does not produce desmoplasia.** So, it is more yielding on palpation and cutting than typical breast carcinomas.

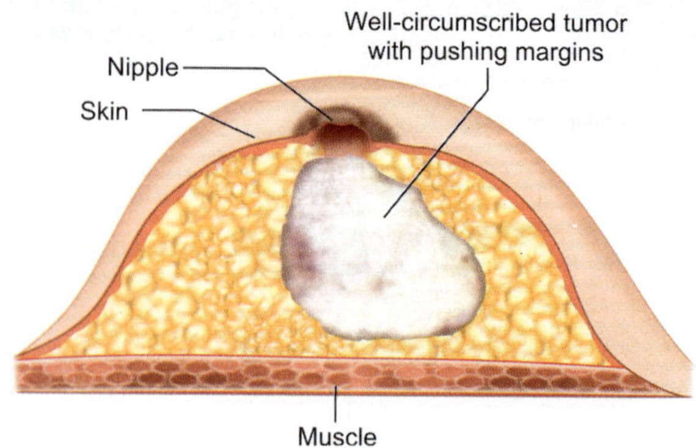

Fig. 23.9: Schematic gross appearance of medullary pattern invasive cancer showing well-circumscribed, soft, and pale-gray tumors in the breast.

Microscopy (Figs. 23.10A and B)

Medullary pattern invasive carcinomas are **poorly differentiated** and their features are:

1. **Syncytial growth pattern** in >75% of the tumor: Tumor cells are arranged in **solid, syncytium-like (cytoplasmic mass containing several nuclei without distinct cell borders) sheets.**
2. **Moderate to marked (intense) lymphoplasmacytic infiltrate** surrounding and within the tumor. Stroma is minimal with lymphoplasmacytic infiltrate.
3. **Solid sheets of large anaplastic cells with highly pleomorphic nuclei:** Tumor cells are **large and pleomorphic.** They have **vesicular, pleomorphic nuclei** (nuclear grades 2–3), **and prominent nucleoli.**
4. **Mitotic figures** are **frequent**.
5. **A pushing (noninfiltrative) border**
6. **No glandular differentiation**
7. **DCIS is minimal or not seen**

Immunohistochemistry: Medullary carcinomas are generally **negative for all biomarkers** [triple-negative breast cancer (TNBC), i.e., ER-negative, PR-negative, HER2-negative].

Prognosis: Pure medullary pattern invasive carcinomas have a **favorable outcome**. However, variant types may not have this prognostic advantage.

Special Histologic Types of Invasive Carcinoma

These are invasive carcinomas with distinctive/unique morphological, biological, genetic, and clinical features. Similar to "no special type", of breast cancer, these special tumors can be grouped depending on the expression of ER and *HER2*. These include lobular carcinoma, mucinous carcinoma (MC), tubular carcinoma (TC), and papillary carcinoma.

Invasive Lobular Carcinoma

Q. Write a short note on invasive lobular carcinoma of the breast.

Invasive lobular carcinoma (ILC) is an invasive breast carcinoma (IBC) **composed of dyscohesive cells.** These tumor cells are **most often individually dispersed or arranged in a single-file linear pattern** (as single cells). The ILC comprises about 15% of all invasive carcinomas. Increased incidence is observed in patients receiving postmenopausal combined hormone replacement therapy (HRT).

Characteristics of ILC: These are as follows:

- **Dysfunction of E-cadherin:** Like LCIS, most ILCs show **biallelic loss (loss of both alleles of the gene) of expression of** ***CDH1*** (a gene that encodes E-cadherin). E-cadherin is a transmembrane protein that is required for the cohesion of normal epithelial cells in the breast and other glandular tissues. Males and females with heterozygous germline mutations in *CDH1* have an increased risk for developing lobular carcinoma and also have an **increased risk for signet ring carcinoma of the stomach.**
- **Sometimes without desmoplastic response:** Sometimes, ILC may not produce a desmoplastic response. This **makes it difficult to detect these cancers by palpation and imaging.**
- **Unique patterns of metastasis:** Lobular carcinomas **often spread to cerebrospinal fluid, serosal surfaces, gastrointestinal tract, ovary, uterus, and bone marrow.**

MORPHOLOGY

Localization: ILC has a higher rate of **multifocality in the ipsilateral breast** and is also **more often bilateral** than other subtypes.

Gross (*refer* online Fig. 23.11)

ILCs may either appear as **irregular and poorly demarcated masses** or only show an area of firm, rubbery breast tissue.

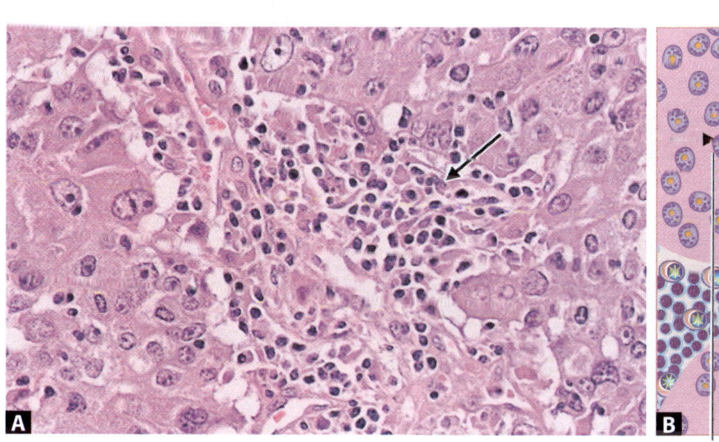

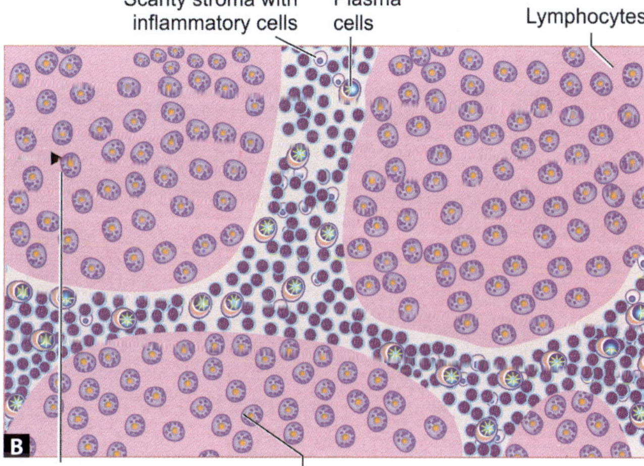

Figs. 23.10A and B: Medullary pattern invasive carcinoma of the breast: (A) H&E shows syncytial masses of large pleomorphic cells separated by stroma with lymphoplasmacytic infiltrate: (B) Diagrammatic representation.

Microscopy (Figs. 23.12A to C)

ILCs may either appear as irregular and poorly demarcated masses or only show an area of firm, rubbery breast tissue.

- **"Indian file" pattern:** Lobular carcinoma is composed of **loose and noncohesive (dyscohesive/lack cohesion). Tumor cells appear individually dispersed and infiltrate in a single "Indian file" pattern** (Indian file means a line of cells arranged one after another) **(Fig. 23.12A and C)** and form linear strands. They **do not form ducts or tubules** but form solid sheets, trabeculae, or nests.
- **Targetoid pattern of growth: Tumor cells may concentrically surround benign epithelial elements**/periductal region known as the targetoid pattern of growth **(Fig. 23.12B).**
- **Tumor cells:** They are **small, uniform (monotonous), and dyscohesive**. The **nuclei are small, regular, oval, or round nuclei with small nucleoli.** They have a **thin rim of cytoplasm. Nuclei are located eccentrically** within a cytoplasm that occasionally shows intracytoplasmic lumen. The lumen represents an intracytoplasmic vacuole containing an eosinophilic mucin droplet **(signet-ring cells).** Mitotes are usually sparse.
- **Minimal or absent desmoplasia.**

Immunohistochemistry: Most ILCs have **reduced or absent expression of E-cadherin.** Up to 95% of ILCs **express ER and PR.** ILCs **usually do not overexpress the *HER2* gene product.**

Mucinous (Colloid) Carcinoma

Mucinous carcinoma (MC) of the breast is an IBC characterized by **clusters of epithelial tumor cells suspended in pools of extracellular mucin.** It is usually seen in **older patients.** Pure MC is slow-growing and is usually associated with a **favorable outcome. Lymph node metastases** are **uncommon.**

MORPHOLOGY

Gross

It shows a **glistening, gelatinous, well-circumscribed nodule with pushing margins.** It has a **soft, viscous, pale gray-blue gelatin consistency** (due to the presence of mucin pools). The size of the tumor ranges from <1 to >20 cm.

Microscopy

It consists of **cuboidal to columnar tumor cells** arranged in **clusters or sheets of neoplastic cells suspended in abundant extracellular mucin** (*refer* **online Fig. 23.13).**

Immunohistochemistry: Tumors typically are positive for ER (>90% of tumors) and PR biomarkers and negative for HER2 overexpression.

Prognosis: Better than infiltrating ductal or lobular carcinoma.

Tubular Carcinoma

Tubular carcinoma is an uncommon, **low-grade** (well-differentiated) invasive carcinoma **composed of exclusively well-formed tubules with open lumina lined by a single layer of neoplastic cells.** It constitutes 5% of invasive carcinoma and has a **favorable prognosis.** Metastasis is rare. It occurs in the late 40s.

MORPHOLOGY

Gross

Tubular carcinomas are **firm to hard in consistency** and **pale gray.** They are usually **smaller than 2 cm** in diameter and irregular.

Microscopy

Tumors are very well-differentiated and are characterized by a **haphazard** (irregularly) **arrangement of small, well-formed round to ovoid or angulated tubules with tapering ends.** The lumens of these tubules are open. These tubules are separated by dense stroma (*refer* **online Fig. 23.14).**

Immunohistochemistry: Typically, it is **positive for ER and PR** in >90% of tumors, but usually **negative for HER2** overexpression.

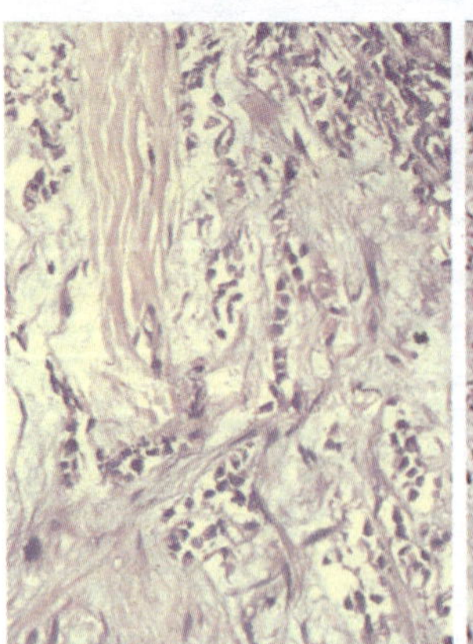

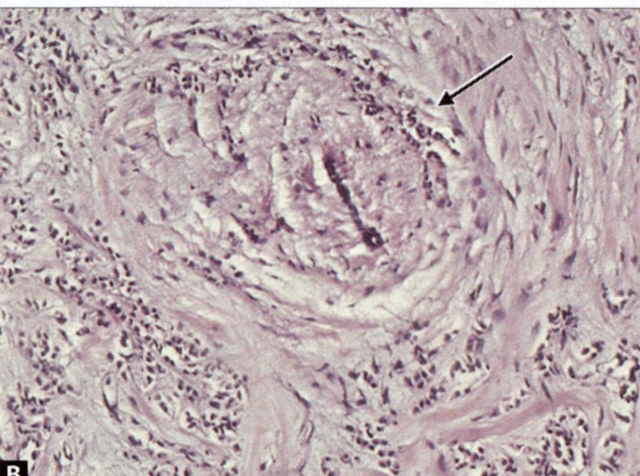

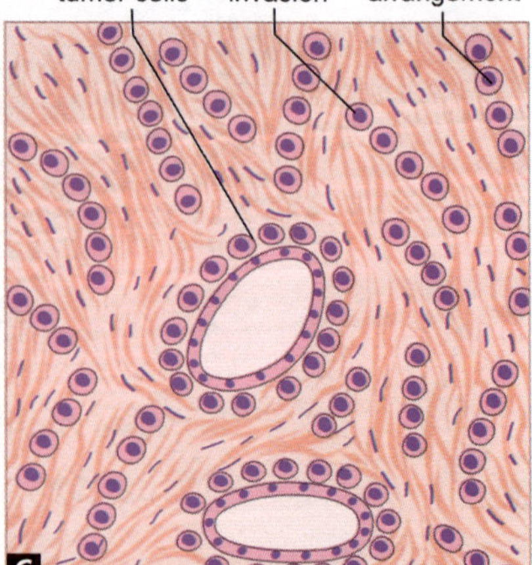

Figs. 23.12A to C: Lobular carcinoma of the breast: (A) The tumor shows small, uniform (monotonous), and dyscohesive cells (loosely cohesive) that infiltrates in a single "Indian file" pattern; (B) Tumor cells concentrically surround the benign periductal region showing a targetoid pattern of growth (arrow); (C) Diagrammatic appearance of Indian file and targetoid pattern.

Special Clinical Scenario

Inflammatory Carcinoma

It is a **clinical-pathologic entity.** It is characterized by **diffuse erythema, induration** (swelling and skin thickening), **and tenderness of breast skin**. The name "inflammatory" is a misnomer because usually, no inflammation is present. The presentation can be **confused with a breast infection.** Hence, its diagnosis may be delayed.

MORPHOLOGY

Gross

Peau d'orange appearance of skin: In inflammatory carcinoma, the edematous skin is attached to the breast by Cooper ligaments. The **skin of the breast shows nonpitting edema** that **mimics the surface of an orange peel (orange skin), an appearance referred to as** ***peau d'orange***. It is due to the involvement of subdermal lymphatics (permeation and blockage/obstruction) of the skin.

Underlying carcinoma: An underlying breast mass **may or may not form a discrete palpable mass.** The underlying carcinoma is usually diffusely infiltrative and of high-grade but does not belong to any particular molecular subtype.

Microscopy

Non pitting edema (*peau d'orange*) is caused by extensive plugging of dermal lymphatic (lymphovascular spaces) by tumor emboli (carcinoma cells). Microscopic diagnosis is necessary to demonstrate invasive carcinoma in the underlying breast tissue.

Immunohistochemistry: Most cases are ER/PR negative, with HER2-positive invasive carcinomas.

Prognosis: Inflammatory carcinoma carries a very poor prognosis. Most patients have distant metastases.

Common Clinical Features of Invasive Breast Carcinoma

- **Palpable mass:** About one-third of breast cancers are first detected as a **palpable mass.**
- **Invasion:** Larger carcinomas **may infiltrate the pectoralis muscle and be fixed to the** underlying **chest wall or invade the dermis and produce dimpling of the skin (skin retraction).**
- **Retraction of the nipple and nipple discharge:** It may occur when the tumor involves the central portion of the breast.
- **Regional lymph node metastasis:** At least 50% of the cancers show spread to regional lymph nodes at the time of presentation. Involved lymphatics may block the local area of skin drainage and cause **lymphedema** and thickening of the skin.
- **Metastasis:** Rarely, breast cancer may first present as metastasis to an axillary node or distant metastasis before cancer is detected in the breast. In these cases, the primary carcinoma may be small.

Mammographically, invasive carcinomas most commonly present as a **radiodense mass.**

PAGET DISEASE OF THE NIPPLE

Q. Write a short note on Paget disease of breast/nipple.

Paget disease of the nipple is a **rare manifestation** (1–4% of cases) **of ductal carcinoma, either in high-grade** ductal carcinoma in situ **(DCIS) or invasive** (occasionally). In Paget disease, **malignant glandular cells (Paget cells) of high-grade DCIS extend into the basal layers of the epidermis of the nipple and areola.** The DCIS is present within the subareolar ducts and extends via the lactiferous sinuses along the basement membrane into the skin of the nipple and areola. It produces a unilateral crusting exudate over the nipple and areolar skin **(Fig. 23.15C).** They do not cross the basement membrane.

MORPHOLOGY

Q. Write a short note on the morphology of Paget disease of the breast.

Gross (Figs. 23.15A and B)

- **Skin of the nipple and areola:** It may show redness or **frank erosion (ulceration)** with oozing **resembling eczema.**
- **It shows underlying ductal carcinoma (in situ or invasive).**

Microscopy (Figs. 23.16A and B)

- **Paget cells in the epidermis of skin lesions in the nipple:** The epidermis contains an **infiltrate of single (or small groups/ closely packed clusters of) large pleomorphic high-grade glandular epithelial tumor cells** known as **Paget cells.** They do not infiltrate the basement membrane. Paget cells **represent extension from underlying ductal carcinoma via the lactiferous sinuses.** The tumor cells allow seepage of extracellular fluid onto the nipple surface.
- **Appearance of Paget cells (Figs. 16A and B):** These are intraepidermal **large spherical cells with abundant clear cytoplasm and contain mucin globules** (stain positively with alcian blue and periodic acid-Shiff reaction). They have

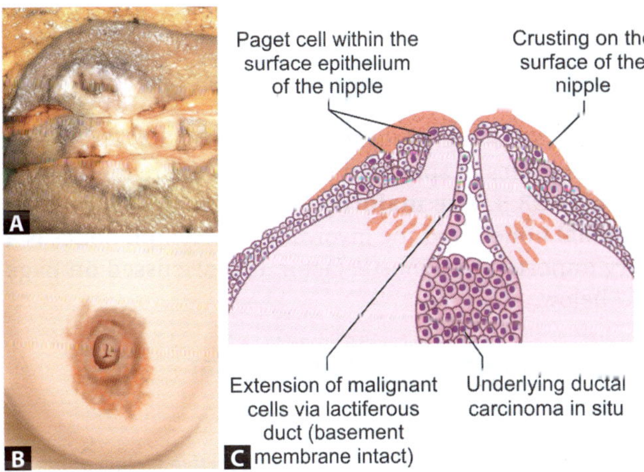

Figs. 23.15A to C: Paget disease of the nipple: (A) and (B) Appearance of nipple and areola with ulceration; (C) Diagrammatic representation of ductal carcinoma in situ with extension along the lactiferous duct into the epidermis of nipple and areola.

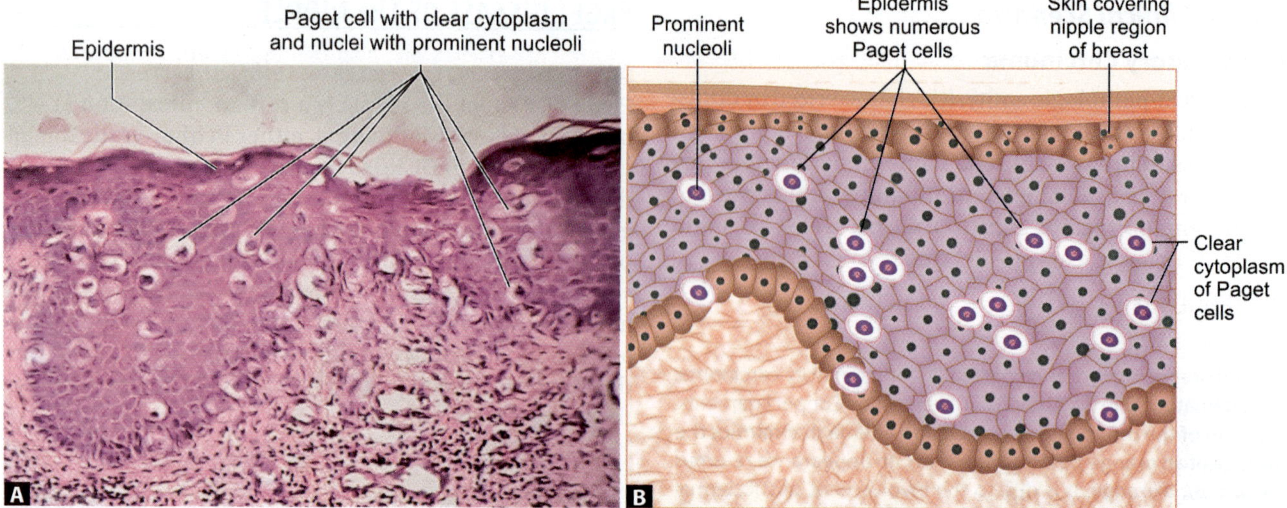

Figs. 23.16A and B: (A) Photomicrograph; (B) Diagrammatic appearance show microscopic features of Paget disease of the breast.

pleomorphic, hyperchromatic nuclei with prominent nucleoli. The Paget cells can be detected by nipple biopsy or cytologic examination of the exudate.

Immunohistochemistry: Underlying carcinoma when present is usually poorly differentiated, **ER-negative, and overexpress *HER2*/neu.**

Clinical Presentation

- Presents as a unilateral **erythematous eruption** in the region of the nipple and areola with a scale crust.
- **Pruritus** (itching) is common, and the lesion may be **mistaken for eczema.**
- **Palpable mass** in the breast is present in 50–60% of women and shows an **underlying invasive carcinoma.**
- Majority of women **without a palpable mass** have only **DCIS.**

Prognosis: Depends on the features of the underlying ductal carcinoma.

Spread of Breast Carcinoma

Q. Write a short answer on the spread of breast cancer.

Various routes of spread of breast cancer are mentioned in **Table 23.3. The majority of cancers first spread to regional nodes,** and the involvement of lymph nodes is a very important prognostic factor. It is discussed on page 857 below.

TABLE 23.3 Various routes of spread of breast carcinoma.

Direct	*Lymphatics*	*Hematogenous*
• Skin, including nipple and areola • Chest wall	• Outer quadrant carcinoma to axillary lymph node • Inner quadrant carcinoma to internal mammary lymph node • Infra- and supra-clavicular lymph node	• Lung • Bone • Liver • Brain

BOX 23.4: Prognostic factors in breast cancer.

- Distant metastases
- Lymph node metastases
- Tumor size
- Histologic grade
- Expression of ER, PR, *HER2*/neu
- Lymphovascular invasion
- Special histologic type
- Response to neoadjuvant chemotherapy
- Locally advanced disease
- Gene expression profiling
- Proliferative index and ploidy
- Molecular subtype

(ER: estrogen receptor; PR: progesterone receptor)

Prognostic and Predictive Factors for Invasive Carcinoma

Q. Write a short note on prognostic and predictive factors of breast carcinoma.

The prognosis of breast cancer is determined by the biological features of the carcinoma (molecular or histologic type) and the extent of cancer spread (stage) at the time of diagnosis. Several factors determine the prognosis of breast cancer **(Box 23.4)**. Prognostic factors help to know about the likely outcome of cancer, select the most appropriate treatment, and design clinical trials. Predictive factors help to determine the possible response of cancer to a specific type of treatment.

- **Distant metastases:** Metastasis beyond regional lymph nodes is the most important prognostic factor. Once distant metastases are present, it has a poor prognosis, and a cure is unlikely. Bone metastases occur in 25% of patients. The most likely site and time of metastasis vary with the biologic type of cancer.
  - **Triple-negative cancers and HER2 cancers:** They are more likely to metastasize to the **brain and viscera**.
  - **ER-positive cancers:** They usually **metastasize to bones** and are likely to have late recurrences.
- **Lymph node metastases:** The **presence or absence of axillary lymph node metastases**, including the number of involved lymph nodes, is the **second most important** prognostic indicator for patients with invasive breast cancer in the absence of distant metastases.
  - **Sentinel node biopsy:** Lymphatic vessels in most breast carcinomas drain first to one or two lymph nodes in the axilla, which are known as **sentinel nodes**. These are **usually examined for metastasis.** If these nodes do not show tumor deposits, the remaining axillary nodes are usually free of carcinoma. Sentinel node biopsy is the standard method for assessing nodal status.
  - **The number and level involved** are directly related to the survival rate.
  - Depending on the size of metastatic foci, they can be divided into:
    - **Macrometastases** mean metastasis greater than 0.2 cm.
    - **Micrometastases** mean metastasis 0.2 cm or less.

  Till recently, the status of lymph nodes was considered a major determinant of treatment choice. After the advent of molecular typing of carcinoma, the information obtained from nodal status is becoming less important. In the future, many women need not undergo sampling of nodes.
- **Tumor size:** Prognosis varies with tumor size (T in the TNM protocol) and is an independent prognostic factor. Women with larger tumors show poorer survival. Only the invasive part is considered while assessing the size of the tumor. The risk of axillary lymph node metastasis increases with the size of the primary tumor. Patients with **node-negative carcinomas <1 cm** in size have a **10-year survival rate of over 90%.** This survival rate drops to 77% for cancers more than 2 cm.
- **Histological grade: Nottingham histologic score** (also referred to as **Scarff–Bloom–Richardson**) is the **most commonly used grading system**, which classifies invasive carcinomas into three groups (grade 1 to grade 3). These grades are highly correlated with survival. This grading system is **based on: (1) tubule formation, (2) nuclear grade, and (3) mitotic rate.**
- **Expression of ER, PR, and HER2:** Survival is highest for the most favorable combination (high ER and PR and absent HER2) and is lowest for the least favorable combination (absent ER, PR, and HER2).
  - **Estrogen (ER) and progesterone receptors (PR) expression:**
    - **ER and PR positive (Figs. 23.17A and B):** These carcinomas **respond to hormonal manipulation.** ER-positive cancers are less likely to respond to chemotherapy.
    - **ER and PR negative:** These carcinomas are more likely to respond to chemotherapy.
  - **HER2/neu expression:** Its **overexpression (Fig. 23.17C)** or gene amplification is associated with **poorer survival**. However, they are a predictor of response to agents that target this receptor.
- **Lymphovascular invasion:** In about 50% of invasive carcinomas, tumor cells are found within vascular spaces (either lymphatics or small capillaries). This is strongly associated with lymph node metastases. It is a poor prognostic factor in cancers without lymph node metastases and is a risk factor for local recurrence. Severe plugging of the lymphovascular spaces of the dermis with carcinoma cells (**inflammatory carcinoma**) also has a very poor prognosis.
- **Special histologic type**: Some histologic types of breast cancer are strongly correlated with very favorable survival, such as tubular and adenoid cystic carcinoma. Inflammatory breast carcinoma is characterized by extensive invasion of dermal lymphovascular channels and has a poor prognosis. In inflammatory carcinoma, the 3-year survival rate is only 3–10%.
- **Response to neoadjuvant chemotherapy:** Preoperative (before surgery) systemic treatment with chemotherapy is called neoadjuvant therapy. It provides the opportunity to observe the tumor response to chemotherapy. It does not by itself enhance survival. However, the response to neoadjuvant therapy is a strong prognostic factor. It can render inoperable tumors resectable and downstage tumors in patients with large tumors.
- **Locally advanced disease** with invasion into the skin or skeletal muscle has a bad prognosis.
- **Gene expression profiling:** Many multigene prognostic proprietary assays have been developed to quantify messenger ribonucleic acid (mRNA) levels in breast cancer cells. Most mainly include genes that are involved in proliferation. Now, they are widely used as both prognostic tools and in predicting responses to various therapies. The main clinical importance of these assays is to identify patients with ER-positive breast cancer that are slowly growing, antiestrogen-responsive cancers.
- **Proliferative index and ploidy:** Cancers with high proliferative indices have a worse prognosis. In breast cancers, proliferation can be measured by counting mitotic figures during histological grading or by immunohistochemical detection of proteins that are specifically expressed by actively dividing cells (e.g.,

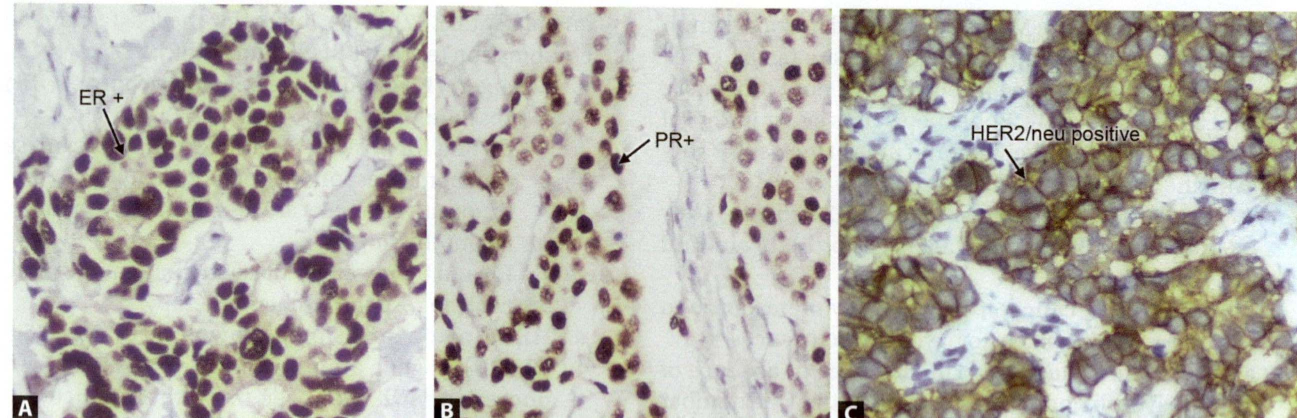

Figs. 23.17A to C: Immunohistochemistry in breast carcinoma: (A) ER-positive; (B) PR positive and (C) HER2/neu positive.

cyclins, Ki-67). Proliferative rate is mainly important for ER-positive and *HER2*-negative carcinomas. Most of the ER-negative and/or *HER2*-positive carcinomas have high proliferative rates. Carcinomas with high proliferation rates have a poorer prognosis, but they may respond better to chemotherapy. This is because rapidly growing cancer cells are more sensitive to agents that damage DNA or otherwise interfere with cell division. Aneuploidy, detected by cell cycle analysis in two-thirds of breast cancers, is associated with a poorer prognosis.

- **Molecular subtype:** It is determined by immunohistochemistry for the expression of ER and HER2 proliferation. It is an important prognostic factor.

SCENARIO-BASED ESSAY QUESTION

Q. A 49-year-old woman came to the surgical outpatient department for a lump in her left breast noticed 1 month back. On physical examination, a 2.5 cm, firm, irregular mass was palpable in the upper outer quadrant of the left breast. There are no overlying skin lesions. Two axillary lymph nodes were palpable. FNAC confirmed the clinical diagnosis and a left mastectomy was done.

a. What is the probable diagnosis? (Ans: Carcinoma of the breast)
b. Discuss the etiopathogenesis of this disease *(refer pages 845-9)*.
c. Mention the classification of these lesions in the breast *(refer Box 23.1 and Table 23.2)*.
d. Describe the morphological features of this disease *(refer pages 850-1)*.

FIBROEPITHELIAL TUMORS OF BREAST

The breast has **two types of stroma** (mesenchyma), **intralobular and interlobular**. Fibroepithelial tumors of the breast are a spectrum of heterogeneous, biphasic neoplasms that show the proliferation of epithelial and stromal (mesenchymal) components. These tumors are termed "biphasic" because they **contain neoplastic stroma and non-neoplastic epithelial components**. Two tumors that arise from intralobular stroma are **fibroadenoma and phyllodes tumor.**

Fibroadenoma

Q. Write a short note on the fibroadenoma of the breast.

Fibroadenoma is the **most common, well-circumscribed, benign fibroepithelial neoplasm** of the female breast. It shows **biphasic proliferation of epithelial and stromal components**.

- **Age-group:** Mostly occurs in females between **20 and 30 years.** Fibroadenomas may grow rapidly during pregnancy and suggest that it has a hormonal influence on their development and growth.
- **Origin:** It arises from **intralobular stroma.**
- **Clinical presentation:** Young women usually present with a **palpable and freely movable mass.** This accounts for its mobility on clinical examination ° known as **'breast mouse'**.

MORPHOLOGY

Q. Write a short note on the morphology of the fibroadenoma of the breast.

Gross (Fig. 23.18)

- Fibroadenomas can be **single or multiple and unilateral or bilateral.**
- **Well-circumscribed tumors:** Fibroadenomas are **solid, round to ovoid in shape, and** usually **well-circumscribed tumors.** The tumor can compress the surrounding breast tissue but is not fixed.
- **Cut section:** It appears **uniform, rubbery, lobulated, glistening, grayish-white** nodule. It bulges above the surrounding tissue and often contains **slit-like spaces.**
- **Size:** Varies, usually **1–4 cm** in diameter.

Microscopy (Figs. 23.19A to D)

Q. Write a short answer on microscopy of fibroadenoma of the breast.

Components: Fibroadenomas **have a mixture of both neoplastic stromal (fibrous connective tissue) and reactive epithelial (duct-like structures) components.** The relationship of the stroma to the epithelium is typically uniform throughout.

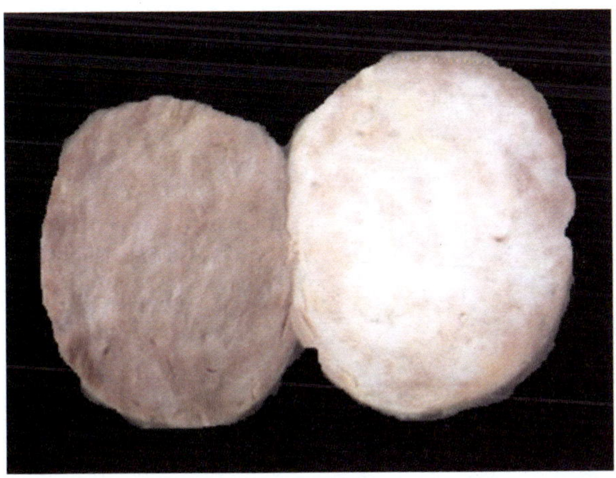

Fig. 23.18: Fibroadenoma of breast showing a well-circumscribed tumor and cut surface grayish-white in color.

- **Neoplastic epithelial component:** The epithelial component **lines the ducts**. Ducts may be either simple and **round or elongated** and **branching.** Epithelium lining the ducts ranges from the **double layer of epithelium** of normal lobules to varying degrees of hyperplasia.
- **Neoplastic stromal component (fibrous connective tissue stroma):** The stromal component is usually **uniform, delicate, and of low cellularity.** It is often myxoid and **resembles a normal** intralobular (peritubular) stroma, **contains spindle cells**, and lacks atypia. It constitutes most of the tumor.
- **Growth patterns**: According to the microscopic appearance, two growth patterns are recognized. These patterns may be seen singly or in combination. Usually, both patterns co-exist. These growth patterns have no prognostic significance.
  - **Pericanalicular (Figs. 23.19A and B):** In this type, **epithelium forms round or oval tubules with patent lumen.** The proliferating **stromal cells grow around** (surrounded) open ducts in a circumferential fashion.
  - **Intracanalicular (Figs. 23.19C and D):** In this, **stromal growth compresses ducts into curvilinear** slits (clefts) or distorts ducts.
- **Hormonal-induced changes:** Similar to normal breast, fibroadenomas can undergo hormonally-induced changes.
  - **Epithelial changes:** During pregnancy, fibroadenomas may grow rapidly in size; the glands may **increase in size** due to lactational changes.
  - **Stromal changes**: In older women (after menopause), the **stroma may become more fibrous** and **densely hyalinized**. It may also calcify and form large, lobulated ("popcorn") calcifications.

Variants of Fibroadenoma

- **Juvenile fibroadenoma:** It is most common in **adolescent girls or young women**. It **grows rapidly** and **may reach 20 cm**, causing breast distortion. Microscopically, it resembles fibroadenomas and commonly shows a pericanalicular growth pattern. The **stroma is uniform but more cellular than fibroadenoma.** It does not recur after excision.
- **Tubular adenoma:** It is a well-circumscribed tumor composed of small, closely packed tubular structures with small lumina and may have scant secretions. These are surrounded by a loosely cellular vascularized very scanty stroma.
- **Lactating adenoma:** It occurs as a palpable mass in pregnancy and lactating women (during the postpartum period). It commonly represents the coalescence of enlarged lobular units with lactational changes. It is composed of normal-appearing breast acini with secretory activity. They represent an exaggerated local response to gestational hormones.

Phyllodes Tumor

Q. Write a short note on phyllodes tumor.

Phyllodes tumor is a generally **circumscribed fibroepithelial (biphasic) neoplasm** that **arises from the intralobular and periductal stroma**. It shows a **prominent intracanalicular architectural pattern** with **leaf-like stromal fronds capped by luminal epithelial and myoepithelial cell layers**. It is accompanied by stromal hypercellularity.

- **Origin:** Arises from **intralobular and periductal stroma** (like fibroadenomas).
- **Terminology:** Originally known as cystosarcoma phyllodes to imply its malignant behavior. Since, most of these tumors behaved in a benign fashion, and most are not cystic, the **term phyllodes tumor is preferred**.
- **Age-group:** Mostly occurs **between 30 and 70 years of age**, with a peak in the fifth decade.
- **Clinical presentation:** The majority are detected as palpable masses.
- **Grading:** Depending on the appearance of the stromal component, phyllodes tumors are divided into (1) benign (2) borderline, and (3) malignant phyllodes.

MORPHOLOGY

Q. Write a short answer on the morphology of phyllodes.

Gross (Fig. 23.20A)

Most phyllodes tumors are benign.

Benign Phyllodes Tumor (Fig. 23.20A)

- **Sharply circumscribed:** It is **round, sharply circumscribed** (clearly defined margins), and **can be shelled out surgically.**
- **Size varies:** Phyllodes tumors **vary from a few centimeters to 20 cm in diameter** (average size is 4–5 cm).
- **Cut surface:** It forms a **solid, firm, glistening, gray-white bulging mass.** Small phyllodes tumors may have a homogeneous appearance. But, in **large tumors**, the characteristic **whorled pattern with curved prominent, cleft-like spaces resemble the leaf-buds (phyllodes** is Greek for "leaflike"). Leaf-like appearance is due to the epithelium which covers the nodules of proliferating stroma.

Malignant phyllodes: It is usually **poorly circumscribed and locally invasive with infiltrative borders.** It may show hemorrhage and necrosis (*refer* **online Fig. 23.20B**).

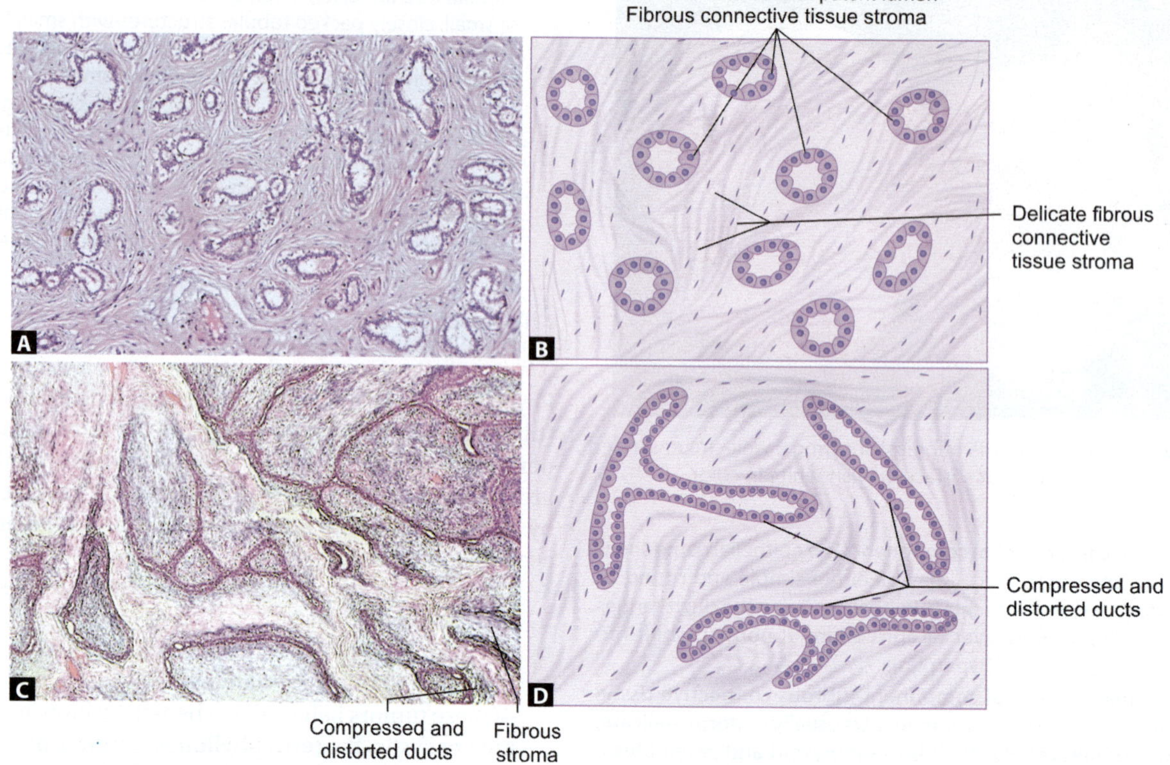

Figs. 23.19A to D: Fibroadenoma of the breast: (A) Hematoxylin and eosin (H&E); and (B) Diagrammatic. Pericanalicular type showing ducts with patent lumen, surrounded by delicate stroma. The border (left) shows sharp demarcation; (C) (H&E); and (D) Diagrammatic. Intracanalicular type composed of slit-like compressed ducts surrounded by fibrous tissue.

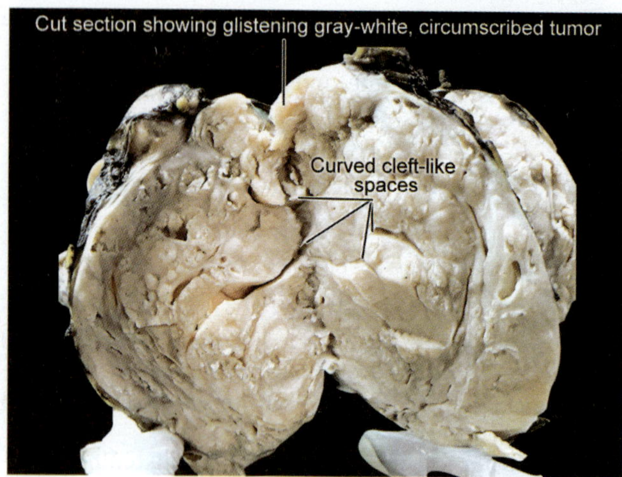

Fig. 23.20A: Gross appearance of phyllodes tumor: (A) Benign phyllodes tumor.

Microscopy [Figs. 23.21B and C (*refer* online Fig. 23.21A)]

- **Biphasic tumor:** Phyllodes tumors have **epithelial and stromal components**, the latter being neoplastic.
- **Exaggerated intracanalicular growth pattern:** Phyllodes tumors typically show an exaggerated intracanalicular growth pattern **with leaf-like projections into the dilated lumens.**
- **Two key features:** (1) the presence of benign epithelial elements and (2) stromal hypercellularity.
  - **Benign epithelial component:** The epithelial component consists of two layers (i) **luminal epithelial and (ii) myoepithelial cells.** They cover large club-like (bulbous)/ leaf-like projections (nodules) of proliferating stroma. In some tumors, these bulbous protrusions push or extend into a cystic space (hence the term cysto).
  - **Stromal hypercellularity:** It is the amount and appearance of the stromal component that determines the biological nature of neoplasm.

Grading: Depending on the appearance of the stromal component, phyllodes tumors are divided into three groups:

- **Benign phyllodes tumor:** It resembles fibroadenomas, but the stroma has the following additional features:
  - **More cellular** (hypercellular): These are mildly cellular and stromal cells resemble fibroblasts. **Stromal cellularity may be more in the region immediately adjacent to the epithelium.**
  - **Mitotic figures:** They show only mild atypia, and **less than 5 mitotic figures/10 HPFs**
- **Malignant) phyllodes tumor** (*refer* **online Fig. 23.22**): Diagnosis of malignant phyllodes requires all the following five features:
  1. **Marked stromal cellularity** (diffuse hypercellular stroma)
  2. **Severe cytologic atypia** with **marked stromal nuclear pleomorphism;** like sarcomas (e.g., malignant fibrous histiocytoma, chondrosarcoma, rhabdomyosarcoma)

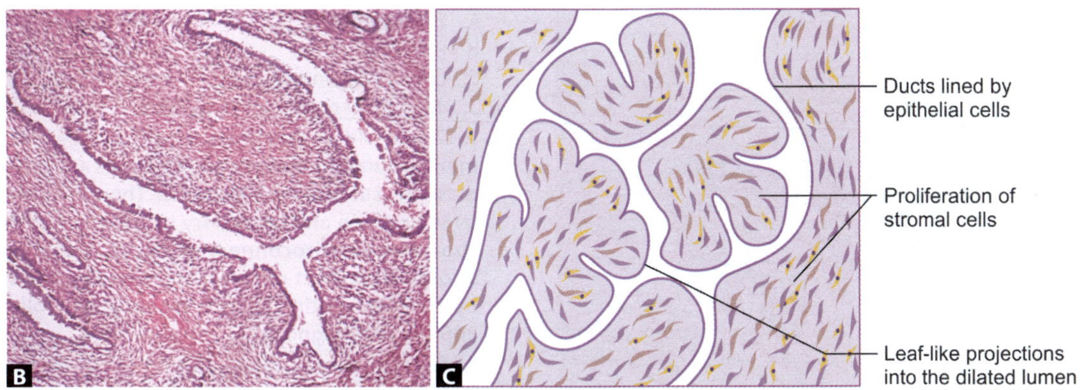

Figs. 23.21B and C: Benign phyllodes tumor (B) H&E, and (C) Diagrammatic. Shows an exaggerated intracanalicular growth pattern, increased stromal cellularity, and overgrowth giving rise to the typical leaf-like architecture.

3. **Numerous mitotic figures** (≥10 mitotic figures/10 HPFs)
4. At least **focal stromal overgrowth**
5. **Infiltrative borders** (permeative margins).

- **Borderline phyllodes tumors:** The diagnostic criteria for benign and malignant phyllodes tumors are relatively well defined. However, these criteria for borderline phyllodes tumors are less clear. Tumors that contain some, but not all, of the five histological features of malignant phyllodes (mentioned above) are called borderline.

Behavior: The grade of phyllodes correlates with behavior. **Malignant phyllodes tumors have the highest risk for local recurrence** and also likely metastatic potential. **Benign tumors usually do not metastasize** and are likely to recur if not excised with wide margins. High-grade lesions frequently recur and may also develop hematogenous metastases. Metastatic deposits contain only the stromal component.

Clinical Features

Age: Phyllodes tumors can occur at any age but are most common in the sixth decade, 10–20 years later than the peak age for fibroadenoma.

Clinical presentation: Most phyllodes tumors present as rapidly growing, palpable breast masses. Few are detected by mammography as well with circumscribed or lobulated lesions. Ultrasound may show internal hyperechoic areas in a hypoechoic mass

MALE BREAST

The male breast consists of the nipple and a rudimentary duct system without lobule formation.

Gynecomastia

PA 31.4 (NC): Enumerate and describe the etiology, hormonal dependency, and pathogenesis of gynecomastia.

Q. Write a short note on gynecomastia.

Gynecomastia (enlargement of the male breast) is a benign **diffuse or focal proliferation of glandular tissue in the male breast.**

Etiology and Pathogenesis

The male breast is subjected to hormonal influences similar to the female breast. Gynecomastia may occur due to an **imbalance between estrogens** (which stimulate breast tissue), **and androgens** (which counteract the effects of estrogens).

- Gynecomastia before 25 years of age is usually due to hormonal changes during puberty.
- Gynecomastia during later years (any time during adult life) may be due to:
  - **Hyperestrinism: Cirrhosis** and hormonally active tumors (Leydig cell tumor of testis, hCG-secreting germ cell tumors, lung carcinoma, or others).
  - Drugs: Examples include, alcohol, marijuana, heroin, antiretroviral therapy, anabolic steroids (used by some athletes and body builders), digitalis, reserpine, phenytoin, and some psychoactive agents.
  - Klinefelter syndrome (XXY karyotype)
  - Idiopathic

MORPHOLOGY

Gross

Gynecomastia appears under the nipple. It forms discrete, soft, rubbery to firm, gray or white, oval (disk-shaped) masses or a poorly defined area of induration.

Microscopy (Fig. 23.23)

- Ducts are lined by multilayered **columnar to cuboidal epithelium** with regular nuclei. The lining shows marked micropapillary epithelial hyperplasia.
- The ducts are surrounded by a **dense collagenous connective tissue stroma.**

Clinical Features

- Unilateral or bilateral.
- Usually centered below the nipple as a button-like subareolar enlargement, an important point in contrast to carcinoma, which tends to be located eccentrically. In advanced cases, it can simulate the adolescent female breast.

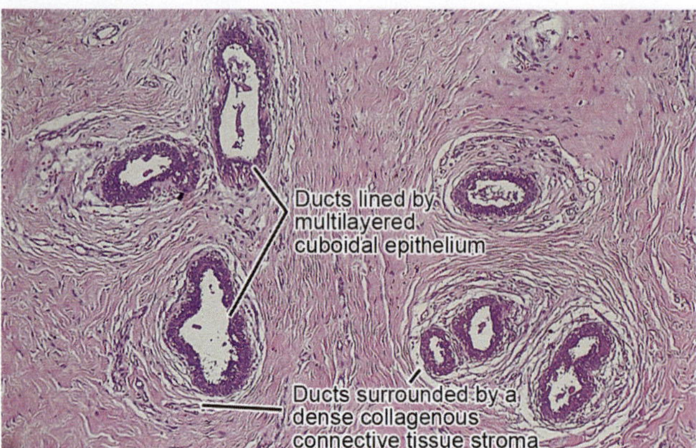

Fig. 23.23: Microscopic appearance of gynecomastia showing ducts lined by a multilayered cuboidal epithelium surrounded by hyalinized fibrous tissue.

SCENARIO-BASED MCQs

1. **A 53-year-old woman presents with a lump in her left breast for the past 1 month. Physical examination shows a palpable, firm, irregular mass in the upper outer quadrant of her left breast. The overlying skin is unremarkable. The gross appearance of the excised tumor shows an irregular, infiltrative gay-white mass. Microscopically shows malignant tumor cells arranged in sheets surrounded by thick fibrous stroma. The most likely diagnosis is:**
   A. Tubular adenoma
   B. Invasive ductal carcinoma
   C. Invasive lobular carcinoma
   D. Medullary pattern of invasive carcinoma
2. **A 45-year-old woman has noticed an enlarging mass in her left breast for the past 6 months. On physical examination, it is 4 cm in diameter and is circumscribed mass, without calcifications. An excisional biopsy shows solid nests and sheets of large, highly pleomorphic cells, with vesicular nuclei and prominent nucleoli. Many mitotic figures are seen. The surrounding stroma shows a dense infiltrate of lymphocytes. Following the biopsy findings, a simple mastectomy is performed with axillary lymph node sampling. On gross sectioning, the mass has a soft, tan, fleshy surface. With noninfiltrative border. No axillary node metastases are present. The most likely diagnosis is:**
   A. Paget disease
   B. Colloid carcinoma
   C. Invasive lobular carcinoma
   D. Medullary pattern of invasive carcinoma
3. **A 45-year-old woman presents with an oozing, reddish scaly area on the skin of her left nipple for the last 3 months. Physical examination shows a 1 cm area of eczematous skin adjacent to the areola. Cytologic examination of fluid oozing from the skin lesion shows neoplastic cells. Excisional biopsy shows large malignant cells with clear cytoplasm in the epidermis of the areola. The most likely diagnosis is:**
   A. Phyllodes tumor B. Paget disease of the breast
   C. Inflammatory carcinoma D. Colloid carcinoma
4. **A 25-year-old woman complains of a lump in her left breast. On physical examination, it is 2 cm in size, discrete, and freely movable beneath the nipple. Microscopy showed ductal structures lined by benign epithelial cells surrounded by delicate fibrous stroma. The most likely diagnosis is:**
   A. Fibroadenoma
   B. Phyllodes tumor
   C. Lobular carcinoma in situ
   D. Medullary pattern of invasive carcinoma
5. **A 52-year-old woman presents with a large breast mass of 3 months duration. Mammography shows a well-circumscribed mass measuring 9 cm in diameter. There are no lesions of the overlying skin and no axillary lymphadenopathy. A biopsy shows loose fibroconnective tissue with a sarcomatous stroma, abundant mitoses, and nodules and ridges lined by cuboidal epithelial cells. Which of the following is the appropriate diagnosis?**
   A. Paget disease
   B. Phyllodes tumor
   C. Fibroadenoma
   D. Medullary pattern of invasive carcinoma

Answers and Explanation

1. **The answer is B: Invasive ductal carcinoma.** The irregular, infiltrative mass is an infiltrating (invasive) ductal carcinoma and is the most common form of breast cancer. Other choices are not associated with the features of this case.
2. **The answer is D: Medullary pattern of invasive carcinoma.** It presents as a fleshy, bulky, circumscribed mass without any calcifications tumors. Microscopically, it is composed of sheets of cells that are highly pleomorphic and have a high mitotic index. The stroma shows a lymphoid infiltrate. A dense lymphoid infiltrate is not characteristic of the other choices. Paget disease involves the nipple and areola. Colloid carcinomas show colloid. Infiltrating lobular carcinomas do not produce large, localized lesions because they are more invasive, and they lack a distinct lymphoid infiltrate.
3. **The answer is B: Paget disease.** Paget disease of the nipple is associated with ductal carcinoma, either in situ or invasive, that extends to involve the epidermis of the nipple and areola. This produces an eczematous change in the skin of the nipple and areola. Microscopically, large cells with clear mucinous cytoplasm (Paget cells) are found singly or in groups within the epidermis. Eczematous changes in the skin of the nipple and areola are not observed in the other choices. Phyllodes tumor does not show the Paget cells. In inflammatory carcinoma, the involvement of dermal lymphatics by infiltrating carcinoma produces thickening and a reddish-orange appearance to the skin. Colloid carcinomas show colloid.
4. **The answer is A: Fibroadenoma.** It is a common tumor. Its small size and freely movable features along with microscopy favor fibroadenoma. Phyllodes tumors are uncommon and are usually larger than 4 cm. Lobular carcinoma in situ is generally an ill-defined lesion without producing a mass. The medullary pattern of invasive carcinomas tends to be large and shows characteristic microscopic features.
5. **The answer is B: Phyllodes tumor.** Phyllodes tumors of the breast are characterized by the proliferation of stromal elements accompanied by a benign growth of ductal structures. Phyllodes tumors may be benign or malignant. Microscopically, the stroma of a benign phyllodes tumor is hypercellular and has mitotic activity. Malignant phyllodes tumors have sarcomatous stroma with abundant mitotic activity, and the stromal component is increased out of proportion to the benign duct elements. They are usually poorly circumscribed, with invasion into the surrounding breast tissue. Sarcomatous elements are not observed in the other choices.

Endocrine Disorders

Chapter Outline

Thyroid Gland
- Autoimmune Thyroid Disease
- Thyrotoxicosis
- Hypothyroidism
- Diffuse and Multinodular Goiters
- Thyroid Neoplasms
- Follicular Cell-derived Neoplasms
- Laboratory Diagnosis of Diabetes

Parathyroid Glands
- Hyperparathyroidism
- Hypoparathyroidism

Adrenal Glands
- Adrenal Cortex
- Adrenal Neoplasms
- Adrenal Medulla
- Multiple Endocrine Neoplasia Syndromes

Various glands that constitute endocrine system located throughout the body is presented along with **Box 24.1**.

THYROID GLAND

Introduction: The thyroid gland is one of the largest endocrine organs in the body. In adults, it consists of two lateral lobes connected anteriorly by a thin isthmus. It is in the lower neck, across the trachea anteriorly, below, and anterior to the larynx (below the level of the cricoid cartilage). The right and left lobes are situated lateral to the trachea. In adults, the thyroid weighs approximately 15–25 g. Each lobe measures about 2–2.5 cm in width and 4–5 cm in length.

AUTOIMMUNE THYROID DISEASE

Autoimmune thyroid diseases are thyroid diseases caused due to autoimmunity. It includes thyroiditis and antibody-mediated disturbances in thyroid function that are not necessarily associated with inflammation (e.g., Graves disease).

Thyroiditis: It is a diverse group of disorders characterized by **inflammation of the thyroid gland (Box 24.2)**. The three most common and clinically significant subtypes are (1): Hashimoto thyroiditis, (2) granulomatous (de Quervain) thyroiditis, and (3) subacute lymphocytic thyroiditis.

BOX 24.2: Various types of thyroiditis.

1. Acute thyroiditis
   - Infectious thyroiditis: Bacterial including mycobacterial, fungal
2. Hashimoto (chronic lymphocytic) thyroiditis
3. Granulomatous (subacute/de Quervain) thyroiditis
4. Reidel's thyroiditis

Hashimoto Thyroiditis

Autoimmune disease: Hashimoto (**chronic lymphocytic**) thyroiditis is an **autoimmune disease that destroys the thyroid parenchyma and gradual and progressive thyroid failure** (gradual failure of thyroid function). First reported in 1912 by Hashimoto; goiter and intense lymphocytic infiltration of the thyroid (struma lymphomatosa).

Depletion of epithelial cells and infiltration by lymphocytes: Hashimoto thyroiditis is characterized by the progressive depletion of thyroid epithelial cells associated with lymphocytic infiltrates and fibrosis. It is the **most common cause of hypothyroidism in regions where iodine levels are sufficient.**

Age and gender: Hashimoto thyroiditis is typically seen in **middle-aged women** and is most prevalent between **45 and 65 years** of age. It is **more common in women** than in men. The female-to-male ratio is 10:1–20:1.

Circulating autoantibodies against thyroid antigens: They are present in almost all patients.

Pathogenesis

Q. Describe the pathogenesis of Hashimoto thyroiditis.

Hashimoto thyroiditis is an autoimmune disease. The **thyroid gland is destroyed by an immune response**

against thyroid antigens. Like most autoimmune disorders, susceptibility to Hashimoto thyroiditis is determined by a combination of immunologic, and genetic factors.

Genetic factors: Hashimoto thyroiditis has a **strong genetic component** and is supported by the following findings:

- **Concordance of disease in monozygotic twins** (40%).
- **Presence of antithyroid antibodies** in about 50% of **asymptomatic siblings** of affected patients.
- **Polymorphism in HLA:** HLA-DR polymorphisms are the genetic risk factors for autoimmune hypothyroidism. These include HLA-DR3, DR4, and DR5 alleles.
- **Polymorphism in T-cell-regulatory genes:** Increased susceptibility to Hashimoto disease is associated with polymorphisms in several immune regulation-associated genes. These genes encode regulators of T-cell responses. It includes cytotoxic T lymphocyte-associated antigen-4 *(CTLA4)* gene and *protein tyrosine phosphatase-22 (PTPN22),* and interleukin 2 receptor subunit alpha (*IL2RA*).
- **Association with other autoimmune diseases:** Examples include Graves disease, type 1 diabetes mellitus (T1DM), Sjögren syndrome, pernicious anemia, Addison disease, and myasthenia gravis.

Molecular Pathogenesis (Fig. 24.1)

Hashimoto thyroiditis is an **autoimmune disease** caused by a **breakdown in self-tolerance to thyroid autoantigens. Failure of self-tolerance** to thyroid autoantigens is the initial event. Probably, it is abnormalities of regulatory T-cells (Tregs), or exposure of normally sequestered thyroid antigens. Probably autoimmunity is triggered by inflammatory events in the gland. Inflammation may be related to infection (viral or bacterial) or injury to the thyroid cells from toxins.

Progressive destruction of thyrocytes (thyroid epithelial cells): Autoimmunity in the thyroid is accompanied by a progressive depletion of thyroid epithelial cells due to the death of follicular cells. It is accompanied by the replacement of the thyroid parenchyma by mononuclear cell infiltration and fibrosis. Immunologic mechanisms involved in thyroid parenchymal cell damage and death are as follows.

1. **Thyroid epithelial cell death by CD8+ cytotoxic T-cells***:* *CD8+ cytotoxic T cells* specific for thyroid antigens are responsible for killing thyroid epithelial cells (type IV hypersensitivity).
2. **Cytokine-mediated cell death: Activation of CD4+ T-cells** (Th1 cell) **produces inflammatory cytokines such as interferon-**γ in the thyroid gland. These locally released cytokines **recruit and activate macrophages and damage thyroid follicles.**

Previously, it was thought that a contributing mechanism of thyroid epithelial cell death is the binding of *antithyroid antibodies* (antithyroglobulin and antithyroid peroxidase antibodies), followed by antibody-dependent cell-mediated cytotoxicity. The antithyroid antibodies can damage follicular cells by complement-dependent mechanisms. However, it is not known whether these antibodies are the cause or consequence of thyroid injury.

MORPHOLOGY

Q. Describe the morphological changes in Hashimoto thyroiditis.

Gross (Fig. 24.2)

- **Diffuse and symmetric enlargement** of the thyroid gland.
- The thyroid gland is **firm and nodular**.
- **The capsule** is **intact**, and the thyroid gland is well-demarcated from adjacent structures.
- **Cut surface** is **pale, gray-tan,** and shows **accentuation of normal lobulation.** It **resembles a hyperplastic lymph node or salivary gland.**

Microscopy (Figs. 24.3A and B)

Q. Write a short answer on oncocyte (Hürthle cell).

1. **Inflammatory infiltrate:**
   - **Widespread infiltration of the parenchyma by a mononuclear inflammatory infiltrate:** The thyroid shows **extensive prominent (dense) mononuclear inflammatory infiltrate.** It consists of small **lymphocytes, plasma cells, and macrophages** in the thyroid parenchyma.

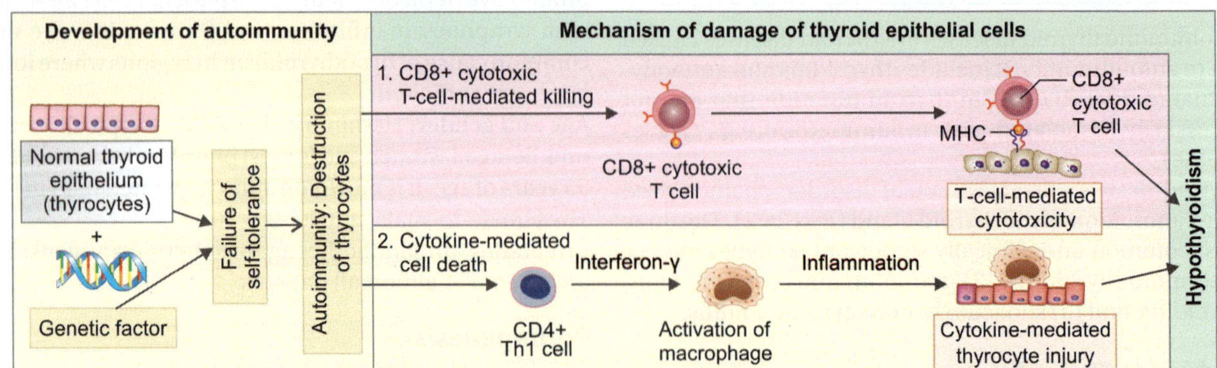

Fig. 24.1: Pathogenesis of Hashimoto thyroiditis. Failure of self-tolerance to thyroid autoantigens results in progressive autoimmune destruction of thyroid epithelial cells by infiltrating cytotoxic T-cells, or through locally released cytokine.

(MHC: major histocompatibility complex)

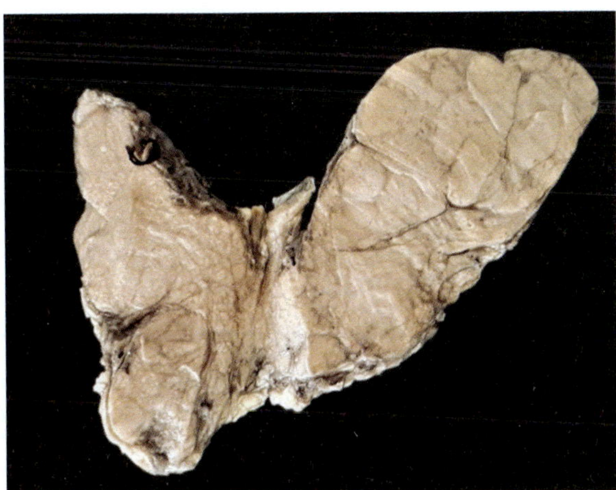

Fig. 24.2: Gross appearance of Hashimoto thyroiditis. The cut section shows an enlargement of the thyroid, a pale gray-tan color, and an accentuation of normal lobulation.

- **Lymphoid follicles with well-formed germinal centers**: The lymphocytes form lymphoid follicles with well-developed germinal centers.

2. **Changes in follicles and epithelial cells:**
   - **Atrophy of thyroid follicles:** The thyroid follicles appear smaller than normal follicles.
   - **Oncocytes (Hürthle cell):** The follicles are lined in many areas by **Hürthle cells (better termed oncocytes)**. These are epithelial cells with **abundant eosinophilic, granular cytoplasm**. They have large, round nuclei with vesicular chromatin and often prominent nucleoli. **Hürthle cells are also called Askanazy, oxyphil cells, or oncocytes**. They line up some of the follicles. It is a metaplastic response to thyroid injury. **Ultrastructurally**, oncocytes have **prominent mitochondria** that are responsible for their appearance.
3. **Increased interstitial connective tissue:** Hashimoto thyroiditis shows increased interstitial connective tissue **(fibrosis)** and may be abundant. Unlike Riedel's thyroiditis, **fibrosis is limited to the thyroid** and does not extend beyond the capsule of the thyroid gland.

Fine-needle aspiration cytology (FNAC): It shows oncocytes (Hürthle cells) with a heterogeneous population of lymphocytes.

Clinical Course

- **Painless diffuse enlargement of the thyroid** in middle-aged women. Generally, the thyroid gland is symmetrically and diffusely enlarged.
- **Some degree of hypothyroidism** gradually develops.
- **Hashitoxicosis:** Early stages may produce transient thyrotoxicosis due to the destruction of thyroid follicles, with secondary release of thyroid hormones (Hashitoxicosis). It is caused by the disruption of thyroid follicles and the release of thyroid hormones. During this phase, serum levels of free T4 and T3 are elevated, TSH is diminished, and radioactive iodine uptake is decreased. As hypothyroidism supervenes, the levels of T4 and T3 decrease, accompanied by compensatory raised TSH levels.

Risk of other autoimmune diseases: Patients with Hashimoto thyroiditis are at an increased risk for developing other autoimmune diseases.

Risk of malignant tumors: Patients with Hashimoto thyroiditis also are at an increased risk for the development of extranodal marginal zone B-cell lymphoma within the thyroid gland. Probably, they are predisposed to papillary thyroid cancer.

Subacute Granulomatous Thyroiditis

Subacute granulomatous thyroiditis is also known as **de Quervain thyroiditis**. It is **less common** than Hashimoto disease. It is characterized by **granulomatous inflammation within the thyroid parenchyma**.

Age and gender: It usually presents between **30 and 50 years** of age. **Affects women** more often than men (4:1).

Pathogenesis

Triggered by upper respiratory viral infection: Subacute thyroiditis is most likely **initiated by a viral infection** or an inflammatory process triggered by viral infections. Points in favor are:

- Majority have an upper respiratory infection just before the onset of thyroiditis.

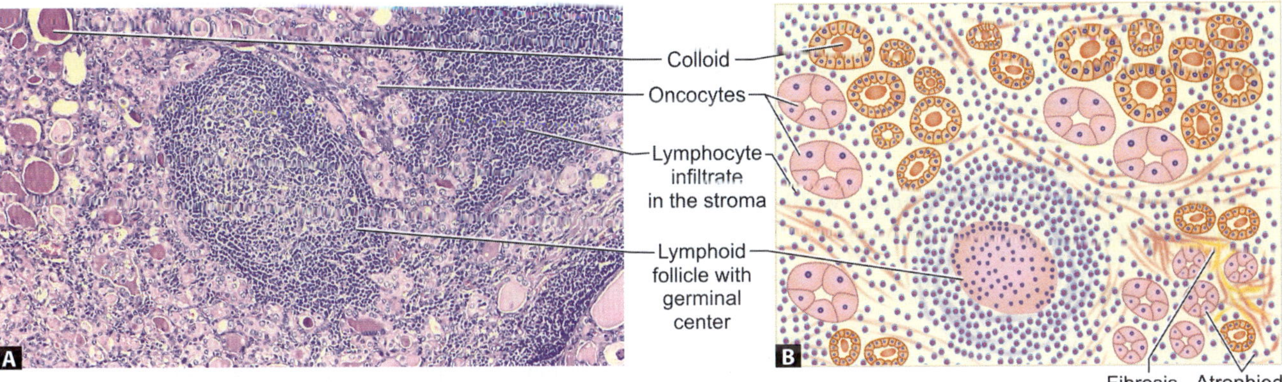

Figs. 24.3A and B: (A) Photomicrograph; (B) Diagrammatic. Microscopy of Hashimoto thyroiditis shows parenchyma densely infiltrated by lymphocytes with germinal centers. Some of the thyroid follicles are lined by deeply eosinophilic oncocytes (Hürthle cells).

- Seasonal variation with peak occurrence in the summer. Association with virus infection (e.g., coxsackie virus, mumps, measles, adenovirus).
- The process spontaneously remits.

Pathogenesis is unclear: It probably results from virus-induced host tissue damage. It stimulates a cytotoxic T-lymphocyte response to one or more thyroid antigens that damage thyroid follicle cells. In contrast to autoimmune thyroid disease, the immune response is virus-initiated and not sustained. Thus, the process is limited and does not progress.

MORPHOLOGY

Gross

- **Enlargement of thyroid**: The thyroid gland is enlarged and **firm with intact capsule**. Enlargement may be **unilateral or bilateral** and **often asymmetrical**.
- **Cut section:** The involved regions are **firm and yellow-white.**

Microscopy

Microscopic changes are patchy.

- **Scattered disruption of follicles with loss of the follicular epithelium and colloid depletion.**
- **Colloid extravasation**: The **colloid escapes from damaged thyroid follicles.**
- **Inflammation:** It is elicited by the escaped colloid seen surrounding the damaged follicles. Initially shows infiltration of **neutrophils** which are later replaced by **lymphocytes, plasma cells, and macrophages.**
- **Granulomatous reaction** (*refer* **online Fig. 24.4**): The extravasated colloid initiates an abundant granulomatous reaction. It shows **multinucleate giant cells** (some containing fragments of colloid) **surrounding** pools or fragments of **colloid**. Hence, the designation **granulomatous thyroiditis.**
- **Healing by fibrosis:** In the late stages, healing occurs by resolution of inflammation and replacing the destroyed area of the gland with fibrous tissue.

Clinical Course

- **Enlargement of the thyroid**: The onset is usually acute. The patient presents with neck pain (particularly with swallowing), fever, malaise, and variable enlargement of the thyroid.
- **Transient hyperthyroidism during the early phase: Hyperthyroidism** with high serum T_4 and T_3 levels and low serum TSH levels may occur during an early stage.
- Increased leukocyte count and raised erythrocyte sedimentation rate.
- **Self-limited disease: Recovery occurs within 6–8 weeks** and thyroid function returns to normal.

Riedel Thyroiditis

It is a rare form of thyroiditis. It is a manifestation of IgG4-related disease.

MORPHOLOGY

Gross: The thyroid is stony hard and fixed which **clinically simulates a thyroid carcinoma.**

Microscopy: It shows **lymphoplasmacytic infiltrates** and **extensive fibrosis involving the thyroid and nearby neck structures.** It encroaches on parathyroid glands or the recurrent laryngeal nerve.

THYROTOXICOSIS

PA 32.2 (CC): Describe the etiology, pathogenesis, manifestations, laboratory, and imaging features, and course of thyrotoxicosis.

Q. Write a short essay on thyrotoxicosis.

Thyrotoxicosis: It is a **hypermetabolic state caused by** exposure to **elevated circulating levels of thyroid hormone** (free T_3 and T_4), irrespective of the source. The elevated thyroid hormone levels may be produced by **thyroid or extrathyroid** sources. Thyrotoxicosis is not synonymous with hyperthyroidism. Thus, **thyrotoxicosis may be associated with or without hyperthyroidism.**

Hyperthyroidism: It is characterized by excessive synthesis and release of thyroid hormone by the thyroid gland.

Causes of Thyrotoxicosis (Box 24.3)

Thyrotoxicosis Associated with Hyperthyroidism

It is the **clinical consequence due to the excessive circulating thyroid hormone** (**excessive thyroid function**/hyperfunction). It is the **most common cause of thyrotoxicosis. Excessive synthesis and secretion of thyroid hormone** may be a primary disorder of the thyroid or secondary to other disorders.

BOX 24.3: Causes of thyrotoxicosis.

Associated with hyperthyroidism

Primary hyperthyroidism

- Graves disease (diffuse toxic hyperplasia of the thyroid)*
- Toxic (hyperfunctioning) multinodular goiter*
- Toxic (hyperfunctioning) adenoma*

Secondary hyperthyroidism

- TSH-secreting pituitary adenoma (rare)

Not associated with hyperthyroidism

- Thyroiditis
  - Granulomatous (de Quervain) thyroiditis (painful)
  - Subacute lymphocytic thyroiditis (painless)
- Struma ovarii (ovarian teratoma with ectopic thyroid)
- Factitious thyrotoxicosis (excessive exogenous intake of thyroxine)

*Three most common causes of hyperthyroidism

- **Primary hyperthyroidism:** It is due to an intrinsic thyroid abnormality.
  - **Abnormal thyroid stimulation:** Diffuse hyperplasia of the thyroid associated with **Graves disease**.
  - **Intrinsic disease of the thyroid gland**.
    - Toxic multinodular goiter
    - Toxic adenoma of the thyroid.
- **Secondary hyperthyroidism:** It is due to processes arising outside of the thyroid, such as increased TSH-secreting **pituitary adenoma** (rare).

Thyrotoxicosis Not Associated with Hyperthyroidism

Excessive release of preformed thyroid hormone from the **thyroid** (e.g., in thyroiditis) or an **extrathyroidal source** (e.g., struma ovarii).

Clinical Manifestations of Hyperthyroidism

The clinical features may be due to the (i) **increased metabolism (hypermetabolic state) caused due to excess levels of thyroid hormone** and (ii) **overactivity of the autonomic (sympathetic) nervous system** to catecholamines (i.e., an increase in the β-adrenergic "tone").

Due to the hypermetabolic state: Excessive thyroid hormone results in an **increase in the basal metabolic rate.** Its manifestations are as follows:

- **Skin: It appears soft, warm, and moist** because of increased blood flow and peripheral vasodilation to increase heat loss. **Heat intolerance** and **sweating** are common.
- **Cardiac manifestations:** These include **increased cardiac output, tachycardia, palpitations, arrhythmias,** and **cardiomegaly**.

Due to the overactivity of the sympathetic nervous system: Its manifestations are as follows:

- **Neuromuscular system:** It manifests as **fine tremors, hyperactivity, nervousness, anxiety, emotional liability,** inability to concentrate, and insomnia.
- **Thyroid myopathy:** The muscle may show weakness of the proximal muscle and decreased muscle mass.
- **Gastrointestinal system: Increased stool frequency,** often with diarrhea, malabsorption, and steatorrhea.
- **Ocular changes: Lid retraction (lag)** causes a staring appearance. It is due to sympathetic overstimulation of the superior tarsal muscle, which raises the upper eyelid. However, **Graves disease is associated with proptosis** which comprises Graves ophthalmopathy.
- **Skeletal system: Osteopenia** and a small increase in fracture rate.
- **Thyroid storm:** It is the **sudden onset of severe hyperthyroidism**. It occurs **most commonly in Graves disease** and is **probably due to sudden elevation in catecholamine levels**. It may occur during infection, surgery, cessation of antithyroid medication, or any form of stress. It is a medical emergency and if untreated may cause death due to cardiac arrhythmias.

The diagnosis of hyperthyroidism depends on clinical features and laboratory findings.

Laboratory findings in hyperthyroidism: Laboratory findings that support the diagnosis of hyperthyroidism include (1) a **low TSH value** and (2) an **increase in free T4.**

- **Serum TSH concentration:** It is the **most useful single screening test** for hyperthyroidism because it is **decreased even at the subclinical stage**.
- **Free T_4:** It is **increased.**
- **Measurement of radioactive iodine uptake** by the thyroid gland to determine the cause. For example, diffusely increased uptake in the whole gland is seen in Graves disease, increased uptake in a solitary nodule in toxic adenoma, or decreased uptake in thyroiditis.

Graves Disease

Graves disease (also known as Basedow disease) is the **most common cause of endogenous hyperthyroidism. Graves disease is an autoantibody-mediated disorder.** It was first reported by Graves as "violent and long-continued palpitations in females" associated with enlargement of the thyroid gland.

Triad of clinical findings in Graves disease is as follows:

1. **Hyperthyroidism:** It is due to diffuse hyperplasia of the thyroid.
2. **Infiltrative ophthalmopathy:** It results in exophthalmos **(Fig. 24.7)**.
3. **Localized, infiltrative dermopathy** (pretibial myxedema) in a few patients.

Age: Peak between **20 and 40 years** of age.

Sex: Females are affected 10 times **more frequently** than males.

Etiology

Graves disease (hyperthyroidism) **and Hashimoto thyroiditis** (hypothyroidism) are considered **two extremes of autoimmune thyroid disorders.**

Genetic Factor

- Graves disease has a **strong genetic component** and is supported by the following observations:
  - Concordance of disease in **monozygotic twins** (60%).
  - **Presence of circulating antithyroid antibodies** in asymptomatic siblings of Graves disease.
  - **Association with other autoimmune diseases.**
- Genetic susceptibility for Graves disease has been associated with polymorphisms in **genes associated with immune regulation**, e.g., cytotoxic T lymphocyte–associated antigen-4 *(CTLA4)* gene and protein tyrosine phosphatase-22 *(PTPN22)*.

Pathogenesis (Refer Online Fig. 24.5)

Q. Describe the pathogenesis of Graves disease.

Failure of self-tolerance to thyroid autoantigens is the initial event.

Production autoantibodies: Graves disease is an **autoimmune disease** characterized by the **presence of multiple autoantibodies.**

1. **Thyrotropin (TSH) receptor antibody: It is the most important autoantibody and** is an immunoglobulin (Ig) G type of antibody.
   - **Characteristics:** Almost **all patients with Graves disease** have detectable amounts of this autoantibody. It is **specific** for Graves disease.
   - **Action:** They bind to the TSH receptor on the plasma membrane of thyroid epithelial cells. It mimics the action of TSH. This leads to increased production and release of thyroid hormones (*refer* **Fig. 6.5C**).
2. **Other TSH receptor–binding antibodies:**
   - **TSH-binding inhibitor immunoglobulin (anti-TSH receptor antibody):** Some antibodies may block TSH binding **to its receptor** on thyroid epithelial cells, thereby inhibiting hormone production.
   - **Coexistence** of **stimulating and inhibiting immunoglobulins:** In some patients, there may be the coexistence of stimulating and inhibiting immunoglobulins in the serum. This may be responsible for intercurrent episodes of hypothyroidism in some patients with Graves disease.

The development of autoimmune reactions against their TSH receptor is not known.

Pathogenesis of infiltrative ophthalmopathy: Autoimmunity may be involved in its development. The TSH receptor is present not only in the thyroid epithelial cells but also present on ocular fibroblasts and fat cells. Activated CD4+ T cells secrete cytokines that cause increased production of extracellular matrix proteins. This accumulates in the retro-orbital space and causes ophthalmopathy.

MORPHOLOGY

Q. Describe the morphological changes in Graves disease.

Gross

- **Diffuse symmetrical enlargement**: The thyroid gland is **symmetrically enlarged** due to **diffuse hypertrophy and hyperplasia** of thyroid follicular epithelial cells. The thyroid is usually smooth and soft, with an intact capsule.
- **The weight** of the gland is **increased.**
- **Cut section**: The parenchyma appears **soft and meaty resembling normal muscle (Fig. 24.6A).**

Microscopy

Changes in Thyroid (Fig. 24.6B)

- **Changes in the thyroid follicular epithelial cells:** In untreated patients, the findings are as follows:
  - **Crowding of epithelial cells:** Epithelial cells lining the thyroid follicles are **tall and more crowded** than normal glands.
  - **Small papillae without fibrovascular cores:** They are formed **due to the crowding of epithelial cells.** These small **papillae project into the lumen** of the follicles and **encroach on the colloid.** These papillae do not have fibrovascular cores. This contrasts with the papillary thyroid carcinoma which has papillae with fibrovascular core.
- **Pale colloid with scalloped margins within the lumen of the follicles.**
- **Lymphocyte (predominantly of T cells) infiltration in the interstitium:** It is seen throughout the gland, along **with mature plasma cells.** These lymphoid aggregates commonly show **germinal centers.**

Changes in Extrathyroidal Tissue

- Generalized lymphoid hyperplasia

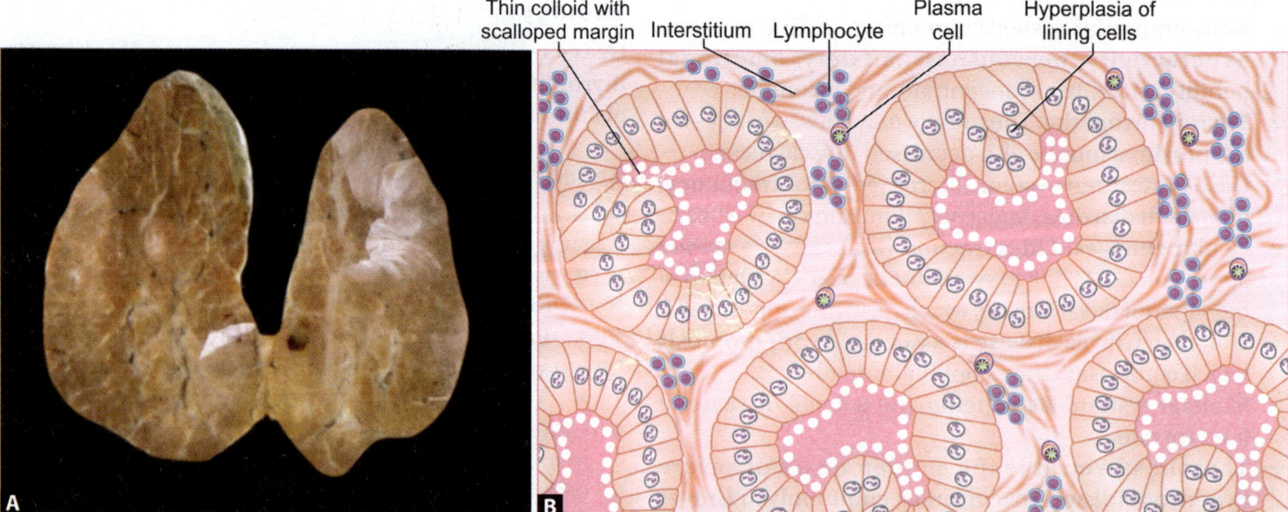

Figs. 24.6A and B: Graves disease: (A) Cut section of thyroid showing meaty appearance; (B) Microscopic view (diagrammatic) showing follicles lined by tall, columnar epithelium that are crowded and project into the lumens.

- **Myocardial hypertrophy** and ischemic changes
- **Ophthalmopathy:** The tissues of the orbit show edema because of the presence of mucopolysaccharides. It is also infiltrated by lymphocytes, mostly T cells, and associated with fibrosis. Initially, orbital muscles show edema and later may undergo fibrosis.
- **Dermopathy**: It is characterized by thickening of the dermis due to the deposition of glycosaminoglycans and lymphocyte infiltration.

Clinical Features

- **Thyrotoxicosis:** The clinical manifestations of Graves disease include features of thyrotoxicosis (discussed above on page 867). The degree of thyrotoxicosis varies.
- **Unique features of Graves:** Apart from features of thyrotoxicosis, other features unique to Graves disease are as follows:
  - **Diffuse hyperplasia of the thyroid:** It is seen in all cases and causes enlargement of the thyroid. Increased blood flow through the hyperactive thyroid gland may produce an audible bruit.
  - **Ophthalmopathy:** The ophthalmopathy causes **abnormal protrusion of the eyeball (exophthalmos)**. Sympathetic overactivity may produce a characteristic **wide, staring gaze and lid lag (Fig. 24.7)**. Infiltrative ophthalmopathy is characterized by an increase in the volume of the retro-orbital connective tissues and extraocular muscles. The exophthalmos may persist or progress even after successful treatment of the thyrotoxicosis. Sometimes, it may cause corneal injury. The extraocular muscles are usually weak.
  - **Infiltrative dermopathy** or **pretibial myxedema:** It is present in a minority of patients. This is most commonly seen in the skin over the **shins**. It presents as a **scaly thickening and induration** of the skin (pretibial edema) due to the deposition of glycosaminoglycans and infiltration by lymphocytes. The skin lesions may appear as lightly pigmented papules or nodules and usually have an orange peel texture.

Laboratory Findings in Graves Disease

- **Elevated free T_4 and T_3 levels**
- **Decreased TSH levels**
- **Radioactive iodine uptake is increased**, and **radioiodine scans show a diffuse uptake of iodine.** This is because of continuous stimulation of the thyroid follicles by thyroid-stimulating immunoglobulins.

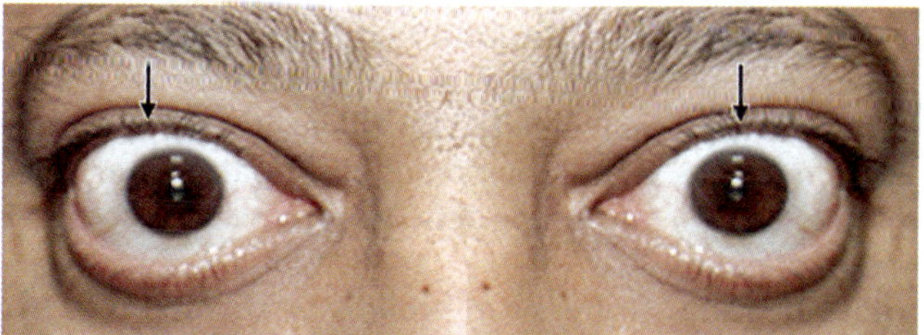

Fig. 24.7: Exophthalmos with wide, staring gaze and lid lag in Graves disease.

HYPOTHYROIDISM

PA 32.3 (CC): Describe the etiology, pathogenesis, manifestations, laboratory, imaging features, and course of hypothyroidism.

Definition: Hypothyroidism is the clinical manifestation due to **reduced secretion of thyroid hormone** (thyroid hormone deficiency).

Hypothyroidism is a common disorder. It is more common in women than in men.

Causes of Hypothyroidism: Hypothyroidism is caused by reduced thyroid hormone production either due to structural or functional derangements in the thyroid. It can be produced due to a defect anywhere in the hypothalamic-pituitary-thyroid axis.

Types of hypothyroidism (Box 24.4): It may be divided into:

1. **Primary hypothyroidism (>90%):** Due to intrinsic abnormality in the thyroid gland itself. There may be enlargement of the thyroid gland (goiter).
2. **Secondary hypothyroidism:** Due to pituitary and hypothalamic disease.

Cretinism

Definition: It is hypothyroidism that develops in infancy or early childhood.

BOX 24.4: Types and causes of hypothyroidism.

Primary
- Autoimmune hypothyroidism (inflammatory destruction of follicles): Hashimoto thyroiditis*
- Iatrogenic
  - Postablative (removal/excision/destruction of thyroid tissue): Surgery, radioiodine therapy, or external irradiation
  - Adverse effect of drugs (interference with thyroid hormone synthesis)*: Lithium, iodides, amiodarone, p-aminosalicylic acid sulfonamides, and phenylbutazone
- Iodine deficiency*: Decreased synthesis of thyroid hormone—a common cause in infants and children
- Genetic defects:
  - Congenital biosynthetic defect (dyshormonogenetic goiter) (rare)*
  - Defect in thyroid development (thyroid dysgenesis) (rare)

Secondary (Central) (Defective TSH production)
- Pituitary failure (rare)
- Hypothalamic failure (rare)

*Associated with enlargement of the thyroid ("goitrous hypothyroidism").

Etiology

- **Endemic cretinism:** Cretinism formerly was fairly common in areas where there was endemic dietary iodine deficiency [e.g., mountainous areas such as the Himalayas and the Andes (endemic cretinism)]. It is now less frequent due to the widespread supplementation of salt with iodine.
- **Sporadic cretinism:** It is caused due to enzyme defects that interfere with thyroid hormone synthesis.
- **Genetic defects:** Rarely cretinism may be due to genetic defects that interfere with the biosynthesis of thyroid hormone (e.g., dyshormonogenetic goiter).

Clinical Features

In cretinism, there is impaired development of the **skeletal system and central nervous system**.

Impaired development of the skeletal system: It manifests as **short stature, coarse facial features, a protruding tongue, and an umbilical hernia**.

Nervous system: Hypothyroidism in pregnancy produces neurologic consequences for the fetus. Normally, maternal hormones namely T3 and T4 cross the placenta. They are important to the development of the brain in the fetus. It manifests as a **severe mental retardation** and the severity of the **mental impairment** depends on the time at which the fetus develops thyroid deficiency in utero.

- If there is a deficiency of the thyroid hormone in pregnant women before the development of the fetal thyroid gland, there will be severe mental retardation in the fetus.
- By contrast, if reduction of thyroid hormones occurs later in pregnancy after the fetal thyroid has developed, the fetal brain may develop normally.

Myxedema

Definition: It is **hypothyroidism** that develops **in older children and adults.**

Clinical Features

Symptoms of hypothyroidism are due to decreased circulating thyroid hormone. In older children with myxedema, the signs and symptoms are intermediate between those of the cretin and those of the adult with hypothyroidism. In the adult, the symptoms of myxedema develop insidiously.

Initial symptoms include generalized fatigue (tiredness), apathy, and mental sluggishness. This may mimic depression. They are listless and frequently overweight.

Skin: Cutaneous signs are almost common.

- **Myxedema:** Connective tissue matrix substances (glycosaminoglycans and hyaluronic acid) accumulate in the extracellular matrix in the skin and subcutaneous tissue. They bind water and produce a peculiar form of nonpitting edema called **myxedema**. Myxedematous patients have **broadening and coarsening of facial features** (boggy facies, puffy eyelids), **edema of the hands and feet, enlargement of the tongue, and deepening of the voice** (due to thickening of laryngeal mucous membranes).
- The **skin is cool and pale** because of decreased blood flow due to cutaneous vasoconstriction. The skin is also dry, coarse, and cold intolerant with **decreased sweating**. Ecchymoses may develop due to increased capillary fragility. Skin wounds heal slowly.

Nervous system: Hypothyroid adults are **lethargic, and show memory loss and slowed mental processes.** Psychiatric symptoms are common and severe agitation termed **myxedema madness**, may develop. Other symptoms include sensory defects (deafness and night blindness), cerebellar ataxia, and slow tendon reflexes.

Cardiovascular system: Reduced cardiac output produces shortness of breath and decreased exercise capacity. Coronary atherosclerosis is common due to an increase in total cholesterol and low-density lipoprotein (LDL) levels.

Gastrointestinal (GI) tract: Decreased sympathetic activity results in **constipation**.

Laboratory Findings in Hypothyroidism

Diagnosis of hypothyroidism depends on laboratory evaluation because of the nonspecific nature of symptoms.

- **Decreased serum T_3/T_4** in patients with hypothyroidism of any origin
- **Increased serum TSH** is observed **in primary hypothyroidism.** It is the most sensitive screening test. TSH is not increased with hypothyroidism caused by primary hypothalamic or pituitary disease.
- **Hypercholesterolemia** caused by decreased synthesis of LDL receptors [type II hyperlipoproteinemia (HLP)].

DIFFUSE AND MULTINODULAR GOITERS

PA 32.1 (CC): Enumerate, classify, and describe the etiology, pathogenesis, pathology, and iodine dependency of thyroid swellings.

Definition: Goiter (from the Latin guttur, which means "throat") is defined as the **enlargement of the thyroid due to any etiology**. It may involve the thyroid gland diffusely, nodular, or multinodular.

Goiter is the **most common manifestation of thyroid disease**. It **is caused by reduced synthesis of thyroid hormone.** Iodine is needed for the synthesis of thyroid hormones; its deficiency leads to impaired hormone production. Dietary **iodine deficiency is the most common cause of goiter.**

Classification: Goiters can broadly be divided into two types: (1) *Diffuse nontoxic* and (2) *multinodular*.

Etiology and Pathogenesis

Q. Describe the etiopathogenesis of goiter.

Types of goiters: It may be (1) endemic and (2) sporadic.

Endemic Goiter

Endemic goiter is the term used **when goiters are present** in **more than 10% of the population in a given region.** It is mainly due to iodine deficiency.

Deficiency of Iodine

This may be due to **low iodine** in the soil, water, and diet (food):

- Common in mountainous areas (e.g., Himalayas) where there is widespread deficiency of iodine.
- Dietary supplementation of iodine has reduced the frequency and severity of endemic goiter.

Consequences of iodine deficiency (Flowchart 24.1)

- **Diffuse goiter:** Iodine is required for the synthesis of thyroid hormones. Iodine deficiency leads to impaired hormone production. **Decreased synthesis of thyroid hormone** in turn results in a compensatory **increase in serum TSH.** This leads to **follicular cell hypertrophy and hyperplasia. Ultimately, the thyroid gland is diffusely enlargement** (diffuse/simple goiter) **without any nodularity.** Microscopically, it consists of large thyroid follicles distended with colloid * also known as **colloid goiter.**
- **Multinodular goiter:** In long-standing diffuse goiter, **recurrent attacks of hyperplasia and involution** occur. These processes combine to produce a **more irregular enlargement of the thyroid gland**, known as *multinodular goiter*.

The extent of thyroid enlargement corresponds directly to the severity and duration of thyroid hormone deficiency. These compensatory changes effectively counteract hormone deficiency, thereby maintaining a **euthyroid metabolic state** in the majority of affected individuals. Nevertheless, in cases of severe underlying disorders such as congenital biosynthetic defects, these compensatory responses may be insufficient, leading to the development of goitrous **hypothyroidism.**

Sporadic Goiter

Sporadic goiter **less frequent** than endemic goiter

Age and gender: Its peak incidence is during **puberty or in young adult life** when there is an increased physiologic demand for thyroxine. It is **more common in females.**

Q. Write a short note on goitrogens.

Causes

Sporadic goiter may be caused by several conditions. But, in **most cases of sporadic goiter, the cause is not known.**

Flowchart 24.1: Sequences of events in the development of goiter.

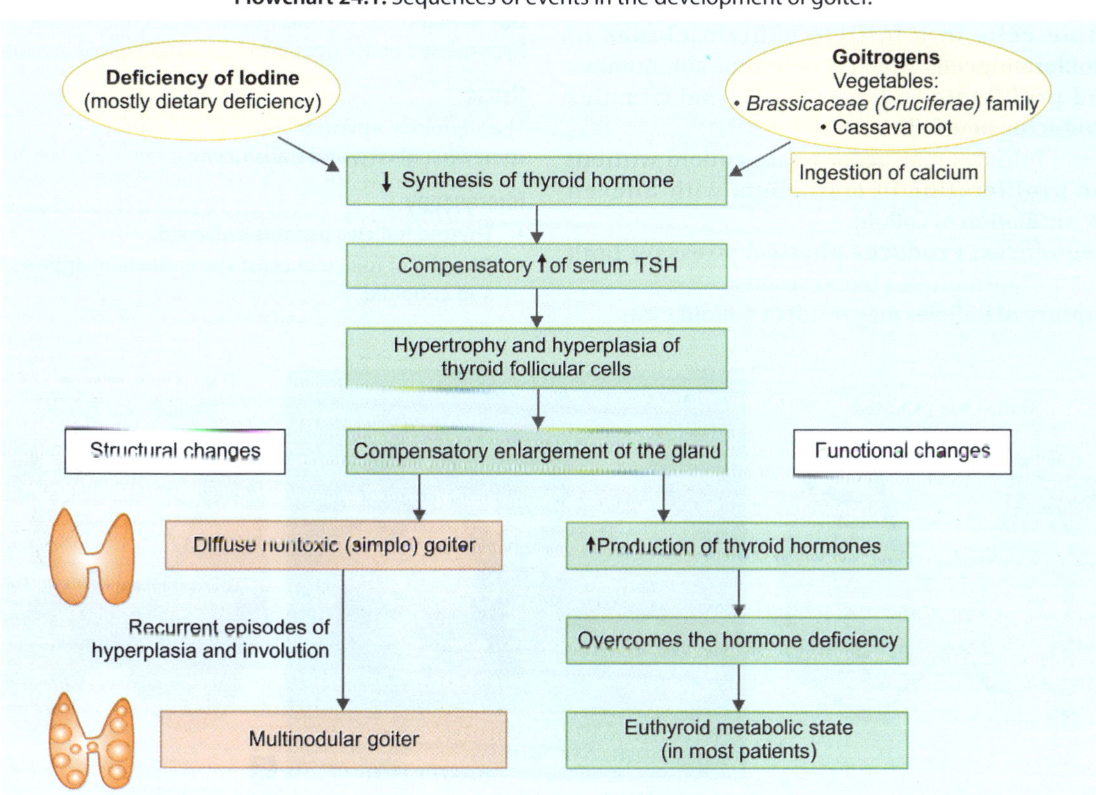

(TSH: thyroid-stimulating hormone)

Excessive ingestion of substances that interfere with thyroid hormone synthesis

- **Goitrogens:** These are **substances, ingestion of which interferes with thyroid hormone synthesis.** Goitrogenic substances include vegetables which belong to:
  - ***Brassicaceae (also called Cruciferae)* family,** e.g., cabbage, cauliflower, Brussels sprouts, and turnips.
  - **Cassava root:** It contains a thiocyanate that inhibits iodide transport within the thyroid. Consumption of this may worsen the concurrent iodine deficiency.
- **Ingestion of calcium**

Inherited enzyme defects that interfere with thyroid hormone synthesis

Hereditary enzymatic defects that interfere with thyroid hormone synthesis. Transmitted as autosomal recessive conditions (e.g., dyshormonogenetic goiter).

Unknown cause: Sequences of events in the development of goiter are shown in **Flowchart 24.1**.

Evolution of Multinodular Goiter

Q. Write a short note on stages in the evolution of multinodular goiter.

- In long-standing simple goiters, due to **variations among follicular cells** in their **response to external stimuli** (such as trophic hormones), multiple nodules are formed.
- **Uneven follicular hyperplasia**:
  - **Some** cells in a **follicle** contain **clones of proliferating cells,** which may become **autonomous and proliferate** without the external stimulus **producing new follicles.**
  - **Some follicles** may **accumulate colloid without the proliferation** of epithelium with **uneven accumulation of colloid.**
- **Consequences: Produces physical stress** on both follicles and surrounding blood vessels.
  - **Rupture of follicles** may result in **colloid cysts.**
  - **Rupture of vessels** may produce **hemorrhages** followed by **scarring,** and sometimes **calcifications.** With scarring, **multiple nodules** appear and these nodules show **varying microscopic appearance.**

MORPHOLOGY

Diffuse Nontoxic (Simple) Goiter

Q. Write a short note on colloid goiter.

The evolution of diffuse nontoxic goiter shows two phases, namely (1) the **hyperplastic phase** and (2) the phase of **colloid involution.**

1. Hyperplastic Phase

Gross (Fig. 24.8A)

The thyroid is **moderately, diffusely, and symmetrically enlarged.** The gland rarely exceeds 100–150 g (normally 10–20 grams). The thyroid gland is soft without any nodules.

Microscopy

- **Hyperplasia of the lining epithelium** of thyroid follicles. The epithelium consists of **crowded columnar cells,** which may pile up to **form pseudopapillae** (Sanderson's Polster) (similar to those seen in Graves disease) and project into the follicular lumen.
- **Colloid content varies** throughout the gland. Some follicles are distended with colloid, whereas others are small with minimal colloid.

2. Phase of Colloid Involution

Subsequently, if the dietary content of iodine increases or if the demand for thyroid hormone decreases, the stimulated hyperplastic phase goes into a phase of colloid involution.

Gross

The thyroid is **enlarged** and the **cut surface** is usually **brown,** somewhat **glassy, and translucent.**

Microscopy

- **Thyroid follicles become enlarged.**
- **Atrophy of follicular cells:** The epithelium appears **flattened and cuboidal.**

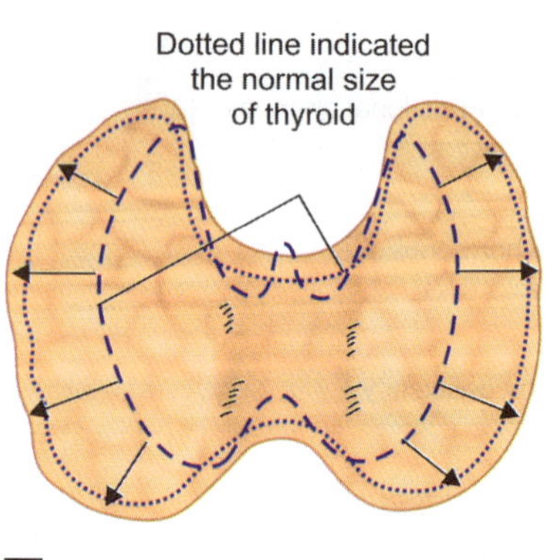

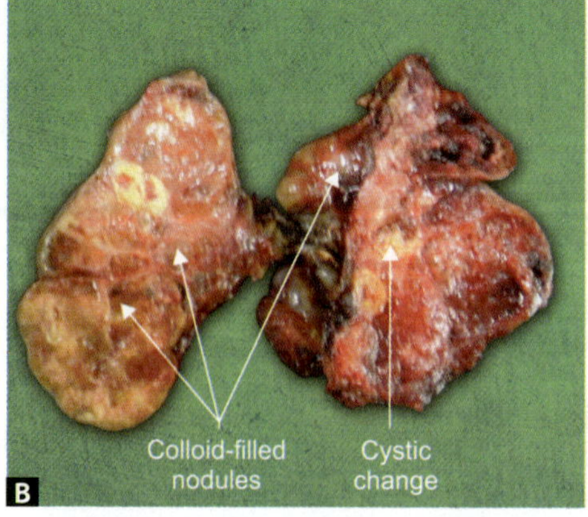

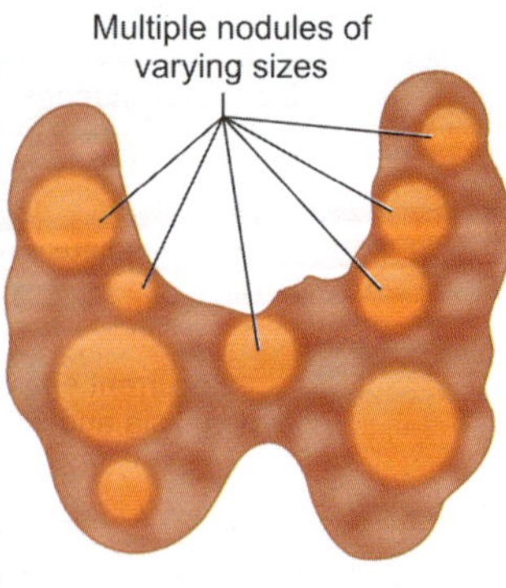

Figs. 24.8A to C: Gross appearance of goiter: (A) Diffuse nontoxic goiter (Size of normal gland is shown in dotted lines); (B) and (C) Multinodular goiter showing nodular thyroid gland, containing numerous colloid-filled nodules (A, and C, diagrammatic appearances).

- **Lumen of follicle filled with abundant colloid:** Massive storage of colloid leads to the formation of a colloid-rich, enlarged thyroid gland **(so-called colloid goiter)**.

Multinodular Goiter

Q. Write a short note on the morphology of multinodular goiter.

Gross (Figs. 24.8B and C)

- **Multiple nodules:** The thyroid is lobulated, **diffusely, asymmetrically** (irregularly) **enlarged**, and **nodular** due to **multiple nodules of varying sizes.**
- **Pattern of enlargement:** Varies
  - **One lobe of the thyroid may be more involved** than the other. It may produce pressure on midline structures, such as the trachea and esophagus.
  - **One nodule may** become so **prominent** and appear as a **solitary nodule.**
  - Goiter may **grow behind the sternum and clavicles** to produce **intrathoracic** or **plunging goiter**.
- **Weight of thyroid:** It is **increased** and varies.
- **Cut section:**
  - Shows **numerous irregular nodules containing variable amounts of colloid.**
  - **When the nodules contain large amounts of colloid,** they appear soft, **glistening, and reddish-brown**, due to gelatinous colloid.
  - **Older lesions** may show areas of **hemorrhage, fibrosis, calcification**, and **cystic change**.

Microscopy (Figs. 24.9A and B)

It shows a spectrum of morphologic changes. It shows heterogeneous **nodules composed of thyroid follicles of variable sizes.** They range from hypercellular, hyperplastic regions to cystic areas filled with colloid.

Thyroid parenchyma

- **Colloid nodules:** They consist of **follicles of varying sizes distended with colloid** and lined by **flat to cuboidal inactive epithelium.**
- **Hypercellular nodules:** Some nodules may show **follicular hyperplasia.** They are composed of tightly packed follicular epithelium **with little colloid.** They **may be mistaken for follicular adenomas.** In contrast to follicular adenoma, no prominent capsule is seen between the hyperplastic nodules and residual compressed thyroid parenchyma (*refer* **online Table 24.2**).
- **Colloid cysts:** They may be formed by **fusion (or rupture)** of large **colloid-containing follicles.**

Stroma

It shows degenerative changes due to physical stress. These include:

- **Areas of fibrosis and dystrophic calcification**
- **Areas of hemorrhage** and **chronic inflammation** are common. The presence of **hemosiderin-laden macrophages and cholesterol granulomas** indicates old hemorrhage.

Clinical Features

Due to mass effects of the enlarged thyroid gland: These are the dominant clinical features of goiter. Large goiters may cause compression of surrounding structures and may cause:

- **Airway obstruction** due to compression of the trachea
- **Dysphagia** by compressing the esophagus
- **Venous congestion of the head and face** (superior vena cava syndrome) due to compression of large vessels in the neck and upper thorax
- **Hoarseness** from recurrent laryngeal nerve compression.

Functional status: Usually, goiters are **hormonally silent** (patients are euthyroid) and T_4, T_3, and TSH at the upper range of normal are normal or **elevated.** Some multinodular goiter may produce the following effects:

- **Subclinical hyperthyroidism** with reduced TSH levels.
- Few may develop **thyrotoxicosis** secondary to the development of autonomous nodules that produce thyroid hormone independent of TSH stimulation (one or more nodules become TSH-independent). This condition is called **toxic multinodular goiter or Plummer syndrome**. This thyrotoxicosis is not associated with infiltrative ophthalmopathy (exophthalmos) and dermopathy (pretibial myxedema) of Graves disease–associated thyrotoxicosis.

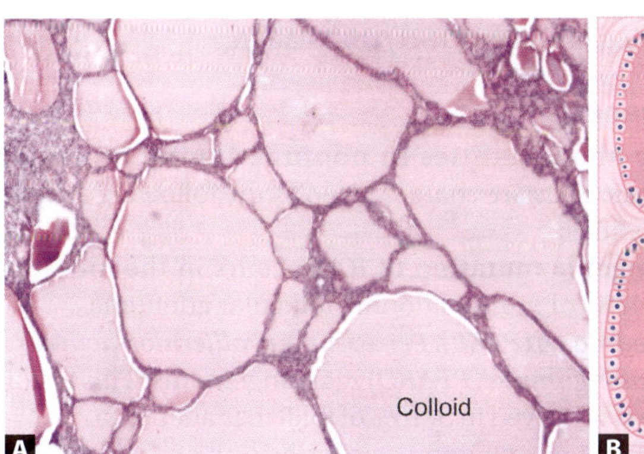

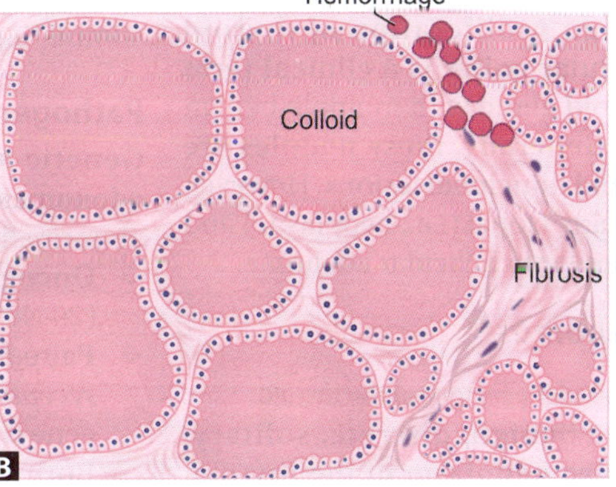

Plunging goiter is: Retrosternal goiter.
Plummer syndrome: Multinodular goiter with hyperthyroidism

Figs. 24.9A and B: (A) Photomicrograph; (B) Diagrammatic. Microscopy of a multinodular goiter composed of thyroid follicles of varying sizes distended with variable amounts of colloid.

Incidence of malignancy in long-standing multinodular goiters: It is low (<5%). Development of malignancy should be suspected when the goiters suddenly increase in size or produce new symptoms (e.g., hoarseness).
Diagnosis: Fine-needle aspiration biopsy is helpful for diagnosis.

THYROID NEOPLASMS

Thyroid neoplasms range from benign adenomas to highly aggressive, anaplastic carcinomas. Thyroid nodule is one of the presenting symptoms. The majority of solitary thyroid nodules are typically benign adenomas or localized, nonneoplastic conditions, such as a dominant nodule in multinodular goiter, simple cysts, or foci of thyroiditis. By contrast, thyroid carcinomas are uncommon and account for less than 1% of solitary thyroid nodules. Some clinical criteria provide a clue to the nature of a given thyroid nodule (*refer* **online Table 24.1**). However, the morphologic evaluation of a thyroid nodule by fine-needle aspiration, combined with the histologic study of surgically resected thyroid tissue, is required for the definitive diagnosis of thyroid nodules.

Q. Classify thyroid tumors.

WHO (2022) classification of thyroid neoplasms is presented in **Box 24.5**.

BOX 24.5: The World Health Organization (WHO) (2022) (abridged) classification of thyroid neoplasms.

Follicular cell-derived neoplasms
- Benign tumors
  - Thyroid follicular nodular disease
  - Follicular thyroid adenoma
  - Follicular thyroid adenoma with papillary architecture
  - Oncocytic adenoma of the thyroid
- Low-risk neoplasms
  - Noninvasive follicular thyroid neoplasm with papillary-like nuclear features
  - Thyroid tumors of uncertain malignant potential
    - Follicular tumor of uncertain malignant potential
    - Well-differentiated tumor of uncertain malignant potential
  - Hyalinizing trabecular tumor of the thyroid
- Malignant neoplasms
  - Follicular thyroid carcinoma
  - Invasive encapsulated follicular variant papillary carcinoma
  - Papillary thyroid carcinoma
  - Oncocytic carcinoma of the thyroid
  - Follicular-derived carcinomas, high-grade
  - Poorly differentiated thyroid carcinoma
  - Differentiated high-grade thyroid carcinoma
  - Anaplastic follicular cell-derived thyroid carcinoma

Thyroid C-cell-derived carcinoma
- Medullary thyroid carcinoma

Mixed medullary and follicular-cell-derived carcinomas
Salivary gland-type carcinomas of the thyroid
Thyroid tumors of uncertain histogenesis
Thymic tumors within the thyroid
Embryonal thyroid neoplasms

FOLLICULAR CELL-DERIVED NEOPLASMS

Follicular cell-derived neoplasms are divided into three classes: benign tumors, low-risk neoplasms, and malignant neoplasms.

Benign Tumors

Benign follicular cell-derived tumors include thyroid follicular nodular disease (FND), follicular adenoma, follicular adenoma with papillary architecture, and oncocytic adenomas.

Thyroid Follicular Nodular Disease

Thyroid follicular nodular disease (FND) is a **multifocal, noninflammatory, benign proliferation of thyroid follicular cells. Multinodular goiter is a clinical term used for an enlarged thyroid gland** with multiple benign nodules caused by FND. **Generally, these nodules are considered hyperplastic and nonclonal lesions.** However, some nodules are molecularly clonal (i.e., neoplastic) and morphologically appear similar to follicular adenoma.

Follicular Thyroid Adenomas

Q. Write a short essay on the follicular adenoma of the thyroid.

A follicular adenoma is a **benign, discrete, solitary, encapsulated, noninvasive neoplasm** of the thyroid. It is the **most common thyroid tumor** and is **derived from follicular epithelial cells, hence called follicular adenomas.** Most follicular adenomas are sporadic.
Toxic adenomas: The majority of follicular adenomas are nonfunctional. Only a minority of them produce thyroid hormones and cause clinically apparent thyrotoxicosis. These hormones producing functional adenomas are called *toxic adenomas.* These are not dependent on thyroid-stimulating hormone (TSH) stimulation.

Pathogenesis

Genetic abnormalities in nonfunctioning follicular adenomas: They are characterized by the following genetic abnormalities:
- **Oncogenic mutation of *RAS*** occurs in the minority (20–40%) of nonfunctioning follicular adenomas.
- **Paired-box 8 (*PAX8*): *Peroxisome proliferator-activated receptor gamma* (*PPARG*) rearrangements:** This fusion gene is observed in 5–10% of follicular adenoma.

Both the above genetic alterations are seen more frequently in follicular carcinomas. This suggests that conventional follicular adenomas carrying these alterations are **precursors to carcinomas**.

Genetic abnormality in toxic adenomas: The most common are somatic mutations that lead to constitutive activation of the TSH receptor signaling pathway.

- **Gain-of-function mutations in the gene encoding the TSH receptor** *(TSHR)*: It is the most common abnormality present in over 50% of toxic adenomas. Such mutations may occur in a few patients with autonomous nodules of toxic multinodular goiters.

MORPHOLOGY

Gross (Fig. 24.10A)

- Follicular adenoma is a **solitary** (single), **spherical** (round, or oval nodule), **solid,** and **encapsulated** tumor. It is completely surrounded by a well-defined, intact fibrous capsule.
- **Size:** It ranges from **1–3 cm in diameter.**
- **Cut surface:**
  - **Appearance:** Tumor is **homogeneous grayish-white to red-brown, fleshy, pale, and very soft in appearance** than the surrounding gland.
  - **Well-demarcated** and surrounded by a **thin intact, well-formed fibrous capsule.** Tumor **compresses the adjacent thyroid gland.**
  - **Cut surface** of the **tumor bulges** when fresh.
- **Secondary changes:** They are common and include **areas of hemorrhage, fibrosis, calcification,** and **cystic change.**

Microscopy

- **Follicular architecture:** The tumor shows a follicular growth pattern usually composed of uniform-appearing follicles containing colloids **(Figs. 24.10B and C).** This architecture is generally quite different from those of the surrounding (adjacent) nonneoplastic thyroid parenchyma of the thyroid. Follicular adenomas show a **variety of architectural growth patterns,** which **do not have any significance. The tumor cells are arranged in uniform follicles that contain colloid and show little variation in cell size, shape, or nuclear morphology.** These follicles may resemble normal thyroid tissue or mimic different stages in the embryonic development of the gland. These include normofollicular (simple), macrofollicular (prominent, large follicles with abundant colloid), microfollicular (common and contains small follicles with colloid), solid, fetal, embryonal, and trabecular.
- **Monotonous cuboidal follicular cells:** The thyroid follicle of follicular adenoma is lined by monotonous, cuboidal, or polygonal cells with little variation in size and shape.
  Mitotic figures are rare. **Oncocytic changes:** Occasionally, the neoplastic cells show brightly eosinophilic granular cytoplasm **(oxyphil** or **oncocytic cell change).**
- **Intact, well-formed fibrous capsule:** It is the hallmark of all follicular adenomas. A thorough, **careful examination of the integrity of the capsule is essential to distinguish follicular adenoma from follicular carcinoma.**
- **Scant stroma:** Follicular adenoma typically contains a scant stroma.

Features that distinguish between follicular adenoma and solitary dominant hyperplastic nodule are listed (*refer* **online Table 24.2).**

Clinical Features

Presentation: Many follicular adenomas present as solitary painless masses. They typically occur sporadically in euthyroid patients. They are "cold" nodules that do not take up radioiodine. They are clinically discovered on the routine physical examination once they grow to palpable size.

Age and gender: They show a **female predominance** and are usually detected in the fifth or sixth decade of life.

Investigations

Radionuclide scanning:

- **Nonfunctioning adenomas:** They **take up less radioactive iodine than normal thyroid parenchyma.** The nonfunctioning adenomas usually **appear as cold nodules. About 10%** of cold nodules **may be malignant** on microscopic examination.
- **Functioning follicular adenomas** (toxic adenomas): They appear as **hot nodules. Malignancy is rare** in hot nodules.
- **Ultrasonography**
- **Fine-needle aspiration biopsy**

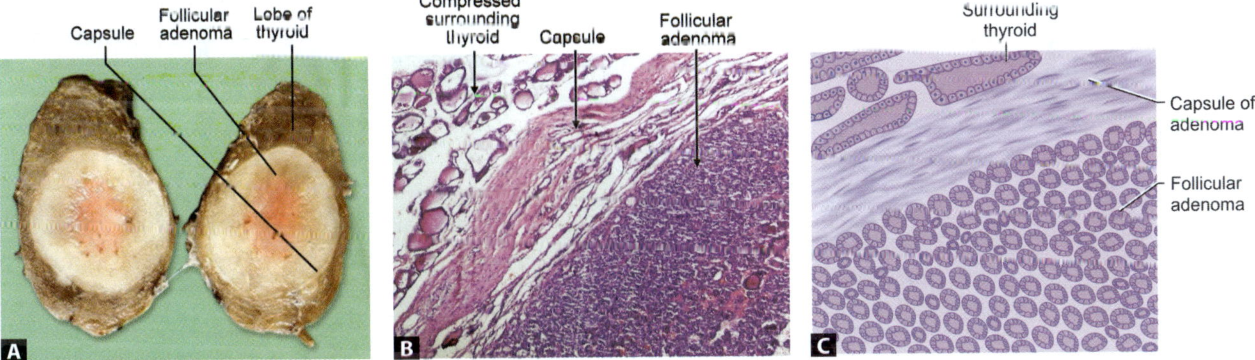

Figs. 24.10A to C: Follicular adenoma of the thyroid: (A) A solitary, well-circumscribed, gray-white nodule is visible in this gross specimen (Cut section); (B) Photomicrograph; (C) Diagrammatic. Microscopic appearance of part of follicular adenoma of the thyroid showing well-differentiated, uniform thyroid follicles, well-formed capsule, and compressed adjacent thyroid follicles.

- **Histological examination** of surgically resected specimens should be evaluated for capsular integrity and definitive diagnosis of adenomas.
- **Prognosis:** Excellent and adenomas do not recur or metastasize.

Malignant Neoplasms

- Carcinomas of the thyroid is **relatively uncommon**.
- **Sex and age:**
  - **Early and middle adult years: Female** predominance.
  - **Childhood and late adult life:** Males and females are **equally** affected.
- **Nature of carcinoma: The majority** of thyroid carcinomas are **well-differentiated**.

Major Subtypes

Q. Write a short essay on major subtypes of carcinoma of the thyroid and genetic alterations in follicular cell-derived neoplasms of the thyroid.

The major subtypes of thyroid carcinoma include three follicular cell-derived neoplasms and one C-cell-derived carcinoma.

Follicular Cell-derived Neoplasms

1. Papillary carcinoma (>85%)
2. Follicular carcinoma (5–15%)
3. Anaplastic (undifferentiated) carcinoma (<5%)

General genetic features in follicular cell-derived carcinoma: Genetic alterations in the three follicular cell-derived malignancies result in **gain-of-function mutations** along components of the **two signaling pathways (Fig. 24.11)** namely:

1. **Mitogen-activated protein (MAP) kinase pathway**, and
2. **Phosphatidylinositol-3-kinase (PI-3K)/AKT pathway.**

Normally, these two signaling pathways are transiently activated by the binding of soluble growth factor ligands to the extracellular domain of receptor tyrosine kinases. This binding leads to autophosphorylation of the cytoplasmic domain of the receptor, and results in intracellular signal transduction. **Mutation** of genes involved in the above two pathways **leads to** oncogenic **constitutive activation** even in the absence of ligands and promotes **carcinogenesis.**

Thyroid C-cell Derived Carcinoma

Medullary thyroid carcinoma (5%).

Conventional Papillary Thyroid Carcinoma

Q. Write a short note on papillary carcinoma of the thyroid.

- Papillary thyroid carcinoma (PTC) is a **malignant epithelial tumor showing evidence of follicular cell differentiation**. They **show a set of distinctive nuclear features and a variety of architectural subtypes.**

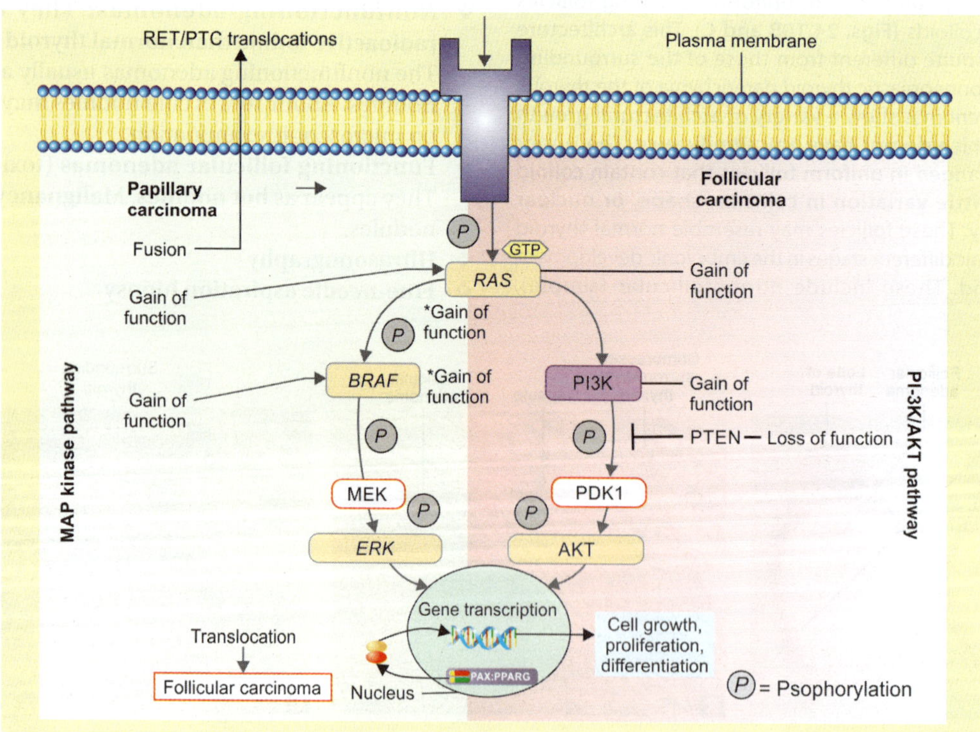

Fig. 24.11: Genetic alterations (driver mutations) in follicular cell-derived malignant tumors of the thyroid gland. The most common mutations are indicated by asterisks.

- PTC is the **most common malignant tumor of the thyroid** and constitutes ~85% of sporadic **thyroid cancer**.
- **Age and gender:** It **can occur at any age**, but is **mostly** found between the ages of **20 and 50 years**. It is the most common thyroid cancer in children and young adolescents. The female-to-male ratio is about 3:1.
- **Risk factor**: It is associated with **previous exposure** to **ionizing radiation**.

Pathogenesis

Activation of MAP kinase pathway: MAP kinase pathways regulate cell growth and division. Activation of the MAP kinase pathway is a major feature of most conventional papillary carcinomas **(Fig. 24.11)**. The three most common mechanisms of unregulated activation of MAPK signaling are (1) point mutations in *BRAF* (40–65%); (2) translocations that result in gene fusions of *RET* or *NTRK* (10–20%); and (3) oncogenic mutations of *RAS* (10–30%). These are driver mutations in PTC.

1. Activating point mutations in BRAF

One of the methods of activation of the MAP kinase pathway is by **activating point mutations in *BRAF*.** The protein product of the *BRAF* gene is a transduction protein and is an intermediate signaling component in the MAP kinase pathway. **Gain of function point mutation of the *BRAF* gene** is observed in ~30–50% of papillary carcinomas. **Significance of *BRAF* mutations:** In conventional PTCs, *BRAF* mutations are **associated with a higher risk of extrathyroidal extension and recurrence.**

2. Translocations that result in gene fusions of RET or NTRK

RET and *NTRK* genes encode transmembrane receptor tyrosine kinase (RTK) growth factor receptors, namely: (1) RET and (2) NTRK1 (neurotrophic tyrosine kinase receptor) respectively. These act through the activation of the:

- ***Translocations resulting in gene fusions of RET* (rearrangement of *RET* gene):** Transmembrane receptor tyrosine kinase (**RTK**) growth factor receptors are **normally not expressed in thyroid follicular cells**. RET (rearranged during transfection) is a receptor tyrosine kinase. In papillary thyroid cancers, chromosomal **(somatic) rearrangements of the *RET* gene** are common. These rearrangements **cause the fusion of the tyrosine kinase domain of RET to various other genes.** They create ***RET::PTC* (*RET*::papillary thyroid carcinoma) fusion oncogenes.** Their product causes constitutive activation of the tyrosine kinase receptor in thyroid follicular cells thereby activating the MAP kinase pathway. *RET::PTC* translocations. It is present in about 5–35% of papillary thyroid cancers and frequency is higher in those following radiation exposure.
- **NTRK (neurotrophic tyrosine kinase) translocation:** Similar to RET::PTC, paracentric inversions or translocations can involve *NTRK*. It is another gene that encodes an RTK. NTRK translocations are present in 5–10% of PTCs. These rearrangements also produce constitutively active NTRK fusion proteins and activate the MAP kinase pathway.

***RET::PTC* rearrangements** and ***BRAF* point mutations** are **not found in follicular adenomas or carcinomas.**

3. Oncogenic mutations of RAS

They also occur in 0–35% of papillary thyroid cancer. They are more common in the follicular variant of papillary thyroid cancer (FVPTC).

Refer **online Table 24.3** for the most relevant genetic alterations (driver mutations) in papillary thyroid carcinoma (PTC).

MORPHOLOGY

Q. Write a short note on the morphology of papillary carcinoma of the thyroid.

Gross

- Conventional papillary carcinomas may be **solitary or multifocal** lesions.
- Tumors may be: (1) **well-circumscribed**, (2) **encapsulated**, or (3) **ill-defined** (infiltrate the adjacent parenchyma).
- **Gray white, firm to hard tumor**, which may show areas of fibrosis and calcification. May also be cystic.
- **Cut surface** may show **papillary foci (Figs. 24.12A and B)**.

Microscopy [Figs. 24.13A to C (*refer* online Fig. 24.13B)]

The microscopic hallmarks of papillary thyroid carcinoma are as follows:

- **Complex branching papillae:** They have a dense central fibrovascular stalk/core.
    - Papillae are covered by **single to multiple layers of uniform cuboidal to columnar** epithelial **cells**.
- **Nuclear features:** These following nuclear features are **sufficient for the diagnosis of papillary thyroid carcinoma**,

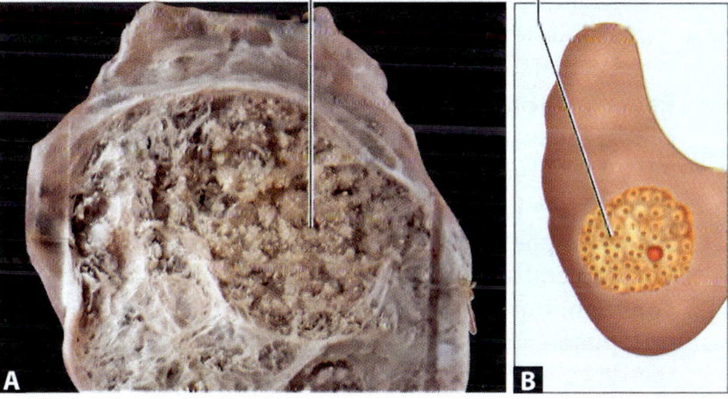

Figs. 24.12A and B: Cut section of papillary carcinoma: (A) Thyroid showing grossly visible papillary structures; (B) Diagrammatic appearance.

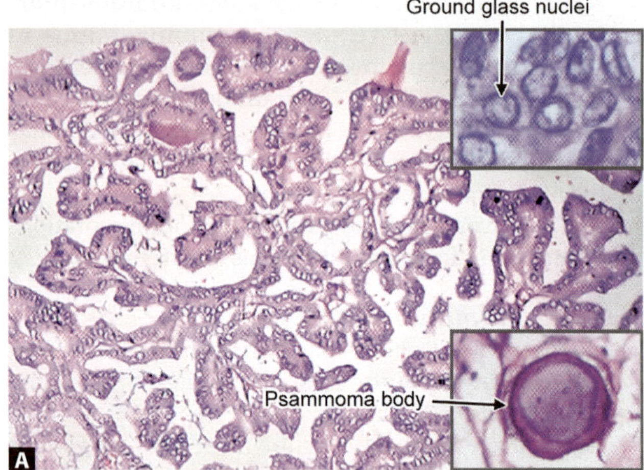

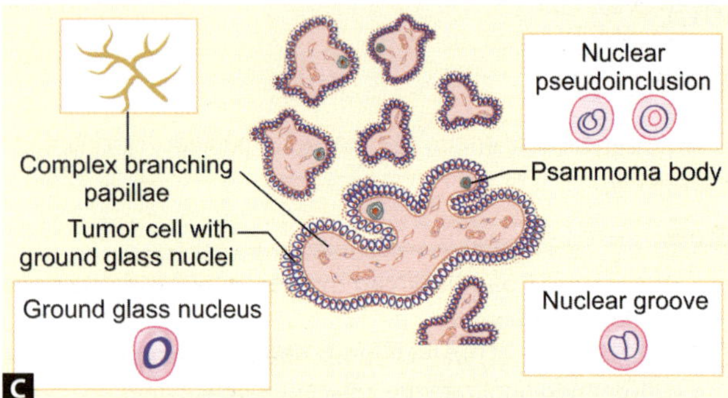

Figs. 24.13A to C: Papillary thyroid carcinoma: (A) Well-formed, complicated, branching papillae lined by cells with characteristic empty-appearing ("Orphan Annie eye") nuclei. Inset in (A) upper right shows Orphan Annie eye nuclei and nuclear groove, and the right lower shows the psammoma body; (C) The diagrammatic appearance of papillary thyroid carcinoma.

even in the absence of papillary architecture. The nuclear features are as follows:
- **Nuclei with finely dispersed chromatin:** This produces an **optically clear or empty appearance** (hypochromatic empty nuclei) giving rise to the designation **ground-glass nuclei** or **Orphan Annie eye nuclei.**
- **Intranuclear inclusions and intranuclear grooves:** Invaginations of the cytoplasm into the nucleus may give the appearance of **eosinophilic intranuclear inclusions** (pseudo-inclusions) or **intranuclear grooves.**

- **Psammoma bodies** (calcospherites): These are **concentrically calcified structures usually** present **within the papillary core.** They are virtually **diagnostic** of papillary carcinoma, and almost **never found in follicular and medullary carcinomas.**
- **Foci of lymphatic invasion and lymphatic spread: Lymphatic invasion** and **spread** to regional cervical lymph nodes are **common**, but **vascular invasion and blood spread are uncommon.** Metastases to adjacent cervical lymph nodes are seen in up to 50% of cases.

Histological Variants of Papillary Thyroid Carcinoma

- **Encapsulated follicular variant:** It is the **most common variant**, in which the **nuclei show characteristic features of papillary carcinoma** but have **follicular architecture.** About one-third of these tumors contain the translocation that creates a *PAX8::PPARG* fusion gene. This is typical of follicular carcinomas.
- **Infiltrative follicular PTC:** It shows infiltrative growth margins. It has many features of conventional PTC.
- **Diffuse sclerosing variant:** It shows prominent papillary projections, admixed with nests of squamous metaplasia, **extensive, diffuse fibrosis** with a **prominent lymphocytic infiltrate.**

Three aggressive forms of PTC are as follows:
- **Tall cell PTC:** It is composed of tall, large columnar cells that are **three times as tall as they are wide.**
- **Hobnail PTC:** It shows papillary and micropapillary (small papillae without fibrovascular cores) structures and dyscohesive tumor cells.
- **Columnar cell PTC:** It consists of thin papillae or glandular-like spaces lined by tall columnar cells that form prominent pseudostratification.

Spread of Papillary Carcinoma

Lymphatic spread: PTC invades lymphatics and spreads to regional cervical lymph nodes. Lymph node metastases vary from tiny foci in a normal-appearing lymph node to large masses. Sometimes, the first manifestation of PTC may be a mass in a cervical lymph node.

Hematogenous metastases: They can occur in PTC but are more common in other thyroid carcinomas, including FTC.

Clinical Course

Most papillary carcinomas present as **asymptomatic thyroid nodules**, sometimes the presenting symptom may be a mass in a cervical lymph node (due to metastasis).

Diagnostic tests: Different diagnostic tests may help to distinguish benign from malignant thyroid nodules. These include **radionuclide scanning and fine-needle aspiration.**
- **Fine-needle aspiration cytology** shows nuclear features characteristic of papillary carcinoma.

Prognosis: Excellent.

Follicular Thyroid Carcinoma

- Follicular thyroid carcinoma (FTC) is a **malignant tumor arising from follicular cells.** It constitutes ~5–15% of primary thyroid cancers.
- **Age and gender:** Develop at **an older age than papillary carcinoma** with a peak incidence between **40 and 60 years** of age. More common in **women** (3:1).
- **Vascular invasion:** Follicular carcinoma has a marked tendency for vascular invasion. Through the

hematogenous route, it disseminates and metastasizes to distant sites such as the bone, lungs, brain, and liver. It avoids lymphatics; hence, true embolic lymph node metastases are very rare.

Etiology: More **frequent in regions** where there is a **dietary deficiency of iodine**.

Pathogenesis

Follicular thyroid carcinomas have mutations in *RAS* or components of the PI3K/AKT signaling pathway (**Fig. 24.11**).

1. Gain-of-function Point Mutations of RAS

RAS is a signal transduction protein. *RAS* mutations are seen in approximately 20–40% of follicular adenomas and 30–50% of follicular carcinomas.

2. Mutations in PI-3K/AKT Cell Signaling Pathway

It is observed in ~30–50% of follicular carcinomas. These mutations result in constitutive activation of this oncogenic pathway. The mutations may involve different subsets of PI-3K/AKT signaling. These include:

- **Gain-of-function mutations in *PIK3CA*:** *PIK3CA* encodes PI3K. Follicular tumors show amplification of *PIK3CA*.
- **Loss-of-function mutations in *PTEN*: *PTEN*** is a **tumor suppressor gene** and negative regulator of PI3K. Follicular carcinoma may show **mutations of *PTEN*** with **loss-of-function of this tumor suppressor gene**.

RAS and *PIK3CA* mutations are also observed in benign follicular adenomas and anaplastic carcinomas. This suggests a shared histogenesis.

3. PAX8::PPARG Fusion Gene

A unique (2;3) (q13; p25) translocation occurs in 30–50% of follicular carcinomas. This translocation produces a fusion gene composed of portions of *PAX8* (the gene involved in thyroid development), and the peroxisome proliferator-activated receptor gene *(PPARG)*. The product of *PPARG* is a nuclear hormone receptor involved in the terminal differentiation of thyroid epithelial cells. [The Nomenclature Committee recommends the separators be replaced with a double colon (: :) (e.g., *PAX8::PPARG*)].

Major driver mutations in follicular carcinoma are listed in **Table 24.4**.

TABLE 24.4 Most relevant genetic alterations (driver mutations) in follicular carcinoma of the thyroid, with prevalence.

Genetic profile	*Follicular carcinoma*
RAS mutations	30–50%
PAX8::PPARG rearrangements	20–30%
PIK3CA	0–10%
PTEN	0–10%

MORPHOLOGY

Gross (Fig. 24.14A)

- Follicular thyroid carcinomas (FTCs) are **single nodules.**
- They may be **either well-circumscribed or infiltrate** into the surrounding thyroid parenchyma.
  - **Circumscribed tumors:** They may be difficult to distinguish from follicular adenomas on gross examination.
  - **Large tumors:** They may penetrate the capsule and infiltrate into the adjacent structures in the neck.
- The **cut section** of the tumor appears **gray to pink** in color.

Microscopy

Follicular Pattern of Tumor Cells

- **Tumor cells:** Tumor consists of **uniform cuboidal to columnar** follicular epithelial **cells.** They are **similar to those of follicular adenoma.**
- **Follicular pattern:** Tumor cells may form **small follicles containing colloid or may be arranged in nests or sheets** without forming follicles.
- **Increased mitotic activity.**
- **Neither the nuclear feature of papillary carcinoma nor psammoma bodies** is seen.
- **Capsular and/or vascular invasion [Fig. 24.14B (*refer* online Figs. 24.14C and D)]:** Follicular thyroid carcinoma is usually surrounded by a thick and irregular capsule. Demonstration of capsular and/or vascular invasion is necessary for the diagnosis of FTC. **The distinction between follicular adenoma and carcinoma requires extensive histologic sampling of the tumor capsule, to look for evidence of capsular and/or vascular invasion.**

Invasion

Depending on the pattern of invasion, follicular carcinoma can be **subdivided into three** variants.

1. **Minimally invasive follicular carcinomas:** Most tumors closely resemble follicular adenoma.
   - Gross: Tumors appear as a **well-defined** and **encapsulated lesion.**
   - Microscopy: **Resemble follicular adenoma** but **shows mitoses, and capsular invasion** (*refer* **online Fig. 24.14C and D).** The tumor extends through the fibrous capsule in a "mushroom"-like pattern into the surrounding tissue.
2. **Encapsulated angioinvasive:** It is an encapsulated tumor that shows **vascular invasion (Figs. 24.14A and B)**
3. **Widely invasive follicular carcinomas:** These tumors are typically large. They **infiltrate the thyroid parenchyma**, its **capsule,** and the surrounding **extrathyroidal soft tissues.**

Spread of Follicular Carcinoma

1. **Lymphatic spread:** In contrast to papillary thyroid carcinomas, **regional lymph node metastases are uncommon.**
2. **Hematogenous spread is common to bone, lungs, and liver.** Well-differentiated metastases may take up radioactive iodine.

Clinical features: Follicular thyroid carcinomas present as **slowly enlarging, solitary, painless, cold thyroid nodules.** Rarely, they may be hyperfunctional.

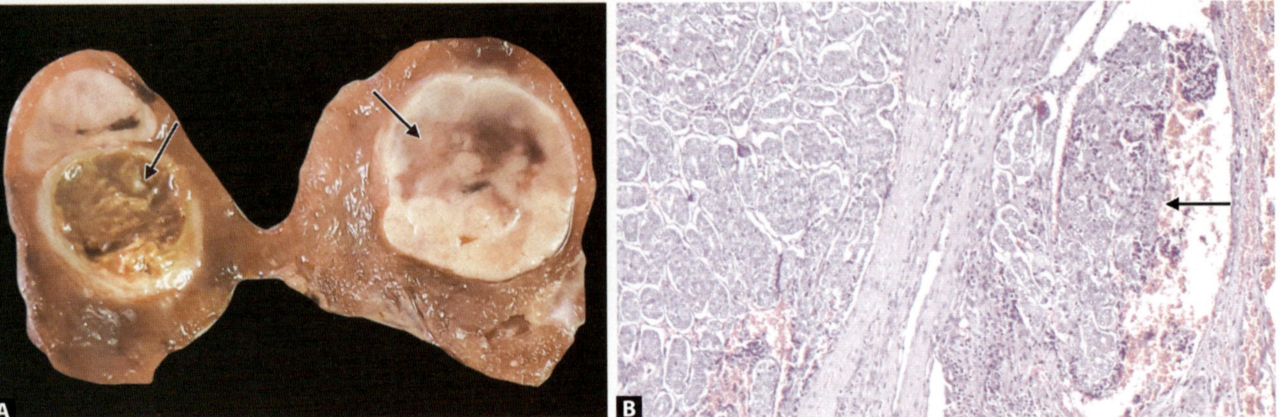

Figs. 24.14A and B: Encapsulated angioinvasive follicular carcinoma: (A) The cut section shows a well-demarcated solid tumor with cystic change (arrow); (B) Vascular invasion. Tumor cells (arrow) are seen in the intracapsular vessel.

Anaplastic (Undifferentiated) Thyroid Carcinoma

- Anaplastic carcinomas are **undifferentiated tumors** of the follicular epithelium. These are highly **aggressive and lethal tumors.**
- They are **composed of undifferentiated follicular thyroid cells** without detectable thyroid differentiation by histomorphology. They **can arise de novo or more commonly by "dedifferentiation" of a well-differentiated follicular or papillary carcinoma**. Constitute less than 5% of thyroid tumors.
- **Age: Elderly** with a mean age of 65 years.

Pathogenesis

- Molecular changes are **similar to those found in well-differentiated carcinomas** [e.g., ***RAS*** **(~20%), or** ***PIK3CA*** **(~10%) mutations**], but occur at a higher rate.
- **Other genetic changes specific to anaplastic carcinoma:** These include **loss-of-function mutations in** ***TP53*** (up to 70%) *or* mutations of β-catenin *(CTNNB1)*.

MORPHOLOGY

Gross

Anaplastic carcinomas manifest as bulky, diffusely infiltrative tumors that usually grow rapidly beyond the thyroid capsule into adjacent neck structures.

Microscopy

These neoplasms are composed of highly anaplastic cells. These include:

- **Spindle-shaped** cells with a sarcomatous appearance
- **Large, pleomorphic giant** cells
- **Mixed** spindle and pleomorphic cells

In some tumors, there may be foci of papillary or follicular differentiation. This may suggest the origin from a better-differentiated carcinoma.

Immunohistochemistry: The tumor cells express epithelial markers like **cytokeratin**, but are usually **negative for thyroglobulin**.

Spread

- **Local spread** into thyroid capsule and adjacent neck structures.
- **Hematogenous spread** to lungs.

Clinical features: Usually, it presents as a rapidly growing bulky neck mass. Symptoms due to compression and invasion of the neck structures may cause dyspnea, dysphagia, hoarseness, and cough.

Prognosis: Aggressive tumor with poor prognosis.

Medullary Thyroid Carcinoma

Q. Write a short note on medullary carcinoma of the thyroid.

- Medullary carcinomas of the thyroid are **malignant neuroendocrine tumors derived from** the **parafollicular cells** or **C-cells** of the thyroid.
- Similar to normal C-cells, they **secrete calcitonin,** the measurement of which is **useful in the diagnosis and postoperative follow-up**. The tumor cells may also secrete other polypeptide hormones such as **somatostatin, serotonin, and vasoactive intestinal peptide**.
- They are rare and comprise <3% of all thyroid cancers.
- **Diagnostic importance:** Medullary carcinoma is an aggressive tumor closely associated with multiple neuroendocrine (MEN) syndromes (MEN 2A and 2B or 3), and its probable precursor lesion is C-cell hyperplasia.

Sporadic or familial medullary carcinoma: Medullary carcinoma occurs in both sporadic and familial forms. Both are strongly associated with RET proto-oncogene.

- **Sporadic:** Constitutes about 70–80% of tumors with a peak incidence in the **40s and 50s**.
- **Familial:** About 20–30% of medullary carcinoma are familial. It may occur:
  - **With associated MEN syndrome 2A or 2B** in younger patients.
  - Without an associated MEN syndrome.

Pathogenesis

1. **Germline *RET* gene mutations in familial medullary thyroid carcinomas occurring in MEN-2:** The ***RET* gene codes for growth factor receptor namely receptor tyrosine kinase. Familial medullary thyroid carcinomas** occur in multiple endocrine neoplasia type 2 (**MEN-2**) and are associated with **germline *RET* gene mutations.** The **oncogenic version** of the *RET* gene (mutated RET) leads to **constitutive activation of the tyrosine kinase receptor and cell proliferation.**
2. **Acquired *RET* mutations:** These are seen in about 50% of nonfamilial (sporadic) medullary thyroid cancers.

Chromosomal rearrangements involving *RET*, such as the *RET/PTC* translocations found in papillary cancers, are **not seen in medullary carcinomas.**

MORPHOLOGY

Gross (Figs. 24.15A and B)

- **Size:** Medullary thyroid carcinomas vary in size from <0.1 cm in diameter to several centimeters.
- **Number: Solitary nodule** in **sporadic** medullary thyroid carcinomas and **multicentric and bilateral** (involving both lobes) **common in familial cases.**
- **Cut surface:** The tumor is **firm and pale gray.** They **may be circumscribed** (but not encapsulated) **or infiltrative. Larger lesions** may show areas of **necrosis and hemorrhage** and they **may extend through the capsule of the thyroid.**

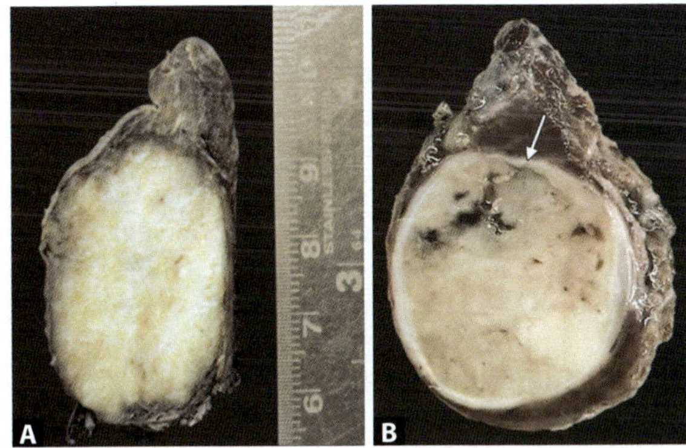

Figs. 24.15A and B: Cut section of medullary carcinoma of the thyroid: (A) Infiltrative pale gray tumor (arrow); (B) Circumscribed tan-colored tumor (arrow).

Microscopy (Figs. 24.16A and B)

Q. Write a short answer on microscopy of medullary carcinoma of the thyroid.

Medullary thyroid carcinomas show a **wide variety of histological appearances.** They can mimic the entire spectrum of thyroid malignancies. They are similar in both sporadic and hereditary types.

Growth pattern: Typically, tumor cells form a **solid, lobular, trabecular, or insular** growth pattern. Tumor cells **may form nests, cord sheets, and even follicles.** These are separated by varying amounts of stroma.

Tumor cells:

- **Cell types:** Individual tumor cells are **variably sized** and can be **round, polygonal, plasmacytoid, or spindle-shaped.**
- **Nuclei:** They are usually **round to oval** in shape. They have **coarsely clumped**, somewhat granular neuroendocrine chromatin. **Mitotic activity is relatively low.**
- **Cytoplasm:** It shows **moderate to generous amounts of eosinophilic to amphophilic cytoplasm.**

Multicentric C-cell hyperplasia: It is seen in the surrounding thyroid of familial medullary cancers, which is not observed in sporadic lesions. They represent the **precursor lesions for medullary thyroid carcinoma.**

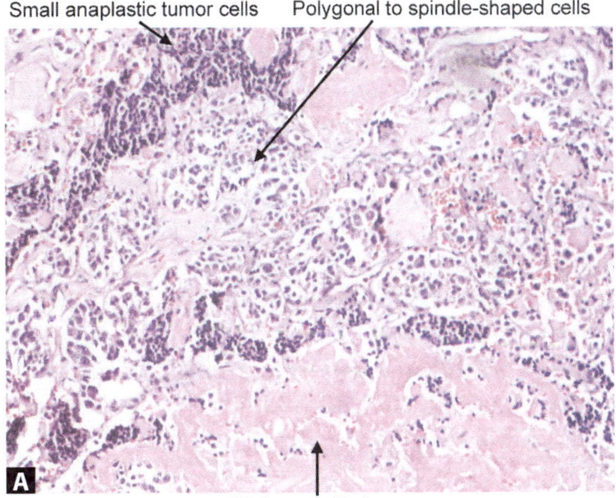

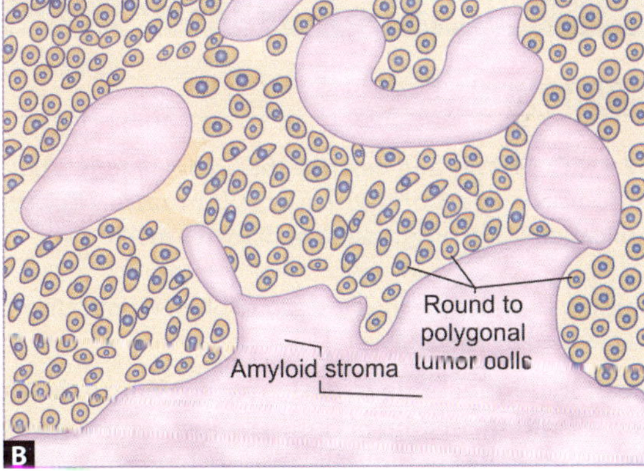

Figs. 24.16A and B: (A) Photomicrography; (B) Diagrammatic. Medullary carcinoma of the thyroid shows nests and trabeculae of round, spindle to polygonal cells separated by abundant homogeneous, extracellular, pink deposits of amyloid.

Stroma with Amyloid Deposits

As many as 90% of medullary thyroid carcinoma show **acellular amyloid deposits** in the stroma (*refer* **Fig. 6.29**). It is formed from the deposition of calcitonin in the peritumoral stroma. Amyloid stains positive by Congo red staining and **gives apple-green birefringence under a polarizing microscope.** Amyloid is not necessary for the diagnosis. Focal calcification may be extensive and may be detected radiologically.

Immunohistochemistry: Calcitonin can be demonstrated within the cytoplasm of the tumor cells and in the stromal amyloid by immunohistochemical methods.

Electron microscopy: It shows **membrane-bound electron-dense granules** within the cytoplasm of the tumor cells. They contain calcitonin.

Clinical Features

Sporadic Medullary Thyroid Carcinoma

- Present as a **painless mass in the neck** that is "cold" on scintigraphy.
- **Paraneoplastic syndrome**: It may occur in some medullary carcinoma caused by the secretion of a peptide hormone. These include diarrhea due to the secretion of VIP or Cushing syndrome due to ACTH.
- **Tumor markers:** These include calcitonin and carcinoembryonic antigen (CEA). They are useful presurgical assessment of tumor load. CEA is useful mainly in calcitonin-negative tumors.

Familial Medullary Thyroid Carcinoma

- Present with **symptoms localized to the thyroid or as a component of familial syndromes** along with neoplasms in other organs (e.g., adrenal, or parathyroid glands).
- Medullary carcinomas arising as a component of MEN- 2B are **more aggressive** and **more frequently metastasize** than sporadic tumors (MEN-2A or FMTC).

Spread: Local invasion into adjacent tissues and lymph node metastases are very common in MTC. Hematogenous spread may also occur in the lungs, bone, and liver.

Treatment: Medullary thyroid carcinoma is treated with total thyroidectomy and lymph node dissection. This is because lymph node metastases are more common in MTC.

Prognosis: The behavior of medullary thyroid carcinoma depends on the stage of the disease.

DIABETES MELLITUS

INTRODUCTION

PA 32.4 (CC): Classify and describe the epidemiology, etiology, pathogenesis, pathology, clinical laboratory features, complications, and progression of diabetes mellitus.

Definition: Diabetes mellitus is a **group of metabolic disorders characterized by hyperglycemia.**

Cause of hyperglycemia in diabetes: It is due to **defects in insulin secretion, insulin action, or**, most commonly, **both.**

Organ systems damaged: The chronic hyperglycemia and associated metabolic abnormalities of diabetes usually damage multiple organ systems. Most commonly it affects the **kidneys, eyes, nerves**, and **blood vessels**.

The prevalence of diabetes is increasing sharply in developing countries because of more sedentary lifestyles. India and China have the largest prevalence of diabetics.

Diagnostic of Diabetes

Diagnosis of Diabetes Mellitus

Normally, the **blood glucose levels** are maintained in a very narrow range of **70–120 mg/dL**. Individuals are euglycemic (blood glucose levels within normal range) when the **fasting glucose** level is **less than 100 mg/dL**, or glucose level **less than 140 mg/dL** following an **OGTT**.

BOX 24.6: Criteria for diagnosis of diabetes according to the American Diabetes Association (ADA) and the World Health Organization (WHO).

1. Fasting plasma glucose >126 mg/dL **or**
2. A random plasma glucose >200 mg/dL with classical signs and symptoms of hyperglycemia **or**
3. A 2-hour plasma glucose ≥200 mg/dL during an oral glucose tolerance test (OGTT) with a loading oral 75 g glucose **or**
4. A glycated hemoglobin (HbA1c) level **≥6.5%.**

Notes:

- In a patient with classic hyperglycemic signs, all tests (mentioned in **Table 24.5**), except the random blood glucose test, must be repeated and confirmed on a separate day.
- Transient hyperglycemia may be observed in many acute conditions associated with stress (e.g., severe infections, burns, or trauma). This is due to the secretion of hormones such as catecholamines and cortisol that oppose the effects of insulin. Thus, diabetes should be diagnosed when there is persistent hyperglycemia following resolution of the acute illness.

Diagnostic criteria for diabetes according to the American Diabetes Association (ADA) and the World Health Organization (WHO) is presented in **Box 24.6**.

Diagnosis of Prediabetes

Impaired glucose tolerance (IGT) or "prediabetes" is defined as **elevated blood sugar that does not reach the criterion used for diagnosis of T2DM**. Criteria for the diagnosis of prediabetes are presented in **Table 24.5**.

Risks in prediabetes: (1) Progression to frank diabetes (T2D) over time (over 5 years) in as many as 25% of individuals and (2) prediabetes has a significant risk for the development of **cardiovascular disease.** Additional factors such as obesity and family history increase this risk.

TABLE 24.5 Diagnosis of prediabetes.

Parameter	*Value*
Diagnosis of prediabetes requires one or more of the following:	
A fasting plasma glucose (FPG) [fasting blood sugar (FBS)]	100 and 125 mg/dL ("impaired fasting glucose")
A 2-hour postprandial plasma glucose (PPPG) [postprandial blood sugar (PPBS)]	140 and 199 mg/dL during a 75-g oral glucose tolerance test (OGTT) ("impaired glucose tolerance")
Glycated hemoglobin (HbA1c) level	5.7% and 6.4%

Note: Glucose tolerance is classified into three broad categories: (1) Normal glucose tolerance; (2) Impaired glucose tolerance, or (3) Diabetes mellitus.

Classification

Q. Classify diabetes mellitus.

Diabetes is classified according to etiopathogenesis into different groups **(Box 24.7),** but the **majority of cases fall into one of two** broad classes namely: **type 1 diabetes** (T1D, a minority of cases) and **type 2 diabetes** (T2D, the vast majority).

Type 1 Diabetes Mellitus

- Type 1 diabetes (T1D) accounts for ~**5–10%** of all cases of diabetes mellitus.
- **Age:** It is most common in **childhood (younger than 20 years** of age). Since it can develop at any age, the term "juvenile-onset diabetes" should be avoided. It was formerly called insulin-dependent diabetes mellitus (IDDM).

General Features

- **Autoimmune disease: Type 1 diabetes mellitus:** It is an **autoimmune disease** characterized by: (1) **destruction of insulin-producing pancreatic β cells in the islets of Langerhans, and (2) an absolute deficiency of insulin.**
- **Islet cell destruction**: It is caused **mainly by immune effector cells.** These immune cells react against endogenous β-cell antigens.
- **Autoimmune attack on β-cells and manifestation:** The clinical onset of T1D is abrupt. But, the autoimmune attack on β-cells usually begins years before the disease becomes evident. The classic features of diabetes occur late in its course, after the destruction of more than 90% of the β-cells.
- **Most patients with T1DM require insulin for survival.**

Pathogenesis of Type 1 Diabetes Mellitus

Q. Write a short note on the pathogenesis of type 1 diabetes mellitus.

Similar to all autoimmune diseases, the pathogenesis of type 1 diabetes involves the interplay of both (1) genetic susceptibility and (2) environmental factors.

Genetic susceptibility: Genetic susceptibility contributes to only a part of diabetes risk.

- **Incidence of type 1 diabetes is greater in twins** of affected individuals than in the general population, and greater in monozygotic (about 50%) than in dizygotic twins.
- **Association with class II MHC (HLA-DR) genes:** Most of the patients with type 1 diabetes have either human leukocyte antigen **(HLA)-DR3 or HLA-DR4, or both,** compared with the general population. However, most individuals with these HLA alleles do not develop diabetes. This indicates that these genes may predispose to the disease, but they do not cause it.

BOX 24.7: Classification of diabetes.

Type 1 diabetes mellitus (β-cell destruction, usually leading to absolute insulin deficiency)
- Immune-mediated β-cell destruction
- Idiopathic (autoantibody-negative)

Type 2 diabetes mellitus (combination of insulin resistance and β-cell dysfunction)

It may range from predominantly insulin resistance with relative insulin deficiency to a predominantly insulin secretory defect with insulin resistance. It is associated with the progressive loss of β-cells.

Specific types of diabetes [monogenic or maturity-onset diabetes of the young (MODY)] due to other causes
- ***Genetic defects of β-cell function or development***
- ***Genetic defects in insulin action***

Exocrine pancreatic defects ("pancreatogenic" or type 3C diabetes)

Any process that diffusely injures the pancreas.
- Chronic pancreatitis with collateral damage to the endocrine pancreas
- Pancreatectomy/trauma
- Pancreatic cancer
- Cystic fibrosis
- Hemochromatosis

Endocrinopathies
- Acromegaly
- Cushing syndrome
- Hyperthyroidism
- Pheochromocytoma
- Glucagonoma

Infections causing β-cell destruction by:
- Cytomegalovirus
- Coxsackie B virus
- Congenital rubella

Drugs- or chemical-induced β-cell dysfunction
- Glucocorticoids
- Thyroid hormone
- Interferon α
- Protease inhibitors
- β-adrenergic agonists
- Thiazides

Other genetic syndromes are sometimes associated with diabetes
- Down syndrome
- Klinefelter syndrome
- Turner syndrome

Gestational diabetes mellitus (GDM)

Diabetes diagnosed in the second or third trimester of pregnancy in a patient who did not have clear overt diabetes before gestation.

- **Non-HLA genes:** Few non-HLA alleles also increase susceptibility to T1D. It includes polymorphism in gene coding insulin.
  - **Polymorphisms in *CTLA4* and *PTPN22* genes:** CTLA-4 is an inhibitory receptor of T cells and PTPN-22 is a protein tyrosine phosphatase. Both these genes inhibit T-cell responses. Polymorphisms in these genes diminish their functional activity and promote excessive T-cell activation (instead of inhibiting T-cell responses). This leads to a **failure to eliminate developing T cells specific for self-protein.**

Environmental factors: Environmental factors probably play a role. Numerous environmental events may trigger the autoimmune process in genetically susceptible individuals.

- **Viral infections:** They **may trigger islet cell destruction** and associations have been found between type 1 diabetes and infection with ***mumps, rubella, coxsackie B, or cytomegalovirus***.

Mechanisms of β-cell Destruction

The clinical onset of T1DM is usually abrupt. However, it shows a lengthy lag period between the initiation of the autoimmune process and the development of symptomatic disease. During this lag period, there is a progressive loss of insulin reserves.

Stages of T1DM (Fig. 24.17)

β-cell destruction in T1DM usually develops slowly over years and progresses through three distinct stages **(Fig. 24.17)**.

Stage 1 (autoimmunity positive, normoglycemia, presymptomatic T1DM): It is characterized by autoimmunity. During this initial stage, individuals have **two or more islet autoantibodies** (antibodies against islet cells). But they are still normoglycemic. This stage is present several years before the start of T1DM.

Stage 2 (autoimmunity positive, dysglycemia, presymptomatic T1DM): During this stage, there is autoimmunity, and there is an **increasingly severe loss of glucose tolerance due to the progressive loss of β-cell mass.** There is mild dysglycemia. But frank symptoms of diabetes are not observed. The 5-year risk of developing symptomatic T1DM increases from <50% in stage 1 to 75% in stage 2.

Stage 3 (autoimmunity positive, dysglycemia, symptomatic T1DM): During this stage, individuals present with **classic manifestations of diabetes**, namely polyuria, polydipsia, polyphagia, hyperglycemia, and ketoacidosis. It is usually clinically evident when there is destruction of >90% of the β-cells, and insulin deprivation is severe.

Autoimmunity (Flowchart 24.2)

Type 1 diabetes mellitus is caused by the autoimmune destruction of β-cells. Triggers for this autoimmune destruction are not known.

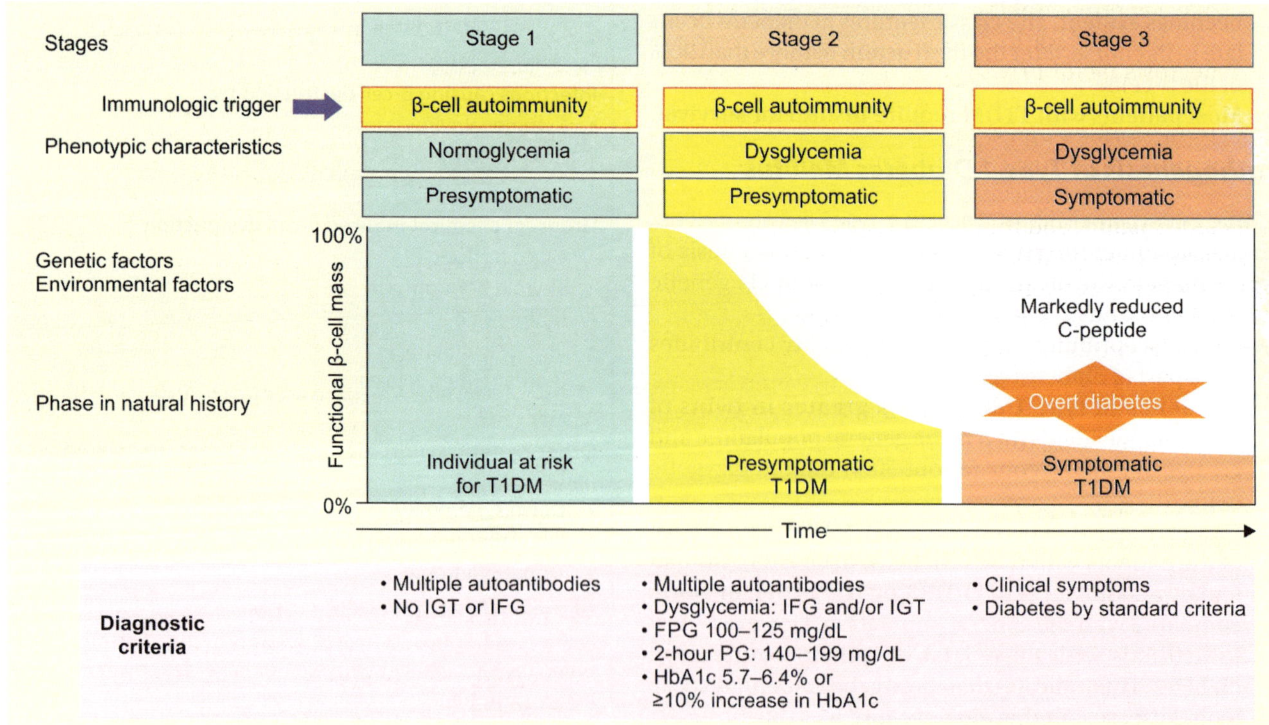

Fig. 24.17: The three pathologic stages in the development of type 1 diabetes mellitus (T1DM).
(FPG: fasting plasma glucose; HbA1c: glycated hemoglobin; IFG: impaired fasting glucose; IGT: impaired glucose tolerance)

Failure of self-tolerance: Self-tolerance is the absence of an immune response to an individual's antigens. It is responsible for our ability to live in harmony with our cells and tissues. The **main immune abnormality in T1DM is a failure of self-tolerance in T cells specific for islet antigens**. This failure of self-tolerance may be a result of some combination of different abnormalities. These abnormalities may be:

1. **Defective clonal deletion of self-reactive T cells** in the thymus.
2. **Defects in the functions of regulatory T cells** that normally reduce the effector T-cell responses, or
3. **Abnormal resistance of effector T cells to suppression by regulatory cells**.

These abnormalities lead to the survival of autoreactive T cells, and these cells are likely to respond to self-antigens.

Mechanisms of injury to β-cells: The destruction of islet cells is mediated mainly by T cells reacting against islet antigens (type IV hypersensitivity).

- **Cell-mediated immune mechanisms:** These are fundamental to the pathogenesis of T1DM. Pancreatic islets of the T1DM often show mild mononuclear infiltration, a process termed insulitis. These inflammatory cells consist of T cells, predominately **CD8+ cytotoxic T lymphocytes** (CTLs) and **type 1 T helper (Th1) cells (CD4+ cells).**
    1. **CD8+ cytotoxic T lymphocytes (CTLs)**: They **kill β-cells directly**.
    2. **Type 1 T helper (Th1) cells (CD4+ cells):** They may **secrete cytokines and injure β-cells**. These cytokines include interferon-gamma (IFN-γ), tumor necrosis factor (TNF), IL-1, IL-6, reactive oxygen species (ROS), and nitric oxide (NO).
- **Autoantibodies against β-cell components:** The islet autoantigens are the targets of immune attack. Autoantigens against which autoantibodies are produced include **insulin**, and the **β-cell enzyme glutamic acid decarboxylase** (GAD). These autoantibodies develop as a response to antigens released due to the destruction of β-cells by cell-mediated immune mechanisms. They are **not responsible for β cell depletion**. However, detection of **these antibodies is useful, especially in obese patients, for differentiating T1DM**, which has an autoimmune basis, **from T2DM** with the autoimmune mechanism.

Pathogenesis of type 1 diabetes mellitus is summarized in **Flowchart 24.2**.

Type 2 Diabetes

Q. Discuss the pathogenesis of type 2 diabetes mellitus. Mention its major long-term complications.

- Type 2 diabetes accounts for ~**90–95% of diabetic patients**.
- **Majority** of patients are **overweight**.

Flowchart 24.2: Pathogenesis of type 1 diabetes mellitus.

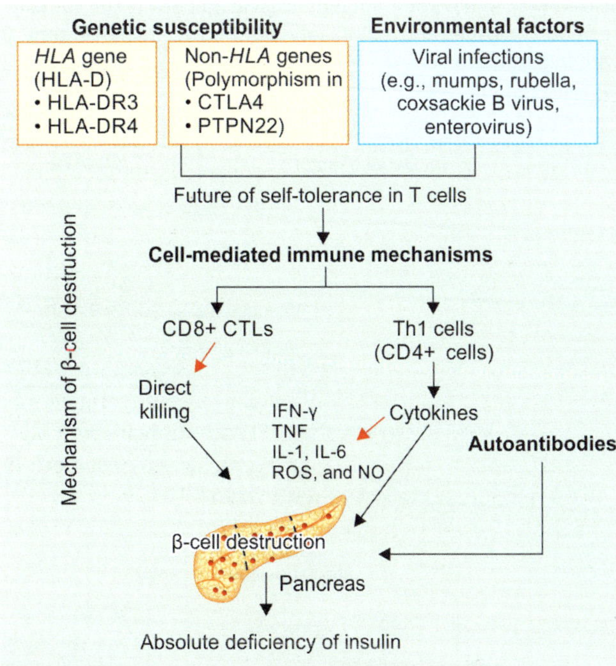

(CTLs: cytotoxic T lymphocytes; IL: interleukin; IFN: interferon; NO: nitric oxide; ROS: reactive oxygen species; TNF: tumor necrosis factor)

- Though formerly known as "adult-onset," it is now found in children and adolescents.

Pathogenesis of Type 2 Diabetes Mellitus (Flowchart 24.3)

Type 2 diabetes is a complex, **multifactorial disease.** It involves interactions of genetic and environmental factors. There is **no evidence of an autoimmune basis.**

- **Environmental factors** play a role and include:
    - **Obesity: The most important environmental risk factor for T2DM** is obesity. The obesity that accompanies T2DM, **particularly central or visceral obesity**, is probably part of the pathogenic process
    - **Sedentary lifestyle.**
    - **Dietary habits and associated obesity particularly central or visceral obesity.**
- **Genetic factors:**
    - Type 2 diabetes has a **concordance rate of 80–90% in monozygotic twins.** This is greater than that for type 1 diabetes (about 50% concordance rates in twins).
    - **Lifetime risk** for type 2 diabetes in an offspring is more than double **if both parents** are **affected**.
    - **Diabetogenic genes:** Several susceptibility loci have been found and are called diabetogenic genes.
    - **Not linked to genes involved in immune tolerance and regulation** (e.g., *HLA, CTLA4*).

Flowchart 24.3: Development of type 2 diabetes mellitus. Insulin resistance associated with obesity is produced by adipokines, free fatty acids (FFAs), and chronic inflammation in adipose tissue. Initially, pancreatic β-cells compensate for insulin resistance by increasing the secretion of insulin and maintaining normoglycemia. Over time, β-cell compensation is followed by β-cell failure, and diabetes develops with hyperglycemia.

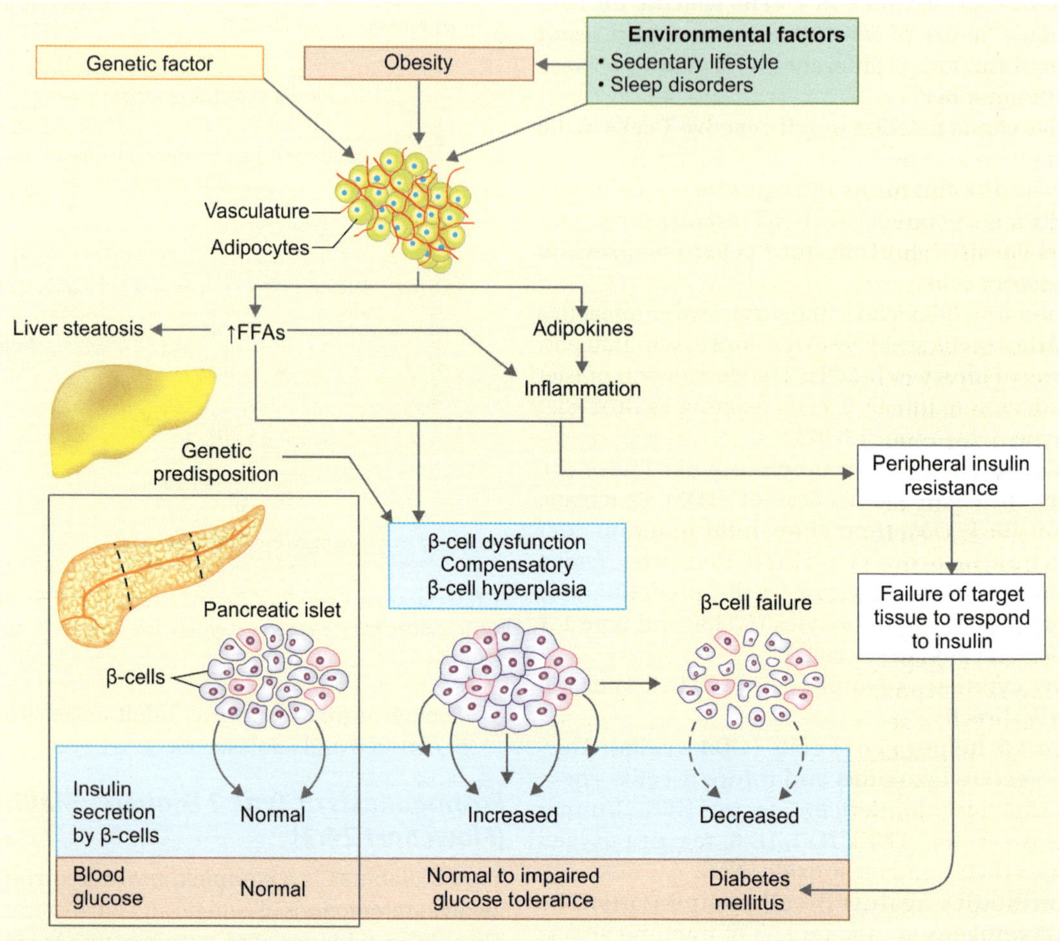

Metabolic defects in type 2 diabetes: The two *important metabolic* defects that are characteristic of T2D are:

1. **Insulin resistance: It is the decreased ability of peripheral tissues to respond to insulin, and**
2. **β-cell dysfunction: It manifests as inadequate insulin secretion in the presence of insulin resistance and hyperglycemia.**

Insulin Resistance

Definition: Insulin resistance is **the failure of the target (peripheral) tissues to respond normally to insulin.** The target peripheral tissues mainly include **skeletal muscle, liver, and fat** (adipose tissue).

Consequences of insulin resistance: It results in the following:

- **Failure to inhibit endogenous glucose production leads to high fasting blood glucose (FBG) levels:** Insulin resistance is associated with **failure to inhibit endogenous glucose production** (gluconeogenesis) in the liver and leads to **increased glucose output from the liver.**
- **Abnormally low glucose uptake and glycogen synthesis in skeletal muscle following a meal leads to high postprandial blood glucose level:** Insulin resistance **decreases the uptake (utilization) of glucose and glycogen synthesis by peripheral tissue**, especially skeletal muscle, and liver, following a meal. There is also reduced glycogen storage by the liver in the postprandial state. All these lead to high postprandial blood glucose levels (postprandial hyperglycemia).
- **Failure to inhibit hormone-sensitive lipase in adipose tissue, leads to high levels of circulating free fatty acids (FFAs):** Insulin resistance leads to **failure to inhibit activation of "hormone-sensitive" lipases in adipose tissue**. The lipases produce **excessive breakdown of triglyceride** in adipocytes and **produce high levels of circulating FFAs.**

Obesity and insulin resistance

Obesity: Of the multiple factors involved in insulin resistance, probably obesity is the most important factor in the development of insulin resistance. Obesity is associated with type 2 diabetes and **visceral obesity is found in more than 80% of patients.** Both the absolute amount of fat and the distribution of fat determine insulin sensitivity.

- **Absolute amount of fat:** Insulin resistance is found even in simple obesity without hyperglycemia. The **risk for diabetes increases as the body mass index** (a measure of body fat content) **increases.**
- **Distribution of body fat:** It affects insulin sensitivity. **Central obesity** (abdominal fat) is **more associated with insulin resistance than peripheral** (gluteal/ subcutaneous) fat depots.

Mechanism of insulin resistance in obesity (Flowchart 24.3): Obesity can affect insulin sensitivity and produce insulin resistance in different ways: (i) nonesterified free fatty acids, (ii) adipokines, and (iii) chronic inflammation in adipose tissue.

- **Excess of free fatty acids (FFAs):** There is an **inverse correlation between fasting plasma FFAs and insulin sensitivity**. The increased adipocyte mass in obesity increases levels of circulating FFAs. High levels of FFAs in the circulation may cause the accumulation of **excess fat (steatosis) in hepatocytes.**
- **Adipokines: Adipose tissue** acts as a functional endocrine organ. It **secretes a variety of proteins** into the systemic circulation, which are **termed adipokines** (or adipose cytokines). Adipokines can divided into:
  - **Prohyperglycemic adipokines:** The increased production of these adipokines promotes hyperglycemia, for example, resisting retinol-binding protein 4 (RBP4).
  - **Antihyperglycemic adipokines**: Leptin and adiponectin improve insulin sensitivity. In obesity, adiponectin levels are reduced, which contributes to insulin resistance.
- **Inflammation:** Inflammation is an important factor in the pathogenesis of T2DM. **Proinflammatory cytokines are secreted as a response to excess FFAs and glucose.** They **cause both insulin resistance and β-cell dysfunction.** Excess FFAs within macrophages and β-cells activate the inflammasome (a multiprotein cytoplasmic complex) and secret cytokine interleukin IL-1β. IL-1β secretes additional proinflammatory cytokines from macrophages, islet cells, and other cells and releases them into circulation. IL-1 and other cytokines act on the major sites of insulin action and produce insulin resistance. Thus, excess **FFAs can directly disturb insulin signaling within peripheral tissues and also indirectly through the secretion of proinflammatory cytokines.**

Metabolic syndrome: This term is applied to a combination of findings namely visceral obesity accompanied by insulin resistance, glucose intolerance, and cardiovascular risk factors such as hypertension and abnormal lipid profiles. These individuals are at high risk for the development of T2D.

β-cell Dysfunction

In type 2 diabetes, **β-cell dysfunction is an important component in the development of overt diabetes.** β-cell dysfunction manifests as **inadequate insulin secretion by the pancreatic β-cells (relative insulin deficiency)** in association with insulin resistance and hyperglycemia. β-cell dysfunction is multifactorial in origin. Various changes in β-cells are as follows:

- **Compensatory β-cell hyperplasia: Initially, pancreatic β-cells respond** to long-term demands of peripheral insulin resistance **by undergoing compensatory hyperplasia in most patients. This leads to increased insulin secretion (hypersecretion).** Thus, the insulin secretion is initially higher for each level of glucose than in controls. This hyperinsulinemic state can compensate for peripheral resistance and maintain normal blood glucose for years.
- **β-cell failure:** However, at some point, β-cells exhaust their capacity to adapt to the long-term demands of peripheral insulin resistance. This leads to relative insulin deficiency and frank diabetes develops.

Molecular mechanisms of β-cell dysfunction

Several mechanisms can cause β-cell dysfunction in T2D. These are as follows:

- **Excess free fatty acids (FFAs):** They **decrease insulin signaling** (lipotoxicity) and decrease the release of insulin. It may be responsible for both insulin resistance and β-cell failure.
- **Chronic hyperglycemia ("glucotoxicity").**
- **An abnormal "incretin effect":** It leads to reduced secretion of hormones that promote insulin release (e.g., GIP and GLP-1).
- **Direct toxicity by amyloid deposits:** In long-standing type 2 diabetes, amyloid deposits in islets are seen in more than 90% of cases. The islet **amyloid protein may be directly cytotoxic to islets** causing β-cell dysfunction.
- **Polymorphisms in genes that control insulin secretion:** These are associated with an increased risk for T2D.

Clinical Features of Diabetes

Diabetes clinically presents with diverse symptoms. The most common initial presentation or mode of diagnosis of two major subtypes is briefly discussed, followed by a discussion of acute and chronic (long-term) complications of diabetes.

Type 1 diabetes mellitus: Its clinical presentations are as follows:

- **Age:** Type 1 diabetes can arise at any age. Most often, it manifests during childhood or young adulthood.

- **Insulin requirement:** Following the onset of overt T1DM, **the requirement of exogenous insulin** may be **minimal** during the **initial 1 or 2 years**. This is because of endogenous insulin secretion. **Later**, insulin requirement suddenly **increases**. β-cell destruction in T1DM is a prolonged process. This usually clinically manifests when the insulin requirements increase (e.g., superimposed stress/acute illness, such as a febrile viral or bacterial infection).

Type 2 diabetes mellitus: Its clinical presentations are as follows:

- **Age:** Usually occurs in older **above the age of 40 years** and frequently in **obese individuals**. Due to the increase in obesity and sedentary lifestyle, it is now detected also in children and adolescents.
- **Presentation:** Some patients present with **unexplained fatigue, dizziness, or blurred vision. Polyuria, polydipsia, unexplained weakness, or weight loss. Ketoacidosis is infrequent** and presentation is usually mild.
- In **asymptomatic individuals**, the **diagnosis** of T2DM **is made after routine blood or urine testing**.
- Routine blood glucose testing is recommended for every individual >45 years of age and in young individuals with obesity, family history, or the presence of metabolic syndrome.

The Classical Classic Triad of Diabetes

Type 1 diabetes mellitus is usually manifested with the **classic triad, namely (1) polyuria, (2) polydipsia, and (3) polyphagia resulting from metabolic derangements. When severe**, the patient may develop **diabetic ketoacidosis (DKA)**.

Consequences of Insulin Deficiency

Insulin is an anabolic hormone and its **deficiency results in a catabolic state**. This **affects glucose metabolism, fat, and protein metabolism (Flowchart 24.4).**

Catabolism of carbohydrates

- **Hyperglycemia: Sharp reduction of transport of glucose** into **muscle cells** and **adipose tissue.**
- **Aggravation of hyperglycemia: Reduction of stored glycogen in the liver and muscle** due to the breakdown of reserves of glycogen into glucose (**glycogenolysis).** This **further aggravates hyperglycemia.**
- **Glycosuria and polyuria**: When **hyperglycemia exceeds the renal threshold** level, glycosuria develops. It leads to osmotic diuresis and **increased quantity of urine known as polyuria,** with **loss of water and electrolytes** (in urine).
- **Depletion of intracellular water and polydipsia**: Water loss through urine along with hyperosmolarity due to increased levels of glucose in the blood causes **depletion of intracellular water.** This **stimulates** the osmoreceptors of the **thirst centers** of the brain resulting in severe thirst known as **polydipsia.**

Catabolism of protein and fat

- **Proteolysis of proteins**: Insulin deficiency causes **catabolism of proteins.** This produces gluconeogenic

Flowchart 24.4: Sequence of metabolic derangements underlying the symptoms and signs of uncontrolled hyperglycemia in type 1 diabetes mellitus. Absolute deficiency of insulin leads to a catabolic state. This causes ketoacidosis and severe volume depletion.

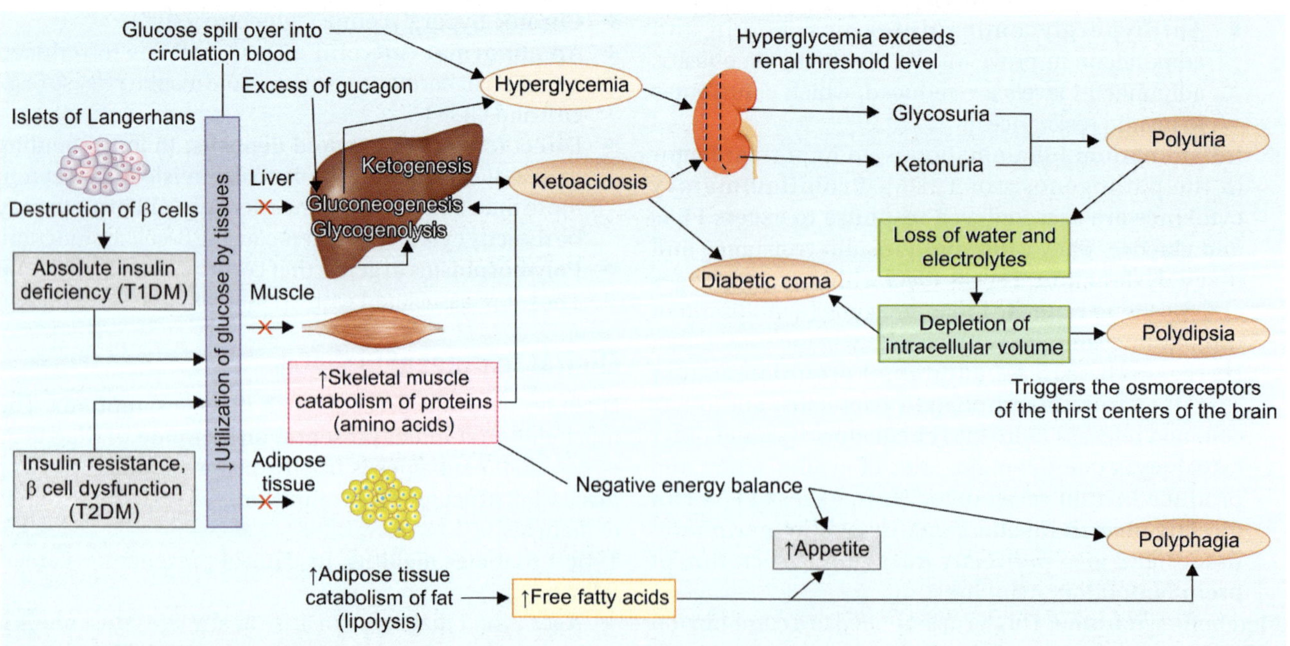

amino acids. They are taken up by the liver and used as building blocks for glucose.

- **Catabolism of proteins and fats:** It produces a **negative energy balance.** This leads to **increased appetite (polyphagia)**. Despite increased appetite, insulin's catabolic effects result in paradoxical **weight loss and muscle weakness.**

When a patient presents with a combination of polyphagia and paradoxical loss of weight, it is necessary to always consider the possibility of diabetes.

Acute Metabolic Complications of Diabetes

Diabetic ketoacidosis and hyperosmolar hyperglycemic nonketotic syndrome are **acute, severe disorders** directly related to diabetes. Both are associated with an **absolute or relative deficiency of insulin, volume depletion, and acid-base abnormalities.** Inflammatory markers (cytokines, C-reactive protein) are raised in both conditions.

Diabetic Ketoacidosis

- **Acute serious complication of diabetes:** Diabetic ketoacidosis is a **serious, acute metabolic complication** of diabetes.
- **More common and marked in type 1 diabetes (T1DM)** but may also occur in T2DM.
- **Precipitating (triggering) factors:** The most frequent precipitating factor is a **failure to take insulin**. Other triggering factors include significant deviations from normal dietary intake, stressors such as infection, and any other forms of stress. It may occur less often in T2DM with serious infections and trauma.

Mechanism (Flowchart 24.5)

- **Insulin deficiency with severe hyperglycemia:** Diabetic ketoacidosis is caused by severe hyperglycemia (plasma glucose ranging from 500 to 700 mg/dL) due to marked insulin deficiency.
- **Release of epinephrine and secretion of glucagon:** Severe hyperglycemia causes the release of the catecholamine epinephrine. This **worsens functional insulin deficiency** by blocking insulin action and stimulating the secretion of the counterregulatory hormone glucagon. **The glucagon decreases peripheral utilization of glucose and increases gluconeogenesis, thereby** causing **severe hyperglycemia.**
- **Hyperglycemia causes osmotic diuresis and dehydration:** Severe hyperglycemia causes osmotic diuresis and dehydration (characteristic features of ketoacidosis).
    - **Formation of free fatty acids:** Insulin deficiency also **stimulates lipoprotein lipase** which produces excessive **breakdown of fat stores** and **increases the free fatty acids levels.**
    - **Formation of ketone bodies: Free fatty acids** are oxidized by the liver to produce **ketone bodies (acetoacetic acid and β-hydroxybutyric acid).**

Flowchart 24.5: Pathogenesis of diabetic ketoacidosis.

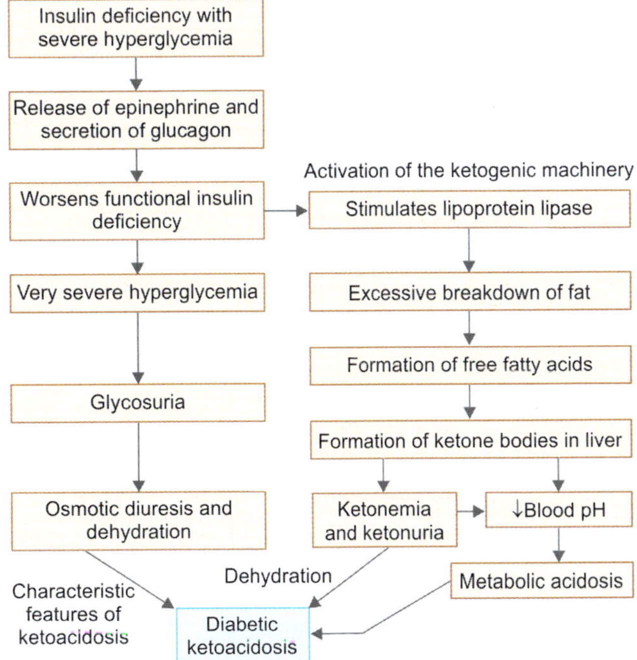

    - **Ketonemia and ketonuria:** When the **rate of production of ketone bodies exceeds the rate of utilization** by peripheral tissues, it results in **ketonemia** and **ketonuria**
    - **Metabolic acidosis:** The accumulation of ketones in blood decreases blood pH, resulting in metabolic acidosis. This is worsened if the urinary excretion of ketones is compromised by dehydration.

Clinical manifestations of diabetic ketoacidosis: These include **fatigue, nausea and vomiting, and severe abdominal pain.** It produces a **characteristic fruity odor and deep, labored breathing** (also known as ***Kussmaul breathing***). If the ketotic state persists, it leads to **depressed consciousness and coma.** Ketoacidosis is treated by insulin, correction of metabolic acidosis, and treatment of any underlying precipitating factors (e.g., infection).

Hyperosmolar Hyperglycemic Nonketotic Syndrome (Flowchart 24.6)

The hyperosmolar hyperglycemic nonketotic syndrome is a dangerous condition. It can affect both types of diabetics but **mainly develops in** the decompensated state in **patients with T2DM**. Typically, it develops in **older adult** diabetics. **Precipitating factors:** It develops in T2DM patients with **severe dehydration resulting from sustained osmotic diuresis due to chronic hyperglycemia.** This occurs particularly in T2DM patients **who do not drink enough water to compensate for urinary losses of water.** This typically occurs in T2DM patients affected by a stroke or an infection and is not able to maintain an adequate intake of water. Relative **deficiency of insulin** and **inadequate fluid intake** are the underlying causes.

Flowchart 24.6: Pathogenesis of hyperglycemic hyperosmolar nonketotic coma.

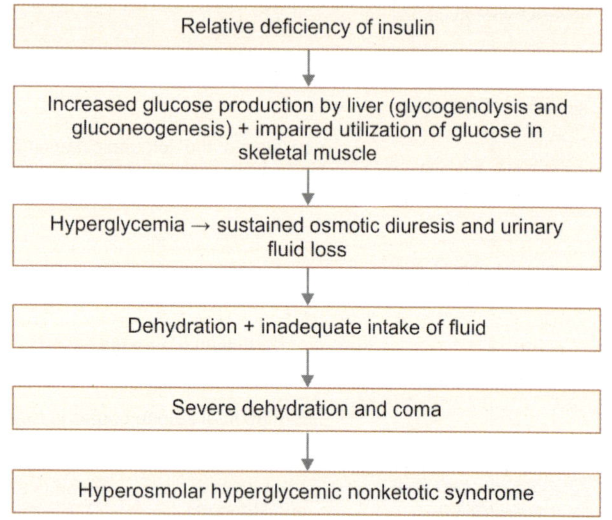

Mechanism (Flowchart 24.6)

Insulin deficiency increases glucose production by the liver (through glycogenolysis and gluconeogenesis) and impairs the utilization of glucose in skeletal muscle. The resulting **chronic hyperglycemia** causes sustained **osmotic diuresis and urinary fluid loss** that leads to intravascular volume depletion (*severe dehydration*). This volume depletion is further exacerbated due to inadequate intake of fluid. The cause for the absence of ketosis/ketoacidosis in hyperosmolar hyperglycemic nonketotic syndrome is not known. Probably, insulin deficiency is only relative and less severe in hyperosmolar hyperglycemic nonketotic syndrome than in diabetic ketoacidosis. Also, the liver is less capable of synthesizing ketone bodies, or the insulin/glucagon ratio does not favor ketogenesis. The absence of ketoacidosis and its symptoms (nausea, vomiting, respiratory difficulties) is responsible for the delay in recognizing HHS until the onset of severe dehydration and coma. Hyperglycemia is usually more severe than diabetic ketoacidosis. It is generally between 600 and 1,200 mg/dL.

Hypoglycemia

Hypoglycemia is one of the **most common acute metabolic complications** that can occur **in either type of diabetes once the treatment is started.** It is the most common acute complication in patients being treated with insulin.

Causes: These include **missing a meal, excessive physical exertion, excessive insulin dose**, or misdosing during the phase of correct insulin dose finding for antidiabetic agents such as sulfonylureas.

Clinical features: The signs and symptoms of hypoglycemia include dizziness, confusion, sweating, palpitations, and tachycardia. If hypoglycemia continues or is not treated, the patient loses consciousness. It is critical to rapidly reverse hypoglycemia by oral or intravenous glucose intake to prevent permanent neurologic damage due to hypoglycemia.

Chronic Complications of Diabetes Mellitus

Q. Write a short note on complications of diabetes mellitus.

Long-standing diabetes-related complications can affect many organ systems and are responsible for the majority of morbidity and mortality associated with the disease. Chronic complications usually develop about 15–20 years after the onset of hyperglycemia. The complications are similar for both T1DM and T2DM. The complications may be delayed or prevented by tight control of hyperglycemia. Hyperglycemic control can be assessed by following laboratory tests:

- **Control of blood sugar level** (glycemic control) **can reduce the long-term complications** of diabetes.
- **Glycemic control is assessed by** estimation of **glycosylated hemoglobins (HbA1c)**. HbA1c is formed by the addition of glucose to hemoglobin in red cells. Hb_{A1C} should be maintained below 7% in diabetic patients and its **measurement is helpful in knowing the glycemic control over the lifespan of a red cell** (120 days).

Classification: The complications can be divided into **vascular and nonvascular complications (Box 24.8). The morbidity in either type of diabetes is mainly due to vascular complications due to damage induced by chronic hyperglycemia to vessels.** The vascular complications are further subdivided into microvascular and macrovascular complications.

- **Microvascular complications:** They involve **small vessels (diabetic microvascular disease)** and are diabetes-specific (in both T2DM and T1DM). The effects of the microvascular disease are most severe in the retina (*diabetic retinopathy*), kidneys (*diabetic nephropathy*), and peripheral nerves (*neuropathy*).

BOX 24.8: Classification of diabetes-related complications.

Vascular complications

- **Microvascular (small vessels)**
  - Retinopathy (nonproliferative/proliferative)
  - Neuropathy
  - Nephropathy (albuminuria and declining renal function)
- **Macrovascular causes accelerated atherosclerosis in large- and medium-sized muscular arteries:**
  - Coronary heart disease
  - Peripheral arterial disease
  - Cerebrovascular disease

Nonvascular complications

- Genitourinary (uropathy/sexual dysfunction)
- Infectious
- Cataracts
- Glaucoma

- **Macrovascular complications:** They involve **large- and medium-sized muscular arteries (diabetic macrovascular disease)**, are not specific to diabetes, and can occur in the general population also. Macrovascular disease causes accelerated atherosclerosis in diabetic patients. This may result in an increased risk of myocardial infarction, cerebrovascular stroke, and lower extremity ischemia (with gangrene). Macrovascular complications are especially common in patients with T2DM. This is because the patients tend to be older and frequently have additional cardiovascular risk factors (e.g., dyslipoproteinemia, hypertension, and hypercoagulability).

Other Complications of Diabetes

Diabetic dyslipidemia: It is a condition in which there are **increased blood levels of triglycerides and LDL and decreased levels of high-density lipoprotein** (protective). This develops due to insulin resistance, which causes increased production of atherogenic lipoproteins by the liver and decreased uptake of circulating lipids in peripheral tissues.

Increased susceptibility to infections: Infections of the skin, tuberculosis, pneumonia, and pyelonephritis are common in diabetes. The increased susceptibility may be due to **defective neutrophil functions** (chemotaxis, adherence to the endothelium, phagocytosis, and microbicidal activity), and **impaired cytokine production by macrophages**.

Pathogenesis of the Complications of Diabetes

Q. Write a short note on the pathogenesis of complications in diabetes mellitus.

Persistent hyperglycemia (glucotoxicity) is most likely responsible for the long-term complications of diabetes. Persistent hyperglycemia produces harmful effects on multiple tissues, mainly by three distinct mechanisms (**Box 24.9**).

Formation of Advanced Glycation End Products (AGEs) (*Refer* Online Flowchart 24.7)

In diabetics, glucose-derived precursors (e.g., glyoxal, methylglyoxal, and 3-deoxyglucosone) bind **to proteins** (intracellular and extracellular proteins) **nonenzymatically** and **are termed nonenzymatic glycosylation.**

- **Initial products:** The initial products of nonenzymatic glycosylation are chemically known as Schiff bases **are labile and can dissociate rapidly.**
- **Later products:** Over time, the initial labile products form **stable advanced glycation end products** (AGEs). **The rate of AGE formation is markedly increased in the presence of hyperglycemia**.

BOX 24.9: Pathways of mechanisms of complications in diabetes mellitus due to chronic hyperglycemia.

- Formation of advanced glycation end products
- Activation of protein kinase C
- Disturbances in metabolic pathways

Harmful effects of AGEs

It may be brought out by the binding of AGEs to its specific receptor (RAGE-receptor for AGE) or by its direct action.

Through RAGE: AGEs bind to RAGE on inflammatory cells (macrophages and T-cells), endothelial cells, and vascular smooth muscle cells. In the vascular compartment, AGE-RAGE has the following actions:

- **Releases proinflammatory cytokines** and **growth factors** from intimal macrophages. For example, transforming growth factor-β (TGF-β) leads to the deposition of excess basement membrane material, and vascular endothelial growth factor (VEGF), is involved in diabetic retinopathy.
- **Production of reactive oxygen species (ROS) in endothelial cells.**
- **Increases procoagulant activity of endothelial cells and macrophages.**
- **Increased proliferation of vascular smooth muscle cells** and **synthesis of extracellular matrix.**

Direct effect of AGE: AGEs can **directly cross-link extracellular matrix proteins.** Trapping of other plasma or interstitial proteins occurs within these cross-linked proteins. Examples are as follows:

- **Trapping of low-density lipoprotein (LDL) within AGE-modified large-vessel walls**: This accelerates atherosclerosis.
- **Trapping of albumin within capillary walls:** This is partly responsible for the basement membrane thickening that is characteristic of diabetic microangiopathy.

Activation of Protein Kinase C (PKC)

Intracellular hyperglycemia stimulates the synthesis of diacylglycerol: In patients with hyperglycemia, intracellular hyperglycemia stimulates the synthesis of diacylglycerol (DAG) from **glycolytic intermediates**.

DAG activates intracellular protein kinase C: Consequences of PKC activation are the production of the following molecules:

- **Proangiogenic molecules:** For example, **vascular endothelial growth factor (VEGF)** causes **neovascularization** characteristic of **diabetic retinopathy**.
- **Profibrogenic factors:** For example, **TGF-β** results in **increased production of extracellular matrix and basement membrane material**.

- **Plasminogen activator inhibitor (PAI-1)**: It **reduces fibrinolysis** and **favors vascular occlusion** (by forming atherosclerotic plaques or thrombus).

Disturbances in Metabolic Pathways

Formation of intracellular fructose from glucose: Some tissues (e.g., nerves, lenses, kidneys, blood vessels) **do not require insulin for glucose transport.**

- **Persistent hyperglycemia increases** the **intracellular glucose in these tissues.** The **excess intracellular glucose is metabolized by the enzyme aldose reductase to sorbitol (polyol) and finally** to **fructose.**
- **Reduction of NADPH**: The above **reaction uses NADPH** (the reduced form of nicotinamide dinucleotide phosphate) as a cofactor. NADPH is also necessary for the regeneration of reduced glutathione (GSH).
- **Oxidative stress**: Reduced NADPH decreases GSH. GSH is one of the important antioxidant mechanisms in the cell that protects against injury by free radicals. Reductions in GSH increase cellular susceptibility to *oxidative stress.*

MORPHOLOGY

Pancreas

Lesions of the pancreas are **not diagnostic** and are **more common with type 1** than with type 2 diabetes. The morphological changes include:

- **Reduced in the number and size of islets:** It is seen in type 1 diabetes which is mild in type 2 diabetes.
- **Leukocytic infiltrates in the islets (insulitis):** Mainly by T lymphocytes **predominantly in type 1 diabetes.**
- **Amyloid deposition within islets in T2D:** It is observed in and around capillaries and between cells. In advanced stages, the islets may be virtually obliterated and may show fibrosis.
- **Increase in the number and size of islets: It may be seen in nondiabetic newborns of diabetic mothers** as a hyperplastic response to maternal hyperglycemia.

Diabetic Macrovascular Disease

The lesions of large- and medium-sized muscular arteries are the **most common causes of mortality** in long-standing diabetes. These include:

- **Accelerated atherosclerosis:** This is the hallmark of diabetic macrovascular disease. Diabetes is one of the major modifiable risk factors for atherosclerosis and other cardiovascular morbidities. It affects the aorta and large- and medium-sized arteries. Atherosclerosis **is more severe and occurs at an earlier age.** Diabetics have **increased levels of** plasminogen activator inhibitor **(PAI-1),** which **inhibits fibrinolysis and favors the development of atherosclerotic plaques. Renal arteries** also develop **severe atherosclerosis.**
- **Myocardial infarction:** It is due to **atherosclerosis of the coronary arteries** and is the **most common cause of death in diabetics.** Diabetics have a greater risk of coronary artery disease and cardiovascular complications than nondiabetics. The risk for cardiovascular disease is more even in prediabetics.
- **Gangrene of the lower extremities:** It **results from advanced vascular disease** and is more common in diabetics.
- **Renal vascular insufficiency** due to severe atherosclerosis
- **Cerebrovascular accidents** (stroke).

Hyaline arteriosclerosis: It can be found in hypertension, elderly nondiabetics without hypertension, and a more severe degree in diabetics also.

- In diabetics, it is **related to the duration of diabetes and the level of blood pressure.**
- **Hyaline arteriolosclerosis** is characterized by **amorphous, hyaline thickening of the wall of the arterioles,** which may **narrow the lumen** of the vessel (*refer* **Figs. 16.11A and B**).

Diabetic Microvascular Disease (Microangiopathy)

Diffuse thickening of basement membrane: It is one of the most consistent morphologic findings of diabetes.

- **Thickening of basement membranes of capillaries:** The thickening is **mostly seen in the capillaries of the skin, skeletal muscle, retina, renal glomeruli, and renal medulla.** Though **capillaries show basement membrane thickening, they are leakier to plasma proteins than normal.** The microangiopathy results in diabetic nephropathy, retinopathy, and some forms of neuropathy.
- **Thickening of basement membranes in nonvascular structures:** It may be seen in nonvascular structures such as renal tubules, the Bowman capsule, peripheral nerves, and the placenta.

Organs involved in microangiopathy: Microangiopathy mainly occurs in kidneys (nephropathy), retina (diabetic retinopathy), and peripheral nerves (neuropathy).

Diabetic Nephropathy

About **30–40% of all diabetics** develop nephropathy refer to pages 735-6, which is the **leading cause of end-stage renal disease.** The different stages of diabetic nephropathy are:

- **Microalbuminuria:** It is the **earliest manifestation** of diabetic nephropathy in which the urine has low amounts of albumin (>30 mg/day, but <300 mg/day). Microalbuminuria is also a marker for increased cardiovascular morbidity and mortality in either type 1 or type 2 diabetics.
- **Nephropathy with macroalbuminuria:** Without specific interventions, diabetics will develop **overt nephropathy with macroalbuminuria** (>300 mg of urinary albumin per day), usually associated with hypertension.
- **End-stage renal disease:** The overt nephropathy may progress to end-stage renal disease.

Diabetic Retinopathy (Fig. 24.18)

The ocular involvement in diabetes may be in the form of (i) retinopathy, (ii) cataract formation, or (iii) glaucoma. Retinopathy is the most common and it develops in **~60–80% of diabetics, about 15–20 years after diagnosis.** Retinopathy may be seen in two forms: nonproliferative retinopathy and proliferative retinopathy. The basic lesion of retinopathy is **neovascularization caused by hypoxia-induced overexpression of VEGF in the retina.**

- **Nonproliferative retinopathy:** The lesions include intraretinal or preretinal hemorrhages, retinal exudates, microaneurysms (appear as small red dots under the ophthalmoscope), venous dilations, edema, and the thickening of the retinal capillaries (microangiopathy). The retinal exudates can be "soft" (microinfarcts) or "hard" (deposits of plasma proteins and lipids).

- **Proliferative retinopathy:** It is a process of neovascularization and fibrosis. If it involves the macula, it **can produce blindness**. Vitreous hemorrhages due to the rupture of newly formed capillaries and their subsequent organization can lead to retinal detachment.

Diabetic Neuropathy

It may involve the **central and peripheral nervous systems.**

- **Distal symmetric polyneuropathy:** It affects **both motor and sensory function** of the lower extremities later, it may involve the upper extremities leading to a **"glove and stocking" pattern of polyneuropathy.**
- **Autonomic neuropathy: Produces disturbances in bowel and bladder function** and sometimes sexual impotence.
- **Diabetic mononeuropathy:** It may manifest as sudden foot drop, wrist drop, or isolated cranial nerve palsies.

Various complications of diabetes are depicted in **Figure 24.18.**

Differences between type 1 and type 2 diabetes mellitus are listed in **Table 24.6.**

LABORATORY DIAGNOSIS OF DIABETES

Q. Write a short essay on laboratory diagnosis of diabetes mellitus.

Hyperglycemia: It is the fundamental basis for the diagnosis of diabetes mellitus.

- **In symptomatic cases**: Diabetes can be confirmed by finding glucosuria and a random plasma glucose level above 200 mg/dL. The severity of clinical symptoms of polyuria, polyphagia, and polydipsia depends on the degree of hyperglycemia.
- **In asymptomatic cases**: Most of these patients have persistently elevated fasting plasma glucose levels. However, in asymptomatic patients (suspected to be suffering from diabetes mellitus) with normal fasting glucose levels in the plasma need an oral glucose tolerance test (GTT).

Investigations for the Diagnosis of Diabetes Mellitus

Urine Examination

Urine examination is an economical and convenient test for the diagnosis of diabetes mellitus. However, urine alone may show false-positive and false-negative results. It can be used as a screening test. Urine is examined for the presence of glucose and ketones.

Glucosuria

- **Benedict's qualitative test** (*refer* pages 455-6): It detects any reducing substance in the urine and is not specific for glucose.
- **Dipstick method** (*refer* page 456): This method is more sensitive and specific for glucose.

Disadvantages: Apart from diabetes mellitus, *glucosuria* may be found in other conditions (*refer* **Box 15.12**).

Ketonuria

Tests for ketone bodies in the urine are needed for assessing the severity of diabetes and not for diagnosis of diabetes. However, if both glucose and ketone bodies are present, the diagnosis of diabetes is almost certain. Rothera's test (nitroprusside reaction) and dipstick methods can be used for the detection of ketonuria (*refer* page 457).

Single Plasma Glucose Estimation

Estimation of plasma glucose is absolutely necessary for the diagnosis of diabetes mellitus. A fasting plasma glucose level above 126 mg/dL is indicative of diabetes. In other cases, oral GTT is performed.

Population Screening by Fasting Plasma Glucose Test for Type 2 DM

Estimation of fasting plasma glucose is a screening test used for type 2DM. It is advisable that all individuals above 45 years of age must undergo screening fasting glucose test every 3 years, and relatively earlier if the person is overweight.

Oral Glucose Tolerance Test (OGTT)

Indication: It is not recommended for routine diagnosis of either type 1 or type 2 DM. This is because fasting plasma glucose identifies abnormal glucose metabolism.

- In patients where the fasting plasma glucose is in the range of impaired fasting glucose (100–125 mg/dL)
- Diagnosis of gestational diabetes mellitus
- Uncertainty about the diagnosis of diabetes

Preparation of the patient: The patient should be taking an unrestricted carbohydrate diet for at least 3 days or more before the test. Because a carbohydrate-restricted diet reduces glucose tolerance, the patient should be with normal physical activity.

- OGTT is performed in the morning after the patient has fasted overnight (at least 8 hours).
- The patient should rest for at least half an hour before starting the test, and refrain from smoking, tea/coffee, or exercise during the test.

Test: A fasting venous sample of blood is drawn to estimate the glucose level.

- Patients are given 75 g of anhydrous glucose dissolved in 250–300 mL of water orally over 5 minutes. The dose in children is 1.75 g of glucose/kg body weight up to a maximum of 75 g. The time of starting glucose is taken as 0 hours.
- A single venous sample of blood is drawn 2 hours after the glucose administration and glucose level is estimated (previously, blood samples were collected at 1/2-hour, 1 hour, 11/2 hour, and 2 hours).

Postprandial Plasma Glucose

Determination of plasma glucose level 2 hours after food has no standardized role in the diagnosis of diabetes mellitus. However, it is useful in patients on treatment.

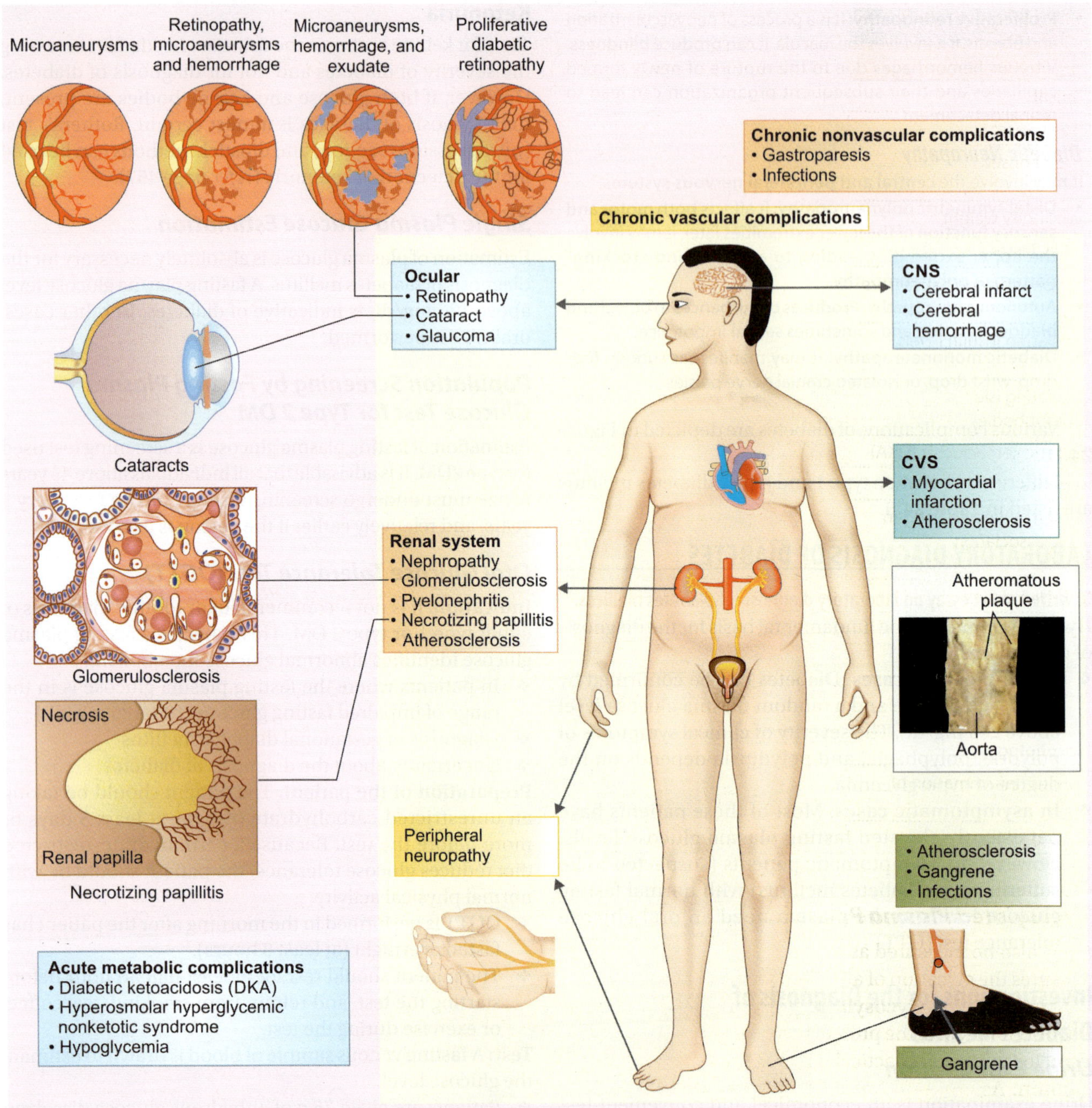

Fig. 24.18: Complications of diabetes.
(CNS: central nervous system; CVS: cardiovascular system)

Glycosylated Hemoglobin (HbA1c)

Nonenzymatic glycosylation is the chemical process whereby glucose attaches to proteins without the help of enzymes. The degree of glycosylation is proportionate to the level of blood glucose. Many proteins, including hemoglobin, undergo nonenzymatic glycosylation. Blood glucose level in diabetics varies with the dietary intake of the previous day of estimating blood glucose. Long-term assessment (for the last 90–120 days) of the degree of glycemic control is assessed by measurement of glycosylated hemoglobin (HbA1c). It is a minor hemoglobin component present in normal individuals. This test does not need any dietary preparation or fasting. The advantages of HbA1c assay are (i) it has a direct relation between poor control and development of complications and (ii) it is also a good measure of prediction of microvascular complications. The reference range is 3.8–6.3% and the target for therapy is <7%.

TABLE 24.6 Differences between type 1 and type 2 diabetes mellitus.

	Type 1 diabetes mellitus	*Type 2 diabetes mellitus*
Clinical		
Age of onset	Childhood and adolescence	Adult, also seen in childhood and adolescence
Type of onset	Abrupt; symptomatic (polyuria, polydipsia, dehydration); often severe with ketoacidosis	Gradual; usually subtle; often asymptomatic
Usual body weight	Normal or present with weight loss	Majority are obese
Family history	<20%	>60%
Precipitating and risk factors	Mostly not known; microbial, chemical, dietary, or other	Age, obesity (central), sedentary lifestyle, previous gestational diabetes mellitus
Circulating insulin levels	Progressive decrease	Increased (early); normal or moderate decrease (late)
Circulating islet autoantibodies	Detected (anti-insulin, anti-GAD, anti-ICA512)	Not found
Diabetic ketoacidosis (DKA)	Develops in the absence of insulin therapy	Nonketotic hyperosmolar coma
Genetics		
Human leukocyte antigen (HLA) association	Major linkage to MHC (major histocompatibility complex) class I and II genes *HLA-DR3* and/-*HLA- DR4*	No HLA association
Non-HLA genes	Polymorphisms in *CTLA4* and *PTPN22*	Diabetogenic and obesity-related genes
Etiopathogenesis		
Mode of development	Autoimmune	Multifactorial
Mechanism	Breakdown in self-tolerance to islet autoantigens	Insulin resistance in peripheral tissues, β-cell dysfunction
Morphology		
Insulitis (inflammation of islets)	Inflammatory infiltrate of T-cells and macrophages in islets	No insulitis; amyloid deposition in islets
β-cell depletion	Moderate to severe	Mild

Glycosylated Plasma Proteins (Fructosamine)

It may also be measured as an index of diabetic control. It measures the glycation of all serum proteins and the major component being **glycosylated albumin**. Since albumin accounts for most of the protein in blood, the measurement of fructosamine, for practical purposes, measures glycated albumin. As albumin has a turnover of about 2 weeks, fructosamine reflects **glycemia over the preceding 2–3 weeks** (shorter period). It is **useful in diabetic patients with anemia or hemoglobinopathy and pregnancy** (when hemoglobin turnover is changeable).

Other Investigations

These are sometimes performed in specific conditions in diabetics and for research purposes. These include:

- **Other GTTs**
  - **Extended GTT:** In this, the oral GTT is extended to 3–4 hours for the appearance of symptoms of hyperglycemia. It is useful in cases of reactive hypoglycemia of early diabetes.
  - **Intravenous GTT:** It is a test performed in individuals suffering from intestinal malabsorption or those who have undergone gastrectomy.
  - **Cortisone-primed GTT:** It is a provocative test and is useful in potential diabetics.
- **Insulin assay:** Deficiency of plasma insulin levels is crucial for type 1 DM but is not essential for making the diagnosis of DM. It can be estimated by radio-immunoassay and ELISA technique.
- **Proinsulin assay:** Insulin is synthesized first as a precursor molecule, namely proinsulin. Normally, it is <20% of total insulin and can be estimated by immunoassay.
- **C-peptide assay:** The A and B chains in insulin are held together by a peptide called C peptide. This C-peptide is released into the circulation during the conversion of proinsulin to insulin in equimolar quantities to insulin. Its levels correlate with insulin levels in the blood except in islet cell tumors and obesity. This test is more sensitive than insulin assay because its levels are not affected by treatment with insulin.

- **Islet autoantibodies:** Markers of cell-mediated autoimmune destruction of islet β-cells can be used as a marker for type 1 diabetes mellitus. **These include (i) islet cell antibodies (ICAs), (ii) autoantibodies to insulin (IAAs), (iii) autoantibodies to glutamic acid decarboxylase** (GAD65) and (iv) autoantibodies to tyrosine phosphatases IA-2α and IA-2β.
- **Screening for diabetes-associated complications:** Apart from making the diagnosis of DM based on the defined criteria, screening tests can be performed for DM-associated complications (e.g., microalbuminuria, dyslipidemia, thyroid dysfunction, etc.).

PARATHYROID GLANDS

The normal anatomy of the parathyroid glands is presented **online, along with Figure 24.19**.

HYPERPARATHYROIDISM

PA 32.5 (NC): Describe the etiology, genetics, pathogenesis, manifestations, laboratory, and morphologic features of hyperparathyroidism.

Hyperparathyroidism is a **condition caused by elevated PTH.**
Classification: Hyperparathyroidism is classified into **primary, secondary, and tertiary** (least common), types.

Primary Hyperparathyroidism

Definition: Primary hyperparathyroidism is a common endocrine disorder. It is **characterized by** excessive **autonomous production and secretion of PTH** from the parathyroid glands. **It is an important cause of hypercalcemia.**

Age and gender: Primary hyperparathyroidism is usually seen in adults. It is more common in women than in men (ratio of 4:1).
Etiology: Usually, the primary hyperparathyroidism is due to a **parathyroid adenoma** (~85–95%) or **diffuse or nodular primary hyperplasia** of parathyroid tissue (~5–10%) or **parathyroid carcinoma** (~1%).

Pathogenesis

Commonly, abnormalities in two genes are associated with parathyroid tumors:

1. ***Cyclin D1* gene rearrangements:** Cyclin D1 is a positive regulator of the cell cycle and *cyclin D1* gene is normally on 11q.
   - **Acquired inversion on chromosome 11:** This **positions the *cyclin D1* gene from** its normal position on **11q to 11p** adjacent to **genomic elements that regulate the *PTH* gene.** This drives **abnormal expression of cyclin D1 in PTH-producing cells** and leads to increased proliferation of these cells. About 10–20% of parathyroid adenomas show this acquired genetic defect of inversion.
   - **Overexpression of cyclin D1:** This is seen in about 40% of parathyroid adenomas.
2. **MEN1 mutations:** About 30–35% of sporadic parathyroid tumors show **mutations in both copies of the *MEN1* tumor suppressor gene.** Germline mutations of *MEN1* are also found in patients with familial parathyroid adenomas.

MORPHOLOGY

In primary hyperparathyroidism, the morphologic changes are found in the parathyroid glands and also in other organs affected by hypercalcemia. In about 75–80% of cases, one of the parathyroid glands shows a solitary adenoma.

Parathyroid Adenoma

- **Gross:** They appear as a **well-circumscribed, soft, tan nodule or red-brown and solitary mass** surrounded by a **thin capsule.** It measures about 1–3 cm and weighs between 0.5 and 2 g. They are **seen in only one gland** and the other glands are either normal in size or somewhat shrunken (due to feedback inhibition by raised serum calcium).
- **Microscopy:** They are composed predominantly of sheets of neoplastic chief cells in a rich capillary network. A rim of compressed, non-neoplastic, normal parathyroid tissue is usually found outside the capsule and helps to distinguish adenomas from parathyroid hyperplasias.

Primary Parathyroid Hyperplasia

It may occur sporadically or familial as a component of MEN syndrome.

- **Gross:** Typically, a **multiglandular process** involving all four parathyroid glands, but sometimes it may be asymmetrical with sparing of one or two glands. In such cases, enlargement may be grossly apparent in only one or two glands, making it difficult to distinguish between hyperplasia and adenoma.
- **Microscopy:** Most commonly there is **chief cell hyperplasia,** which may involve the glands in a diffuse or multinodular pattern.

Parathyroid Carcinomas

- **Gross:** They **may be circumscribed** lesions similar to adenomas **or may be clearly invasive** neoplasms. They enlarge one parathyroid gland. They appear as **gray-white, firm, irregular** masses and are usually larger than adenomas (sometimes exceeding 10 g in weight).
- **Microscopy:** The tumor **cells are usually uniform** and resemble normal parathyroid cells. These cells are arranged in nodular or trabecular patterns. The tumor is usually enclosed by a dense, fibrous capsule and occasionally invades capsules or blood vessels. The diagnosis of carcinoma based on cytologic features is not reliable. The only definitive criteria for malignancy are **invasion into the surrounding tissues** and metastasis. Local recurrence and distant dissemination can occur.

Morphologic Changes in Other Organs

- **Skeletal changes:** Bone shows increased osteoclastic activity. It is characterized by erosion of bone matrix and mobilization of calcium salts, especially in the metaphyses of long tubular bones. Bone resorption is associated with increased osteoblastic activity and the formation of new bone trabeculae.

- **Osteitis fibrosa cystica:** In more severe cases, there may be gross thinning of the cortex and the bone marrow shows increased fibrous tissue with foci of hemorrhage and cysts. This is termed as generalized osteitis fibrosa cystica (von Recklinghausen disease of bone).
- **Brown tumors of hyperparathyroidism:** Aggregates of osteoclasts, reactive giant cells, and hemorrhagic debris may form masses that may be mistaken for neoplasms. These are termed brown tumors of hyperparathyroidism.

- **Renal changes:** Hypercalcemia induced by PTH results in the formation of stones in the urinary tract (**nephrolithiasis**) and calcification of the renal interstitium and tubules (**nephrocalcinosis**).
- **Metastatic calcification:** It develops due to hypercalcemia and can be found in other sites such as the stomach, lungs, myocardium, and blood vessels.

Clinical Features

Age and gender: Primary hyperparathyroidism is usually manifest in adults. It is more frequent in women than in men (4:1).

Primary hyperparathyroidism may be (1) asymptomatic and detected during routine blood chemistry profile, or (2) symptomatic with the classic clinical manifestations of primary hyperparathyroidism.

- **Asymptomatic primary hyperparathyroidism with hypercalcemia:** The most common manifestation is hypercalcemia (increase in serum ionized calcium). Routinely serum calcium levels are assessed in most patients who need blood tests for unrelated conditions. Hence, most patients with primary hyperparathyroidism are diagnosed incidentally when clinically silent hypercalcemia is found. The most common cause of asymptomatic hypercalcemia is primary hyperparathyroidism.
  - **Hypercalcemia in cancer patients**: Apart from primary hyperparathyroidism, clinically apparent hypercalcemia in adults is due to cancer. In cancer patients, hypercalcemia **may be part of a paraneoplastic syndrome** caused by the secretion of PTH-like polypeptides (PTHrP) from tumor cells or may be due to **osteolytic metastatic malignancy to bone.**
- **Symptomatic primary hyperparathyroidism:** The signs and symptoms of hyperparathyroidism are due to the combined effects of increased PTH secretion and hypercalcemia. These include painful bones, renal stones, abdominal groans (deep inarticulate sounds in response to pain), and psychic moans (long, low sounds made by a person expressing physical or mental suffering).
- **Bone disease and bone pain:** It is secondary to fractures of bones (pathologic fractures) that are weakened by osteoporosis or osteitis fibrosa cystica.
- **Nephrolithiasis (renal stones):** It causes renal colic and obstructive uropathy. Chronic renal insufficiency and abnormal renal function produce polyuria and secondary polydipsia.
- **Gastrointestinal:** Constipation, nausea, peptic ulcers (hypercalcemia increases serum gastrin, thus stimulating gastric acid secretion), pancreatitis, and gallstones.
- **Central nervous system:** Depression, lethargy, memory defects and seizures.
- **Neuromuscular abnormalities:** Weakness, hypotonia, and fatigue.
- **Cardiac manifestations:** Aortic or mitral valve calcifications (or both).

Laboratory Findings

- Increased serum PTH
- Increased serum calcium
- Decreased serum 1, 25-(OH) 2D (hypovitaminosis D): Hypercalcemia decreases the synthesis of 1-α-hydroxylase in the proximal renal tubule, which decreases the synthesis of 1, 25-(OH) 2D.

Secondary Hyperparathyroidism

Secondary hyperparathyroidism is due to compensatory parathyroid hypersecretion of the PTH. The hypersecretion of PTH.

Etiology and Pathogenesis

Secondary hyperparathyroidism is commonly caused by **chronic hypocalcemia**, most often because of **chronic renal failure.** This leads to **compensatory hyperplasia of the parathyroid**. It can also develop in association with **vitamin D deficiency, intestinal malabsorption, Fanconi syndrome, and renal tubular acidosis.**

Mechanisms of secondary hyperparathyroidism in chronic renal failure (Flowchart 24.8): Chronic renal insufficiency is associated with decreased excretion of phosphate. This raises the levels of serum phosphate (hyperphosphatemia).

Flowchart 24.8: Mechanism of hypocalcemia and secondary hyperparathyroidism in chronic renal failure.

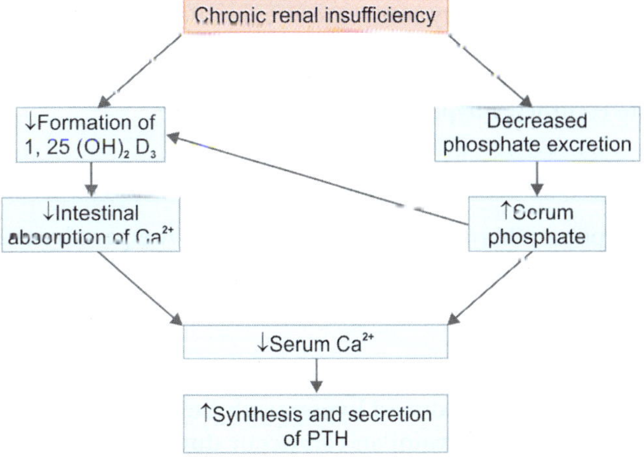

Hyperphosphatemia directly depresses the levels of serum calcium. Renal α1-hydroxylase activity is required for the synthesis of the active form of vitamin D (1, 25(OH) 2D). In a diseased kidney, there is also a loss of renal α1-hydroxylase activity, which reduces the synthesis of the active form of vitamin D (1, 25(OH) 2D). This reduces the intestinal absorption of calcium. All these alterations cause chronic hypocalcemia. This in turn stimulates the parathyroid glands to undergo secondary hyperplasia. Hyperplasia causes increased secretion of PTH.

MORPHOLOGY

Parathyroid glands in secondary hyperparathyroidism: They show **hyperplastic changes.** The degree of enlargement of the parathyroid need not be symmetric. Microscopically, the hyperplastic glands show an increased number of chief cells, or cells with more abundant, clear cytoplasm (water-clear cells). It shows fewer fat cells.

Skeletal/bone changes and metastatic calcification: Similar to primary hyperparathyroidism (*refer* pages 896-7).

Clinical Features

Related to chronic renal failure: The clinical features of secondary hyperparathyroidism are usually due to chronic renal failure.

Bone abnormalities (renal osteodystrophy): Excess levels of PTH produce skeletal pain and deformities, osteomalacia, and osteitis fibrosis cystica. The osseous manifestations are similar to primary hyperparathyroidism (*refer* pages 896-7). They are usually less severe than those seen in primary hyperparathyroidism. Rarely, metastatic calcification of blood vessels (secondary to hyperphosphatemia) may produce significant ischemic damage to the skin and other organs (a process termed calciphylaxis).

Laboratory findings: Serum calcium remains near normal. This is due to the compensatory increase in PTH levels which sustains serum calcium.

Tertiary hyperparathyroidism: Long-standing secondary parathyroid hyperplasia in renal failure may be followed by autonomous parathyroid hyperplasia with resultant hypercalcemia. In such cases, parathyroid hyperplasia persists and may not regress even after the cause of prolonged hypocalcemia is corrected, for example, after renal transplant. Such patients require parathyroidectomy to control the hyperparathyroidism.

HYPOPARATHYROIDISM

Hypoparathyroidism is hypofunction of the parathyroid glands leading to hypocalcemia.

Etiology

The major causes of hypoparathyroidism are as follows:

- **Surgically induced hypoparathyroidism:** Acquired hypoparathyroidism can occur due to inadvertent removal of parathyroid glands during thyroidectomy or during radical neck dissection (parathyroid glands are mistaken for lymph nodes).
- **Congenital absence of parathyroid glands:** This may be seen in association with thymic aplasia (Di George syndrome) and cardiac defects. It occurs secondary to deletions on chromosome 22q11.2.
- **Autoimmune hypoparathyroidism:** It may be associated with a syndrome known as autoimmune polyendocrine syndrome type 1 (APS1) and is caused by mutations in the autoimmune regulator (AIRE) gene.
- **Autosomal-dominant hypoparathyroidism:** It is due to gain-of-function mutations in the calcium-sensing receptor (CaSR) gene.
- **Familial isolated hypoparathyroidism (FIH):** It is a rare disorder that may be inherited as either autosomal dominant or autosomal recessive.

Clinical Features

The major clinical features are produced due to hypocalcemia and depend on its severity and chronicity.

Tetany (hypocalcemia): It is the hallmark of hypocalcemia. It is characterized by **neuromuscular irritability, resulting from decreased serum calcium levels**. The symptoms range from circumoral numbness or paresthesias (tingling) of the distal extremities and sustained carpopedal spasm to life-threatening laryngospasm and generalized seizures.

Features of chronic hypoparathyroidism: These are as follows:

- **Calcification of the basal ganglia**: Caused by metastatic calcification. Increased serum phosphates in primary hypoparathyroidism cause calcification of the cerebral basal ganglia.
- **Cataracts** (opacification of the lens) and **dental abnormalities**

Laboratory findings in hypoparathyroidism: These include hypocalcemia, hyperphosphatemia, and a decrease in serum PTH.

ADRENAL GLANDS

The adrenal (or suprarenal) glands are paired endocrine organs. They consist of two independent regions namely the outer cortex and inner medulla. They differ in structure, function, and development

ADRENAL CORTEX

The adrenal cortex consists of three layers (zones) of distinct cell types namely the (i) **zona glomerulosa** (outermost layer), **(ii) zona fasciculata** (middle), and (iii) **zona reticularis (innermost layer)**. The hormones produced by the adrenal cortex are called steroids and it contains **three different types of steroids.**

1. **Glucocorticoids (named for their primary effect on glucose metabolism):** Glucocorticoids mainly consist of cortisol and it opposes the effects of insulin. It is produced primarily in the zona fasciculata, with a small amount from the zona reticularis.
2. **Mineralocorticoids:** Principally, it is aldosterone and is synthesized in the zona glomerulosa. They **maintain normal salt and water balance** by promoting sodium retention and potassium excretion at the distal renal tubules.
3. **Sex steroids (estrogens and androgens):** They are synthesized mainly in the zona reticularis.

Note: The stimulus for the synthesis and secretion of both cortisol and androgen is ACTH; whereas that for aldosterone is angiotensin II (AII). The activities of these three steroids (hormones) regulate the "three S's": sugar, salt, and sex.

Diseases of the adrenal cortex: They can be divided into two major groups namely those associated with (i) **hyperfunction or (ii) hypofunction**.

Adrenocortical Hyperfunction (Hyperadrenalism)

Syndromes of adrenal hyperfunction are caused by the overproduction of one or more of the three major hormones produced by the three layers of the adrenal cortex.

1. **Cushing syndrome:** Due to an excess of cortisol
2. **Hyperaldosteronism:** Due to excess of mineralocorticoid (aldosterone).
3. **Adrenogenital or virilizing syndromes:** Due to an excess of androgens.

In some of these syndromes, the clinical features may show some similarities because of the shared functions of adrenal steroids.

Hypercortisolism (Cushing Syndrome)

PA 32.8 (NC): Describe the etiology, pathogenesis, manifestations, laboratory, morphologic features, and complications of Cushing's syndrome.

Definition: The term Cushing syndrome is used to describe the **clinical features/abnormalities due to hypercortisolism** (excessive production of glucocorticoid/cortisol) **from any cause.**

The term Cushing disease is reserved for pituitary-dependent excessive ACTH secretion by pituitary corticotroph tumors.

Etiopathogenesis

Cushing syndrome is produced by conditions that produce raised glucocorticoid levels.

Causes (Fig. 24.20)

Exogenous causes: The majority of cases are the result of the administration of exogenous glucocorticoids ("iatrogenic" Cushing syndrome). Exogenous steroids may be used for the management of diseases such as allergic and autoimmune diseases.

Endogenous causes: The most common endogenous causes are:

- **ACTH dependent** (~80%)
  - **Primary hypersecretion of ACTH by pituitary diseases (Cushing disease):** About 70% of cases of endogenous hypercortisolism are due to **ACTH-secreting pituitary corticotroph adenomas/ corticotroph hyperplasia.**
  - **Secretion of ectopic ACTH by nonpituitary neoplasms:** It accounts for 10–15% of Cushing syndrome. It is most common in *small cell carcinoma of the lung*. Other neoplasms include carcinoid, medullary thyroid carcinoma, and PanNET. The adrenal glands undergo bilateral cortical hyperplasia secondary to elevated ACTH.
- **ACTH independent (~20%) Cushing syndrome: Primary adrenal tumors such as adrenal adenoma and carcinoma**, and, rarely, ***primary cortical hyperplasia,*** cause 15–20% of cases of endogenous Cushing syndrome. They are termed *ACTH-independent Cushing syndrome* because the tumors or hyperplastic glands function autonomously. The biochemical hallmark of adrenal Cushing syndrome is elevated serum levels of cortisol and low levels of ACTH.

MORPHOLOGY

The main lesions of Cushing syndrome are observed in the **pituitary and adrenal glands.**

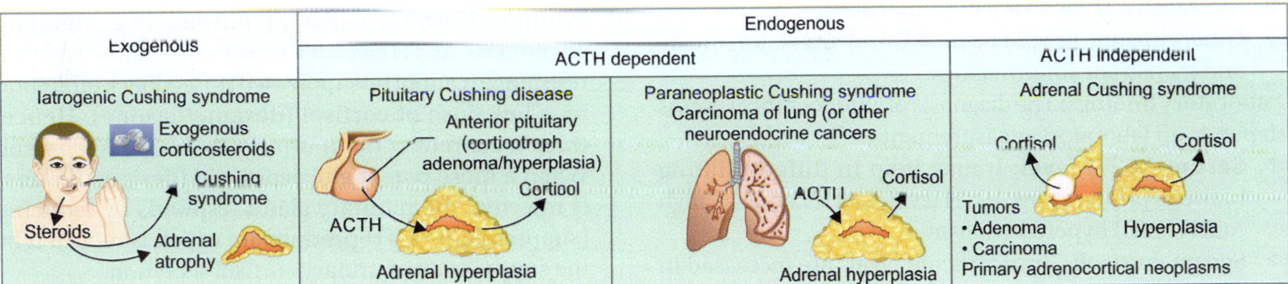

Fig. 24.20: Various causes of Cushing syndrome. (ACTH: adrenocorticotropic hormone).

Pituitary: Most common changes are due to high levels of endogenous or exogenous glucocorticoids and are called **Crooke hyaline changes.** This is characterized by the replacement of the normal granular, basophilic cytoplasm of the ACTH-producing cells in the anterior pituitary by homogeneous, pale basophilic material in the anterior pituitary. This is due to the accumulation of intermediate keratin filaments in the cytoplasm.

Adrenals: Changes depend on the cause of the hypercortisolism the adrenals may show one of the following abnormalities.

1. **Cortical atrophy:** Bilateral cortical atrophy is seen in cases due to exogenous glucocorticoid, suppression.
2. **Diffuse hyperplasia:** Found in ACTH-dependent Cushing syndrome.
3. **Macronodular or micronodular hyperplasia.**
4. **Functional adenoma or carcinoma of the adrenal cortex** (*refer pages 903-4*).

Clinical Features (Fig. 24.21)

Cushing syndrome develops slowly and the clinical features are as follows:

- **Weight gain** caused by hyperinsulinism from **hyperglycemia.** There is also **glucosuria and polydipsia** (secondary diabetes). More characteristic features are due to fat deposition/accumulation in the trunk (**truncal obesity), in the face (moon facies)**, and in the posterior neck and upper back (**buffalo hump**).
- Hypertension
- **Muscle weakness:** Cortisol breaks down muscles in the extremities (**decreased muscle mass) and produces proximal limb weakness.**
- **Secondary diabetes:** Glucocorticoids stimulate gluconeogenesis and inhibit the uptake of glucose by cells. This causes secondary diabetes, hyperglycemia, glycosuria, and polydipsia.
- **Purple abdominal stria (stretch marks):** The glucocorticoids cause loss of collagen. **Skin is thin, fragile, and easily bruised**; and cutaneous striae are particularly common in the abdominal area.
- **Osteoporosis:** Hypercortisolism causes increased breakdown and resorption of bone leading to **osteoporosis** and associated with increased susceptibility to fractures.
- Increased risk for a variety of infections.
- Others include several mental disturbances, hirsutism, and menstrual abnormalities.

Laboratory findings: The diagnosis of adrenocortical excess depends on laboratory measurements.

- **Serum ACTH level:** It may help in differentiating between primary (low ACTH level) and secondary (high ACTH level) hypercortisolism.
- **Serum cortisol:** Glucocorticoid levels are increased in all forms of Cushing syndrome.
- **Urinary free cortisol levels:** It is elevated in all forms of hypercortisolism. Usually, a 24-hour urine collection is done to exclude diurnal variations in cortisol production.
- **Dexamethasone suppression test:** It helps in the differentiation of pituitary causes and ectopic causes of excessive ACTH production. If the ACTH level is increased or normal and the 24-hour urinary-free cortisol level is raised, a dexamethasone suppression test may be done.

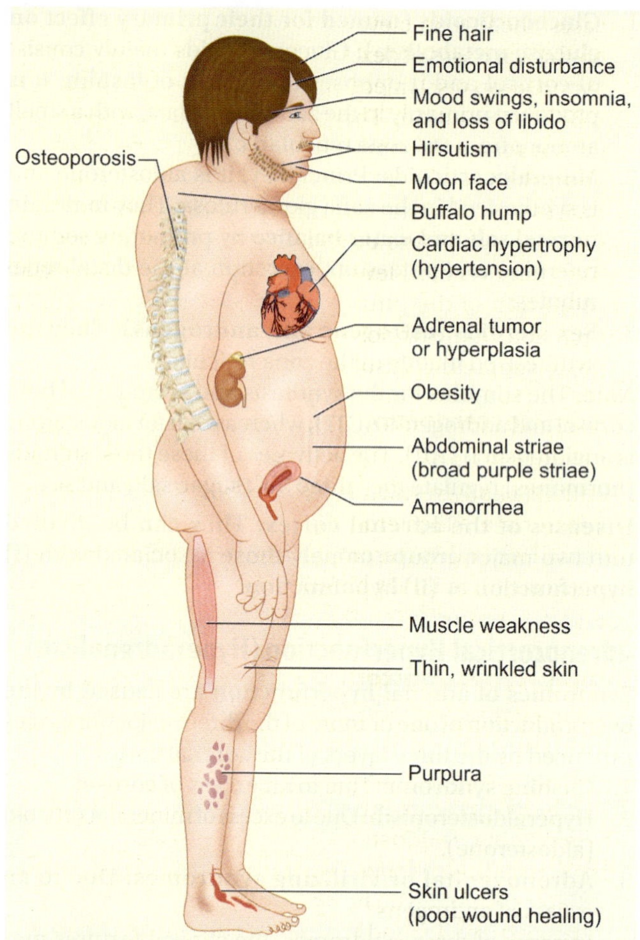

Fig. 24.21: Clinical manifestations of Cushing syndrome.

The results of the above tests can fall into the following three general patterns:

1. **Pituitary Cushing disease/syndrome** (e.g., pituitary adenomas): ACTH levels are elevated and show a relative resistance (cannot be suppressed) to feedback inhibition by a low dose of cortisol (dexamethasone). Hence, there is no reduction in urinary excretion of cortisol. When a more potent glucocorticoid (dexamethasone) is injected, the pituitary gland responds by reducing (suppressing) ACTH production, which is reflected by the suppression of urinary cortisol secretion.
2. **Ectopic ACTH secretion:** Cushing syndrome may be produced due to ectopic production of ACTH by cancer cells (e.g., small cell carcinoma of the lung). In such

cases, there is an elevated level of ACTH. Neither low nor higher doses of dexamethasone (in dexamethasone suppression test) injection in these cases fail to reduce ACTH production. This is because the cancer cells do not respond (completely insensitive) to feedback control. When the suppression test is negative, it is necessary to find the ectopic cancer source.

3. **Cushing syndrome due to adrenal cortical tumors:** They have very low levels of ACTH because of feedback inhibition of the pituitary. Similar to ectopic ACTH secretion, both low-dose and high-dose dexamethasone fail to suppress cortisol excretion.

Hyperaldosteronism

Hyperaldosteronism is a group of closely-related conditions **characterized by chronic excessive secretion of aldosterone**. Aldosterone is not under pituitary control. **Causes:** Hyperaldosteronism may be primary (due to adrenal cause), or it may be secondary to an extra-adrenal cause.

Primary Hyperaldosteronism

It is characterized by the **autonomous excessive production of aldosterone**. This, in turn, suppresses the renin-angiotensin system and decreases plasma renin activity. **Raised blood pressure is the most common manifestation of primary hyperaldosteronism.** The causes of primary hyperaldosteronism (*refer* **online Fig. 24.22**) are as follows:

- **Bilateral idiopathic hyperaldosteronism (IHA):** It is characterized by nodular hyperplasia of both adrenal glands and is the most common (about 60%) cause of primary hyperaldosteronism. Its exact pathogenesis is not known. Usually, it occurs in older individuals who have less severe hypertension than those with adrenal neoplasms.
- **Adrenocortical neoplasm:** This may be an aldosterone-producing adrenocortical adenoma (cause about 35%) or, rarely, an adrenocortical carcinoma. Primary hyperaldosteronism caused by a solitary aldosterone-secreting adenoma is called Conn syndrome. This occurs mostly in adult middle life and the female-to male ratio is 2:1.
- **Familial hyperaldosteronism**: It is due to a rare genetic defect that leads to overactivity of the aldosterone synthase gene, *CYP11B2*.

Secondary Hyperaldosteronism

In secondary hyperaldosteronism, there is the release of aldosterone in response to activation of the renin-angiotensin system. There are increased levels of plasma renin due to an extra-adrenal cause such as:

- **Decreased renal perfusion:** For example, in renal artery stenosis, arteriolar nephrosclerosis
- **Arterial hypovolemia and edema:** For example, in congestive heart failure, cirrhosis, nephrotic syndrome
- **Pregnancy:** Estrogen increases plasma renin substrate in pregnancy

Clinical Features of Hyperaldosteronism

- **Hypertension**: It is a common symptom. The long-term hyperaldosteronism-induced hypertension can lead to cardiovascular complications (e.g., left ventricular hypertrophy, reduced diastolic volumes, and myocardial infarction) and an increased incidence of stroke.
- **Hypokalemia**: Potassium moves from the blood into the renal tubule and is lost through the kidneys. This causes hypokalemia (decreased potassium in blood). Hypokalemia can produce neuromuscular manifestations such as weakness, paresthesias, visual disturbances, and occasionally frank tetany.

Adrenogenital Syndromes

The adrenal cortex can secrete excess androgens due to either of the following:

- Adrenocortical neoplasms (usually *virilizing* carcinomas).
- Congenital adrenal hyperplasia (CAH): It consists of a group of autosomal recessive disorders characterized by defects in steroid biosynthesis, usually cortisol. Reduced secretion of cortisol causes a compensatory increase in ACTH secretion, which in turn stimulates androgen production.

Androgens have virilizing effects. These effects include masculinization in females (ambiguous genitalia, oligomenorrhea, hirsutism), and precocious puberty in males.

Adrenocortical Insufficiency/Hypofunction (Hypoadrenalism)

PA 32.7 (NC): Describe the etiology, pathogenesis, manifestations, laboratory, morphologic features, and complications of adrenal insufficiency.

Adrenocortical insufficiency/hypofunction is the lack of or reduced production of glucocorticoids or mineralocorticoids by the adrenal cortex.

Etiology and Pathogenesis

Adrenocortical insufficiency (hypofunction or hyposecretion of adrenocortical hormones can be due to disease of the adrenal cortex (primary adrenocortical insufficiency, Addison disease) or due to the inadequate secretion of ACTH from the anterior pituitary gland (secondary adrenal insufficiency). Though hypofunction can affect all the adrenocortical hormones, the most severe clinical manifestations of adrenocortical insufficiency are because of low/inadequate levels of circulating cortisol.

The causes of adrenocortical insufficiency are listed in **Box 24.10.**

BOX 24.10: Causes of adrenocortical insufficiency or hypofunction.

Primary Adrenocortical Insufficiency (Hypoadrenalism)

It is due to adrenal disease and can be acute or chronic.

- **Acute:** Characterized by acute adrenal crisis
  - Sudden or abrupt withdrawal of corticosteroids in a patient with adrenal atrophy due to long-term corticosteroid therapy and is the most common cause of acute adrenal insufficiency.
  - Massive adrenal hemorrhage, e.g., anticoagulation therapy, in postoperative patients who develop disseminated intravascular coagulation, in patients with overwhelming sepsis (Waterhouse–Friderichsen syndrome).
  - Stress of infection or surgery in patients with chronic adrenal insufficiency
- **Chronic (Addison disease)**
  - Autoimmune adrenalitis
  - Infections: Tuberculosis, acquired immunodeficiency syndrome, fungal infections *(Histoplasma capsulatum and Coccidioides immitis)*
  - Amyloidosis, sarcoidosis, hemochromatosis
  - Metastatic carcinoma to the adrenals: Carcinomas of the lung and breast

Secondary Adrenocortical Insufficiency (Hypothalamic-Pituitary Dysfunction)

Decreased stimulation of the adrenals due to a deficiency of ACTH (secondary hypoadrenalism).

- Hypothalamic pituitary disease: Destruction of the pituitary with loss of pituitary function by—
  - Inflammation (sarcoidosis, tuberculosis, pyrogens, fungi) and infections due to opportunistic pathogens associated with the human immunodeficiency virus
  - Pituitary tumors, craniopharyngioma. Metastatic tumors to the pituitary, pituitary infarction, trauma, surgery, and radiation therapy
- Hypothalamic pituitary suppression
  - Long-term steroid administration

Primary Adrenocortical Insufficiency

Acute Adrenocortical Insufficiency

Definition: A sudden lack of production of glucocorticoids or mineralocorticoids by the adrenal cortex is termed acute adrenocortical insufficiency or adrenal crisis. There is a sudden loss of adrenal cortical function.

The causes of acute adrenocortical insufficiency are listed in **Box 24.10**.

Waterhouse–Friderichsen syndrome: It is a catastrophic syndrome characterized by an acute, adrenal crisis due to bilateral, hemorrhagic infarction of the adrenal cortex. It is usually secondary to *meningococcus* (*Neisseria meningitidis*) or *Pseudomonas septicemia*. Waterhouse–Friderichsen syndrome is more common in children.

Clinical feature: Adrenal crises are usually manifested with hypotension and shock. Nonspecific symptoms include fatigue, weakness, and gastrointestinal disturbances which may progress to coma.

Chronic Adrenocortical Insufficiency: Addison Disease

Chronic adrenal insufficiency (Addison disease) is characterized by decreased production of glucocorticoids and mineralocorticoids, with a corresponding increase in ACTH.

Etiology: Addison disease is an uncommon disorder resulting from progressive destruction of the adrenal cortex. The causes of chronic adrenocortical insufficiency are listed in **Box 24.10**. More than 90% of cases are due to one of four disorders namely: autoimmune adrenalitis, tuberculosis, acquired immune deficiency syndrome (AIDS), or metastatic cancer.

Clinical features and complications: Usually, the clinical manifestations may not appear until at least 90% of the adrenal cortex has been compromised.

- **Nonspecific symptoms:** These include—progressive weakness, tiredness, fatigue, and anorexia.
- **Gastrointestinal disturbances:** These include—anorexia, nausea, vomiting, weight loss, and diarrhea.
- **Diffuse hyperpigmentation of skin and mucosal surfaces:** In primary adrenal disease, increased plasma levels of ACTH hormone stimulate melanocytes. This causes hyperpigmentation of the skin and mucosal surfaces. In contrast, hyperpigmentation does not occur in secondary adrenocortical insufficiency because there is a low level of ACTH and melanotropic hormone levels are not increased.
- **Electrolyte disturbances and hypotension:** Decreased mineralocorticoid (aldosterone) in primary adrenal insufficiency results in potassium retention and sodium loss. This leads to hyperkalemia, hyponatremia, volume depletion, and hypotension (blood pressure around 80/50 mm Hg). In secondary hypoadrenalism, there is deficient cortisol and androgen output but normal or near-normal aldosterone synthesis.
- **Hypoglycemia:** It may be occasionally observed in infants and children and is due to glucocorticoid deficiency and impaired gluconeogenesis.

Laboratory findings in Addison disease

- Increased plasma ACTH
- Short and prolonged ACTH stimulation test: There is no increase in serum cortisol in both tests.
- Electrolyte findings: These include hyponatremia and hyperkalemia.
- Anemia
- Increased serum blood urea nitrogen (BUN) and creatinine (azotemia) caused by volume loss of fluid and electrolytes in urine.
- Fasting hypoglycemia: This is because cortisol is a gluconeogenic hormone and there is a loss of gluconeogenesis.

Other investigations: Abdominal computerized tomography (CT) or magnetic resonance imaging (MRI) to determine the size of the adrenal glands. In autoimmune adrenalitis, the adrenal glands are smaller; in tuberculosis, glands are large and calcified.

Secondary Adrenocortical Insufficiency

Secondary adrenal insufficiency reflects a lack of ACTH. Thus, any disorder of the hypothalamus and pituitary that reduces the output of ACTH can cause secondary adrenal insufficiency.

Causes of secondary adrenocortical insufficiency: Destruction of the pituitary and consequent panhypopituitarism result in secondary adrenal insufficiency and its causes are listed in **Box 24.10**. ACTH deficiency may occur alone or sometimes as one component of panhypopituitarism (deficiencies of multiple pituitary hormones).

Differentiation of Primary and Secondary Adrenocortical Insufficiency

Response to exogenous ACTH:

- **No response to ACTH: In primary adrenocortical insufficiency**, there is destruction of the adrenal cortex. This prevents increased plasma levels of cortisol response when an exogenous ACTH is administered.
- **Response to ACTH:** In contrast, **in secondary adrenocortical insufficiency**, there is low serum ACTH and there will be a rise in plasma cortisol levels (due to secretion of glucocorticoids by adrenal) in response to exogenous ACTH administration.

Hyperpigmentation (no raised levels of melanocyte-stimulating hormone) and **electrolyte abnormalities** (hyponatremia and hyperkalemia) of primary Addison disease are typically absent in secondary adrenal insufficiency because these processes are not regulated by ACTH.

MORPHOLOGY

The appearance of the adrenal glands in adrenocortical insufficiency depends on the underlying cause.

Secondary hypoadrenalism: It is due to hypothalamic or pituitary disease and the appearance of the adrenals depends on the severity of ACTH deficiency. The adrenal glands are small and flattened (moderate to marked reduction in size). A thin rim of atrophic yellow cortex surrounds a central, unaffected/Intact medulla.

Microscopically shows atrophy of cortical cells with loss of cytoplasmic lipid (mainly in the zona fasciculata and zona reticularis).

Primary autoimmune adrenalitis: It shows irregular shrinkage of adrenal glands. Microscopically, the adrenal cortex shows only scattered residual cortical cells in a collapsed network of connective tissue. A variable amount of lymphocyte infiltrates in the cortex may extend into the subjacent normal adrenal medulla.

Tuberculosis or fungal diseases: The architecture of the adrenal gland may be effaced by a granulomatous inflammatory reaction (similar to that observed in other sites of infection).

Metastatic carcinoma: The adrenals are enlarged, and their normal architecture is distorted by the infiltrating neoplasm.

ADRENAL NEOPLASMS

Adrenal neoplasms may arise either from the adrenal cortex or adrenal medulla and they may be functional or nonfunctional.

Adrenocortical Neoplasms

PA 32.9 (NC): Describe the etiology, pathogenesis, manifestations, laboratory, and morphologic features of adrenal neoplasms.

Adrenocortical neoplasms include adenomas and carcinomas. Most cortical neoplasms are sporadic. They may be functional (producing steroid hormones) or nonfunctional. Functional adrenocortical neoplasms produce steroid hormones. To determine whether a cortical neoplasm is functional or not, it is necessary to clinically evaluate the patient and measure the hormone or its metabolites in the laboratory.

Adrenocortical Adenoma

Adenomas and carcinomas are about equally common in adults. Adrenal cortical adenoma is a **benign epithelial tumor derived from adrenal cortical cells**.

Etiopathogenesis: Adenomas are frequently seen as part of syndromes such as MEN1 (multiple endocrine neoplasias 1), Carney complex, and McCune-Albright syndrome.

MORPHOLOGY

Most adrenocortical adenomas are nonfunctional and usually are discovered as incidental ("adrenal incidentaloma") findings at the time of autopsy or during abdominal imaging for an unrelated cause.

Gross

A typical adenoma is small measuring about 1–4 cm, encapsulated, firm, yellow, and slightly lobulated. They usually weigh 10–50 g. Cut surfaces are usually yellow to yellow brown, due to the presence of lipids within the neoplastic cells

Microscopy

It is composed of clear, lipid-laden (fasciculate type) tumor cells arranged in sheets or nests. These tumor cells appear similar to the cells of the normal adrenal cortex. As with other endocrine tumors, pleomorphism may be seen in benign tumors and is not a reliable marker of malignancy.

Clinical Features

Functional adenomas commonly produce hormones, the most common being cortisol and aldosterone. Thus, they are associated with hyperaldosteronism and Cushing's syndrome.

Adrenocortical Carcinomas

They are rare and may occur at any age and are predominant in children.

Etiopathogenesis: Two rare inherited causes of adrenal cortical carcinomas are Li-Fraumeni syndrome and Beckwith-Wiedemann syndrome.

MORPHOLOGY

Gross

They are large, invasive lesions and may be more than 20 cm in diameter and efface the native adrenal gland. Cut surfaces are variegated pink, brown, or yellow and poorly demarcated lesions. They usually show areas of necrosis, hemorrhage, and cystic change.

Microscopy

They are composed of well-differentiated cells similar to that of cortical adenomas or bizarre, pleomorphic cells, monstrous giant cells, which may be difficult to distinguish from those of an undifferentiated carcinoma metastatic to the adrenal gland. It is to be kept in mind that carcinomas metastatic to the adrenal cortex are more frequent than primary adrenocortical carcinoma. Adrenal carcinomas have a strong tendency to invade the adrenal vein, vena cava, and lymphatics. It can metastasize to regional and periaortic nodes and through blood to the lungs and other viscera. Bone metastases are not common.

Clinical Features

Functional adrenal cortical carcinomas secrete glucocorticoids and androgens and are associated with virilization.

Laboratory Findings in Adrenocortical Neoplasm

- **Blood and urine tests:** To measure the amount of adrenal hormones (if it is a functional tumor that secrets hormones)
- Biopsy
- **Radiological:** CT or CAT scan and MRI

ADRENAL MEDULLA

The adrenal medulla is entirely surrounded by the adrenal cortex. It is embryologically, functionally, and structurally distinct from the adrenal cortex. It consists of neuroendocrine cells, or **chromaffin cells derived from the neural crest** (neuroendocrine) and their supporting (sustentacular) cells. The chromaffin cells are so named because **catecholamines in their cytoplasmic granules bind chromium (chromium affinity) salts.** These granules darken and develop a brown-black color after exposure to potassium dichromate (causes oxidation). The adrenal medulla is the major source of catecholamines (epinephrine, norepinephrine).

The most important diseases of the adrenal medulla are neoplasms. These include both neuronal neoplasms (including neuroblastomas and more mature ganglion cell tumors) and neoplasms composed of chromaffin cells (pheochromocytomas).

Tumors of the Adrenal Medulla

PA 32.9 (NC): Describe the etiology, pathogenesis, manifestations, laboratory, and morphologic features of adrenal neoplasms.

Pheochromocytoma

Q. Write a short note on pheochromocytoma.

- Pheochromocytomas are **neoplasms composed of chromaffin cells**.
- The **tumor cells synthesize and release catecholamines** and some may produce peptide hormones.
- These tumors are the rare cause of surgically correctable **hypertension**.

Rule of 10s (Box 24.11)

- 10% of pheochromocytomas are **extra-adrenal**: They occur in the organs of Zuckerkandl (present at the bifurcation of the aorta or the origin of the inferior mesenteric artery) and the carotid body. Extra-adrenal pheochromocytomas are called **paragangliomas.**
- 10% of sporadic adrenal pheochromocytomas are **bilateral**. In pheochromocytomas associated with familial syndromes up to 50% may be bilateral.
- 10% of adrenal pheochromocytomas are **malignant and metastasize.** Malignancy is more common in extra-adrenal paragangliomas, and tumors developing due to germline mutations.
- 10% of adrenal pheochromocytomas are **not associated with hypertension.**
- 10% occur in children.

The 10% rule has been modified to apply only to familial cases of pheochromocytoma.

Etiology

About 25% of individuals with pheochromocytomas and paragangliomas harbor a germline mutation in one of six known genes *RET, NF1, VHL,* and three succinate dehydrogenase complex subunit genes, i.e., *SDHB, SDHC,* and *SDHD.*

BOX 24.11: Rule of 10s in pheochromocytoma.

- 10% extra-adrenal as sympathetic paragangliomas
- 10% bilateral
- 10% malignant
- 10% not associated with hypertension
- 10% occur in children

MORPHOLOGY

Gross [Fig. 24.23B (*refer* online Fig. 24.23A)]

- **Size: Varies** and may range from small, circumscribed lesions to large hemorrhagic masses.
- **Weight:** Average **100 g**, but may range from 1–4,000 g.
- Larger tumors are **well-demarcated** and **may** produce a **lobular pattern.** Part of the adrenal gland can be seen over the surface of the tumor.
- **Cut surface**: Small tumors have a **yellow tan.** Large tumors show areas of **hemorrhage, necrosis, and cystic changes and typically efface the adrenal gland.**
- **Chromaffin reaction:** When the **fresh tumor tissue is incubated in potassium dichromate solution**; the **tumor turns dark brown in color (Fig. 24.23B)** due to oxidation of stored catecholamines. This is termed as a positive **chromaffin reaction.**

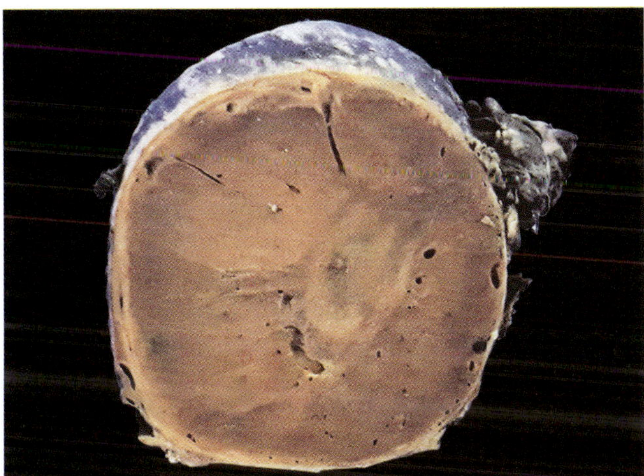

Fig. 24.23B: Cut sections of pheochromocytomas: Chromaffin reaction showing dark brown color after incubation in potassium dichromate solution.

Microscopy (Figs. 24.24A and B)

Tumor cells: The tumor is composed of **polygonal to spindle-shaped chromaffin cells** and their supporting cells.

- **Cytoplasm:** It has a **fine granular appearance due to** the presence of granules containing **catecholamines.** It is best **demonstrated with silver stains.**
- **Nuclei:** They are **round to oval**, with a stippled **"salt and pepper"** chromatin that is characteristic of neuroendocrine tumors.

Zellballen pattern: The **polygonal to spindle-shaped chromaffin cells**, clustered with the sustentacular (supporting) cells **into small nests or alveoli (Zellballen)** separated by a **rich vascular network (Fig. 24.24).**

Electron microscopy: It shows **membrane-bound, electron-dense secretory granules.**

Immunohistochemistry: Neuroendocrine markers (chromogranin and synaptophysin) are positive in the chief cells**.** The peripheral sustentacular cells stain with antibodies against S-100, a calcium-binding protein expressed by a variety of mesenchymal cell types.

Criteria for Malignancy

- None of the histologic features can reliably predict clinical behavior.
- **Histologic features associated with aggressive behavior and increased risk of metastasis** include:
  - **Numbers of mitoses**
  - **Confluent tumor necrosis**
  - **Spindle cell morphology**
- **Capsular and vascular invasion may be found in benign lesions.**

Spread

- **Definitive diagnosis of malignancy in pheochromocytomas is made only when they develop metastases.**
- The tumor may metastasize to regional lymph nodes as well as more distant sites, including liver, lung, and bone.

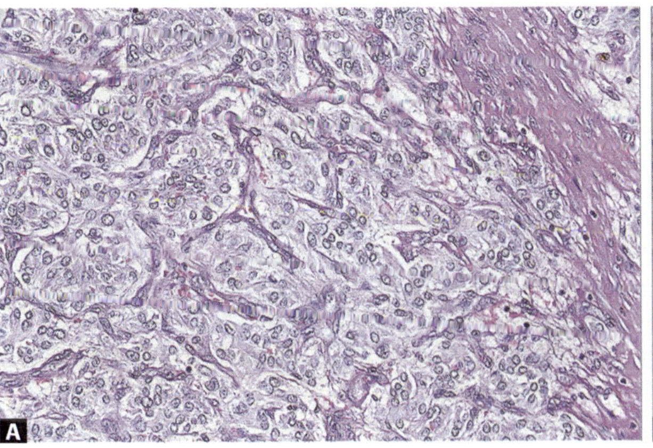

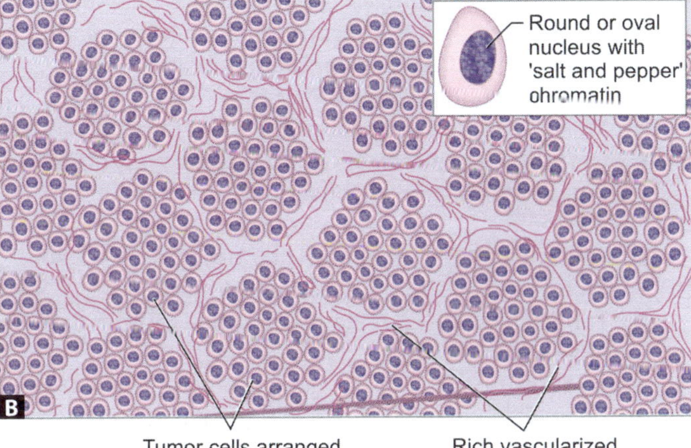

Figs. 24.24A and B: (A) H&E and (B) Diagrammatic**.** Pheochromocytoma is composed of characteristic nests of tumor cells (Zellballen) with abundant cytoplasm. Inset of (B) shows nucleus with salt and pepper chromatin.

Clinical Features

Catecholamines (dopamine, epinephrine, and norepinephrine) mediate the functions of the sympathetic nervous system. Their release from pheochromocytoma produces symptoms that mimic sympathetic nervous hyperactivity. The dominant clinical manifestation is **hypertension in 90% of patients.**

- **Chronic:** Sustained elevation in blood pressure punctuated by paroxysms.
- **Paroxysmal hypertensive episodes:** It is characterized by an abrupt, precipitous elevation in blood pressure, associated with tachycardia, palpitations, headache, sweating, tremors, and a sense of apprehension.
- **Isolated paroxysmal episodes:** Less common.

The elevations of blood pressure are induced by the sudden release of catecholamines. This may precipitate congestive heart failure, pulmonary edema, myocardial infarction, ventricular fibrillation, and cerebrovascular accidents.

Complications

Cardiac complications are called **catecholamine cardiomyopathy**, or catecholamine-induced myocardial instability and ventricular arrhythmias.

Laboratory diagnosis

Demonstration of **increased urinary excretion of free catecholamines and their metabolites**, such as vanillylmandelic acid and metanephrines.

Neuroblastoma

Q. Write a short note on neuroblastoma.

- Neuroblastoma is the most **important neuroblastic tumor.** Neuroblastic tumors are a group of tumors of the sympathetic ganglia and adrenal medulla that are derived from primordial neural crest cells.
- **Age:** Neuroblastoma is the **most common extracranial childhood solid tumor**. It is most frequently diagnosed during infancy. It is the second most common solid malignancy of childhood after brain tumors.
- **Sporadic and familial types**:
  - Mostly occur sporadically, but 1–2% is familial.
  - **Germline mutations in** the **anaplastic lymphoma kinase** ***(ALK)*** gene are observed in familial neuroblastoma.
  - Somatic gain-of-function *ALK* mutations are also found in a few sporadic neuroblastomas.
  - Tumors having *ALK* mutations respond to drugs that target their activity.
- Amplification of *N-MYC* (*MYC* family of proto-oncogenes) is found in about 30% of neuroblastomas (*refer* **Fig. 7.14** and page 233).

MORPHOLOGY

Gross

- **Site:** About 40% of neuroblastomas occur in the **adrenal medulla.**
  - **Other sites:** It may develop along the sympathetic chain.
    - **Paravertebral region of the abdomen** (25%).
    - **Posterior mediastinum** (15%).
    - Pelvis, the neck, and brain (**cerebral neuroblastomas**).
- **Size: Vary** from minute nodules (as in situ lesions) to large tumors weighing 1 kg.
- **Nature: The majority** are **silent** and **regress spontaneously**.
- May be **sharply demarcated** by a fibrous pseudocapsule **or infiltrate** the surrounding structures (kidneys, renal vein, vena cava, and aorta).
- **Cut section: Soft, brain-like tissue and gray-tan. Large tumors** may show areas of **necrosis, cystic change,** and **hemorrhage**.

Microscopy (Figs. 24.25A and B)

Q. Write a short answer on microscopic features of neuroblastoma.

Tumor cells: They are arranged in solid sheets. The tumor cells appear as **small, primitive tumor cells containing dark nuclei.** They have **scant cytoplasm with poorly defined cell borders.**

- **Mitotic activity, karyorrhexis** (breakdown of nuclear material), and pleomorphism may be prominent.
- These tumors may be **difficult to differentiate morphologically from** other **small round blue cell tumors.**

Homer–Wright pseudorosettes: May be seen which consist of tumor cells concentrically arranged about a central space filled with neuropil. Because of the absence of an actual central lumen, they are called pseudorosettes.

Background: Shows a faintly **eosinophilic fibrillary material** (**neuropil**), which represents the neuritic processes of the primitive neuroblasts.

Immunohistochemistry: Neuron-specific enolase positive.

Electron microscopy: It shows **small, membrane-bound, catecholamine-containing secretory granules in the cytoplasm.**

Maturation: Neuroblastomas have several unique features in their natural history. Some neoplasms may show **spontaneous or induced** (by therapy) **maturation**. These differentiated lesions include ganglioneuroblastoma and ganglioneuroma. Maturation is **characterized by the presence of Schwannian stroma** composed of organized fascicles of neuritic processes, mature Schwann cells, and fibroblasts. This type of stroma is required for the designation of ganglioneuroblastoma and ganglioneuroma. The presence of ganglion cells is not a criterion for maturation.

- **Ganglioneuroblastoma:** It consists of **primitive neuroblasts** that may be **admixed with ganglion cells** in various stages

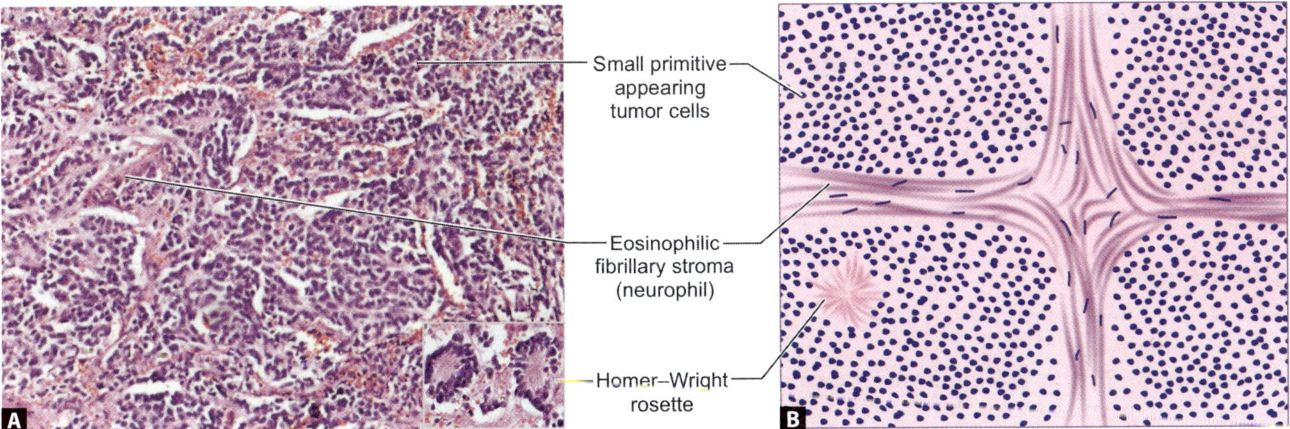

Figs. 24.25A and B: (A) Photomicrograph; and (B) Diagrammatic. Neuroblastoma consists of small primitive appearing cells with scant cytoplasm embedded in a finely fibrillar matrix. Inset of A shows two Homer–Wright rosettes.

of maturation. The ganglion cells appear as large cells with abundant cytoplasm having large vesicular nuclei and a prominent nucleolus.

- **Ganglioneuroma** (*refer* **online Fig. 24.26**): It is a **more mature tumor than ganglioneuroblastoma.** It contains many **more large cells resembling mature ganglion cells** with few, if any, residual neuroblasts. The maturation of neuroblasts into ganglion cells is usually accompanied by the appearance of **Schwann cells.** The presence of **Schwannian stroma is associated with** a **favorable outcome.**

Spread of Tumor

- Local infiltration
- Lymph node spread
- Blood spread: Liver, lungs, bone marrow, and bones.

Clinical Features

- **Children below 2 years of age:** Usually present as **large abdominal masses, fever, and weight loss.**
- **Older children:** Symptoms develop due to metastases such as bone pain, respiratory symptoms, or gastrointestinal complaints.
- Ganglioneuromas may present either as asymptomatic mass or symptoms related to compression.

Laboratory finding

- **Majority** (~90%) of neuroblastomas, **secrete catecholamines** (similar to pheochromocytomas) leading to raised blood levels of catecholamines (hypertension is less frequent).
- **Raised urine levels** of the **metabolites vanillylmandelic acid** (VMA) and **homovanillic acid** (HVA).

Course: It is extremely variable.

Prognostic factors

Many factors influence prognosis the most important being the stage of the tumor and the age of the patient.

- **Staging of neuroblastomas:** It is important in establishing a prognosis.
- **Morphology:** It is an **independent prognostic factor.** Accordingly, tumors are divided into favorable and unfavorable histologic subtypes.
- **Age and stage:** Children **younger than 18 months of age** have **excellent prognosis** regardless of the stage of the neoplasm.
- **Amplification of the *N-MYC* oncogene high-risk category**, irrespective of age, stage, or histology.
- **Ploidy of the tumor cells:** It is of **prognostic value in children younger than 2 years** and loses its prognostic significance in older children.

MULTIPLE ENDOCRINE NEOPLASIA SYNDROMES

Q. Write a short note on MEN (multiple endocrine neoplasia).

The MEN syndromes are a group of inherited diseases characterized by proliferative lesions (hyperplasia, adenomas, and carcinomas) of multiple endocrine organs.

Characteristic Features

- **Age:** These tumors **develop at a younger age** compared to sporadic cancers.
- **Multiple:** They occur in multiple endocrine organs, either synchronously (at the same time) or metachronously (at different times).
- **Multifocal:** Even in one organ involved, the tumors are often multifocal.
- **Clinical features:** They are usually preceded by an **asymptomatic stage of endocrine hyperplasia** of the cell of origin of the tumor (e.g., in MEN-2 there is C cell hyperplasia in the thyroid parenchyma adjacent to medullary thyroid carcinomas).
- **Nature of tumor**: Usually, these tumors are more aggressive and recur compared to sporadic endocrine tumors.

There are two main types of MEN namely MEN type 1 and MEN type 2.

Multiple Endocrine Neoplasia Type 1

MEN-1 syndrome is caused due to germline mutations in the *MEN1* tumor suppressor gene. MEN1 gene encodes a protein called menin that is a component of several different transcription factor complexes. Loss of menin function causes deregulation of the corresponding binding partners and leads to endocrine neoplasia.

Organs Involved

3 Ps: Most commonly involves (1) parathyroid, (2) pancreas, and (3) pituitary.

1. **Parathyroid: Primary hyperparathyroidism** is the most common feature of MEN-1 (80–95%) and is the presenting feature in most patients. Usually, it is detected by 40–50 years of age. **Parathyroid shows hyperplasia and adenomas.**
2. **Pancreas: Endocrine tumors of the pancreas** are the leading cause of death in patients with MEN-1. These tumors usually are aggressive and present with metastatic disease. Pancreatic endocrine tumors often are functional (i.e., secrete hormones). Zollinger-Ellison syndrome associated with gastrinomas, and hypoglycemia, associated with insulinomas, are common endocrine manifestations.
3. **Pituitary:** The most frequent pituitary tumor in patients with MEN-1 syndrome is a **prolactin-secreting macroadenoma**. In some cases, acromegaly develops in association with somatotropin-secreting tumors.

Multiple Endocrine Neoplasia Type 2

MEN-2 syndrome consists of two distinct groups/types of disorders (type 2A and 2B) characterized by the presence of activating (i.e., gain-of-function) **mutations of the *RET*** proto-oncogene at chromosomal locus 10q11.2. MEN-2 is inherited in an **autosomal dominant disorder**. All persons with germline RET mutations should undergo prophylactic thyroidectomy to prevent the inevitable development of medullary carcinomas.

Multiple Endocrine Neoplasia Type 2A

Commonly affected organs in MEN-2A are:

- **Medullary carcinoma of the thyroid:** It is found in almost all untreated cases. It usually manifests during the first 2 decades of life. The tumors are usually multifocal and associated with foci of C cell hyperplasia in the adjacent thyroid.
    - **Familial medullary thyroid cancer:** It may be seen in a variant of MEN-2, without the other features of MEN-2A. They usually occur at an older age and follow a more indolent course.
- **Pheochromocytomas of adrenal medulla:** Observed in 50% of the patients and no more than 10% of these are malignant.
- **Hyperplasia of parathyroid gland:** Found in about 10–20% of patients and they manifest with features of primary hyperparathyroidism.

Multiple Endocrine Neoplasia Type 2B

In MEN type 2B, there is a single amino acid change in RET, which is distinct from the mutations observed in MEN-2A.

Features

- **Medullary thyroid carcinomas**: These patients have medullary thyroid carcinomas, that are usually multifocal and more aggressive than in MEN-2A.
- **Pheochromocytomas**
- **No primary hyperparathyroidism in MEN-2B.**
- **Extraendocrine manifestations:** These are characteristic of MEN-2B. These include ganglioneuromas of mucosa (e.g., gastrointestinal tract, lips, tongue) and a **marfanoid habitus** (long bones appear similar to that in Marfan syndrome).

SCENARIO-BASED MCQs

1. **A 22-year-old woman and her twin sister both complain of increasing diplopia. She has noted increasing fatigue and a 7-kg weight loss without dieting over the past 3 months. She also has anxiety and nervousness with diarrhea. Physical examination shows exophthalmos and weak movement of extraocular muscles. In both, the thyroid gland is diffusely enlarged but painless and has no lymphadenopathy. A fine tremor is observed in her outstretched hands. A radionuclide scan of the thyroid shows a diffuse increase in uptake. The serum is most likely to show the following features on laboratory examination:**
   A. Decreased free thyroxine level
   B. Increased triiodothyronine level
   C. Antibodies against TSH receptor
   D. Increased thyrotropin-releasing hormone (TRH) level
2. **A 45-year-old woman living in the Himalayan region complains of a feeling of fullness in her neck. The enlargement has been gradual and painless for more than 1 year. Physical examination shows a diffuse enlargement of the thyroid gland without any apparent nodular masses or lymphadenopathy. Laboratory studies of thyroid function show a normal free T4 level and a slightly elevated TSH level. The most likely cause of these findings is:**
   A. Follicular adenoma
   B. Diffuse nontoxic goiter
   C. Toxic multinodular goiter
   D. Hashimoto thyroiditis
3. **A 34-year-old, woman complains of a small lump on the left side of her neck for 4 months. On physical examination, a firm, painless, 1.5 cm cervical lymph node is palpable. The thyroid gland is not enlarged. Laboratory studies show no thyroid autoantibodies in her serum, and the T4 and TSH levels are normal. A fine-needle aspiration biopsy of the thyroid gland is done. After the characteristic cytologic finding, thyroidectomy is performed. The tumor cells showed**

ground glass nuclei in the tumor cells and psammoma bodies. The most likely diagnosis is:

A. Papillary carcinoma
B. Follicular carcinoma
C. Anaplastic carcinoma
D. Medullary carcinoma

4. **A 12-year-old girl collapses in the school while playing on the ground. She is semiconscious when brought to the emergency department. On physical examination, she is hypotensive and tachycardic with deep, rapid, labored respirations. Laboratory studies show plasma glucose of 510 mg/dL. Urinalysis shows 4+ glucosuria and 4+ ketonuria levels, but no protein, blood, or nitrite. The most likely underlying disease that is associated with complication is:**

A. Type 1 diabetes
B. Acute pyelonephritis
C. Cerebral hemorrhage
D. Acute pancreatitis

5. **A 52-year-old man with fasting blood glucose >160 mg/dL on two occasions is put on a restricted caloric diet and started on antidiabetic drugs. Of the following laboratory studies, the most likely useful method of monitoring disease control is:**

A. Microalbuminuria
B. Cholesterol, total
C. Fasting plasma glucose
D. Glycosylated hemoglobin

Answers and Explanation

1. **The answer is C: Antibodies against TSH receptor.** Exophthalmos is seen in about 40% of patients with Graves disease. Other clinical features also favor the diagnosis of Graves disease. In this condition, the hyperfunctioning thyroid gland leads to an increased T4 level. There is positive feedback from the pituitary to decrease thyroid-stimulating hormone (TSH) secretion. Graves disease is an autoimmune with about 50% concordance among identical twins. It is characterized by the presence of an autoantibody against the TSH receptor and mimics the action of TSH. Thus, it increases the secretion of T4. An increased thyrotropin-releasing hormone (TRH) level would increase the TSH level and increase the T4. However, feedback typically occurs at the level of the pituitary and the hypothalamus, and abnormal increases in TRH are uncommon. T3 levels are less likely to be elevated than T4 levels.
2. **The answer is B: Diffuse nontoxic goiter.** It is most commonly caused by dietary deficiency of iodine. This is endemic in regions of the world where iodine is deficient (e.g., Himalayan areas); it also may occur sporadically. The patients are usually euthyroid. A follicular adenoma produces a solitary nodule and does not involve the thyroid diffusely. Toxic multinodular goiter (Plummer disease) occurs when there is a hyperfunctioning nodule in a goiter. Hashimoto thyroiditis initially can produce thyroid enlargement, but atrophy eventually occurs leading to hypothyroidism.
3. **The answer is A: Papillary thyroid carcinomas may present initially with metastases.** The most common sites for metastases are local lymph nodes. The primary site may not be detectable as a palpable nodule. Papillary carcinoma is the most common thyroid malignancy. The tumor cells that have clear nuclei are a pattern typical for papillary carcinoma along with psammoma bodies. These nuclear changes, even if the pattern is follicular, confirm the diagnosis of papillary carcinoma. Follicular and medullary carcinomas tend to spread hematogenously; they do not show ground glass nuclei. Anaplastic carcinomas are uncommon, but are very aggressive, locally invasive lesions.
4. **The answer is A: Type 1 diabetes mellitus.** The girl has ketoacidosis. Acute pyelonephritis is associated with fever and microscopically shows pus cells and WBC casts. Cerebral hemorrhage occurs usually in older patients with hypertension and the clinical and laboratory findings do not support it. Acute pancreatitis presents with acute severe abdominal pain and the clinical features and laboratory findings are not supportive of this lesion.
5. **The answer is D: Glycosylated hemoglobin.** Nonenzymatic glycosylation is the chemical process whereby glucose attaches to proteins without the help of enzymes. The degree of glycosylation is proportionate to the level of blood glucose. Many proteins, including hemoglobin, undergo nonenzymatic glycosylation. Since RBCs have a normal life span of about 120 days, the amount of glycosylated hemoglobin indicates the blood glucose level over the previous 120-day period. The level of glycosylated hemoglobin is not affected by short-term changes in plasma glucose levels. Measurements of cholesterol have no value in managing diabetes mellitus. Microalbuminuria may precede the development of diabetic renal disease. Fasting glucose testing provides a better way to diagnose diabetes mellitus initially.

Papillary carcinoma:
- The most common malignant tumor of the thyroid.
- Most common endocrine malignancy.
- Most common thyroid cancer in children and persons exposed to external radiation.

Complications of diabetes mellitus:
Vascular complications
- Microvascular (small vessels)
- Macrovascular causes accelerated atherosclerosis in large and medium-sized muscular arteries: Nonvascular complications

Glycosylated hemoglobin (HbA1c): Marker of glycemic control.

Tumors of adrenal medulla:
- Pheochromocytoma
- Neuroblastoma

Pheochromocytoma:
- Rule of 10%
- Zellballen pattern.

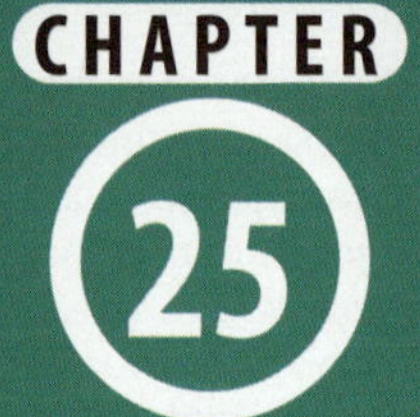

Bones, Joints, and Soft Tissue Tumors

Chapter Outline

- Infections—Osteomyelitis
- Paget Disease of Bone (Osteitis Deformans)
- Bone Tumors
- Rheumatoid Arthritis
- Osteoarthritis
- Gout and Gouty Arthritis
- Healing of a Fracture
- Soft Tissue Tumors
- Tumors of Adipose Tissue
- Fibroblastic/Myofibroblastic Tumors
- Skeletal Muscle Tumors
- Smooth Muscle Tumors
- Peripheral Nerve Sheath Tumors
- Tumors of Uncertain Origin

INTRODUCTION

The skeletal system consists of the bones, their associated cartilages, and the joints. Bone is a specialized connective tissue that has structural, protective, metabolic, and hematopoietic functions (produces blood cells).

Different regions in the bone (Fig. 25.1): The anatomy of bone is defined in relation to the growth plate (physis). The growth plate is a transverse structure in the growing child. Long bones (and some short bones such as metacarpal bones) are topographically divided into three regions—(1) epiphysis, (2) metaphysis, and (3) diaphysis. These regions are defined in relation to the growth plate.

1. **Epiphysis:** It is the area of the bone that extends from the base of the articular surface (the site of close approximation of two bones) to the region of the growth plate.
2. **Metaphysis:** It is the region that extends from the region of the growth plate to the area where the diameter of the bone becomes significantly narrow (becomes funnel-shaped).
3. **Diaphysis (shaft):** It is the zone that extends from the base of one metaphysis to the base of the opposing metaphysis.

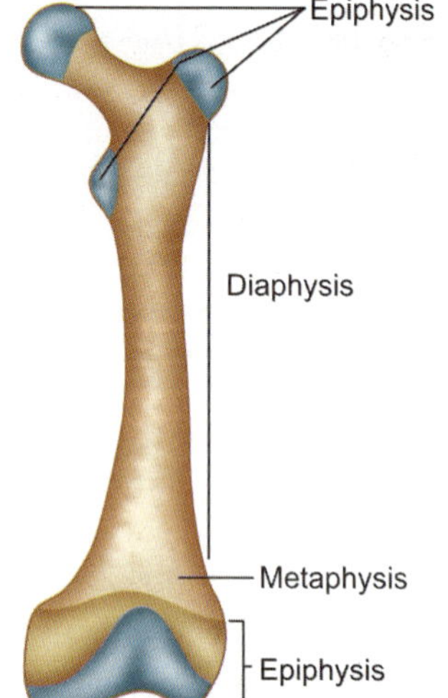

Fig. 25.1: Different regions of bone.

Cells of the bone tissue: There are three types of cells in the bone.

1. **Osteoblasts:** These cells produce osteoid and are thus bone-forming cells. Osteoid is an unmineralized organic bone matrix.
2. **Osteocytes:** When an osteoblast is enveloped by bone matrix it becomes an osteocyte. With time osteocytes lose the capacity for matrix synthesis.
3. **Osteoclasts:** These are mature multinucleated cells (on an average they have 6–12 nuclei) that are responsible for bone resorption (removal by absorption).

INFECTIONS—OSTEOMYELITIS

PA 33.1 (CC): Classify and describe the etiology, pathogenesis, manifestations, radiologic and morphologic features, and complications of osteomyelitis.

Q. Write a short essay on osteomyelitis.

Osteomyelitis is defined as **inflammation of the bone and marrow**. It is **almost always secondary to infection.**

Classification: Osteomyelitis may be classified as primary or secondary. Osteomyelitis **usually manifests as a primary solitary focus of the disease**. But it can also develop as a complication of any systemic infection. Any infectious agent can produce osteomyelitis. These include bacteria, viruses, parasites, and fungi. But, the most common pathogens are pyogenic bacteria and mycobacteria.

- **Primary:** Where bone is the primary solitary focus of disease.
- **Secondary:** Develops as a complication of any systemic infection.

Pyogenic Osteomyelitis

Q. Write a short essay on pyogenic osteomyelitis.

Q. Write a short note on the etiology of osteomyelitis.

Etiology: Pyogenic osteomyelitis is almost always caused by bacterial infection.

- ***Staphylococcus* species:** The most common pathogens are *Staphylococcus* **species** (*Staphylococcus aureus* in 80–90% of the cases).
- **Other organisms:**
  - *Escherichia coli, Pseudomonas, Klebsiella, Neisseria gonorrhoeae, Haemophilus influenzae,* and *Salmonella* species.
  - *Escherichia coli* in patients with genitourinary tract infections or intravenous drug abusers.
  - **Neonatal period:** *Haemophilus influenzae* and group B streptococci.
  - **Patients with sickle cell disease:** *Salmonella* infection.
- **Mixed bacterial infections:** It is due to direct spread or surgery or open fractures.
- **No specific organism:** In about 50%, no organisms can be isolated.

Portal of entry of organism: Causative organisms may reach the bone through the **bloodstream, directly** or extend **from a contiguous site.**

- **Hematogenous spread:** It is the most common portal of entry of organisms.
- **Direct implantation:** Organisms may enter into the bone through penetrating wounds, open fractures, or surgical procedures (staphylococci, streptococci, anaerobic organisms).
  - **Spread from adjacent (contiguous) site:** For example, infections of the feet may spread into the bone in diabetics.

Location of osteomyelitis: The site of bone infections depends on the nature of blood circulation to the bone, which varies with age.

- **In children**, the most common sites affected by hematogenous osteomyelitis are the **metaphyseal area of the long bones (e.g., in the knee, ankle, and hip).** This is because of the unique vascular supply in this region (refer to pathogenesis underneath). In healthy children, most osteomyelitis is hematogenous in origin and more commonly occurs in the long bones.
- **In neonates**, metaphyseal vessels penetrate the growth plate. This results in frequent infection of the **metaphysis, epiphysis, or both.**
- **In adults, the epiphyses and subchondral regions** are more commonly involved. In adults, after growth plate closure, there is a merger of metaphyseal and epiphyseal vessels. This provides a route for bacterial spread to the epiphysis and subchondral regions. In adults, osteomyelitis most commonly develops as a complication of open fractures, surgical procedures, or diabetes (e.g., infections of the feet).

Pathogenesis of Hematogenous Osteomyelitis (Figs. 25.2A to D)

Q. Write a short note on pathogenesis and morphology of pyogenic osteomyelitis.

Age and gender affected: Hematogenous osteomyelitis usually affects **boys aged 5–15 years**. In otherwise healthy children, osteomyelitis is most commonly due to hematogenous spread.

Source of organisms: It may be a **focus of infection anywhere in the body** (e.g., skin pustule or infected teeth and gums, intestinal mucosa).

The sequence of events in osteomyelitis is as follows:

- **Transient bacteremia: Minor injuries** to the mucosa (such as may occur during defecation, vigorous chewing of hard foods, and brushing of teeth) or minor infections of the skin can initiate bacteremia by **releasing the causative organisms into the blood** (e.g., *Staphylococcus aureus*). This produces **temporary bacteremia, and the organism reaches the bone.**
- **Infection reaches metaphysis of long bone:** In the metaphysis, capillaries form a loop and drain into the medullary cavity without forming a capillary bed. This loop system causes slowing and prevents the smooth flow of blood. During bacteremia, this loop allows bacteria to penetrate blood vessel walls to initiate and establish infective foci within the marrow.
- **Inflammatory reaction**: Once in bone, the bacteria grow and induce an **acute neutrophilic inflammatory reaction with exudates.**
- **Necrosis of bone and marrow within the first 48 hours: Exudate increases the pressure** on the adjacent vessels which further **decreases the blood supply** and causes **bone necrosis.** The necrotic areas coalesce and allow **further bacterial proliferation.**
- **Spread of bacteria and inflammation**: The bacteria and inflammation spread longitudinally and radially throughout the haversian systems. The infection reaches the periosteum.
- **Formation of a subperiosteal abscess**: In children, the periosteum is loosely attached to the cortex. Bacterial **infections and pus may spread into the cortex** and collect beneath the periosteum. The periosteum may be detached from the underlying cortex by the inflammatory infiltrate. This may lead to the formation of a subperiosteal abscess that may be dissected along the bone surface.

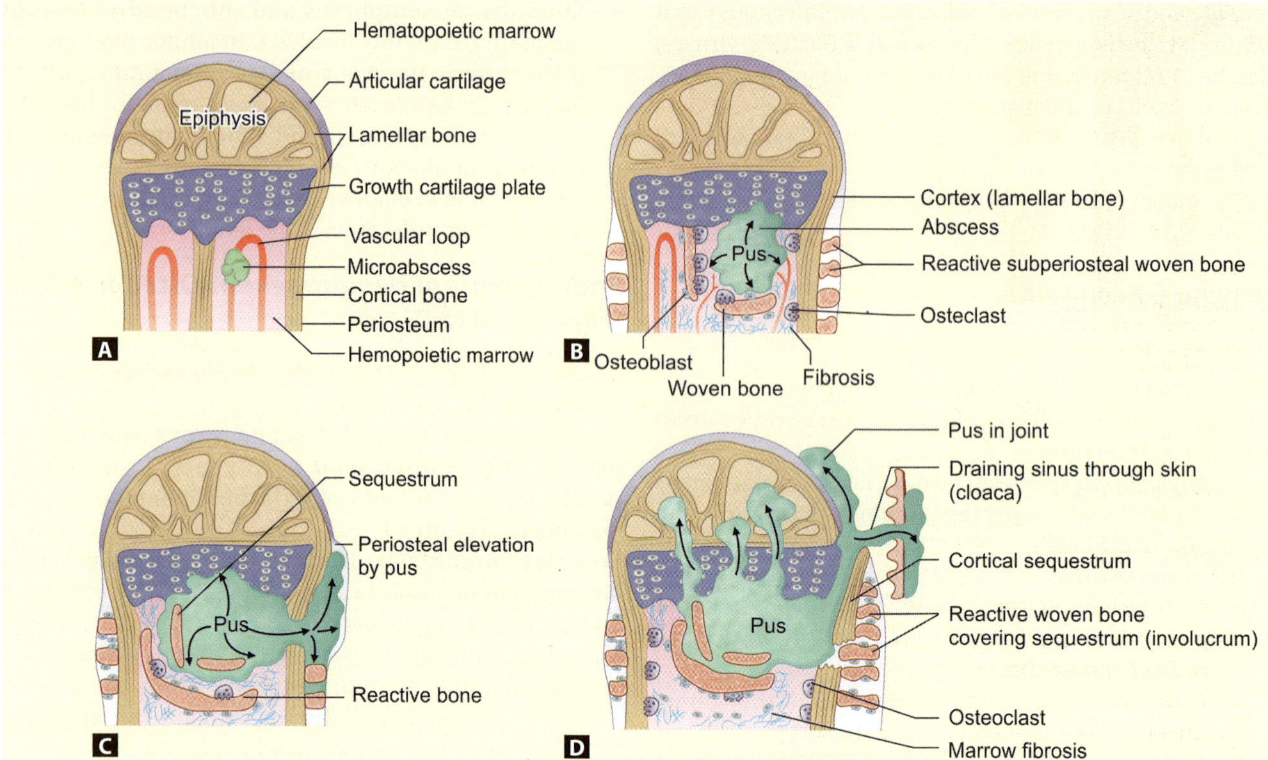

Figs. 25.2A to D: Pathogenesis of hematogenous osteomyelitis: (A) A small, septic microabscess is formed at the capillary loop; (B) Expansion of the septic focus stimulates resorption of adjacent bony trabeculae. The abscess expands and stimulates reactive bone formation by the periosteum; (C) The abscess continues to expand through the cortex into the subperiosteal tissue; and (D) The extension of this process into the skin produces a draining sinus.

Q. Write a short answer on sequestrum.

- **Formation of sequestrum: Pus** may **lift the periosteum** and **reduce the blood supply** to the affected region. This results in **segmental necrosis of the bone** due to both suppuration and ischemia. The fragment of a **dead necrotic piece of bone**, which is embedded in the pus, is known as a **sequestrum (Figs. 25.3B and D).**
- **Soft tissue abscess:** The **pus may rupture the periosteum** and lead to a **soft-tissue abscess.**
- **Draining sinus**: The soft tissue abscess may penetrate the skin to form a **draining sinus. A hole formed in the bone** during the formation of a draining sinus is known as a **cloaca**. The sinus tract may become epithelialized and may remain open, continually draining pus, necrotic bone, and bacteria.

Q. Write a short answer on involucrum.

- **Involucrum**: After the first week, chronic inflammatory cells become more numerous and the cytokines released stimulate osteoclastic bone resorption and **deposition of reactive bone in the periphery**. Reactive new bone forms a sheath around the necrotic (segment of devitalized infected bone) sequestrum. This **reactive new bone formed is known as involucrum (Fig. 25.3C).**

MORPHOLOGY

Q. Write a short essay on the morphology of pyogenic osteomyelitis.

The morphologic features **depend on the stage** (acute, subacute, or chronic) and location of the infection.

Gross

Sequestrum appears as a fragment of bone with ragged brownish-to-black colored margins **(Fig. 25.3B)**.

Microscopy (*refer* online Fig. 25.3A)

- **Acute osteomyelitis:** In the **initial stages**, only the **neutrophils** are seen.
- **Chronic osteomyelitis**: As the disease become chronic, the histologic findings are more variable. The neutrophils are admixed with chronic inflammatory cells (lymphocytes and plasma cells). But typically, it shows marrow fibrosis and sequestrum. Sequestrum does not show osteocytes and has empty lacunae.

Morphologic Variants of Osteomyelitis

- **Brodie abscess:** It is a distinctive form of **subacute pyogenic osteomyelitis.** It appears as a **small, solitary, intraosseous abscess localized to the metaphysis** and is surrounded by reactive bone. It may be **due to inadequate treatment of infection by less virulent organisms.**
- **Sclerosing osteomyelitis of Garré**: It is characterized by **extensive new bone formation,** which obscures the underlying structure of the bone and **typically develops in the jaw.**

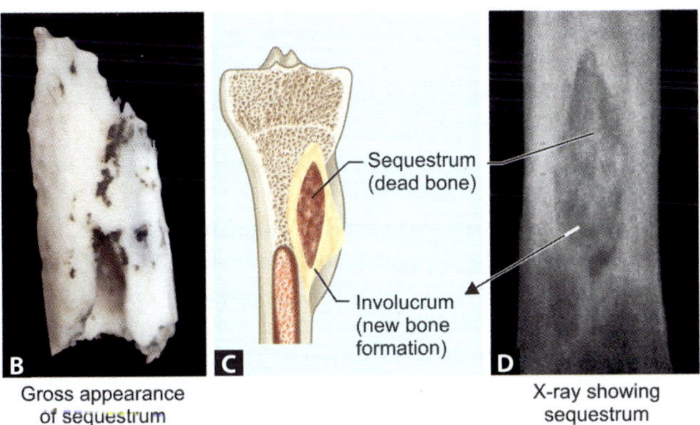

Figs. 25.3B to D: (B) Gross appearance of the necrotic bone in osteomyelitis is called a sequestrum; (C) The viable bone surrounding a sequestrum is termed the involucrum; (D) X-ray showing sequestrum.

Complications

Q. Write a short note on complications of pyogenic osteomyelitis.

- **Septicemia**: From infection in the bone, organisms may disseminate through the bloodstream and cause septicemia.
- **Acute suppurative arthritis**: Epiphyseal infection may spread through the articular surface or along capsular and tendoligamentous insertions into a joint. This may produce suppurative or septic arthritis. It may destroy the articular cartilage and lead to permanent disability. It is more common in infants.
- **Pathologic fractures:** Osteomyelitis may weaken the involved region and lead to fractures.
- **Squamous cell carcinoma:** It may arise from the epithelialized sinus tract, rarely sarcoma of bone may develop.
- **Secondary amyloidosis:** This was a common consequence of chronic osteomyelitis but is now rare in industrialized countries.
- **Chronic osteomyelitis:** It may develop due to delay in diagnosis, extensive bone necrosis, and inadequate therapy.

Clinical Features

Hematogenous osteomyelitis in children may present with malaise, **fever, chills, leukocytosis,** and **throbbing pain over the affected region**. On examination, it characteristically shows swelling, erythema, and tenderness over the involved bone.

Diagnosis

- **Imaging studies:** They are very helpful. These include conventional radiography, computed tomography (CT), magnetic resonance imaging (MRI), and bone scan. The characteristic radiographic finding suggestive of osteomyelitis is the lytic focus of bone destruction surrounded by a zone of sclerosis **(Figs. 25.3C and D)**.
- **Blood cultures** are positive.
- **Biopsy** and bone cultures.
- **Erythrocyte sedimentation rate (ESR) and C-reactive protein** are usually elevated but are not specific.

Tuberculous Osteomyelitis

Q. Write a short note on tuberculous osteomyelitis.

Tuberculous (mycobacterial) osteomyelitis is **usually solitary** but in patients with acquired immunodeficiency syndrome, it is frequently multifocal. It tends to be **more destructive and resistant to control** than pyogenic osteomyelitis.

- **Age**: Usually **adolescents or young adults** in developing countries.
- **Source of infection: Pulmonary or extrapulmonary** tuberculosis.
- **Predisposing factors:** Diabetes, elderly, immune compromised states, and general debility.
- **Mode of infection:**
  - **Blood borne**: Usually blood-borne infection, which is from a focus of **active pulmonary or extrapulmonary disease**.
  - **Direct extension**: From the lung into a rib or tracheobronchial nodes into adjacent vertebrae.

Sites Affected

Q. Write a short answer on Pott's spine.

- **Spine** (thoracic and lumbar vertebrae) commonly known as **Pott disease (tuberculous spondylitis).** The **infection breaks through intervertebral discs** to involve multiple vertebrae and **extends down into the soft tissues** forming abscesses (**cold abscess—psoas abscess**).
- **Knees and hips**.

MORPHOLOGY

Microscopy

It shows a dead bone surrounded by **tuberculous granuloma**. The granuloma consists of a central area of caseous necrosis surrounded by epithelioid cells and Langhans giant cells, which in turn are surrounded by lymphocytes (*refer* **online Fig. 25.4**). The epithelioid cells have a pale-pink granular cytoplasm with indistinct cell boundaries, often appearing to merge into one another. The nucleus is oval or elongate in shape.

Clinical features: It presents with low-grade fever with an evening rise in temperature, pain in motion, localized tenderness, and weight loss.

Complications: These include the following:

- **Spine:**
  - **Destruction of vertebrae**: Causes severe **scoliosis or kyphosis** and neurologic deficits due to spinal cord and nerve compression.
  - **Psoas abscess:** Infection from the spine may rupture into the soft tissue anteriorly and pus and necrotic

debris may drain along the spinal ligaments and form a **cold abscess, i.e., an abscess lacking acute inflammation.** **Psoas abscess** is the condition in which infection from lower lumbar vertebrae dissects along the pelvis, and appears as a draining sinus of the skin in the inguinal region. It may be the first manifestation of tuberculous spondylitis.

- **Tuberculous arthritis**
- **Sinus tract formation**
- **Amyloidosis**

PAGET DISEASE OF BONE (OSTEITIS DEFORMANS)

PA 33.4 (NC): Classify and describe the etiology, pathogenesis, manifestations, radiologic and morphologic features, and complications of Paget disease of the bone.

Q. Write a short note on Paget disease of bone.

Paget disease is a chronic progressive disorder characterized **by disordered bone remodeling**. In Paget disease, there is an **imbalance of osteoclastic and osteoblastic activities. Initially, it shows** predominantly **excessive** osteoclastic **bone resorption** that results in lytic lesions, **followed by osteoblastic activity** persisting late in the disease. This leads to **increased but disordered and structurally unsound bone mass.**

Age and gender: Paget disease usually presents in **late adulthood** and becomes progressively more common with increasing age. Paget disease often affects men and women older than 50 years of age. **Many** affected individuals **are asymptomatic.**

Pathogenesis: The cause of Paget's disease is unknown, but current evidence suggests both genetic and environmental contributions. It is considered an infectious (viral) etiology in genetically predisposed individuals.

- **Genetic predisposition:** About 50% are familial cases and 10% of sporadic cases show mutations in the *SQSTM1* gene. This gene encodes a protein known as sequestosome-1. These mutations increase the activity of NF-κB, which increases osteoclast activity. Some juvenile Paget diseases are due to activating mutations in *RANK* and inactivating mutations in *OPG.*
- **Environmental factors:** Infection of osteoclast precursors with viruses (e.g., measles or other RNA viruses) alters vitamin D sensitivity and IL-6 secretion. Both of them can lead to increased bone resorption.

MORPHOLOGY

Monostotic or polyostotic: The lesions of Paget disease may be solitary (monostotic) or involve multiple bones (polyostotic).

Bones involved: Paget disease tends to localize in **bones of the axial skeleton**. These include the **spine, skull, and pelvis**. In approximately 70% of cases, it involves the skull and temporal bones. In the polyostotic form of Paget's disease, the proximal femur and tibia may be involved.

Paget disease shows histologic variation throughout its course of disease and from site to site.

Phases (Fig. 25.5): Paget disease develops in three sequential phases.

1. **Initial osteolytic (osteoclastic) phase:** It is characterized by **numerous large osteoclasts** and resorption pits. The osteoclasts may have 100 or more nuclei. The findings are not specific.
2. **Mixed osteoclastic–osteoblastic stage: In this phase, there is both osteoclastic–and osteoblastic activity.** Osteoclasts persist but many of the bone surfaces are also lined by prominent osteoblasts. It progresses to the predominance of osteoblastic activity and evolves into the next final phase.
3. **Final burned-out quiescent osteosclerotic stage: The hallmark is a mosaic pattern of lamellar bone during the sclerotic phase.** The unusually **prominent cement lines,** which join haphazardly oriented units of lamellar bone produce a **jigsaw puzzle-like appearance.** During the sclerotic phase, the **bone is thickened but without structural stability.** Thus, the bone is **susceptible to deformation and fracture.**

Clinical Features

Paget disease may involve one bone (*monostotic)* in about 15% and multiple bones (*polyostotic)* in about 85% of cases. The axial skeleton or proximal femur is affected in up to 80% of cases. Most cases are asymptomatic. It usually begins in late adulthood. It is usually detected as an incidental radiographic finding.

Symptoms

- **Pain:** Commonly complains of pain localized to the involved bone. Pain may be due to microfractures or by bone overgrowth which may compress spinal and cranial nerve roots.
- **Enlargement of the craniofacial skeleton:** It may produce *leontiasis ossea* (lion face). The cranium becomes heavy and it becomes difficult to hold the head erect. The weakened Pagetic bone may cause invagination of the skull base *(platybasia)* and compression of the posterior fossa.
- **Leg bones:** Weight-bearing produces anterior bowing of the femurs and tibiae and may distort the femoral heads. It may result in severe *secondary osteoarthritis. Chalk stick–type fractures* may develop in the long bones of the lower extremities.
- **Compression fractures of the spine:** It may produce injury to the spinal cord and kyphosis.

Diagnosis

- **Radiological findings:** Diagnosis is usually done by the radiographic findings.
- **Raised serum alkaline phosphatase levels** but normal serum calcium and phosphorus.

Complications

Most of the patients have mild symptoms which are suppressed by treatment with calcitonin and

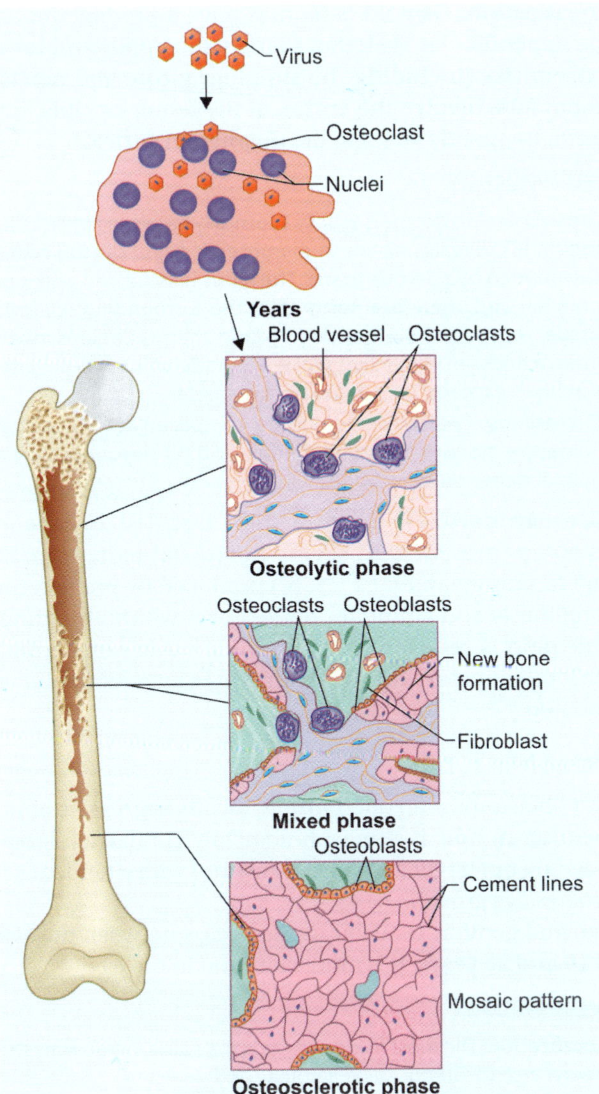

Fig. 25.5: Pathogenesis and schematic representation of three stages of Paget's disease of bone. Probably, a viral infection of osteoclastic progenitors or osteoclasts in a genetically predisposed individual stimulates osteoclastic activity. This leads to excessive resorption of bone. Over the years, the bone develops a characteristic mosaic pattern. This pattern is produced by haphazardly arranged units of lamellar bone that form irregular cement lines. The adjacent marrow usually undergoes fibrosis, and the surface of the bone shows a mixture of osteoclasts and osteoblasts.

bisphosphonates. However, a **variety of tumor and tumor-like conditions may develop in Pagetic bone. Secondary osteosarcoma may develop** in less than 1% of cases and about 5–10% in patients with severe polyostotic disease.

BONE TUMORS

PA 33.2 (CC): Classify and describe the etiology, pathogenesis, manifestations, radiologic and morphologic features, and complications and metastases of bone tumors.

Primary bone tumors and tumorlike lesions of bone are rare in daily clinical practice. Though certain bone lesions are common, they are usually without symptoms and indolent. Benign bone tumors are usually asymptomatic and identified incidentally. Bone tumors mainly constitute metastatic neoplasms and hematopoietic tumors. Bone sarcomas account for only 0.2% of neoplasms. Bone malignancies often require disfiguring surgery as a treatment, and they have poor survival rates.

Age: Bone sarcomas are mainly related to age. For example, the first peak of sarcoma is during the second decade of life, in which age-group osteosarcoma (during adolescence most frequently involves the knee) and Ewing sarcoma are most frequent. The second peak occurs in patients older than 60 years when chondrosarcoma forms the most frequent bone sarcoma and affects the pelvis and proximal extremities.

Distribution of bone tumors: The anatomic site of the bone lesion is essential. This is because some specific tumor types of bone preferentially affect particular areas of the skeleton. Most bone neoplasms have a tendency for the long bones of the extremities. *Refer* **online Fig. 25.6** for the specific location of a few bone tumors in the long bones.

Classification of Bone Tumors

The World Health Organization (WHO) (2020) classification of bone tumors **(Box 25.1)** is based on the normal cell types recapitulated (i.e., the differentiation of the tumor cells) and the extracellular matrix that is deposited (produced) by the tumor (e.g., chondrogenic tumors deposit cartilaginous matrix, and osteogenic tumors deposit osteoid).

Q. Classify bone tumors.

Q. Enlist bone forming and chondrogenic/cartilaginous tumors.

Osteogenic (Bone-forming) Tumors

Osteogenic (bone-forming) tumors are characterized by the production of unmineralized osteoid or mineralized woven bone by the tumor cells.

Osteoma

Osteoma is a **benign, slow-growing tumor arising on the surface of a bone**. It is **composed of the lamellar/dense, compact cortical-type bone**. Osteomas are usually asymptomatic and seldom require surgical treatment.

Localization: Osteomas mainly arise in the **calvarial, facial, and jaw bones**. They are rare outside the skull.

MORPHOLOGY

Gross: Osteomas **arise on the surface of the bone** and are usually **well-circumscribed** tumors with a **broad attachment to the underlying bone.**

Microscopy: Osteomas are mainly composed of mature lamellar/cortical-type bone.

BOX 25.1: World Health Organization (WHO) (2020) (abridged) classification of bone tumors.

Osteogenic (bone-forming) tumors

Benign

- Osteoma not otherwise specified (NOS)
- Osteoid osteoma NOS

Intermediate (locally aggressive)

- Osteoblastoma NOS

Malignant

- Low-grade central osteosarcoma (LGCOS)
- Osteosarcoma NOS
  - Conventional osteosarcoma
  - Telangiectatic osteosarcoma
  - Small cell osteosarcoma
- Parosteal osteosarcoma
- Periosteal osteosarcoma
- High-grade surface osteosarcoma
- Secondary osteosarcoma

Chondrogenic (cartilaginous) tumors

Benign

- Enchondroma
- Osteochondroma
- Chondroblastoma NOS
- Chondromyxoid fibroma

Intermediate (locally aggressive)

- Synovial chondromatosis
- Central atypical cartilaginous tumor/chondrosarcoma, grade 1 (ACT/CS1)
- Secondary peripheral atypical cartilaginous tumor/chondrosarcoma, grade 1 (ACT/CS1)

Malignant

- Central chondrosarcoma, grades 2 and 3
- Secondary peripheral chondrosarcoma, grades 2 and 3
- Periosteal chondrosarcoma
- Dedifferentiated chondrosarcoma

Osteoclastic giant cell-rich tumors

Benign

- Aneurysmal bone cyst
- Nonossifying fibroma

Intermediate (locally aggressive, rarely metastasizing)

- Conventional giant cell tumor of bone

Malignant

- Giant cell tumor of bone, malignant

Undifferentiated small round cell sarcomas of bone

- Ewing sarcoma of bone

Osteoid Osteomas

Q. Write a short note on osteoid osteoma.

Osteoid osteoma is a **benign, bone-forming** (bone-producing), **painful tumor** characterized by small size (<2 cm) and limited growth potential.

Age: Osteoid osteomas are most common in **young men in their teens and 20s**. Males are affected more often than females (3:1).

Localization: Osteoid osteomas have a predilection for the **appendicular skeleton, namely the upper and lower extremities (including the shoulder girdle and pelvis).** About **50% involve the cortex of the femur or tibia**. The lesion frequently arises in the **diaphyseal cortex.**

MORPHOLOGY

Gross: Osteoid osteoma is usually a cortically based and hyperemic tumor. It is usually **<2 cm in diameter.** It has a **central nidus surrounded by sclerotic tissue. The nidus is small, red gritty, or granular and, therefore, softer than the surrounding sclerotic tissue.** The nidus is **surrounded by (and sharply circumscribed from) a thick rim of reactive, ivory-white sclerotic, cortical bone. It seldom exceeds 1 cm in greatest diameter.**

Microscopy: Osteoid osteomas are composed of—**(i) central immature osseous tissue (the nidus) and (ii) surrounded by a halo of dense reactive bone.**

Clinical features: Despite their small size, osteoid osteomas present with **severe nocturnal pain** probably due to prostaglandin E2 (PGE_2) produced by proliferating osteoblasts and abundant nerve fibers within the tumor. This **pain is relieved by aspirin** and other nonsteroidal anti-inflammatory drugs. Treatment is by radiofrequency ablation.

Osteoblastoma

Osteoblastoma is an **uncommon, locally aggressive bone-forming tumor**. It is morphologically similar to osteoid osteoma but larger (usually >2 cm) and with a tendency to progressive growth.

Age and gender: Osteoblastoma occurs between the ages of **10 and 35 years**. It is more common in males.

MORPHOLOGY

Localization: The **most frequent site is the spine**, particularly the neural arch [posterior spine (laminae and pedicles)].

Gross

Osteoblastomas are usually **red to tan lesions** due to their intense vascularity. They have well-defined pushing borders. Osteoblastomas are **larger than 2 cm** (generally 3–10 cm).

Microscopy

Osteoblastoma is microscopically similar to osteoid osteoma.

Trabeculae of haphazardly arranged woven bone: Composed of randomly interconnecting delicate trabeculae of woven bone rimmed by a single layer of osteoblasts.

Loose and highly vascularized stroma: It is present between the trabeculae of woven bone and shows dilated and congested capillary-type blood vessels.

Clinical features: It is less painful and is not accompanied by the characteristic **nocturnal pain of osteoid osteoma.** The **pain does not respond to aspirin.** Treatment is by either curettage or excision.

Osteosarcoma

Q. Write a short note on osteosarcoma.

Osteosarcoma, or osteogenic sarcoma (OS), is a **highly malignant and the most common primary malignant tumor of bone**. It accounts for approximately 20% (one-fifth) of all bone cancers.

Formation (production) of bone matrix or osteoid (bone matrix) directly by malignant tumor cells: It is the hallmark of osteosarcoma.

Age and gender: Males are affected slightly more often than females (1.6:1). Osteosarcoma has a bimodal age distribution.

- **About 75%** occur in adolescents **between 10 and 20 years**.
- A **smaller peak occurs in older adults**. In these older adults, it is frequently associated with predisposing conditions such as **Paget disease, bone infarcts,** and **prior radiation** (sometimes called **secondary osteosarcomas**).

Classification (Box 25.2)

Q. Write a short note on the types of osteosarcoma.

Osteosarcoma is a collective name given to a **group of sarcomas** characterized by the production of osteoid directly by malignant tumor cells. Osteosarcoma can be **subdivided according to the site of origin** (intraosseous, surface, or soft tissue), **grade of malignancy** (low or high grade), and **differentiation** (e.g., osteoblastic, fibroblastic, and chondroblastic). Conventional osteosarcoma is described in detail. Conventional osteosarcoma is an **intramedullary high-grade malignant neoplasm** in which the **tumor cells produce bone**.

Localization

Conventional osteosarcoma is the prototypical osteosarcoma. Most of the information refers to this type. It can arise in any bone, but the **majority originate in the long bones of the extremities** which are the sites of the most proliferative growth plates. It usually arises near the knee or shoulder. Common sites include the following:

- **Lower end of the femur (30%)**
- **Upper end of the tibia (15%)** or fibula
- **Proximal humerus (15%),**

Usually metaphysis: In long bones, the tumor is usually found in the metaphysis (90%) and only infrequently in the diaphysis (9%) or rarely in the epiphysis.

BOX 25.2: Classification of osteosarcoma.

Low grade central osteosarcoma

Osteosarcoma

- Conventional osteosarcoma (classical, medullary, intramedullary, textbook)
  - Osteoblastic osteosarcoma
  - Chondroblastic osteosarcoma
  - Fibroblastic osteosarcoma
- Telangiectatic osteosarcoma
- Small cell osteosarcoma

Parosteal (juxtacortical) osteosarcoma arise on the surface of the cortex

Periosteal osteosarcomas arise on the surface of periosteum

High-grade surface osteosarcoma

Secondary osteosarcoma

Pathogenesis

Q. Describe the etiology and pathogenesis of osteosarcoma.

Based on the pathogenesis, osteosarcoma is divided into primary and secondary.

Primary osteosarcomas

In this type, the underlying bone is unremarkable.

Occurs during the speed of growth in adolescence: The **peak incidence of osteosarcoma is during the speed of growth in adolescence.** The tumor **occurs most frequently in the growth plate of rapidly growing bones**. These regions show increased proliferation and may predispose to mutations that drive oncogenesis.

Etiology unknown: The etiology of osteosarcoma is unknown.

Genetic abnormalities: There is an increased incidence of primary osteosarcoma associated with several genetic abnormalities or syndromes. Conventional osteosarcomas have complex karyotypes with multiple nonspecific numerical and structural chromosomal aberrations. Increased incidence is observed with several genetic syndromes, including **Li-Fraumeni and hereditary retinoblastoma**. Genetic abnormalities are usually associated with mutations in well-known tumor suppressor genes and oncogenes.

Mutations in tumor suppressor genes: These include the following:

- ***RB* (Retinoblastoma) gene mutations: RB protein is** a cell cycle regulator. Retinoblastoma gene mutations are observed in up to 70% of sporadic osteosarcomas. Germline mutations in the *RB* gene are associated with a 1,000-fold increased risk of osteosarcoma.
- **Inactivation of tumor protein 53 (*TP53*) gene:** Many patients show mutations in the *TP53* gene. Individuals with **Li-Fraumeni syndrome have inactivation of the *TP53* gene due to germline mutations**. These individuals have a greatly increased incidence of osteosarcoma. Abnormalities that interfere with p53 function are **also common in sporadic osteosarcomas.**
- **Inactivation of *CDKN2A* (cyclin-dependent kinase inhibitor 2A) gene (also known as INK4α):** This gene encodes two tumor suppressors, p16 (a negative regulator of cyclin-dependent kinases) and p14(it augments the function of tumor suppressor gene *p53*). *CDKN2A* is **inactivated in many osteosarcomas.**

- **Overexpression of *MDM2* and *CDK4*:** They are cell cycle regulators. *MDM2 inhibits* the function of p53 and *CDK4* inhibits the RB function. They are over-expressed in many low-grade osteosarcomas.

***MYC* amplification:** It is seen in up to 50% of osteosarcomas and may be associated with a poor prognosis.

Secondary osteosarcomas

Osteosarcomas in older persons almost always develop in association with pre-existing bone disorders (secondary osteosarcoma). These include:

- **Paget disease of bone:** Osteosarcoma occurs in the areas of active growth of **Paget disease.**
- **Following radiation exposure:** Radium watches dial painters, who wetted their brushes by licking them, developed osteosarcomas many years later. Presently, secondary osteosarcoma usually develops in adults and children previously subjected to **external therapeutic radiation for some other malignancy (e.g., lymphoma).**
- **Pre-existing benign bone lesions.** Several preexisting benign bone lesions are associated with an increased risk of developing osteosarcoma. These include **fibrous dysplasia, osteomyelitis, and bone infarcts.** Trauma may call attention to an existing osteosarcoma rather than causing the tumor.

MORPHOLOGY

Q. Describe the gross, microscopy, and radiological appearance of osteosarcoma.

Conventional Osteosarcoma

Gross (Figs. 25.7A and B)

- The gross appearance is highly variable. It **depends on the proportions of bone, cartilage, stroma, and blood vessels.**
- **Region of the bone involved:** Usually arises in the **metaphyseal region of the long bones** of the extremities.
- **Sites:** It usually arises near the knee or shoulder. The common sites include the lower femur, upper tibia, or fibula, and proximal humerus.
- **Big bulky tumor:** Conventional osteosarcoma usually presents as a **large** (bulky **>5–10 cm**) **intramedullary mass.**
- **Cut surface: Gray-white, gritty,** and shows **areas of hemorrhage and cystic degeneration.** It tends to destroy the surrounding cortices and invade into soft tissue.

Microscopy (Figs. 25.8A and B)

Q. Write a short note on microscopic types of osteosarcoma.

Malignant Tumor Cells

- **High-grade hypercellular tumor:** Osteosarcomas are high-grade hypercellular tumors.
- **Anaplasia, pleomorphic neoplastic cells:** Tumor cells vary in size and shape (severe anaplasia, pleomorphic neoplastic cells).

  The tumor cells may be fusiform, plasmacytoid, epithelioid, polygonal, or spindle-shaped. **Bizarre tumor giant cells** are common.
- **Large, atypical, pleomorphic,** and **hyperchromatic nucleus:** The tumor cells usually show large, atypical, pleomorphic, and hyperchromatic nuclei. The tumor cells show a **high nucleus-to-cytoplasmic ratio.**
- **Numerous mitoses,** including **numerous atypical mitotic figures (e.g., tripolar),** are commonly seen.

Neoplastic Bone Formation

Production of **osteoid** (unmineralized/noncalcified) **or bone** (calcified osteoid) **by malignant tumor cells:** Diagnosis of osteosarcoma requires the presence of malignant tumor cells directly **producing unmineralized osteoid or mineralized bone.**

- **Unmineralized osteoid:** It appears as a **dense, uniform, eosinophilic glassy intercellular material.**
- **Mineralized bone:** It usually has a fine and lace-like architecture.

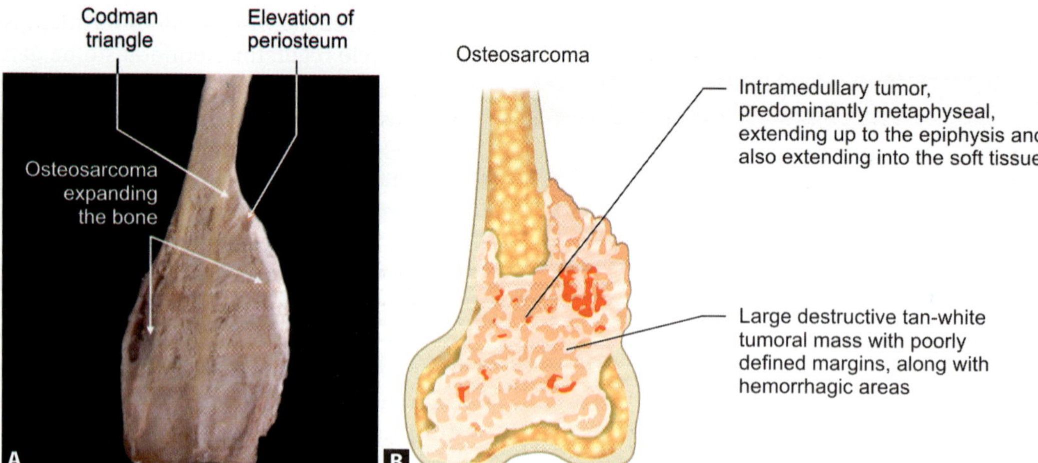

Figs. 25.7A and B: (A) Specimen; and (B) Diagrammatic. The gross appearance of the conventional osteosarcoma from the distal femur shows a tan-white tumor, filling most of the medullary cavity of the metaphysis and proximal diaphysis. The tumor has infiltrated through the cortex and lifted the periosteum, and this region on X-ray appears as a Codman triangle.

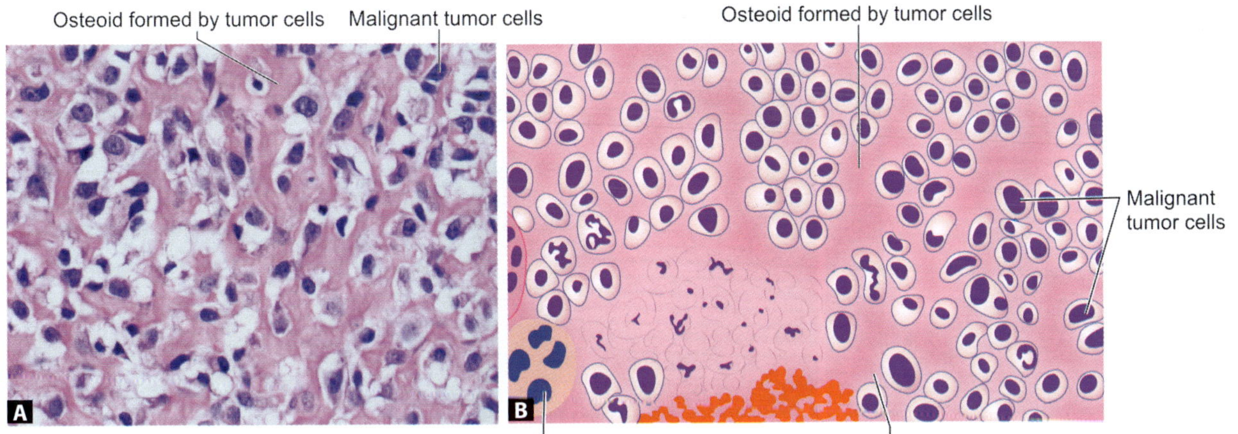

Figs. 25.8A and B: Microscopy of osteosarcoma: (A) H&E and (B) Diagrammatic. Conventional osteosarcoma showing pleomorphic tumor cells separated by osteoid.

Other features: Extensive **necrosis** and intravascular invasion are also common.

Histological Patterns (Subtypes) of Conventional Osteosarcoma

Osteosarcomas may show different histological patterns, and historically, it has been subclassified based on the predominant matrix (osteoblastic, chondroblastic, or fibroblastic). However, there is no relationship between histological patterns, treatment, and prognosis. Most tumors contain a **mixture of cells with varying amounts of matrices. Depending on the one predominant matrix**, conventional OS is **divided into**:

- **Osteoblastic (70–80%)**: In this type, neoplastic bone is the principal matrix (a **large amount of osteoid and bony trabeculae**).
- **Chondroblastic (10–13%):** It contains **abundant malignant cartilage**.
- **Fibroblastic (10%):** In this, the malignant cells are usually spindle-shaped and less frequently epithelioid.

Other Osteosarcomas

Telangiectatic: It shows many **large, cystic spaces filled with blood clots** separated by highly cellar **large septae** and it is **more aggressive**.

Small cell: The tumor **cells are small, and uniform** and simulate the appearance of Ewing's sarcoma and malignant lymphoma.

Immunohistochemistry: The malignant tumor cells **stain prominently for alkaline phosphatase** and **osteonectin**.

Radiological Appearance (Figs. 25.9A to C)

Q. Write a short note on radiological features/Codman triangle.

Radiographically, the enlarging osteosarcoma forms a **large, destructive, mixed lytic** (bone destruction) and **blastic mass** (neoplastic bone formation) with infiltrative margins.

Codman triangle: Osteosarcoma frequently **infiltrates** and **breaks through the cortex. The tumor lifts the periosteum from the bone** and produces a **space between the cortex and the lifted ends of the periosteum**. Radiologically, the **triangular shadow between the cortex and raised (lifted) periosteal ends is known as a Codman triangle**. The Codman triangle is a radiologic sign seen **characteristically in osteosarcoma but is not diagnostic** of this sarcoma. The Codman triangle indicates an aggressive tumor most commonly on musculoskeletal plain films. The **space** mainly contains **reactive new bone, which is arranged perpendicular to the bone surface**, but it may also contain malignant tumors.

Codman triangle may also be seen in aggressive lesions such as Ewing sarcoma, osteomyelitis, active aneurysmal bone cyst, giant cell tumor, metastasis, chondrosarcoma (especially juxtacortical chondrosarcoma), and malignant fibrous histiocytoma

Sunburst appearance: When the malignant **tumor extends into soft tissue, parallel lines of mineral deposition** in the **periosteal region** give an appearance of rays of the sun called a "sunburst" appearance **(Figs. 25.9A to C)**.

Spread of Osteosarcoma

Local spread

Spread along the medullary (marrow) cavity: Tumor often spreads within the marrow cavity and may show extensive involvement of the medullary canal, and replace hematopoietic marrow.

Invasion of the adjacent cortex and destroys the nearby cortex.

Elevation or perforation of the periosteum and extension into the soft tissues: The tumor frequently breaks through the cortex, invading adjacent soft tissues to produce soft tissue masses. This usually forms an eccentric or circumferential soft tissue mass that elevates the periosteum peripherally or perforates the periosteum.

Extension into the epiphysis: Tumors infrequently penetrate the epiphyseal plate or even reach the joint space.

Blood spread

Osteosarcoma is an aggressive tumor, which may spread through the bloodstream to the **lungs**. Less commonly, it may metastasize to other bones, the pleura, the brain, and the heart.

Clinical Features

- **Pain in the involved regions:** Osteosarcoma often presents with **mild or intermittent pain around the**

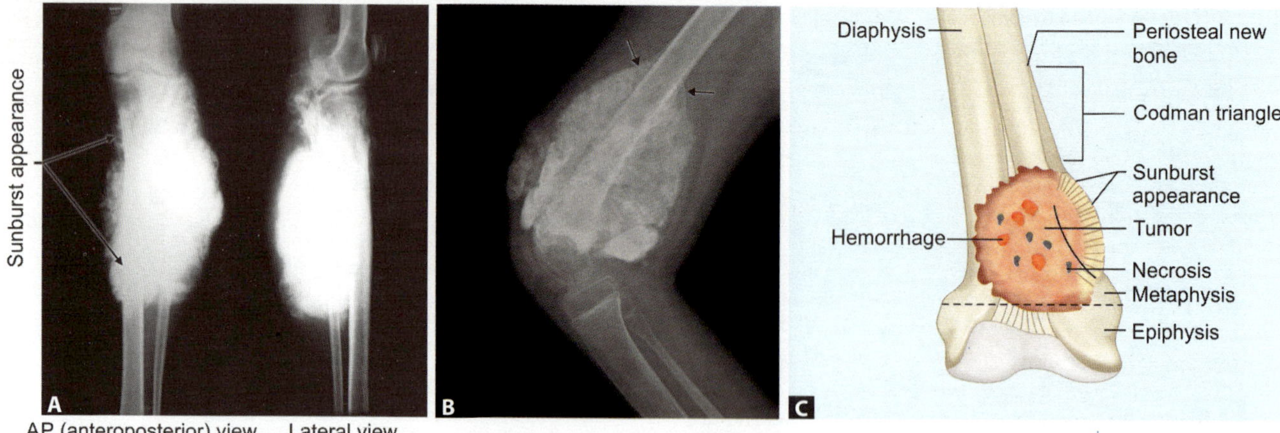

Figs. 25.9A to C: Radiological features of osteosarcoma: (A) X-ray of the osteosarcoma involving proximal tibia extending into the soft tissue with parallel lines of mineral deposition giving rise to sunburst appearance; (B) Radiologic appearance of osteosarcoma showing Codman's triangle (arrows); (C) Diagrammatic representation of Codman's triangle and sunburst appearance of osteosarcoma involving the metaphysis of the lower end of the femur.

involved area. Sometimes, the pain may be due to pathologic fractures.

- **Progressively enlarging mass:** As the pain intensifies, **the area becomes swollen and tender and produces a palpable mass**. The function of the adjacent joint becomes limited.
- **Serum alkaline phosphatase is increased in 50% of patients.** It may decrease after amputation, only to increase again with recurrence or metastasis.

Treatment: All osteosarcoma patients may have occult metastases at the time of diagnosis. Hence, treatment generally includes neoadjuvant chemotherapy, surgery, and postoperative adjuvant chemotherapy.

Surface Osteosarcoma

Surface osteosarcomas occur in association with the bone surface rather than in the medullary cavity. The majority of these are low-grade tumors. These **include parosteal osteosarcoma and periosteal osteosarcoma.**

- **Parosteal osteosarcoma** is a rare, **low-grade malignant bone-forming neoplasm** that arises on the cortical surface of a bone. It **grows along the external surface** of the bone, **both linearly and longitudinally**, without involving the medullary cavity. **The prognosis for this type of osteosarcoma is excellent.**
- **Periosteal osteosarcoma** is an **intermediate-grade malignant cartilage and bone-forming sarcoma that arises on the surface of the bone**, typically **below the periosteum** (between the cortex and periosteum). Microscopically, it is a **high-grade osteosarcoma** and characteristically has a predominant cartilage component.

SCENARIO-BASED ESSAY QUESTION

Q. An 18-year-old male presented to the orthopedic department with a complaint of pain and progressive swelling around his right knee for the past 3 months. Physical findings showed a diffuse hard swelling with local pain over the area of the distal right femur. An X-ray of the right knee showed an ill-defined mass involving the metaphyseal region of the distal right femur with elevation of the adjacent periosteum. A bone biopsy specimen was obtained and it confirmed the provisional clinical diagnosis.

a. **What is the probable diagnosis? (Ans: Osteosarcoma lower end of femur).**
b. **Describe the morphological appearance of the lesion (*refer pages 918-9*).**
c. **What are the salient radiological appearances of this disease? (*refer page 919*).**

Chondrogenic (Cartilaginous) Tumors

Cartilaginous tumors constitute the majority of benign and malignant primary bone tumors. These tumors **form hyaline cartilage.** Benign cartilage tumors are much more common than malignant lesions.

Osteochondroma

- **Most common benign tumor:** Osteochondroma (exostosis) is the most common benign cartilage-capped tumor. **It arises from the bone surface.**
- **Sessile or pedunculated**: It may be sessile or pedunculated (attaches to the underlying bone by a bony stalk). It is **covered by a cartilage cap.**
- **Age and gender:** About **85% of osteochondromas are solitary and sporadic**. The remaining 15% are multiple and hereditary and occur as part of autosomal dominant multiple hereditary exostosis syndromes. Solitary osteochondroma usually presents **during late adolescence and early adulthood**. Multiple osteochondromas are usually apparent during childhood. **Males are affected three times** more often than females.

Pathogenesis: Hereditary exostoses are associated with germline loss-of-function **mutations in either the *EXT1* or**

the *EXT2* gene. Reduced expression of EXT1 or EXT2 may also occur in sporadic osteochondromas.

MORPHOLOGY

Site and location: Arise from the **metaphysis near the growth plate** of **long tubular bones**, especially about the knee (the **distal femur and proximal tibia**).

Gross: Osteochondromas show a **bony stalk with underlying cortical and cancellous bone covered by a cartilage cap (Fig. 2510A).** It may be **sessile, or pedunculated** and range in size from 1 to 20 cm. The **cap is composed of benign hyaline cartilage and the underlying bone is lamellar in nature.**

Microscopy (Fig. 25.10B): Osteochondroma has cartilage cap, and bone and is covered by perichondrium.

1. **Cartilage cap:** It is composed of benign **hyaline cartilage**.
2. **Bone:** The bony stalk comprises of **cortical lamellar bone**, and the medullary cavity contains lamellar bone trabeculae with fatty and/or hematopoietic marrow.

Clinical features: Most osteochondromas are **asymptomatic** and many are detected incidentally. Osteochondromas **present as slow-growing masses**.

Chondrosarcoma

Q. Write a short note on chondrosarcoma.

Chondrosarcomas are **malignant tumors** characterized by the **production of neoplastic cartilage.** After osteosarcoma, chondrosarcoma is the second most common primary malignant matrix-producing tumor of bone. They account for about 20% of all primary malignant tumors of the bone.

Age and gender: Chondrosarcoma is most frequently seen in individuals between 5th to 7th decades (usually around **40 years or older**). Men are affected twice as frequently as women.

Subclassification: The term *chondrosarcoma* describes a heterogeneous group of tumors with diverse morphologic features and clinical behavior. World Health Organization (2020) subclassification of malignant cartilaginous tumors is presented in **Box 25.3**. Chondrosarcoma may be primary (without known pre-existing lesion) or secondary chondrosarcoma (developing in a pre-existing lesion such as enchondroma, solitary osteochondroma, and hereditary multiple osteochondromas). According to the anatomic site, it may be termed central (intramedullary about 90%) or peripheral (juxtacortical and surface), which is common and arises outside the bone.

BOX 25.3: Subclassification of malignant cartilaginous tumors.

- Central atypical cartilaginous tumor/chondrosarcoma, grade 1
- Secondary peripheral atypical cartilaginous tumor/chondrosarcoma, grade 1
- Central chondrosarcoma, grades 2 and 3
- Secondary peripheral chondrosarcoma, grades 2 and 3
- Periosteal chondrosarcoma
- Dedifferentiated chondrosarcoma

Pathogenesis

Chondrosarcomas are genetically heterogeneous. Few of them produce reproducible abnormalities. Chondrosarcomas arising in multiple osteochondroma syndrome show mutations in the *EXT* genes. Sporadic chondrosarcomas may show *IDH1* and *IDH2* mutations, mutation of the collagen *COL2A1* gene, and silencing of the *CDKN2A* tumor suppressor gene by DNA methylation.

MORPHOLOGY

Q. Write a short note on the morphology of chondrosarcoma.

Central conventional chondrosarcoma: It consists of malignant hyaline and myxoid cartilage.

Location

Chondrosarcomas commonly arise in the **central medullary cavity** of **pelvic bones, shoulder, ribs, and long bones.**

Gross (Fig. 25.11A)

Large bulky tumors, and consist of **nodules of gray-white/light-blue with translucent glistening areas (represents cartilage).**

Cut section:

- **Mucoid/myxoid feel** and the matrix may ooze from the cut surface.

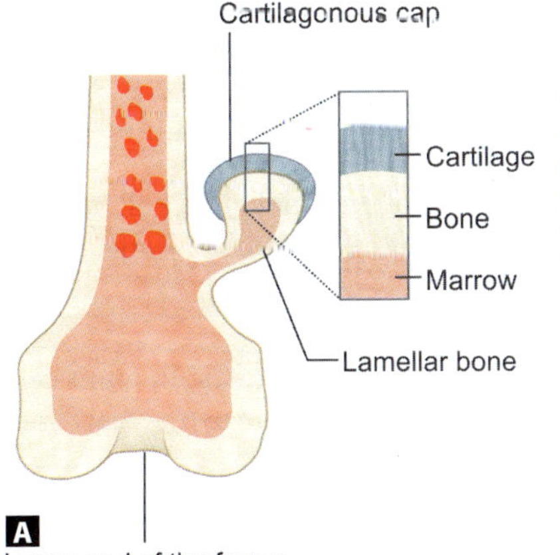

Figs. 25.10A and B: (A) Osteochondroma appears as a mushroom-shaped tumor covered by cartilage; (B) Microscopy of osteochondroma showing a cap composed of benign hyaline cartilage and underlying lamellar bone.

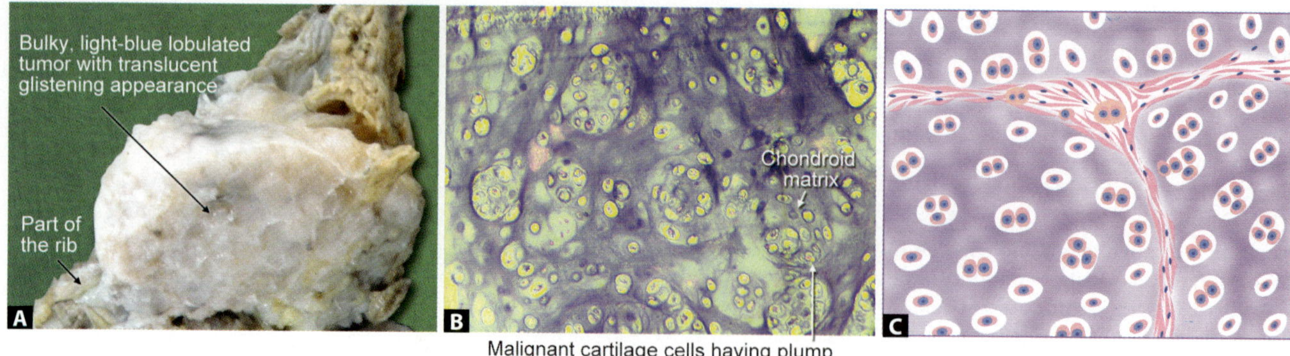

Figs. 25.11A to C: (A) Gross appearance of grade 1 chondrosarcoma of rib. The cut section shows typical translucent, bluish-gray, or grayish-white lobular tumor tissue; (B) H&E and (C) Diagrammatic. Chondrosarcoma grade 1 showing a lobular growth pattern, with abundant predominantly hyaline cartilaginous matrix and low cellularity.

- **Spotty calcifications** are common and appear as white gritty areas.
- **Central area of necrosis** may produce cystic spaces. The adjacent cortex may show thickening or erosion.

Microscopy

It consists of **malignant cartilage cells** in **various stages of maturity.** Tumors vary in cellularity, cytologic atypia, and mitotic activity and are graded from 1 to 3.

Low-grade or Grade 1 (Fig. 25.11B)

- Mild hypercellularity with lobular growth pattern.
- **Cells: Chondrocytes show plump vesicular nuclei with small nucleoli. Binucleate cells** are **few** in number.
- **Mitotic figures** are **rare.**
- **Matrix:** Portions of the matrix frequently mineralize, and the cartilage may undergo endochondral ossification.

Grade 2

It is separated from grade 1 predominantly based on **increased cellularity, a greater degree of nuclear atypia,** hyperchromasia, and nuclear size. Mitoses, although scarce, can be seen. The matrix appears more myxoid.

Grade 3

The tumor is **highly cellular and more pleomorphic with nuclear atypia.** Mitoses can be more easily identified. The cells at the periphery of the mostly myxoid tumor lobules are spindled (spindle cell change) and less differentiated.

Radiological appearance

Shows a tumor in the **medullary cavity** with **poorly defined borders.** The shaft is thickened and the tumor perforates the cortex. The calcified matrix (**popcorn calcification**) appears as foci of **flocculent densities** with **ring-like ossifications.**

Clinical features: Chondrosarcomas usually manifest as **painful, progressively enlarging masses.** The biologic behavior of the tumor depends on the histological grade. Most conventional chondrosarcomas are grade 1 tumors.

Spread

- **Local spread:** Locally aggressive tumor. It may **infiltrate the marrow space** and may grow with broad pushing fronts into the **surrounding soft tissue.**
- **Hematogenous spread:** Lungs and skeleton.

Osteoclastic Giant Cell-rich Tumors

Osteoclastic giant cells can be found in several different bone lesions. These include neoplastic (benign and malignant), reactive, and metabolic lesions (*refer* **Box 25.1**). The mononuclear cell compartment, combined with the size and distribution of the giant cells, helps diagnose these lesions.

Giant-cell Tumor of Bone

Q. Write a short note on giant-cell tumor/osteoclastoma.

A giant cell tumor (GCT) of bone is a **locally aggressive, relatively uncommon,** and **rarely metastasizing tumor.** It is composed of **neoplastic mononuclear stromal cells, and numerous, randomly and uniformly distributed multinucleate osteoclast-like giant cells. It was also called *osteoclastoma*, and this terminology is not recommended.** It is **usually a benign** tumor, but **small subsets** of giant cell tumors **are malignant.**

Age and gender: It usually arises in the **third through fifth decades** (between **20 and 40 years**) of life. In the elderly, it may be secondary to irradiation. It has a slight predilection for women.

Subtype(s): These are—(1) conventional giant cell tumors of bone and (2) malignant giant cell tumors of bone.

Pathogenesis

The majority are nonneoplastic osteoclasts: In giant cell tumors, most of the cells are **nonneoplastic osteoclasts and their precursors.**

Neoplastic cells are primitive osteoblast precursors: The neoplastic cells of giant cell tumors are **primitive**

osteoblast precursors. They **form only a minority of the cells**. These neoplastic cells produce RANKL and **express high levels of RANKL. RANKL** promotes the **proliferation of osteoclast precursors** and **their differentiation into mature osteoclasts.**

Absence of normal regular feedback between osteoblasts and osteoclasts: This results in localized, highly destructive, bone resorption.

MORPHOLOGY

Q. Write a short essay on gross, microscopy, and radiological features of giant cell tumors.

Localization: Giant-cell tumors occur in the **epiphyses but may extend into the metaphysis** of a **long bone**.

Bones involved: Any bone can be involved, the majority arise in:

- **Knee area: Distal femur and proximal tibia.**
- **Lower end of radius, humerus, and fibula.**

Gross (Figs. 25.12A and B)

The gross appearance of a giant cell tumor is usually **quite characteristic.**

- It is a **circumscribed lesion**. It **often lies eccentrically within the end of a long bone**, which is typically **asymmetrically expanded**. They **frequently undergo a cystic change.**
- **Cut surface:** It is **soft and dark brown (red-brown) and has a hemorrhagic appearance** without bone or calcification. **Numerous hemorrhagic areas** give it the **appearance of a sponge full of blood.**

Microscopy (Figs. 25.13A and B)

Two types of cells: A giant cell tumor is a highly cellular tumor with two main types of cells—(1) the mononuclear ("stromal") cells and (2) large osteoclast-like multinucleated cells.

1. Mononuclear (Stromal) Cells

They are of two types.

i. **Neoplastic mononuclear cells:** They are **uniform oval and plump** with **large nuclei, prominent nucleoli,** and **scanty cytoplasm.** Tumor mostly consists of these neoplastic cells. Mitotic activity is common in these cells but not found in the giant cells. **Diagnosis of malignancy depends upon the morphology of the mononuclear cells rather than that of the multinucleated giant cells.** The nuclei of these cells and the osteoclasts are similar. Thus, it is difficult to identify the neoplastic osteoblast precursors on routine histology. The tumor cells do not synthesize bone or cartilage.
ii. **Nonneoplastic macrophages:** These are mononuclear cells derived from macrophage–monocyte.

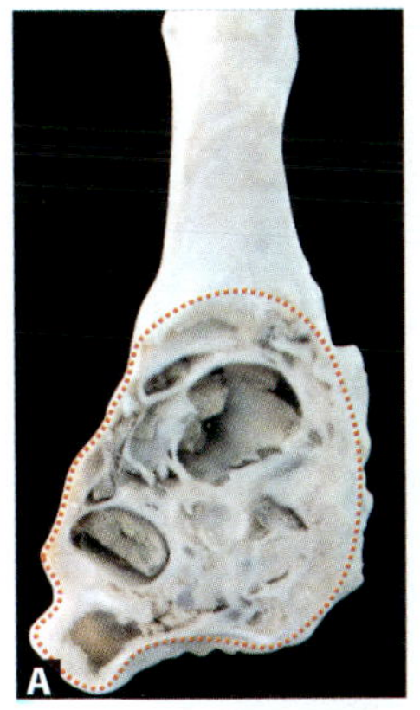
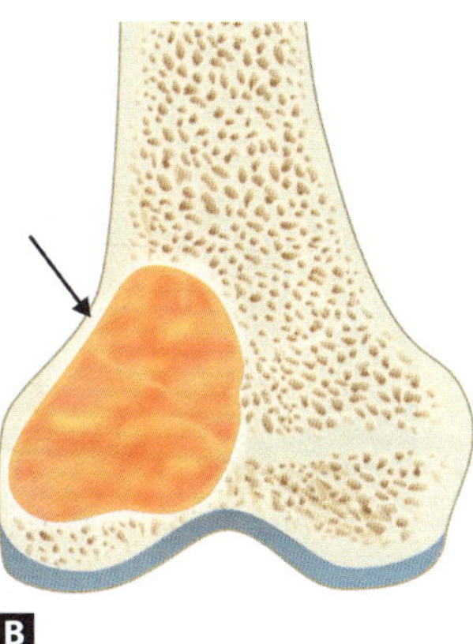

Figs. 25.12A and B: Gross appearance of giant-cell tumor of bone: (A) Grossly shows a circumscribed, eccentrically placed tumor with hemorrhage and cystic spaces (within dotted lines); (B) Diagrammatic appearance.

2. Large Multinucleated (Osteoclastic) Giant Cells

- The **background** shows **numerous large osteoclast-type giant cells** throughout the richly vascularized stroma.
- These **cells have 100 or more nuclei**, which resemble those of the mononuclear cells.

An area of cystic degeneration, necrosis, and mitotic figures may be seen.

Secondary features: These include areas of **hemorrhage, necrosis**, hemosiderin deposition, and reactive bone formation.

Radiological appearance

Q. Write a short answer on the radiological features of giant cell tumors.

- Giant cell tumors cause eccentric, expansile, and **lytic lesions.** It **grows slowly, expands the bone,** and **destroys the overlying cortex.**

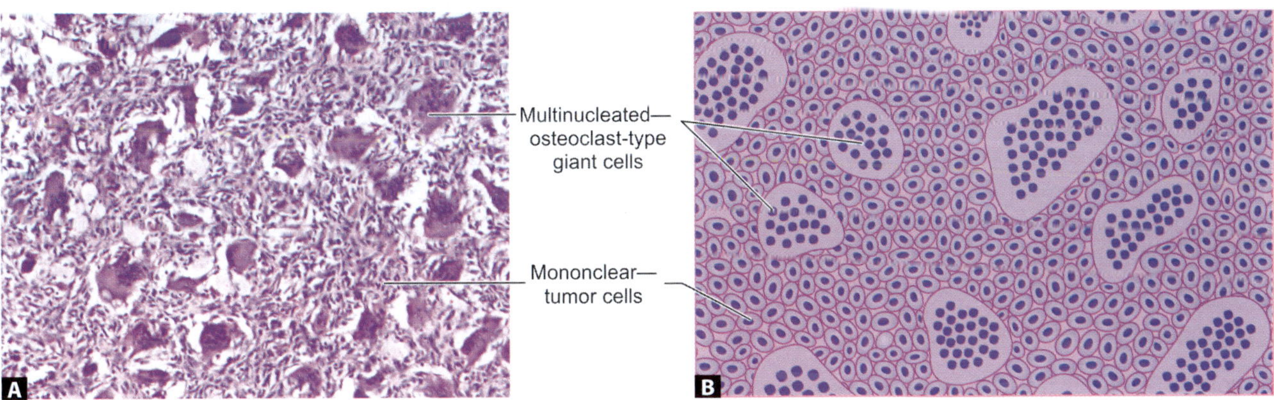

Figs. 25.13A and B: Microscopic appearance of giant-cell tumor of bone: (A) Photomicrograph; (B) Diagrammatic shows numerous multinucleated giant cells. The background shows mononuclear stromal cells.

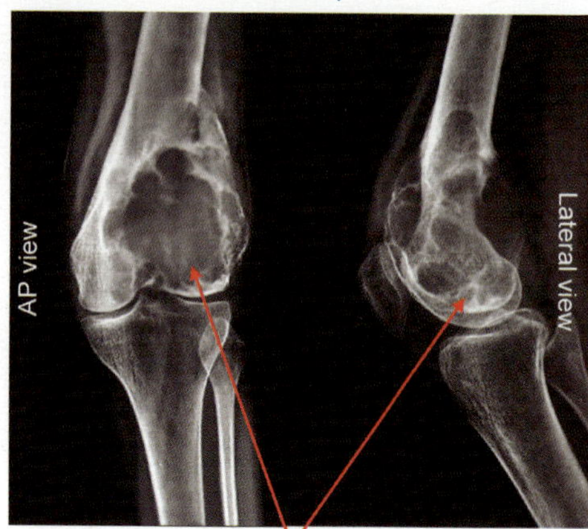

Fig. 25.14: X-ray of the knee joint. Giant cell tumor of the distal femur showing soap-bubble appearance.

- The tumor produces a bulging **soft tissue mass surrounded by a thin, shell of reactive bone** due to periosteal reaction. This on radiology has a multiloculated or **soap-bubble** appearance **(Fig. 25.14)** due to endosteal resorption of the bone.

Primary malignancy giant cell tumor: It is uncommon. It typically appears as an area of high-grade sarcoma containing highly pleomorphic, neoplastic mononuclear cells within an otherwise conventional giant cell tumor of bone.

Refer **online Box 25.4** for giant cell lesions of bone and synovium.

Q. Write a short answer on giant cell lesions of bone and synovium.

Clinical Features

- Most commonly occurs in the **distal femur and proximal tibia**.
- Giant cell tumors present with **pain and swelling**, usually in the joint adjacent to the tumor. They typically arise near joints and may cause arthritis-like symptoms.
- Microfractures and pathologic fractures may develop due to thinning of the cortex.

Biologic behavior: The majority of GCTs behave in a **benign fashion**, but **locally aggressive tumors may locally recur**. However, **all GCTs** must be **considered as potentially malignant**, because they may metastasize.

Spread

- **Local spread**: Tumor is usually restricted within the involved bone surrounded by periosteum. Aggressive tumors may penetrate the cortex and the periosteum and may involve the joint capsule and the synovial membrane.
- **Hematogenous spread:** The common site is the lung.

SCENARIO-BASED ESSAY QUESTION

Q. A 30-year-old female complains of pain in the region of her left knee for the past month. On physical examination, there is tenderness on palpation of the distal left thigh. The area is firm, but there is no erythema or warmth. An X-ray showed a five-centimeter mass involving the distal femoral epiphyseal region with a "soap bubble" appearance. The biopsy confirmed the clinical diagnosis.

a. **What is the probable diagnosis? (Ans: Giant cell tumor of the lower end of the femur)**
b. **Describe the morphological appearance of the lesion** *(refer pages 923-4)*.
c. **What are the salient radiological appearances of this disease?** *(refer pages 923-4)*.

Undifferentiated Small Round Cell Sarcomas of Bone

Ewing sarcoma is an undifferentiated small round cell sarcoma of bone.

Ewing Sarcoma of Bone

Q. Write a short note on Ewing sarcoma.

Ewing sarcoma (EWS) is an **uncommon** (only 5% of all bone tumors), **high-grade small round cell sarcoma characterized by primitive small, uniform, round cells without obvious differentiation.**

Uncommon tumor: Ewing sarcomas account for approximately 6–10% of primary malignant bone tumors.

Age and gender: It occurs in **children and adolescents** (between **10 and 15 years** of age), and **approximately 80% of patients are younger than 20 years of age**. It forms the **second most common group of bone sarcomas in children**, the first being osteosarcoma. Boys are affected slightly more often than girls (2:1).

Pathogenesis

Ewing sarcoma shows **gene fusions** involving **one member of the FET** (FUS, EWSR1, and TAF15) family of genes (usually EWSR1) **and a member of the ETS** (*FLI1*/friend leukemia integration 1) family of transcription factors.

EWSR1/FLI1* fusion genes**: About >95% of Ewing sarcoma are associated with structural rearrangements in genes producing pathognomonic recurrent **balanced reciprocal translocation between the *FLI1 gene on **chromosomes 11** and the *EWSR1* gene **on chromosome 22** [t(11;22)(q24;q12)]. This **translocation generates a novel *FET-ETS (EWSR1/FLI1)* fusion gene** that is crucial to the pathogenesis of Ewing sarcoma. This **fusion activates the C-myc promoter leading to abnormal cell proliferation and survival**.

***EWS/ERG* fusion gene**: It is a less common translocation, t(21;22)(q22;q12).

MORPHOLOGY

Q. Write a short note on the morphology of Ewing sarcoma.

Localization: Ewing sarcoma may arise in bones or extraskeletal regions. **Skeletal Ewing sarcoma** arises in the **diaphysis** (midshaft) **and diaphyseal-metaphyseal portions of the medullary cavity of long tubular bones** (especially the **femur, humerus,** and **tibia**).

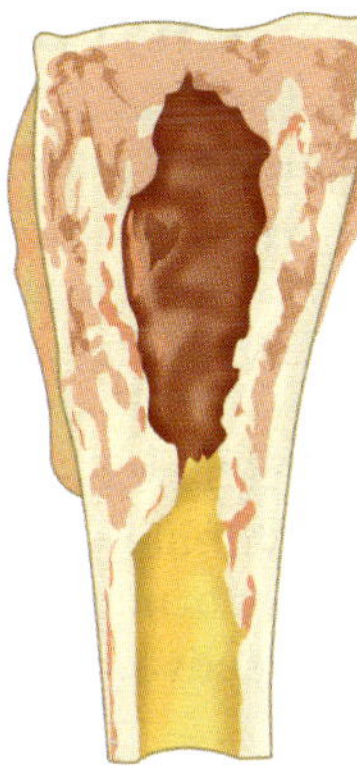

Ewing sarcoma: Highly aggressive small round cell tumor affecting the diaphysis. Onion-skin appearance on X-ray.

Tumors with Homer–Wright rosette: Ewing sarcoma, neuroblastoma, and medulloblastoma.

Fig. 25.15: Diagrammatic representation of the gross appearance of Ewing sarcoma of the tibia. The tumor appears soft, grayish-white, and shows areas of hemorrhage.

Gross

- **Arises in the diaphysis:** Skeletal Ewing sarcoma usually arises in the **diaphysis** and **may infiltrate the medullary spaces** without destroying the bony trabeculae.
- **Diffusely infiltrate the cortex** and the tumor **may also penetrate the periosteum** and spread into the soft tissues.
- **Soft, grayish-white (tan-white) appearance** and frequently show areas of **hemorrhage and necrosis (Fig. 25.15).**

Microscopy (Figs. 25.16A and B)

- **Uniform, small, round tumor cells**: Ewing sarcoma comprises **sheets of closely packed, uniform, small, and round cells.**
  - **Tumor cell size:** Tumor cells are up to **twice the size of a lymphocyte and are more cohesive.**
  - **Scanty cytoplasm: Tumor cells have scant (little) cytoplasm.** The cytoplasm **appears clear** because it is **rich in glycogen,** which is an important diagnostic feature. The glycogen **stain is positive** with the **periodic acid-Schiff (PAS) stain.**
  - The **nuclei are round and contain finely stippled chromatin and inconspicuous nucleoli. Mitoses are infrequent** even though the tumor is highly cellular.

Q. Write a short answer on Homer–Wright rosette.

- **Homer–Wright rosettes:** In some areas, the neoplastic cells tend to form Homer–Wright rosettes. They consist of **tumor cells arranged in a circle about a central fibrillary space (round cell clusters with** a **central fibrillary core)**. This is **indicative of neural differentiation.**
- **Interstitial stroma: Little or absent.** The fibrous strands separate the sheets of tumor cells into irregular **nests or sheets.** Geographic **necrosis** may be prominent.

Immunohistochemistry

EWS cells express characteristic antigens, some of which are part of the translocation product (e.g., **FLI-1 and CD99**).

Radiographic Appearance

- It produces **destructive lytic lesions** in which the border between normal bone and the tumor is indistinct. The tumor may extend into the surrounding soft tissues.
- Characteristic circumferential, **discontinuous layers of periosteal new bone formation** produce an **onion-skin pattern** (Fig. 25.17).

Clinical Features

- Ewing sarcoma usually presents as a **painful, enlarging mass** and the affected site is **tender, warm, and swollen.**
- **Systemic features**: It may develop in some and be **mistaken for an infection like osteomyelitis.**
  - Fever, weakness, and bone pain.
  - Hematological findings: Anemia, leukocytosis, and raised erythrocyte sedimentation rate.

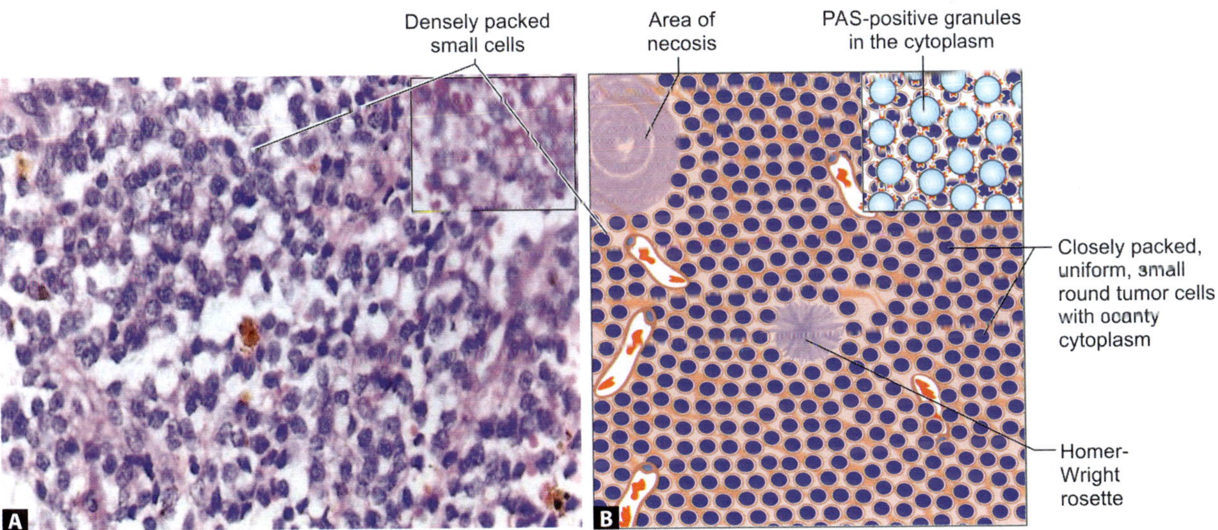

Figs. 25.16A and B: (A) Photomicrograph; (B) Diagrammatic; Ewing sarcoma composed of sheets of closely packed uniform small round cells with scanty cytoplasm. The inset of A and B shows PAS-positive granules in the cytoplasm.

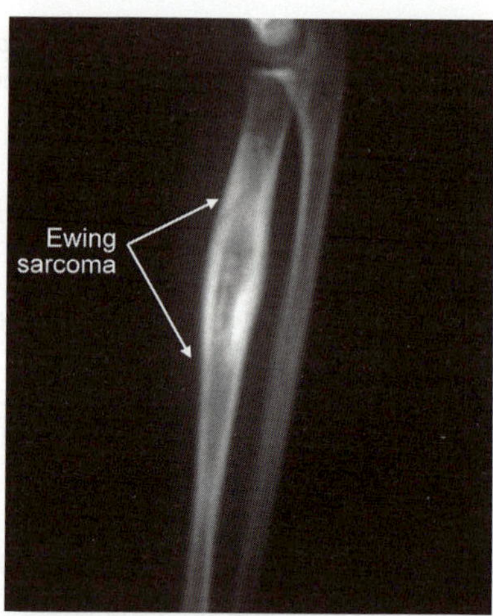

Fig. 25.17: X-ray of Ewing sarcoma involving the diaphysis of tibia.

Spread

- **Local spread:** It may spread from the medullary cavity **into the cortex, periosteum, and surrounding soft tissue.**
- **Blood spread:** Lungs, brain, and other bones (skull).

Treatment includes chemotherapy and surgical excision with or without irradiation. **The prognosis is dismal.**

RHEUMATOID ARTHRITIS

PA 33.5 (NC): Classify and describe the etiology, immunology, pathogenesis, manifestations, radiologic and laboratory features, diagnostic criteria, and complications of rheumatoid arthritis.

Q. Write a short essay on rheumatoid arthritis.

Definition: Rheumatoid arthritis (RA) is a **systemic, chronic inflammatory disorder**, that mainly **affects the joints** but can affect many **other tissues and organs.**

Joints affected: RA involves diarthrodial joints, symmetrically and bilaterally. Most commonly affected are the proximal interphalangeal and metacarpophalangeal joints, elbows, knees, ankles, and spine. RA often progresses to produce destruction of articular cartilage and, in some cases, joint fusion *(ankylosis)*.

Age and gender: RA may occur at any age, but its incidence peaks in the second to fourth decades. Its prevalence increases until the age of 70 years. RA is three times more common in women (especially premenopausal) than men.

Etiology

Q. Write a short note on the etiopathogenesis of rheumatoid arthritis.

The cause of rheumatoid arthritis remains **unknown**. As in other autoimmune diseases, genetic predisposition, and environmental and immunological factors contribute to RA's development, progression, and persistence.

1. **Genetic factors:** Genetic susceptibility is a **major factor** in the pathogenesis of rheumatoid arthritis.
   - **HLA genes:** RA is linked to a specific set of **HLA-DR alleles** (DR4, DR1, DR10, and DR14). The *HLA-DR4* allele is associated with anticitrullinated protein antibody (ACPA) positive RA. An epitope on a citrullinated protein, vinculin, mimics an epitope on many microbes and can be presented by the class II HLA-DR4 molecule.
   - **Non-HLA genes:** Several non-HLA loci have been linked to RA. These include a region of chromosome 18q21 that encodes the receptor activator of nuclear factor kappa B (NF-κB), or receptor activator of nuclear factor κB (RANK).
2. **Environmental arthritogenic agents:** They are thought to **initiate the disease** process. **Smoking,** infection (including periodontitis), and several **microbial agents** (e.g., viruses, mycobacteria, and *Mycoplasma)* may promote the citrullination of self-proteins. This creates new epitopes that trigger autoimmune reactions.
3. **Autoimmunity:** The initial inflammatory synovitis, an autoimmune reaction with T cells is responsible for the chronic destructive nature of rheumatoid arthritis.

Pathogenesis (Fig. 25.18)

- **Breakdown of self-tolerance**: Rheumatoid arthritis is initiated in a **genetically susceptible individual** by **exposure to an unknown joint (arthritogenic) antigen.** It results in a breakdown of immunological self-tolerance.
- **CD4+ helper T cells initiate the autoimmune response: The CD4+ helper T cells react against a joint antigen.** The pathologic changes in rheumatoid arthritis are due to inflammation caused by CD4+ T cells and perhaps antibodies.
- **Joint antigens**: Several joint antigens have been proposed as initiators and targets of the pathologic immune response in rheumatoid arthritis. These include collagen and chemically modified peptides.
- **Cytokine-mediated inflammation (cell-mediated immunity): CD4+** helper **T cells** (Th1 and Th17). and other cells (**macrophages and other inflammatory cells)** produce multiple cytokines. These cytokines produce joint injury as well as activate resident synovial cells (synoviocytes). These cytokines include:
  - **TNF, IL-1, and IL-6 from macrophages:** They recruit and activate leukocytes and other cells and stimulate the secretion of proteases. These proteases **destroy hyaline cartilage.** The cytokine TNF is the key mediator of inflammation and joint damage.
  - **IL-17 from Th17 cells:** This cytokine recruits' **neutrophils and monocytes**.
  - **RANKL expressed on activated T cells:** This stimulates osteoclasts, and causes **resorption of bone**.
- **Antibodies (humoral immunity)**: Antibodies may also be responsible for damage to the joint. The synovium in

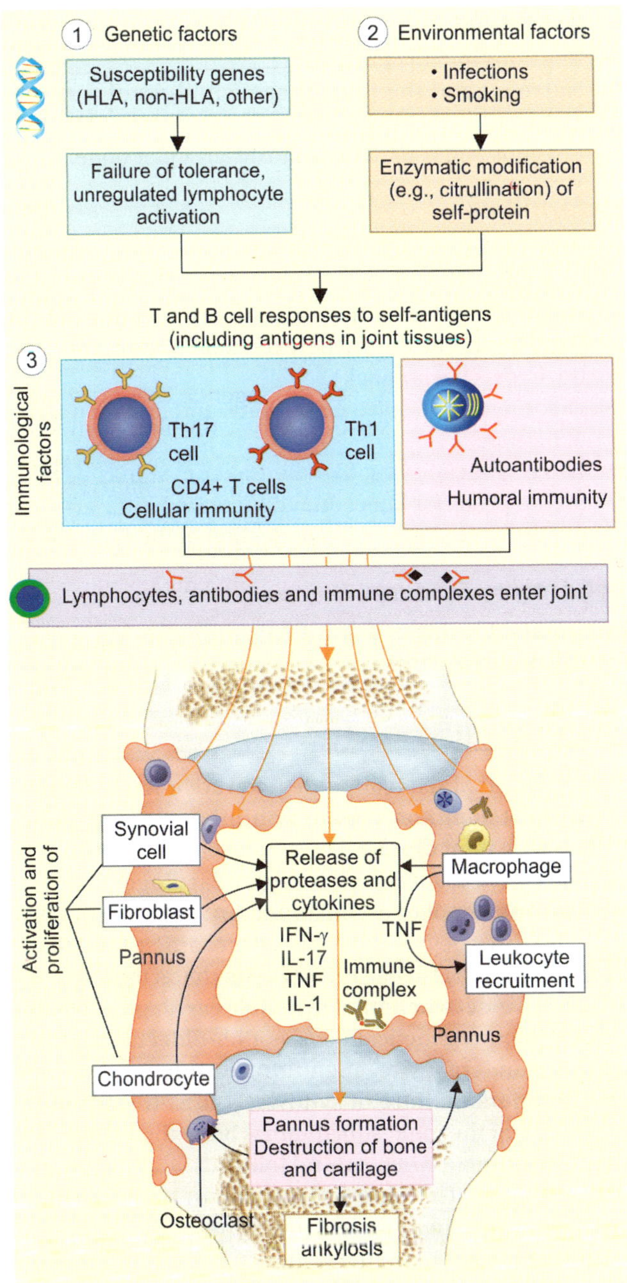

Fig. 25.18: Pathogenesis of rheumatoid arthritis.

(HLA: human leukocyte antigen; IFN: interferon; IL: interleukin; Th1: type 1 T helper; Th17: T helper 17 cells; TNF: tumor necrosis factor)

rheumatoid arthritis usually shows lymphoid follicles with germinal centers and abundant plasma cells.

- **Anticitrullinated peptide antibody:** Many patients have serum **antibodies against cyclic citrullinated peptides (CCPs).** In this, arginine residues are post-translationally converted to citrulline. Protein citrullination, a post-translational modification, can be induced by tobacco smoke and other environmental agents. These modified epitopes are found in several proteins found in joints, including fibrinogen, type II collagen, α-enolase, and vinculin. These modified CCPs may elicit antibodies, namely anticitrullinated peptide antibody (ACPA). It forms immune complexes and deposits in various tissues, the main being the joints. These antibodies are **useful for diagnosis** and may be involved in tissue injury. *Anticitrullinated peptide antibody* is a diagnostic marker and can be found in the serum of up to 70% of patients. ACPAs may contribute to the severity of the disease and its persistence.
- **Rheumatoid factor:** About 80% of rheumatoid arthritis patients also have serum IgM or IgA autoantibodies that bind to the Fc portions of IgG. This autoantibody is called a **rheumatoid factor.** Its role in disease progression is unclear. This antibody may also be detected in some individuals without rheumatoid arthritis. Rheumatoid factor is absent in some patients with rheumatoid arthritis (seronegative).

❖ **Release of proteases and cytokines:** Inflammation causes tissue injury and activation of synoviocytes.

Activated synoviocytes produce proteolytic enzymes, which **along with antigen-antibody complexes destroy the articular cartilage, ligaments, and tendons of the joint.** The TNF family of cytokines may cause increased activity of osteoclasts and produce destruction of bone.

❖ **Consequences**: The above actions bring out **edema, hyperplasia of synoviocytes,** and **inflammatory infiltration in the synovium, which forms pannus.** The pannus adheres and grows over the articular surface destroying **cartilage and erosion of adjacent subchondral bone.**

MORPHOLOGY

Joints

Rheumatoid arthritis causes **most severe changes in the joints.**

- **Joints involved**: **Symmetrical and bilateral arthritis.** Most affected are **diarthrodial joints,** such as **proximal interphalangeal** and **metacarpophalangeal joints, elbows, knees, ankles, and spine.**
- **Joint lesions**: They produce **chronic nonsuppurative proliferative polyarthritis** and inflammatory **synovitis**. As it progresses, it **destroys the articular cartilage** and causes **ankylosis of the joints.**

Synovium

Gross

The involved synovium shows **edema, thickening, and hyperplasia of lining synoviocytes.** This results in the conversion of smooth-surfaced **synovium** into **delicate and bulbous papillary structures.**

Microscopy (refer online Figs. 25.19A to E)

The characteristic histologic features of rheumatoid arthritis include:

- **Synovial cell hyperplasia:** The lining synovial shows 6–10 layers of synoviocytes compared to normal 2–3 layers. These hyperplastic synoviocytes **may form villus or finger-like structures.**

- **Dense inflammatory infiltrate:** The synovium shows edema and dense infiltration of **lymphocytes** (mostly CD4+helper T cells), **B cells**, **plasma cells**, and **macrophages.** Lymphocytes may **aggregate to form lymphoid follicles.** Neutrophils can be seen in the synovial fluid and on the synovial surface.
- **Increased vascularity due to angiogenesis:** Vascularity of synovium increases in RA.
- **Neutrophils and aggregates of organizing fibrin on the synovial and joint surfaces:** Increased vascularity is associated with the exudation of fibrin into the joint space. Fibrin, along with inflammatory cells, covers the synovium and joint surfaces. They may **form small fibrin nodules that float in the joint space** as **rice bodies.**
- **Osteoclastic activity in underlying bone:** This results in periarticular erosions and subchondral cysts.
- **Pannus formation:** Pannus is a **mass of synovium** and **synovial stroma** consisting of **inflammatory cells, granulation tissue,** and **synovial fibroblasts.** Pannus grows **over the articular cartilage and destroys it.**
- **Ankylosis:** After the destruction of cartilage, the **pannus bridges the opposing bones** to form **fibrous ankylosis,** which may ossify resulting in **bony ankylosis. Destruction of joint followed by fusion is termed ankylosis.**
- **Osteoporosis:** Osteoclastic activity in underlying bone causes erosions and osteoporosis of the underlying bone.

Skin

Rheumatoid nodules are the **most common cutaneous lesion.**

- **Sites:** Develops **at sites subjected to pressure.** For example, the ulnar aspect of the forearm, elbows, occiput, and lumbosacral area.
- **Gross: Round to oval, firm, nontender,** nodules in the **subcutaneous tissue.**
- **Microscopy:** It consists of a **central zone of fibrinoid necrosis surrounded by epithelioid histiocytes (activated macrophages), lymphocytes, and plasma cells.**

Blood Vessels

Rheumatoid **vasculitis** is a dangerous complication of rheumatoid arthritis, especially when it affects vital organs. It may also affect the heart, lungs, and muscles.

Clinical Features

- **Age:** RA can occur at any age, but is most common between **40 and 70 years.**
- **Sex:** Three to five times more often in **women than men** (3:1).
- **Slow and insidious in onset** and presents with malaise, fatigue, and generalized musculoskeletal pain.
- **Usually, small joints are involved before larger ones** and are **symmetrical.** It affects the hands (metacarpophalangeal and proximal interphalangeal joints) and feet, followed by the wrists, ankles, elbows, and knees. The affected joints are swollen, warm, painful, and stiff on arising or following inactivity.

Radiography

- Effusions into the joint.
- Narrowing of the joint space with loss of articular cartilage.
- Erosions and osteopenia of juxta-articular bone.

Deformities

- Destruction of tendons, ligaments, and joint capsules produces characteristic deformities. These consist of **radial deviation of the wrist, ulnar deviation of the fingers,** and flexion-hyperextension abnormalities of the fingers (**swan neck**).
- Deformed joints have no stability, and lose their range of motion.
- Large synovial cysts, like the **Baker cyst** may develop on the posterior knee, due to increased intra-articular pressure causing outside projection of the synovium.

Laboratory Findings

Rheumatoid factor and anti-CCP antibodies are **specific for rheumatoid arthritis.**

OSTEOARTHRITIS

Osteoarthritis (also called degenerative joint disease) is the **most common type of noninflammatory, slowly progressive joint disease.**

Degenerative disorder of articular cartilage: The term osteoarthritis implies an inflammatory disease. However, it is primarily a degenerative disorder of articular cartilage.

Characteristics: Osteoarthritis (OA) is characterized by the **progressive destruction of articular cartilage** of weight-bearing joints of **genetically susceptible older persons.** The **cartilage undergoes degeneration, resulting in structural and functional failure of synovial joints.** It leads to the narrowing of the joint, subchondral bone thickening, and finally **nonfunctioning, painful joint.**

Joints affected: The joints affected are:

- **Weight-bearing joints:** Knee, hips, and cervical and lumbar segments of the spine.
- **Nonweight-bearing joints:** These include **proximal and distal interphalangeal joints** of the fingers, first carpometacarpal joints, and first tarsometatarsal joints of the feet.

Types: Osteoarthritis constitutes a group of conditions that have in common the mechanical destruction of a joint. It may be divided into primary and secondary osteoarthritis.

- **Primary (idiopathic) osteoarthritis:** Most cases of osteoarthritis appear **insidiously, without apparent initiating cause,** as an aging phenomenon. It develops as an aging process and may affect a few (oligoarticular) or many joints.

- **Secondary osteoarthritis:** In about 5% of cases, osteoarthritis appears in younger individuals with predisposing conditions or underlying causes. These include
  - **Local conditions**, e.g., joint deformity, a previous joint injury (trauma), crystal deposits, infection, osteonecrosis, and hemarthrosis
  - **Secondary to systemic disease**, e.g., diabetes, hemochromatosis, endocrinopathies, chronic inflammatory diseases, or marked obesity.

Pathogenesis and Morphology (Figs. 25.20A to C)

OA is characterized by **degeneration of articular cartilage and disordered repair of cartilage.** Osteoarthritis (OA) is a multifactorial disease having biochemical stress and genetic factors.

Genetic factors: These include polymorphisms in genes encoding components of the matrix and signaling molecules. These may predispose to chondrocyte injury and matrix alterations. Mechanical stress is the triggering factor.

Biomechanical Stress

Chondrocyte injury: Aging, together with genetic and biochemical factors, initiates chondrocyte injury.

Proliferation of chondrocytes: In the early stages of osteoarthritis, chondrocytes of articular cartilage proliferate and form clusters. It occurs in response to the loss of the matrix.

Secretion of matrix metalloproteinases by chondrocytes and degradation of collagen: The proliferated chondrocytes secrete matrix metalloproteinases (MMPs) that degrade the type II collagen network.

Decreased concentration of proteoglycans: Simultaneously, the water content of the matrix increases (leads to swelling of osteoarthritic cartilage) and the concentration of proteoglycans decreases.

Formation of fissures and clefts at the articular surface: Normally, collagen type II fibers are horizontally arranged. Cleaving these collagen fibers produces fissures and clefts at the articular surface. Thus, the articular surface **of the involved bone** becomes **granular and soft.**

Death of chondrocytes and formation of loose bodies: As the disease progresses, chondrocytes die. Later, full-thickness of cartilage is sloughed into the joint. The **broken pieces of cartilage form loose bodies(joint mice**) in the synovial cavity.

Fibrillation of articular cartilage: OA may be arrested at this stage for many years before progressing to the next stage. In this stage, fibrillation occurs, and it may persist for many years. **Fibrillation is the development of surface cracks parallel to the long axis of the articular surface.**

Leakage of synovial fluid into cracks: As fibrillations grow, synovial fluid begins to flow into the defects or cracks in the articular cartilage. The cracks are progressively oriented more vertically, parallel to the long axis of the collagen fibrils. Along these cracks, synovial fluid penetrates deeper into the articular cartilage.

Subchondral bone cyst: In some areas, the synovial fluid extends from the joint surface into the subchondral bone region. It may produce a subchondral bone cyst.

Damage to articular cartilage: Cytokines and diffusible factors are secreted from chondrocytes, synovial cells, and macrophages recruited in response to the joint damage. These molecules include TGF-β (which stimulates the production of MMPs), IL-1, IL-6, prostaglandins, and nitric oxide.

Chronic, low-level inflammation: It contributes to cartilage damage and progression of osteoarthritis.

Formation of osteophytes at the periphery of the articular surface: Bone morphogenetic proteins and TGF-β play the main role in the development of osteophytes, bony outgrowths at the periphery of the articular surface.

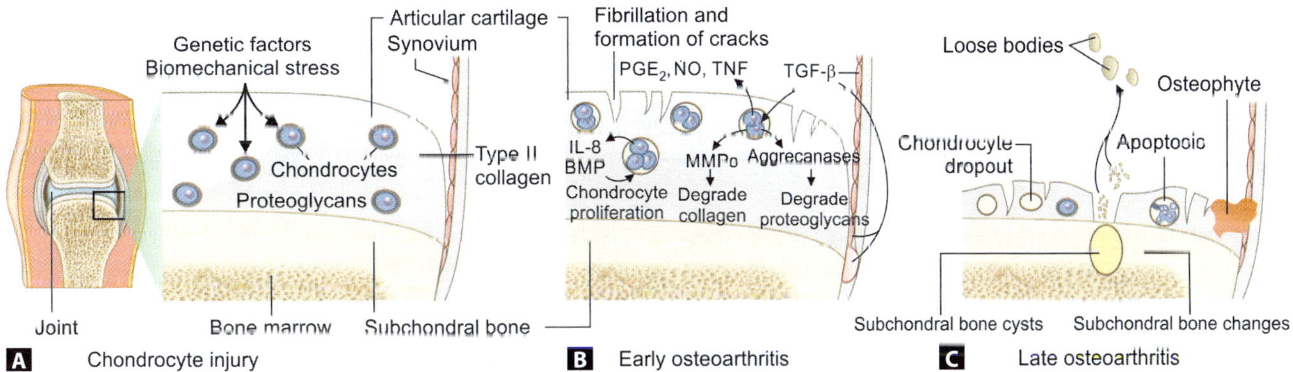

Figs. 25.20A to C: Pathogenesis of osteoarthritis (OA): (A) OA begins with biomechanical injury to cartilage injury. It can be accelerated in genetically predisposed individuals. It results in changes in the extracellular matrix; (B) In early osteoarthritis; chondrocytes may proliferate in an attempt to repair the damaged matrix. Later there is a loss of chondrocyte. The degradation of proteoglycans exceeds its synthesis. Matrix metalloproteinases (MMPs) degrade collagen, and aggrecanases (extracellular proteolytic enzymes) degrade proteoglycans; (C) Late OA shows loss of both matrix and chondrocytes with subchondral bone damage.

MORPHOLOGY

Gross (Figs. 25.21A to E)

The most significant gross changes in an osteoarthritic joint are—(i) damage to the articular cartilage, (ii) bone loss, and (iii) an alteration in the shape of the articulating surface.

Damage to the articular cartilage: The normal cartilage has a smooth and shiny appearance. In osteoarthritis, the cartilage may be absent in the weight-bearing joints. The remaining cartilage shows tan **discoloration, and it appears rough and velvety**.

Bone changes: These include the following:

- **Bone eburnation:** The friction of the opposing articular surface smoothens and burnishes the exposed subchondral bone. The subchondral bone appears thick, shiny, and smooth giving it the appearance of polished ivory and known as **bone eburnation** (eburnated means ivory-like). New vessels growing from the epiphysis and fibrocartilage get deposited.
- **Subchondral bone cyst:** The eburnated bone may crack in some areas (fracture gaps) and force synovial fluid from the joint surface into the subchondral bone marrow regions but cannot exit. Because of this one-way ball valve-like mechanism, a **subchondral bone cyst** filled with synovial fluid is formed. The loculated fluid collection increases in size surrounded by a reactive bone wall.
- **Development of osteophytes:** Mushroom-shaped pearly grayish bony outgrowths (spurs) known as **osteophytes** develop at the periphery of the joint surface. The synovium shows mild fibrosis and chronic inflammatory cells.

Microscopy (Figs. 25.21A to E)

Microscopic changes follow a well-described sequence.

Loss of proteoglycans from the surface of the articular cartilage: This is the earliest microscopic feature of OA. This is seen as decreased metachromatic staining.

Changes in chondrocytes: During the **early stages of OA, chondrocytes proliferate. As the disease progresses, chondrocytes die.** Later, full-thickness portions of cartilage are sloughed into the joint, forming **loose bodies.**

Fibrillation of articular cartilage: Fibrillation is the development of surface cracks parallel to the long axis of the articular surface.

Leakage of synovial fluid into cracks: Along these cracks, synovial fluid penetrates deeper into the articular cartilage.

Inflammation and a foreign body giant cell reaction: Eventually, fragments of articular cartilage break off and lodge in the synovium, inducing inflammation and a foreign body giant cell reaction.

Eburnation: This appears like polished ivory and is called bone eburnation (hard and dense ivory-like).

Development of osteophytes: In the fingers, osteophytes at the distal interphalangeal joints are called **Heberden's nodes.**

Changes in the synovium: The synovium is usually only mildly congested and fibrotic. It shows few chronic inflammatory cells.

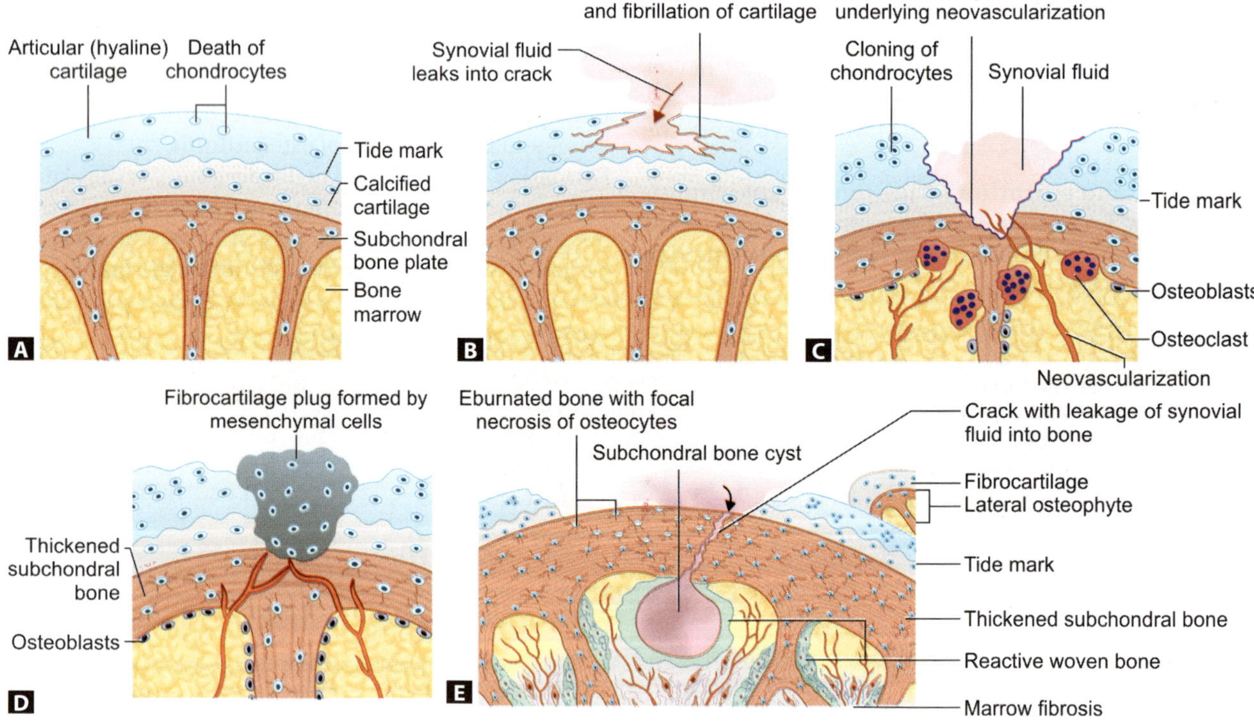

Figs. 25.21A to E: Histogenesis and changes in osteoarthritis: (A) Death of chondrocytes in the articular cartilage; (B) A crack in the articular cartilage is formed, followed by an influx of synovial fluid and further cartilage loss and degeneration; (C) Articular cartilage gradually wears away, forming deep cracks through tide marks. Below the tidemark, new vessels grow (neovascularization); (D) The mesenchymal cells form fibrocartilage plugs over the cracks; (E) The fibrocartilage plug is not mechanically sufficient and may be worn away. This exposes the subchondral bone plate, which becomes thickened and eburnated (i.e., ivory-like). If a crack forms in the subchondral bone, synovial fluid leaks into the bone and produces a subchondral bone cyst. Focal regrowth of the articular surface leads to the formation of osteophytes.

Radiologic findings: OA is characterized by—(i) narrowing of the joint space due to loss of articular cartilage, (ii) increased thickness of the subchondral bone, (iii) subchondral bone cysts, and (iv) large peripheral growths of bone and cartilage (osteophytes).

Clinical Features

- Osteoarthritis is an **insidious slowly progressive disease** and causes long-term disability.
- Present with **deep, aching pain**, which worsens with joint movement and is relieved by rest.
- Involved **joints may be swollen, and tender**, and may demonstrate crepitus.
- Osteophytes in the spine can cause nerve root compression and neurologic deficits.
- **Prominent osteophytes** at the **distal interphalangeal joints** are known as **Heberden nodes** and are seen commonly in women.

Currently, no treatments prevent or arrest the progression of primary OA. Therapy is directed at specific orthopedic conditions. It includes pain management by nonsteroidal anti-inflammatory drugs (NSAIDs) to reduce inflammation, intra-articular corticosteroids, exercise, weight loss, and other supportive measures. In severe disabling OA, arthroplasty or joint replacement may be necessary.

GOUT AND GOUTY ARTHRITIS

Q. Write a short note on gout/gouty tophi.

Definition: Gout is a **heterogeneous group of diseases** characterized by **increased serum uric acid** (**hyperuricemia** with plasma urate level above 6.8 mg/dL) and **urate crystal deposition in joints and kidneys.**

Arthritis: Gout is associated with acute and chronic arthritis. The **transient attacks of acute arthritis** are **initiated by depositing monosodium urate crystals within and around joints.**

Q. Write a short note on the causes/etiology of gout.

Classification (Box 25.5): Gout is classified as primary or secondary, depending on the etiology of hyperuricemia.

- **Primary (idiopathic):** Hyperuricemia occurs without any other disease and constitutes approximately 90% of cases of gout. Primary gout usually affects **adult men,** and only 5% occurs in women. The **peak incidence of gout is in the fifth decade.**
- **Secondary:** Hyperuricemia occurs in association with another illness.

BOX 25.5: Classification of gout.

Primary gout (90%)
- Increased production of uric acid
  - Increased dietary intake of purine
  - Due to inborn errors in purine metabolism
- Decreased excretion of uric acid with normal production

Secondary gout (10%)
- Increased production of uric acid with increased urinary excretion
  - Increased catabolism of nucleic acid due to increased cell turnover (e.g., leukemias, cancers, and during tumor lysis induced by chemotherapy)
- Decreased excretion of uric acid with normal production
  - Chronic renal disease

Pathogenesis (Fig. 25.22)

Q. Write a short essay/note on the pathogenesis of gouty arthritis.

Uric acid: It is the **end product of purine metabolism,** which is eliminated only in the urine. Humans do not have uricase, an enzyme which degrades uric acid. Usually, there is a balance between uric acid production and tissue deposition of urates.

Hyperuricemia: The **plasma urate level above 6.8 mg/dL** is called hyperuricemia. It is necessary, but not sufficient for the development of gout.

Mechanism of hyperuricemia: Elevated uric acid can be due to overproduction, reduced excretion, or both. Several factors determine uric acid levels. These are as follows:

- **Increased synthesis of uric acid:** It is usually due to some abnormality in purine production. Purines are the product of two interlinked pathways:
  1. **The de novo pathway:** In this pathway, purine nucleotides are synthesized **from nonpurine precursors.**
  2. **The salvage pathway:** In this pathway, purine nucleotides are synthesized **from free purine bases in the diet or** produced **during the degradation of DNA and RNA.**
- **Reduced excretion:** Uric acid is filtered from the circulation by the glomerulus and almost completely resorbed by the proximal tubule of the kidney. A small amount of the resorbed uric acid is secreted by the distal nephron and excreted in the urine. Defective excretion can lead to hyperuricemia. Reduced excretion of uric acid may result from chronic renal disease. Dehydration and diuretics increase tubular reabsorption of uric acid and cause hyperuricemia

Hyperuricemia in primary gout: Elevated uric acid in primary gout is most commonly due to reduced excretion, the basis of which is not known in most patients. In a few patients, primary gout is caused by uric acid overproduction due to enzymatic defects. For example, a partial deficiency of hypoxanthine-guanine phosphoribosyltransferase (HGPRT) interferes with the salvage pathway, and purine metabolites cannot be recycled and are instead degraded into uric acid.

Hyperuricemia in secondary gout: Secondary gout is associated with medications or conditions that cause

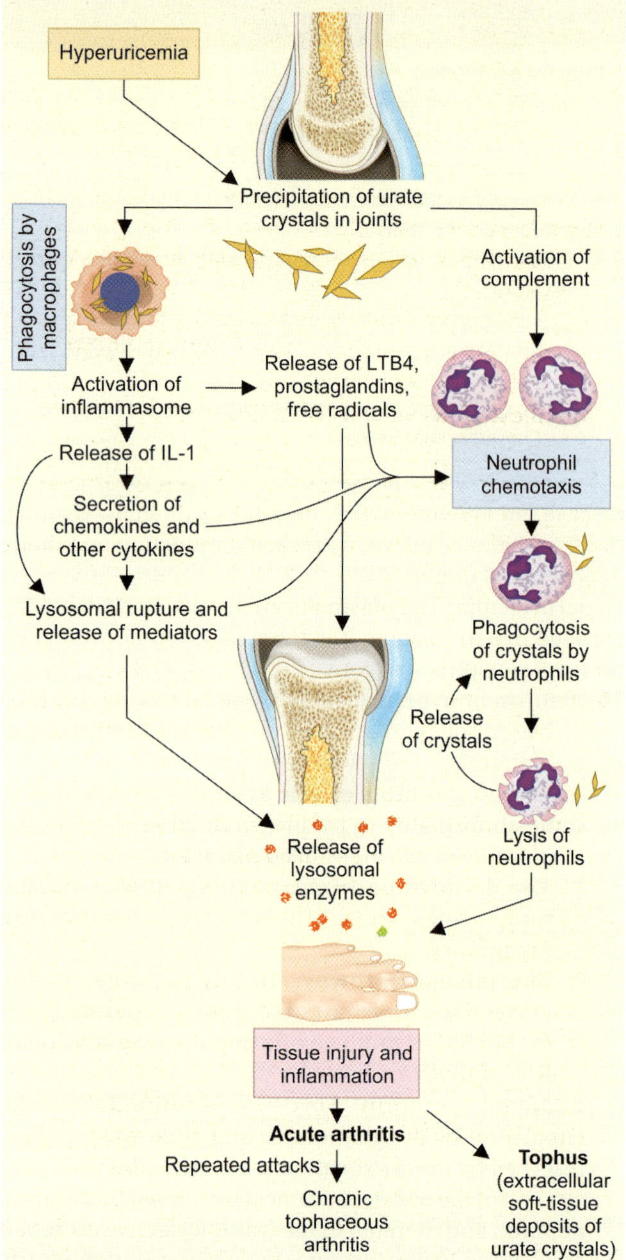

Fig. 25.22: Pathogenesis of acute and chronic gouty arthritis. Urate crystals are phagocytosed by macrophages and lead to the production of various inflammatory mediators. They elicit the inflammation characteristic of gout. IL-1 stimulates the production of chemokines and other cytokines from various cells.

(IL-1: interleukin 1; LTB4: leukotriene B4)

hyperuricemia. The complete absence of HGPRT causes not only hyperuricemia but also produces neurologic manifestations *(Lesch-Nyhan syndrome)*. Lesch-Nyhan syndrome is classified as a form of secondary gout. Secondary gout can also occur when there is increased production (rapid lysis of tumor cells killed by chemotherapy, so-called *tumor lysis syndrome*) or decreased excretion (chronic renal disease).

Arthritis in Gout

- **Precipitation of monosodium urate** (MSU) **crystals in the joints:** It triggers arthritis in gout. The solubility of urate in a joint is dependent on the intra-articular concentration of urate and the temperature (less soluble in low temperature). Monosodium urate is less soluble in synovial fluid compared to plasma. So, they become easily supersaturated in the peripheral joints (ankles and toes), where temperatures are usually low. With hyperuricemia, precipitation of urate crystals develops in the synovium and in the joint cartilage.
- **Production of mediators and recruitment of leukocytes: The precipitation of urate crystals stimulates the production of mediators that recruit leukocytes.**
- **Phagocytosis of the MSU crystals by resident macrophages**: Macrophages in the synovium phagocytose the crystals, and **activate** a cytosolic sensor called the **inflammasome.**
- **Recruitment and accumulation of neutrophils in the joint**: The inflammasome activates caspase-1. This produces active IL-1β and stimulates the recruitment and accumulation of neutrophils in the joint.
- **Inflammation and release of other molecules:** As in other acute inflammatory reactions, neutrophils release other cytokines, free radicals, and proteases.
- **Acute arthritis:** Crystals ingested by macrophages and neutrophils also damage the membranes of phagolysosomes. This causes leakage of lysosomal enzymes and produces acute arthritis. Arthritis usually remits spontaneously in days to weeks.
- **Formation of tophi:** Repeated attacks of acute arthritis led to the formation of tophi. Tophi is characterized by aggregates of urate crystals and inflammatory tissue, in synovial membranes and periarticular tissue. Severe damage to the cartilage produces functional impairment of the joints.

Gout develops in only about 10% of patients with hyperuricemia. Thus, other factors contribute to the development of symptomatic gout. These are as follows:

- **Age:** Gout usually presents after 20–30 years of age.
- **Duration of the hyperuricemia: Usually not** <20–30 years.
- **Genetic predisposition:** Gout is associated with X-linked abnormalities of *HGPRT.* Gout is also associated with polymorphisms in genes involved with urate or ion transport and inflammation.
- **Alcohol consumption.**
- **Obesity.**
- **Drugs** (e.g., thiazides) **that reduce excretion of urate.**
- **Lead toxicity.**

MORPHOLOGY

Q. Write a short note on acute gout/gouty arthritis.

Four distinctive patterns of gout are—(i) acute arthritis, (ii) chronic arthritis, (iii) accumulation of tophi in extra-articular sites, and (iv) urate (gouty) nephropathy.

Acute Gouty Arthritis

It is generally **monoarticular** and usually affects the **lower extremities**, particularly the first metatarsophalangeal joint.

- **Intense acute inflammation**: Acute arthritis is characterized by edema, congestion, and dense infiltration of synovium by neutrophils. Few lymphocytes, plasma cells, and macrophages may also be seen.
- **Monosodium urate (MSU) crystals:** The synovium shows negatively birefringent urate crystals.
  - They are **long, slender, and needle-shaped** and arranged in small clusters in the synovium.
  - They are found in the cytoplasm of the neutrophils.
  - As the acute attack subsides, they may be resolubilized.

Chronic Tophaceous Arthritis

Q. Write a short note on gouty tophi.

- Chronic tophaceous arthritis follows the repeated precipitation of urate crystals during acute attacks.
- The urates may heavily coat (encrust) the articular surfaces and form chalky deposits in the synovium.
- The synovium shows hyperplasia, fibrosis, thickening, and infiltration by inflammatory cells. It forms a pannus, destroys the cartilage, and causes juxta-articular bone erosions.
- When severe, fibrous, or bony ankylosis may lead to loss of joint function.

Tophi (Figs. 25.23 and 25.24)

A tophus (plural: tophi) is a lesion consisting of large aggregates of urate crystals, surrounded by the inflammatory reaction. It is **pathognomonic of gout**.

- **Sites:** Tophi are commonly found in the **articular cartilage** of joints and the periarticular ligaments, **tendons** (e.g., Achilles tendon), bursae, and earlobes. It may also occur in **extra-articular sites such as soft tissues.**
- **Microscopy**: They consist of aggregations of **urate crystals surrounded by macrophages, lymphocytes, and foreign body giant cells.**

Gouty Nephropathy

It is the renal complications due to the deposition of urate crystals or tophi in the renal medullary interstitium or tubules. The complications include uric acid nephrolithiasis (kidney stones), and pyelonephritis.

Clinical Features

The gout has four stages:

1. **Asymptomatic hyperuricemia:** Appears at puberty in males and after menopause in females. It usually precedes clinically evident gout by many years.

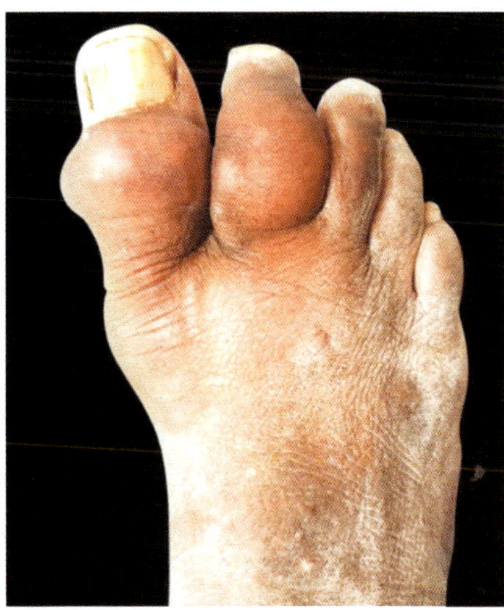

Fig. 25.23: Usual site of gouty tophus showing swollen great and second toe.

2. **Acute gouty arthritis:** It appears as sudden excruciating joint pain with tenderness. Even if not treated, acute attacks of gout are usually self-limited.
3. **Asymptomatic intercritical gout:** The intercritical period is the asymptomatic interval between the first acute attack and subsequent attacks.
4. **Chronic tophaceous gout:** After several years (about 12 years) of acute gouty arthritis, chronic tophaceous gout may develop, which may lead to severe crippling disease.

Treatment: The main aim of the treatment of gout is to (1) reduce the severity of acute attacks; (2) reduce serum urate levels; (3) prevent future attacks; (4) promote the dissolution of urate deposits, and (5) alkalinize the urine to prevent renal stone formation. Treatment includes lifestyle modification (e.g., weight loss, avoiding alcohol consumption, dietary changes to reduce purine intake) and medication to reduce inflammation (e.g., NSAIDs) and lower serum urate levels (e.g., xanthine oxidase inhibitors).

Prognosis: Gout does not reduce the life span, but may cause morbidity.

HEALING OF A FRACTURE

Q. Discuss the healing of fractured bone (or long bone) and its complications.

Fracture is defined as **loss of bone integrity** or a **discontinuity of the bone resulting from mechanical injury and/or diminished bone strength.** Fracture is the most common pathologic condition (lesion) affecting bone. Fractures can range from a thin crack to a complete break in the bone. The term *pathologic* is used for fractures involving bone weakened by an underlying disease process, such as a tumor.

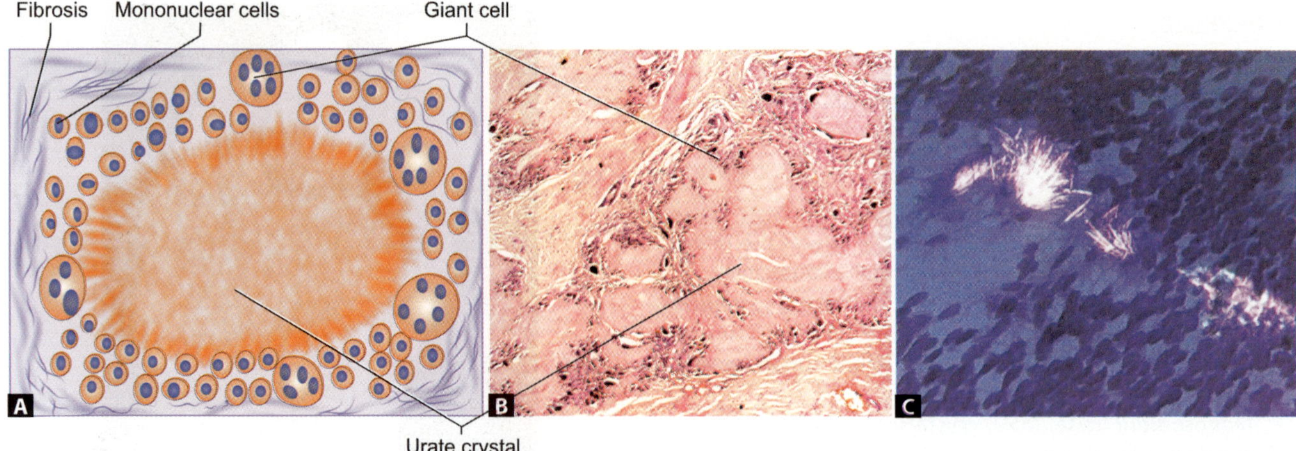

Figs. 25.24A to C: (A) Diagrammatic; (B) H&E. Microscopy of a gouty tophus showing aggregates of dissolved urate crystals surrounded by fibroblasts, mononuclear inflammatory cells, and giant cells; (C) Urate crystals are needle-shaped and negatively birefringent under polarized light.

Phases of fracture healing: Bone can be repaired by reactivating processes that normally take place during embryogenesis. Fracture healing is a complex process. There are three major phases of fracture healing **(Figs. 25.25A to E)** namely: (1) inflammatory phase, (2) reparative phase, and (3) remodeling phase.

1. Inflammatory Phase (1–3 Days)

- **Hemorrhage and formation of hematoma:** Immediately **after fracture, blood vessels** (in the periosteum, cortex, and medullary cavity) **rupture** which leads to the formation of a hematoma (clot) at the fracture site and surrounding area of bone injury. **Necrosis of bone** also occurs at the fracture site.
- **Formation of fibrin meshwork:** The clotted blood seals off the fracture site and creates a fibrin meshwork. **Fibrin meshwork** in the clotted blood **helps.**
  - To seal the fracture site
  - Guides the entry of inflammatory cells (neutrophils and macrophages) to the area.
  - Ingrowth of fibroblasts and new capillary vessels (neovascularization) to the site, producing granulation tissue between the fracture fragments.
- **Migration of inflammatory cells**: Damage to tissue and cells promotes the initiation of the inflammatory cascade. The inflammatory cells migrate to the site of fracture.
- **Formation of granulation tissue**: Granulation tissue consists of proliferating capillaries and fibroblasts. It is formed at the site of fractures.

2. Reparative Phase

The reparative phase follows the first week after a fracture. By this time, acute inflammation subsides. Repair proceeds from the periphery toward the center of the fracture site.

Activation of osteoprogenitor cells: Degranulated platelets and inflammatory cells at the site of fracture release platelet-derived growth factor (PDGF), TGF-β, fibroblast growth factor (FGF), and other growth factors. They activate osteoprogenitor cells in the periosteum, medullary cavity, and surrounding soft tissues to stimulate osteoclastic and osteoblastic activity. The periosteum is an important source of repair tissue (callus) following a fracture. Pluripotent **osteoprogenitor cells differentiate into fibroblasts and osteoblasts.**

Formation of callus: Repair tissue following fracture consists of **granulation tissue containing bone** (mineralized or unmineralized) **or cartilage and is called a *callus*.** Callus is of two types—(1) soft tissue callus and (2) the bony callus.

1. **Formation of soft tissue callus (procallus): Uncalcified tissue** forms at the site of the fracture, known as *soft tissue callus* or *procallus*. It bridges the ends of the fractured bones without structural rigidity for weight bearing at the fracture site. The soft callus **consists of new connective tissue, blood vessels, cartilage, and soft spongy bone** (unmineralized bone is called osteoid).
2. **Formation of bony callus:** Within 2 weeks of injury, the soft callus is converted to a *bony callus.* The activated osteoprogenitor cells give rise to the **osteoblasts** that **synthesize and deposit subperiosteal trabeculae** of **woven bone**. The woven bone consists of **osteoid collagen in a haphazard pattern.** These processes transform the procallus into a *bony callus* consisting of granulation tissue and woven bone. Since bone formation requires a good blood supply, woven bone spicules begin to appear at the periphery of the clot. The callus depending on its site and appearance can be divided into external and internal callus.
   - **External callus:** The callus formed on the surface of the bone is called the external callus, which

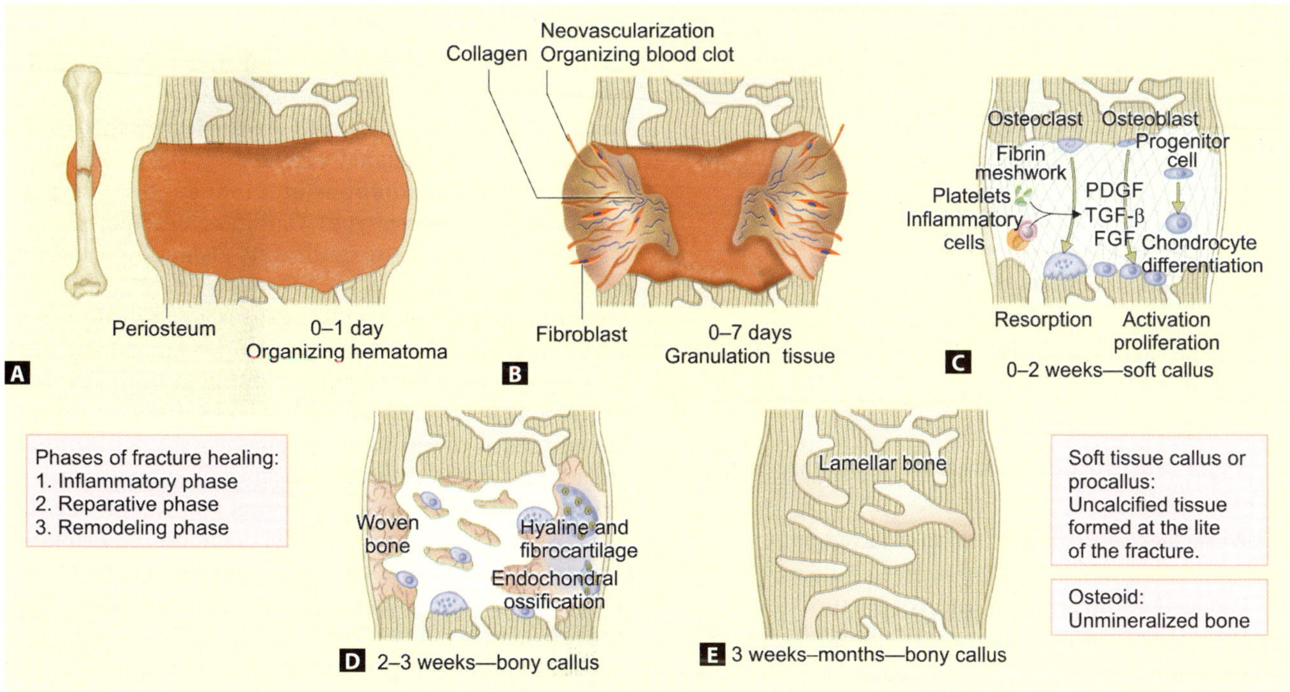

The rate of newly synthesized osteoid mineralization is best estimated by: Tetracycline labeling.

Figs. 25.25A to E: Various fractures in the healing stages. Repair of a fractured bone occurs through several steps: (A) Immediately after fracture, the blood vessels torn within the fracture release blood that clots to produce a large fracture hematoma in the subperiosteal and soft tissue, as well as in the marrow cavity; (B) The inflammatory phase of fracture healing is characterized by inflammatory cell infiltration, neovascularization and early organization of the blood clot. The blood clot is gradually removed by macrophages and replaced by granulation tissue; (C) Within 2 weeks, the two ends of the bone are bridged by a fibrin meshwork in which osteoclasts, osteoblasts, and chondrocytes differentiate from osteoprogenitor cells. These cells produce cartilage and bone matrix. The reparative phase of fracture healing is characterized by the formation of a callus of cartilage called procallus tissue and woven bone near the fracture site. The procallus is invaded by regenerating blood vessels and proliferating osteoblasts; (D) In the next few weeks, the fibrocartilage is gradually replaced by woven bone that forms a hard callus in the original area of the fracture; (E) Extensive osteoclastic and osteoblastic cellular activity is maintained. The woven bone is then remodeled as compact and cancellous bone in continuity with the adjacent uninjured areas. The fracture site remodels into normal lamellar bone if it is adequately immobilized.

arises from the periosteum and the soft-tissue mesenchymal cells. It continues to grow toward the fracture site.

- **Internal callus:** Simultaneously, an endosteal or internal callus forms within the medullary cavity and grows outward toward the fracture site. The bony callus reaches the maximal size at the end of the second or third week and helps stabilize the fracture site.

3. Remodeling Phase

In the early stages of the callus formation, an excess amount of fibrous tissue, cartilage, and woven bone is produced. After the ingrowth of the callus has sealed the bone ends, the bone at the fracture site becomes reorganized such that the structure of the original cortex is restored. This is called the *remodeling phase*.

Formation of lamellar bone: As the callus matures, the portions of the callus that are not subjected to physical stress are resorbed by osteoclasts. With the continued migration of osteoblasts and osteoclasts, the hard callus undergoes repeated remodeling. This reduces the size of the healing bone and recreates lamellar bone. The lamellar bone is stronger and consists of **parallel collagen fibers**. The center of the callus is ultimately replaced by compact bone, while the callus edges become replaced by lamellar bone. The healing process is completed by restoration of the medullary cavity and regeneration of the normal bone structure.

The remodeling phase **substitutes the trabecular bone with compact bone**. The remodeling phase continues till the original bone shape (contour), outline, and strength of the fractured bone are re-established. The **whole process of healing** of a bone fracture usually takes **about 6–8 weeks**.

TABLE 25.1 Major causes of delayed fracture healing.

Local factors	*General factors*
Excessive movement of a fractured bone during the healing process	Old age
Infection of the fractured site	Poor general health
Severe local soft-tissue injury	Drugs, e.g., corticosteroids
Wide separation of fracture ends	
Extensive necrosis of the fractured bone	
Poor or impaired blood supply (e.g., tibia, head of femur)	

Major causes of delayed fracture healing are presented in Table 25.1.

Q. Mention the complications of healing of fracture bone.

Complications of healing: These are as follows:

- **Delayed union and nonunion** of fracture.
- **Pseudoarthrosis:** In the case of nonunion, too much movement along the fracture gap can cause cystic degeneration in the callus, creating a false joint or pseudoarthrosis.
- **Large callus with deformity**.

SOFT TISSUE TUMORS

PA 33.3 (CC): Classify and describe the etiology, pathogenesis, manifestations, radiologic and morphologic features, and complications and metastases of soft tissue tumors.

Soft tissue is the term used for nonepithelial tissue excluding the skeleton, joints, central nervous system, hematopoietic and lymphoid tissues.

- Soft tissue tumors are mesenchymal neoplasms and **include tumors of skeletal muscle, fat, fibrous tissue peripheral nerve, or blood vessels.** These neoplasms may arise anywhere in the body, but **most soft tissue occurs in the extremities,** especially the **thigh.**
- Soft tissue tumors may be **benign, locally aggressive, or malignant. Benign soft tissue** tumors are **more** (100 times) **common** than malignant counterparts, except skeletal muscle neoplasms. **Malignant soft tissue tumors** are **termed sarcomas.** Locally aggressive tumors (e.g., fibromatosis) invade the surrounding tissue and may recur locally. **Sarcomas** (malignant soft tissue tumors) **can metastasize to the lungs or bone** through blood vessels. Generally, **patients die of metastatic disease rather than local invasion** at the primary tumor site.

Age and gender: Soft tissue sarcomas may occur at any age and, as with carcinomas, are more common in older patients. **Approximately 15% of soft tissue tumors arise in children**, and their incidence increases with age.

Etiology and Pathogenesis

Most sarcomas are sporadic and there are no known precursor lesions for soft tissue sarcomas.

Genetic disorders: A **small minority of soft tissue neoplasms** are associated with genetic disorders. These include **germline mutations in tumor suppressor genes** (e.g., neurofibromatosis type1, Gardner syndrome, tuberous sclerosis, Li-Fraumeni syndrome, Osler-Weber Rendu syndrome).

Environmental factors: Exposures to radiation (e.g., angiosarcoma, osteosarcoma, or undifferentiated sarcoma), burns (fibroblastic tumors developing in burn scars), or toxins may be associated with a few soft tissue tumors. Trauma has no role in the development of soft tissue tumors, and it merely draws attention to a pre-existing tumor.

Origin: The origin of sarcomas is not known and does not usually arise from recognized precursor lesions. **Probably**, they **arise from pluripotent mesenchymal stem cells** that reside in soft tissues and bone marrow. These stem cells acquire somatic "driver" mutations. Few generalizations can be made based on the genomic complexity of soft tissue tumors.

- **Simple karyotype (15–20% of sarcomas):** Similar to many leukemias and lymphomas, sarcomas may be **euploid** (presence of chromosome number which is the multiple of the basic chromosome set) tumors with a single or limited number of chromosomal changes occurring during early tumorigenesis. They may be specific and useful as diagnostic markers. Such tumors usually arise in younger patients and microscopically have a monomorphic appearance. For example, Ewing sarcoma and synovial sarcoma.
- **Complex karyotype (80%–85% of sarcomas):** Usually, these tumors are **aneuploid or polyploid**. They show multiple chromosomal gains and losses, indicating genomic instability. For example, leiomyosarcoma and undifferentiated pleomorphic sarcoma. Such tumors usually arise in adults and microscopically have a pleomorphic appearance.

WHO classification (2020) of soft tissue tumors is presented in Box 25.6.

General principles of soft tissue tumors are presented in **Box 25.7.**

TUMORS OF ADIPOSE TISSUE

Lipoma

Q. Write a short note on lipoma.

- Lipoma is the **most common benign tumor composed of mature fat (with adipocyte differentiation).**
- **Age:** It shows a wide age range (40–60 years most common). It is the **most common soft tissue tumor in adults.**

BOX 25.6: The World Health Organization (WHO) (2020) (abridged) classification of soft tissue tumors.

Adipocytic tumors

Benign:

- Lipoma

Malignant:

- Dedifferentiated liposarcoma
- Myxoid liposarcoma
- Pleomorphic liposarcoma
- Myxoid pleomorphic liposarcoma

Fibroblastic and myofibroblastic tumors

Benign:

- Nodular fasciitis
- Proliferative fasciitis and proliferative myositis

Intermediate (locally aggressive):

- Palmar fibromatosis and plantar fibromatosis
- Desmoid fibromatosis

Intermediate (rarely metastasizing):

- Dermatofibrosarcoma protuberans NOS
- Solitary fibrous tumor NOS

Malignant:

- Solitary fibrous tumor, malignant
- Adult fibrosarcoma

So-called fibrohistiocytic tumors

Benign:

- Tenosynovial giant cell tumor NOS

Intermediate (rarely metastasizing):

- Giant cell tumor of soft parts NOS

Malignant:

- Malignant tenosynovial giant cell tumor

Vascular tumors

Benign:

- Hemangioma
- Lymphangioma NOS

Intermediate (rarely metastasizing)

- Kaposi sarcoma

Malignant:

- Angiosarcoma

Smooth muscle tumors

Benign and intermediate:

- Leiomyoma

Malignant:

- Leiomyosarcoma

Skeletal muscle tumors

Benign:

- Rhabdomyoma NOS

Malignant:

- Embryonal rhabdomyosarcoma NOS
- Alveolar rhabdomyosarcoma
- Pleomorphic rhabdomyosarcoma NOS

Contd...

Contd...

Peripheral nerve sheath tumors

Benign:

- Schwannoma NOS
- Neurofibroma NOS

Malignant:

- Malignant peripheral nerve sheath tumor NOS

Tumors of uncertain differentiation

Benign:

- Angiomyolipoma

Malignant:

- Synovial sarcoma NOS
- Epithelioid sarcoma
- Alveolar soft part sarcoma
- Undifferentiated sarcoma

(NOS: not otherwise specified)

BOX 25.7: General principles of soft tissue tumors.

Location: Superficial tumors usually tend to be benign and deep lesions are often malignant

Size: Large tumors are more likely malignant than small ones

Growth: Rapidly growing tumors are more likely to be malignant than tumors that grow slowly

Calcification: It may be seen in both benign and malignant tumors

Vascularity: Benign tumors are relatively avascular, whereas most malignant tumors tend to be highly vascular

MORPHOLOGY

Localization: Lipoma can arise from any site in the body that contains adipose tissue. Usually arises in the **subcutaneous tissues of the proximal extremities**, neck, back, shoulder, and trunk. Infrequently, lipomas are large and intramuscular.

Morphological variants: There are several morphological variants such as conventional lipoma, fibrolipoma, angiolipoma, spindle cell lipoma, and myelolipoma. Conventional lipoma is the most common subtype.

Gross (Fig. 25.26A)

Lipoma is usually a **well-encapsulated** (may be poorly circumscribed), **small, round to oval mass.** The cut surface is **soft, yellow, greasy, and often lobulated.** They vary in size and may become very large. Infrequently, lipomas may be large, intramuscular, and poorly circumscribed.

Microscopy (Figs. 25.26B and C)

Lipoma shows **lobules of mature** (well-differentiated) **adipocytes** separated by delicate fibrous septa. The adipocytes **closely resemble normal fat.** A thin fibrous capsule is usually found surrounding the tumor.

Presentation: Lipomas are usually single, soft, mobile, and painless (except angiolipoma). Lipomas are completely benign tumors. Adequate treatment is the local excision of the tumor.

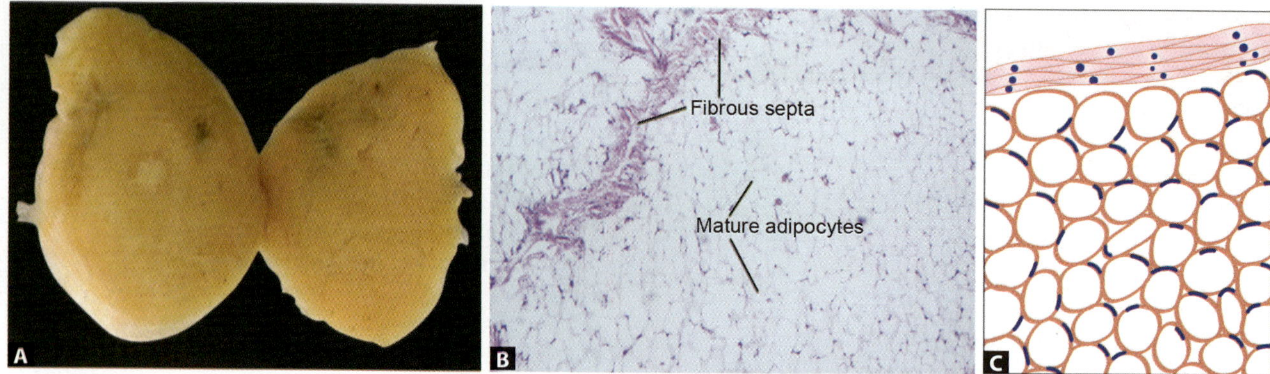

Figs. 25.26A to C: Lipoma; (A) Gross; (B and C) Microscopically a well-differentiated tumor composed of lobules of fat cells that are identical in appearance to normal fat cells.

Liposarcoma

Liposarcoma is a malignant tumor of adipose tissue.
Age: It occurs mainly during the 5–7th decades of life. It is one of the **most common soft tissue sarcomas** (15–25% of malignant soft tissue tumors) in adulthood.

Molecular Pathogenesis

Liposarcomas are divided into four distinct subtypes. These are histologically, biologically, and cytogenetically distinct from one another.

1. **Atypical lipomatous tumor/well-differentiated liposarcomas is** characterized by the presence of a **giant marker chromosome** or a **supernumerary ring chromosome**. Both supernumerary rings and giant markers chromosomes are **associated with the amplification of** the **12q13-15 region**. This region is the **site of several genes** (e.g., ***MDM2****, GLI, SAS, CDK4, HMGIC*). MDM2 encodes a potent inhibitor of p53.
2. **Dedifferentiated liposarcoma**: Dedifferentiation is a **histologic progression of a tumor to a higher grade**, and the **tumor appears less well differentiated**. Dedifferentiated liposarcoma is an **atypical lipomatous tumor/well-differentiated liposarcomas with adjacent areas of high-grade nonlipogenic sarcoma.** It is genetically like an atypical lipomatous tumor/well-differentiated liposarcomas characterized by consistent amplification of *MDM2* and *CDK4* (12q14-q15).
3. **Myxoid liposarcomas:** They have a reciprocal translocation between chromosomes 12 and 16, [t (12;16) (q13; p11)]. It is characterized by a fusion of the *TLS/FUS* gene on chromosome 16 with the *DDIT3* gene on chromosome 12. The resultant fusion gene arrests adipose differentiation. The *TLS/FUS* gene product is like the EWS protein of Ewing sarcoma.
4. **Pleomorphic liposarcoma**: It is a **pleomorphic, high-grade sarcoma demonstrating evidence of lipoblastic differentiation and contains variable numbers of pleomorphic lipoblasts.** Pleomorphic liposarcomas have complex karyotypes. It has no reproducible genetic abnormalities.

MORPHOLOGY

Localization: Deep soft tissues of the proximal extremities (deep thigh) and in the **retroperitoneum.**

Gross

The gross appearance of liposarcoma depends on the subtypes. Usually, liposarcomas appear as nodular masses of 5 cm or more in diameter. Tumors usually appear circumscribed but infiltrate into surrounding tissue. The cut section shows a gray-white to yellow color with a myxoid and gelatinous appearance. The gross appearance depends on the proportions of adipose, mucinous, and fibrous tissue.

- **Atypical lipomatous tumor/well-differentiated liposarcomas:** They are **usually large, well-circumscribed, multilobulated masses.** They usually measure 5–10 cm in diameter. The retroperitoneal tumors may be large up to 40 cm in diameter. They may resemble normal fat or may show fibrotic or gelatinous cut surfaces.
- **Dedifferentiated liposarcoma**: It usually presents as a **large (>5 cm) multinodular mass** that ranges in color from **yellow to yellow-tan, admixed with firm tan-gray areas.**
- **Myxoid liposarcoma**: They usually arise in the proximal extremities and are rare in the retroperitoneum. They are **nonencapsulated, multinodular, gelatinous tumors with ill-defined margins.**
- **Pleomorphic liposarcoma**: Most tumors are large, with a median size of 8–10 cm. They are well demarcated but nonencapsulated, or irregular and infiltrative.

Microscopy (Figs. 25.27A to C)

Lipoblasts may be seen microscopically in all types of liposarcoma. Lipoblasts are early adipocytes. They may be uninucleated or multinucleated having univacuolated or multivacuolated cytoplasmic fat vesicles indenting the nucleus. Lipoblasts are frequently seen in liposarcoma. However, **lipoblasts may be seen in reactive or regenerative conditions and are neither necessary nor sufficient for the diagnosis of liposarcoma.**

Liposarcomas are histologically divided into four subtypes:

1. **Atypical lipomatous tumor/well-differentiated liposarcoma (Fig. 25.27A):** Contains large amounts of mature adipocytes (fat cells) with scattered atypical spindle cells and lipoblasts. These may be confused with lipomas if inadequately sampled.

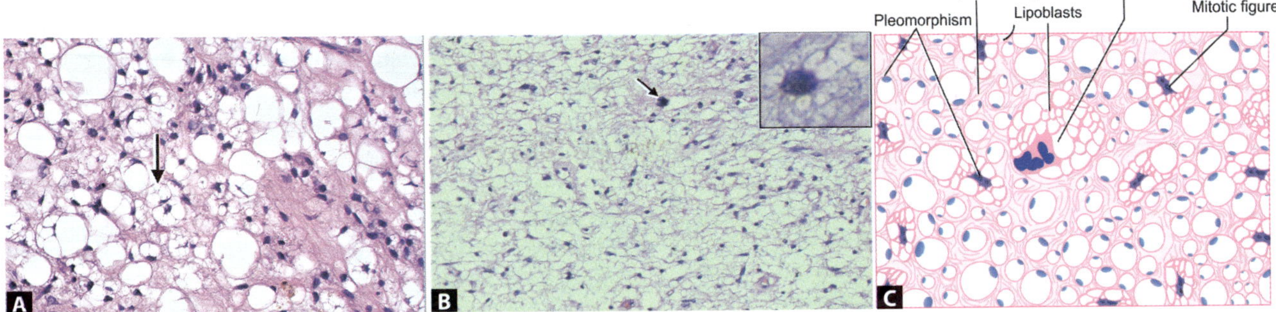

Figs. 25.27A to C: (A) Atypical lipomatous tumors/well-differentiated liposarcoma showing atypical stromal cells and few multivacuolated lipoblasts (arrow). The adipocytes show variation in size; (B) Myxoid liposarcoma with an abundant myxoid matrix. The neoplastic cells are small, round to ovoid, and bland. Few lipoblasts (arrows and inset) are seen. Few delicate capillaries are seen; (C) The diagrammatic appearance of myxoid liposarcoma.

2. **Dedifferentiated liposarcoma:** It is an **atypical lipomatous tumor/well-differentiated liposarcomas with adjacent areas of high-grade nonlipogenic sarcoma** (resembles undifferentiated pleomorphic sarcoma).
3. **Myxoid liposarcoma (Fig. 25.27B):** Most common histological subtype. The tumor is characterized by an **abundant myxoid matrix** (abundant basophilic extracellular matrix), **scattered lipoblasts, relatively bland primitive round to oval cells, and a delicate curvilinear to plexiform capillary network** (arborizing capillaries with **chicken-wire pattern).**
   - **Progression to round cell areas:** As myxoid liposarcomas lose their differentiation, the cells assume an increasingly round cell appearance. The primitive round cells may form sheets. These cells have a high nuclear/cytoplasmic ratio and a prominent nucleolus.
4. **Pleomorphic liposarcoma:** It is highly undifferentiated/anaplastic liposarcoma and consists of sheets of large, anaplastic cells, with bizarre nuclei. These are admixed with variable numbers of immature adipocytes (lipoblasts).

Clinical features and behavior: All histological subtypes of liposarcoma recur locally and often repeatedly unless excised adequately. Well-differentiated liposarcoma is relatively indolent and almost never metastasizes. The pleomorphic variant usually is aggressive and frequently metastasizes with the worst outcome. The myxoid liposarcoma is intermediate in its malignant behavior with a risk of local recurrence and metastasis.

FIBROBLASTIC/MYOFIBROBLASTIC TUMORS

Nodular Fasciitis

Nodular fasciitis is a **rapidly growing but self-limited mesenchymal (fibroblastic and myofibroblastic) neoplasm.** It presents as a rapidly growing tumor (several weeks or months).

Age and gender: Most tumors occur in **young adults.** It is more frequent between the ages of 20 and 50 years. Men and women are equally affected.

Pathogenesis: It is characterized by a **translocation (17;22) (p13; q13)** producing a *MYH9USP6* fusion gene. The fusion results in the overexpression of USP6, an oncogenic protein.

MORPHOLOGY

Localization: Nodular fasciitis usually arises **on the surface of the fascia, deep dermis, subcutis, or muscle.** It **typically affects superficial tissues of the upper extremities** (forearm, trunk, and back).

Gross

Grossly, it is <5 cm, **circumscribed, or slightly infiltrative but is not encapsulated.**

Microscopy

Well-demarcated lesion: Usually, nodular fasciitis is a spherical nodule with a well-demarcated peripheral border.

Tumor cells: It is a highly cellular tumor composed of **plump, uniform, elongated, spindle-shaped, immature-appearing fibroblasts and myofibroblasts.** The tumor cells vary in size and shape (spindle to stellate) and contain nuclei with conspicuous nucleoli. Mitosis is variable and may be numerous. But it does not show atypical forms. Nonetheless, nodular fasciitis is the **classic example of a dictum,** i.e., **benign lesions may be quite mitotically active.**

Architecture: Nodular fasciitis has a characteristic architecture. It has a gradient, termed the **zonation effect, in which there are transitions from hypercellular regions with myxoid stroma to hypocellular areas with fibrous stroma.**

Stroma: It shows a myxoid appearance. Lymphocytes and extravasated red blood cells are common.

Prognosis: Nodular fasciitis is a self-limited lesion and can regress spontaneously. It is cured by surgical excision and it rarely recurs. Malignant transformation does not occur.

Fibromatoses

Fibromatosis (singular: fibromatosis; plural: fibromatoses) comprises a **broad group of benign fibroblastic proliferation** and has similar microscopic appearances. These tumors are characterized by infiltrative growth and a tendency toward recurrence, but they never metastasize.

Groups: Fibromatosis can be grouped into two distinct forms: (1) palmar/plantar and (2) desmoid fibromatosis.

1. Palmar and Plantar Fibromatoses

Palmar and plantar fibromatoses are **benign nodular fibroblastic/myofibroblastic proliferations** on the hands and feet, respectively. These are grouped under superficial fibromatosis.

MORPHOLOGY

Localization

Palmar fibromatosis: Typically, it arises in the volar or flexor aspect of the hands and fingers.

Plantar fibromatosis: Typically involves nonweight-bearing areas, such as the aponeurosis of the medial plantar arch (plantar aponeuroses).

Both palmar and plantar fibromatoses have a similar morphologic appearance.

Gross

Tumors are **small, firm, poorly defined** 0.5–3.0 cm **nodules.** They are **closely associated with a tendon or aponeurosis** and extend into subcutaneous tissue. The cut surface appears grayish-yellow or white (depending on the collagen content) and slightly whorled.

Microscopy

Typically, tumors **involve thickened palmar/plantar aponeurosis.** They form **single to multiple discontinuous, moderately cellular spindle cell nodules** in a **collagenous stroma.**

Tumor cells: The fibroblasts are **bland, plump, elongated, relatively uniform, and spindle-shaped. They have tapering, monomorphic nuclei** (devoid of nuclear atypia) with vesicular chromatin and small or inconspicuous nucleoli.

Cellularity: Some plantar fibromatoses are hypercellular and can mimic spindle cell sarcomas, but they do not show atypical features.

Minimal stromal collagen: The tumor shows a variable amount of collagen in the stroma, which is usually minimal.

Behavior: Palmar and plantar fibromatoses progress in about 50% of patients; the remainder stabilize and do not progress. Some resolve spontaneously. They may recur locally after excision. However, these are localized lesions without the same potential for destructive growth and infiltration seen in desmoid tumors.

2. Desmoid Fibromatosis

Desmoid fibromatosis (desmoid tumor) is a **locally aggressive but nonmetastasizing** (does not metastasize), **deep-seated (myo)fibroblastic neoplasm**. These **tumors form large, infiltrative masses** and have a high **frequency** of **recurrence**. Desmoid fibromatosis (plural fibromatoses) is also called **deep fibromatosis** and involves deep structures. Their biological behavior is more aggressive than that of the superficial fibromatoses.

Subtypes: It may be **extra-abdominal desmoid or abdominal fibromatosis**.

Age and gender: Extra-abdominal fibromatosis occurs between puberty and 40 years of age, with a peak incidence between 25 and 35 years. **Abdominal fibromatosis occurs in women of childbearing**.

Pathogenesis

Most desmoid fibromatoses are sporadic, and 10% are familial.

Increased activation of the Wnt/β-catenin signaling pathway: This may occur due to the activating mutations in *CTNNB1* or inactivating mutations in *APC*. This promotes cell proliferation and survival and appears to drive tumorigenesis.

- **Activating mutation of *CTNNB1* (*β-catenin*) gene:** The majority (90–95%) of sporadic desmoid fibromatoses have activating mutations in the *CTNNB1* (*β-catenin*) gene.
- **Inactivating mutation of *APC* gene:** Few desmoid tumors arise in the setting of Gardner syndrome (individuals with familial adenomatous polyposis). These patients harbor **germline inactivate mutations** in the *APC* tumor suppressor gene.

MORPHOLOGY

Localization

Extra-abdominal fibromatosis: It mainly arises from the connective tissue of muscle and the overlying fascia or aponeurosis. It mainly occurs in the shoulder, pelvic girdle, and thigh muscles of adolescents and young adults.

Abdominal fibromatosis: It occurs in young, gravid, or parous women during gestation or, more commonly, during the first year following childbirth. Abdominal fibromatosis usually arises in the musculoaponeurotic structures of the **anterior abdominal wall.**

Gross

Desmoid fibromatosis appears as a **solid, poorly circumscribed, firm mass.** The size varies from 1 to 15 cm in diameter (usually 5–10 cm in diameter). The cut surface shows a **whitish-tan, fibrous or gelatinous, coarsely trabecular or whorled tumor.**

Microscopy (Fig. 25.28)

Poorly circumscribed: Most fibromatosis are poorly circumscribed with ill-defined margins. They infiltrate the adjacent adipose tissue, nerve, or skeletal muscle.

Architecture: The tumor **grows in long, "sweeping" fascicles or graceful arcs.** The tumor cells appear parallel, **a pattern sometimes likened to a school of fish.**

Tumor cells: It is composed of **elongated, spindle-to-stellate-shaped uniform, bland fibroblasts** (wiry cells), **and myofibroblasts.** These cells have pale eosinophilic cytoplasm and pale staining small vesicular nuclei with 1 or several (usually one to three) pinpoint (tiny) nucleoli. They lack nuclear hyperchromasia, pleomorphism, and atypical mitotic figures. Mitotic figures are typically absent or rare.

Cellularity: The overall cellularity of the tumor is low to intermediate (cellularity is never marked).

Stroma: The uniform cells are separated from one another by a collagenous stroma. The tumor shows thin-walled staghorn or hemangiopericytoma-like blood vessels.

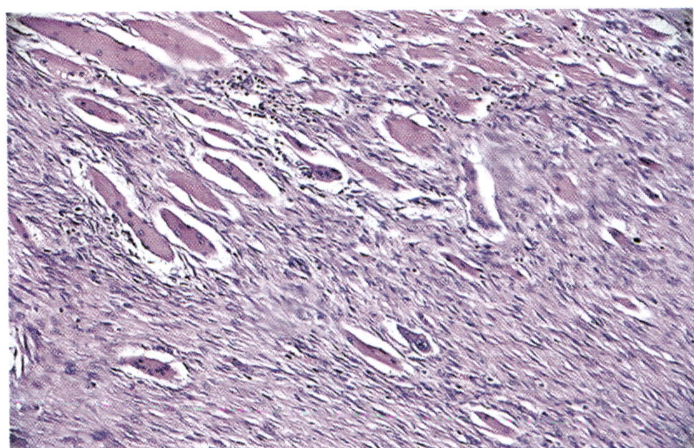

Fig. 25.28: Desmoid fibromatosis showing elongated, spindle-to-stellate-shaped uniform cells. The tumor is poorly circumscribed and shows infiltration into the adjacent skeletal muscle.

Behavior: The natural course of desmoid fibromatosis is variable, with unpredictable growth, stabilization, and regression. It often recurs, but if left alone, it may stop growing or regress. The *CTNNB1* mutation may predict recurrence.

Fibrosarcoma

The term fibrosarcoma is used for two tumor types: **Infantile fibrosarcoma (IFS)** and **adult fibrosarcoma.**

Infantile fibrosarcoma: It is a malignant fibroblastic tumor most commonly occurring in infancy. It often grows as a large mass in the extremities or trunk wall. It is a locally aggressive and rapidly growing tumor that rarely metastasizes. Microscopically, it is composed of intersecting, highly cellular fascicles of primitive-appearing, mitotically active spindle cells. Most frequently, it harbors an *ETV6-NTRK3* rearrangement giving rise to an *ETV6-NTRK3 fusion*. Recently, alternate gene fusions have been identified (e.g., *NTRK1, BRAF*, or *MET*).

Adult fibrosarcoma: It is a rare sarcoma composed of relatively monomorphic (uniform) fibroblastic tumor cells. They show variable collagen production and often herringbone architecture. The median age is 5 years. In the past, tumors in adults labeled as fibrosarcomas formed a high percentage of soft tissue sarcomas. Recently, the total number of tumors labeled fibrosarcoma has significantly decreased. This is mainly because of the following two reasons: (i) **pleomorphic tumors in adults** are currently termed undifferentiated pleomorphic sarcoma (UPS), and (ii) the **use of IHC and molecular genetic analysis** have identified several distinct tumor types that mimic fibrosarcoma in adults. **Diagnosis of adult fibrosarcoma** is a diagnosis of exclusion, and true fibrosarcomas are very rare.

MORPHOLOGY

Localization: Adult fibrosarcoma usually arises in the deep soft tissues of the extremities, trunk, and head and neck region.

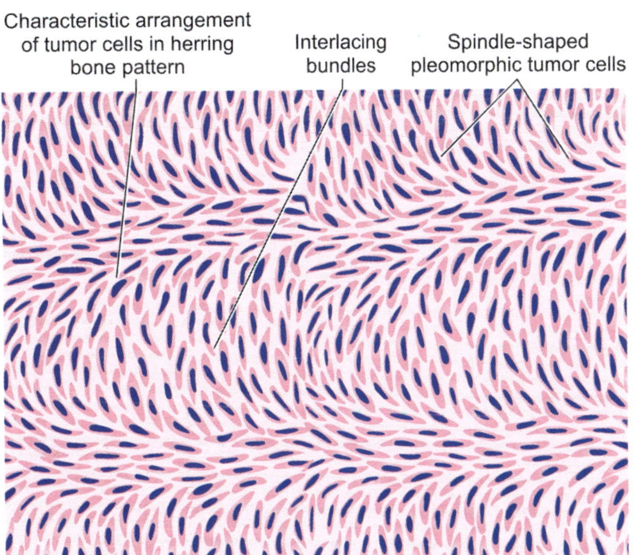

Fig. 25.29: Fibrosarcoma composed of spindle-shaped fibroblasts arranged in intersecting fascicles (characteristic herringbone pattern).

Gross

Adult fibrosarcoma is a circumscribed, firm, white, or tan mass. The median size is 6.5 cm. Hemorrhage and necrosis can be seen in high-grade tumors.

Microscopy (Fig. 25.29)

- **Uniform spindle-shaped tumor cells:** Adult fibrosarcoma is composed of relatively uniform (monomorphic) fusiform/spindle cells. The cells have tapering hyperchromatic nuclei with variably prominent nucleoli. The cytoplasm is scant. These cells show only a mild-to-moderate degree of pleomorphism. Mitotic figures are almost always present but variable.
- **Herringbone pattern (Fig. 25.29):** The tumor cells are characteristically (but nonspecific) arranged in long, sweeping fascicles. These may be angled in a chevron-like or herringbone pattern.
- **Stroma:** The stroma has variable collagen. These collagen fibers are seen between tumor cells and run parallel.

Prognosis. More than 80% of adult fibrosarcomas are high-grade. The overall survival rate is <70% at 2 years and <55% at 5 years. They metastasize to lungs and bone, especially the axial skeleton. The local recurrence is related to the completeness of excision.

SKELETAL MUSCLE TUMORS

Skeletal muscle neoplasms unlike other mesenchymal tumors, are almost all malignant. The benign tumor namely, rhabdomyoma occurs in individuals with tuberous sclerosis.

Rhabdomyosarcoma

Rhabdomyosarcoma (RMS) is a malignant mesenchymal tumor that shows **skeletal muscle differentiation.**

Rhabdomyosarcomas **do not arise in the extremities**, where the bulk of skeletal muscle resides.

Subtypes: There are four major subtypes namely: (1) embryonal (50%), (2) alveolar (20%), (3) pleomorphic (20%), and (4) spindle cell/sclerosing (10%).

Age: Alveolar and embryonal subtypes of RMS are the most common soft tissue sarcoma in childhood (children between 3 and 12 years), and adolescence. They usually appear before 20 years of age. Pleomorphic RMS occurs in adults, while the spindle cell/sclerosing type can manifest at all ages.

Localization

- **Embryonal rhabdomyosarcoma:** It shows morphological and immunophenotypic **features of embryonic skeletal muscle**. It **often arises in locations that do not normally contain much skeletal muscle** (arises in the sinuses, head and neck, and genitourinary tract). Thus, sarcomas seem to not arise from mature, terminally differentiated cells. Botryoid-type RMS has a characteristic exophytic, polypoid appearance with clusters of small, sessile, or pedunculated (grapelike) nodules adjacent to an epithelial surface.
- **Alveolar rhabdomyosarcoma:** It is less frequent than the embryonal type. It is mainly found in young individuals between 10 to 25 years of age and rarely in elderly patients. The most common site is the upper and lower extremities.
- **Pleomorphic rhabdomyosarcoma:** It occurs in the skeletal muscles of older individuals (e.g., thigh).
- **Spindle cell rhabdomyosarcoma**: The most common site of involvement is the head and neck region.

MORPHOLOGY

1. **Embryonal (50%):**

   Gross: It presents as a **soft, fleshy, friable, gray, poorly demarcated, infiltrative mass.**

   Microscopy (*refer* **online Fig. 25.30A)**

   - The tumor cells mimic skeletal muscle at various stages of embryogenesis. It consists of sheets of both primitive round and spindled cells in a myxoid stroma.
   - Well-differentiated tumors may show **rhabdomyoblasts with strap-like eosinophilic cytoplasm and cross-striations** [better seen with phosphotungstic acid (PTAH) stain]. Poorly differentiated tumors show small cells.

   Sarcoma botryoides (botryoid embryonal rhabdomyosarcoma): It is a variant of embryonal rhabdomyosarcoma and is distinguished by the formation of **polypoid, grape-like tumor masses.** It occurs in the walls of hollow, mucosal-lined structures (e.g., nasopharynx, urinary bladder, common bile duct, vagina).

   - **Microscopy:** The malignant cells are scattered in an abundant myxoid stroma. Where the tumors abut (touch) the mucosa of an organ, they form a submucosal zone of hypercellularity called the **cambium layer.**

2. **Alveolar (20%):**

   Gross: Alveolar RMS is soft, fleshy, and gray. It contains variable amounts of fibrous tissue and occasional areas of necrosis and hemorrhage.

   Microscopy (*refer* **online Fig. 25.30B)**

   - **Tumor cells:** It is a highly cellular tumor composed of **primitive, relatively uniform** (monomorphic), **medium-sized round cells** with **scant (minimal or little) cytoplasm.**
   - **Alveolar pattern:** Tumor cells are arranged in nests and sheets separated by a network of fibrovascular septa of variable thickness. These septae divide the cells into clusters or aggregates, creating a crude resemblance to pulmonary alveoli.

3. **Pleomorphic (20%)**

   Gross: Pleomorphic RMSs are usually large and measure >10 cm, which occur in deep skeletal muscle (intramuscular). They are well-circumscribed, with a pseudocapsule.

   Microscopy: It is characterized by numerous, large, sometimes multinucleated, bizarre eosinophilic tumor cells. Microscopically, it can resemble other pleomorphic sarcomas.

4. **Spindle cell/sclerosing (10%)**

   Gross: Spindle cell/sclerosing rhabdomyosarcomas appear as variably circumscribed tumors. Their sizes range from 1.5 to 35 cm.

   Microscopy: Tumor cells appear as **primitive round, ovoid, or spindle cells.** They have **scant, pale, eosinophilic, or clear cytoplasm.** The cells contain **blunted, ovoid, or fusiform, centrally located nuclei with small inconspicuous nucleoli.** Tumor cells are arranged predominantly in **cords, nests, microalveoli, or trabeculae in a pseudovascular growth pattern.**

Immunohistochemistry: All rhabdomyosarcoma shows immunohistochemical evidence of skeletal muscle (rhabdomyoblastic) differentiation. These include nonspecific myoid markers (e.g., actin and desmin) and skeletal muscle-specific markers (at least focal expression), such as the transcription factors myogenin and MyoD1.

Prognosis: Rhabdomyosarcomas are **aggressive malignant tumors.** They may be treated with surgery and chemotherapy, with or without radiation therapy. Factors that indicate a worse prognosis include age older than 10, tumor size more than 5 cm, alveolar and pleomorphic histologic subtypes, and advanced stage of disease. The botryoid rhabdomyosarcoma has the best prognosis, whereas the pleomorphic subtype is often fatal.

SMOOTH MUSCLE TUMORS

Smooth muscle cells are spindled cells with brightly eosinophilic cytoplasm and contain cylindrical nuclei. Immunohistochemically they **express smooth muscle actin, muscle-specific actin, and desmin.**

Leiomyoma

Leiomyoma of deep tissue is a benign soft tissue tumor of smooth muscle origin. However, leiomyoma arising from the smooth muscles of the uterus (*refer* page 816) is the most common neoplasm in women.

Age and gender: They most commonly occur during the 4–6th decades. Deep soft tissue (somatic) leiomyomas occur equally in both sexes.

Localization: It usually arises in sites associated with normal smooth muscle. It can arise in any site having soft tissue (e.g., dermis, blood vessel walls in subcutaneous or deep somatic tissues, and the muscular wall of the esophagus).

MORPHOLOGY

Gross

They appear as firm, gray-white, well-circumscribed nodules and usually measure 1–2 cm in diameter. Dermal or subcutaneous tumors may be painful.

Microscopy (*refer* Fig. 22.24)

Uniform spindle cells: They are composed of intersecting (intersecting each other at right angles) fascicles of uniform densely eosinophilic spindled cells with cigar-shaped (blunt-ended, elongated) nuclei. Tumor cells show minimal atypia and few (very low) mitotic figures.

Treatment: Simple excision is curative.

Leiomyosarcoma

Leiomyosarcoma is a **malignant smooth muscle tumor that** accounts for about 10–20% of soft tissue sarcomas. They can spread to the lungs via a hematogenous route.

Age and gender: They occur most commonly in middle-aged to older adults. Retroperitoneal and pelvic LMSs show clear female predilection.

Site: Most common in the **deep soft tissues of the extremities and retroperitoneum**. Leiomyosarcomas **present as painless firm masses**. Retroperitoneal tumors may be large and bulky and cause abdominal symptoms.

MORPHOLOGY

Gross

Leiomyosarcomas of soft tissue appear as a fleshy, gray to white to tan tumor. The cut surface may show a whorled appearance. Large tumors usually show areas of hemorrhage, necrosis, or cystic change.

Microscopy (*refer* online Figs. 25.31A and B)

The tumor border frequently appears well-circumscribed and "pushing." It may be irregular and infiltrative. They are composed of **eosinophilic spindle cells with blunt-ended, hyperchromatic nuclei.** Mitotic activity and necrosis are common. The tumor **cells are arranged in broad, interweaving fascicles.**

Immunohistochemistry: They are positive for smooth muscle actin, desmin, and caldesmon.

Treatment: It depends on tumor size, location, and grade.

PERIPHERAL NERVE SHEATH TUMORS

Common types of peripheral nerve sheath tumors are schwannoma, neurofibroma, and malignant peripheral nerve sheath tumor (MPNST).

Schwannoma (Neurilemmoma)

Schwannoma or neurilemmoma **is a benign encapsulated tumor of peripheral nerve sheath origin that shows Schwann cell differentiation. These tumors often arise directly from peripheral nerves.** Most schwannomas are sporadic. However, about 10% are associated with *familial neurofibromatosis type 2 (NF2).*

Localization: It **arises from the soft tissues, internal organs, or** cranial or **spinal nerve roots. Most common in the vestibular portion of the eighth cranial nerve** (acoustic schwannoma).

MORPHOLOGY

Gross

Most schwannomas appear as a solitary, **solid, well-circumscribed, encapsulated tumor (Fig. 25.32).**

The nerve of origin, if large enough, may be identifiable in <50% of cases. In these cases, the tumors are attached loosely to the associated nerve without invading it. They are firm and gray.

Microscopy

Well-circumscribed tumor: It appears as a nodular mass with a fibrous capsule.

Schwann cells: Schwannoma is a tumor of Schwann cells. These cells are characterized by the presence of a **spindled elongated nucleus** with a **wavy or buckled shape.**

A biphasic tumor (Figs. 25.33A to C): Microscopically, a helpful clue to the diagnosis is the dimorphic growth pattern. The majority are biphasic (dimorphic) tumors with an admixture of compact (dense) areas (Antoni A tissue) alternating with loosely arranged, acellular foci (Antoni B tissue). The tumor cells are neoplastic Schwann cells of the peripheral nerve sheath.

- **Antoni A areas:** These are **dense, cellular, and eosinophilic areas.** The spindle-shaped cells are arranged in **intersecting fascicles.** The cells show **palisading of nuclei and alternating bands of "nuclear-free zones."** These nuclear free zones between the regions of nuclear palisading are termed **Verocay bodies.**

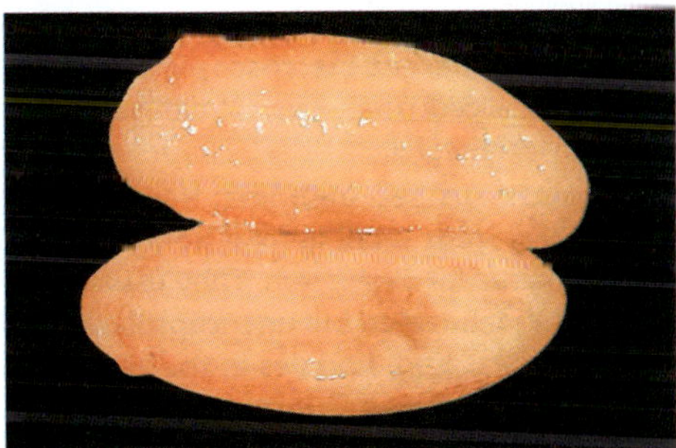

Fig. 25.32: Bisected schwannoma showing a circumscribed firm tumor with a tan-to-gray color.

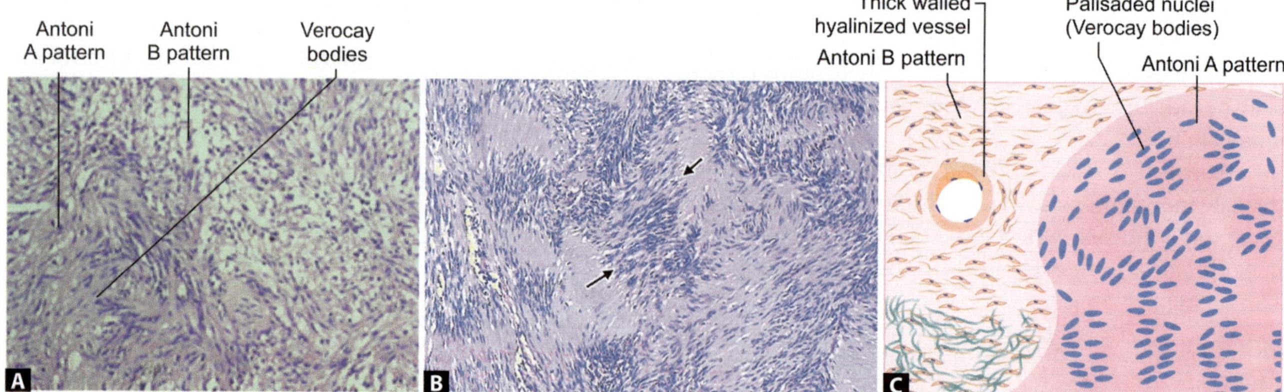

Figs. 25.33A to C: Microscopic appearance of Schwannoma (neurilemmoma): (A) It shows densely cellular (Antoni A) and loosely cellular (Antoni B) areas with characteristic nuclear palisading (Verocay bodies) in the Antoni A area (B) Shows densely cellular (Antoni A) area with characteristic nuclear palisading (Verocay bodies) (arrows); (C) Diagrammatic appearance.

Antoni B areas: Antoni A areas alternate with **loosely arranged** foci referred to as Antoni B tissue. Antoni B pattern has a spindle or oval Schwann cells with indistinct cytoplasm. The Antoni B areas are **loose, hypocellular, and lack orientation of the Schwann cells.** A **prominent vacuolated, myxoid extracellular matrix separates the spindle cells.** Antoni B tissue commonly contains a **cobweb-like network of tumor processes** with collections of **lipid-laden histiocytes.** Antoni B areas may be associated with microcyst formation.

Thick-walled hyalinized vessels: Blood vessels show thickening of the wall and hyalinization. Hemorrhage or cystic changes may be sometimes seen.

Neurofibromas

Neurofibroma is a **benign, slowly growing peripheral nerve sheath tumor**. It is more heterogeneous than schwannoma. It consists of differentiated **neoplastic Schwann cells admixed with perineurial/perineurial-like cells, fibroblasts, mast cells, and CD34+ spindle cells.** It may be either sporadic or NF1-associated.

Age: It shows a wide age range (most common in young to middle-aged adults). Plexiform and diffuse variants occur more often in younger age groups, including children.

MORPHOLOGY

Gross

Neurofibroma has **different macroscopic forms.** The most common are (1) localized cutaneous, (2) diffuse neurofibroma, and (3) plexiform intraneural.

1. **Localized cutaneous neurofibroma:** Neurofibromas most commonly arise from small dermal nerves in the dermis and subcutaneous fat in the skin. They usually present as **small, soft, well-delineated but unencapsulated nodular or polypoid** (pedunculated) **nodules in the skin** of the trunk, head/neck, and extremities.
2. **Diffuse neurofibroma:** They have a **variety of gross appearances.** These include flat, sessile, globular, and pedunculated. These tumors may diffusely infiltrate the dermis and subcutaneous connective tissue, trapping fat and appendage structures.
3. **Plexiform intraneural neurofibroma:** These may be deep or superficially located in association with nerve roots or large nerves. They are commonly observed in the head and neck, trunk, and extremities. They grow within and expand nerve fascicles entrapping associated axons. The ropy thickening of multiple nerve fascicles produces a "bag of worms" appearance.

Microscopy [Figs. 25.34A and C (*refer* online Fig. 25.34B)]

- **Spindle tumor cells with wavy nuclei:** Neurofibromas are characterized by **bland, scattered spindle cells.** These cells have thin **wavy nuclei, "buckled" or "S-shaped" nuclei** (*refer* **online Fig. 25.34B**). These spindle cells represent the neoplastic Schwann cell. The tumor cells are typically smaller than that of schwannoma. Other constituent cells in neurofibroma include perineurial and perineurial-like cells, endoneurial fibroblasts, and mast cells.
- **Loose extracellular stroma:** The cells of neurofibroma are within a **variably loose extracellular myxoid matrix** (stroma). Scattered small vessels and mast cells are common.
- **Pattern:** The tumor cells are arranged **haphazardly or in a vaguely storiform configuration.**
- **No capsule (Fig. 25.34A):** Neurofibromas may appear well demarcated from adjacent connective tissue, but they are not encapsulated (lack a capsule). The neurofibroma frequently merges and often extends beyond the nerve fascicle into adjacent tissue.
- **Nerve fibers course through a neurofibroma.**

Malignant Peripheral Nerve Sheath Tumors

Malignant peripheral nerve sheath tumor (MPNST) is a poorly differentiated, aggressive, spindle cell sarcoma of the peripheral nerve of uncertain histogenesis. MPNST **often arises from a peripheral nerve**. It may occur sporadically (50%), from a pre-existing benign nerve sheath tumor, in patients with NF1 (40%), or following therapeutic radiation therapy (10%). Sporadic cases may arise de novo. MPNSTs are prone to local recurrence and blood-borne metastasis.

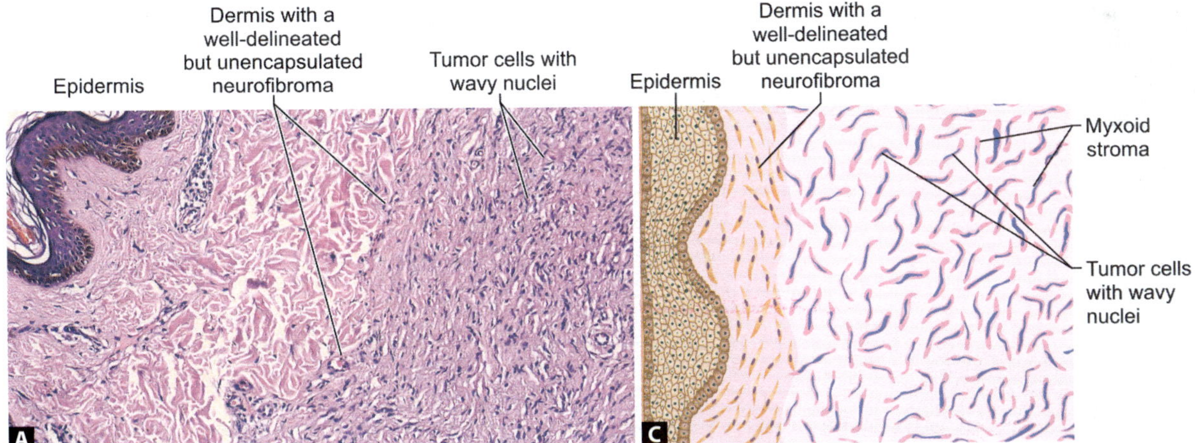

Figs. 25.34A and C: Microscopic appearance of neurofibroma: (A) Cutaneous localized neurofibroma composed of interlacing bundles of spindle-shaped Schwann cells with wavy nuclei; (C) Diagrammatic appearance.

Age: MPNST is most common in adults (20–50 years).
Localization: Commonly arises in larger nerves of the trunk or proximal limbs. They may arise from the transformation of neurofibroma in patients with neurofibromatosis.

MORPHOLOGY

Gross

When MPNSTs arise in a nerve, they appear as **unencapsulated, fusiform enlargements**. MPNSTs are **unencapsulated and usually >5 cm in size.** The surface is **fleshy or gelatinous with a tan–white appearance.**

Microscopy

They are **highly cellular tumors** composed of **spindle cells with buckled nuclei** (*refer* **online Figs. 25.35A and B**). The tumor cells show cytological features of malignancy, including anaplasia (pleomorphism, nuclear atypia, mitotic figures/high proliferative activity), foci of necrosis, and infiltrative growth pattern.

MPNSTs may recur locally and metastasize through blood.

TUMORS OF UNCERTAIN ORIGIN

Many soft tissue tumors do not recapitulate any known mesenchymal lineage. One of the examples is synovial sarcoma.

Synovial Sarcoma

Synovial sarcoma (SS) is a **monomorphic blue spindle cell mesenchymal sarcoma showing variable epithelial differentiation (including gland formation). It** accounts for about 10%of all soft tissue sarcomas.

Synovial sarcoma was so-named because the first few cases described were observed in the soft tissues near the knee joint and were thought to arise from synovium. However, this term is a misnomer, because despite the name **these tumors do not arise from synovial tissues** and can occur in locations without synovium (e.g., chest wall, head, and neck), and morphologically they do not show synoviocyte differentiation.

Age and gender: It typically occurs most commonly in **young adults (majority 10–40 years)**. It has a slight male predominance. Individuals often present with a deep-seated mass that has been present for several years.

Localization: Synovial sarcoma can occur in locations that lack synovium. The majority (70%) of SS arises in the **deep soft tissue of the lower and upper extremities**. Most commonly, they occur **near joints** (juxta-articular or para-articular region), particularly the knee, in association with tendon sheaths, bursae, and joint capsules.

Presentation: They usually present as a deep-seated painless mass of several years duration.

Pathogenesis

Translocation t(X;18)(p11.2;q11.2): Most synovial sarcomas show a characteristic balanced chromosomal translocation involving chromosomes X and 18 [t(x;18)(p11.2; q11.2)]. This translocation involves the **fusion of the *SS18* (also known as SYT synteny) gene** on chromosome 18 **and the *SSX* gene** on the X chromosome (at Xp11). *SSX* gene may be either the *SSX1* (approximately two-thirds of SSs) or *SSX2* gene (one-third of cases), or rarely, *SSX4*. This leads to the production of a hybrid protein, SS18-SSX1, SS18-SSX2, or, rarely, SS18-SSX4. These fusion genes encode chimeric transcription factors that derail the cell cycle.

MORPHOLOGY

Gross (Fig. 25.36)

Synovial sarcoma usually **appears as well-circumscribed, round, or multilobular masses** attached to tendons, tendon sheaths, or the exterior wall of the joint capsule. The tumors may be surrounded by a glistening pseudo capsule and may show cystic areas. The cut surface appears **soft to firm, and the color may be tan, gray, yellow, or pink.** Areas of hemorrhage, necrosis, and calcification may be seen. Their size ranges from small nodules to tumors measuring 15 cm or more in diameter (average 3–5 cm).

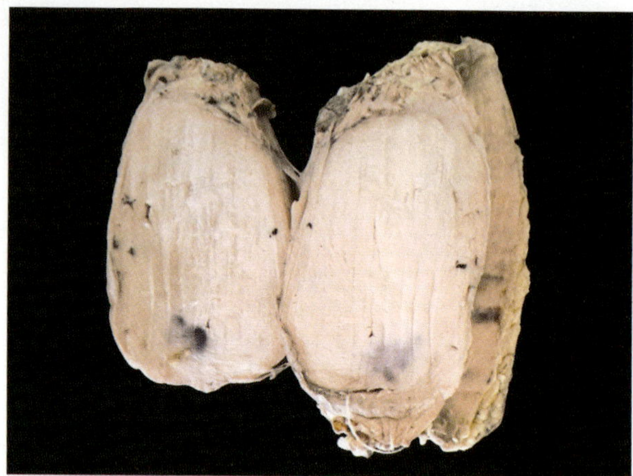

Fig. 25.36: Synovial sarcoma. Grossly appears as a nodular, circumscribed mass. The cut surface shows pink with focal hemorrhage.

Microscopy

Subtypes: Histologically, synovial sarcoma may be (1) spindle cell (monophasic in the majority); (2) biphasic (in approximately one-quarter to one-third of cases); and (3) poorly differentiated.

- **Monophasic (spindle cell) synovial sarcoma:** It consists of **relatively uniform spindle cells** with scant cytoplasm. The **nucleus is ovoid and hyperchromatic** with regular granular chromatin and inconspicuous nucleoli. These tumor cells **grow in short, tightly packed fascicles**. Calcifications may be observed within the tumor. It shows a variable amount of collagenous stroma.
- **Biphasic synovial sarcoma:** It consists of varying proportions of **epithelial and spindle cell components.**
- **Epithelial cell component (Figs. 25.37A and B):** The epithelial cells are **arranged in solid nests or cords or glands** with a tubular architecture. In glandular areas, the **epithelial cells are cuboidal to columnar with distinctly outlined cellular borders.** These cells have **ovoid vesicular nuclei** and typically have more abundant palely eosinophilic cytoplasm than in the dark blue spindle cell component.
- **Spindle cell component (Fig. 25.37):** This comprises the same spindle cell population as in monophasic SS (at least focally). The **epithelial tumor cells are embedded in these plump spindle cells in swirling fascicles that appear like a "school of fish."**
- **Poorly differentiated SS:** In an otherwise typical biphasic or monophasic SS, there may be poorly differentiated areas. They may be focal or extensive. These areas show increased cellularity, high-grade nuclear atypia, and increased mitoses. These are disproportionately more common in elderly patients.

Immunohistochemistry: It helps in differentiating them from many other sarcomas. The tumor cells, especially in the biphasic type, are positive for epithelial antigens (e.g., keratins or epithelial membrane antigens). This supports the evidence of epithelial differentiation.

Treatment and prognosis: Synovial sarcoma is usually an **aggressive neoplasm**, similar to other common adult sarcomas. They are treated aggressively with limb-sparing surgery and frequently chemotherapy. The recurrence rate is high, and metastases occur in more than 60% of cases. Common sites of metastases are the lungs.

Undifferentiated (Unclassified) Sarcoma

Undifferentiated soft tissue sarcoma (USTS) shows **no identifiable line of differentiation** with the use of presently available technology, namely histomorphology, immunohistochemistry (IHC), and molecular genetics. It is a heterogeneous group of malignant mesenchymal tumors with **high-grade pleomorphic cells**. Its **diagnosis is by exclusion**.

Molecular genetics: Most USTSs are aneuploid with multiple structural and numerical chromosomal changes.

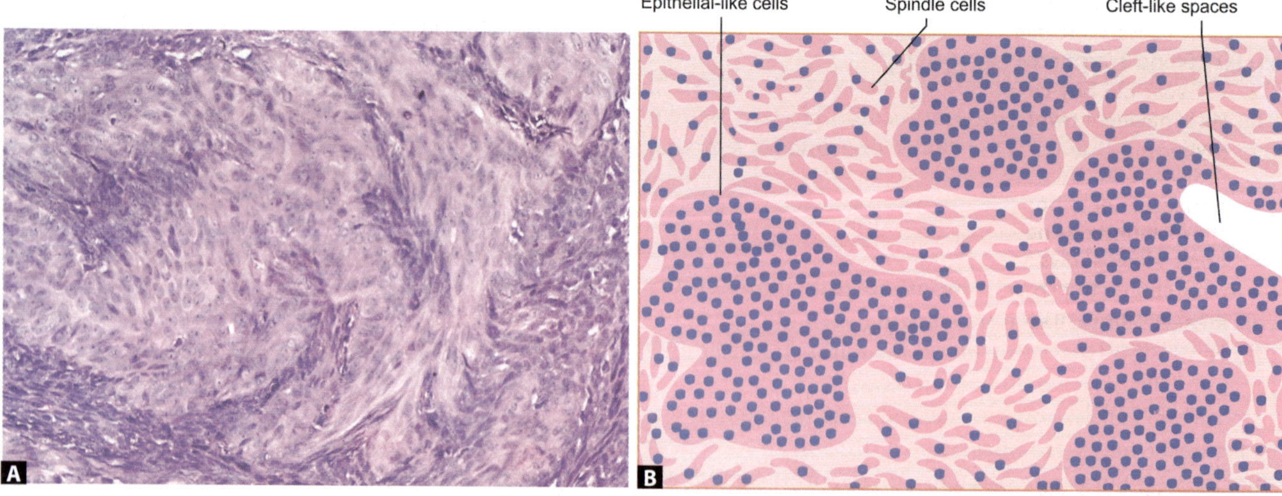

Figs. 25.37A and B: Biphasic synovial sarcoma: (A) The tumor shows glandular areas composed of nests of cohesive, cuboidal to columnar epithelial cells separated by dark blue spindle cells. The epithelial cells have ovoid vesicular nuclei and typically have more abundant palely eosinophilic cytoplasm than in the dark blue spindle cell component; (B) Diagrammatic appearance.

Localization: USTS may arise at any location. It most commonly occurs in the deep soft tissues of the extremities, especially the thigh.
Age: It usually occurs in middle-aged or older adults (50–70 years).

MORPHOLOGY

Gross

They usually appear as **large, gray-white fleshy masses.** The size varies and may be as large as 10–20 cm. **Areas of necrosis and hemorrhage are common.**

Microscopy

They are composed of sheets of large, anaplastic, spindled to polygonal cells with hyperchromatic irregular, sometimes bizarre nuclei (*refer* **online Fig. 25.38**). There will be numerous mitotic figures (including atypical mitotic figures) and areas of necrosis. Tumor cells do not show differentiation along any of the recognized lineages or characteristic genetic defects.

Clinical features: Undifferentiated sarcomas are aggressive malignancies and usually of high grade. They are treated with surgery and adjuvant chemotherapy and/or radiation.
Prognosis: It is generally poor. Local recurrence occurs in up to 30% of cases, and distant metastases develop in 30–50% of cases. The 5-year survival rate is approximately 50%.

SCENARIO-BASED MCQs

1. **An 8-year-old boy has had pain in the right knee for the past 3 weeks. On physical examination, he is having a fever. There is swelling with marked tenderness to palpation in the right knee, pain, and reduced range of motion. Radiographs of the knee region show areas of osteolysis and cortical erosion involving the tibial metaphysis. There is also adjacent soft-tissue swelling extending from the subperiosteal region, and apparent abscess formation. The most likely organisms that can produce these findings are:**
   A. *Neisseria gonorrhoeae*
   B. *Salmonella enterica*
   C. *Staphylococcus aureus*
   D. Group B *Streptococcus*
2. **A 9-year-old boy complains of 2 weeks of pain in the hip. He is having a fever. Laboratory studies show an elevated erythrocyte sedimentation rate. An X ray shows a mottled radiolucent defect in the upper femur, with abundant periosteal new bone formation. Fine-needle aspiration shows numerous neutrophils and cocci. Cultured from the bone lesion shows *Staphylococcus aureus*. A biopsy shows a fragment of necrotic bone embedded in fibrinopurulent exudate. The term used for the necrotic bone in this condition is:**
   A. Cloaca
   B. Involucrum
   C. Sequestrum
   D. Brodie abscess
3. **An 18-year-old boy complains of pain around the right knee for the past 3 months. Physical examination shows local pain over the area of the distal right femur. A radiograph of the right leg shows an ill-defined lytic mass involving the metaphyseal region of the distal right femur, and there is elevation of the adjacent periosteum. Serum levels of alkaline phosphatase are markedly elevated. A bone biopsy is taken. It shows large, hyperchromatic, pleomorphic spindle cells forming an osteoid matrix. Molecular studies of this tumor would most likely reveal a mutation in the tumor suppressor gene:**
   A. *RB*
   B. *APC*
   C. *BRCA1*
   D. *PTEN*
4. **A 30-year-old woman complains of pain in the region of the left knee for 1 month. Physical examination, reveals tenderness to palpation at the distal left thigh and knee. The area is firm in consistency, but there is no erythema or warmth. A radiograph of the left leg shows a 6 cm mass in the distal femoral epiphyseal area, with a "soap bubble" appearance. Microscopic examination of a curettage shows numerous spindle-shaped mononuclear cells and uniformly distributed osteoclast-type giant cells. The lesion recurs in the next year; it is excised and does not recur again. The most likely diagnosis is:**
   A. Chondrosarcoma
   B. Giant cell tumor
   C. Ewings sarcoma
   D. Osteosarcoma
5. **A 14-year-old, previously healthy boy complains of pain in the right leg for the past month. There is no history of trauma or any illness. Physical examination shows warmth and tenderness over the right lower thigh anteriorly. The circumference of the right thigh is slightly more than that of the left. A radiograph of the right leg shows a 5 cm expansile mass in the diaphyseal region of the right lower femur. It extends into the soft tissue and is covered by layers of reactive bone giving rise to an "onion skin" pattern. A biopsy of the mass is done. Microscopically it shows sheets of closely packed primitive cells with small, uniform nuclei and only scant cytoplasm. A PAS stain demonstrates abundant intracellular glycogen Karyotypic analysis of the tumor cells shows a t(11;22) translocation. The most likely diagnosis is:**
   A. Chondrosarcoma
   B. Ewing sarcoma
   C. Giant cell tumor
   D. Osteosarcoma
6. **A 32-year-old man has noticed a painless lump over his right forearm. The lump has enlarged slowly over the past 3 years. On physical examination, the lesion is soft, movable, and 2 cm in diameter in the subcutis of the right forearm. The lesion is excised. Grossly, it is circumscribed and has a uniformly yellow-cut surface. The cell types that are most likely to comprise this lesion is:**
   A. Fibroblast
   B. Adipocyte
   C. Skeletal muscle
   D. Smooth muscle
7. **A 56-year-old woman complains of pain in the area around the left knee for the past 6 weeks. She did not have any trauma to the leg. On physical examination, no warmth or swelling, no palpable mass, and the range of motion is normal. MRI shows a well-circumscribed 2.5 cm mass**

superior and inferior to the patella. The mass is seen within soft tissue, without any bony erosion. A biopsy of the mass is performed. Microscopic examination shows a biphasic pattern of spindle cells and cuboidal epithelial cells forming glands. Karyotypic analysis of tumor cells shows a t(X;18) translocation. The most likely diagnosis is:

A. Liposarcoma
B. Osteosarcoma
C. Leiomyosarcoma
D. Synovial sarcoma

Answers and Explanation

1. **The answer is C: *Staphylococcus aureus*.** It is a case of pyogenic osteomyelitis that may develop due to hematogenous dissemination of an infection. In children without any history of previous illnesses, *Staphylococcus aureus* is the most common causative organism. Gonorrhea occasionally may disseminate and involve the bones (osteomyelitis) or joints (septic arthritis). It occurs in sexually active individuals. Salmonella infection of bone is infrequent, except in patients with sickle cell anemia. Group B streptococcal infections are most common in the neonatal period.
2. **The answer is C: Sequestrum.** Infectious organisms causing osteomyelitis may reach the bone through the bloodstream. If the infection is not treated, pus and bacteria extend underneath the periosteum leading to devitalizing the cortex. The bone undergoes necrosis and this necrotic bone is called a sequestrum. Cloaca (option A) is the hole in the bone during the formation of a draining sinus. Involucrum (option B) refers to a lesion in which periosteal new bone formation forms a sheath around the necrotic sequestrum. Brodie abscess (option D) consists of reactive bone from the periosteum and the endosteum that surrounds and contains the infection.
3. **The answer is A: RB.** This is a case of osteosarcoma involving the metaphyseal region of the distal femur. This is the most common location. Osteosarcoma is most frequent in adolescents between the ages of 10 and 20. On an X-ray, it produces a Codman triangle and a "sunburst" periosteal reaction. Almost two-thirds of osteosarcoma show mutations in the retinoblastoma (Rb) gene. APC mutations are observed in association with colonic adenocarcinomas. BRCA1 mutations are seen in association with breast and ovarian cancers. PTEN mutations are usually associated with endometrial and prostate cancers.
4. **The answer is B: Giant cell tumors.** It typically arises in the epiphyses of long bones of individuals 20–40 years old. It shows slight female predominance. Giant cell tumors may recur after curettage. Microscopically it shows multinucleated cells in a stroma predominantly composed of spindle-shaped mononuclear cells. Microscopic and radiological features are against other options. Chondrosarcoma (option A) is usually larger destructive lesions. Ewings sarcoma (option C) affects the diaphyseal region. Osteosarcoma involves metaphysis.
5. **The answer is B: Ewing sarcoma.** The histologic appearance, radiologic features, and t(11;22) translocation are characteristic of an Ewing sarcoma. The two most common malignant bone tumors in children are osteosarcoma and Ewing sarcoma. Osteosarcomas usually arise in the metaphyseal region, whereas Ewing sarcoma arises in the diaphyseal region of long tubular bones. Chondrosarcoma (option A) shows a cartilaginous matrix on microscopic examination. A giant cell tumor (option C) arises in the epiphysis of the long bones of young adults and has a "soap bubble" radiographic appearance. An osteosarcoma (option D) typically arises in the metaphyseal region, and the malignant spindle cells produce an osteoid matrix.
6. **The answer is B: Adipocyte.** The most common neoplasm is a lipoma, composed of mature adipocytes. They are slow-growing tumors. Fibroblasts (Option A) may form reactive lesions such as fibromatoses, which are firm and immovable. Smooth muscle cells (Option C) form firm leiomyomas. Neoplasms resembling skeletal muscle (rhabdomyoma) (option D) are rare.
7. **The answer is D: Synovial sarcomas.** Synovial sarcoma is a highly malignant soft tissue tumor that accounts for 10% of all adult sarcomas. It occurs mainly in adolescents and young adults as a painful or tender mass in the region of a large joint, particularly the knee. The neoplasm consists of spindle-shaped cells and cuboidal epithelial-like cells. Most synovial sarcomas show the t(X;18) translocation. Liposarcoma (option A) does not show t(X;18) translocation and is more common in the deep soft tissues and retroperitoneal region. An osteosarcoma (Option B) is common in children and involves the metaphyseal region of bone. The tumor cells produce osteoid. Leiomyosarcoma (option C) microscopically does not have a biphasic pattern and is rarely seen in soft tissues.

Psoas abscess: This may be the first manifestation of tuberculous spondylitis.

Osteosarcoma:
- Mutton leg appearance
- Codman's triangle
- Sun burst appearance

Osteosarcoma: Microscopy.
- Malignant pleomorphic tumor cells
- Production of osteoid by tumor cells

Giant cell tumor: Soap bubble appearance on X-ray.

Giant cell tumor of bone: Microscopy
- Neoplastic mononuclear cells
- Large multinucleated giant cells

Ewing sarcoma of bone: Microscopy
- Uniform, small, round tumor cells
- Cytoplasm appears clear (rich in glycogen)
- Homer–Wright rosettes may be seen

Ewing sarcoma: Onion peel appearance on X-ray.

CHAPTER 26

Skin Disorders

Chapter Outline

- Carcinoma Precursors
- Squamous Cell Carcinoma
- Basal Cell Carcinoma
- Melanocytic Neoplasms

CARCINOMA PRECURSORS

Q. Write a short note on precancerous lesions of the skin.

Malignant epidermal tumors may be preceded by precursor lesions, similar to squamous cell carcinoma of the uterine cervix. Premalignant keratoses and precursors are listed in **Box 26.1**.

Actinic Keratosis

Develops in sun-damaged skin: Actinic (solar) keratosis (pleural actinic keratoses) (as the name indicates from the sun's rays) is a keratinocyte **intraepithelial neoplasm with atypia of keratinocytes** [squamous cell carcinoma (SCC) in situ]. These lesions are usually due to chronic exposure to sunlight and are associated with hyperkeratosis. Hence, they are called *actinic* (sun-related). Exposure to **ionizing radiation**, **industrial hydrocarbons**, and **arsenicals** may produce similar lesions.

More frequent in light-pigmented individuals: It is a common sun-induced lesion. Its incidence is high in lightly pigmented individuals.

A premalignant lesion that may show progressive dysplastic changes: Actinic keratosis may show progressively dysplastic changes that may evolve into squamous carcinomas in situ and finally into cutaneous invasive SCC.

Age: Usually, it arises in **middle-aged to older individuals**.

Caused by UV-induced DNA damage: It is associated with mutations in *TP53* and other genes that are frequently mutated in squamous cell carcinoma of the skin.

BOX 26.1: Premalignant keratoses and precursors.

- Actinic keratosis
- Arsenical keratosis
- Psoralen plus ultraviolet A (PUVA) radiation keratosis
- Squamous cell carcinoma in situ (Bowen's disease)

MORPHOLOGY

Gross

- **Size:** It is usually **less than 1 cm** in diameter.
- **Appearance: Tan-brown, red, or skin-colored.**
- **Consistency:** Rough, **sandpaper-like consistency** and rough to the touch.
- **Sites: Sun-exposed sites,** such as the face, arms, and dorsum of hands.

Microscopy

- **Cytologic atypia** is seen in the **epidermis's lowermost basal cells; these** atypical cells have pink or reddish cytoplasm. It is often associated with hyperplasia of basal cells or with atrophy and diffuse thinning of the epidermal surface.
- **Superficial dermis** shows **thickened blue-gray elastic fibers** (solar elastosis).
- **Thicken stratum corneum with parakeratosis**: The stratum corneum is thickened and shows abnormal retention of nuclei (parakeratosis).
- **Squamous cell carcinoma in situ**: Rarely, full-thickness epidermal atypia may occur and these are considered squamous cell carcinoma in situ.

Clinical features: Actinic keratoses occur in fair-skinned individuals and their incidence increases with age and sun exposure. Local eradication with cryotherapy (superficial freezing) or topical agents is effective for these lesions.

PA 34.4 (NC): Identify, distinguish, and describe common tumors of the skin.

Squamous Cell Carcinoma In Situ (Bowen's Disease)

Squamous cell carcinoma (SCC) in situ also known as Bowen's disease is characterized by the involvement of the full-thickness of the epidermis by dysplastic squamous cells. It is confined to the epidermis and superficial adnexal epithelium.

Etiology: Most cases of SCC in situ (Bowen's disease) are caused by exposure to UV radiation, including UVB and UVA radiation.

MORPHOLOGY

Localization: It mainly occurs in sun-exposed skin, but is also seen in nonsun-exposed skin. Usual sites of involvement include the lower limbs, head, neck, and hands.

Gross: SCC in situ usually presents as a **solitary, slow-growing, scaly, erythematous patch or plaque.**

Microscopy: SCC in situ is characterized by **dysplasia involving the full-thickness of the epidermis without invasion of the underlying dermis.** Dysplasia shows enlarged and pleomorphic atypical squamous cells with hyperchromatic nuclei. They replace the full-thickness of the epidermis and usually show a loss of polarity. Increased mitotic figures are seen and typically extend to the epidermal surface. The basal layer of the epidermis may be retained (the so-called eyeliner sign).

SQUAMOUS CELL CARCINOMA

PA 34.1 (CC): Describe the risk factors pathogenesis, pathology, and natural history of squamous cell carcinoma of the skin.

Q. Write a short note on squamous cell carcinoma of the skin.

- Cutaneous squamous cell (epidermoid) carcinoma is a **malignant tumor of epidermal keratinocytes. The second** (the first being basal cell carcinoma) **most common tumor** arising **on sun-exposed sites**. It shows varying degrees of differentiation that partially recapitulate the cytology of the stratum spinosum squamous cells of the epidermis. They are most **common on the skin of fair individuals with light hair** and **often arise in actinic keratoses**. They are rare on normal black skin.
- **Age and gender:** It typically arises in older adults with lighter skin types. More **common in men** than in women.
- **Localization:** SCC may arise anywhere on the skin and mucous membranes lined by squamous epithelium. Characteristically, they occur in chronically sun-exposed areas such as the **backs of the hands, face, lips, and ears.**
- **Clinical presentation:** Appear as sharply defined, red, scaling plaques.

Etiology and Pathogenesis

Q. Write a short note on the etiology of squamous cell carcinoma of the skin.

Risk Factors

- **Exposure to UV light:** Cutaneous SCCs have multiple causes. **The most important and common cause is deoxyribonucleic acid (DNA) damage produced by exposure to UV light** (UVB is the most important, and UVA plays a minor role). Apart from DNA damage, sunlight probably causes a transient defect in cutaneous innate immunity that may reduce the immune-mediated elimination of sun-damaged keratinocytes. The incidence of SCC is proportional to the degree of lifetime sun exposure.
- **Chronic immunosuppression:** A second common association of SCCs is with immunosuppression. Most commonly, it is associated with **chronic immunosuppression** because of **chemotherapy or organ transplantation**, particularly renal transplantation. Immunosuppression may contribute to carcinogenesis mainly in two ways: (1) By reducing host surveillance of epidermal Langerhans cells and (2) by increasing the susceptibility of keratinocytes to infection and transformation by oncogenic viruses, particularly human papillomavirus (HPV) subtypes HPV-5 and HPV-8.
- **Cutaneous scars of varying types:** These include chronic scarring processes, such as **sinus tracts draining chronic osteomyelitis, old burn scars** ("Marjolin ulcers"), and hidradenitis suppurativa.
- **Other risk factors:** These include ionizing radiation, industrial chemical carcinogens (tars and oils), ingestion of arsenicals, and areas of radiation dermatitis. In the oral cavity, the risk factors include tobacco and betel nut chewing. More than 90% of SCCs, and many actinic keratoses, have mutated *TP53* genes.

Genetic Aspects

As in all other cancers, cutaneous SCC develops from **multiple driver mutations.**

- **Mutations in tumor suppressor *TP53* gene**: The incidence of *TP53* mutations in actinic keratoses and cutaneous SCCs is high. This suggests that **p53 dysfunction is an early event** in tumors induced by sunlight. *TP53* is a tumor suppressor gene, and its protein product is p53. **Cells with DNA damage is arrested in the G_1** phase of the cell cycle by normal *TP53*. This promotes either DNA repair by DNA repair genes or cells undergoing apoptosis if the damage is beyond repair. These protective functions of p53 are lost when *TP53* is mutated and DNA mutations induced by UV light are passed down to daughter cells. *TP53* mutations are unique in that they occur at pyrimidine dimers. This indicates that *TP53* mutations are also caused by UV light.
- **Loss of expression of *CDKN2A*:** The *CDKN2A* gene plays an active role in the p53 and retinoblastoma (Rb) tumor suppressor pathways. Apart from *TP53* gene mutations, loss of expression of *CDKN2A* via deletion also plays a role in the pathogenesis of SCCs. These deletions in *CDKN2A* may occur spontaneously during tumor progression.
- **Mutations in DNA repair genes:** Patients with **xeroderma pigmentosum** are remarkably susceptible to

SCC. **Xeroderma pigmentosum** is caused by **inherited mutations in genes in the nucleotide excision repair pathway**. This gene is required for the accurate repair of pyrimidine dimers. These **patients are susceptible to squamous cell carcinoma**.

- **Other genes**: These include activating mutations in *RAS* and loss of function mutations in Notch receptors. They also contribute to the transformation process involved in SCCs.

MORPHOLOGY

Q. Write a short note on the morphology of squamous cell carcinoma.

Gross

Invasive lesions are more advanced lesions, which

Early lesions: They are small, scaly, or ulcerated, erythematous papules.

More advanced invasive SCC (Fig. 26.1): It appears as **nodular growth and may ulcerate**. The ulcer is **surrounded by a wide, elevated, indurated border**. The ulcer is often covered by a crust that conceals a red, granular base.

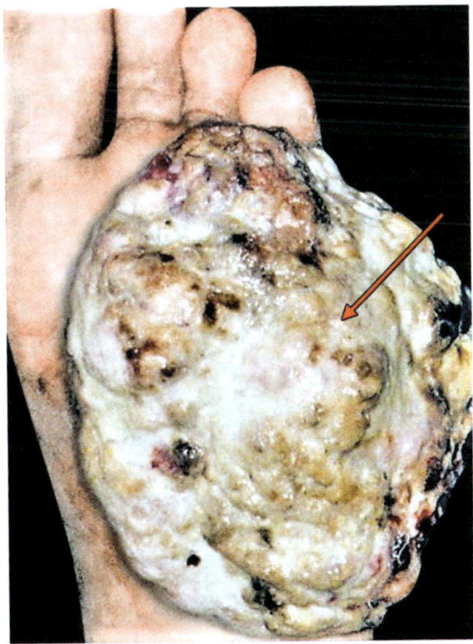

Fig. 26.1: Gross appearance of advanced squamous cell carcinoma showing a cauliflower-like growth in the foot (arrow).

Microscopy

The tumor consists of **irregular masses or nests of atypical (malignant) squamous cells** that **proliferate downward into the dermis**. They show variable degrees of differentiation, ranging from well to poorly differentiated.

- **Well-differentiated squamous cell carcinoma** (**Figs. 26.2A and B**): They are composed of **polygonal squamous tumor cells arranged in orderly lobules** and **produce large amounts of keratin**. Some of this keratin forms **epithelial or squamous/keratin pearls** and is characteristically seen in well-differentiated tumors. The keratin "pearls" consist of **cells forming localized concentric whorls of squamous cells** showing gradually increasing keratinization toward the center. The central region of the pearl usually shows incomplete or rarely complete keratinization and consists of deposits of anucleated or parakeratotic keratin.
- **Moderately differentiated squamous cell carcinoma (Fig. 26.2C)**: They consist of **anaplastic squamous cells, which show single-cell keratinization** (dyskeratosis). These dyskeratotic cells are **large and round with a deep eosinophilic cytoplasm and a hyperchromatic nucleus**. It may be associated with areas of geographic necrosis.
- **Poorly differentiated squamous cell carcinoma:** They consist of **highly anaplastic cells** with foci of necrosis Poorly differentiated tumors **may require immunohistochemical stains for keratins to confirm the diagnosis.**

Clinical features: Invasive squamous cell carcinomas of the skin are usually detected while they are small and easily resected. They may metastasize to regional lymph nodes.

Treatment: SCCs are usually treated by excision. Some cases require electrosurgery, topical chemotherapy, or radiation therapy.

BASAL CELL CARCINOMA

PA 34.2 (CC): Describe the risk factors pathogenesis, pathology, and natural history of basal cell carcinoma of the skin.

Q. Write a short note on basal cell carcinoma (rodent ulcer) of skin.

- Basal cell carcinoma is the most common, **distinctive, slow-growing, locally invasive cancer of skin** that **rarely metastasizes.**

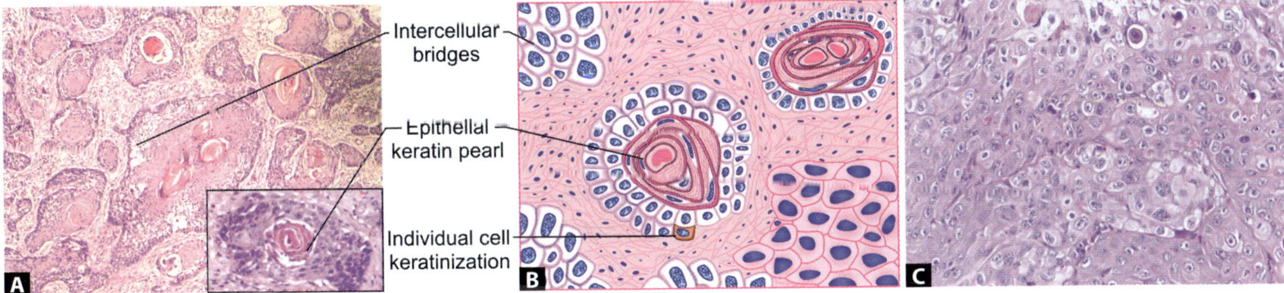

Figs. 26.2A to C: (A) Photomicrograph; (B) Diagrammatic representation of well-differentiated squamous cell carcinoma composed of polygonal squamous tumor cells arranged in orderly lobules and produce large amounts of keratin. Some of this keratin forms epithelial or squamous pearls (inset of A); (C) Moderately differentiated squamous cell carcinoma composed of anaplastic squamous cells, which show single-cell keratinization.

- **Localization:** It occurs at **sun-exposed sites** and in fair-skinned people, especially on the face. It was classically described as a tumor that occurs **above a line drawn from the angle of the mouth to the pinna of the ear**.
- **Origin:** Basal cell carcinoma derives its name from the cytological similarity of the tumor cells to the normal basal cells of the epidermis. However, it is thought to **be derived from pluripotential basal cells of the interfollicular epidermis and/or bulge region of the hair follicle**.
- **Age:** It usually occurs in adults.

Etiology and Pathogenesis

Q. Write a short note on the etiology of basal cell carcinoma of the skin.

Like SCC, the incidence of BCC is higher in the **setting of exposure to UV radiation, immunosuppression**, and **disorders of DNA repair**, such as **xeroderma pigmentosum**. Other risk factors include ionizing radiation and systemic arsenic exposure.

Genetic Aspects

Increasing evidence indicates that genetic factors play a role in the susceptibility to BCC in some individuals.

Mutation in Tumor Suppressor Gene

Loss-of-function mutations in the *PTCH* gene: *PTCH 1* (patched homolog 1) gene is a tumor suppressor gene that negatively regulates Hedgehog signaling. This signaling pathway has diverse functions in embryonic development and tissue homeostasis. *PTCH* gene encodes patched-1, a protein (PTCH1 protein). **Loss of function mutations in PTCH leads to constitutive activation of the Hedgehog pathway.** BCC is associated with **mutations that activate the hedgehog signaling pathway**. This in turn activates many downstream genes involved in cell proliferation and survival. Mutations of genes belonging to the *PTCH* signaling pathway are important for the development of both common **sporadic and inherited** forms of basal cell carcinoma.

1. **Sporadic form:** *PTCH* mutations are found in ~30% of sporadic basal cell carcinomas, and may be due to UV light-induced DNA damage.
2. **Germline mutation: Nevoid basal cell carcinoma syndrome** (NBCCS; also known as **basal cell nevus or Gorlin syndrome**) is an autosomal dominant disorder characterized by multiple basal cell carcinomas. Patients with NBCCS are born with a germline mutation in one of the *PTCH* alleles; the second normal allele is inactivated in tumors by exposure to mutagens (such as UV light).

Acquired *TP53* mutations: It is caused by UV light and is common in both familial and sporadic basal cell carcinoma.

Defect in DNA Repair Genes

Xeroderma pigmentosum is a disorder of DNA repair, associated with an increased incidence of basal cell carcinoma.

MORPHOLOGY

Q. Write a short note on the morphology of basal cell carcinoma.

Gross

Appearance varies and may be **nodular, ulcerative (Figs. 26.3A and B), superficial, pigmented, or erythematous.**

- **Nodulo-ulcerative basal cell carcinoma:** It is the **most common type.** It presents as a pearly papule that slowly increases in size and undergoes central ulceration often with prominent, dilated subepidermal blood vessels **(telangiectasia)**. A **typical lesion** consists of a **slowly enlarging ulcer surrounded by a pearly, rolled border**. This represents the so-called rodent ulcer, which **erodes the underlying structures like a rodent**. Rodents include mice, squirrels, or beavers (the second-largest living rodents) that have a single pair of incisors with a chisel-shaped edge in both jaws. On the face, BCCs can destroy the eyes and nose.

Microscopy (Figs. 26.4A and B)

Basal cell carcinoma shows considerable variability in the morphology, and several histopathological subtypes have been defined. However certain features are common for these subtypes.

Pattern: BCCs are composed of **islands or nests** of deeply **basaloid epithelial cells (Fig. 26.4)**. These nests, in many cases, are attached to the epidermis and protrude into the underlying papillary dermis.

- **Peripheral palisading:** The periphery of each **island or nest** has an **organized layer of polarized, columnar, deeply basophilic keratinocytes.** These cells have a **large, oval, or elongated nucleus with a narrow rim of cytoplasm.** The **long axis of the peripheral cells is perpendicular to the surrounding stroma** (known as **"peripheral palisading"**). Usually, the peripheral palisading of tumor cells resembles the basal layer of the epidermis. No intercellular bridges are seen on routine light microscopy. There are numerous mitotic figures, sometimes atypical.
- **Center of islands of closely packed keratinocytes:** The central part of each **island contains closely packed keratinocytes that are haphazardly arranged.** These cells are slightly smaller than normal epidermal basal keratinocytes. They may show occasional apoptosis and mitoses.

Clefting artifact between tumor islands and adjacent stroma: Clefting at the stromal–tumor interface is common. It may **sometimes help distinguish BCC from other adnexal neoplasms displaying basaloid cell proliferation.**

Two common patterns of growth:

1. **Multifocal superficial growths:** These tumors originate from the epidermis and extend over several square centimeters or more of the skin surface (multifocal superficial type).
2. **Nodular lesions:** These tumors grow deeply downward into the dermis as cords and islands of variably basophilic cells with hyperchromatic nuclei.

Clinical features: BCC is more common in sunny climates near the equator, such as Australia. It **appears as pearly papules often containing prominent, dilated subepidermal blood vessels.** Some tumors may contain melanin and may resemble melanocytic nevi or melanomas. Advanced tumors may ulcerate locally invade, and erode the underlying bone or facial sinuses like a rodent and are known as rodent ulcers.

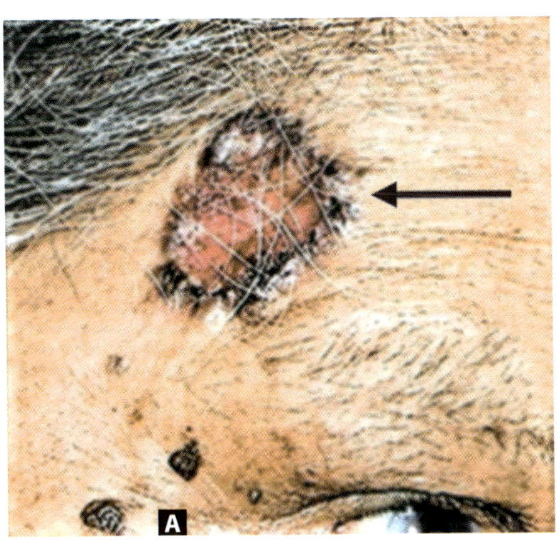

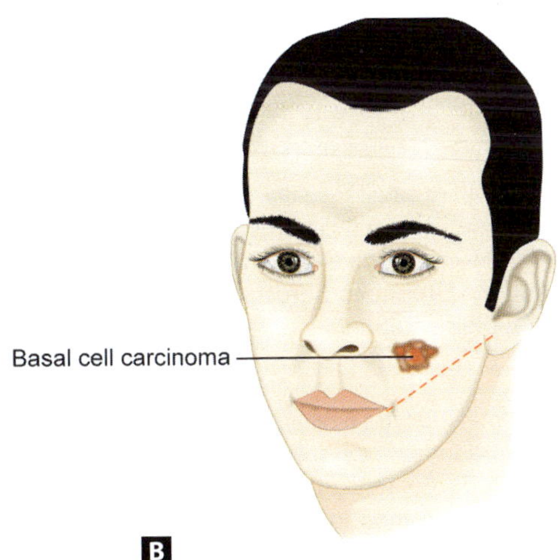

Figs. 26.3A and B: Basal cell carcinoma of the skin: (A) Gross appearance of basal cell carcinoma; (B) Common location and macroscopic appearance of basal cell carcinoma (diagrammatic). Basal cell carcinoma occurs above a line drawn from the angle of the mouth to the pinna of the ear.

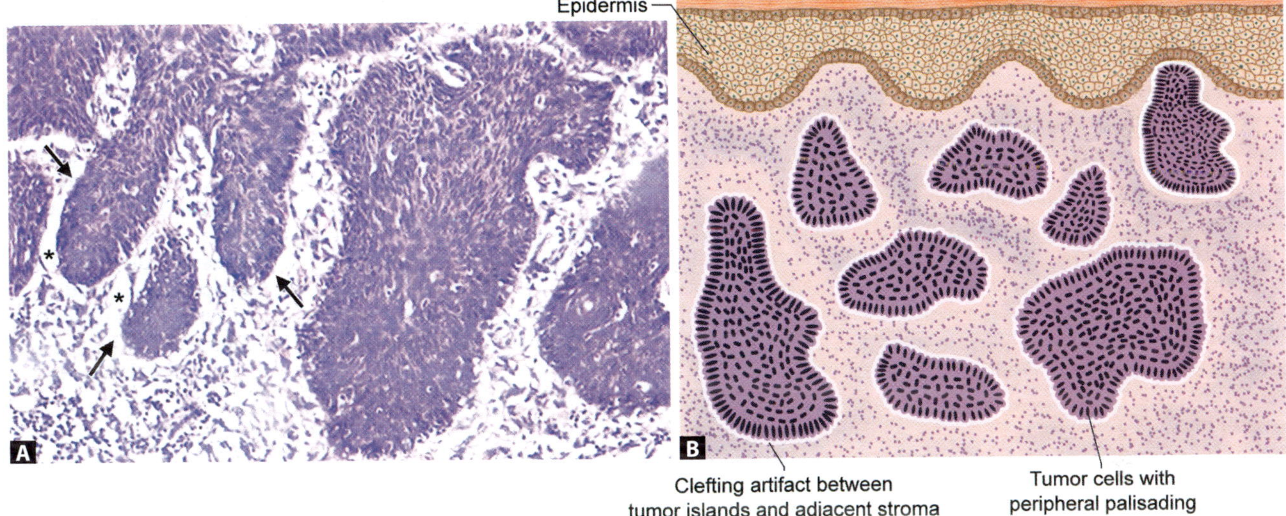

Figs. 26.4A and B: Basal cell carcinoma. Composed of nests of uniformly atypical basaloid cells within the dermis, that are often separated from the adjacent stroma by thin clefts (arrows in A): (A) Photomicrograph; (B) Diagrammatic representation.

MELANOCYTIC NEOPLASMS

Nevi

Q. Write a short note on nevus.

Nevi **(acquired melanocytic nevi, pigmented nevus, moles)** that occur in intermittently sun-exposed skin are **neoplasms or precursors derived from epidermal melanocytes** (singular, nevus; plural nevi).

The term "nevus" may be used for various hamartomatous and/or neoplastic lesions in the skin, but the unqualified term refers to a *melanocytic nevus*. The acquired melanocytic nevus is a common benign melanocytic neoplasm found in virtually all individuals. Melanocytic nevi are diverse, dynamic, and biologically fascinating neoplasms. Some nevi may transform into melanoma or have an increased risk for melanoma.

Subtypes of nevi: These are junctional, compound, and dermal nevi. Junctional, compound, and dermal nevi are benign localized clonal proliferations of nevus cells (a type of melanocyte).

Epidemiology: Acquired nevi appear during childhood and reach maximum number in adolescence. Thereafter, they decline in number.

Common sites of occurrence: These include the head and neck, sun-exposed trunk, and extremities.

Etiology: Exposure to UV radiation, particularly intermittent exposure in childhood, is associated with the formation of melanocytic nevi. They result in mutations of a single oncogene in a single cell. This cell expands to form a clone.

MORPHOLOGY

Q. Write a short note on junctional/compound/intradermal nevus.

Gross

Common acquired melanocytic nevi are small (usually <6 mm in diameter) localized, usually symmetrical, well-circumscribed, and uniformly pigmented lesions. They are relatively flat macules or elevated papules with well-defined, rounded borders. They appear tan to brown with uniform pigmentation.

Microscopy

Histologic subdivision: Acquired melanocytic nevi are divided into junctional, compound, and intradermal nevi subtypes. But melanocytic nevi are thought to progress through a series of morphologic changes over time. The designations *junctional*, *intradermal*, and *compound* do not necessarily refer to different melanocytic lesions but rather represent the transitional stages in the "life cycle" of nevi **(Figs. 26.5A to E)**.

Junctional Nevus (refer online Fig. 26.6A)

The junctional nevus is believed to be the earliest stage of intra-epidermal melanocytic proliferation. It consists of **multiple discrete aggregates or nests of round cells at the tips of epidermal rete ridges. These cells grow along the dermo-epidermal junction (Fig. 26.5B)**. The nuclei of nevus cells are uniform and rounded in contour, contain inconspicuous nucleoli, and show little or no mitotic activity. They retain pigment in their cytoplasm.

Compound Nevus (refer online Fig. 26.6B)

Eventually, most junctional nevi grow into the underlying dermis as nests or cords of cells. This forms a compound melanocytic nevus. In compound nevus, **nests of melanocytes are seen in the epidermis (junctional component), and the nevus cells also migrate into the dermis, distributed singly and in nests (Fig. 26.5C)**. It shows features of both a junctional and an intradermal nevus.

Dermal Nevus (refer online Figs. 26.6C and D)

As the compound nevus grows older, the **epidermal nests of nevus cells may be lost,** retaining only the intradermal component to form pure **intradermal nevi (Fig. 26.5D)**. Thus intradermal (dermal) nevi no longer show an intraepidermal melanocytic growth (i.e., junctional component) and have no junctional activity. The nevomelanocytes are present only in the dermis. Pigment tends to be lost at this stage. Clinically, compound and intradermal nevi appear as elevated lesions compared to junctional nevi.

Maturation

It is a process in which progressive growth of nevus cells occurs from the dermo-epidermal junction into the underlying dermis.

- **Superficial (type A) nevus cells** are larger, produce melanin, and grow in nests.
- **Deeper (type B) nevus cells** are smaller, produce little or no pigment, and appear as cords and single cells.
- **Deepest (type C) nevus cells** are seen in the lower dermis. These nevus cells often have a fusiform appearance and are usually elongated with a spindle-shaped nucleus. They grow in fascicles or strands resembling neural tissue (neurotization) or Schwann cells.

This sequence of maturation of nevus cells is of diagnostic use in differentiating benign nevi from melanomas. Melanoma usually does not show maturation. Melanocytic nevi are common and may be confused with melanoma.

Melanoma

PA 34.3 (NC): Describe the distinguishing features between a nevus and melanoma. Describe the etiology, pathogenesis, risk factors morphology clinical features, and metastases of melanoma.

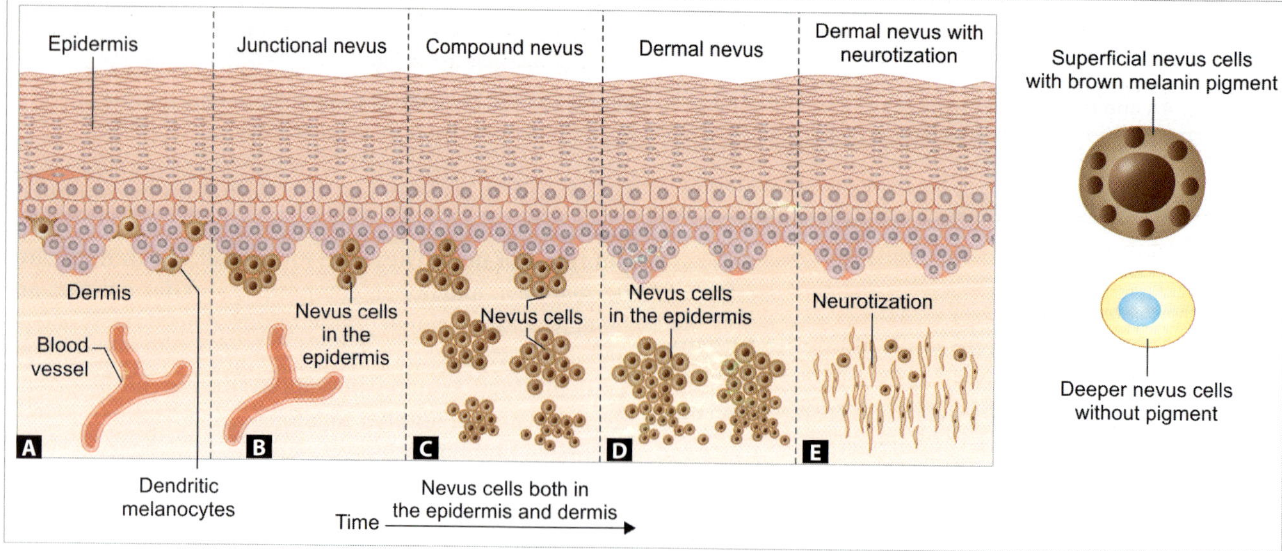

Figs. 26.5A to E: Schematic representation of maturation sequence of melanocytic nevi. (A) Normal skin showing scattered dendritic melanocytes within the basal layer of the epidermis; (B) Junctional nevus showing nests of nevus cells at the dermo-epidermal junction; (C) Compound nevus showing nests of nevus cells in both the dermo-epidermal junction and dermis; (D) Dermal nevus showing only intradermal nests of nevus cells; (E) Dermal nevus with neurotization and this change is also called maturation.

BOX 26.2: Sites of origin of melanoma.

Skin (most common site): It may develop in the trunk, leg, face, sole, palm, and nail beds

Other sites:

- Oral and anogenital mucosal surfaces [i.e., oropharynx, gastrointestinal (anus), and genitourinary tracts (vulva, vagina, urethra)]
- Esophagus
- Meninges
- Uvea of the eye

Q. Write a short note on malignant melanoma.

Malignant melanoma is a relatively common, malignant neoplasm of melanocytes. The term "melanoma" is synonymous with "malignant melanoma." It is the deadliest of all skin cancers. However, melanoma can be cured surgically if it is detected and treated when it is in its earliest stages.

Age: Melanoma is a leading cause of cancer mortality in young adults. Melanoma is rare in adolescence and exceedingly rare in childhood.

Q. Write a short note on sites of melanoma.

Sites of origin of melanoma: Various sites of melanoma are presented in **Box 26.2**.

Cell of origin: Malignant melanoma originates from melanocytes.

Etiology and Pathogenesis

Q. Write a short essay on the etiology and pathogenesis of malignant melanoma.

Melanoma may arise de novo or from precursor lesion: The neoplastic transformation of melanocytes to melanoma may occur de novo or through a precursor lesion (e.g., common acquired nevus, dysplastic nevus).

- **Evolution from a precursor to frank melanoma:** About 30–50% of melanomas show histologic remnants of a benign nevus. Most benign melanocytic lesions show *BRAF* or *NRAS* mutations. The adjacent intermediate lesions or frank melanoma show an accumulation of additional mutations. These include p16/*CDKN2A*, phosphatase and tensin homolog (*PTEN*), *TP53*, and telomerase expression (*TERT*). This suggests that the development of melanoma is an evolutionary path from a benign precursor to frank melanoma **(Figs. 26.7A to E)**.

Familial melanoma: In about 10–15% of melanoma, the risk of melanoma is inherited (hereditary predisposition) as an autosomal dominant trait with variable penetrance. The genetic abnormalities in these melanomas are as follows:

Sporadic melanoma: In 85–90% of patients, melanoma is sporadic.

- **Sun exposure:** A single predisposing environmental factor in these cases is **exposure to UV radiation from sunlight**. Melanomas **most commonly occur on sun-exposed surfaces**, particularly the upper back in men and the back and legs in women. **Lightly-pigmented individuals (e.g., Australians) are at higher risk than darkly-pigmented individuals.** Exposure to UV radiation from sunlight **damages the DNA which leads to the stepwise acquisition of driver mutations** in melanocytes over time. Intense intermittent sun exposure at an early age may carry the highest risk. The relationship between sun exposure and melanoma is not as straightforward as with other skin cancers (e.g., squamous cell carcinoma). Thus, sunlight is not always an essential predisposing factor, and other environmental factors may also contribute to the risk of melanoma.

Molecular Pathogenesis (Figs. 26.7A to E)

Activating mutation in *BRAF* or *RAS* (oncogene activation): The initiating event in the development of melanoma is probably an activating mutation in *BRAF* or (less commonly) *RAS*. The protein products of these genes are involved in signal transduction. In most cases, this produces only a benign nevus unless other mutations occur. An aberrant increase in RAS signaling may occur due to **mutations in** *RAS* or *BRAF*, which promote cell **growth and survival.**

- **Activating mutations in *RAS*** leads to melanoma in 10–15% of tumors. *RAS* downstream regulator RAS/RAF/MAP kinase cascade resulting in cell proliferation.
- **Activating mutations in *BRAF*** are seen in 60–70% of melanomas. *BRAF* (one of the members of the RAF family) is an **intermediate signaling component in the MAP kinase pathway** (*refer* **Fig. 24.11**).

Mutations that activate the expression of telomerase: Telomerase is an enzyme that preserves telomeres and protects cells from senescence (*refer* pages 247-8). *TERT* is a gene that encodes the catalytic subunit of telomerase. Reactivation of telomerase preserves telomeres and is important in cancer. These are commonly observed in nevi with "atypical" morphologic features and melanomas in the radial phase. These mutations break senescence (the usual fate of benign nevi). TERT is the most mutated gene in 70% of sporadic melanomas. Rare melanoma-prone families may show germline *TERT* promoter mutations.

Loss of *CDNK2A* and its encoded tumor suppressor p16: *CDKN2A* is a complex locus, which encodes three different **tumor suppressors** namely, (1) *p15/INK4b*, (2) *p16/INK4a*, and (3) *p14/ARF*. **p16** is a cyclin-dependent kinase inhibitor. It regulates the G_1-S transition of the cell cycle by maintaining the retinoblastoma tumor suppressor protein in its active state. **p14** increases the activity of the p53 tumor suppressor by preventing its degradation.

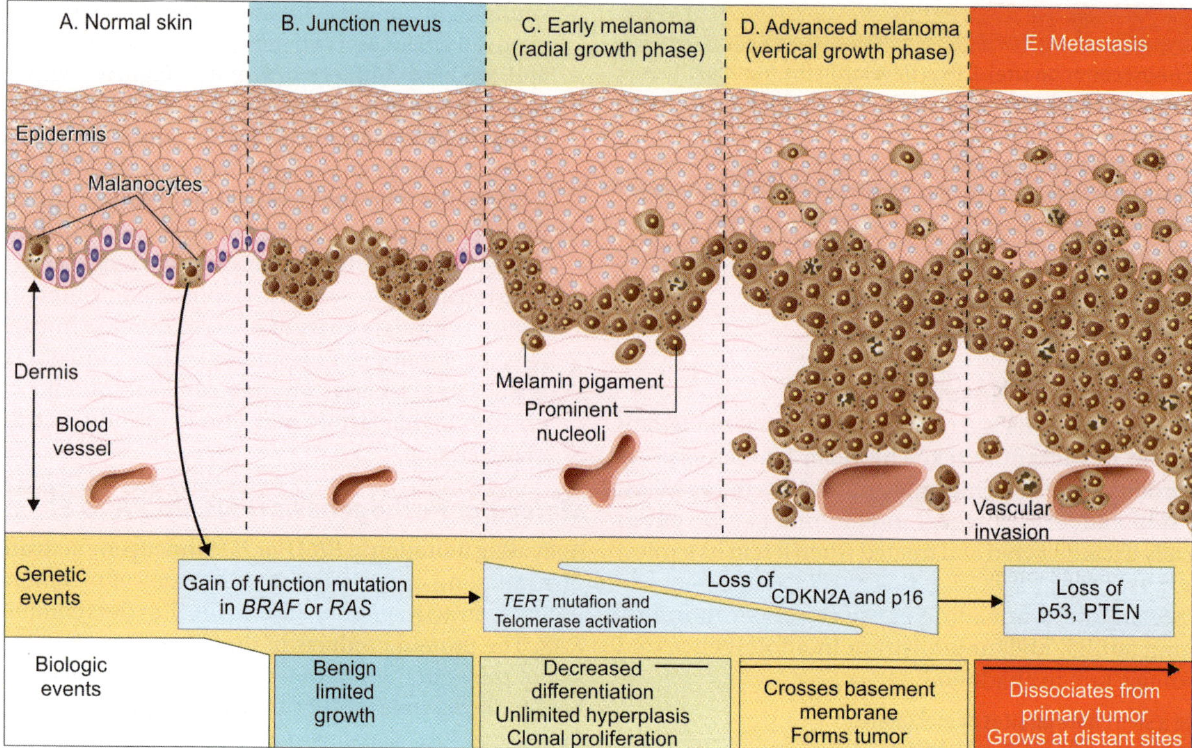

Figs. 26.7A to E: Biologic event and major molecular changes in the progression of melanoma: (A) Normal skin shows only scattered melanocytes in the basal layer of the epidermis; (B) Gain of function mutation in *BRAF* or *RAS* drives the proliferation of junctional melanocytes. *BRAF* mutation and activation of the mitogen-activated protein kinase (MAPK) pathway leads to the formation of junctional nevus; (C) Mutations that activate telomerase expression, lead to transformation and development of early melanoma. This tumor spreads laterally (radial growth phase); (D) Additional genetic events such as the loss of the tumor suppressor p16 produce more invasive growth (vertical growth phase); (E) Metastatic spread is associated with mutations that lead to loss of function of the tumor suppressors PTEN (phosphatase and tensin homolog) and p53.

- **Mutations in *CDKN2A* gene**: Additional mutations or epigenetic aberrations lead to loss of *CDNK2A* and its encoded tumor suppressor p16. *CDKN2A* mutation is observed in 40% of familial melanoma (germline mutations of *CDKN2A*) as well as in a few (about 10%) sporadic melanomas. These mutations result in increased melanocytic proliferation and escape from oncogene-induced cellular senescence. In this stage, the melanoma develops the invasive vertical phase of growth. Throughout the cutaneous phase of the evolution of the tumor, exposure to UV light adds to the mutational burden and increases the chances of tumor progression.

Mutations in *TP53* and *PTEN* tumor suppressor genes: Finally, additional mutations occur in tumor suppressor genes such as *TP53* and *PTEN*. At this stage, the tumor gains the ability to metastasize. This phase is characterized by the appearance of aneuploidy and genomic copy number alterations.

- **Silencing of tumor suppressor PTEN gene:** PTEN normally downregulates PI-3K/AKT signaling (*refer* **Fig. 24.11**). *PTEN* is **epigenetically silenced** in ~20% of melanomas, which leads to **activation of PI-3K/AKT signaling and proliferation of cells.**

The less common melanomas that develop in **nonsun-exposed acral and mucosal sites** have different molecular courses. One common initiating genetic alteration in these tumors is a **gain-of-function mutation in the *KIT* receptor tyrosine kinase gene**. The melanomas that develop in the uvea of the eye also show a distinct set of driver gene mutations, most important being mutually exclusive mutations that activate the GTP-binding proteins GNAQ or GNA11.

In melanomas that occur in sun-exposed regions, UV light produces a high burden of mutations. Some of these mutations create neoantigens. In melanoma, tumor cells acquire the capacity to either suppress or escape the host immune response. **This property of immune evasion is made use for treating many advanced melanomas with immune checkpoint inhibitors.**

Classification of Melanomas

The World Health Organization (WHO 2023) (abridged) classification of melanomas is presented in **Box 26.3**.

BOX 26.3: World Health Organization (WHO) (2023) (abridged) classification of melanomas.

Melanomas associated with cumulative solar damage (CSD)
- **Melanoma intermittently sun-exposed skin**
  - Low-CSD (cumulative solar damage) melanoma [including superficial spreading melanoma (SSM)]
- **Melanocytic neoplasms in chronically sun-exposed skin**
  - Lentigo maligna melanoma (LMM)

Melanomas not consistently associated with CSD
- Acral melanomas
- Mucosal melanomas

Nodular, and metastatic melanomas
- **Nodular melanomas**
- **Metastatic melanomas**

Ocular and CNS melanomas
- Conjunctival melanoma
- Uveal melanoma
- CNS melanoma (meningeal melanoma)

Notes:
- Melanomas associated with CSD arise in the sun-exposed skin.
- Melanomas not consistently associated with CSD arise at sun-shielded sites or without known etiological association with ultraviolet (UV) radiation exposure.
- Nodular melanoma has a vertical growth pattern that can occur with other types of melanomas.

MORPHOLOGY

Q. Write a short note on the morphology of malignant melanoma. Mention its growth phases.

Gross (Figs. 26.8A to C)

Unlike benign melanocytic nevi, melanomas show **striking variations in color**. Melanoma shows **shades of black, brown, red, dark blue, and gray color**. Melanocytic nevi have smooth, round, and uniform borders, whereas **the borders of melanomas are irregular and often notched.**

Growth Patterns

Melanomas may progress through stages. The growth pattern of melanoma can be divided into two categories (phases or stages): (1) "Radial growth phase" (RGP) and (2) "vertical growth phase" (VGP).

1. Radial Growth Phase

During this phase, the **melanoma spreads horizontally or radially within the epidermis and superficial dermis.**

- **Slow growing:** RGP melanoma represents the **initial stage** where the tumor cells **lack the capacity to metastasize.** It is a slow-growing lesion and may be present for months to years before its identification.
- **Tumors with RGP:** Tumors in the radial growth phase **fall into different clinicopathologic classes.**
  - **Superficial spreading:** It is the **most common type** of melanoma, and **usually** involves the **skin exposed to sun.**
  - **Lentigo maligna:** It usually **presents as an indolent lesion** on the **face of older men.** The tumor may remain in the radial growth phase for **several decades.**
  - **Acral/mucosal lentiginous melanoma:** It is **not related to sun exposure** and is usually seen in the **palm, sole, or mucosa.**

2. Vertical Growth Phase

After a variable and unpredictable period, melanoma from the radial phase develops a **vertical growth phase.**

Characteristics: During this phase:
- Tumor cells **invade downward** into the deeper dermis.
- **Melanoma may appear as a nodule and develop a clone of cells with metastatic potential.**
- **Maturation is absent from the deep invasive portion** of melanoma.
- **Risk of metastasis** correlates with the **depth of invasion,** which is the distance from the superficial epidermal granular cell layer to the deepest intradermal tumor cells. This measurement is known as the **Breslow thickness.**

Microscopy (Figs. 26.9A and B)

Q. Write a short note on the microscopy of melanoma.

1. **Tumor cells:** The tumor cells of melanoma have a **similar appearance in both the radial and vertical phases** of growth.
   - **Size:** Tumor cells are usually **larger than normal melanocytes** or nevus cells found in melanocytic nevi.
   - **Nuclei:** They are **large with irregular shapes, clumped chromatin at the periphery of the nuclear membrane,** and **prominent "cherry red" eosinophilic nucleoli. Mitotic figures** are often seen.
2. **Architecture:** Tumor cells are arranged in **solid masses, sheets, islands,** poorly formed nests, or as individual cells at all levels of the epidermis (pagetoid spread) (constitute the radial spread). The tumor cells may form expansile dermal nodules (vertical growth phases). Tumor invades the upper epidermis as well as the deeper dermis.
3. **Melanin pigment:** It is **seen in melanoma.** The melanoma, **which does not show the pigment,** is known as **amelanotic melanoma.** Melanin is present **in the cytoplasm as uniform brown fine granules.**
4. **Tumor-infiltrating lymphocytes (TILs):** They may be seen in the **tissue surrounding the tumor.**

Special stain for melanin: Masson–Fontana or DOPA-oxidase reaction.

HMB 45 is a tumor marker for Malignant melanoma.

Clinical Features

- Melanoma of the skin is **usually asymptomatic** but may present with itching or pain at the site of the lesion. The incidence of melanoma on the skin is inversely related to the extent of skin pigmentation. Melanoma is more common in individuals of lighter skin types. Melanoma in individuals with darker skin types most commonly occurs on the sole (so-called acral melanoma), palm, or nail bed.

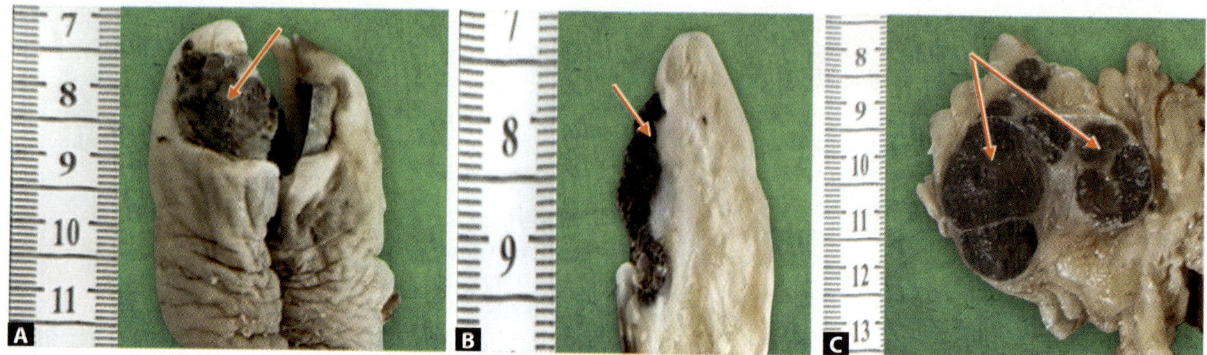

Figs. 26.8A to C: Gross features of malignant melanoma (arrows): (A) Nodular growth projecting from the skin; (B) Cut section of the same shows blackish pigmentation in the tumor; (C) Lymph node with extensive metastasis from malignant melanoma (black color).

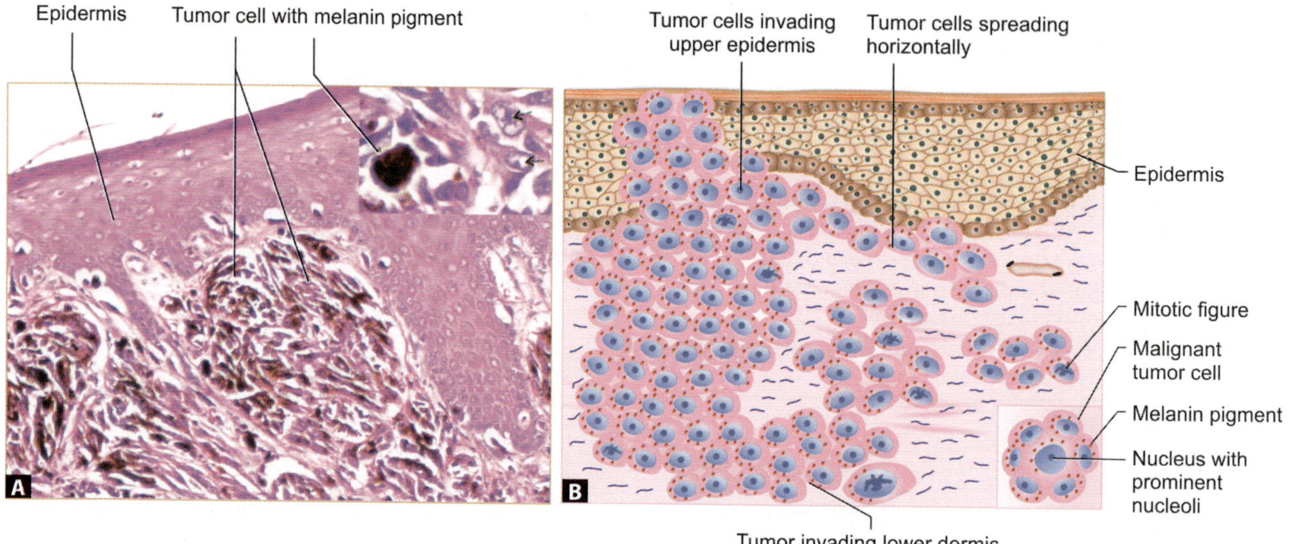

Figs. 26.9A and B: (A) Photomicrograph of malignant melanoma showing nests of tumor cells in the upper dermis containing melanin pigment. Inset shows tumor cells with melanin pigment; (B) Diagrammatic microscopic appearance of malignant melanoma showing nests of tumor cells infiltrating epidermis (radial growth phase) and dermis (vertical growth phase).

- **Changes in pigmented lesions:** These are the **most important clinical signs** of melanoma and include:
- **Color:** Unlike benign nevi, **melanomas show color variations**, ranging from shades of black, brown, red, dark blue, and gray.
  - **Size:** The majority are **larger than 10 mm** in diameter at the time of diagnosis. But, if a pigmented lesion is greater than 6 mm in diameter, any change in appearance, and new onset of itching or pain should raise the suspicion of malignancy.
  - **Border:** The borders of melanomas are **irregular and often notched**, whereas they are smooth, round, and uniform in melanocytic nevi. The main warning signs of melanoma are listed in **Box 26.4**.

Q. What is the ABCDE of melanoma?

BOX 26.4: ABCDE warning signs of melanoma.

- Asymmetry of shape
- Borders of a pigmented lesion (irregularity or poorly defined)
- Color (variegation in color within a pigmented lesion)
- Diameter increased: Rapid enlargement of a preexisting nevus
- Evolving or change over time, especially if rapid (appears different from the rest, or changes in size, shape, or color) or E can stand for elevation
- Others
  - Development of a new pigmented lesion during adult life
  - Development of itching or pain in a lesion

BOX 26.5: Pathologic variables that predict the outcome of melanoma.

- Tumor thickness: Tumor depth of invasion (Breslow thickness)
- Ulceration of overlying skin
- Number of mitoses
- Levels of invasion
- Presence and number of tumor-infiltrating lymphocytes
- Evidence of tumor regression (presumably due to the host immune response)
- Microsatellites, clinical satellites, and "in-transit metastases"
- Sentinel lymph node involvement
- Location (central body or extremity)

Favorable prognosis: Thinner tumor depth, no or few mitoses (<1/mm^2), a brisk tumor-infiltrating lymphocyte (TIL) response, absence of regression, and lack of ulceration

Probability and Risk of Metastasis

- **Breslow thickness:** The probability of metastasis is predicted by Breslow thickness. This is the **measurement of the depth of invasion in millimeters of the vertical growth phase nodule. It is the distance from the top of the granular cell layer of the** superficial **epidermis to the deepest intradermal tumor cells.**
- **Tumors with high mitotic rate**: It also increases the risk of metastasis.
- **Tumors that fail to induce a local immune response: It also increases the risk.**

Sites of Metastasis

Sentinel lymph node biopsy: The sentinel lymph node is the first draining node[s] of a primary melanoma. Most melanomas metastasize to regional lymph nodes. As in breast cancer, sentinel lymph node biopsy may provide additional prognostic information. The presence of even a small number of melanoma cells (micrometastases) indicates a worse prognosis. The degree and number of lymph nodes involved correlate well with overall survival. **Other sites:** These include the liver, lungs, brain, and almost any other site.

Prognostic factors

The prognosis for a patient with melanoma depends on many factors Various pathologic variables that predict the outcome of melanoma are listed in **Box 26.5**.

Distinguishing features between a nevus and melanoma are presented (*refer* **online Table 26.1**).

SCENARIO-BASED MCQs

1. **A 7-year-old boy was brought by his mother for an enlarging nodule on his ear during the past month. Physical examination shows a 1.2 cm, flesh-colored, dome-shaped nodule on his left ear lobe. The nodule is excised and microscopically shows nests of poorly differentiated islands of squamous epithelium invading the dermis. The boy continues to develop similar lesions. The most likely genetic mutation in this boy involves the following:**
   A. Involved in apoptosis
   B. Growth factor signaling
   C. Amplification of oncogenes
   D. Nucleotide excision repair
2. **A 72-year-old farmer presents with a slowly enlarging nodule on his right upper eyelid near the lateral limbus of the right eye for 4 years. On physical examination, there is a 0.4 cm pearly nodule. A biopsy of the lesion shows nests of deeply basophilic epithelial cells with narrow rims of cytoplasm that are attached to the epidermis. They protrude into the subjacent papillary dermis. The nests of tumor cells show peripheral palisading with Clefting artifacts. The most probable diagnosis is:**
   A. Junctional nevus B. Melanoma
   C. Basal cell carcinoma D. Squamous cell carcinoma
3. **A 39-year-old woman complains of a nodule on her right big toe that has become larger over the past 2 months. Physical examination shows a 2.5 cm pigmented lesion with irregular borders and irregular brown-to-black areas. An excisional biopsy with wide margins is done. Microscopically, it shows malignant melanoma composed of epithelioid cells that extend 2 mm into the reticular dermis. It shows a band of lymphocytes beneath the lesion. The most important determinant of prognosis for this woman is:**
   A. Location on the skin B. Depth of the lesion
   C. Extent of radial growth D. Inflammatory response

Answers and Explanation

1. **The answer is D: Nucleotide excision repair.** The appearance of squamous cell carcinoma in a child in a sun-exposed area favors the diagnosis of a rare disorder known as xeroderma pigmentosum (XP). It is an inherited disorder resulting from a mutation in one of the DNA repair genes. The DNA damage induced by UV radiation is repaired by the nucleotide excision repair system. Individuals with XP are prone to develop skin malignancies related to sun exposure. This includes squamous cell carcinoma, basal cell carcinoma, and melanoma. Other options are not true.
2. **The answer is C: Basal cell carcinoma.** Basal cell carcinoma (BCC) is locally aggressive, but metastases are exceedingly rare. It usually develops on the sun damaged skin of individuals with fair skin, particularly the face. Basaloid keratinocytes are not seen in other tumors. The gross and microscopic features do not fit into the diagnosis of junctional nevus (option A). Melanomas (option B) are usually pigmented, and they are composed of polygonal or spindle cells. These tumor cells tend to grow in sheets and infiltrate to produce a grossly irregular border to the lesion. Squamous cell carcinoma (option D) does not contain basaloid cells and does not show clefting artifact.
3. **The answer is B: Depth of the lesion.** Extension downward into the reticular dermis indicates vertical (nodular) growth. Although the tumor shows a lymphocytic response, it is insufficient to destroy or contain the tumor completely. Most melanomas are sporadic, nonfamilial, and related to sun exposure. Other options are not correct.

Disorders of the Central Nervous System and Eye

Chapter Outline

- Meningitis
- Interpretation of Cerebrospinal Fluid Findings
- Tumors of Central Nervous System
- Gliomas
- Embryonal Tumors
- Meningiomas
- Metastatic Tumors
- Eye

MENINGITIS

PA 35.1 (CC): Describe the etiology, types, and pathogenesis, differentiating factors, and CSF findings in meningitis.

Q. Write a short note on meningitis.

Meninges have three layers and from the inside out are **pia, arachnoid, and dura mater.**

Leptomeningitis: Meningitis is the term usually used for **inflammation within the subarachnoid space between the pia and the arachnoid mater** and is known as leptomeningitis. Thus, meningitis is an **infection confined to the leptomeninges with exudate in the subarachnoid space**.

Meningitis can spread into parenchyma: In leptomeningitis (meningitis), the inflammatory response and most causative microorganisms are within the subarachnoid space containing CSF. The inflammatory response may spread from the meninges leading to parenchymal involvement (cerebritis). *Meningoencephalitis* is the term used for inflammation of the meninges and brain parenchyma.

Long-term complications of meningitis: These include effusions, obstruction of CSF flow resulting in hydrocephalus, and cranial nerve palsies (particularly deafness from VIII nerve involvement) from the thick basal exudate.

Causes

Infectious meningitis: Meningitis is a **dangerous infection and is usually** caused by a variety of microorganisms. Cerebrospinal fluid (CSF) is an excellent culture medium for most causative organisms. Infectious meningitis may be acute or chronic. Each type of meningitis shows characteristic changes in the CSF. Depending on the etiology and clinical evolution of the illness, infectious meningitis is broadly classified into the following types:

- **Acute:** It may be (1) acute pyogenic (usually bacterial) or (2) aseptic (usually acute or subacute viral) meningitis.
- **Chronic:** These include (1) tuberculous, (2) syphilitic (spirochetal), and (3) cryptococcal.

Chemical meningitis: Meningitis can also be a response to a nonbacterial irritant introduced into the subarachnoid space (e.g., debris from a ruptured epidermoid cyst).

Carcinomatous meningitis: It is inflammation caused by metastatic cancer cells that have spread to the subarachnoid space.

Acute Pyogenic (Bacterial/Purulent) Meningitis

Q. Write a short note on acute pyogenic meningitis.

Acute meningitis is an acute inflammatory process of the leptomeninges and CSF within the subarachnoid space. Acute pyogenic meningitis is the most common pyogenic infection of the CNS. It carries high morbidity and mortality. Since most bacteria initiate purulent responses, the presence of neutrophils in the CSF is strong evidence of meningitis.

Etiology

Different microorganisms cause acute pyogenic meningitis. The causes of bacterial meningitis depend on the age of the patient. The causative bacteria are different in different age groups **(Table 27.1)**.

Routes of Spread (refer online Fig. 27.1)

Most commonly, a bacterial infection of the meninges occurs through the **hematogenous route**. But it can also complicate **trauma and neurosurgical operations** and **spread from adjacent foci of infection**. It may be iatrogenic through lumbar puncture.

TABLE 27.1 Etiology of acute bacterial meningitis.

Age group	*Common causative microorganisms*
Neonate (<1 month)	***Escherichia coli*, β-hemolytic *Streptococcus* species**, *Klebsiella* species, *Citrobacter* species, *Listeria monocytogenes, Staphylococcus epidermidis, Staphylococcus aureus*
Children (1 month to 16 years)	***Haemophilus influenzae* type b** (in unvaccinated young children), ***Neisseria meningitidis*** *(meningococcus), Streptococcus agalactiae* (group B β-hemolytic streptococci), *Streptococcus pneumoniae (pneumococcus)*
Adults	*Streptococcus pneumoniae (pneumococcus),* ***Neisseria meningitides*** *(meningococcus)*, gram-negative bacilli *(E. coli, Klebsiella* species, *Pseudomonas* species), *Listeria monocytogenes*
Elderly	***Streptococcus pneumoniae*** *(pneumococcus),* ***Listeria monocytogenes***
Immunosuppressed individual	*Klebsiella* or anaerobic organisms

Note: Common causative organs are in bold.

Pathogenesis

Cerebrospinal fluid is an excellent culture medium for most bacteria. Bacteria stimulate an inflammatory reaction by recruiting polymorphonuclear leukocytes/neutrophils to the site of infection. This response, called leptomeningitis, occurs between the pia and the arachnoid layers of the meninges. The inflammatory response to infections in the CSF varies with the virulence of the organism and the severity of the infection. A vigorous host response is necessary to clear the infection. The inflammatory cells release several cytokines, chemokines, and cytotoxic substances such as free radicals. These produce significant vascular and neuropil damage and tissue injury. Corticosteroids may be given with antibiotics to reduce host response-induced damage. The inflammatory cells may compete with the brain for glucose.

MORPHOLOGY

Gross

Purulent exudate (*refer* **online Fig. 27.2): Thick creamy** (purulent) **exudate** is seen within the subarachnoid space (leptomeninges) **over the surface of the brain** (cerebral hemispheres). The **meninges** appear **opaque**. The **meningeal vessels are engorged and appear prominent** over the surface of the brain. The brain is usually swollen and edematous.

Anatomic distribution of the exudate: It can vary depending on the organism.

- *H. influenzae* meningitis: The exudate is usually basal.
- Pneumococcal meningitis: The exudate is often densest over the cerebral convexities near the sagittal sinus.

Microscopy

Acute meningitis

- **Exudates:** It shows dense collections of neutrophils and fibrin **within the subarachnoid space** and along perivascular Virchow–Robin (VR) spaces. VR spaces surround the vessels as they travel through the subarachnoid space through the brain parenchyma.
- **Gram stain:** It shows variable numbers of causative bacteria, particularly in untreated meningitis. It may show intra- or extracellular bacteria.

Fulminant meningitis: The inflammatory cells infiltrate the walls of the leptomeningeal veins. It may spread focally into the brain parenchyma (**cerebritis**).

With time, the neutrophils are replaced by chronic inflammatory cells, and the exudate gets transformed into fibrous tissue.

Complications

The complications of acute bacterial meningitis include the following.

Cerebritis: In fulminant meningitis, the inflammatory cells infiltrate the walls of the veins of the leptomeninges. The inflammation may extend focally into the brain's substance (cerebritis).

Hemorrhagic cerebral infarction: Severe meningitis may produce **secondary vasculitis and venous thrombosis,** which can lead to hemorrhagic cerebral infarction.

Obstructive or communicating hydrocephalus: Leptomeningeal fibrosis may follow pyogenic meningitis. This may cause hydrocephalus. Particularly in pneumococcal meningitis, a large amount of the organism's capsular polysaccharide produces a gelatinous exudate. This promotes arachnoid fibrosis, and this condition is referred to as ***chronic adhesive arachnoiditis***. However, hydrocephalus is a more common complication of tuberculous meningitis.

Waterhouse Friderichsen syndrome: It results from **meningitis-associated septicemia and hemorrhagic infarction of the adrenal glands.** It most often develops with meningococcal and pneumococcal meningitis.

Other complications: These include subdural hygroma, cerebral abscess, and subdural empyema. However, cerebral abscesses rarely occur as a complication of meningitis. **Epilepsy may develop following meningitis.**

Clinical Features

Systemic symptoms of infection: Affected individuals develop systemic signs of infection. These are superimposed on symptoms related to meningeal irritation and neurologic impairment. Symptoms of meningitis include **headache, vomiting, fever, photophobia, irritability, clouding of consciousness** (altered mental status), **convulsions** (especially in children)**, and neck stiffness**.

Classic signs of meningeal inflammation: These include
- **Cervical rigidity/neck stiffness**
- **Kernig sign: Knee pain with hip flexion**
- **Brudzinski sign: Knee/hip flexion when the neck is flexed.**

Cerebrospinal Fluid (CSF) Changes

Q. Write a short note on CSF changes in pyogenic meningitis.

The presence of polymorphonuclear leukocytes in the CSF is the most definitive feature of meningitis (**Table 27.2**).
- **Gross appearance:** Normally CSF is clear. In acute meningitis, it becomes **cloudy or frankly purulent**.
- **CSF pressure: Increased** (>180 mm of water).
- **Microscopy:** CSF shows marked **pleocytosis** (increased cell count) containing **predominantly neutrophils** (as many as 90,000 neutrophils per cubic millimeters) as cellular constituents. **Gram staining** may be useful in identifying bacteria. The organisms can be identified and characterized by culture, antigenicity, and in some cases, polymerase chain reaction (PCR).
- **Biochemical findings:** These are as follows:
  - **Reduced glucose levels:** CSF shows markedly **reduced glucose levels** (<40 mg/dL), mostly due to the consumption of glucose by inflammatory cells.
  - **Raised CSF protein***:* The concentration of CSF protein is increased (>50 mg/dL) due to the leakage of proteins from damaged vessels.
  - **Chlorides:** It may be slightly reduced.

Prognosis: Effective treatment with antibiotics markedly reduces mortality. Untreated pyogenic meningitis can be fatal.

Aseptic (Viral) Meningitis

Aseptic meningitis is a clinical term used for the patient who manifests with features of meningitis in the absence of any organisms by bacterial culture (no identifiable organisms). The features of meningitis include meningeal irritation, fever, and alterations of consciousness of relatively acute onset. It is common in children and young adults. Most often transmitted by fecal-oral route.

Etiology: Aseptic meningitis is **generally caused by a wide range of viruses** but may be nonviral (e.g., rickettsial) infections or autoimmune in origin. The viruses include **enteroviruses** in 80% of cases (e.g., *echovirus, coxsackie B virus*), ***herpes simplex virus*** *(HSV) 2*, ***mumps virus, human immunodeficiency virus (HIV)****, lympho choriomeningitis virus, arboviruses, measles virus, parainfluenza virus, adenovirus.* The causative agent is identified in only a minority of cases. However, the use of more sensitive and specific detection techniques (such as DNA sequencing) may detect the etiologic agent.

MORPHOLOGY

It is characterized by a **scanty infiltrate of chronic inflammatory cells within the leptomeninges** around superficial cortical blood vessels and choroid plexus.

Clinical features: Aseptic meningitis (viral meningitis) is mainly a disease of children and young adults. It manifests with a **sudden febrile illness with a severe headache**. The viral aseptic meningitides are treated symptomatically.

CSF Findings (Table 27.2)

- **Gross appearance**: CSF is clear.
- **Microscopy**: CSF in aseptic meningitis shows pleocytosis containing **predominantly lymphocytes** (lymphocytic pleocytosis) (10–100 lymphocytes/mL).
- **Biochemical findings:** These are as follows:
  - **Protein:** Mild to moderately elevated (>40 mg/100 mL).
  - **Glucose**: There is no decrease in CSF glucose, and glucose content is nearly always normal.

Prognosis: It is usually a **benign self-limited condition**. Its clinical course is less fulminant than that of pyogenic meningitis and usually resolves without sequelae.

Chronic Meningitis

Types: It may be bacterial or fungal.
- **Bacterial:** Chronic bacterial infection of the meninges may be caused by (1) *Mycobacterium tuberculosis, (2) Treponema pallidum,* and *Borrelia* species.
- **Fungal:** Cryptococcal.

Tuberculous Meningitis

Q. Write a short note on tuberculous meningitis.

Tuberculous meningitis is the **infection of the meninges by tubercle bacilli**. It is more common in developing nations, particularly in Asia and Africa.

Etiology: *Mycobacterium tuberculosis* **human type is the most common cause.**

Mode of infection: Tuberculous meningitis occurs through the following routes:
- **Hematogenous (miliary) spread** from other site (most commonly from a primary in the lung) and it is the usual mode. It may be reactivation of latent infection elsewhere in the body.
- **Direct spread** from adjacent sites such as the vertebral body. It develops when intraparenchymal granulomas rupture into the CSF.

TABLE 27.2 Cerebrospinal fluid findings in meningitis.

	Normal	*Acute pyogenic*	*Acute viral*	*Tuberculous*
Physical examination	Clear and colorless	Turbid and forms coagulum	Clear	Clear and colorless, forms cobweb on standing due to the coagulation of fibrinogen
CSF pressure	60–150 mm of H_2O	Raised above 180 mm of H_2O	Raised above 250 mm of H_2O	Raised above 300 mm of H_2O
Total protein	20–40 mg/100 mL	50–200 mg/100 mL	>40 mg/100 mL	50–150 mg/100 mL
Glucose	45–80 mg/100 mL	0–20 mg/l00 mL	Normal	20–50 mg/100 mL
Chlorides	720–750 mg/100 mL	600–700 mg/100 mL	Normal	450–600 mg/100 mL
Cells				
Polymorphs	Usually absent	150–2,000/μL	Absent	0–5 cells/μL
Lymphocytes	0–5 cells/μL	5–50 cells/μL	10–100 cells/μL	500–700 cells/μL
Gram stain/ZN stain	–	Bacteria +	–	AFB +

Bacterial meningitis: Most organisms originate in the nasopharynx.

MORPHOLOGY

Gross

- Diffuse **meningoencephalitis** is the most common pattern of tuberculous involvement in the CNS.
- **Subarachnoid space** contains a **greenish, gelatinous, or fibrinous exudate**, most **prominent at the base of the brain surrounding cranial nerves.**
- Leptomeninges may show discrete, white granules of the tubercle.

Microscopy

- Tuberculous meningitis is a **chronic infection**. The involved areas show a mixed inflammatory infiltrate composed of lymphocytes, plasma cells, and macrophages. **Severe cases produce a well-formed granulomatous host response.**
- **Granuloma** consisting of epithelioid cells, Langhans giant cells surrounded by lymphocytes. It may show the central area of caseous necrosis.
- **Ziehl–Neelsen stain** (acid-fast stain) may show variable numbers of acid-fast bacilli.
- **Confirmation** of tuberculosis is by either culture (takes around 6–8 weeks) or PCR testing based on the amplification of ribosomal ribonucleic acid (rRNA) derived from *Mycobacterium tuberculosis* (takes about 6–8 hours).

Clinical Features

Tuberculous meningitis usually presents with **headache, malaise, mental confusion, and vomiting**. On examination, there will be neck rigidity. Untreated tuberculous meningitis is generally fatal in 4–6 weeks. However, it may progress more rapidly in immunocompromised patients.

Complications

- **Spread of infection:** The inflammation can also affect the arteries that run through the subarachnoid space. They may show **obliterative endarteritis** (endarteritis obliterans) and marked thickening of intima-producing arterial occlusion. This results in **ischemic complications** (cause infarcts). These **brain infarcts** are usually in the distribution of the penetrating striate and brainstem arteries. The infectious process may travel through the CSF and spread to the choroid plexus and ependymal surface.
- **Communicating hydrocephalus:** The most serious complication is **arachnoid (meningeal) fibrosis**. In long-standing cases, a dense, fibrous adhesive arachnoiditis may develop. This is most prominent around the base of the brain. It may produce communicating hydrocephalus.
- **Damage to the nerve root.**

Cerebrospinal Fluid Findings

Q. Write a short note on CSF changes in tuberculous meningitis.

- **Physical examination: Clear and colorless, forms cobweb on standing** due to coagulation of fibrinogen.
- **CSF pressure: Raised above 300 mm of H_2O**
- **Biochemical findings:** These are as follows:
  - **Protein:** It is **raised** and ranges from **50 to 150 mg/100 mL**.
  - **Glucose:** Moderately reduced or normal (20–50 mg/100 mL).
  - **Chloride: Decreased (450–600 mg/100 mL).**

Microscopy: It shows **moderate CSF pleocytosis** (500–700 cells/μL) made up of mononuclear cells (**mainly lymphocytes**).

Tuberculoma

It is another manifestation of tuberculosis of CNS. CNS involvement by tuberculosis may also appear as one or more well-circumscribed intraparenchymal masses termed **tuberculomas**.

MORPHOLOGY

Gross

- **Number:** Tuberculoma may be **single or multiple well-circumscribed intraparenchymal mass.**
- **Size:** Varies and may be as large as several centimeters in diameter, and may present as an intracranial space-occupying lesion.

Microscopy

Shows **epithelioid granuloma** consisting of the central core of caseous necrosis surrounded by epithelioid cells, Langhans giant cells, and lymphocytes. Calcification may occur in inactive lesions. Tubercle bacilli can be difficult to detect in these lesions.

CSF findings in various types of meningitis are summarized in **Table 27.1.**

Neurosyphilis

Syphilis is caused by a spirochete, *T. pallidum*. Neurosyphilis **develops in the tertiary stage of syphilis** and occurs in about 10% of untreated patients.

Major Patterns of CNS Involvement

Meningovascular neurosyphilis

- Syphilitic meningitis is a chronic meningitis.
- **Sites affected:** It involves the **base of the brain,** more variably **the cerebral convexities** and **spinal leptomeninges.**

MORPHOLOGY

Obliterative endarteritis (heubner arteritis): In *meningovascular syphilis,* the inflammation involves arteries causing obliterative endarteritis. This is accompanied by a **distinctive perivascular** (surrounding the arterioles of the cerebral cortex) **inflammatory reaction rich in plasma cells and lymphocytes (hallmark of syphilis).** These changes may produce ischemic lesions **resulting in multiple small infarcts** in the cerebral cortex or brainstem.

Cerebral gummas (plasma cell-rich mass lesions) in parenchyma may also occur in the meninges.

Luetic dementia: The spirochete, *T. pallidum,* may remain latent in the brain for decades. The spirochetes replicate sluggishly and escape eradication. This results in dementia and psychosis several years after the initial infection.

Paretic neurosyphilis

Paretic neurosyphilis is caused by the invasion of the brain by *Treponema pallidum*. It manifests as insidious but progressive cognitive and motor disturbances with mood alterations (including delusions of grandeur). It may terminate in severe dementia (termed **general paresis of the insane**) and may lead to death.

MORPHOLOGY

The brain appears atrophic and firm with opaque leptomeninges.

Sites affected: Parenchymal damage of the cerebral cortex commonly occurs in the **frontal lobe.**

Microscopy: The lesions show the following features:

- **Loss of cortical neurons,** disfigurement of residual nerve cells ("windblown appearance").
- **Proliferation of microglia (rod cells), gliosis,** and conversion of microglia into elongated forms encrusted with iron ("rod cells") associated with nodular ependymitis (ependymal granulations). The iron deposits can be demonstrated by the Prussian blue stain in the perivascular region and in the neuropil. These are probably the sequelae of small bleeds caused due to microvascular damage. Occasionally, the spirochetes can be demonstrated in tissue sections using silver stain or immunohistochemistry using *Treponema* antibody.

Tabes dorsalis

Tabes dorsalis is an **impairment of dorsal (posterior) spinal column function.** It is due to damage to the sensory nerves in the dorsal roots and is manifested by loss of joint position sense and fine touch.

MORPHOLOGY

Microscopy

- The spinal cord shows **loss of both axons and myelin in the dorsal roots** and the corresponding pallor and atrophy in the dorsal columns. The spirochetes are absent in these lesions in the spinal cord.
- A **gumma** is a round, firm, rubbery lesion with central necrosis surrounded by a granulomatous reaction. Gumma is similar to that seen in tuberculomas.

Clinical features: These include impaired joint position sense and resultant ataxia (locomotor ataxia), and loss of pain sensation, leading to skin and joint damage (Charcot joints). Other sensory disturbances include lightning pains and the absence of deep tendon reflexes.

INTERPRETATION OF CEREBROSPINAL FLUID FINDINGS

PA 35.3 (CC): Identify the etiology of meningitis based on given cerebrospinal fluid (CSF) parameters.

Case 1

History: A 24-year-old male presented to an emergency department with the complaint of fever and severe headache of 1-day duration. The headache has rapidly become more intense. He had vomited twice and appears drowsy and confused. He finds bright lights uncomfortable. There was no significant previous medical history.

Examination: His temperature is 39.2°C. He has stiffness on passive flexion of his neck. His consciousness level is decreased, but he is rousable to command; there are no focal neurological signs.

Investigations

Hematological tests: WBC count of 16,200/µL (normal 4,000–11,000/µL) and platelet count of 310,000/µL (150,000–450,000/µL).

Cerebrospinal Fluid (CSF) Findings

Physical appearance	Turbid and formed coagulum (clear and colorless)
Pressure	210 mm of H_2O (60–150 mm of H_2O)
Protein	150 mg/100 mL (20–40 mg/100 mL)
Glucose	8 mg/100 mL (45–80 mg/100 mL)
Chlorides	645 mg/100 mL (720–750 mg/100 mL)
Microscopy	
• Leukocytes	1,500 cells/µL (Usually absent)
• Lymphocytes	8 cells/µL (0–5 cells/µL)
• Gram stain	Demonstrated intracellular diplococci

Note: Reference values in brackets.

Questions

1. What is the probable diagnosis?
2. What is/are the cause/s of this condition?
3. What are the complications?

Answers

1. A probable diagnosis is **acute bacterial meningitis**. The clinical features that favor the diagnosis are sudden onset of severe headache, vomiting, confusion, photophobia, and neck stiffness. The presence of leukocytosis suggests acute bacterial infection rather than viral meningitis. Normally CSF is clear. In acute meningitis, it becomes **cloudy or frankly purulent**. The combination of 1,500 neutrophils/µL CSF (the most definitive feature of pyogenic meningitis), decreased CSF glucose (8 mg/100 mL) and a raised CSF protein of 150 mg/100 mL is strongly suggestive of bacterial meningitis. Glucose is reduced because the organisms use glucose for their multiplication. The gram stain and culture will give the definitive diagnosis. In this case, the gram stain demonstrated gram-negative cocci consistent with *Neisseria meningitidis* infection.
2. The most likely causative bacteria are *Neisseria meningitidis* (meningococcal meningitis), *Haemophilus influenzae,* and *Streptococcus pneumoniae*. Meningitis may be caused by viruses, fungi, and *Mycobacterium tuberculosis* apart from bacteria.
3. Complications (*refer* page 961).

Case 2

History: A 10-year-old male child presented to an emergency department with the complaints of fever and severe headache of 1-day duration. He had vomited twice and appears drowsy and confused. He finds bright lights uncomfortable. There was no significant previous medical history.

Examination: His temperature is 38.8°C. He has stiffness on passive flexion of his neck. His consciousness level is decreased, but he is rousable to command; there are no focal neurological signs.

Investigations

Cerebrospinal Fluid (CSF) Findings

Physical examination	Clear
CSF pressure	270 mm of H_2O (60–150 mm of H_2O)
Total protein	80 mg/100 mL (20–40 mg/100 mL)
Glucose	50 mg/mL (45–80 mg/100 mL)
Chlorides	730 mg/mL (720–750 mg/100 mL)
Cells	
Polymorphs	Absent (usually absent)
Lymphocytes	70 cells/µL (0–5 cells/µL)
Gram stain/ZN stain	No organism detected

Note: Reference values in brackets.

Questions

1. What is the probable diagnosis?
2. What are the features that help in diagnosis?
3. What is/are the cause/s of this condition?

Answers

1. Probable diagnosis is **acute aseptic (viral) meningitis**. It is common in children and young adults.
2. Features that favor the diagnosis: The clinical features that favor the diagnosis of meningitis are sudden onset of severe headache, vomiting, confusion, photophobia, and neck stiffness. The presence of lymphocytes in CSF suggests acute viral infection rather than bacterial meningitis. The combination of 70 lymphocytes/µL in CSF, normal CSF glucose (50 mg/100 mL), and a moderate increase of CSF protein of 80 mg/100 mL are strongly suggestive of acute viral meningitis. Symptoms of acute meningitis with **no identifiable organisms** on Gram stain/ZN stain will give the definitive diagnosis. Culture will be negative for bacteria.
3. The **etiological agents include** enterovirus, HIV, mumps virus, EB virus, and herpes simplex virus.

Case 3

History: A 10-year-old boy was brought to an emergency department for a complaint of fever and severe headache for 2 days duration. The headache has rapidly become more intense. He had vomited twice and appears drowsy and confused. He finds bright lights uncomfortable. His father has had a chronic cough, an evening rise in temperature, and taking treatment for the past 3 months for a chronic disease of the lung.

Examination: His temperature is 38.0°C. He has stiffness on passive flexion of his neck (on neck rigidity). His consciousness level is decreased, but he is rousable to command; there are no focal neurological signs.

Investigations

Cerebrospinal Fluid (CSF) Findings

Physical examination	Clear and colorless, forms cobweb on standing due to the coagulation of fibrinogen
CSF pressure	320 mm of H_2O (60–150 mm of H_2O)
Total protein	130 mg/100 mL (20–40 mg/100 mL)
Glucose	40 mg/100 mL (45–80 mg/100 mL)
Chlorides	550 mg/100 mL (720–750 mg/100 mL)
Cells	
Polymorphs	2 cells/μL (usually absent)
Lymphocytes	600 cells/μL (0–5 cells/μL)
ZN stain	AFB +

Note: Reference values in brackets.

Questions

1. What is the probable diagnosis?
2. What are the features that help in diagnosis?
3. What are the complications?

Answers

1. A probable diagnosis is **tuberculous meningitis**. It is caused by the *Mycobacterium tuberculosis* **human type**.
2. **Features that favor the diagnosis:** The clinical features that favor the diagnosis of meningitis are sudden onset of severe headache, vomiting, confusion, photophobia neck stiffness, and raised **CSF pressure. Physical examination of clear and colorless CSF which forms cobweb on standing** due to coagulation of fibrinogen and the presence of lymphocytes (600 cells/μL) in CSF (which is more than seen in acute viral infection) suggests tuberculous meningitis. The combination of 600 lymphocytes/μL CSF, mildly reduced CSF glucose (40 mg/100 mL) an increase of CSF protein of 130 mg/100 mL and **decreased chloride** is strongly suggestive of tuberculous meningitis. ZN stain for AFB will give the definitive diagnosis.
   Mode of infection: (i) **Hematogenous route** from other site (most commonly from the lung); (ii) **Miliary spread** or (iii) **Direct spread** from an adjacent site such as vertebral body.
3. **Complications:** (1) Hydrocephalus, (2) nerve root damage, and (3) tuberculous encephalitis.

TUMORS OF CENTRAL NERVOUS SYSTEM

PA 35.2 (CC): Classify and describe the etiology, genetics, pathogenesis, pathology, presentation, sequelae, and complications of CNS tumors.

Introduction

Tumors of the central nervous system (CNS) represent **around 3% of all malignancies.**

Primary versus secondary: Most **CNS tumors are primary** and represent 1.5% of all primary malignant tumors. **Metastatic tumors of the CNS** occur **more commonly than primary** tumors.

Children versus adults: Different types of brain tumors tend to arise at particular ages. Some tumors may be most common in adults but can occur in any age group. For example, glioblastomas, the most common and malignant gliomas, can occur at any age.

- **Children**: The primary brain tumors of the CNS are **second** only to leukemias as the **most common type of malignant tumors in children and young adults.** They are the most common solid tumors in children, accounting for nearly 20% of childhood cancers. **Seventy percent of childhood CNS tumors** arise in the **posterior fossa. Certain tumors are more common in childhood, the most prominent being medulloblastomas, ependymomas, pilocytic astrocytomas, craniopharyngiomas, choroid plexus tumors, and diffuse pontine astrocytoma.**
- **Adults:** Most brain tumors occur in adults, mainly within the cerebral hemispheres above the tentorium. The frequency of each type of tumor varies with age and gender. For example, gliomas are more common in men, and meningiomas are more common in women. Metastatic lung, breast, and colon carcinomas are mainly seen in older adults.

Wide range of tumors: CNS has a broad spectrum of cellular constituents. Tumors can arise from these diverse cell types. It produces a wide range of tumor types in the brain and spinal cord and their overlying meninges.

Unique characteristics of central nervous system tumors: These are as follows:

1. **No premalignant or in situ lesions**: Compared to carcinomas, CNS tumors do not have premalignant or in situ lesions.
2. **Low-grade lesions may be infiltrative**: Even if the tumor appears low-grade, it may infiltrate large brain areas. This may cause serious clinical deficits, tumors become unresectable and carry a poor prognosis.
3. **The anatomic site of the tumor can influence outcome**: Irrespective of tumor type and grade, the anatomic location of the tumor can produce local effects and influence the outcome. For example, a benign meningioma may cause cardiorespiratory arrest due to compression of the medulla.
4. **Few malignant tumors of CNS rarely spread outside the CNS**: For example, highly malignant gliomas, rarely spread outside of the CNS.

Classification of tumors of CNS: It is based on the presumed **cell of origin and biological grade of malignancy and**

newer molecular analyses. The biological grade is derived from the microscopic appearances. The most commonly used is the World Health Organization (WHO) classification system **(Box 27.1)**. **A key change in the most recent WHO (2021) classification** is the introduction of **genetic abnormalities into the classification system**.

BOX 27.1: World Health Organization (WHO) (2021) (abridged) classification of central nervous system (CNS) tumors.

Gliomas, glioneuronal tumors, and neuronal tumors
- *Adult-type diffuse gliomas*
  - Astrocytoma, IDH-mutant
    - Astrocytoma, IDH-mutant, grade 2
    - Astrocytoma, IDH-mutant, grade 3
    - Astrocytoma, IDH-mutant, grade 4
  - Oligodendroglioma, IDH-mutant and 1p/19q-codeleted
    - Oligodendroglioma, IDH-mutant and 1p/19q-codeleted, grade 2
    - Oligodendroglioma, IDH-mutant and 1p/19q-codeleted, grade 3
  - Glioblastoma, IDH-wildtype tumors
- *Pediatric-type diffuse low-grade gliomas*
  - Diffuse astrocytoma, *MYB*- or *MYBL1*-altered
- *Pediatric-type diffuse high-grade gliomas*
  - Diffuse midline glioma, H3 K27-altered
  - Diffuse pediatric-type high-grade glioma, H3-wildtype and IDH-wildtype
- *Circumscribed astrocytic gliomas*
  - Pilocytic astrocytoma
  - Pleomorphic xanthoastrocytoma
  - Subependymal giant cell astrocytoma
- *Glioneuronal and neuronal tumors*
  - Ganglioglioma
  - Gangliocytoma
- *Ependymal tumors*
  - Supratentorial ependymoma, NOS
  - Posterior fossa ependymoma, NOS
  - Spinal ependymoma, NOS
  - Myxopapillary ependymoma
  - Subependymoma

Choroid plexus tumors
- Choroid plexus papilloma
- Atypical choroid plexus papilloma
- Choroid plexus carcinoma

Embryonal tumors

Medulloblastoma
- *Medulloblastomas, molecularly defined*
  - Medulloblastoma, WNT-activated
  - Medulloblastoma, SHH-activated and *TP53*-wildtype
  - Medulloblastoma, SHH-activated and *TP53*-mutant
  - Medulloblastoma, non-WNT/non-SHH
- *Medulloblastomas, histologically defined*
  - Medulloblastoma, histologically defined
  - Classic medulloblastoma

Contd...

Contd...

Other CNS embryonal tumors

Pineal tumors

Cranial and paraspinal nerve tumors

Meningioma
- **Meningioma**

Mesenchymal, nonmeningothelial tumors involving the CNS

Melanocytic tumors

Hematolymphoid tumors involving the CNS

Germ cell tumors

Tumors of the sellar region

Metastases to the CNS

(CNS: central nervous system; IDH: isocitrate dehydrogenase; NOS: not otherwise specified)

GLIOMAS

Gliomas are the **most common group of primary brain tumors** of the brain parenchyma. They are divided into six groups **(Box 27.1)**. The recent WHO (2021) classification has included molecular features, specifically mutations of the *IDH* gene and deletion of the chromosomal segments 1p and 19q, into the previous histology-based classification. The meaning of **1p/19q codeletion** is the combined loss of the short arm of chromosome 1 (i.e., 1p) and the long arm of chromosome 19 (i.e., 19q). In the present WHO classification, **diffuse gliomas are grouped into "adult-type"** (that occur primarily in adults) **and "pediatric-type"** (that occur primarily in children) **diffuse gliomas.** These tumors are subdivided into one of four grades according to their biological behavior, ranging from grade 1 to grade 4.

Adult-type Diffuse Gliomas

Adult-type diffuse gliomas are subdivided into three distinct types—astrocytoma, *IDH*-mutant; oligodendroglioma, *IDH*-mutant and 1p/19q-codeleted; and glioblastoma *IDH*-wild-type **(Box 27.2)**. These tumors are the most common malignant tumors of the adult central nervous system.

BOX 27.2: Three distinct adult-type diffuse gliomas.

1. **Astrocytoma, IDH-mutant**
   - Astrocytoma, IDH-mutant, grade 2
   - Astrocytoma, IDH-mutant, grade 3
   - Astrocytoma, IDH-mutant, grade 4
2. **Oligodendroglioma, IDH-mutant and 1p/19q-codeleted**
   - Oligodendroglioma, IDH-mutant and 1p/19q-codeleted, grade 2
   - Oligodendroglioma, IDH-mutant and 1p/19q-codeleted, grade 3
3. **Glioblastoma, IDH-wild type tumors**

Astrocytoma, IDH-Mutant

Q. Write a short note on astrocytoma.

Astrocytoma, IDH-mutant, is a **diffusely infiltrating *IDH1*- or *IDH2*-mutant glioma that arises from astrocytes.**

Grading: Based on the histologic and molecular features, of astrocytoma, IDH-mutant is graded into WHO grade 2, WHO grade 3, and CNS WHO grade 4. All diffuse gliomas are considered malignant. Grade 1 indicates a benign behavior. Hence, grade 1 is not used for diffuse gliomas.

Age: Astrocytoma, IDH-mutant, generally presents in individuals **younger than 55 years** and usually in their 30s or 40s (younger than GLIOBLASTOMA, *IDH*-wild type). The **higher-grade tumors occur more often in older patients.**

Sites: Astrocytomas with *IDH1* or *IDH2* mutation can occur at **any region of the CNS**. They are most **commonly seen in the supratentorial compartment** and are usually **near or within the frontal lobes.**

Pathogenesis

The classic triad of *IDH1* or *IDH2* mutation with additional mutations in *TP53* and *ATRX* is the characteristic molecular signature of "astrocytoma, IDH-mutant."

Driver mutations in IDH: The *IDH1* and *IDH2* genes encode for isoforms of the isocitrate dehydrogenase (IDH) enzyme. Astrocytoma and IDH-mutant are characteristically associated with gain of function driver mutations of the isocitrate dehydrogenase 1 gene *IDH1*, or (**much less commonly**) its homologue *IDH2*. These mutations occur early in gliomagenesis (formation and development of glioma). It favors the **development or maintenance of a stem cell-like state** subjected to **self-renewal and tumorigenesis.**

Inactive mutations in *TP53* and *ATRX* gene: IDH-mutant astrocytomas also show **loss-of-function mutations in *TP53* and *ATRX*. *ATRX* gene encodes an essential chromatin-binding protein, namely ATRX protein.** *ATRX* mutations lead to **ATRX protein deficiency** and are associated with **generalized genomic instability**. This **can cause p53-dependent cell death.** Therefore, ***TP53* mutations in IDH-mutant astrocytomas may facilitate the survival of tumor cells when there is ATRX loss.**

Homozygous deletion of *CDKN2A* and/or *CDKN2B*: It is associated with **shorter survival** in patients with IDH-mutant astrocytomas. It corresponds to CNS WHO grade 4 behavior.

MORPHOLOGY

Gross Appearance of IDH-mutant Astrocytomas

Grade 2 and grade 3 astrocytoma: These are **poorly defined, gray, infiltrative tumors** that expand and distort the involved area of the brain. They do not form a discrete mass.

Grade 4 astrocytoma (Fig. 27.3): It **diffusely infiltrates brain parenchyma without any delineated borders.** Unlike *IDH-wild-type* glioblastomas, it usually does not contain large areas of central necrosis and hemorrhage.

Microscopy

CNS WHO grade 2 IDH-mutant astrocytoma (Figs. 27.4A to C): These are **well-differentiated** tumors with **low-cell density.** They are **slow-growing** tumors.

- **Mild to moderate cellularity:** These tumors show a **mild-to-moderate increase** in the number of glial cell nuclei **(increased cellularity).**
- **Neoplastic fibrillary astrocytes (glial cells):** These tumors are composed of **fibrillary glial cells** that diffusely infiltrate the CNS parenchyma individually.

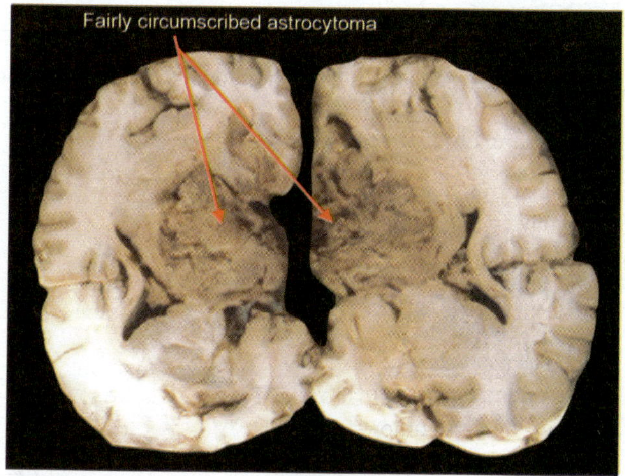

Fig. 27.3: Coronal section of cerebral hemispheres showing astrocytoma.

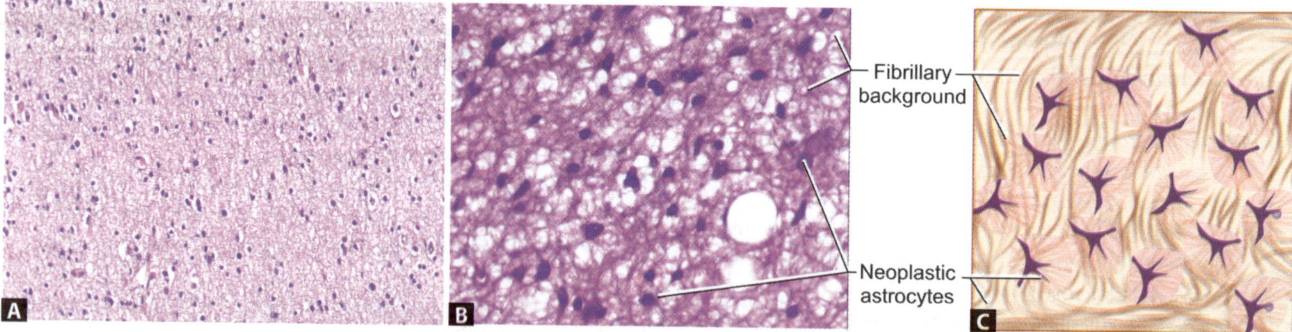

Figs. 27.4A to C: Microscopic appearance of diffuse astrocytoma, IDH-mutant, grade 2: (A) and (B) H&E, and (C) diagrammatic. Astrocytoma showing diffusely infiltrative astrocytic glioma without microscopic features of anaplasia; (B) Higher magnification; (C) Diagrammatic appearance.

- **Nuclear features:** Microscopically, the **recognition of neoplastic astrocytes is principally based on nuclear characteristics.** Compared to normal astrocytes, the nuclei in IDH-mutant astrocytomas are **enlarged.** They **characteristically show mild nuclear atypia,** variable nuclear pleomorphism, **irregular nuclear outlines, an uneven chromatin pattern,** and **hyperchromasia.** Typically, **nucleoli are indistinct** and are usually **not visible. Mitotic activity is absent or uncommon.**
- **Fibrillary background:** The background shows an intervening network of fine, glial fibrillary acidic protein (GFAP)-positive astrocytic cell processes. This gives a fibrillary appearance to the background.
- **Indistinct transition between neoplastic and normal tissue:** The tumor cells infiltrate healthy tissue many centimeters from the main tumor.

CNS WHO grade 3 IDH-mutant astrocytoma (Fig. 27.5A): The main features differentiating grade 3 astrocytomas from grade 2 astrocytomas are as follows:

- **More densely cellular:** WHO grade 3 tumors also often show increased cell density.
- **Greater nuclear pleomorphism, and increased mitotic activity: It shows** histological **anaplasia** and **more significant nuclear atypia.** The features of nuclear atypia are **variations in nuclear size and shape** and **coarsely dispersed chromatin.** It shows **increased mitotic activity.** It may show multinucleated tumor cells and abnormal mitoses.
- **Absence of microvascular proliferation and necrosis:** By definition, there is the **absence of microvascular proliferation (MVP; multilayered endothelia within vessels) and necrosis.**

CNS WHO grades 4 IDH-mutant astrocytoma (Figs. 27.5B and C): The main feature is:

- **Densely cellular:** These are **hypercellular, showing greater cellular crowding.** These are **rapidly progressive tumors.**
- **Highly anaplastic:** The tumor cells show marked cytological atypia.
- **Increased proliferative activity;** Tumor shows **increased mitotic activity.**
- **Necrosis and/or MVP:** In addition to the features of CNS WHO grade 3 lesions mentioned above, grade 4 tumors must have areas of **necrosis and/or microvascular proliferation (MVP).** However, the tumor should be called CNS WHO grade 4 IDH-mutant astrocytoma **if the tumor shows homozygous deletion of *CDKN2A* and/or *CDKN2B*, even in the absence of necrosis or MVP.**

Differential Diagnosis

Glioblastoma versus CNS WHO grade 4 IDH-mutant astrocytoma: The term "glioblastoma" is no longer used for WHO grade 4 **IDH-mutant astrocytoma.** Morphologically, however, the microscopic appearance of individual cells of WHO grade 4 IDH-mutant astrocytoma has considerable overlap with that of IDH-wild type glioblastoma. Distinguishing between these two tumors **requires testing for IDH mutations.** However, there are certain differentiating features.

- **Areas of ischemic zonal and/or palisading necrosis:** They are seen **in 50% of WHO grade 4 IDH-mutant astrocytomas.** They are less frequent than in **IDH-wild type glioblastoma, where they occur in up to 90% of cases. Focal oligodendroglioma-**like components are more **common in WHO grade 4 IDH-mutant astrocytoma** than in IDH-wildtype glioblastoma.

Immunohistochemistry

GFAP: Individual tumor cells of IDH-mutant astrocytoma **variably express GFAP.**

IDH1: It is a sensitive and specific marker of infiltrating gliomas, both astrocytic and oligodendroglial. It recognizes only the most common mutation (*IDH1* p.R132H), which accounts for 90% of all glioma-associated *IDH* mutations. It is rare in children <14 years.

Clinical features: Astrocytoma, IDH-mutant is commonly present with gradual onset of symptoms such as headache, seizures (common in cerebral hemispheric lesions), and changes in behavior or personality (especially in frontal lobe tumors).

Glioblastoma, IDH-Wild-type

Q. Write a short note on glioblastoma.

Glioblastoma is an adult-**type diffuse glioma (grade 4 astrocytic glioma)** with **IDH-wild-type** (wild type is a gene that predominates in a natural population). It arises from astrocytes. These tumors are grade 4 tumors and do not have lower-grade precursors. They have a very poor prognosis.

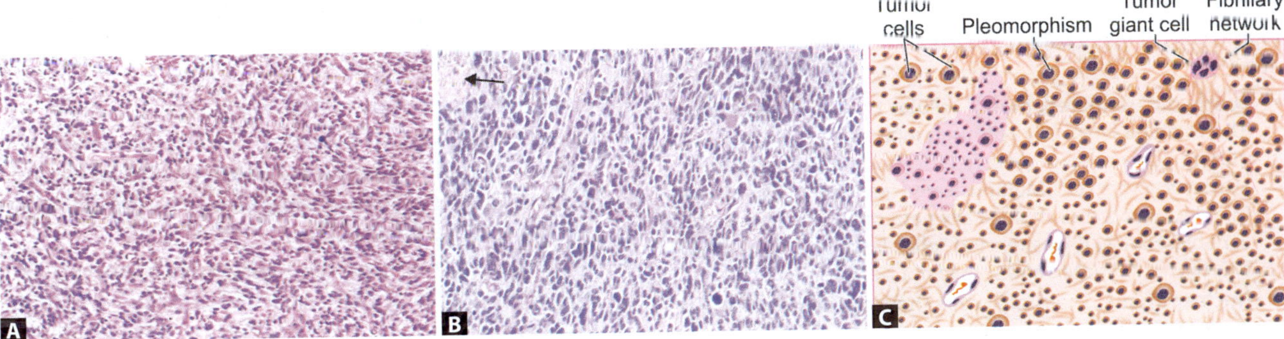

Figs. 27.5A to C: Microscopic appearance of diffuse astrocytoma, IDH-mutant: (A) Astrocytoma grade 3 shows a diffusely hypercellular, infiltrative astrocytic glioma with anaplasia. The cells show nuclear polymorphism and have less cytoplasm than normal astrocytes. No necrosis is seen; (B) H&E; (C) Diagrammatic astrocytoma grade 4 shows a highly anaplastic, hypercellular tumor and area of necrosis (arrow in B).

Age: Glioblastoma is the most frequent malignant brain tumor in adults. It accounts for about 15% of all intracranial neoplasms and 45–50% of all primary malignant brain tumors. It can manifest at any age but mainly occurs in older adults. The peak incidence is between **55 and 85 years**.

Pathogenesis

Glioblastomas, IDH-wild-type, show many genetic alterations that lead to cancer hallmarks. These include the following:

- **Evasion of senescence**: Most glioblastomas have genetic aberrations that lead to evasion of senescence. This may be due to telomerase mutations or mutations that lead to alternative lengthening of telomeres.
- **Escape from normal growth controls:** It may be due to biallelic deletion of *CDKN2A*. The *CDKN2A* gene encodes the cyclin-dependent kinase inhibitor p16.
- **Activation of growth factor signaling pathways**: This may be due to *EGFR* or *PDGFR* gene amplification.
- **Resistance to apoptosis**: This may be due to *TP53* mutation.
- **Methylation of the promoter of the *MGMT* gene: The** *MGMT* gene encodes a DNA repair enzyme and influences sensitivity to chemotherapeutic agents.

MORPHOLOGY

Localization: Glioblastoma, IDH wild-type, commonly occurs in the **supratentorial regions in the subcortical white matter and deeper gray matter of the cerebral hemispheres** (temporal, parietal, and frontal lobes; basal ganglia, and thalamus).

Gross

Glioblastomas are **usually large at presentation**. Most glioblastomas in the cerebral hemisphere are **intraparenchymal and centered in the white matter**. Rapid infiltration of the corpus callosum with growth in the contralateral hemisphere produces a bilateral, symmetrical lesion (butterfly glioma).

Cut section: Glioblastomas are **poorly outlined (ill-defined)**. The cut surface is **variable in color**. It shows variation in the appearance of the tumor from region to region is characteristic. The periphery appears **gray to pink and central areas show** soft **yellowish necrosis** or **red due to hemorrhage**. It may show cystic degeneration.

Microscopy [Figs. 27.6A and B (*refer* online Figs. 27.6C and D)]

- **Poorly differentiated, highly cellular tumor:** Glioblastoma, IDH-wildtype, is typically a **diffusely infiltrating, highly cellular** glioma composed of poorly differentiated pleomorphic astrocytic tumor cells. Multinucleated giant cells may be seen. Glioblastoma is morphologically heterogeneous and highly variable. Hence, it was termed **"glioblastoma multiforme."** This term is **outdated** and should not be used.
- **Nuclear atypia**: The tumor cells show **nuclear atypia and marked pleomorphism.**
- **Frequent (brisk) mitotic activity: is often brisk**. Some tumors show marked cellular and nuclear polymorphism, with numerous cells; others may be markedly cellular but relatively monomorphic.
- **Necrosis [Figs. 27.6A and B (*refer* online Fig. 27.6C)]:** The characteristic diagnostic features of glioblastoma microvascular proliferation and necrosis. The necrosis can be geographic, **with or without perinecrotic palisading** [serpentine **(snake-like)** pattern].. The **edges of the** central **necrotic area** are surrounded by the palisading tumor cells, which is known as **pseudo palisading (garlanding).**
- **Microvascular proliferation (MVP)** (*refer* **online Fig. 27.6D):** It is rapid blood vessel growth and appears as **multilayered small-caliber blood vessels.** It produces tufts of cells (at least two layers) that pile up and bulge into the lumen of small blood vessels. In some glioblastomas, endothelial and smooth muscle cell/pericyte overgrowth is so prominent that the vessels assume a **glomeruloid (like glomerulus in the kidney) appearance.**

In an IDH- and H3-wildtype diffuse glioma, the presence of either **microvascular proliferation or (2) necrosis** is sufficient for the diagnosis of glioblastoma.

Molecular features: Molecular features are also used for grading. These include **(1) *TERT* promoter mutation, (2) *EGER* gene amplification, and (3) gain of chromosome 7 (+7) and loss of chromosome 10 (–10)**. These are used for the diagnosis of glioblastoma grade 4 even in the absence of necrosis or microvascular proliferation.

Clinical features: Glioblastoma, IDH-wild-type, usually affects older patients (6–8th decades of life). It typically presents with symptoms of short duration (<3 months in about 68% of patients). The signs and symptoms depend on the tumor's location. It manifests with **focal neurological deficits such as hemiparesis, aphasia, visual field defects, and/or seizures** (in about 50% of patients). Symptoms of raised intracranial pressure may manifest with **headache, nausea, and vomiting. Imaging studies** show a large lesion with an **irregular often ring of contrast enhancement**. This is due to abnormal "leaky" vessels with an abnormally permeable blood-brain barrier.

Prognosis: It is very poor, even with treatment. Treatment modalities include resection, radiotherapy, and chemotherapy. The median survival is only about 15–18 months.

Oligodendroglioma, IDH-Mutant, and 1p/19q-Codeleted

Q. Write a short note on oligodendroglioma.

- Oligodendroglioma, IDH-mutant, and 1p/19q-codeleted is the **third major subtype of adult-type diffuse glioma.** It is an infiltrating gliomas **composed of tumor cells that resemble oligodendrocytes.**
- **Defined using morphologic and genetic features:** It is a diffusely infiltrating glioma defined using **morphologic and genetic features.** It is with *IDH1* or *IDH2* mutation and codeletion of chromosome arms 1p and 19q.
- Oligodendrogliomas **constitute 5–15% of gliomas.**
- **Age**: Oligodendroglioma is most common during the **fourth and fifth decades of life**.

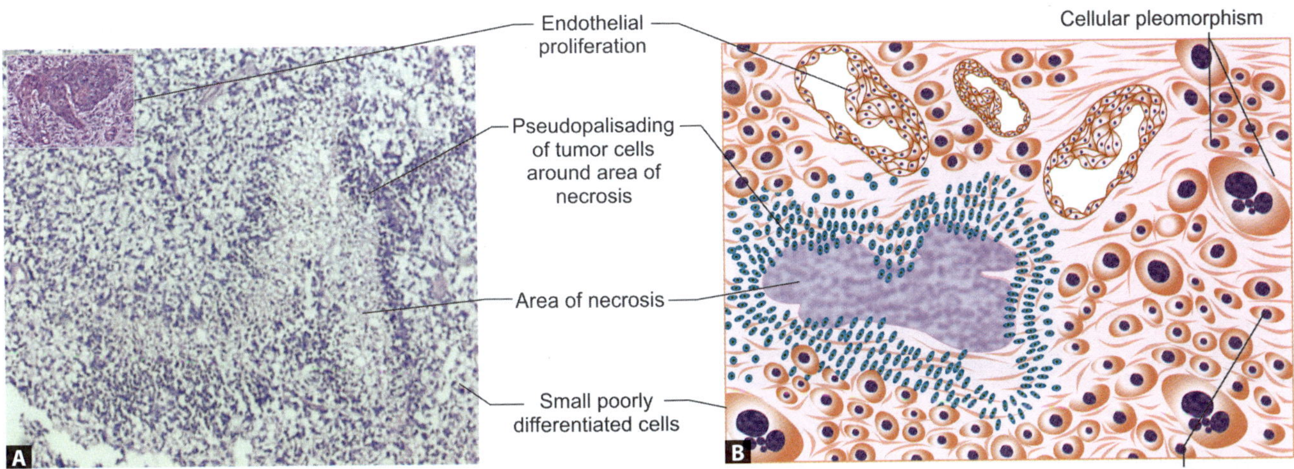

Figs. 27.6A and B: Microscopic features of glioblastoma: (A) Photomicrograph; (B) Diagrammatic. Foci of necrosis with pseudopalisading of tumor nuclei and endothelial cell proliferation are seen. Inset in A shows vascular endothelial proliferation. The microscopic features of glioblastoma are Increased cellularity, pleomorphism, serpentine necrosis, pseudopalisading, and endothelial cell proliferation.

- **CNS WHO grade 2, 3 tumors**: Oligodendrogliomas are graded into 2 (well-differentiated) and 3. These tumors have the best prognosis among diffuse glial tumors.

Pathogenesis

Defining genetic alterations in oligodendroglioma: These are missense **mutations involving the isocitrate dehydrogenase gene** (*IDH1* and *IDH2*), **along with whole-arm deletions of 1p and 19q** an IDH mutation and 1p/19q codeletion are both required for the diagnosis of oligodendroglioma.

Mutations in the promoter of the *TERT* gene: Most oligodendrogliomas also have mutations in the promoter of the *TERT* gene. It leads to increased activity of telomerase.

MORPHOLOGY

Well-differentiated Oligodendroglioma (WHO Grade 2)

Gross

- **Site:** Common in the **white matter of the cerebral hemispheres** (particularly the frontal or parietal lobe).
- They form **well-circumscribed, gelatinous, and gray mass** They may show **cysts, focal areas of hemorrhage**, and calcification.

Microscopy (Figs. 27.7A and B)

Cellular Features

- **Sheets of uniform round cells:** Tumor shows sheets of **small, round, and regular cells.**
- **Spherical nuclei: Spherical nuclei with fine granular chromatin** (similar to that in normal oligodendrocytes).
- **Clear halo of cytoplasm:** Nuclei are surrounded by a **clear halo of cytoplasm** giving rise to a **fried egg appearance** to the cell.
- **Mitotic activity is low or absent.**

Stroma with "chicken-wire"-like anastomosing capillaries: the stroma of the tumor consists of a **delicate network of anastomosing capillaries (chicken-wire appearance).**

Calcification (calcospherites) is common: It is observed in up to 90% of tumors. It ranges in extent from microscopic foci to massive deposits.

WHO Grade 3 Tumors

Gross: They may show areas of necrosis.

Microscopy: Grade 3 oligodendroglioma is a more aggressive subtype. It shows higher cell density, nuclear atypia, and increased mitotic activity, and may show microvascular proliferation and/or necrosis.

Clinical features: Patients may have had several years of neurologic complaints. About two-thirds of patients present with seizures. Other symptoms depend on anatomic location. These include headaches, focal neurologic deficits, or altered cognitive/mental status. They are typically located in the cortex and subcortical white matter. They commonly show calcifications but are not diagnostic.

Prognosis: Generally, oligodendroglioma has a better prognosis than astrocytomas. Current treatment consists of surgery, chemotherapy, and radiation. It has an average survival of 10–20 years for grade 2 oligodendrogliomas and 5–10 years for grade 3 oligodendrogliomas.

Circumscribed Astrocytic Gliomas

Pilocytic Astrocytoma

Pilocytic astrocytoma is a **WHO grade 1 astrocytic neoplasm (relatively benign grade 1)**, that grows very slowly and has an **excellent prognosis.**

Age: It usually occurs in **children and young adults**.

Pathogenesis

Activation of the mitogen-activated protein kinase (MAPK) signaling pathway: Pilocytic astrocytoma in the

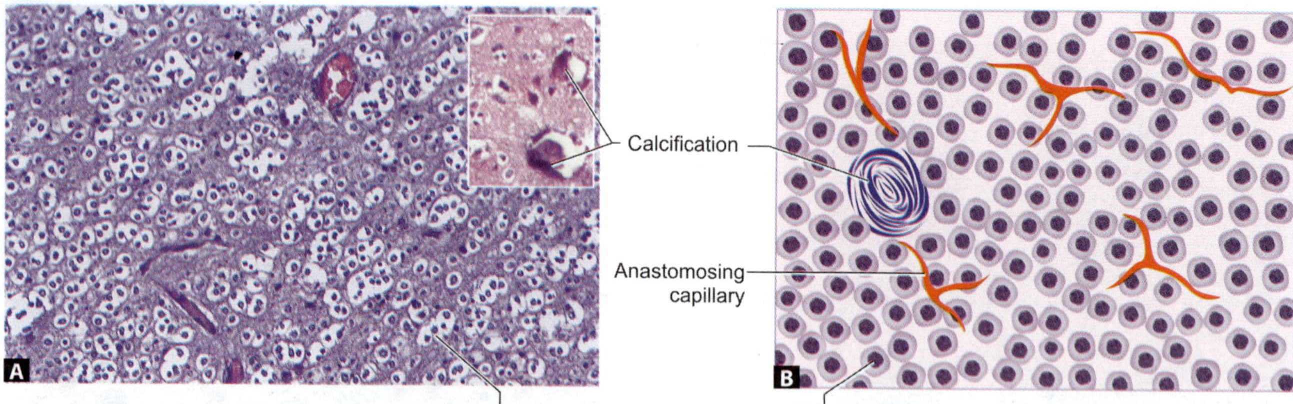

Figs. 27.7A and B: (A) (Photomicrograph); (B) (Diagrammatic), microscopy of oligodendroglioma. Tumor cells are small, round, and regular, having clear cytoplasm forming "halos" around nuclei. The stroma shows thin-walled capillaries and foci of calcification (inset in A).

cerebellum is mostly associated with *KIAA1549::BRAF fusion* (75% of cases). This gene fusion leads to increased BRAF kinase activity and cell proliferation.

Absence of *IDH1* and *IDH2* mutations in pilocytic astrocytomas.

MORPHOLOGY

Localization: Usually arises in the **cerebellum.** Other sites include the floor and walls of the third ventricle and optic nerves.

Gross

Pilocytic astrocytoma is **usually a cystic or solid** and **well-circumscribed tumor.** The cystic tumor shows a mural nodule in the wall of the cyst.

Microscopy (*refer* online Figs. 27.8A and B)

Cellularity: It has low-to-moderate cellularity. The tumor cells have round to elongate nuclei. Mitotic figures are rare, and their presence indicates aggressive behavior.

Biphasic architectural patterns: The biphasic pattern is common in cerebellar tumors. It shows the combination of:

1. **Compact, densely fibrillar areas rich in elongated bipolar cells.** These cells have **abundant, long, thin hair-like** cytoplasmic **processes (pilocytes/piloid cells)** which form dense fibrillary meshworks. These **processes are GFAP-positive.** They also contain Rosenthal fibers.
2. **Loose and "microcystic" regions** rich in oligodendrocyte-like cells.

Rosenthal fibers and eosinophilic granular bodies: They are common and are characteristic findings and histologic hallmarks of pilocytic astrocytoma.

- **Rosenthal fibers:** These are eosinophilic, corkscrew-shaped, granular inclusions and represent hyaline accumulations of filamentous material.
- **Granular bodies:** These are mulberry-like eosinophilic inclusions.

Do not show infiltration into the surrounding brain.

Clinical features: Pilocytic astrocytoma is the most common glioma in **children** and the most common glioma during the **first two decades of life.** They **grow and expand very slowly.** The signs and symptoms are usually due **to mass effect or ventricular obstruction.** These include macrocephaly, obstructive hydrocephalus, headache, endocrinopathy, and evidence of increased intracranial pressure. Usually, these can be treated by resection alone. Symptomatic recurrence and incompletely resected tumors may be treated with repeat surgery, chemotherapy, or targeted therapies.

Ependymal Tumors

Normally, ependymal cells line the ventricular system or central canal of the spinal cord. Ependymomas are tumors that are **derived from ependymal lining cells.** Hence, they usually **arise in near (proximity) to the ependyma-lined ventricular system**, including the central canal of the spinal cord.

Localization: It depends on age.

- **During the first 2 decades of life**: It occurs **near the fourth ventricle.** It constitutes 5–10% of the primary brain tumors during this age.
- **Adults**: Most commonly, it arises in the **spinal cord.** These tumors are frequent in patients with neurofibromatosis type 2 (NF2).

Classification and grading of ependymoma: Is based on histopathological features, anatomical sites (i.e., supratentorial, posterior fossa, and spinal), and molecular changes (e.g., ZFTA fusion, YAP1 fusion, MYCN amplification, etc.). Other ependymal tumors include subependymoma (CNS WHO grade 1) and myxopapillary ependymoma (CNS WHO grade 2). Ependymomas can be WHO grade 2–3.

MORPHOLOGY

Gross

Ependymoma of the fourth ventricle: They are usually **solid and homogeneous** or papillary masses. They extend from the ventricular floor. They are **moderately well-demarcated** from adjacent brain parenchyma.

Microscopy (Figs. 27.9A to C)

Tumor cells: They **resemble normal ependymal cells. Cells are regular** having well-defined cell membranes. **Nuclei are round to oval having abundant granular chromatin.**

Background: Between the nuclei of tumor cells, a **variable amount of dense fibrillary background is seen.**

Rosettes (Figs. 27.9A to C): Tumor cells may form rosettes. They may be true rosettes or pseudo rosettes.

- **True ependymal rosettes:** Tumor **cells may form round or elongated gland-like structures (rosettes, canals)** that surround a central lumen. **They resemble the embryologic ependymal canal** known as ependymal rosettes or canals. They show long, delicate processes extending into a lumen. They are true rosettes.
- **Perivascular pseudorosettes:** Tumor **cells are arranged around vessels** with an intervening zone containing thin ependymal processes. These are termed perivascular pseudorosettes. They are **more frequent** than true ependymal rosettes.

Special stain: Phosphotungstic acid hematoxylin (PTAH) may reveal **PTAH-positive blepharoplasts**, which represent basal bodies of cilia of ependymal cells.

Immunohistochemistry: GFAP is positive in most ependymomas.

Anaplastic ependymomas

It shows increased cellularity, high mitotic rates, necrosis, microvascular proliferation, and minimal ependymal differentiation.

Spread: Through CSF is common and **is associated with a poor prognosis.**

EMBRYONAL TUMORS

Embryonal tumors are a large category of CNS tumors (*refer* **Box 27.1**). They are **mostly pediatric tumors** that almost always **occur in infants or children**. They are termed embryonal because these **tumors appear primitive or undifferentiated and multipotential**. But some resemble embryonic stages of CNS. The most common is the medulloblastoma.

Medulloblastoma

Q. Write a short note on medulloblastoma.

- **Medulloblastoma is a highly malignant undifferentiated or embryonal tumor.** Neuronal and glial markers may be expressed.
- **Age:** Medulloblastomas occur **predominantly in children** (the majority at the end of the first decade). Constitutes about 20% of the brain tumors in children.
- **WHO grade 4 tumors:** All medulloblastomas are considered embryonal tumors and belong to WHO grade 4. However, some molecular groups and subgroups of medulloblastoma (e.g., WNT-activated tumors) respond very well to current therapeutic regimens, and almost all these patients can be cured.

Molecular Subtypes

Depending on the molecular alterations (activation of WNT, activation of SHH, and mutant *TP53*), medulloblastoma can be divided into four main groups:

1. **Medulloblastoma, WNT-activated:** It is characterized by mutations in the WNT signaling pathway. It develops in older children and shows classic histological features of medulloblastoma. It shows the monosomy of chromosome 6 and nuclear expression of β-catenin. It has the best prognosis.
2. **Medulloblastoma, SHH-activated and *TP53*-wildtype:** It is characterized by gain-of-function mutations involving the sonic hedgehog signaling pathway (important role

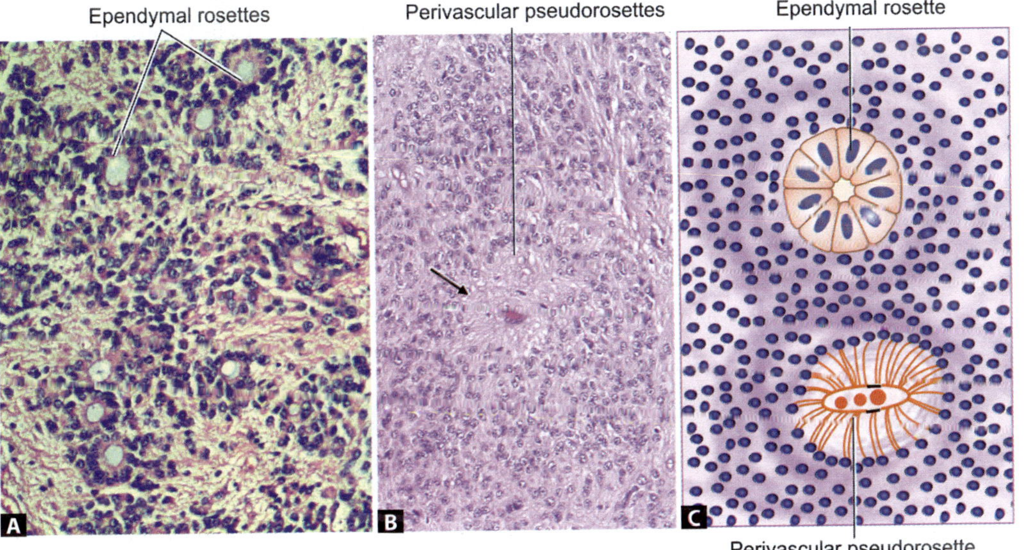

Homer–Wright rosette:
- Medulloblastoma
- Neuroblastoma
- Ewing sarcoma

Medulloblastoma
- Occurs exclusively in the cerebellum.
- Most radiosensitive brain tumors.
- Dissemination through CSF is common leading to drop metastasis

Figs. 27.9A to C: Microscopic appearance of ependymoma: (A and B) Hematoxylin and eosin (H & E); and (C) diagrammatic, showing ependymal rosettes and perivascular pseudorosettes.

in normal cerebellar development). It is seen in infants or young adults and histologically shows a nodular desmoplastic appearance. It may show amplification of MYCN. Prognosis is intermediate between the WNT subtype and groups 3 and 4.

3. **Medulloblastoma, SHH-activated and *TP53*-mutant**: It usually shows MYC amplification and isochromosome 17 (i17q). It is usually found in infants and children. Microscopically, it may show a classic or large cell histology and has the worst prognosis.
4. **Medulloblastoma, non-WNT/non-SHH**: It is characterized by an i17q cytogenetic alteration, classic or large cell histology, and without MYC amplification. The prognosis is intermediate.

Medulloblastoma, Histologically Defined

It consists of four subtypes: (1) Classic medulloblastoma, (2) desmoplastic/nodular medulloblastoma, (3) medulloblastoma with extensive nodularity, and (4) large-cell/anaplastic medulloblastoma.

MORPHOLOGY

Site

Exclusively occurs in the **cerebellum.**

- **Children:** In the midline of the cerebellum
- **Adults:** Lateral locations in the cerebellar hemispheres.

Gross

Medulloblastoma is well-circumscribed, gray, and friable. It may extend to the surface of the cerebellar folia and involve the leptomeninges.

Microscopy (Figs. 27.10A and B)

- **Highly cellular, small blue cell tumor**: Medulloblastoma is one of several "small blue cell" tumors of childhood. It is densely cellular composed of **sheets of monomorphic (small blue) cells.**
- **Tumor cells:** Individual **tumor cells are small. They have little cytoplasm** and **hyperchromatic nuclei** (elongated or crescent-shaped).
- **Numerous mitotic figures**
- **Homer–Wright (neuroblastic) rosette:** It is seen in some classic medulloblastomas. It is characterized by **central neuropil** (delicate pink material formed by neuronal processes) **surrounded by primitive tumor cells.** They resemble the rosettes found in neuroblastomas. These represent focal neuronal differentiation.

Immunohistochemistry: GFAP+

Nodular/desmoplastic variant: Characterized by nodular, reticulin-free zones (pale islands) surrounded by densely packed highly proliferative tumor cells. These tumor cells have hyperchromatic and moderately pleomorphic nuclei and they produce a collagen and dense intercellular reticulin fiber network.

Large cell variant: It is characterized by monomorphic cells with large, round, vesicular nuclei, prominent nucleoli, and frequent mitoses and apoptotic cells. These cells show variable amounts of eosinophilic cytoplasm.

Spread: Medulloblastomas can spread to the subarachnoid space. **Spread through the CSF** is common and can produce either extensive growth along the surface likened to "icing" or nodular **"drop metastases,"** which tend to involve the cauda equina.

Clinical features: Rapid growth of medulloblastoma may **occlude the flow of CSF and cause noncommunicating hydrocephalus.** Therefore, most patients present with symptoms and signs of raised intracranial pressure. Medulloblastomas are **highly malignant and highly radiosensitive.**

Prognosis: The prognosis **for untreated patients is bad.** The molecular and histologic subtype greatly influences prognosis. WNT-activated medulloblastomas are associated with nearly 100% survival at 5 years. More aggressive subtypes have a 5-year survival rate of 20–30%.

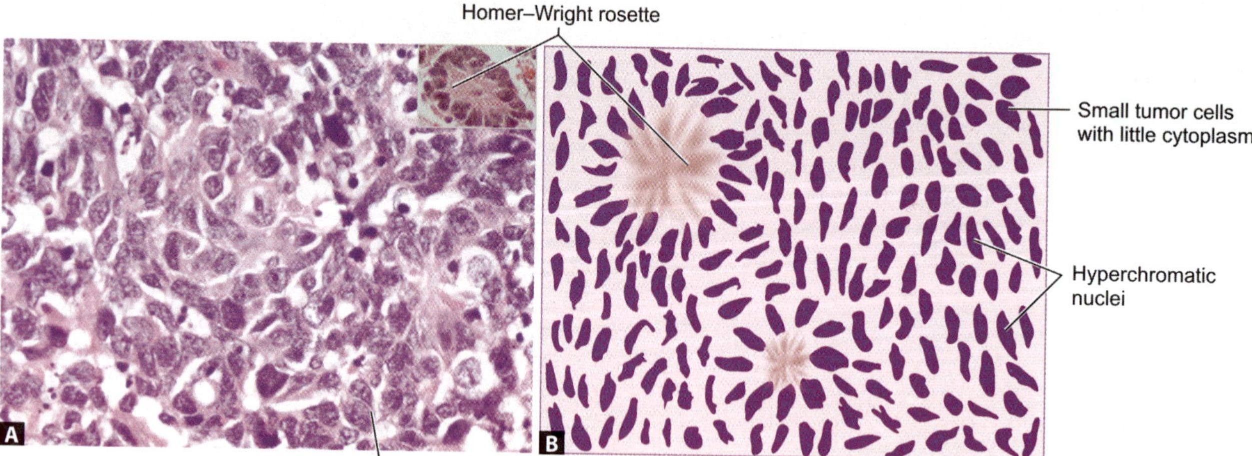

Figs. 27.10A and B: Microscopic: (A) Photomicrograph; (B) Diagrammatic appearance of medulloblastoma showing densely crowded, small, malignant cells. Inset of (A) shows Homer–Wright rosette.

MENINGIOMAS

Q. Write a short note on meningioma.

Meningiomas are a family of neoplasms that most likely **arise from the meningothelial cells of the arachnoid mater.** Meningiomas are **benign intracranial tumors (WHO grades 1–3)**. These tumors are **usually attached to the dura (dural-based extra-axial lesion)**. It accounts for 20% of all primary intracranial neoplasms.

Age and gender: Peak during the **fourth to fifth decades of life**. Grade 1 meningioma is 2.32 times more common in women than in men.

Pathogenesis

Meningiomas can arise in one of three settings:

1. **Sporadic:** *The majority of meningiomas occur sporadically.*
    - **Somatic loss-of-function mutations in the *NF2* tumor suppressor gene:** The *NF2* gene encodes the protein merlin. Approximately 50–60% of meningiomas carry mutations in the *NF2* gene. These mutations are observed in all grades of meningioma, suggesting that they are involved in tumor initiation.
    - **Other genetic alterations:** These include mutations in ***TRAF7*** [involved in tumor necrosis factor (TNF) signaling], ***KLF4*** (encodes a transcription factor that regulates proliferation and migration), ***AKT1*** (encodes a kinase that regulates proliferation and cell survival), and ***SMO*** (encodes smoothened, a G-protein-coupled receptor in the SHH pathway). Most of these occur in the **meningiomas of the skull base** and have a **lower risk of malignant progression**.
    - ***TERT* promoter mutations:** These are associated with more aggressive behavior in meningiomas. Higher-grade meningiomas usually have chromosomal losses involving several chromosomes (2p/q, 3p, 4p/q, 7p, and 8p/q), *TERT*-promoter mutations, and homozygous *CDKN2A* gene deletions.
2. **Iatrogenic:** Meningiomas can develop as a complication of radiation therapy. They generally occur after a latent period of a decade or more and are directly related to radiation dosage.
3. **Tumor predisposition syndromes.** Several genetic tumor predisposition syndromes increase the risk of meningioma development, the most important being neurofibromatosis type 2 (NF2). These individuals may have multiple meningiomas. Meningiomas can occur in families with germline defects in *NF1, VHL, PTEN, PTCH1, BAP1, SUFU, SMARCE1,* and *CREBBP* genes.

MORPHOLOGY

Q. Write a short note on the morphology of meningioma.

Localization

Anatomic locations in which meningiomas occur are **parallel to the distribution of the arachnoid membrane**. Meningiomas can arise at any CNS site where arachnoid cells are present. They typically occur in **intracranial** (both on external surfaces of the brain as well as within the ventricular system), **intraspinal, or orbital locations. Most common sites** include **parasagittal regions of the cerebral hemispheres**, dura over the **lateral convexity, olfactory grooves**, etc.

Meningioma (WHO Grade 1)

Gross

- **External surface:** It appears as a **well-circumscribed** (usually encapsulated), **smooth, rounded, bosselated,** or polypoid, dura-based mass **(Fig. 27.11). It may extend** into the overlying bone and may be present.
- **Size:** Variable
- **Consistency:** Range from **firm** and fibrous to finely gritty (in the presence of psammoma bodies).
- **Broad dural attachment: The base is usually attached to the dura.**
- **Cut surface: Gray without necrosis or hemorrhage.**
- **Compression of the underlying brain (Fig. 27.11):** Most **grade 1 meningiomas compress the adjacent (underlying) brain** but can be easily separated from the brain, **but do not infiltrate.**

Microscopy (Figs. 27.12A and B)

General features of meningioma: Whorls and psammoma bodies are characteristic features of meningiomas. Whorls are characterized by **concentric wrapping of tumor cells around one another.** Psammoma bodies consist of **concentrically laminated, spherical calcifications.**

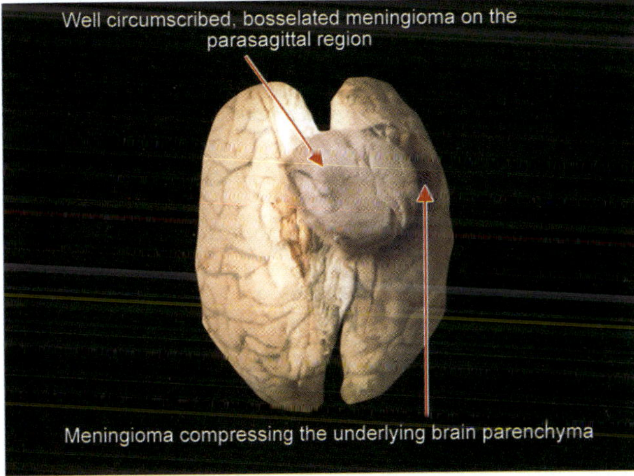

Fig. 27.11: Meningioma on the parasagittal region of the cerebral hemispheres.

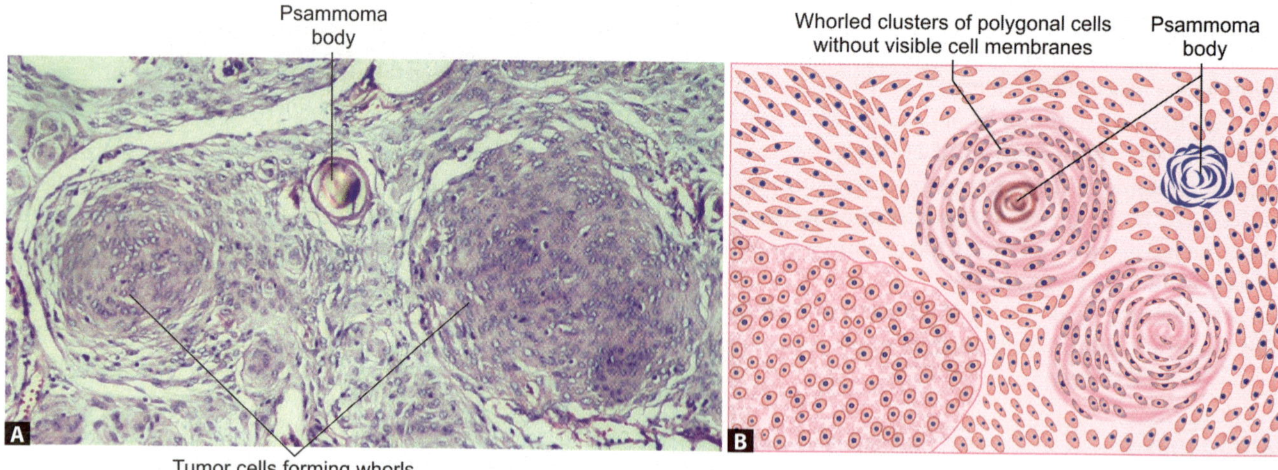

Figs. 27.12A and B: Microscopy of meningothelial meningioma: (A) Hematoxylin and eosin (H & E); (B) Diagrammatic, showing a tumor cell forming whorls. The tumor cells have syncytium like appearance due to poorly defined cell borders.

Histologic Subtypes

Q. Write a short note on histological subtypes of meningioma.

Meningioma shows a wide morphological spectrum, and 15 subtypes have been described (**Box 27.3**). Most subtypes follow a benign course and are WHO grade 1. Chordoid and clear cell subtypes of meningiomas have a higher risk of recurrence than the WHO grade 1 meningioma and are therefore considered WHO grade 2.

- **Syncytial (meningothelial) (Figs. 27.12A and B): Syncytial appearance** is a **peculiar feature of meningothelial meningiomas** and a focal feature of other subtypes of meningioma. In this subtype, whorled clusters of epithelioid (polygonal) cells with fuzzy or indiscernible cell membranes are arranged as syncytia-like lobules (cytoplasmic mass without visible cell membranes containing several nuclei). The tumor cells are largely **monomorphic** and have **abundant eosinophilic cytoplasm** with **centrally placed round to oval nuclei**.
- **Fibroblastic:** It consists of **spindle-shaped elongated cells,** which are **arranged in interlacing or parallel bundles. These cells are separated by varying amounts of the intercellular collagen-rich matrix.**
- **Fibroblastic:** It consists of **spindle-shaped elongated cells,** which are **arranged in interlacing or parallel bundles. These cells are separated by varying amounts of the intercellular collagen-rich matrix.**
- **Transitional/mixed** (*refer* **online Fig. 27.13A):** It is composed of **mixed syncytial (meningothelial) and fibroblastic components.** The tumor cells show a whorled pattern often around a central capillary-sized blood vessel. The center of some of the whorls **may show psammoma bodies.**
- **Psammomatous** (*refer* **online Fig. 27.13B):** It shows **numerous, conspicuous, concentrically laminated psammoma bodies.** These psammoma bodies represent concentric rings of calcification deposited over preexisting whorls.

  Angiomatous: It has features typical of a benign meningioma but, in addition, **contains many variable hyalinized small or large vascular channels.**

BOX 27.3: Subtypes of meningioma.

- Meningothelial meningioma*
- Fibrous meningioma*
- Transitional meningioma*
- Psammomatous meningioma
- Angiomatous meningioma
- Microcystic meningioma
- Secretory meningioma
- Lymphoplasmacyte-rich meningioma
- Metaplastic meningioma
- Chordoid meningioma†
- Clear cell meningioma†
- Rhabdoid meningioma
- Papillary meningioma
- Atypical meningioma†
- Anaplastic (malignant) meningioma#

*Most common subtype.
†Grade 2
#Grade 3

- **Microcystic:** It is composed of **microcystic spaces** with a loose, spongy appearance. It produces a cobweb-like background.
- **Secretory:** It consists of **gland-like PAS-positive, eosinophilic secretions** (pseudo psammoma bodies).

Immunohistochemistry: Negative for GFAP and keratins, but **positive for epithelial membrane antigen.**

Atypical Meningioma (Grade 2)

Features of more aggressive growth can arise in any of the subtypes. Atypical meningioma shows an increased mitotic rate, clear-cut brain invasion; certain microscopic features, such as prominent nucleoli or foci of necrosis. The chordoid or clear cell subtype belongs to grade 2 tumors. Atypical meningiomas show either 4–19 mitoses/10 high power fields or at least 3 of 5 atypical features [increased cellularity, small cells with a high nuclear-to-cytoplasmic ratio, prominent nucleoli, sheeting (uninterrupted patternless or sheet-like growth) or necrosis]. Atypical meningioma (grade 2) has **more aggressive local growth and a higher rate of recurrence.** They may require therapy in addition to surgery.

Anaplastic (Malignant) Meningioma (Grade 3)

Anaplastic (malignant/grade 3) meningioma is a high-grade (highly aggressive) meningioma and accounts for 1–3% of meningiomas. It shows frank cytomorphologic features (anaplasia) of malignancy and is highly aggressive. Criteria for diagnosis are markedly elevated mitotic activity (20 or more mitotic figures/10 HPF), **or** frank anaplasia (morphologically resembles high-grade sarcoma, carcinoma, or melanoma), **or** *TERT* promoter mutation, **or** homozygous deletion of *CDKN2A* and/or *CDKN2B*. Most of these tumors show extensive necrosis and can invade the brain.

Clinical features: Meningiomas are **usually slow-growing tumors**. They produce **symptoms by compressing underlying brain** tissue and depend on the site.

METASTATIC TUMORS

Metastatic tumors are the **most common intracranial neoplasms.**

Primary site: The tumors that are most likely to give rise to brain metastasis are mostly carcinomas. The **five most common primary sites are (1) lung, (2) breast, (3) kidney, (4) melanoma of the skin, and (5) gastrointestinal tract (particularly colon).**

Route of spread: Through the bloodstream, generally in patients with advanced cancer.

MORPHOLOGY

Localization: About 80% of all brain metastases are in the cerebral hemispheres, 15% occur in the cerebellum, and 5% occur in the brainstem. The meninges can also be involved in metastatic disease.

Gross

- Intraparenchymal metastases in contrast with a primary glioma, form **multiple, sharply demarcated masses (Fig. 27.14)**, usually surrounded by a prominent zone of edema.
- The **boundary between metastatic tumor and surrounding brain parenchyma is sharp** and well-defined both grossly and microscopically.
- They are **usually seen at the junction of gray matter and white matter**.

Microscopy

It is similar to that of a primary tumor.

Discussion on "Brain Abscees" and" Cerebrovascular Diseases" (along with **Figs. 27.15 and 27.16**) are presented online.

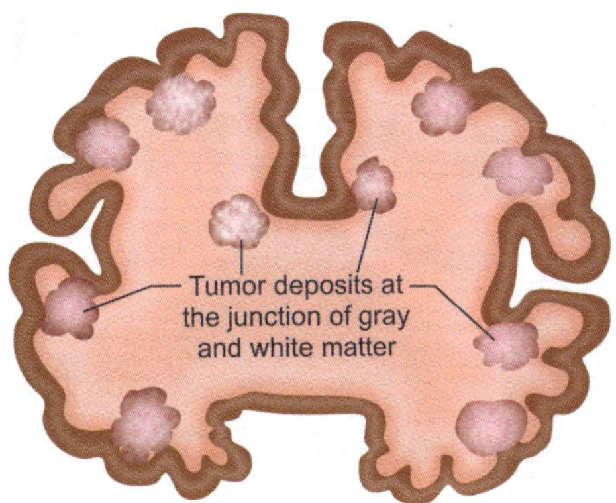

Fig. 27.14: Sites of deposit of metastatic tumors in the brain.

EYE

Retinoblastoma

PA 36.1 (NC): Describe the etiology, genetics, pathogenesis, pathology, presentation, sequelae, and complications of retinoblastoma.

Q. Write a short note on retinoblastoma.

Retinoblastoma is the **most common primary intraocular malignant tumor occurring in children.**

The cell of origin of retinoblastoma: It is a **neuronal progenitor**. Retinoblastoma arises when the retinal progenitor suffers a second somatic mutation, and the *RB* gene function is lost.

Age: It occurs most frequently within the **first 2 years of life**. It may even be found at birth.

Etiology and Pathogenesis

Retinoblastoma may be sporadic or familial. Most retinoblastomas occur sporadically and are unilateral.

***RB* gene:** Nearly all retinoblastomas are related to inherited or acquired deletions of, or mutations in, the retinoblastoma (*RB*) gene (biallelic inactivation). It is a tumor suppressor gene located on the long arm of chromosome 13 (13q14).

- **Familial cases**: Features of familial retinoblastoma are:
  - About **40% of cases** occur as familial/hereditary cases in individuals who **inherit a germline mutation of one *RB* allele.**
  - **Usually is associated with the** development of **multiple tumors (multifocal)** that are **bilateral**, but may be unifocal and unilateral.
  - Have an **increased risk for** the development of second tumors, such as **osteosarcoma** and other soft tissue tumors.
- **Sporadic cases**: The remaining **60%** of the tumors develop sporadically. In these cases, **both RB alleles are lost by somatic mutations**. All the sporadic, nonheritable tumors are **unilateral and unifocal.**

***MYCN*-amplified retinoblastoma:** Recently, a form of retinoblastoma without mutations in the *RB* gene has been described. These tumors are associated with the amplification of the *MYCN* gene. This gene is a member of the Myc family of oncogenes. Tumors due to *MYCN* amplification are typically unilateral, manifest at an earlier age, and are more invasive.

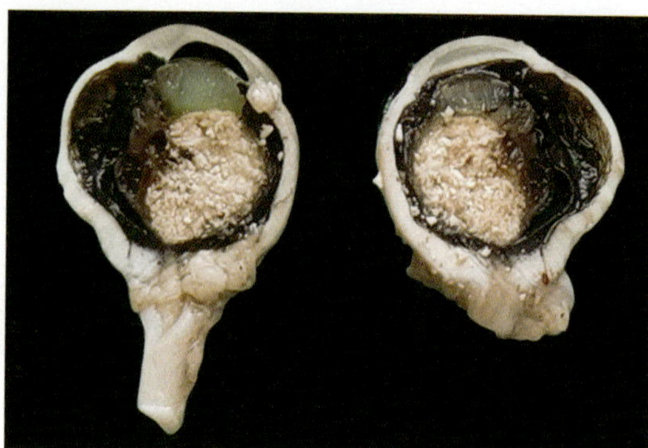

Fig. 27.17: Retinoblastoma. Bisected eyeball showing a cream-colored tumor in the retina.

MORPHOLOGY

Morphological features are the **same in both hereditary and sporadic retinoblastoma.**

Gross (Fig. 27.17)

Retinoblastomas appear as **nodular,** cream-colored (creamy white) **masses**, usually in the **posterior retina**, often with satellite seedings.

Microscopy (Figs. 27.18A and B)

Cellularity: Retinoblastomas are **highly cellular** tumors.

Cellular elements: Tumors may contain **both undifferentiated and differentiated elements.** However, the degree of tumor differentiation does not appear to be associated with the prognosis.

- **Undifferentiated elements:** It consists of collections of **small, round cells with large hyperchromatic nuclei and scant cytoplasm.** They resemble undifferentiated retinoblasts. Thus, it belongs to the "small round blue cells" group of tumors.
- **Well-differentiated tumors:** Differentiated structures are found within many retinoblastomas. However, the degree of tumor differentiation does not have any prognostic value. The most characteristic is **Flexner–Wintersteiner rosettes** and **fleurettes** that reflect photoreceptor differentiation.
  - **Flexner–Wintersteiner rosettes:** These structures **consist of clusters of cuboidal or short columnar cells arranged around a central lumen (true rosette).** This is in contrast with the pseudorosettes of neuroblastoma which does not have a central lumen. The nuclei are displaced away from the lumen and microscopically appear to have a limiting membrane resembling the external limiting membrane of the retina.
  - **Fleurette:** The tumor cells are aligned in patterns reminiscent of the fleur-de-lis (a small flower composed of three petals bound together near their bases).

Focal zones of dystrophic calcification: These are characteristic of retinoblastoma.

Spread: Retinoblastoma spreads through the optic nerve (and extends into the intracranial CNS) or subarachnoid space. The most common sites of distant metastases are the CNS (brain), skull, distal bones, bone marrow, and lymph nodes. Because of the absence of a lymphatic supply to the eye, retinoblastomas do not spread to lymph nodes of the head and neck.

Clinical features: It presents with poor vision, strabismus, pain, and tenderness in the affected eye. On examination, it shows a whitish hue to the pupil ("cat's eye reflex").

Prognosis: Some tumors spontaneously regress. If not treated, they are usually fatal. Survival is the rule when treated with chemotherapy, radiotherapy, and (in locally advanced tumors) enucleation.

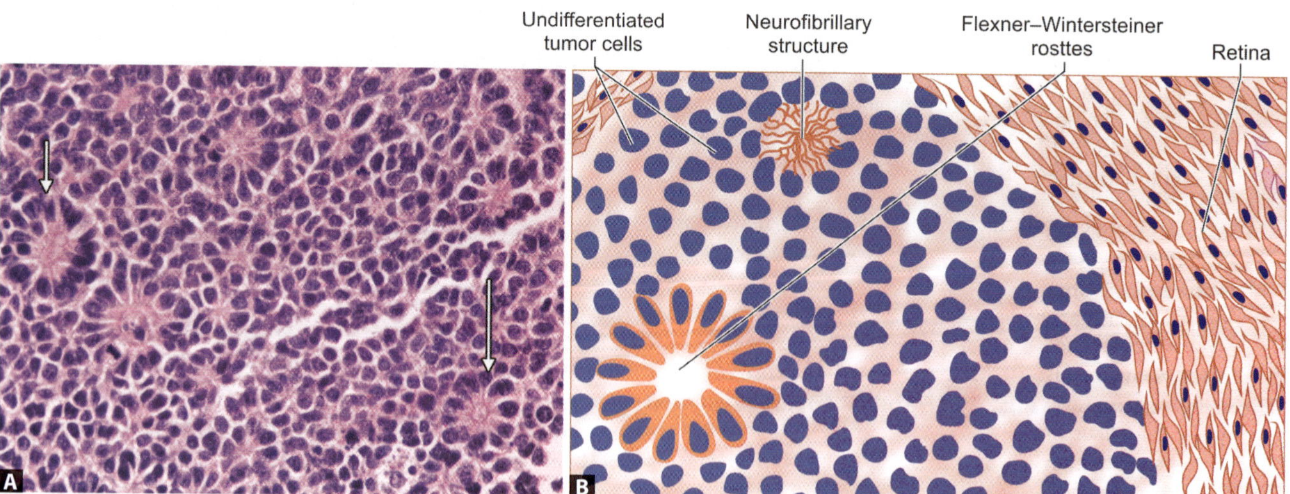

Figs. 27.18A and B: Retinoblastoma: (A) H&E and (B) Diagrammatic. Shows undifferentiated, small, round, neoplastic cells with hyperchromatic nuclei and scant cytoplasm. The tumor also shows the typical Flexner–Wintersteiner rosette. Homer Wright (short arrow) rosettes are shown in (A).

SCENARIO-BASED MCQs

1. A 30-year-old woman complains of headache, vomiting, and fever for the last 3 days. Physical examination shows neck rigidity and knee pain with hip flexion. Lumbar puncture shows numerous neutrophils and decreased levels of glucose in the CSF. The most likely organism associated with these clinical and laboratory findings is:
   A. Viral (aseptic) meningitis
   B. Meningococcal meningitis
   C. Staphylococcal meningitis
   D. Tuberculous meningitis
2. A 17-year-old man complains of a sore throat followed a day later by the sudden onset of a severe headache. Physical examination shows mild pharyngitis, fever, petechial hemorrhages in the skin, and neck rigidity. His blood pressure is 95/50 mm Hg. The CSF examination shows numerous neutrophils, reduced glucose, and increased proteins. The most likely infectious organisms that produced this disease are:
   A. *Escherichia coli* B. *Neisseria meningitidis*
   C. Viral (aseptic) meningitis D. *Mycobacterium tuberculosis*
3. A 4-day-old infant develops fever and convulsions. The infant is started on broad-spectrum antibiotics and antiviral medications but slips into a coma and expires. At autopsy, the brain shows a purulent exudate in the subarachnoid space at the base of the brain. The most likely cause of suppurative meningitis in this neonate is:
   A. *Escherichia coli* B. *Neisseria meningitidis*
   C. *Haemophilus influenzae* D. Tuberculous meningitis
4. A 26-year-old woman complains of headaches for 4 weeks along with increasing malaise. Physical examination shows no significant findings. No abnormalities are seen on the CT scan of the head. A lumbar puncture shows clear, and colorless CSF. Laboratory analysis of the CSF shows a normal glucose level and a minimal increase in the protein level. Microscopically, CSF shows few lymphocytes without any neutrophils. A Gram stain on smears prepared and Indian ink preparations on CSF are negative. She gradually recovers within the next 3 months. The most likely diagnosis is:
   A. Acute viral meningitis B. Acute pyogenic meningitis
   C. Fungal meningitis D. Tuberculous meningitis
5. A 4-year-old girl has been brought to the hospital for worsening headache and irritability for the past week. Now she has nausea, vomiting, and diminished responsiveness to verbal commands. On physical examination, she is febrile and her eyes do not move laterally. A lumbar puncture is done and CSF shows 110 leukocytes/mm^3 and 75% of them are mononuclear cells. The CSF glucose is decreased, but the protein is markedly elevated. The infectious agents that are most likely to cause this condition are:
   A. Virus B. *Treponema pallidum*
   C. *Haemophilus influenzae* D. *Mycobacterium tuberculosis*
6. A 55-year-old man is brought to the hospital for headaches that developed for the first time in his life beginning 2 months ago. He also develops a generalized tonic-clonic seizure. On physical examination, there is weakness on his left side. An MRI of his brain shows a large, irregular, 6-cm mass in the right cerebral hemisphere that extends across the corpus callosum. A stereotaxic biopsy of the mass is done. Microscopically, it shows pleomorphic cells, serpentine necrosis with characteristic palisading of tumor cells around necrotic areas, and microvascular proliferation. The most likely diagnosis is:
   A. Glioblastoma B. Medulloblastoma
   C. Pilocytic astrocytoma D. Meningioma
7. A 9-year-old boy is brought to the hospital with a history of persistent headaches for the past 3 months. On physical examination, he has an ataxic gait. CT scan of the head shows a 4-cm cystic mass in the right cerebellar hemisphere. And enlargement of cerebral lateral ventricles. Neurosurgery is performed, and the mass is removed. Grossly, it is a cyst filled with gelatinous material. The cyst has a thin wall and a 1-cm mural nodule. Microscopically, it is composed of cells with long, hairlike processes and they stain positive for glial fibrillary acidic protein (GFAP). The probable diagnosis is:
   A. Meningioma B. Ependymoma
   C. Medulloblastoma D. Pilocytic astrocytoma
8. A 43-year-old man complains of headaches for the past 5 months and seizures for 2 days. On physical examination, there are no remarkable findings. MRI of the brain shows a solitary, circumscribed 3-cm mass in the right parietal region. The mass has small cysts and areas of calcification. The mass is removed. Microscopically, it consists of sheets of cells with round nuclei that have granular chromatin. The cells show a moderate amount of clear cytoplasm and stroma with the chicken-wire appearance of blood vessels. Immunohistochemistry shows GFAP positivity. The probable diagnosis is:
   A. Astrocytoma B. Oligodendroglioma
   C. Medulloblastoma D. Meningioma
9. A 10-year-old girl is brought to the hospital for increasing headaches upon awakening for the past month. On examination, shows bilateral papilledema. An MRI of the brain shows a 3-cm solid circumscribed mass within the fourth ventricle. There is dilatation of the third and lateral ventricles. The mass is excised. Macroscopically, it shows a cellular tumor composed of round and regular tumor cells. These cells are arranged around vessels forming perivascular pseudorosettes. Which of the following tumors she is most likely to have?
   A. Ependymoma B. Glioblastoma
   C. Pilocytic astrocytoma D. Medulloblastoma
10. A 5-year-old boy has had headaches for the past week and has an ataxic gait. He suddenly develops vomiting, and he is brought to the emergency department, where he becomes comatose. On physical examination, he is afebrile. A lumbar puncture is performed and cytologic examination of the CSF shows anaplastic cells with dark blue nuclei and scant cytoplasm. The most likely location of this tumor is:
    A. Fourth ventricle
    B. Cerebellar vermis
    C. Parietal lobe gray-white junction
    D. Dura covering the cerebral hemisphere
11. A 47-year-old woman complains of unilateral headaches on the left for the past 4 months. Physical examination does not reveal any remarkable findings. A CT scan shows a circumscribed mass on the surface of the left cerebral hemisphere in the parasagittal location. The mass is surgically removed and grossly appears solid, globular, circumscribed, and tan-yellow. Microscopic examination shows elongated cells with pale, oblong nuclei, and pink

cytoplasm with occasional psammoma bodies. The tumor cells are arranged in a whorled pattern. What is the most likely diagnosis?

A. Metastasis
B. Glioblastoma
C. Ependymoma
D. Meningioma

Answers and Explanation

1. **The answer is B: Meningococcal meningitis.** The presence of numerous neutrophils in the CSF is the most definitive feature of bacterial meningitis. The lymphocytes in CSF are the characteristics of tuberculosis (Choice D) and the viral meningitides (choice A). The classic signs of meningitis are neck rigidity, knee pain with hip flexion (Kernig sign), and knee/hip flexion when the neck is flexed (Brudzinski sign). Staphylococcus (choice C) is rarely a cause of meningitis. CSF does not show predominant neutrophils in tuberculous meningitis (choice D).
2. **The answer is B: *Neisseria meningitidis.*** It is a case of acute pyogenic meningitis, due to bacterial infection. **Neisseria meningitidis** is the common etiologic agent at his age. It initially presents as pharyngitis, and if untreated it may proceed to Waterhouse-Friderichsen syndrome with disseminated intravascular coagulopathy. *Escherichia coli* (option A) is the main cause of meningitis in the newborn. Viral meningitis (option C) shows lymphocytes in the CSF rather than neutrophils. Tuberculous meningitis ((option D) does not manifest acutely, and the CSF shows lymphocytes.
3. **The answer is A: *Escherichia coli.*** E. coli is the main cause of meningitis in the newborn. The transplacental transfer of maternal IgG protects the newborn against many bacteria, but *E. coli* requires IgM for neutralization. At autopsy, the brain shows a creamy exudate in the leptomeninges Neisseria meningitides (choice B), *Haemophilus influenzae* (choice C), and tuberculous meningitis (Choice D) causes meningitis at a later age.
4. **The answer is A: Acute viral (aseptic) meningitis.** It is termed aseptic meningitis because routine Gram staining and bacterial cultures are negative. Most cases are self-limited and occur in immunocompetent individuals. Acute pyogenic meningitis shows numerous neutrophils in the CSF. Fungal meningitis can occur in immunocompromised patients, but the India ink test would be positive. Tuberculous meningitis shows cobweb formation on the gross and contains many lymphocytes.
5. **The answer is D: *Mycobacterium tuberculosis.*** Tuberculous meningitis occurs as a complication of disseminated tuberculosis and is seen in young children. It usually produces a more chronic course. Cranial nerves, such as the abducens in this case, can be involved. It is responsible for the inability to move eyes laterally. Viral "aseptic" meningitis (option A) shows mononuclear cells, but the protein is not usually markedly elevated. *Treponema pallidum* (Option B) causes chronic meningitis with a long, insidious course. Bacterial meningitis by *Haemophilus influenzae* (Option C) usually has a low glucose, and the inflammatory response is predominantly polymorphonuclear on CSF examination.
6. **The answer is A: Glioblastoma.** History of headache for first time in life, MRI finding and microscopic features are those of glioblastomas. These are aggressive tumors and have a poor prognosis. Medulloblastomas (Option B) and pilocytic astrocytomas (option C) are usually childhood brain tumors arising in the posterior fossa. Meningiomas (option C) are dural-based tumors and consist of whorls and psammoma bodies.
7. **The answer is D: Pilocytic astrocytoma.** The two most common neoplasms at this site (cerebellum) in children are pilocytic (cystic cerebellar) astrocytoma and medulloblastoma. Pilocytic astrocytoma is slow-growing and has a better prognosis than glial neoplasms in adults. Both may enlarge and block CSF flow, causing hydrocephalus. The cystic nature of the tumor and the presence of long, hairlike processes is characteristic of pilocytic astrocytoma. Meningiomas (option A) occur in adults; they are circumscribed, solid mass lesions adjacent to the dura. Ependymomas (Option B) can occur in childhood but most commonly arise in the fourth ventricle. Medulloblastomas (Option C) occur in the cerebellar midline, are composed of primitive round blue cells, and have a poor prognosis.
8. **The answer is B: Oligodendrogliomas.** Oligodendrogliomas arise in the white matter and are slow-growing tumors with better prognosis than most other glial neoplasms. They consist of uniform cells with clear cytoplasm (fried egg appearance) with small rounded nuclei similar to normal oligodendrocytes. The stroma shows chicken-wire pattern of blood vessels. These features along with MRI findings (calcospherites/calcification) favor oligodendroglioma. Other options do not have the microscopic features mentioned in this case.
9. **The answer is A: Ependymoma.** In children, ependymomas most commonly arise on the floor of the fourth ventricle. Ependymoma originates in the lining of the cavities that contain cerebrospinal fluid. It can obstruct the flow of CSF producing obstructive, noncommunicating hydrocephalus. The tumor cells of an ependymoma characteristically have an "epithelial" appearance, similar to that of normal ependymal cells. They may arrange around blood vessels forming perivascular pseudorosettes. Glioblastomas (option B) are adult neoplasms arising in the cerebral hemispheres. Pilocytic astrocytomas (option C) arise in the cerebellar hemisphere and appear as a cystic mass with a mural nodule and tumor cells with hairlike processes. Medulloblastomas (option D) are also childhood tumors, and they arise in the midline cerebellum. They are composed of undifferentiated, primitive blue cells.
10. **The answer is B: Cerebellar vermis.** The tumor in this boy is medulloblastoma, which arises from cerebellar vermis in children. Medulloblastoma is the most common intracranial neoplasm in the posterior fossa of children. Medulloblastoma is one of the "blue cell tumors" of childhood, and the tumor cells can seed into the CSF. A glioblastoma is also a high-grade CNS tumor that can seed the CSF, but it occurs in adults in the cerebral hemisphere. Ependymomas can occur in children, but they usually arise in the ventricles (option A). Metastatic tumors may involve the gray-white junction (Option C) but are uncommon in children. Meningiomas are benign tumors that are a dural-based tumor (option D) and are rare in children.
11. **The answer is D: Meningioma.** The meningioma is a circumscribed tumor that arises from meningothelial cells of the arachnoid. It is grossly attached to the overlying dura and is most common in parasagittal regions of the cerebral hemispheres. They are most common in women. Most meningiomas are benign. Metastasis to the brain (Option A) is usually multiple and involves the gray-white junction. The parasagittal location is unusual for a metastatic lesion. Glioblastomas (option B) are found within the cerebral hemisphere in an adult. Ependymomas (option C) occur within the ventricles or on the distal spinal cord.

Bibliography

1. Bain BJ, Bates I, Laffan MA. Dacie and Lewis practical hematology, 12th edition. London: Churchill Livingstone; 2017.
2. Fenderson BA, Strayer DS, Rubin R, Rubin E. Lippincott's Illustrated Review of Rubin's Pathology, 2nd edition. Philadelphia: Wolters Kluwer; 2011.
3. Goldblum JR, Lamps LW, McKenney JK, et al. Rosai and Ackerman's surgical pathology (2 vols), 11th edition. Philadelphia: Elsevier; 2018.
4. Goljan EF. Rapid review of pathology, 5th edition. Mosby: Elsevier; 2019.
5. Klatt EC, Kumar V. Robbins and Cotran Review of Pathology, 4th edition. Philadelphia: Saunders Elsevier; 2015.
6. Kumar V, Abbas AK, Aster JC, Deyrup AT, Das A. Robbins and Kumar's Basic Pathology, 11th edition. Philadelphia: Saunders Elsevier; 2023.
7. Kumar V, Abbas AK, Aster JC, Turner JR. Robbins and Cotran pathologic basis of disease, 10th edition. Philadelphia: WB Saunders; 2021.
8. Longacre TA, Greenson JK, Hornick JL, Reuter VE. Mills and Sternberg's Diagnostic Surgical Pathology, 7th edition. Philadelphia: Wolter Kluwer; 2022.
9. Mohan H. Textbook of Pathology, 9th edition. New Delhi: Jaypee Brothers Medical Publishers (P) Ltd; 2023.
10. Nayak R, Rai S. Essentials in Hematology and Clinical Pathology, 2nd edition. New Delhi: Jaypee Brothers Medical Publishers (P) Ltd; 2017.
11. Nayak R, Nayak R. Manual of Transfusion Medicine, 1st edition. New Delhi: Jaypee Brothers Medical Publishers (P) Ltd; 2020.
12. Nayak R, Nayak R. Review of Postgraduate Pathology-General Pathology. New Delhi: Jaypee Brothers Medical Publishers (P) Ltd; 2022.
13. Nayak R, Nayak R. Review of Postgraduate Pathology-Systemic Pathology. New Delhi: Jaypee Brothers Medical Publishers (P) Ltd; 2024.
14. Penman ID, Ralston SH, Strachan MWJ, et al. Davidson's Principles and Practice of Medicine, 24th edition. Edinburgh: Churchill Livingstone; 2023.
15. Roberts F, MacDuff E. Pathology illustrated, 8th edition. Philadelphia: Elsevier; 2019.
16. Singh T. Atlas and Text of Hematology, New Delhi: Arya Publications; 2022.
17. Strayer DS, Saffitz JE. Rubin's Pathology: Mechanism of Human Disease, 8th edition. Philadelphia: Wolters Kluwer; 2020.
18. Suvarna SK, Layton C, Bancroft JD. Bancroft's theory and practice of histopathological techniques, 8th edition. London: Churchill Livingstone; 2019.
19. Walter JB, Talbot IC. General pathology, 7th edition. Edinburgh: Churchill Livingstone; 2009.
20. WHO Classification of Tumors Editorial Board. Breast tumors [Internet]. Lyon (France): International Agency for Research on Cancer; 2019 [cited 2014 May 21]. (WHO Classification of tumors series, 5th edition; vol. 2). Available from: https://tumourclassification.iarc.who.int/chapters/32.
21. WHO Classification of Tumors Editorial Board. Breast tumors. Lyon (France): International Agency for Research on Cancer; 2019. (WHO Classification of tumors series, 5th edition; vol. 2). https://publications.iarc.fr/581.
22. WHO Classification of Tumors Editorial Board. Central nervous system Tumors [Internet]. Lyon (France): International Agency for Research on Cancer; 2021 [cited 2024 May 21]. (WHO Classification of Tumors series, 5th edition; vol. 6). Available from https://Tumorclassification.iarc.who.int/chapters/45.
23. WHO Classification of Tumors Editorial Board. Central nervous system Tumors. Lyon (France): International Agency for Research on Cancer; 2021. (WHO Classification of Tumors series, 5th edition; vol. 6). https://publications.iarc.fr/601.
24. WHO Classification of Tumors Editorial Board. Digestive system Tumors [Internet]. Lyon (France): International Agency for Research on Cancer; 2019 [cited 2024 May 21]. (WHO Classification of Tumors series, 5th edition; vol. 1). Available from: https://Tumorclassification.iarc.who.int/chapters/31.
25. WHO Classification of Tumors Editorial Board. Digestive system Tumors. Lyon (France): International Agency for Research on Cancer; 2019. (WHO classification of Tumors series, 5th edition; vol. 1). https://publications.iarc.fr/579
26. WHO Classification of Tumors Editorial Board. Endocrine and neuroendocrine tumors [Internet]. Lyon (France): International Agency for Research on Cancer; 2022 [cited 2024 May 21]. (WHO classification of tumors series, 5th edition; vol. 10). Available from: https://tumourclassification.iarc.who.int/chapters/53.

27. WHO Classification of Tumors Editorial Board. Endocrine and neuroendocrine tumors. Lyon (France): International Agency for Research on Cancer; 2022. (WHO classification of tumors series, 5th edition; vol. 10). https://publications.iarc.fr.
28. WHO Classification of Tumors Editorial Board. Eye tumors [Internet; beta version ahead of print]. Lyon (France): International Agency for Research on Cancer; 2023 [cited 2024 May 21]. (WHO classification of Tumors series, 5th edition; vol. 13). Available from: https://Tumorclassification.iarc.who.int/chapters/??.
29. WHO Classification of Tumors Editorial Board. Female genital Tumors [Internet]. Lyon (France): International Agency for Research on Cancer; 2020 [cited 2024 May 21]. (WHO classification of Tumors series, 5th edition; vol. 4). Available from: https://Tumor classification.iarc.who.int/chapters/34.
30. WHO Classification of Tumors Editorial Board. Female genital Tumors. Lyon (France): International Agency for Research on Cancer; 2020. (WHO Classification of Tumors series, 5th edition; vol. 4). https://publications.iarc.fr/592.
31. WHO Classification of Tumors Editorial Board. Genetic Tumor Syndrome. WHO Classification of Tumors Series, 5th edition. Lyon (France): International Agency for Research on Cancer; 2023. [online] Available from https://Tumorclassification.iarc.who.int/ chapters/67. [Last accessed August, 2023].
32. WHO Classification of Tumors Editorial Board. Head and neck Tumors [Internet; beta version ahead of print]. Lyon (France): International Agency for Research on Cancer; 2022 [cited 2024 May 21]. (WHO Classification of Tumors series, 5th edition; vol. 9). Available from: https://Tumorclassification.iarc.who.int/chapters/52.
33. WHO Classification of Tumors Editorial Board. Head and neck Tumors. Lyon (France): International Agency for Research on Cancer; forthcoming. (WHO Classification of Tumors series, 5th edition; vol. 9). https://publications.iarc.fr.
34. WHO Classification of Tumours Editorial Board. Haematolymphoid tumours [Internet]. Lyon (France): International Agency for Research on Cancer; 2024 [cited 2024 May 21]. (WHO classification of tumours series, 5th edition; vol. 11). Available from: https://tumourclassification.iarc.who.int/chapters/63.
35. WHO Classification of Tumours Editorial Board. Haematolymphoid tumours. Lyon (France): International Agency for Research on Cancer; Forthcoming 2024. (WHO classification of tumours series, 5th edition; vol. 11). https://publications.iarc.who.int/.
36. WHO Classification of Tumors Editorial Board. Pediatric Tumors [Internet]. Lyon (France): International Agency for Research on Cancer; 2022 [cited 2024 May 21]. (WHO Classification of Tumors series, 5th edition; vol. 7). Available from: https://Tumorclassification. iarc.who.int/chapters/44.
37. WHO Classification of Tumors Editorial Board. Pediatric Tumors. Lyon (France): International Agency for Research on Cancer; 2022. (WHO Classification of Tumors series, 5th edition; vol. 7). https://publications.iarc.fr/608.
38. WHO Classification of Tumors Editorial Board. Pediatric Tumors. Lyon (France): International Agency for Research on Cancer; 2023. (WHO Classification of Tumors series, 5th edition; vol. 13). https://publications.iarc.fr.
39. WHO Classification of Tumors Editorial Board. Skin Tumors [Internet; beta version ahead of print]. Lyon (France): International Agency for Research on Cancer; 2023 [cited 2024 May 21]. (WHO classification of Tumors series, 5th edition; vol. 12). Available from: https://Tumorclassification.iarc.who.int/chapters/64.
40. WHO Classification of Tumors Editorial Board. Skin Tumors. Lyon (France): International Agency for Research on Cancer; forthcoming. (WHO classification of Tumors series, 5th edition; vol. 12). https://publications.iarc.fr.
41. WHO Classification of Tumors Editorial Board. Soft tissue and bone Tumors [Internet]. Lyon (France): International Agency for Research on Cancer; 2020 [cited 2023, Sep 1]. (WHO Classification of Tumors series, 5th edition; vol. 3). Available from: https://Tumorclassification.iarc.who.int/chapters/33.
42. WHO Classification of Tumors Editorial Board. Soft tissue and bone Tumors. Lyon (France): International Agency for Research on Cancer; 2020. (cited 2024 May 21) (HO Classification of Tumors series, 5th edition; vol. 3). https://publications.iarc.fr/588.
43. WHO Classification of Tumors Editorial Board. Soft tissue and bone Tumors. Lyon (France): International Agency for Research on Cancer; 2020. (WHO Classification of Tumors series, 5th edition; vol. 3). https://publications.iarc.fr/588.
44. WHO Classification of Tumors Editorial Board. Thoracic Tumors [Internet]. Lyon (France): International Agency for Research on Cancer; 2021 [cited 2024 May 21]. (WHO Classification of Tumors series, 5th edition; vol. 5). Available from: https://Tumorclassification. iarc.who.int/chapters/35.
45. WHO Classification of Tumors Editorial Board. Thoracic Tumors. Lyon (France): International Agency for Research on Cancer; 2021. (WHO classification of Tumors series, 5th edition; vol. 5). https:// publications.iarc.fr/595.
46. WHO Classification of Tumors Editorial Board. Urinary and male genital Tumors [Internet]. Lyon (France): International Agency for Research on Cancer; 2022 [cited 2024 May 21]. (WHO classification of Tumors series, 5th edition; vol. 8). Available from: https://Tumor classification.iarc.who.int/chapters/36.
47. WHO Classification of Tumors Editorial Board. Urinary and male genital Tumors. Lyon (France): International Agency for Research on Cancer; 2022. (WHO classification of Tumors series, 5th edition; vol. 8). https://publications.iarc.fr/610.

Index

Page numbers followed by *b* refer to box, *f* refer to figure, *fc* refer to flowchart, and *t* refer to table

A

- Abdomen
  - fullness of 379
  - mesenchymal tumor of 611
  - pain 764
- Abdominal aorta, popliteal artery 487
- Abdominal fat 887
  - aspirates, examination of 212*s*
- Abdominal mass 490, 764
  - palpable 762
- Abdominal pain 364, 618, 626, 701, 756
  - lower 628, 825
  - repeated attacks of 703
  - severe 290, 839, 889
- Abdominal stria, purple 900
- Abnormal cell 443
  - proliferation 924
- Abnormal endogenous substance, accumulation of 43
- Abnormal exogenous substance
  - accumulation of 44
  - deposition of 44
- Abnormal transforming growth factor-beta 489
- ABO
  - antibodies 422
    - acquired 422
    - natural 422
  - antigens 422
  - blood group system 422, 423, 425*b*
  - grouping, methods of 424
  - hemolytic disease 359
  - incompatibility 358, 420
  - system 422
- Abortions
  - criminal 159
  - previous 838
  - risk of spontaneous 292
- Abrasive techniques 307, 309
- Abscess 19, 81, 82, 526, 618, 743
  - amebic 682
  - central 121
  - lacking acute inflammation 914
  - local 696
  - metastatic 545
  - myocardial 526
  - pericholecystic 694
  - perinephric 740
  - psoas 913, 914
  - pulmonary 582
  - pyogenic 682
  - ring 526
  - suppurative 548*f*
- Absorption 332
- Abundant commensal bacteria 622
- Abundant eosinophilic cytoplasm 808, 865, 976
- Abundant reactive small lymphocytes 395
- Acalculous cholecystitis, acute 693, 694
- Acanthocytosis 672
- Acanthosis 590
  - nigricans 263
- Accidental death, causes of 289
- Acellular amyloid deposits 881
- Acellular collagen 394*f*
- Acellular connective tissue 99*f*
- Acetaldehyde 666, 666*f*, 667
  - formation of 664
  - toxicity 293
- Acetaminophen 652
- Acetate 45, 667
- Acetic acid 666*f*
  - application of 807
  - formation of 666
  - test 454
- Acetoacetic acid 457, 889
- Acetone 457
  - free methyl alcohol 441
- Achalasia cardia 596
- Achondroplasia 279
- Achycardia 515
- Acid 605
  - aerosols 288
  - hematin 48
    - method 438
  - production 599
  - secretion 599, 600
- Acid-base abnormalities 889
- Acid-fast
  - bacilli 110*f*, 314, 560, 567
    - demonstration of 110
  - stain 109, 110
  - tubercle bacilli 567
- Acidic urine 453, 453*t*
- Acid-Schiff reaction 855
- Acinar adenocarcinoma 793
- Acinar cell 699, 702, 703
  - carcinoma 704
  - injury 702*f*
    - primary 699
  - mass 703
- Acinar necrosis 700*f*
- Acini per lobule, number of 844
- Acini, size of 703
- Acquired atelectasis 585
  - types of 585
- Acquired immunodeficiency syndrome 165, 197, 203, 449
  - clinical features of 203
  - diagnosis of 203
  - pathogenesis of 199
- Acral lentiginous melanoma 957
- Acromegaly 456
- Actinic keratosis 949, 950
- *Actinomycetes israelii* 121
- Actinomycetoma 120
- Actinomycosis 121
  - abdominal 121
  - microscopy of 121*f*
- Activated partial thromboplastin time 324, 419
- Activating complement system 173, 174
- Acute bacterial meningitis 965
  - etiology of 961*t*
- Acute decompression sickness 159
  - mechanism of 159, 160*fc*
- Acute hemolytic transfusion reaction 431, 432, 432*fc*
- Acute inflammation 60, 60*t*, 63, 65, 68, 69, 77, 78, 80, 80*t*, 82, 82*fc*, 83, 700, 933
  - Acute inflammation, causes of 60
  - characteristic of 86
- Acute inflammatory
  - infiltrate 163, 518*f*
  - process 72, 960
  - reaction 80, 82, 518
- Acute kidney injury 712, 737, 742, 744
  - causes of 743, 744
  - complications of 744*b*
  - types of 743
- Acute leukemia 371, 372
  - classification of 372
  - French, American, and British classification of 372
  - group of 371
- Acute myeloid leukemia 372, 375, 376
  - classification of 376
  - general features of 375
- Acute nonhemolytic transfusion reactions 432
- Acute pancreatitis 20, 20*f*, 59, 645, 693, 696, 697, 699, 702, 709
  - causes of 697*b*
  - classification of 700
  - complications of 701, 701*t*
- Acute pericarditis 532, 533
  - clinical features of 533
- Acute poststreptococcal glomerulonephritis
  - etiopathogenesis of 717
  - light microscopic appearance of 718*f*
- Acute pyelonephritis 736, 737, 773
  - complications of 772
  - etiopathogenesis of 737
  - gross appearance of 740*f*
- Acute respiratory distress syndrome 144, 159, 161, 585
  - changes of 159
  - etiological factors of 585*b*
- Acute transfusion reaction 431
  - division of 432*f*
  - nonimmunological 433
- Acute tubular injury 144, 737, 744
  - microscopic appearance of 746*f*
- Adapter protein 26
- Adaptive immune
  - cells 140
  - responses, cytokine of 169
  - system, deficiencies of 196
- Adaptive immunity 166, 166*t*, 196
  - general features of 166*b*
  - types of 166
- Addison's disease 10, 48, 901, 902
- Adenine 426
  - replaces thymidine 273*f*
- Adenocarcinoma 218, 262, 316*f*, 574, 576-578, 584, 597, 640, 641*f*, 645, 687, 798, 801, 806, 844
  - development of 596
  - in situ 577, 578*f*
  - invasive 578
  - mucin-secreting 781
  - risk factors for 793
- Adenofibroma 819
- Adenolymphoma 593
- Adenoma 217, 270, 611, 845, 903
  - adrenocortical 217, 903
  - benign 874
  - carcinoma sequence 637, 638*f*
  - fulminant 900, 903
  - nonfunctioning 875
  - pedunculated 632
- Adenomatous polyposis coli 607, 633, 638
  - gene, mutations of 636
- Adenomyosis 810, 810*f*
- Adenosine
  - diphosphate, oxidative phosphorylation of 29
  - triphosphate 29
    - depletion of 29
- Adenosis 843, 843*f*, 844, 845

Adenovirus 557, 738, 866, 962
Adhesins 585, 599
Adipocytes 297, 673
Adipokines 887
 antihyperglycemic 887
Adipose
 cytokines 887
 tissue 44, 158, 886*f*
 tumors of 936, 938
Adrenal adenoma 899
Adrenal cortex 898
 carcinoma of 245, 900
 disease of 899
Adrenal cortical
 adenoma 903
 carcinoma, causes of 904
 cells 903
 tumors 901
Adrenal glands 416, 898, 899, 961
Adrenal hyperplasia, congenital 901
Adrenal insufficiency
 chronic 902
 secondary 901
Adrenal medulla 904, 906, 908
 normal 903
 tumors of 904, 909
Adrenal neoplasms 903
Adrenal tumors, primary 899
Adrenocortical insufficiency 901
 acute 902
 causes of 901, 902*b*, 903
 chronic 902
 primary 901-903
 secondary 902, 903
Adrenocortical neoplasm 901, 903, 904
Adrenogenital syndromes 901
Adult respiratory distress syndrome 143
Advanced glycation end products, formation of 891, 735
Advanced squamous cell carcinoma, gross appearance of 951*f*
Adventitial fibrosis 496
Adverse transfusion reaction 431
Aerobic glycolysis 245, 389
Aerosolized droplets, inhalation of 541
Aflatoxin 229, 684
Agammaglobulinemia 546
 X-linked 196
Aganglionic megacolon, congenital 630
Agenesis 280
Agglutination 424, 468
Aggressive fibromatoses 102
Agnogenic myeloid metaplasia 320
Agranular casts 745
Agranulocytosis 367
Air
 embolism 159
 pollution 288, 554, 556, 575
Air-dried smears 312, 314
Airway 552, 555, 569
 chronic inflammation of 552
 epithelium 552
 hyperresponsiveness 554
 infection 550
 inflammation 554
 obstruction 550, 552, 557, 873
 chronic 552
 remodeling 554, 555
Alanine aminotransferase 654, 656
Albinism 48
Albumin 132, 324, 722, 725
 bilirubin complex 646
 loss of 132
 serum levels of 194, 294
 synthesis, reduced 132
 trapping of 891
Albuminuria 132
Alcohol 530, 666, 667, 697, 699
 abuse 230, 474, 702
 chronic 683
 effects of 677
 activates hepatic stellate cells 668
 consumption 482, 590, 637, 932, 933
 chronic excessive 702
 heavy 847
 dehydrogenase 664, 666*f*
 direct toxic action of 678
 effects of 292
 intake, duration of 666
 intoxication 542
 metabolism of 292, 293
Alcoholic abuse 44, 45
Alcoholic cirrhosis 600, 670, 672, 689
 end-stage 670
 gross appearance of 671*f*
 microscopic appearance of 671*f*
Alcoholic liver disease 47, 653, 666, 709
 end-stage of 670
 etiology of 666
 pathogenesis of 666, 667*f*
Alcoholism
 acute 293
 chronic 292, 293, 294*t*
Aldehyde dehydrogenase 666*f*
Aldosterone 901, 903
 compensatory secretion of 723
Aldosteronism, primary 451
Alimentary system 337
Alimentary tract 195
Alkaline
 causes of 453*t*
 phosphatase 649, 672, 688, 919
 urine 453
Alkaptonuria 49
Alkylating agents 254, 255, 371
Allergen 170, 553, 554
 binding of 554
 triggering environmental 553
Allergic bronchopulmonary aspergillosis 120
Allergic diseases 83, 553, 899
Allergic reactions 69, 432
 mild 433
Allergic transfusion reactions 432
Allergic tubulointerstitial nephritis 748
Allergic vascular disease 407
Allografts 182, 184
 failure, chronic 186
 recognition and rejection of 183
Alpha-1-antitrypsin deficiency 600
Alpha-fetoprotein 473, 475, 687, 779, 830
Alpha-gene, deletion of 352
Alpha-globin chains
 absent synthesis of 352
 production of 364
Alpha-methylacyl-coenzyme A-racemase 795
Alpha-thalassemia 352
Alport's syndrome 746
Altered cellular metabolism 245
Altered protein homeostasis 56
Alternative complement pathway 355
 activation of 716, 732
Alveolar capillaries, wall of 134
Alveolar fibrosis 545
Alveolar macrophage 570, 571
Alveolar rhabdomyosarcoma 942
Alveolar septa, thickened 135
Alveolar space 134
Alveolar walls, destruction of 550
Alveolitis, allergic 120
Alzheimer disease 23, 27, 47, 208
Amebiasis 617
 complications of 619*f*
Amebic colitis 618
Amebic dysentery, complications of 682
Amebic liver abscess 618, 682
 Anchovy sauce appearance of 682*f*
 clinical features of 619
Amebic liver abscess, spread of 618
Amebic ulcer
 microscopic appearance of 619*f*
 multiple 619*f*
Ameboma 618
Ameloblast-like cells 595
Ameloblastoma 594, 595*f*
Amenorrhea 832
Ames test 255
Amides 255
Amino acid 273*f*, 274*f*, 755
 disorder 452, 452*t*
Aminotransferases 473
Ammonia, increased blood level of 474
Ammonium 756
 oxalate 323
Amniotic fluid 160
 embolism 160, 160*f*
Amorphous electron-dense, deposition of 713
Amphibole 572
Amphophilic cytoplasm 390, 881
Amplicon length analysis 287
Amyloid 205, 207*f*, 209-211
 biochemical forms of 206
 chemical nature of 206
 deposit 208, 209, 212, 881, 887, 892
 forms of 205
 kidney 211*f*
 cut section of 211*f*
 light chain protein 206
 physical nature of 205
 protein 206, 887
 properties of 205
 special stains for 211*b*
 staining properties of 210
 types of 205
Amyloidosis 165, 205, 207, 209, 212, 263, 382, 401, 532, 723, 736, 914
 categories of 206
 classification of 207, 208*t*
 familial 209
 hemodialysis-associated 208
 hereditary 209
 pathogenesis of 206, 207*f*
 primary 207, 208
 secondary 548, 567, 913
Analgesics 768
Anaphylactic transfusion reactions 432
Anaphylatoxin 79
Anaplasia 220, 221, 620, 764, 918
 microscopic features of 221, 222*b*, 222*f*
Anaplastic large cell lymphoma 385
Anaplastic lymphoma kinase 906
Anasarca 129, 722
Anchovy paste 618, 682
Anchovy sauce appearance 682*f*
Ancillary diagnostic test 473, 475
Ancillary studies, applications of 314
Ancillary techniques 307
 special and 314
Androgen 793, 831, 861, 899
 receptor 790
 role of 789
Anemia 44, 159, 203, 261, 295, 304, 324, 325, 334, 342, 348, 361*b*, 366, 374, 412, 438, 444, 445*f*, 496, 672, 748, 895
 alloimmune hemolytic 357, 358
 chronic 433
 classification of 325
 clinical features of 325, 327*f*
 effects of 327*f*
 etiological classification of 324, 326*b*
 features of 438
 hemolytic 174, 319, 326, 342, 344, 349, 355, 362*fc*, 429, 459, 460
 hypoplastic 429
 investigation of 325, 327*b*
 morphological classification of 325*t*
 severe 333, 429
 severity of 325, 326*b*
 speed of onset of 325
 type of 325
Anesthesia 541
Aneuploidy 151, 233, 275
Aneurysm 487, 497
 atherosclerotic 292, 488
 formation 485
 gross types of 488*f*
 rupture of 137
Angina
 history of 522
 pectoris 509, 511
 variants of 511
 stable 485, 509, 510, 512
Angiogenesis 95, 96*f*, 251, 254
 induction of 248
 mechanism of 248
 promote 760
 significance of 95
 steps in 95
 sustained 248
Angiogenic stimuli 96*f*
Angiolipoma 937
Anisocytosis 346*f*, 351, 441
 moderate 332
Anitschkow cells 505, 505*f*
Ankles 130, 506, 911
Ankylosis 926, 928
Ann Arbor staging classification 397*t*
Anogenital mucosal surfaces 955
Anorexia 671, 694

Anoxia 44, 542
Antemortem venous thrombi 154, 154*t*
Antiandrogens 793
Antiapoptotic proteins
  blocking function of 26
  overexpression of 247
Antibody 63, 166, 188, 191, 196, 214, 371, 409*f*, 423, 475, 926
  absence of 79
  binding of 181
  formation of 176
  glomerulonephritis 714*f*
  mediated rejection, acute 185, 186*f*
  salient features of 168*t*
  screening 425
  tests for 468
  types of 191
Anticardiolipin 192
  antibody 192, 195
Anticitrullinated peptide antibody 927
Anticoagulant 302, 321, 322*t*, 324
  effects 147, 149
  preservative solution 426*t*
  types of 321
Anticoagulated blood, centrifugation of 324
Anti-deoxyribonuclease B 717
Antiendothelial cell antibodies 495, 496
Antifibrinolytic effect 149, 150
Antigen 106, 170, 172, 176, 181, 188, 385
  antibody complexes 174, 715, 718
    formation of 191
  bacterial 623
  derivatives, prostate-specific 797
  nature of 169
  origin of 714
  presenting cells 166-168, 172*f*, 179*f*, 183
  process 168
  prolonged exposure to 715
  recognition of 167
  short-lived exposure to 715
  specific 475
  type of 553
Antiglobulin test 359
  direct methods of 359*f*
  indirect methods of 359*t*
  types of 359
  uses of indirect 360
Anti-glomerular basement membrane 714*f*
  antibody 716, 720
    deposition of 716
Antiglycolytic agent 323
Anti-human globulin test 329
Anti-human immunodeficiency virus antibodies 202
Anti-hyaluronidase 717
Anti-inflammatory cytokines
  expression of 599
  liberation of 72
Antimicrobial peptides 563, 622
Antimitochondrial antibodies 680, 681
Antimycobacterial effects 562
Anti-myeloperoxidase 496
Antineutrophil cytoplasmic antibodies 495, 496, 720
Anti-nicotinyl adenine dinucleotidase 717
Antinuclear antibodies 191
Antioxidant 31, 230, 302
  defense mechanisms, reduction of 54
  mechanisms 71
  nonenzymatic 32
  properties 301
  reduction of 54
  types of 32*b*
Antiphospholipid antibody 191
  syndrome 152, 192
Antiplatelet antibodies 420
Anti-proteases 72
Anti-proteinase 496
Antiretroviral drug therapy, effects of 203
Antisperm antibodies, tests for 468
Antistreptococcal antibody titers 719
Anti-streptokinase 717
Anti-streptolysin O 717
  antibody titer 540
Antithrombin deficiency 429
Antithrombotic properties 147, 149, 149*t*
Antithyroglobulin 864
Antithyroid peroxidase antibody 470, 864
Antitreponemal antibody tests 114
Antiviral defense 166
Antiviral drugs 658*f*
Antler horn configuration 314, 315*f*
Antral gastritis 599, 600
Anuria 451
Anus 801
Aorta 46, 530, 539
  ascending 491
  dissecting aneurysm of 53
  intimal surface of 485*f*
Aortic aneurysm 157
  abdominal 489
Aortic dissection 491
  classification of 492*f*
  complications of 491
  fate of 491
Aortic stenosis 514
Aortic valve 507, 527*f*
  dilation 490
  stenosis 538
Aortic wall 491
Aphasia 970
Aplasia 280
Aplastic anemia 341, 408, 449
  causes of 341*b*
  pathogenesis of 341*f*
Aplastic crises 346, 354
Apocrine metaplasia 843, 843*f*
Apoproteins, decreased synthesis of 45
Apoptosis 16, 22, 24, 24*f*, 25*f*, 26, 27, 35*f*, 36, 59, 190, 191, 223, 231, 232, 244, 247, 390, 515*f*
  causes of 23
  diagnosis of 27
  execution phase of 27
  extrinsic pathway of 26
  inhibition of 233
  initiators, regulated 25
  intrinsic pathway of 24, 247
  mechanisms of 22, 24, 25*f*
  pathways of 247
  phases of 24, 27
Apoptotic bodies, formation of 24
Apoptotic cells
  inadequate clearance of 191
  phagocytosis of 24
  removal of 27
  secrete soluble factors 27
Appendicitis
  acute 642, 643*f*, 644
    gangrenous 643
    suppurative 643
Appendicular skeleton 916
Appendix 197, 833
  neuroendocrine tumor of 620*f*
Appetite 298, 889
  loss of 363
  suppresses 77
Apple core appearance 641
Arachidonic acid 74
  metabolites 73, 74, 74*f*, 75, 75*t*
    production of 75
  products 178
Arachnoid
  fibrosis 963
  membrane 975
Arachnoiditis, chronic adhesive 961
Arboviruses 962
Architectural disorder, mild 766
Areola 855
  epidermis of 855*f*
Aristolochia 767
Armanni-Ebstein lesions 737
Aromatic amines 255
  mechanism of action of 768*f*
Arrhythmias 151, 212, 507, 519, 521
Arrhythmogenic right ventricular cardiomyopathy 531
Arsenic 289, 290, 575, 768
  interferes 290
  poisoning
    acute 290
    chronic 48
Arterial air embolism 159
Arterial blood 324
  gas analysis 323
Arterial circulation 151, 159
Arterial dissection 488
Arterial occlusion 21, 162
Arterial oxygen saturation 381
Arterial system, thrombosis in 150
Arterial thrombi 152, 153, 153*t*, 155
  grow retrograde 154
Arterial thrombosis, causes of 150
Arterial vasodilation 140, 141
Arteriolar vasoconstriction 145
Arterioles 749
  capillaries, rupture of 749
  dilation of 74
Arteriolosclerosis, hyperplastic 494, 495*f*
Arteriopathy, transplant-associated 479
Arteriosclerosis 97, 479
  hyperplastic 749
Arteritis, healed 479
Artery 46, 151, 152, 479, 487, 682
  obstruct 155
  tunica media of 51*f*
Arthritis 412, 508, 931, 932
  acute 932
    suppurative 913
  chronic tophaceous 933
  suppurative 545
Arthus reaction 178
Articular cartilage 929, 930, 933
  degeneration of 929
    disorder of 928
  fibrillation of 929, 930
Articular surface 929, 930
Arylamines 767
Asbestos 255, 575, 586
  bodies 51, 573, 573*f*, 574
  diseases 572
  types 572
  use 572
  white 572
Asbestosis 476, 572, 573*f*
  clinical features of 574
  pathogenesis of 573*f*
Ascaris lumbricoides 692, 697
Aschoff body 4, 505, 505*f*, 506
  formation of 505
  multiple 506
Aschoff nodule 505
Ascites 130, 675, 688
  causes of 464, 464*t*
  pathogenesis of 675, 677*f*
Ascitic fluid 316*f*, 825
  examination of 465
Ascorbic acid 301, 455
Aseptic meningitis, acute 965
Askanazy zones 604
Aspergilloma 120, 567
Aspergillosis 119
  invasive 120
Aspergillus 739
  flavus 684
Aspermia 468
Aspiration 547
  method of 313
  pneumonia 542
Aspirin 410, 598, 602, 916
  protective effect of 636
  sensitive asthma 556
Assisted reproductive technology 536
Asterixis 652
Asteroid bodies 568
Asthma 548, 553, 556*f*
  bronchial 83
  characteristics features of 553*b*
  classification of 553*b*
  drug-induced 556
  non-atopic 556
  occupational 556
  pathogenesis of 555*f*
  subtypes of 556
  trigger 556
  type of 553
Asthmatic attack, acute 556
Astrocytoma 967, 968, 968*f*
Ataxia-telangiectasia 54, 232, 253
Atelectasis 582, 585
  acquired 585
Atheroembolism 485, 486
Atherogenesis, injury hypothesis of 483*f*
Atheroma formation 483
Atheromatous emboli 161
Atheromatous plaque 484, 485*f*, 486, 513
  microscopy of 486*f*
  structure of 510
  surface of 485

Atherosclerosis 46, 50, 83, 292, 479, 481, 484, 486f, 487f, 488, 489, 494
accelerated 892
chronic coronary 514
clinical consequences of 486b
clinicopathologic manifestations of 485
complications of 485
coronary 486f, 509, 723
development of 481, 482
pathogenesis of 482
risk factors of 480, 480t, 512
severe 892
Atherosclerotic abdominal aortic aneurysm 489
Atherosclerotic occlusion
degree of 509
severity of 509
Atherosclerotic plaque 484, 486b, 486f, 510, 510f, 512, 892
basic structure of 486f
Atherothrombosis 513
Atmospheric pressure 159
Atomic bomb explosion 261
Atopic asthma 553, 554
etiology of 554
pathogenesis of 554
Atopic disorders 724
Atopic march 173
Atopic triad 173
Atresia 280
Atrial fibrillation 150-502, 507, 531
Atrial natriuretic
factor 39
peptide, release of 500
Atrial septal defect 537
Atrophic endometrium 815
Atrophic gastritis 598
chronic 230, 333, 336
multifocal 599
Atrophic glossitis 337
Atrophy 41, 42t, 59, 775
physiological 41
Atypia 811, 813, 847
Auer rods 405
Autoantibody 188, 191, 326, 680, 885, 896
development of 283
multiple 868
persistent production of 191
presence of 681
specificity of 191
spectrum of 191
tests for 193
Autoantigen 726
Autocatalytic reactions 30
Autocrine signaling 92
Autohemolysis
spontaneous 346
test 346
Autoimmune 557
adrenalitis, primary 903
cholangiopathies 680
disease 27, 82, 83, 170, 183, 188, 188t, 189, 194, 283, 369, 382, 714, 726, 734, 863, 864, 867, 868, 883, 899
risk of 865
disorder 178, 188, 194, 408, 447, 680
gastritis 598
hemolytic anemia 174, 188, 357, 360, 385, 398, 459
hepatitis 652
hypoparathyroidism 898
hypothyroidism 869
injury 702
pancreatitis 703
response 732
states, presently complicates 208
thrombocytopenia 188
thyroid
disease 863
disorders 867
Autoimmunity 15, 170, 188, 195, 884, 926
mechanisms of 188
Autoinflammatory syndromes 63
Autologous blood
donation 435
transfusion
advantages of 435b
contraindications of 436b
disadvantages of 435b
types of 436, 436b, 437
Autologous collections, preoperative 436b
Autolysis 28, 28t
Autophagy 56, 246
Autopsy 6, 10
Autosomal dominant
adult polycystic kidney disease 753f
cancer syndromes 232
disorder 279t, 650, 908
hypoparathyroidism 898
syndrome 631
trait 242
Autosomal recessive 279
disorder 279t, 209, 353
hereditary disorder 348
polycystic kidney disease 753, 754f
Autosplenectomy 354, 355
Avascular necrosis 160
Axial skeleton
bone of 795
metastasis to 795
Axillary lymph node 133
metastases, absence of 857
Ayre's spatula 311, 311f
Azo dyes 255
Azoospermia 468
Azotemia 471, 472, 712, 716, 732, 902
postrenal 472
Azurophil 72
Azurophilic granules 167
Azzopardi effect 582

B

Babesiosis 443
Bacillary dysentery 617, 617f
Bacilli, isolation of 615
Bacillus anthracis 128
Bacillus Calmette-Guerin 560
Back pain 567, 741, 742
Bacteremia 82, 115, 525, 545, 562, 613
massive 613
temporary 911
transient 613, 911
Bacteria 69f, 259, 308, 523, 557, 719
anaerobic 121, 547
intestinal 88
killing of 562
pleuritis 533
spread of 911
Bacterial diseases 114
Bacterial enzyme
actions of 691
beta-glucuronidases 691
hydrolyze bile salts 691
Bacterial infections 204, 678, 737
recurrent 197
secondary 546
Bacterial phospholipases hydrolyze phospholipids 691
Bacteriuria 741, 742
Bacteroides 547
Baker cyst 928
Balanced reciprocal translocation 233, 275, 379, 379f
Balloon cells 590
Barr body 276, 277f
buccal smear for 276
number of 277
Barrett esophagus 42, 224, 230, 595, 596f, 597, 645
Basal cell 578f, 790, 801
carcinoma 260, 951, 953f, 959
development of 290
gross appearance of 953f
morphology of 952
noduloulcerative 952
hyperplasia 577
layer 794
nevus 952
Basal ganglia, calcification of 898
Basal metabolic rate 867
Basal plasmacytosis 627
Basaloid 785
epithelial cells 952
squamous cell carcinoma 786
Basement membrane 730f, 767, 892
breaching of 249
rupture of 745
thickening of 713
Basket cells 386
Basket-weave pattern 574
Basophilia 368, 380
Basophilic cytoplasm 390
moderate amount of deeply 390
Basophils 79, 319, 321, 369f, 554, 555f
Bean-shaped nuclei 84
Beck's triad 536
Beckwith-Wiedemann syndrome 763
Bed sores 98
Bence-Jones proteins 208, 398, 400, 405, 454, 455
Benedict's qualitative test 456, 893
Benedict's reagent 455
chemistry of 456
Benign epithelial
component 860
lesions 842, 843t
proliferations 845
tumors 217f, 635, 903
Benign neoplasms 229, 284
characteristics of 220, 229
diagnosis of 307
Benign nodular
fibroblastic proliferations 940
myofibroblastic proliferations 940
Benign prostatic acini 794
Benign prostatic
hyperplasia 789, 791f, 792f
complications of 792b
hypertrophy 739, 757
Benzidine 255
test 458
Beriberi 303
Bernard-Soulier syndrome 410
Berry aneurysm 488, 753
Beta-cell 166, 191, 194
antigens 883
destruction, mechanisms of 884
dysfunction 883, 886, 887
molecular mechanisms of 887
enzyme 885
failure 887
function 201
hyperplasia, compensatory 887
lymphoid malignancies 259
lymphoma 203, 385
neoplasms 373
precursor 373
produce antibodies against self-antigens 191
stimulate 167
Beta-globin chains
diminished synthesis of 348
production of 364
Beta-hydroxybutyric acid 889
Beta-lymphocytes, immortalization of 259
Beta-naphthylamine 767
Beta-thalassemia 348, 350f, 691
major 348, 350, 351, 398
diagnosis of 351
pathogenesis of 349
pathophysiology of 349
minor 351, 352, 352t
syndromes 352t
trait 351, 352t
Bethesda system 309, 309t, 803
Bicarbonate 601f
secretion 601, 602
Big bulky tumor 918
Bile acid 473, 691
deficiencies of 649
produce, blood levels of 473
retention of 649
synthesis 690
Bile constituents 691
Bile ducts 693
adenocarcinoma of 260
common 697
Bile peritonitis 694
Bile pigment 459
Bile salts 460, 473, 690, 693
Biliary cholangitis, primary 680, 690
Biliary cholesterol secretion 690
Biliary cirrhosis, primary 680
Biliary enteric fistula 696
Biliary fistulas 693
Biliary lecithin 690
Biliary obstruction 693
Biliary system 687
Biliary tract 691
chronic infections of 687
obstruction of 302
Biliary tree 613, 687
Bilirubin 459, 473, 649, 652
blood levels of 647
calcium salts 688

    conjugation 648
    diglucuronide, water-soluble 646
    estimation of 324
    formation 646
    glucuronides, deconjugation of 647
    hepatic processing of 646
    increased production of 648
    metabolism 473, 646, 647*f*, 651
        intestinal phase of 647
    production 646
    reduced hepatic uptake of 648
    renal excretion of 647
    retention of 649
    sources of 646
    tests for 459*b*
    transport of 646
    unconjugated 646, 649,650, 691, 692
Bilirubinuria 660, 672
    causes of 459
Biliverdin 459, 646
Bioaerosols 289
Biochemical injury 158, 158*fc*
Biochemical tests 338, 660
Biopsy 212
    interpretation, pitfalls in 265
    sediment cytology 315
Biosynthesis, tests of 473, 474
Biphasic reaction 650
Biphasic synovial sarcoma 945*f*, 946
Births, preterm 292
Bitot spots 299
Bizarre cells 221, 222
Black pigment stones 688, 689, 691, 692
Black tarry stool 362
Bladder 757
    cancer 255, 743
        clinical course of 770
        history of 768
    carcinoma 243, 458
    compression of 817
    diverticula 792
    hypertrophy of 791
    stones 458
    symptoms 758
    wash 310
Bland fibroblasts 940
Blast phase 380
Blastocyst, inner cell mass of 93
Blastomas 219
Blastomyces 120
Bleeding 141, 197, 303, 376, 407, 414, 429, 604, 678
    abnormal 817
    diatheses 137
    disorders 98, 406, 407, 416, 417*fc*, 417*t*
        broad classification of 407*b*
        classification of 406, 407, 407*b*
        diagnosis of 417
        laboratory diagnosis of 416
    excessive 413
    internal 138
    life-threatening 411
    severity of 408
    spontaneous 413
    tendency 416
        causes of 416
    time 399, 416, 418
        template method for 418
Blindness 893
    irreversible 299
Blisters 116
Blood 267, 319*t*
    ammonia estimation 672
    and anticoagulant, ratio of 446
    bag, storage of 425
    bank 323, 422
    basophils 74
    borne 913
        metastasis 263, 944
    cells 460
        excessive destruction of 137
        functions of 319
        normal development of 320
        type of 319
    chemistry 471
    cholesterol, lowers 480
    chronic loss of 138
    clot 99, 99*f*, 934*f*
        formation of 99
    collection 324, 425, 426, 426*f*
        perioperative 436
    colloid osmotic pressure of 723
    components 11, 428, 428*fc*, 428*t*, 437
        preparation of 428
    culture 615
    disease of 11
    disorders 458
    donors, selections of 425, 438
    films 11
        stain for peripheral 11
    findings 719
    flow 15, 64, 136, 150, 355, 744
        normal 66, 144, 150
        slowing of 64, 137
    from ventricles, outflow of 139
    glucose
        fasting 882, 886
        levels 882
        postprandial 886
    group 422, 425, 425*f*, 432, 435
        classification of 422
        gel card method of 425*f*
        interpretation of 424*f*
        methods of 422
        system 422, 422*b*
    hypercoagulability of 149
    inadequate oxygenation of 15
    loss 139, 326, 429
        acute 361
        anemia of 361
        chronic 332, 361, 362
    overnight, incubation of 449
    oxygen content of 162
    parasites, detection of 443
    pressure 493, 493*f*, 902
        diastolic 480
        elevation of 906
        raised 901
        regulation of 493
        systolic 480
    process of transferring 425
    products 425, 430, 430*t*
    recurrent loss of 138
    sample 323
        hemolysis of 324
        post-transfusion 435
        type of 323
    smear 11
        fixation of 441
        preparation of 440, 440*f*
        stains for 440
    spread 591, 610, 642, 686, 706, 878, 919
    stained fluid 463
    sugar 882
        estimation of 323
        level, control of 890
    supply 143, 712, 912
    tests 458*b*, 904
    transfusion 112, 198, 422, 425
        anticoagulant for 323
        complications of 431*b*
        cross-matching for 360
        mismatched 49
        reactions 431
        sequential steps for 425
        supervision of 425
    types, incompatibility of 358
    urea 400
        nitrogen 472*b*, 743, 750
        raised 719
    vessels 112, 137, 157, 158, 192, 198, 217, 226, 495*t*, 928, 720, 749, 729, 838, 772, 892
        abluminal surface of 95
        bifurcation of 151*f*
        central 830
        destruction of 700
        dilation of 80
        disorder of 407
        gradual narrowing of 186
        reactions of 63
        wall of 21*f*
    volume 64, 493*f*, 494
Bloodstream 613
    metastasize through 830
Bloody diarrhea 290, 618, 626
    attacks of 628
    causes of 616
Bloom syndrome 54, 232, 253
Blue asbestos 572
Blurred vision 888
B-lymphoblastic
    leukemias 373
    lymphomas 374
B-lymphocyte 167, 190, 207*f*, 405, 503
Body cavity 81, 129, 228, 307
    lining of 81
    seeding of 228
Body fat
    distribution of 887
    progressive loss of 261
Body fluids 267, 307, 308, 310, 462
Body mass index 297, 297*t*, 887
Boggy facies 870
Bombay blood group 423
Bone 217, 350, 354, 583, 610, 642, 784, 809, 830, 910, 910*f*, 936
    abnormalities 898
    changes 301, 350
    chronic bacterial infection of 86
    dactylitis of 354
    disease 301, 897
    eburnation 930
    Ewing sarcoma of 924
    forming tumors 916
    giant cell tumor of 922, 923*f*
    infarcts 917, 918
    lesions, benign 918
    long 910, 911
    malignant tumor of 917
    marrow 84, 93, 187, 208, 277, 287, 296, 319, 332, 338, 342, 344, 346, 349, 351, 356, 357, 373, 375, 377, 378, 380, 381, 386, 396, 399, 408, 409, 613, 614, 838, 915
        aspiration 306, 339*f*, 400*f*, 410, 448, 448*b*
        dysfunction 408
        examination 329, 447
        failure 197, 373, 374, 376
        hematopoietic cells of 91
        iron 332, 338, 351
        necrosis of 911
        needles 448
        normal adult 322*t*
        smear, evaluation of 449*b*
        transplantation, frequent complication of 188
        trephine biopsy 448
    matrix 917
    metastasis 228, 369, 904
    mineralization 300
    morphology 449
    necrosis 911
    necrotic piece of 912
    pain 374, 376, 897
    reactive new 919
    resorption 400, 914
    segmental necrosis of 912
    short 910
    small round cell sarcomas of 916, 924
    strength 933
    surface of 920
    tissue
        cell of 910
        destruction of 51
        resorption of 51
    tumors 915
        classification of 915
        distribution of 915
Bony callus 934
    formation of 934
Borderline leprosy 109
Borderline tuberculoid 109
Bordetella pertussis 115
Botryoid embryonal rhabdomyosarcoma 942
Bouveret's syndrome 693
Bowel 693
    infarctions of 158
Bowen's disease 785, 786, 949, 950
Bowenoid papulosis 786
Bowman capsule 710, 710, 721*f*, 736
Bowman space 711
Bradykinin 65, 80
    actions of 80
Brain 158, 286, 416, 583, 679, 680, 784, 809, 837, 838, 964
    abscesses of 682
    edema 133
    infarcts 963
    parenchymal edema 133
    tumors 245
        primary 967
Bread-and-butter pericarditis 506
Breast 41, 687, 833, 843
    adenocarcinoma of 249
    benign epithelial lesions of 843*t*

- cancer 233, 243, 245, 262, 268, 283, 301, 846-848, 848*f*, 856*b*
  - development of 846*f*
  - familial 847
  - invasive 844, 845
  - pathways of 848
  - prognosis of 856
  - risk, reduce 847
  - subsequent development of 843
- carcinoma 217*f*, 225*f*, 227, 245, 260, 264*f*, 833, 843-845, 850, 853*f*, 858*f*
  - invasive 845, 846*t*, 850
  - risk factors for 847*b*
  - spread of 856, 856*t*
  - types of 849
- change, nonproliferative 843, 843*f*
- density 847
- disease
  - benign 847
  - proliferative 847
- disorders 842
- epithelial
  - cells, proliferation of 848
  - tumors of 844
- female 842
- fibroadenoma of 225*f*, 314, 859*f*, 860*f*
- fibroepithelial tumors of 845, 858
- fine-needle aspiration cytology of 315*f*
- invasive
  - carcinoma of 851*f*, 852*f*
  - ductal carcinoma of 225*f*
- irradiation of 133
- lesions, biopsy techniques of 842
- lobular carcinoma of 854*f*
- lymphedema of 133
- male 861
- malignant tumor of 844
- skin 855
  - tenderness of 855
- stroma 842
  - invasion of 225*f*
- structure 842*f*
- tumors 232
  - classification of 844

Breath, shortness of 501
Breathlessness 333, 501
Brenner tumor 818, 819, 825, 825*f*
- benign 825

Breslow thickness 959
Bridging necrosis 661
Bright's disease 10
Brittle fibers 572
Brittle nails, spoon-shaped 362
Brodie abscess 912
Bromosulfthalein excretion 473
Bronchi 552, 565
- infiltration of 544*f*

Bronchial aspirate 309
Bronchial brush 309
Bronchial mucosa, dysplasia of 230
Bronchial neoplasm 547
Bronchial submucosa 553*f*
Bronchial surface epithelium 552
Bronchial wall 558
- destruction 588
- elastic tissue of 556
- fibrosis of 558
- thickness of 553*f*

Bronchial wash 309
Bronchiectasis 547, 548, 556, 557, 559*f*, 582, 585
- complications of 558, 558*b*
- etiopathogenesis of 556
- focal nonobstructive 557
- gross appearance of 559*f*
- microscopic
  - features of 559*f*
  - pathology of 557
- morphological types of 558*f*
- nonobstructive 556
- pathogenesis of 557*fc*

Bronchioalveolar stem cells 576
Bronchioles 544*f*
Bronchitis
- chronic 502, 548, 551, 552, 553*f*
- pathogenesis of chronic 552*fc*

Bronchoalveolar lavage 309
Bronchoconstriction 288, 621
Bronchopleural fistula 567
Bronchopneumonia 542, 542*f*, 543, 544*f*, 545, 545*t*
Bronchospasm 75, 621
Bronchus 231
Brown asbestos 572
Brown pigment stones 688, 691, 692
Brudzinski sign 962
Brussels sprouts 793
Bruton disease 69
Bruton tyrosine kinase gene 196
B-thalassemia
- clinical classification of 348*t*
- genetic classification of 348*t*
- pathogenesis of 348, 349*f*

Buccal mucosa 194, 292
Buckled nuclei 945
Buerger disease 292
Buffalo hump 900
Buffy coat 445
Bullous emphysema 551
Bullous eruption 114
Burkitt lymphoma 233, 238, 258, 259, 261, 385, 389, 390*f*, 405
Burns 81, 158, 598
- severe 139, 459, 597

Burst forming unit 321
Busulfan 254
Butterfly rash over face 193
Bypass 676
- surgery 159

C

Cachexia 77, 296, 350
Cadmium 289, 290, 575
- exposure, chronic 290
- inhalation, short-term 290

Cäfe-au-lait spots 48
Caffeine 847
Caisson disease 160
Cajal interstitial cells 611
Calcification 485
Calcinosis 194
- cutis 51

Calciphylaxis 898
Calcitonin level 470
Calcium
- biliary 691
- bilirubin 688
- bilirubinate 688, 692
  - salts 688
  - water-insoluble 692
- carbonate 688
- chelating agents 321
- flux 699
- homeostasis 34
- influx 37
- ingestion of 872
- ions 323
- mechanism of damage by 34
- metabolism 50
- oxalate 755, 756
  - stone 756, 756*f*
- palmitate 688
- phosphate 755, 756
  - stone 756, 756*f*
- reabsorption, stimulates 300
- salts 691
  - deposition of 50, 51
- stimulates intestinal absorption of 300
- stones 755, 756*f*

Call-Exner bodies 832, 832*f*
Callus 934
- formation of 934

Caloric restriction 56
Calyces 740, 741, 757
Cancer 27, 230, 231*t*, 232, 232*t*, 233, 248, 251, 260, 263, 267, 292, 848*f*
- advanced 611
- anal 203
- cachexia 261
- cells 55*f*, 215, 234, 239, 247, 248, 249, 251
  - cytological characteristics of 266
  - telomerase reactivation in 56
- colonic 637
- colorectal 628, 634, 636*fc*, 637, 640
- cure for 226
- death, causes of 226
- detection of 267
- diagnosis of 306
- eight hallmarks of 234*b*
- epidemiology of 229
- etiology of 254
- formation of 638*f*
- fundamental features of 215
- genes 231
  - classification of 231
  - functional classes of 231*b*
  - mutations in 231, 232
- grading of 262, 263
- hallmarks of 215, 234, 240
- invasive 577
- laboratory diagnosis of 264
- management of 306, 307
- molecular basis of 234
- occupational 10
- prognosis and behavior of 268
- promoting inflammation 234
- promotion of 256*f*
- staging of 262
- testis antigens 251
- well-differentiated 220

Candida 682, 739
- *albicans* 7, 118, 800
- dissemination of 119
- esophagitis 118
- infections 118
- *vaginitis* 118

Candidiasis 118, 204
- cutaneous 118
- invasive 119
- superficial 118

Cannonball metastases 584
Capillary 150, 195, 227
- basement membranes of 892
- blood 324
- congestion of 135
- distension of 135
- fragility test 418
- growth of 95
- hemangioma 498, 499*f*

Capsule creates 225
Carbohydrate 303, 635
- catabolism of 888
- diet 893
- metabolism 475
- restricted diet 893

Carbon 49
- laden macrophages 570
- monoxide 288
- pigment 570
  - accumulation of 43*f*

Carbonate 688
Carcinoembryonic antigen 267, 706
Carcinogenesis 876
- mechanisms of 606, 684

Carcinogenic agents 254
- classes of 254
- types of 254*fc*

Carcinogenic polycyclic aromatic hydrocarbons 289
Carcinogens 230, 291, 575, 590, 696
- endogenous synthesis of 229

Carcinoid 581
- atypical 581
- heart disease 621
- syndrome 620, 621, 621*f*
- tumor 581, 620*f*

Carcinoma 218, 223, 223*t*, 224, 271, 781, 877, 899, 903
- adrenocortical 901, 904
- anal 204
- anaplastic 880
- cells 267, 855
- cervix 800
  - spread of 805, 806
- colon, morphology of 640
- colonic 637
- colorectal 635
- development of 626
- esophagus, gross types of 597*f*
- ex pleomorphic adenoma 593
- familial medullary 880
- gastric 607, 608
- in situ 224, 577, 768, 769, 799, 803*f*, 804, 844, 849
  - system 804
- infiltrative ulcerative type of 609*f*
- lung, gross types of 579*f*
- nature of 876
- nomenclature of 218*t*
- noninvasive 849
- poorly differentiated 218, 851
- precursors 949
- stomach
  - development of 606*fc*
  - diffuse infiltrative type of 609*f*
  - spread of 610
- subdivision of 218
- type of 578
- ulcerative type of 787*f*
- well-differentiated 851

- Carcinosarcoma 218
- Cardiac amyloidosis 212
- Cardiac arrhythmia 290, 433
- Cardiac cirrhosis 135
- Cardiac dilation, secondary causes of 530
- Cardiac diseases 529
- Cardiac edema
  - mechanism of 131
  - pathogenesis of 131
- Cardiac emboli 156
- Cardiac failure 44, 151
  - congestive 463
- Cardiac hypertrophy 492
- Cardiac lesions 504
- Cardiac manifestations 867, 897
- Cardiac muscle 508
  - cells 91
  - fibers, coagulative necrosis of 514
  - hypertrophy of 38, 500
- Cardiac myocytes, coagulative necrosis of 540
- Cardiac myxoma 539, 539*f*
- Cardiac sclerosis 135
- Cardiac tamponade 139, 491, 533-536
- Cardiac thrombi 152
- Cardiac troponins 520
- Cardiac tumor, primary 539
- Cardiac valve 513
  - small thrombi on 150
- Cardiac valvular fibrosis 621
- Cardiobacterium 524
- Cardiogenic shock 139, 139*fc*, 144, 145, 519, 521
  - causes of 139
- Cardiomyopathy 150, 151, 528, 529
  - hypertrophic 529, 531
  - morphologic patterns of 530*f*
  - primary 529
  - restrictive 532
  - secondary 529
- Cardiovascular anomalies 283
- Cardiovascular disease 600, 748
- Cardiovascular disorders 479
- Cardiovascular dysfunction 303
- Cardiovascular surgery 437
- Cardiovascular system 112, 502, 870, 894
- Carditis 507
- Carnification 545
- Cartilage 217, 929
  - injury 929*f*
- Cartilaginous tumors 916, 920
  - subclassification of malignant 921*b*
- Cartridge-based nucleic acid amplification test 567
- Casal's necklace 304
- Caseating granuloma 560, 564
- Caseous necrosis 19
  - gross appearance of 20*f*
  - microscopic appearance of 20*f*
- Caseous pericarditis 534
- Casoni test 126
- Cassava root 872
- Castleman's disease 382
- Casts 461, 748
  - classification of 461*b*
- Catalase 32
- Cataracts 898
- Catarrhal inflammation 82
- Catecholamine 142
  - cardiomyopathy 906
  - release 904
  - secrete 907
- Cathepsin 249
  - histamine 552
- Catheter trauma 150
- Cationic trypsinogen gene, mutation in 697
- Cat-scratch disease 88
- Causative exogenous factors 556
- Causative organism 524, 547
  - identification of 476
- Caval lymph nodes 763
- Cecal tuberculosis, hyperplastic 616
- Celiac disease 596
- Cell 31, 78, 84, 319, 460, 464, 476, 484, 748, 749, 922
  - appearance of 369*f*
  - block technique 312, 314
  - chromosomal constitution of 277
  - counts 323, 463, 465
  - cycle 91, 92*f*, 235, 238*f*
    - arrest of 36
    - control of 238
    - dysregulation of 239
    - governor of 241
    - phases of 91
    - regulators 239
  - damage
    - mechanism of 34*f*
    - sensors of 62
  - death 16, 231, 254, 789
    - evasion of 247
    - mechanisms of 28
    - pathways of 27
  - derived mediators 73
  - destruction, antibody-mediated 174
  - division 233
  - free circulating tumor 267
  - function, antibody-mediated stimulation of 174
  - genome of 252
  - growth, stimulate 760
  - infection of 199, 200
  - injury 14, 15, 29*f*, 30, 32*f*, 36
    - biochemical mechanism of 28
    - causes of 15
    - etiology of 15
    - general principles of 28
    - mechanisms of 28
    - reversible 16
    - types of 16
  - loss 226
    - rate of 226
  - lung carcinomas, non-small 584
  - lysis 79
  - malignant 133, 251, 315*f*, 316*f*, 460, 464, 476, 852*f*
  - medium-sized 782
  - membrane 22, 173, 200
    - phospholipids 71
  - monotonous 766, 850
  - mummified 393
  - necrosis of 29
  - normal 247
  - oncogenes stimulate proliferation of 240
  - origin 70, 217, 218, 392, 592, 595, 611, 759, 955
    - normal products of 223
  - pleomorphism of 229
  - populations of 275
  - primary granules of mature 373
  - production 226
    - rate of 226
  - proliferation 91, 240, 602, 713, 881
    - prevent uncontrolled 240
    - steps in normal 234
    - sustained 256
    - uncontrolled 233
  - proportion of 226
  - regulatory 885
  - replicative senescence of 55*f*
  - shrinkage 24
  - surfaces, membrane receptors on 78
  - turnover, rapid 755
  - types of 91, 393*t*, 476, 476*t*, 764, 923
- Cell-mediated immunity 561, 562
  - development of 562
- Cellular adaptations 14, 38
  - types of 43*f*
- Cellular aging, mechanisms of 54, 57, 57*f*
- Cellular atypia 221
- Cellular cytotoxicity, antibody-dependent 167
- Cellular dysfunction, antibody-mediated 174, 176
- Cellular dysplasias 684
- Cellular elements 460, 468, 978
- Cellular enzymes 17
- Cellular hypoxia 141
- Cellular immunity 166, 504*f*
- Cellular masses 844
- Cellular membranes 666
- Cellular pathology 10
- Cellular pleomorphism 221, 222, 224, 766, 767*f*, 782
- Cellular proliferation 240, 721*f*, 789
- Cellular proteins 56, 667
- Cellular protrusions 460
- Cellular rejection, acute 185
- Cellular response 28, 61
  - types of 14*b*
- Cellular senescence 55, 247
  - mechanisms of 55
- Cellular swelling 16
- Cellularity 332, 338, 351, 380, 386, 449
  - mild-to-moderate 968
- Cellulitis 82
- Central conventional chondrosarcoma 921
- Central nervous system 19, 112, 119, 199, 201, 293, 333, 337, 679, 870, 894, 897, 966, 967
  - disease 203
  - disorder of 263, 960
  - pathogenesis of 201
  - primary tumors of 226
  - tumors of 634, 966
- Central processing system 297
- Central vein sclerosis 670
- Central venous congestion 136
- Centriacinar emphysema 548
- Centrifugation 324, 443
- Centrilobular emphysema 548
- Centrilobular regions 135, 670
  - congested 135
- Centroblasts 387
- Centrocytes 273, 387
- Cerebellar ataxia 870
- Cerebellar vermis 980
- Cerebellum 972, 974
- Cerebral arterial circulation 159
- Cerebral convexities 964
- Cerebral edema 159, 466
- Cerebral gummas 964
- Cerebral hemispheres 970, 975, 975*f*
  - coronal section of 968*f*
  - white matter of 971
- Cerebral vessels 144
- Cerebritis 961
- Cerebrospinal fluid 8, 228, 308, 310, 465, 960, 961
  - changes 962
  - collection, sites of 465
  - examination 375, 465, 466
  - findings 962, 963, 963*t*, 964, 965, 966
  - parameters 964
  - pleocytosis, moderate 963
  - pressure 466
  - protein 962
- Cerebrovascular accidents 892
- Cerebrovascular disease 292
- Cerebrovascular dysfunction 303
- Cerebrovascular stroke 891
- Ceruloplasmin 679
- Cervical cancer 203, 805
  - early detection of 12
  - etiology of 800
  - invasive 743
  - pathogenesis of 800
  - prevention 807
  - screening 807
- Cervical conization 807
- Cervical cytology 309, 311
- Cervical intraepithelial neoplasia 802, 805*f*
  - classification 803, 804
  - spectrum of 803*f*
- Cervical lymphadenitis 383
- Cervical precancer lesions, classification of 803
- Cervical smear 308, 311*f*
- Cervicitis 799, 800
  - acute 800
  - chronic 800
  - nonspecific 800
- Cervicofacial actinomycosis 121
- Cervix 42, 91, 799
  - barrel-shaped 805
  - carcinoma of 805
  - inflammations of 799
  - invasive carcinoma of 805
  - invasive squamous cell carcinoma of 806*f*
  - malignant neoplasms of 800
  - morphology of carcinoma of 805
  - premalignant neoplasms of 800
  - squamous cell carcinoma of 807*f*
- Cestode parasites 124
- Chalk stick-type fractures 914
- Chancre, primary 112*f*
- Charcot-Leyden crystals 555, 556, 556*f*
- Chédiak-Higashi syndrome 70
- Cheilosis, angular 304
- Chemical
  - adducts 667
  - agents 15
  - analysis 467

  carcinogenesis 254
  carcinogenicity of 255
  carcinogens 254, 255b, 256f, 684
    classification of 254
    mechanism of action of 255
    molecular targets of 255
  dust 556
  induced beta-cell dysfunction 883
  inflammation 693
  injury 61
  mediators 65, 67, 72, 74
    general properties of 73
  meningitis 960
  pathology 6
  substance 266
Chemokines 73, 76, 77, 86, 483, 484, 554, 668
Chemotactic factors 68
Chemotaxis 68, 69, 75, 77, 78, 891
Chemotherapeutic 36
Chemotherapeutic drugs 254
Chemotherapy 187, 261, 950
  effects 750
Chest
  barrel-shaped 551
  deformity 301
  pain 519, 541, 548, 583
  radiography 159
  syndrome, acute 354
  tightness, mild degree of 556
  wall injuries 159
Chicken-wire pattern 939
Chief cell hyperplasia 896
Child-Pugh classification 653
Child-Pugh score 653
Chills 432, 740
Chimeric antigen receptor T-cell therapy 140, 252
Chipmunk face 350
Chlamydia 800
  pneumoniae 481
  trachomatis 117, 788
Chlamydial infections 117
Chloasma 48
Chloride 962, 963
Chokes 160
Cholangiocarcinoma 260, 687
  risk of 681
Cholangitis 680
  acute 693
  chronic 680
Cholecystenteric fistula 695, 696
Cholecystitis 615, 693
  acute 693
    calculous 694
    emphysematous 694
    gaseous 694
    on chronic 695
  chronic 86, 693, 695
  gangrenous 694, 694f
  glandularis 695
Choledochoceles 698
Choledocholithiasis 689
Cholelithiasis 346, 688
Cholestasis 473, 474, 648, 662
  consequence of 649
Cholesterol 44, 46, 446, 480, 681, 688, 689, 690
  amounts of 692
  clefts 486f
  crystal 482
    nucleation, accelerated 691
    precipitation of 689
  esters 46
  excretion of 690
  gallstones, mixed 688, 692
  granulomas 873
  intracellular accumulation of 46
  lowering drug 480
  mixture of 688
  monohydrate 688
    crystals 691
  nucleation of 691
  rich macrophages 681
  stones 688, 689, 692
    mixed 689
    pathogenesis of 689, 690f
    pure 688, 692
    risk factors for 689
  supersaturation 690
  synthesis of 689
Cholesterolosis 46
Chondrocytes 922, 929, 929f, 930, 934f
  death of 929, 930f
  die 929
  injury 929
  proliferation of 929
Chondroid matrix 219f
Chondrosarcoma 218, 860, 921, 922f
Chordoid meningioma 976
Choriocarcinoma 227, 830, 834, 836, 838, 838f
Chorion villous biopsy samples 277
Chorionic gonadotropins 830
Chorionic villi 836
Choristoma 219, 283
Choroid plexus tumors 966, 967
Christmas disease 412
Chromaffin cells 904
  spindle-shaped 905, 945f
Chromaffin reaction 905
Chromatin
  components 72
  condensation 24
  fragmentation 24
  salt and pepper appearance of 620f
  texture 766
Chromium 290, 904
Chromogranin 267, 582, 620
Chromophobe renal cell carcinoma 761, 762, 762f
Chromosomal aberrations 275
  numerical 275
Chromosomal alterations 268
Chromosomal translocation 232, 390f, 399
Chromosomes 760, 763, 783, 896
  classification of 277
  complete set of 277
  ends 273
  non-disjunction of 282
  normal number of 275
  number 233, 275
  small segment on 181
  source of 277
  structural changes in 278
  total number of 275, 278
Chronic cholecystitis 86, 693, 695
  gross appearance of 695f
Chronic gastritis 598, 601f, 602
  complications of 600
Chronic glomerulonephritis 53, 734, 747
  causes of 734t
  gross appearance of 734f
Chronic granulomatous disease 559
Chronic hemolytic anemia 354
  features of 355
Chronic hepatitis 475, 656f, 659, 661, 662, 665f
  B 653, 663, 663f, 708
  C 653, 663
  causes of 662t
  clinical features of 663
Chronic immune thrombocytopenic purpura 408
  clinical features of 408
Chronic inflammation 60, 60t, 83, 84, 86, 91, 230, 260, 696, 873
  causes of 83
Chronic inflammatory
  cells 558, 559f, 740f, 962
  diseases, treatment of 77
  disorder 926
  infiltrate 627, 703, 741
  reaction 84, 253
  state 230
Chronic kidney disease 712, 736, 746, 746b, 747
  causes of 746
  complications of 748
Chronic liver disease 475, 653, 683, 684
  frequency of 660
Chronic obstructive pulmonary disease 548, 553, 600, 602
Chronic pancreatitis 696, 702, 702f, 703
  complications of 703, 704b
Chronic rheumatic heart disease 503, 504f, 506, 525
  complications of 507
Chrysotile 572
Churg-Strauss syndrome 496
Chylomicrons 44
Chylous 463
  fluid 463
Chyluria 451
Chymotrypsinogen 697
Cicatrization, zone of 604
Ciliary dyskinesia, primary 557
Ciliary function, lack of 557
Circulation, invasion of 250
Cirrhosis 474, 653, 664, 673, 673f, 675, 676f, 677, 677f, 679, 680, 681, 861
  alcoholic 600, 670, 672, 689
  alcohol-related 602, 665f
  classification of 674b
  complications of 708
  mechanisms of 667, 668
  micronodular 670, 674, 679
  microscopic features of 709
  mixed 674
  morphological classification of 674f
  risk of 659, 666
Cirsoid aneurysm 488
Cisplatin 254
Cisternal puncture 465
Citrate phosphate dextrose 426
  adenine 323, 426
Classical macrophage activation, mediators of 85
Clean surgical wound, healing of 99
Clean-catch specimen 451
Clear cell 818
  carcinoma 760, 819
  meningioma 976
  renal cell carcinoma 761, 762f
    cut section of 761f
  renal tumors 759
  solid alveolar arrangement of 762f
  tumors 818
Clofibrate 689
Clonal hematopoiesis 481, 482
Clonorchis sinensis 692, 697
Clostridium
  difficile 82
  perfringens 21
Clot 153
  formation 137, 466
  retraction test 418
  stabilization 147
Cloudy purulent 962, 965
Clubbing 537
Coagulation 420t
  abnormalities 416
  component 417
    tests for 418
  defect 413
  disorders 409, 413, 419
    acquired 410, 414
    classification of 410b
  factors, consumption of 421
  pathway 79
    activation of 513
  products of 79
  studies 323
  system, activation of 37, 141, 142, 698
  systemic activation of 414
  tests 414
Coagulative necrosis 17, 59, 163, 515f, 740
Coagulopathy 429, 652
Coal dust 49
Coal macule 570
Coal nodule 570
Coal-worker's pneumoconiosis 548, 570, 570f
  pathogenesis of 570
Cobalamin 334
Cobblestone appearance 625f
Cobra venom 79
Cob-web appearance 466
Cocarcinogens 801
Coccidioides immitis 902
Coccidioidomycosis 204
Codman's triangle 918f, 919, 920f
Codons 272
Cohesive neoplastic epithelial cells 849
Cola-colored urine 718, 719
Cold
  abscess 913, 914
  antibody 357
    immunohemolytic anemia 360
  common 289
  hemolysin 357, 360
  sores 116
  thyroid nodules 879
Colicky abdominal pain 621
Colicky flank, severe 756
Colitis, progressive 627
Collagen 105
  bands 394
  degradation of 487, 929
  formation 571
    stimulates 679

  progressive deposition of 195
  synthesis of 487, 489
  vascular diseases 188
Collagenous connective tissue 832
Collagenous scar 604
Collar-stud abscess 383
Colliquative necrosis 18
Colloid 754
  accumulation of 872
  cysts 872, 873
  extravasation 866
  goiter 871, 872
  involution, phase of 872
  nodules 873
  osmotic pressure 130, 722
Colon 618, 619, 626, 640
  adenocarcinoma of 249, 635
  cancer 301, 638*f*
    investigation of 640
  carcinogenesis 639*f*
  carcinoma of 245, 635, 641*f*
  familial polyposis of 636
  polyps of 630
  precancerous lesions of 637*f*
  villous adenoma of 230
Colonic adenocarcinoma, risk of 631
Colonic adenomas 632, 634
Colonic cancer 637
  pathogenesis of 645
Colonic epithelial cell 618
Colony forming unit 321
Colony stimulating factors 169
Colorectal adenocarcinoma 635
Colorectal adenomas 632
Colorectal cancer 628, 634, 636*fc*, 637, 640
  incidence of 635
  risk factors for 635*b*
Colton system 422
Columnar cells 593, 872
Columnar epithelial cells 556
Columnar metaplasia 42, 59
Columnar mucosa 224, 596
Columnar tumor cells 854
Coma 541, 889
Commensal flora breaches skin, normal 118
Commissures, fusion of 507
Compact bone 935
Complement fixation, antibody-mediated 213
Complement system 78
  activation, pathways of 78
  functions of 78*f*
  regulation of 79
Complementary recurrent driver mutations 371
Complete blood counts 325, 327*t*
Complete hydatidiform mole 836*f*, 838
Complete mole 834, 836, 837
  complications of 836
Complex branching papillae 821, 877
Complex polysaccharides 79
Complex sclerosing lesion 844
Compound nevus 954
Compression atelectasis 585
Concentration tests 471, 472
Condyloma acuminatum 801
Condylomata lata 113
Cone biopsy 805
Confusion 890
Congenital cardiac anomaly 281, 537
Congenital fibropolycystic diseases 687
Congenital heart disease 525, 536
  causes of 536
  classification of 536*b*
  late cyanotic 537
  type of 536
Congestion 134-136, 155, 355, 543
  acute 134
    pulmonary 134
  chronic
    passive 164
    venous 134, 134*fc*, 135, 135*f*, 135*fc*, 136*f*, 136*fc*, 501
Congestive splenomegaly, chronic 398
Conjugated bilirubin 646, 647, 649, 650
  level 648
  part of 647
Conjugation 646
Conjunctivitis 617
Connective tissue
  abnormal synthesis of 489
  cells 76
  degradation 489
  deposition of 91, 94, 96
  disease 188, 195, 491
  metaplasia 42
  mucin 53
  remodeling of 97
  replacement 82*fc*, 83
  stroma 551
Conservative missense mutation 273
Constipation 870
Constrictive pericarditis 130, 534, 535
Consumptive coagulopathy 414
Contact dermatitis 179
Contraceptive drugs, use of 816
Contractile dysfunction 521
Contractile proteins, increased risk of 39
Contraction
  atelectasis 585
  band necrosis 519
Contractures 412
Contralateral ovary 823, 833
Conventional cytogenetics 277
Conventional osteosarcoma 917, 918
  gross appearance of 918*f*
  histological patterns of 919
Conventional papillary thyroid carcinoma 876
Convulsions 962
Coomb's test 329, 346, 359, 359*f*
Copious foul-smelling sputum 558
Copper
  increased urinary excretion of 680
  metabolism 491
    disorder of 679
  sulfate 455
Cor pulmonale 502, 551
Coronary artery 159, 509, 515*f*
  atherosclerosis 511*f*, 512, 530, 892
  disease 134, 509
  occlusion 513
Coronary blood flow 509, 510
Coronary lumen, complete occlusion of 513
Coronary ostia 490
Coronary syndrome, acute 509, 511, 511*f*
Coronary vessels 144
Cortical atrophy 900
Cortical fibrosis 741
Cortical hyperplasia, primary 899
Cortical necrosis 748
Cortical neurons, loss of 964
Cortical surface 749
Corticosteroids 75, 98
  high-dose 602
  therapy 727
Corticotroph hyperplasia 899
Cortisone 895
Corynebacterium diphtheriae 82, 115
Cotton emboli 161
Cough 502, 551, 556, 583
  persistent productive 552
  prominent 547
  reflex 541
Councilman body 661
COVID-19 pandemic 546
Coxsackie
  B 884
  virus 866
C-peptide assay 895
Cranial nerve tumors 967
Craniofacial skeleton, enlargement of 914
Craniopharyngiomas 966
Craniotabes 300
C-reactive protein 90, 141, 481, 508, 701, 889
Creatine kinase 514, 520
Creatinine 324, 750
  clearance 472
  serum levels of 194
Creola bodies 556, 556*f*
Crescendo angina 512
Crescentic glomerulonephritis 721*f*
  electron microscopic appearance of 721*f*
Cretinism 869
Crigler-Najjar syndrome 650
Crisis, types of 354
Critical proteins, secretion of 47
Critical stenosis 485, 510
Crohn disease 5, 88, 600, 621, 622, 624, 624*f*, 625, 625*f*, 626*f*, 629, 629*t*, 645, 689, 690
Crooke hyaline changes 900
Crossmatch techniques 427, 427*b*
Crowded gland architecture 811, 812
Crush
  cytology 307
  injuries 158
  preparation 307
  smear cytology 315
Cryoglobulinemic vasculitis 496
Cryoprecipitate 428, 429
  indications for 429
Crypt 627
  abscess 627, 628*f*
  destructive, chronic 626
Cryptitis 627
Cryptococci, polysaccharide capsule of 119
Cryptococcosis 119, 204
Cryptococcus neoformans 119
Cryptogenic lung abscesses, primary 547
Cryptorchid testes 776
Cryptorchidism 774, 774*f*, 776, 798
  diagnosis of 774
Cryptosporidiosis 204
Crystalline 571
  cholesterol monohydrate 688
Cuboidal epithelium 821*f*
Culture-negative endocarditis 524
Cumulative solar damage, melanomas with 957
Cupric sulfate 456
Curling ulcers 597
Curschmann's spirals 556*f*
Cushing's disease 899
Cushing's syndrome 262, 263, 407, 456, 762, 899, 899*f*, 900, 901, 904
  clinical manifestation of 900*f*
Cushing's ulcers 597
Cutaneous squamous cell 950
Cyanmethemoglobin 439, 440
  method 439, 440
Cyanosis 134, 558
  mild 553
Cyclic citrullinated peptides, antibody against 927
Cyclin-dependent kinase inhibitor 238, 258, 917
Cyclins
  D genes, overexpression of 239
  normal role of 238
  role of 238*f*
Cyclooxygenase 74, 75, 638
  inhibitors 75
  pathway 74*f*
    products of 75
Cyclophosphamide 254, 767
Cylindrical aneurysm 488, 488*f*
Cylindrical bronchiectasis 557
Cylindroids 461
Cyst 752, 843
  amebic 618
  formation, mechanisms of 752*f*
  medullary diseases with 753
  numerous 752
  rupture of 126
  simple 843
  spherical 127
  stage 618
  wall 821*f*
Cystadenocarcinoma 841
Cystadenofibroma 819
Cystadenoma 217, 819
  benign
    mucinous 823
    serous 820
Cystic duct, obstruction of 693
Cystic fibrosis 53, 557, 702
  transmembrane regulator gene 697
Cystic kidneys 753
Cystic larvae 125
Cystic medial degeneration 489
Cystic spaces 573, 593, 923*f*
Cystic structure 758, 843
Cystic teratoma
  benign 826, 827
  mature 826
Cysticerci, ingestion of 125
Cysticercosis 124
Cysticercus cellulosae 125
Cystine 755
  stones 755, 756, 756*f*
Cystitis 737, 792
Cystocele 757
Cytocentrifuge 312

Cytochemistry 266, 372, 374, 378, 378*t*
Cytochrome C 24, 59
prevent leakage of 25
Cytogenetics 277, 307, 377, 387, 389
abnormalities 281
assays 287
disorder 281, 283
techniques of 277
Cytogenomic array technology 287
Cytokeratin 266, 880
Cytokines 73, 75-77, 94, 140, 150, 169, 172, 183, 261, 391, 484, 668, 889
effects of 140
interleukin-1, stimulates production of 63
mediated cell death 864
mediated inflammation 926
production 62
release syndrome 140
secretion of 554
storm 141
Cytologic atypia 781, 811, 815, 821, 824, 949
low-grade 766, 766*f*
severe 860
Cytological disorders 766
Cytological examination 265
disadvantages of 266
Cytology
applications of 306
diagnostic role of 306
techniques 315
Cytomegalovirus 187, 204, 481, 598, 738, 884
Cytopathology 7, 306
Cytoplasm 87, 336, 387, 582, 761, 769, 777, 778, 804, 843, 881, 905
abundant 84, 505, 778, 829
clear halo of 971
ranges 795
Cytoplasmic blebs, formation of 24
Cytoplasmic membranes 778*f*
Cytoskeletal abnormalities 33
Cytoskeletal proteins 725
accumulation of 47
Cytosolic calcium 34, 34*f*
mechanism of increased 34
Cytosolic enzyme 474
Cytotoxin 260, 599
Cytotrophoblasts 837

D

Damage associated molecular patterns 62, 165
Damaged gastric epithelial cells, restitution of 601
Daughter cell 93
D-dimer test 416
De novo pathway 931
De Quervain thyroiditis 865
Dead tissue, indistinct outline of 17
Deafness 870
Death
causes of 194, 412, 492, 672*f*, 678, 681, 892
inducing proteins 25
receptor 26
pathway 24, 27, 247
Debakey classification 491
Debris 69, 487
Decompression sickness 159
forms of 160
Decubitus ulcers 98
Deep fibromatosis 940
Deep leg veins 156
Deep soft tissues 938, 943
Deep tissue, leiomyoma of 942
Deep venous thrombosis 130, 134, 150, 164, 611
Deeper nevus cells 954
Deep-seated cancers, complications of 155
Defensins 563
Degenerative calcific valvular diseases 525
Dehydration 99, 889
severe 889, 890
Delayed hemolytic transfusion reactions 433
Delayed hypersensitivity reaction 214, 560
Delayed nonimmunological iron overload 434
Dementia 113
Den Bergh Diazo reaction 473
Dendritic cells 73, 76, 166, 168, 191, 200, 202, 202*f*, 554
Dendritic melanocytes 954*f*
Denervation atrophy 41
Dense collagen bundles 686
Dense deposit disease 728, 729, 730, 730*f*, 731
electron microscopic appearance of 730*f*
Dense fibromatous stroma 825
Dense inflammatory infiltrate 928
Dense lymphoplasmacytic inflammation 490
Dense stromal fibrosis 705
Dental
abnormalities 898
lamina 595
Denys-Drash syndrome 763
Deoxyribonucleic acid 656
damage 33, 34, 54, 244, 260
methylation 234
microarray 269
mismatch repair gene, role of 638
molecular analysis of 351
repair 54
genes 252, 253
segment of 272
sequencing 269
synthesis 334
virus 251, 259
Deoxythymidine monophosphate 336
Deoxyuridine monophosphate, conversion of 336
Depression 304
Dermal nevus 954, 954*f*
Dermatologic disorders 263
Dermatopathic lymphadenitis 382
Dermis, superficial 949
Dermo-epidermal junction 954, 954*f*
Dermoid cyst 817, 826, 827*f*, 828
Dermopathy 869
Desçemet's membrane 680
Desmin 266, 267
Desmoid 102
fibromatosis 940, 941*f*
tumors 634
Desmoplasia 216, 687, 850, 852*f*, 854
Desmosomal junctional proteins 531
Desmosome 531
Destructive free radical 71
Destructive lytic lesions 925
Destructive stromal invasion 819
Dexamethasone 900
suppression test 900
Dextrocardia 557
Dextrose 426
Diabetes insipidus 451, 453
Diabetes mellitus 47, 53, 98, 180, 209, 292, 299, 451, 455, 456, 481, 679, 689, 703, 716, 723, 735, 737*f*, 813, 882, 883, 884, 884*f*, 885, 887-889, 891, 891*f*, 892, 893, 895, 895*t*, 896, 909
chronic
complications of 890
manifestations of 884
classification of 883*b*, 890*b*
clinical features of 887
complications of 890, 891, 896
development of 886*fc*
diagnosis of 882, 888, 893
gestational 883
laboratory diagnosis of 893
long-standing 892
pathogenesis of 883, 885, 885*fc*
prevalence of 882
renal changes in 735
secondary 900
stages of 884
types of 883, 890
Diabetic dyslipidemia 891
Diabetic glomerulopathy, sign of 736
Diabetic glomerulosclerosis 737*f*
Diabetic ketoacidosis 457, 888-890
pathogenesis of 889*fc*
Diabetic ketonuria 457
Diabetic kidney 735
Diabetic macrovascular disease 891, 892
Diabetic microvascular disease 890
Diabetic mononeuropathy 893
Diabetic nephropathy 735, 736, 736*f*, 737*b*, 890, 892
glomeruli 735*f*
pathognomonic of 736
Diabetic neuropathy 893
Diabetic retinopathy 890-892
Diabetic ulcers 103
Diacetic acid 457
Diaphragm 574, 618
Diaphysis 910
Diarrhea 212, 290, 304, 621
bloody 290, 618, 626
mild 626
Diego system 422
Dietary carcinogens, consumption of 605
Dietary fiber, low intake of 635
Differential leukocyte count 443
Diffuse alveolar damage 160, 585, 586, 734
Diffuse astrocytoma, microscopic appearance of 968*f*, 969*f*
Diffuse idiopathic pulmonary neuroendocrine cell hyperplasia 577
Diffuse large B-cell lymphoma 388, 388*f*
Diffuse mesangial sclerosis 735
Diffuse nontoxic goiter 872, 872*f*
Diffuse pontine astrocytoma 966
Diffuse pulmonary interstitial fibrosis 573, 574
Diffuse systemic sclerosis 194
DiGeorge syndrome 197
Digest cell 17
Digestive enzymes 699
Dihydrotestosterone 789
synthesis of 789, 790*f*
Dilated duct 843, 844
Dilated subepidermal blood vessels 952
Dilution test 471, 472
Dimethylaminoazobenzene 255
Diminished glomerular filtration rate 716
Dimorphic anemia 340
peripheral blood smear of 341*f*
Dimorphic fungi 120
Diphtheria 115
cutaneous 115
toxoid 115
Diploid chorionic epithelial cells 834
Dipstick method 893
Dipyridamole 410
Direct antiglobulin test 346 , 360
uses of 360
Direct endothelial injury 65
Direct hyperbilirubinemia 650*t*
Direct mucosal injury 602
Direct trauma 699
Direct Van Den Bergh reaction 473
Directly injure mucosal epithelium 598
Dissecting hematoma 488, 488*f*
Disseminated cancers 152
Disseminated intravascular coagulation 142, 143, 155, 324, 414, 414*b*, 415*f*, 421
consequence of 415
Distal acinar emphysema 549
Distal bile duct tumors 687
Distal convoluted tubule 712, 760
Distal femur 924
giant cell tumor of 924*f*
Distal interphalangeal joints 928, 931
Distal symmetric polyneuropathy 893
Distal ulcers 603
Distal urethra 738
Distant metastasis 642, 857
Distinct cell membrane 778
Distinctive germ cell tumor 782
Disulfide bonds 32
Disuse atrophy 41
Diuretic therapy 451
Divalent metal transporter 331
Diverse genetic aberrations 576
Diverse microorganisms 140
Dizziness 888, 890
Dombrok system 422
Dominant cells 85
Dominant disorders, X-linked 280
Donath-Landsteiner antibodies 360
Donor
blood, testing of 425
sample 435
selection 425
testing 430
Dopa-oxidase reaction 957
Double-barreled aorta 491
Double-contrast barium enema 641

Down syndrome 5, 275, 281, 282, 371, 536, 883
  clinical features of 282*f*
Downstream pathways, activation of 236
D-penicillamine 190
Drabkin solution
  constituents of 440*t*
  detergent-modified 439
Driver mutations 232, 371, 575, 876*f*, 879*t*, 968
Dropout necrosis 661
Drug-induced hemolytic anemia 174
Drugs 15, 541, 652
  hypersensitivity vasculitis 496
Dry fixation 312
Dry gangrene 21, 22, 22*f*, 22*t*
Dry tap 448
  causes of 448
Dubin-Johnson syndrome 651
  diagnosis of 473
Ductal adenocarcinoma 793
Ductal breast cancer, development of 848*f*
Ductal carcinoma 855
  in situ 845, 848, 848*f*, 849, 850*f*, 855*f*
Ductal hyperplasia, atypical 844, 848*f*
Ductal reserve cell 592
Ducts
  adenocarcinoma 704
  epithelium 703
  lining of 842
  obstruction 703
  smaller 681
Ductular reactions 653
Ductus arteriosus, normal function of 538
Duffy system 422
Duke criteria, modified 527
Duodenal epithelial cell 331*f*
Duodenal peptic ulcer 605*t*
Duodenal ulcer 597, 602, 603*f*, 605
Duodenum 600, 603, 694
Durck granuloma 128
Dyscohesive cells 853, 854*f*
Dysfunctional cardiac valves 326
Dysgerminoma 218, 778, 826, 828, 830
  morphology of 829
Dysglycemia 884
Dyshormonogenetic goiter 870, 872
Dyskinetic ciliary syndromes 557
Dyslipidemia 896
Dysmenorrhea 810
Dysmorphic red cells 719
Dysmorphology 280
Dyspareunia 810
Dysphagia 873
Dysplasia 224, 230, 553, 578*f*, 590, 596, 597, 600, 794, 799
  low-grade 633*f*
  severe 578*f*
Dysplastic epithelium 634*f*
Dysplastic nodules 684
  high-grade 684
  low-grade 684
Dysplastic squamous epithelium 785
Dyspnea 159, 325, 433, 501, 551, 553, 556, 558, 574
Dystrophic calcification 50, 52*t*, 59, 485
  focal zones of 978
  significance of 51
Dysuria 797, 810

E

Early gastric carcinoma 607
  subclassification of 608*f*
E-cadherin
  dysfunction of 853
  function, loss of 249, 607
  gene 270, 849
   mutations of 849
  lack of 849
Ecchymosis 138, 324
Echinococcosis 125
Echinococcus granulosus 125
  life cycle of 125*f*
E-cigarette 292
Ectocervix 799
Ectocyst 126
Ectoderm 219, 779
Ectodermal derivatives 781
Ectopic adrenocorticotropic hormone secretion 900
Ectopic gastric mucosa 600
Ectopic hormones 223
Ectopic pregnancy 437, 838, 839
  sites of 839
Ectopic thyroid 866
Ectopic tissues, tumors of 574
Eczema 197
Edema 64, 95*f*, 129, 131, 133, 134, 144, 155, 195, 295, 542, 552, 722, 901, 927
  causes of 129
  fluid 133
   types of 129
  impairs tissue perfusion 142
  mechanism of generalized 131*fc*, 132*fc*
  nonpitting 855
  pathogenesis of 130
  pathophysiologic of 129, 130*t*
  peripheral 296
  special forms of 129*t*
Effusions 310, 462
  lymphoma, primary 259
Eggshell calcification 571
Ehlers-Danlos syndrome 491
Ehrlich's aldehyde
  reagent 11, 460
  test 11, 460
Eicosanoids 74, 75
Eikenella 524
Eisenmenger syndrome 537
Ejection murmur, systolic 531
Elastase 552
  from neutrophils, release of 588
Elastin
  stain 97
  synthesis of 489
Elbows 506
Electrolyte disturbances 145, 628, 902
Electron
  dense deposits 733
  microscope 24, 267, 718
   examination 226
  microscopy 5, 178, 205, 267, 286, 581, 582, 721, 724, 725, 727, 729, 733, 736, 905
Electrophoresis 323
  monoclonal spike on 398
Elephantiasis 126, 126*f*, 132*f*, 133
Elevated serum transaminases, causes of 473*t*
Ellipsoid cytoplasmic inclusions 127*f*
Emboli 156, 514
  classification of 156*t*
  flow of 156
  formation of 525
  physical nature of 155
  small 526
  types of 155
Embolism 155, 485, 490
Embolization 155
Embryo 10
  dies 834
Embryonal carcinoma 777, 779, 826, 830
Embryonal cells 779
Embryonal rhabdomyosarcoma 942
Embryonal tumor 219, 219*t*, 967, 973
  malignant primary 763
  type of 219
Embryonic skeletal muscle 942
Embryonic stem cells 93
Embryonic yolk sac 84
Emotional stress 509
Emphysema 502, 548, 551*f*
  classification of 550
  etiopathogenesis of 549
  focal 582
  forms of 551
  microscopy of 551*f*
  pathogenesis of 550*f*
  types of 548, 549*b*, 549*f*
Empty ovum, fertilization of 834, 835*f*
Empyema 545
Encapsulated angioinvasive follicular carcinoma 879, 880*f*
Encephalopathy, ischemic 485
Encrustation hypothesis 482
Endarteritis, proliferative 112
Endemic cretinism 870
Endemic mycoses 118
Endobronchial tuberculosis 565
Endocardial fibroelastosis 532
Endocardial mural plaque 531
Endocarditis 150, 504*f*, 505, 545
  acute 524, 524*t*
   infective 524
  bacterial 150, 527*f*
  subacute 524*t*
  type of 529
Endocardium 150, 505
Endocervical cells, malignant 806
Endocrine
  abnormalities 748
  amyloid 209
  disorders 156, 748, 863
  gland 209
  hyperplasia, asymptomatic stage of 907
  insufficiency 261
  organs 679
  pancreas 619
  stimulation, loss of 41
  tumors 209, 908
Endocrinopathies 263, 883
Endocyst 126
Endocytosis 561
Endoderm 219, 779
  elements 781
Endodermal sinus tumor 829, 830
Endogenous anticoagulants, actions of 415
Endogenous antigens 170, 173, 716
Endogenous antioxidants 32
Endogenous glucose production 886
Endogenous hormone exposure 845
Endogenous toxic plasma lipid components 83
Endometrial adenocarcinomas 815
Endometrial aspiration smear 311
Endometrial atypical hyperplasia 811, 812*f*
Endometrial carcinoma 260, 812
  clinical features of 815
  precursor of 810
  soil for 810
Endometrial cavity 815*f*
Endometrial epithelial tumors 812
Endometrial glands 807, 808, 810, 810*f*
  proliferation of 811
Endometrial hyperplasia 230, 810, 811, 811*b*, 811*f*, 813, 841
  classification of 810
  types of 810
Endometrial implants 809
Endometrial intraepithelial neoplasia 811
Endometrial stroma 808
Endometrial stromal precursor cells 817
Endometrioid carcinoma 813*f*, 814, 819, 824, 825
  pathogenesis of 825
Endometrioid endometrial
  adenocarcinoma 814*f*
   development of 813*f*
  carcinoma 813
Endometrioid intraepithelial neoplasia 811, 812*f*
Endometrioid tumors 818
Endometriosis 808, 809, 818, 825
  development of 819*f*
  proposed origin of 809
  sites of 809*b*
  types of 808
Endometrium 41, 228, 845
  background 812
  endometrioid adenocarcinoma of 814*f*
Endomyocardial fibrosis 532
Endonucleases 35
Endophytic cervical carcinoma 806*f*
Endoplasmic reticulum 16, 23, 34, 35, 35*f*
  stress 35
Endoscopy biopsy 265
Endothelial activation 76, 150
Endothelial anticoagulant factors, reduce production of 142
Endothelial cell 67, 75, 57, 96*f*, 143*f*, 147, 150, 185*f*, 510, 513, 891
  activation 142, 142*fc*, 143*f*, 151
  bind thrombin 147
  contraction of 65
  damage, widespread 415
  ingrowth of 155
  injury 585
  proliferation of 730*f*
  surface of 77
  swelling of 718
  synthesize tissue factors 149
  tight junctions 142
Endothelial damage 148, 150, 186*f*
Endothelial dysfunction 482, 483, 749

Endothelial injury 149, 149*f*, 150, 482, 483*f*
produce 482
sites of 152
triggers of 482
widespread severe 415
Endothelial leukocyte adhesion 68*t*
Endothelial protein C receptor 147
Endothelin 510
Endothelium 66, 67, 77, 151, 711, 891
antithrombotic
activities of 150
properties of 149*t*
functions of normal 147
gene expression in 150
increase procoagulant activity of 76
prothrombotic
activities of 150
properties of 149*t*
Endotoxin release 293
Endotracheal tuberculosis 565
End-stage renal disease 433, 731, 740, 892
Energy balance 297
Engulfment 70
Entamoeba histolytica 3, 475, 617, 682
Enteric fever 613
Enteric infections, frequency of 622
Enterobacter 738, 772
Enterohepatic circulation 649
Enteropathy, protein-losing 132
Enteroviruses 962
Envelope glycoproteins 654
Environmental antigens 554
reactions against 170
Environmental arthritogenic agents 926
Environmental diseases 288
Environmental pollution 288
Environmental toxins 846
Enzymatic antioxidants 32
Enzymatic defects, hereditary 872
Enzymatic fat necrosis 20, 700, 700*f*
Enzyme 119, 120, 473, 474, 784, 790
defects 872
deficiencies 326
formation of 79
glucocerebrosidase, deficiency of 286
glucuronidase 255
marker, nonspecific 520
rich fluid 699
system 664
Enzyme-linked immunosorbent assay 205
Eosinophilia 368, 368*f*, 380
causes of 368*t*
Eosinophilic cytoplasm 593, 805
moderate amount of 816
Eosinophilic epithelial cells 594*f*
Eosinophilic fibrillary material 906
Eosinophilic granular bodies 972
Eosinophilic granulomatosis 496
Eosinophilic intranuclear inclusions 878
Eosinophilic nucleoli, prominent 392
Eosinophils 86, 166, 319, 321, 393, 394*f*, 554, 555*f*, 556, 556*f*, 748
cationic protein 554
count 556
numerous 555
recruitment of 555*f*
Ependymal tumors 972
Ependymoma 228, 966, 972, 980
anaplastic 973
classification of 972
grading of 972
microscopic appearance of 973*f*
Epicardial coronary arteries 509
Epidemic typhus 117
Epidermal cysts 103, 634
Epidermal growth factor 242, 790
receptor 576
Epidermal keratinocytes, malignant tumor of 950
Epidermal melanocytes 953
Epidermal tumors, malignant 949
Epidermis 92*f*, 110*f*, 391, 855*f*
basal layer of 956*f*
epithelial cells of 127*f*
Epigenetic abnormalities 637, 639
acquired 793
Epigenetic alterations 215, 371
Epigenetic changes 234, 597
Epigenetic modifications 233
Epilepsy 961
Epinephrine 889, 904
Epiphysis 910, 911, 919
Epistaxis 408
Epithelial barrier 165, 601
Epithelial cells 127, 218, 219*f*, 314, 315*f*, 460, 550, 585, 593*f*, 616, 721*f*, 760, 791, 793, 813, 846, 865, 868, 946*f*
atypical 794
component 946
crowding of 868
death of 790, 790*f*
depletion of 863
increased number of 789
layers of 710
necrosis of 617
proliferation of 792*f*, 819
specialized 299
stratification of 824
Epithelial changes 100, 859
Epithelial damage 696
Epithelial defects 622
Epithelial dysplasia 632, 633
Epithelial elements 592
combinations of 683
Epithelial hyperplasia 844
degree of 844
Epithelial keratin pearls 580
Epithelial metaplasia 42, 299, 625
Epithelial mucin 53
Epithelial myoepithelial tumors 845
Epithelial proliferation 99*f*
Epithelial regeneration 602, 745
Epithelial stem cells 93
Epithelial stratification 821*f*
Epithelial tissues 224
components 592
Epithelial tumors 217, 574, 577, 801, 818, 819*f*
cells
clusters of 854
primitive 830, 830*f*
classification of 818
malignant 596, 635, 876
mixed 812, 818
Epithelioid cells 20*f*, 87, 87*f*, 315*f*, 563
aggregates of 180*f*
Epithelioid granuloma 964
noncaseating 680
Epithelioid macrophages 564, 568
Epithelium 601*f*, 842
bronchial 582
differentiation of 818
endocervical type of 824*f*
hyperplastic 632*f*
intestinal type of 824*f*
nests of 595
proliferation of 818, 843
superficial layers of 804*f*
thickened 785
Epstein-Barr nuclear antigen 259, 371
Epstein-Barr virus 251, 258, 259*b*, 389, 405, 590, 606
Erosion 565, 643
superficial 511
Erythema 855
marginatum 504*f*, 506
nodosum leprosum 110
Erythematous eruption 856
Erythroblastosis 358
Erythroblasts 334
Erythrocyte 321
count 324
sedimentation rate 383, 401, 445, 446*f*, 447, 447*t*, 489, 661, 913
estimation, indications for 447, 447*b*
stages of 446
Erythrocytosis 381, 687
Erythroferrone 350
Erythroid 379
hyperplasia 342, 351
precursors 320
Erythroplakia 589, 590
Erythropoiesis 320, 332, 338, 338*f*, 340, 351, 380, 386, 409, 449
megaloblastic type of 338*f*
normal 320
stages of 322*f*
Erythropoietin 320
levels 382
Esbach's albuminometer 454*f*
Escherichia coli 738, 772, 911, 961, 980
Esophageal cancer 596
type of 596
Esophageal dysmotility 194
Esophageal squamous mucosa 595
Esophageal varices 678
Esophageal webs 333
Esophagogastric junction 676
Esophagus 575, 595, 955
gastroesophageal junction of 603
middle-third of 596
squamous epithelium of 42
Estrogen 260, 689, 790*f*, 813, 814, 831, 845, 847, 899
antagonists, benefits of 848
endogenous source of 811
exogenous source of 811
nuclear receptors for 267
receptor 848
reduced hepatic catabolism of 677
role of 790, 847
secretion 831
Estrogenic stimulation, produce prolonged 845
Ethanol 664, 666
impairs 667
metabolism 664, 666*f*
oxidizing system 666
Ethylenediaminetetraacetic acid 321, 444
Eumycetoma 120
Euthyroid metabolic state 871
Ewing sarcoma 924, 925*f*
gross appearance of 925*f*
X-ray of 926*f*
Excision biopsy 265
Excretion, reduced 931
Exertional angina 510
Exfoliated cells
sampling of 309
sources of 308*b*
Exfoliative cytology 12, 265, 271, 306, 307
basis of 307
Exocrine glands 194
Exocrine pancreatic defects 883
Exocrine parenchyma 702
Exoerythrocytic stage 122
Exogenous antigens 170, 173, 716, 717
Exogenous antioxidants 32
Exogenous carcinogen 229
Exogenous drugs, enzymatic metabolism of 30
Exogenous glucocorticoids 98
Exogenous hormone exposure 846
Exogenous insulin, requirement of 888
Exogenous pigments 48, 49
Exogenous substances 553, 683, 684
Exophthalmos 869*f*, 873
Exophytic carcinoma cervix 806*f*
Exophytic growth 579, 591*f*
Exophytic tumor, large 769*f*
Expression 183
Extensive mucinous ascites 824
External callus 934
External therapeutic radiation 918
Extra-abdominal fibromatosis 940
Extracardiac lesions 506
Extracellular collagenous matrix 713
Extracellular fibrillar networks 72
Extracellular fluid 743
Extracellular hyaline 52
Extracellular lipid 484
Extracellular matrix 77, 91, 96, 148, 173, 249, 484, 486*f*
excessive amounts of 102
invasion of 249
proteins 891
proteolysis of 550*f*
synthesis of 891
Extracellular mucin 854
Extracellular proteolytic enzymes 929*f*
Extracellular stroma, loose 944
Extracorpuscular abnormalities 326, 343
Extragenital tumors 833
Extraglandular disease 194
Extragonadal germ cell tumors 283
Extrahepatic biliary tract 696
Extrahepatic disorders 136
Extraintestinal disease 618
Extraintestinal lesions 614
Extralobular terminal duct 842
Extraluminal obstruction 743
Extramedullary disease 374

Extramedullary hematopoiesis 320, 350, 356, 380, 381
Extramedullary infiltration 374, 376
Extranodal lymphoma 384
Extranodal sites 389
Extrapancreatic fat 700
Extrapancreatic lesions 700
Extraparenchymal renal cysts 751
Extrapulmonary disease 913
Extrathyroidal tissue 868
Extrauterine stem 809
Extravascular hemolysis 343, 44, 344t, 345, 349
Extravascular red cell hemolysis 648
Extravascular tissue 68, 80
Extremities 485
Extrinsic abnormalities 326, 343
Extrinsic pathway 247, 415
  functions of 27, 27b
Extrinsic vessel compression 161
Exuberant granulation 102, 102f
Exudate 64, 65, 65t, 463, 464, 961
Eyeball, abnormal protrusion of 869
Eyes 194, 628, 679, 882, 977
  lesions 680
  disorder of 960
  uvea of 955

F

Face, venous congestion of 873
Facial edema 621
Fainting 324
Falciparum malaria 459
Fallopian tube 228, 819f, 833, 839
  epithelium 818
  pregnancy, pathogenesis of 839
False aneurysm 488, 488f
Familial adenomatous polyposis 633, 636, 636f, 638f
  variants of 634
Familial medullary thyroid
  cancer 908
  carcinoma 882
Fanconi anemia 253
Fanconi syndrome 897
Fasting plasma glucose 884, 893
  test 893
Fat 635
  absolute amount of 887
  accumulation of 669
  catabolism of 888, 889
  cell 217
  demonstration of 265
  destruction, focal areas of 20
  emboli, sites of arrest of 159
  embolism 158
    consequences of 159
    demonstration of 159
    pathogenesis of 158f
  metabolism 44, 303
  necrosis 20, 20f
    foci of 700
    traumatic 20
  stores, breakdown of 889
Fatal arrhythmias, causes of 522
Fatal disseminated intravascular coagulation 160
Fatigue 376, 496, 681, 687, 888
Fatty acid 689
  increased risk of 45
  oxidation of 45
  synthesis 667
Fatty casts 725
Fatty change 135, 680
Fatty liver 44, 45, 45f, 46f, 295, 671, 672
  microscopy of 45
  pathogenesis of 44
Feathery degeneration 681
Febrile nonhemolytic transfusion reaction 432
Fecal-oral route 654
Feces 473
Feet 130
Female genital tract 155
  disorders 799
Femur 916, 924
  head of 160
  lower end of 917
Fenestrated glomerular endothelial cells 711
Fenton reaction 679
Ferric chloride test 457, 459
Ferroptosis 28
Ferruginous bodies 574
Fertilization 835f
Fertilized ovum, implantation of 839
Fetal cells 160
Fetal hemoglobin 348, 351
  synthesis of 350
Fetal proteins, production of 223
Fetal red cells 359
Fetal tobacco syndrome 292
Fever 89, 140, 193, 432, 432f, 479, 496, 508, 547, 548, 615, 626, 682, 718, 740-742
  blisters 116
  familial mediterranean 209
  low-grade 566
  mild 694
Fiberoptic colonoscopy 641
Fibril protein 206, 208
Fibrillary glial cells 968
Fibrillary myxoid stroma 315f
Fibrin 412
  caps 736
  clot, causes of 466
  degradation 416
  deposition 81, 415
  meshwork 934
  thrombi activate secondary fibrinolytic system 416
Fibrinogen 90, 446
  degradation products 412
Fibrinoid necrosis 21, 21f, 749
Fibrinolysis, reduce 142
Fibrinolytic factors, activation of 415
Fibrinolytic system 698
  activation of secondary 416
Fibrinous exudate 81
Fibrinous inflammation 81
  mechanism of 81
Fibrinous pericarditis 506f, 533, 533f
  causes of 533, 533b
Fibroadenoma 316, 858, 859, 862
  juvenile 859
  variants of 859
Fibroblastic proliferation
  benign 939
  stimulate 571
Fibroblastic tumors 937, 939
Fibroblasts 91, 95f, 155, 162, 832, 934, 939, 944
  activation of 96
  growth factor receptor, amplification of 576
  outer rim of 87
  proliferate 519
  proliferation of 668f
Fibrocartilage 934f
Fibrocystin 753
Fibrogenic agent 101
Fibrogenic cytokines 586, 703
Fibrohistiocytic tumors 937
Fibroids 815
Fibrolamellar carcinoma 686, 686f
Fibroma 832
Fibromatosis 936, 939
  abdominal 940
Fibromatous stroma 831
  prominent 821f
Fibromuscular intimal hyperplasia 479
Fibrosarcoma 941, 941f
  adult 941
Fibrosis 83-85, 97, 98, 135, 195, 395, 618, 653, 663, 670, 674, 675, 680, 702, 843, 865, 866, 873, 878
  absence of 669
  broad bands of 670
  cysts 843f
  mechanisms of 668
  pathogenesis of 668f
  prolongation of 570
  promote 703
  regression of 653, 674
  stimulate 133
Fibrothecomas 832
Fibrotic disorders 101
Fibrous ankylosis 928
Fibrous capsule, thickened 137
Fibrous connective tissue
  mature 595f
  stroma 859
Fibrous dysplasia 918
Fibrous histiocytoma, malignant 860
Fibrous meningioma 976
Fibrous scar 157, 517
Fibrous stroma 825f, 829
Fibrous tissue 217, 535, 604, 671f, 860f, 866
  deposition of 675
  septa 674
Fibrovascular cores 868
Filariasis 126, 132, 443
Fine-needle aspiration
  biopsy 313, 875
  cytology 265, 306, 309, 313, 396, 783, 865, 870
    advantages of 313, 313b
    applications of 313
    complications of 313b
    contraindications of 313b
Fingers, clubbing of 548
Fissures 624
  formation of 929
Fistula 624, 695
  formation 626
Fite-Faraco stain 108, 109, 110f
Fixatives, special purpose 312
Flagella 598, 599
Flame cells 399
Flank pain 752
Flat dysplasia 611
Flat invasive carcinoma 769f
Flat noninvasive urothelial carcinoma in situ 768, 769f
Flattened atrophic epithelium 843
Flattened epidermis 109
Flea-bitten kidney 749
  causes of 750b
Flexible sigmoidoscopy 640
Flexner-Wintersteiner rosette 978, 978f
Florid duct lesion 680
Flow cytometry 267, 314, 361
Fluid 700
  accumulation 535
    mechanism of 81
  balance, normal 129
  conservation 144
  increased risk of 752
  intake 889
  loss of 139
  samples, preservation of 312
  significant volumes of 585
  volume, reduced 743
Fluorescence
  in situ hybridization 287
  microscopy 12
Foam cells 484
  formation of 484
Foamy macrophages 110, 725
Focal granulomas, formation of 614
Focal neurological deficits 970
Folate 672
Folic acid 304, 334
  deficiency 336, 338
    tests for 338
  metabolism 335
  role of 335
Follicles
  filled, lumen of 873
  rupture of 872
  scattered disruption of 866
  stimulating hormone 282
Follicular adenoma 873-875, 875f, 877, 879
Follicular architecture 875, 878
Follicular carcinoma 875, 876, 878, 879, 879t
  spread of 879
Follicular cell 872, 878
  atrophy of 872
  benign 874
  derived
    carcinoma 876
    neoplasms 874, 876
  hypertrophy 871
Follicular center cell lymphoma, morphology of 387
Follicular cervicitis 800
Follicular dendritic cell 168, 201, 874, 879
Follicular growth pattern 387
Follicular hyperplasia 872, 873
Follicular lymphoma 233, 385, 386, 387f, 405
  pathogenesis of 386
  survival of 387
Follicular thyroid
  adenomas 874
  carcinoma 878, 879
  cells 880
Forensic pathology 6
Fouchet's test 459
Foveolar cells, neck regions of 598
Fracture
  blood vessels 934
  healing 933, 934f
    inflammatory phase of 934, 934f

Fragile leukemic cells 386
Fragmentation 460
  syndrome 343, 360
Fragmented nuclei 661
Frameshift mutation 274
Frank diabetes, progression to 882
Frank melanoma 955
Frankly purulent 962, 965
Frank-Starling mechanism 500
Free fatty acids 482, 673, 689, 691, 886, 886*f*, 887, 889
  excessive entry of 45
  formation of 889
  increased release of 673
  metabolism of 44
Free light chains 398
Free radicals 30
  accumulation of 30
  generation of 30
  injury 30
    causes of 30
  neutralization of 31
  pathologic effects of 32
  production of 288
  types of 30
Free thyroxine 470
Fresh frozen plasma 428, 429
  indications for 429*b*
Frozen section 6, 11, 159, 265
  concept of 11
  uses of 265, 265*b*
Fructosamine 895
Fructosuria 456
Functional adrenocortical neoplasms 903
Fungal abscess 682
Fungal disease 903
  chronic granulomatous 120
Fungal disorders 448
Fungal infections 118, 203, 204
  acute 366
  types of 118
Fungemia 525
Fungi 572
Fungicides 255
Fungus 308
Fusiform 558
  aneurysm 488, 488*f*
  enlargements 945
Fusion gene 684
Fusobacterium 547

G

Gain-of-function mutations 232, 235, 239, 274, 576, 607, 764, 875, 879
Gaisböck's syndrome 381
Gallbladder 613-615, 688, 691, 693
  bacilli 613
  calcification of 696
  carcinoma 693, 696
    precursor lesions of 696
  disease of 695
  empties 689
  empyema of 693, 694
  hydrops of 693
  hypomotility 690
  perforation of 693, 694, 696
  rupture 696
  stasis 689, 690
  stones 689
Gallstone 299, 346, 688, 691, 693, 695-698
  classification of 688, 688*b*
  ileus 693, 695
  pathogenesis of 689
  risk factors for 689*b*
  types of 686*f*
Gamete 124
Gamma globulin 196
Gamma-glutamyl transpeptidase 671
Gamna-Gandy bodies 50, 137, 137*f*
Ganglion
  cell 906
    tumors, mature 904
  myxoid change in 53
Ganglioneuroblastoma 906, 907
Ganglioneuroma 267, 907
Gangliosidosis 286
Gangrene 21, 22, 22*f*, 22*t*, 891
Gangrenous necrosis 21
Gardner syndrome 634
Gas gangrene 21
Gasometric method 438
Gastrectomy 609*f*
Gastric
  acid, hypersecretion of 599
  adenocarcinoma 260, 605, 606, 610
  antrum 625
  bicarbonate transporters 598
  cancer 600, 606, 611
    characteristic of 603
    familial 606
    macroscopic subtypes of advanced 608*f*
    sporadic intestinal-type 607
  carcinoma 607, 608
    advanced 607
    classification of 607, 607*b*
    diffuse type of 610*f*
    etiology of 605
    intestinal type of 609*f*
    morphology of 607
    pathogenesis of 605
    risk factors of 606*b*
  contents, aspiration of 547
  damage 293
  endoscopy 841
  epithelial cells 601
  foveolar 823, 824*f*
  glands 599*f*
  lumen 601*f*
  lymphoma 260
  mucosa 598, 605
    inflammation of 597
  mucosal blood flow 602
  mucus barrier 601*f*
  outlet obstruction 604, 611
  peptic ulcers 603
  surgery 598
  ulcer 597, 602, 605, 605*t*
    chronic 604*f*
    complications of 604
    pathogenic mechanism of 598
  wall 608*f*
Gastrin secreting tumors 605
Gastrinomas 605, 908
Gastritis 597, 598, 598*b*
  acute 293, 598, 601*f*, 602
    erosive hemorrhagic 598
  chronic 598, 601*f*, 602
  mild acute 598
  severe 363, 598
Gastroesophageal junction 595, 603
Gastroesophageal reflux
  diseases 597
  complications of, chronic 596
Gastrointestinal amyloidosis 212
Gastrointestinal bleeding 688
Gastrointestinal diseases 689
Gastrointestinal disorders 696
Gastrointestinal disturbances 762, 902
Gastrointestinal epithelium 828*f*
Gastrointestinal hamartomatous polyps, multiple 631
Gastrointestinal polyps, classification of 631*b*
Gastrointestinal stromal tumor 611, 612, 612*f*
Gastrointestinal system 867
Gastrointestinal tract 145, 188, 290, 309, 496, 589, 595, 624, 687, 870, 908, 977
  cancers 610*f*
  carcinoma of 833
  columnar epithelium of 91
  lesions of 309
  malignant tumor of 635
  precancerous lesions of 231*b*
Gastropathy 597
Gaucher's cells
  accumulation of 287
  appearance of 287*f*
Gaucher's disease 286, 369, 398
Gelatinous tumor 938
General pathology 1, 3
Genes 231, 232, 240, 246, 272
  amplification 233, 236
  encode proteins 272
  expression of 790
  fusions 924
  loci of 181
  mismatch repair 634
  mutation 876
    causes of 273
  point mutations in 232
  products 235
  pro-survival 793
  rearrangements 232
  regions of 272
  standard 199
  structure of 272, 272*f*
Genetic
  abnormalities 190, 376, 637, 917
    acquired 793
    nature of 273
  alterations, multiple 696
  basics of 272
  code 272
  defects 869, 870
  derangements 15
  diseases 272
  disorder 215, 278, 287*b*, 371, 531, 536, 936
    classification of 278*b*
    molecular diagnosis of 287
  factors 885
  lesions 232
  pathways 637
  predisposition 549, 554, 689, 720, 914, 932
  profile 879
  susceptibility 170, 732
  tumor syndrome 633
Genital herpes 116
Genital hygiene 787
Genital tract 155, 586
  disorders 774
Genital tumors 833
Genitalia 283
Genitourinary tracts 955
Genome
  alterations, molecular analysis of 287
  guardian of 243, 244
Genomic damage 259
Genomic instability 234, 253
Genotype 348
Gerhardt's test 457
Germ cell 55*f*, 782, 830, 830*f*
  differentiation of 780
  layers 93, 218, 779, 780
  mutations 273
  neoplasia
    in situ 774-777, 780, 782
    noninvasive 775, 777
  postpubertal-type 782
  sex cord-stromal tumors 826
  telomerase active in 56
  tumors 775-777, 780, 782, 784, 819, 826, 829, 830, 967
    development of 776, 776*f*
    extragonadal site of 777*b*
    invasive 776
    malignant 777, 828, 829
    mixed 780, 826, 830
    progression of 776*f*
    sites of 777
  type of 780, 780*t*
Germinal centers, underdeveloped 197
Germline inactivate mutations 940
Germline mutation 242, 245, 607, 634, 846, 906, 936, 952
  prevalence of 284
Gestation, abnormal 834
Gestational choriocarcinoma, treatment of 838
Gestational disorders 833
Gestational sac 836
Gestational trophoblastic
  disease 833
    classification of 834
  neoplasia 834, 837
Ghon complex 563, 563*f*
  fate of 563
Ghon focus 563
Ghrelin 297
Giant cell 87, 88, 564, 783, 923, 934*f*
  arteritis 496, 497*f*
  reaction 930
  tumor 922, 923
    primary malignancy 924
  types of 88, 88*f*, 89*b*
Giant granules 70
Giardia lamblia 197
Giemsa stain 277, 441, 599*f*
Gilbert syndrome 650
Gingival hypertrophy 376
Gingival tissues 212
Gingivostomatitis 116
Glands 552
  architecture, loss of 824
  cystic dilatation of 811*f*
  formation 945
  irregular distribution of 811
  late secretory endometrium saw-tooth appearance of 808*f*

malignant 795f
periurethral part of 791f
recognizable 814
Glandular cell
abnormalities 309
malignant 855
Glandular fever 370
Glandular lesions, benign 801
Glandular structures 217, 619
Glandular tissue, focal proliferation of 861
Glandular tumors 801
Glans penis 112f, 787f
Glanzmann thrombasthenia 410
Gleason grading 796
Gleason pattern 796
Gleason score 796
Gleason system 796
Glial cell 968
neoplasms 267
Glial fibrillary acidic protein 267
Glioblastoma 236, 967, 969, 980
microscopic features of 971f
Gliomas 967, 967b, 970
astrocytic 969, 971
Glioneuronal tumors 967
Gliosis 964
Globin, alpha-chains of 348
Globulin 324, 446, 725
Glomerular antigens 713
Glomerular basement membrane 711, 711f, 714, 719, 722, 728, 728f, 730, 730f, 731f, 737f
duplication of 186
thickening of 729
Glomerular capillary 711
lumens 718
rupture of 749
wall 717, 722, 727
Glomerular cells 717
Glomerular damage 455
mechanism of 717
Glomerular disease 460, 712, 713b, 747
mechanism of 713
primary 720, 723
secondary 712
Glomerular filtration rate 471, 757
Glomerular function 471
Glomerular hyperfiltration 747
Glomerular hypertrophy 735
Glomerular injury 713, 714b, 714f, 728
causes of 716
mechanism of 713, 714, 727
nonimmune 714, 716
severe 720
Glomerular involvement 713, 725
Glomerular lesions 734, 735, 737
Glomerular proteinuria, types of 455, 722b
Glomerular syndromes 712
Glomerular tufts 712
Glomeruli 210, 496, 726f
sclerosis of 749
Glomerulocystic disease 751
Glomeruloid appearance 970
Glomerulonephritis 712, 713, 713b, 714-716, 748
acute 458
diffuse proliferative 718
proliferative 717
antibody-mediated 714f
chronic 53, 734, 747
nonstreptococcal acute 719
primary 712, 713
proliferative 713
type of 728
Glomerulopathy 186, 712, 713, 713f, 725, 729, 730f, 731f, 746
Glomerulosclerosis 736
focal segmental 723, 725, 726f
Glomerulus 18f, 193f, 710, 718f, 726f, 729f, 742f, 970
light microscopic appearance of 710f
periphery of 736f
Glossitis 304
angular 333
Glucagon, secretion of 889
Glucagon-like peptide-1 298
Glucocerebrosides 286
accumulation of 286
Glucocorticoids 261, 899
production 142
Gluconeogenesis 886, 889
loss of 902
Glucose 296, 455, 889, 892, 962, 963
amounts of 456
estimation 463
intolerance 735
levels, reduced 962
metabolism 899
oxidase, specific 456
reduced renal threshold for 456
tolerance 884
transport, insulin of 892
Glucose-6-phosphate dehydrogenase 444
deficiency 346
Glucosuria 893, 900
Glucotoxicity 887, 891
Glucuronic acid 646, 767
Glutamic acid decarboxylase 885, 896
Glutathione
depletion of 667
peroxidase 31
S-transferases 646
Glycated hemoglobin 884
Glycemia 895
Glycemic control 890
Glycogen 47, 778, 799
storage disease 47
Glycolysis, anaerobic 29, 144
Glycolytic enzyme deficiencies 326
Glycolytic pathway 745
Glycoprotein 268, 489, 693, 823
Glycosaminoglycans 206, 486f
Glycosuria 453, 456, 701, 747, 888
alimentary 456
causes of 456, 456b
Glycosylated albumin 895
Glycosylated hemoglobin 890, 894
Glycosylated plasma proteins 895
Glycosylation, nonenzymatic 735, 891, 894
Goblet cells 595, 596f
loss of 627
Goiter 870, 871
development of 871fc
endemic 871
etiopathogenesis of 871
gross appearance of 872f
sporadic 871
Goitrogens 871, 872
Gomori's methenamine silver stain 120
Gonadal failure 678
Gonads, direct toxic action of 678
Goodpasture antigen 716, 720
Goodpasture disease 716
Goodpasture syndrome 176, 188, 716, 720, 721, 721f
Gorlin syndrome 952
Gout 462, 748, 755, 931, 932
asymptomatic intercritical 933
chronic tophaceous 933
classification of 931b
pathognomonic of 933
primary 931
secondary 931
Gouty arthritis 931
acute 933
pathogenesis 931
acute 932f
chronic 932f
Gouty nephropathy 933
Gouty tophus 931
microscopy of 934f
usual site of 933f
Graft 186
alloantigens
pathways of 184
recognition of 184
antigens 184
arteriosclerosis 186
blood vessels, endothelium of 185f
damage 186f
increasing survival of 187
ischemic necrosis of 185f
rejection, mechanisms of 184
Graft-versus-host disease 187, 434
acute 187
chronic 188
Gram's smear 464
Gram's stain 465, 961, 962
Gram-negative bacilli 737, 961
Gram-negative bacteria 668
infections 115
Granular bodies 972
Granular casts 748
Granular contracted kidney 747, 747t
causes of 750
Granular cytoplasm 84, 686, 761
Granular immunofluorescence 919
Granular lumpy deposits 178
Granulation tissue 95, 95f, 99f, 101f, 163, 519, 604, 618, 928, 934f
formation 102, 934
granular appearance of 95f
ingrowth of 543
Granules
bind chromium 904
contents, release 146
types of 72
Granulocyte 319, 321
decreased production of 367
Increased destruction of 367
macrophage colony-stimulating factor 320
Granuloma 19, 86-88, 108, 180f, 315f, 384f, 449, 564, 963
formation 105, 563
mechanisms of 86, 86f, 179, 180f
high power of 625f
microscopic appearance of 87f
noncaseating 109f, 564, 568, 625, 625f
types of 87
Granulomatosis 497
Granulomatous inflammation 86, 88t, 179, 180f, 384f, 496, 563
Granulomatous lesion 505
Granulomatous lymphadenitis 86, 314
Granulomatous prostatitis 789
nonspecific 789
Granulomatous reaction 121, 866
Granulomatous thyroiditis 866
subacute 865
Granulomatous vasculitis 497
Granulopoiesis 320, 336
Granulosa cell
component 831
tumor 260, 831, 831f
adult 831, 832f
juvenile 832
Granulosa theca cell tumor 841
Graves disease 176, 188, 863, 867, 868, 868f, 869, 869f, 873
Gravity, specific 452
Great veins, punctures of 159
Griseofulvin 255
Grocott's methenamine-silver stain 546
Gross pathology, era of 9
Ground-glass hepatocytes 661f, 663, 663f
Growth 350
autonomous 215
controls 970
factors 38, 92, 235, 236
actions of 236
excessive production of 236
increased production of 40
receptor 92, 235, 236, 237f, 239
release of 484
signaling pathways, activation of 970
stimuli proliferation 94
fraction 226
inhibitors 242f
inhibitory signals 239, 240
patterns 95, 223, 395, 832, 957
retardation 283
signaling pathway 576
signals, self sufficiency in 234
stimulating signals, absence of 41
suppressors, removal of 254
Guaiac test 640, 645
Guanosine
diphosphate 237
triphosphate 237
Gum bleeding 408
Gut
lumen 622
microbiome, role of 294
mucosa, immune response of 622
peristalsis 611
Gynecologic exfoliative cytology 307
Gynecologic malignancy 817
Gynecomastia 708, 861
microscopic appearance of 862f

H

H antigens 423
H genes 423
role of 423*f*
Haemophilus influenzae 201, 355, 557, 911, 961, 965
Hairlike cytoplasmic projections 391
Hairy cell 391
leukemia 391
Hairy leukoplakia 590
Halogenation 71
Halts atrial blood flow 150
Ham's acidified serum test 361
Hamartoma 219, 283
Hamartomatous polyps, multiple 632*f*
Hand-foot syndrome 354
Hansen's disease 128
Haploid numbers, multiple of 233
Haptoglobin 359
Harrison's sulcus 301
Hart's test 457
Hashimoto thyroiditis 307, 863, 864, 867
gross appearance of 865*f*
microscopy of 865*f*
pathogenesis of 863, 864*f*
Hashitoxicosis 865
Hay's sulfur test 460
Head 441
defects 468
injury 597
venous congestion of 873
Headache 479, 496, 621, 963, 970
severe 962
Healing 60, 83, 91, 93, 99, 565, 866
complications of 936
whole process of 935
Heart 45, 145, 193, 195, 210, 281, 496, 501
brown atrophy of 49
compression of 139
defects, congenital 536
disorders 499
dysfunction of 529
morphology of 504
sound, third 502
tissue, mechanism of damage to 503
transverse section of 39*f*
valves 50, 523, 545
thrombi on 157
Heart disease
acquired 525
acute rheumatic 504, 505
chronic 499
ischemic 485, 522
rheumatic 503, 504*f*, 506, 525
coronary 3, 492, 509
cyanotic congenital 537
hypertensive 492
ischemic 131, 481, 492, 500, 508, 509*b*, 511*f*
obstructive congenital 536, 537
pre-existing 433
type of 536
Heart failure 129, 131, 134, 135, 499, 500, 501*f*, 502
acute 499
causes of 500*b*, 501*b*, 502*b*
cells 134, 136
chronic 499
compensated 500
congestive 130, 131, 131*fc*, 132, 134, 157, 212, 333, 492, 499, 507, 551, 743, 906
pathophysiology of 500, 501*fc*
progressive late 521
stages of 500
Heat and acetic acid test 454
Heberden's nodes 930, 931
Heinz bodies 347*f*
Helicobacter pylori 259, 598, 606, 645
gastritis 598, 599
infection 598, 600, 602, 605, 606
acute 598
chronic 598
mechanism of action of 599
role of 598, 602
source of 598
Heller's test 454
Helminthic infections 204
Helper T cells 167, 194, 926
Helter-skelter pattern 219, 781
Hemangioma 225, 284, 498
cavernous 498, 499*f*
types of 498
Hemarthrosis 138
Hematin 49
Hematocrit 337, 355, 443
estimation of 444
Hematocrit, uses of 444
Hematogenous infection 738*f*, 739
Hematogenous osteomyelitis, pathogenesis of 911, 912*f*
Hematogenous route 739, 960
Hematogenous spread 227, 583, 618, 788, 795, 922
Hematologic diseases 514
treatment of 93
Hematological tests 323, 660, 672, 964
Hematology 8, 317, 319
Hematolymphoid disorders, primary 448
Hematoma 138, 324, 406
formation of 934
Hematopoiesis 320, 320*t*
normal 320
qualitative state of 447
regulation of 320
sites of 320
stages of 321*f*
Hematopoietic cells, erythropoietin receptors of 381
Hematopoietic diseases, diagnosis of 306
Hematopoietic islands 320
Hematopoietic neoplasms 268
Hematopoietic stem cell 84, 93, 187, 319, 448, 481
sources of 187
transplantation 187
complications of 187
types of 187
Hematopoietic system 279, 284, 319
components of 319
Hematosalpinx 839
causes of 839
Hematoxylin and eosin stain 209, 312, 312*b*
Hematuria 194, 716, 718, 719, 731, 732, 750, 756, 762, 764, 797
asymptomatic 712
causes of 458, 458*b*
painless 770
Hemazoin 49
Heme
iron 330
synthesis 364
Hemiparesis 970
Hemochromatosis 49, 532, 678, 679, 702
idiopathic 475
primary 678
secondary 350, 678
Hemodialysis, long-term 208
Hemodilution, acute normovolemic 436
Hemodynamic disorders 129
Hemoglobin 273*f*, 323, 337, 344, 345, 348, 352*f*, 355, 386, 399, 455, 745
abnormal 357
breakdown product of 459
catabolism of 646
concentration 8, 324, 436
derived pigments 48
electrophoresis 328, 351, 352, 356
estimation 438
indications for 438*b*
methods of 438, 438*t*
formation 348, 440
pipette 439
S, solubility test for 356
synthesis, disorder of 326, 343
types of 439
Hemoglobinemia 343, 433
confirmation of 324
Hemoglobinization, degree of 325
Hemoglobinopathy 895
Hemoglobinuria 433, 458
causes of 459
Hemogram 325
complete 323
Hemojuvelin 678
Hemolysis 348, 350, 354, 427, 648
susceptible to 354
Hemolytic anemia 174, 319, 326, 342, 344, 349, 355, 362*fc*, 429, 459, 460
causes of 343, 343*b*
classification of 343, 343*b*
confirmation of 362*b*
diagnosis of 361, 361*fc*
mechanism of severe 349
moderate-to-severe 354
Hemolytic crisis 354
Hemolytic disease 358, 360, 424, 648
Hemolytic transfusion reaction 424
investigation of 360
Hemolytic uremic syndrome 617, 743
Hemoparasites 441, 443, 445
Hemopericardium 138, 465, 535
Hemoperitoneum 138
Hemophilia 411, 411*f*, 412, 421
A 411, 412, 412*t*, 413, 421
B 412, 413
features of 411
treatment of 412
Hemopoietic system 319
Hemoptysis 567, 583
Hemorrhage 135, 137, 138, 138*t*, 142, 361, 411, 485, 486, 615, 628, 694*f*, 701*f*, 824, 872, 873, 923*f*, 925*f*, 934
focal 144, 193, 946*f*
intracranial 292
intraperitoneal 839
massive 139, 491
intraperitoneal 839
produce minute 134
severe 613
site of 138
small 159
speed of 138
subarachnoid 466
Hemorrhagic cerebral infarction 961
Hemorrhagic diathesis 137, 138, 406
Hemorrhagic disease 303, 414
Hemorrhagic fluid 463
Hemorrhagic infarcts 162, 163, 961
Hemorrhagic necrosis, massive 144
Hemosiderin 48, 59, 343, 458
laden macrophages 134, 135*f*, 873
Hemosiderinuria 343, 458
Hemosiderosis 350, 434, 678
Hemostasis 145, 146*f*
normal 145, 406
primary 147
secondary 147
steps in 145
Hemostatic disorders 417*t*
Hemostatic plug 94
primary 145, 147, 406
secondary 147, 406
Hemothorax 138
Hemozoin 48
pigment 122
Henle loop 711, 746*f*
Henoch-Schönlein purpura 407, 720
Hepar lobatum 114
Heparin 323
disadvantages of 323
induced thrombocytopenia syndrome 152
Hepatic angiosarcomas 255
Hepatic blastomatous tumor, malignant primary 683
Hepatic congestion, acute 134
Hepatic decompensation 681
Hepatic destruction, massive 652
Hepatic ducts 687
Hepatic dysfunction 677
Hepatic encephalopathy 474, 652, 678
Hepatic failure 651
Hepatic fibrosis 673
congenital 753
Hepatic ischemia 648
Hepatic lymph flow 676
Hepatic metastases, primary tumor producing 687
Hepatic necrosis, massive 652
Hepatic steatosis 664, 669*f*
causes of 44*b*
Hepatic stellate cells, activation of 675, 679
Hepatic vein 135
Hepatitis 447, 663
A 648, 653
infections 652
virus 653, 654
acute 654, 654*f*, 656*f*, 660, 661, 665*f*
fulminant 474
viral 652, 660, 661, 662*b*, 707, 708
alcoholic 669, 670*f*

- B 648, 653, 655, 657
  - core 475, 655, 656, 663*f*
  - infection 652, 656*fc*
  - serological markers of chronic 664*b*
  - surface antigen 475, 654, 656, 663*f*
  - treatment of chronic 657
- B E antigen 656
- B virus 259, 496, 653, 654, 655*f*, 656, 714
  - genome of 683
  - infection 656, 656*b*, 683
  - structure of 654
- C 653
  - life cycle of 657, 658*f*
- C virus 259, 653, 657, 658
  - antigens 714
  - infection 659*b*, 687
- chronic 475, 656*f*, 659, 661, 662, 665*f*
  - viral 683
- D 653
  - virus 653, 659
- E 653
  - infections 652
  - virus 653, 659
- lobular 661
- microscopic features of chronic 663*f*
- mild 663
- severe 662*f*
  - acute 659, 665*f*
- sporadic acute 659
- virus 654, 659
  - features of 660*t*
  - infection 652

Hepatobiliary disease 474
Hepatobiliary disorders 646
Hepatoblastoma 683, 709
Hepatocellular adenoma 684
Hepatocellular cancer, risk of 659, 666
Hepatocellular carcinoma 228, 255, 259, 681-683, 683*b*, 685*f*, 686*f*, 764
- development of 678
- gross patterns of 685*f*
- precursor lesions of 684
- spread of 686

Hepatocellular disorder, primarily 649
Hepatocellular injury 473, 665*f*
Hepatocellular necrosis, mechanism of 652, 666
Hepatocellular steatosis 669
Hepatocytes 59, 135, 657, 661, 666*f*, 673
- ballooning degeneration of 670*f*
- cytoplasm of 669
- damage 44
- death of 259, 666
- injury 662
- massive necrosis of 662
- necrosis of 661
- nuclei 661*f*, 663*f*
- paraffin 687
- proliferation of remaining 94
- swelling of 661

Hepatoma 218
Hepatomegaly 379
Hepatorenal syndrome 652
Hepatosplenic T-cell lymphoma 385
Hepatosplenomegaly 285, 374, 376
Hepatotoxin 666
Hepatotropic viruses 653, 683
Hepcidin
- increased production of 90
- role of 331
- synthesis, suppression of 350

Herbicides 290
Hereditary autosomal recessive disorder 260
Hereditary coagulation disorders 410, 413*t*
Hereditary hemochromatosis 678, 679
- pathogenesis of 678

Hereditary nonpolyposis
- colon cancer 232
- colorectal cancer 634, 636

Hereditary spherocytosis 344, 363, 450, 450*f*, 689
- pathogenesis of 345*f*
- peripheral blood smear of 346*f*

Hernia, incisional 102
Heroin abusers 208
Herpes simplex 800
- virus 116, 204, 962

Herpes stromal keratitis 116
Herpesvirus 258
- infections 116

Herringbone pattern 941
Hess test 418
Heterocyclic aromatic hydrocarbons 255
Heterophile antibodies, demonstration of 371
Heterotopia 283
Heterozygosity, loss of 240, 638, 639
Heterozygote 278
Heubner arteritis 964
Hexose monophosphate shunt enzyme deficiencies 326
Hidradenitis suppurativa 950
High-density lipoprotein 480, 891
Highly active antiretroviral therapy 203
Highly anionic macromolecules 715
Highly cellular tumor 945, 970
High-performance liquid chromatography 351, 357
Hilar lymph nodes 571
Hip 911
- flexion 962

Hirschsprung disease 630, 630*f*
Histamine 64, 65, 73, 105, 172, 620
- from mast cells, release of 79

Histidine, metabolism of 336
Histiocytes 393
Histochemistry 266
Histocompatibility complex 181, 183*f*, 259
- molecules 181

Histoid leprosy 107
Histones 72, 234
- modifications 234

Histopathology 50*t*, 308
Histoplasma 120
- capsulatum 789, 902

Histoplasmosis 204
Hoarseness 873, 874
Hodgkin cell 393, 395
- mononuclear 393

Hodgkin lymphoma 4, 252, 391, 392, 393*t*, 394*f*-396*f*, 397, 397*t*, 724
- classic 392, 393
- clinical presentation of 397*f*
- distinctive features of 392*b*
- microscopy of mixed cellularity classical 395
- mixed cellularity classical 395
- pathognomonic of 392
- staging of 396
- subtypes of 393
- types of 392

Homan sign 155
Homeopathic medicine 290
Homer-Wright pseudorosettes 906
Homer-Wright rosette 907, 925, 974, 974*f*
Homocysteine 336, 482
Homogentisic acid 49
Homovanillic acid 907
Homozygote 278
Homozygous deletion 968
Honeycomb pattern 571, 574
Hormesis 57
Hormonal status, assessment of 307
Hormonal stimulation 226
Hormones 40, 98, 223, 256, 260, 899
- adrenocortical 901
- adrenocorticotropic 899
- anabolic 888
- antidiuretic 472
- dependent tumors 260
- secrete 784, 908
- stress-induced 142

Horseshoe kidney 751, 751*f*
Host cell 232
- cytoplasm of 200
- genome of 200
- membrane, penetration of 200

Host immune response, abnormal 503
Human anatomy 9, 10
Human chorionic gonadotropin 841
Human genome project 12
- uses of 12*b*

Human immunodeficiency virus 198, 202, 203, 214, 557, 962
- genome 199
- infection 200, 201, 203, 728
  - Centers for Disease Control classification of 203
  - clinical manifestations of 202
  - diagnosis of 203, 205*b*
  - pathogenesis of 199, 202*f*
- life cycle of 199, 201*f*
- properties of 190
- structure of 198, 198*f*
- syndrome, acute 202
- tropism of 199

Human leukocyte antigen 183, 724, 733, 883, 927
- complex 181, 183*f*

Human muscles 10
Human papillomavirus 230, 251, 257, 258, 596, 799, 800, 801, 950
- associated squamous cell carcinoma 786
- carcinogenicity of 802
- classification of 801
- genome
  - episomal form of 258
  - integration of 802
- independent squamous cell carcinoma 786
- infection 786, 800
- low-risk 802
- oncogenic effects of 802*f*
- protein 841
- role of 800
- types of 257
- vaccine, nature of 807

Human peripheral lymphoid cells 167
Human retrovirus, non-transforming 198
Human T-cell leukemia virus 256
Human tumors 257*t*, 258
Humerus 924
- head of 160

Huntington's disease 23, 27, 275*f*, 279
Hürthle cells 865, 865*f*
Hyaline 52
- alcoholic 47, 52
- arteriolosclerosis 494, 495*f*, 736
- arteriosclerosis 736, 749, 892
- cartilage 920, 926
- change 52, 53*t*
- droplets 52, 830
- membrane 53, 145, 586
  - formation of 585
- thickening 195

Hyalinosis 713
Hyaluronic acid 870
Hydatid cysts 126
Hydatid disease 125
Hydatidiform mole 834, 837
- etiopathogenesis of 834
- laboratory diagnosis of 837
- morphology of 834
- partial 835*f*, 837*t*

Hydralazine 190
Hydrocephalus 961, 963
- noncommunicating 974

Hydrogen peroxide 31, 71
Hydrolyze bilirubin glucuronides 691
Hydronephrosis 41, 757, 792
- bilateral 757
- unilateral 757
  - complete 759
  - partial 759

Hydroperoxy eicosatetraenoic acid 74
Hydrostatic pressure 130, 131, 131*f*, 132
- regional increase in 130

Hydrothorax 833
Hydroureter 792
Hydroxyapatite crystals 52
Hydroxyeicosatetraenoic acid 74
Hydroxyl radical 31, 71, 71*f*
Hydroxytryptamine 74
Hygiene hypothesis 554
Hyperacute rejection 184, 185, 185*f*
Hyperadrenalism 899
Hyperaldosteronism 899, 901
- bilateral idiopathic 901
- clinical features of 901
- familial 901
- primary 901
- secondary 901

Hyperbilirubinemia 343, 647, 650*t*, 652, 672
- conjugated 651
- hereditary 650, 651*t*
- unconjugated 650

Hypercalcemia 262, 263, 400, 401, 687, 755, 897, 897
- causes of 51

Hypercalciuria 755
Hypercapnia 553
Hypercellular glomeruli 729, 730*f*, 731
Hypercellular nodules 873
Hypercellular tumor, high-grade 918
Hypercholesterolemia 480, 681, 870
  familial 481
Hyperchromatic nuclei 221, 767*f*, 769, 918, 978*f*
Hypercoagulability 151
  acquired 151
  primary 151
  secondary 151
Hypercoagulable state, causes of 151, 152*t*
Hypercortisolism 899
Hyperdynamic circulation 676
Hyperemesis gravidarum, prolonged 303
Hyperemia 134, 552
Hyperestrinism 861
Hyperestrogenism 677
Hyperfunction, adrenocortical 899
Hypergastrinemia 605
Hyperglobulinemia 672
Hyperglycemia 142, 451, 456, 735, 882, 888-890, 893, 900
  aggravation of 888
  causes of 882
  chronic 887, 889, 890, 891*b*
  severe 889
Hyperglycemic hyperosmolar nonketotic coma, pathogenesis of 890*fc*
Hyperhomocysteinemia 481
Hyperinflation, compensatory 551
Hyperinsulinemia 299
Hyperkalemia 261, 745, 902
Hyperlipidemia 44, 480-482, 721, 723, 732
Hypermetabolic state 867
Hypernephroma 759
Hyperosmolar hyperglycemic nonketotic syndrome 889
Hyperparathyroidism 896
  asymptomatic primary 897
  brown tumors of 897
  primary 896, 897, 908
  secondary 734, 897, 897*f*, 898
  symptomatic primary 897
  tertiary 898
Hyperphosphatemia 261, 897, 898
Hyperphosphorylated state 241
Hyperpigmentation 903
  alternating zones of 295
  causes of 48*t*
Hyperplasia 40, 41, 42*t*, 552, 578*f*, 749, 868, 871, 900, 927
  atypical 847
    adenomatous 577
    lobular 844
  compensatory 40, 320
  micronodular 900
  nodular
    primary 896
    prostatic 798
  pathological 40
  physiological 40
  reactive 227
Hyperplastic phase 872
Hyper-reactive malarial splenomegaly syndrome 398
Hypersecretory states 600
Hypersegmentation 729
Hypersegmented neutrophils 337*f*, 363
Hypersensitivity 83, 169, 173, 560
  antibody-mediated 173
  delayed-type 178
  diagnosis of 173
  diseases 169, 176*t*
  disorders, general features of 169
  reaction 15, 69, 169, 173, 173*t*, 174, 175*f*, 178, 179*f*, 180*f*, 182*t*, 560, 563
    causes of 170
    cell mediated 179
    classification of 170, 171*t*
    mediators of 172
    type of 171
Hypersplenism 137, 366, 398, 676
Hypertension 52, 134, 480-482, 488, 490, 495*f*, 499, 500, 515, 716, 734, 749, 813, 901, 904
  causes of 492, 492*f*
  chronic 480
  essential 455
  malignant 493, 495*f*, 743, 744-750
  mechanisms of primary 494
  mild-to-moderate 716, 718
  obesity-related 299
  pathogenesis of 494
  primary 492, 748-750
  secondary 493
  severe 494, 750
  types of 492*f*
  uncontrolled 436
  vascular pathology in 494
Hypertensive vascular disease 492
Hyperthyroidism 470, 866, 867
  clinical manifestations of 867
  monitoring treatment of 470
  primary 866, 867, 869, 870
  secondary 867
  subclinical 873
  transient 866
Hypertriglyceridemia 299
Hypertrophic scar 102
Hypertrophied bladder, gross appearance of 792*f*
Hypertrophy 38, 39*f*, 41, 42*f*, 58, 552, 661
  causes of 38*b*
  mechanisms of 38
Hyperuricemia 261, 755, 931, 932
  asymptomatic 933
  mechanism of 931
Hyperviscosity syndromes 151
Hypervolemia 130
Hypoadrenalism 901, 902
  secondary 903
Hypoalbuminemia 305, 664, 672, 676, 721, 722, 732, 771
Hypoalbuminemic edema 703
Hypocalcemia 261, 301, 701, 898
  chronic 897
  mechanism of 897*f*
Hypocalcemic tetany 301
Hypochlorite 31
  radical 71
Hypochromia 351
Hypocomplementemia 717, 719, 731*fc*
Hypofibrinogenemia 447
Hypogammaglobulinemia 385
Hypoglycemia 263, 687, 890, 895, 902, 908
  signs of 890
  symptoms of 890
Hypogonadism 282, 678
Hypokalemia 672, 745, 901
Hypomagnesemia 672
Hypomethylation 234
Hyponatremia 672, 902
Hypoparathyroidism 898
  chronic 898
  familial isolated 898
  surgically induced 898
Hypophosphatemia 301, 672
Hypopigmentation 295
  acquired focal 48
  causes of 48*t*
Hypoplasia 280
Hypoproteinemia 130, 463
Hyposthenuria 453
  causes of 453
Hypotension 902
  produce systemic 142
Hypothalamic pituitary
  disease 902
  dysfunction 902
  suppression 902
Hypothalamus 297
Hypothesis
  multistep 256
  response-to-injury 482
Hypothyroidism 133, 283, 470, 869, 870
  causes of 869, 869*b*
  degree of 865
  diagnosis of 870
  secondary 869
  symptoms of 870
  types of 869, 869*b*
Hypotonic saline 449
Hypovolemia 429, 743
  arterial 901
Hypovolemic shock 139, 144, 145, 164
  causes of 139
  pathogenesis of 139*fc*
Hypoxemia 433, 553
Hypoxia 15, 29, 36, 37*f*, 162
  chronic 355
  consequences of 37*f*
  severe central 135
Hypoxic damage 668
Hypoxic encephalopathy 502

I

Icteric phase, symptomatic 660
Icterus 652
Idiopathic nephrotic syndrome 728
Idiopathic thrombocytopenic purpura 408
Ileocecal valve 612
Ileoileal intussusception 630*f*
Ileum 616*f*
Iliac spine, superior 644
Iliac veins 156
Immature basal epithelial cells 801
Immature cells 826
  primary granules of 373
Immature elements 781, 828
Immature epithelial component 764
Immature fetal tissue 827
Immature granulocytic progenitors 380
Immature megakaryocytes 409, 410*f*
Immature neuroepithelium 828
Immature squamous cells 257, 804
Immature teratoma 826, 827, 828*f*
Immature tissue 780, 783, 828
  stroma 781*f*
Immotile cilia syndrome 541, 557, 798
Immune complex 174, 192, 481, 732
  deposits 717
    in glomeruli, sites of 715
  diseases 176*t*, 178, 717
  endocytosis of 191
  formation of 170, 176, 732
  in situ, formation of 714, 715
  large circulating 715
  mechanisms 527
Immune deficiency 295, 300
  diseases, classification of primary 196*b*
Immune deposits, fate of 715
Immune destruction, evasion of 254
Immune dysregulation 385
Immune effector
  cells 883
  mechanisms, resisting 252
Immune function, alteration of 261
Immune granulomas 87
Immune mechanisms 171, 171*t*, 713, 714
  cell mediated 885
Immune mediated
  acute hemolytic transfusion reaction, causes of 432
  diseases 557
  hepatocyte destruction 652
  injury 367
  vasculitis, causes of 496
Immune reactions 61, 88, 129, 251
Immune regulation 622, 867
Immune response 251, 252, 655
  normal 165
  types of 165
Immune responsiveness 40
Immune suppression, mechanisms for 141
Immune surveillance 251
  evasion of 251
Immune system 83, 165, 166, 199, 251, 622
  cell of 166
  messenger molecules of 169
Immune thrombocytopenic purpura 408, 419, 421
  acute 408
  chronic 408, 409*f*
Immunity 11, 165, 295, 664
  adaptive 166, 166*t*, 196
  cell mediated 107, 166, 168, 560-562, 716, 926
  cellular 166, 504*f*
  effective 659
  humoral 166, 168, 401, 504*f*, 926
  innate 165, 196
Immunization 724
  basis of 11
Immunocytochemistry 314
Immunodeficiency 188, 389, 557
  manifestations of 196
  primary 196
  secondary 197, 197*b*

states 230, 231
syndromes 196
Immunoelectrophoresis 212
Immunofluorescence 5, 724, 729, 731
diffuse linear pattern of 716
microscopy 178, 715, 716, 718, 721, 725, 727, 736
Immunoglobulin 46, 168*t*, 324, 455, 474, 725, 727, 868
A nephropathy 731*f*, 732
pathogenesis of 733*fc*
G 654, 656, 721*f*
light chains, produces free 207
M 654, 656
molecules, produce abnormal 207
Immunohemolytic anemias 343, 357
classification of 357, 357*b*
Immunohistochemical markers 267, 795
Immunohistochemistry 5, 226, 266, 582, 925, 969, 974, 976
uses of 266
Immunologic inflammatory disorders 397
Immunologic tests 473, 475
Immunological defects, acquired 541
Immunological phenomena 527
Immunology 8
Immunopathology 6, 165
Immunophenotype 386, 387, 389, 390, 394, 395
Immunosuppression
chronic 950
complications of 187
Immunosuppressive agent 541, 767
Impaired red cell production, anemia of 319, 329
In situ hybridization 12
In situ immune complexes 715-717
nephritis 719*f*
In utero infections 536
Inactivate tumor suppressor genes 374, 637, 683
Inadequate blood flow, prerenal causes of 744
Incision biopsy 265
Incompatible blood transfusion 459
Indeterminate leprosy 107, 110
Indirect antiglobulin test 360
Indirect immunofluorescence assay 193
Indoor air pollution 289
Inducible nitric oxide synthase 71
Industrial hazards 575
Industrial hydrocarbons 919
Indwelling nasogastric tube 598
Ineffective erythropoiesis 336, 349
consequences of 349
Ineffective megakaryopoiesis 408
Infarction 161, 162, 162*t*, 354
causes of 161
microscopy of 163
patterns of 515
produce 162
Infections 35, 70, 97, 101, 106, 118, 127, 162, 163, 188, 194, 196, 201, 355, 369, 397, 434, 488, 530, 725, 726, 767, 792, 889, 373, 910
absence of 162
acute 369
bacterial 366
ascending 682
asymptomatic acute 660
biliary 691
chronic 369, 666, 963
persistent 557
life-threatening 376
mixed 124
mode of 682, 966
productive 200, 258
role of 189, 552
route of 738
secondary 295, 557
site of 72, 560
source of 106, 111, 525, 564, 565, 654, 655, 738
spread of 565, 963
suppurative 19, 740
symptomatic acute 660
systemic symptoms of 962
treatment of 912
type of 383
Infectious agents 15, 150, 230, 532
Infectious diseases 369, 398
Infectious virus 200
releases new 200
Infective endocarditis 507, 523, 526*f*, 527, 529*f*, 739
complications of 526, 527*b*
diagnosis of 528*b*
etiology of 524
morphology of 525
pathogenesis of 524
subacute 524, 526*f*
Infertility 775
Infiltrative dermopathy 869
Infiltrative ophthalmopathy 867
pathogenesis of 868
Infiltrative tumors 640
Inflammasome 62, 63, 572
activation of 62
Inflammation 37, 60, 61, 63, 72, 73*t*, 76, 76*t*, 79, 81, 85, 94, 129, 130, 134, 166, 174, 481, 666, 747
absence of 669
activated immune cells of 259
activation of 62
acute 60, 60*t*, 63, 65, 68, 69, 77, 78, 80, 80*t*, 82, 82*fc*, 83, 700, 933
suppurative 543, 737
bacterial 693
cardinal signs of 61, 61*t*
causes of 61
chemical mediators of 72
chronic nonspecific 86
complement-mediated 174
elevated markers of 299
endogenous causes of 61*b*
excessive 61
exogenous causes of 61*b*
gangrenous 82
general features of 60
macrophage events in 84
markers of acute 141
mediators of 73, 79, 84
pathways in acute 61
plasma-derived mediators of 78
prolongation of 570
prolonged 61
promote 179
role of 78, 552
signs of 61
spread of 911
systemic reactions of 75
types of 60, 68, 86
vascular reactions of acute 63
Inflammatory abdominal aortic aneurysm 489, 490
Inflammatory bowel disease 369, 621, 635, 636, 645, 681
hypothesis of 623*f*
pathogenesis of 621*b*, 623*f*
Inflammatory carcinoma 855, 857
Inflammatory cells 254, 513, 549, 550, 598, 618, 663, 727, 891, 928, 934
attraction of 550
infiltrate, reactive 392
migration of 934
Inflammatory changes
nonspecific 308
specific 308
Inflammatory chemokines, production of 77
Inflammatory cytokines 142, 668
Inflammatory diseases 183, 369
Inflammatory lesions 137, 757
diagnosis of 307
Inflammatory mediators 549
local production of 703
massive outpouring of 140
release of 571
Inflammatory myopathies 195
Inflammatory polyps 627, 631
Inflammatory reactions 17, 61, 85, 140, 216, 643, 911
initiation of 85
propagation of 85
Influenza virus 557
Inguinal hernia 775
Inguinal lymph nodes, superficial 788
Injury
antibody-mediated 713, 714
chronic 41, 702
consequences of 28
irreversible 23*t*, 514
resolution of 586
site of 66
Innate immune system 143*f*
deficiencies of 196
Innate immunity 165, 196
components of 165
cytokine of 169
general features of 165*b*
Inner epithelium 842
Inner tunica media 490
Innervation atrophy, loss of 41
Inorganic salts 726
Insane, general features of 113, 964
Insecticides 255, 290
Insoluble fibrin 147
Insulin 889, 895
deficiency 735, 883, 887, 889, 890
consequences of 888
excessive 890
requirement 748, 888
resistance 142, 299, 636, 886, 887
consequences of 886
mechanism of 887
secretion 887
signaling 887
treatment of 895
Insulin-like growth factor 39, 790
inhibition of 57
Insulinomas 908
Insulitis 892
Intact tumor suppressor gene, role of 240
Integrin, distribution of 68
Intercellular connections, loosening of 249
Interferon 562, 927
gamma 623
Interleukin 76, 143, 169, 623, 885, 927, 932
Internal callus 935
Internal organs 21, 195
Interphalangeal joints, proximal 928
Interstitial connective tissue 249, 865
Interstitial diseases, classification of 737*b*
Interstitial emphysema 551
Interstitial fibrosis 186, 195, 573, 747
Interstitial fluid 133*f*
colloid osmotic pressure 130
pressure 130
Interstitial inflammation 757
Interstitial inflammatory reaction 546
Interstitial lung disease 196
Interstitial pancreatitis, acute 700
Interstitial pressure 745
Interstitial pulmonary inflammation 573
Interstitial stroma 774, 925
Interstitial tissue, migration through 250
Interstitium 144, 712, 737, 749
Interventional cytology 306
Interventricular septum, posterior third of 516
Intestinal amebiasis
clinical features of 618
complications of 618
Intestinal complications 615
Intestinal defensins, abnormal 622
Intestinal disturbances 810
Intestinal epithelium 93, 823
benign neoplasms of 632
Intestinal lesions 614, 616
Intestinal lumen 622
Intestinal metaplasia 42, 595, 596, 596*f*, 599, 600, 606
Intestinal microbiota 622
Intestinal microflora 622
Intestinal obstruction 613, 824
gallstone-induced 696
Intestinal tuberculosis 560, 615
primary 615
secondary 615
Intestinal wall, fibrotic thickening of 624
Intestine 158, 563, 564, 612, 612*f*, 693, 694, 829
healed tuberculosis of 5
neoplastic polyps of 632
segment of 629
tuberculosis of 616*f*
Intimal tear 491
site of 491
Intra-abdominal testes, failure of 774
Intracardiac mural thrombi 157
Intracellular accumulation 14, 43
causes of 35
mechanism of 43, 43*f*
Intracellular glucose 892
Intracellular granules 73
Intracellular hyaline 52
Intracellular hyperglycemia 891

Intracellular infections 182
Intracellular ions 261
Intracellular lipid 832
Intracellular mucin production 704
Intracellular proteins, leakage of 22
Intracellular signal transduction 234
Intracellular tight junctions 602
Intracellular water, depletion of 888
Intracranial bleed 408
Intracranial disease 597
Intracranial neoplasms 977
Intracytoplasmic myelin figures 17
Intraductal carcinoma 849
Intraepithelial neoplasm 949
Intrahepatic bile
  destruction, mechanism of 680
  ducts 680
    small 681
Intrahepatic obstruction 136
Intrahepatic stones 689
Intralobular stroma 858
Intralobular terminal duct 842
Intraluminal growth 581
Intraluminal obstruction 743
Intraluminal pressure 642
Intramedullary high-grade malignant neoplasm 917
Intramucosal carcinoma 633
Intranuclear inclusions 878
Intraosseous abscess 912
Intraparenchymal mass 964
Intraprenchymal growth 579
Intrarenal reflux 739
Intratubal hematoma 839
Intratubular germ cell neoplasia 777
Intratubular nonseminoma 777
Intratubular seminoma 777
Intratumoral vessels, abnormal 248
Intrauterine death 114, 536
Intrauterine growth retardation 292
Intravascular hemolysis 343, 344, 344*t*
Intravascular microthrombi, formation of 144
Intravenous drug abusers 198, 524
Intrinsic glomerular
  antigens 715, 716
  cells, proliferation of 718*f*
Intrinsic myocardial damage 139
Intrinsic pathway 24, 247, 415
Intrinsic red cell defect 433
Introitus 738
Intussusception 629, 630*f*
  mechanism of 630*f*
  nomenclature of 630*f*
Inulin clearance test 472
Invasion 226, 248, 254, 879
  depth of 607, 642
  mechanism of 248
Invasive breast carcinoma 845, 846*t*, 850
  clinical features of 855
Invasive carcinoma 705*f*, 849, 850, 856
  common features of 850
  medullary pattern of 852, 852*f*, 862
  types of 853
Invasive ductal carcinoma 225*f*, 851, 862
Invasive hydatidiform mole 837
Invasive lobular carcinoma 853
Invasive papillary carcinoma 769*f*
Invasive prostatic cancer, precursor of 794
Invasive squamous cell carcinoma 578*f*, 786, 806*f*
Invasive tumors, high-grade 768, 769
Invasive urothelial
  carcinoma 767, 769*f*, 770*f*
  neoplasms 765
Involucrum 912
Iodine
  deficiency 871, 879
    consequences of 871
  low 871
  solution produces 211
Ionizing radiation 260, 371, 575, 949
Iron 334
  absorption 330
    metabolism of 331*f*
    molecular aspect of 330
    regulation of 331*f*
  balance, regulation of 331
  deficiency anemia 329, 332, 333*t*, 334, 352, 361, 362, 372*t*, 604, 611, 626
    causes of 332*b*
    clinical features of 333
    etiology of 331
    pathogenesis of 331
    stages of 332*fc*
  distribution 330, 330*t*
  excretion 330
  loss of 344
  metabolism 329
  overload 350
    classification of 678, 678*b*
  preparations 598
  status 356
  storage 409
  store 448, 449
  transport of 330
Irradiation 187
Irritability 304, 479
Irritable bowel syndrome 5
Irritation, chronic 41, 696, 767
Ischemia 15, 17, 29, 36, 37*f*, 61, 415, 490, 521, 602, 743, 744, 749
  consequences of 37*f*
  reperfusion injury 37
  sudden 511
Ischemic acute tubular injury 744, 745
Ischemic cell injury, mechanism of 37
Ischemic heart disease 131, 481, 492, 500, 508, 509*b*, 511*f*
  causes of 509*b*
  pathogenesis of 509
  risk of 490
Ischemic injury 19, 27, 643, 694, 750
Ischemic necrosis 158, 160
Ischemic tissue damage 354, 415*f*
Islet autoantibodies 884, 896
Islet cell destruction 883, 884
Isochromosome 275, 776
Isocitrate dehydrogenase 967
  encode isoforms of 372
Isoenzymes 268
Isohemagglutinins 326
Isolated-organ tuberculosis 566
Isoniazid 190
Isosporidiosis 204
Isosthenuria 453
Itching 681, 856

J

Jamshidi trephine biopsy needle 448*f*
Jarisch-Herxheimer reaction 114
Jaundice 138, 343, 346, 359, 647, 649, 652, 681, 688
  cholestatic 648
  classification of 648, 648*f*
  hemolytic 459, 648
  hepatic 648
  hepatocellular 459, 648, 707
  mechanism of 648
  mild 363
  nonobstructive 649
  surgical 648
  types of 651*t*
Jaw bones 915
Jenner stain 441
Jigsaw puzzle appearance 681
Joints 545, 910, 927, 931, 932
  antigens 926
  articular cartilage of 933
  deformity 929
  immobilization of 195
  lesions 927
  mice 929
  nonweight-bearing 928
  painful 928
  peripheral 193
  space 928
  weight-bearing 928
Jones criteria, revised 508*t*
Junctional nevus 954, 954*f*
Juvenile polyposis syndrome 631

K

Kala-azar 398
Kallikreins 80
Kaposi sarcoma 203, 259
Karyolysis 17
Karyorrhexis 17, 906
Karyotypic abnormalities 283
Karyotyping 277
  uses of 278
Kawasaki disease 496
Kayser-Fleischer rings 680
Kell and Duffy system 422
Keloid 102, 102*f*
  formation 105
Keratin pearls 805, 805*f*, 806*f*
  formation 786
Keratinization 299
Keratinizing squamous cell carcinoma 805, 806*f*
Keratinocyte 949
  atypical 786
  growth factor 790
Keratoconjunctivitis sicca 194
Keratomalacia 299
Keratoses, premalignant 949*f*
Keratosis, arsenical 949
Kernicterus 359
Kernig sign 962
Ketoacidosis 888, 889
Ketone, reaction for 457
Ketone bodies 44, 45, 457, 889, 890
  formation of 889
  increased production of 457
  tests for 457*b*, 893
Ketonemia 889
Ketonuria 889, 893
  causes of 457, 457*b*
Kidd system 422
Kidney 158, 178, 192, 195, 210, 300, 401, 496, 498, 545, 575, 679, 710, 744, 763, 882, 890, 892, 931
  acute suppurative inflammation of 737
  amyloidosis of 211*f*
  carcinoma of 228
  collecting system of 754
  cut section of 742*f*
  cystic diseases of 751
  disease of 712
    chronic 712, 736, 746, 746*b*, 747
    end-stage 101, 747
  histology of 710
  infarct of 18*f*
  injury, acute 712, 737, 742, 744
  intrinsic diseases of 743
  involvement 52
  malignant
    neoplasms of 759
    tumor of 759
  marked hydronephrosis of 759*f*
  morphology of 718
  nephroblastoma of 764*f*
  poles of 739
  role of 493
  stones 933
  tumor 759, 763
  vascular diseases of 748
Killing microbes, mechanism of 72
Kimmelstiel-Wilson
  disease 736
  lesion 736
Kingella 524
Kininogens 80
Kinins 64, 73, 80
Klatskin tumors 687
Klebsiella 738, 772
  infection 115
  pneumoniae 547
Klinefelter's syndrome 5, 277, 281, 282, 282*f*, 776, 798, 861, 883
Knee 506, 911
  joint, X-ray of 924*f*
  pain 962
Knudson's two-hit hypothesis 240
Koch's disease 559
Koch's phenomena 11
Koch's postulate 11
Koilocytes 804
Koilocytic atypia 804
Koilocytic halos 805*f*
Koilonychia 333, 362
Koplik spots 117
Korsakoff syndrome 303
Krukenberg tumor 611, 645, 833, 833*f*
Kupffer cells
  hyperplasia of 661
  hypertrophy of 661
Kussmaul breathing 889
Kwashiorkor 295, 295*f*, 296, 296*t*
Kyphosis 913

L

Lacerations 595
Lacrimation 621

- Lactate
  - dehydrogenase 473, 474, 514, 520, 520*f*, 784, 784
  - hydrogenase 359
- Lactic acid 144, 514
- Lactic acidosis 143, 144, 261, 457
- Lactiferous sinus 842
- Lactose 245
- Lactosuria 457
- Lacunar cell 393, 394
- Laennec cirrhosis 670
- Lamellar bone 921*f*
  - formation of 935
- Lamina densa 711
- Lamina propria 618, 623
  - inflammation of 643
- Landsteiner's rule 423
- Langerhans
  - cells 87, 168, 950
  - islets 209, 883
- Lardaceous spleen 210
- Large cell 778
  - carcinoma 580, 580*f*
- Large duct
  - inflammation 681
  - papillomas 844
  - system 842
- Large intestine 637*b*, 833
  - tumors of 635
  - ulcerative lesions of 616
- Laryngeal tuberculosis 565
- Larynx 575
- Latency 260
- Latent infection 200, 258
  - reactivation of 196, 564
- Latent membrane protein 1 259
- Latent viruses, reactivation of 187
- Late-phase reaction 172, 554
- Lead 289
  - toxicity 932
- Leather bottle appearance 609*f*
- Lectin pathway 79
- Lee-White method 418
- Left atrial appendage 150
- Left atrium 530, 538
- Left ventricle 530, 538
- Left ventricular
  - failure 521
  - hypertrophy 39*f*, 734, 901
- Leg
  - bones 914
  - bowing of 301
  - elephantiasis of 126*f*
- Legionnaires' disease 289
- Leiomyoma 817, 817*b*, 841, 942
  - different sites of 814*f*
  - growth of 815
  - microscopic appearance of 817*f*
  - microscopy of 816
  - morphology of 816
- Leiomyosarcoma 262, 817, 943
- Leishman stain 11, 192*f*, 333*f*, 337*f*, 339*f*, 346*f*, 356*f*, 377*f*, 380*f*, 386*f*, 400*f*, 410*f*, 441
- *Leishmania donovani* 443
- Lenses 892
- Lentigo 48
  - maligna 957
- Leonine facies 109, 109*f*
- Lepra bacilli 106, 110
- Lepra cells 109, 110*f*
  - collections of 110*f*
- Lepromatous leprosy 7, 108, 110, 110*f*, 111, 111*t*
  - leonine facies of 109*f*
  - microscopic appearance of 110*f*
- Lepromin test 110
- Leprosy 88, 106, 107, 107*fc*, 128
  - classification of 128
  - diagnosis of 110
  - reactions of 110
- Leptin 297
- Leptomeninges, acute inflammatory process of 960
- Leptomeningitis 960
- Lesch-Nyhan syndrome 932
- Lesion 127, 257, 566, 819, 892, 933
  - atherosclerotic 509, 510
  - depth of 959
  - low-grade 966
  - proliferative 757
  - sites of 109
  - small benign 765
  - well-demarcated 939
- Lesionsm, multiple 624
- Lethal tumors 880
- Leucine-rich repeat proteins 62
- Leukemia 218, 226, 245, 260, 267, 371, 372, 373, 384, 398, 448, 724, 755
  - acute 371, 372
    - lymphoblastic 261, 372-374, 375*f*, 402, 404
    - lymphoid 372
    - myeloblastic 402
    - myeloid 372, 375, 376
    - promyelocytic 375
  - childhood 373
  - chronic 372
    - lymphocytic 261, 384, 385, 386*f*, 404
    - myelogenous 237, 402, 405
    - myeloid 268, 367, 367*t*, 378, 380, 380*f*, 398
  - incidence of 261
  - risk factors for acute 371*b*
  - traditional classification of 372*b*
- Leukemoid reaction 366, 367, 367*t*, 379, 404
  - causes of 367*b*
  - types of 367*b*
- Leukocyte 65, 66, 66*f*, 67, 70, 70*t*, 71*f*, 72, 75, 77, 80, 89, 277, 323, 402*t*, 482, 483, 718, 721*f*, 729, 742
  - accumulation of 68, 80
  - activation of 65, 69, 76
  - adhesion 66, 75, 484
    - deficiency, types of 69
    - molecules, clinical importance of 69
  - arrest 67
  - casts 460, 742
  - chemotaxis of 66, 68
  - common antigen 267
  - emigration of 63*f*
  - events 64, 72
  - granule contents 71
  - granules of 72
  - infiltrates, nature of 68
  - infiltration 84, 728
  - infiltration of 713
  - inhibit recruitment of 75
  - large numbers of 81
  - mediated tissue injury 72
  - membrane 69*f*
  - migration 66, 66*f*, 67
  - movement of 68
  - normal range of different 365*t*
  - plasma membrane of 70
  - qualitative disorders of 370
  - quantitative disorders of 365, 370*f*
  - receptors 70, 77
  - recruitment 65, 75, 76, 79, 554, 555*f*, 732, 932
    - steps in 66
  - specific types of 77
  - type of 66
- Leukocytic infiltrate 99*f*, 892
- Leukocytosis 140, 365, 445, 701
  - causes of 366*b*
  - marked 380
  - mild 643
  - reactive 366
- Leukoderma 48
- Leukoerythroblastic reaction 369
  - causes of 369*b*
- Leukopenia 140, 365, 541, 615, 672
  - causes of 366*b*
- Leukoplakia 230, 589
- Leukotriene 65, 68, 73-75, 172, 550, 932
  - receptor antagonists 75
- Lewis system 422
- Lewy bodies 47
- Leydig cell 775, 831
  - prominent 774
- Leydig gonad 831
- Libman-Sacks endocarditis 150, 528, 529*f*
- Lichen sclerosus et atrophicus 787
- Lichtheimia 120
- Lid lag 869
- Lid retraction 867
- Li-Fraumeni syndrome 245, 917
- Ligamentum arteriosum 538
- Ligand, expression of 67, 68
- Light chain deposition 401
- Limbic encephalitis 827
- Linear chromosomes 55*f*
- Lining epithelial cells 765, 766
- Lining epithelium, type of 823
- Linitis plastica 608, 609
- Lip 908
  - cancer of 292
- Lipid 44, 49, 484
  - accumulation 483, 484
  - breakdown products 33
  - content, lower 761
  - defective metabolism of 45
  - droplets 832
  - envelope 199
  - laden histiocytes 944
  - mediators 141
  - metabolism 45*f*
    - abnormalities 748
    - products of 673
  - peroxidation 71, 33, 668, 679
  - release 484
- Lipiduria 451, 721, 723, 732
- Lipoblasts 938, 939*f*
- Lipofuscin 49, 59
- Lipolytic enzymes 697
- Lipoma 269, 936, 938*f*
- Lipopolysaccharide 62, 166, 668
- Lipoprotein 324, 482, 483
  - defective excretion of 45
  - formation of 44
  - lipase, stimulates 889
  - low-density 480, 891
  - metabolism 475
  - secretion of 667
  - very low-density 44
- Liposarcoma 218, 938, 939, 939*f*
  - diagnosis of 938
  - well-differentiated 938, 939
- Lipotoxicity 887
- Lipoxin 74, 75
- Lipoxygenase
  - actions of 75
  - inhibitors 75
  - pathway 75
- Liquefaction 467
- Liquefactive necrosis 18, 19, 19*f*, 59
- Liquid
  - based cytology 266, 311
  - biopsies 250, 267
- *Listeria monocytogenes* 961
- Lithiasis 458
- Lithogenic bile 691
- Liver 44, 45, 114, 126, 136*f*, 145, 162, 188, 210, 228, 293, 335, 350, 354, 496, 498, 502, 583, 610, 614, 628, 646, 678, 679, 682*f*, 696, 763, 784, 829, 830, 838
  - abscess 682
  - angiosarcoma of 261
  - biopsy 419, 475, 661, 663, 671, 673, 681
    - indications for 475
  - cancer 120
  - carcinoma of 674
  - chronic venous congestion of 135, 136*f*, 136*fc*
  - cirrhosis of 101, 129, 130, 136, 463, 668*f*
  - damage, chronic 663
  - hepatic malignant tumor of 687
  - injury, chronic 94
  - malignant neoplasms of 682
  - mechanism of regeneration of 94
  - metastasis to 709
  - percutaneous needle biopsy of 475
  - pigmentation of 49
  - primary tumors of 687
  - proinflammatory cytokine in 673
  - regeneration 94
  - tumors of 709
- Liver cell 92*f*, 658*f*, 663*f*
  - cytoplasm of 657
  - death of 675
  - injury, tests of 473
  - necrosis, repeated cycles of 683
  - regeneration, compensatory 259
  - ruptures 122
  - swollen 669
- Liver disease 414, 460
  - advanced chronic 653
  - alcoholic 47, 653, 666
  - alcohol-related 664, 665*f*, 666, 672*b*, 709
  - causes of 664
  - chronic 475, 653, 683, 684
    - sclerotic 10
  - coagulopathy of 429
  - severe 132
  - symptoms of chronic 673
  - type of 672

Liver failure 651, 653
acute 652, 653, 662, 680
chronic 653
types of 652
Liver function 419, 459
interpretation of 706
tests 94, 472, 473b, 648, 649, 660, 706-708
Lobar pneumonia 542, 542f, 543, 544f, 545, 545t, 588
four stages of 543b
Lobe
hypertrophy, median 791
lower 549
upper 548
Lobular architecture, accentuation of 729
Lobular carcinoma in situ 844, 847, 849
Lobular distortion 729
Lobular inflammation 661
Lobular neoplasia, noninvasive 845
Lobule
consists of 842
lining of 842
Lodgment of emboli, site of 155
Loeffler endomyocarditis 532
Loose bodies, formation of 929
Loss-of-function mutations 232, 242, 274, 252, 607, 679, 879, 880
Low albumin levels, consequences of 132
Low columnar epithelial
cells 687
lining 794
Lower extremity 892, 945
ischemia 891
Lower urinary tract 228, 458
infection 737, 739
obstruction 739
Low-molecular-weight proteins 722
Luetic dementia 964
Luetic vasculitis 112
Lumbar lordosis 301
Lumbar puncture 465
complications of 466b
contraindications for 466, 466b
indications for 466, 466b
needle 465, 465f
Lumen, occlusions of 161
Luminal bacterial components 623
Luminal obstruction by casts 744
Luminal spaces, slit-like 815
Lung 114, 159, 162, 195, 228, 231, 354, 501, 563, 573, 610, 618, 619, 642, 687, 696, 809, 830, 837, 899, 900, 936
abscess 83, 542, 543, 547, 588, 682
adenocarcinoma of 579f
asbestosis of 573f
brown induration of 48, 134, 135f
carcinoma of 227, 245, 255, 290, 575, 583t, 584
chronic venous congestion of 134, 134fc, 135f
collapse of 582, 585
disorder of 502
fibrosis of 574
gray hepatization of 544f
infections 289, 572
interstitium of 135
involvement, massive 52
large cell carcinoma of 580f
lesions, spectrum of 570
malignant epithelial tumor of 580
metastasis in 574
microvasculature of 159
miliary tuberculosis of 565f
morphology 543
neuroendocrine tumor of 581
opacification of 159
parenchyma 548, 571, 579f
peripheral carcinoma of 579f
primary tuberculosis of 561f, 562f, 567t
secondary tuberculosis of 566f, 567t
small-cell carcinomas of 243
squamous cell carcinoma of 580f
tumors 228, 574
Lung cancer 261, 289-292, 574, 575
classification of 574
clinical subgroups of 584
development of 291
local effects of 583t
location of 577
pathogenesis of 578f
risk of 290, 573, 575
spread of 583f
Lung disease 10, 569t
asbestos-related occupational 572, 572b
chronic 157
obstructive 548
occupational 569
Lung injury
acute 570, 585
prolongation of 570
transfusion-related acute 432, 433
Lupus anticoagulant syndrome 152, 192
Lupus erythematous
bodies 192
cell 192
test 445, 447
Lupus nephritis 193, 193f, 734, 735
Luteinizing hormone 282
Luteinizing hormone-releasing hormone 797
Lutheran system 422
Lymph node 197, 202, 202f, 205, 320, 350, 382, 384f, 386, 389, 394f, 568, 591, 614, 616
biopsy of 383
cells of 91
cut section of 384f
disorder of 365
enlargement of 227, 382
fine-needle aspiration cytology of 383
involvement, pattern of 227
matted 383
medulla of 387f
mesenteric 613, 614
metastases 607, 642, 854, 857
significance of 227
normal 593
structure of 382f
peripheral 395
periumbilical 610, 610f
sarcoidosis of 569f
section of 180f
status 264
tuberculosis of 316
Lymphadenitis 126, 227, 566
Lymphadenopathy 113, 374, 382
bilateral hilar 569
causes of 382, 382b
Lymphangiomas 284
Lymphatic drainage 130f
Lymphatic invasion, foci of 878
Lymphatic obstruction 130, 131f, 132
causes of 132
Lymphatic spread 227, 583, 596, 610, 642, 686, 706, 779, 795, 823, 879
Lymphatic vessels 857
Lymphedema 132, 164, 855
Lymphoblast 375f, 378, 378t
cytochemistry of 374
Lymphoblastic leukemias 373
Lymphoblastic lymphoma 404
Lymphochoriomeningitis virus 962
Lymphocyte 20f, 87, 166, 167, 180f, 194, 259, 316f, 319, 323, 369f, 394f, 449, 464, 467, 505, 552, 555f, 558, 564, 571f, 598, 614, 661, 663, 669, 741, 778, 829f, 866, 868
activated 76
depleted classical Hodgkin lymphoma 395
mature 386
predominant cell 393
reactive 393, 396f
rich classical Hodgkin lymphoma 395
role of 85
size of background 392
Lymphocyte-depleted classical Hodgkin lymphoma, microscopy of 395
Lymphocyte-rich classical Hodgkin lymphoma, microscopy of 395
Lymphocytic infiltrate 386, 778f
prominent 878
Lymphocytic lymphoma tumor, small 384, 385
Lymphocytopenia 369
causes of 369b
Lymphocytosis 368, 370, 615
absolute 386
atypical 370
causes of 369b
relative 660
Lymphogranuloma venereum 118, 133
Lymphoid
activation marker 393
cells, medium-sized 390
elements 594f
follicles 614, 865
malignant 387f
malignancy, staging of 448
neoplasms 384
classification of 384
miscellaneous 391
organs 117
stroma, reactive 594f
stromal tissue 593
tissue 202f, 319, 936
spread to 202
tumor cells 384
Lymphoma 218, 226, 267, 373, 383, 384, 398, 449, 600, 918
acute lymphoblastic 373
develops 259
malignant 267
Lymphopenia 660
Lymphoplasmacyte-rich meningioma 976
Lymphoplasmacytic infiltrate 853f, 866
Lymphoplasmacytic sclerosing pancreatitis 703
Lymphotoxin 183
Lymphovascular invasion 857
Lynch syndrome 634, 636, 812
Lyon hypothesis 276
Lysolecithin, production of 693
Lysosomal compartment 699
Lysosomal enzymes 72
deficiency of 285
release 178
Lysosomal granules 70
Lysosomal membrane 33, 34
Lysosomal storage
diseases 43f
disorder 286
Lysosome 72, 286
prevention of fusion of 561
Lysozyme 455
Lytic infection 258

M

M proteins 398
MacCallum plaques 505
Macroalbuminuria 892
Macroangiopathic hemolytic anemia 360
Macrocyte 441
round 340
Macrocytic anemia 339
nonmegaloblastic causes of 339
Macrocytosis, investigation of 340
Macrogamete 124
Macrometastases 857
Macromethods 443
Macromolecular substrate 285
Macronodular cirrhosis 674, 679
Macronodular hyperplasia 900
Macro-ovalocytes 337f, 341f
Macrophage 66, 72, 75, 84, 107, 110f, 143f, 168, 207f, 321, 385, 394f, 395f, 496, 505, 506, 552, 561, 571f, 614, 720, 741, 866, 891
activation of 85, 85f, 286, 484, 562
aggregates of 661
appearance of 518
differentiation of 563
engulfs lipoproteins 484
functions of 85
in repair, role of 97
lysosomes of 286
modified 564
origin of 84
products of activated 85
role of 84
tissue-resident 84
Macrovascular complications 891
Macrovesicular steatosis 669, 669f
Maculopapular rash 434
Madura foot 120, 121f
Madurella
grisea 120
mycetomatis 120

Magnesium 756
stones 755
Main pulmonary artery, bifurcation of 156
Malabsorption 132, 212, 300, 626
Malaise 671, 687, 718, 740, 963
Malaria 122, 123, 430, 443, 719
chronic 49, 398
Malarial parasite
appearance of 124f
life cycle of 123f
Malarial pigment 49, 122
Male infertility 557, 797
causes of 798b
Malformation 280
congenital 283
Malignancy
characteristic of 221
criteria for 905
diagnosis of 268
enabler of 253
hematologic 254, 262, 369, 410
risk for 633
tendency of 284
Malignant melanoma 266, 955, 957, 958f
etiology of 955
Malignant mesenchymal
component 815
tumor 217t, 941
Malignant neoplasm 218, 220, 244f, 284, 534, 874, 876
characteristics of 220
Malignant ovarian
germ cell tumors 828
tumors 825
Malignant tumor 216-217, 218t, 220, 225, 229, 229t, 248, 262, 284, 307, 683, 726, 759, 817, 819, 832, 838, 844, 921
cells 917, 918
constitute 283
grading of 262
invasive 133
pathways of spread of 226
Mall pancreatic ductules and ducts 699
Mallory body 47, 52, 52f, 670f
form of 668
Mallory's hyaline 53, 669, 686
Mallory-Denk bodies 669
Mallory-Weiss tears 595
Malnutrition 293, 546, 668
deficiencies 668
pathogenesis of severe acute 294
primary 293
severe acute 41, 293
Mandatory screening tests 430
Mandible, skull, and long bones, osteomas of 634
Mannose-rich oligosaccharides 62
Mantle cell lymphoma 391
Mantoux test 179, 560
Marasmus 294, 296, 296t, 305
Marcello Malpighi 10
March hemoglobinuria 459
Marfan syndrome 279, 489, 491
Marfanoid habitus 908
Marjolin ulcers 950
Marrow
by tumor, severe replacement of 367
hypoplasia 367
replacement 326
trephine biopsy 448
Mass
bilateral abdominal 752
red-blue 284
spectroscopy 212
Massive fibrosis, progressive 571, 572f
Masson trichrome 671f
Masson-Fontana reaction 957
Mast cell 73-75, 79, 86, 554, 944
activation of 172
granules of 74, 172, 554
Maternal chromosomes, complete absence of 834
Maternal imprinting 276
Maternal smoking 292
Matrix metalloproteinases 96, 97, 249, 809, 929f
inflammation-associated release of 489
Maturation 954, 954f
abnormal 785
Mature B-cell
neoplasms 373, 384
origin 384
Mature epithelium, hyperplastic 632
McBurney's point 644
McBurney's sign 644
McCune-Albright syndrome 903
Mean corpuscular volume 334
Measles 117, 557, 866
rash 117
virus 962
Mechanical inflammation 693
Meckel's diverticulitis 613
Meckel's diverticulum 612, 613f
Mediastinal germ cell tumors, development of 776
Mediastinal mass 374
Mediastinal nodes 784
Mediastinal thymic mass 374
Mediastinopericarditis, adhesive 535
Medulla, compresses renal vasculature of 757
Medullary carcinoma 208, 852, 881
atypical 852
development of 908
Medullary cavity 934
spread along 919
Medullary cystic disease 746, 751
Medullary pattern invasive carcinoma, characteristic features of 852b
Medullary sponge kidney 754
Medullary thyroid carcinoma 876, 880-882, 899, 907, 908
Medulloblastoma 228, 967, 973, 974, 974f
Megakaryocyte 321, 410f
Megakaryocytic disorders 448
Megakaryopoiesis 320, 332, 336, 338, 351, 380, 386, 409, 449
stages of 322f
Megaloblast 338, 339
Megaloblastic anemia 334, 337, 337f, 338, 340f, 363
bone marrow aspirate of 339f
causes of 336, 336t
clinical features of 339
indicative of 363
Megaloblastic marrow 340
Megaloblastic precursors 339f
Megaloblasts 338, 339t
Meigs syndrome 833
Meiotic division 826
Melanin 48, 260
pigment 957
production 119
protective mantle of 260
Melanocytes 955
malignant neoplasm of 955
tumors of 48
Melanocytic neoplasms 953, 957
Melanocytic nevus 953
acquired 953
maturation sequence of 954f
Melanocytic tumors 967
Melanoma 218, 232, 260, 262, 954, 955, 957, 959b
ABCDE warning signs of 958b
classification of 956
familial 955
morphology of malignant 957
pathogenesis of malignant 955
progression of 956f
sites of origin of 955, 955b
sporadic 955
Melanosis coli 48
Membrane attack complex 78f, 727
formation of 79
Membrane cofactor protein 730
Membrane damage 33
effects of 33f, 34
mechanism of 33f
Membrane defect 326, 343
Membrane filter preparations 312
Membrane lipids, peroxidation of 32
Membrane-bound
electron-dense granules 881
polysomes 16
Membranoproliferative glomerulonephritis 728, 728b, 729f, 730f
Membranous glomerulopathy 723, 726
causes of 726b
electron microscopy of 728f
secondary 726
Membranous inflammation 82
Membranous lupus nephritis 193
Membranous nephropathy 716, 726, 727f
electron microscopic appearance of 728f
light microscopy of 727f
Memory loss 870
Mendelian disorders 278, 279
Meningeal fibrosis 963
Meningeal vessels 961
Meninges 81, 545, 955, 960
Meningioma 51f, 967, 975, 975f, 976, 980
anaplastic 976, 977
angiomatous 976
atypical 976
malignant 976, 977
microcystic 976
morphology of 975
subtypes of 976, 976b
transitional 976
Meningitis 355, 465, 466, 545, 960, 961, 963t, 965
acute 960, 961
bacterial 965
pyogenic 467, 960
viral 980
aseptic 962, 980
bacterial 963
carcinomatous 960
chronic 962
complications of 960
fulminant 961
infectious 960
Meningococcal meningitis 965, 980
Meningococcus 902, 961
Meningoencephalitis 960, 963
Meningothelial meningioma 976
microscopy of 976f
Meningovascular disease, chronic 113
Meningovascular neurosyphilis 964
Meningovascular syphilis 964
Menopause 481, 512
late 845
Menorrhagia 408, 817, 832
Menstrual bleeding, heavy 362
Menstrual cycle 807
Menstrual flow, excessive 362
Menstrual phase 808
Menstruation, painful 810
Mental confusion 963
Mental impairment 870
Mental processes 870
Mental retardation, severe 870
Mental status 281
Mercury 289
binds 289
Merozoites 123
Mesangial cell 728, 731f, 737f
activation of 732
proliferation of 729f, 730f, 735
swelling of 718
Mesangial hypercellularity 728
Mesangial matrix 711, 711f, 737f
Mesangial proliferation 731
Mesangial proliferative lupus nephritis 193
Mesangiocapillary glomerulonephritis 728
Mesangium 711, 715, 733
Mesenchyma 858
Mesenchymal cells 76, 91, 765f, 930f
Mesenchymal elements, combinations of 683
Mesenchymal neoplasm 939
Mesenchymal stem cells 93, 936
Mesenchymal tissue type 780
Mesenchymal tumor 217, 801, 812, 818, 967
Mesenchyme 829
Mesenteric occlusion 485
Mesoderm 219, 779
Mesodermal derivatives 781
Mesothelial cells, malignant tumor of 586
Mesothelial tumors 819
Mesothelioma 218, 255, 574, 586
MET gene 760
Metabolic abnormalities 140, 142, 143f, 261, 689, 748
Metabolic acidosis 145, 745, 889
Metabolic bone disease 748
Metabolic byproducts, large amounts of 261
Metabolic complications, acute 889, 890
Metabolic defects 735
Metabolic derangements 141, 888
Metabolic diseases 746

Metabolic disorders 697
Metabolic dysfunction 672
Metabolic enzyme 372
Metabolic fatty liver disease 672
Metabolic liver diseases 678
Metabolic pathways 892
Metabolic status 98
Metabolic syndrome 283, 299, 481, 672, 684, 887
Metabolism
inherited errors of 183
rate of 293
tests of 473, 474
Metabolite produced, type of 72
Metabolites vanillylmandelic acid 907
Metabolome 269
Metanephric tumors 759
Metaphysis 910, 911, 917
Metaplasia 41, 59, 224, 553
causes of 42
types of 42
Metaplastic apocrine cells 843
Metaplastic columnar epithelium 595
Metaplastic meningioma 976
Metaplastic theory 809
Metastasis 226, 248, 250, 254, 581, 781, 819, 825, 837, 855, 857, 967
mechanism of 248
morphological appearance of 226
resemble primary tumor 226
retrograde 227
risk of 957, 959
significance of 226
sites of 959
skip 227
target organ for 228
theory, benign 809
to lung, sources of 584
unique patterns of 853
Metastatic calcification 51, 52*t*, 59, 401, 897
Metastatic cancer, multiple 228*f*
Metastatic carcinoma 649, 903
to ovary 833
Metastatic deposits, morphology of 228
Metastatic disease 262, 620, 779
Metastatic hydatidiform mole 837
Metastatic melanomas 957
Metastatic mole, diagnosis of 837
Metastatic neoplasm 397
Metastatic tumor 465, 584, 687, 775, 833, 966, 977, 977*f*
Methionine 336
Methyl violet 211
Metrorrhagia 817, 832
MGMT gene, promoter of 970
MHC gene 181
Microalbuminuria 455, 736, 892, 896
causes of 455
Microangiopathic hemolytic anemia 326, 343, 360, 416, 429, 750
Microangiopathy 892
Microbe
and damaged cells, recognition of 62
cellular receptors for 62
derived substances containing, recognize 141
intracellular destruction of 69, 70
reactions against 170
Microbial agents 623, 926
Microbial carcinogenesis 256
Microbial carcinogens 259
Microbial cell wall constituents 141
Microbial products 76
Microbial sensors 165
Microbial surface molecules 79
Microbiological examination 464, 465
Microbiology 8
Microbiota 622
control of 622
Microcytes 341*f*
Microcytic hypochromic anemia 304, 334*t*, 351
causes of 333, 334*b*
diagnosis of 333
Microcytosis 351
Microfilaria 126*f*, 443
Microgametes 124
Microglia, proliferation of 964
Microhemorrhages 134
Microlithiasis 691
Micrometastases 857
formation of 251
local growth of 251
Micromethods 443
Microorganisms 83, 165
adherence of 525
identification of 11
Micropapillary serous borderline tumors 821
Microplate method 424
Micrornas 233
Microsatellite instability 253, 634, 639
causes of 639
consequences of 639
pathway 638, 639*f*
Microscope 10
Microscopy, light 24, 46, 210, 581, 718, 724, 725, 727, 729, 730
Microtubules 666
Microvascular complications 890
Microvascular proliferation 969, 970
Microvascular thrombosis, pathogenesis of 415
Microvesicular steatosis 669, 669*f*
Midstream specimen 451
Miliary pulmonary disease 565
Milky fluid 463
Millionaire's antibody 168
Milroy's disease 133
Mineralocorticoids 899
Minimal change disease 721*f*, 723, 771
Minimal inflammatory reaction 662
Minimal residual disease, detection of 268
Minimal stromal collagen 940
Minimal-change disease
etiology of 724
morphology of 724
pathogenesis of 724
Minimally invasive
adenocarcinoma 578
follicular carcinomas 879
Miscellaneous disorders 448
Misfolded proteins, normal processing of 206
Missense mutations 273
Missense point mutation 353
Mitochondria 16, 17, 29, 29*f*, 667
alcohol produces dysfunction of 666
changes 23
dysfunction 29, 667
enzyme 474
injury, causes of 26*b*
Mitochondria damage 29, 143, 667
consequences of 29
effects of 29*f*
role of 29*f*
Mitochondrial membrane 33
damage of 34
Mitochondrial pathway 25*f*, 35*f*, 247
activates initiator caspase-9 27
critical initiator caspase of 26
Mitochondrial permeability 24, 26
transition pore, opening of 34
Mitochondrial proteins, leakage of 26, 29
Mitochondrial respiratory chain 666
Mitochondrial succinate dehydrogenase 612
Mitogen-activated protein kinase 237
pathway 876
signaling pathway, activation of 971
Mitoses 778, 804
atypical 221
rare 220
Mitotic activity 224, 821, 906
Mitotic catastrophe 247
loss of 248
Mitotic figures 795, 813, 816, 945
numerous atypical 918
Mitotic index 612
Mitral incompetence 507
Mitral stenosis 5, 134, 157, 507*f*
consequences of 507
Mitral valve 506, 507, 527*f*
gross appearance of 505
posterior leaflet of 506
prolapse 525, 753
Mitsuda reaction 110
Modern pathology 12
Moist tissues 21
Molar chorionic villi 837
Mole, partial 836, 837
Molecular classification 844
Molecular cytogenetic assays 287
Molecular cytogenetics 277
Molecular diagnosis, uses of 268
Molecular genetics 387, 946
Molecular mimicry 189, 214
Molecular pathogenesis 374, 389, 776, 823, 864, 938, 955
Molecular pathology 8, 348
Molecular subtype 858, 973
Molecular techniques 314
Molecules favor gluconeogenesis 142
Moles 953
Molluscum
body 127
contagiosum 127, 127*f*
Monckeberg's medial
calcific sclerosis 50, 51*f*
sclerosis 479
Monoclonal antibodies 385*t*
Monoclonal hypothesis 482
Monoclonal immunoglobulins 208
Monoclonal plasma cells serve, secretions of 398
Monocyte 84, 165, 179, 319, 323, 369, 385, 554, 555*f*, 720
adhesion 483
differentiation of 84
migration of 483*f*
Monocytosis 368
causes of 369*b*
Monodermal teratoma 826, 828
Monogenic disorders 278
Monomorphic blue spindle cell 945
Monomorphic cells, sheets of 974
Monomorphic lymphocytes 386
Mononuclear cells 370, 481, 923
aggregates of 572
infiltrate 83
Mononuclear infiltration 112
Mononuclear inflammatory
cells 661
infiltrate 112
Mononuclear phagocyte
maturation of 84*f*
system 84
part of 168
Mononuclear stromal cells 923*f*
Mononucleosis, infectious 370
Monophasic synovial sarcoma 946
Monosodium urate crystals 933
precipitation of 932
Monosomy 275
Monotonous cuboidal follicular cells 875
Monotonous tumor cells 829
Monozygotic twins 864, 867
Moon facies 900
Morbidity, causes of 288, 479
Morphologic classification 674
Morphologic precursor epithelial lesions 577*b*
Morphological classification 325, 674
Mortality, causes of 288, 479
Morula cells 399
Mosaicism 275
Mosquito cycle 123
Motile flagellate protozoa 443
Motile spermatozoa sticking 468
Motor neuron disease 41
Mott cells 399
Mouth 575
M-proteins, production of 401
Mucin 268, 691
depletion 627
globules 855
glycoprotein 688, 689
Mucinous adenocarcinomas 640
Mucinous borderline tumors 824
Mucinous carcinoma 819, 854
prognosis of 824
spread of 824
Mucinous cystadenoma 841
Mucinous tumor 818, 823, 824*f*
cells 824
Mucocele 693
Mucociliary apparatus 541
Mucociliary clearance 546
Mucocutaneous
hyperpigmentation 632*f*
Mucocutaneous lesions 113, 116
Mucoepidermoid carcinoma 594, 594*f*
Mucoid contents 824
Mucoid degeneration 53

Mucopurulent secretions 558
Mucormycosis 120
Mucosa 603, 607, 614, 626, 627
chemical irritation of 602
superficial inflammation of 623
Mucosal aphthous ulcers 624
Mucosal atrophy 626, 627
Mucosal bleeding 408
Mucosal blood flow 602
Mucosal crypt architecture, distortion of 625
Mucosal edema 624
Mucosal epithelium 695
Mucosal immune responses, abnormal 622, 623
Mucosal lentiginous melanoma 957
Mucosal lesions 624
Mucosal lymphoid tissue 201
Mucosal neutrophils 643
Mucosal prostaglandin synthesis, suppresses 602
Mucosal ulceration 616
Mucous membrane 552, 589, 655
catarrhal inflammation of 53
Mucus 53
excessive secretion of 53
hypersecretion of 552, 691
secreting
cells 594
tumors 53
Müllerian epithelium 818
Müllerian tumors 815
Multicentric castleman disease 259
Multicystic renal dysplasia 751
Multidrug resistance protein, complete absence of 651
Multifactorial disease 885
Multifactorial disorder 494
Multiglandular process 896
Multinodular goiter 871, 872*f*, 873, 874
evolution of 872
microscopy of 873*f*
morphology of 873
Multinodular mass 938
Multinodular tumor 938
Multinucleate giant cells 180*f*, 564*f*, 866, 923, 923*f*
Multiorgan failure 143
end-stage 143*f*
Multiparous women 184
Multiple endocrine neoplasia 908
syndromes 907
Multiple myeloma 207, 214, 398, 399, 400, 400*t*, 455
laboratory diagnosis of 399
Multiple nodules 584, 873
Multiple pituitary hormones, deficiencies of 903
Multiprotein cytoplasmic complex 887
Multistep carcinogenesis 256
Multistix reagent strip 460, 461*f*
Multisystem disease 193
Multivalvular rheumatic disease 507*f*
Multivitamin deficiencies 295
Mumps 699, 866, 884
virus 962
Mural endocarditis 505
Mural thrombi 507, 530
and embolism 521
Muscle
abdominal 614
mass 295, 900
specific actin 267
weakness 889, 900
Muscular arteries, media of 50
Muscularis mucosae 600
Muscularis propria, inflammation of 643
Musculoskeletal system 195, 279
Mutant gene, location of 279
Mutant protein 206
production of normal amount of 206
Mutant transthyretin 209
Mutated genes, products of 251
Mutation 215, 273, 348, 955
accumulation of 848
acquired 231, 232, 242, 245
acquisition of 36
classification of 273
functional effects of 274
spontaneous 273
Mutator phenotype 253
Myasthenia 263
gravis 174, 176, 188
MYC gene, translocations of 389
Mycetoma 120, 121*f*
foot 120
Mycobacteria 106, 561, 572, 926
atypical 560
characteristics of 560
entry of 561
ingestion of 107
proliferation of 561
Mycobacterial antigen 560
Mycobacterial cell wall 107
Mycobacterial infection 106, 448
Mycobacteriosis 204
Mycobacterium 562*f*, 567
bovis 560, 615
hominis 615
leprae 88, 106, 128
Mycobacterium avium
complex 106, 398, 542, 560
intracellulare 204
Mycobacterium tuberculosis 3, 87, 88, 106, 170, 557, 559, 561, 562, 567, 572, 588, 800, 965, 980
hominis 560
Mycoplasma 788, 800, 926
Mycosis
fungoides 391
superficial 118
Mycotic abdominal aortic aneurysm 490
Mycotic aneurysm 155, 158, 161, 488, 526
Myeloblast 373, 377*f*, 378, 378*t*, 380
Myelodysplastic syndromes 448, 449
Myelofibrosis 378, 448
Myeloid
leukemia, natural history of chronic 379
sarcoma 376, 378
series 373
tissue 319
Myeloma 401*fc*
cell 399
diagnosis of 402*b*
kidney 401
Myeloperoxidase 71, 71*f*, 373, 377*f*
Myelopoiesis 320, 332, 338, 351, 380, 386, 409, 449
stages of 322*f*
Myeloproliferative neoplasms 366, 378, 378*b*, 448, 449
Myocardial cell 162
vacuolization of 518
Myocardial contractile function worsens 144
Myocardial damage, severe 520*f*
Myocardial demand 509, 513
Myocardial hypertrophy 509, 869
massive 531
mechanisms of 39*f*
Myocardial infarction 150, 157, 292, 492, 509, 512, 517, 517*t*, 518, 519, 520*f*, 520*t*, 522*f*, 892, 906
acute 151, 518*f*, 520*f*, 743
causes of 512*b*
classification of 514
complications of 520, 521*b*
consequences of 520
development of 518*f*
diagnosis of 519
etiopathogenesis of 512
massive 139
pathogenesis of 513
pattern of 516*f*
risk of 480
site of acute 152
Myocardial ischemia 113, 508, 522
acute 522
causes of 509
Myocardial necrosis 513, 515*f*
Myocardial response to ischemia 514
Myocardial rupture 521
Myocardial structural changes 500
Myocarditis 504*f*, 506
Myocardium 505, 508, 515*f*, 679
noninfarcted 517
thickness of 514
Myocytes, marked hypertrophy of 531
Myocytolysis 518
Myoepithelial cells 219*f*, 592, 842, 842*f*, 844, 860
Myoepithelial elements 592
Myofiber disarray 531
Myofibroblastic tumors 937, 939
Myofibroblasts 100, 702*f*, 939
Myoglobin 455, 520, 520*f*, 745
in urine 458
tests for 457
Myoglobinuria 458
Myomas 815
Myometrial smooth muscle
hyperplasia 59
hypertrophy 59
Myometrium 810*f*, 817, 838
Myopathy, proximal 301, 748
Myopericarditis 533
Myosin-binding protein c 531
Myositis ossificans 42
Myxedema 53, 133, 870
madness 870
Myxoid
degeneration 53
liposarcoma 938, 939, 939*f*
stroma 593*f*

N

Nails, spoon-shaped 362
Naïve lymphocytes 167
Nasal cavities, cancer of 290
Nasal sinuses 547
Nasopharynx, rhinosporidiosis of 127*f*
Natural killer cell 166, 167, 169*f*, 321
neoplasms 373, 385
precursors 319
Natural microbial product 255
Nausea 694, 718, 890, 970
Neck
defect 468
great arteries of 492
stiffness 962
Necroptosis 27
Necrosis 16, 17, 27, 28*t*, 36, 87, 144, 223, 824, 970
causes of 17
coagulative type of 161
laboratory detection of 22
morphologic patterns of 18*b*
Necrotic bone, gross appearance of 913*f*
Necrotic cells 18*f*, 62, 76, 514, 700*f*
fate of 17
Necrotic fat cells 20*f*
Necrotic foam cells 484
Necrotic smooth muscle cell debris 486*f*
Necrotic tissue 50
Necrotic uterine mass 838
Necrotizing granulomas 497, 498
Necrotizing inflammation 82
Necrotizing papillitis 736
causes of 737, 773
Needle biopsy 265, 796
Negative energy balance 889
Neisseria
gonorrhoeae 911
meningitidis 902, 961, 965, 980
Neoangiogenesis, effects of 248
Neoantigens 251
Neoplasia 103, 215, 743
clinical aspects of 261
role in 243
Neoplasm 204, 204*t*, 215, 414, 953
anaplastic 221
basic microscopic components of 216
benign 229, 284
diagnosis of 266*t*
epithelial odontogenic neoplasm 594
low-risk 874
nomenclature of 216
premalignant 230
produced 259
pure 783
Neoplastic blast cells 371
Neoplastic bone formation 918, 919
Neoplastic cartilage, production of 921
Neoplastic cells 393, 534, 922, 939*f*
minority of 392
Neoplastic cuboidal cytotrophoblast, dimorphic population of 838*f*
Neoplastic epithelial
cell 593
abnormalities 308
component 859
Neoplastic fibrillary astrocytes 968
Neoplastic follicles 387*f*
Neoplastic glands 794
Neoplastic leukocytosis 366
Neoplastic lymphoid cells, features of 390

Neoplastic mononuclear cells 923
Neoplastic polyps 632
Neoplastic squamous cells 788*f*
Neoplastic stroma 858
 component 859
Neoplastic transformation 256
 suppression of 243
 target for 257
Neoplastic villous trophoblastic cells 838
Nephrin 725
Nephritic syndrome 712, 713, 716, 716*b*, 719, 732, 732*t*, 771, 773
Nephritis
 acute 719
 tubulointerstitial 743
Nephritogenic strains 717
Nephroblastoma 763, 765*f*
 morphology of 764
Nephrocalcinosis 52, 897
Nephrogenic rests 764
Nephrolithiasis 600, 754, 897
Nephron 710, 725
 different components of 710*f*
Nephronophthisis-medullary cystic disease complex 753
Nephropathy 892
 obstructive 757
Nephrosclerosis 747, 749, 750
Nephrotic syndrome 129, 132, 212, 401, 451, 712, 721, 722*fc*, 723*f*, 724, 727, 729, 731, 732, 732*t*, 736, 901
 causes of 721, 723, 723*t*, 724, 773
 complications of 723
Nephrotic-nephritic picture 729
Nephrotoxic acute tubular injury 744, 745
Nephrotoxicity 290
Nephrotoxins 743
Nerve 882, 892
 and muscle syndromes 263
 biopsy 111
 fibers 108, 944
 sheath tumors, malignant peripheral 944
Nervous system 116, 279, 284, 748, 870
NESTROF test 352
Neural crest cells, migration of 630
Neurilemmoma 269, 943, 944*f*
Neuroblastic tumor 906
Neuroblastoma 233*f*, 238, 267, 764, 906, 907*f*
 staging of 907
Neuroblasts, primitive 906
Neurocysticercosis 125
Neurodegenerative diseases 27
Neuroendocrine 904
 carcinoma 576, 580, 619
 low-grade 581
 cell hyperplasia 577
 markers 582
 neoplasms 580, 845
 tumor 267, 576, 619, 828
Neurofibrillary tangle 47
Neurofibroma 944
 microscopic appearance of 945*f*
Neurofibromatosis 230, 279
Neurofilament proteins 267
Neurogenic bladder 757, 768
 dysfunction 739
Neurohumoral mechanisms 297
Neurohumoral systems, activation of 500
Neurologic symptoms 159
Neuromuscular abnormalities 897
Neuromuscular irritability 898
Neuromuscular system 867
Neuromuscular transmission 300
Neurons 91, 92*f*, 162
 second-order 298
Neuron-specific enolase 267, 906
Neuropathy 890
 autonomic 893
 familial amyloidotic 209
 peripheral 303, 304
Neuropeptides 80
Neurosurgical operation 960
Neurosyphilis 113, 964
Neurotoxicity 290
Neurotrophic tyrosine kinase 877
Neutral charge, molecules of 715
Neutropenia 174, 203, 342, 367, 373, 374, 660
 causes of 367, 368*b*, 366*b*
Neutrophil 66, 68, 72, 79, 86, 98, 104, 105, 143*f*, 165, 179, 179*f*, 319, 323, 380, 393, 464, 467, 552, 554, 555*f*, 614, 739, 866, 928, 962
 activator of 75
 aggregates of 739
 alkaline phosphatase 373
 bactericidal system of 71
 disorder of 366
 extracellular traps 72
 extravasation of 585
 function 142, 891
 granules of 71*f*
 infiltrates of 540
 infiltration 99
 production, selective suppression of 367
 recruitment and accumulation of 932
Neutrophilia 366, 366*f*, 645
 causes of 366
Neutrophilic infiltration 669, 670*f*
Neutrophilic tubulitis 739
Nevoid basal cell carcinoma syndrome 952
Nevus cells 954*f*
 superficial 954
Newer cancer diagnostics 269
Next-generation sequencing 269, 287
Niacin 303
 to nicotinic acid 303
Nickel 290, 575
Nicotinamide adenine dinucleotide 303
 depletion of 293
 phosphate 666
Nicotine 291
Niemann-Pick disease 46, 285, 369
Night blindness 299, 870
Nipple 855
 and nipple discharge, retraction of 855
 appearance of 855*f*
 epidermis of 855*f*
 retraction 851
 tumors of 845
Nitric oxide 54, 64, 71*f*, 143, 147, 148, 510, 805
 production of 142
 synthase, stimulates inducible 563
Nitrogen
 derived molecules 71
 dioxide 551, 552
 oxides of 289
Nitroprusside 457
 reaction 893
Nitroprusside test 457
Nitrosamine 229, 255, 291, 596
Nocardiosis 204
Nocturia 741, 759
Nocturnal pain, severe 916
Nodular fasciitis 939
Nodular glomerulosclerosis 736, 736*f*
Nodular lesions 952
Nodular lymphocyte 396*f*
 predominant Hodgkin lymphoma 392, 396
Nodular melanomas 957
Nodular sclerosis 405
 classical Hodgkin lymphoma 392, 393, 394, 394*f*
Nodular silicosis, simple 571, 572*f*
Nodular thyroid gland 872*f*
Nodules 789
 composition of 791
 hyperplastic 791*f*
 types of 791
Nonalcoholic fatty liver disease 299, 653, 672, 673, 684
Nonalcoholic steatohepatitis 672
Nonatheromatous causes 509
Nonbacterial thrombotic endocarditis 150, 262, 263, 528
Nonclonal lesions 874
Nonconservative missense mutation 273
Noncrystalline amorphous deposits 52
Nondiabetic ketonuria 457
Nonendemic Burkitt lymphoma, mechanism of 259
Non-endocrine diseases 456
Nonenzymatic mechanism 32
Nongerm cell 781
Nongestational choriocarcinoma 826
 of ovary 830
Nonglomerular antigens 715
Nonglomerular causes 458
Non-hematopoietic solid tumors 233
Nonheme iron 330
 promotes absorption of 301
Non-Hodgkin lymphoma 384, 392*b*, 397, 397*t*
Nonimmune-mediated
 hemolysis 433
 red cell hemolysis, causes of 433
Nonimmunocyte-derived tumors 208
Nonimmunological destruction 408
Noninfectious complications 431
Noninfectious disorders, complications of 140
Noninvasive papillary
 carcinoma 767*f*
 tumors 765, 768, 769*f*
 urothelial carcinoma 765*f*
Non-ionic detergent 440
Nonlethal genetic damage 252
Nonlipogenic sarcoma, high-grade 939
Nonmegaloblastic macrocytic anemia, etiology of 340*b*
Nonmegaloblastic marrow 340
Nonmucin glycoproteins 691
Non-neoplastic
 cells 393
 diseases 292
 disorders 230
 epithelial components 858
 hematological disorders 397
 lesions, diagnosis of 307
 osteoclasts 922
 polyps 631
Non-nephrotic proteinuria 736
Nonpituitary neoplasms 899
Nonreplicative senescence 240
Nonseminomatous germ cell tumors 775, 779, 783
Nonseminomatous tumors 777, 779, 782*t*
Nonsense mutation 274
Non-ST elevated myocardial infarct 515
Nonsteroidal anti-inflammatory drug 724, 410, 598, 602, 931
Nonstratified mucinous epithelium 823
Nonstructural protein 658
Nonsyndromic nephroblastomas, molecular abnormalities in 764
Nonthrombocytopenic purpura 407, 407*b*
Nontreponemal antibody tests 114
Nonvascular complications 890
Norepinephrine 500, 904
Normal architecture, loss of 386
Normoblast 339, 339*t*
Normocytic normochromic anemia 325, 380
Nottingham histologic score 851, 857
NTRK3 fusion 941
Nuclear
 changes 17
 characters 378
 factor, activation of 392
 grooves 825
 hyperchromasia 578*f*
 maturation 334, 336
 morphology, abnormal 221
 plant accidents 261
 pleomorphism 221, 222, 224
 regulatory proteins 239
 self-antigens 191
 transcription factors 237
Nuclear atypia 766, 812, 819, 922, 945, 970
 mild-to-moderate 824
Nuclear-cytoplasmic asynchrony 338
Nuclear-free zones 943
Nucleic acid 255, 431
 amplification test 431
 test 431
Nucleoli, prominent 777
Nucleolus 582
 prominent 843
Nucleotide
 base pairs 272
 excision repair 959
 pathway 260
 oligomerization binding domain 622

Nucleus 16, 87, 582, 777, 778, 804, 813
cigar-shaped 816
delayed maturation of 336
large 392, 829
pleomorphism of 229
Numerous mitoses 767, 918
Numerous mitotic figures 390, 769, 861, 974
Numerous polymorphonuclear leukocytes 547
Nutmeg liver 502
Nutritional cirrhosis 670
Nutritional deficiencies 15
Nutritional derangements 61
Nutritional diseases 288
Nutritional excesses 15
Nutritional factors 536
Nutritional imbalances 15
Nutritional status 98

O

Obesity 230, 296, 297, 482, 637, 689, 813, 886*fc*, 887
central 297, 887
classification of 297*t*
clinical consequences of 298, 298*b*
complications of 298
development of 673
etiology of 297
genes 297
metabolic complications of 299
pathogenesis of 297
prevalence of 297
types of 297
Obliterated capillary lumina 725
Obliterative endarteritis 963, 964
Obstruction
bilateral partial 759
causes of 743, 757, 758
complete bilateral 759
consequences of 792
level of 758
Obstructive bronchiectasis 557
Obstructive disease 548
Obstructive hydrocephalus 961
Obstructive jaundice 459, 649, 705, 707
causes of 649*f*
Obstructive proteinaceous casts 401
Occlusion, rate of 162
Occult
blood loss 640
neoplasm 610
Ocular changes 867
Oddi sphincter 699
Odontogenic tumor 594
Odor 452
Old burn scars 950
Oligodendroglioma 967, 970, 972*f*, 900
well-differentiated 971
Oligospermia 468
Oligospermic infertility 776
Oliguria 451, 716, 718, 719, 732, 742, 743
produce 744
severe 719
Omega-3 fatty acids 480
Omentum 20*f*
Oncocytes 593, 865
Oncocytic cell change 875
Oncocytic changes 875
Oncofetal antigens 268
Oncogene 235
activation of 576, 577, 705, 955
categories of 239
group of 235
products of 235
Oncogenesis, Knudson's two-hit hypothesis of 240
Oncogenic
damage 252
DNA viruses 257
gain-of-function mutations 576
mechanisms, specific 684
mutations 705, 877
ribonucleic acid viruses 256
Oncogenic virus 204, 251, 256
classification of 257*fc*
types of 257*fc*
Oncometabolism 246
Oncoprotein 235
production 235
One nucleotide, replacement of 273
Onion skin fibrosis 681
Oocyst 124
Ookinete stage 124
Ophthalmic lesions 116
Ophthalmopathy 869
Opisthorchis sinensis 687
Opportunistic infections 118, 203, 204
Opportunistic mycoses 118
Opsonin 69, 70, 79
receptors for 69
Opsonization 69
Optic nerve head, swelling of 133
Oral anticoagulant therapy, monitor 419
Oral cancer 291, 292
Oral candidiasis 118
Oral cavity 91, 118, 589
precancerous lesions of 589
premalignant lesions of 589
Oral contraceptive 689
use 152, 512
Oral glucose tolerance test 893
Orchiectomy 783
Organ damage 750
chronic 354, 355
evidence of 399
Organ dysfunction 140, 143, 143*f*
Organ failure 141
Organ systems 495
Organ toxicity 188
Organ transplantation 181, 950
Organic materials, smoke from burning of 289
Organic mercury 290
Orientia tsutsugamushi 117
Oropharyngeal contents, aspiration of 541
Oropharynx 801
Orphan Annie eye 878, 878*f*
Orthopnea 501, 558
Orthotoluidine test 458
Osmotic diuresis 889, 890
Osmotic fragility 323, 346, 449, 450
test 323, 346, 362, 449, 450*f*
Osmotic pressure 164
Osseous metaplasia 42
Ossifications, ring-like 922
Osteitis
deformans 914
fibrosa cystica 897, 898
Osteoarthritic cartilage 929
Osteoarthritis 299, 928, 929*f*, 930*f*
pathogenesis of 929*f*
primary 928
secondary 914, 929
Osteoarthropathy, hypertrophic 537
Osteoblast precursors 922, 923
Osteoblastic activity 914
Osteoblastic lesion 228
Osteoblastic metastases, detection of 797
Osteoblastoma 916
Osteoblasts 910, 915*f*, 934, 934*f*
Osteochondroma 920, 921*f*
microscopy of 921*f*
Osteoclastic activity 928
Osteoclastic giant cell 923
rich tumors 916, 922
Osteoclastic-osteoblastic stage, mixed 914
Osteoclastoma 922
Osteoclasts 910, 915*f*, 934*f*
mature 923
numerous large 914
Osteocytes 910
Osteogenesis imperfecta 279
Osteogenic tumors 915, 916
Osteoid 919*f*
osteomas 916
production of 918
unmineralized 918
Osteolytic lesion 228
Osteoma 915
Osteomalacia 301, 449, 681
Osteomyelitis 86, 355, 910, 913*f*, 918
acute 912
chronic 83, 86, 912, 913
etiology of 911
location of 911
morphologic variants of 912
Osteonectin 919
Osteopenia 867
Osteophytes 930
development of 930
formation of 929, 930*f*
prominent 931
Osteoporosis 449, 681, 900, 928
Osteoprogenitor cells 934, 934*f*
activation of 934
Osteosarcoma 227, 242, 764, 916-919, 920*f*
classification of 917*b*
etiology of 917
high-grade 920
microscopy of 919*f*
pathogenesis of 917
primary 917
radiological features of 920*f*
secondary 915, 917, 918
spread of 919
sunburst appearance of 920*f*
surface 920
type of 917, 920
X-ray of 920*f*
Outdoor air pollution 288, 288*b*
Oval blue cells 764
Oval fat bodies 725
Oval typhoid ulcers 614
Ovarian cancer 817
Ovarian endometrioid 809
Ovarian fibroma 833
Ovarian germ cell tumors 826
Ovarian neoplasms 818, 823, 826, 831
Ovarian serous carcinoma, spread of 823
Ovarian teratoma 826, 866
Ovarian tumors 232, 817, 826
Ovary 817
adult granulosa cell tumor of 832*f*
benign cystic teratoma of 826
dermoid cyst of 827*f*
dysgerminoma of 778, 829*f*
epithelial tumors of 818, 819*f*
germ cell tumors of 818, 826
granulosa cell tumor of 260, 831*f*
high-grade serous carcinomas of 822*f*
immature teratoma of 828*f*
mucinous
carcinoma of 824
cystadenoma of 823*f*, 824*f*
tumors of 823
opened mature cystic teratoma of 827*f*
routes of spread to 833
serous
borderline tumor of 821*f*
cystadenoma of 820*f*
epithelial tumors of 820
tumors of 820, 823
sex cord-stromal tumors of 818
teratoma of 826
Overweight, classification of 297*t*
Oxidant air pollutants 288
Oxidation reactions 304
Oxygen
delivery 144
intoxication 542
Oxygen-derived free radicals 30
Oxyntic cells 297
Oxyphil 875
cells 865
Ozone 288

P

P53 gene 243
P53 tumor suppressor gene, mutation of 590
Pacemaker cells 611
Packed cell volume 443
Packed red blood cells 428, 429, 429*b*
Paget's cells, appearance of 855
Paget's disease 862, 914, 917
causes of 914
of bone 914, 915*f*, 918
of breast 856*f*
of nipple 855, 855*f*
Pagetic bone 915
Pagetoid infiltration 226
Pain 80, 193, 705, 914
acute abdominal 354
and fever 75
crises 354
with intercourse 810
Palisading, peripheral 952
Palmar erythema 677
Palmar fibromatosis 940
Palmitate 688
Palpable mass 855, 856
Palpable nodularity 843
Palpation, abdominal 708
Palpitations 890

Panacinar emphysema 548
Pancarditis 504*f*
Pancoast tumors 583
Pancreas 155, 575, 678, 679, 687, 696, 700, 702, 892, 908
cystic fibrosis of 53
parenchyma of 700
pseudocyst of 703, 704*f*
Pancreatic acinar cells, loss of 702*f*
Pancreatic acini 700*f*
Pancreatic beta-cells 887
Pancreatic cancer 698, 704
Pancreatic carcinogenesis, genetic progression of 705*f*
Pancreatic carcinoma 704, 707
risk factors for 704*b*
Pancreatic disorders 646
Pancreatic duct 697, 702
obstruction 698, 703
variable dilation of 703
Pancreatic ductal
adenocarcinoma 704
cells 702
Pancreatic endocrine
insufficiency 703
tumors 908
Pancreatic enzymes, activation of 697
Pancreatic exocrine insufficiency 703
Pancreatic fibrosis 679
Pancreatic intraepithelial neoplasia 704
low-grade 705*f*
Pancreatic necrosis 700
Pancreatic parenchyma 700
extensive necrosis of 700
Pancreatic secretions 699
Pancreatic stellate cells, proliferation of 703
Pancreatic trypsin inhibitor gene, mutation in 697
Pancreatitis 668, 696
acute 20, 20*f*, 59, 645, 693, 696, 697, 699, 702, 709
hemorrhagic 700, 701*f*
necrotizing 700, 700*f*
alcoholic-induced chronic 703
alcohol-induced 699
chronic 696, 702, 702*f*, 703
edematous 700
nonobstructive chronic 703
obstructive chronic 703
pathogenesis 698, 698*f*, 702*f*
recurrent acute 703
sporadic acute 698
Pancytopenia 342, 342*b*
Paneth cell metaplasia 625, 627
Panlobular emphysema 548
Pannus formation 928
Pap smear 307, 807
applications of 308
examination 807
Pap test 807
abnormal 804
Papanicolaou
method 807
smear 307, 805*f*, 807*f*
stain 312, 312*b*, 316*f*
Papillae with fibrovascular core 820
Papillary carcinoma 762*f*, 876, 878, 880, 909
cut section of 877*f*
spread of 878
Papillary cystadenoma 217
lymphomatosum 593
Papillary growth pattern 762
Papillary meningioma 976
Papillary muscle
dysfunction 521
rupture of 521
Papillary necrosis 736, 739
Papillary neoplasms 765, 845
Papillary renal
cell carcinoma 760, 760*f*, 761
tumors 759
Papillary serous
cystadenofibroma 821*f*
Papillary structures 766, 821
Papillary thyroid carcinoma 877, 878, 878*f*
Papillary urothelial neoplasm 765
Papilledema 133
Papilloma 217, 843, 844
Paracentric inversions 275
Paracetamol 648
Paracrine
action 236
signaling 92
Paradoxical embolism 156-158, 537
Parafollicular cells 880
Paragangliomas 904
Parainfluenza virus 962
Parakeratosis 590
Parallel collagen fibers 935
Paraneoplastic hypercalcemia 582
Paraneoplastic syndrome 261, 262, 263*t*, 582, 583*t*, 584, 687, 762, 882
part of 897
types of 262
Paraplegia 567
Parasitemia
low levels of 122
produces high levels of 122
Parasites 260, 308, 361*b*, 692, 719
Parasitic diseases 121
Parasitic disorders 448
Parasitic infestations 132
Paraspinal nerve tumors 967
Parathyroid 908
adenoma 896, 908
carcinoma 896
compensatory hyperplasia of 897
hyperplasia 40, 896, 898, 908
Parathyroid gland 896, 898
congenital absence of 898
hyperplasia of 908
Parathyroid hormone 687
increased risk of 51
related protein 262
Paratyphoid 366
Parenchyma 216, 669, 960
adjacent 663
destruction of 701*f*
Parenchymal cells 91
Parenchymal fibrosis 703
Parenchymal inflammation and necrosis 663
Parenchymal liver disease, consequence of 648
Parenchymal organs 101
Parenteral transmission 198
Paretic neurosyphilis 964
Parietal cell 718
hyperplasia of 602
mass 599
Parietal epithelium 711, 736
Parkinson disease 23, 27, 680
Parosteal osteosarcoma 920
Parotid gland, superficial 593
Parotid tumors 591
Parotitis 533
Paroxysmal cold
hemoglobinuria 360, 459
Paroxysmal hypertensive
episodes 906
Paroxysmal nocturnal
dyspnea 501
hemoglobinuria 361, 459
Passenger mutations 232
Patchy distribution 716, 777
Patchy mucosal atrophy 599
Patent ductus arteriosus 537, 538, 538*f*
Patent foramen ovale 538
Paternal genetic material 834
Paternal imprinting 276
Pathogen-associated molecular patterns 62, 141, 143, 165
Pathogenesis, genetic basis of 834, 836
Pathology 3
calcification 50
evolution of 9
fractures 400
history of 9
subdivisions of 5
Patient's own fecal flora 738
Patterson-Kelly syndrome 333
Pauci-immune 720
Peau d'orange 133, 855
appearance 855
Pectus carinatum 301
Pediatric diseases 272
Pellagra 304
Pelvic
actinomycosis 121
bones, cavity of 921
inflammatory disease 839
mass 833
pain 810
syndrome, chronic 789
sonography 834
Penicillin 496
sensitivity 447
Penile intraepithelial neoplasia 784, 785
Penis 784, 801
carcinoma of 787*f*
invasive epithelial tumors of 785
squamous cell carcinoma of 788*f*
tumors of 784
Pentosuria 457
Pepsin 605
activity 601
Peptic enzymes 601
Peptic ulcer 83
gross appearance of 603*f*
microscopic features of 604*f*
morphology of 603
pathogenesis of 600
pathogenic mechanism of 598
recurrent 605
Peptic ulcer disease 292, 600, 603, 645
complications of 604, 604*b*
risk factors for 602*b*
sites of 603*b*
Peptic ulcerogenesis 602
Peptide YY 297
Peptidoglycans 62
Peptostreptococcus 547
Percutaneous membrane 655
Perfusion, disorder of 134
Periacinar myofibroblasts 703
Periampullary carcinomas 687
Periampullary neoplasms 698
Peribronchial growth 579
Pericardial effusion 465, 532, 535
diagnosis of 536
types of 535, 535*t*
Pericardial injury 534
Pericardiectomy, total 535
Pericarditis 135, 504*f*, 506, 521, 532, 545, 582
acute 532, 533
adhesive 507, 535
causes of 532*b*
chronic 533-535
classification of 532, 533*b*
healed 535
hemorrhagic 534
primary 532
secondary 532
Pericardium 81, 505, 545, 586, 618
Pericentric inversions 275
Periglomerular fibrosis 741, 742*f*
Perihilar tumors 687
Perimenopausal women 813
Perinatal death 114
Perinephric fat 763
Perineural inflammation 108
Perineural invasion 226, 706, 706*b*, 795*f*
Perineural tumor invasion 795
Perinodal tissue, infiltration of 387*f*
Periodic acid-Schiff
reaction 211
stain 373, 375*f*, 721*f*, 726*f*, 925
Periorbital edema 718
Periosteal osteosarcoma 920
Periosteum 912
Peripancreatic tissue 700
Peripartum cardiomyopathy 530
Peripheral arteries, atherosclerosis of 103
Peripheral blood 167, 187, 332, 337, 342, 344, 347, 350, 351, 355, 357, 359, 374, 376, 380, 381, 386, 399, 409
film 441
picture 332, 672
smear 323, 337*f*, 340, 347*f*, 351*f*, 358, 375*f*, 378, 386*f*, 440, 445*t*
examination of 441
Peripheral nerve 108, 109, 944
sheath tumors 943
Peripheral nervous systems 893
disorder of 263
Peripheral smear 322, 332, 337, 342, 344, 346*b*, 347, 351, 352*b*, 356, 357, 359, 380, 386, 374, 396, 409, 416
examination 441
reporting of 443
Periportal region 135
Periprostatic fat 795
Periprostatic tissue 795
Peritoneal adhesions 824
Peritoneal cavities 228, 490, 502, 682, 700

Peritoneal fluid 464
Peritoneum 586, 618, 824
Peritonitis 682
Peritubular capillaritis 186
Peritubular capillary basement membranes 186
Periurethral region 789
Perivascular infiltrates 195
Perivascular niches 93
Perl's stain 48, 49*f*, 134
Pernicious anemia 336, 337, 340*f*, 648, 689
  autoimmune atrophic gastritis of 188
  diagnostic tests for 338
  etiopathogenesis of 336
  morphology of 337
Peroxidase method 456
Peroxide 54
Peroxisome 666*f*
  proliferator-activated receptor gamma 874
Persistent bacterial infections 740
Persistent hyperglycemia 891, 892
Persistent intravascular hemolysis 344
Persistent lymphedema 126
Persistent productive cough, severe 558
Pertussis 115, 557
Petechiae 406
Petechial hemorrhages 145
Peutz-Jeghers syndrome 48, 631
Peyer's patches 197, 614
Phagocyte 166
  oxidase 70
    enzyme 71*f*
Phagocytic cells 165
Phagocytic leukocyte 31, 447
Phagocytic receptor 69
Phagocytic vacuole 69, 69*f*, 84, 561
Phagocytosis 11, 27, 69, 69*f*, 72*b*, 79, 85, 168, 173, 176, 409*f*, 891
  steps in 69
  targeting cells for 173
Phagolysosomal membranes 572
Phagolysosome 69*f*, 70
  function 70
Phagosome 69*f*, 70
  membrane of 71*f*
Pharyngeal cultures 508
Pharyngeal pouches 197
Pharyngeal webs 333
Pharyngitis 504*f*
Pharynx 575
Phenacetin 768
Phenol 256, 455
Phenotypic female 283
Phenytoin 536
Pheochromocytoma 904, 904*b*, 905*f*, 908, 909
  cut section of 905*f*
Philadelphia chromosome 378, 379, 379*f*, 380
Phlebothrombosis 153, 155
Phlebotomy 425
Phorbol esters 256
Phosphate 688
  stones 756
    triple 755
Phosphatidylinositol 3-kinase 237, 876
Phosphatidylserine 27
Phospholipases 35, 120
Phospholipid 44, 49
  breakdown 33
  synthesis 33
Phosphotungistic acid hematoxylin stain 21*f*
Photoelectric method 438
Photophobia 479
Photosensitivity 193
Phyllodes tumor 858, 859, 860, 862
  benign 859, 860, 860*f*, 861*f*
  gross appearance of 860*f*
  malignant 859, 861
Physical injury 74, 75, 150
Physical stress, produces 872
Piecemeal necrosis 663
Pigeon breast 301
  deformity 301
Pigment 48
  gallstones 354, 363, 688, 692
  nevus 283, 953
  stones 343, 688, 689
    pathogenesis of 691
  types of 48, 48*t*
Pilocytic astrocytoma 966, 971, 980
Pineal tumors 967
Pink frothy fluid 546
Pink puffers 553
Pinocytosis 46
Pinpoint petechial hemorrhages 749
Pitting edema 133*f*
  peripheral 131
Pituitary adenoma 867, 900
Pituitary corticotroph adenomas 899
Pituitary Cushing disease 900
Pituitary gland 899
  injury 41
PKD1 gene mutations 752
PKHD1 gene, mutation in 753
Placental alkaline phosphatase 777
Placental site trophoblastic tumor 839
Placental tissue, formation of 839
Plakoglobin 531
Plantar aponeurosis 940
Plantar fibromatosis 940
Plaque 589
  change, acute 486, 511
  fissuring of 511
  stability of 487
  stable 510
Plasma 324, 749
  albumin 722
    reduced 132
  colloid osmotic pressure 130, 132
  derived mediators 73, 78
  loss of 139
  osmotic pressure 130, 130*f*, 132
  renin 749
  unconjugated bilirubin 328
Plasma cell 86, 208, 393, 394*f*, 400*f*, 449, 505, 558, 614, 663, 741, 747, 778, 866
  clonal proliferation of 207, 208
  immature forms of 399
  infiltrate 598
  mature 399
  morphological features of 399
  myeloma 398, 399
  neoplasms 398, 399, 448
  proliferation 207*f*
  rich mass lesions 964
Plasma glucose
  determination of 893
  estimation of 893
  postprandial 893
Plasma membrane 16, 33, 62, 345*f*
  ATP-dependent sodium pump, reduced activity of 29
  damage of 34
  phospholipids 74
Plasma protein 63, 73, 722, 725, 745, 749
  excessive reabsorption of 52
  synthesis 474
Plasmacytoma 399
Plasmin 416
Plasminogen activator inhibitor 143, 892
Plasmodium
  falciparum 122, 124*f*, 443, 714
    infection 389
  infectious stage of 122
  merozoites bind 122
  species of 122, 124
  vivax 124*f*, 443
Platelet 74, 79, 80, 145, 173, 319, 332, 338, 344, 420*t*, 441, 443, 445, 749
  activation of 513
  adhesion 146, 484
    disorder of 410
  aggregation 147, 417
    disorder of 410
    potent inhibitor of 75
    production of inhibitors of 147
  antibody-coated 421
  component 417
    tests for 417, 418
  concentrate 428, 429
    indications for 429*b*
  congenital qualitative disorders of 417
  count 398, 416, 417
  decreased production of 408
  deficiencies of 407
  deposition 749
  derived growth factor 236
  destruction of 408, 409*f*
  disorder 413, 418
    qualitative 409
  distribution, abnormal 408
  emboli 161
  function 412
  functional disorders 409, 410*f*
    classification of 410*b*
  inhibitory effects 147
  number 443
  production, selective impairment of 400
  reduced number of 407
  secretion 146
    disorder of 410
Platelet-activating
  effect 148
  factor 73, 79, 143
Platelet-activation 146, 749
Platelet-derived growth factor 242, 702*f*
Platelet-vessel wall interactions 418
Platybasia 914
Pleocytosis 467, 962
Pleomorphic adenoma 219*f*, 314, 592, 593*f*
Pleomorphic cells 880
  high-grade 946
Pleomorphic epithelial cells 850*f*
Pleomorphic giant cells 880
Pleomorphic lipoblasts 938
Pleomorphic liposarcoma 938, 939
Pleomorphic malignant squamous cells 788*f*
Pleomorphic neoplastic cells 918
Pleomorphic nucleus 767, 918
Pleomorphic rhabdomyosarcoma 942
Pleomorphic sarcoma 936
Pleomorphic tumor 941
  cells 919*f*
Pleura 81, 577, 586
  inflammation of 545
Pleural biopsy 464
Pleural cavity 228, 585, 618
  spread of infection to 545
Pleural effusion 464*t*, 545
  causes of 463, 463*t*
  malignant 464
Pleural fibrosis 585
Pleural fluid 463, 464
  examination of 463
  hemorrhagic 464
  protein 463
Pleural plaques 574
Pleural surfaces 558
Pleural tumor 586
Pleuritic chest pain 193
Pleuritic pain 567
Pleuritis 545, 582
Plexiform intraneural neurofibroma 944
Plummer syndrome 873
Plummer-Vinson syndrome 333, 596, 645
Plump spindle cells 832
Pluripotent germ cells 818
Pneumococcus 355, 542, 961
Pneumoconiosis 101, 569
  progressive 571
Pneumocystis
  jirovecii 542, 546
  pneumoniae 546
Pneumocystosis 204
Pneumonia 201, 355, 533, 541, 542, 546, 547, 615, 891
  chronic 542
    necrotizing 557
  classification of 541, 542*f*
    bacterial 542
  community-acquired
    acute 541
    bacterial 542
    viral 542, 546
  complications of 543, 545*b*
  etiology of 541
  healthcare-associated 542
  hospital-acquired 542, 546
  necrotizing 542
  pathogenesis of 541
Pneumothorax, produce 551
Podocin 725
Podocytes 725
Poikilocytosis 351, 441
Poisons 744
Poliomyelitis 41
Poliovirus infection 115
Polyangiitis 496, 497
  microscopic 496, 744
Polyarteritis nodosa 196, 496
  acute phase of 497*f*

Polyarthritis 504f
chronic nonsuppurative proliferative 927
migratory 506, 508, 628
Polychromasia 442
Polychromatophilia 442
Polyclonal hypergammaglobulinemia 568
Polycyclic aromatic hydrocarbons 254, 255, 291, 305, 575
Polycyclic hydrocarbons 575, 596
Polycystic kidney
disease 751, 752f
adult 753
hepatic disease 753
Polycystic liver disease 753
Polycythemia 263, 381, 537, 687
absence of 444
decreases ESR 446
pathophysiologic classification of 381b
screening for 438
secondary 444
vera 378, 381, 444, 445f, 447
Polydipsia 888, 900
Polyelectrolyte 452
Polygonal cells 593, 686
Polyhedral tumor cells 829f
Polymerase chain reaction 12, 268, 287, 430
Polymorphisms 273, 666, 887
Polymorphonuclear leukocytes 68f, 962
Polymorphonuclear neutrophils 518f
Polyneuromyopathy 762
Polyol pathways 735
Polyomavirus 187, 737, 738
Polyp 217, 629
adenomatous 633
classification of 631
colorectal 631
hamartomatous 631
hyperplastic 632
juvenile 631, 631f
nature of 634
number of 634
size of 633
Polyphagia 888, 889
Polyploid 936
Polypoid
appearance 608f
tumor 814f
Polyposis coli 633, 636
Polyunsaturated fats 480
Polyuria 451, 741, 759, 888
Polyvinyl chloride 255
Poor dietary intake 303
Popcorn
calcification 922
cells 396f
Porcelain gallbladder 695, 696
Pores of Kohn 550
Portal cirrhosis 670
Portal hypertension 397, 398, 652, 675, 676, 676f, 681, 688
causes of 675
consequences of 675, 676b
in cirrhosis, pathogenesis of 675
Portal inflammation 663
Portal tracts 669
Portal vein 682
thrombosis 136
Posthepatic causes 675
Postinfectious
glomerulonephritis 717, 719, 720
Postmenopausal
bleeding 812, 832
hormonal replacement therapy 846
obese 845
vaginal bleeding 815
women 814, 817, 831
Postmortem clots 153, 154
Postpubertal teratoma 784
cut section of 780f
microscopic features of 781f
prognosis of 781
Postpubertal testicular germ cell tumors 777
Postrenal causes 743
Poststreptococcal
glomerulonephritis 132, 715, 717, 719, 719f
pathogenesis of 717fc
Postural edema 130
Potassium
cyanide 440
dichromate solution 904, 905f
dihydrogen phosphate 440
ferricyanide 440
loss of 745
oxalate 323
Potent oxidant 71
Potentially toxic
chemicals 573
injurious agents, prolonged exposure to 83
Pott's disease 10, 566, 567, 913
Precancerous lesions
histologic diagnosis of 807
removal of 807
Precursor glandular lesions 574, 577
Precursor lesions 230, 577, 683, 768, 812, 815
Precursor neuroendocrine lesion 577
Precursor squamous lesions 784, 785
Prediabetes
diagnosis of 882, 882t
risks in 882
Predominant cell 84, 380
type 442
Predominant fibromuscular stroma 791
Predominant glands 791
Predominantly conjugated hyperbilirubinemia 648
Predominantly fibrous areas 819
Predominantly lymphocytes 962
Predominantly neutrophilic inflammatory infiltrate 604
Predominantly unconjugated hyperbilirubinemia 648
Pre-erythrocytic schizogony 122
Pregnancy 152, 757, 895
complications 750
first-term 845
healthy 838
normal 838
Prehepatic causes 675
Prehepatic jaundice 648
Preicteric phase, symptomatic 660
Premalignant lesions 687
detection of 306
Premenopausal women 481
Prerenal azotemia 472, 502, 743
Prerenal causes 743
Pressure
atrophy 41
sores 103
Pretibial edema 869
Pretibial myxedema 869, 873
Pretransfusion testing 426, 436
protocol 427b
Prevotella 547
Primary membranous
glomerulopathy 726
nephropathy 726
Primitive sex cords 831
Primordial germ cell 776, 826
Prinzmetal angina 511, 512
Prion diseases 47
Proangiogenic molecules 891
Proapoptotic genes 232
Proapoptotic protein, prevents upregulation of 247
Procainamide 190
Procalcitonin 141
Procallus tissue 934f
Procarcinogens 254, 255
Procoagulant state, induction of 142
Procoagulant substances into circulation, release of 415
Procollagen, hydroxylation of 301
Proelastase 697
Proenzymes 699
defective intracellular transport of 699
Progenitor cell 385
theory 809
Progesterone, nuclear receptors for 267
Pro-growth genes 793
Prohyperglycemic adipokines 887
Proinflammatory cytokines 887
actions of 142
increased expression of 599
increased production of 668
releases 891
Proinflammatory mediators
production of 141
release of 141
Proinflammatory responses, triggering of 141
Proinsulin assay 895
Prolactin-secreting macroadenoma 908
Proliferating cells, clones of 872
Prolonged bleeding 409
following trauma 412
Prophylaxis 654
Propylthiouracil 496
Prostacyclin 75, 147, 148
Prostaglandin 64, 73, 74, 74f, 75, 105, 143, 172, 602, 620, 693
secretion of 602
Prostate 40f, 228, 231, 301, 788
adenocarcinoma of 792
pathogenesis of 794
benign hyperplasia of 792f, 797
cancer 795f, 796
carcinoma of 227, 458, 794, 795f, 797
cut section of 794f
cut section of 40f, 791f, 794f
epithelial tumors of 793
glands 224
benign 794
malignant 794
infarct of 797
mesenchymal tumors to 793
Prostate-specific antigen, causes of raised 797b
Prostatic acid phosphatase 797
Prostatic adenocarcinoma 268
Prostatic cancer 793
diagnostic of 797
grading of 796
staging of 796
Prostatic carcinoma 225f, 260
Prostatic diseases 458
Prostatic ducts, preexisting 794
Prostatic epithelium cells 797
Prostatic hyperplasia, pathogenesis of benign 790f
Prostatic intraepithelial neoplasia, high-grade 794
Prostatitis 788, 797
acute 788, 789
bacterial 788, 789
chronic
bacterial 788, 789
nonbacterial 788
clinical features of 789
Prosthetic cardiac valves 152
Protease 35, 120, 199
activated receptors 80
antiprotease imbalance 550
release of 927
specific 80
Proteasome function 668
Protein 32, 46, 49, 235, 246, 289, 296, 303, 324, 692, 891, 962, 963
abnormal 47
amounts of normal 206
accumulation of 46, 669
acute phase 89, 90
catabolism of 88, 888, 889
categories of 206
coding genes, mutations in 273
compartments 294
concentrations 703
deficiency 98
estimation 463
excretion 454
extracellular accumulation of 47
folding of 35
homeostasis, abnormal 56
in urine 453
increased uptake of 46
intracellular accumulation of 46
kinase
A, aberrant activity of 684
C, activation of 891
malnutrition 132
matrix 199
misfolding of 206
misfolding within cells 36
mutations of 245
normal folding of 56
parathormone-related 582
plugging, promotes 702
plugs 699
precursor 208
products 240
proteolysis of 888
rich fluid, escape of 64
rich in iron 573
serum electrophoresis of 324
small 77
specific 268

synthetic apparatus, structural disruption of 29
tests for 454*b*
types of 454
tyrosine phosphatase 864
Proteinaceous casts, formation of 745
Proteinuria 52, 212, 453, 716, 719, 724, 725, 732, 742, 747
amounts of 455*b*
asymptomatic 712
categories of 455
causes of 455, 455*b*
heavy 455
hemodynamic 455
highly selective 722
massive 721, 722
mechanism of 724
mild 455, 750
moderate 455, 721
nonselective 455, 722, 723, 727
overflow 455
qualitative categories of 455
quantification 455
selective 455, 725
tests for 454
Proteoglycans 77, 206
concentration of 929
degradation of 929*f*
loss of 930
Proteolytic enzymes, release 100
Proteus 738, 772
infections 741
vulgaris 755
Prothrombin 323
mutation 151
Prothrombin time 8, 414, 419, 664, 672
interpretation of 419
Prothrombotic tissue factors, release 150
Proto-oncogene 204, 232, 235, 239, 255
overexpression of 232
point mutations in 232
Protozoa 121, 682
Protuberance 827
Proximal colon, carcinoma of 641*f*
Pruritus 678, 681, 856
Prussian blue stain 679
Psammoma bodies 50, 51, 51*f*, 820, 821, 821*f*, 822, 878, 878*f*, 975
Psammomatous meningioma 976
Pseudoaneurysm 488
Pseudohyphae 118
Pseudomembrane 115
Pseudomembranous inflammation 82
Pseudomonas 557, 911
bacteria 68
septicemia 902
species 547, 772, 961
Pseudomyxoma peritonei 228, 824
Pseudopapillae 872
Pseudopodia 96*f*
Pseudopolyps 627, 627*f*
Pseudopyloric metaplasia 625
Pseudorosettes, perivascular 973
Psoralen plus ultraviolet A radiation keratosis 949
Psychologic stress 602
PTH gene 896
Pubic hair 283
Puffy eyelids 870
Pulmonary alveolar basement membranes 720
Pulmonary anthracosis 570
Pulmonary artery 538
Pulmonary blood flow 536
Pulmonary chondroid hamartoma 219
Pulmonary circulation 156, 501
Pulmonary congestion 500, 542
Pulmonary disease 433, 913
diagnosis of 567
Pulmonary dysfunction 570
Pulmonary edema 133, 134, 140, 160, 521, 906
Pulmonary emboli
miscellaneous 161
multiple recurrent 157
Pulmonary embolism 139, 156, 159, 463
Pulmonary embolus, large 156
Pulmonary epithelial cells 575
Pulmonary fibrosis 585
Pulmonary hemorrhage 157
life-threatening 721
Pulmonary hypertension 135, 157, 195, 196, 536, 537, 570
primary 502
Pulmonary infarction 157
Pulmonary infections, secondary 300
Pulmonary neuroendocrine cells 577
Pulmonary thromboembolism 164
mechanism of 157*fc*
recurrent 502
Pulmonary tuberculosis
primary 563*f*
progressive 565
secondary 565*f*
systemic symptoms of secondary 566
Pulmonary valvular stenosis 538, 539
Pulsating hematoma 488
Pulsus paradoxus 535
Puncture, traumatic 466
Purified protein derivative, injection of 179
Purine metabolism, end product of 931
Purine, synthesis of 336
Purulent inflammation 81
Purulent pericarditis 533
Pus 740, 912
cells 740
production of 81
Pyelonephritis 736, 737, 738*f*, 740, 751, 756, 772, 792, 891
acute 736, 737, 773
on chronic 740*f*
bacterial 401
chronic 86, 736, 737, 740, 741, 741*f*, 742*f*, 747, 750, 792*f*
obstructive 740, 741
reflux associated 740
classification of 737
infection of 738
microscopic appearance of chronic 742*f*
pathogenesis of 738, 738*f*
reflux-associated 741
Pyemia 82, 115
Pyknosis 17
Pyknotic nuclei 661
Pyloric obstruction 604
Pyloric valve 603
Pyogenic bacteria 114, 163, 533
infection 78
Pyogenic meningitis 962
Pyogenic organisms 115
Pyogenic osteomyelitis 911
complications of 913
morphology of 912
subacute 912
Pyonephrosis 740, 756
Pyothorax 545
Pyrexia of unknown origin 449, 475
Pyridoxine 304
Pyrimidine dimers, formation of 260
Pyroptosis 28
Pyruvate kinase deficiency 326
Pyuria 460, 740-742

Q

Queyrat erythroplasia 785, 786
Quinacrine fluorescent stain 277

R

Rabies 116
Rachitic rosary 300
Radial growth phase 957
Radial scar 843
Radiation 36
carcinogenesis 260
exposure 846
therapy 767
types of 260
Radioactive gas derived from uranium 289
Radioactive iodine uptake 471
measurement of 867
use of 471*b*
Radiodense mass 855
Radiolucent lesion 595
Radionuclide bone scans 795
Rapamycin
activity, molecular target of 57
mammalian target of 237
Rapidly progressive glomerulonephritis 712, 719
classification of 720*b*
morphology of 720
Rash 114
Raynaud phenomenon 194, 195
Reaction
positive 179
reduction 304
severe 433
systemic acute-phase 76
Reactive leukocytosis, classification of 365
Reactive nitrogen species 30, 71
Reactive oxygen species 29, 54, 56, 57, 70, 71, 143, 178, 252, 667, 668, 679, 885
degradation of 30
generation of 293, 563
mechanism of production of 70
production of 37, 71*f*, 141, 891
type of 70, 70*t*
Reagent 439
strip 452, 456-459
method 454
to cuprous oxide 456
Recapitulates hepatic ontogenesis 683
Receptor tyrosine kinase 881
Recessive disease, X-linked 197, 411
Recessive disorders, X-linked 280*t*
Recessive traits, X-linked 280
Recombinant DNA technique 12
Rectum 619, 626
tissues 212
Red blood cell 8, 319, 329*t*, 333*f*, 441, 442*f*-444*f*, 460, 648, 836
count 398
disorders 319, 324
lifespan of 320
nucleated 442
shrinks 323
spherical 345
swelling of 323
Red cell 173, 385, 748
aplasia 263
casts 719, 748
complement-mediated lysis of 213
concentrate 428, 429
destruction 319, 326, 342, 433
disorders 448
enzyme studies 323
exposure 434
folate 328
indices 326, 337, 345
infections of 343
mechanical trauma to 326, 343
membrane
abnormalities 326, 343
damage 354
morphology 443
production 326
sensitization, drug-induced 360
shape, variations in 441
size 325
transfusion of 422
Red hepatization 543
Reduction-oxidation reactions 30
Reed-Sternberg cell 4, 392, 393, 393*f*, 394*f*, 395, 395*f*, 405
plenty of 395
variants of 393
Reflux nephropathy 740
Refractometer method 452
Regenerating nodules 670, 674, 675
Regenerating parenchymal nodules 675
Regeneration, variation of 94
Regional lymph node 263, 565
metastasis 855
Regional lymphadenitis 113, 563
Regional mesenteric lymph nodes 616
Regional node involvement 227
Regurgitation theory 809
Reinfarction 521
Reiter syndrome 617
Renal arterioles 52
sclerosis of 749
Renal artery 712, 892
stenosis 748
Renal atrophy 757
Renal azotemia 472, 750
Renal biopsy 472, 733
complications of 472*t*
contraindications of 472*t*
indications for 472*b*
Renal bladder stones 300
Renal blood vessels 495*f*
Renal calculi 754

Renal capsule, invasion of 764
Renal causes 743
Renal cell carcinoma 227, 228, 741, 759, 761, 763*b*
classification of 759
morphology of 761
risk factors for 759*b*
Renal cell tumors 759
Renal changes 897
Renal clearance tests 471
Renal colic 752, 756
Renal cystic disease, classification of 751, 751*b*
Renal damage 756
Renal disease 196, 401, 458, 748
clinical manifestation of 712*t*
hypertensive 748
indicative of 461
Renal dysfunction 401, 757
Renal edema, pathogenesis of 132
Renal failure 52, 131*f*, 194, 212, 261, 290, 410, 433, 493, 652, 735, 736, 753
acute 132, 742
chronic 40, 208, 449, 451, 600, 702, 712, 736, 753, 897, 897*fc*, 898
Renal function 747
irreversible worsening of 746
progressive deterioration of 747
tests 400, 471
Renal glomerulus 711*f*, 892
Renal glycosuria 456
Renal hypoperfusion 743
Renal infarcts 748
Renal infection, risk of 751
Renal insufficiency 145
Renal lesions 498
Renal medulla 892
Renal mesenchymal tumors 759
Renal osteodystrophy 748, 898
Renal parenchyma 41, 743, 752, 756
thinning of 759*f*
Renal pelvis 42, 739, 740, 741, 757
and calyces 758
Renal perfusion 901
Renal pyramids 758
Renal sinus 763
Renal status 452
Renal stone 712, 754, 897
causes of 755*b*
clinical features of 756
complications of 756
formation 933
general features of 755
pathogenesis of 755
types of 755, 755*b*, 773
Renal tubular
acidosis 897
epithelial cell injury 743
epithelium 759
Renal tumors 712, 759
Renal vascular
insufficiency 892
lesions 737
Renin 493
Renin-angiotensin
aldosterone system 676
activation of 500
system 493, 749
Renovascular diseases 746
Renovascular hypertension, mechanism of 494
Reperfused infarct, morphology of 519
Reperfusion injury 59
mediators of 519
Reproductive history 230
Reproductive life, long duration of 845
Resemble colon cancer 618
Resemble spermatogonia 778
Resident stromal cells 254
Resorption atelectasis 585
Respiratory difficulties 890
Respiratory diphtheria 115
Respiratory disorders 541
Respiratory distress 160
syndrome 290, 414
Respiratory infections 556
Respiratory lining cells 546
Respiratory symptoms 159
Respiratory system 291, 502
Respiratory tract 42, 290, 309, 541, 548
bronchoconstriction of 288
infection 551
inflammation of 288
lower 497, 498
Response-to-neoadjuvant chemotherapy 857
Restrictive disease 548
Reticular cystic pattern 830*f*
Reticulin
fibers 570
stain 97, 831
Reticulocyte
hemoglobin 333
smear shows 328*f*
Reticulocyte count 328, 328*t*, 332, 340, 350
methods of 328
normal 328
uses of 328
Reticulocytopenia 328
Reticulocytosis 328, 342
Retina 286, 892
Retinal hemorrhages 493
Retinoblastoma 241, 242, 258, 764, 977, 978*f*
cell of origin of 977
develops 242
familial 241, 242
gene 241
mutations 917
hereditary 241, 917
pathogenesis of 241, 243*f*
role of 241
sporadic 242
Retinoic acid 299, 536
Retinoids, metabolic effects of 299
Retinopathy
nonproliferative 892
proliferative 354, 893
Retroperitoneal fibrosis 743
Retroperitoneal tissues 490
Retroperitoneum 676, 943
Retrovirus, spherical enveloped 198
Reverse transcriptase 199
polymerase chain reaction 205
Reversible injury 14, 23*t*, 514
Reversible irreversible injury 16
Rh
antibodies 424
antigens 424
blood group system 424
hemolytic disease 358, 358*f*
incompatibility 358
between donor and recipient 424
between mother and fetus 424
negative mother 358
positive 424
fetus 358
system 422, 424
typing techniques 424
Rhabdoid meningioma 976
Rhabdomyosarcoma 860, 941
Rheumatic carditis 504, 504*f*
Rheumatic fever 503, 506*f*
acute 503, 505, 506, 529*f*
diagnosis of 508*t*
pathogenesis of acute 504*f*, 504*fc*
sequelae of acute 504*f*
stage of 508
Rheumatic heart disease 4, 5, 189, 503, 529*f*
complications of 503, 507
pathology of 503
Rheumatic myocarditis, pathognomonic of 505
Rheumatic valvular disease 507*f*
Rheumatoid arthritis 83, 194, 208, 382, 447, 926, 927
etiopathogenesis of 926
pathogenesis of 926, 927*f*
Rheumatoid factor 927
Rheumatoid nodules 928
Rhinocerebral mucormycosis 120
Rhinosporidiosis 127
Rhinosporidium seeberi 127
Rhizopus 120
Rib, chondrosarcoma of 922*f*
Riboflavin 303
Ribonucleic acid 444, 658
genome of virus, reverse transcription of 200
viruses 256
Rickets 300, 301*f*
X-ray of 301*f*
Rickettsia prowazekii 117
Rickettsial infections 117
Ridley-Jopling classification 107, 107*fc*
Riedel thyroiditis 866
Right atrium 530, 538, 539
Right upper quadrant pain 695
Right ventricle 131, 530, 538
Right ventricular
hypertrophy 538
infarction 521
Ring chromosome 275
Robertsonian translocation 275, 281
Rocky mountain spotted fever 117
Rod cells 964
Rokitansky nodules 827
Rokitansky-Aschoff sinus 695, 695*f*
Romanowsky stains 312, 440, 441*b*
Rose spots 615
Rosenthal fibers 972
Rothera's test 457, 893
Rotor syndrome 651
Rouleaux formation 446
Round blue cell tumors 906
Round cell 939
Rubeola 117
Rubner's test 457
Rupture 486, 490, 511, 934
Russell bodies 46, 52, 52*f*

S

Saber shin 114
Saccular aneurysm 113, 488, 488*f*, 753
Saccular bronchiectasis 558
Sacrococcygeal teratomas 284
Sacroiliitis 628
Saddle embolus 156
Saddle nose deformity 114
Sago spleen 210
Sahli's hemoglobinometer 439*f*
Sahli's method 438
Sahli's pipette 439
Saint Vitus' dance 506
Salah bone marrow aspiration needle with stilette 448*f*
Salicylates 455
Salivary gland 124, 194, 592, 594, 845
minor 592
neoplasm 591, 593
pleomorphic adenoma of 315*f*, 592*f*
tumors 591, 591*t*
classification of 591
Salmonella 355, 613
infection 204, 911
osteomyelitis 615
paratyphi 613
typhi 613
typhimurium 355
Salt and pepper chromatin 905*f*
Sanded nuclei 663
Sanderson's polster 872
Sanger sequencing 287
Sanguineous sputum 547
Sarcoidosis 88, 369, 382, 398, 568
Sarcoma 218, 223, 223*t*, 245, 781, 936
botryoides 942
group of 917
undifferentiated 946
Saturated fats 480
Scalene node 583
Scant and pink granular cytoplasm 620
Scant stroma 875
Scanty cytoplasm 764, 925
Scar 94, 97
endometriosis 809
formation 85, 91
steps in 94
nature of 741
Scattered Hodgkin cells 395
Scattered inflammatory cells 95
Scattered spindle cells 944
Schaumann body 568, 569*f*
Schiller-Duval body 830, 830*f*
Schilling test 338
Schistocytes 416
Schistosoma 260
haematobium infections 768
Schistosomiasis 161
Schizogony 122
Schizont 122
Schwann cells 907, 943, 944
neoplastic 944
Schwannian stroma 907
Schwannoma 943
acoustic 943
microscopic appearance of 944*f*
Scintigraphy 212
Sclera, coloration of 647
Sclerodactyly 194

Scleroderma 194
Sclerosing adenosis 844
Sclerosing cholangitis, primary 681, 687, 696
Sclerosing osteomyelitis of Garré 912
Sclerosis 395, 713, 741, 913
Scrape cytology 307
Screening tests 417
Scrotal mass, progressively growing 779
Scrotal sac 774
Scrotal skin 783
  cancer of 10
Scrub typhus 117
Scuba and deep-sea divers 159
Scurvy 407, 489
Secretion increases 808
Secretory meningioma 976
Segmental duct 842
Seizures 304
Selectin 67, 105
  distribution of 67
  type of 67
Self-limited disease 866
Sellar region, tumors of 967
Semen
  analysis 467
    indications for 467*b*
  examination of 467
  pH 467
  viscosity 467
  volume 467
Seminal vesicles 795
Seminiferous tubules, atrophy of 774
Seminoma 218, 777, 779, 783, 798
  cells 778, 778*f*
  classical 782
  microscopy of 778*f*
  prognosis of 779
Semiquantitative test 456
Semitranslucent fluid 843
Senescence 244
  evasion of 970
Senile
  cardiac amyloidosis 209
  purpura 407
  systemic amyloidosis 209
Sense genomic damage 240
Sensitive test 418
Sensitivity 287
Sensitization 554
  against antigen 554
Sentinel cells in tissues, recognition by 62
Sentinel lymph node 227
  biopsy 959
Sentinel node 788
  biopsy 857
Sepsis 140, 142, 597, 743
  transfusion-associated 432
Septal hypertrophy, asymmetric 531
Septal walls, destruction of 551
Septic
  embolus 163, 488, 526
  infarctions 162, 163, 526
  peritonitis 704
Septic shock 140, 141, 141*f*, 142*fc*, 143*f*, 145, 164
  hallmarks of 141
  pathogenesis of 140, 140*b*, 143*f*
  pathogenic
    mechanism of 140*fc*
    pathways in 140
Septicemia 82, 115, 355, 682, 739, 913
  meningitis-associated 961
Sequelae 5
Sequestration crisis 354
Serofibrinous pericarditis 533
  causes of 533, 533*b*
Serologic testing 436
Serological crossmatch techniques 427
Serological markers, sequence of 656
Serological tests 114, 371, 430, 615
Seromucinous tumors 818
Serotonin 65, 73, 74, 620, 880
Serous carcinoma 812, 815, 821
  grade of 820
  high-grade 818, 819, 822, 822*f*
  low-grade 819, 821, 822*f*
Serous cystadenoma, microscopic appearance of 821*f*
Serous endometrial carcinoma 814, 815
  development of 815*f*
Serous endometrial intraepithelial carcinoma 814, 815
Serous exudate 81
Serous inflammation 80, 105
Serous intraepithelial carcinoma 819
Serous pericarditis 533
Serous tubal intraepithelial carcinoma 819*f*, 822
Serous tumors 818, 820, 823
  malignant 821
Serpentine 572
Sertoli
  cell 775
  gonad 831
Serum 324, 328, 398, 654, 870
  adrenocorticotropic hormone level 900
  alanine transaminase 474
  albumin 400, 646, 672, 722
  ammonia 474
  amylase 701
  and urine protein electrophoresis 212
  antinuclear antibody test 214
  aspartate transaminase 474
  calcium levels 898
  ceruloplasmin 680
  concentrations, monitoring 837
  copper levels 680
  cortisol 900
  electrolytes 672
  electrophoresis 400*f*
  enzymes, estimation of 473
  gamma globulins 475
  globulin 672
  haptoglobin, reduced 356
  ionized calcium 897
  lipase 701
  lipids 480
  sickness 176, 178
  soluble transferrin receptors 334
  uric acid 375, 931
Serum alkaline phosphatase 474, 649, 660, 664, 672, 920
  elevation of 681
  levels of 681, 797
Serum aminotransferase 660, 664, 672
  levels, elevation of 664
Serum amyloid 207
  A protein 90
  P 206
Serum bilirubin 356, 647, 649, 660, 664, 672
  estimation 473
  level, normal 647
Serum cholesterol
  level 480
  total 475
Serum creatinine 400, 719, 743, 745
  causes of raised 472*b*
Serum iron
  indices 328
  profile 332, 333*t*
Serum protein 660, 664, 672
  ratio 463
Serum thyroid
  hormones 470
  stimulating hormone
    concentration 867
Serum transaminases 649, 652, 672
  incidental elevation of 673
Sesmoplasia 705
Sessile serrated adenomas 633
Sex chromatin 276
  demonstration of 276
Sex chromosome 278, 281, 283
Sex cord
  derivatives 831
  stromal
    cells 818
    tumors 775, 818, 831
  tumors, pure 831
Sex hormones 190
  female 689
Sex steroids 899
Sex-linked recessive disorders 411
Sexual contact, unprotected 655
Sexual forms 123
Sexual transmission 198
Sexually transmitted infection 793
Sézary syndrome 391
Shaggy hyperparakeratosis 590
Sheehan postpartum pituitary necrosis 416
Shigella 616
  organisms 617
  species 616
Shigellosis-bacillary dysentery 616
Shock 129, 138, 156, 290, 597, 602
  bacteremic 144
  cardiogenic 139, 139*fc*, 144, 145, 519, 521
  characteristic features of 138*fc*
  hemorrhagic 839
  hypotensive 140
  hypovolemic 139, 144, 145, 164
  initiation of 140
  morphological features of 144*t*
  stages of 143
  types of 139, 139*t*
Shoulder 485
  girdle and pelvis 916
Shunt
  fatty acid 667
  left-to-right 536, 537
  portosystemic 676
  right-to-left 156, 536-538
Sicca syndrome 194
Sickle cell 446
  anemia 151, 273*f*, 352, 354, 355, 355*f*, 356, 363, 689, 739
    pathogenesis of 353, of 353*f*
  disease 8, 347, 355, 447, 458, 514, 615, 911
  irreversible 353
  nephropathy 748
  trait 357
Sickle hemoglobin 347, 352
  production of abnormal 353
Sickled red cells 357*f*
Sickling
  molecular basis of 353
  pathologic consequence of 354
  reversal of 353
  test 356, 357, 357*f*, 362
Sickness
  chronic decompression 160
  chronic serum 178
Sideroblastic anemia 334, 678
Signal transduction
  pathways, activation of 38
  proteins 235, 236, 239
Signet-ring cell 609, 610*f*
  adenocarcinoma 645
  carcinoma 609, 610*f*, 640
Silencing genes 234
Silica 552
  forms of 571
Silica-Laden macrophages 571*f*
Silicosis 571, 572*f*
  causes of 571
  chronic 571
  pathogenesis of 571*f*
Silicotic nodule 571, 571*f*
  coalesce of 571
Silver impregnation
  method 51
  stain 721*f*, 727*f*, 729*f*
Single distinct nodule 685
Single germ layer 218
Single large mass 157
Single plasma glucose estimation 893
Single-base primer extension 287
Single-gene 278
Sinus formation 383
Sinus tract
  draining chronic osteomyelitis 950
  formation 914
Sinusitis 557
Sinusoidal hypertension 676
Sinusoidal vascular resistance 675
Sirtuins 57
  functions of 57
  promote 57
Sister Mary Joseph nodule 610, 610*f*, 823
Situated bland nuclei 823
Sjögren syndrome 194
Skeletal abnormalities 114
Skeletal changes 896
Skeletal deformities 350
Skeletal Ewing sarcoma 924
Skeletal muscle 160, 217, 474, 673, 892, 941*f*, 942
  cells 91
  differentiation 941
  hypertrophy of 30
  neoplasms 941
  tumors of 936, 937, 941
Skeletal system 867
Skin 120, 188, 193, 195, 221*f*, 563, 564, 628, 693, 855, 867, 870, 891, 892, 928, 955
  basal cell carcinoma of 226, 951, 953*f*

biopsy 111
blistering formed 81
cancer of 260, 290
consists of 827
diffuse hyperpigmentation of 902
disorders 949
flushing of 621
lesions 295
melanoma of 977
pigmentation 679
pustule 911
rashes 113
retraction 855
squamous cell carcinoma of 950
surface epithelia of 91
test 553, 556
antigens 568
tumors, arsenic-induced 290
wounds, healing of 98
Skinfold thickness, reduced 294
Skull, X-ray of 350f
Sleep apnea, obstructive 299
Slide technique 424
Slight antigen excess 715
Small airway 552
disease 573
obstruction 550
Small artery 195, 749
Small blood vessels, dilation of 80
Small cell
carcinoma 575-577, 582, 899, 900
microscopic appearance of 582f
lung carcinoma 581, 584
Small duct papillomas 844
Small intestine 619, 632
disease, chronic 302
ileum of 615f
serosal aspect of 625f
stricture 625f
ulcerative lesions of 613
Small opaque plaques 299
Small quantity required 287
Small ventricular septal defect 537
Small vessel diseases 494
Small-caliber blood vessels, multilayered 970
Small-cell change 684
Smear
preparation of 314
staining of 312, 314
triple 308
Smoke, second-hand 575
Smoking 575, 590
passive 554
related carcinoma 576
Smoky colored urine 718, 719
Smooth endoplasmic reticulum 661f, 663f
Smooth muscle 217, 484
actin 942
contraction of 80, 172
fibers 632
hyperplasia 588
hypertrophy of 38
neoplasms, benign serous 815
reactions 75
tumors 937, 942, 943
Smooth muscle cell 96f, 100, 155, 483f, 486f, 489
proliferation 484
into intima, migration of 484
loss of 496
Smooth painful tongue 363
Smudge cells 386
Snake bite 459
Soap-bubble appearance 924f
Sodium
active reabsorption of 711
and water retention 132, 723
biphosphate 426
chloride, concentrations of 449
citrate binds 323
dithionite 356
fluoride 323
homeostasis 494
increased retention of 132
loss of 745
low 672
metabisulfite 356, 357f
reabsorption 744
retention of 130, 131f, 676
Soft spongy bone 934
Soft tissue 255, 284, 411, 913, 919, 922, 936
abscess 912
benign 936
callus, formation of 934
neoplasms, minority of 936
procallus 934
sarcomas 242, 267, 938, 945
trauma 158
tumors 910, 936, 945
general principles of 937b
malignant 936
well-circumscribed 852
Soldier's plaque 535
Solid islet 619
Solid malignancies 254
Solid organs, parenchymal cells of 91
Solid tumor, unilateral 832
Solitary fibrous tumor 586
Soluble factors, secretion of 27
Somatic cell 56
mutations 273
Somatic mutation, spontaneous 242
Somatic protein compartment, depletion of 294
Somatic stem cells 56
Somatic tissue
elements 779
mature 826
resembling 781
Somatic-type
malignancy, teratoma with 781
tumors 828
Somatostatin 880
secreting tumors 908
Southern blotting 287
Space of Disse 668f
Specimen
collection 310
methods for obtaining 307
Sperm
aggregation 467
count
normal range of 468
total 468
dysmotility 557
free fluids 468
morphology 468, 469f
abnormal 468
motility, assessment of 468
vitality 468
Spermatocytes, primary 782
Spermatocytic seminoma 782
Spermatocytic tumor 782, 782f
Spermatogenesis 282, 782
Spermatogonia 782
Spermatozoa 468
tests for antibody coating of 468
Spherical nuclei 971
Spherocytes 345, 363, 446
causes of 346b
Spherocytic red cells 450
Sphincter of Oddi 699
Spinal cord 490
involvement 116
Spinal leptomeninges 964
Spindle cell 259, 612, 808, 832, 942, 944, 946
component 946
rhabdomyosarcoma 942
Spindle tumor cells 944
fascicles of 612f
Spine 913
compression fractures of 914
tuberculosis of 10
Spirochete 111
Splanchnic vasodilation 676
Spleen 91, 158, 173, 210, 354, 380, 382, 408, 545, 613-615
blood in 354
chronic venous congestion of 137f
disorder of 365
enlarged 363, 397
enlargement of 136
hypofunction of 355
in amyloid 210
with multiple infarcts, reduced size of 354
Splenectomy 345
Splenic cysts 398
Splenic disease 396
Splenic function 542
Splenic vein obstruction 398
Splenomegaly 343, 346, 379, 397, 676, 688
absence of 342
causes of 397, 397b
congestive 136, 398, 502, 676, 677f
massive 398, 398b
mild 397
moderate 354, 398
Spondylitis, ankylosing 183, 628
Spoon nails 333
Sporadic breast cancers 847
Sporadic cancers 246, 246t
Sporadic clear cell carcinomas 760
Sporadic colonic cancers 637
Sporadic cretinism 870
Sporadic diffuse gastric cancers 607
Sporadic juvenile polyps 631
Sporangia 127
Sporozoite 122
migrate 124
spindle-shaped 124
Spray fixation 312
Spray paints 289
Spurious polycythemia 381
Sputum 309, 552, 567
collection 476
culture of 567
examination of 476
processing of 312
SQSTM1 gene 914
Squamocolumnar junction 799, 802
Squamous cell 575, 594, 768, 799, 802, 951
abnormalities 309, 309t
large malignant 806f
mature 802, 804
type 260
Squamous cell carcinoma 218, 260, 262, 574, 576, 579, 579f, 584, 588, 590, 591, 591f, 596, 597f, 756, 784, 786, 787, 788f, 798, 801, 805, 841, 913, 920f, 950, 951
cytology of 807f
development of 290
in situ 949
moderately differentiated 951
morphology of 951
nonkeratinizing 806f
well-differentiated 221f, 223, 591, 951
Squamous cell tumors
etiology of 800
pathogenesis of 800
Squamous dysplasia 577
Squamous epithelial
cells 221f
tumors 801
Squamous epithelium 224, 578f, 801
mature 841
Squamous intraepithelial lesion 785, 800, 802-804, 841
cytology of 805f
high-grade 803, 805f
low-grade 803, 804f, 805f
morphology of 804
Squamous metaplasia 42, 42f, 230, 299, 559f, 577, 578f, 799
Squamous papilloma 269, 270f
microscopic appearance of 270f
Squamous precursor lesions 574, 577
Squamous tumor cells, polygonal 920f
ST elevated myocardial infarct 515
Staghorn calculus 756f
Stain, pour undiluted 441
Staphylococcus
aureus 81, 524, 542, 547, 557, 911, 961
epidermidis 524, 961
species 911
Starling's hypothesis 130
Starling's law 500
Starry sky
appearance 390f
pattern 390
Starvation 296
metabolic changes in 296
Stasis 64, 151, 739
Static image-based systems 13
Status asthmaticus 556
Steatofibrosis, alcoholic 670
Steatohepatitis 665f, 667, 669, 671, 683
alcoholic 669
mechanism of 667
microscopic features of 670b
Steatorrhea 681
Steatosis 16, 44, 671, 680, 887
liver 44
mechanism of 45
Stellate cell 709
activation 668

- Stem cell 55*f*, 93, 94, 385, 592
  - abnormal 341*f*
  - niches 93
  - research 12
  - varieties of 93
- Stenosis 509
  - atherosclerotic 485
- Sterile
  - arthritis 617
  - gallbladder 692
  - thrombus, formation of 525
- Sterility 775
- Sternal tenderness 374
- Steroid
  - anabolic 260
  - androgenic 260
  - hormones, producing 903
  - types of 898
- Stiffness 195
- Stimulus 74, 76
  - mature of 14
- Stomach 597, 600, 603, 619, 833
  - adenocarcinoma of 599
  - benign ulcers of 611*t*
  - chronic inflammation of 598
  - fundus of 297
  - malignant ulcers of 611*t*
  - normal process in 600
  - peptic ulcer of 603*f*
  - risk factors for carcinoma of 605
  - signet ring carcinoma of 853
- Stomatitis 304, 363
  - angular 333
- Stone 754
  - facies 195
- Stool cultures 615
- Stop codon 274
- Storage diseases 397
- Storage disorders 369
- Storage pool deficiency 410
- Stratified squamous epithelium 589
- Streptococcal antigens 717
  - antibody against 717
- Streptococcal glyceraldehyde-3-phosphate dehydrogenase 717
- Streptococcal infection 508, 717
  - primary 717
- Streptococcal pyogenic exotoxin B 717
- *Streptococcus* 503
  - *agalactiae* 961
  - *bovis bacteremia* 635, 636
  - *faecalis* 738
  - *pneumoniae* 355, 542, 588, 961, 965
  - *pyogenes* 517
  - *viridans* 524, 540
- Streptokinase 496
- Streptomycin 455
- Stress 38
  - acute hemodynamic 499
  - biomechanical 929
  - oxidative 30, 550, 666, 668, 702, 892
  - ulcers 597
- Stressful lifestyle 482
- Striking basophilia 380
- Striking nuclear pleomorphism 769
- Stroke 354, 490, 492
  - ischemic 292
  - risk of 480
  - volume, reduced 531
- Stroma 216, 581, 761, 781, 783, 823, 851, 873, 881, 916, 939-941, 971
  - amounts of 640
  - components of 216
  - types of 858
- Stromal cells 249, 789, 790, 848, 923
  - activated 254
  - atypical 939*f*
  - increased number of 789
  - proliferation of 789, 790
  - role of 848
- Stromal component 831
- Stromal hypercellularity 860
- Stromal invasion 824
  - absence of 821, 824
- Stromal proliferation 844
- Stromal tumors, pure 832
- Structural chromosomal
  - aberration 275
  - mutations 273
- Structural heart diseases 529
- Struma ovarii 828, 866, 867
- Strumal carcinoids 828
- Struvite stones 755, 756
- Subarachnoid space 960, 963
- Subchondral bone cyst 929, 930
- Subclavian artery 492, 492*f*
- Subcutaneous fat 295
- Subcutaneous mycoses 118
- Subcutaneous nodules 504*f*, 506
- Subcutaneous tissue 120, 502
- Subdiaphragmatic region 682
- Subendocardial infarct 514, 516
- Subendocardial lesions 505
- Subendothelial deposits 715, 718
- Subendothelial immune complex 192, 729
- Subepithelial barrier 602
- Subepithelial deposits 715, 718
- Subepithelial inflammatory infiltrate 589
- Subepithelial region 589
- Submucosa 597, 607, 627, 790
- Submucosal glands
  - hyperplasia of 552, 553*f*
  - hypertrophy of 552
- Subnuclear vacuoles 808
- Subperiosteal abscess 911
- Subpulmonary stenosis 539
- Subpulmonic stenosis 538, 539*f*
- Subsegmental duct 842
- Subsequent scarring 506
- Subserosal fibrous tissue 695
- Substances
  - release of 261
  - secretion of normal 223
- Sucrose hemolysis test 361
- Sudden cardiac death 509, 522, 531
- Sudden death 157
- Sudden febrile illness 962
- Suicidal death, causes of 289
- Sulfinpyrazone 410
- Sulfosalicylic acid test 454
- Sulfur
  - dioxide 288, 551, 552
  - granules 121
  - powder sinks 460
- Sun exposure 955
- Sunburst appearance 919
- Superantigens 143
- Superinfection 659
  - bacterial 696
- Superoxide 54
  - anion 31, 70
  - dismutase 31, 32
- Suppurative pericarditis 526, 533
- Supraclavicular lymph node 227
- Supraclavicular
  - lymphadenopathy 383
- Supraclavicular nodes 784
- Supraclavicular sentinel node 610
- Surface epithelial
  - carcinomas 819
  - tumors
    - biochemical markers of 825
    - clinical presentation of 825
- Surface mucus secretion 601
- Susceptibility genes 622
  - role of 189
- Suture 101
  - materials 87
- Swan neck 928
- Sweating 621, 740, 870, 890
- Swelling 552
- Sydenham's chorea 504*f*, 506
- Sympathetic nervous system 867
- Synaptophysin 267, 582, 620
- Syncope 324
- Syncytiotrophoblast 837, 838*f*
- Synovial cell hyperplasia 927
- Synovial fibroblasts 928
- Synovial fluid 308, 462, 930*f*
  - leakage of 929
- Synovial sarcoma 945, 946*f*
- Synovial tissues 945
- Synoviocytes 926, 927
- Synovitis 927
- Synovium 927, 930
- Synthesis 75
  - excessive 46, 207
- Synthesized de novo 73
- Syphilis 111, 114, 128, 964
  - acquired 112
  - benign tertiary 113
  - cardiovascular 113
  - congenital 114, 128
  - early 114
  - manifestations of 112*f*
  - primary 112, 128
  - secondary 113, 128
  - stages of 112
  - tertiary 113, 128, 488, 489, 964
- Syphilitic aneurysm 488, 490
- Syphilitic aortitis 113
- Syphilitic osteochondritis 114
- Syphilitic periostitis 114
- Systemic amyloidosis 208, 626, 762
- Systemic anaphylaxis 173
- Systemic arterial emboli 157*f*
- Systemic arteries 156
- Systemic arteriolar vasodilation 141
- Systemic diseases 448, 713, 746, 929
- Systemic disorder 653
- Systemic edema, pathogenesis of 131
- Systemic emboli, sources of 157
- Systemic hypertension 489
- Systemic hypotension 142
- Systemic immune complex disease 176
  - pathogenesis of 177*f*
- Systemic immunological
  - abnormalities 568
  - diseases 496
- Systemic inflammatory response syndrome 76, 90, 140
- Systemic lupus erythematosus 188, 189, 191, 214, 496, 528, 714, 716, 717, 720, 723, 735
  - clinical manifestations of 193*b*
  - pathogenesis of 189, 190, 190*f*
- Systemic mastocytosis 600
- Systemic miliary tuberculosis 566
- Systemic sclerosis 194, 195, 750
- Systolic failure 500
- Systolic pressure 493

T

- T cells, regulatory 885
- T lymphocytes 167, 190, 483, 496, 552
- Tabes dorsalis 113, 964
- Tachycardia 140, 144, 159, 433, 890
- Tachykinins 620
- Tachypnea 140, 159
- *Taenia solium* 124, 125
  - life cycle of 125*f*
- Talc emboli 161
- Tamm-Horsfall
  - glycoprotein 453
  - protein 461, 745
- Tandem repeats, variable number of 253
- Tapeworms 124
- Tardive syphilis 114
- Target cell 351, 441
  - destruction of 173
  - opsonization of 173
  - phagocytosis of 173
- Tattooing 49
- Tau protein 47
- Tay-Sachs disease 286
- T-banding 277
- T-cell 188, 374, 562, 868, 884, 891
  - activated 623, 926
  - autoreactive 495, 496
  - cytotoxic 167, 252, 864
  - depletion, mechanism of 200
  - immature 374
  - immunity 108
  - immunodeficiency disorder 197
  - killer 167
  - leukemia, adult 257, 391
  - malignant 374
  - mature 373, 385
  - neoplasm 372, 373, 385
  - reactions, types of 178
  - regulatory genes 864
  - self-reactive 885
  - significant depletion of 201
- T-cell lymphoma 724
  - adult 391
  - cutaneous 391
  - peripheral 385, 391
- T-cell mediated
  - diseases 170
  - hypersensitivity 181*t*
  - immune response 496, 503
  - immunity 560
    - loss of 197
  - macrophage activation 562
  - reactions 503
  - rejection 185
- T-cell receptor
  - antigen-specific 167
  - loci 374

Tear
- characteristic of 491
- site of 595

Tearing pain, sudden onset of severe 492
Telangiectasia 194, 952
Telepathology 13
Telomerase 56, 248
- activation of 258, 638
- expression of 638

Telomere 55, 273
- attrition 55, 55*f*
- progressive shortening of 247
- role of 55*f*
- shortening of 55

Tender hepatomegaly 682
Teratoma 219, 284, 779, 780, 826, 828, 830
- benign 826
- containing mature neural tissue 827
- malignant 826, 827
- mature 826
- origin of 826
- postpubertal 780, 783
- prepubertal 783, 784, 798
- pure 780
- solid 827

Terminal duct-lobular unit 842, 842*f*
Terminal hepatic veins 669
Terminal ileum 615
Terminal-deoxynucleotidyl-transferase 375
TERT gene 768
Testicular atrophy, causes of 775
Testicular cancer, increased risk of 775
Testicular causes 798
Testicular dysfunction 775
Testicular dysgenesis syndrome 776
Testicular germ cell tumors 777
- clinical features of 783
- markers of 784*t*

Testicular mass 780
Testicular neoplasm 783
- diagnosis of 784
- management of 784

Testicular teratomas, classification of 780*b*
Testicular tumors 775, 776
- etiology of 775
- mode of spread of 784

Testis 774, 775, 782*t*
- cut section of 778*f*
- mixed germ cell tumors of 782
- normal descent of 774
- painless enlargement of 783
- region of 781
- seminoma of 778*f*, 828
- seminomatous tumors of 782*t*
- sites of arrest of 774
- teratoma of 784*t*
- tunica vaginalis of 586
- undescended 230, 776

Testosterone 790*f*
- conversion of 789
- reduced levels of 282

Tetany 898
Tetrahydrofolate 335
Tetralogy of Fallot 537, 538, 539*f*
Thalassemia 347, 648
- major 363
- minor 334
- peripheral blood picture of 347

Thalassemic face 350
Theca cell 831
Thecomas 832
Thecomatous stroma 831
T-helper cells 554, 560, 562, 623
Therapeutic radiation 261
Thiamine 303, 668, 672
Thiazides 883, 932
Thin-walled venules 227
Thioflavin T 211
Thoracic actinomycosis 121
Thoracic aortic aneurysm 490, 490*t*
Thoracic duct 130*f*, 613
Thoracocentesis 159
Three enzyme systems 664
Thrombin 323
- cleaves circulating fibrinogen 147
- systemic activation of 142
- time 419

Thrombocythemia, essential 378
Thrombocytopenia 159, 174, 197, 203, 342, 374, 380, 407, 408, 672, 750
- causes of 408, 408*b*

Thromboemboli 155, 507
Thromboembolic complications 723
Thromboembolic phenomena 628
Thromboembolism 129, 155, 157
Thrombomodulin 147
Thrombophlebitis 155
- migrans 155
- migrating 611
- migratory 155, 706

Thrombopoiesis 320
Thrombopoietin 90, 320
Thrombosis 145, 149, 151, 354, 485, 487
- elevated risk for 152
- signs of 416
- symptoms of 416

Thrombospondin 27
Thrombotic complications 723
Thrombotic episodes, recurrent 155
Thrombotic microangiopathies 748, 750
Thrombotic process, triggering factors of 415
Thrombotic thrombocytopenic purpura 750, 751
Thromboxane A2 75
Thrombus 149, 153
- appearance of 153*f*
- consequences of 155
- dissolution of 154
- fate of 154, 154*f*
- formation 155
  - mechanism of 415
- mechanism of 150
- types of 152

Thymic hypoplasia 197
Thymidine synthesis 334
Thymoma 724
Thymus, development of 197
Thyrocytes, progressive destruction of 864
Thyroglobulin 267, 470, 880
Thyroid 868, 881
- and genetic alterations, subtypes of carcinoma of 876
- antigens 863, 864
- autoantibody
  - measurement, uses of 471*b*
  - tests 470
- autoantigens 864*f*
- carcinoma 866, 880
  - anaplastic 880
- C-cell 880
  - derived carcinoma 874, 876
- cut section of 868*f*
- diffuse hyperplasia of 869
- dysfunction 896
  - screening for 468
- enlargement of 866
- epithelial cells 864, 864*f*, 868
- failure 863
- follicle 742*f*, 864, 865*f*, 872, 873*f*, 875*f*
  - atrophy of 865
  - cells 866, 874, 877
- follicular
  - adenoma of 874, 875*f*
  - carcinoma of 879*t*
  - epithelial cells 868
  - nodular disease 874
- function
  - gradual failure of 863
  - tests 468, 469*t*, 471, 471*t*
- functional state 471
- gland 863, 867, 871
  - enlarged 873
  - follicular cell-derived malignant tumors of 876*f*
  - inflammation of 863
- goiter of 50
- hormone 866, 867, 883
  - levels 470
  - synthesis 870, 872
- medullary carcinoma of 209, 211*f*, 880, 881, 881*f*, 908
- myopathy 867
- neoplasms 874
  - classification of 874
- nodule 874
  - asymptomatic 878
- painless diffuse enlargement of 865
- papillary carcinoma of 261, 876, 877
- parenchyma 863, 865, 873
- scintiscanning 471
  - use of 471*b*
- stimulating hormone 470, 871, 874
  - estimation, uses of 470*b*
- stimulation, abnormal 867
- storm 867
- tissue 869
- tumor 634, 874
- weight of 873

Thyroiditis 863, 866, 867
- acute 863
- types of 863*b*

Thyroidization 741, 742*f*
Thyrotoxicosis 866, 867, 869, 873
- causes of 866, 866*b*

Thyrotrophin 470
Thyrotrophin-releasing hormone 470
- stimulation test 470

Thyrotropin 868
Tibia 916, 924
- diaphysis of 926*f*
- head of 160
- proximal 924
- upper end of 917

Tile techniques 424
Tiny dark granules adjacent 276
Tissue 226, 261
- architecture, maintenance of 77
- components 779
- damage 22, 61, 71, 84, 178, 563
  - mechanism of 679
  - pathogenesis of 191
- derivatives 780
- destruction 83, 560
  - leading 563
- diagnosis, methods of 797
- dysfunction 155
- edema 142
- expression, normal 266
- factor activates 415
- factor pathway inhibitor 143, 148
- forming cavity, dissolution of 19*f*
- hypoperfusion 141
  - widespread 144
- injured, type of 98
- injury 173, 180
  - extent of 91
  - massive 414
  - mechanism of 170, 192
- intrinsic proliferative capacity of 91
- invasion of adjacent 225
- ischemia 160, 485
- loose textured 162
- macrophage 73, 165
- mature 631, 828
- necrosis 61
  - types of 17
- perfusion, impairment of 142
- peripheral 677
- plasminogen activator 147, 148
- reaction 88
- repair 85, 91, 98, 101
  - initiation of 85
- sampling, techniques for 265
- stable 91
- stem cells 93
- to hypoxia, vulnerability of 162
- toxicity 679
- types of 97, 780
- uncalcified 934
- with dual blood supply 162

T-lymphoblastic
- leukemia 373
- lymphoma 373

T-lymphocytes 196
- autoreactive 680
- classes of 167
- cytotoxic 180, 180*f*, 251, 885

Tobacco 291
- products 590
  - and smoking 291, 590
- smoke 289, 291*t*, 542, 552, 573, 575, 576, 596, 637
- smokeless 291, 589, 590
- types of 291
- use of 589

Toes, clubbing of 548
Toll-like receptor 62, 62*f*, 141, 166
- signals 190

Tomb stones 17
Tongue 292, 763, 908
Tonsil 197, 563, 564, 801
Tophi 933
- formation of 932

Total cell
- count 467
- cycle 226

Total leukocyte count 463, 615
Totipotent germ cells 219
Touch cytology 307
Tourniquet test 409, 418
Toxic
adenomas 874, 875
effects 290
granulation 366*f*
industrial inhalants 551
injury 744, 745
lysolecithin, release 693
megacolon 628
multinodular goiter 873
shock syndrome 143
Toxins 15, 120, 530, 652, 744
Toxoplasmosis 204, 719
TP53 mutations 576, 606
Trabecular bone 935
Trabecular structure 619
Trace elements 98
Trachea 552
Tracheobronchial mucosa 291
Tracheobronchial tree 619
Traditional cancer typing 269
Transabdominal phase 774
Transaminase 473
estimations, significance of 474
Transbronchial needle aspiration 584
Transcoelomic spread 642
Transcription factor mutations 371
Transepithelial influx 623
Transforming growth factor 39, 242, 586, 639, 702*f*, 790
Transfusion hemosiderosis 434
Transfusion medicine 6, 8, 425
Transfusion reaction 431, 431*f*, 435*b*
Transfusion-transmitted
diseases 430, 437
infectious agents 430*t*
Transmural infarcts 516
Transmural inflammation 626
Transplacental transmission 112
Transplant rejection 180, 183
characteristics of 184*t*
Transthyretin 206, 207
Transudate 65, 65*t*, 463, 464
Trauma 151, 597
operation 960
severe 158, 597
Trephine biopsy 448
indications for 449, 449*b*
sites of 449
Treponema
demonstration of 112
pallidum 88, 112*f*, 128, 714, 964
Trichloroacetic acid 459
Trichomonas vaginalis 308, 800
Trichrome stain 97
Tricuspid
stenosis 135
valve 507
Triglycerides 45*f*
formation of 44
Triiodothyronine 470
Trinucleotide 274
repeat disorder 275*f*
Triphasic growth pattern 765*f*
Triple stones 756
Triplet codon 272
Trisodium citrate 446
uses of 321
Trisomy 21 281, 536
Troisier's sign 610, 611
Trophic hormones 872
Trophoblast proliferation 835
Trophoblastic disease 834
morphology of 833
pathogenesis 833
Trophoblastic hyperplasia 836
Trophozoite 122, 618*f*
clusters of 618
kill hepatocytes 618
late 122
stage 618
Tropical pulmonary eosinophilia 126
Troponin 520*f*, 531
Trousseau's sign 611, 706
Trousseau's syndrome 155
True aneurysm 488
True ependymal rosettes 973
Truncal obesity 900
Trypanosoma cruzi 430
Trypanosomes 443
Trypsin
actions of 698
inadequate oxygenation of 698
Trypsinogen 697
Tubal pregnancy 839, 839*f*
Tubercle 564, 616
bacilli 962
Tuberculin
reaction 179
skin testing 562*f*
test 560
Tuberculoid leprosy 108, 111, 111*t*
microscopy of 109*f*
Tuberculoma 963
Tuberculosis 88, 106, 369, 449, 559-561, 564, 588, 891, 903
complications of secondary 567
course of 292
fate of secondary 565
intestinal 560, 615
oropharyngeal 560
pathogenesis of 560
primary 561, 563, 565, 567
progressive primary 564
secondary 564, 567
spread of 566*b*
types of secondary 564
Tuberculous
arthritis 914
granuloma 20*f*, 87*f*
infections 560
lung, microscopic appearance of 564*f*
lymph node 315*f*
lymphadenitis 314, 383, 384*f*
meningitis 466, 567, 962, 963, 966
osteomyelitis 913
salpingitis 567
spondylitis 913
ulcer 616*f*, 617, 617*t*
Tuberous sclerosis 279
Tubular adenoma 633, 633*f*, 859
Tubular adenomatous polyp, pedunculated 633*f*
Tubular bronchiectasis 557
Tubular carcinoma 854
Tubular casts 745
Tubular damage 455
patterns of 746*f*
Tubular diseases, classification of 737*b*
Tubular endometrial glands 808*f*
Tubular epithelial
alterations 745
cells 744
Tubular glands 633, 633*f*
Tubular injury
ischemic acute 746*f*
toxic acute 746*f*
Tubular lesions 736, 737
Tubular lumens, occlusion of 745
Tubular necrosis 290, 746*f*
acute 290, 743, 744
Tubules 144, 711, 729, 749, 758
Tubuloglomerular feedback, triggering of 744
Tubulointerstitial nephritis 737
Tubulointerstitial pattern 185
Tubulorrhexis 745
Tubulovillous adenomas 633
Tumor 182, 203, 215, 218, 218*t*, 219*t*, 237, 238, 238*t*, 239, 268, 283, 285*b*, 581, 739, 757, 813, 815, 831, 879, 973
adipocytic 937
aggressive 814, 830, 942
anatomic site of 966
antigens 251
atypical lipomatous 938, 939, 939*f*
benign 216, 220, 223, 225, 226, 229, 229*t*, 269, 539, 799, 819, 874
endometrioid 824
mesenchymal 217
serous 820
biphasic 860, 943
borderline 217, 819
serous 821
bulky mass of 389
cells, adjacent 248
childhood 241
chondrogenic 915, 916, 920
classification of 267, 966
common benign 498, 592, 920
consistency 216
degree of differentiation 7
develop 256
diagnosis of 266*t*
edges of 7
effects of 261
elements 592
excision, adequacy of 7
germinoma family of 775, 777
giant cells 221, 229
grade of 7, 220
gross types of 218*f*
hematolymphoid 571, 967
hemorrhagic 838
high-grade 768
infiltrating lymphocytes 852, 957
invasion 705
large 879
low-grade 262, 766
lysis syndrome 261
malignant mixed 593
masses 942
microenvironment 236
mixed 218, 592
molecular profiling of 269
nature of 907
neuronal 967
nonencapsulated 938
nonmeningothelial 967
origin of 582
painful 916
peripheral 581
poorly differentiated 221
predisposition syndromes 975
primary 262
malignant 594
rare 782
risk of malignant 865
size 857
solid 261, 448
source of primary 833
sporadic 760
spread of 582, 907
malignant 226, 227*b*, 262
staging of 262, 264*f*
type 262, 583, 784
ulcerating 640
undifferentiated 880
well-circumscribed 858, 943
well-differentiated 978
wide range of 966
Tumor cell 27, 167, 180, 232, 249, 249*f*, 250, 250*f*, 251, 262, 267, 391, 575, 580, 612*f*, 620, 620*f*, 621, 686*f*, 759, 761, 762*f*, 765*f*, 777, 779, 782, 795, 813, 821, 825*f*, 829, 830, 831, 832*f*, 850, 851, 879, 880*f*, 881, 896, 905*f*, 906, 932, 939, 942, 957, 973, 974, 976*f*
attachment of 249
breakdown products of 261
characteristics of 581
colon composed of 641*f*
death, rate of 226
doubling time of 226
follicular pattern of 879
homing of 250
killing of 251
locomotion of 250
mass of 784
migration, stimulation of 249
movement of 250
ploidy of 907
primitive appearing 284
produce bone 917
resemble 782
size 925
synthesize 904
Tumor emboli 155, 161, 855
formation of 250
Tumor marker 267, 268, 268*t*, 398, 671, 640, 784, 797, 830, 882
tissue-related 226
types of 267
Tumor necrosis factor 76, 141, 143, 183, 261, 562, 623, 885, 927
antagonists 77
receptor family 26
system 263, 796
Tumor progression 215
molecular pathways of 768
Tumor suppressor gene 232, 235*f*, 239, 240, 241*b*, 243, 253, 255, 576, 607, 637, 638, 705*f*, 813, 879, 896, 936
activation of 56
deletion of 586
group of 240
inactivation of 576, 705
loss of 240
mutations of 240, 952
normal functions of 240

P53, degradation of 258
point mutations in 232
Tumor-like lesions 283, 834
Tumor-nodes-metastasis classification 642
Tumor-promoting inflammation 253
facilitates malignancy 254
Tunica albuginea 778
Tunica media 485
Turbid fluid 463
Turbulence contributes 151
Turner syndrome 275, 277, 282, 283, 283*f*, 634, 883
Two cell layers 844
Typhoid 366, 617*t*
bacillus 613
cells 614
cholecystitis 614
nodules 614
Typhoid fever 52, 613
chronic carriers of 613
pathogenesis of 614*f*
Typhoid ulcer 617
characteristics of 614
gross appearance of 615*f*
Tyrosinase 251
Tyrosine kinase 877
receptor 881
signaling 576

U

Ulcer 81, 615, 617
aphthous 624
arterial 103
benign 611, 611*t*
flask-shaped 618
malignant 611
multiple 603
neuropathic 102, 103
oval 614
perforations of 615
proximal 603
trophic 102, 103
Ulcerated atherosclerotic plaques 151, 157
Ulceration, nonhealing 98
Ulcerative bronchitis 582
Ulcerative colitis 224, 621, 622, 626, 628*f*, 628*t*, 629, 629*t*, 681
complications of 628*f*
gross appearance of 627*f*
morphology of 626
Ultraviolet radiation 190
Ultraviolet rays 260
type of 260
Umbilical cord blood 187
Umbilical metastasis 823
Umbilicus 676
Unconjugated bilirubin 354
levels of 359
Undernutrition, secondary 296
Underwater construction workers 159
Uniform round cells, sheets of 971
Uniform spindle cells 943
Uniform tumor cells, solid islands of 620*f*
Unilocular hydatid cysts, multiple 126*f*
Unstable angina 509, 512
Untracranial disease 597
Upper abdominal
discomfort 671
pain 687
Upper extremities 945
Upper respiratory tract 497
infection 724, 533
lesions 498
viral infections 554
Upper respiratory viral infection 865
Uranium 575
Urate
crystals stimulates, precipitation of 932
reduce excretion of 932
stones 755
Urea
clearance test 472
increased production of 472
Ureaplasma urealyticum 788
Urease 599
Uremia 212, 600, 712, 746, 806
Uremic
complications 734
gastroenteritis 734
pericarditis 734
pneumonitis 734
Ureter 739, 740, 756, 757, 806, 757
Ureteral stones 743
Ureteric colic 756
Ureteropelvic junction 757
Urethra 791*f*, 955
compression of 791
proximal 790
shorter 738
Urethral valves, posterior 741
Urethritis 617, 737
Uric acid 324, 382, 755, 931
increased risk of 931
levels 400
nephrolithiasis 933
stone 756, 756*f*
Urinary abnormalities 770
Urinary bladder 40*f*, 42, 575, 738, 806
carcinoma of 260
infection 738*f*
stones 300
tumors of 765
urothelial carcinoma of 769*f*
Urinary calculi 757
Urinary casts 462*f*, 745
Urinary citrate 754
Urinary crystals 462*f*
Urinary flow, complete obstruction of 789
Urinary fluid loss 890
Urinary free cortisol levels 900
Urinary frequency 817
Urinary infection 740
bacterial 748
Urinary obstruction 791
risk of 751
Urinary rectum 806
Urinary symptoms 797
Urinary tract 255, 310, 615, 757
disorders 710
infection 460, 712, 737
obstruction 712, 739, 757
causes of 757*b*
obstructive lesions of 758*f*
Urinary urobilinogen 660
Urine 255, 458, 660, 664, 672, 706, 707, 721
analysis 450, 471
culture 615
examination 451, 770, 771, 893
findings 649, 721, 725
formation, near-complete suppression of 451
levels 907
markers 797
microscopy of 732, 748
odor 452
of low specific gravity, secretion of 453
outflow 745
pH 453
preservation of 451
reduced volume of 743
retention of 791
sample
post-transfusion 435
processing of 310
specific gravity 472
tests 460, 904
for blood in 457
for hemoglobin in 457
urobilinogen in 459
volume 755
Urinometer 452, 452*f*
Urobilinogen 11, 356, 460, 647
absent 649
excretion of 647
reabsorption of 647
tests for 460*b*
Urokinase plasminogen activator 249
Urolithiasis 754
Uropathy, obstructive 757
Urothelial carcinoma 767, 768
pathogenesis of 767
Urothelial cells 766, 770*f*
Urothelial epithelium 825
Urothelial neoplasms 765, 765*b*
Urothelial papilloma 765
Urothelial tumors 764
Urothelium 224, 825
normal 766
thickened 765, 766
Urticarial allergic reactions 433
Uterine
bleeding, abnormal 810
cavity 814*f*
cervix 575
carcinoma of 308
squamous epithelial lining of 224
corpus, endometrial surface of 814*f*
endometrium 809
leiomyoma 52, 815
leiomyosarcoma 817
lesions 838
myometrium, leiomyoma of 814*f*
prolapse 757
wall 837
Uterus 807, 833, 834, 837
body of 814*f*
columnar epithelium of 91
leiomyoma of 53*f*, 225
mesenchymal tumors of 812
myometrium of 51*f*
Uveitis 628

V

Vacuum tubes 324
types of 324*f*
Vagina 91, 801, 838, 955
adenocarcinoma of 260
normal 800
Vaginal bleeding 806
irregular 815
Vaginal flora 800
Vaginal smear 307, 311
Vaginitis 119, 800
Vaguely storiform configuration 944
Valve
abnormal 524
leaflet, thickening of 507
severe stenosis of 507
Valvular ball-valve obstruction 539
Valvular dysfunction 526
Valvular endocarditis 505
Valvular heart disease 499
Valvular inflammation 506
Valvular regurgitation 525
van den Bergh reaction 473, 650
Van Gieson stains 211
Vaping fluid 292
Variant angina 512
Varicella-zoster virus 204
Varicose
bronchiectasis 558
veins 98
Vasa vasorum 489
lumen 489
Vascular amyloidosis 212
Vascular complications 890, 909
Vascular component, tests for 418
Vascular congestion 354
Vascular damage 195, 406
Vascular disease 137
classification of 748*b*
Vascular disorder 413, 414, 418, 479
Vascular dissemination 249
Vascular emboli 156
Vascular endothelial
cells 91
growth factor 95, 96, 809, 891
Vascular hydrostatic pressure 130
Vascular injury, site of 146, 147
Vascular invasion 686, 879, 880*f*
Vascular leakage 64, 140, 141
Vascular neoplasm 259
Vascular obstructions 354
Vascular occlusion
chronic 509
effects of 355*f*
Vascular pattern 185
Vascular permeability 64, 65, 75, 79, 80, 104, 172
Vascular purpura 407
Vascular reactions 79
Vascular smooth muscle
cells 749, 891
relaxation of 142
Vascular stroma 762*f*
Vascular tumors 267, 498
classification of 498*b*
Vasculitides 196
Vasculitis 495, 514, 716, 743, 748
acute necrotizing 192
classification of 495*f*
consequences of 497
immune complex-associated 496
necrotizing 110
noninfectious 495
pathogenesis of 495
plural of 496
secondary 961

Vasoactive amines 73, 172
secretion of 581
Vasoactive inflammatory mediators 142
Vasoactive intestinal peptide 880
Vasoactive substances, secretion of 620
Vasoconstriction 75, 487, 510, 675
severe 75
Vasodilation 64, 75, 172
Vaso-occlusive crises 354, 355, 364
Vasospasm 513
Vater ampulla 687
Vegetative endocarditis 529*t*
Vein 151, 676
compression of 134
obstruction of 129
Vena cava
inferior 228
superior 228, 582
syndrome, superior 582, 873
Venous air embolism 159
Venous blood
flow 98
pooling 140, 141
Venous emboli 155
effects of 156*f*
sources of 156*f*
Venous invasion 761
tumors with affinity for 228
Venous leg ulcers 103
Venous obstruction 130
Venous occlusions 162
Venous pressure, systemic increase in 131
Venous system, thrombosis in 150
Venous thrombosis, cause of 151
Venous thrombus 130, 152, 153, 153*t*, 155, 961
Ventricular aneurysm 521
Ventricular arrythmias 139
Ventricular chamber, dilatation of 521
Ventricular free wall, rupture of 521
Ventricular puncture 465
Ventricular septal defect 537, 538, 539*f*
Ventricular septum 516
rupture of 521
Venules, increased permeability of 75
Verocay bodies 943
Verrucous carcinoma 591, 591*f*, 787, 788
Vertebrae, destruction of 913
Vertebral column 228
Vertebral metastases 797
Vertical growth phase 957
Vesalius dissected human body 10
Vesicles 690
Vesicoureteral reflux 737, 738*f*, 739
acquired 739
congenital 739, 740
Vesicular mole 834
Vessel
external compression of 161
maturation of 96*t*
neoplastic invasion of 137
Vessel wall 66
abnormalities 407, 407*b*
inflammatory lesions of 137
weakening of 489
VHL gene 760
VHL gene mutations 760
Vhromophobe renal tumors 759
Villous adenoma 633, 634*f*
Villous papilloma 633
Villous trophoblasts, proliferation of 834
Vim Silverman's needle showing prongs 475*f*
Vimentin 266, 267
Vinyl chloride 255, 575
Viral capsid antigens, antibody against 371
Viral core 199
Viral cytokine 259
Viral diseases 115
Viral genome, entry of 200
Viral hepatitis 412, 653, 706
causes of 653, 653*b*
clinical course of 660*b*
mimic acute 680
Viral inclusions 476
Viral infection 35, 41, 68, 81, 167, 204, 598, 865, 884
direct detection of 205
gastrointestinal 733
vasculitis secondary to 496
Viral meningitis 962, 965
Viral pneumonia 289
Viral protease 251, 657
Viral replication 200, 202, 202*f*
high level of 655, 803
Viral ribonucleic acid 199
Viral set point 203
Viral transmission 198
Virchow's lymph node 11, 227
Virchow's node 583
Virchow's triad 11, 149*f*
constituents of 149*b*
Virchow-Robin spaces 119, 961
Viremia 202, 202*f*
Virtual slide systems 13
Virulence factors 119
Virulent organism 524
Virus 308, 557, 662, 699, 719, 738, 926
direct inoculation of 198
dissemination of 202
induced tumors 187
infected cells 27
replication 655
type of 257, 660
Viscera, abdominal 354
Visceral cancer, sign of 155
Visceral compartment 294
Visceral epithelial cells 721*f*, 724, 728*f*
Visceral epithelium 711
Visceral metastasis 795
Visceral protein compartment
marginal depletion of 294
reduced 294
Viscid watery secretion 53
Viscous fluid 463
Vision, maintenance of normal 299
Visual error 440
Visual field defects 970
Visual method 328
Vitalism, theory of 9
Vitamin 305, 305*t*
A 32, 299, 636
deficiency, effects of 299
B_1 303
B_{12} 304, 335
antibody blocking binding of 174
concentrations 328
delivery of 335
metabolism of 334
role of 335
serum 382
source of 334
B_{12} absorption 338
mechanism of 335*f*
B_{12} deficiency 334, 336, 338, 364
diagnostic tests of 338
neurologic complications of 335
B_2 303
B_3 303
B_6 304
deficiency, severe 304
C 32, 301
deficiency 98, 105, 302*f*, 407, 491
D 300, 898, 914
insufficiency 300
malabsorption of 681
nonskeletal effects of 301
related disorders 51
D deficiency 300
skeletal effects of 300
deficiency 295, 299, 668
pathological effects of 300*f*
E 32, 302
fat-soluble 299, 300
K 302, 414, 652
K deficiency 414, 419, 429
diagnosis of 414
water-soluble 299
Vitiligo 48
Voided urine specimen 310
Vomiting 479, 595, 963, 694, 890, 970
severe 139
von Hippel- Lindau
disease 760
gene mutations, consequences of 760
protein 760
von Willebrand disease 412, 413
von Willebrand factor 146, 148, 411
complex 410
Vulnerable plaque 487, 510
Vulva 801, 955

W

Warburg metabolism, regulator of 389
Warfarin 302
Warm antibody
immunohemolytic anemia 360
type 357
Warm autoantibodies 385
Warthin's tumor 591, 593, 594*f*
gross appearance of 593*f*
Warthin-Finkeldey giant cells 117
Warthin-Starry stain 599*f*
Warty carcinoma 786
Water 289
accumulation of 669
loss of 745
retention 132
urinary losses of 889
Waterhouse-Friderichsen syndrome 143, 144, 416, 902, 961
Wavy nuclei 944
Webbed neck 283
Wegener's granulomatosis 720
Weight gain 900
Weight loss 295, 548, 583, 618, 671, 687, 689, 888, 889, 933
Well-formed fibrous capsule 875
Werner syndrome 54
Wernicke's encephalopathy 303
Westergren method 323, 446
Westergren pipette 446
Westergren rack 446
Western blot 205
Wet fixed smear 314
Wheal-and-flare reaction 553
Wheezing 556, 558
White blood cell 8, 319, 344, 441, 442, 460
count 398
disorder of 365, 443
type of 365
White cell
disorders 448
neoplasms of 371
Whole blood 323
Whooping cough 115
Widal reaction 615
Widely invasive follicular carcinomas 879
Willebrand factor 417
Willis circle 753
Wilms tumor 763
Wilson disease 679
Wintrobe method 443, 446
Wintrobe tube 443, 445*f*
uses of 444
Wire-loop lesions 192
Wiskott-Aldrich syndrome 197
Wood preservatives 290
Worsens functional insulin deficiency 889
Wound 98
chronic 103
contracture 103*f*
dehiscence 102
healing 94, 97, 98, 98*t*, 103*fc*
complications of 101
cutaneous 133
infection of 103
nature of 101
size and type of 97, 98
strength 100
increase of 97
tensile strength of 100
Woven bone 934
Wright stain 441
Wrinkled epidermis 027
Wrist 506
radial deviation of 920
Wuchereria bancrofti 126, 132, 132*f*, 451
embryo of 126*f*

X

X chromatin 276
X gene 683
Xanthine oxidase inhibitors 933
Xanthochromia 466
Xanthogranulomatous cholecystitis 695
Xanthogranulomatous pyelonephritis 741
Xanthoma 46
X-chromosome 276

missing of 283
monosomy of short arm of 283
number of 277
paired normal 411
structural abnormalities of 283
Xeroderma pigmentosum 232, 253, 260, 951, 952
Xerophthalmia 194, 299
Xerosis conjunctivae 299
Xerostomia produces dry mouth 194

Y

Yeasts 118
Yolk sac tumor 826, 829, 830, 830*f*
Young's syndrome 557

Z

Z allele 550
Zahn lines 153, 153*f*
Zellballen pattern 905
Zenker's degeneration 52, 614
Ziehl-Neelsen stain 110, 314, 464, 465, 476, 560, 963
Zollinger-Ellison syndrome 600, 602, 605, 908
Zona
fasciculata 898
glomerulosa 898
reticularis 898
Zoonotic disease 659
Zygomycosis 120
Zygote 124